Shackelford's

Surgery of the Alimentary Tract

Section Editors
Volume I

Jeffrey H. Peters, MD

Seymour I. Schwartz Professor and Chairman
Department of Surgery
University of Rochester School of Medicine and Dentistry
Rochester, New York

Section I
Esophagus and Hernia

Daniel T. Dempsey, MD

Professor and Chairman of Surgery
Temple University School of Medicine
Philadelphia, Pennsylvania

Section II
Stomach and Small Intestine

Volume II

Andrew S. Klein, MD, MBA

Esther and Mark Schulman Chair in Surgery and Transplant Medicine
Director, Cedars-Sinai Comprehensive Transplant Center
Professor of Surgery, University of California at Los Angeles School of Medicine
Los Angeles, California

Section III
Pancreas, Biliary Tract, Liver, and Spleen

John H. Pemberton, MD

Professor of Surgery
Mayo Clinic College of Medicine
Consultant in Colon and Rectal Surgery
Mayo Clinic and Mayo Foundation
Rochester, Minnesota

Section IV
Colon, Rectum, and Anus

Shackelford's
Surgery of the Alimentary Tract

Sixth Edition

Charles J. Yeo, MD

Samuel D. Gross Professor and Chair
Department of Surgery
Thomas Jefferson University
Philadelphia, Pennsylvania

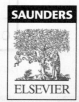

SAUNDERS

ELSEVIER

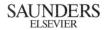

SAUNDERS
ELSEVIER

1600 John F. Kennedy Blvd.
Ste 1800
Philadelphia, PA 19103-2899

SHACKELFORD'S SURGERY OF THE ALIMENTARY TRACT

ISBN-13: 978-1-4160-2357-9
ISBN-10: 1-4160-2357-7
Vol 1 PN: 9996026507
Vol 2 PN: 9996026566

Notice

Knowledge and best practice in this field are constantly changing. As new research and experience broaden our knowledge, changes in practice, treatment and drug therapy may become necessary or appropriate. Readers are advised to check the most current information provided (i) on procedures featured or (ii) by the manufacturer of each product to be administered, to verify the recommended dose or formula, the method and duration of administration, and contraindications. It is the responsibility of the practitioner, relying on his or her own experience and knowledge of the patient, to make diagnoses, to determine dosages and the best treatment for each individual patient, and to take all appropriate safety precautions. To the fullest extent of the law, neither the Publisher nor the editors assumes any liability for any injury and/or damage to persons or property arising out of or related to any use of the material contained in this book.

The Publisher

Previous editions copyrighted 2002, 1996, 1991, 1986, 1983, 1982, 1981, 1978, 1955

Library of Congress Cataloging-in-Publication Data

Shackelford's surgery of the alimentary tract / [edited by] Charles J. Yeo . . . [et al.].–6th ed.
p. ; cm.
Includes bibliographical references and index.
ISBN 1-4160-2357-7 (set)
1. Alimentary canal–Surgery.   I. Title: Surgery of the alimentary tract.   II. Yeo, Charles J.
[DNLM: 1. Digestive System Surgical Procedures–methods.   2. Digestive System Diseases–surgery. WI 900 S9617 2007]
RD540.S476 2007
617.4'3–dc22

Publishing Director: Judith Fletcher
Developmental Editor: Kim Davis
Publishing Services Manager: Tina Rebane
Project Manager: Amy L. Cannon
Design Director: Ellen Zanolle

Printed in China
Last digit is the print number: 9 8 7 6 5 4 3 2 1

To my wife, Theresa, and my children, William and Katerina;
to my many mentors (alive and deceased) who contributed to the science of surgery;
and to the many colleagues and friends whose work made this sixth edition possible.

CHARLES J. YEO

To my wife, Barbara, and my son, Patrick.

DANIEL T. DEMPSEY

To my wife, Julia, and my sons, Jeffrey, David, and Alexander
for their support, their understanding, and their willingness to savor life's adventures.

ANDREW S. KLEIN

To my mentors, Ollie Beahrs, Bob Beart, Keith Kelly, Roger Dozois, and Sid Phillips,
who each challenged me from the start to aim high;
to my colleagues who supported wordlessly (usually!) these desires,
and to my family, who put up with all of this for so long—my deepest respect, profound thanks, and love.

JOHN H. PEMBERTON

To the hard work and dedication of surgeons
struggling with esophageal disease throughout the world
and to those few who have generously shared their wisdom and experience
in my personal education toward the successful management
of diseases of the esophagus.

JEFFREY H. PETERS

Contributors

Herand Abcarian, MD
Turi Josefsen Professor of Surgery, University of Illinois at Chicago College of Medicine; Head, Department of Surgery, University of Illinois at Chicago Medical Center, Chicago, Illinois
Complete Rectal Prolapse

Waddah B. Al-Refaie, MD
Fellow, Department of Surgical Oncology, The University of Texas M. D. Anderson Cancer Center, Houston, Texas
Multimodality Treatment of Esophageal Cancer

Hisami Ando, MD
Professor, Chairman, and Chief of Pediatric Surgery, Department of Pediatric Surgery, Nagoya University Graduate School of Medicine, Nagoya, Japan
Cystic Disorders of the Bile Ducts

Cletus A. Arciero, MD
Teaching Fellow, Temple University; Fellow, Surgical Oncology, Fox Chase Cancer Center, Philadelphia, Pennsylvania
Gastrointestinal Carcinoid Tumors

Joanna C. Arcuni, MD
Formerly of Department of Radiology, Baystate Medical Center, Springfield, Massachusetts
Small Intestinal Diverticula

Stanley W. Ashley, MD
Frank Sawyer Professor of Surgery, Harvard Medical School; Vice Chairman, Brigham and Women's Hospital, Boston, Massachusetts
Operations for Peptic Ulcer

Itzhak Avital, MD
Surgical Oncology Fellow and Hepatobiliary Fellow, Memorial Sloan-Kettering Cancer Center, New York, New York
External Biliary Fistula

Leah M. Backhus, MD
Resident, Department of Surgery, Keck School of Medicine, University of Southern California, Los Angeles, California
pH and Bilirubin Monitoring

H. Randolph Bailey, MD
Clinical Professor of Surgery and Chief, Division of Colon and Rectal Surgery, The University of Texas Health Science Center, Houston, Texas
Pilonidal Disease

Dimitra G. Barabouti, MD
Clinical Assistant Professor, Department of Surgery, James H. Quillen College of Medicine, East Tennessee State University; Attending Colorectal Surgeon, James H. Quillen VA Medical Center, Johnson City, Tennessee
Ultrasonographic Diagnosis of Anorectal Disease

John M. Barlow, MD
Instructor in Radiology, Mayo Clinic College of Medicine; Staff Radiologist, Mayo Clinic, Rochester, Minnesota
Imaging in Esophageal Disease

Stephen T. Bartlett, MD
Barbara Baur Dunlap Professor and Chairman, Department of Surgery, Surgeon-in-Chief, University of Maryland; Chairman, Department of Surgery, University of Maryland Medical Center, Baltimore, Maryland
Pancreas Transplantation

Amir L. Bastawrous, MD
Assistant Clinical Professor of Surgery, The University of Illinois at Chicago College of Medicine; Associate Program Director, Cook County Colon and Rectal Surgery Residency Training Program, Stroger Hospital of Cook County, Chicago, Illinois
Complete Rectal Prolapse

David E. Beck, MD
Clinical Associate Professor of Surgery, F. Edward Herbert School of Medicine, Uniformed Services University of the Health Sciences, Bethesda, Maryland; Chairman, Department of Colon and Rectal Surgery, Ochsner Clinic Foundation, New Orleans, Louisiana
Miscellaneous Disorders of the Rectum and Anus

Jacques J. G. H. M. Bergman, MD, PhD
Assistant Professor, Department of Gastroenterology, Academic Medical Center, Amsterdam, The Netherlands
Endoscopic Evaluation of the Esophagus

Adil E. Bharucha, MD
Associate Professor of Medicine, Mayo Clinic College of Medicine; Consultant in Gastroenterology, Mayo Clinic, Rochester, Minnesota
Physiology of the Colon and Its Measurement

David Binion, MD
Associate Professor of Medicine, Medical College of Wisconsin; Director, IBD Center, Division of Gastroenterology and Hepatology, Froedtert Hospital, Milwaukee, Wisconsin
Small Intestine

John Blebea, MD
Professor of Surgery, Temple University School of Medicine; Chief of Vascular Surgery, Temple University, Philadelphia, Pennsylvania
Aortoenteric Fistula and Visceral Artery Aneurysms

Ronald Bleday, MD
Associate Professor of Surgery, Harvard Medical School;
Chief, Section of Colorectal Surgery, Brigham and Women's
Hospital, Boston, Massachusetts
Local Excision of Rectal Cancer

Dennis Blom, MD
Associate Professor of Surgery, Indiana University Medical
Center, Indianapolis, Indiana
Perforation of the Esophagus

Leslie H. Blumgart, MD, FRCS(Engl, Edin), FRCPS(Glas)
Enid A. Haupt Chair in Surgery and Professor of Surgery,
Weill Medical College, Cornell University; Chief,
Hepatobiliary Service and Director, Hepatobiliary Disease
Management Program, Memorial Sloan-Kettering Cancer
Center, New York, New York
External Biliary Fistula

Dale E. Bockman, PhD
Professor and Chairman Emeritus, Department of Cellular
Biology and Anatomy, Medical College of Georgia, Augusta,
Georgia
Anatomy, Physiology, and Embryology of the Pancreas

Scott J. Boley, MD
Montefiore Medical Center, Bronx, New York
Colonic Bleeding and Ischemia

Luigi Bonavina, MD
Associate Professor of Surgery, University of Milano School of
Medicine; Chief, Surgical Unit, Policlinico San Donato,
IRCCS, San Donato Milanese, Milan, Italy
Surgical Management of Esophageal Diverticula

Robin P. Boushey, MD, PhD, CIP, FRCSC
Assistant Professor of Surgery, University of Ottawa; Assistant
Professor of Surgery, Clinical Investigator at the Ottawa
Health Research Institute in the Cancer Centre Program and
Director of Research in the Division of General Surgery, The
Ottawa Hospital, Ottawa, Ontario, Canada
Colonic Intussusception and Volvulus

Jan Brabender, MD
Department of Surgery, University of Cologne, Cologne,
Germany
*Epidemiology, Risk Factors, and Clinical Manifestations of
Esophageal Carcinoma*

Cedric G. Bremner, MD
Co-Director, University of Southern California University
Hospital, Swallowing Center; Professor, Clinical Surgery;
Director, Clinical Research, Department of Surgery, Keck
School of Medicine, University of Southern California, Los
Angeles, California
*Diffuse and Segmental Esophageal Spasm, Nutcracker Esophagus,
and Hypertensive Lower Esophageal Sphincter*

Ross M. Bremner, MD, PhD
Chief, General Thoracic Surgery, The Heart and Lung
Institute, St. Joseph's Hospital and Medical Center, Phoenix,
Arizona
pH and Bilirubin Monitoring

Timothy J. Broderick, MD
Associate Professor of Surgery and Biomedical Engineering,
University of Cincinnati College of Medicine; Chief, Division
of Gastrointestinal/Endocrine Surgery, University Hospital,
Cincinnati, Ohio
Vagotomy and Drainage

Robert E. Brolin, MD
Adjunct Professor, Department of Surgery, University of
Pittsburgh Medical Center, Pittsburgh, Pennsylvania; Director
of Bariatric Surgery, Department of Surgery, University
Medical Center at Princeton, Princeton, New Jersey
Operations for Morbid Obesity

Michael R. Burgdorf, MD
Tulane Center for Abdominal Transplantation, New Orleans,
Louisiana
Cysts and Tumors of the Spleen

Sathyaprasad C. Burjonrappa, MD, FRCS(Edin)
Staff, Department of Pediatric Surgery, Children's Hospital of
Boston, Boston, Massachusetts
Basic Features of Groin Hernia and Its Repair

R. Cartland Burns, MD
Associate Professor, Surgery and Pediatrics, University of
Virginia Health System, Charlottesville, Virginia
Congenital Disorders of the Esophagus

Molly M. Buzdon, MD
Laparoscopic Surgery, Union Memorial Hospital, Baltimore,
Maryland
Benign Tumors and Cysts of the Esophagus

John L. Cameron, MD
Alfred Blalock Distinguished Service Professor of Surgery,
Department of Surgery, Johns Hopkins Medical Institutions,
Baltimore, Maryland
Pancreatic and Periampullary Carcinoma

Michael Camilleri, MD
Atherton and Winifred W. Bean Professor, Professor of
Medicine and Physiology, Mayo Clinic College of Medicine;
Consultant in Gastroenterology, Mayo Clinic, Rochester,
Minnesota
Physiology of the Colon and Its Measurement

E. Ramsay Camp, MD
Fellow, Department of Surgical Oncology, The University of
Texas M. D. Anderson Cancer Center, Houston, Texas
Unusual Pancreatic Tumors

Cheri M. Canon, MD
Associate Professor of Radiology, Vice Chair for Education,
and Chief, Gastrointestinal Radiology, University of Alabama
at Birmingham, Birmingham, Alabama
Liver Abscess

Peter W. G. Carne, MBBS
Cabrini Medical Centre, Malvern, Victoria, Australia
Rare Colorectal Malignancies

Riaz Cassim, MD
Assistant Professor, Department of Surgery, West Virginia
University; Surgeon, West Virginia University Hospitals,
Morgantown, West Virginia
Ileostomy

Donald O. Castell, MD
Professor of Medicine and Director, Esophageal Disorders
Program, Medical University of South Carolina, Charleston,
South Carolina
*Physiology of the Esophagus and Its Sphincters; Multichannel
Intraluminal Impedance*

Peter Cataldo, MD
Associate Professor of Surgery, University of Vermont College
of Medicine; Colon and Rectal Surgeon, General Surgeon,
Fletcher Allen Health Care, Burlington, Vermont
Ostomy Management

Samuel Cemaj, MD
Assistant Professor of Surgery and Attending Surgeon,
Creighton University, Omaha, Nebraska
Basic Features of Groin Hernia and Its Repair

Parakrama Chandrasoma, MD
Professor of Pathology, Keck School of Medicine, University
of Southern California; Chief of Anatomic and Surgical
Pathology, LAC+USC Medical School, Los Angeles,
California
The Pathology of Gastroesophageal Reflux Disease

Andrew C. Chang, MD
Assistant Professor, Section of Thoracic Surgery, The
University of Michigan Medical School, Ann Arbor, Michigan
Complications of Esophageal Surgery

Eugene Y. Chang, MD
Research Fellow, Department of Surgery, Oregon Health and
Science University, Portland, Oregon
Medical Therapy for Gastroesophageal Reflux Disease

George J. Chang, MD
Assistant Professor of Surgery, The University of Texas M. D.
Anderson Cancer Center, Houston, Texas
Surgery in the Immunocompromised Patient

David B. Chessin, MD
Research Fellow, Memorial Sloan-Kettering Cancer Center,
New York, New York
*Colorectal Polyps, Polyposis Syndromes, and Hereditary Nonpolyposis
Colorectal Cancer*

Clifford S. Cho, MD
Chief Fellow, Surgical Oncology, Memorial Sloan-Kettering
Cancer Center, New York, New York
Biliary Tract Tumors

Karen A. Chojnacki, MD
Assistant Professor of Surgery, Thomas Jefferson University,
Philadelphia, Pennsylvania
Foreign Bodies and Bezoars of the Stomach and Small Intestine

Michael A. Choti, MD, MBA
Professor of Surgery, Johns Hopkins University; Consultant,
Johns Hopkins Hospital, Baltimore, Maryland
*Management of Malignant Hepatic Neoplasms Other Than
Hepatocellular Carcinoma*

Rashad Choudry, MD
Instructor in Surgery, Temple University School of Medicine;
Section of Vascular Surgery, Temple University, Philadelphia,
Pennsylvania
Aortoenteric Fistula and Visceral Artery Aneurysms

Donald O. Christensen, DO
Resident, Department of Pathology, University of Arizona
Health Sciences Center, Tucson, Arizona
Anatomy and Physiology of the Spleen

Albert K. Chun, MD
Physician, Department of Radiology, The George Washington
University, Washington DC
Imaging and Intervention in the Biliary System

James M. Church, MD
Staff Endoscopy, Department of Colorectal Surgery, The
Cleveland Clinic, Cleveland, Ohio
Diagnosis of Colon, Rectal, and Anal Disease

Robert R. Cima, MD
Assistant Professor, Mayo Clinic College of Medicine; Senior
Associate Consultant, Mayo Clinic and Mayo Foundation,
Rochester, Minnesota
Inflammatory Bowel Disease

Pierre-Alain Clavien, MD, PhD, FRCS
Professor and Chairman, Department of Visceral and
Transplantation Surgery, University Hospital Zurich, Zurich,
Switzerland
Benign Hepatic Neoplasms

Alfred M. Cohen, MD
Professor of Surgery, University of Kentucky College of
Medicine; Director, Lucille P. Markey Cancer Center,
Lexington, Kentucky
Operations for Colorectal Cancer: Low Anterior Resection

Jeffrey L. Cohen, MD
Associate Clinical Professor of Surgery, University of
Connecticut, Farmington; Lead Physician, Division of General
and Colorectal Surgery, Connecticut Surgical Group,
Hartford, Connecticut
Diverticular Disease

Paul M. Colombani, MD
Chief, Pediatric Surgery; Professor of Surgery, Oncology, and
Pediatrics; and Children's Surgeon-in-Charge, Johns Hopkins
University School of Medicine, Baltimore, Maryland
Management of Splenic Injury in Children

Steven D. Colquhoun, MD
Associate Clinical Professor, Liver and Pancreas
Transplantation, University of California at Los Angeles;
Director, Liver Transplantation, Cedars-Sinai Medical Center,
Los Angeles, California
*Perioperative Management and Nutrition in Patients with Liver and
Biliary Tract Disease; Hepatic Transplantation*

Anthony J. Comerota, MD
Clinical Professor of Surgery, University of Michigan, Ann
Arbor, Michigan; Director, Jobst Vascular Center and Section
Head, Peripheral Vascular Surgery, The Toledo Hospital,
Toledo, Ohio
Mesenteric Ischemia

Willy Coosemans, MD, PhD
Professor in Surgery, Abdominal Transplantation Surgery
Section, Catholic University Leuven; Clinical Head, University
Hospital Gasthuisberg, Leuven, Belgium
Pathophysiology and Treatment of Zenker's Diverticulum

Edward E. Cornwell III, MD
Professor of Surgery and Chief of Adult Trauma, Johns
Hopkins Hospital, Baltimore, Maryland
Pancreatic Trauma

Daniel A. Craig, MD
Assistant Professor of Radiology, Mayo Clinic College of
Medicine; Staff Radiologist, Mayo Clinic, Rochester,
Minnesota
Imaging in Esophageal Disease

Peter F. Crookes, MD
Associate Professor of Surgery, Keck School of Medicine,
University of Southern California; Attending Physician,
University of Southern California University Hospital, Los
Angeles, California
Esophageal Caustic Injury

Felix Dahm, MD
Surgical Resident, Department of Visceral and
Transplantation Surgery, University Hospital Zurich, Zurich,
Switzerland
Benign Hepatic Neoplasms

John M. Daly, MD
Dean, Temple University School of Medicine, Philadelphia,
Pennsylvania
Adenocarcinoma of the Stomach, Duodenum, and Small Intestine

Jarrod Day, MD
General Surgery Resident, Virginia Commonwealth University
Health System, Richmond, Virginia
Anatomy and Physiology of the Duodenum

Georges Decker, MD
Consultant, University Hospital Gasthuisberg, Leuven,
Belgium
Pathophysiology and Treatment of Zenker's Diverticulum

Thomas C. B. Dehn, MS, FRCS, MBBS, LRCP
Consultant Surgeon, Royal Berkshire Hospital, Reading,
Berkshire, England
Palliative Treatment of Carcinoma of the Esophagus

Paul De Leyn, MD
Professor in Surgery, Thoracic Surgery Section, Catholic
University Leuven; Clinical Head, University Hospital
Gasthuisberg, Leuven, Belgium
Pathophysiology and Treatment of Zenker's Diverticulum

Eric J. DeMaria, MD
Professor of Surgery and Vice Chair and Chief, Network
General Surgery; Director, Endosurgery and Bariatric Surgery,
Duke University Medical Center, Durham, North Carolina
Internal Hernias—Congenital and Acquired

Steven R. DeMeester, MD
Associate Professor, Department of Cardiothoracic Surgery,
University of Southern California, Los Angeles, California
Pathophysiology of the Columnar-Lined Esophagus

Tom R. DeMeester, MD
The Jeffrey P. Smith Professor of General and Thoracic
Surgery and Chairman, Department of Surgery, Keck School
of Medicine, University of Southern California; Chief of
Surgery, Department of Surgery, University of Southern
California University Hospital, Los Angeles, California
*Perspectives on Esophageal Surgery; The Gastroesophageal
Barrier*

Achilles A. Demetriou, MD, PhD
Executive Vice President and Chief Operating Officer,
University Hospitals Health System, Cleveland, Ohio
Fulminant Hepatic Failure and Bioartificial Liver Support

Daniel T. Dempsey, MD
Professor and Chairman of Surgery, Temple University School
of Medicine, Philadelphia, Pennsylvania
*Miscellaneous Benign Lesions and Conditions of the Stomach,
Duodenum, and Small Intestine*

L. Christopher DeRosier, MD
General Surgery Resident, University of Alabama at
Birmingham School of Medicine, Birmingham, Alabama
Liver Abscess

James P. Dolan, MD
Keesler Medical Center, Keesler Air Force Base, Biloxi,
Mississippi
Zollinger-Ellison Syndrome

John H. Donohue, MD
Professor of Surgery, Mayo School of Medicine; Consultant,
General Surgery, Mayo Clinic, Rochester, Minnesota
Splenectomy for Conditions Other Than Trauma

Eric J. Dozois, MD
Assistant Professor of Surgery and Program Director, Colon
and Rectal Surgery, Mayo Clinic College of Medicine;
Consultant, Colon and Rectal Surgery, Mayo Clinic and Mayo
Foundation, Rochester, Minnesota
Retrorectal Tumors

Stephen Dunn, MD
Professor of Surgery, Thomas Jefferson Medical College,
Philadelphia, Pennsylvania; Chief, Division of Pediatric
Surgery, Alfred I. duPont Hospital for Children, Wilmington,
Delaware
Biliary Atresia, Biliary Hypoplasia, and Choledochal Cyst

André Duranceau, MD
Professor, Thoracic Surgery Service, University of Montreal,
Montreal, Canada
Disorders of the Pharyngoesophageal Junction

Jonathan E. Efron, MD
Associate Professor of Surgery, Mayo Clinic College of
Medicine, Rochester, Minnesota; Senior Associate Consultant,
Division of Colon and Rectal Surgery, Mayo Clinic Scottsdale,
Scottsdale, Arizona
Neoplasms of the Anus

Burton L. Eisenberg, MD
Professor of Surgery, Dartmouth Medical School, Hanover;
Professor of Surgery, Surgical Oncology, Dartmouth-
Hitchcock Medical Center; Deputy Director, Norris Cotton
Cancer Center, Lebanon, New Hampshire
Gastrointestinal Stromal Tumors

Scott A. Engum, MD
Associate Professor of Surgery, Indiana University School of
Medicine; Clinical Associate Professor of Surgery, James
Whitcomb Riley Hospital for Children, Indianapolis, Indiana
Anorectal Anomalies

Warren E. Enker, MD
Professor, Department of Surgery, Albert Einstein College of Medicine; Vice Chairman and Chief, Division of Colorectal Surgery and Gastrointestinal Surgical Oncology, Department of Surgery and Director, Institute for Gastrointestinal Cancer, Continuum Cancer Centers of New York, Beth Israel Medical Center, New York, New York
Abdominoperineal Resection of the Rectum for Cancer

Douglas B. Evans, MD
Professor of Surgery, Department of Surgical Oncology, The University of Texas M. D. Anderson Cancer Center, Houston, Texas
Unusual Pancreatic Tumors

B. Mark Evers, MD
Professor and Robertson-Poth Distinguished Chair in General Surgery, Department of Surgery; Interim Director, Sealy Center for Cancer Cell Biology, The University of Texas Medical Branch, Galveston, Texas
Gastrointestinal Lymphomas

Victor W. Fazio, MD
Professor of Surgery, Lerner College of Medicine, Case Western Reserve University; Chairman, Colorectal Surgery, The Cleveland Clinic, Cleveland, Ohio
Reoperative Pelvic Surgery

Edward L. Felix, MD
Assistant Clinical Professor of Surgery, University of California at San Francisco, San Francisco; Medical Director, Advanced Bariatric Centers of California, Fresno, California
Femoral Hernia

Charles J. Filipi, MD
Professor of Surgery, Creighton University, Omaha, Nebraska
Endoscopic Antireflux Repairs

David R. Fischer, MD
Assistant Professor, Department of Surgery, and Associate Director, Residency Program in General Surgery, University of Cincinnati Medical Center, Cincinnati, Ohio
Gastric, Duodenal, and Small Intestinal Fistulas

Robert J. Fitzgibbons, Jr., MD
Dr. Harry E. Stuckenhoff Professor of Surgery and Chief, Division of General Surgery, Department of Surgery, Creighton University Medical Center, Omaha, Nebraska
Basic Features of Groin Hernia and Its Repair; Laparoscopic Inguinal Hernia Repair

Evan L. Fogel, MD
Associate Professor of Clinical Medicine and ERCP Fellowship Director, Indiana University Medical Center, Indianapolis, Indiana
Endoscopic Retrograde Cholangiopancreatography in the Evaluation and Management of Hepatobiliary and Pancreatic Disease

Yuman Fong, MD
Professor of Surgery, Weill Cornell Medical College; Murray F. Brennan Chair in Surgery and Chief, Gastric and Mixed Tumor Service, Memorial Sloan-Kettering Cancer Center, New York, New York
Biliary Tract Tumors

Debra Holly Ford, MD
Associate Professor and Head, Section of Colon and Rectal Surgery, Department of Surgery, Howard University College of Medicine, Howard University Hospital, Washington, DC
Pilonidal Disease

Karl-Hermann Fuchs, MD
Professor and Doctor of Medicine, Department of Gastrointestinal, Vascular, and Thoracic Surgery, Markus Krankenhaus, Frankfurt, Germany
Tests of Gastric Function and Their Use in the Evaluation of Esophageal Disease

Thomas R. Gadacz, MD
Professor, Department of Surgery, Medical College of Georgia; Staff Surgeon, MCG Health Incorporated, Augusta, Georgia
Anatomy, Embryology, Anomalies, and Physiology

Susan Galandiuk, MD
Professor of Surgery, University of Louisville School of Medicine; Director, Section of Colon and Rectal Surgery and Director of Price Institute of Surgical Research, University of Louisville; Staff, University of Louisville Hospital, Louisville, Kentucky
Traumatic Colorectal Injuries, Foreign Bodies, and Anal Wounds

Henry Gale, PhD
Assistant Professor, Department of Biomedical Sciences, Creighton University, Omaha, Nebraska
Endoscopic Antireflux Repairs

Scott F. Gallagher, MD
Assistant Professor, Department of Surgery, University of South Florida College of Medicine (USF Health); Attending Physician and Surgeon, Tampa General Hospital, Tampa, Florida
Acute Pancreatitis

Tasha A. K. Gandamihardja, MBBS, MRCS(Edin)
London, United Kingdom
Diffuse and Segmental Esophageal Spasm, Nutcracker Esophagus, and Hypertensive Lower Esophageal Sphincter

Amy J. Goldberg, MD
Professor of Surgery, Temple University School of Medicine; Director, Trauma Program, Temple University Hospital, Philadelphia, Pennsylvania
Injuries to the Stomach, Duodenum, and Small Bowel

Steven B. Goldin, MD, PhD
Assistant Professor of Surgery and Clerkship Director, University of South Florida; Assistant Professor of Surgery and Clerkship Director, Tampa General Hospital, Tampa, Florida
Anatomy and Physiology of the Mesenteric Circulation

Henry F. Gomez, MD
Supervisor, Data Analysis, Department of Surgical Oncology, The University of Texas M. D. Anderson Cancer Center, Houston, Texas
Unusual Pancreatic Tumors

Gregory J. Gores, MD
Reuben P. Eisenberg Professor of Medicine and Chair, Division of Gastroenterology and Hepatology, Mayo Clinic College of Medicine, Rochester, Minnesota
Primary Sclerosing Cholangitis

Jacob A. Greenberg, MD
Clinical Fellow in Surgery, Harvard Medical School; Resident in General Surgery, Brigham and Women's Hospital, Boston, Massachusetts
Local Excision of Rectal Cancer

Harsh Grewal, MD
Associate Professor, Surgery and Pediatrics, Temple University School of Medicine, Philadelphia; Chief, Section of Pediatric Surgery, Temple University Children's Medical Center, Philadelphia; Attending Surgeon, Abington Memorial Hospital, Abington, Pennsylvania
Surgical Diseases of the Stomach and Duodenum in Infants and Children

Jay L. Grosfeld, MD
Lafayette F. Page Professor of Pediatric Surgery, Emeritus, Indiana University School of Medicine; Surgeon-in-Chief, Emeritus, J. W. Riley Hospital for Children, Indianapolis, Indiana
Anorectal Anomalies

José G. Guillem, MD, MPH
Professor of Surgery, Weill Medical College, Cornell University; Attending Surgeon, Memorial Sloan-Kettering Cancer Center, New York, New York
Colorectal Polyps, Polyposis Syndromes, and Hereditary Nonpolyposis Colorectal Cancer

Jeffrey A. Hagen, MD
Associate Professor of Surgery, Division of Thoracic/Foregut Surgery, Keck School of Medicine, University of Southern California, Los Angeles, California
Carcinoma of the Esophagus and Gastroesophageal Junction

Sean P. Harbison, MD
Associate Professor of Surgery, Temple University School of Medicine; Associate Professor, Department of Surgery, Temple University Hospital, Philadelphia, Pennsylvania
Intubation of the Stomach and Small Intestine

Andrew G. Harrell, MD
Clinical Fellow, Division of Gastrointestinal and Minimally Invasive Surgery, Carolinas Medical Center, Charlotte, North Carolina
Ventral Herniation in Adults

Elliott R. Haut, MD
Assistant Professor of Surgery, Johns Hopkins Hospital, Baltimore, Maryland
Pancreatic Trauma

Richard F. Heitmiller, MD
Thoracic Surgery, Union Memorial Hospital, Baltimore, Maryland
Benign Tumors and Cysts of the Esophagus

J. Michael Henderson, MBChB, FRCS(Edin)
Professor of Surgery, The Cleveland Clinic Lerner College of Medicine; Chairman, Quality and Patient Safety Institute, The Cleveland Clinic, Cleveland, Ohio
Multidisciplinary Approach to the Management of Portal Hypertension

B. Todd Heniford, MD
Chief, Division of Gastrointestinal and Minimally Invasive Surgery and Director, Carolinas Medical Center, Charlotte, North Carolina
Ventral Herniation in Adults

Doris Henne-Bruns, MD
Chairperson, Department of General Surgery, University of Ulm, Ulm, Germany
Radiation Enteritis

H. Franklin Herlong, MD
Associate Professor of Medicine, Johns Hopkins School of Medicine; Physician, Division of Gastroenterology, Johns Hopkins Hospital, Baltimore, Maryland
Approach to the Patient with Abnormal Hepatic Laboratory Tests

Wayne L. Hofstetter, MD
Assistant Professor, The University of Texas M. D. Anderson Cancer Center, Houston, Texas
Multimodality Treatment of Esophageal Cancer

Arnulf H. Hölscher, MD
Department of Surgery, University of Cologne, Cologne, Germany
Epidemiology, Risk Factors, and Clinical Manifestations of Esophageal Carcinoma

Philip Huber, Jr, MD
Dallas Surgical Group, Dallas, Texas
Fissure-in-Ano

Eric S. Hungness, MD
Assistant Professor of Surgery, University of Chicago Medical Center, Chicago, Illinois
Management of Common Bile Duct Stones

John G. Hunter, MD
MacKenzie Professor and Chair, Department of Surgery, Oregon Health and Science University, Portland, Oregon
Laparoscopic and Open Nissen Fundoplication

James E. Huprich, MD
Assistant Professor of Radiology, Mayo Medical School; Consultant, Mayo Clinic, Rochester, Minnesota
Imaging in Esophageal Disease

Hero K. Hussain, MD
Assistant Professor of Radiology and Director of Body Magnetic Resonance Imaging, Department of Radiology/MRI, University of Michigan, Ann Arbor, Michigan
Hepatic Cyst Disease

Matthew M. Hutter, MD, MPH
Instructor in Surgery, Harvard Medical School; Assistant Surgeon, Massachusetts General Hospital, Boston, Massachusetts
Paraesophageal and Other Complex Diaphragmatic Hernias

Neil H. Hyman, MD
Samuel B. and Michelle D. Labow Professor of Surgery, University of Vermont College of Medicine; Chief, Division of General Surgery, Fletcher Allen Health Care, Burlington, Vermont
Ostomy Management

Roberto C. Iglesias, MD
General Surgery Resident, Virginia Commonwealth University Health System, Richmond, Virginia
Anatomy and Physiology of the Duodenum

Elizabeth A. Ignacio, MD
Assistant Professor of Radiology, Department of Radiology, The George Washington University, Washington, DC
Imaging and Intervention in the Biliary System

Gerald Isenberg, MD
Professor of Surgery, Thomas Jefferson Medical College; Program Director, Colorectal Residency, Thomas Jefferson University Hospital, Philadelphia, Pennsylvania
Coloanal Anastomosis

Atif Iqbal, MD
Resident, Department of Surgery, University of Missouri Columbia, Columbia, Missouri
Endoscopic Antireflux Repairs

Rao R. Ivatury, MD
Professor of Surgery, Emergency Medicine, and Physiology, Virginia Commonwealth University; Chief, Division of Trauma, Critical Care, and Emergency General Surgery, Virginia Commonwealth University Medical Center, Richmond, Virginia
Mesenteric Arterial Trauma

Jakob R. Izbicki, MD
Professor of Surgery, University of Hamburg; Head, Department of Surgery, University Medical Center Hamburg-Eppendorf, Hamburg, Germany
Chronic Pancreatitis

Lindsey N. Jackson, MD
Research Fellow and Resident, General Surgery, The University of Texas Medical Branch, Galveston, Texas
Gastrointestinal Lymphomas

Danny O. Jacobs, MD, MPH
Professor and Chair, Department of Surgery, Duke University Medical Center, Durham, North Carolina
Volvulus of the Stomach and Small Bowel

Colleen E. Jaffray, MD
Assistant Professor of Surgery, University of South Florida College of Medicine (USF Health), Tampa; Staff Surgeon, Bay Pines VA Medical Center, Bay Pines, Florida
Acute Pancreatitis

Mohammad K. Jamal, MD
Assistant Professor of Surgery, Department of Surgery, University of Iowa Hospitals and Clinics, Iowa City, Iowa
Internal Hernias—Congenital and Acquired

Catherine Jephcott, MRCP, FRCR, BMCh
Consultant Oncologist, Department of Oncology, Peterborough and Addenbrookes Hospital, Peterborough, Cambridgeshire, England
Palliative Treatment of Carcinoma of the Esophagus

Blair A. Jobe, MD
Assistant Professor, Oregon Health and Science University; Director, Swallowing Center, Division of Surgery, Portland VA Medical Center, Portland, Oregon
Medical Therapy for Gastroesophageal Reflux Disease

Michael A. Jobst, MD
Staff Surgeon, St. Elizabeth Regional Medical Center, Lincoln, Nebraska
Anal Sepsis and Fistula

Michael Johnston, MB, BS, FRACS
St. Vincent's Consulting Suites, Fitzroy, Victoria, Australia
Rare Colorectal Malignancies

Jeffrey R. Jorden, MD
Assistant Professor of Colorectal Surgery, University of Louisville School of Medicine; Staff, University Hospital, Louisville, Kentucky
Traumatic Colorectal Injuries, Foreign Bodies, and Anal Wounds

Ronald Kaleya, MD
Montefiore Medical Center, Bronx, New York
Colonic Bleeding and Ischemia

Seth J. Karp, MD
Assistant Professor, Surgery, Beth Israel Deaconess Medical Center, Harvard Medical School, Boston, Massachusetts
Small Intestine

Elika Kashef, MBBS, MRCS
Specialist Registrar in Diagnostic Radiology, King's College Hospital, London, England
Hepatocellular Carcinoma

Werner K. H. Kauer, MD
Privatdozent and Resident, Klinikum rechts der Isar, Technischen Universität München, Munich, Germany
Esophageal Mucosal Injury and Duodenal Reflux

Howard S. Kaufman, MD, MBA
Associate Professor of Surgery and Obstetrics/Gynecology, Department of Surgery, Keck School of Medicine and Chief, Division of Colorectal and Pelvic Floor Surgery, Department of Surgery, University of Southern California; Chief, General Surgery, University of Southern California University Hospital, Los Angeles, California
Lumbar and Pelvic Hernias

Mark L. Kayton, MD
Assistant Member, Memorial Sloan-Kettering Cancer Center; Assistant Attending Surgeon, Division of Pediatric Surgery, Department of Surgery, Memorial Hospital for Cancer and Allied Diseases, New York, New York
Pancreatic Problems in Infants and Children

John M. Kellum, MD
Professor of Surgery, Virginia Commonwealth University Health System, Richmond, Virginia
Small Intestinal Diverticula; Anatomy and Physiology of the Duodenum

Kent W. Kercher, MD
Clinical Assistant Professor of Surgery, University of North Carolina, Chapel Hill; Teaching Faculty, Department of Surgery, Carolinas Medical Center, Charlotte, North Carolina
Ventral Herniation in Adults

Soo Y. Kim, MD
Assistant Professor of Surgery, Temple University School of Medicine; Attending Surgeon and Associate Program Director, Department of General Surgery Residency, Temple University Hospital, Philadelphia, Pennsylvania
Small Bowel Obstruction

Contributors

Andrew S. Klein, MD, MBA
Esther and Mark Schulman Chair in Surgery and Transplant Medicine and Director, Cedars-Sinai Comprehensive Transplant Center; Professor of Surgery, University of California at Los Angeles School of Medicine, Los Angeles, California
Hepatic Transplantation

Mark J. Koruda, MD
Chief, Gastrointestinal Surgery, Professor and Vice Chair, University of North Carolina, Chapel Hill, North Carolina
Crohn's Disease: General Considerations, Medical Management, and Surgical Treatment of Small Intestinal Disease

Christopher Kowalski, MD
Assistant Professor of Surgery, Division of Bariatric, Advanced Laparoscopic, and General Surgery; Clinical Assistant Professor, Department of Urology; Director of Laparoscopic Donor Nephrectomy Program, Temple University Hospital and School of Medicine, Philadelphia, Pennsylvania
Operations for Morbid Obesity

Richard A. Kozarek, MD
Clinical Professor of Medicine, University of Washington; Director of GI Institute and Chair of GI Research, Virginia Mason Medical Center, Seattle, Washington
New Developments in Chronic Pancreatitis: Before Head Resection, Try Endoscopic Treatment First

David Kuwayama, MD, MPhil
Fellow, Department of Surgery, Johns Hopkins Hospital, Baltimore, Maryland
Pancreatic Trauma

Daniela Ladner, MD
Fellow, Multi-Organ Transplant Surgery, Department of Surgery, Stanford University School of Medicine, Stanford, California
Neuroendocrine Tumors of the Pancreas

Dave R. Lal, MD
Senior Fellow and Acting Instructor, Center for Videoendoscopic Surgery and Swallowing Center, Department of Surgery, University of Washington, Seattle, Washington
Laparoscopic Esophageal Myotomy: Techniques and Results

Alan N. Langnas, DO
Professor of Surgery and Chief, Organ Transplant Program, University of Nebraska Medical Center, Omaha, Nebraska
Short-Bowel Syndrome

David W. Larson, MD
Assistant Professor of Surgery, Mayo Clinic College of Medicine; Consultant, Department of Surgery, Division of Colon and Rectal Surgery, Mayo Clinic, Rochester, Minnesota
Surgery for Inflammatory Bowel Disease: Crohn's Disease

Simon Law, MBBChir, FCSHK, FHKAM, FRCS(Edin)
Clinical Professor, Department of Surgery and Honorary Consultant, Department of Surgery, University of Hong Kong Medical Centre, Queen Mary Hospital, Hong Kong
Esophageal Cancer: Current Staging Classifications and Techniques, Endoscopic Ultrasound, and Laparoscopic and Thoracoscopic Staging

L. P. Lawler, MD
Johns Hopkins Medical Institutions, Baltimore, Maryland
Minimally Invasive Surgical and Image-Guided Interventional Approaches to the Spleen

Konstantinos N. Lazaridis, MD
Assistant Professor of Medicine, Division of Gastroenterology and Hepatology, Mayo Clinic College of Medicine, Rochester, Minnesota
Primary Sclerosing Cholangitis

David B. Leeser, MD
Organ Transplant Center, Walter Reed Army Medical Center, Washington, DC
Pancreas Transplantation

Glen A. Lehman, MD
Professor of Medicine and Radiology, Indiana University Medical Center, Indianapolis, Indiana
Endoscopic Retrograde Cholangiopancreatography in the Evaluation and Management of Hepatobiliary and Pancreatic Disease

Toni Lerut, MD
Professor in Surgery, Thoracic Surgery Section, Catholic University Leuven; Chairman, Department of Thoracic Surgery, University Hospital Gasthuisberg, Leuven, Belgium
Pathophysiology and Treatment of Zenker's Diverticulum

David M. Levi, MD
Associate Professor of Clinical Surgery, University of Miami Miller School of Medicine; Attending, Transplant Surgery, Jackson Memorial Medical Center, Miami, Florida
Vascular Diseases of the Liver

Anne Lidor, MD
Assistant Professor, Department of Surgery, Johns Hopkins University School of Medicine, Baltimore, Maryland
Management of Splenic Trauma in Adults

Dorothea Liebermann-Meffert, MD
Professor, Surgical Clinic and Policlinic, Department of Surgery, Technische Universität, München, Munich, Germany
Human Foregut Anatomy, Prenatal Development and Abnormalities, and Their Relation to Surgical Approaches; Esophageal Mucosal Injury and Duodenal Reflux

Keith D. Lillemoe, MD
Jay L. Grosfeld Professor and Chairman, Department of Surgery, Indiana University School of Medicine; Surgeon-in-Chief, Indiana University Hospital, Indianapolis, Indiana
Pseudocysts and Other Complications of Pancreatitis; Operative Management of Strictures and Benign Obstructive Disorders of the Bile Duct

Edward V. Loftus, Jr., MD
Associate Professor of Medicine, Mayo Clinic College of Medicine; Consultant, Gastroenterology and Hepatology, Mayo Clinic, Rochester, Minnesota
Inflammatory Bowel Disease

Reginald V. N. Lord, MD, FRACS
Associate Professor of Surgery, St. Vincent's Hospital, Conjoint University of New South Wales, Sydney, Australia
History and Definition of Barrett's Esophagus

Brian E. Louie, MD, FRCSC
Director of Education, Thoracic Oncology Program, Swedish Cancer Institute, Seattle, Washington
Carcinoma of the Esophagus and Gastroesophageal Junction

Val J. Lowe, MD
Associate Professor of Radiology, Mayo Clinic College of Medicine; Associate Professor of Radiology and Radiologist, Mayo Clinic, Rochester, Minnesota
Imaging in Esophageal Disease

Matthew L. Lynch, MD
Chief Resident, Department of Surgery, Rush University Medical Center, Chicago, Illinois
Radiation Injuries of the Rectum

Robert L. MacCarty, MD
Professor of Radiology, Mayo Clinic College of Medicine; Staff Radiologist, Mayo Clinic, Rochester, Minnesota
Imaging in Esophageal Disease

Robert D. Madoff, MD
Professor of Surgery, University of Minnesota, Minneapolis, Minnesota
Diagnosis and Management of Fecal Incontinence

Anurag Maheshwari, MD
Instructor in Medicine, Johns Hopkins University School of Medicine, Baltimore, Maryland
Drug-Induced Liver Disease

Massimo Malagó, MD, PhD
The Ilse Bagel Chair and Professor of Surgery and Transplantation; Director of Transplantation and Hepato-Biliary-Pancreatic Surgery, Department of General Surgery and Transplantation, University Hospital Essen, Essen, Germany
Anatomy and Physiology of the Liver

Ahmed Mami, MD
Research Resident, Department of Surgery, Drexel University College of Medicine, Philadelphia, Pennsylvania
Surgical Conditions of the Small Intestine in Infants and Children

Oliver Mann, MD
Associate Professor, Department of Surgery, University of Hamburg; Senior Associate, Department of Surgery, University Medical Center Hamburg-Eppendorf, Hamburg, Germany
Chronic Pancreatitis

Peter W. Marcello, MD
Staff Surgeon, Department of Colon and Rectal Surgery, Lahey Clinic, Burlington, Massachusetts
Laparoscopic Colorectal Surgery

Jeffrey M. Marks, MD
Assistant Professor, Department of Surgery, Case Western Reserve University; Chief, Division of Regional Surgery, University Hospitals of Cleveland, Cleveland, Ohio
Diagnostic and Therapeutic Endoscopy of the Stomach and Small Bowel

Michael R. Marohn, MD
Associate Professor of Surgery, Johns Hopkins University School of Medicine; Program Director, Minimally Invasive Surgery Fellowship, Johns Hopkins Medical Institutions, Baltimore, Maryland
Minimally Invasive Surgical and Image-Guided Interventional Approaches to the Spleen

David J. Maron, MD
Clinical Fellow, Department of Colorectal Surgery, The Cleveland Clinic Florida, Weston, Florida
Surgical Treatment of Constipation

Joseph Martz, MD
Attending, Department of Surgery, Beth Israel Medical Center, New York, New York
Abdominoperineal Resection of the Rectum for Cancer

Rodney John Mason, MBBCh, PhD, FRCS, FCS(SA)
Associate Professor of Surgery, Keck School of Medicine, University of Southern California; Service Chief, Emergency Surgery Service, LAC+USC Medical Center, Los Angeles, California
Esophageal Motility

Douglas J. Mathisen, MD
Grillo Professor of Surgery, Harvard Medical School; Chief, Thoracic Surgery, Massachusetts General Hospital, Boston, Massachusetts
Techniques of Esophageal Reconstruction

Jeffrey B. Matthews, MD
Christian R. Holmes Professor and Chairman, Department of Surgery, University of Cincinnati College of Medicine; Surgeon-in-Chief, University Hospital, Cincinnati, Ohio
Vagotomy and Drainage; Small Intestine

David W. McFadden, MD
Professor and Chairman, Department of Surgery, West Virginia University; Surgeon-in-Chief, West Virginia University Hospitals, Morgantown, West Virginia
Ileostomy

Lee McHenry, MD
Associate Professor of Medicine, Indiana University Medical Center, Indianapolis, Indiana
Endoscopic Retrograde Cholangiopancreatography in the Evaluation and Management of Hepatobiliary and Pancreatic Disease

Paul J. McMurrick, MBBS
Victorian Colorectal Clinic, Cabrini Medical Centre, Malvern, Victoria, Australia
Rare Colorectal Malignancies

Anthony S. Mee, MD, FRCP, MBBS
Consultant Gastroenterologist, Royal Berkshire Hospital, Reading, Berkshire, England
Palliative Treatment of Carcinoma of the Esophagus

John E. Meilahn, MD
Associate Professor of Surgery, Temple University School of Medicine; Director, Bariatric Surgery, Temple University Hospital, Philadelphia, Pennsylvania
Motility Disorders of the Stomach and Small Intestine

David W. Mercer, MD
Professor and Vice Chairman, Department of Surgery, The University of Texas Medical School at Houston; Chief of Surgery, LBJ General Hospital, Houston, Texas
Anatomy and Physiology of the Stomach

John Migaly, MD
Assistant Professor, Colon and Rectal Surgery, Department of Surgery, Temple University School of Medicine, Philadelphia, Pennsylvania
Suturing, Stapling, and Tissue Adhesives

Matthew Todd Miller, MD
Senior Resident, Jobst Vascular Center, The Toledo Hospital, Toledo, Ohio
Mesenteric Ischemia

Thomas A. Miller, MD
Ammons Professor of Surgery, Virginia Commonwealth University School of Medicine; Chief of Surgery, McGuire VA Medical Center; Attending Surgeon, Medical College of Virginia Hospitals, Richmond, Virginia
Postgastrectomy Syndromes

Ernesto P. Molmenti, MD, PhD, MBA
Professor of Surgery, University of Arizona; Chief, Section of Abdominal Transplantation, Department of Surgery, Arizona Health Sciences Center, Tucson, Arizona
Anatomy and Physiology of the Liver; Anatomy and Physiology of the Spleen

Jon B. Morris, MD
Professor, Department of Surgery, University of Pennsylvania School of Medicine; Attending Surgeon and Program Director, Department of General Surgery Residency; Medical Director, Admissions, Hospital of the University of Pennsylvania, Philadelphia, Pennsylvania
Small Bowel Obstruction

Christopher R. Morse, MD
Cardiothoracic Fellow, Division of Thoracic Surgery, Massachusetts General Hospital, Boston, Massachusetts
Techniques of Esophageal Reconstruction

Neal James McCready Mortensen, MBChB, MD, FRCS
Professor of Surgery, University of Oxford Clinical Medical School; Professor and Consultant Colorectal Surgeon, Department of Colorectal Surgery, John Radcliffe Hospital, Oxford, England
Anatomy of the Colon

Ruth Moxon, RGN, RM, MSc
Upper GI Cancer Nurse Specialist, Department of Upper GI Surgery and Oncology, Royal Berkshire Hospital, Reading, Berkshire, England
Palliative Treatment of Carcinoma of the Esophagus

Michael W. Mulholland, MD
Professor of Surgery, Chairman, and Surgeon-in-Chief, Department of Surgery, University of Michigan, Ann Arbor, Michigan
Gastric Resection and Reconstruction; Hepatic Cyst Disease

Edward C. Mun, MD
Director, Faulkner Hospital Bariatric Surgery Program, Boston, Massachusetts
Small Intestine

Michel M. Murr, MD
Associate Professor of Surgery, University of South Florida College of Medicine (USF Health); Attending Physician and Surgeon, Tampa General Hospital, Tampa, Florida
Acute Pancreatitis

Philippe Nafteux, MD
Joint Clinical Head, Department of Thoracic Surgery, University Hospital Gasthuisberg, Leuven, Belgium
Pathophysiology and Treatment of Zenker's Diverticulum

Alexander P. Nagle, MD
Assistant Professor, Department of Surgery, Feinberg School of Medicine, Northwestern University, Chicago, Illinois
Epidemiology and Natural History of Gastroesophageal Reflux Disease

David M. Nagorney, MD
Professor of Surgery, Mayo Medical School; Consultant in Surgery, Division of Gastroenterologic and General Surgery, Mayo Clinic, Rochester, Minnesota
Splenectomy for Conditions Other Than Trauma; Resection and Ablation of Metastatic Colorectal Cancer to the Liver

Atta Nawabi, MD
Chief Resident, General Surgery, Louisiana State University Health Sciences Center, Shreveport, Louisiana
Management of Hepatobiliary Trauma

Heidi Nelson, MD
Professor of Surgery, Mayo Medical School; Chair, Division of Colon and Rectal Surgery and Consultant, Mayo Foundation, Rochester, Minnesota
Recurrent and Metastatic Colorectal Cancer

Gregg K. Nishi, MD
Associate Clinical Professor in Surgery, University of California at Los Angeles; Staff Surgeon, Cedars-Sinai Medical Center, Los Angeles, California
Laparoscopic Management of Common Bile Duct Stones

Nicholas N. Nissen, MD
Cedars-Sinai Medical Center, Los Angeles, California
Hepatic Transplantation

C. Joe Northup, MD
Assistant Professor, University of Virginia Health System, Charlottesville, Virginia
Reoperative Surgery of the Stomach and Duodenum

Jeffrey A. Norton, MD
Professor of Surgery and Chief of Surgical Oncology, Stanford University Medical Center, Stanford, California
Zollinger-Ellison Syndrome; Neuroendocrine Tumors of the Pancreas

Yuri W. Novitsky, MD
Clinical Fellow, Division of Gastrointestinal and Minimally Invasive Surgery, Carolinas Medical Center, Charlotte, North Carolina
Ventral Herniation in Adults

Michael S. Nussbaum, MD
Associate Professor, Department of Surgery and Vice Chairman, Clinical Affairs, University of Cincinnati Medical Center; Chief of Staff, The University Hospital, Cincinnati, Ohio
Gastric, Duodenal, and Small Intestinal Fistulas

Brant K. Oelschlager, MD
Assistant Professor; Director, Swallowing Center; Director, Center for Videoendoscopic Surgery, University of Washington, Seattle, Washington
Laparoscopic Esophageal Myotomy: Techniques and Results

Daniel S. Oh, MD
Resident in General Surgery, Department of Surgery, University of Southern California, Los Angeles, California
Pathophysiology of the Columnar-Lined Esophagus

Robert W. O'Rourke, MD
Assistant Professor, Department of Surgery, Oregon Health and Science University, Portland, Oregon
Laparoscopic and Open Nissen Fundoplication

Mark B. Orringer, MD
Professor and Head, Section of Thoracic Surgery, University of Michigan Medical School, Ann Arbor, Michigan
Reflux Strictures and Short Esophagus; Complications of Esophageal Surgery

Mary F. Otterson, MD, MS
Professor of Surgery and Associate Professor of Physiology, Department of Surgery, Medical College of Wisconsin; Staff Surgeon, Froedtert Hospital; Staff Surgeon, Zablocki VA Hospital, Milwaukee, Wisconsin
Small Intestine

James R. Ouellette, MD
Assistant Professor of Surgery, Division of Surgical Oncology, Wright State University, Dayton, Ohio
Perioperative Management and Nutrition in Patients with Liver and Biliary Tract Disease

D. Wayne Overby, MD
Clinical Instructor and Fellow in Advanced Gastrointestinal Surgery and Endoscopy, University of North Carolina, Chapel Hill, North Carolina
Crohn's Disease: General Considerations, Medical Management, and Surgical Treatment of Small Intestinal Disease

Charles N. Paidas, MD
Professor of Surgery, Department of Surgery, University of South Florida; Chief, Pediatric Surgery, Tampa General Hospital, Tampa, Florida
Pancreatic Problems in Infants and Children

Harry T. Papaconstantinou, MD
Assistant Professor of Surgery and Chief, Section of Colon and Rectal Surgery, The Texas A&M University System Health Science Center Scott and White Hospital, Temple, Texas
Fissure-in-Ano

Theodore N. Pappas, MD
Professor of Surgery, Duke University Medical Center, Duke University School of Medicine, Durham, North Carolina
Operative Management of Cholecystitis and Cholelithiasis

Rolland Parc, MD
Centre de Chirurgie et Réanimation Digestives, Hôpital Saint Antoine, Paris, France
Coloanal Anastomosis

Alexander A. Parikh, MD
Assistant Professor of Surgery, Division of Surgical Oncology, Vanderbilt University School of Medicine, Nashville, Tennessee
Adenocarcinoma of the Stomach, Duodenum, and Small Intestine

Susan C. Parker, MD
Adjunct Associate Professor, University of Minnesota, Minneapolis, Minnesota
Diagnosis and Management of Fecal Incontinence

Abhijit S. Pathak, MD
Associate Professor of Surgery, Temple University School of Medicine; Attending Surgeon and Director of Surgical ICU, Temple University Hospital, Philadelphia, Pennsylvania
Injuries to the Stomach, Duodenum, and Small Bowel

Marco G. Patti, MD
Associate Professor of Surgery, Department of Surgery, University of California at San Francisco School of Medicine, San Francisco, California
Epidemiology, Pathophysiology, and Clinical Features of Achalasia

Walter Pegoli, Jr., MD
Associate Professor of Surgery and Pediatrics and Section Chief, Pediatric Surgery, Golisano Children's Hospital at Strong, University of Rochester Medical Center, Rochester, New York
Hernias and Congenital Groin Problems in Infants and Children

John H. Pemberton, MD
Professor of Surgery, Mayo Clinic College of Medicine; Consultant in Colon and Rectal Surgery, Mayo Clinic and Mayo Foundation, Rochester, Minnesota
Embryology and Anatomy of the Colon; Surgery for Inflammatory Bowel Disease: Chronic Ulcerative Colitis

Christophe Penna, MD
Hôpital Ambroise Paré, Billancourt, France
Coloanal Anastomosis

Jeffrey H. Peters, MD
Seymour I. Schwartz Professor and Chairman, Department of Surgery, University of Rochester School of Medicine and Dentistry, Rochester, New York
Assessment of Symptoms and Approach to the Patient with Esophageal Disease; The Gastroesophageal Barrier; Surgical Treatment of Barrett's Esophagus; Endoscopic Ablation of Barrett's Metaplasia and Dysplasia

Edward H. Phillips, MD
Clinical Associate Professor of Surgery, University of Southern California; Director of Endoscopic Surgery and Director of Breast Center, Cedars-Sinai Medical Center, Los Angeles, California
Laparoscopic Management of Common Bile Duct Stones

Allan Pickens, MD
Assistant Professor of Surgery, Department of Surgery, Section of Thoracic Surgery, University of Michigan Medical School, Ann Arbor, Michigan
Reflux Strictures and Short Esophagus

Henry A. Pitt, MD
Vice Chairman and Professor, Department of Surgery, Indiana University School of Medicine; Vice Chairman, Department of Surgery, Indiana University Medical Center, Indianapolis, Indiana
Anatomy, Embryology, Anomalies, and Physiology; Operative Management of Strictures and Benign Obstructive Disorders of the Bile Duct

Hiram C. Polk, Jr., MD
Ben A. Reid Sr. Professor of Surgery, Department of Surgery, University of Louisville School of Medicine; Staff, University Hospital, Louisville, Kentucky
Traumatic Colorectal Injuries, Foreign Bodies, and Anal Wounds

Jeffrey L. Ponsky, MD
Oliver H. Payne Professor and Chairman, Department of Surgery, Case Western Reserve University School of Medicine; Chairman, Department of Surgery, University Hospitals of Cleveland, Cleveland, Ohio
Diagnostic and Therapeutic Endoscopy of the Stomach and Small Bowel; Management of Splenic Abscess

Emil L. Popa, MD†
Department of Surgery, Temple University School of Medicine, Philadelphia, Pennsylvania
Miscellaneous Benign Lesions and Conditions of the Stomach, Duodenum, and Small Intestine

Mitchell C. Posner, MD
Professor and Chief, Section of General Surgery and Surgical Oncology, University of Chicago, Chicago, Illinois
Adenocarcinoma of the Colon and Rectum

Brent J. Prosser, MD
Physician, Division of Gastroenterology, Johns Hopkins Bayview Medical Center, Baltimore, Maryland
Approach to the Patient with Abnormal Hepatic Laboratory Tests

Varun Puri, MBBS, MS
Resident in Surgery, Creighton University Medical Center, Omaha, Nebraska
Laparoscopic Inguinal Hernia Repair

Florencia G. Que, MD
Associate Professor of Surgery, Mayo Clinic College of Medicine; Consultant, Division of Gastroenterologic and General Surgery, Department of Surgery, Mayo Clinic, Rochester, Minnesota
Resection and Ablation of Metastatic Colorectal Cancer to the Liver

Arnold Radtke, MD
Department of General Surgery and Transplantation, University Hospital Essen, Essen, Germany
Anatomy and Physiology of the Liver

Rudra Rai, MD
Assistant Professor of Medicine, Johns Hopkins University School of Medicine, Baltimore, Maryland
Drug-Induced Liver Disease

Jan Rakinic, MD
Associate Professor of Surgery, Division of General Surgery, Southern Illinois University School of Medicine; Attending Surgeon, Colorectal Surgery, Memorial Medical Center and St. John's Hospital, Springfield, Illinois
Antibiotics, Approaches, Strategy, and Anastomoses

David W. Rattner, MD
Professor of Surgery, Harvard Medical School; Chief, Division of General and Gastrointestinal Surgery, Massachusetts General Hospital, Boston, Massachusetts
Paraesophageal and Other Complex Diaphragmatic Hernias

Dan J. Raz, MD
Resident, General Surgery, University of California at San Francisco, San Francisco, California
Epidemiology, Pathophysiology, and Clinical Features of Achalasia

Thomas William Rice, MD
Professor of Surgery, The Cleveland Clinic, The Cleveland Clinic Lerner College of Medicine of Case Western Reserve University; The Daniel and Karen Lee Chair in Thoracic Surgery and Head, Section of General Thoracic Surgery, The Cleveland Clinic Foundation, Cleveland, Ohio
Endoscopic Esophageal Ultrasonography

John P. Roberts, MD
Professor of Surgery, University of California at San Francisco; Chief, Transplant Services, University of California at San Francisco Medical Center, San Francisco, California
Hepatocellular Carcinoma

Patricia L. Roberts, MD
Associate Professor of Surgery, Tufts University School of Medicine, Boston; Chair, Department of Colon and Rectal Surgery, Lahey Clinic, Burlington, Massachusetts
Rectovaginal and Rectourethral Fistulas

Rolando Rolandelli, MD
Temple University Hospital, Philadelphia, Pennsylvania
Suturing, Stapling, and Tissue Adhesives

Ernest L. Rosato, MD
Associate Professor of Surgery and Director, Division of General Surgery, Jefferson Medical College, Thomas Jefferson University, Philadelphia, Pennsylvania
Pseudocysts and Other Complications of Pancreatitis

Alexander Rosemurgy, MD
Professor of Surgery and Medicine and Reeves/Culverhouse Chair for Pancreatic Cancer, University of South Florida; Director, Digestive Disorders Center, Department of Surgery, Tampa General Hospital, Tampa, Florida
Anatomy and Physiology of the Mesenteric Circulation

Kari M. Rosenkranz, MD
Breast Oncology Fellow, Department of Surgery, The University of Texas M. D. Anderson Cancer Center, Houston, Texas
Gastrointestinal Stromal Tumors

Adheesh A. Sabnis, MD
Resident, General Surgery, The George Washington University Medical Center, Washington, DC
Management of Splenic Abscess

Theodore J. Saclarides, MD
Professor of Surgery, Rush University Medical Center; Head, Section of Colon and Rectal Surgery, Rush University Medical Center, Chicago, Illinois
Radiation Injuries of the Rectum

Rainer K. Saetzler, MD
Universität Ulm, Ulm, Germany
Radiation Enteritis

Peter M. Sagar, MD, FRCS
Honorary Senior Lecturer, The University of Leeds; Consultant Surgeon, Department of Colon and Rectal Surgery, The General Infirmary at Leeds, Leeds, England
Surgery for Inflammatory Bowel Disease: Chronic Ulcerative Colitis

---

†Deceased.

George H. Sakorafas, MD, PhD
Consultant, Surgeon, 251 Hellenic Air Force Hospital, Athens, Greece
Primary Cystic Neoplasms of the Pancreas

Leonard B. Saltz, MD
Professor of Medicine, Weill Medical College, Cornell University; Attending Physician and Member, Memorial Sloan-Kettering Cancer Center, New York, New York
Adenocarcinoma of the Colon and Rectum

Michael G. Sarr, MD
James C. Masson Professor of Surgery, Mayo Clinic College of Medicine; Consultant, Division of Gastroenterologic and General Surgery, Mayo Clinic, Rochester, Minnesota
Primary Cystic Neoplasms of the Pancreas

Jeannie F. Savas, MD
Associate Professor of Surgery, Virginia Commonwealth University School of Medicine; Attending Surgeon, McGuire VA Medical Center; Attending Surgeon, Medical College of Virginia Hospitals, Richmond, Virginia
Postgastrectomy Syndromes

Bruce Schirmer, MD
Stephen H. Watts Professor of Surgery, Vice Chair, and Program Director, Department of Surgery, University of Virginia Health System, Charlottesville, Virginia
Reoperative Surgery of the Stomach and Duodenum

Paul M. Schneider, MD
Department of Surgery, University of Cologne, Cologne, Germany
Epidemiology, Risk Factors, and Clinical Manifestations of Esophageal Carcinoma

David J. Schoetz, Jr., MD
Professor of Surgery, Tufts University School of Medicine, Boston; Chairman Emeritus, Department of Colon Rectal Surgery and Chairman of Medical Education, Lahey Clinic, Burlington, Massachusetts
Colonic Intussusception and Volvulus

Richard D. Schulick, MD
Associate Professor of Surgery, Oncology, and Gynecology and Obstetrics; Chief, Cameron Division of Surgical Oncology; and John L. Cameron Professor of Surgery, Johns Hopkins University, Baltimore, Maryland
Pancreatic and Periampullary Carcinoma; Diagnostic Operations of the Liver and Techniques of Hepatic Resection

Marshall Z. Schwartz, MD
Professor of Surgery and Pediatrics, Drexel University College of Medicine; Surgeon-in-Chief, Chief of Pediatric Surgery, and Surgical Director, Pediatric Renal Transplantation, St. Christopher's Hospital for Children, Philadelphia, Pennsylvania
Surgical Conditions of the Small Intestine in Infants and Children

Mark Seamon, MD
Clinical Instructor, Temple University School of Medicine; Chief Resident, Temple University Hospital, Philadelphia, Pennsylvania
Injuries to the Stomach, Duodenum, and Small Bowel

Anthony J. Senagore, MD, MBA, MS
Professor and Chairman; Department of Surgery, Medical University of Ohio, Toledo, Ohio
Hemorrhoids

A. M. James Shapiro, MD, PhD, FRCS(Engl), FRCSC
Clinical Research Chair in Transplantation and Director, Clinical Islet Transplant Program, University of Alberta, Edmonton, Alberta, Canada
Islet Transplantation

Stuart Sherman, MD
Professor of Medicine and Radiology, Clinical Director of Gastroenterology and Hepatology, and Director of ERCP, Indiana University Medical Center, Indianapolis, Indiana
Endoscopic Retrograde Cholangiopancreatography in the Evaluation and Management of Hepatobiliary and Pancreatic Disease

Ketan R. Sheth, MD
Instructor of Surgery, Harvard Medical School, Cambridge, Massachusetts
Operative Management of Cholecystitis and Cholelithiasis

Jason K. Sicklick, MD
Surgical Resident, Johns Hopkins Hospital, Baltimore, Maryland
Management of Malignant Hepatic Neoplasms Other Than Hepatocellular Carcinoma

Elin R. Sigurdson, MD
Professor, Temple University; Head of Surgical Research and Attending Surgeon, Surgical Oncology, Fox Chase Cancer Center, Philadelphia, Pennsylvania
Gastrointestinal Carcinoid Tumors

Diane M. Simeone, MD
Attending Surgeon and Associate Professor of Surgery and Molecular and Integrative Physiology, University of Michigan Medical Center, Ann Arbor, Michigan
Hepatic Cyst Disease

Clifford L. Simmang, MD
Dallas Surgical Group, Dallas, Texas
Fissure-in-Ano

Cuthbert O. Simpkins, MD
Professor, Department of Surgery, Louisiana State University Health Sciences Center; Trauma Medical Director, Louisiana State University Hospital, Shreveport, Louisiana
Management of Hepatobiliary Trauma

James V. Sitzmann, MD
Department of Surgery, Indiana University School of Medicine, Indianapolis, Indiana
Perioperative Management and Nutrition in Patients with Liver and Biliary Tract Disease

Douglas P. Slakey, MD
Tulane Center for Abdominal Transplantation, New Orleans, Louisiana
Cysts and Tumors of the Spleen

Amy P. Soltes, RN, MSN, ACP-BC
Nurse Practitioner, Department of Radiology, The George Washington University, Washington DC
Imaging and Intervention in the Biliary System

Contributors

Christopher J. Sonnenday, MD
Assistant Chief of Service and Instructor, Department of Surgery, Johns Hopkins University School of Medicine; Attending Surgeon, Johns Hopkins Hospital, Baltimore, Maryland
Pseudocysts and Other Complications of Pancreatitis

Nathaniel J. Soper, MD
James R. Hines Professor of Surgery, Feinberg School of Medicine, Northwestern University; Director, Minimally Invasive Surgery; Chief, Gastrointestinal/Endocrine Surgery; and Vice Chair, Clinical Affairs, Northwestern Memorial Hospital, Chicago, Illinois
Epidemiology and Natural History of Gastroesophageal Reflux Disease; Management of Common Bile Duct Stones

George C. Sotiropoulos, MD
Department of General Surgery and Transplantation, University Hospital Essen, Essen, Germany
Anatomy and Physiology of the Liver

David I. Soybel, MD
Senior Staff Surgeon, Division of General and Gastrointestinal Surgery, Brigham and Women's Hospital, Boston, Massachusetts
Small Intestine

Stuart Jon Spechler, MD
Berta M. and Cecil O. Patterson Chair in Gastroenterology and Professor of Medicine, The University of Texas Southwestern Medical Center; Chief, Division of Gastroenterology, Dallas VA Medical Center, Dallas, Texas
Endoscopic Evaluation of the Esophagus

Kimberley E. Steele, MD
Department of Surgery, Johns Hopkins University School of Medicine, Baltimore, Maryland
Minimally Invasive Surgical and Image-Guided Interventional Approaches to the Spleen

Hubert J. Stein, MD
Professor, Paracelsus Medical University, Salzburg, Austria
Human Foregut Anatomy, Prenatal Development and Abnormalities, and Their Relation to Surgical Approaches; Esophageal Mucosal Injury and Duodenal Reflux

F. Dylan Stewart, MD
University of Maryland School of Medicine, Baltimore, Maryland
Management of Splenic Injury in Children

Luca Stocchi, MD
Associate Staff, Department of Colorectal Surgery, The Cleveland Clinic Foundation, Cleveland, Ohio
Embryology and Anatomy of the Colon; Recurrent and Metastatic Colorectal Cancer

Michael C. Stoner, MD
Assistant Professor of Surgery, The Brody School of Medicine, East Carolina University, Greenville, North Carolina
Small Intestinal Diverticula

Tim G. Strate, MD
Associate Professor, Department of Surgery, University of Hamburg; Senior Associate, Department of Surgery, University Medical Center Hamburg-Eppendorf, Hamburg, Germany
Chronic Pancreatitis

Scott A. Strong, MD
Staff, Departments of Colorectal Surgery and Pathobiology, The Cleveland Clinic, Cleveland, Ohio
Diagnosis of Colon, Rectal, and Anal Disease

James W. Suliburk, MD
Resident, Department of Surgery, The University of Texas Medical School at Houston, Houston, Texas
Anatomy and Physiology of the Stomach

Lee L. Swanström, MD
Clinical Professor of Surgery, Oregon Health Sciences University; Director, Division of Minimally Invasive Surgery, Legacy Health System, Portland, Oregon
Partial Fundoplications

Daniel E. Swartz, MD
Attending Surgeon, Community Medical Centers, St. Agnes Hospital, and Fresno Surgery Hospital, Fresno, California
Femoral Hernia

Tadahiro Takada, MD
Professor, Chairman, and Chief of HBP Division, Department of Surgery, Teikyo University School of Medicine, Tokyo, Japan
Cystic Disorders of the Bile Ducts

Eric P. Tamm, MD
Associate Professor of Radiology, The University of Texas M. D. Anderson Cancer Center, Houston, Texas
Unusual Pancreatic Tumors

Ali Tavakkolizadeh, MBBS
Instructor in Surgery, Harvard Medical School; Minimally Invasive Surgery Fellow, Department of Surgery, Brigham and Women's Hospital, Boston, Massachusetts
Operations for Peptic Ulcer

Pietro Tedesco, MD
Fellow in Gastrointestinal Surgery, University of California at San Francisco, San Francisco, California
Epidemiology, Pathophysiology, and Clinical Features of Achalasia

Swee H. Teh, MD, FRCSI
Instructor in Surgery, Department of Surgery, Oregon Health and Science University, Portland, Oregon
Laparoscopic and Open Nissen Fundoplication

Gordon L. Telford, MD
Professor of Surgery, Medical College of Wisconsin; Chief of Surgery, Zablocki VA Medical Center, Milwaukee, Wisconsin
Appendix

Julie K. Marosky Thacker, MD
Colon and Rectal Surgeon, Exempla Good Samaritan Hospital, Boulder; Northwest Surgical Associates, Wheat Ridge, Colorado
Diagnosis of Colon, Rectal, and Anal Disease

Jon S. Thompson, MD
Professor and Vice Chairman, University of Nebraska Medical Center, Omaha, Nebraska
Short-Bowel Syndrome

Alan G. Thorson, MD
Clinical Associate Professor of Surgery and Program Director, Section of Colon and Rectal Surgery, Creighton University; Clinical Associate Professor of Surgery, University of Nebraska, Omaha, Nebraska
Anal Sepsis and Fistula

L. William Traverso, MD
Clinical Professor of Surgery, University of Washington;
Attending Surgeon, Section of General, Thoracic, and
Vascular Surgery, Virginia Mason Medical Center, Seattle,
Washington
*New Developments in Chronic Pancreatitis: Before Head Resection,
Try Endoscopic Treatment First*

Wayne Truong, MD
Faculty of Medicine, Department of Surgery, University of
Alberta, Edmonton, Alberta, Canada
Islet Transplantation

Douglas J. Turner, MD
Assistant Professor of Surgery, University of Maryland,
Baltimore, Maryland
Gastric Resection and Reconstruction

Radu Tutuian, MD
Head, Gastrointestinal Function Unit, Division of
Gastroenterology and Hepatology, University of Zurich,
Zurich, Switzerland
*Physiology of the Esophagus and Its Sphincters; Multichannel
Intraluminal Impedance*

Andreas G. Tzakis, MD, PhD
Professor of Surgery, University of Miami Miller School of
Medicine; Co-Director, Division of Transplantation and
Director, Liver/Gastrointestinal Transplant Program, Jackson
Memorial Medical Center, Miami, Florida
Vascular Diseases of the Liver

David Utley, MD
Chief Medical Officer, BARRx Medical Incorporated,
Sunnyvale, California
Endoscopic Ablation of Barrett's Metaplasia and Dysplasia

Daniel Vallböhmer, MD
Department of Surgery, University of Cologne, Cologne,
Germany
*Epidemiology, Risk Factors, and Clinical Manifestations of
Esophageal Carcinoma*

Dirk Van Raemdonck, MD, PhD
Professor in Surgery, Thoracic Surgery Section, Catholic
University Leuven; Clinical Head, Department of Thoracic
Surgery, University Hospital Gasthuisberg, Leuven, Belgium
Pathophysiology and Treatment of Zenker's Diverticulum

Anthony C. Venbrux, MD
Professor of Radiology and Surgery, Department of
Radiology, The George Washington University, Washington
DC
Imaging and Intervention in the Biliary System

Selwyn M. Vickers, MD
Professor and Chief, Section of Gastrointestinal Surgery,
University of Alabama at Birmingham, Birmingham, Alabama
Liver Abscess

Hugo V. Villar, MD
Professor of Surgery and Professor of Radiation Oncology,
University of Arizona; Interim Head, Department of Surgery
and Chief, Section of Surgical Oncology, Arizona Health
Sciences Center, Tucson, Arizona
Anatomy and Physiology of the Spleen

James R. Wallace, MD, PhD
Associate Professor, Medical College of Wisconsin; Director,
Bariatric Surgery Program, Froedtert Memorial Lutheran
Hospital/Medical College of Wisconsin, Milwaukee,
Wisconsin
Appendix

Huamin Wang, MD, PhD
Assistant Professor, Gastrointestinal and Liver Pathology,
Department of Pathology, The University of Texas M. D.
Anderson Cancer Center, Houston, Texas
Unusual Pancreatic Tumors

Nir Wasserberg, MD
Assistant Professor of Clinical Surgery, Department of
Surgery, Division of Colorectal and Pelvic Floor Surgery, Keck
School of Medicine, University of Southern California;
Assistant Professor of Clinical Surgery, LAC+USC Medical
Center, Los Angeles, California
Lumbar and Pelvic Hernias

James L. Watkins, MD
Associate Professor of Clinical Medicine, Indiana University
Medical Center, Indianapolis, Indiana
*Endoscopic Retrograde Cholangiopancreatography in the Evaluation
and Management of Hepatobiliary and Pancreatic Disease*

Thomas J. Watson, MD
Associate Professor of Surgery, Division of Thoracic and
Foregut Surgery, University of Rochester School of Medicine
and Dentistry; Chief, Thoracic Surgery, University of
Rochester Medical Center, Strong Memorial Hospital,
Rochester, New York
Esophageal Replacement for End-Stage Benign Esophageal Disease

William H. Weintraub, MD
Abington Memorial Hospital, Abington, Pennsylvania
*Surgical Diseases of the Stomach and Duodenum in Infants and
Children*

Martin R. Weiser, MD
Assistant Member, Memorial Sloan-Kettering Cancer Center;
Assistant Professor of Surgery, Weill Medical College, Cornell
University, New York, New York
Adenocarcinoma of the Colon and Rectum

John P. Welch, MD
Clinical Professor of Surgery, University of Connecticut
School of Medicine, Farmington; Adjunct Professor of
Surgery, Dartmouth Medical School, Hanover; Lead
Physician, General Surgery Division, Connecticut Surgical
Group, Hartford; Senior Attending Surgeon, Hartford
Hospital, Hartford, Connecticut
Diverticular Disease

Mark L. Welton, MD
Associate Professor, Stanford University; Chief, Colon and
Rectal Surgery, Stanford University Medical Center, Stanford,
California
Surgery in the Immunocompromised Patient

Contributors

Steven D. Wexner, MD
Associate Professor of Surgery, Ohio State University Health Sciences Center, The Cleveland Clinic Foundation, Cleveland, Ohio; Clinical Professor, Department of Surgery, University of South Florida College of Medicine, Tampa; Chairman, Department of Colorectal Surgery and Chief of Staff, The Cleveland Clinic Florida, Weston, Florida
Surgical Treatment of Constipation

James M. D. Wheeler, MD, FRCS
Consultant Colorectal Surgeon, Cheltenham General Hospital, Cheltenham, Gloucestershire, England
Anatomy of the Colon

Rebekah R. White, MD
Surgical Oncology Fellow, Memorial Sloan-Kettering Cancer Center, New York, New York
Volvulus of the Stomach and Small Bowel

Thomas Wiegel, MD
Universität Ulm, Ulm, Germany
Radiation Enteritis

Bruce G. Wolff, MD
Professor of Surgery, Mayo Clinic College of Medicine; Consultant, Department of Surgery, Division of Colon and Rectal Surgery, Mayo Clinic and Mayo Foundation, Rochester, Minnesota
Surgery for Inflammatory Bowel Disease: Crohn's Disease

Herbert C. Wolfsen, MD
Associate Professor of Medicine, Mayo Clinic College of Medicine, Rochester, Minnesota; Consultant, Division of Gastroenterology and Hepatology, Mayo Clinic, Jacksonville, Florida
Endoscopic Ablation of Barrett's Metaplasia and Dysplasia

W. Douglas Wong, MD
Professor of Surgery, Weill Medical College, Cornell University; Chief, Colorectal Service, Department of Surgery, Memorial Sloan-Kettering Cancer Center, New York, New York
Ultrasonographic Diagnosis of Anorectal Disease

M. Jonathan Worsey, MA, MBBS, FRCS
Chief, General Surgery, Scripps Memorial Hospital, La Jolla, California
Reoperative Pelvic Surgery

Alene J. Wright, MD
Instructor of Surgery, Creighton University Medical Center, Omaha, Nebraska
Laparoscopic Inguinal Hernia Repair

Francis Yao, MD
Professor of Clinical Medicine and Surgery, University of California at San Francisco, San Francisco, California
Hepatocellular Carcinoma

Emre F. Yekebas, MD
Associate Professor of Surgery, University of Hamburg; Senior Associate, Department of Surgery, University Medical Center Hamburg-Eppendorf, Hamburg, Germany
Chronic Pancreatitis

Charles J. Yeo, MD
Samuel D. Gross Professor and Chair, Department of Surgery, Thomas Jefferson University, Philadelphia, Pennsylvania
Pseudocysts and Other Complications of Pancreatitis; Operative Management of Strictures and Benign Obstructive Disorders of the Bile Duct

Y. Nancy You, MD
Senior Resident, Department of Surgery, Mayo Clinic, Rochester, Minnesota
Splenectomy for Conditions Other Than Trauma

Tonia M. Young-Fadok, MD, MS
Associate Professor of Surgery, Mayo Clinic College of Medicine, Rochester, Minnesota; Chair, Division of Colon and Rectal Surgery, Mayo Clinic, Scottsdale, Arizona
Neoplasms of the Anus; Retrorectal Tumors; Laparoscopic Colorectal Surgery

Gazi B. Zibari, MD
Professor, Louisiana State University School of Medicine; Director, Willis-Knighton/Louisiana State University Health Sciences Center Regional Transplant Program; Courtesy Staff, Chrustus Schumpert Health System; Courtesy Staff, VA Medical Center, Shreveport, Louisiana
Management of Hepatobiliary Trauma

Gregory Zuccaro, Jr., MD
Head, Section of Gastrointestinal Endoscopy, The Cleveland Clinic Foundation, Cleveland, Ohio
Endoscopic Esophageal Ultrasonography

Preface

It is with great delight that the section editors and I present the sixth edition of *Shackelford's Surgery of the Alimentary Tract*. This encyclopedic set has served as an invaluable resource for surgeons, internists, gastroenterologists, residents, medical students, and other medical professionals over the past 50 years. I know that you will find this sixth edition educationally fulfilling, nicely illustrated, and up-to-date.

The first edition of *Surgery of the Alimentary Tract* was written by Dr. Richard T. Shackelford and published in 1955. Following the success of that first edition, the W. B. Saunders Company urged Dr. Shackelford to produce a second edition. Between 1978 and 1986 consecutive volumes were released, culminating in a five-volume set that had been expanded substantially from the first edition. Dr. George D. Zuidema was added as a co-editor. It was this second edition that served as my "bible" for alimentary tract diseases during my surgical residency and early faculty appointment.

The third edition, edited by Dr. Zuidema, was published in 1991 and proved to be an important step forward. The field of alimentary tract surgery had advanced, and many emerging techniques and new research findings were included in that edition. For that third edition, Dr. Zuidema enlisted the help of a guest editor for each of the five volumes.

The fourth edition, which was published in 1996, was encyclopedic in scope, breadth, and depth of coverage. This led it to be consulted as the classic reference source for surgeons, internists, gastroenterologists, and others involved in the care of patients with alimentary tract diseases.

In 2002, the fifth edition was published. I was delighted that Dr. Zuidema asked me to join him as a co-editor for that edition. Its publication nicely presented numerous changes in surgical practice, operative techniques, molecular biology, and noninvasive therapies. The world of alimentary tract surgery had continued to change, and the textbook reflected these changes.

This current sixth edition represents even more change, both for the field of alimentary tract surgery and for the textbook itself. All involved listened to the book's many users and have made substantial changes in the look and content of the text. The book has gone from five volumes to two volumes, while adding material and including a four-color production scheme. The authors have emphasized new procedures, including endoscopic and minimally invasive ones, and advances in technology. Dr. Zuidema, who was involved with the second through the fifth editions, has passed the baton, but he remains an inspiration to all those in the field of alimentary tract surgery. I am delighted to keep this project moving forward and have done so with his blessings and oversight from afar.

This sixth edition has been completed with an enormous amount of help from four colleagues, who have served as section editors for the four major sections of the book. These section editors have worked tirelessly planning, organizing, and developing this massive textbook. They have incorporated numerous changes in surgical practice, operative approaches, and noninvasive therapies within the text. Each area retains extensive sections on anatomy and physiology but then directs attention to both standard and cutting edge innovations. This sixth edition includes the contributions of two new and two retained section editors, in order to provide both innovation and stability.

Section I, "Esophagus and Hernia," is now edited by Dr. Jeffrey H. Peters, the Seymour I. Schwartz Professor and Chairman of the Department of Surgery at the University of Rochester School of Medicine and Dentistry in Rochester, New York. Dr. Peters is a world-renowned expert who brings his detailed knowledge of the esophagus and esophageal diseases to the textbook. He has put together a spectacular section on esophageal diseases, focusing on esophageal pathology and ambulatory diagnostics, gastroesophageal reflux disease, esophageal motility disorders, and esophageal neoplasia. This represents an entirely new presentation of esophageal diseases in *Shackelford's Surgery of the Alimentary Tract*, sixth edition.

For Section II, "Stomach and Small Intestine," Dr. Daniel T. Dempsey has expanded his previous contribution by taking on the jejunoileum as part of his section. Dr. Dempsey is Professor and Chairman of the Department of Surgery at Temple University School of Medicine in Philadelphia, Pennsylvania. He has done a superb job of merging both standard and innovative areas in this field. New to the section are discussions of upper gastrointestinal foreign bodies and bezoars, as well as entirely redone sections dealing with neoplasia, gastrointestinal stromal tumors, and vascular diseases. Dr. Dempsey's section is an outstanding contribution to this area, advancing the field to new heights.

For Section III, "Pancreas, Biliary Tract, Liver, and Spleen," we have a new section editor, Dr. Andrew S. Klein. Dr. Klein is the Esther and Mark Schulman Chair in Surgery and Transplant Medicine and Director of the Cedars-Sinai Comprehensive Transplant Center in Los Angeles. Dr. Klein has put together a tremendous hepatopancreaticobiliary (plus spleen) section, including new contributions about acute pancreatitis, chronic pancreatitis, cystic neoplasia of the pancreas, and laparoscopic approaches to biliary and liver diseases. Also included are top level discussions of fulminant hepatic failure and the bio-artificial liver, drug-induced liver damage, and extensive operative sections dealing with liver resection and liver transplantation. Dr. Klein has taken a previously very well done section and made it even better.

The last section, Section IV, "Colon, Rectum, and Anus," has again been supervised by Dr. John H. Pemberton, Professor of Surgery at the Mayo Clinic College of Medicine in Rochester, Minnesota. Dr. Pemberton is a world-renowned figure in his field, and his section has been nicely reworked. Included are new developments in the field, a better understanding of pelvic floor anatomy and physiology, updates regarding diagnosis and interventions for inflammatory bowel disease, as well as the addition of more extensive laparoscopic interventions and their outcomes.

This sixth edition would have been impossible without the hard work of each of these section editors. They have been helped immensely by their colleagues, staff, and all of the chapter contributors. I would like to thank each of these section editors for their hard work, vision, and skill in bringing this project to its fruition.

Very importantly, I would like to express my appreciation to the more than 300 individuals who have contributed chapters to this new, sixth edition. I understand how difficult it is to produce superb chapters, and I wish to recognize these individuals and thank them for their dedication and commitment. Many of the contributors here are topnotch, world class leaders in their fields, and I am deeply indebted to them for sharing their knowledge and enthusiasm, culminating in an outstanding product.

I would also like to thank the production team at Elsevier/W.B. Saunders, who have been instrumental in making this edition a reality. My thanks go out to Judith Fletcher, Kim Davis, Amy Cannon, and many others, who have been instrumental in overseeing this project. This edition represents an immense amount of new work, redesign, and illustration. These professionals have made it a labor of love to work on this project.

Finally, I must thank individuals who helped me during this process over the past 3 years. The majority of the early correspondence, mailings, and editorial oversight originated in the Department of Surgery at the Johns Hopkins University School of Medicine in Baltimore. My thanks go out to Janet Romanelli and Irma Silkworth for providing me with this support. Additionally, within the past year, Mary Toelke in my office here at the Thomas Jefferson University Hospital and the Jefferson Medical College has been an outstanding assistant and editor, providing me with tremendous support here in Philadelphia.

Charles J. Yeo, MD
Philadelphia, Pennsylvania

Contents

Contributors vii

Preface xxiii

VOLUME I

Section

I Esophagus and Hernia

Section Editor: Jeffrey H. Peters

Part

1 The Normal Esophagus

Chapter

1 Perspectives on Esophageal Surgery 3

Tom R. DeMeester

Chapter

2 Human Foregut Anatomy, Prenatal Development and Abnormalities, and Their Relation to Surgical Approaches 9

Dorothea Liebermann-Meffert and Hubert J. Stein

Chapter

3 Physiology of the Esophagus and Its Sphincters 48

Radu Tutuian and Donald O. Castell

Part

2 Evaluation of Esophageal Pathology and Ambulatory Diagnostics

Chapter

4 Assessment of Symptoms and Approach to the Patient with Esophageal Disease 56

Jeffrey H. Peters

Chapter

5 Imaging in Esophageal Disease 63

John M. Barlow, Daniel A. Craig, James E. Huprich, Val J. Lowe, and Robert L. MacCarty

Chapter

6 Endoscopic Evaluation of the Esophagus 100

Stuart Jon Spechler and Jacques J. G. H. M. Bergman

Chapter

7 Endoscopic Esophageal Ultrasonography 111

Thomas William Rice and Gregory Zuccaro, Jr.

Chapter

8 Esophageal Motility 128

Rodney John Mason

Chapter

9 pH and Bilirubin Monitoring 164

Leah M. Backhus and Ross M. Bremner

Chapter

10 Multichannel Intraluminal Impedance 175

Radu Tutuian and Donald O. Castell

Chapter

11 Tests of Gastric Function and Their Use in the Evaluation of Esophageal Disease 184

Karl-Hermann Fuchs

Part

3 Gastroesophageal Reflux Disease

Chapter

12 Epidemiology and Natural History of Gastroesophageal Reflux Disease 197

Alexander P. Nagle and Nathaniel J. Soper

Chapter

13 The Pathology of Gastroesophageal Reflux Disease 206

Parakrama Chandrasoma

Chapter

14 The Gastroesophageal Barrier 223

Jeffrey H. Peters and Tom R. DeMeester

Contents

Chapter

15 Esophageal Mucosal Injury and
Duodenal Reflux 230

Hubert J. Stein, Werner K. H. Kauer, and
Dorothea Liebermann-Meffert

Chapter

16 Reflux Strictures and Short Esophagus 234

Allan Pickens and Mark B. Orringer

Chapter

17 Medical Therapy for Gastroesophageal
Reflux Disease 252

Eugene Y. Chang and Blair A. Jobe

Chapter

18 Laparoscopic and Open Nissen
Fundoplication 265

Swee H. Teh, Robert W. O'Rourke, and John G. Hunter

Chapter

19 Partial Fundoplications 276

Lee L. Swanström

Chapter

20 Esophageal Replacement for End-Stage Benign
Esophageal Disease 285

Thomas J. Watson

Chapter

21 Endoscopic Antireflux Repairs 306

Atif Iqbal, Charles J. Filipi, and Henry Gale

Part

4 Barrett's Esophagus

Chapter

22 History and Definition of Barrett's
Esophagus 334

Reginald V. N. Lord

Chapter

23 Pathophysiology of the Columnar-Lined
Esophagus 341

Daniel S. Oh and Steven R. DeMeester

Chapter

24 Surgical Treatment of Barrett's
Esophagus 354

Jeffrey H. Peters

Chapter

25 Endoscopic Ablation of Barrett's Metaplasia
and Dysplasia 365

Herbert C. Wolfsen, David Utley, and Jeffrey H. Peters

Part

5 Esophageal Motility Disorders and
Diverticula of the Esophagus

Chapter

26 Disorders of the Pharyngoesophageal
Junction 374

André Duranceau

Chapter

27 Pathophysiology and Treatment of
Zenker's Diverticulum 391

Toni Lerut, Willy Coosemans, Georges Decker,
Paul De Leyn, Philippe Nafteux, and
Dirk Van Raemdonck

Chapter

28 Epidemiology, Pathophysiology, and Clinical
Features of Achalasia 405

Dan J. Raz, Pietro Tedesco, and Marco G. Patti

Chapter

29 Laparoscopic Esophageal Myotomy:
Techniques and Results 411

Dave R. Lal and Brant K. Oelschlager

Chapter

30 Diffuse and Segmental Esophageal Spasm,
Nutcracker Esophagus, and Hypertensive
Lower Esophageal Sphincter 419

Tasha A. K. Gandamihardja and Cedric G. Bremner

Chapter

31 Surgical Management of Esophageal
Diverticula 427

Luigi Bonavina

Part

6 Neoplasms of the Esophagus

Chapter

32 Epidemiology, Risk Factors, and Clinical
Manifestations of Esophageal Carcinoma 441

Daniel Vallböhmer, Jan Brabender, Paul M. Schneider,
and Arnulf H. Hölscher

Chapter

33 Esophageal Cancer: Current Staging Classifications and Techniques, Endoscopic Ultrasound, and Laparoscopic and Thoracoscopic Staging 448

Simon Law

Chapter

34 Carcinoma of the Esophagus and Gastroesophageal Junction 465

Jeffrey A. Hagen and Brian E. Louie

Chapter

35 Palliative Treatment of Carcinoma of the Esophagus 487

Thomas C. B. Dehn, Anthony S. Mee, Catherine Jephcott, and Ruth Moxon

Chapter

36 Multimodality Treatment of Esophageal Cancer 499

Waddah B. Al-Refaie and Wayne L. Hofstetter

Chapter

37 Benign Tumors and Cysts of the Esophagus 513

Richard F. Heitmiller and Molly M. Buzdon

Part

7 Miscellaneous Esophageal Conditions

Chapter

38 Perforation of the Esophagus 528

Dennis Blom

Chapter

39 Esophageal Caustic Injury 540

Peter F. Crookes

Chapter

40 Paraesophageal and Other Complex Diaphragmatic Hernias 549

Matthew M. Hutter and David W. Rattner

Chapter

41 Congenital Disorders of the Esophagus 563

R. Cartland Burns

Chapter

42 Techniques of Esophageal Reconstruction 578

Christopher R. Morse and Douglas J. Mathisen

Chapter

43 Complications of Esophageal Surgery 598

Andrew C. Chang and Mark B. Orringer

Part

8 Hernia

Chapter

44 Femoral Hernia 623

Daniel E. Swartz and Edward L. Felix

Chapter

45 Basic Features of Groin Hernia and Its Repair 632

Sathyaprasad C. Burjonrappa, Samuel Cemaj, and Robert J. Fitzgibbons, Jr.

Chapter

46 Laparoscopic Inguinal Hernia Repair 656

Varun Puri, Alene J. Wright, and Robert J. Fitzgibbons, Jr.

Chapter

47 Ventral Herniation in Adults 671

Andrew G. Harrell, Yuri W. Novitsky, Kent W. Kercher, and B. Todd Heniford

Chapter

48 Lumbar and Pelvic Hernias 687

Nir Wasserberg and Howard S. Kaufman

Chapter

49 Hernias and Congenital Groin Problems in Infants and Children 705

Walter Pegoli, Jr.

Section

II Stomach and Small Intestine

Section Editor: Daniel T. Dempsey

Chapter

50 Anatomy and Physiology of the Stomach 717

David W. Mercer and James W. Suliburk

Chapter

51 Diagnostic and Therapeutic Endoscopy of the Stomach and Small Bowel 733

Jeffrey M. Marks and Jeffrey L. Ponsky

Contents

Chapter

52 Intubation of the Stomach and
Small Intestine 749

Sean P. Harbison

Chapter

53 Injuries to the Stomach, Duodenum, and
Small Bowel 760

Amy J. Goldberg, Mark Seamon, and Abhijit S. Pathak

Chapter

54 Small Intestinal Diverticula 775

Michael C. Stoner, Joanna C. Arcuni, and
John M. Kellum

Chapter

55 Operations for Peptic Ulcer 791

Ali Tavakkolizadeh and Stanley W. Ashley

Chapter

56 Vagotomy and Drainage 811

Timothy J. Broderick and Jeffrey B. Matthews

Chapter

57 Gastric Resection and Reconstruction 831

Douglas J. Turner and Michael W. Mulholland

Chapter

58 Zollinger-Ellison Syndrome 862

James P. Dolan and Jeffrey A. Norton

Chapter

59 Postgastrectomy Syndromes 870

Thomas A. Miller and Jeannie F. Savas

Chapter

60 Miscellaneous Benign Lesions and Conditions
of the Stomach, Duodenum, and Small
Intestine 882

Emil L. Popa and Daniel T. Dempsey

Chapter

61 Adenocarcinoma of the Stomach, Duodenum,
and Small Intestine 904

Alexander A. Parikh and John M. Daly

Chapter

62 Motility Disorders of the Stomach and
Small Intestine 920

John E. Meilahn

Chapter

63 Operations for Morbid Obesity 928

Robert E. Brolin and Christopher Kowalski

Chapter

64 Foreign Bodies and Bezoars of the Stomach
and Small Intestine 940

Karen A. Chojnacki

Chapter

65 Surgical Diseases of the Stomach and
Duodenum in Infants and Children 947

Harsh Grewal and William H. Weintraub

Chapter

66 Anatomy and Physiology of
the Duodenum 964

John M. Kellum, Roberto C. Iglesias, and Jarrod Day

Chapter

67 Small Intestine 988

Mary F. Otterson, David Binion, Seth J. Karp,
David I. Soybel, Edward C. Mun, and Jeffrey B. Matthews

Chapter

68 Small Bowel Obstruction 1025

Soo Y. Kim and Jon B. Morris

Chapter

69 Volvulus of the Stomach and
Small Bowel 1035

Rebekah R. White and Danny O. Jacobs

Chapter

70 Crohn's Disease: General Considerations,
Medical Management, and Surgical Treatment
of Small Intestinal Disease 1041

D. Wayne Overby and Mark J. Koruda

Chapter

71 Ileostomy 1070

Riaz Cassim and David W. McFadden

Chapter

72 Suturing, Stapling, and Tissue Adhesives 1083

John Migaly and Rolando Rolandelli

Chapter

73 Gastric, Duodenal, and Small Intestinal
Fistulas 1092

Michael S. Nussbaum and David R. Fischer

Chapter

74 Internal Hernias—Congenital and
Acquired 1120

Mohammad K. Jamal and Eric J. DeMaria

Chapter

75 Mesenteric Arterial Trauma 1128

Rao R. Ivatury

Chapter

76 Reoperative Surgery of the Stomach and
Duodenum 1133

Bruce Schirmer and C. Joe Northup

Chapter

77 Radiation Enteritis 1150

Rainer K. Saetzler, Thomas Wiegel,
and Doris Henne-Bruns

Chapter

78 Short-Bowel Syndrome 1162

Jon S. Thompson and Alan N. Langnas

Chapter

79 Gastrointestinal Carcinoid Tumors 1179

Cletus A. Arciero and Elin R. Sigurdson

Chapter

80 Gastrointestinal Stromal Tumors 1189

Burton L. Eisenberg and Kari M. Rosenkranz

Chapter

81 Gastrointestinal Lymphomas 1199

Lindsey N. Jackson and B. Mark Evers

Chapter

82 Surgical Conditions of the Small Intestine in
Infants and Children 1213

Marshall Z. Schwartz and Ahmed Mami

Chapter

83 Anatomy and Physiology of the
Mesenteric Circulation 1234

Steven B. Goldin and Alexander Rosemurgy

Chapter

84 Mesenteric Ischemia 1247

Anthony J. Comerota and Matthew Todd Miller

Chapter

85 Aortoenteric Fistula and Visceral Artery
Aneurysms 1269

John Blebea and Rashad Choudry

VOLUME II

Section

III Pancreas, Biliary Tract, Liver, and Spleen

Section Editor: Andrew S. Klein

Part

1 Pancreas

Chapter

86 Anatomy, Physiology, and Embryology of
the Pancreas 1287

Dale E. Bockman

Chapter

87 Acute Pancreatitis 1296

Scott F. Gallagher, Colleen E. Jaffray, and Michel M. Murr

Chapter

88 Chronic Pancreatitis 1310

Jakob R. Izbicki, Tim G. Strate, Emre F. Yekebas,
and Oliver Mann

Chapter

89 New Developments in Chronic Pancreatitis:
Before Head Resection, Try Endoscopic
Treatment First 1321

L. William Traverso and Richard A. Kozarek

Chapter

90 Pseudocysts and Other Complications of
Pancreatitis 1329

Ernest L. Rosato, Christopher J. Sonnenday,
Keith D. Lillemoe, and Charles J. Yeo

Chapter

91 Pancreatic and Periampullary
Carcinoma 1358

Richard D. Schulick and John L. Cameron

Chapter

92 Neuroendocrine Tumors of
the Pancreas 1375

Daniela Ladner and Jeffrey A. Norton

Chapter

93 Primary Cystic Neoplasms of
the Pancreas 1387

George H. Sakorafas and Michael G. Sarr

Contents

Chapter

94 Pancreatic Trauma 1400

Edward E. Cornwell III, Elliott R. Haut,
and David Kuwayama

Chapter

95 Pancreatic Problems in Infants
and Children 1407

Charles N. Paidas and Mark L. Kayton

Chapter

96 Pancreas Transplantation 1415

David B. Leeser and Stephen T. Bartlett

Chapter

97 Islet Transplantation 1422

Wayne Truong and A. M. James Shapiro

Chapter

98 Unusual Pancreatic Tumors 1431

E. Ramsay Camp, Eric P. Tamm, Henry F. Gomez,
Huamin Wang, and Douglas B. Evans

Part
2 Biliary Tract

Chapter

99 Anatomy, Embryology, Anomalies,
and Physiology 1440

Henry A. Pitt and Thomas R. Gadacz

Chapter

100 Imaging and Intervention in
the Biliary System 1460

Anthony C. Venbrux, Elizabeth A. Ignacio,
Amy P. Soltes, and Albert K. Chun

Chapter

101 Operative Management of Cholecystitis
and Cholelithiasis 1471

Ketan R. Sheth and Theodore N. Pappas

Chapter

102 Laparoscopic Management of Common Bile
Duct Stones 1482

Edward H. Phillips and Gregg K. Nishi

Chapter

103 Endoscopic Retrograde
Cholangiopancreatography in the Evaluation
and Management of Hepatobiliary and
Pancreatic Disease 1490

Stuart Sherman, James L. Watkins, Lee McHenry,
Evan L. Fogel, and Glen A. Lehman

Chapter

104 Biliary Tract Tumors 1519

Clifford S. Cho and Yuman Fong

Chapter

105 External Biliary Fistula 1537

Itzhak Avital and Leslie H. Blumgart

Chapter

106 Biliary Atresia, Biliary Hypoplasia, and
Choledochal Cyst 1545

Stephen Dunn

Chapter

107 Cystic Disorders of the Bile Ducts 1552

Tadahiro Takada and Hisami Ando

Chapter

108 Primary Sclerosing Cholangitis 1560

Konstantinos N. Lazaridis and Gregory J. Gores

Chapter

109 Operative Management of Strictures
and Benign Obstructive Disorders of
the Bile Duct 1573

Keith D. Lillemoe, Charles J. Yeo, and Henry A. Pitt

Chapter

110 Management of Common Bile Duct
Stones 1590

Eric S. Hungness and Nathaniel J. Soper

Part
3 Liver

Chapter

111 Anatomy and Physiology of the Liver 1597

Ernesto P. Molmenti, Arnold Radtke,
George C. Sotiropoulos, and Massimo Malagó

Chapter

112 Approach to the Patient with Abnormal
Hepatic Laboratory Tests 1610

Brent J. Prosser and H. Franklin Herlong

Chapter

113   Perioperative Management and Nutrition
       in Patients with Liver and Biliary
       Tract Disease   1618
       James R. Ouellette, James V. Sitzman, and
       Steven D. Colquhoun

Chapter

114   Hepatic Cyst Disease   1630
       Michael W. Mulholland, Hero K. Hussain,
       and Diane M. Simeone

Chapter

115   Liver Abscess   1640
       L. Christopher DeRosier, Cheri M. Canon,
       and Selwyn M. Vickers

Chapter

116   Management of Hepatobiliary Trauma   1659
       Cuthbert O. Simpkins, Atta Nawabi, and Gazi B. Zibari

Chapter

117   Diagnostic Operations of the Liver and
       Techniques of Hepatic Resection   1670
       Richard D. Schulick

Chapter

118   Hepatic Transplantation   1685
       Steven D. Colquhoun, Nicholas N. Nissen,
       and Andrew S. Klein

Chapter

119   Fulminant Hepatic Failure and Bioartificial
       Liver Support   1702
       Achilles A. Demetriou

Chapter

120   Vascular Diseases of the Liver   1711
       David M. Levi and Andreas G. Tzakis

Chapter

121   Drug-Induced Liver Disease   1717
       Anurag Maheshwari and Rudra Rai

Chapter

122   Benign Hepatic Neoplasms   1726
       Felix Dahm and Pierre-Alain Clavien

Chapter

123   Hepatocellular Carcinoma   1732
       Elika Kashef, Francis Yao, and John P. Roberts

Chapter

124   Management of Malignant Hepatic
       Neoplasms Other Than Hepatocellular
       Carcinoma   1743
       Jason K. Sicklick and Michael A. Choti

Chapter

125   Multidisciplinary Approach to the Management
       of Portal Hypertension   1751
       J. Michael Henderson

Part

4   Spleen

Chapter

126   Anatomy and Physiology of the Spleen   1771
       Ernesto P. Molmenti, Donald O. Christensen,
       and Hugo V. Villar

Chapter

127   Minimally Invasive Surgical and Image-Guided
       Interventional Approaches to the Spleen   1780
       Michael R. Marohn, Kimberley E. Steele, and L. P. Lawler

Chapter

128   Management of Splenic Trauma in
       Adults   1798
       Anne Lidor

Chapter

129   Management of Splenic Injury in
       Children   1805
       Paul M. Colombani and F. Dylan Stewart

Chapter

130   Cysts and Tumors of the Spleen   1813
       Michael R. Burgdorf and Douglas P. Slakey

Chapter

131   Management of Splenic Abscess   1818
       Adheesh A. Sabnis and Jeffrey L. Ponsky

Chapter

132   Splenectomy for Conditions Other
       Than Trauma   1822
       Y. Nancy You, John H. Donohue, and David M. Nagorney

Contents

Section

IV Colon, Rectum, and Anus

Section Editor: John H. Pemberton

Part 1 Anatomy, Physiology, and Diagnosis of Colorectal and Anal Disease

Chapter
133 Anatomy of the Colon 1845
James M. D. Wheeler and Neal James McCready Mortensen

Chapter
134 Embryology and Anatomy of the Colon 1857
Luca Stocchi and John H. Pemberton

Chapter
135 Physiology of the Colon and Its Measurement 1871
Adil E. Bharucha and Michael Camilleri

Chapter
136 Diagnosis of Colon, Rectal, and Anal Disease 1883
Julie K. Marosky Thacker, Scott A. Strong, and James M. Church

Chapter
137 Ultrasonographic Diagnosis of Anorectal Disease 1899
Dimitra G. Barabouti and W. Douglas Wong

Part 2 Benign Colon, Rectal, and Anal Conditions

Chapter
138 Diagnosis and Management of Fecal Incontinence 1917
Susan C. Parker and Robert D. Madoff

Chapter
139 Surgical Treatment of Constipation 1929
David J. Maron and Steven D. Wexner

Chapter
140 Rectovaginal and Rectourethral Fistulas 1945
Patricia L. Roberts

Chapter
141 Complete Rectal Prolapse 1958
Amir L. Bastawrous and Herand Abcarian

Chapter
142 Pilonidal Disease 1966
Debra Holly Ford and H. Randolph Bailey

Chapter
143 Traumatic Colorectal Injuries, Foreign Bodies, and Anal Wounds 1972
Susan Galandiuk, Jeffrey R. Jorden, and Hiram C. Polk, Jr.

Chapter
144 Colonic Intussusception and Volvulus 1980
Robin P. Boushey and David J. Schoetz, Jr.

Chapter
145 Colonic Bleeding and Ischemia 1987
Ronald Kaleya and Scott J. Boley

Chapter
146 Diverticular Disease 2012
Jeffrey L. Cohen and John P. Welch

Chapter
147 Hemorrhoids 2029
Anthony J. Senagore

Chapter
148 Fissure-in-Ano 2038
Harry T. Papaconstantinou, Philip Huber, Jr., and Clifford L. Simmang

Chapter
149 Anal Sepsis and Fistula 2045
Michael A. Jobst and Alan G. Thorson

Chapter
150 Miscellaneous Disorders of the Rectum and Anus 2062
David E. Beck

Part 3 Inflammatory Diseases

Chapter
151 Inflammatory Bowel Disease 2080
Edward V. Loftus, Jr. and Robert R. Cima

Chapter

152 Surgery for Inflammatory Bowel Disease: Chronic Ulcerative Colitis 2101

Peter M. Sagar and John H. Pemberton

Chapter

153 Surgery for Inflammatory Bowel Disease: Crohn's Disease 2127

David W. Larson and Bruce G. Wolff

Chapter

154 Appendix 2141

Gordon L. Telford and James R. Wallace

Part

4 Neoplastic Disease

Chapter

155 Colorectal Polyps, Polyposis Syndromes, and Hereditary Nonpolyposis Colorectal Cancer 2152

David B. Chessin and José G. Guillem

Chapter

156 Adenocarcinoma of the Colon and Rectum 2183

Martin R. Weiser, Mitchell C. Posner, and Leonard B. Saltz

Chapter

157 Local Excision of Rectal Cancer 2208

Jacob A. Greenberg and Ronald Bleday

Chapter

158 Operations for Colorectal Cancer: Low Anterior Resection 2218

Alfred M. Cohen

Chapter

159 Abdominoperineal Resection of the Rectum for Cancer 2234

Joseph Martz and Warren E. Enker

Chapter

160 Coloanal Anastomosis 2245

Gerald Isenberg, Christophe Penna, and Rolland Parc

Chapter

161 Recurrent and Metastatic Colorectal Cancer 2255

Luca Stocchi and Heidi Nelson

Chapter

162 Resection and Ablation of Metastatic Colorectal Cancer to the Liver 2274

Florencia G. Que and David M. Nagorney

Chapter

163 Neoplasms of the Anus 2288

Jonathan E. Efron and Tonia M. Young-Fadok

Chapter

164 Retrorectal Tumors 2299

Tonia M. Young-Fadok and Eric J. Dozois

Chapter

165 Rare Colorectal Malignancies 2312

Paul J. McMurrick, Peter W. G. Carne, and Michael Johnston

Chapter

166 Radiation Injuries of the Rectum 2320

Matthew L. Lynch and Theodore J. Saclarides

Part

5 Techniques and Pearls

Chapter

167 Antibiotics, Approaches, Strategy, and Anastomoses 2327

Jan Rakinic

Chapter

168 Laparoscopic Colorectal Surgery 2340

Tonia M. Young-Fadok and Peter W. Marcello

Chapter

169 Ostomy Management 2362

Peter Cataldo and Neil H. Hyman

Chapter

170 Surgery in the Immunocompromised Patient 2375

George J. Chang and Mark L. Welton

Chapter

171 Anorectal Anomalies 2387

Scott A. Engum and Jay L. Grosfeld

Chapter

172 Reoperative Pelvic Surgery 2409

M. Jonathan Worsey and Victor W. Fazio

Index i

Esophagus and Hernia

Jeffrey H. Peters

1

Perspectives on Esophageal Surgery

Tom R. DeMeester

To write a perspective on a subject is to clearly view a subject through a medium, usually an optical glass such as spectacles or some form of scope. In this instance the scope is history or, if you prefer, the retrospective scope. The accumulation of human experience makes up history and, according to C. S. Lewis, "authority, reason and experience; on these three, mixed in varying proportions all our knowledge depends."[1] If today's esophageal surgeon desires to stand on the shoulders of those who went before us and not repeat their mistakes, the knowledge and appreciation of important milestones in esophageal surgery must be appreciated and embraced.

To understand a surgical disease requires the capacity to see and touch the affected tissue. Until the science of surgery was translated to human patients, autopsy reports provided most of our understanding of esophageal disease. They consisted largely of spontaneous perforations (Boerhaave's syndrome)[2] and tumors of the esophagus and provided little to the understanding of benign inflammatory disease, such as esophagitis. This is because autolysis of the distal esophageal mucosa by digestive enzymes occurred during the interval between death and autopsy. Any tissue injury around the gastroesophageal junction was assumed to be a postmortem change, much like the organism *Helicobacter pylori* was assumed to not be a pathogen in the stomach. Consequently, the existence and pathologic description of esophagitis and inflammatory strictures were not appreciated until Heinrich

Quincke, a German internist, brought attention to them through his publication on esophageal ulcers in 1879.[3]

Further, the remote inaccessibility of the esophagus in the posterior mediastinum surrounded by the lungs and heart deterred understanding of diseases that affect the organ until the introduction of rigid esophagoscopy 130 years ago by Bevan in 1868,[4] Kussmaul in 1868,[5] and Mikulicz in 1881.[6] Subsequently, several breakthroughs in technology permitted complete and safe endoscopic examination of the entire esophagus, stomach, and duodenum. First was the invention of the incandescent light bulb by Thomas Edison in the 1870s. Second was the introduction of the rod-lens system by Hopkins in the 1950s. Third was the development of fiberoptic cold-light transmission in the 1960s. Last was the evolution of the computer chip video camera in the 1980s.[7] Combined, these technologic advancements provided reliable clinical esophagoscopy with the ability to directly examine and biopsy the esophageal mucosa. This ability opened the door to understanding the pathophysiology of esophagitis, stricture, and Barrett's esophagus with its inherent cancer risk.

ESOPHAGEAL CANCER

Cancer of the esophagus was a unique challenge for the surgeon. For decades, surgical pioneers have struggled with safe removal of the diseased organ. Emslie in his "Perspectives in the Development of Esophageal Surgery" states, "the history of esophageal surgery is the tale of men repeatedly losing to a stronger adversary yet persisting in this unequal struggle until the nature of the problems became apparent and the war was won."[8] The major obstacles were the continuation of respiration with an open thorax and the restoration of alimentary tract continuity after esophageal resection.

The first successful esophagectomy for squamous cell carcinoma was performed by Franz Torek.[9] General anesthesia was administered by a new technique called insufflation, in which ether was delivered through a woven silk tube used to intubate the patient. The existing technique of a differential pressure chamber was not considered because the rubber cuff around the patient's neck, used to create subatmospheric pressure about the body, prevented construction of a cervical esophagostomy. The esophagus with a cancer abutting the left main bronchus was removed by a transthoracic transpleural exposure. Dr. Torek avoided injury to the vagi and the possibility of "sudden death due to vagal collapse" by carefully dissecting them off the esophagus. His fear of vagal circulatory collapse is reflected in his statement: "At the site of the tumor the dissection of the vagi was more difficult, and some of the branches crossing over in front of it had to be cut in order to permit liberating the tumor without undue roughness in handling the vagi. To my great satisfaction the pulse never wavered during the procedure, remaining between 93 and 96. The dreaded vagus collapse had, therefore, been safely avoided."[9] A pleural infection from an esophageal leak was circumvented by carefully closing the cardia and performing a cervical esophagostomy. The reported existence of extensive adhesions between the left lung and the parietal pleura in all probability prevented collapse of the left lung and contributed as much to the success of the procedure as Torek's surgery. The patient recovered and survived for another 13 years, with continuity between the cervical esophagostomy and gastrostomy established by an external "rubber tube."

The fact that 20 barren years intervened between the first and second successful procedure testifies to the challenge that removal of the esophagus posed to surgeons. Wolfgang Denk took up the challenge and developed a totally different approach to resection of the thoracic esophagus.[10] He showed in cadavers that the esophagus could be removed by blunt dissection through the combination of an abdominal transhiatal and a cervical transthoracic inlet approach. This technique, knowingly or unknowingly, was used in the second successful esophagectomy reported by Grey Turner in 1933.[11] As suggested by Denk, the procedure was performed without opening the chest by blunt burrowing from the abdomen and neck. The esophagus with a midconstricting neoplasm was successfully removed. Alimentary tract continuity was re-established 7 months after the esophagectomy by a second procedure connecting the cervical esophageal and abdominal gastric stomas by a subcutaneous skin tube.

While surgeons struggled with esophagectomy, advances in anesthesia continued. The description of an intratracheal tube with an inflatable cuff by Theodore Tuffeir in 1896[12] and its introduction into clinical practice in 1928 by Magill[13] allowed the development of positive pressure anesthesia and the direct transthoracic approach to the esophagus. Similarly, experimental work on restoration of the alimentary tract after esophageal resection continued. Claude Beck in 1905 showed in animals that a tube constructed along the greater curvature of the stomach could be used to replace a portion of the esophagus.[14] Cesar Roux in 1907 developed the technique of using the jejunum to replace the distal end of the esophagus.[15] G. Kelling devised a method of using an isoperistaltic segment of transverse colon to completely replace the thoracic esophagus.[16]

In the wake of these accomplishments, it is not surprising that the final successful step of performing an esophagectomy with an intrathoracic esophagogastric anastomosis was reported by Tatsuo Ohsawa from Japan in 1933.[17] He successfully performed a simultaneous esophagogastrectomy and esophagogastrostomy in eight patients with carcinoma of the lower esophagus and cardia. No follow-up is available on Ohsawa's patients, and unfortunately his paper did not reach the attention of the Western world for 5 years. Samuel Marshall from the United States reported a similar procedure in one patient in 1938. However, this patient was plagued by persistent esophageal obstruction and esophagitis that required repetitive dilation.[18]

With initial success, surgeons realized that performing a dependable intrathoracic esophagogastric anastomosis was a major part of the challenge. Infection of the mediastinum and pleural cavities because of disruption of the anastomosis was the most frequent cause of failure of the operation. Adams and Phemister took the problem to the laboratory, and only when a high degree of success was attained in dogs was a similar anastomotic procedure applied to humans with carcinoma of the thoracic esophagus. Their report in 1938 popularized the one-stage resection for esophageal cancer with an intrathoracic esophagogastrostomy.[19]

Today, challenges still remain in the surgical treatment of esophageal cancer. Questions of temporal interest include the following: Does en bloc esophagogastrectomy reduce the incidence of local recurrence of cancer that occurs after more limited resections? Are limited resections for early cancer sufficient to eradicate the disease and are they superior to endoscopic methods of resection? Is a vagal-sparing esophagectomy without lymphadenectomy a less morbid and safer procedure, and is it adequate therapy for early disease?

In the history of surgical practice, therapy for carcinoma of the esophagus carries an aura of pessimism with an attitude that cure is a chance phenomenon. This setting has given rise to two current treatment philosophies. First is that surgical removal of the primary tumor is the goal of therapy and the need for lymph node dissection is of limited benefit. Second, is that surgery alone is insufficient therapy and neoadjuvant or adjuvant radiation therapy or chemotherapy (or both) is necessary to achieve cure. This philosophy persists even though contemporary surgical experience has validated that complete surgical resection of an early tumor and limited nodal disease can cure a patient of esophageal cancer with an effectiveness better than that achieved by any other single or combined therapy.

ESOPHAGEAL MOTILITY DISORDERS

Surgical therapy for esophageal motility disorders started with the treatment of achalasia. *Megaesophagus*, or *achalasia* as it later came to be known, was first described by Willis in 1674. He advocated the use of a small sponge attached to a long strip of whalebone to force impacted food through the narrow distal esophagus.[20] Arthur Hurst showed that an abnormality of the intermuscular nerve plexus was responsible for the disease. He named the disease achalasia of the cardia because the continued tonic contraction of the cardiac sphincter prevented esophageal emptying. Hurst devised rubber tubes of various size with blunt tips filled with mercury to dilate the tonic sphincter. They are now referred to as Hurst dilators and were subsequently modified with tapered tips and called Maloney dilators.[21]

The initial surgical procedures used to relieve a spastic cardia were designed to enlarge the narrowed gastroesophageal junction with various cardioplasties of the Heineke-Mikulicz or Finney pyloroplasty type or to bypass the junction with an esophagogastrostomy. Ernst Heller in 1914 described a simple myotomy for the treatment of achalasia with the suggestion that it replace the more dramatic operation being performed.[22] The operation was based on Ramstedt's pyloromyotomy developed in 1912. Ramstedt's operation was immediately accepted by other surgeons for the treatment of congenital pyloric stenosis.[23] In contrast, despite knowledge of Heller's myotomy for achalasia, the procedure was seldom used and largely ignored in Germany, England, and the United States. Part of the problem of acceptance was the unknown etiology of achalasia, the absence of a histologic lesion, and disagreement over the nature of the physiologic abnormality and hence the purpose of the operation. According to Ravitch[24] this situation was changed dramatically by a paper from Norman Barrett in 1949 in which he described dismal results after esophagogastrostomy or cardioplasty operations.[25] Phillip Allison,[26] Barrett, and others were studying reflux esophagitis at the time and pointed out that destroying or bypassing the gastroesophageal junction encouraged esophagitis of such severity that patients suffered heartburn, would not eat, and bled seriously. Barrett proposed Heller's operation as an alterative and reported success with it. Barrett encouraged the use of Groeneveldt's modification of Heller's operation, specifically, performing only one myotomy instead of two. Barrett's paper and the increased awareness and interest in esophagitis led to widespread acceptance of the Heller procedure as the primary mode of operative therapy for achalasia. Dor in 1962[27] and Toupet in 1963[28] developed antireflux repairs to be used in conjunction with Heller myotomy to provide further protection against the sequelae of esophagitis. Eventually, gastroenterologists were able to rupture the muscle of the cardia with pneumatic dilators and obtain results close to those of surgery. This, along with the fear of surgery and the custom of patients first

contacting the gastroenterologist, led to a decrease in referral of patients for surgical myotomy. The recent introduction of laparoscopic myotomy with its greater safety and minimal morbidity has reversed this trend.

Franz Ingelfinger[29] in 1959 and Charles Code[30] in 1958 introduced esophageal manometry to clarify the diagnosis of achalasia and identify other esophageal motility disorders such as diffuse spasm and hypertensive lower esophageal sphincter. These latter conditions very rarely require myotomy of the esophageal body or lower esophageal sphincter.

Today, laparoscopic myotomy is the accepted therapy for achalasia. The procedure has been standardized in that most esophageal surgeons perform a myotomy that extends at least 3 cm onto the stomach and add a partial fundoplication to reduce the reflux of gastric juice into the esophagus. The location of the myotomy, either in the anterior quadrant between the "clasps" and "oblique" fibers or in the left lateral quadrant in line with the greater curvature and cutting only the "oblique" fibers, is still debated. The performance of a surgical myotomy is the creation of a defect to correct a defect and, consequently, can never restore the function of the cardia to normal. Therefore, a modified Heller myotomy is a palliative procedure.

ESOPHAGEAL DIVERTICULUM

The first description of a pharyngoesophageal diverticulum is attributed to Abraham Ludlow. He observed the abnormality at an autopsy he performed and reported the finding to William Hunter, John's brother, in 1764. Ludlow eventually published the observation in 1767.[31] Today, Ludlow's autopsy specimen is registered in the Hunterian Museum. Sir Charles Bell, a surgeon who described Bell's palsy, was the first to define the abnormalities necessary for the development of a pharyngoesophageal diverticulum.[32] Before Bell's publication in 1816, the diverticulum was thought to be congenital or traumatic in origin. The two components that Bell identified as necessary for a diverticulum to form were discoordination of the inferior pharyngeal constrictors and the cricopharyngeus muscle and a preexisting anatomic defect between these muscles. These observations predated our modern acceptance of them by 100 years.

The first successful resection of a pharyngoesophageal diverticulum was performed in 1886 by a surgeon with the last name of Wheeler on a patient named Captain E.[33] Diverticulectomy became the standard form of treatment, but the incidence of salivary fistulas and late recurrence was high. This prompted Girard from France in 1896 to treat two patients by invagination of the diverticulum into the lumen of the esophagus and oversewing the resultant dimple.[34] This approach was apparently successful, but in subsequent follow-up of the patients, at least one had a complete recurrence. Diverticulopexy was also described during this early period as a means of avoiding contamination of the wound and fistula formation.

The dangers of surgical therapy for pharyngoesophageal diverticula were reported in 1906 by Zesas,[35] who collected 42 patients from published reports and noted that primary healing occurred in only 6, fistulization in 26, and death in 8, for a mortality rate of 19%. To avoid the devastating results, Goldmann in 1909[36] devised a two-stage method of repair that was later modified by Lahey and Warren in 1954.[37] The modified procedure consisted of diverticulopexy and mediastinal packing in the first stage and resection of the diverticulum in the second. In 1945 the one-stage operation was readvocated by Harrington.[38] The battle between the protagonists of one-stage and two-stage resection continued for years and diverted attention from identifying the etiology of the diverticulum. Aubin, in 1936, was the first to propose, based on Bell's observations, a rational treatment of a pharyngoesophageal diverticulum that consisted of cricopharyngeal myotomy combined with diverticulectomy.[39] His publication refocused attention on the underlying pathology in the skeletal muscle of the cricopharyngeal sphincter and cervical esophagus. His report lead to the gradual abandonment of the two-stage operation. In 1966 Ronald Belsey,[40] in keeping with the desire to avoid contamination of the wound and fistula formation, advocated cricopharyngeal and cervical esophageal myotomy with diverticulopexy for all but very large diverticula.

The story of the pharyngoesophageal diverticulum is an object lesson from the history of surgery. It illustrates that medicine is a science often forced to be practiced before it is understood. It is not uncommon for observations, which form the bases for successful therapy, to be initially ignored or overlooked, rediscovered, and then adopted years later, in this example 2 centuries later!

In 1840 Rokitansky[41] described traction diverticula of the thoracic esophagus but was uncertain about their etiology. He thought that they were due to pressure from ingested food or obstruction of the distal esophagus by a stricture or extrinsic compression. Excision of an intrathoracic diverticulum was rarely reported, probably because of the disastrous results from leakage and fatal mediastinal and pleural sepsis. Moreover, considerable confusion existed during the middle of the 19th century regarding the etiology of the different diverticula affecting the esophagus. The confusion was resolved largely by the pathologist Albert Zenker, who with von Zeimssen in 1877 published "Krankheiten des Oesophagus," the best compendium of information on the esophagus in the latter part of the 19th century.[42] They introduced for the first time the separation of diverticula into two etiologic categories: traction and pulsion. The former is caused by inflammatory adhesions and the latter by forces within the esophageal muscular tube. The concept was quickly accepted, but confusion persisted with regard to terminology. The concept was further supported when esophageal manometry confirmed that development of a pulsion diverticulum was a complication of a motility disorder rather than a primary anatomic abnormality.[43] The major obstacle to accepting the concept was the inconsistency in identifying a motility disorder in all patients with a pulsion diverticulum. This inconsistency led to controversy over the necessity for primary correction of the motility abnormality before any direct attack

was made on the diverticulum. With technical improvements in esophageal manometry, 24-hour ambulatory motility studies became possible and showed, in all patients who had a pulsion diverticulum, a disordered motility pattern distal to the diverticulum. Today, the combination of myotomy of the esophagus distal to the diverticulum, including the lower esophageal sphincter, resection of the diverticulum, and a Dor partial fundoplication has become the standard procedure.[27]

HIATAL HERNIA AND GASTROESOPHAGEAL REFLUX DISEASE

In 1853 Henry Ingersoll Bowditch commented on hiatal hernia in his published monograph titled *A Treatise on Diaphragmatic Hernia:* "Owing to the ignorance of most of the observers in regard to the true nature of the affection, their modes of treatment have been entirely empirical and generally very absurd, and not a few times absolutely hurtful to the patient."[44] Even though Heinrick Quinche described esophagitis in 1879,[3] symptoms of the abnormality were poorly understood and no consideration was given to reflux of gastric contents up into the esophagus as its cause. In 1928 Harrington reported on 51 patients with a diaphragmatic hernia and concentrated only on describing the anatomic defect and closure of the hiatus for therapy without discussing symptomatology.[38] It was not until Philip Allison's publication in 1951[26] that the symptoms associated with a hiatal hernia were linked to the reflux of gastric contents into the esophagus. Allison used the term reflux esophagitis to describe the cause of the symptoms and emphasized correction of the defect at the cardia as the proper therapy. The term reflux esophagitis was confusing to gastroenterologists, who emphasized increased gastric acidity as the major problem and advocated reduction of gastric acid and peptic secretion as a means of treating the esophagitis rather than stopping the reflux. This started a lasting controversy between gastroenterologists and surgeons. Gastroenterologists emphasized the use of bougies, antacids, and advice on posture, and surgeons devised operations to restore sphincter competence and sought methods to objectively select patients for the procedure.

Allison described the first logical hiatal hernia repair by emphasizing repositioning of the gastroesophageal junction into its normal intra-abdominal location in the hope of improving its function.[26] Recognition of the high incidence of symptomatic and anatomic recurrence after the Allison repair led to the development of procedures designed to place and anchor the lower esophagus in the intra-abdominal position in a more effective manner. A posterior gastropexy in which the phrenoesophageal membrane and the cardioesophageal junction are anchored to the median arcuate ligament of the aortic hiatus was devised, used, and reported by Lucious Hill in 1967.[45] Two additional operations, the Nissen fundoplication introduced in 1956[46] and the Belsey Mark IV introduced in 1967,[47] were designed to augment the lower esophageal sphincter with a cuff of stomach, as well as re-establish an intra-abdominal segment of esophagus.

An important contribution was made in 1957 by Lee Collis in the management of advanced gastroesophageal reflux disease when reflux-induced intramural fibrosis causes esophageal shortening. He worked out a technique to add 4 cm to the length of the esophagus by the creation of a proximal gastroplasty tube, around which later surgeons applied a partial or full fundoplication.[48]

Norman Barrett in 1950[49] opened a whole new era in esophageal disease that ultimately connected benign gastroesophageal reflux disease with esophageal adenocarcinoma, one of the most devastating cancers known to affect humans. He reported his experience on columnar-lined esophagus with accompanying esophagitis and ulceration. He thought that the condition was due to congenital shortening of the esophagus but was subsequently proved wrong by Allison and Johnstone in 1953, who noted normal esophageal musculature and esophageal submucosal glands underneath the columnar epithelium. They reported that the change in epithelium was acquired as a result of erosive injury of the squamous mucosa.[50] In 1975 Naef and Ozzello[51] cautioned that the acquired columnar epithelium had a predisposition to malignant change. In 1978 Haggitt[52] suggested and subsequently Skinner[53] and Reid[54] confirmed that only intestinalized columnar mucosa was associated with malignant degeneration.

The Nissen fundoplication, because of its simplicity and effectiveness, was rapidly adopted worldwide as the procedure of choice for gastroesophageal reflux disease. Dorothea Liebermann-Meffert, a personal friend of Nissen, archived the historical development of the Nissen fundoplication.[55] The first step toward the operation occurred in 1937 when Rudolf Nissen, then in Istanbul, Turkey, operated on a 28-year old man with a chronic bleeding ulcer in the distal esophagus. He resected the cardia and anastomosed the esophageal stump into the gastric fundus. To protect the anastomosis he covered the esophagogastrostomy with a cuff of stomach. Sixteen years latter Nissen had the opportunity to re-examine the patient, and in contrast to the usual experience after resection of the cardia and esophagogastrostomy, the patient was free of symptoms and signs of gastroesophageal reflux. The second step toward fundoplication occurred in 1946 when Nissen, then in New York, performed a transabdominal reduction of a paraesophageal hernia in a patient who refused a thoracotomy. He was surprised by the ease with which the hernia could be reduced and the degree of exposure of the esophageal hiatus through a transabdominal incision. The third and final step occurred in 1954 when Nissen, then in Basel, Switzerland, combined the two previous observations into a planned antireflux procedure in a patient suffering from severe gastroesophageal reflux disease. He formed a fold from the anterior and posterior gastric fundic walls and attached both to each other on the lesser curvature side of the stomach above the gastroesophageal junction. The clinical outcome, a complete success, could be reproduced in a subsequent patient. In the publication of the procedure in *Schweizer Medizinische Wochenschrift* in 1956 he termed the operation "gastroplication" and described it as a "simple and effective operation for reflux esophagitis."

During the 1960s and 1970s gastroesophageal reflux disease was accepted as a distinct disease entity independent of hiatal hernia. With the introduction of water perfusion esophageal manometry in 1956, the lower esophageal sphincter was identified as the major barrier against the reflux of gastric contents, and the physiology of barrier augmentation by a surgical antireflux procedure was clarified. The availability of 24-hour pH monitoring in 1974 allowed gastroesophageal reflux disease to be defined quantitatively and improved the selection of patients for antireflux surgery.[56] In 1991 Bernard Dallemagne of Liege, Belgium, performed the first known human laparoscopic Nissen fundoplication.[57] Successful laparoscopic ligation of the short gastric vessels and safe posterior dissection of the abdominal portion of the esophagus were the significant accomplishments at the time. Today, laparoscopic Nissen fundoplication has become commonplace. Its safe, effective, and user-friendly characteristics have positioned surgical therapy for earlier application in the treatment of gastroesophageal reflux disease.

THE ESOPHAGEAL SURGEON

The esophagus has never had a sizable patronage. This is well illustrated in a vignette recorded by Earle Wilkins about Dr. Willy Meyers, who reported successful esophageal resection at the annual meeting of the American Medical Association in 1903. The report was met with indifference and no discussion. The obvious lack of interest among physicians for problems concerning the esophagus was the direct impetus for Dr. Meyer to take the lead, with a small group of "interested" surgeons, and form the American Association for Thoracic Surgery, the founding organization in the clinical specialty of thoracic surgery.[58] Esophageal surgery, despite being the spark that ignited the first society for thoracic surgery, was soon crowded out by the burgeoning business of coronary bypass surgery. Consequently, over the years the esophagus has been used, sometimes ill-used and sometimes ignorantly used, by gastroenterologists, otolaryngologists, thoracic surgeons, general surgeons, and oncologic surgeons. There have been no specialty hospitals erected to care exclusively for esophageal illnesses. There have been no departments or clinics devoted exclusively to the diagnosis and treatment of esophageal diseases. Many hospitals did not have staff familiar with the postoperative care of esophageal patients. Surprisingly, such clinics are developing today, probably aided by the necessity for an esophageal laboratory to unsnarl complex esophageal disease, an awareness of the relationship of esophageal to pulmonary disease, and the metaplasia-dysplasia-carcinoma sequence in Barrett's esophagus. Virtual esophageal motility, wireless esophageal pH monitoring, esophageal impedance measurements, endoscopic ultrasound, and a variety of endoscopic diagnostic and therapeutic procedures are now commonplace and have accelerated the status of individual esophageal units. If the anatomic demarcation of the gastrointestinal and cardiothoracic surgeons could give way and the pharynx, esophagus, lungs, and stomach be coalesced, there could be the advent of a new therapist—a foregut or esophageal surgeon who is competent at endoscopy, as skilled in transthoracic as in transabdominal operations, at home in the esophageal laboratory, and an expert at unsnarling complex foregut problems.

REFERENCES

1. Lewis CS: Religion: Reality or substitute. In Hooper E (ed): Christian Reflections. Grand Rapids, MI, Eerdmans, 1967, p 41.
2. Boerhaave H: Atrocis nec descripti prima morbid historia. Lugd Batavia, 1704.
3. Quincke H: Ulcus oesophagi ex digestione. Dtsch Arch Klin Med 24:72, 1879.
4. Rosenthal DJ, Dickman CA: The history of thoracoscopic spine surgery. In Dickman CA, Rosenthal DJ, Perin NI (eds): Thoracoscopic Spine Surgery. New York, Thieme, 1999, p 1.
5. Kussmaul A: Zur Geschicte der Oesophago und Gastroskipie. Dtsch Arch Klin Med 6:456, 1868.
6. Mikulicz J: Uber Gastroskipie und Oesophagoskopie mit Demonstration am Lebender. In Verhandl Deutsche Gesellsch Chir, XI Congress, 1882, p 30.
7. Davis CJ, Filipi CJ: A history of endoscopic surgery. In Arregui MC, Fittzgibbons RJ, Katkhouda N, et al (eds): Principles of Laparoscopic Surgery. New York, Springer-Verlag, 1995, p 3.
8. Elmslie RG: Perspectives in the development of oesophageal surgery. In Jamieson GG (ed): Surgery of the Oesophagus. Melbourne, Australia, Churchill Livingstone, 1988, p 3.
9. Torek E: The first successful case of resection of the thoracic portion of the esophagus for carcinoma. Surg Gynecol Obstet 16:614, 1913.
10. Denk W: Zur Radikaloperation des Oesophaguskarzinoms. Zentralbl Chir 40:1065, 1913.
11. Turner GG: Excision of the thoracic oesophagus for carcinoma with construction of an extra-thoracic gullet. Lancet 2:1315, 1933.
12. Tuffeir T: Regulation de la pression intrabronchique et de la narcose. Compte-Rendu Soc Biol 3:1086, 1896.
13. Magill I: Endotracheal anaesthesia. Proc R Soc Med 22:83, 1928.
14. Beck C: Demonstration of specimens illustrating a method of formation of a prethoracic esophagus. Ill Med J 7:463, 1905.
15. Roux C: L'Esophago-jejuno-gastromie, nouvelle operation pour retrecissement infranchisable de l'esophage. Semaine Med 27:37, 1907.
16. Kelling G: Osophagoplastik mit Hilfe des Querkolon. Zentralbl Chir 38:1209, 1911.
17. Ohsawa T: [Esophageal surgery.] J Jpn Surg Soc 34:1518, 1933.
18. Marshall SE: Carcinoma of the esophagus: Successful resection of lower end of esophagus with re-establishment of esophageal and gastric continuity. Surg Clin North Am 18:643, 1938.
19. Adams WE, Phemister DB: Carcinoma of the lower esophagus. Report of a successful resection and esophagogastrostomy. J Thorac Surg 7:621, 1938.
20. Willis T: Pharmaceutice Rationalis: Siva Diatriba de Medicamentorum Operationibus in Humano Corpore. London, Hagae-Comitis, 1674.
21. Hurst AF: Treatment of achalasia of the cardia (so-called cardiospasm). Lancet 1:618, 1927.
22. Heller E: Extramukose Cardiaplastik beim chronischen Cardiospasmus mit Dilatation des Osophagus. Mitt Grenzgeb Med Chir 27:141, 1914.
23. Rammstedt WC: Berichte über krankheitsfälle und behandlungsverfahren. Med Klin 8:1702, 1912.
24. Ravitch MM: The reception of new operations. In Zeppa R (ed): Transactions of the One Hundred and Fourth Meeting of the American Surgical Association. Philadelphia, JB Lippincott, 1984, p 25.
25. Barrett NR, Franklin LH: Concerning the unfavourable late results of certain operations performed in the treatment of cardiospasm. Br J Surg 37:194, 1949.
26. Allison PR: Reflux esophagitis, sliding hiatal hernia, and the anatomy of repair. Surg Gynecol Obstet 92:149, 1951.
27. Dor J, Humbert P, Dor V, et al: L'intétét de la technique de Nissen modifee dans la prevention de reflux après cardiomyotomie extramuqueuse de Heller. Mem Acad Chir (Paris) 88:877, 1962.
28. Toupet A: Technique l'oesophago-gastroplastic avec phrenogastropexie appliquee dans la cure radicale des herniahiatales et comme complement de l'operation d'Heller dans les cardiospasmes. Mem Acad Chir 89:394, 1963.
29. Ingelfinger FJ: Esophageal motility. Physiol Rev 38:533, 1959.
30. Code CF, Creamer B, Schlegel JF, et al: Atlas of Oesophageal Motility. Springfield, IL, Charles C Thomas, 1958.
31. Ludlow A: A case of obstructed deglutition, from a preternatural dilatation of, and bag formed in, the pharynx. Med Observ Inquiry 3:85, 1767.
32. Bell C: Surgical observations. London, Longmans, Greene, 1816, p 64.
33. Wheeler WI: Pharyngocele and dilatation of the pharynx, with existing diverticulum at lower part of pharynx lying posterior to the oesophagus. Dublin J Med Sci 82:349, 1886.
34. Girard C: Du traitement des deverticules de l'oesophage. Congres Franc Chir 10:392, 1896.
35. Zesas DG: Beitrag zur chirurgischen Behandlung der speiserohren Divertikels. Dtsch Z Chir 82:575, 1906.
36. Goldmann EE: Die zweideutige Operation von pulsion Divertikelm der Speiseröhre. Beitr Klin Chir 61:741, 1909.
37. Lahey FH, Warren K: Esophageal diverticula. Surg Gynecol Obstet 98:1, 1954.
38. Harrington SW: Pulsion diverticulum of the hypopharynx at the pharyngoesophageal junction. Surgery 18:66, 1928.
39. Aubin A: Un cas de diverticule de pulsion de l'oesophage traite par la resection de la poche associee à l'oesopfagotomie extramuqueuse. Ann Otolaryngol 2:167, 1936.
40. Belsey R: Functional disease of the esophagus. J Thorac Cardiovasc Surg 52:164, 1966.
41. Rokitansky C: Divertikel am Pharynx. Jahrb Dkk Osterr Staates 30:22, 1840.
42. Zenker FA, von Ziemssen H: Krankheiten des Osophagus. Handbuch Spezillen Pathol Ther 7:50, 1877.
43. Mondiere JT: Notes sur quelques maladies de l'oesophage. Arch Gen Med Paris 3:28, 1833.
44. Bowditch HI: A Treatise on Diaphragmatic Hernia. Buffalo, NY, Jewett, Thomas, 1853.
45. Hill LD: An effective operation for hiatal hernia: An eight year appraisal. Ann Surg 166:681, 1967.
46. Nissen R: Eine einfache Operation zur Beeinflussung der Refluxoesophagitis. Schwiez Med Wochenschr 86:590, 1956.
47. Skinner DB, Belsey RHR: Surgical management of esophageal reflux and hiatus hernia: Long-term results with 1,030 patients. J Thorac Cardiovasc Surg 53:33, 1967.
48. Collis JL: An operation for hiatus hernia with short esophagus. J Thorac Cardiovasc Surg 34:768, 1957.
49. Barrett NR: Chronic peptic ulcer of the oesophagus and "oesophagitis." Br J Surg 38:174, 1950.
50. Allison PR, Johnstone AS: The oesophagus lined gastric membrane. Thorax 8:87, 1953.
51. Naef AP, Ozzello L: Columnar-lined lower esophagus: An acquired lesion with malignant predisposition: Report on 140 cases of Barrett's esophagus with 12 adenocarcinomas. J Thorac Cardiovasc Surg 70:826, 1975.
52. Haggitt RC, Tryzelaar J, Ellis FH, Colcher H: Adenocarcinoma complicating columnar epithelium-lined (Barrett's) esophagus. Am J Clin Pathol 70:1, 1978.
53. Skinner DB, Walther BC, Riddell RH, et al: Barrett's esophagus. Comparison of benign and malignant cases. Ann Surg 198:554, 1983.
54. Reid BJ, Weinstein WM: Barrett's esophagus and adenocarcinoma. Annu Rev Med 38:477, 1987.
55. Liebermann-Meffert D, Stein HJ: Rudolf Nissen and the World Revolution of Fundoplication. St. Louis, Quality Medical, 1999.
56. Johnson LF, DeMeester TR: 24-hour pH monitoring of the distal esophagus. A quantitative measure of gastroesophageal reflux. Am J Gastroenterol 62:325, 1974.
57. Dallemagne B, Weerts JM, Jehaes C, et al: Laparoscopic Nissen fundoplication: Preliminary report. Surg Laparosc Endosc 1:138, 1991.
58. Wilkins E: The historical evolution of esophageal surgery. In Pearson FG, Cooper JD, Deslauriers J, et al (eds): Esophageal Surgery, 2nd ed. New York, Churchill Livingstone, 2002, p 1.

Human Foregut Anatomy, Prenatal Development and Abnormalities, and Their Relation to Surgical Approaches

Dorothea Liebermann-Meffert · Hubert J. Stein

Anatomy of the Esophagus

MACROSCOPIC FEATURES

General Aspects

The esophagus is a midline structure lying on the anterior surface of the spine. It descends through three compartments: the neck, the chest, and the abdomen. This progression has led to its classic anatomic division into cervical, thoracic, and abdominal segments (Fig. 2–1). Two new subdivisions more useful for clinicians have recently been proposed (see Fig. 2–1). One refers to functional aspects and makes a distinction between the esophageal body and the upper and lower sphincters.[1] The other refers to oncosurgery and distinguishes between the proximal and the distal esophagus, with the tracheal bifurcation used as a partition.[2] This concept integrates the features of embryologic development, in particular, the differently oriented pathways of lymphatic drainage (see the section "Lymphatic Drainage" later in this chapter).

The topographic relationships of the esophagus to its neighboring structures have been studied extensively by the authors and other experts using different technical approaches. The conclusions are as follows:

Joining the pharynx, the esophagus begins at the cricoid cartilage in front of the sixth cervical vertebra. It passes into the chest at the level of the sternal notch and travels within the chest cavity on the anterior limit of the posterior mediastinum. Between the thoracic inlet and the diaphragm, the esophagus remains in close relationship with the spine (Fig. 2–2). It ends at the inlet of the stomach, in front of the 12th thoracic vertebra. On radiologic evaluation, the esophageal axis is virtually straight. Unaffected by scoliotic curves of the vertebral column, the esophagus maintains a straight course; in contrast, the large neurovascular structures, because of their origin at the posterior body wall, follow the deformity of the skeleton.[3] Vascular anomalies or mediastinal masses, on the other hand, may displace, bow, or indent the esophagus. However, any distortion of its axis strongly suggests mediastinal invasion and retraction, usually by a malignancy.[4]

A healthy esophagus has three minor deviations along its trajectory (see Fig. 2–1). The first is toward the left at the base of the neck (see Fig. 2–2); hence surgical approaches to the esophagus are easier from the left than from the right when performing intestinocervical esophageal anastomoses after esophagectomy. The second deviation is at the level of the seventh thoracic vertebra, where the esophagus turns slightly to the right of the spine (see Fig. 2–1). Because of the third deviation, the terminal esophagus and the esophagogastric junction are positioned slightly lateral to the xiphoid process of the sternum and to the left of the spine. At this point, the fundus and proximal part of the stomach extend anterolateral to the body of the vertebra (see Fig.

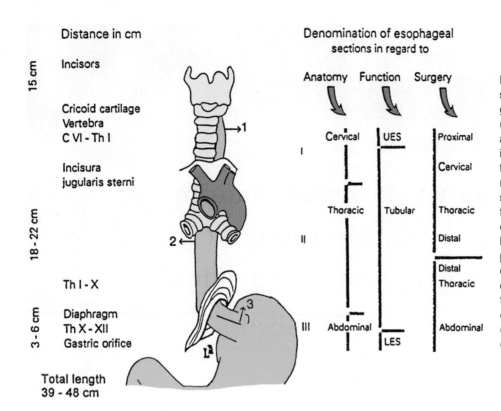

Figure 2–1. Classic anatomic division of the esophagus and its topographic relationship to the cervical (C) and thoracic (Th) vertebrae. The approximate length of each segment is given, and the three narrowings of the esophagus are shown. More recently, the esophagus has been subdivided according to its different functions by Diamant.[1] Based on the embryology and main direction of lymphatic flow, Siewert (1990) proposed a subdivision of the thoracic esophagus at the level of the tracheal bifurcation for determining treatment strategies in patients with esophageal cancer. LES, lower esophageal sphincter; UES, upper esophageal sphincter.

2–2); as a result, the greater curvature faces the posterior subdiaphragmatic space, and the anterior gastric wall faces laterally. This topographic feature is not well displayed in standard anatomy textbooks but is definitely clarified by computed tomographic studies (see Fig. 2–2). A better understanding of the function of the cardia and interpretation of pressure measurement data of the lower esophageal sphincter (LES) are based on this topography.

Measured Dimensions

Length of the Esophagus

The length of the esophagus is defined anatomically as the distance between the cricoid cartilage and the gastric orifice. In adults, it ranges from 22 to 28 cm (24 ± 5 SD), 3 to 6 cm of which is located in the abdomen (see "Suggested Readings").[5,6] In contrast to the previous assumption about the incidence of sex differences (see Lerche in "Suggested Readings"), Liebermann-Meffert et al.[6] found the length of the esophagus to be related to the subject's height rather than sex.

Identification and marking of the cricoid cartilage are rather difficult in a living individual. For practical reasons, therefore, clinicians measure the length of the esophagus by including the oropharynx and the pharynx and using the incisors as a direct macroscopic landmark during endoscopic procedures (see Savary and Miller in "Suggested Readings"). The distances are shown in Figure 2–1.

Length of the Orthotopic Bypass

Esophagectomy for cancer requires transfer of the substitute to the position formerly occupied by the esophagus. To measure the length required for esophageal replacement, the shortest distance between the cricoid cartilage and the celiac axis was found to be the orthotopic route in the posterior mediastinum (30 cm). The retrosternal location (32 cm) and the subcutaneous route (34 cm) proved to be longer.[7] There were no differences between men and women.

Diameter of the Esophagus

The esophagus is the narrowest tube in the intestinal tract. It ends by widening into its most voluminous part, the stomach. At rest, the esophagus is collapsed; it forms a soft muscular tube that is flat in its upper and middle parts, with a diameter of 2.5 × 1.6 cm. The lower esophagus is rounded, and its diameter is 2.5 × 2.4 cm.[6,8]

Compression or constriction by adjacent organs, vessels, or muscles may cause narrowing, which can be visualized by means of fluoroscopy and endoscopy (see "Suggested Readings"). The aortic compression, which is left sided and anterolateral, is caused by crossing of the aortic arch, the left atrium, and the left main bronchus at a location 22 cm from the incisors. Occasionally, a mechanical imprint of the diaphragm exists, but more apparent are two functional muscular constrictions: the upper and the lower esophageal sphincters. They are found manometrically at the esophageal opening, 14 to 16 cm distant from the incisors, and at the entrance into

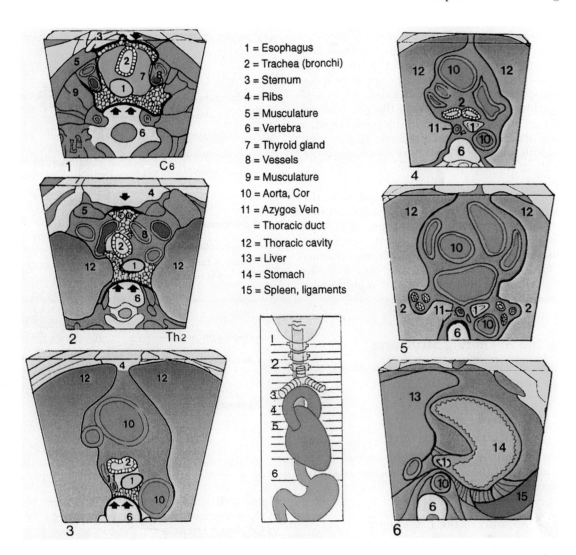

1 = Esophagus
2 = Trachea (bronchi)
3 = Sternum
4 = Ribs
5 = Musculature
6 = Vertebra
7 = Thyroid gland
8 = Vessels
9 = Musculature
10 = Aorta, Cor
11 = Azygos Vein
  = Thoracic duct
12 = Thoracic cavity
13 = Liver
14 = Stomach
15 = Spleen, ligaments

Figure 2–2. Topographic anatomy of the esophagus shown from the cervical level (1) to the esophagogastric junction (6). A transverse section through the mediastinum shows the esophagus and its surrounding structures in a computed tomographic aspect. The close positional relationship among the esophagus, trachea, and vertebrae and the fascial planes is displayed. The *thick dark lines* are the prevertebral and previsceral fascia (*arrows*); the net-like pattern represents the respective areolar connective tissue. (Modified after Wegener OH: Neuromuscular organization of esophageal and pharyngeal motility. Arch Intern Med 136:524, 1976, with permission.)

the stomach, between 40 and 45 cm from the incisors (see Fig. 2–1) (see the section "Esophageal Sphincters" later in this chapter).

Periesophageal Tissue, Compartments, and Fascial Planes

Unlike the general structure of the digestive tract, the esophageal tube has neither mesentery nor serosal coating. Its position within the mediastinum and a complete envelope of loose connective tissue allow the esophagus extensive transverse and longitudinal mobility.[9,10] Respiration may induce craniocaudal movement over a few millimeters, and swallows may result in excursion over as much as the height of one vertebral body. This mobility is also the reason why the esophagus may be sub-

jected to easy blunt stripping from the mediastinum. Invasion by malignant tumor and fixation to the surroundings, however, strictly contraindicate the use of this technique.[4,6,11]

Another anatomic peculiarity is of clinical relevance: the connective tissues in which the esophagus and trachea are embedded are bounded by fascial planes, the pretracheal fascia anteriorly and the prevertebral fascia posteriorly. In the upper part of the chest, both fascias unite to form the carotid sheath, and the anterior and posterior spaces between these fascias form a communicating compartment between the neck and the chest that provides a plane for rapid spread of infection through the mediastinum (see Fig. 2–2).

The anterior space coincides with the previsceral (i.e., pretracheal) space. Infections spreading from anterior lesions of the esophagus may follow this route, but they are limited distally by the strong fibrous tissue of the pericardium. The posterior space, which is the retrovisceral (i.e., prevertebral) space, extends from the base of the skull to the diaphragm. It is formed by the buccopharyngeal fascia spreading downward via a sheath that separates the esophageal tissue bed from the prevertebral fascia. This space is clinically of greater importance than the previsceral space. The reason is that most instrument perforations with subsequent outflow of esophageal contents occur above the narrowing of the cricopharyngeal sphincter in the posterior hypopharynx (see Savary and Miller in "Suggested Readings"). At this level, as in the chest, there is no barrier to the spread of infection into the mediastinum. Rupture of the esophagus or leakage of an esophageal anastomosis may result in descending mediastinitis along these planes as well. Prompt diagnosis is vital for the patient because the prognosis for esophageal perforation depends on the rapidity with which treatment is initiated!

Stabilizing and Anchoring Structures

The esophagus is stabilized by bony, cartilaginous, and membranous structures (Fig. 2–3).

Anchorage in the Neck

Through the exterior longitudinal layer of its muscle coat the cranial end of the esophagus fastens at the posterior ridge of the cricoid cartilage via the cricoesophageal tendon (Fig. 2–4).

Anchorage of the Body of the Esophagus

The tubular esophagus lies in the loose areolar tissue bed of the mediastinum (see Fig. 2–2). The claim that broad fibrous tissue or muscle strings connect the trachea and esophagus, as depicted by Laimer[10] and later adopted in Netter's atlas,[13] could not be substantiated by the authors' studies.[8,10] Instead, there were numerous delicate, slightly undulated membranes mostly 170 μm in thickness and approximately 3 to 5 mm in length (Fig. 2–5A and B). They connected the esophagus with the trachea (see Fig. 2–5A) and the surrounding tissue (see Fig. 2–5B). Consisting of collagen and elastic fiber elements and occasional interpositioned sparse muscle fibers, the membranes are stretchable to some extent and accumulate around the tracheal bifurcation.[10] A few individuals possess membranes up to 700 μm in thickness, together with firm intramural insertion (see Fig. 2–5A).

Anchorage of the Cardia

When the distal end of the esophagus traverses the diaphragm through the esophageal hiatus, it is bounded by the two diaphragmatic crura and the phrenoesophageal membrane (Figs. 2–6 and 2–7; see also Fig. 2–3).

The muscular portion of the diaphragm is inserted on the lumbar vertebrae, the ribs, and the sternum. The central membranous portion is frequently larger than that described in the literature, and the left crus of the

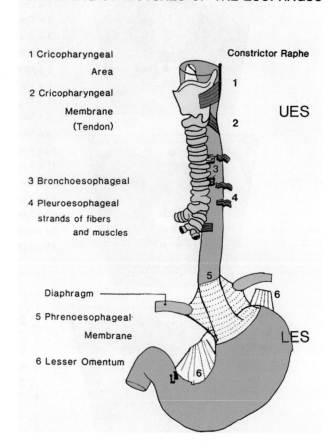

ANCHORING STRUCTURES OF THE ESOPHAGUS

1 Cricopharyngeal Area

2 Cricopharyngeal Membrane (Tendon)

Constrictor Raphe

UES

3 Bronchoesophageal

4 Pleuroesophageal strands of fibers and muscles

Diaphragm

5 Phrenoesophageal Membrane

6 Lesser Omentum

LES

Figure 2–3. Attachments of the esophagus. The upper end of the esophagus obtains firm anchorage by the insertion of its longitudinal muscle into the cartilaginous structures of the hypopharynx (1) via the cricoesophageal tendon (2). The circular muscle is stabilized by its continuity with the inferior laryngeal constrictor muscles (1), which insert via the raphe to the sphenoid bone. Tiny membranes connect the esophagus with the trachea, bronchi, pleura, and prevertebral fascia (3 and 4). The attachment at the lower end by the phrenoesophageal membrane (5) is rather mobile, whereas the posterior gastric ligaments, such as the gastrosplenic, phrenicolienal, and phrenicogastric ligaments (6), and the lesser omentum (6) yield a tight adherence. LES, lower esophageal sphincter; UES, upper esophageal sphincter.

diaphragm may consist of membranous tissue rather than a significant muscular mass (see Fig. 2–6) (see also Williams and Warwick in "Suggested Readings"). The subdiaphragmatic and endothoracic aponeuroses blend at the central margin of the diaphragm to constitute the phrenoesophageal membrane (PEM), also known as Laimer's ligament or Allison's membrane. Intraoperatively, the PEM can be recognized by its well-defined lower edge (Fig. 2–7) and its slightly yellow color, even in the presence of severe periesophagitis. The PEM is composed of elastic and collagenous fiber elements, which guarantee sufficient pliability. Because of its origin

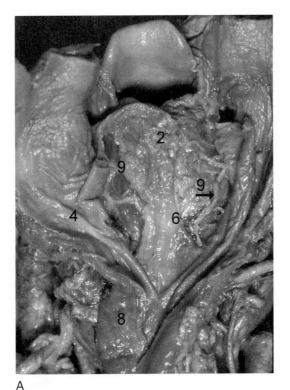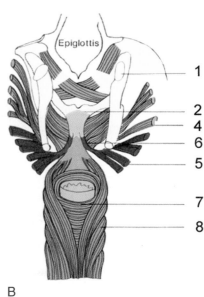

Figure 2–4. The posterior walls of the pharynx (4) and the esophagus (7 and 8) have been cut open in the midline, as shown in a specimen (**A**) and half-schematically (**B**). The structures of the hypopharynx are exposed by retracting the overlying incised tissue and removing the mucosa. In the center lies the cricoesophageal tendon (6), which attaches the longitudinal muscle layer of the esophagus (8) to the cricoid cartilage (2). The terminal branches of the left laryngeal recurrent nerve (9) are dissected and are seen lateral to the crico-esophageal tendon. 1, Thyroid cartilage. (Specimen and photo courtesy of Liebermann-Meffert, Munich.)

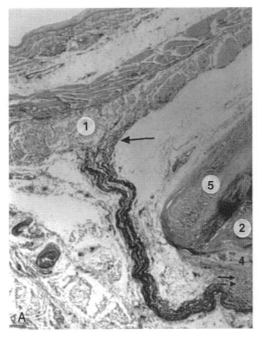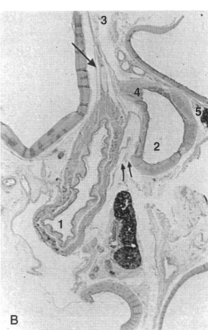

Figure 2–5. **A** and **B**, Example of the tiny fiber membranes that connect the esophagus (1), trachea (2), pleura (3), tracheal membrane (4), and cartilaginous structures (5). At their insertions, the fiber elements fan out to deep finger-shaped extensions between the muscular bundles of the esophagus (*arrow*) and into the membranous part of the trachea (*double arrows*). This texture, in conjunction with the elasticity of the membranes, certainly provides adequate adjustment during movement of the esophagus. In case of rapid pull, the fibers eventually tear off the tissues in which they are anchored (human esophagus, transverse section, hematoxylin and eosin stain). (Courtesy of Huber, Haeberle, and Liebermann-Meffert, Munich.)

from a fascia, the PEM in general is relatively strong. It splits into two sheets (Fig. 2–8). One sheet extends 2 to 4 cm upward through the hiatus, where its fibers traverse the esophageal musculature to insert on the submucosa.[10,14] The other sheet passes down across the cardia up to the level of the gastric fundus, where it blends into the gastric serosa, the gastrohepatic ligament, and the dorsal gastric mesentery (see Figs. 2–3 and 2–7).

Although there are sparse attachments via elastic cords in the pattern shown in Figure 2–8, the PEM is clearly some distance away and separated by loose connective tissue and fat accumulation from the musculature of the gastroesophageal junction (see Fig. 2–7). This structural arrangement allows the terminal esophagus and the junction to move in relation to the diaphragm and to "slip through the hiatus like in a tendon sheath."[15] With advancing age, the elastic fibers are replaced by inelastic collagenous tissue, and the adhesion of the PEM to the lower portion of the esophagus loosens,[14] which leads to loss of pliability. Disruption of the anchoring structures

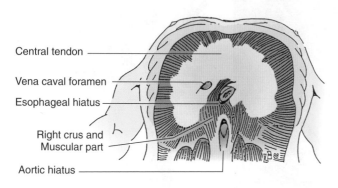

Figure 2–6. Diaphragm and esophageal hiatus viewed from the abdominal aspect.

of the cardia and the proximal part of the stomach in conjunction with a wide hiatus may result in herniation of the gastroesophageal junction and the cardia, or even parts of the stomach, into the mediastinum. Abnormal anchoring of the PEM in youth and pathologic accumulation of adipose tissue in the separating connective tissue space between the PEM and the cardia musculature are thought to contribute to the development of a hiatal hernia.[14]

Selected Topographic Relationships and Surgical Risk Areas

Neck

Ventral to the cervical esophagus lie the fibrous membranes that unite the adjacent hoops of the tracheal cartilage (Fig. 2–9). Note that only an inconspicuous amount of areolar connective tissue—if any—separates the two structures (see Figs. 2–5 and 2–9). Malignant

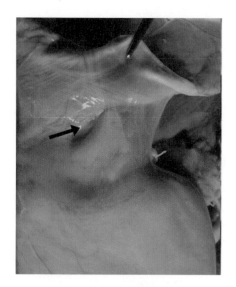

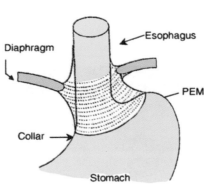

Figure 2–7. The phrenoesophageal membrane (PEM). The lower component of the membrane inserts on the gastric fundus. On the *left*, the diaphragm is held up with forceps. Diaphragmatic decussating fibers (*long arrow*) and a submembranous inlay of adipose tissue (*short arrow*) are seen. The PEM wraps the esophagogastric junction with a wide membranous collar. (Specimen and photo courtesy of Liebermann-Meffert, Munich.)

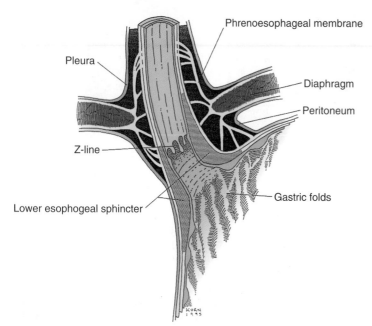

Figure 2–8. Diagram of the tissue organization and supporting structures at the esophagogastric junction. The esophagus is opened alongside the greater and lesser curvatures. The luminal aspect is displayed from the left side. The fiber elements that attach the phrenoesophageal membrane to the muscle wall of the terminal esophagus are shown. The fibers equal those shown in Figure 2–5. (Courtesy of Dr. Owen Korn, Munich and Santiago di Chile.)

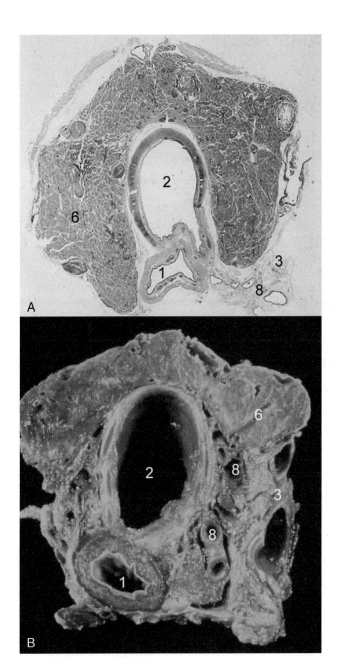

Figure 2–9. Transverse section through the neck and upper part of the chest of a human autopsy specimen viewed from a cranial aspect. 1, Esophagus; 2, trachea; 3, pleura; 6, thyroid gland; and 8, vessels. The histologic section shows the esophagus still in the midline posterior position (**A**), whereas on the more distal level of the macroscopic cut surface (**B**), the esophagus has shifted toward the left. Note the intimate local relationship between the esophagus and the trachea. (From Liebermann-Meffert D: Funktionsstörungen des pharyngoösophagealen Übergangs: Funktionelle und chirurgisch orientierte Anatomie. In Fuchs KH, Stein HJ, Thiede A [eds]: Gastrointestinale Funktionsstörungen. Berlin, Springer, 1997, with permission.)

THE AZYGOS VEIN

From Lateral = RIGHT THORACIC APPROACH

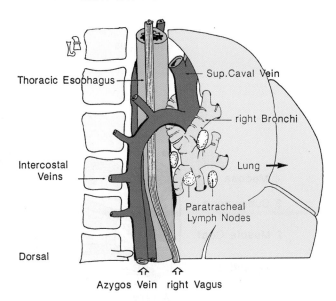

Figure 2–10. The position and relationships of the azygos vein, the thoracic duct, and the vagus nerve are shown from a right lateral aspect.

tumors are known to spread from the trachea to the esophagus and vice versa. Clinically, such spread results in an "acquired fistula."[16-18] Unfortunately, it appears that the lack of interposed connective tissue between the two organs predisposes to this unlucky event. Remember that a tracheoesophageal fistula after either an instrumental perforation, esophagectomy, or chemotherapy and irradiation in this inherently weak area is a catastrophic problem for both the patient and physician.[16-19]

Chest

Between the thoracic inlet and the tracheal bifurcation (which lies at the level of the fifth thoracic vertebra), the esophagus retains its intimate relationship to the trachea ventrally and to the prevertebral fascia posteriorly (see Fig. 2–2). The mediastinal pleura, the lungs, and their hila are positioned on both sides. On the right lies the subclavian artery and the azygos vein, which arches over the right main bronchus to end in the superior vena cava (Fig. 2–10). When performing transthoracic esophagectomy, surgical access for safe removal of the esophagus is preferably through the right side of the chest, and the azygos vein must usually be divided before the esophagus can be dissected free (see "Suggested Readings"). The primarily right side–positioned thoracic duct crosses behind the esophagus just above the arch of the azygos vein at the level of T4 to T5. Structures on the left of the esophagus are the aortic arch and the aorta, which subsequently turns to the midline and travels in a posterior course behind the esophagus (see Fig. 2–2). In front of

TISSUE TEXTURE OF THE ESOPHAGOGASTRIC JUNCTION

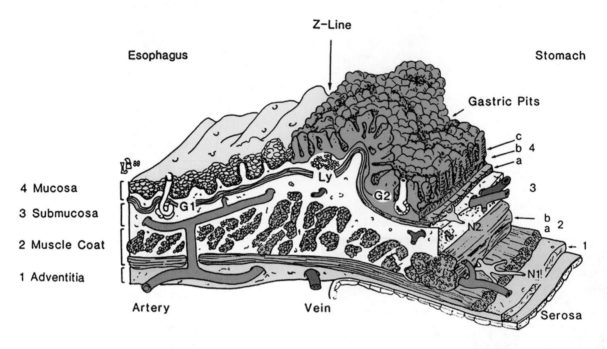

Figure 2–11. Wall structure at the esophagogastric junction. The tunica muscularis is composed of both a longitudinal (2a) and a circular layer (2b). a, muscularis mucosae; b, lamina propria; c, epithelium; G1, esophageal glands; G2, gastric glands; Ly, lymph vessels; N1, myenteric plexus; N2, submucous nerve plexus.

the esophagus are the lung hilum and the heart. The pleura on the left side of the mediastinum may occasionally extend behind the esophagus. Both vagi accompany the esophagus as it passes through the hiatus at the level of the 10th thoracic vertebra.

Abdomen

In the abdomen, part of the left lobe of the liver lies ventral to the esophagus. The two diaphragmatic crura are lateral and posterior. The inferior vena cava is lateral to the right crus, whereas the aorta is posterior to the left crus. The cranial pole of the spleen is in close relationship to the terminal esophagus (see Fig. 2–2). Other vessels and nerves that supply the esophagus and the adjacent organs are discussed later in this chapter.

Constituents and Tissue Organization of the Foregut

The basic tissue organization of the esophagus and cardia is shown in Figure 2–11.

TISSUES

Tunica Adventitia

This thin coat of loose connective tissue envelops the esophagus, connects it to adjacent structures, and

contains small vessels, lymphatic channels, and nerves (see Fig. 2–11).

Tunica Muscularis

Esophageal Body

Muscular Arrangement The tunica muscularis coats the lumen of the esophagus in two layers, the fibers of which follow a diametric course: the external muscle layer parallels the longitudinal axis of the tube, whereas the muscle fibers of the inner layer are arranged in the horizontal axis (Fig. 2–12). For this reason, these muscle layers are classically called longitudinal and circular, respectively.

The *longitudinal layer* originates from the dorsal plane of the cricoid cartilage as shown earlier in Figure 2–4. Its muscular bundles fan out in a posterior direction, with an area of circular muscle left vacant—Laimer's triangle—before they wrap the esophagus entirely (Figs. 2–13 and 2–14; see also Fig. 2–11).[8,20] As long bundles, they run in a straight course down the esophageal tube and cross the gastric inlet (see Fig. 2–12).

The *circular layer* begins at the level of the cricoid cartilage. In their descent, the short fibers of the inner muscular layer form imperfect circles with overlapping ends, as illustrated in Figures 2–12 and 2–13.[8,20]

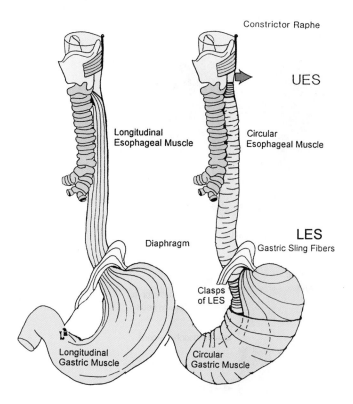

Constrictor Raphe

UES

Longitudinal
Esophageal Muscle

Circular
Esophageal Muscle

LES

Diaphragm

Gastric Sling Fibers

Clasps
of LES

Longitudinal
Gastric Muscle

Circular
Gastric Muscle

Figure 2–12. Architecture of the longitudinal and circular muscle layers across the esophagus, stomach, and respective junctions. LES, lower esophageal sphincter; UES, upper esophageal sphincter.

Muscle Types: Striated Versus Smooth It is generally accepted that the striated musculature behaves different from smooth muscle. Both types of muscle are present in the esophagus. The question has been raised of how the striated and smooth muscle is distributed in the wall of the esophagus. When systematically examining serial histologic sections of the esophagus from 15 individuals,[21] the authors found exclusively striated musculature in the pharynx and particularly in the cricopharyngeal muscle, which of course is the upper esophageal sphincter muscle (UES). The first sparse smooth muscle fascicles appear 2 to 3 mm caudal to the UES. Farther caudally, progressively more and more smooth muscle bundles replace the striated muscle in both the external and internal layers. The transition between both types is neither abrupt nor confined to individual muscle bundles and lacks any distinct anatomic border (Fig. 2–16).[10,21] Caudal to the tracheal bifurcation, no striated muscle elements are seen any more. With regard to sphincter function, it might be of interest to be aware that the muscle type of the UES differs completely from that of the LES!

The muscularis mucosa is composed uniquely of smooth muscle fibers throughout the entire esophagus.

Esophageal Sphincters

Zones of increased pressure in the esophagus have been verified, one at the upper and the other at the lower end.

Diverse factors and mechanisms are suggested as the cause of the sphincter pressure, but ultimately, all remain disputable. This has prompted us to reinvestigate the human muscle morphology of the esophagus and both sphincters with special techniques. The results have been published previously in detail,[8,9,20,22] and the findings are presented in abridged version in the following two sections.

Structural Counterpart of the High-Pressure Zone: The Upper Esophageal Sphincter The UES is manometrically a 2- to 4-cm-long zone of elevated pressure[23] and marks the entrance into the esophagus. The high pressure results from contraction of the cricopharyngeus muscle. This semicircular muscle originates from the lateral cricoid processes (see Figs. 2–13 and 2–14) and closes the esophageal opening by exerting pressure toward the posterior plane of the cricoid cartilage. This arrangement accounts for the asymmetric pressure profile in manometric measurements.[23-25] The position of the cricopharyngeal muscle at the end of the pharynx implies that the structure is a "lower pharyngeal" rather than an "upper esophageal" sphincter.

Muscular Counterpart of the High-Pressure Zone: The Lower Esophageal Sphincter The LES is manometrically a 3- to 5-cm-long zone of elevated pressure and marks the end of the esophagus and the entry into the stomach.[26] Biochemically, the muscle of this area behaves differently from the muscle above and below it.[2,24,27] Markers applied surgically to these muscles in a simultaneous radiomorphologic study have shown that this high-pressure zone correlates with the thickened musculature at this site.[20,22] The high pressure results from contraction of the special muscle organization at this location.

It is unfortunate that fresh muscle tissue inevitably retracts when cut through, in particular, hollow organs such as the intestinal tube. Distorted muscle architecture escapes critical examination; sphincters can neither be palpated nor compared with the neighboring muscle wall. To circumvent this dilemma, the authors used en bloc fixation of the chest and upper abdominal organs to study this anatomic situation in autopsy specimens.[20,22] Such study allowed macroscopic measurement of the muscle thickness of the LES in order to compare it with that of the esophageal body and stomach. Another group of specimens was used to study the respective muscle arrangement.[20,22] The results indicated that the muscular sphincter was the equivalent of the physiologic high-pressure zone (Fig. 2–15).

We described in this paper and depicted in detail[20] that approximately 3 cm cranial to the junction with the stomach, the imperfect muscle circles of the circular layer (see Fig. 2–12) increase in number and result in a stepwise, significant thickening ($P < .001$) of the terminal esophageal musculature.[10,20] This transition is consistent with conspicuous remodeling of the muscle architecture, specifically, asymmetric rearrangement of the muscle fibers of the inner layer (see Figs. 2–12 and 2–15). The bundles on the side of the lesser curvature retain their orientation and form short muscle clasps, whereas those on the greater curvature change to

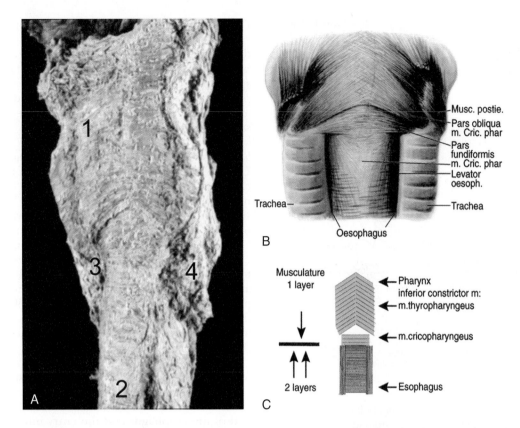

Figure 2–13.   Structures at the pharyngoesophageal junction viewed from a posterior aspect. They are shown in a human dried-fiber specimen (**A**) (by Liebermann-Meffert), of a schematic drawing of an anteriorly opened and unfolded specimen (**B**) (by Killian), and in a simplified diagram of the muscle organization (**C**). The muscular arrangement of the inferior constrictor of the pharynx (1) confirms Killian's observation of the tile-shaped arrangement of the bundles of the inferior constrictor muscle (Killian G: Z Ohrenheilk 55:1, 1908). With respect to the junction, two features should be emphasized: (a) the change of one muscle layer at the pharynx (1) into two at the esophagus (2) just caudal to the cricopharyngeal muscle (3) (upper esophageal sphincter); (b) the cricopharyngeal muscle is part of the pharynx by position and anatomic characteristics. 4, Residual tissue from the removed thyroid gland. (From Liebermann-Meffert D: Funktionsstörungen des pharyngo-ösophagealen Übergangs: Funktionelle und chirurgisch orientierte Anatomie. In Fuchs KH, Stein HJ, Thiede A [eds]: Gastrointestinale Funktionsstörungen, Berlin, Springer, 1997, with permission.)

become the oblique gastric sling fibers. It has been suggested that myotomy for achalasia should preferably be performed between the muscle clasps and gastric sling fibers to preserve the complete strength of the sling (i.e., maintain sphincter competence).[28]

The specific arrangement of the musculature, which we have shown in Figures 2–12 and 2–15, also accounts for sphincter asymmetry.[9,20,22,29] Asymmetry of the high-pressure zone at this position has likewise been proved manometrically.[26] The manometric pressure image of the lower esophageal high-pressure zone, obtained by a three-dimensional computerized vector diagram, matches the muscular asymmetry at the human cardia perfectly (see Fig. 2–15).[30-32] Surgical removal of these structures by partial or total myectomy was shown to significantly reduce the specific sphincter pressure values of this muscle arrangement as recorded on manometry.[2,28,33] Displacement of the LES into the chest through the diaphragm or dissection of the PEM produced no effect on the pressure values of the sphincter in long-lasting animal experiments.[22]

Tela Submucosa

The submucosa is the connective tissue layer that lies between the muscular coat and the mucosa. It contains a meshwork of small blood and lymph vessels, nerves, and mucous glands. The deep esophageal glands are small branching glands of a mixed type, and their ducts pierce the muscularis mucosae (see Fig. 2–11).

Tunica Mucosa

The mucous layer is composed of three components: the muscularis mucosae, the tunica propria, and the inner lining of nonkeratinizing stratified squamous epithelium (see Fig. 2–11). The muscularis mucosae forms the long mucosal folds that run in the longitudinal axis of the tube and shapes the small transverse ripple folds at the cardia.[20,34] All these folds disappear on distention of the esophageal lumen. The tunica propria contains areolar connective tissue, blood vessels, and lymph channels derived from the lower level of the mucosa. At

MUSCULAR ARCHITECTURE OF UPPER ESOPHAGEAL SPHINCTER

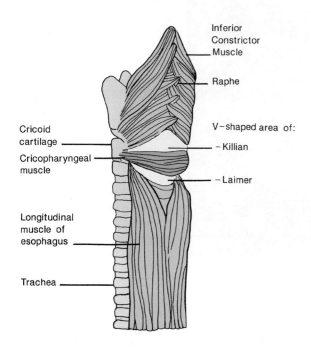

Figure 2–14. Schematic drawing of the structures at the pharyngoesophageal junction seen from the posterior aspect. The location of Killian's and Laimer's triangles is indicated; Zenker's diverticula develop cranial to the cricopharyngeal muscle, and the upper esophageal sphincter is located caudal to the V-shaped area of Killian.

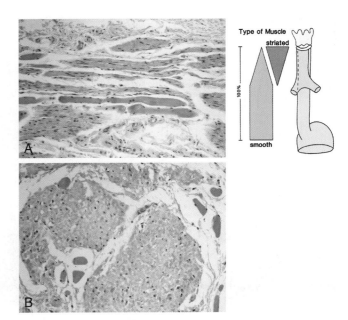

Figure 2–16. Histologic specimens of the human esophagus taken in transverse (**A**) and longitudinal (**B**) sections 4 cm above the tracheal bifurcation cranial to the transition between striated and smooth muscle. Individual striated muscle fibers are interspersed among smooth muscle strands. The diagram shows the distribution of striated and smooth muscle in adult esophagus as evaluated from consecutive serial histologic sections of 13 esophagi. (Specimen and photo courtesy of Liebermann-Meffert, Geissdörfer, and Winter, Munich.)

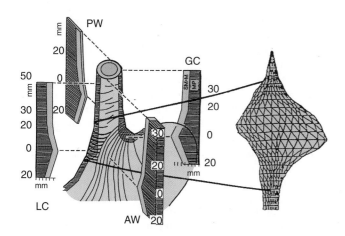

Figure 2–15. Schematic drawing showing the correlation between radial muscle thickness (*left*) and a three-dimensional manometric pressure image (*right*) at the gastroesophageal junction. Muscle thickness across the gastroesophageal junction at the posterior gastric wall (PW), greater curvature (GC), anterior gastric wall (AW), and lesser curvature (LC) is shown in millimeters. Radial pressure at the gastroesophageal junction (in mm Hg) is plotted around an axis representing atmospheric pressure. Note the marked radial and axial asymmetry of both the muscular thickness coinciding with the manometric pressure profile.

the esophagogastric junction, a short 0.5- to 1.0-cm area of superficial (mucous) glands that resemble cardiac glands is a consistent finding.[35,36] Heterotopic gastric mucosa may occasionally also be found at the upper end of the esophagus.[37]

Clinically, the surface of the esophageal mucosa is reddish but becomes paler toward the lower third of the esophagus. The smooth esophageal mucosa can easily be distinguished from the dark mammillated gastric mucosa. The mucosal transition at the squamocolumnar junction is an objectively recognizable reference point for the endoscopist (see Savary and Miller in "Suggested Readings"). On fresh anatomic specimens, the transition is characterized by a serrated, but abrupt demarcation line. The so-called Z-line is located at or immediately above the gastric orifice. Any proximal extension of gastric- or intestinal-type columnar epithelium is considered pathologic and attributed to long-standing reflux of gastric contents causing chronic, severe esophageal mucosal damage.[38] The transition between the two types of mucosa is a "mucosal junction" wherever it is positioned. By no means should it be considered a "sphincter" (as the mucosal transition at the cardia is occasionally termed by gastroenterologists). The term *sphincter* by traditional anatomic definition is restricted to the presence of muscular constrictor structures.

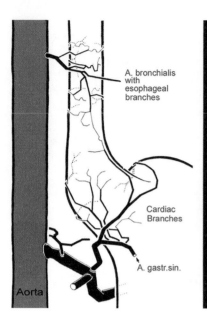

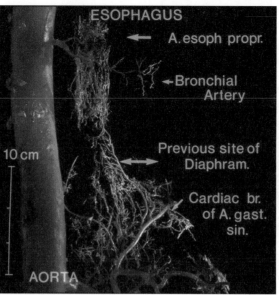

Figure 2–17. Arterial cast showing the vascular supply to the middle and lower portions of the esophagus. Note that the esophageal branch derives from the bronchial artery. During esophageal resection, it should be ligated close to the esophageal wall so that the blood supply of the left main bronchus is not jeopardized. In this context, it should be mentioned that the esophagus shares its blood supply with other organs: the thyroid gland, the trachea, the stomach, and the spleen.

STRUCTURES SUPPLYING THE ESOPHAGUS

Arterial Supply

Extraparietal Sources

Knowledge of the blood supply of the foregut assumes increasing importance. Adequate display of the esophageal vessels is technical difficult, and inadequate technique has caused errors in evaluation and description. Angiograms do not outline the arterial pattern well because of the overlying arteries associated with other structures. Large en bloc corrosion casts, however, produce realistic three-dimensional replicas of the macrovascular and microvascular systems, as seen in Figures 2–17 and 2–18. Such casts establish that the esophagus is an organ of "shared vasculature" because it receives its blood through vessels feeding mainly other organs such as the thyroid gland, trachea, and stomach.[6] There are three principal extraparietal arterial sources for the esophagus (Fig. 2–19). In the neck, the upper superior and inferior thyroid arteries send small descending arteries to the cervical esophagus. At the level of the aortic arch, a group of three to five tracheobronchial arteries arise from the concavity of the arch and give rise to several tracheoesophageal tributaries. Small proper esophageal arteries most often arise from the anterior wall of the thoracic aorta via a larger bronchial artery (see Fig. 2–17). At the cardia, the left gastric artery gives off up to 11 branches that ascend and supply the anterior and right aspects of the lower part of the esophagus (see Fig. 2–17).[6,39] Vessels arising from the splenic artery supply the esophageal wall and parts of the greater curvature from the posterior aspect as seen in Figures 2–17 and 2–19. Two facts became obvious through Liebermann-Meffert and colleagues' studies[6] that had not been appreciated before: all the major arterial vessels divide into minute branches at some distance

from the esophageal wall (see Fig. 2–17), and it appears that such small esophageal tributaries, when torn from the esophagus, have the benefit of contractile periesophageal hemostasis.

Intraparietal Vascularity

Previous claims that essential nutritional vessels arise from the intercostal or phrenic arteries or directly from the aorta could not be confirmed.[6] The minute extraesophageal branches enter the esophageal wall, pass through the tunica muscularis, and give off branches to the muscle before they form the wide vascular plexus within the submucosa and mucosa as seen in Figure 2–18. The clear continuity of the vessels and the rich anastomosing intramural vascularity[6,40,41] explain why a mobilized esophagus retains an excellent blood supply over a long distance[42]; on the other hand, the extremely small caliber of the nutritional vessels also explains leaks after esophagointestinal anastomosis in the event of mechanical damage to the microvascular circulation.

Blunt pull-through stripping of the esophagus without thoracotomy for cancer of the cardia has found an increasing number of advocates.[4,6,11,41] It is described as a relatively safe procedure[6,11,41] that involves minor blood loss, provided that dissection is undertaken close to the esophagus. When hemorrhage has occurred after stripping of the esophagus, it was most often from the site of malignant tumor fixation and, in particular, from injury to the azygos vein.

Venous Drainage

Intraparietal Veins and Plexuses

The most comprehensive macroscopic description of esophageal venous drainage was presumably presented by Butler[43] in 1951. He classified the esophageal veins

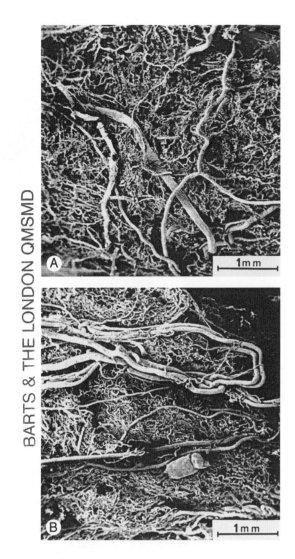

Figure 2–18. Scanning electron micrographs of complete vascular casts using a specially created resin without particles. The microvascular supply in the esophageal submucosa in the midesophagus (**A**) and in the cardia (**B**) is displayed. The vessels form a polygonal meshwork overlying the mucosa. (Courtesy of Duggelin and Liebermann-Meffert, Basel.)

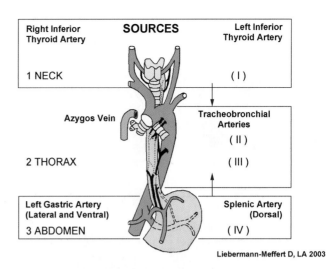

Figure 2–19. Extravisceral sources of arterial blood supply to the esophagus, intramural anastomoses (*dotted line*), and topographic relationship of the azygos vein to the esophagus and tracheal bifurcation. The *arrows* indicate the direction of flow.

into *intrinsic* and *extrinsic* veins, referring to intra-esophageal and extraesophageal wall veins. The intra-esophageal veins include a subepithelial plexus in the lamina propria mucosa that receives blood from the adjacent capillaries. Aharinejad et al.[40] described two small veins that usually accompany the arteries in the lamina submucosa, pierce the muscular wall of the esophagus together with the perforating arteries, and then form the extramural veins at the surface of the esophagus.[40] No valves were found within the esophageal venous circulatory system.[40,43]

It is clinically noteworthy that two clearly delineated venous plexuses are present beneath the mucosa of the hypopharynx. These plexuses had been described in 1918 by Elze and Beck,[8] but their report had not hitherto been well appreciated (Fig. 2–20). One plexus lies on the dorsal aspect of the inferior constrictor muscle, and the other is in the midline posterior to the cricoid cartilage. This is exactly at the level of the pharyngo-esophageal junction. In the 10 specimens restudied by Liebermann-Meffert,[8] the plexuses were located within an extremely thin submucosa; both were 2 to 3 cm broad and 4 cm long. The veins were up to 4 mm thick and of mostly longitudinal orientation, similar to Figure 2–20. The plexuses receive blood from the mucosa of the laryngopharynx and esophagus and drain into the thyroid and jugular veins. Considered to account for the postcricoid impression on the esophagus (for reference, see legend for Fig. 2–20), they may be involved in the "globus sensation" in patients with venous stasis and tissue swelling. It is tempting to postulate that the plexuses also contribute to some extent to the competence and action of the UES.

It may be of further clinical interest that a specialized venous arrangement, clearly documented by Vianna et al., is present at the terminal esophagus (Fig. 2–21). It has been suggested that these venous anastomoses possibly constitute a communication between the azygos and the portal systems. The intermediate "palisade zone" (see Fig. 2–21) is thought to act as a high-resistance watershed between both systems that provides bidirectional flow. Anastomoses between the systemic and the portal systems are found in the submucosa and lamina propria of the lower end of the esophagus and may enlarge in patients with portal venous obstruction to form varices.

Extraparietal Veins

The extrinsic veins drain into the locally corresponding large vessels: the inferior and superior thyroid veins, the azygos and hemiazygos veins, and the gastric and splenic veins. One point of surgical interest is that because of the

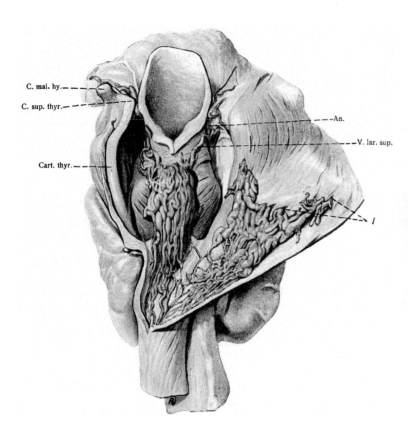

C. mai. hy.

C. sup. thyr.

An.

V. lar. sup.

Cart. thyr.

l

Figure 2–20. The hypopharyngeal-endoesophageal venous plexuses, which are located just underneath the mucosa. Original drawing. (From Elze C, Beck K: Die venösen Wundernetze des Hypopharynx. Z Ohrenheilk 77:185, 1918.)

proximity to the hilum of the lung and its lymph nodes, the azygos vein is one of the initial structures to become involved by extramural spread of tumors of the midesophagus (see Fig. 2–10). In this situation, the azygos vein may easily be injured during esophageal resection. In particular, during blunt pull-through stripping, injury to this vein is a high-risk factor for fatal hemorrhage. Collateral circulation between the azygos vein and the hemiazygos vein is well known. However, the hemiazygos, the accessory hemiazygos, and the superior intercostal trunks may also form a vessel that does not connect with the azygos vein. The hemiazygos vein, if not ligated out, can be a source of severe bleeding when the esophagus is resected through a right thoracotomy.

Lymphatic Drainage

Initial Lymphatic Pathways

The lymphatic drainage in healthy individuals has been sparsely investigated. At present, the authors are conducting a study to demonstrate the pathways of the lymphatic drainage of the esophagus. The histologic picture of the initial lymphatics (as demonstrated by electron microscopy) resembles that elegantly shown by Lehnert in Figure 2–22 concerning the stomach.

Lymph capillaries may commence in the tissue spaces of the mucosa and then unite to form blind endothelial sacculations or channels (see Fig. 2–22). These initial lymphatics appear to originate exclusively in the region between the mucosa and the submucosa and form a

network of collecting channels within the submucosa that run parallel to the organ axis (Fig. 2–23). Eventually, the plexuses give off branches that pass the muscle layers and empty into the collecting subadventitial and surface trunks. In contrast to the esophageal veins, all these channels possess valves (see Fig. 2–23).

Clinical Implication   The concept that lymph flows in the submucosal channels more readily longitudinally than through the few transverse connections in the muscle (see Fig. 2–23) and that only finally does lymph flow through the subadventitial lymphatics and small ducts into the mediastinal lymph nodes is supported by the clinical observation that initial tumor spread follows the longitudinal axis of the esophagus within the submucosa rather than extending in a circular manner. A paucity of lymphatics within the lamina mucosa and the abundance of submucosal lymphatic channels[10] may explain why intramural cancer spreads predominantly within this layer. Unappreciated malignant mucosal lesions may be accompanied by extensive tumor spread underneath an intact mucosa, and tumor cells may follow the lymphatic channels for a considerable distance before they pass the muscular coat to empty into the lymph nodes. A tumor-free margin at the resection line, as confirmed from the anatomic point of view, does not guarantee radical tumor removal. This may be consistent with the relatively high postoperative recurrence rate at the resection line, including satellite tumors and metastases in the submucosa far distant from the primary tumor,[4] even if the margins at the resection line were previously tumor-free.

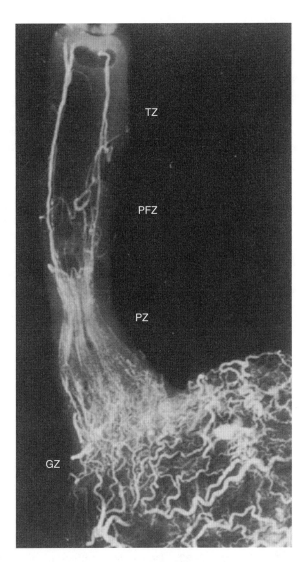

Figure 2–21. Radiograph of the venous circulation at the esophagogastric junction and the esophagus after injection with barium gelatin. This example shows the various zones of different venous architecture, such as the gastric zone (GZ), the palisade zone (PZ), the perforating zone (PFZ), and the truncal zone (TZ), as well as the irregular polygonal network of the proper gastric veins. (From Vianna A, Hayes PC, Moscoso G, et al: Normal venous circulation of the gastroesophageal junction: A route of understanding varices. Gastroenterology 93:876, 1987, with permission.)

From clinical observations in cancer patients,[4] one may deduct (see Fig. 2–24) that lymph from above the carina flows in a cranial direction into the thoracic duct or subclavian lymph trunks whereas lymph from below the carina flows mainly toward the cisterna chyli via the lower mediastinal, left gastric, and celiac lymph nodes. Flow may, however, change under pathologic conditions. When lymph vessels become blocked and dilated because of tumor invasion, the valves become incompetent and the flow reverses (see Figs. 2–22 and 2–23). This explains the retrograde and unexpected spread of some malig-

nant tumors but limits the value of establishing pathways of normal flow.

Lymphatic Ducts and Lymph Nodes

The lymphatic ducts at the surface of a healthy esophagus are thought to empty into the regional lymph nodes. As has been postulated,[13] the thoracic esophagus drains into the paratracheal, tracheobronchial, carinal, juxtaesophageal, and intra-aorticoesophageal lymph nodes, and the abdominal esophagus empties into the superior gastric, pericardiac, and inferior diaphragmatic lymph nodes. Large, often dark lymph nodes normally accumulate around the tracheal bifurcation (Fig. 2–24). However, the author's study failed to display the classic chain of lymph nodes surrounding the esophagus as described in textbooks and illustrated by Netter.[13] Instead, 17 noncancerous autopsy specimens revealed only a small number of lymph nodes being prominent in the periesophageal tissue. This observation coincides with the report of Wirth and Frommhold,[44] who found mediastinal lymph nodes in only 5% of 500 normal lymphograms. Moreover, the authors microscopically identified multiple tiny lymph nodes with a diameter less than 1 mm located in the entire tracheoesophageal sulcus. It is conceivable that such small lymph nodes could increase in size when involved in inflammatory processes or tumor disease, thus augmenting the number of visible nodes. Furthermore, regional differences may potentially prevail.

Thoracic Duct

The thoracic duct begins at the proximal end of the cisterna chyli, at the level of the 12th thoracic vertebra, and passes up through the diaphragm via the aortic foramen. It then ascends through the posterior mediastinum, between the aorta on its left and the azygos vein on its right aspect, and continues left dorsal to the esophagus (Fig. 2–25; see also Fig. 2–10). At the level of the fifth thoracic vertebra and just above the arch of the azygos vein, the thoracic duct inclines to the left to become left side positioned with regard to the esophagus and spine.[44] Then it ascends lateroposteriorly parallel to the trachea and esophagus to convey the lymph into the bloodstream and terminates at the confluence between the left subclavian and jugular veins. There are, however, numerous anatomic variations.[13,44] The close local relationship of the delicate thoracic duct to the esophagus and trachea accounts for the occasional injury causing chylothorax during esophagectomy and cervical anastomosis.[11]

Innervation

Innervation of the esophagus is through the visceral (splanchnic) component of the autonomic nervous system. It consists of two parts, the sympathetic and the parasympathetic systems, that exert antagonistic influences on the viscera. The various pathways have been described in detail elsewhere.[24] The nerve trunks and the

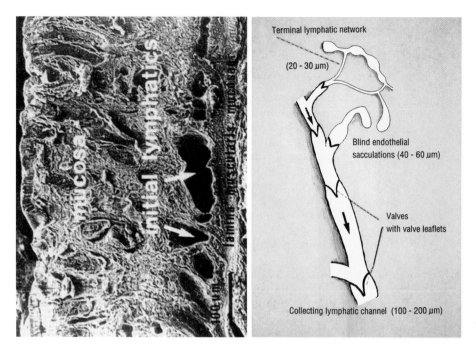

Figure 2–22. Initial lymphatics (*arrows*) between the lower border of the tunica mucosa and the tela submucosa seen on a histologic photomicrograph and in a schematic drawing. This view is taken from the gastric wall, but it also seems to be of relevance for the esophagus. (*Left*, from Lehnert T, Erlandson RA, Decosse JJ, et al: Lymph and blood capillaries of the human gastric mucosa. Gastroenterology 89:939, 1985.)

LOCAL LYMPHATIC DRAINAGE OF ESOPHAGEAL WALL

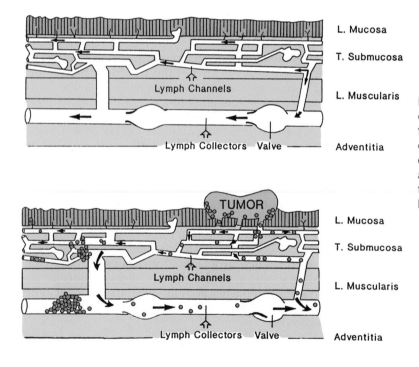

Figure 2–23. Lymphatic pathways in the esophageal wall. The suggested pattern of lymph flow is shown to explain the possible local and distal spread of tumor cells, including the block of distal lymphatics. The embryologic development and the presence and alignment of valves suggest this pattern of lymph flow, although it has never been substantiated experimentally up to now.

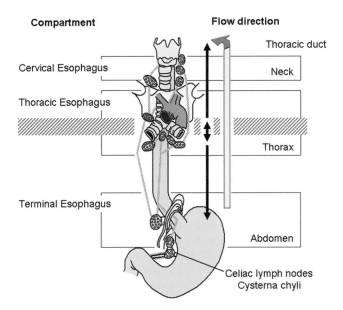

Figure 2–24. Knowledge of the direction of lymph flow and the position of major lymph nodes is essential for understanding the potential spread of an esophageal malignancy. Lymph from areas above the tracheal bifurcation drains mostly toward the neck, and that below the tracheal bifurcation flows preferentially toward the celiac axis. Lymph flow at the bifurcation appears to be bidirectional. The dimensions of the lymph nodes are out of scale. In the normal, nonmalignant condition, esophageal and mediastinal lymph nodes are difficult to discern because of their small diameter of only 3 to 7 mm. Lymph nodes that drain the lung are usually bigger and can be easily visualized by their carbon particle content.

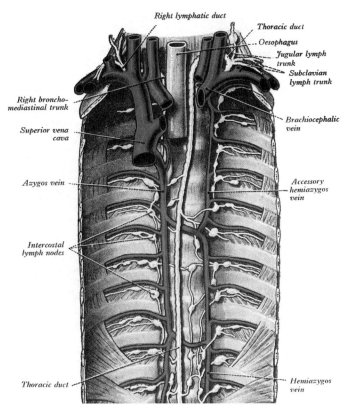

Figure 2–25. The upper thoracic and right lymphatic ducts. (From Warwick R, Williams RL [eds]: Gray's Anatomy, 35th ed. Edinburgh, Longman, 1973, p 727.)

principal branches are composed of parallel nerve bundles that contain efferent or afferent axons. The epineurium, a dense connective tissue sheath, surrounds the nerve trunk.

Extramural Innervation

The *sympathetic nerve* supply, according to the classic description, is via the cervical and thoracic sympathetic chain, which runs downward lateral to the spine (Fig. 2–26). The other sources of sympathetic supply to the middle and lower portions of the esophagus are the cardiobronchial and periesophageal splanchnic nerves, which derive from the celiac plexus.[13] Interconnecting with fibers of the parasympathetic cervical and thoracic plexus, the sympathetic nervous system also uses the vagus nerve as a carrier for some of its fibers.[13,24]

The *vagus nerve* is the 10th cranial nerve and is derived from the dorsal vagal nucleus. The fibers that supply the striated musculature in the pharynx and esophagus, however, derive from the nucleus ambiguus. The vagus is a mixed nerve that also carries sensory fibers from the superior ganglion and inferior ganglion (nodose ganglion). As thick trunks, the right and left vagus nerves descend bilaterally (see Fig. 2–26); they reduce their

diameters by giving off fibers in the neck to the superior laryngeal nerves (SLNs), which innervate the pharynx and larynx musculature. The inferior (recurrent) laryngeal nerves (RLNs) originate within the chest. The right RLN leaves the vagus and turns dorsally around the subclavian artery (see Fig. 2–26). The left RLN leaves the vagus and circles around the aortic arch. On both sides, the RLNs ascend as slack cords that sinuously pass upward within the lateral peritracheal loose connective tissue, the left being closer to the tracheal groove than the right (Figs. 2–27 and 2–28).[12] The left RLN lies closer to the esophagus than the right does. Both RLNs give off 8 to 14 branches to the esophagus and trachea in equal distribution.[12] When stretched, they are 2.5 mm to 1 cm long. Toward the cranial aspect, the RLNs "disappear" beneath the thyroid glands, where the thyroid vessels, in an unpredictable manner, encircle the RLNs in the fashion displayed in Figure 2–29. They enter the larynx laterocaudad to the cricopharyngeal muscle (see Figs. 2–28 and 2–29; see also Fig. 2–4A). Except for the cricothyroids, they innervate all the muscles of the larynx via small branches.[12,45] Injury to the RLN is an unwelcome and not infrequent complication of operations on or near the upper thoracic and cervical esophagus. Because the RLN and SLN supply the same laryngeal

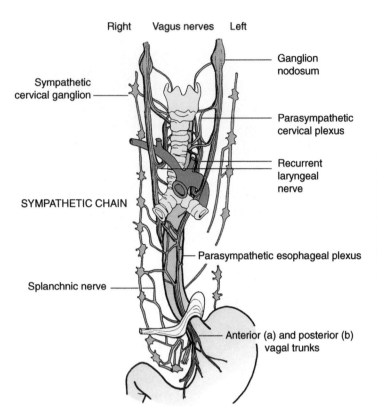

Figure 2–26. Sympathetic and parasympathetic nerve systems. The sympathetic system forms a chain of ganglia from the base of the skull to the coccyx. In the neck, the sympathetic chain is posterior to the carotid sheath. In the chest, it is found anterolateral to the bodies of the vertebrae. Both vagus nerves carry the parasympathetic innervation and travel along the esophagus. The locations of the right and left superior and inferior recurrent laryngeal nerves are shown.

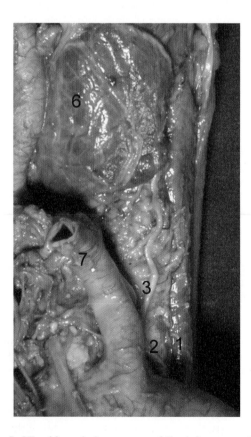

Figure 2–27. Meandering course of the left recurrent laryngeal nerve (3) shown before its dissection from the underlying peritracheal tissues (2). The thyroid gland (6) is still in place. 1, Esophagus; 7, left common carotid artery.

muscles, this twofold innervation may compensate for some sequelae of RLN injury. Displaying the RLNs (an important step in a number of neck operations[12,18,45]), dissecting the RLN branches close to the esophagus, and placing intestinocervical anastomoses as low as possible will certainly reduce RLN injury.[45]

The vagal trunks, at the level of the tracheal bifurcation and posterior to the lung hilum, give off numerous branches to form pulmonary plexuses. More distally, the vagal trunks separate into the coarse network of the anterior and posterior esophageal plexuses (see Fig. 2–26). Before they cross the diaphragm through the esophageal hiatus, these plexuses join again to form the anterior and posterior vagus nerves. The anterior branch has a number of anatomic variants and is usually found on the anterior esophageal wall, where it is visible underneath the PEM. The posterior vagus nerve is usually at some distance from the esophagus and to its right.

Intramural Innervation

The fine structure of the esophageal innervation is composed of a dense network of nerve fibers containing numerous groups of ganglia. The ganglia are located either between the longitudinal and circular muscle layers (Auerbach's plexus) or in the submucosa (Meissner's plexus). The ganglia of Auerbach's plexus are scattered throughout the entire esophagus and have a variable number of cells. However, the concentration of ganglion cells is greatest in the terminal esophagus and at the gastroesophageal junction.[13,24,34]

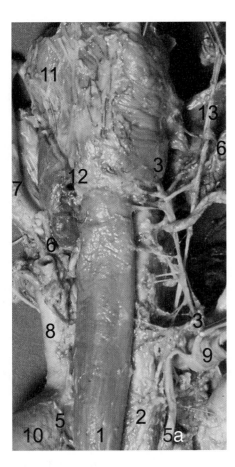

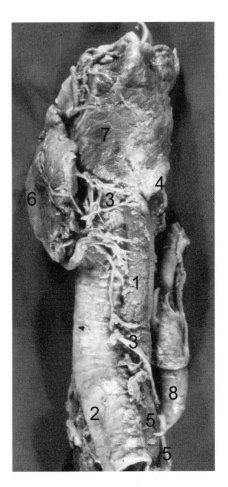

Figure 2–28. Posterior aspect of the muscular wall of the esophagus (1) and pharynx (11). The right recurrent laryngeal nerve (3), largely removed from its peritracheal tissue bed, is pulled down toward the lateral aspect behind its turning point (forceps) around the subclavian artery (9). The rami of the recurrent laryngeal nerve enter the lateral wall of the esophagus (1) and trachea (2). The left thyroid gland (6) is in its natural position, with the right gland displaced posteriorly. Underneath the lower lobe, the thyroid artery and its branches encircle the recurrent laryngeal nerves. The turning point of the left recurrent laryngeal nerve (5) is seen under the aortic arch (10). 7, Common carotid artery; 8, brachiocephalic trunk. Note the venous network on top of the pharyngeal muscle (11), the upper esophageal sphincter (12), the right vagus nerve (5a), and the phrenic nerve (13).

Figure 2–29. The course of the left recurrent laryngeal nerve (3) between the turning point from the vagus nerve (5) and its entry into the larynx is photographed from the left lateral aspect after removal from the peritracheal tissues. The attachments of the thyroid gland (6) are removed, and the gland is shifted posteriorly to display the left recurrent laryngeal nerve (3) and the vascular arrangement underneath. 1, Esophagus; 2, trachea; 8, subclavian artery; 11, inferior constrictor muscle of the pharynx wall. Note the Zenker diverticulum on the right (4).

SUGGESTED READINGS

Lerche W: The Esophagus and Pharynx in Action: A Study of Structure in Relation to Function. Charles C Thomas, Springfield, IL, 1950.

Liebermann-Meffert D: Anatomy, embryology, and histology. In Pearson FG, Cooper JD, Delauriers J, et al (eds): Esophageal Surgery, 2nd ed. Philadelphia, WB Saunders, 2000.

Postlethwait RW: Surgery of the Esophagus. Norwalk, CT, Appleton-Century-Crofts, 1987.

Savary M, Miller G: The Esophagus: Handbook and Atlas of Endoscopy. Solothurn, Switzerland, Gassmann, 1978.

Williams PL, Warwick R: Gray's Anatomy. Edinburgh, Churchill Livingstone, 1980.

REFERENCES

1. Diamant NE: Physiology of esophageal motor function. Gastroenterol Clin North Am 18:179, 1989.
2. Siewert JR, Jennewein HM, Waldeck F: Experimentelle Untersuchungen zur Funktion des unteren Oesophagussphinkters nach Intrathorakalverlagerung, Myotomie und zirkulärer Myektomie. Bruns Beitr Klin Chir 22:818, 1973.
3. Nathan H: Relations of the soft structures of the posterior mediastinum in the scoliotic spine. Acta Anat (Basel) 133:260, 1988.
4. Akiyama H: Surgery for carcinoma of the esophagus. Curr Probl Surg 17:53, 1980.
5. Enterline H, Thompson JJ: Pathology of the Esophagus. New York, Springer, 1984.
6. Liebermann-Meffert D, Lüscher U, Neff U, et al: Esophagectomy without thoracotomy: Is there a risk of intramediastinal bleeding? A study on blood supply of the esophagus. Ann Surg 206:184, 1987.
7. Ngan SYF, Wong J: Lengths of different routes for esophageal replacement. J Thorac Cardiovasc Surg 91:790, 1986.
8. Liebermann-Meffert D: The pharyngoesophageal segment: Anatomy and innervation. Dis Esophagus 8:242, 1995.
9. Korn O, Stein HJ, Richter TH, et al: Gastroesophageal sphincter: A model. Dis Esophagus 10:105, 1997.
10. Liebermann-Meffert D, Duranceau A, Stein HJ: Anatomy and embryology. In Orringer MB, Heitmiller R (eds): The Esophagus, vol 1. In Zuidema GD, Yeo CJ (series eds): Shackelford's Surgery of the Alimentary Tract, 5th ed. Philadelphia, WB Saunders, 2002, pp 3-39.
11. Orringer MB, Orringer JS: Esophagectomy without thoracotomy: A dangerous operation? J Thorac Cardiovasc Surg 85:72, 1983.
12. Liebermann-Meffert D, Walbrun B, Hiebert CA, et al: Recurrent and superior laryngeal nerves—a new look with implications for the esophageal surgeon. Ann Thorac Surg 67:212, 1999.
13. Netter FH: The Ciba Collection of Medical Illustrations, vol 3, Digestive System. Part 1: Upper Digestive Tract. New York, Ciba Pharmaceutical Embassy, 1971.
14. Eliska O: Phreno-oesophageal membrane and its role in the development of hiatal hernia. Acta Anat (Basel) 86:137, 1973.
15. Hayek HV: Die Kardia und der Hiatus Oesophagus des Zwerchfells. Z Anat Entwickl Gesch 100:218, 1933.
16. Baisi A, Bonavina L, Narne S, Peracchia A: Benign tracheoesophageal fistula: Results of surgical therapy. Dis Esophagus 12:209, 1999.
17. Bartels H, Stein HJ, Siewert JR: Tracheobronchial lesions following oesophagectomy: Predisposing factors, respiratory management and outcome. Br J Surg 85:403, 1998.
18. Ferguson MK, Altorki NK: Malignant esophagorespiratory fistula. Postgrad Gen Surg 5:107, 1993.
19. Hosoya Y, Yokoyama T, Arai W, et al: Tracheoesophageal fistula secondary to chemotherapy for malignant B-cell lymphoma of the thyroid: Successful surgical treatment with jejunal interposition and mesenteric patch. Dis Esophagus 17:266, 2004.
20. Liebermann-Meffert D, Allgöwer M, Schmid P, et al: Muscular equivalent of the lower esophageal sphincter. Gastroenterology 76:31, 1979.
21. Liebermann-Meffert D, Geissdörfer K: Is the transition of striated into smooth muscle precisely known? In Giuli R, McCallum RW, Skinner DB (eds): Primary Motility Disorders of the Esophagus: 450 Questions—450 Answers. Paris, Libbey Eurotext, 1991.
22. Liebermann-Meffert D, Heberer M, Allgöwer M: The muscular counterpart of the lower esophageal sphincter. In DeMeester TR, Skinner DB (eds): Esophageal Disorders: Pathology and Therapy. New York, Raven Press, 1985.
23. Winans CS: The pharyngoesophageal closure mechanism: A manometric study. Gastroenterology 63:768, 1972.
24. Goyal RK, Cobb BW: Motility of the pharynx, esophagus and esophageal sphincters. In Johnson LR (ed): Physiology of the Gastrointestinal Tract. New York, Raven Press, 1981.
25. Ekberg O, Lindström C: The upper esophageal sphincter area. Acta Radiol 28:173, 1987.
26. Winans CS: Manometric asymmetry of the lower esophageal high pressure zone. Gastroenterology 62:830, 1972.
27. Preiksaitis HG, Tremblay L, Diamant NE: Regional differences in the in vitro behaviour of muscle fibers from the human lower esophageal sphincter. J Gastrointest Motility 3:195, 1991.
28. Bombeck CT, Nyhus LM, Donahue PE: How far should the myotomy extend on the stomach? In Giuli R, McCallum RW, Skinner DB (eds): Primary Motility Disorders of the Esophagus. Paris, Libbey Eurotext, 1991, p 455.
29. Friedland GW: Historical review of the changing concepts of lower esophageal anatomy, 430 B.C.-1977. AJR Am J Roentgenol 131:373, 1978.
30. Stein HJ, DeMeester TR, Naspetti R, et al: Three-dimensional imaging of the lower esophageal sphincter in gastroesophageal reflux disease. Ann Surg 214:374, 1991.
31. Stein HJ, Liebermann-Meffert D, DeMeester TR, et al: Three-dimensional pressure image and muscular structure of the human lower esophageal sphincter. Surgery 117:692, 1995.
32. Stein HJ, Korn O, Liebermann-Meffert D: Manometric vector volume analysis to assess the lower esophageal sphincter function. Ann Chir Gynaecol 84:151, 1995.
33. Samuelson SL, Bombeck CT, Nyhus LM: Lower esophageal sphincter competence: Anatomic-physiologic correlation. In DeMeester TR, Skinner DB (eds): Esophageal Disorders: Pathophysiology and Therapy. New York, Raven Press, 1985.
34. Eckardt VF, LeCompte PM: Esophageal ganglia and smooth muscle in the elderly. Dig Dis Sci 23:443, 1978.
35. DeHertogh G, van Eyken P, Ectors N, et al: On the existence and location of the cardiac mucosa: An autopsy study in embryos, fetuses, and infants. Gut 52:791, 2003.
36. Marsman WA, van Sandick JW, Tytgat GNJ: The presence and mucin histochemistry of cardiac type mucosa at the esophagogastric junction. Am J Gastroenterol 99:212, 2004.
37. von Rahden BHA, Stein HJ, Becker K, et al: Heterotopic gastric mucosa of the esophagus: Literature-review and proposal of a clinicopathologic classification. Am J Gastroenterol 99:543-553, 2004.
38. Chandrasoma PT, Der R, Ma Y, et al: Histology of the gastroesophageal junction: An autopsy study. Am J Surg Pathol 24:204, 2000.
39. Liebermann-Meffert D, Siewert JR: Arterial anatomy of the esophagus: A review of literature with brief comments on clinical aspects. Gullet 2:3, 1992.
40. Aharinejad S, Böck P, Lametschwandtner A: Scanning electron microscopy of esophageal microvasculature in human infants and rabbits. Anat Embryol 186:33, 1992.
41. Liebermann-Meffert D, Meier R, Siewert JR: Vascular anatomy of the gastric tube used for esophageal reconstruction. Ann Thorac Surg 54:1110, 1992.
42. Williams DB, Payne WS: Observations on esophageal blood supply. Mayo Clin Proc 57:448, 1982.
43. Butler H: The veins of the esophagus. Thorax 6:276, 1951.
44. Wirth W, Frommhold H: Der Ductus thoracicus und seine Variationen. Lymphographische Studie. Fortschr Roentgenstr 112:450, 1970.
45. Hiebert CA, Liebermann-Meffert D, Kraus D: Laryngeal nerve palsy. In Pearson FG, Cooper JD, Deslauriers J, et al (eds): Thoracic Surgery, vol 2, 2nd ed. New York, Churchill Livingstone, 2002, pp 331-340.

Clinically Related Prenatal Development

PRENATAL FOREGUT DEVELOPMENT AND ABNORMALITIES

The first stages of life take place in the embryonic period, which extends from fertilization to the fetal period. The fetal period starts at the ninth week of gestation and ends at birth. The age of the embryo is estimated by the number of somites and by the crown-rump length (CRL) when this measure becomes adequate at the end of the fifth week.[1] The events that take place during the various stages of development are shown in Table 2–1.

Because species differences have caused erroneous conclusions in the past, we omit accounts of development obtained from animals as much as possible. The

Table 2–1 Progression of Various Stages of Esophageal Development

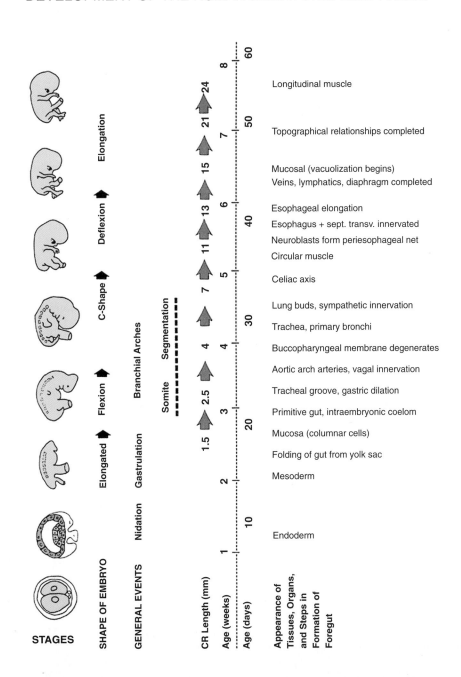

DEVELOPMENT OF THE HUMAN EMBRYONIC ESOPHAGUS

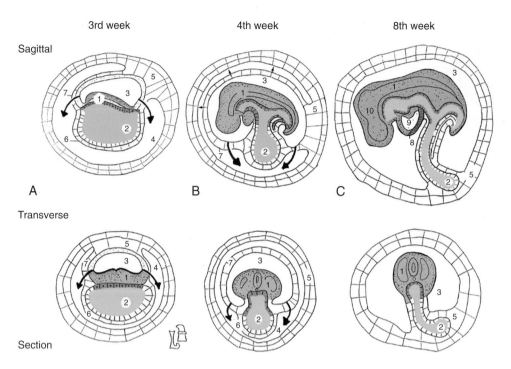

Figure 2–30. The primitive intestinal tube is shown at three stages of its development (**A** to **C**) during the third, fourth, and eighth weeks of gestation. Before formation of the head fold, during the third week the yolk sac is an ovoid cavity. Its roof is the endoderm, which is the underlayer of the embryonic disk. With formation of the head fold during the fourth week, a portion of the yolk sac becomes included within the embryo. This process results in an endodermal tube dorsal to the pericardial cavity and the septum transversum; it adopts a medial position. The tissues of the cranial foregut form the buccopharyngeal membrane, which separates the future digestive tube from the primitive mouth, the stomodeum. Laterally, the foregut is bounded by the bronchial mesoderm. Rapid growth of the brain with transverse and sagittal folding during the fifth week results in apparent flexion of the embryo. Simultaneous constriction at the junction between the embryo and the yolk sac separates the primitive midgut from the yolk sac remnant. The amniotic cavity expands and obliterates the extraembryonic coelom. 1, Embryo; 2, yolk sac cavity; 3, amniotic cavity; 4, extraembryonic coelom; 5, cytotrophoblast and extraembryonic mesenchyme; 6, somatopleure; 7, splanchnopleure; 8, septum transversum; 9, cardiac tube; 10, developing brain.

information presented in the following pages is based on original research, includes personal studies,[2-4] and uses the teaching of established embryology textbooks (see "Suggested Readings").

Basic Tissue and Organ Development

During the first to second week, the embryo develops in its blastocyst cavity from the inner cell mass. It forms a flattened plate of cells, the embryonic disk, that initially consists of two layers, the ectoderm (which gives rise to the nervous system and the epidermis) and the endoderm (which gives rise to the epithelial lining of the respiratory tract and the gut and its derivatives). The precursor tissue of the mucosa, the endoderm, is recognizable by the eighth day of the embryonic period, when its cells rapidly form the lining of the yolk sac (Fig. 2–30A). A third embryonic layer, which appears to develop between the two initial layers on the 15th day, is the mesoderm. According to its position it is classified into paraxial, intermediate, and lateral intraembryonic mesoderm. Mesodermal cells give rise to the mesenchyme, the loosely organized embryonic connective tissue. The pluripotential mesenchymal cells have the ability to differentiate into the material necessary for connective tissues, muscles, blood and lymph cells, and the serous coverings. By the 21st day, the mesenchyme has thickened on both sides lateral to the neurotube and the notochord. It forms longitudinal masses called paraxial mesoderm, which segments progressively in a cranial/caudal direction into cubes of tissue called somites (Fig. 2–31; see also Table 2–1). This process ends by the 31st embryonic day (≈5-mm CRL).

Congenital Malformations and Anomalies

Arrest in development of the foregut may be caused by defective embryogenesis as a result of

- Environmental factors (viruses, drugs, alcohol, etc.)
- Genetic factors (chromosomal abnormalities)
- Multifactorial inheritance
- Unknown etiology

For more information, see Moore and Skandalakis in "Suggested Readings."

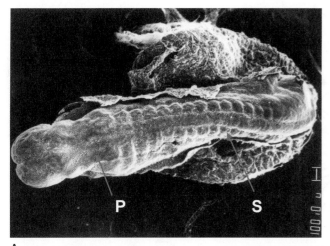

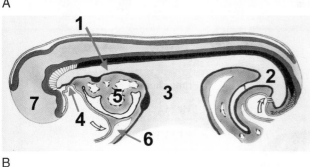

Figure 2–31. Formation of the gut in the human embryo, 3-mm crown-rump length, at the end of the first month of gestation. **A,** Scanning electron micrograph showing an embryo with paired somites (S) that develop from the mesenchymal plate (P). **B,** Schematic counterpart in the sagittal plane showing the developing structures: 1, foregut; 2, hindgut; 3, yolk sac cavity; 4, stomodeum and buccopharyngeal membrane; 5, developing heart; 6, septum transversum; and 7, brain. (**A** From Jirásek JE: Atlas of Human Prenatal Morphogenesis. Boston, Nijhoff, 1983, with permission; **B** from Hinrichsen KV: Human Embryologie. Heidelberg, Springer-Verlag, 1990, with permission. Modified from Liebermann-Meffert D: Anatomy, embryology, and histology. In Pearson FG, Delauriers J, Ginsberg RJ, et al [eds]: Esophageal Surgery. New York, Churchill Livingstone, 1995, with permission.)

Mesenchymal Clefts and Development of the Intraembryonic Body Cavity (Coelom)

Isolated small spaces appear in the lateral and cardiogenic mesenchyme in the 21-day-old embryo and subsequently form the intraembryonic coelom. Partial degeneration of the mesenchyme results in fusion of the paired cavities and the development of clefts that will allow growth of the foregut derivatives. The coelom enlarges to extend from the thorax to the pelvis. The common body cavity can now be subdivided into three parts: (1) the pericardial cavity, (2) the channel-like pericardioperitoneal cavity, and (3) the peritoneal cavity. The

mesothelium derived from the somatic mesoderm lines the parietal wall, and the mesothelium from the splanchnic mesoderm lines the visceral wall.

FORMATION OF THE PRIMITIVE DIGESTIVE SYSTEM

The digestive tube is derived from the endoderm and the mesoderm. The appearance of mesoderm allows the endoderm to undergo the extensive changes needed for establishment of the primitive gut during the fourth week (see "Suggested Readings").

Formation of the somites curves the embryonic disk ventrad into a C shape (see Fig. 2–31). Excessive growth of the brain, heart, tail, and lateral folds and expansion of the amniotic cavity simultaneously narrow the dorsal portion of the yolk sac so that it becomes incorporated stepwise and channel-like into the embryo (see Fig. 2–31A and B). The resulting compression of the yolk stalk divides the yolk sac successively into (1) an extraembryonic portion, which regresses and disappears at about the 12th week, and (2) an intraembryonic portion, which represents the developing digestive tract and its accessory glands (Figs. 2–32 and 2–33, see also Fig. 2–30C). The early digestive system at this point is divided into the foregut, the midgut, and the hindgut (see Fig. 2–33). The tubular structures are attached to the posterior body wall by a relatively broad and strong mass of mesenchyme.

SHAPING THE FOREGUT AND ITS DERIVATIVES

As part of the intraembryonic portion of the yolk sac, the primitive foregut tube is initially nearly uniform in shape (see Fig. 2–32A). It then gives rise to pouches or buds (diverticula) through which develop the paired pharyngeal pouches, the ventral laryngotracheal tube and lungs, the stomach and duodenum, the liver bud, the biliary system, and the pancreatic buds (see Fig. 2–33).

Pharynx, Hypopharynx, Larynx, and Respiratory System: Cranial Foregut Segment

The pharynx, larynx, trachea, and lungs originate from the wide cranial portion of the foregut (i.e., from the branchial apparatus).[5] The primordium of the aditus into the larynx is bounded by the hypobranchial eminence, which becomes the epiglottis. Caudal to the primitive aditus, T-shaped arytenoid swellings develop from the anterior pharyngeal wall and constrict the lumen. The swellings fuse with the lateral margins of the epiglottis to form the aryepiglottic folds. Development of the lower respiratory system is marked by a ventral outgrowth in the wall of the pharyngoesophageal foregut (Figs. 2–34 and 2–35).[5-7] Called the tracheal bud, this protrusion gives rise to the trachea and the lungs and appears during the fourth week, as early as the 25-somite stage.[8]

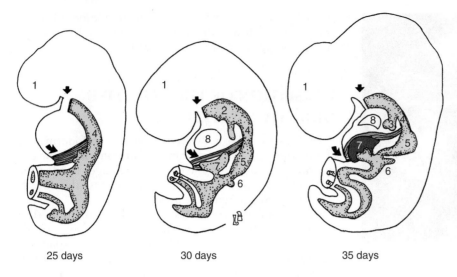

Figure 2–32. Diagrams of sagittal sections through human embryos of different stages. The digestive tract and its accessory glands undergo rapid development between the 25th and 35th days. 1, Head; 2, pharynx; 3, tracheal bud; 4, esophagus; 5, stomach; 6, pancreas; 7, liver; 8, heart. The septum transversum and the buccopharyngeal membrane are indicated by *short* and *curved arrows*, respectively. (Diagram by Liebermann-Meffert.)

25 days　　　30 days　　　35 days

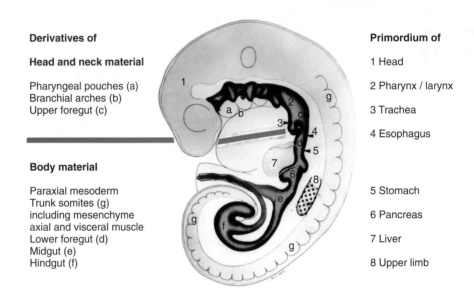

Derivatives of

Head and neck material

Pharyngeal pouches (a)
Branchial arches (b)
Upper foregut (c)

Body material

Paraxial mesoderm
Trunk somites (g)
including mesenchyme
axial and visceral muscle
Lower foregut (d)
Midgut (e)
Hindgut (f)

Primordium of

1 Head

2 Pharynx / larynx

3 Trachea

4 Esophagus

5 Stomach

6 Pancreas

7 Liver

8 Upper limb

Figure 2–33. Schematic drawing of a sagittal section through the body of a 28-day-old human embryo. The foregut, midgut, and hindgut are differentiated. The stomach, however, is still an asymmetric tubal segment. The initially elongated body bends because of the increasing number of somites and the prominence of the head. This gives the embryo a C shape. The *horizontal line* at the left indicates the limits between the branchial derivatives and those of the somites. The *dotted area* in the gut marks the caudal border of the foregut, which is disproportionately large when compared with the midgut and hindgut. (After Hinrichsen KV: a. Intestinaltrakt, b. peripheres Nervensystem, c. Venen. In Hinrichsen KV [ed]: Human Embryologie: Lehrbuch und Atlas der vorgeburtlichen Entwicklung des Menschen. Berlin, Springer-Verlag, 1990, pp 105, 449, 516, with permission.)

It forms a tube, half the diameter of the pharynx, that rapidly elongates downward within the anterior mesenchyme of the foregut before it bifurcates into the lung buds in the 4-mm CRL embryo (see Fig. 2–35). The elongating tracheal tube immediately approaches the esophagus, but in my extensive embryologic material never was found to fuse with it. By the end of the seventh week, the lung tissue has developed and distinct rings of cartilage are seen within the tracheal wall (Fig. 2–36A and B).

Malformations: The Myth of Esophageal Atresia

Downward growth of the tracheal bud has been described in detail in newer anatomic and scanning electron microscopic studies (see Fig. 2–34).[6-9] These studies contradict the misleading concept initiated in 1887 by His,[10] who taught that the trachea "pinches off" the primitive foregut by means of wall folding.[7] Although this claim has not been substantiated, it is still wrongly regarded as one cause for the formation of esophageal atresia.[8]

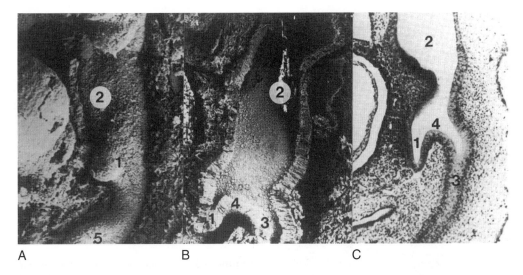

Figure 2–34. Sprouting of the tracheal bud (1) from the foregut. The primitive pharynx (2), esophagus (3), tracheoesophageal fold (4), and stomach (5) are shown. Although this is a photograph of a chick embryo, it strongly resembles the wax plate reconstructions of 3- to 5-mm crown-rump length human embryos studied by Zwa-Tun,[7] who used the material of the Carnegie collection. Sagittal sections; scanning electron micrographs from the external (**A**) and internal (**B**) aspects and histologic section (**C**). (Courtesy of D. Kluth, M.D., Hamburg, Germany.)

Figure 2–35. Diagram showing the event of separation of the trachea from the foregut. After formation of the primitive foregut, the appearance and downward elongation of the tracheal and lung bud make the trachea and esophagus two different entities. Both structures become intimately positioned but do not fuse. Sagittal sections. (Diagram by Liebermann-Meffert.)

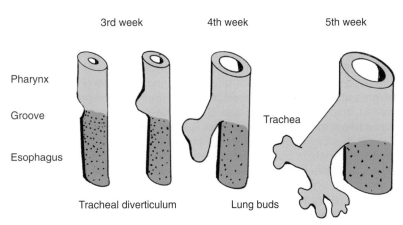

Congenital anomalies of the esophagus are uncommon. The most frequently encountered are congenital atresia, usually combined with a fistula from the distal segment into the trachea, or a fistula without atresia.

Recent Concepts of the Development of Atresia

Different factors are thought to cause esophageal atresia, such as failure in folding the trachea from the esophageal tube,[8,10] epithelial occlusion caused by the lack of recanalization,[11] a growth potential difference secondary to genetic defects,[12] and teratogenic agents[12] (see also Moore in "Suggested Readings").

Recent researchers suggest that tracheoesophageal anomalies are not a failure of organogenesis. They are believed to be due to secondary lesions of the already differentiated organs.[7,12] Local disorders of the microcirculation in utero can explain partial necrosis of the wall

of the esophagus because interruption of the blood supply, as found in animal experiments, induces atresia of the intestines.[6,9] The same authors emphasize that fistula formation is due to mechanical injury caused by too close proximity of the epithelia of both organs. This event is known to occur in normal development during organ regression.

Esophagus: Intermediate Foregut Segment

During incorporation of the endodermal yolk sac material into the body, tubular structures—the primitive esophagus and hindgut—are formed in the head and tail area of the embryo[13] (see Patten in "Suggested Readings"). The esophagus is recognizable at the 2.5-mm stage.[14] It begins at the tracheal groove, lies between the heart and neural tube, follows the curvature of the

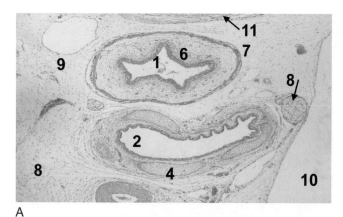

A

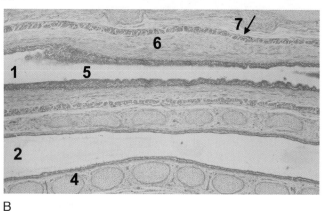

B

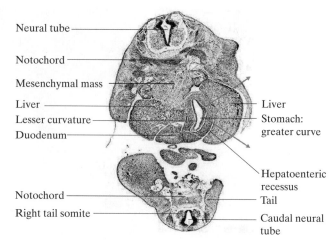

Figure 2–37. A histologic transverse section through an 8.5-mm crown-rump length embryo, 8 μm, hematoxylin and eosin staining, shows the attachment of the developing stomach. The stomach is attached to the posterior wall by the mesenchymal mass. *Arrows* indicate the asymmetric growth of the gastric wall toward the left lateral aspect. The neural tube is cut twice because of the C-shaped bending of the young embryo. (From the collection of Liebermann-Meffert.)

Figure 2–36. Histologic sections, hematoxylin and eosin staining, 5 μm, through two human embryos of similar age, 44-mm (**A**) and 46-mm (**B**) crown-rump length, and similar level, which is at the entry into the chest. **A** is in the transverse plane viewed from caudal aspect, and **B** is in the sagittal plane viewed from the left. The esophagus is in the posterior position. Both slices show developing tissues but definite adult organ relationships, such as the intimate location of the esophagus (1) relative to the trachea (2). 3, Tracheal membrane; 4, tracheal cartilages; 5, developing mucosa (note the difference of the cell layers between 1 and 2); 6, esophageal submucosa (note the dimension of the tissue portion when compared with 7); 7, muscle coat with large circular and small longitudinal layer; 8, future inferior laryngeal (recurrent) nerves; 9, primitive mediastinum with undifferentiated tissue of the previsceral and retrovisceral spaces; 10, pleural cavities (coelom); 11, primitive vertebral fascia. (From the collection of Liebermann-Meffert.)

embryo, and extends down to the dilatation of the foregut, which is to become the stomach (see Fig. 2–32). By the end of the sixth week, the esophagus stretches and lengthens by two means: (1) extensive growth of the embryonic head and (2) deflection of the body backward away from the pericardium (see Table 2–1).[13] The shift of the head and vertebral column away from the heart at this stage of 6 to 8 weeks accounts for the classic misinterpretation that organs migrate upward or downward within the body. In reality, the esophagus elongates by extension in conjunction with prominent growth processes of its wall. The esophagus attains its definite topographic relationships to adjacent structures by the end of the seventh week (18- to 22-mm CRL stage).

Cardia, Stomach, and Duodenum: Lower Foregut Segment

Having passed the septum transversum at the level of the yolk stalk, the lower part of the foregut lies embedded in the ventral portion of the huge posterior mesenchymal mass (Fig. 2–37).[3,4] This part of the foregut represents the developing cardia, stomach, and duodenum with its derivatives. Even in the very early stages of development, the subdiaphragmatic foregut is locally fixed: (1) ventrally by the septum transversum, the yolk stalk tissue, the ducts of the growing liver, and the pancreas and (2) dorsally by the branches of the celiac vessels.

At the time when the tracheal bud pushes downward, a one-sided dilatation of the foregut, the primitive stomach, appears caudal to the septum transversum at the 6- to 7-mm CRL stage (see Fig. 2–32).[2-4] The protrusion extends in a laterodorsal direction and successively shapes the greater gastric curvature (Fig. 2–38).[4,5] The greater gastric curvature grows at a much faster rate with age than does the wall of the opposite right side, which is to become the lesser gastric curvature (see Fig. 2–37). The tissue dilatation coincides with extensive local mitotic activity.[15] This in particular concerns the area of the future gastric fundus. The growing fundus delineates the initially ill-defined gastroesophageal junction (Fig. 2–39; see also Fig. 2–38A through D).[3,4] Individual varia-

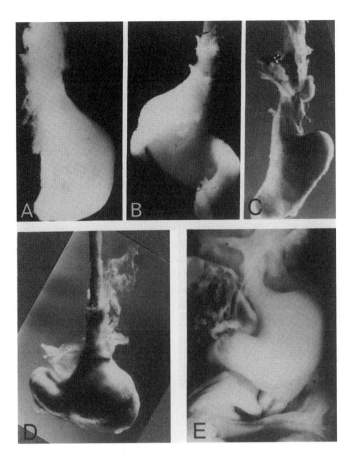

Figure 2–38.   A to **E,** Macroscopic view of human stomachs of embryos between 8- and 22-mm crown-rump (CR) lengths. Because of localized cell proliferation, the greater curvature undergoes extensive growth toward the left during the 5- through 25-mm stages. This growth will also give rise to the gastric fundus, the cardiac angulation, and the esophagogastric junction. Both the cardia and pylorus are connected by the stalk of the celiac and superior mesenteric vessels. Thereafter, growth processes will occur mainly at the free margin of the stomach, at the greater curvature. The lesser curvature does not take part in this excessive growth stimulation, which causes the gastric asymmetry. This event is illustrated by the series of human embryos of different CR length: **A,** 8 mm; **B,** 14 mm (posterior view); **C,** 18 mm; **D,** 19 mm; **E,** 22 mm.

tions in the height of the fundus and the acuteness of the angle of His (cardiac angle) persist during the subsequent fetal period (see Fig. 2–38). Finally, the stomach, limited by the prospective cardia and pylorus, assumes its definite shape.

The Myth of Gastric Rotation

The asymmetric growth of the gastric wall[3,4,15] simulates positional changes of the stomach; in fact, there is no evidence at all of any esophageal[16] or gastric mechanical rotation.[2,3,15] Instead, the differences between the vertical and oblique axes show little change with age (Fig. 2–39), and their curves remain almost parallel. This means that the future cardia and pylorus are definitely fixed at the

posterior wall.[3,15] However, despite the lack of evidence for the concept of gastric rotation, the embryologic enigma continues.

Congenital Malformation of the Stomach

With the exception of congenital pyloric stenosis (2.4 per 1000 live births), malformations of the stomach are rare. According to Skandalakis et al.[17] and Moore (see "Suggested Readings"), anomalies include microgastria and agastria, atresia and stenosis, duplication, defects of the gastric musculature, malposition (situs inversus), and other even less frequent abnormalities.

MEDIASTINUM AND DIAPHRAGM

The cranial foregut lies in the mesenchymal mass of embryonic connective tissue that extends from the heart to the primordium of the spine. This tissue forms the primitive ventral and dorsal mediastinum that holds the foregut in place. Caudally, the ventral portion is bounded by a transverse mesenchymal plate separating the primordium of the heart from the liver. This plate is the septum transversum (see Fig. 2–32). Within the umbilical cord and caudal to the septum transversum course the omphaloenteric and umbilical veins.

As mentioned earlier, the lung buds grow into the mesenchyme that surrounds the pericardioperitoneal spaces. Yet the developing trachea maintains close tissue contact with the esophagus (see Figs. 2–36 and 2–44). During the sixth week, bulges extend ventrally and medially. These bulges develop mesentery-type folds that later become membranes, the free ends of which fuse with the mesoderm located ventral and dorsal to the esophagus and with the septum transversum (see Fig. 2–32). Supported by the rapid growth of the liver, the partitions that will become the diaphragm isolate the caudal portion of the pericardioperitoneal channel, thus closing the pleural and peritoneal cavities (Fig. 2–40).

The diaphragm develops from four sources (Fig. 2–41).[18,19] The largest portion derives from the septum transversum, which has already fused with the ventral mesenchyme of the esophagus in the 7-mm embryo. It eventually forms the central tendon of the diaphragm. The median portion derives from the dorsal mesenchyme of the esophagus and gives rise to the crura of the diaphragm. The crura are formed at a point where the septum transversum and the pleuroperitoneal membrane fuse. The peripheral muscular diaphragm originates from the dorsolateral body wall tissue. What is initially the largest portion of the primitive diaphragm eventually forms the small intermediate muscular portion of the diaphragm. It is derived from the pleuroperitoneal membranes at the point where they have fused with the dorsal mesenchyme of the esophagus and the septum transversum (see Fig. 2–41). Rapid growth of the dorsal body of the embryo, as opposed to the more slowly growing pericardium, causes an apparent descent of the diaphragm.[19] By the end of the sixth week, the diaphragm is complete and is located at the level of the thoracic somites. By the end of the seventh week, it

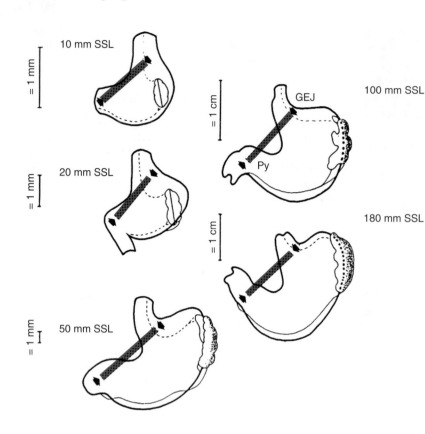

Figure 2–39.   The asymmetric growth process involves the greater curvature and is caused by extensive mitotic activity within the wall.[2,3,15] The cardia and the pylorus remain in place anterior to the spine, where they are held because of their firm dorsal attachment (GEJ and Py) and their relationship to the vessel stalks. GEJ, Gastroesophageal junction; Py, = pylorus; SSL, crown-rump length of the embryo (i.e., fetus).

reaches its final position at the level of the first lumbar vertebra. The future diaphragm can already be easily identified by its distinctive musculature at the 12- to 15-mm CRL stage (see Fig. 2–40).

The phrenoesophageal membrane, which holds the esophagus in place within its diaphragmatic hiatus (see Fig. 2–40), differentiates when the muscle of the esophagus has specialized.

By the end of the embryonic period, in the early ninth week, the definite shape of all the main organ systems are established. The external appearance of the organs is now less affected by further development. During the fetal period, maturation and growth of the various tissues and organs take place.

Anomalies: Congenital Diaphragmatic Hernias and Deformations

An enlarged esophageal hiatus and a congenital defect of the phrenoesophageal membrane are considered predisposing factors for sliding and paraesophageal hernia in childhood.[17,20]

Occasionally, and mainly on the left, the pleuroperitoneal cavity remains open and a posterolateral defect is created. This is the congenital foramen of Bochdalek, which allows free communication between the chest and abdomen. The abdominal contents may then herniate into the thorax (mostly during return of the intestines from the umbilicus) and cause neonatal problems. The foramen of Morgagni, a rare parasternal defect, is the result of a persisting gap from the costosternal origin of the diaphragm; it permits herniation into the anterior

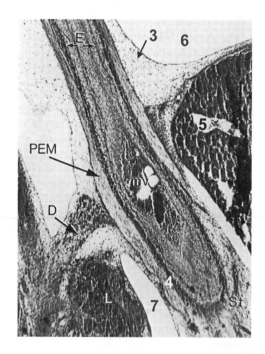

Figure 2–40.   Anchoring structures above the esophagogastric junction (sagittal section through a 15-mm crown-rump length human embryo). The axial section parallels but does not cut the esophageal and gastric lumen. Developing structures: D, diaphragm; E, esophagus; 3, PEM, phrenoesophageal membrane; 4, stomach; 5, liver; 6, pleural cavity; 7, abdominal cavity; mv, vacuoles in the mucosa. The *small arrows* show the differentiated muscular wall. (Courtesy of Fernandez de Santos, MD, Madrid, with permission.)

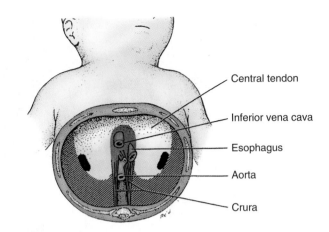

Figure 2–41. Tissue origin of the diaphragm and its four sources. (From Moore KL: The Developing Human. Philadelphia, WB Saunders, 1988.)

Septum transversum

Mesentery of the esophagus

Pleuroperitoneal membranes

Body wall

Central tendon

Inferior vena cava

Esophagus

Aorta

Crura

mediastinum. Incomplete development of the musculature deriving from the lateral body wall may lead to congenital eventration of the diaphragm. The rare diaphragmatic agenesis is due to failure of formation of the diaphragmatic components or failure to join properly.[18,21] For more information, see Skandalakis et al.[17]

TISSUE ORGANIZATION OF THE FOREGUT

Formation of the Foregut Muscular Systems

The esophageal musculature develops from myoblasts originating in the splanchnic mesenchyme that surrounds the endoderm of the early gut. The myoblasts give rise to the cells that constitute the muscular system of the esophagus. At first a ring-shaped condensation of elongated, fusiform nuclei can be distinguished around the external aspect of the entire esophageal tube in the 8- to 10-mm CRL embryo (Fig. 2–42A). Similar muscular precursor cells are present in the esophageal wall of the 12- to 14-mm CRL embryo (see Fig. 2–42B) and appear as a ring-shaped cellular condensation on the outer surface of the tube. The muscular nuclei, however, are arranged in the opposite (i.e., longitudinal) direction from the upper toward the terminal esophagus. Thereafter, the surface of each precursor nucleus acquires a lamellar tissue cover and develops into bundles and sheets of tissue that resemble smooth muscle. These cells constitute the circular and the longitudinal layers of the esophagus. They form complete sheets surrounding the epithelial lumen of the esophagus at the 20-mm CRL stage (see Fig. 2–42C). However, at this stage the musculature is very thin in comparison to the extent of the submucosa and mucosa. By the 24-mm CRL stage (see Fig. 2–42D), the muscularis mucosae becomes apparent, and it is well defined in the 65-mm CRL stage.

Striated musculature can be distinguished only much later in the fetal stage (about 40-mm CRL) and is found in the pharynx, larynx, and upper half of the esophagus. The striated muscle derives from the caudal branchial arches and is innervated by the branchiomotor branches of the vagus nerves. The smooth foregut muscle rises from the visceral splanchnopleural mesoderm and is innervated by the sympathetic nervous system.

The muscle bundles of the esophagus can be distinguished and the fibers seen macroscopically in the 76- to 90-mm fetus. The fiber arrangement of the muscle layers in the esophagus and at the esophagogastric junction[2,3] is comparable at that point to the arrangement seen in the adult.[2,22,29] This is also the case for the sphincter at the cardia, the structures of which have been discussed previously[22] (see Liebermann-Meffert in Pearson et al. in "Suggested Readings").

Formation of the Lamina Mucosa, Submucosa, and Esophageal Lumen

Discussion about the developmental changes of the mucosa of the human esophagus dates back to the turn of the 19th to the 20th century.[11,23-25] Up to the present, however, these changes have been a matter of debate (Table 2–2).[26-28] New attention arose because of the diversity of opinion about the histopathologic background in the development of gastric metaplasia of the esophageal mucosa in connection with Barrett's esophagus.

Differentiation from Endoderm to Mature Foregut Mucosa: Sequence of Events

Proliferation of the Precursor Mucosa Differentiation of the intraembryonic epithelium from the endoderm has been identified at about the third week of gestation (see Patten in "Suggested Readings" and Table 2–1). By the fifth week, when the embryo is 6- to 8-mm in CRL, the internal coat of the foregut is lined with two or three layers of pseudostratified columnar epithelium; this layer is uniformly thick, spreads along the entire esophageal tube, and is surrounded by undifferentiated mesenchymal cells (Figs. 2–43 and 2–44; see also Fig. 2–42). This aspect of the developing mucosa lasts until the 10- to 12-mm CRL stage.[13,27] At that time, the embryonic mucosa becomes multilayered and thickens as a result of excessive cell proliferation (see Fig. 2–43 and Table 2–2). This thickening of the mucosa narrows the esophageal lumen considerably.

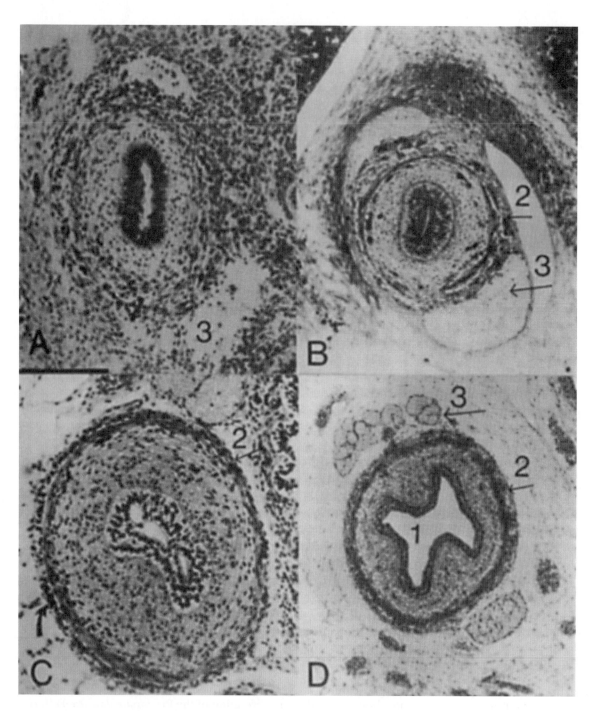

Figure 2–42. Transverse section through the upper chest level of the esophagus in embryos of 8.5-mm (**A**), 12.5-mm (**B**), 20-mm (**C**), and 23-mm (**D**) crown-rump length (CRL). The mucosal epithelium lining the lumen (1) is stratified columnar in the 8.5-mm CRL embryo and will become vacuolized between 12.5- and 20-mm CRL and multilayered columnar in the 25- to 40-mm CRL stage. The tissue that surrounds the mucosal epithelium consists mainly of undifferentiated mesenchyme in the 8.5-mm CRL embryo. Differentiation of the inner muscle coat is identified in the 8.5-mm CRL embryo but more prominent by the cell condensation around the mucosal ring seen in the 12.5-mm CRL embryo in **A** (2). Pale areas of neural cells that are precursors to the vagal nerves are seen exterior to the foregut tube (3). In the 12.5- and 20-mm CRL stages, the inner and outer muscular layer is further advanced. The muscularis mucosae, however, can be identified only at the 23-mm CRL stage. During this development, the extrinsic innervation, in particular, the recurrent laryngeal nerve, has become conspicuous in size (3). The developmental changes in luminal diameter and the shape of the esophagus are caused by submucosal protrusions toward the lumen (mesenchymal proliferation). (**A, B**, and **D** From the collection of Liebermann-Meffert; **C** from Enterline H, Thompson J: Pathology of the Esophagus. Heidelberg, Germany, Springer, 1984, with permission.)

Table 2–2	Prenatal Development of the Mucosa in the Human Esophagus

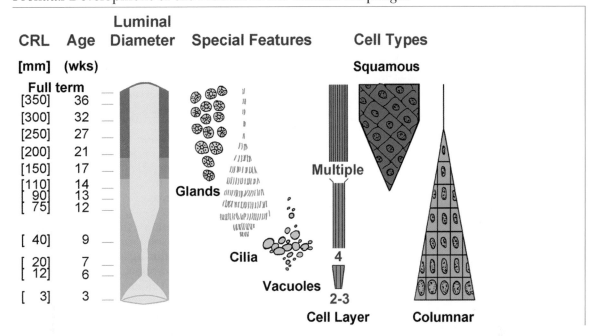

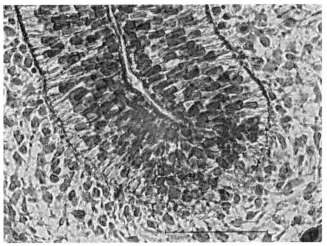

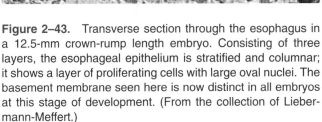

Figure 2–43. Transverse section through the esophagus in a 12.5-mm crown-rump length embryo. Consisting of three layers, the esophageal epithelium is stratified and columnar; it shows a layer of proliferating cells with large oval nuclei. The basement membrane seen here is now distinct in all embryos at this stage of development. (From the collection of Liebermann-Meffert.)

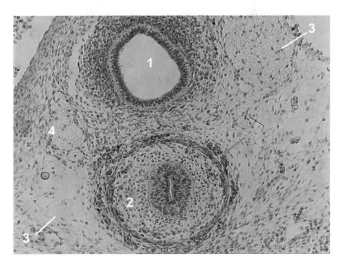

Figure 2–44. Transverse section through the upper part of the esophagus of a 12.5-mm crown-rump length embryo above the level of the developing tracheal bifurcation with narrowing of the lumen because of extreme cell proliferation. The *arrow* shows the differentiating circular muscle layer of the esophagus. 1, Primordium of the trachea; 2, esophagus; 3, vagus; 4, recurrent laryngeal nerve). (From the collection of Liebermann-Meffert.)

Vacuolization of the Epithelium When the embryo is at the 12-mm CRL stage, thin-walled hollow spaces appear in the proliferating epithelium (Fig. 2–45A; see also Table 2–2); subsequently, when the embryo is about 6 weeks old and has attained 13- to 14-mm CRL, the spaces form differently sized cellular vacuoles. The vacuoles increase to a huge number. They may also become much larger than the esophageal lumen itself (see Fig. 2–45B) because the vacuoles fuse through rupture of their thin membranes. In the embryologic material examined by the authors, vacuoles are most conspicuous in the 14- to 22-mm CRL stage. This feature occurs in our own serial sectioned specimens earlier than claimed previously by others.[13] Condensation and size of the vacuoles vary individually. They are smaller and less frequent in the upper portion of the esophagus, but largest and most numerous at levels close to the tracheal bifurcation, followed by those at the junction into the stomach. Small circular vacuoles are found in a far smaller amount in the mucosa of the trachea, but never in the stomach. Vacuolization

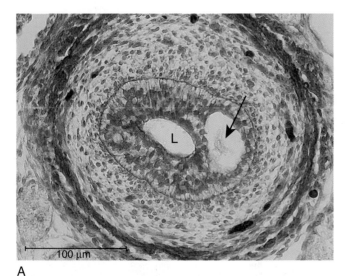

A

B1

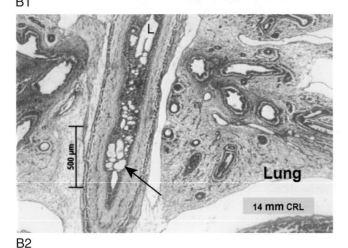

B2

Figure 2–45. Transverse section of the middle portion of the esophagus at the vacuolated stages of the mucosa in 12.5-mm crown-rump length (CRL) (**A**) and 14.5-mm CRL (**B**) embryos. The vacuoles are located within the epithelial cells. Some are multichambered and large because of fusion and occasionally have a diameter greater than that of the esophageal lumen. Some of the vacuoles contain aggregated fiber material (*arrows* in **A** and **B**). L, esophageal lumen. (From the collection of Liebermann-Meffert.)

is an indicator of cell death. At first, the vacuoles seem to be empty; at second look, however, it becomes evident that many of the larger vacuoles contain lysate (cytolytic content) (see Fig. 2–45A). Finally, the vacuoles rupture and discharge their contents into the esophageal lumen. At a stage of 32-mm CRL (month 3), the vacuoles have disappeared, except that very occasionally small ones have been observed by us until the 75-mm CRL embryo (late 12th week).[13,29]

Lumen Occlusion Secondary to Vacuoles: Fact or Myth? Histologic sections made in the sagittal plane of the embryo during the period of vacuolization eventually cut parts of the muscular layers of the wall instead of the lumen; an image of "occlusion" may result as shown in Figures 2–40, 2–45, and 2–49. This picture is probably what led Kreuter[11] in 1905 to suggest, erroneously, that a physiologic solid occlusion of the esophageal lumen takes place during this stage of development. He concluded that esophageal atresia results if "recanalization" of the lumen does not occur. Although no subsequent investigator has ever reconfirmed Kreuter's claim,[5,13,20] his opinion[11] is still a dogma presented in a number of current surgery and anatomic textbooks. It is better to remember that vacuolization in the esophageal mucosa occurs long before the trachea and lungs are already fully developed. From this observation and the normally patent lumen, recent researchers have emphasized that atresia of the esophagus, as well as esophagotracheal fistula formation, is mostly due to a congenital growth defect of the esophagus or trachea (or both).[6,9,12]

Ciliated Columnar Epithelium and Goblet Cells Large, darker-stained cells appear in the basal epithelial cell layer of the 30- to 40-mm CRL embryo. The stratified columnar epithelium is generally four to six cells deep. The surface epithelial cells show a clear affinity to eosin and project toward the lumen to increasingly become ciliated columnar cells (Fig. 2–46; see also Table 2–2). These cells progress from the middle third of the esophagus in a cranial and caudal direction and are usually interspersed among nonciliated cuboidal surface cells. Ciliated cells line the entire mucosa of the esophagus of the 60 mm CRL fetus.[13,27] Successively, the epithelium now consists of a single layer of large columnar cells containing mucin-bearing cells (goblet cells).[27] In the 70- to 90-mm CRL fetus, the cells below the surface layer become squamous and some in the proliferative zones are vacuolated. In 100- to 150-mm CRL fetuses, alternating patches of ciliated cells and nonciliated cells are seen in the squamous epithelium. In the 200-mm CRL fetus, the area of these cells is reduced by cell degeneration[27,28] (Fig. 2–47B and C), and in large areas they are lost at about the 240-mm CRL stage. Stratified columnar epithelium persists in the upper part of the esophagus only, which is consistent with our own results.[27]

An interesting aspect of the mechanisms of the developing esophageal mucosa was studied by Menard and Arsenault.[30] These investigators were able to study explants of the esophagus from early-stage human fetuses maintained in organ culture. Using this fresh material, they charted the ultrastructural changes that

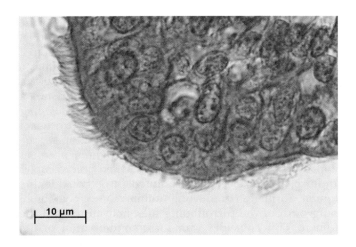

Figure 2–46. Transverse section through the surface mucosa of a 25-mm crown-rump length embryo showing a border of ciliated and nonciliated columnar epithelial cells. (From the collection of Liebermann-Meffert.)

occurred in esophageal epithelialization during maturation of the tissue. They observed that during replacement of the epithelium, islets of ciliated cells actually developed into squamous epithelium.

Stratified Squamous Epithelium Squamous cells are markedly flattened. Stratified epithelium can be seen in patches in the 60-mm CRL fetus and progressively increases in the 90- to 130-mm CRL fetus[13,27] (see Fig. 2–47C). Replacing the ciliated cells, this epithelium spreads from the middle third of the esophagus craniad and caudad until squamous epithelium has progressively and almost completely replaced the ciliated columnar epithelium in the 250-mm CRL fetus.[13] Some patches of ciliated columnar cells, however, occasionally remain until birth. They are usually also found in the proximal part of the esophagus in the newborn.

Glands

The first superficial glands have been observed to develop during the 160-mm CRL stage (see Table 2–2). They contain acini. These glands are superficial to the muscularis mucosa and are numerous in the esophagus of 210-mm CRL fetuses; they are located mostly at the level of the cricoid cartilage and at the lower end of the esophagus.[27,31] Not before the last 3 months of gestation does the downward growth of the surface epithelium begin to generate deep submucosal glands (Fig. 2–48).

The Specialized Cardia Mucosa: Acquired or Congenital?

The presence of a small area of specialized so-called cardiac mucosa has been identified at the junction between the squamous mucosa of the esophagus and the pure oxyntic cells of the stomach. In full-term specimens the zone of superficial glands was limited to a 5-mm distance.[27,31] Some authors regard this cardiac mucosa as a

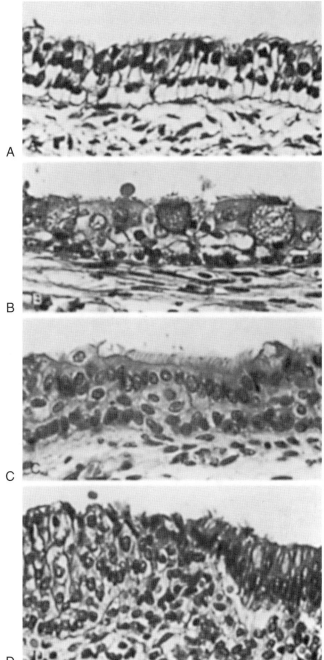

Figure 2–47. Transverse sections through the esophagus at different stages of mucosal development. **A,** Ciliated pseudostratified columnar epithelium at the 28-mm crown-rump length (CRL) stage. **B,** Ciliated columnar cells. Goblet cells are present on top of several layers of polygonal cells and represent the early squamous replacement found in the 190- to 230-mm CRL fetus. **C,** A later stage in the process of squamous replacement in which patchy remnants of ciliated epithelium may remain until birth. **D,** A residual island of mucin-secreting cells in the esophagus of a newborn. (From Enterline H, Thompson J: Diseases of the Esophagus. Heidelberg, Germany, Springer-Verlag, 1984, with permission.)

pathologic condition acquired by acid and bile gastro-esophageal reflux,[32-34] whereas others deny such an etiology and consider the cardiac mucosa to be a normal development.[31,35-37]

Shaping the Esophageal Lumen

The shape of the esophageal lumen is greatly influenced by the development of the mucosa. Because of cell pro-

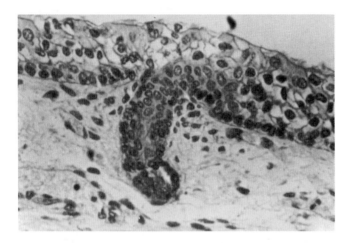

Figure 2–48. During the last trimester of fetal development, downward growth of the surface epithelium begins to generate submucosal glands. A few short ciliated cells are present on the surface above the squamous epithelium. (From Enterline H, Thompson J: Diseases of the Esophagus. Heidelberg, Germany, Springer-Verlag, 1984, with permission.)

liferation and the appearance of vacuoles between the 10- and 21-mm CRL stages, the initially oblong (Fig. 2–49; see also Figs. 2–42 and 2–44) or elliptical lumen of the embryonic esophagus narrows and then assumes a bizarre configuration (see Figs. 2–36, 2–42C, and 2-49). This phenomenon is more pronounced at levels between the tracheal bifurcation and the cardia than in the upper part of the esophagus (see Fig. 2–49). As the process of vacuolization continues and larger vacuoles appear, the deformation of the entire esophageal lumen becomes apparent. During the next stages when the vacuoles rupture, this space is incorporated into the widening lumen. Formation of the longitudinal folds appears as an outgrowth of the surrounding mesenchyme toward the lumen. This coincides with local condensation of the mesenchyme at the 23-mm CRL stage (see Fig. 2–42D). These events lead to the bizarre form of the upper esophagus and the star-like shape present in the cross-sectional view of the lower esophagus (Fig. 2–50). These folds parallel the longitudinal axis of the esophagus and constitute the definite configuration of the esophageal lumen. The muscularis mucosa follows the protrusions of the mesenchyme, but the main external muscular layer of the esophagus never follows these folds at any time.

Formation of the Foregut Vascular System

The vasculature is formed in the early somite stage in the somatopleural mesenchyme of the body wall. Two major arterial sources supply the foregut. One is located in the

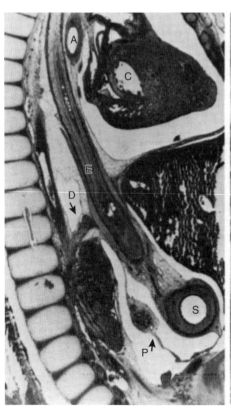
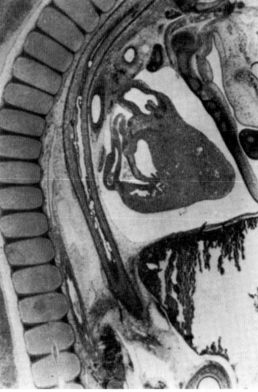

Figure 2–49. Sagittal sections through the curved esophagus of a 15-mm crown-rump length embryo seen here at two consecutive levels. **A,** The muscular wall of the esophagus is cut partially at its peripheral limits; the lumen therefore appears to be obliterated and the musculature mimics a solid structure. **B,** A deeper slice through the esophageal wall displays the vacuolated, but patent esophageal lumen. A, aorta; C, heart; D, diaphragm; E, esophagus; P, pancreas; S, stomach. (Courtesy of Fernandez de Santos, M.D., and Tello Lopez, M.D., Madrid, with permission.)

A

B

mesenchyme of the fourth to the sixth pharyngeal arches and represents the arterial system of the aortic arches that partly encircle the pharynx (Fig. 2–51). These vessels supply the thyroid diverticula (the future thyroid glands) and the tissues of the upper half of the esophagus. At the end of the somite period (5-mm CRL), a pair of pharyngeal arch arteries develop in the mesenchyme of the sixth branchial arch and give rise to vascular branches that descend to supply the primordium of the trachea and the lung buds. The second major source develops at the level where the initially paired dorsal aortas fused caudally to form a single midline vessel, the infradiaphragmatic aorta. The second visceral blood vessel forms the celiac axis, which gives off tributaries to the

lower portion of the foregut. These vessels supply the developing stomach, duodenum, liver, pancreas, and greater omentum (see Fig. 2–51).

During this period a number of changes alter the primitive original vascular pattern to result in establishment of the final arterial pattern of the fetus. As shown in Figure 2–52, vessels deriving from the branchial pharyngeal region maintain blood and lymph flow in a caudal direction, whereas vessels deriving from the celiac axis contribute the arterial vascular supply to the esophagus in a cranial direction of flow. Venous and lymphatic drainage follows the same bidirectional pattern of flow, but in a reverse orientation (Fig. 2–52). This orientation never changes from the fetal pattern throughout adult life. In light of this, one must keep in mind that the esophagus originates from two different tissue sources: (1) one from the branchial apparatus (head and neck material) and (2) the other from body tissues. The two sources maintain a delimitation at the level of the tracheal bifurcation (see Fig. 2–52) throughout life.

The lymphatic system itself appears concurrently with the venous system 2 weeks after the cardiovascular system. Lymph sacculations develop in the jugular region (Fig. 2–53), and definitive lymph vessels are identified in the 11-mm CRL embryo during the sixth week and supply the foregut and trachea.[6,14]

Formation of the Foregut Nervous System

The nervous system develops during the third week from the neural plate. This is an area where the dorsal embryonic ectoderm thickens by cell proliferation and, during the fourth week, folds into the neural tube. The tissue of the neural tube then gives rise to the brain cranially and the spinal cord caudally.

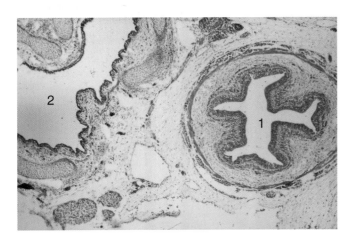

Figure 2–50. Transverse section through the esophagus of a 25-mm crown-rump length embryo showing the bizarre shape of the lumen caused by fold formation of the submucosal mesenchyme 1, esophagus; 2, trachea.

Figure 2–51. Schematic drawing of a sagittal section through an embryo of month 2. The foregut and its blood vessels are displayed. Two of the three main sources of the adult blood supply of the foregut are derived from branchial arch arteries. These are the esophageal branches from source I, the later thyroid arteries, and from source II, the tracheobronchial arteries. The third source (III) derives from the gastric and splenic branches of the celiac artery. The septum transversum is related to the position of the celiac vessels. (Modified from Moore KL: The Developing Human. Philadelphia, WB Saunders, 1988.)

ARTERIAL VASCULARIZATION OF THE 28 DAY EMBRYO

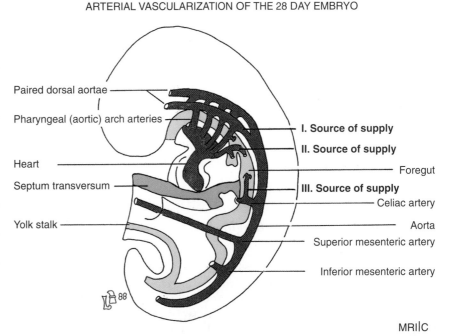

ESOPHAGUS IN FINAL STAGE OF DEVELOPMENT

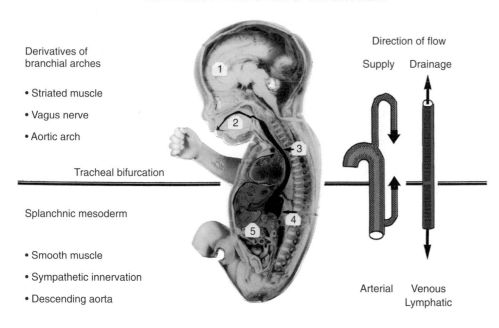

Derivatives of
branchial arches

• Striated muscle

• Vagus nerve

• Aortic arch

Tracheal bifurcation

Splanchnic mesoderm

• Smooth muscle

• Sympathetic innervation

• Descending aorta

Direction of flow

Supply   Drainage

Arterial   Venous
        Lymphatic

Figure 2–52.   The esophagus in the fetus and its topographic development. Structures above the line of the tracheal bifurcation (vessels, nerves, and lymphatics) originate from the tissue of the branchial arches and pharyngeal pouches (branchial apparatus). Below this line, the structures derive from the lateral plate of the body mesenchyme. This border, located at the level of the tracheal bifurcation, permanently defines the direction of vascular flow (see *arrows*). 1, Head; 2, oral cavity and pharynx; 3, esophagus; 4, stomach; 5, bowel.

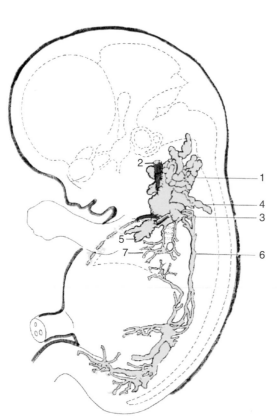

Figure 2–53.   Schematic illustration of the saccular lymphatic system at the 30-mm crown-rump length stage, eighth week of gestation. The branchiogenic part into which the upper foregut drains is far more voluminous than that of the lower foregut, midgut, and hindgut. The saccus jugularis (1); the jugular vein (2); the suprascapular (3), supraclavicular (4), and axillary lymphatic protrusions (5); the thoracic duct (6); and the bronchoesophago-mediastinal lymphatics (7) are seen. (Modified after von Gaudecker B: Lymphatische Organe. In Hinrichsen KV [ed]: Human Embryologie: Lehrbuch und Atlas der vorgeburtlichen Entwicklung des Menschen. Berlin, Springer-Verlag, 1990, p 340, with permission.)

The Cranial Nerves: Their Origin and Distribution

The cranial nerves develop during weeks 5 and 6. According to their embryologic origin they are classified into "somatic efferent cranial nerves" and "nerves of the branchial arches." The structures that derive from the branchial arches maintain their respective innervation throughout life. One of the branchial arch nerves (i.e., the cranial nerve) is the vagus nerve.

The Vagus Nerve: The Major Foregut Nerve

The vagus nerve is the 10th cranial nerve and is formed by the early fusion of nerves from the last three branchial arches (Fig. 2–54). Large efferent and afferent compo-

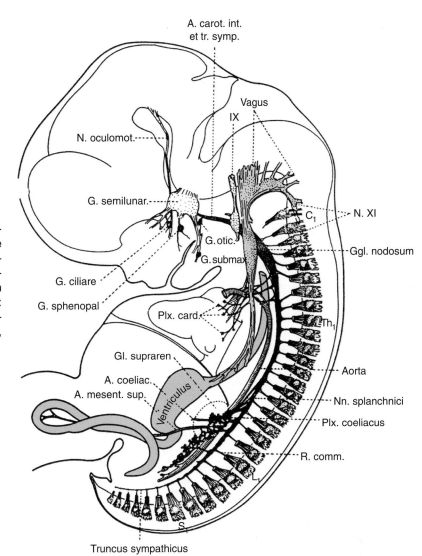

A. carot. int.
et tr. symp.

Vagus
IX

N. oculomot.

G. semilunar.

C₁

N. XI

G. otic.

Ggl. nodosum

G. submax.

G. ciliare

G. sphenopal

Plx. card.

Th₁

Gl. supraren

A. coeliac.

Ventriculus

A. mesent. sup.

Aorta

Nn. splanchnici

Plx. coeliacus

R. comm.

L₁

S₁

Truncus sympathicus

Figure 2–54. The parasympathetic and sympathetic nervous systems in relation to the foregut in a human embryo of 18-mm crown-rump length. (From Hinrichsen KV: a. Intestinaltrakt, b. peripheres Nervensystem, c. Venen. In Hinrichsen KV [ed]: Human Embryologie: Lehrbuch und Atlas der vorgeburtlichen Entwicklung des Menschen. Berlin, Springer-Verlag, 1990, pp 305, 449, 516, with permission.)

nents of the vagus nerve are distributed to the heart, the foregut and its derivatives, as well as part of the midgut.[14,17,38,39] The efferent fibers arise from the specialized dorsal motor nucleus, whereas the afferent fibers derive from neuroblasts of the neural crest. Removal of the neural crest at an early stage of development has been shown to result in an absence of ganglia in the esophagus.[14,40]

Smith and Taylor[41] reviewed the subject of vagal system development and emphasized the diverse opinions that exist on the issue. Liebermann-Meffert has clearly identified the two precursor vagal trunks in the 8.5-mm CRL embryo[3] (see Fig. 2–42). The superior laryngeal nerves can be distinguished at 7- to 9-mm CRL; the inferior laryngeal (recurrent) nerves can be seen at almost the same stage (see Fig. 2–42A). The vagus nerves are extremely large at the 12- to 20-mm CRL stage (see Figs. 2–42 and 2–44). Both vagal nerves (see Fig. 2–54) and the recurrent laryngeal nerves keep their definite position alongside and attached to the esophagus at an early stage of development when the embryonal body straightens by the end of the sixth week (14-mm CRL).[29]

The fibers of the superior laryngeal nerves derive from the mesenchyme of the fourth branchial arches,

whereas the nerves of the sixth branchial arches become the inferior (laryngeal) recurrent nerves (see Moore in "Suggested Readings").

Congenital Malformation: The Nonrecurrent Inferior Laryngeal Nerve

This anomaly occurs as a result of the embryologic interrelationships of development of the inferior RLN and the subclavian artery. In the presence of an aberrant retroesophageal right subclavian artery, the nerve passes to the larynx without recurring. This is related to abnormal degeneration of the sixth and fifth aortic arteries (see Skandalakis and Moore in "Suggested Readings").

Origin of the Sympathetic (Thoracolumbar) Nervous System, the Phrenic Nerve

Neural crest cells of the sympathetic nervous system migrate along the rami of the thoracic spinal nerves in the late somite stage (week 5) (see Hamilton and Mossman and Moore in "Suggested Readings"). The nerve fibers then leave their medial position and form segmentally arranged paired cell masses behind the aorta. They constitute the primordium of the sympathetic nervous system (see Fig. 2–54). The precise origin of these cells has not yet been clarified.

The phrenic nerve, which is responsible for innervation of the developing diaphragmatic muscle, is formed from the anterior primary rami of the third to the fifth cervical nerves.[41]

Distribution of the Developing Periesophageal Nerves

van Campenhout[38] observed that neuroblasts from the periesophageal plexus enter the esophageal wall very early in development, before the embryo has reached 10-mm CRL. The neuroblasts form a complete periesophageal network at the outer limits of the circular muscle layer of the esophagus before the longitudinal muscle differentiates. In the 40-mm CRL embryo, 8 to 12 nerve bundles cover the mid and terminal portions of the esophagus. By the time that the embryo reaches 65-mm CRL, the periesophageal plexus of the lower esophagus consists of large, interlacing vagal bundles that contain ganglia.

The Myenteric Plexus

The myenteric plexus is identifiable in the 10-week-old fetus.[14,41,42] At this stage, ganglion cells are not positively identifiable but are represented by numerous pale areas in the myenteric plexus. The number of cells, cell size, and nerve density peak at the 16th to 20th week of gestation.[39] Sparse submucosal nerve fibers can be discerned in the 35-mm CRL embryo. These fibers become the submucosal plexus. According to Hewer,[42] this plexus is not well developed until the 67-mm CRL stage, but it is complete in the 80-mm CRL fetus.[41] In the 90-mm CRL fetus, the submucosal plexus is extensive and consists of fine nerve fibers and ganglia. The innervation of the muscularis mucosae is particularly rich in the fetus at the 140-mm CRL stage.

SUGGESTED READINGS

Hamilton WJ, Mossman HW: Hamilton, Boyd and Mossman's Human Embryology. Prenatal Development of Form and Function, 4th ed. London, Williams & Wilkins, 1972.

Moore KL: The Developing Human: Clinically Oriented Embryology, 4th ed. Philadelphia, WB Saunders, 1988.

Patten BM: Human Embryology, 3rd ed. New York, McGraw-Hill, 1968.

Pearson FG, Cooper JD, Deslauriers J, et al: Esophageal Surgery, vol 1, 2nd ed. New York, Churchill Livingstone, 2002.

Skandalakis JE: Skandalakis' Surgical Anatomy, vol 1, in The Embryologic and Anatomic Basis of Modern Surgery. Athens, Paschaldis Medical Publications, 2004.

Tuchmann-Duplessis H, Haegel P: Organogenesis, vol 2, in Illustrated Human Embryology. New York, Springer, 1972.

REFERENCES

1. Heuser CH, Corner GW: Developmental horizons in human embryos—age groups xi to xxiii. Collected Papers from the Contributions to Embryology. Washington, DC, Carnegie Institution of Washington, 1951.
2. Liebermann-Meffert D: Die Muskelarchitektur der Magenwand des menschlichen Föten im Vergleich zum Aufbau der Magenwand des Erwachsenen. Morphol Jb 108:391, 1966.
3. Liebermann-Meffert D: Form und Lageentwicklung des menschlichen Magens und seiner Mesenterien. Acta Anat 72:376, 1969.
4. Liebermann-Meffert D: Die Frühentwicklung der Milz menschlicher Feten mit Befunden zur Problematik der Erythropoese. Embryonic development of the human spleen and erythropoiesis. In Lennert K, Harms D (eds): Die Milz/The Spleen. Berlin, Springer, 1970, pp 222-236.
5. O'Rahilly R, Tucker JA: The early development of the larynx in staged human embryos. Part I: Embryos of the first five weeks (to stage 15). Ann Otol Rhinol Laryngol 82(Suppl 7):1, 1973.
6. Kluth D, Habenicht R: The embryology of usual and unusual types of esophageal atresia. Pediatr Surg Int 2:223, 1987.
7. Zwa-Tun HA: The tracheo-esophageal septum—fact or fantasy? Acta Anat (Basel) 114:1, 1982.
8. Smith EI: The early development of the trachea and esophagus in relation to atresia of the esophagus and tracheoesophageal fistula. Contrib Embryol Carnegie Inst 36:43, 1956.
9. Kluth D, Steding G, Seidl W: The embryology of foregut malformations. J Pediatr Surg 22:389, 1987.
10. His W: Zur Bildungsgeschichte der Lungen beim menschlichen Embryo. Arch Anat Entwickl Gesch 17:89, 1887.
11. Kreuter E: Die angeborenen Verschliessungen und Verengerungen des Darmkanals im Lichte der Entwicklungsgeschichte. Dtsch Z Chir 79:1, 1905.
12. Merei JM, Farmer S, Hasthorpe BQ, et al: Timing and embryology of esophageal atresia and tracheo-esophageal fistula. Anat Rec 249:240, 1997.
13. Mueller-Botha GS: Organogenesis and growth of the gastro-esophageal region in man. Anat Rec 133:219, 1959.
14. Hinrichsen KV: a) Intestinaltrakt, b) peripheres Nervensystem, c) Venen. In Hinrichsen KV (ed): Human Embryologie. Lehrbuch und Atlas der vorgeburtlichen Entwicklung des Menschen. Berlin, Springer, 1990, pp 516, 449, 305.
15. Dankmeijer J, Miete M: Sur le développement de l'estomac. Acta Anat 47:384, 1961.
16. Kanagasuntheram R: Development of the human lesser sac. J Anat (Lond) 91:188, 1957.
17. Skandalakis JE, Gray SW, Ricketts R: Various anomalies. In Embryology for Surgeons: The Embryological Basis for the Treatment of Congenital Anomalies, 2nd ed. Baltimore, Williams & Wilkins, 1994, pp 65-112, 154-183, 355-392, 491-539.
18. Keith A: The nature of the mammalian diaphragm and pleural cavities. J Anat (Lond) 39:243, 1905.
19. Wells LJ: Development of the human diaphragm and pleural sacs. Contrib Embryol Carnegie Inst 24:93, 1954.
20. Kluth D, Teubrinck R, von Ekesparre M, et al: The natural history of congenital diaphragmatic hernia and pulmonary hypoplasia in the embryo. J Pediatr Surg 28:456, 1993.
21. Keith A: Human Embryology and Morphology, 5th ed. London, Arnold, 1933, p 303.
22. Liebermann-Meffert D, Allgöwer M, Schmid P, et al: Muscular equivalent of the lower esophageal sphincter. Gastroenterology 76:31, 1979.
23. Boerner-Patzelt D: Die Entwicklung der Magenschleimhautinseln im oberen Anteil des Oesophagus von ihrem ersten Auftreten bis zur Geburt. Anat Anz 55:162, 1922.
24. Johnson FD: The development of the mucous membrane of the esophagus, stomach and small intestine in the human embryo. Am J Anat 10:521, 1910.
25. Schridde H: Ueber die Epithelproliferationen in der embryonalen menschlichen Speiseröhre. Virchows Arch Pathol Anat 191:178, 1908.

26. Enterline H, Thompson J: Pathology of the Esophagus. New York, Springer, 1984, pp 1-6.
27. Johns BAE: Developmental changes in the esophageal epithelium in man. J Anat (Lond) 86:431, 1952.
28. Sakai N, Suenaga T, Tanaka K: Electron microscopic study on the esophageal mucosa in human fetuses. Auris Nasus Larynx (Tokyo) 16:177, 1989.
29. Liebermann-Meffert D, Duranceau A, Stein HJ: Anatomy and embryology. In Zuidema GD, Yeo CJ: Shackelford's Surgery of the Alimentary Tract, 5th ed. WB Saunders, Philadelphia, 2002, pp 3–39.
30. Menard D, Arsenault P: Maturation of human fetal esophagus maintained in organ culture. Anat Rec 217:348, 1987.
31. Kilgore SP, Ormsby AH, Gramlich TL, et al: The gastric cardia: Fact or fiction. Am J Gastroenterol 95:921, 2000.
32. Chandrasoma PT, Der R, Ma Y, et al: Histology of the gastroesophageal junction: An autopsy study. Am J Surg Pathol 24:402, 2000.
33. Oberg S, Peters JH, DeMeester TR, et al: Inflammation and specialized intestinal metaplasia of cardiac mucosa is a manifestation of gastroesophageal reflux disease. Ann Surg 226:522, 1997.
34. Park YS, Park HJ, Kang GH, et al: Histology of gastroesophageal junction in fetal and pediatric autopsy. Arch Pathol Lab Med 127:451, 2003.
35. de Hertogh G, van Eyken P, Ectors N, et al: On the existence and location of cardiac mucosa: An autopsy study in embryos, fetuses, and infants. Gut 52:791, 2003.
36. Marsman WA, van Sandick JW, Tytgat GNJ, et al: The presence and mucin histochemistry of cardiac type mucosa at the esophagogastric junction. Am J Gastroenterol 99:212, 2004.
37. Zhou H, Greco MA, Daum F, et al: Origin of cardiac mucosa, ontogenic considerations. Pediatr Rev Pathol 4:358, 2001.
38. van Campenhout E: Le développement du système nerveux sympathique chez le poulet. Arch Biol (Paris) 42:479, 1931.
39. Hitchcock RJI, Pemble MJ, Bishop AE, et al: Quantitative study of the development and maturation of human oesophageal innervation. J Anat 180:175, 1992.
40. Jones DS: Origin of the vagi and the parasympathetic ganglion cells of the viscera of the chick. Anat Rec 582:185, 1942.
41. Smith RB, Taylor JM: Observations on the intrinsic innervation of the human fetal esophagus between the 10-mm and 140-mm crown-rump length stages. Acta Anat 81:127, 1972.
42. Hewer E: Development of nerve endings in the foetus. J Anat (Lond) 69:369, 1934.

3

Physiology of the Esophagus and Its Sphincters

Radu Tutuian · Donald O. Castell

The esophagus is a muscular tube whose major role is transporting nutrients from the mouth to the stomach. It also allows evacuation of gas (belching) or gastric content (vomiting) from the stomach. In humans, the musculature of the esophagus transitions from (1) predominantly striated at the level of the upper esophageal sphincter (UES) and proximal 1 to 2 cm of the esophagus through (2) a mixed striated–smooth muscle transition zone spanning 4 to 5 cm to (3) an entirely smooth muscle structure in the distal 50% to 60% of the esophagus, including the lower esophageal sphincter (LES) (Fig. 3–1).[1] Recognizing this difference in the muscular sequence of the esophagus is important to understanding swallowing and the pathophysiology of diseases affecting the esophagus.

SWALLOWING PROCESS

Normal human subjects swallow on average 500 times a day.[2] The act of swallowing can be divided into three stages: the oral (voluntary) stage, the pharyngeal (involuntary) stage, and the esophageal stage. These stages are a continuous process closely coordinated through the medullary swallowing centers.[3]

Oral Stage

The oral stage of the swallowing process involves the tongue and the extrinsic oropharyngeal muscles and is the phase during which the swallowing mechanism is primed. During the oral phase, the tongue changes its three-dimensional configuration to allow contraction of the tongue to push the bolus backward and upward toward the hard palate. The configuration of the tongue is changed so that it forms an "expulsion chamber" in which the bolus is contained by the base of the tongue (anterior and inferior), the peripheral edges of the tongue (lateral), the hard palate (superior), and the

closed glossopalatal gate (posterior). The size of the bolus-loading chamber varies with the size of the bolus. The loading time of the expulsion chamber also varies with the size of the bolus. However, expulsion time is independent of the size of the bolus and lasts around 0.5 second. Volume-independent oral expulsion and clearance are achieved by increases in glossopalatal gate opening, lingual propulsion velocity, and contraction amplitude with increasing bolus volumes. Once the bolus passes through the glossopalatal opening, swallowing enters the pharyngeal phase and the process becomes involuntary.

Pharyngeal Stage

In the pharyngeal stage of swallowing, food passes from the oral cavity into the pharynx, across the UES, and into the proximal end of the esophagus. This involuntary phase consists of a series of rapid, carefully coordinated striated muscular contractions (Fig. 3–2). Aside from propelling the food bolus from the mouth into the esophagus, the muscular activity in the pharyngeal phase of deglutition has to prevent food from entering the airways (i.e., a "safe" swallow). Once the food is inserted into the mouth and masticated, the swallowing reflex is initiated by stimulating receptors at the base of the tongue, tonsils, anterior and posterior pillars, soft palate, posterior pharyngeal wall, epiglottis, and larynx.[4] The afferent information from these receptors is carried through the maxillary branch of the trigeminal nerve (cranial nerve V), the glossopharyngeal nerve (cranial nerve IX), and the superior laryngeal branch of the vagus nerve (cranial nerve X).[5] Swallowing can also be initiated voluntarily from the cerebral cortex, but some additional sensory input is required because voluntary deglutition is difficult when the pharynx is anesthetized or no bolus is present in the pharynx.[6] Sensory and cortical input is integrated in the swallowing center located in the brainstem. The swallowing center includes neurons in the

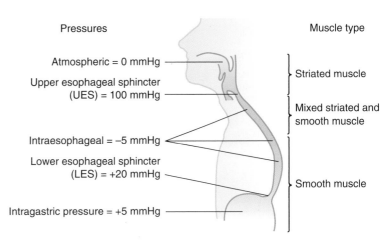

Figure 3–1. Pressures recorded in the upper esophageal sphincter, esophagus, lower esophageal sphincter, and stomach in reference to atmospheric pressure. The type of musculature varies from striated in the pharynx and proximal part of the esophagus, through a transition zone of mixed striated and smooth muscle, to only smooth muscle in the distal part of the esophagus.

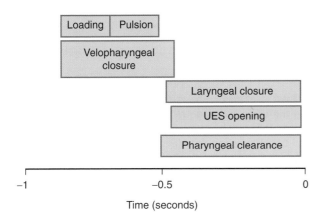

Figure 3–2. Time course of events during swallowing of liquid boluses. The timing of events is presented in reference to closure of the upper esophageal sphincter (UES) (time zero).

nucleus tractus solitarius, the nucleus ambiguus, and the adjacent reticular formation. These centers send efferent information to the oropharyngeal musculature via the trigeminal nerve (cranial nerve V), facial nerve (cranial nerve VII), glossopharyngeal nerve (cranial nerve IX), vagus nerve (cranial nerve X), and hypoglossal nerve (cranial nerve XII).

Just before the beginning of the pharyngeal stage, in anticipation of the arrival of a food bolus, respiration is temporarily suppressed and the pharynx is converted from a respiratory to a swallowing pathway.[7] Conversion of the pharynx into a swallowing pathway requires (1) closure of the openings of the pharynx to the nasal passages, oral cavity, and laryngeal vestibule; (2) opening of the UES; and (3) shortening and widening of the pharyngeal chamber. The following steps are involved in these processes:

1. Pulling up the soft palate and closing the posterior nares
2. Medial pulling of the palatopharyngeal folds, leading to closure of the velopharyngeal junction

(this process limits the opening through the pharynx, which can impair the passage of larger boluses)
3. Closing the vocal cords and a backward and downward swing of the epiglottis to close the larynx
4. Upward and forward movement of the larynx, leading to stretching of the esophageal and UES opening
5. Active relaxation of the UES from the usually tonic cricopharyngeus
6. Passive opening of the UES created by the laryngeal movement
7. Contraction of the superior constrictor muscle of the pharynx, which represents the beginning of pharyngeal peristalsis to clear the food into the esophagus

Combined videofluoroscopic and manometric studies indicate that the pharyngeal peristaltic contraction begins by apposition of the soft palate and contraction of the posterior pharyngeal wall. During the progression of peristalsis toward the esophagus, the posterior pharyngeal wall sequentially comes in contact with the posterior surface of the tongue; the epiglottis; the laryngeal, arytenoid, and interarytenoid muscles; and the cricoid cartilage.[8] Before complete occlusion occurs, the anatomic structure of the pharynx, epiglottis, and cricoid cartilage occludes the medial part of the swallowing chamber and thereby splits the bolus into two lateral halves. Pharyngeal clearance has very rigorous timing and does not vary much with the size of the bolus. The propagation velocity of the tail end of the bolus overlaps the propagation velocity of the pharyngeal contraction and does not vary with the volume of the bolus. This constancy is achieved by earlier opening of the UES and higher bolus-head velocity as the size of the bolus increases.

Anatomically, the UES is composed of the cricoid cartilage ventrally and the cricopharyngeal muscle laterally and dorsally. The insertion of the cricopharyngeal muscle on the cricoid cartilage results in an asymmetric pressure profile of the UES. Normal UES pressure is approximately 100 mm Hg in the anterior-posterior direction and approximately 50 mm Hg laterally.

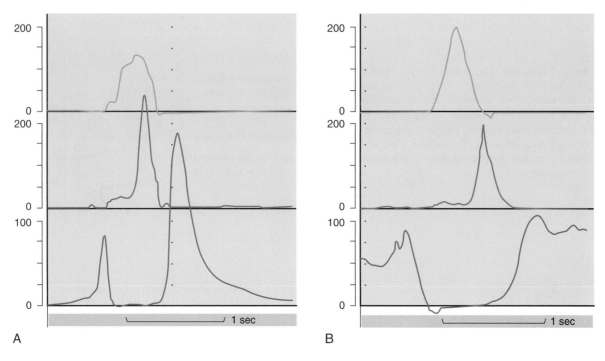

Figure 3–3. Oropharyngeal manometry tracings recorded with the distal transducer above the upper esophageal sphincter (UES) (**A**) and in the UES (**B**). When the distal sensor is placed above the UES, a typical "M" pattern is identified in the distal channel. Initially, the pressure rises as the UES ascends on the transducer, followed by relaxation of the UES. The pressure will then rise again once the UES closes and will return to the pharyngeal baseline when the UES descends back into the initial position. If the distal pressure transducer is placed in the UES, during deglutition it will "drop" into the esophagus and thereby actually lead to overestimation of UES relaxation duration (because it also includes ascent and descent of the UES) and misinterpretation of UES residual pressure (because esophageal baseline pressure is actually being measured).

In view of the asymmetric pressure profile, timing of the pharyngeal-UES transfer and vertical movement of the UES during deglutition are important details when performing UES manometry studies. To obtain accurate information on UES dynamics, circumferential solid-state pressure transducers are preferred because of the rapid response time of the transducers and the capability of evaluating radial forces over the entire 360 degrees.[9] Because the UES ascends approximately 1 cm during deglutition, we prefer placing the UES pressure transducer about 1 cm above the sphincter. During deglutition, the sphincter will initially rise onto the transducer, then open, let the bolus move through, close, and then descend into the initial position. It is our opinion that this approach allows more accurate determination of UES dynamics. When the distal sensor is placed above the UES, a typical "M" pattern is identified in the distal channel. Initially, the pressure rises as the UES ascends onto the transducer, followed by UES relaxation (Fig. 3–3). The pressure will then rise again once the UES closes and will return to the pharyngeal baseline when the UES descends back into the initial position. If the distal pressure transducer is placed in the UES, it will "drop" into the esophagus during deglutition and therefore lead to an overestimation of the duration of UES relaxation (because it also includes ascent and descent

of the UES) and misinterpretation of UES residual pressure (because the transducer is actually measuring esophageal baseline pressure).

Esophageal Stage

The esophageal stage of swallowing starts once the food is transferred from the oral cavity through the UES into the esophagus. The main function of the esophagus is to transport the ingested bolus from the pharynx into the stomach. This active process is achieved by contractions of the circular and longitudinal muscles of the tubular esophagus and coordinated relaxation of the LES. Sequential contraction of the esophageal circular muscle in a proximal-to-distal direction generates a peristaltic clearing wave (Fig. 3–4). Esophageal peristalsis is controlled by afferent and efferent connections of the medullary swallowing center via the vagus nerve (cranial nerve X). The proximal striated esophageal musculature is directly innervated by the nucleus ambiguus, whereas innervation of the distal, smooth musculature of the esophagus and LES comes from the dorsal motor nucleus of the vagus. The vagus nerve carries both stimulating (cholinergic) and inhibitory (noncholinergic, nonadrenergic) information to the esophageal muscula-

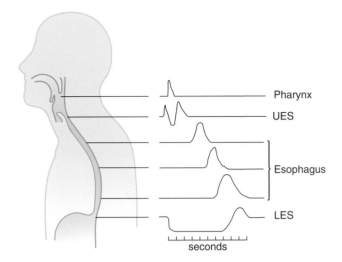

Figure 3–4. Schematic representation of pressure changes recorded in the pharynx, upper esophageal sphincter (UES), esophagus, and lower esophageal sphincter (LES) during esophageal peristalsis.

ture. In addition to the central nervous system control, the myenteric (Auerbach) plexus located between the circular and longitudinal muscle layers plays a major role in coordinating peristalsis in the smooth muscle portion of the distal esophagus. The importance of the myenteric plexus in controlling distal, smooth muscle peristalsis is shown by observations that bilateral cervical vagotomy in animals does not abolish peristalsis in this portion of the gastrointestinal tract.

Esophageal Peristalsis

Esophageal peristalsis is the result of sequential contraction of the circular esophageal muscle. Three distinct patters of esophageal contractions have been described: primary and secondary peristalsis and tertiary contractions.

Primary peristaltic contractions are the usual form of the contraction waves of circular muscles that progress down the esophagus; they are initiated by the central mechanisms that follow the voluntary act of swallowing. The contraction wave begins in the pharynx and requires approximately 8 to 10 seconds to reach the distal part of the esophagus. During primary peristalsis, the LES is relaxed, starting at the initiation of swallowing and lasting until the peristalsis reaches the LES.

Secondary peristaltic contractions are the contraction waves of the circular esophageal muscle occurring in response to esophageal distention. They are not a result of central mechanisms and can be experimentally demonstrated by distending a balloon in the proximal section to midsection of the esophagus. The role of secondary peristaltic contractions is to clear the esophageal lumen of ingested material not cleared by primary peristalsis or material that is refluxed from the stomach. Secondary peristaltic contractions are not accompanied by pharyngeal peristalsis or UES relaxation. However, in

the distal part of the esophagus, secondary peristaltic contractions resemble those of primary peristalsis.

Tertiary contractions are primarily identified during barium x-ray studies and represent nonperistaltic contraction waves that leave segmental indentations on the barium column. The physiologic role of these contractions is unknown, and obliteration of the lumen is their only potential pathologic consequence.

The amplitudes of contractions vary throughout the esophagus. Contraction amplitudes are higher in the proximal and distal parts of the esophagus, with a mid-esophageal low-pressure zone located at the junction of the striated and smooth muscle portion of the esophagus (Fig. 3–5). High-resolution manometry studies using catheters with pressure sensors at each centimeter in the esophagus suggest the existence of two distinct pressure waves, proximally and distally, in the midesophageal low-pressure zone (Fig. 3–6). In healthy individuals, primary esophageal peristalsis during wet swallows of the same volumes is very reproducible. There is little swallow-by-swallow variation in amplitude and velocity when swallows are spaced at least 20 to 30 seconds apart (see later). There is no "fatigue" of the esophageal musculature inasmuch as similar amplitudes have been recorded during as many as 50 consecutive swallows. Esophageal contraction amplitudes are lower in the upright position,[10] and the velocity is higher in the proximal than in the distal esophagus.[11] The amplitude and duration of contraction are increased and the velocity decreased when fluid swallows are given as opposed to dry swallows.[12] Larger bolus volumes elicit stronger peristaltic contractions,[13] warm boluses augment[14] and cold boluses inhibit peristaltic contractions,[15] and the osmolality of the bolus has no influence on esophageal peristalsis.[16] Contrary to popular belief regarding "presbyesophagus," esophageal peristalsis is not affected by age in healthy volunteers.[17]

In vitro studies on sections of esophageal smooth muscle from the opossum have increased our understanding of the activities of circular and longitudinal esophageal muscle during peristalsis.[18] Circular and longitudinal muscles differ not only in the orientation of their fibers but also in their response to electrical stimuli (Fig. 3–7). A stimulus applied to an isolated section of longitudinal esophageal muscle will lead to a sustained contraction of the muscle ("duration response") lasting as long as the stimulus is applied. This response is mediated by acetylcholine because it can be blocked with both atropine and tetrodotoxin. In contrast, circular muscle will show a brief contraction ("on response") at the onset of the electrical stimulus, followed by a period of relaxation lasting as long as the stimulus is applied. Once the stimulus is discontinued, a much larger contraction occurs ("off response"). Furthermore, smooth muscle strips taken from different segments of the esophagus show progressively longer time intervals (latency) from the termination of the stimulus to the onset of the "off response" as one progresses more distally in the esophagus (Fig. 3–8).

Based on these observations, the following model of esophageal peristalsis has been proposed. When a swallow is initiated, the longitudinal muscle contracts

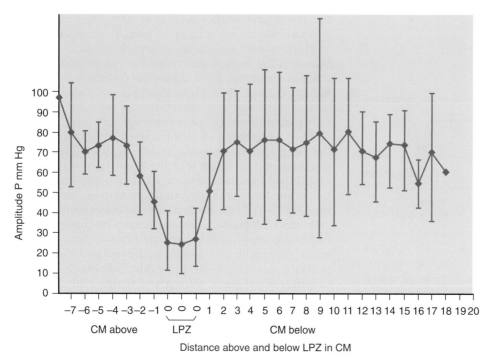

Figure 3–5. Esophageal pressure profile in the esophagus during contractions.

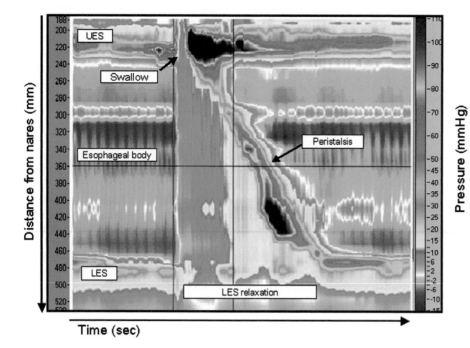

Figure 3–6. Spatial-temporal plots of esophageal peristalsis recorded by high-resolution manometry. The 32 pressure channels located every 1 cm span the entire esophagus, including the pharynx, upper esophageal sphincter (UES), lower esophageal sphincter (LES), and proximal part of the stomach. Intraesophageal pressures of the same amplitude are coded with the same color, starting at –10 mm Hg (blue) and ranging through 110 mm Hg (black).

and "stiffens" the walls of the esophagus to provide support for the circular muscle contractions. The circular muscle responds by a short contraction ("on response"), followed by relaxation of the entire esophagus, including the LES. The increase in the latency gradient, as one progress more distally in the esophagus, is responsible for the delay in esophageal contractions that generates the peristaltic wave. This model does not entirely explain all the phenomena that have been observed in human esophageal peristalsis, but the aforementioned in vitro observations are consistent with many aspects of normal human physiology.

One example is deglutitive inhibition. Although pharynx and UES dynamics last less than 1 second, which allows them to respond with a 1:1 ratio to closely spaced swallows, it takes 8 to 10 seconds for a single food bolus to pass through the esophagus into the stomach. When swallows are very closely spaced (i.e., between 2 and 5

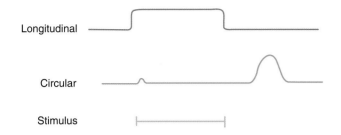

Figure 3–7. Differences in response of longitudinal and circular esophageal musculature to electrical stimuli. Longitudinal muscle exhibits sustained contractions ("duration contraction") lasting as long as the stimulus is present. Circular muscle has a brief contraction ("on response") at the onset of the stimulus, followed by a period of relaxation lasting as long as the stimulus is present. A second, stronger response ("off response") is noted after a lag period once the stimulus is discontinued.

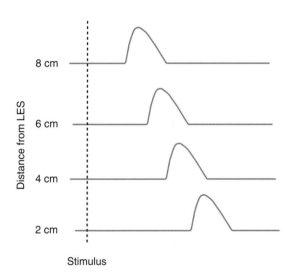

Figure 3–8. Increase in the lag period between the end of the stimulus to the onset of the "off response" in circular muscle fibers harvested at different levels above the lower esophageal sphincter (LES).

seconds), contraction of the distal part of the esophagus is inhibited by the inhibitory neural impulses sent by the subsequent swallow. This phenomenon of "deglutitive inhibition" is physiologically beneficial in that an improperly timed contraction that impairs bolus transit is avoided during subsequent swallows (Fig. 3–9). The off-response and latency period will then produce one peristaltic contraction at the end of a series of closely spaced swallows to allow proper clearance of the esophagus.[19]

The presence of the inhibitory relaxation wave can be demonstrated by measuring the pressure in an inflated balloon in the distal esophagus.[20] Positioning an inflated balloon at either 3 or 8 cm above the LES, Sifrim et al. have documented a decrease in pressure in the artificially balloon-created high-pressure zone starting at the time of swallowing and lasting until the peristaltic contraction reaches the segment. The same investigators found this phenomenon to be absent in patients with achalasia and distal esophageal spasm.[21]

Nonadrenergic, noncholinergic mediators are thought to control in part the latency phase responsible for esophageal peristalsis. From this group of substances, vasointestinal peptide (VIP) and nitric oxide (NO) appear to play an important role in the human esophagus. With the use of NO scavengers (recombinant human hemoglobin) during esophageal contractions, Murray et al.[22] evaluated the role of NO in human esophageal peristalsis. Studying healthy volunteers, they documented altered esophageal peristalsis and simultaneous contractions (resembling esophageal spasm) during the administration of recombinant human hemoglobin.

In addition to peristaltic contractions, clinical studies support the existence of an esophageal propulsive force. This was first reported by Winship et al.[23] during swallowing studies in healthy volunteers when they noticed a steady, aborally directed force of up to 200 g exerted on a balloon that was inflated in the esophagus and prevented from moving distally. The esophageal propulsive force increases with an increase in the diameter of the bolus and is greatest in the distal end of the esophagus. The propulsive force is produced by tonic and phasic contractions of the longitudinal and circular muscle just above the balloon.[24] Once the balloon is released, the propulsive force is converted into a peristaltic sequence that progresses distally and pushes the balloon ahead of it.

Lower Esophageal Sphincter

The LES can be located during manometric stationary pull-through as a tonically contracted region at the esophagogastric junction. Normal LES resting pressure ranges from 10 to 45 mm Hg above the gastric baseline level and results from the tonic (intrinsic) LES component augmented by the phasic (extrinsic) diaphragmatic pressure, which varies with respirations. The function of the LES is to prevent gastroesophageal reflux and to relax with swallowing to allow movement of ingested food into the stomach.

The mechanism by which the circular musculature in the LES maintains tonic closure has been investigated considerably. At present, it is believed to be predominantly due to intrinsic muscle activity because the resting LES tone persists even after surgical or pharmacologic destruction of all neural input.[25] Calcium channel blockers that exert their effect directly on circular muscle can reduce resting LES pressure,[26] and there appears to be some cholinergic tone because resting LES pressure can be reduced with anticholinergic agents.[27] In addition, LES tone can be influenced by a series of hormones and pharmacologic agents (Table 3–1).

The LES relaxes to allow passage of food from the esophagus into the stomach or to allow material from the stomach to come back into the esophagus. Even though

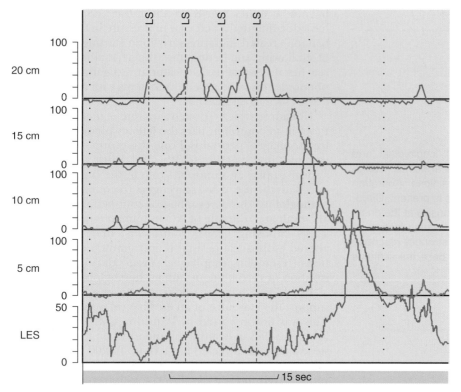

Figure 3–9. Manometric example of deglutitive inhibition. Distal esophageal body contractions of the first three swallows are inhibited when swallows are given 5 seconds apart. The last (fourth) swallow produces a peristaltic contraction that will clear the esophageal lumen. The lower esophageal sphincter is relaxed the entire time during closely spaced swallows.

Table 3–1	Hormonal and Pharmacologic Agents Influencing Lower Esophageal Sphincter Resting Pressure	

Increase LES Pressure	Decrease LES Pressure
Gastrin	Secretin
Motilin	Cholecystokinin (CCK)
Substance P	Glucagon
Pancreatic polypeptide	Gastric inhibitory peptide (GIP)
Bombesin	Vasointestinal peptide (VIP)
Angiotensin II	Progesterone
Cholinergic agents (e.g., bethanechol)	Atropine
Metoclopramide	Nitrates
Dopamine	Calcium channel blockers
Cisapride	Morphine

the relaxations are transient in both instances, many clinicians and investigators attribute the term *transient lower esophageal sphincter relaxation* (tLESR) to the inappropriate LES relaxations resulting in belching or gastroesophageal reflux. Therefore, the term *deglutitive lower esophageal sphincter relaxation* (dLESR) has been used to describe the relaxations that allow material to pass from the esophagus into the stomach.

dLESRs are reflex relaxations starting less than 2 seconds after the initiation of a swallow. Liquid boluses, especially when assisted by gravity in the upright position, may reach the LES before it relaxes and may therefore be slightly delayed in their passage into the stomach. The relaxation usually lasts 8 to 10 seconds and is followed by an after-contraction in the proximal part of the LES. The after-contraction is a continuation of esophageal peristalsis and lasts 7 to 10 seconds. Therefore, after a swallow at least 15 to 20 seconds elapse before the LES reaches the preswallow steady state.

Relaxation of the LES is the most sensitive component of the swallowing reflex. Isolated dLESRs can be provoked by pharyngeal tactile stimulation that is at a subthreshold for producing a full swallowing response. LES relaxations induced by primary peristalsis or pharyngeal tactile stimuli are mediated via the vagus nerve and can be abolished by bilateral vagal nerve section or cooling.[28,29] LES relaxations can also be produced by esophageal distention. Distention of the striated portion of the esophagus leads to a centrally mediated LES relaxation that can be abolished by vagal nerve section. In contrast, vagal nerve sectioning does not abolish LES relaxations triggered by distention of the smooth muscle portion of the esophagus, which suggests that this reflex is mediated via the intramural nerves.[30]

tLESRs occur in response to proximal gastric fundus distention and permit gastroesophageal reflux, belching, retching, and vomiting. Not all tLESRs are accompanied by gastroesophageal reflux, and the proportion of tLESRs associated with reflux varies from 10% to 93%.[31,32] tLESRs are vagally mediated and controlled by the same central structures that control swallow-induced LES relaxations. Pharmacologic interventions that affect the vagal pathways of the medullary center can influence the frequency of tLESRs, and vagotomy or vagal cooling can block tLESRs.[33] Noncholinergic, nonadrenergic mediators such as NO and VIP can facilitate tLESRs.

LES relaxation is different from LES opening. LES relaxation is required for the LES to open, but there is a slight delay in opening of the LES during both dLESRs and tLESRs. Most recently, combined multichannel intraluminal impedance and manometry have been adapted to evaluate the relationship between these two phenomena without the use of radiation.[34]

SUMMARY

During food ingestion, the primary function of the esophagus is to facilitate the passage of boluses from the oral cavity into the stomach. This process can be separated into transfer of food from the oral cavity through the pharynx into the proximal part of the esophagus, where it is transported distally into the stomach. The initial part of the swallowing reflex is voluntary, after which carefully coordinated contractions transform swallowing into an involuntary series of events. Functional changes of the pharynx during deglutition transiently transform this airway conduit into a digestive conduit to ensure that food is not aspirated into the lungs. Once food passes into the esophagus, peristaltic contractions transport the bolus into the stomach while the LES is temporary relaxed and opened. In between swallowing, the esophagus and its sphincters prevent food from coming back from the stomach into the pharynx and oral cavity.

Recognizing the functional organization of each stage of swallowing and reflux prevention is important for understanding the pathophysiology of esophageal and esophagus-related diseases.

REFERENCES

1. Meyer GW, Austin RM, Brady CE III, Castell DO: Muscle anatomy of the human esophagus. J Clin Gastroenterol 8:131-134, 1986.
2. Lear CS, Flanagan JB, Moorrees CF: The frequency of deglutition in man. Arch Oral Biol 10:83-100, 1965.
3. Weisbrodt NW: Neuromuscular organization of esophageal and pharyngeal motility. Arch Intern Med 136:524-531, 1976.
4. Jean A, Car A: Inputs to the swallowing medullary neurons from the peripheral afferent fibers and the swallowing cortical area. Brain Res 178:567-572, 1979.
5. Sessle BJ, Henry JL: Neural mechanisms of swallowing: Neurophysiological and neurochemical studies on brain stem neurons in the solitary tract region. Dysphagia 4:61-75, 1989.
6. Jean A: Brain stem control of swallowing: Neuronal network and cellular mechanisms. Physiol Rev 81:929-969, 2001.
7. Dua KS, Ren J, Bardan E, et al: Coordination of deglutitive glottal function and pharyngeal bolus transit during normal eating. Gastroenterology 112:73-83, 1997.
8. Kahrilas PJ, Logemann JA, Lin S, Ergun GA: Pharyngeal clearance during swallowing: A combined manometric and videofluoroscopic study. Gastroenterology 103:128-136, 1992.
9. Olsson R, Castell JA, Castell DO, Ekberg O: Solid-state computerized manometry improves diagnostic yield in pharyngeal dysphagia: Simultaneous videoradiography and manometry in dysphagia patients with normal barium swallows. Abdom Imaging 20:230-235, 1995.
10. Tutuian R, Elton JP, Castell DO, et al: Effects of position on oesophageal function: Studies using combined manometry and multichannel intraluminal impedance. Neurogastroenterol Motil 15:63-67, 2003.
11. Sears VW Jr, Castell JA, Castell DO: Comparison of effects of upright versus supine body position and liquid versus solid bolus on esophageal pressures in normal humans. Dig Dis Sci 35:857-864, 1990.
12. Hollis JB, Castell DO: Effect of dry swallows and wet swallows of different volumes on esophageal peristalsis. J Appl Physiol 38:1161-1164, 1975.
13. Janssens J, Valembois P, Hellemans J, et al: Studies on the necessity of a bolus for the progression of secondary peristalsis in the canine esophagus. Gastroenterology 67:245-251, 1974.
14. El Ouazzani T, Mei N: Electrophysiologic properties and role of the vagal thermoreceptors of lower esophagus and stomach of cat. Gastroenterology 83:995-1001, 1982.
15. Meyer GW, Castell DO: Human esophageal response during chest pain induced by swallowing cold liquids. JAMA 246:2057-2059, 1981.
16. Winship DH, Viegas de Andrade SR, Zboralske FF: Influence of bolus temperature on human esophageal motor function. J Clin Invest 49:243-250, 1970.
17. Hollis JB, Castell DO: Esophageal function in elderly man. A new look at "presbyesophagus." Ann Intern Med 80:371-374, 1974.
18. Christensen J, Lund GF: Esophageal responses to distension and electrical stimulation. J Clin Invest 48:408-419, 1969.
19. Tutuian R, Jalil S, Katz PO, Castell DO: Effect of interval between swallows on oesophageal pressures and bolus movement in normal subjects—studies with combined multichannel intraluminal impedance and oesophageal manometry. Neurogastroenterol Motil 16:23-29, 2004.
20. Sifrim D, Janssens J, Vantrappen G: A wave of inhibition precedes primary peristaltic contractions in the human esophagus. Gastroenterology 103:876-882, 1992.
21. Sifrim D, Janssens J, Vantrappen G: Failing deglutitive inhibition in primary esophageal motility disorders. Gastroenterology 106:875-882, 1994.
22. Murray JA, Ledlow A, Launspach J, et al: The effects of recombinant human hemoglobin on esophageal motor functions in humans. Gastroenterology 109:1241-1248, 1995.
23. Winship DH, Zboralske FF: The esophageal propulsive force: Esophageal response to acute obstruction. J Clin Invest 46:1391-1401, 1967.
24. Williams D, Thompson DG, Heggie L, Bancewicz J: Responses of the human esophagus to experimental intraluminal distension. Am J Physiol 265:G196-G203, 1993.
25. Goyal RK, Rattan S: Genesis of basal sphincter pressure: Effect of tetrodotoxin on lower esophageal sphincter pressure in opossum in vivo. Gastroenterology 71:62-67, 1976.
26. Richter JE, Spurling TJ, Cordova CM, Castell DO: Effects of oral calcium blocker, diltiazem, on esophageal contractions. Studies in volunteers and patients with nutcracker esophagus. Dig Dis Sci 29:649-656, 1984.
27. Dodds WJ, Dent J, Hogan WJ, Arndorfer RC: Effect of atropine on esophageal motor function in humans. Am J Physiol 240:G290-G296, 1981.
28. Reynolds RP, El-Sharkawy TY, Diamant NE: Lower esophageal sphincter function in the cat: Role of central innervation assessed by transient vagal blockade. Am J Physiol 246:G666-G674, 1984.
29. Ryan JP, Snape WJ Jr, Cohen S: Influence of vagal cooling on esophageal function. Am J Physiol 232:E159-E164, 1977.
30. Paterson WG, Rattan S, Goyal RK: Esophageal responses to transient and sustained esophageal distension. Am J Physiol 255:G587-G595, 1988.
31. Dent J, Dodds WJ, Friedman RH, et al: Mechanism of gastroesophageal reflux in recumbent asymptomatic human subjects. J Clin Invest 65:256-267, 1980.
32. Mittal RK, McCallum RW: Characteristics of transient lower esophageal sphincter relaxation in humans. Am J Physiol 252:G636-G641, 1987.
33. Mittal RK, Holloway RH, Penagini R, et al: Transient lower esophageal sphincter relaxation. Gastroenterology 109:601-610, 1995.
34. Pandolfion JE, Shi G, Zhang Q, et al: Measuring EGJ opening patterns using high-resolution intraluminal impedance. Neurogastroenterol Motil 17:200-206, 2005.

4

Assessment of Symptoms and Approach to the Patient with Esophageal Disease

Jeffrey H. Peters

A careful, detailed, and structured assessment of the patient's symptoms is critical to any medical treatment, even more so in the decision to perform esophageal surgery. Accordingly, such evaluation should not be left to the referring physician or gastroenterologist. Experienced clinicians soon realize that many symptoms of esophageal disease can be confused or accompanied by non–esophageal-related gastrointestinal and respiratory symptoms that will not improve or may be worsened by specific therapy. This is particularly true of functional disorders, including gastroesophageal reflux disease (GERD) and esophageal motility abnormalities. Symptoms consistent with irritable bowel syndrome, such as alternating diarrhea and constipation, bloating, and crampy abdominal pain, should be sought and detailed separately from GERD symptoms. Likewise, symptoms suggestive of gastric disorders, including nausea, early satiety, epigastric abdominal pain, anorexia, and weight loss, are important to note and discuss with the patient.

SYMPTOMS OF FOREGUT DISEASE

Heartburn, regurgitation, dysphagia, and chest pain are the most prevalent symptoms of esophageal disease. A myriad of other foregut symptoms may or may not be present, including dyspepsia, anorexia, epigastric pain, nausea, vomiting, and early satiety. These symptoms are considerably more nonspecific and may indicate concomitant gastric or intestinal disease.

Heartburn is generally defined as a substernal burning-type discomfort beginning in the epigastrium and radiating upward. It is often aggravated by meals, spicy or fatty foods, chocolate, alcohol, and coffee and can be worse in the supine position. It is commonly, though not universally, relieved by antacid or antisecretory medications. Epidemiologic studies have shown that heartburn occurs monthly in as many as 40% to 50% of the Western population. The occurrence of heartburn at night and its effect on quality of life have recently been highlighted by a Gallup poll conducted by the American Gastroenterologic Society (Box 4–1).[1]

Regurgitation, the effortless return of acid or bitter gastric contents into the chest, pharynx, or mouth, is highly suggestive of foregut disease. It is often particularly severe at night when supine or when bending over and can be secondary to either an incompetent or an obstructed gastroesophageal junction. With the latter, as in achalasia, the regurgitant is often bland, as though the food were put into a blender. When questioned, most patients can distinguish the two. It is the regurgitation of gastric contents that may result in associated pulmonary

---

Box 4–1 **Nighttime Heartburn Is an Underappreciated Clinical Problem**

50 million Americans have nighttime heartburn at least once per week

80% of heartburn sufferers had nocturnal symptoms—65% both day and night

63% report that it affects their ability to sleep and has an impact on their work the next day

72% are taking prescription medications

Nearly half (45%) report that current remedies do not relieve all the symptoms

---

symptoms, including cough, hoarseness, asthma, and recurrent pneumonia. Bronchospasm can be precipitated by esophageal acidification and cough by either acid stimulation or distention of the esophagus.

Dysphagia, or difficulty swallowing, is a relatively nonspecific term but arguably the most specific symptom of foregut disease. It is often a sign of underlying malignancy and should be aggressively investigated until a diagnosis is established. Dysphagia refers to the sensation of difficulty in passage of food from the mouth to the stomach and can be divided into oropharyngeal and esophageal causes. Oropharyngeal dysphagia is characterized by difficulty transferring food out of the mouth into the esophagus, nasal regurgitation, aspiration, or any combination of these symptoms. Esophageal dysphagia refers to the sensation of food sticking in the lower part of the chest or epigastrium. It may or may not be accompanied by pain (odynophagia), which will be relieved by passage of the bolus.

Chest pain, though commonly and appropriately attributed to cardiac disease, is frequently secondary to esophageal disease as well. As early as 1982, DeMeester et al. showed that nearly 50% of patients with severe chest pain, normal cardiac function, and normal coronary arteriograms had 24-hour pH studies with positive results, implicating gastroesophageal reflux as the underlying cause.[2] Exercise-induced gastroesophageal reflux is a well-known occurrence and may result in exertional chest pain similar to angina.[3] It can be quite difficult if not impossible to distinguish the two causes, particularly on clinical grounds alone.[4,5] Nevens et al. evaluated the ability of experienced cardiologists to differentiate pain of cardiac versus esophageal origin.[6] Of 248 patients initially seen by cardiologists, 185 were thought to have typical angina and 63 to have atypical pain. Forty-eight (26%) of those thought to have classic angina had normal coronary angiograms, and 16 of the 63 with atypical pain had abnormal angiograms. Thus, the cardiologists' clinical impression was wrong 25% of the time. Finally, Pope et al. investigated the ultimate diagnosis in 10,689 patients going to an emergency department with acute chest pain.[7] Seventeen percent were found to have acute ischemia; 6%, stable angina; 21%, other cardiac causes; and 55%, noncardiac causes. They concluded

that the majority of people going to the emergency department with chest pain do not have an underlying cardiac cause for their symptoms. Chest pain that is precipitated by meals, occurring at night while supine, nonradiating, responsive to antacid medication, or accompanied by other symptoms suggesting esophageal disease, such as dysphagia or regurgitation, should trigger the thought of possible esophageal origin. Furthermore, the distinction between heartburn and chest pain is also difficult and largely dependent on the individual patient. One person's heartburn is another's chest pain.

MECHANISMS OF ESOPHAGEAL SYMPTOMS

The precise mechanisms accounting for the generation of symptoms secondary to esophageal disease remain unclear. Considerable insight has been acquired, however. Investigations into the effect of luminal content,[8,9] esophageal distention[9-11] and muscular function,[12] neural pathways, and brain localization[13,14] have provided a basic understanding of the stimuli responsible for the generation of symptoms. It is also clear that the visceroneural pathways of the foregut are complexly intertwined with those of the tracheobronchial tree and heart. This fact accounts for the common overlap of clinical symptoms with diverse disease processes in the upper gastrointestinal, cardiac, and pulmonary systems.

Early investigations of the pathogenesis of esophageal symptomatology studied the effects of balloon distention or esophageal acid infusion (or both) on symptom generation. Classic studies, reported as early as the 1930s, investigated the type and location of symptom perception in patients after balloon distention at 5-cm increments in the esophagus.[15] These data revealed highly variable patient responses (Fig. 4–1). Patients rarely localized the origin of the stimulus accurately, often perceiving the symptom in areas above, below, or quite distant from the location of the distending balloon. Some patients perceived chest pain, some heartburn, and others nausea. Symptoms between the shoulder blades and at the base of the neck, as well as retrobulbar eye pain, were also observed. These findings underscore the highly variable nature of symptom generation secondary to foregut epithelial stimuli. More recent studies have confirmed these findings. Taken together, they suggest considerable variability in individual sensory sensitivity or cerebral cortical processing, or both.

Esophageal perfusion with either acid or bile salts can elicit various degrees of symptoms ranging from mild heartburn to severe angina-like chest pain. Symptom perception is dependent on both the concentration and contact time of the offending agent and is highly variable from individual to individual. In general, discomfort becomes reproducible below pH 4, a fact demonstrated in the early years of esophageal pH testing. This was, in part, responsible for the selection of pH 4 as the threshold pH below which acid reflux was considered present on ambulatory esophageal pH testing. Acid perfusion was the basis for the Bernstein test used historically as a

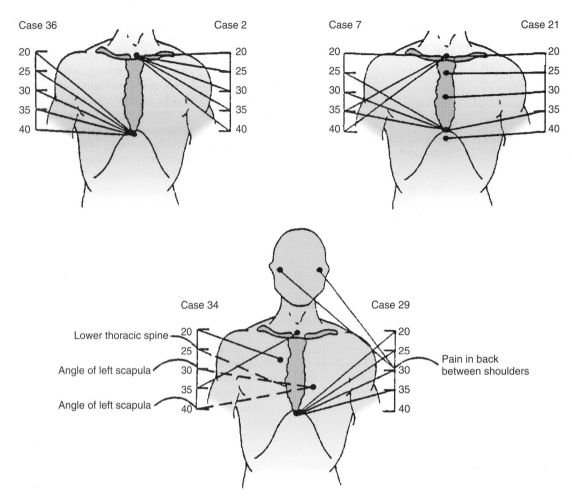

Figure 4–1.   Location of symptoms with esophageal balloon distention in six patients. The *legend* indicates the level (20 to 40 cm) of balloon distention within the esophagus and the *circles* denote the location of the referred symptom. (From Polland WS, Bloomfield AL: Experimental referred pain from the gastrointestinal tract. Part I; the esophagus. J Clin Invest 10:435-452, 1931.)

means to diagnose GERD. The test has largely fallen by the wayside, in part because of its poor sensitivity and specificity. Similarly, studies of the effects of bile salt perfusion of the esophagus have shown nociception with perfusion. Simultaneous measurement of pH and motility and ultrasound have shown that sustained contraction of the esophageal longitudinal muscle correlated with the onset of chest pain.[13]

A number of studies have investigated the cortical response to esophageal balloon distention and acid perfusion. Responses have been detected via cortical evoked potential, positron emission tomography, and magnetic resonance imaging (MRI). Kern et al. recently reported the cerebral cortical MRI response to esophageal acid exposure and balloon distention in 10 healthy volunteers.[13] Intraesophageal perfusion of 0.1 N HCl for 10 minutes increased functional MRI signal intensity in all subjects, with an average 6.7% increase in signal occurring approximately 5 minutes after perfusion without inducing heartburn or chest pain. Saline perfusion elicited no detectable change. Similar changes were seen with balloon distention, although the response times were significantly longer for acid perfusion. Responses were seen in the posterior cingulate, parietal, and anterior frontal lobes. The authors concluded that esophageal mucosal acid contact produces a cerebral cortical response detectable by functional MRI and that the temporal characteristics of the acid response are different from those of balloon distention.

APPROACH TO A PATIENT WITH SUSPECTED GASTROESOPHAGEAL REFLUX DISEASE

GERD-related symptoms can be divided into "typical" symptoms, consisting of heartburn, regurgitation, and dysphagia, and "atypical" symptoms, consisting of cough, hoarseness, asthma, aspiration, and chest pain. Because there are fewer mechanisms for their generation, typical symptoms are more likely to be secondary to increased esophageal acid exposure than atypical symptoms are. The patient's perception of what each symptom means should be explored in an effort to avoid their misinterpretation.[16] Of equal importance is to classify them as primary or secondary for prioritization of therapy and to allow an estimate of the probability of relief of each of the particular symptoms. The response to acid-suppressing medications predicts success and symptom relief after surgery.[17] In contrast to the widely held belief that failure of medical therapy is an indication for surgery, a good response to proton pump inhibitors is desirable because it predicts that the symptoms are actually due to reflux of gastric contents.

The relationship of atypical symptoms such as cough, hoarseness, wheezing, or sore throat to heartburn or regurgitation, or both, should be established. Other more common factors that may contribute to respiratory symptoms should also be investigated. The patient must be made aware of the relatively diminished probably of success of surgery when atypical symptoms are the primary symptoms.[18] Of note is the comparatively longer duration needed for improvement of respiratory symptoms after surgery.[19] It has become increasingly recognized that oral symptoms such as mouth and tongue burning and sore throat rarely improve with antireflux surgery.

The initial diagnostic evaluation should include videoesophagography, upper gastrointestinal endoscopy, stationery esophageal manometry, and 24-hour esophageal pH monitoring (distal ± proximal). These four tests allow the surgeon to determine the presence of gastroesophageal reflux in an objective fashion; the underlying reasons for its presence, such as hiatal hernia or a deficient lower esophageal sphincter; and its severity, including the presence or absence of complications. Although it has been argued that one or more of these studies are superfluous, experience constantly reminds us that they are complementary and that all add useful information before antireflux surgery. Further investigations, in particular, gastric emptying studies or pancreaticobiliary testing or both, are added depending on the findings of the other tests.

Radiographic assessment of the anatomy and function of the esophagus and stomach is one of the most important elements of the preoperative evaluation. A carefully performed videoesophagogram not only provides information about the underlying anatomic defects, such as the presence or absence of a stricture and the size and reducibility of a hiatal hernia, but is also one of the few ways to assess actual bolus transport. A standardized protocol is advised to ascertain different aspects of esophagogastric function during different phases of the study. Given routine review before antireflux surgery, its value becomes increasingly clear. A hiatal hernia is present in more than 80% of patients with gastroesophageal reflux. It is best demonstrated with the patient in the prone position, which causes increased abdominal pressure and promotes distention of the hernia above the diaphragm. The presence of a hiatal hernia is an important component of the underlying pathophysiology of gastroesophageal reflux. Other relevant findings include a large (>5 cm) or irreducible hernia, which suggests the presence of a shortened esophagus[20]; a tight crural "collar" that inhibits barium transit into the stomach, which sug-

gests a possible cause of dysphagia; and the presence of a paraesophageal hernia, which is likely to influence the surgeon's decision on the operative approach.

One of the key goals before taking a patient to the operating room is to connect the patient's complaints to gastroesophageal reflux. Antireflux surgery will reliably and reproducibly prevent the return of gastric contents into the esophagus, but it does little else. If the symptoms that drove the patient to seek surgical treatment are not secondary to reflux, there will be no benefit. Indeed, one will have a patient who is not only no better but often also unusually focused on normally trivial side effects such as bloating and flatulence. The single best way to prevent this scenario is to use 24-hour pH monitoring to prove the presence of pathologic esophageal acid exposure before surgery. The study not only provides for an objective diagnosis but also contributes other useful information. A multivariate analysis of the factors that predict a successful outcome after laparoscopic Nissen fundoplication was recently published.[17] One hundred ninety-nine consecutive patients undergoing laparoscopic Nissen fundoplication were studied, and a variety of demographic, anatomic, clinical, and physiologic factors were analyzed. The three most important predictors of a successful clinical outcome, in order of importance, were an abnormal pH score, a typical primary symptom, and a complete or partial (>50%) response to medical therapy. When all three were present, the patient was 90 times more likely to have relief of symptoms than when they were not!

The choice of treatment of GERD in present-day practice ideally should take into account the underlying severity of the disease and the patient's risk for complications of end-stage reflux disease. This is particularly true given the rising incidence of Barrett's esophagus and adenocarcinoma of the gastric cardia. Studies of the natural history of GERD have shown that although the vast majority of the patients have limited disease and respond well to lifestyle modifications and medical therapy, a substantial proportion (22% to 50%) progress to complications of GERD.[21] This group should be identified early and offered antireflux surgery. The following factors, when identified during the work-up of patients, will help in detecting those at risk: (1) anatomic and physiologic markers of severe disease, such as a defective lower esophageal sphincter, poor contractility of the esophageal body, large hiatal hernias, or bile reflux; (2) severe erosive esophagitis on initial evaluation or the development of esophagitis or peptic strictures during the course of medical therapy; (3) Barrett's esophagus; (4) young age, particularly in patients with the aforementioned characteristics; and (5) progressive respiratory symptoms, aspiration, or pneumonia.

Patients seen for the first time with symptoms suggestive of gastroesophageal reflux may be given initial therapy with H_2 blockers. In view of the availability of over-the-counter medications, many patients will have already self-medicated their symptoms. Failure of H_2 blockers to control the symptoms or immediate return of symptoms after stopping treatment suggests that either the diagnosis is incorrect or the patient has relatively severe disease. Endoscopic examination at this stage of the patient's evaluation provides the opportunity for assessment of the severity of mucosal damage and the presence of Barrett's esophagus. Finding both of these factors on initial endoscopy predicts a high risk for medical failure. The degree and pattern of esophageal exposure to gastric and duodenal juice should be determined at this point via 24-hour pH and bilirubin monitoring. The status of the lower esophageal sphincter and the function of the esophageal body should also be evaluated. These studies identify features that predict a poor response to medical therapy, frequent relapses, and the development of complications; risk factors include supine reflux, poor esophageal contractility, erosive esophagitis or a columnar-lined esophagus at initial evaluation, bile in the refluxate, and a structurally defective sphincter. Patients who have these risk factors should be given the option of surgery as a primary therapy with the expectation of long-term control of symptoms and complications.

APPROACH TO A PATIENT WITH BARRETT'S ESOPHAGUS

Management of Barrett's esophagus is becoming an increasingly common health problem. Long-segment Barrett's esophagus has been estimated to be present in 4% to 6% of patients with reflux symptoms, 1% of all patients who undergo upper endoscopy, and 0.3% of the U.S. population. Short-segment Barrett's esophagus (<3 cm) is probably even more prevalent and has accounted for half to two thirds of all patients with Barrett's esophagus identified in most recent studies. It is commonly argued that most patients with Barrett's esophagus are asymptomatic and therefore need no treatment at all. Although epidemiologic studies suggest that a large reservoir of undiagnosed asymptomatic or minimally symptomatic patients with Barrett's esophagus does exist, there are hundreds of thousands if not millions of symptomatic patients undergoing treatment.

Barrett's esophagus represents severe end-stage GERD, which without surgical prevention of reflux will almost certainly require high-dose, lifetime drug therapy. The severity of the disease has been shown in numerous epidemiologic, clinical, and physiologic studies. Case-controlled epidemiologic studies have shown that patients with Barrett's esophagus have reflux symptoms at an earlier age and have more severe symptoms and that severe complications of reflux, including esophagitis, stricture, and ulceration, occur more frequently in patients with Barrett's esophagus than in age- and gender-matched GERD or upper endoscopy control patients.[22] Physiologic studies reveal markedly abnormal esophageal acid exposure,[23,24] an incompetent lower esophageal sphincter,[25,26] and impaired esophageal body motility in a large majority of patients.[27] The pattern, frequency, and duration of reflux episodes are increased in comparison to patients with no intestinal metaplasia.[28] Contractility of the esophageal body may be profoundly reduced in patients with Barrett's esophagus, and this decreased contractility results in prolonged contact times. The clinical and physiologic severity in patients

with short-segment Barrett's esophagus is generally intermediate between that of patients with long-segment Barrett's esophagus and those with erosive esophagitis.[29,30] Most patients with Barrett's esophagus have a hiatal hernia that is often larger than in patients with reflux esophagitis without Barrett's esophagus.[31]

Studies of the constituents of the refluxate provide further indications that patients with Barrett's esophagus differ significantly from those with GERD without Barrett's esophagus; in addition, such studies have a bearing on the decision regarding medical versus surgical treatment. Patients with Barrett's esophagus are more likely to have mixed reflux of both gastric and duodenal contents into the esophagus.[32] Direct measurement of aspirated bile or measurement of esophageal bilirubin in the distal esophagus as a marker for duodenal juice has shown that duodenoesophageal reflux is significantly more frequent in those with Barrett's esophagus than in those with GERD without Barrett's esophagus.[33] A study of 100 patients with GERD found a significant association between the degree of mucosal injury and the presence of duodenogastroesophageal reflux rather than gastroesophageal reflux only.[34] Some animal model studies indicated that duodenal reflux plays a significant role in esophageal tumor promotion.[35]

Second, there is a growing consensus that the ideal end point of treatment has shifted away from simple symptomatic relief toward the elimination of pathologic esophageal acid exposure. This shift has been stimulated by the desire to prevent neoplastic development, together with the results of basic studies on the biology of Barrett's epithelium. These studies have shown disconcerting reflux-induced cellular changes in a Barrett's mucosa organ culture system. Fitzgerald et al., for example, found that a dramatic increase in cellular proliferation resulted after Barrett's tissues were exposed to short pulses of acid at pH 3.5.[36,37] Interestingly, continuous acid exposure had minimal effect. Cellular differentiation was also assessed by quantifying expression of the apical membrane cytoskeletal protein villin, which is important for brush border microvillus assembly. Increased villin expression was found with exposure to acid in a pH range of 3 of 5. Although these in vitro findings may not reflect the situation in vivo, the finding that short pulses of acid induce proliferation suggests that complete and continuous acid suppression is necessary to prevent these abnormal cellular biologic changes. Though theoretically possible with both medical and surgical treatments, complete esophageal acid control is more reliably provided by antireflux surgery.

Finally, it is increasingly being recognized that using medication to normalize esophageal acid exposure is difficult in patients with Barrett's esophagus, even with proton pump inhibitors. Sampliner et al. reported that a mean dose of 56 mg of omeprazole was necessary to normalize 24-hour esophageal pH studies after multipolar electrocoagulation.[38] Several studies have shown that nocturnal acid breakthrough resulting in supine GERD is common, even with 20 mg of proton pump inhibitor therapy twice daily.[39,40] Although this nocturnal acid breakthrough period can be reduced by adding a histamine H_2 receptor antagonist before sleep, short

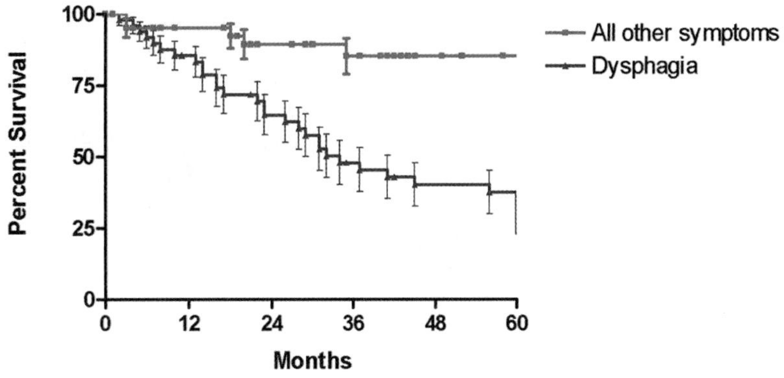

Figure 4–2. Kaplan-Meier actuarial survival curve for patients with esophageal adenocarcinoma with and without dysphagia.

pulses of esophageal acid exposure still occur in some patients.[41]

APPROACH TO A PATIENT WITH A MOTOR DISORDER

Dysphagia, or difficulty swallowing, is the primary symptom of esophageal motor disorders. Its perception by the patient is a balance between the severity of the underlying abnormality causing the dysphagia and the adjustment made by the patient in altering eating habits. Consequently, any complaint of dysphagia must include an assessment of the patient's dietary history. It must be known whether the patient experiences pain, choking, or vomiting with eating; whether the patient requires liquids with the meal, is the last to finish, or has interrupted a social meal; or whether the patient has been admitted to the hospital for food impaction. These assessments, in addition to the ability to maintain nutrition, help quantify the dysphagia and are important in determining the indications for surgical therapy.

Depending on the underlying cause of the nonobstructive dysphagia, the surgeon has a number of options designed to improve the patient's swallowing ability. The results can profoundly improve the patient's ability to ingest food but rarely return the function of the foregut to normal. In most situations, the principle of the operation is to make a defect in order to correct a defect to improve the patient's ability to swallow.

To apply surgical therapy to the problem of dysphagia, the surgeon needs to know the precise functional abnormality causing the symptom. Such knowledge usually entails a complete esophageal motility evaluation. A clear understanding of the physiologic mechanism of swallowing and determination of the abnormality in motility giving rise to the dysphagia are essential for deciding on the choice of surgery. Endoscopy is necessary only to exclude the presence of tumor or inflammatory changes as the cause of dysphagia.

APPROACH TO A PATIENT WITH ESOPHAGEAL CANCER

Dysphagia and weight loss are, by far, the most common symptoms at the time of diagnosis of esophageal cancer. A complaint of dysphagia in patients of any age should be investigated thoroughly because carcinoma is the most common cause of dysphagia. Occasionally, symptoms may arise from invasion of the primary tumor into adjacent structures or from metastasis. Extension of the primary tumor into the tracheobronchial tree can cause stridor, and if a tracheoesophageal fistula develops, coughing, choking, and aspiration pneumonia result. Severe bleeding from erosion into the aorta or pulmonary vessels occurs on rare occasion. Vocal cord paralysis may result from invasion of either recurrent laryngeal nerve. Metastases are usually manifested as jaundice or bone pain.

A surprisingly high proportion of patients with resectable esophageal adenocarcinoma are now identified before the development of dysphagia. In fact, survival in this group of patients is significantly better than if dysphagia heralds the diagnosis (Fig. 4–2). Twenty-five percent of the patients in our recent study were enrolled in a surveillance program for Barrett's esophagus or had a long history of GERD symptoms, and in another 30% of these patients, occult bleeding, anemia, or abdominal symptoms such as pain or discomfort prompted the physician visit leading to a diagnosis of cancer.[42]

Unfortunately, dysphagia usually occurs late in the natural history of the disease because the lack of a serosal layer in the esophagus allows the smooth muscle to dilate with ease. As a result, the dysphagia becomes severe enough to motivate the patient to seek medical advice only when more than 60% of the esophageal circumference is infiltrated with cancer and the lumen is reduced to less than 12 mm in diameter. Because of this insidious onset, the disease is usually advanced at the time of diagnosis. Tracheoesophageal fistula occurs in up to 10% of patients on their first visit to the hospital, and greater than 40% will have evidence of distant metastases or recurrent nerve paralysis. With tumors of the cardia, anorexia and weight loss usually precede the onset of dysphagia.

SUGGESTED READINGS

Frank L, Kleinman L, Ganoczy D, et al: Upper gastrointestinal symptoms in North America; prevalence and relationship to healthcare utilization and quality of life. Dig Dis Sci 45:809-818, 2000.

Kern MK, Birn RM, Jaradeh S, et al: Identification and characterization of cerebral cortical response to esophageal mucosal acid exposure and distention. Gastroenterology 115:1353-1362, 1998.

Shaker R, Castell DO, Schoenfeld PS, Spechler SJ: Nighttime heartburn is an underappreciated clinical problem that impacts sleep and daytime function; the results of a Gallup survey conducted on behalf of the American Gastroenterologic Association. Am J Gastroenterol 98:1487-1493, 2003.

REFERENCES

1. Shaker R, Castell DO, Schoenfeld PS, Spechler SJ: Nighttime heartburn is an underappreciated clinical problem that impacts sleep and daytime function; the results of a Gallup survey conducted on behalf of the American Gastroenterologic Association. Am J Gastroenterol 98:1487-1493, 2003.
2. DeMeester TR, O'Sullivan GC, Bermudez G, et al: Esophageal function in patients with angina-type chest pain and normal coronary angiograms. Ann Surg 196:488-498, 1982.
3. Schofield PM, Bennett DH, Whorwell PJ, et al: Exertional gastroesophageal reflux; a mechanism for symptoms in patients with angina pectoris and normal coronary angiograms. BMJ 294:1459, 1987.
4. Alban-Davies H, Jones DB, Rhodes J, Newcombe RJ: Angina like esophageal pain; differentiation from cardiac pain by history. J Clin Gastroenterol 7:477 1985.
5. Davies HA, Jones DB, Rhodes J: Esophageal angina as the cause of chest pain. JAMA 248:2274-2278, 1982.
6. Nevens F, Janssens J, Piessens J, et al: Prospective study on the prevalence of esophageal chest pain in patients referred on an elective basis to a cardiac unit for suspected myocardial ischemia. Dig Dis Sci 36:229-235, 1991.
7. Pope JH, Aufderheide TP, Ruthazer R, et al: Missed diagnosis of acute cardiac ischemia in the emergency department. N Engl J Med 342:1207-1210, 2000.
8. Harding R, Titchen DA: Chemosensitive vagal endings in the esophagus of the cat. J Physiol 247:52P-53P, 1975.
9. Fass R, Naliboff B, Higa L, et al: Differential effect of long term esophageal acid exposure on mechanosensitivity and chemosensitivity in humans. Gastroenterology 115:1363-1373, 1998.
10. Peghini PL, Johnston BT, Leite LP, Castell DO: Esophageal acid exposure sensitizes a subset of normal subjects to intraesophageal balloon distention. Eur J Gastroenterol Hepatol 8:979-983, 1996.
11. Castell DO, Wood JD, Freiling T, et al: Cerebral electrical potential evoked by balloon distention of the human esophagus. Gastroenterology 98:662-666, 1990.
12. Pehlivanov N, Liu J, Mittal RK: Sustained esophageal contraction; a major correlate of heartburn symptom. Am J Physiol 281:G743-G751, 2001.
13. Kern MK, Birn RM, Jaradeh S, et al: Identification and characterization of cerebral cortical response to esophageal mucosal acid exposure and distention. Gastroenterology 115:1353-1362, 1998.
14. Aziz Q, Anderson JLR, Valind S, et al: Identification of human brain loci processing esophageal sensation using positron emission tomography. Gastroenterology 113:50-59, 1997.
15. Polland WS, Bloomfield AL: Experimental referred pain from the gastrointestinal tract. Part I; the esophagus. J Clin Invest 10:435-452, 1931.
16. Costantini M, Crookes PF, Bremner RM, et al: Value of physiologic assessment of foregut symptoms in a surgical practice. Surgery 114:780-786, 1993.
17. Campos GMR, Peters JH, DeMeester TR, et al: Multivariate analysis of factors predicting outcome after laparoscopic Nissen fundoplication. J Gastrointest Surg 3:292-300, 1999.
18. Ritter MP, Peters JH, DeMeester TR, et al: Outcome after laparoscopic fundoplication is not dependent on a structurally defective lower esophageal sphincter. J Gastrointest Surg 2:567-572, 1998.
19. Demeester TR, Bonavina L, Iascone C, et al: Chronic respiratory symptoms and occult gastroesophageal reflux. A prospective clinical study and results of surgical therapy. Ann Surg 211:337-345, 1990.
20. Horvath KD, Swanstrom LL, Jobe BA: The short esophagus: Pathophysiology, incidence, presentation, and treatment in the era of laparoscopic antireflux surgery. Ann Surg 232:630-640, 2000.
21. Ollyo JB, Monnier P, Fontolliet C, Savary M: The natural history of erosive esophagitis in patients with GERD. Gullet 3:3010, 1993.
22. Eisen GM, Sandler RS, Murray S, Gottfried M: The relationship between gastroesophageal reflux disease and its complications with Barrett's esophagus. Am J Gastroenterol 92:27-31, 1997.
23. Iascone C, DeMeester TR, Little AG, Skinner DB: Barrett's esophagus. Functional assessment, proposed pathogenesis, and surgical therapy. Arch Surg 118:543-549, 1983.
24. Stein HJ, Hoeft S, DeMeester TR: Functional foregut abnormalities in Barrett's esophagus. J Thorac Cardiovasc Surg 105:107-111, 1993.
25. Öberg S, DeMeester TR, Peters JH, et al: The extent of Barrett's esophagus depends on the status of the lower esophageal sphincter and the degree of esophageal acid exposure. J Thorac Cardiovasc Surg 117:572-580, 1999.
26. Stein HJ, Barlow AP, DeMeester TR, Hinder RA: Complications of gastroesophageal reflux disease. Role of the lower esophageal sphincter, esophageal acid and acid/alkaline exposure, and duodenogastric reflux. Ann Surg 16:35-43, 1992.
27. Singh P, Taylor RH, Colin-Jones DG: Esophageal motor dysfunction and acid exposure in reflux esophagitis are more severe if Barrett's metaplasia is present. Am J Gastroenterol 89:349-356, 1994.
28. Campos GM, Peters JH, DeMeester TR, et al: The pattern of esophageal acid exposure in gastroesophageal reflux disease influences the severity of the disease. Arch Surg 134:882-887, 1999.
29. Hirota WK, Loughney TM, Lazas DJ, et al: Specialized intestinal metaplasia, dysplasia and cancer of the esophagus and esophagogastric junction; prevalence and clinical data. Gastroenterology 116:277-285, 1999.
30. Öberg S, Ritter MP, Crookes PF, et al: Gastroesophageal reflux disease and mucosal injury with emphasis on short-segment Barrett's esophagus and duodenogastroesophageal reflux. J Gastrointest Surg 2:547-553, 1998.
31. Cameron AJ: Barrett's esophagus: Prevalence and size of hiatal hernia. Am J Gastroenterol 94:2054-2059, 1999.
32. Kauer WK, Burdiles P, Ireland AP, et al: Does duodenal juice reflux into the esophagus of patients with complicated GERD? Evaluation of a fiberoptic sensor for bilirubin. Am J Surg 169:98-103, 1995.
33. Gillen P, Keeling P, Byrne PJ, et al: Implication of duodenogastric reflux in the pathogenesis of Barrett's oesophagus. Br J Surg 75:540-543, 1988.
34. Kauer WK, Peters JH, DeMeester TR, et al: Mixed reflux of gastric and duodenal juices is more harmful to the esophagus than gastric juice alone. The need for surgical therapy re-emphasized. Ann Surg 222:525-531, 1995.
35. Attwood SE, Smyrk TC, DeMeester TR, et al: Duodenoesophageal reflux and the development of esophageal adenocarcinoma in rats. Surgery 111:503-510, 1992.
36. Fitzgerald RC, Omary MB, Triadafilopoulos G: Dynamic effects of acid on Barrett's esophagus. An ex vivo proliferation and differentiation model. J Clin Invest 98:2120-2128, 1996.
37. Ouatu-Lascar R, Fitzgerald RC, Triadafilopoulos G: Differentiation and proliferation in Barrett's esophagus and the effects of acid suppression. Gastroenterology 117:327-335, 1999.
38. Sampliner RE, Fennerty B, Garewal HS: Reversal of Barrett's esophagus with acid suppression and multipolar electrocoagulation: Preliminary results. Gastrointest Endosc 44:532-535, 1996.
39. Katzka DA, Castell DO: Successful elimination of reflux symptoms does not insure adequate control of acid reflux in patients with Barrett's esophagus. Am J Gastroenterol 89:989-991, 1994.
40. Ouatu-Lascar R, Triadafilopolous G: Complete elimination of reflux symptoms does not guarantee normalization of intraesophageal acid reflux in patients with Barrett's esophagus. Am J Gastroenterol 93:711-716, 1998.
41. Peghini PL, Katz PO, Castell DO: Ranitidine controls nocturnal gastric acid breakthrough on omeprazole: A controlled study in normal subjects. Gastroenterology 115:1335-1339, 1998.
42. Portale G, Peters JH, Hsieh CC, et al: Can clinical and endoscopic findings accurately predict early-stage esophageal adenocarcinoma? Surg Endosc 20:294-297, 2006.

Imaging in Esophageal Disease

John M. Barlow · Daniel A. Craig · James E. Huprich ·
Val J. Lowe · Robert L. MacCarty

NORMAL ANATOMY, FUNCTION, AND RADIOGRAPHIC TECHNIQUES OF EXAMINATION

Although endoscopy has largely replaced contrast studies of the stomach and colon, barium examination is still considered a valuable diagnostic tool for evaluation of the esophagus. Indeed, as we have seen a precipitous drop in the number of upper gastrointestinal (UGI) studies and barium enemas in our practice, the number of barium swallows has remained virtually constant over the past 30 to 40 years. The ability of the barium examination to demonstrate the structure and function of the esophagus has stood the test of time. Its relatively low cost and universal availability add to its value in the management of patients with esophageal disease. Although the introduction of newer imaging modalities such as computed tomography (CT), magnetic resonance imaging (MRI), and positron emission tomography (PET) has proved valuable in special circumstances, barium examination remains the mainstay of esophageal imaging.

PET has largely replaced CT in initial cancer staging and evaluation of recurrent tumor, but CT remains a useful tool for evaluating early complications after esophageal surgery. MRI is of limited usefulness in the management of esophageal disease, but it is likely to become more important in the future. These specialized imaging techniques are discussed in appropriate sections of this chapter.

Normal Anatomy and Function

The esophagus is a muscular tube, 20 to 24 cm in length, that is bounded by a sphincter at both ends. The upper esophageal sphincter (UES), made up of striated muscle and known anatomically as the cricopharyngeus, consists of the thickened horizontal portion of the inferior pharyngeal constrictor. The lower esophageal sphincter (LES) consists of an ill-defined high-pressure zone at the esophagogastric junction (EGJ). The proximal third of the esophagus is made up of striated muscle with a gradual transition to smooth muscle in the middle third. The distal third is composed exclusively of smooth muscle. Because of these anatomic differences, diseases affecting striated and smooth muscle have different regional distributions.

The function of the esophagus is to transport material from the mouth to the stomach and to prevent entry of swallowed material into the airway. The UES and LES act as valves and remain closed at each end of the esophagus until a swallow is initiated. This process prevents inspired air from entering the gastrointestinal (GI) tract from above and gastric contents from entering the esophagus from below. When swallowing is initiated, both sphincters relax to allow passage of the bolus into the stomach. Beginning at the pharyngoesophageal junction, peristaltic contractions traverse the entire esophagus and push the swallowed bolus into the stomach. As the bolus passes into the stomach, the sphincters close again.

The swallowed bolus must be of sufficient volume to consistently sustain peristalsis. If the bolus is too small, the peristalsis may die away and result in stasis in the esophageal body. Secondary peristalsis occurs below the pharyngoesophageal junction as a response to esophageal distention.

In the upright position, a liquid bolus is propelled primarily by gravity, and peristalsis plays almost no role, which explains why motility testing needs to be performed with the subject in the recumbent position. Solid boluses require peristaltic contractions (usually multiple swallows) to be transported effectively in the upright position.

Examination Techniques and Normal Radiographic Appearance

The equipment necessary to perform barium esophageal studies can be found in virtually all radiology departments. Digital spot devices are now in common use and facilitate rapid acquisition of high-quality static images. The addition of a large image intensifier (12 inches and larger) allows the fluoroscopist to see and record events though the entire length of the esophagus. This is especially important when evaluating esophageal function because clinically important motor activity may occur outside the field of view if a small image intensifier is used. A motion-recording device, such as a VCR or digital recorder, is desirable so that rapidly occurring swallowing events are more easily observed when viewed at a slower rate. Motion recording captures the dynamic nature of events far better than rapid sequential spot films do. The tape recording also provides a valuable educational tool during discussions with the patient.

Proper barium swallow technique includes a multiphasic examination, including air-contrast, full-column, and mucosal relief techniques.[1] Each technique has unique advantages and disadvantages.

The air-contrast technique allows detailed evaluation of the esophageal mucosa. Maximum distention of the esophageal body is achieved by the administration of an effervescent solution that produces CO_2. With the esophagus distended with gas, high-density barium is quickly administered to coat the mucosal surfaces. When performed in the upright position, the distended esophageal wall, with its thin coating of barium, is displayed in exquisite detail. The normal esophageal mucosa appears featureless on air-contrast views. Occasionally, tiny filling defects, representing undissolved effervescent crystals, are seen (Fig. 5–1). In patients with normal motility, the esophagus may remain distended only for a short time. Incomplete distention of the esophagus, especially the distal portion, may mask the presence of segmental narrowing and prevent visualization of mucosal detail.

As the esophagus empties of gas, the lumen collapses. Barium is caught in the redundant longitudinal folds, and this constitutes the mucosal relief examination. Mucosal folds should appear as continuous linear structures less than 3 mm thick (Fig. 5–2). Mild thickening and irregularity of the folds in the distal end of the esophagus may be the only sign of reflux esophagitis.

The full-column technique is performed in the prone oblique position and requires rapid swallowing of barium. Patients are encouraged to drink as much and as rapidly as possible to produce maximal distention. By maximally distending the esophagus, areas of fixed narrowing become visible. Should the patient not be able to drink rapidly enough to sufficiently distend the lumen, areas of segmental narrowing may go undetected.[2]

On full-column films, the margins of the esophagus should appear smooth with no areas of fixed irregularity (Fig. 5–3). Normal extrinsic impressions occur at the level of the transverse aorta, the left main stem bronchus, and the esophageal hiatus (Fig. 5–4). Extrinsic impres-

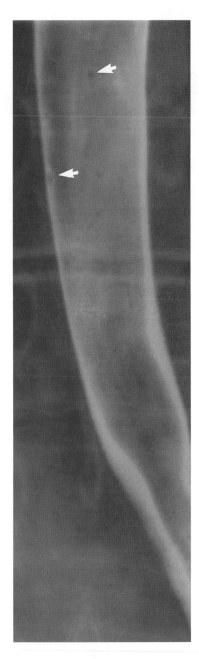

Figure 5–1. Normal air-contrast esophagogram. The mucosa is featureless except for the occasional tiny filling defect caused by undissolved effervescent crystals (*arrows*).

sions occurring elsewhere and areas of fixed irregularity should be viewed with suspicion.

Esophageal motility should be tested with single swallows of barium while the patient is in the prone oblique position. Patients should be instructed to swallow up to five single swallows of barium. During each swallow, the tail of the bolus is observed as the bolus is carried from the cervical esophagus to the stomach. The peristaltic contraction should traverse the entire esophagus from the cervical portion to the stomach. To avoid the effect of deglutitive inhibition, subjects are asked to not swallow between boluses. The temperature and viscosity should

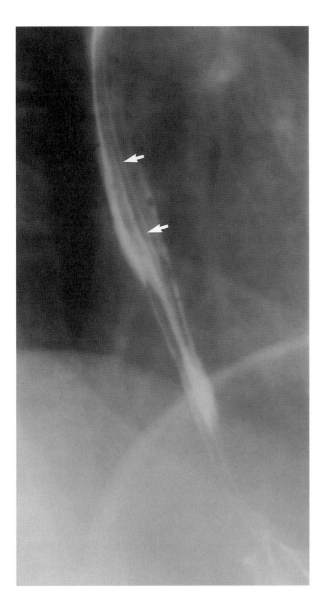

Figure 5–2. Normal mucosal relief esophagogram. The mucosal folds (*arrows*) appear smooth, continuous, and less than 3 mm in thickness.

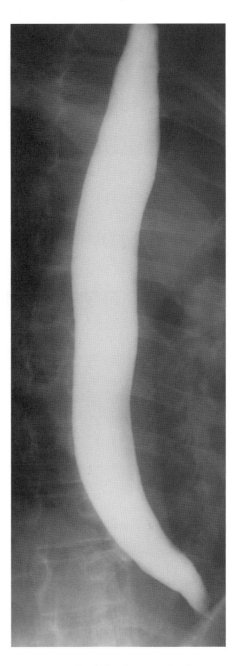

Figure 5–3. Normal full-column esophagogram. The margins of barium are smooth without any fixed irregularities.

be controlled to avoid inducing abnormal motility. A normal swallow should be accompanied by an effective peristaltic wave that strips the esophagus of all barium. The leading edge of the wave resembles an inverted V, with the apposing walls of the esophagus obliterating the lumen and pushing the bolus ahead. Frequently, a small amount of stasis is seen in the middle third of the esophagus as a result of nonocclusive peristalsis and should not be interpreted as abnormal motility. This is the area of transition from striated to smooth muscle and is normally the zone of lowest normal contraction amplitude. Frequent nonocclusive peristalsis in the distal third or failure of peristalsis to traverse the entire length of the esophagus may indicate a motility disorder. Completion of the peristaltic contraction is accompanied by relaxation of the LES as the bolus is emptied into the stomach. Three out of five swallows should result in complete

clearance of barium. Three or more swallows out of five that result in stasis in the esophageal body may reflect abnormal motility.[3] Abnormal contractions include incomplete or ineffective peristalsis that causes incomplete clearance of the barium bolus, tertiary contractions, simultaneous contractions, and failure of the LES to relax.

In normal young patients, 95% of swallows are accompanied by normal peristalsis.[4] Though not universally accepted, the incidence of failed and low-amplitude peristaltic contractions probably increases with age.[5] Whether this is a normal aging process or represents subclinical disease is not known. Therefore, abnormal

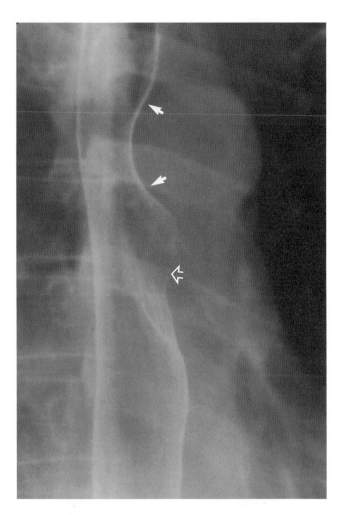

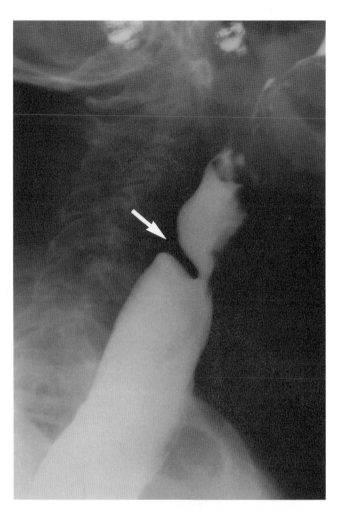

Figure 5–4.   Left posterior oblique air-contrast view demonstrating normal extrinsic impressions on the esophagus from the aorta (*closed arrows*) and left main bronchus (*open arrow*).

Figure 5–5.   Cricopharyngeal bar—a smooth posterior defect (*arrow*) at the level of the cricopharyngeus muscle (usually C5-C6).

peristaltic function, especially tertiary contractions, should be interpreted with caution in older individuals.

Patients with dysphagia and a normal barium examination should be challenged with a solid bolus. Those complaining of difficulty swallowing pills should be challenged to swallow a 12.5-mm barium tablet with 60 ml of water in the 45-degree upright position. In normal subjects, the tablet should pass into the stomach within 60 seconds.[6] A marshmallow cut in half or thirds, swallowed with thin barium, may hang up at areas of narrowing not otherwise visible on the routine examination.[7,8] Single bites of cooked hamburger may be used to assess the functional severity of dysphagia. With severe dysphagia caused by structural narrowing, the patient may chew excessively to pulverize the bolus before swallowing. In these patients, the bolus may be swallowed piecemeal to avoid symptomatic holdup at an area of stenosis. Most patients with motility disorders chew and initiate swallowing normally.

All examinations should include at least a brief look at the oropharyngeal phase of swallowing. Symptoms in patients with dysphagia are frequently difficult to local-

ize; therefore, all areas, from the oropharynx to the stomach, should be examined. In addition, structural abnormalities at the pharyngoesophageal junction occasionally accompany more distal disease and may contribute to the dysphagia (Fig. 5–5).[9] The radiographic findings may provide clues to which abnormalities may account for the symptoms.

Examination of the stomach should be included in patients complaining of dysphagia or gastroesophageal reflux disease (GERD). Neoplasms of the gastric cardia can cause dysphagia and would otherwise be overlooked if the stomach were not evaluated.[10] In patients with GERD, gastric dysfunction may be an important contributory factor, so evidence of delayed gastric emptying (e.g., retained secretions, dilated stomach, previous surgery) and hypersecretion (retained secretions, abnormal gastric folds, gastritis) should be noted.

Common Normal Variants

The esophageal ampulla appears as a smoothly marginated short segmental dilatation of the esophagus just above the hiatus (Fig. 5–6). It is sometimes confused with

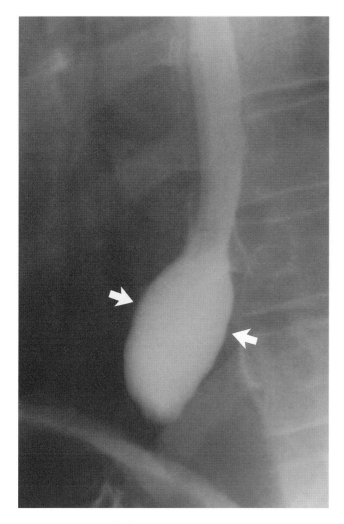

Figure 5–6. Esophageal ampulla—normal slight widening of the distal end of the esophagus (*arrows*).

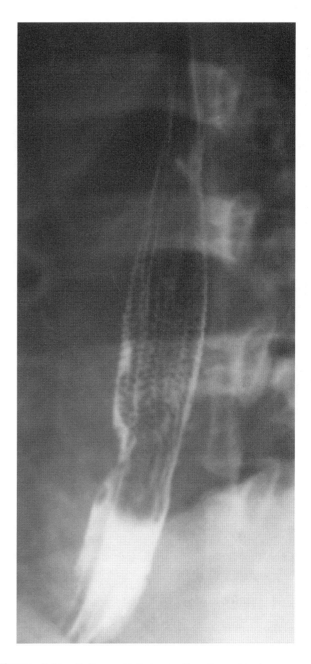

Figure 5–7. Feline esophagus. Regular, closely spaced transverse ridges occurring transiently in the esophageal body are thought to be related to longitudinal muscle contractions.

a small hiatal hernia; however, the absence of gastric folds and the presence of typical esophageal peristalsis within the ampulla distinguish it from a herniated stomach.

The occasional appearance of fine, evenly spaced transverse folds that occur transiently in normal patients is called *feline esophagus* (Fig. 5–7). This condition has reported to be more frequent in patients with GERD but is more commonly seen in asymptomatic patients. It is thought to be due to contraction of the longitudinal muscle layer.

GASTROESOPHAGEAL REFLUX DISEASE

One of the earliest reports of abnormal reflux of gastric contents into the esophagus was based on observations made during GI contrast studies.[11] Barium studies were considered so important that the diagnosis of GERD was synonymous with the presence of reflux on barium studies. Until the introduction of endoscopy and ambulatory pH monitoring, the barium UGI study remained a cornerstone in the evaluation of GERD patients. Today,

the importance of the barium examination has diminished, but it remains useful in evaluating GERD patients, especially those considering surgical intervention.

GERD is extremely common, especially in Western cultures, and it occurs in approximately 15% to 20% of the U.S. population. The popularity of over-the-counter acid-suppression medications testifies to the widespread nature of the condition. In mild, uncomplicated cases, the annoying symptoms of heartburn and regurgitation may not cause permanent changes but may have a significant impact on quality of life. More severe cases may be complicated by permanent esophageal injury and even malignancy.

GERD consists of a constellation of signs and symptoms produced by abnormal exposure of the esophageal lining to gastric contents. The cause of GERD is multifactorial. The most common etiologic factor is abnormality of the LES leading to loss of the normal antireflux barrier. Contributory factors include the volume and composition of the gastric refluxate, altered esophageal mucosal resistance, the effectiveness of esophageal clearance, and abnormal gastric emptying. Although other tests are more accurate in quantifying these etiologic factors, barium studies may provide clues that point to the need for further studies. For example, the demonstration of a hiatal hernia on a barium study suggests alteration of the normal antireflux barrier, which can be confirmed with LES manometry. Radiographic signs of abnormal esophageal motility point to poor esophageal clearance of refluxed material, which can be evaluated with esophageal body manometry. Radionuclide studies may be useful to confirm delayed gastric emptying in patients with a dilated atonic stomach seen during a UGI study.

Role of Barium Examination in Gastroesophageal Reflux Disease

Exclude Motility Disorder The classic symptoms of GERD, namely, heartburn and regurgitation, are nonspecific and may be seen with a variety of esophageal diseases, including motility disorders. A small group of patients (less than 10%) with motility disorders may have symptoms suggestive of GERD, namely, heartburn and regurgitation. Dysphagia and chest pain, typical symptoms in patients with motility disorders, may be absent. Symptoms of heartburn are, in fact, common and occur in 40% of achalasia patients. In the majority of patients with classic achalasia, the barium examination is characteristic. In these patients, the correct diagnosis is easily made and a potential catastrophe resulting from inappropriate antireflux surgery can be avoided.

Detection of Gastroesophageal Reflux The role of barium studies in detecting abnormal gastroesophageal reflux (GER) is controversial. The sensitivity of barium examination in the diagnosis of GERD ranges from 20% to 74% (average, 39%). Many early studies reported favorable results in correlating the presence of radiographically demonstrated GER with symptoms of heartburn or the presence of esophagitis. However, as mentioned earlier, heartburn is a nonspecific symptom seen with many other esophageal disorders, and endoscopic esophagitis occurs in only half the patients with positive pH monitoring. Therefore, one cannot rely on the accuracy of early studies published before the introduction of ambulatory pH testing. We also know that spontaneous GER occurs normally as a result of transient lower esophageal sphincter relaxation (tLESR), which if interpreted as pathologic GER will lead to a false-positive diagnosis. Furthermore, the absence of GER episodes during the short observation period of a barium examination may be erroneously interpreted as evidence against the diagnosis of GERD.

Ambulatory pH monitoring is the gold standard for the diagnosis of GER. A pH of 4 or less for greater than 5% of the 24-hour monitoring period is considered a positive test.[12] A few studies have correlated pH results with radiographic detection of GER. One study[13] demonstrated favorable results and showed a radiographic sensitivity of 70% and specificity of 74% with both spontaneous reflux and the water siphon test. A subsequent study[14] failed to confirm the earlier findings and concluded that barium radiography lacks sufficient sensitivity and specificity to be used as a screening procedure for GERD. In general, the response to trials of proton pump inhibitors in patients with typical symptoms of heartburn and regurgitation and the presence of a hiatal hernia are more predictive of pH test results than the presence of radiologically detectable GER.

GER is diagnosed radiographically when barium is seen to reflux into the distal part of the esophagus from the stomach. A small amount of refluxed barium that occurs infrequently is probably not significant and may reflect normal tLESR. However, frequent episodes of reflux that reach high into the esophagus, particularly in the presence of a large hiatal hernia, are often predictive of a high pH score.

Provocative tests, such as the water siphon test, increase the sensitivity of radiologic detection of reflux disease but result in lower specificity. The water siphon test is performed by having the recumbent subject take a single swallow of water while the gastric fundus is filled with barium.[15,16] A positive test result consists of reflux of barium into the distal esophagus just after the water bolus traverses the gastroesophageal junction (GEJ). Additional provocative testing to increase intra-abdominal pressure and thus promote GER includes the Valsalva maneuver and having the patient ingest a bolus while supine.

Evaluation of Esophageal Clearance Abnormal motility causing poor clearance of refluxed material may promote esophageal damage by prolonging exposure of the esophageal lining to the noxious effects of the refluxate. Before the advent of esophageal motility testing, barium swallows were used to evaluate esophageal motor function. Studies have shown relatively good correlation between the results of stationary manometry and barium swallows and suggest that barium examination may provide accurate estimates of esophageal function.[17] Radiographic evidence of poor esophageal body function may help identify patients who will be resistant to conventional-dose antisecretory therapy. This information is also helpful in selection of the appropriate surgical approach and type of antireflux repair.

Motility disturbances associated with GERD usually involve the distal half of the esophagus. Failed propagation of peristalsis and ineffective contractions resulting in significant stasis of barium in the esophageal body are commonly associated with GERD. In the most severe cases, the pattern of disease is similar to that of scleroderma (discussed later).

Detect Evidence of Esophageal Injury Esophageal injury is manifested by esophagitis, scarring, stricture, Barrett's changes, and alterations in esophageal motility.

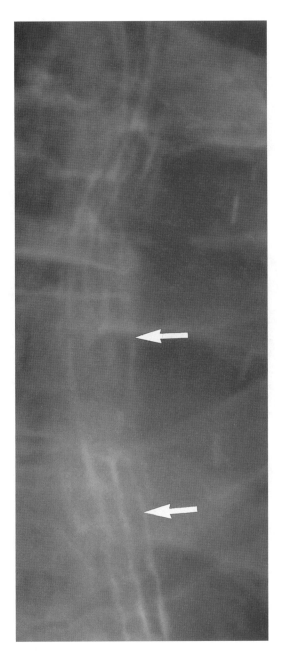

Figure 5–8. Acute reflux esophagitis. Mucosal relief views demonstrate thickened, slightly irregular folds (*arrows*) in the distal end of the esophagus.

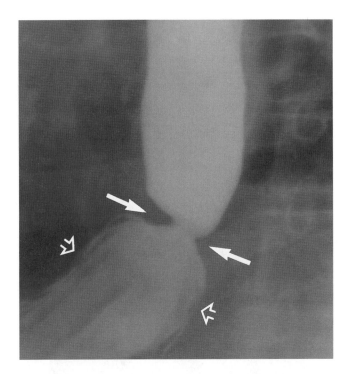

Figure 5–9. Esophageal stricture secondary to gastroesophageal reflux disease. Asymmetric narrowing (*closed arrows*) is evident at the gastroesophageal junction above a hiatal hernia (*open arrows*).

Radiographic detection of esophagitis depends on the severity of changes. Mild to moderate degrees of inflammation are frequently not obvious radiographically.[18] Severe esophagitis is more readily diagnosed, but such cases have become less prevalent as a result of the widespread use of acid-suppression therapy.

Signs of acute esophagitis include thickening and irregularity of the distal esophageal folds, best seen on mucosal relief images (Fig. 5–8). Less frequently, nodularity and erosions are visible on air-contrast films. Occasionally, edema or spasm may produce areas of segmental narrowing that improve after successful treatment.

Scarring and stricture represent more severe and permanent changes of injury from GERD and are generally visible radiographically. Their appearance is typical enough to exclude malignancy.[19] Strictures usually occur at the GEJ and may be smoothly tapered or irregular (Fig. 5–9). When compared with mucosal rings, strictures are generally eccentric and involve a longer segment of the esophagus. Scarring can occur without esophageal narrowing and may be seen as areas of fixed irregularity of the esophageal contour. Air-contrast views may show them as transverse linear defects (Fig. 5–10).

Barium studies are superior to endoscopy in detecting areas of segmental narrowing,[2,20] especially for larger-diameter strictures and those that taper gradually. The latter type may not be appreciated endoscopically, particularly with small-diameter endoscopes.

Radiographic technique is important in detecting areas of segmental narrowing. The examination must be performed with the patient in the recumbent position. Up to half of strictures and rings may be missed if patients are examined only in the upright position.

Initial reports suggested high sensitivity of air-contrast esophagograms for the detection of columnar epithelium in Barrett's esophagus.[21] The changes are described as a reticular mucosal pattern best appreciated on air-contrast views (Fig. 5–11). Others found this radiographic feature to be present in only 23% of cases.[22] Barrett's changes are seen in a large percentage of patients with hiatal hernia, esophageal stricture, and thickened, irregular folds.[23,24] Midesophageal strictures are a relatively specific sign of Barrett's esophagus.

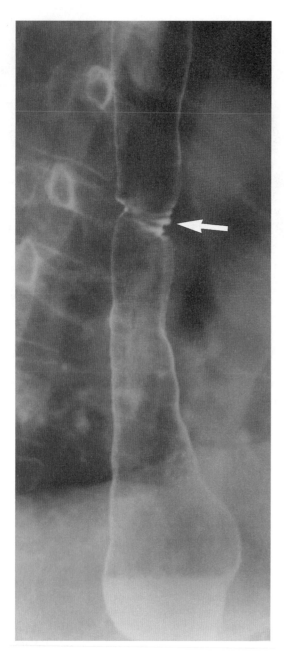

Figure 5–10. Scarring secondary to gastroesophageal reflux disease (GERD). Transverse scars (*arrow*) are typical for a benign stricture caused by GERD.

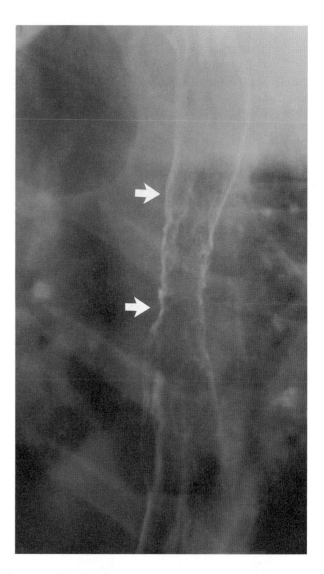

Figure 5–11. Barrett's esophagus. Mild narrowing and a reticular mucosal pattern are apparent in a segment of the midesophagus (between *arrows*)

Preoperative Planning The presence of a large hiatal hernia (>5 cm) or evidence of a shortened esophagus may influence the type of surgical repair and operative approach. Failure to recognize these conditions may lead to surgical failure as a result of an inappropriate surgical approach or type of repair.

The size of a hiatal hernia is best estimated during a barium study. Hernia size is determined by measuring the distance from the GEJ to the esophageal hiatus during maximum filling of the hernia. Our experience suggests that hernia size is underestimated with endoscopy, probably because of partial reduction of the hernia by passage of the endoscope.

Esophageal shortening is the result of injury, usually from severe reflux disease, producing fibrosis in the periesophageal tissue. In such cases, inadequate surgical dissection during laparoscopic fundoplication may leave the repair under tension and lead to early surgical failure. Clues to the diagnosis of esophageal shortening include esophageal scarring, stricture, and the size and shape of the hiatal hernia. A hiatal hernia with tapered shoulders, especially in the presence of scarring or stricture, suggests shortening (Fig. 5–12).

Postoperative Complications Anatomic failure of an antireflux repair occurs in 5% to 15% of cases. Barium examination along with endoscopy and pH monitoring is used to evaluate this group of patients. Findings related to failure of fundoplication are discussed in another section.

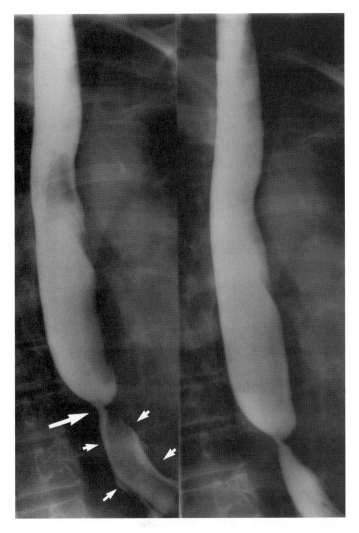

Figure 5–12. Scleroderma with esophageal shortening. A tight stricture at the gastroesophageal junction (*large arrow*) with proximal dilatation is indicative of poor motility. The hiatal hernia demonstrates tapered shoulders with an elongated body (*small arrows*). Compare the appearance with the hiatal hernia in a normal-length esophagus in Figure 5–35.

ESOPHAGEAL MOTILITY DISORDERS

Conditions associated with abnormal esophageal motor function are classified as motility disorders. Common to all these disorders are definable abnormalities demonstrated on manometric examination. Established manometric criteria exist for all of the motility disorders,[25] and the diagnosis is based on a combination of manometric and clinical findings. Barium swallows may suggest the diagnosis and help select patients who would benefit from further functional evaluation.

Simultaneous manofluorography has confirmed the accuracy of barium studies for the evaluation of esophageal function. Agreement between the two studies, when performed simultaneously, is as high as 96%.[17] Agreement is somewhat less (approximately 80%) in studies correlating manometry and barium swallows when they are performed separately.[17]

The efficacy of the barium swallow is dependent on the type of motility disorder. Although the examination is very sensitive for the detection of achalasia (95%), it is less sensitive for diffuse esophageal spasm (71%) and nonspecific esophageal motility disorder (NEMD) (46%).[26] In a group of patients with dysphagia, the overall sensitivity of barium swallow for the detection of a motility disorder was 56%. The sensitivity increased to 89% when patients with nutcracker esophagus and NEMD were excluded.[27]

Symptoms in motility disorders are nonspecific and include dysphagia, regurgitation, chest pain, and heartburn. Dysphagia to both liquids and solids is more common in motility disorders, and this symptom is sometimes helpful in distinguishing motility disorders from conditions that cause esophageal narrowing. When present, regurgitation is usually described as bland rather than acidic as a result of its origin from the esophagus rather than the stomach. Chest pain may vary from intermittent and sharp to constant and pressure-like. It may mimic pain of cardiac origin and trigger a work-up for coronary artery disease. When dysphagia accompanies chest pain, an esophageal origin is more likely. Heartburn is a common complaint, especially in patients with achalasia. The heartburn may be due to esophageal distention or fermentative esophagitis, commonly seen with a massively dilated atonic esophagus. The nonspecific nature of the symptoms in motility disorder makes additional diagnostic studies necessary to clarify the nature of the disease.

Primary Motility Disorders

Motility disorders are classified as either primary or secondary. This distinction is based on whether the esophagus is primarily involved or whether the esophageal involvement is part of a systemic process.

The nature of the motility disorder in an individual patient may not fit into one of the defined classifications. Indeed, this group of diseases represents a continuous spectrum of motor abnormalities. Patients may have characteristics of more than one motility disorder. Furthermore, over time, the character of the motor disturbance may change from one disease to another. It is probably better to describe the nature of the motor abnormalities rather than force a patient into a defined disease category.

Achalasia is a disease of unknown cause characterized manometrically by absent esophageal body peristalsis and abnormally high LES resting pressure or incomplete relaxation of the LES. Histologic findings in the dorsal motor nucleus, vagus nerve, and myenteric plexus suggest a process causing smooth muscle denervation.

In classic achalasia, the esophageal body is markedly dilated. Little or no motor activity is visible except in the proximal third. Sometimes, weak tertiary contractions are visible as minute undulations along the barium column margins. As the patient drinks, barium produces an irregular pattern as it falls through a column of retained food material within the lumen. This produces incomplete opacification of the lumen and mimics the

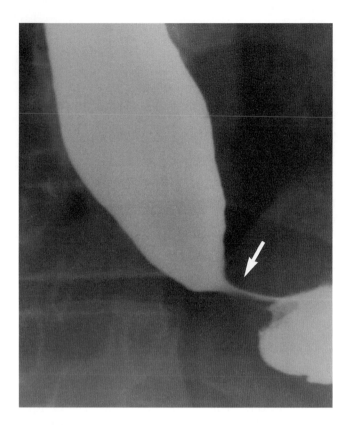

Figure 5–13. Classic achalasia—a markedly dilated atonic esophageal body with tapered narrowing (i.e., "bird's beak" deformity) (*arrow*) at the gastroesophageal junction.

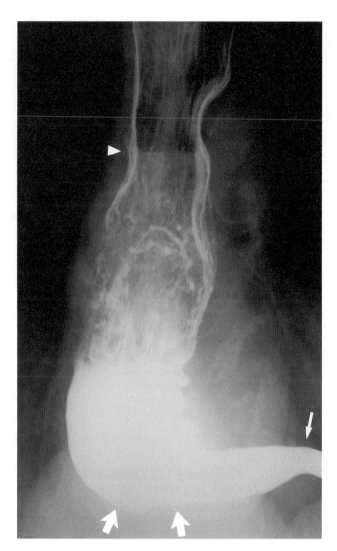

Figure 5–14. "Sigmoid" esophagus. Long-standing achalasia has resulted in an elongated, tortuous esophagus with a dependent segment (*large arrows*) with respect to the esophageal outlet (*small arrow*) that is the cause of poor drainage into stomach. Note the retained debris and air-fluid level (*arrowhead*) near the aortic arch.

appearance of extraluminal contrast. Initially, little if any barium exits the esophagus into the stomach. The lower end of the obstructed contrast column is tapered to a point and resembles a "bird's beak" (Fig. 5–13). The barium-fluid level within the esophagus rises with the addition of more barium from above. Intermittent opening of the lower part of the esophagus causes small amounts of barium to squirt into the stomach, thereby maintaining a relatively constant barium-fluid level. The height of the barium-fluid level is usually characteristic for each patient—the more severe the obstruction, the higher the level. With extreme degrees of dilatation, the esophagus becomes tortuous and nondependent segments are visible (i.e., the so-called sigmoid esophagus) (Fig. 5–14). In the erect position, fluid within these nondependent areas is unable to drain into the stomach, and the constant weight of the fluid within the nondraining segment may accelerate the process of dilatation.

In early or mild achalasia, esophageal body abnormalities may predominate. The esophagus may drain well in the erect position, but poor bolus transport is seen in the recumbent position as a result of ineffective peristalsis. Mild dilatation of the esophageal body and increased tertiary contraction may also be seen. These changes are nonspecific and may occur with other motility disorders. However, in the appropriate clinical setting, these findings should lead to manometric examination to identify LES abnormalities consistent with achalasia.

A less common variant, vigorous achalasia, is characterized by strong tertiary contractions of the esophageal body instead of the atonic esophageal body seen with classic achalasia (Fig. 5–15). Like the classic type, LES abnormalities are seen. The appearance of the esophageal body contractions resembles the findings seen in diffuse esophageal spasm. However, unlike diffuse esophageal spasm, the esophageal body is slightly dilated and the esophagus drains poorly.

Pseudoachalasia may result from malignancies at the GEJ that infiltrate the submucosa. Associated aperistalsis of the esophageal body and narrowing of the GEJ simulate the findings of classic achalasia. In many cases, no mucosal lesion is visible endoscopically, and the diagnosis is suspected only because of the older age of the patient and the recent onset of dysphagia. One paper suggests that the length of the "bird's beak" is greater in

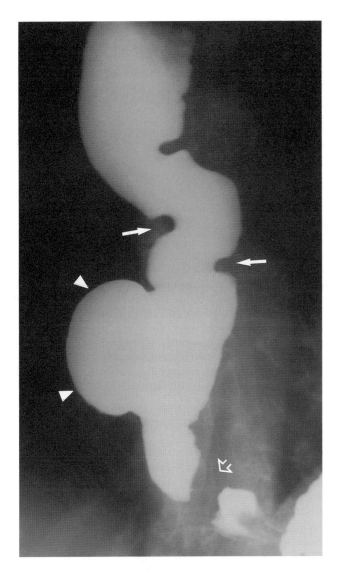

Figure 5–15. Vigorous achalasia identified by a dilated esophageal body with prominent tertiary contractions (*arrows*) and a narrowed gastroesophageal junction (*open arrow*) above a small hiatal hernia. A large pulsion diverticulum (*arrowheads*) arises from the distal esophageal body.

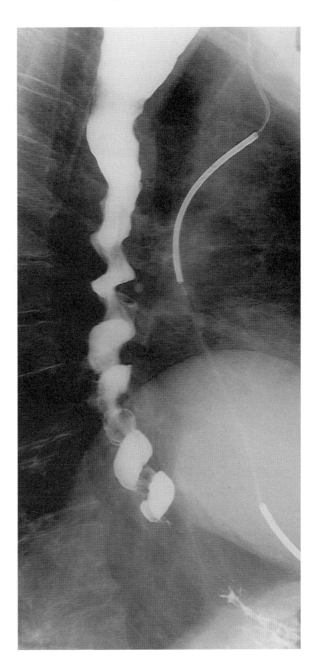

Figure 5–16. Diffuse esophageal spasm. Multiple tertiary contractions are producing a "corkscrew" appearance of the esophageal body.

patients with pseudoachalasia associated with malignancy than in those with classic achalasia.[28]

Diffuse esophageal spasm is a disorder of unknown cause characterized by intermittently abnormal motility associated with symptoms of chest pain and dysphagia. Dysphagia is variably present and does not necessarily accompany the chest pain. Chest pain and dysphagia may be exacerbated by the ingestion of cold liquids.

Manometrically, simultaneous contractions are seen in greater than 10% of wet swallows. Radiographic features reflect the manometric findings—peristalsis is intermittently replaced by tertiary contractions, and a "corkscrew" or "rosary-bead" appearance is produced (Fig. 5–16). Normal peristalsis is usually present in the proximal end of the esophagus. A recent report has suggested that abnormalities of the LES producing delayed esophageal emptying may be more common than a "corkscrew" appearance of the esophageal body.[29]

Radiographic sensitivity in the diagnosis of diffuse esophageal spasm is low in comparison to its sensitivity in the diagnosis of achalasia, probably because of the intermittent nature of the motility disturbance and the nonspecific nature of the radiographic findings. Tertiary contractions are common in both normal patients and those with motility disorders and should not be interpreted as indicative of diffuse esophageal spasm unless accompanied by appropriate symptoms and confirmed with manometry.

Nutcracker esophagus is a term coined for a condition characterized by chest pain in patients with high-amplitude peristaltic contractions in the distal part of the esophagus. The existence of the condition is disputed. Peristaltic wave propagation is otherwise normal and is not accompanied by simultaneous or multipeaked contractions. Precise manometric criteria for diagnosis are not universally agreed on, and overlap between normal and abnormal manometric findings exists.

Radiographically, patients with nutcracker esophagus have normal findings on barium swallow. Because the peristaltic wave is normal except for amplitude, barium peristalsis appears to be normal.

NEMD is a "waste basket" category used to describe motility disorders that do not meet established manometric criteria. Manometric abnormalities include failed peristalsis, low-amplitude contractions, prolonged duration of peristalsis, simultaneous contractions, tertiary contractions, and incomplete relaxation of the LES. Symptoms are nonspecific and include chest pain and dysphagia. Radiographic findings are frequently normal. When present, abnormalities are nonspecific and include ineffective peristalsis causing stasis and tertiary contractions.

Recently, a subgroup of patients with NEMD has been classified as having ineffective esophageal motility. These patients have defined manometric criteria demonstrating hypocontraction of the distal end of the esophagus. GERD is a common accompaniment in these patients. Radiographic findings are nonspecific and are similar to those of NEMD.[30]

Secondary Motility Disorders

Secondary motility disorders include systemic disorders that secondarily affect the esophagus. The list of diseases is diverse and includes collagen vascular disease, diabetes, alcoholism, hypothyroidism, amyloidosis, Chagas' disease, and chronic intestinal pseudo-obstruction. With a few exceptions, the radiographic appearance is nonspecific.

Of the collagen vascular diseases, scleroderma most often involves the esophagus and occurs in 80% of cases. Mixed connective tissue disease, dermatomyositis, polymyositis, systemic lupus, and Behçet's disease have similar findings but involve the esophagus less often. Abnormal motility is due to smooth muscle atrophy and fibrosis. These pathologic changes result in hypomotility in the distal esophageal body and a hypotensive LES. The combined disorders set the stage for severe reflux disease because of profound loss of the antireflux barrier and poor acid clearance.

The radiographic changes reflect a combination of poor esophageal peristalsis and esophageal injury caused by severe reflux disease. Ineffective peristalsis in the distal third of the esophageal body is indicated by nonocclusive peristalsis and stasis. Hiatal hernias with scarring and stricture are common (see Fig. 5–12). In severe cases, signs of esophageal shortening may be seen. Similar but less severe changes may be seen with other collagen vascular disorders.

Chagas' disease is caused by the tropical protozoan *Trypanosoma cruzi*. It is endemic to South and Central America and is rarely seen in the United States. Cardiac muscle and smooth muscle of the GI tract are commonly involved. The radiographic appearance of the esophagus is identical to that of classic achalasia.

Changes in the esophagus as a result of diabetes, hypothyroidism, alcoholism, amyloidosis, and intestinal pseudo-obstruction are similar and usually mild. Increased tertiary contractions and nonocclusive peristalsis resulting in bolus stasis are common but nonspecific findings.

ESOPHAGEAL NEOPLASMS

Esophageal neoplasms are generally found by means of barium esophagography or upper endoscopy. Most malignancies are discovered in symptomatic patients and are high stage with a poor prognosis. The majority of benign tumors are incidental findings, but when they are symptomatic, excision is usually curative. CT can occasionally suggest the diagnosis of esophageal neoplasm, but it is more useful in staging esophageal malignancies, along with newer, more specific modalities such PET imaging and endoscopic ultrasound (EUS).

Carcinoma

Esophageal carcinoma accounts for about 1% of all malignancies and 5.6% of GI malignancies. In 2004, the American Cancer Society estimated that esophageal cancer would be diagnosed in 14,250 people in the United States and that 13,300 would die of this malignancy.[31] The symptoms causing patients with esophageal malignancy to seek medical care are typically significant dysphagia of recent onset (1 to 4 months) and weight loss. The prognosis for symptomatic patients is dismal. Historically, more than 95% of esophageal cancers have been due to squamous cell carcinoma, with adenocarcinoma accounting for most of the rest. In recent decades, the incidence of adenocarcinoma arising in the columnar-lined epithelium of Barrett's esophagus has risen dramatically, with estimates of up to 34% of all esophageal cancers in some series[32] and more than 70% in others. This increase in prevalence is widespread regardless of race and gender, but its relative increase is greatest in white men. The radiographic appearance and clinical features of these two main esophageal cancers are similar regardless of the pathologic subtype. However, the preponderance of adenocarcinomas occurs in the distal esophagus within regions of Barrett's esophagus. Squamous cell carcinoma, by comparison, tends to occur in the upper two thirds of the esophagus. Other primary malignancies of the esophagus, such as sarcomas, melanoma, and lymphoma, are rare.

Radiologic Appearance

Barium studies of the esophagus are useful in the initial diagnosis of esophageal cancer. They can aid in characterizing the size, location, and morphology of the

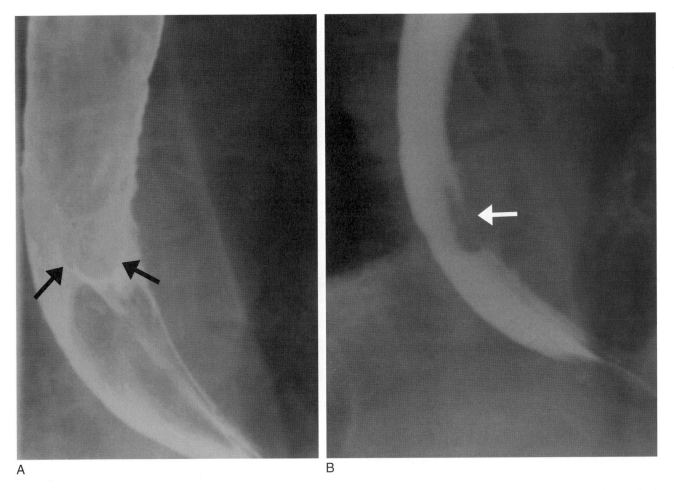

A   B

Figure 5–17. T2 adenocarcinoma within a region of Barrett's esophagus in a 71-year-old man. **A,** An air-contrast image in the left posterior oblique projection shows barium outlining subtle areas of mucosal irregularity (*arrows*) in this sessile 1-cm cancer seen en face. **B,** A single-contrast image in the anteroposterior projection shows a plaque-like lesion (*arrow*) in profile along the left side of the lower part of the esophagus.

disease, both before and after radiation or chemotherapeutic treatment. They can demonstrate complications of unresectable cancer, such as a fistula to the tracheobronchial tree, either primarily or after treatment. Coexistent disorders can be identified, such as benign strictures, hiatal hernias, motility disorders, and rare synchronous second tumors. They are also useful in postoperative evaluation, as discussed later.

Early resectable esophageal carcinomas can be detected or suggested on double-contrast barium esophagograms performed with careful radiographic technique. Single-contrast barium evaluation is not as sensitive but may be complementary to the air-contrast technique. Early disease has a variety of subtle radiographic appearances, including fixed mucosal irregularity, irregular strictures, polypoid filling defects, or plaque-like filling defects (Fig. 5–17). When radiographic findings of a smooth benign-appearing stricture are seen, they can reliably be considered benign.[19] Endoscopy may still be useful to search for signs of esophagitis or Barrett's disease. When radiographically equivocal or malignant-appearing strictures are seen,

endoscopy is required for definitive diagnosis of possible malignancy. It has been said that barium studies of the esophagus are highly accurate for the detection of esophageal neoplasm, but this has been found to be true only in symptomatic (therefore high-risk) patients.[33] Furthermore, detection of esophageal malignancy in symptomatic patients is usually associated with high-stage malignancy and its associated poor prognosis. Early, curable esophageal malignancy is best found by endoscopy in high-risk patients (such as those with known Barrett's esophagus).

More advanced esophageal cancer can readily be detected with a single- or double-contrast barium technique, although the double-contrast technique is nearly always more revealing of mucosal abnormalities. Advanced esophageal cancer is usually manifested as a focal ulcerated or fungating mass extending into the lumen with irregular, eccentric luminal narrowing (Fig. 5–18). The luminal caliber is often narrowed by 50% to 75%, frequently with at least two thirds of the circumference involved.[34] The transition from normal esophagus to carcinoma is usually abrupt, as

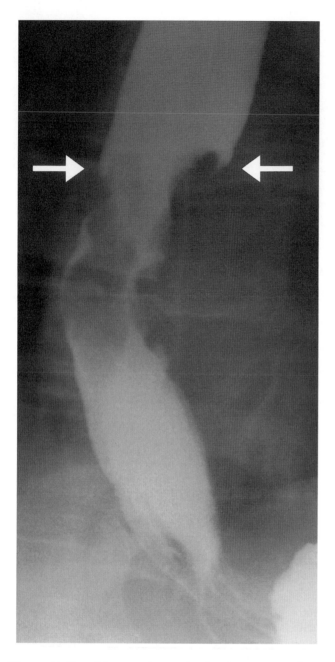

Figure 5–18. Adenocarcinoma in the lower part of the esophagus in a 54-year-old man. An esophagogram shows asymmetric circumferential luminal narrowing, mucosal ulceration, and an abrupt transition (*arrows*) from normal to abnormal mucosal contours.

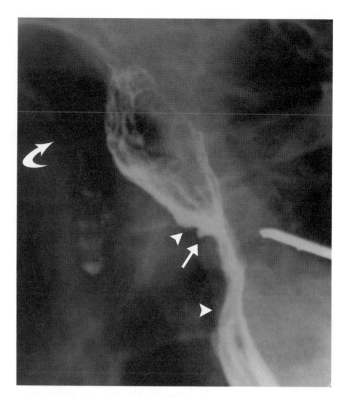

Figure 5–19. Adenocarcinoma in the upper thoracic esophagus arising from the right anterior surface in an 83-year-old man. This is a broad-based eccentric mucosal mass (*arrowheads*) with ulceration (*arrow*). Note the aspirated barium in the trachea (*curved arrow*) related to the dysphagia caused by this tight malignant stricture.

Barium studies can detect some complications of high-stage disease, such as the formation of a fistula to the tracheobronchial tree (Fig. 5–21). The ability of barium studies to give a "global" view of the esophagus, even in the presence of tight strictures, makes it useful in detecting coexistent disorders, including benign strictures, hiatal hernia, motility disorders, and synchronous neoplasms (Fig. 5–22).

Staging

The depth of invasion of esophageal cancer within the wall of the esophagus determines whether a tumor is T1 (limited to the lamina propria or submucosa), T2 (invading the muscularis propria), or T3 (invading the adventitia). Whereas lesions that are T2 or lower have a 5-year survival rate of 40%, T3 (or higher) lesions have a 5-year survival rate of 4%.[35] Additionally, involvement beyond the mucosa is associated with nodal disease in 50% of patients,[35] which also reduces survival. Obviously, the presence of direct invasion of adjacent structures (T4) or the presence of distant metastases (M1) portends a poor prognosis. Unfortunately, many esophageal cancers are unresectable at the time of initial evaluation, thus precluding curative therapy.

A multimodality imaging approach, often including barium studies, CT, endoscopy, EUS, and PET imaging,

demonstrated on barium esophagograms. Aspiration can be seen as a result of partial esophageal obstruction, particularly in high esophageal lesions (Fig. 5–19). A carcinoma near the EGJ can cause high-grade obstruction with dilatation of the proximal esophagus, retention of barium, and significant fixed narrowing of the lumen at the EGJ. This appearance is called *secondary achalasia* because of an appearance and functional behavior similar to that of true achalasia (Fig. 5–20).

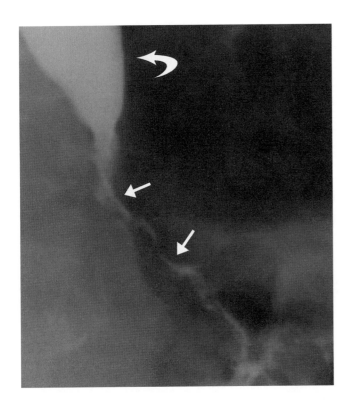

Figure 5–20. Seventy-seven-year-old man with grade 4 adenocarcinoma within Barrett's esophagus located at the esophagogastric junction causing the appearance of secondary achalasia. Note the retained barium in the dilated esophagus (*curved arrow*) above the fixed, narrowed esophagogastric junction from this nearly obstructive carcinoma (*arrows*).

is usually necessary to demonstrate that an esophageal cancer is resectable. CT and PET/CT cannot determine the depth of invasion and are not useful in confirming low-stage disease. However, they are useful in demonstrating the presence of metastatic disease, which confirms high-stage disease, or suggesting the absence of high-stage disease. PET/CT fusion scans are the more useful of these two modalities, but PET is not nearly as available as CT in many regions at this time.

Barium Studies Barium examination has little role in the staging of recently diagnosed esophageal cancer, unless it happens to show the unusual finding of direct invasion of the tracheobronchial tree (see Fig. 5–21), thereby demonstrating a T4 lesion. If a newly diagnosed esophageal cancer is thought to possibly be early stage (see Fig. 5–17), EUS is useful to determine the depth of invasion within the esophageal wall.

Computed Tomography CT can often detect primary changes of esophageal cancer and suggest its diagnosis, but it is inferior to barium studies and endoscopy in this role. CT can sometimes detect esophageal wall thickening, particularly when it is large enough or when esophageal contrast has been used and wall thickening is seen to be asymmetric about the lumen (Fig. 5–23). However, this is particularly difficult near the EGJ (where

many adenocarcinomas develop in the setting of Barrett's esophagus) because of the oblique course that the esophagus takes as it passes through the diaphragmatic hiatus toward the stomach; in such cases, a normal esophagus often appears abnormal on standard axial images. CT is also poor in demonstrating the length of involvement by esophageal cancer, which is quite obvious on barium studies and endoscopy.

CT's greatest contribution is its ability to demonstrate high-stage, often unresectable disease. CT can demonstrate stranding into adjacent fat (confirming invasion beyond the adventitia), direct invasion of adjacent structures (see Fig. 5–21), and worrisome adenopathy (greater than 1 cm in diameter) in adjacent and subdiaphragmatic locations (see Fig. 5–23). Most lymph nodes detected by CT with a minimum diameter greater than 1 cm will represent metastatic adenopathy (in the setting of known esophageal cancer). Unfortunately, lymph nodes that are less than a centimeter in size are frequently metastatic in this setting as well yet could represent benign reactive lymph nodes. These subcentimeter lymph nodes can sometimes be confirmed as metastatic when PET/CT fusion scans show activity in these smaller nodes. When PET/CT is not available, these small nodes may remain indeterminate in the staging process. EUS biopsy techniques can be used to prove metastatic involvement in localized adenopathy. These and other areas of adenopathy can be treated with neoadjuvant chemotherapy or surgical excision (or both), if palliative or definitive surgery is undertaken.

Distant metastases, such as liver, omental, or adrenal involvement, are often well demonstrated by CT. CT is also an appropriate modality to use to guide percutaneous biopsy of suspected metastatic disease. Lymph nodes can be sampled by percutaneous biopsy, which can be useful if it confirms metastatic involvement. However, understaging of lymph nodes because of the limited sampling process can be a problem for accurate staging, particularly with micrometastases in small lymph nodes. MRI has most of the same advantages and disadvantages as CT but often suffers from problems with motion artifact (especially respiratory and cardiac motion), is more expensive than CT, and is an impractical modality to use to provide image-guided percutaneous biopsy. MRI has no routine role in esophageal cancer staging.

Positron Emission Tomography The usefulness of PET is in evaluating documented high-grade malignancies of the esophagus. There is no documented role for PET in differentiating benign tumors or inflammatory conditions such as Barrett's esophagus from malignancy. Generally, some mild inflammation in such cases can result in PET uptake that is indistinguishable from that seen in early malignancy.

PET staging of documented esophageal cancer can provide additive information in several respects. One potential PET contribution is detection of metastatic disease in lymph nodes smaller than the standard CT criteria for nodal enlargement. Additionally, in enlarged lymph nodes without metastasis, PET can improve specificity by excluding some nodes that may be enlarged because of inflammation or reactivity alone. PET

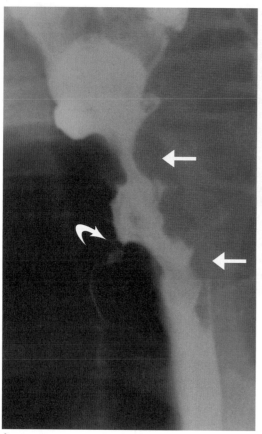

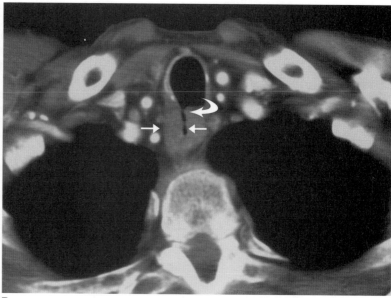

Figure 5–21. Grade 3 (of 4) squamous cell carcinoma of the low cervical and upper thoracic esophagus in a 60-year-old man. **A,** Esophagogram showing irregular luminal narrowing with ulceration (*arrows*) and a fistula to the trachea (*curved arrow*). **B,** CT confirms the tracheoesophageal fistula (*curved arrow*) within the thick-walled (*arrows*) malignant esophagus.

findings can be falsely negative when the burden of nodal disease is below the detection ability of PET, such as in micrometastases. Certainly, some highly active inflammatory lymph nodes that do not harbor malignancy can have elevated uptake on a PET scan as well. The current data have demonstrated such to be the case, but, even so, some variation in the accuracy of assessing nodal disease has been noted in publications. Variation in the ability of PET to detect lymph node metastasis depends a great deal on how close the nodal regions are to the primary tumor—with those adjacent to a metabolically active tumor being more difficult to detect—and what patient groups are included in the analysis. In one study, PET demonstrated a sensitivity for predicting local nodal disease of 76% (22/29) versus 45% (13/29) for CT in patients who all underwent curative surgery.[36] The sensitivity for detection of nodal metastasis by PET has also been reported to be as low as 33% for local nodal disease elsewhere, however.[37-39] These studies have often been performed in different patient groups. Some authors looked only at patients who were determined to be clinically resectable (i.e., negative on CT for metastasis) before performing PET. This subset selection of patients and the use of some variable PET imaging methods could explain the differences. In our experience, local nodal staging has been roughly equivalent between EUS, CT, and PET when all of the referred patients are included. In about 10% of cases, one imaging method does identify disease not seen by the other, however.

Identifying distant metastatic disease has some important caveats for PET. Relative to distant nodal disease, identification of M1a disease can be difficult without the use of CT fusion imaging to provide anatomic guidance on location of the celiac axis. For M1b disease, having CT fusion with PET may not be as uniformly important but can help in locating metastases in bone versus soft tissue, for example. These issues make the use of PET with CT fusion of significant importance when performing PET imaging for esophageal cancer.

For distant disease staging, PET can be quite enlightening. It can improve distant disease staging, and, in addition, identification by PET of other sites of metastatic disease not previously noted may help facilitate confirmation of disease. In one study, of seven patients who did not undergo surgery, PET detected distant metastases that were not identified on CT in five. Another patient had an unsuspected concomitant primary lung tumor discovered by PET alone. In another study of 35 patients with potentially resectable esophageal cancer as determined by CT, PET identified distant metastatic disease in 20%. The accuracy of PET in determining distant metastatic disease in this group was 91%.[40] Others have reported similar findings. Figure 5–24 illustrates a patient with esophageal cancer in whom widespread distant disease was identified by PET that was underestimated on other imaging modalities.

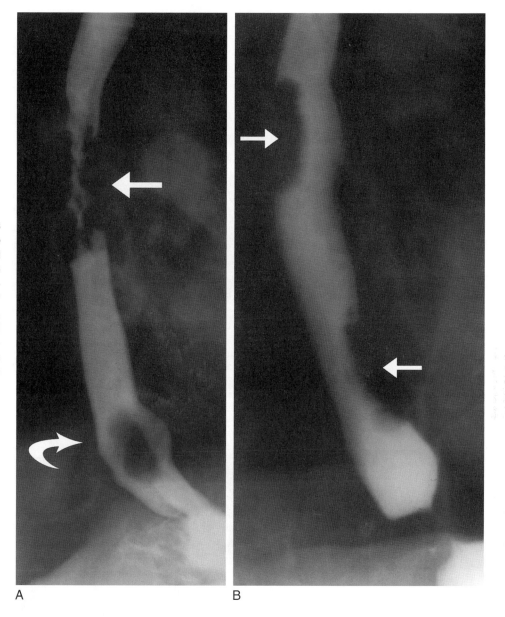

Figure 5–22. Two synchronous squamous cell carcinomas in two separate patients. **A,** Ulcerated infiltrating mass (*arrow*) in the midesophagus with a rare polypoid intraluminal mass (*curved arrow*) in the lower esophagus. **B,** Broad-based sessile polypoid masses (*arrows*) arising eccentrically from opposite sides of the mid and lower portions of the esophagus.

A   B

Evaluation of Therapy for Esophageal Cancer

Attempts to improve the survival of patients with esophageal cancer are leading to multimodality treatment regimens. Time will tell whether survival will be extended, but the use of PET in selecting successful treatment paradigms early in the course of therapy holds the promise of more rapid discovery of a treatment combination that may improve survival. Recent work has shown that PET is able to detect which tumors are responding as early as 14 days into therapy. In a group of 40 patients with locally advanced adenocarcinoma of the EGJ, Weber et al. showed that reduction of tumor fluorodeoxyglucose (FDG) uptake after 14 days of therapy was significantly different between responding and nonresponding tumors. Optimal differentiation was achieved by a cutoff value of 35% reduction of initial FDG uptake. Applying this cutoff value as a criterion for a metabolic response predicted clinical response with a sensitivity and specificity of 93% (14 of 15 patients) and 95% (21 of 22),

respectively. Patients without a metabolic response were also characterized by significantly shorter time to progression/recurrence ($P = .01$) and shorter overall survival ($P = .04$).[41]

Assessment of Recurrent Esophageal Cancer

At the present time, there is little benefit to additional therapy after esophageal cancer recurs following curative resection or multimodality therapy. In patients with a suspicion of recurrence from radiographic or other clinical indicators, PET imaging is able to detect more sites of recurrence than conventional tests can. Whether this is important is still a reasonable question. Flamen et al. showed that PET detected 100% of the documented recurrences in a group of 40 patients who were suspected of having disease recurrence.[42] No data are yet available on the potential role that PET could play in disease surveillance. Hopefully, early detection of recurrence could

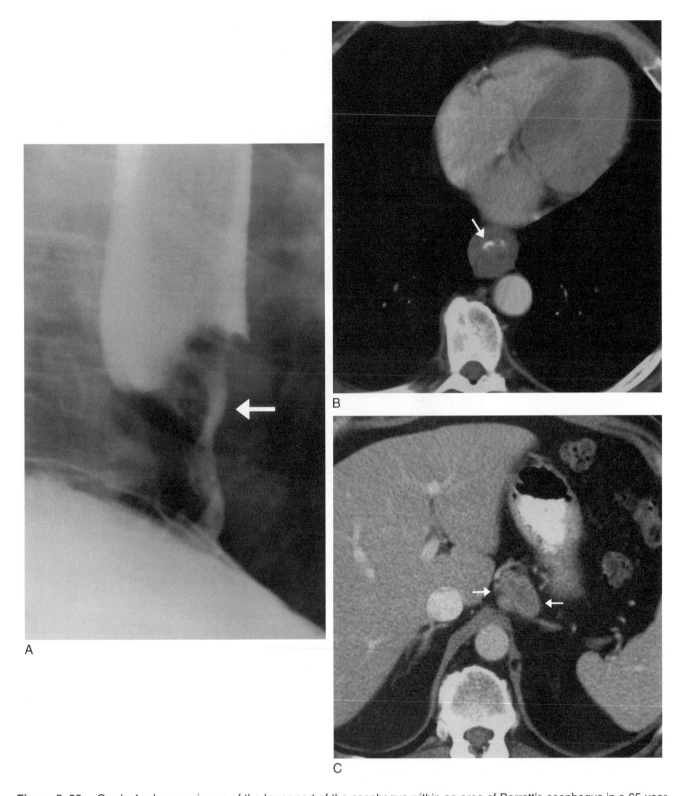

Figure 5–23. Grade 4 adenocarcinoma of the lower part of the esophagus within an area of Barrett's esophagus in a 65-year-old man. **A,** An esophagogram shows an abrupt fungating mass with ulceration and asymmetric luminal narrowing (*arrow*). **B,** An axial CT image shows asymmetric esophageal wall thickening, confirmed by the presence of esophageal luminal contrast (*arrow*) within the eccentrically narrowed lumen. **C,** Enlarged (2.7 × 4 cm) celiac lymphadenopathy (*arrows*) is seen on this axial CT image. Fine-needle aspiration of these nodes by endoscopic ultrasound confirmed adenocarcinoma metastases, thus making this lesion M1a.

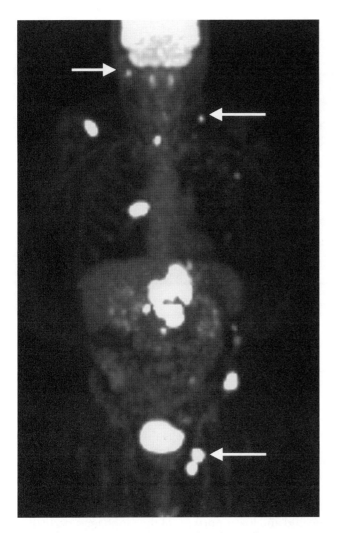

Figure 5–24. Coronal PET in a patient with esophageal cancer. Endoscopic ultrasound had revealed the tumor and suspicious peritumoral nodes, but no biopsy of the nodes could be performed. CT also demonstrated the tumor and suspicious gastrohepatic nodes. PET showed multiple distant metastasis not otherwise described, some of which, right neck, left supraclavicular, and left groin areas (*arrows*), would be easily accessible for biopsy.

play some role in improving survival from recurrent esophageal cancer, and PET could make a contribution in this respect based on its ability to detect recurrence with high sensitivity.

Other Esophageal Malignancies

Other primary malignancies of the esophagus are rare and generally have a poor prognosis. Lymphoma is exceedingly rare as a primary esophageal lesion. Esophageal lymphoma represents less than 1% of lymphoma cases. When it involves the esophagus, it is more likely an extension of gastric lymphoma (causing abnormal thickened longitudinal folds) or due to direct compression from mediastinal lymphoma (with associated luminal narrowing as a result of a mass effect of the

tumor arising outside the esophagus). The most common nonepithelial neoplasm of the esophagus is leiomyosarcoma. Like other sarcomas of the GI tract, it usually has a bulky exophytic component, so much so that it may show up on a chest radiograph. The intraluminal component is often a polypoid mass expanding the lumen, frequently ulcerated but sometimes smooth and relatively benign in appearance. Melanoma accounts for 0.1% to 0.2% of all primary esophageal malignancies. It is usually polypoid but can be plaque-like. These and other unusual primary esophageal malignancies are usually definitively diagnosed in symptomatic patients after endoscopic biopsy. Their imaging characteristics are generally nonspecific.

Metastatic disease to the esophagus is most commonly from stomach, lung, or breast cancer. The method of spread to the esophagus can be by way of direct invasion, lymphatic spread, or hematogenous spread. For example, malignancy from the gastric cardia can spread across the GEJ to directly involve the lower part of the esophagus. Lymphatic spread to the mediastinal lymph nodes can be seen with lung, breast, head/neck, and pancreas cancer. This is seen on barium esophagograms as an extrinsic mass compressing, narrowing, and displacing the esophageal lumen and is readily apparent on CT (Fig. 5–25). Hematogenous spread of metastatic disease to the esophagus is very rare; the appearance can be variable.

Benign Esophageal Neoplasms

Benign neoplasms of the esophagus are rare, with the exception of leiomyoma, which is the most common esophageal neoplasm. Most benign esophageal tumors are asymptomatic and found incidentally. Symptoms, when they occur, are usually those of obstruction, often partial or intermittent. Some of these lesions can be confidently diagnosed on the basis of their CT characteristics. The remainder can be diagnosed by EUS or endoscopy with biopsy. Treatment of these rare benign lesions is based on the severity of symptoms, if present.

The presence and type of symptoms are related to the size and location of these benign tumors. Intraluminal masses usually arise from the esophageal mucosa or protrude through the mucosa to reside within the esophageal lumen. On barium studies, a well-circumscribed intraluminal mass is seen (Fig. 5–26) that often expands the lumen and causes a filling defect in the surrounding barium. These lesions need to be differentiated from an impacted foreign body, such as retained food above a stricture. This is usually easily accomplished fluoroscopically or endoscopically.

Intramural lesions occur within the wall of the esophagus and generally have normal, intact overlying mucosa. An intramural lesion appears as a smooth convex impression on the esophagus that causes focal narrowing of the lumen. These lesions form a right angle or slightly obtuse angle with the normal esophageal wall as they protrude into the lumen. EUS with biopsy capability is useful for diagnosing these lesions because a simple "pinch" biopsy of the overlying mucosa will show only normal esophageal mucosa.

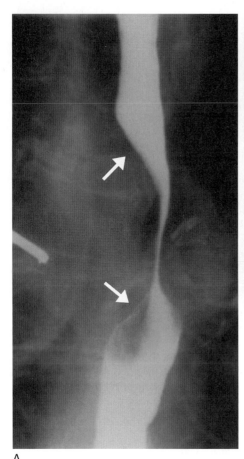

A

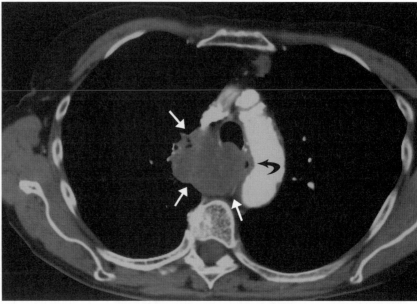

B

Figure 5–25. Grade 4 adenocarcinoma of the right lung in a 78-year-old woman. **A,** An esophagogram shows a long extrinsic impression on the right side of the midesophagus (*arrows*) with intact esophageal mucosa. **B,** CT shows bulky metastatic mediastinal adenopathy (*arrows*) compressing and displacing the esophagus (*curved arrow*) to the left.

Extrinsic lesions arise outside the normal confines of the wall of the esophagus. On barium studies (or endoscopically), an extrinsic mass appears as a smooth convex impression narrowing the esophageal lumen. The main distinction from intrinsic masses is that extrinsic masses cause a more shallow, longer, obtuse impression on the lumen, whereas intrinsic masses are more focal with an abrupt onset of luminal narrowing.

Specific benign lesions deserve some discussion. Fibrovascular polyps (see Fig. 5–26) arise from the submucosa yet are manifested as an intraluminal mass. Typically they arise from the upper part of the esophagus but can occur anywhere. They are frequently quite mobile within the esophagus and are tethered to the esophageal wall by a relatively long, narrow pedicle or point of attachment. Papillomas are smooth-walled polyps, sometimes multiple, arising from the mucosa. They protrude into the lumen, often with a wide base of attachment. Hemangiomas, though rare, may result in esophageal hemorrhage. Inflammatory esophagogastric polyps are actually clubbed, bulbous gastric folds that arise from the gastric cardia and protrude into the lower part of the esophagus at the EGJ. They usually represent inflamed mucosal hypertrophy secondary to GERD.

Leiomyomas (Fig. 5–27) are the most common benign esophageal neoplasm. They are often asymptomatic and discovered incidentally and can be multiple. Leiomyoma is the classic intramural lesion and appears as a focal narrowing with a smooth contour arising from one side of the esophageal wall. They are most commonly seen in the mid and lower portions of the esophagus, particularly near the EGJ. Despite being the most common esophageal neoplasm, leiomyomas often go undetected on most imaging studies because of their frequent lack of symptoms, intact overlying mucosa, and often-subtle impression on the esophageal lumen. Occasionally, they can be quite large and have their epicenter located outside the esophageal wall. In such cases, sarcoma needs to be excluded. EUS can demonstrate a benign-appearing mass, usually arising from the muscularis mucosa, and biopsy is not generally necessary for small, asymptomatic incidental lesions. Other benign lesions, such as lipoma, fibroma, neurofibroma, hamartoma, and hemangioma, have a similar radiographic appearance but are far less common.

The main extrinsic mass arising from the esophagus is an esophageal duplication cyst. Technically, it is a congenital lesion and not a true neoplasm. On CT, an esophageal duplication cyst appears as a well-circumscribed, benign-appearing, thin-walled cystic structure with a CT density value (Hounsfield units) slightly higher than that of water. Other structures that frequently cause an extrinsic impression on the esophagus and potentially narrow the lumen include normal anatomic structures such as the left atrium (particularly if enlarged) on the lower part of the esophagus and the aortic arch (particularly if tortuous and ectatic) on the midportion of the esophagus. They have a

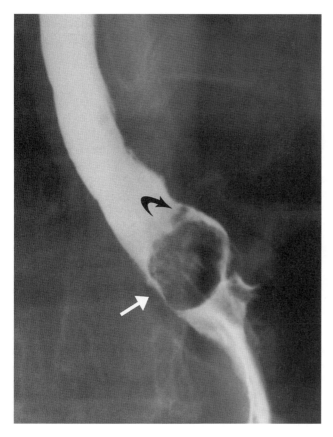

Figure 5–26. Forty-five-year-old woman with a pedunculated fibrovascular polyp seen as an intraluminal filling defect (*arrow*) expanding the lower part of the esophagus. At fluoroscopy, it was noted to move several centimeters within the lower esophagus, tethered by a thin stalk (*curved arrow*).

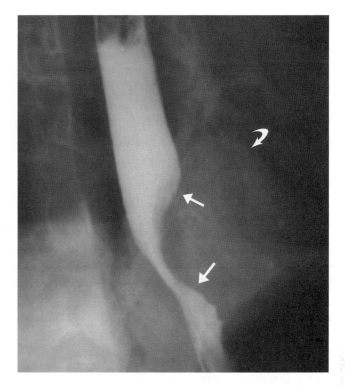

Figure 5–27. Asymptomatic 52-year-old woman with an abnormal chest radiograph. A barium esophagogram shows a mass effect in the lower esophagus on the left that is causing a smooth, sharply obtuse impression on the esophageal lumen (*arrows*). This was shown by biopsy to be a large benign leiomyoma with a prominent exophytic component (*curved arrow*).

characteristic appearance on barium studies and can be confirmed with CT if necessary. Mediastinal neoplasms or adenopathy (see Fig. 5–25), if in direct contact with the esophagus, can also cause extrinsic narrowing of the esophageal lumen, and CT of the chest can identify these mediastinal abnormalities.

POSTOPERATIVE ESOPHAGUS

Goals and Techniques of Postoperative Esophageal Imaging

Radiologic evaluation of a postoperative esophagus is performed to demonstrate the postoperative anatomy, judge the effectiveness of the surgery, and detect postoperative complications.[43] Postoperative images also establish a baseline for comparison of future radiographic studies. The effectiveness of the surgery may not be fully revealed by a radiographic examination performed in the early postoperative period because of transient changes of edema and hematoma. During the early postoperative period (less than 4 weeks), the most common complications after esophageal surgery include leakage, obstruction, and stasis. During the late postoperative period (longer than 4 weeks), the most common

complications include GER, stricture, and recurrent carcinoma.[43]

Techniques: Imaging Modalities

Chest radiography plays an important role in the early postoperative period, especially after esophagectomy, because of the high incidence of respiratory complications in these patients, particularly those who have undergone thoracotomy.[44] Complications such as pneumothorax, pleural effusion, and pneumonia are the most frequent cause of morbidity after esophagectomy.[45] Additionally, chest radiographs can provide indirect evidence of esophageal leakage. Findings such as pneumomediastinum, mediastinal widening, or a rapidly growing pleural effusion suggest esophageal leaks. However, chest radiographic findings are relatively insensitive in the diagnosis of leaks. A normal chest radiograph in the appropriate clinical setting should not discourage further investigation.[43]

Esophagography is the major imaging modality for evaluation of a postoperative esophagus. This fluoroscopic esophagogram is performed as the patient drinks contrast material to opacify the esophageal lumen. Radiographs obtained during (spot films) and after (overhead films) fluoroscopy tell only part of the story. The

Table 5–1   Barium Versus Water-Soluble Contrast Material for Postoperative Esophagograms

	Barium	Water-soluble Contrast Material
Advantages	Increased density shows leaks missed by water-soluble contrast material	Leakage into the mediastinum does not cause mediastinitis
	Aspiration does not cause pulmonary edema	Reabsorption from the mediastinum makes future esophagograms easier to interpret
Disadvantages	There is a risk of mediastinitis with leakage into the mediastinum	Aspiration can cause pulmonary edema
	Barium remaining in the mediastinum may suggest persistent leakage on future esophagograms	Leaks can be missed because of decreased density in comparison to barium

radiologist who observed the dynamic fluoroscopic images may report findings that are not included or poorly demonstrated on the radiographic films.

In the early postoperative period, esophagograms are often limited to examination in the recumbent position. Decreased ability to swallow and poor patient mobility add to the difficulty of performing the examination. These early postoperative esophagograms are carried out, at least initially, with water-soluble contrast material in case of leaks. Later in the postoperative period, esophagograms are typically performed as upright, air-contrast images obtained with high-density barium and recumbent, single-contrast images with low-density barium.[43]

CT is not a primary imaging modality in the early postoperative period after esophageal surgery. However, as a secondary modality, CT provides important additional information after the discovery of a postoperative esophageal leak by esophagography. Chest CT demonstrates the severity and extent of mediastinal inflammation associated with such a leak. It also demonstrates the size and location of any mediastinal fluid collection or abscess. This information is especially helpful in planning further treatment. CT images can guide the placement of drains into these collections by surgeons or interventional radiologists.[46] In the later postoperative period, CT or MRI can detect mediastinal cancer recurrence and metastases.

Techniques: Contrast Materials

Two types of contrast material are used during esophagography: barium and water soluble. Each of these contrast materials has advantages and disadvantages (Table 5–1). The type of contrast material used is at least partially dependent on the time since surgery. Water-soluble contrast material is used, at least initially, for early postoperative esophagograms (less than 4 weeks). Barium is used later in the postoperative period (longer than 4 weeks).

Leaks can occur after any esophageal surgery, but they are most common after esophagectomy. The appearance of pain and fever after esophagectomy warrants emergency esophagography.[44] The examination should be performed initially with water-soluble contrast material. If this initial esophagogram is negative, the examination should be immediately repeated with barium. As a result

of the superior opacity of barium, small leaks may be diagnosed only with barium. Because many postoperative esophageal leaks are asymptomatic, many institutions perform routine esophagography between 7 and 10 days after surgery.

In a recent retrospective study of 24 esophagectomy patients with postoperative leaks, 16 (67%) of these leaks were demonstrated only with use of high-density (250% weight per volume [w/v]) barium.[47] This percentage of esophageal leaks demonstrated only with barium is higher than in previous studies performed with 60% w/v and 100% w/v barium solutions. The authors speculate that the higher rate of leak detection resulted from the use of higher-density barium. The benefit of demonstrating a leak usually outweighs the risk for mediastinitis secondary to barium leakage.[48]

The risk for pulmonary edema after the aspiration of water-soluble contrast material depends on the volume and osmolarity of the material aspirated. Aspiration of high-osmolar water-soluble contrast material, such as diatrizoate meglumine (Gastrografin) or diatrizoate sodium (Gastroview), is more likely to cause pulmonary edema than is aspiration of a similar amount of low-osmolar water-soluble contrast material, such as iohexol (Omnipaque) or metrizamide (Amipaque). Therefore, the use of low-osmolar water-soluble contrast material should be considered in postoperative patients to reduce the risk for pulmonary edema after aspiration.[48]

Specific Findings

Cricopharyngeal Myotomy

Cricopharyngeal myotomy for Zenker's diverticulum is typically combined with diverticulectomy or diverticulopexy. Postoperative esophagography in successfully treated patients shows resolution of the prominent cricopharyngeus muscle and nonfilling of the diverticulum (Fig. 5–28). Mild irregularity with outpouching of the pharyngoesophageal segment posteriorly, superior to the level of the cricopharyngeus muscle—referred to as "mucosal beaking"—is not a worrisome finding.[49]

Because the major complication of cricopharyngeal myotomy is leakage, the postoperative esophagogram should be performed initially with water-soluble contrast material. This contrast material needs to be administered

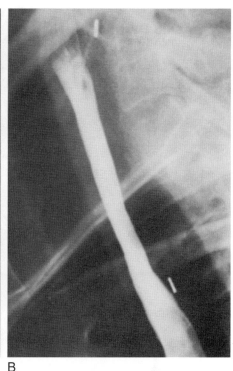

Figure 5–28. Cricopharyngeal myotomy. Frontal and lateral views from a postoperative barium esophagogram demonstrate extended cervical esophagomyotomy. The surgical clips mark the superior and inferior limits of the myotomy. An obstructing posterior cricopharyngeal muscle is not evident.

A   B

cautiously because transient postoperative pharyngeal dysfunction predisposes these patients to aspiration (low-osmolar water-soluble contrast material can be considered for these examinations). If the water-soluble contrast study is negative, re-examination with high-density barium should be performed. Leaks often appear as blind-ending tracts extending from the esophagus posteriorly into the prevertebral space.[49]

Cardiomyotomy

Normally, a postcardiomyotomy esophagogram demonstrates good esophageal emptying and no widely patent GEJ.[43] Eccentric ballooning of the esophageal mucosa through the myotomy defect is a common finding post-operatively (Fig. 5–29) and occurs in 50% of patients after cardiomyotomy.[50] Frequently, an antireflux procedure is performed in conjunction with cardiomyotomy, and radiographic evidence of this procedure may be seen on the postoperative esophagogram.

An early complication of cardiomyotomy is leakage secondary to perforation. Evaluation for this complication should begin with water-soluble esophagography followed by barium to more confidently evaluate for a perforation. Late complications include dysphagia secondary to inadequate myotomy or tight fundoplication. Demonstration of reflux esophagitis suggests the need for an antireflux procedure.[43]

Antireflux Procedures

The appearance of a normal esophagogram after antireflux procedures reflect the goals of these procedures: reduction of esophageal hiatal hernia, diaphragm repair,

restoration of an intra-abdominal esophageal segment, and gastric fundal wrap around the proximal part of the stomach. Common antireflux surgeries include the Nissen, Belsey Mark IV, and Hill procedures.[43] The Nissen procedure results in a 360-degree wrap of the gastric fundus around the esophagus. Radiographic findings include a wrap creating a smooth, symmetrical mass within the fundus. With a Nissen procedure, the esophagus passes through the center of the mass (Fig. 5–30). The Belsey Mark IV procedure uses a 240-degree fundal wrap with suturing of the esophagus to the gastric fundus to recreate an acute angle at the GEJ (angle of His). On barium swallow, this procedure results in a smaller soft tissue mass in the fundus and angulation of the intra-abdominal esophagus. During the Hill procedure, the GEJ is sutured to the median arcuate ligament posteriorly. No fundoplication is performed. By means of esophagography, one sees lengthening of the intra-abdominal esophagus and exaggeration of the angle of His. Regardless of the specific antireflux procedure, one should not see a hiatal hernia or evidence of reflux esophagitis.[43]

The most common early complication of fundoplication demonstrated by esophagography is obstruction of the distal end of the esophagus secondary to self-limited edema of the fundal wrap. This process usually resolves in a matter of weeks, and the esophagus will then drain well. Late complications include (1) esophageal obstruction caused by a tight fundal wrap or tight esophageal hiatus, (2) recurrent hiatal hernia and GER caused by disruption of fundoplication sutures (fundal soft tissue density not visible), and (3) recurrent hiatal hernia (fundal soft tissue density visible) caused by dehiscence of diaphragmatic sutures.[43]

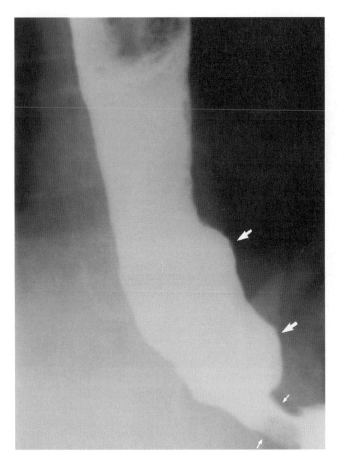

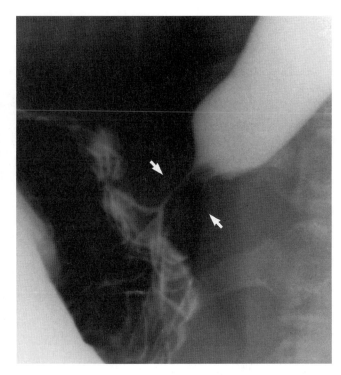

Figure 5–30. Nissen fundoplication—prone, oblique, single-contrast view of the gastroesophageal junction from a barium esophagogram performed 6 weeks after laparoscopic Nissen fundoplication. A smooth, symmetrical, and extrinsic fundal mass resulted from the 360-degree fundal wrap around the intra-abdominal esophagus (*arrows*). The esophagus passes through the center of this mass.

Figure 5–29. Cardiomyotomy (Heller myotomy). An upright, frontal view from a postoperative barium esophagogram demonstrates a common distal esophageal deformity after cardiomyotomy. The distal esophageal mucosa "ballooned" through the myotomy defect and has created a wide-mouthed, false diverticulum (*arrows*). Decreased caliber of the esophagus distal to the myotomy deformity (*small arrows*) should result from partial anterior fundoplication (Dor procedure).

Esophageal Resection

The radiographic appearance after esophagectomy depends on the bowel segment used as an esophageal substitute. Stomach, colon, and jejunum are used as esophageal substitutes, with gastric substitution being most common. Gastric substitution requires resection of the esophagus and cardia, mobilization of the stomach, and anastomosis of the esophagus to the stomach. Pyloromyotomy, or pyloroplasty, and partial resection of the gastric fundus may also be performed to facilitate drainage of the denervated stomach.[43] (Vagotomy is unavoidable during this surgery.) Therefore, a normal postoperative esophagogram should demonstrate patency of the esophagogastrostomy (Fig. 5–31), patency of the stomach as it passes through the esophageal hiatus, and patency of the pylorus.

Leakage is the most feared early postoperative complication of esophagectomy and esophagogastros-tomy. The leak may occur at the esophagogastric anastomosis, at the pyloroplasty or pyloromyotomy, or along the gastric staple line resulting from partial gastric resection.[43] Pain and fever after esophagectomy warrant emergency esophagography[44] with water-soluble contrast material and barium. High-density barium has been reported to be more effective in demonstrating leaks.[47]

Early postoperative obstruction may result from edema at the esophagogastrostomy or pyloroplasty/pyloromyotomy sites. Obstruction may also be seen as a result of diaphragmatic compression of the distal part of the stomach or may be due to gastric volvulus.[43] Gastric atony can cause similar obstructive symptoms.

Late complications after esophagectomy and esophagogastrostomy include GER, stricture, and tumor recurrence. GER can cause reflux esophagitis, stricture (above the esophagogastric anastomosis), Barrett's esophagus, and adenocarcinoma.[43] Postesophagectomy patients with dysphagia should be initially evaluated with a barium swallow. Anastomotic strictures are usually well demonstrated (Fig. 5–32). Reflux esophagitis and Barrett's esophagus are best evaluated with endoscopy. CT and PET are best for detection of recurrent tumor and are discussed in another section of this chapter.

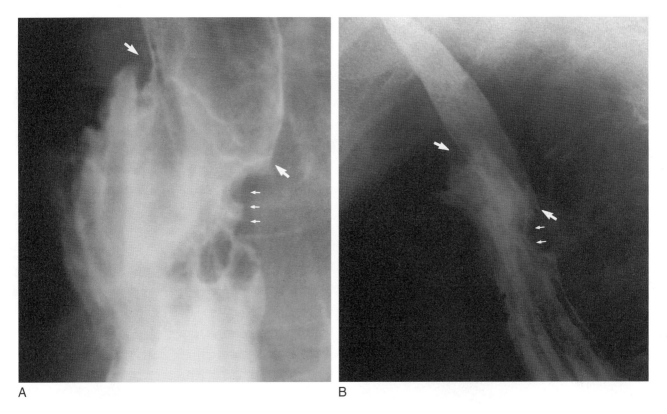

A   B

Figure 5–31.   Esophagogastrostomy. Upright, frontal (magnified) **(A)** and lateral air-contrast images **(B)** from a barium esoph-agogram performed 1 month after esophagectomy for T1N0 adenocarcinoma of the lower esophagus demonstrate a side-to-side esophagogastric anastomosis along the greater curve (*arrows*). The mass along the left posterior margin of the gastrostomy, just distal to the anastomosis (*small arrows*), should represent a benign postoperative finding (the patient had no evidence of recurrent or metastatic disease 10 months after this esophagogram).

MISCELLANEOUS CONDITIONS

Hiatal Hernias

Hiatal hernias can be classified into several types depending on their appearance. By far, the most common type is a sliding hiatal hernia (type I) (Fig. 5–33). Strictly speaking, a sliding hiatal hernia should be transient and is diagnosed when a portion of the stomach is fluoroscopically seen to enter the thorax through the esophageal hiatus of the diaphragm and later to return to the abdomen. Not uncommonly, however, large sliding hernias remain in the chest during the entire fluoroscopic examination. Such hernias should still be considered the sliding type, as long as there is no evidence of esophageal shortening. The observation that sufficient esophageal redundancy exists to allow reduction of the hernia is important to the surgeon in planning hiatal hernia repair. Although the correlation between GER and sliding hiatal hernias is far from perfect, such hernias are thought to predispose to reflux.[51]

The second major type of hiatal hernia (type II) (Fig. 5–34) is a paraesophageal hernia, in which the EGJ remains within (or very near) the esophageal hiatus and a portion or all of the stomach herniates superiorly through the esophageal hiatus and comes to lie adjacent to the esophagus. Such hernias are important to recog-nize because although they are not strongly associated with GER, they are more likely than sliding hernias to be associated with symptomatic gas entrapment, incarceration, obstruction, and strangulation. These important symptoms are more common with large paraesophageal hernias, in which the greater curvature of the stomach rotates superiorly 180 degrees to lie above the lesser curvature ("upside-down, intrathoracic stomach"). At this point, elective surgical repair should be considered to prevent severe complications, especially those resulting from obstructive gastric volvulus.[52,53]

When the EGJ is located above the esophageal hiatus and a portion of the stomach is located adjacent to the esophagus, the term combined (or "mixed") sliding and paraesophageal hernia is sometimes used. These hernias can be considered to essentially be sliding hiatal hernias until the paraesophageal component becomes dominant. When superior rotation of the greater curvature is observed, they should be treated as paraesophageal hernias.

A third type of hernia is a short esophagus hiatal hernia (Fig. 5–35). Sometimes considered to be congenital in origin, most are now believed to be acquired secondary to chronic reflux esophagitis. Although GER is often difficult to elicit in patients with sliding hiatal hernias, it is usually readily apparent in those with a short esophagus hiatal hernia.

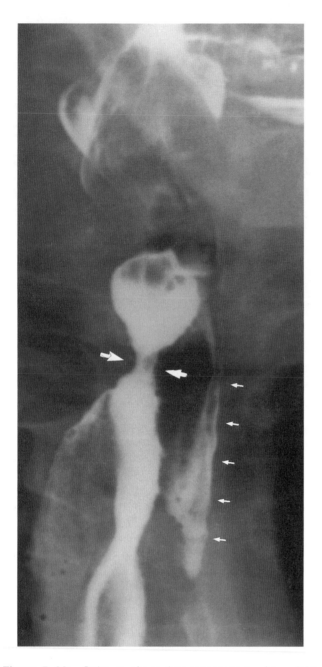

Figure 5–32. Stricture of esophagogastrostomy. An upright, frontal air-contrast view from a barium esophagogram was performed 6 weeks after esophagectomy for T2N0 adenocarcinoma of the proximal third of the esophagus associated with Barrett's mucosa of the distal esophagus. An anastomotic stricture (*arrows*) is causing aspiration of barium into the trachea (*small arrows*) secondary to obstruction of barium and overflow into the trachea.

Esophageal Rings and Web

Mucosal rings are short (2 to 3 mm), diaphragm-like, circumferential indentations commonly observed in the lower part of the esophagus. They are visible only when they are located above the esophageal hiatus and when the esophagus is well distended (see Figs. 5–33 and

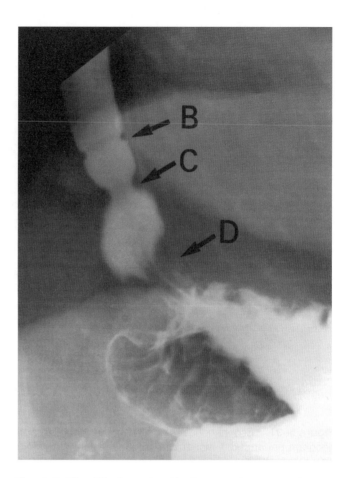

Figure 5–33. Single-contrast barium esophagogram demonstrating a small sliding hiatal hernia. B, mucosal ring; C, muscular ring; D, diaphragmatic impression.

5–35). As a marker of the transition between esophageal squamous epithelium above and columnar gastric epithelium below, they are a useful sign that a hiatal hernia is present. Most have a luminal diameter of at least 2 cm and are asymptomatic. When the diameter is less than 2 cm, patients may have dysphagia. In Schatzki's original article,[54] all patients with ring diameters less than 14 mm were symptomatic. Although some investigations have used the term "Schatzki ring" and "mucosal ring" interchangeably, the term Schatzki ring should be reserved for stenotic rings (<14 mm in diameter) (Fig. 5–36) that are associated with dysphagia and the risk of food impaction to avoid inappropriate interventions in patients with nonobstructive mucosal rings.

Schatzki's rings are idiopathic and not thought to be causally related to reflux esophagitis. Occasionally, however, a peptic stricture from reflux esophagitis may resemble a Schatzki ring. Such rings can usually be distinguished from Schatzki's rings by their more superior location relative to the EGJ and the associated changes of reflux esophagitis (Fig. 5–37). Congenital or idiopathic esophageal webs may also occasionally occur in the lower part of the esophagus (Fig. 5–37), but again are located more superiorly than Schatzki's rings.

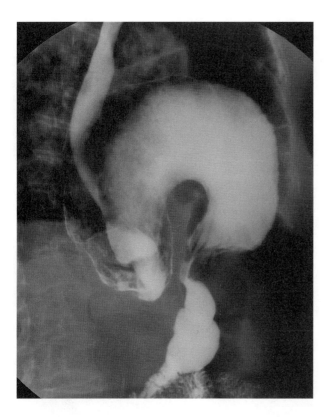

Figure 5–34. Double-contrast upper gastrointestinal examination showing a large paraesophageal hiatal hernia. The greater curvature of the stomach has rotated 180 degrees superiorly ("upside-down, intrathoracic stomach"). The esophagogastric junction has remained within the esophageal hiatus of the diaphragm.

The classic esophageal web occurs in the cervical esophagus, just below the cricopharyngeal muscle (Fig. 5–38). In contradistinction to Schatzki's rings and lower esophageal mucosal rings, cervical esophageal webs are not usually circumferential; rather, they are ∪ shaped and indenting the anterior and lateral walls but sparing the posterior wall. Most cervical esophageal webs measure 1 to 2 mm in thickness, do not narrow the esophageal lumen significantly, and are asymptomatic. They are easily overlooked at fluoroscopy and require maximum luminal distention with large boluses of barium to be detected reliably. Some do narrow the lumen, however, may become circumferential, and may be associated with obstructive symptoms. The common observation of cervical esophageal webs as incidental findings in asymptomatic, otherwise healthy individuals calls into question the classic association of cervical esophageal webs with iron deficiency, splenomegaly, and an underlying predisposition to hypopharyngeal and esophageal cancer (Plummer-Vinson or Paterson-Kelly syndrome).[55,56] Cervical esophageal webs should be differentiated from ectopic gastric mucosa (Fig. 5–39), which produces indentations that may be confused with laterally positioned, incomplete webs. Ectopic gastric mucosa has a classic appearance and location and is asymptomatic.

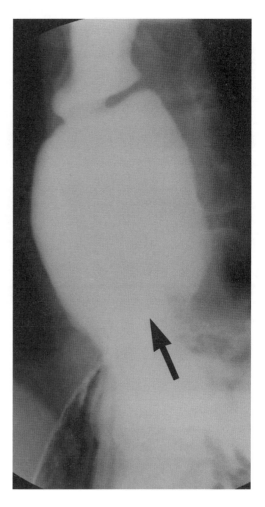

Figure 5–35. Double-contrast upper gastrointestinal examination demonstrating a moderate-sized short esophagus hiatal hernia. Barium is refluxing freely (*arrow*) into the lower part of the esophagus above a mucosal ring.

Muscular rings may be observed in the lower esophagus as transient ring-like narrowings that are longer than mucosal rings and are not normally associated with obstruction (see Fig. 5–33). They occur within the LES mechanism and are considered to be physiologic, unless associated with symptomatic esophageal motility disorders, including achalasia, in which case failure of relaxation of the LES effectively results in a fixed obstructive muscular ring.

Miscellaneous Strictures

The blistering skin diseases cicatricial pemphigoid and epidermolysis bullosa occasionally involve the esophagus.[57,58] Webs and strictures of various length are typical findings (Fig. 5–40), usually more common in the upper part of the esophagus. The skin lesions are the key to diagnosis of the esophageal lesions. The rare skin disorder lichen planus may also involve the esophagus. Strictures may be seen in any portion of the esophagus

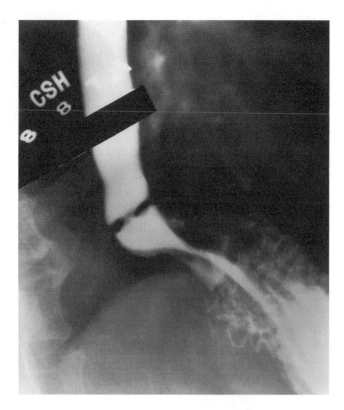

Figure 5–36. Single-contrast barium esophagogram in a patient with dysphagia. A Schatzki ring and a short, stenotic diaphragm-like indentation can be seen in the lower part of the esophagus. The diameter of the ring is less than 1 cm.

and are typically long and smoothly tapered; they may be difficult to detect without adequate luminal distention (Fig. 5–41).

Prolonged nasogastric intubation may result in esophageal strictures. These are, classically, long, smoothly tapered strictures in the mid and lower portions of the esophagus. Reflux esophagitis is thought to be the underlying mechanism of stricture formation, but the nasogastric tube is potentiating and results in a more aggressive, rapidly progressive stricture. In the differential diagnosis of long strictures in the lower part of the esophagus are other conditions that predispose to severe reflux esophagitis, such as severe mental handicap and neglected Zollinger-Ellison syndrome. Ingestion of caustic substances is another important cause of long smooth strictures in the mid and lower esophagus. In patients with lifelong dysphagia and a long smooth stricture of the esophagus, the rare condition of congenital esophageal stenosis should be considered (see Fig. 5–37).[59,60]

Smooth strictures of the midesophagus are often the result of radiation therapy in patients with central lung carcinoma or lymphoma when the midesophagus must be included in the radiation field. Similar strictures may also be the result of extrinsic involvement by adjacent mediastinal lymph nodes in malignant neoplasm or granulomatous infection (Fig. 5–42).

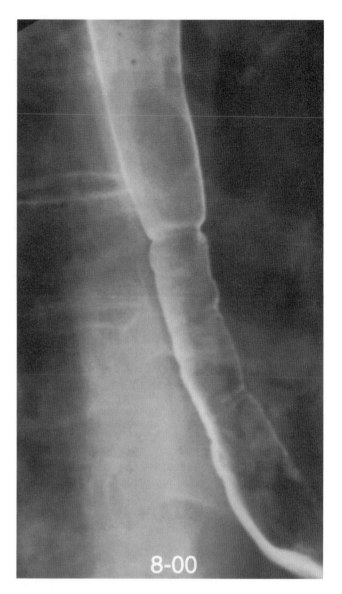

Figure 5–37. Double-contrast barium esophagogram in a 45-year-old woman who had surgery at birth for congenital diaphragmatic hernia. She had medically refractory gastroesophageal reflux disease, mild diffuse narrowing of the lower 3 to 4 cm of the esophagus, and several web-like indentations, findings thought to be due to congenital stenosis of the esophagus with a possible gastroesophageal reflux–related structure.

Eosinophilic esophagitis is a rare cause of esophageal stricture that may be a component of the more generalized condition eosinophilic gastroenteritis, but it is increasingly being recognized as a disorder confined to the esophagus.[61] Strictures usually involve the upper portion or midportion of the esophagus and often have a "corrugated or multiring" appearance, sometimes referred to as "trachealization" of the esophagus (Fig. 5–43). A history of allergy and peripheral eosinophilia is an important clue to the diagnosis.

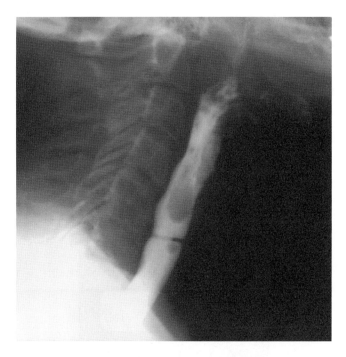

Figure 5–38. Single-contrast barium swallow, lateral view, demonstrating a cervical esophageal web, nonobstructive, and a 1-mm-long indentation in the upper cervical esophagus, most prominent anteriorly.

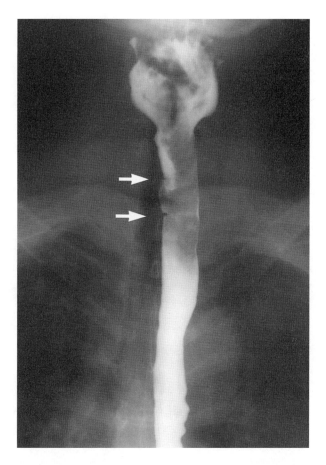

Figure 5–39. Single-contrast barium esophagogram showing ectopic gastric mucosa. Two indentations are evident along the right lateral aspect of the cervical esophagus (*arrows*). Endoscopic biopsy between the indentations confirmed ectopic gastric mucosa.

Patients with Crohn's disease may rarely have esophageal involvement. Manifestations of esophageal Crohn's disease are highly variable, as is true elsewhere in the GI tract, and include ulceration, fold thickening, and stricture (Figs. 5–44 and 5–45). Involvement elsewhere in the colon or small intestine is almost always present, so the diagnosis is usually established when esophageal lesions are discovered.

Caustic Injury

Caustic esophagitis has been a significant medical problem in the United States since the mid-1960s, when liquid solutions of concentrated lye became available as drain cleaners. In children, caustic esophageal injuries result from accidental ingestion, whereas in adults, they usually result from attempted suicide.

The degree of injury varies with the volume and concentration of the caustic agent and the duration of tissue contact.[62] Mild injuries may be confined to the mucosa and heal with little or no sequelae. Severe injuries may result in esophageal perforation, mediastinitis, and death. Patients who survive severe injury are typically left with long, irregular strictures beginning in the mid to upper part of the esophagus. The entire esophagus may be affected, with marked narrowing of the lumen producing a threadlike appearance.[63]

Less severe injury to the esophagus may result from the ingestion of other household products, including ammonium chloride, as well as a variety of medications,[64] such as tetracycline, doxycycline, potassium chloride, quinidine, nonsteroidal anti-inflammatory drugs, and alendronate sodium (Fosamax). Medication-induced esophagitis is a contact esophagitis. Patients at increased risk include those with esophageal motility disorders and those who ingest medications in the recumbent position with insufficient water to propel the medication into the stomach. The diagnosis should be considered in the appropriate clinical context when superficial ulcers are encountered in the midesophagus. In rare instances, deep ulcers and strictures may be seen.

Esophageal Perforation

In addition to caustic ingestion, esophageal perforation may follow blunt or penetrating chest trauma, foreign body ingestion, instrumentation, or breakdown of a surgical anastomosis. Spontaneous perforation (Boerhaave's syndrome) is the result of a sudden, violent increase in intraluminal pressure, usually from extreme

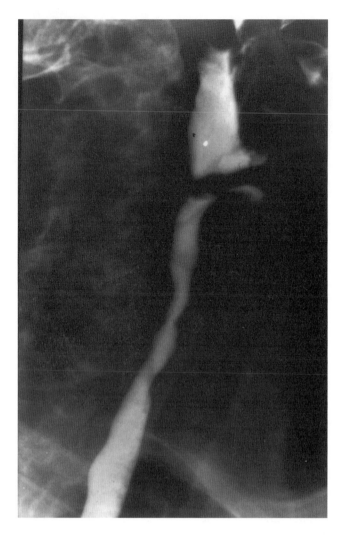

Figure 5–40. Single-contrast barium swallow, left oblique view, from an 86-year-old man with cicatricial pemphigoid and a moderate stricture involving the hypopharynx and upper cervical esophagus. (Note the laryngeal penetration of barium.)

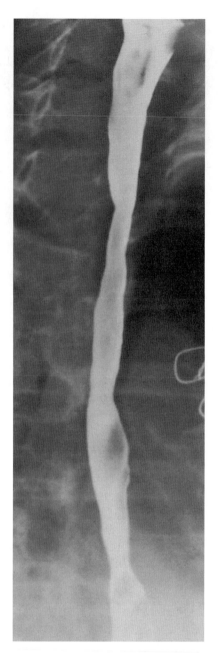

Figure 5–41. Single-contrast barium esophagogram in a 73-year-old woman with oral lichen planus and a moderate, smooth stricture in the mid to upper part of the esophagus, approximately 10 cm in length. Endoscopic biopsies were consistent with lichen planus involving the esophagus.

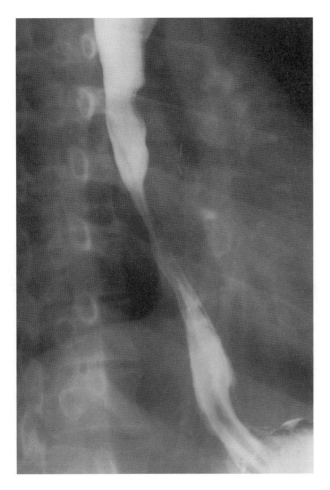

Figure 5–42. Single-contrast barium esophagogram in a 26-year-old man with mediastinal histoplasmosis. Extrinsic narrowing of the midesophagus is due to mediastinal lymphadenopathy.

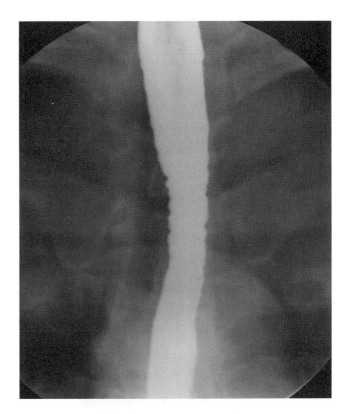

Figure 5–43. Single-contrast barium esophagogram in a 38-year-old man with a long history of dysphagia and food impaction. A midesophageal stricture with a corrugated appearance ("trachealization" of the esophagus) is apparent. Biopsies demonstrated eosinophilic esophagitis.

retching or vomiting, classically after alcoholic binge drinking.

Regardless of cause, esophageal perforations are potentially life threatening and require immediate attention. Localized perforations, especially of the cervical esophagus, may be managed nonoperatively, but perforations of the thoracic esophagus almost always require surgical intervention.[65]

Plain film findings of esophageal rupture include retropharyngeal gas, cervical subcutaneous emphysema, widening of the mediastinum, pneumomediastinum, pleural effusion, and hydropneumothorax (more commonly on the left) (Fig. 5–46A). Rarely, lower esophageal perforations may occur below the diaphragm and produce pneumoperitoneum or retroperitoneal gas collections.

Because plain films are relatively insensitive and often nonspecific, contrast esophagograms should be used early in the investigation of clinically suspected esophageal perforations (Fig. 5–46B). Water-soluble con-

trast agents, either high or low in osmolarity, taken by mouth or injected into a nasogastric tube are the agents of first choice. For patients who are at risk for aspiration (or airway fistula), low-osmolar agents should be used to avoid pulmonary edema, which may result when high-osmolar agents enter the lung.

When water-soluble agents are extravasated into the mediastinum, they are rapidly absorbed and do not incite an inflammatory response. This confers a margin of safety over barium contrast agents, which are nonabsorbable and may incite foreign body granuloma formation.[66,67] Whenever an initial study with water-soluble contrast material is negative, however, it should be immediately followed by a barium esophagogram, which because of its higher density has been reported to increase the sensitivity for detecting esophageal leaks by 15% to 25%.[68,69] The low risk for mediastinal complications from barium extravasation is more than offset by the benefits of earlier diagnosis.

Chest CT is more sensitive in detecting pneumomediastinum than plain films are and is useful after a negative contrast esophagogram in high-risk patients or when contrast esophagograms are difficult to perform in seriously ill patients. With modern, fast scanners, chest

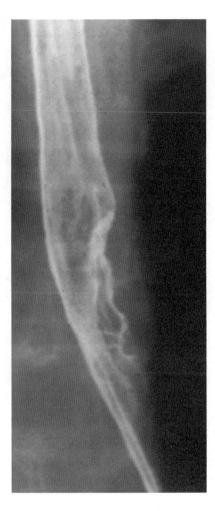

Figure 5–44. Double-contrast barium esophagogram showing Crohn's disease of the esophagus in a 25-year-old man with Crohn's colitis. Thickened, irregular folds can be seen in the lower part of the esophagus. Biopsies demonstrated granulomatous inflammation.

CT can be combined with contrast esophagography to expedite the diagnosis of esophageal rupture.[70]

Diverticula

Esophageal diverticula vary greatly in size, shape, location, cause, and significance. Even incidentally discovered diverticula are important to document because they may predispose the patient to injury during instrumentation.[71]

Traditionally, esophageal diverticula are classified as either traction diverticula, which occur primarily in the midesophagus, or pulsion diverticula, which typically occur in the upper or lower esophagus. In practice, many midesophageal diverticula are pulsion type[72] and are due to increased intraluminal pressure causing "ballooning" of localized weak areas of the esophageal wall around the aortic arch and left main stem bronchus. True traction

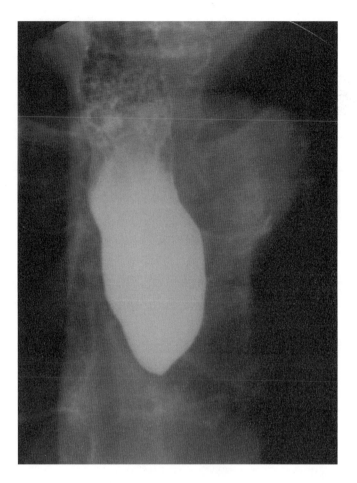

Figure 5–45. Water-soluble contrast esophagogram in a 78-year-old woman with Crohn's disease and an esophageal stricture causing complete obstruction.

diverticula are recognized by elongation, or "tenting," of the diverticulum (Fig. 5–47), typically the result of fibrosis in adjacent lymph nodes involved by granulomatous inflammation.

Pulsion diverticula of the mid and lower part of the esophagus are often associated with an underlying esophageal motor disorder, especially those that are characterized by strong, nonperistaltic tertiary contractions of the muscularis propria, and they are often multiple. In this clinical setting, the motor disorder is more likely to be the cause of symptoms than the diverticula. When large, especially when located near the diaphragm (epiphrenic), pulsion diverticula may empty poorly, thereby serving as a reservoir of ingested food, and become symptomatic (Fig. 5–48).[73]

Zenker's diverticula are pulsion diverticula occurring at the junction of the hypopharynx and cervical esophagus.[74] They are the result of posterior outpouching of the hypopharynx through a weak area near the superior aspect of the cricopharyngeus muscle (Killian's dehiscence) (see Fig. 5–17). Large Zenker's diverticula may retain food and put patients at risk for regurgitation, aspiration, hoarseness, and halitosis. Dysphagia is a common symptom and is usually attributed to a promi-

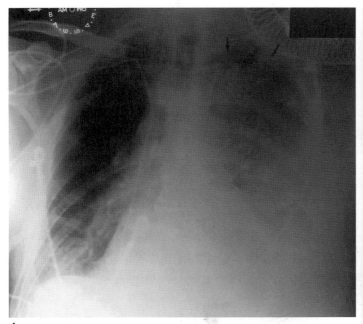

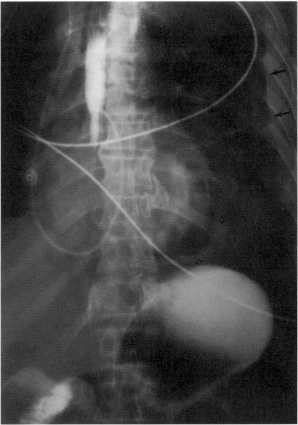

Figure 5–46. **A,** Anteroposterior portable chest radiograph in a patient with Boerhaave's syndrome and left apical pneumothorax (*arrows*). Increased density was noted over the left hemothorax as a result of a left pleural effusion. **B,** Water-soluble contrast upper gastrointestinal examination showing a left pleural effusion (*closed arrows*). A retrocardiac mediastinal collection of gas and contrast medium (*open arrows*) is indicative of esophageal rupture.

nent cricopharyngeus muscle that compromises the hypopharyngeal lumen (Fig. 5–49). Treatment planning should take into account the contribution of a prominent, poorly relaxing (or prematurely closing) cricopharyngeus muscle to the patient's symptoms and formation of the diverticulum.

Just inferior to the cricopharyngeus muscle, in the lateral aspect of the cervical esophagus, is a second area of anatomic weakness. Pulsion diverticula occurring in this region are referred to as lateral cervical esophageal diverticula, or Killian-Jamison diverticula. They can be distinguished from Zenker's diverticula by their location below the cricopharyngeus muscle and their lateral orientation. Most are asymptomatic.

Varices

Though less sensitive than endoscopy, barium esophagography, carefully performed, may demonstrate esophageal varices as undulating, sometimes nodular defects, often easily effaced and transient. They are more commonly seen in the lower part of the esophagus as the result of portal hypertension, usually secondary to cirrhosis ("uphill varices") (Fig. 5–50). Rarely, they may be seen in the upper part of the esophagus secondary to obstruction of the superior vena cava ("downhill varices") (Fig. 5–51).

Esophageal varices are identifiable on contrast-enhanced CT scans as enhancing structures in the esophageal wall supplied by collateral veins. Large varices in and around the lower part of the esophagus may simulate a mediastinal mass or adenopathy on chest films or unenhanced CT scans. CT is well suited to displaying the venous anatomy (in two- or three-dimensional rendering) in addition to providing important related information concerning its cause and associated conditions—such as cirrhosis, splenomegaly, ascites, and hepatocellular carcinoma—as well as superior vena cava obstruction, a mediastinal mass, or adenopathy in patients with "downhill" varices.

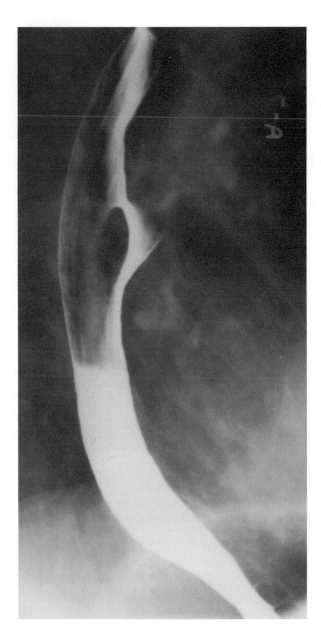

Figure 5–47. Double-contrast barium esophagogram demonstrating a midesophageal traction diverticulum. Note the elongated, "tented" appearance of the diverticulum.

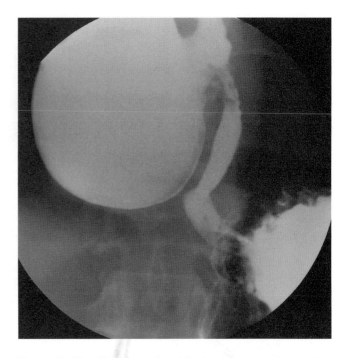

Figure 5–48. Double-contrast barium esophagogram in a 62-year-old man with dysphagia and regurgitation. A large epiphrenic diverticulum is projecting to the right. Barium preferentially filled the diverticulum, with reflux from the diverticulum into the proximal part of the esophagus.

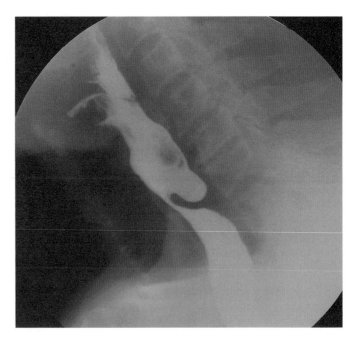

Figure 5–49. Single-contrast barium swallow, lateral view, showing Zenker's diverticulum and a prominent cricopharyngeus muscle encroaching on the lumen. (Note the laryngeal penetration of barium.)

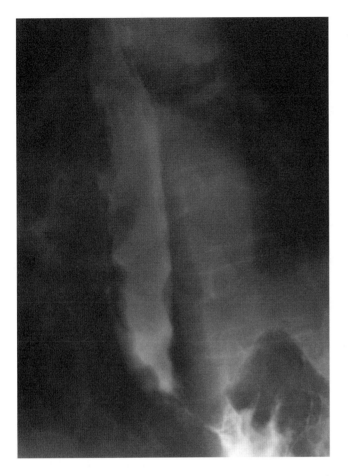

Figure 5–50. Single-contrast barium esophagogram revealing "uphill" varices. Nodular serpentine filling defects are present in the lower part of the esophagus.

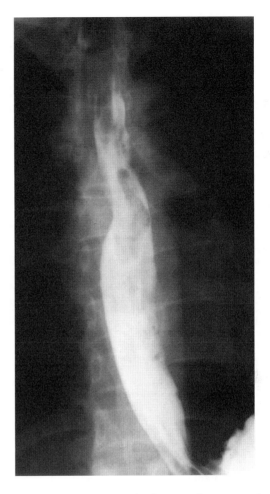

Figure 5–51. Single-contrast barium esophagogram demonstrating "downhill" varices in a 26-year-old man with mediastinal histoplasmosis and superior vena caval obstruction. Smooth, wavy filling defects are present in the upper part of the esophagus.

SUGGESTED READINGS

Enzinger PC, Mayer RJ: Medical progress: Esophageal cancer. N Engl J Med 349:2241-2252, 2003.

Levine MS: Radiology of the Esophagus. Philadelphia, WB Saunders, 1989.

Levine MS: Esophageal cancer: Radiologic diagnosis. Radiol Clin North Am 35:265-279, 1997.

Ott DJ: Motility disorders of the esophagus. Radiol Clin North Am 32:1117-1134, 1994.

Ott DJ: Gastroesophageal reflux disease. Radiol Clin North Am 32:1147-1166, 1994.

Rubesin S, Williams N: Postoperative esophagus. In Gore RM, Levine MS (eds): Textbook of Gastrointestinal Radiology. Philadelphia, WB Saunders, 2000, pp 495-508.

Saunders HS, Wolfman NT, Ott DJ: Esophageal cancer: Radiologic staging. Radiol Clin North Am 35:281-294, 1997.

REFERENCES

1. Gelfand DW: The multiphasic upper gastrointestinal examination. Radiol Clin North Am 32:1067-1081, 1994.
2. Ott DJ, Chen YM, Wu WC, et al: Radiographic and endoscopic sensitivity in detecting lower esophageal mucosal ring. AJR Am J Roentgenol 147:261-265, 1986.
3. Fuller L, Huprich JE, Theisen J, et al: Abnormal esophageal body function: Radiographic-manometric correlation. Am Surg 65:911-914, 1999.
4. Richter JE, Wu WC, Johns DN, et al: Esophageal manometry in 95 healthy adult volunteers. Variability of pressures with age and frequency of "abnormal" contractions. Dig Dis Sci 32:583-592, 1987.
5. Khan TA, Shragge BW, Crispin JS, Lind JF: Esophageal motility in the elderly. Am J Dig Dis 22:1049-1054, 1977.
6. Gallo SH, McClave SA, Makk LJ, Looney SW: Standardization of clinical criteria required for use of the 12.5 millimeter barium tablet in evaluating esophageal luminal patency. Gastrointest Endosc 44:181-184, 1996.
7. Ott DJ, Kelley TF, Chen MY, Gelfand DW: Evaluation of the esophagus with a marshmallow bolus: Clarifying the cause of dysphagia. Gastrointest Radiol 16:1-4, 1991.
8. Ott DJ, Kelley TF, Chen MY, et al: Use of a marshmallow bolus for evaluating lower esophageal mucosal rings. Am J Gastroenterol 86:817-820, 1991.

9. Ekberg O, Lindgren S: Gastroesophageal reflux and pharyngeal function. Acta Radiol 27:421-423, 1986.

10. Levine MS, Chu P, Furth PP, et al: Carcinoma of the esophagus and esophagogastric junction: Sensitivity of radiographic diagnosis. AJR Am J Roentgenol 168:1423-1426, 1997.

11. Robins S, Jankelson IR: Cardioesophageal relaxation. JAMA 87:1961-1964, 1926.

12. DeMeester T, Johnson LF: The evaluation of objective measurements of gastroesophageal reflux and their contribution to patient management. Surg Clin North Am 56:39-53, 1976.

13. Thompson JK, Koehler RE, Richter JE: Detection of gastroesophageal reflux: Value of barium studies compared with 24-hr pH monitoring. AJR Am J Roentgenol 162:621-626, 1994.

14. Johnston BT, Troshnisky MB, Castell JA, Castell DO: Comparison of barium radiology with esophageal pH monitoring in the diagnosis of gastroesophageal reflux disease. Am J Gastroenterol 91:1181-1185, 1996.

15. Crummy A: The water test in the evaluation of gastroesophageal reflux. Its correlation with pyrosis. Radiology 87:501-504, 1966.

16. Linsman J: Gastroesophageal reflux elicited while drinking water (water siphonage test): Its clinical correlation with pyrosis. AJR Am J Roentgenol 94:325-332, 1965.

17. Hewson EG, Ott DJ, Dalton CB, et al: Manometry and radiology. Complementary studies in the assessment of esophageal motility disorders. Gastroenterology 98:626-632, 1990.

18. Ott DJ, Gelfand DW, Wu WC: Reflux esophagitis: Radiographic and endoscopic correlation. Radiology 130:583-588, 1979.

19. Gupta S, Levine MS, Rubesin SE, et al: Usefulness of barium studies for differentiating benign and malignant strictures of the esophagus. AJR Am J Roentgenol 180:737-744, 2003.

20. Ott DJ, Chen YM, Wu WC, et al: Endoscopic sensitivity in the detection of esophageal strictures. J Clin Gastroenterol 7:121-125, 1985.

21. Glick SN, Teplick SK, Amenta PS: The radiologic diagnosis of Barrett esophagus: Importance of mucosal surface abnormalities on air-contrast barium studies. AJR Am J Roentgenol 157:951-954, 1991.

22. Chen M, Frederick MG: Barrett esophagus and adenocarcinoma. Radiol Clin North Am 32:1167-1181, 1994.

23. Glick SN: Barium studies in patients with Barrett's esophagus: Importance of focal areas of esophageal deformity. AJR Am J Roentgenol 163:65-67, 1994.

24. Yamamoto AJ, Levine MS, Katzka DA, et al: Short-segment Barrett's esophagus: Findings on double-contrast esophagography in 20 patients. AJR Am J Roentgenol 176:1173-1178, 2001.

25. Spechler SJ, Castell DO: Classification of esophageal motility abnormalities. Gut 49:145-151, 2001.

26. Ott DJ: Motility disorders of the esophagus. Radiol Clin North Am 32:1117-1134, 1994.

27. Ott DJ, Richter JE, Chen YM, et al: Esophageal radiography and manometry: Correlation in 172 patients with dysphagia. AJR Am J Roentgenol 149:307-311, 1987.

28. Woodfield CA, Levine CA, Rubesin SE, et al: Diagnosis of primary versus secondary achalasia: Reassessment of clinical and radiographic criteria. AJR Am J Roentgenol 175:727-731, 2000.

29. Prabhakar A, Levine MS, Rubesin S, et al: Relationship between diffuse esophageal spasm and lower esophageal sphincter dysfunction on barium studies and manometry in 14 patients. AJR Am J Roentgenol 183:409-413, 2004.

30. Shakespear JS, Blom D, Huprich JE, Peters JH: Correlation of radiographic and manometric findings in patients with ineffective esophageal motility. Surg Endosc 18:459-462, 2004.

31. Jemal A, Tiwari RC, Murray T, et al: Cancer statistics 2004. CA Cancer J Clin 54:8-29, 2004.

32. Blot WJ, Devesa SS, Kneller RW, Fraumeni JF Jr: Rising incidence of adenocarcinoma of the esophagus and gastric cardia. JAMA 265:1287-1289, 1991.

33. Levine MS, Chu P, Furth EE, et al: Carcinoma of the esophagus and esophagogastric junction: Sensitivity of radiographic diagnosis. AJR Am J Roentgenol 168:1423-1426, 1997.

34. Gore RM: Esophageal cancer: Clinical and pathologic features. Radiol Clin North Am 35:243-263, 1997.

35. Iyer RB, Silverman PM, Tamm EP, et al: Diagnosis, staging, and follow-up of esophageal cancer. AJR Am J Roentgenol 181:785-793, 2003.

36. Flanagan FL, Dehdashti F, Siegel BA, et al: Staging of esophageal cancer with ^{18}F-fluorodeoxyglucose positron emission tomography. AJR Am J Roentgenol 168:417-424, 1997.

37. Flamen P, Lerut A, Van Cutsem E, et al: Utility of positron emission tomography for the staging of patients with potentially operable esophageal carcinoma. J Clin Oncol 18:3202-3210, 2000.

38. Rasanen JV, Sihvo EI, Knuuti MJ, et al: Prospective analysis of accuracy of positron emission tomography, computed tomography, and endoscopic ultrasonography in staging of adenocarcinoma of the esophagus and the esophagogastric junction. Ann Surg Oncol 10:954-960, 2003.

39. Rice TW: Clinical staging of esophageal carcinoma. CT, EUS, and PET. Chest Surg Clin N Am 10:471-485, 2000.

40. Luketich JD, Schauer PR, Meltzer CC, et al: Role of positron emission tomography in staging esophageal cancer. Ann Thorac Surg 64:765-769, 1997.

41. Weber WA, Ott K, Becker K, et al: Prediction of response to preoperative chemotherapy in adenocarcinomas of the esophagogastric junction by metabolic imaging. J Clin Oncol 19:3058-3065, 2001.

42. Flamen P, Lerut A, Van Cutsem E, et al: The utility of positron emission tomography for the diagnosis and staging of recurrent esophageal cancer. J Thorac Cardiovasc Surg 120:1085-1092, 2000.

43. Rubesin S, Williams N: Postoperative esophagus. In Gore RM, Levine MS (eds): Textbook of Gastrointestinal Radiology, 2nd ed. Philadelphia, WB Saunders, 2000, pp 495-508.

44. Orringer M: Complications of esophageal surgery. In Orringer M, Heitmiller R (eds): Shackelford's Surgery of the Alimentary Tract, 5th ed. Philadelphia, WB Saunders, 2002, pp 443-571.

45. Kim SH, Lee KS, Shim YM, et al: Esophageal resection: indications, techniques, and radiologic assessment. Radiographics 21:1119-1137, discussion 1138-1140, 2001.

46. Maher M, Lucey BC, Boland G, et al: The role of interventional radiology in the treatment of mediastinal fluid collections caused by esophageal anastomotic leaks. AJR Am J Roentgenol 178:649-653, 2002.

47. Swanson JO, Levine MS, Redfern RO, Rubesin SE: Usefulness of high-density barium for detection of leaks after esophagogastrectomy, total gastrectomy, and total laryngectomy. AJR Am J Roentgenol 181:415-420, 2003.

48. Levine MS: Miscellaneous Abnormalities of the Esophagus. Philadelphia, WB Saunders, 2000, pp 465-483.

49. Sydow BD, Levine MS, Rubesin SE, Laufer I: Radiographic findings and complications after surgical or endoscopic repair of Zenker's diverticulum in 16 patients. AJR Am J Roentgenol 177:1067-1071, 2001.

50. Rubesin SE, Kennedy M, Levine MS, et al: Distal esophageal ballooning following Heller myotomy. Radiology 167:345-347, 1988.

51. Ott DJ, Gelfand DW, Chen YM, et al: Predictive relationship of hiatal hernia to reflux esophagitis. Gastrointest Radiol 10:317-321, 1985.

52. Hill LD: Incarcerated paraesophageal hernia: A surgical emergency. Am J Surg 126:286-291, 1973.

53. Dunn DB, Quick G: Incarcerated paraesophageal hernia. Am J Emerg Med 8:36-39, 1990.

54. Schatzki RGJ: Dysphagia due to diaphragm-like localized narrowing in the lower esophagus (lower esophageal ring). Radiology 70:911, 1953.

55. Waldenström J, Kjeulberg SR: The roentgenological diagnosis of sideropenic dysphagia (Plummer-Vinson's syndrome). Acta Radiol 20:618-638, 1939.

56. Chisholm M: The association between webs, iron and postcricoid carcinoma. Postgrad Med J 50:215-219, 1974.

57. Mauro MA, Parker LA, Hartley WS, et al: Epidermolysis bullosa: Radiographic findings in 16 cases. Am J Radiol 149:925-927, 1987.

58. Naylor MF, MacCarty RL, Rogers RS 3rd: Barium studies in esophageal cicatricial pemphigoid. Abdom Imaging 20:97-100, 1995.

59. Dominiquez R, Zarabi M, Oh KS, et al: Congenital esophageal stenosis. Clin Radiol 36:263-266, 1985.

60. Pokieser P, Schima W, Schober E, et al: Congenital esophageal stenosis in a 21-year-old man: Clinical and radiographic findings. AJR Am J Roentgenol 170:147-148, 1998.

61. Croese J, Fairley SK, Masson JW, et al: Clinical and endoscopic features of eosinophilic esophagitis in adults. Gastrointest Endosc 58:516-522, 2003.

62. Goldman LP, Weigert JM: Corrosive substance ingestion: A review. Am J Gastroenterol 79:85-90, 1984.

63. Franken EA: Caustic damage of the gastrointestinal tract: Roentgen features. AJR Am J Roentgenol 118:77-85, 1973.

64. Bova JG, Dutton NE, Goldstein HM, et al: Medication-induced esophagitis: Diagnosis by double-contrast esophagography. AJR Am J Roentgenol 148:731-732, 1987.

65. Port JL, Kent MS, Korst RJ, et al: Thoracic esophageal perforations: A decade of experience. Ann Thorac Surg 75:1071-1074, 2003.

66. James AE, Montali RJ, Chaffee V, et al: Barium or Gastrografin: Which contrast media for diagnosis of esophageal tears? Gastroenterology 68:1103-1113, 1975.

67. Vessal K, Montali RJ, Larson SM, et al: Evaluation of barium and Gastrografin as contrast media for the diagnosis of esophageal ruptures or complications. AJR Am J Roentgenol 123:307-319, 1975.

68. Buecker A, Wein BB, Neuerburg JM, et al: Esophageal perforation: Comparison of use of aqueous and barium-containing contrast media. Radiology 202:683-686, 1997.

69. Foley MJ, Ghahremani GG, Rogers LF: Reappraisal of contrast media used to detect upper gastrointestinal perforations. Radiology 144:213-237, 1982.

70. Fadoo F, Ruiz DE, Dawn SK, et al: Helical CT esophagography for the evaluation of suspected esophageal perforation or rupture. AJR Am J Roentgenol 182:1177-1179, 2004.

71. Nutter KM, Ball OG: Esophageal diverticula: Current classification and important complications. J Miss State Med Assoc 45:131-135, 2004.

72. Schima W, Schober E, Stacher G, et al: Association of mid esophageal diverticula with oesophageal motor disorders: Videofluoroscopy and manometry. Acta Radiol 38:108-114, 1997.

73. Fasano NC, Levine MS, Rubesin SE, et al: Epiphrenic diverticulum: Clinical and radiographic findings in 27 patients. Dysphagia 18:9-15, 2003.

74. Perrott JW: Anatomical aspects of hypopharyngeal diverticula. Aust N Z J Surg 31:307-317, 1962.

6

Endoscopic Evaluation of the Esophagus

Stuart Jon Spechler · Jacques J. G. H. M. Bergman

The endoscopist who examines the esophagus evaluates a muscular tube whose primary function is to convey swallowed material from the mouth to the stomach. The esophagus is approximately 25 cm in length measured from its origin in the neck just below the cricoid cartilage (C6 level, approximately 15 cm from the incisor teeth as measured by the endoscopist) to its termination in the abdomen at the gastric cardia (T10-T11 level, approximately 40 cm from the incisor teeth).[1] Proximally, the upper esophageal sphincter (UES) separates the pharynx from the esophagus. The UES extends approximately 3 cm in length and comprises three skeletal muscle groups, including the distal portion of the inferior pharyngeal constrictor, the cricopharyngeus, and the circular muscle of the proximal esophagus.[2] Introduction of the endoscope into the UES often causes gagging, and the muscles relax only briefly during a swallow. Consequently, the endoscope is typically passed quickly through the UES, and endoscopic visualization of its mucosal lining is frequently limited.

The esophagus passes from the chest into the abdomen through the diaphragmatic hiatus, a canal-shaped opening in the right crus of the diaphragm. Approximately 2 cm of the distal end of the esophagus normally lies within the abdomen.[3] The lower esophageal sphincter (LES) comprises both the skeletal muscle of the crural diaphragm (external LES muscle) and the circular smooth muscle of the distal esophagus itself (internal LES muscle), although endoscopists often refer only to the latter when describing the LES. Unlike the UES, endoscopic examination of the LES region is not generally limited either by sustained sphincter muscle contraction or by patient discomfort.

The esophageal lumen is collapsed at rest and must be distended with air during endoscopy so that the stratified squamous epithelial lining can be visualized well. When so distended, the squamous epithelium appears pale, glossy, and relatively featureless. Within the chest at about the T4 level, the esophagus is indented on its left side by the aortic arch. This pulsating indentation can be noted during endoscopic examination at a distance of approximately 23 cm from the incisor teeth (Fig. 6–1).[4] Just below the arch at approximately 25 cm, the left main bronchus causes a subtle indentation on the left anterior aspect of the esophagus (see Fig. 6–1). Below the bronchus, the esophagus abuts the left atrium. The heart normally causes no prominent indentation of the esophageal lumen, but atrial pulsations can often be visualized at a level approximately 30 cm from the incisor teeth.

ENDOSCOPIC EVALUATION OF THE GASTROESOPHAGEAL JUNCTION

The gastroesophageal junction (GEJ) is the level at which the esophagus ends and the stomach begins. Unfortunately, there are no universally accepted landmarks that clearly delimit the distal end of the esophagus and the proximal part of the stomach, and the GEJ has been defined differently by anatomists, radiologists, physiologists, and endoscopists.[5] Landmarks suggested by anatomists, such as the peritoneal reflection or the character of the muscle bundles in the esophageal wall, are not useful for endoscopists. Radiologists refer to the region of the GEJ as the vestibule, and they seldom attempt to localize the precise point at which the esophagus joins the stomach.[6] Physiologists have used the distal border of the LES (determined manometrically) to define the GEJ,[7] but it is difficult to identify this border precisely by endoscopic techniques. Indeed, one study has shown that manometric and endoscopic localization of the LES often differs by several centimeters.[8]

When considering any proposed landmark for the GEJ, it is important to appreciate that there is no clear-cut "gold standard" for the structure and, consequently, all of the suggested landmarks can be considered arbitrary. Furthermore, for most disorders of the esophagus and stomach that are diagnosed endoscopically, it is not

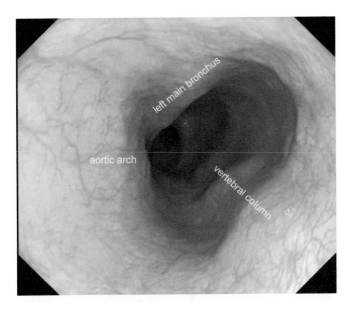

Figure 6–1. Endoscopic photograph of the proximal end of the esophagus showing the normal indentations caused by the aortic arch, the left main bronchus, and the vertebral column.

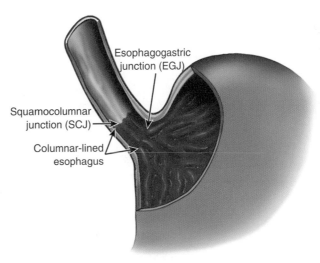

Figure 6–2. Endoscopic landmarks. The squamocolumnar junction (SCJ or Z-line) is the visible line formed by the juxta-position of squamous and columnar epithelia. The esopha-gogastric junction (EGJ) is the imaginary line at which the esophagus ends and the stomach begins. The most proximal extent of the gastric folds has been proposed as a marker for the EGJ. When the SCJ is located proximal to the EGJ, there is a columnar-lined segment of esophagus. (From Spechler SJ: The role of gastric carditis in metaplasia and neoplasia at the gastroesophageal junction. Gastroenterology 117:218-228, 1999.)

important that the GEJ be identified with great precision. For some disorders, most notably Barrett's esophagus, for which the endoscopist must determine the extent of esophageal columnar lining, precise localization of the GEJ can be critical for establishing the diagnosis.

Suggested endoscopic criteria for the GEJ include the level at which the tubular esophagus flares to become the sack-like stomach,[9] the proximal margin of the gastric folds when the esophagus and stomach are partially dis-tended,[10] and the distal end of the esophageal palisade vessels.[11,12] Although these landmarks may be readily recognized in still photographs of the junction region, the distal esophagus in vivo is a dynamic structure whose appearance changes from moment to moment. The loca-tion of the point of flare changes with respiratory and peristaltic activity. The proximal gastric folds can pro-lapse transiently up into the esophagus. The appearance of the junction region also varies with the degree of dis-tention of the esophagus and stomach, and the palisade vessels can be difficult to identify with conventional endoscopes.

The proximal extent of the gastric folds is the land-mark for the GEJ used frequently by Western endos-copists (Figs. 6–2 to 6–4).[13] This landmark was proposed by McClave et al. in 1987 based on their endoscopic observations in only four subjects who were identified as normal controls because they had "no clinical evidence of esophageal disease."[10] The junction between squa-mous and columnar epithelia (the SCJ) was located within 2 cm of the gastric folds in all of these four sub-jects, and thus the authors concluded that the diagnosis of columnar-lined esophagus should be considered only when the SCJ is located more than 2 cm above the GEJ (i.e., the proximal level of the gastric folds). This study can be criticized both for the small number of control subjects and for the lack of documentation that the four

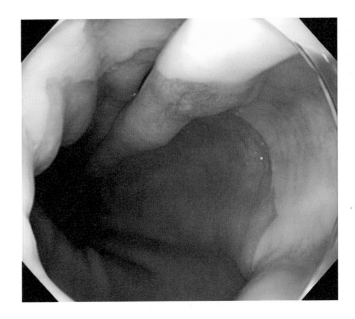

Figure 6–3. Endoscopic photograph of the gastro-esophageal junction region in a patient who has a hiatal hernia. The squamocolumnar junction (SCJ) is located above some of the gastric folds (i.e., there is a columnar-lined segment of esophagus), whereas for others the SCJ seems to coincide with the proximal extent of the folds.

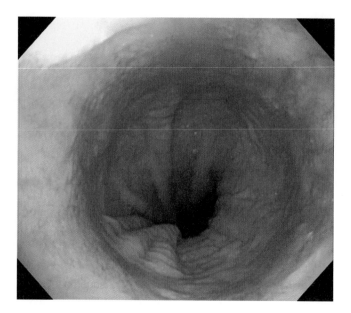

Figure 6–4. Endoscopic photograph of the gastro-esophageal junction region in a patient with long-segment Barrett's esophagus. Columnar epithelium extends above the tops of the gastric folds to involve the distal end of the esophagus in a circumferential fashion.

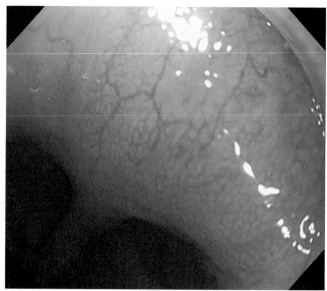

Figure 6–5. The palisade vessels in the distal part of the esophagus are fine, longitudinal veins in the lamina propria. The distal end of the palisade vessels has been proposed as an endoscopic landmark for the gastroesophageal junction.

controls were indeed normal. Esophageal pH monitoring studies were not performed, and therefore it is not clear that the control subjects had normal esophageal acid exposure. Biopsy specimens of the columnar-lined esophagus were not taken, and thus short-segment Barrett's esophagus was not excluded (see later). Furthermore, three of the four control subjects had hiatal hernias and one had reflux esophagitis. It seems surprising that a proposed landmark based on such questionable data has been so widely accepted by endoscopists.

A number of Asian investigators use the end of the esophageal palisade vessels as their landmark for the GEJ (Fig. 6–5).[12] Elegant anatomic studies of the GEJ have revealed four distinct zones of venous drainage, including a gastric zone, a palisade zone, a perforating zone, and a truncal zone.[14] The palisade zone comprises a group of fine, longitudinal veins located largely within the lamina propria of the distal esophagus. The palisade vessels pierce the muscularis mucosae distally to join the submucosal vessels of the gastric zone and proximally to join the submucosal vessels of the perforating zone. The palisade vessels can be difficult to visualize by conventional endoscopy, especially if there is distal esophageal inflammation. The appearance of these vessels can be enhanced by narrow-band imaging endoscopy, which uses primarily blue light that penetrates only the superficial layers of the mucosa (where the palisade vessels are found) and is absorbed by the hemoglobin within the vessels. Presently, narrow-band imaging is not widely available. Furthermore, even in autopsy studies in which blood vessels of the GEJ region are injected with resins that provide exquisite detail of the venous structures, it

is difficult to precisely identify the termination of the palisade vessels.[14] Finally, it is not clear conceptually why the distal end of the palisade vessels should be considered the precise end of the esophagus.

Few studies have specifically addressed the problem of endoscopic localization of the GEJ, and even in those that have done so, the accuracy of the criteria used cannot be assessed meaningfully in the absence of a gold standard. It is not clear which is the best diagnostic criterion for the GEJ, and reproducibility of the various criteria has not been established. If one cannot determine with certainty where the esophagus ends and the stomach begins, any assessment of the extent of esophagus lined by columnar epithelium will be inherently imprecise. This unresolved problem continues to confound clinicians and investigators who deal with Barrett's esophagus.

CONVENTIONAL ENDOSCOPIC DIAGNOSIS OF BARRETT'S ESOPHAGUS

Endoscopic examination is required to establish a diagnosis of Barrett's esophagus, and the endoscopic impression must be confirmed by histologic evaluation of biopsy specimens from the columnar-lined esophagus. Specifically, the endoscopist must ensure that the following two criteria are fulfilled[13]: (1) columnar epithelium lines the distal esophagus, and (2) biopsy specimens of the columnar-lined esophagus show specialized intestinal metaplasia. To document that columnar epithelium lines the esophagus, the endoscopist must identify both the SCJ and GEJ (see Fig. 6–2). Columnar epithelium has

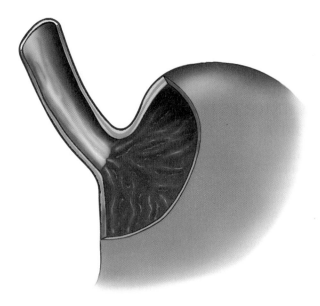

Figure 6–6. In this drawing, the gastroesophageal junction and the Z-line coincide, and there is no columnar-lined segment of esophagus.

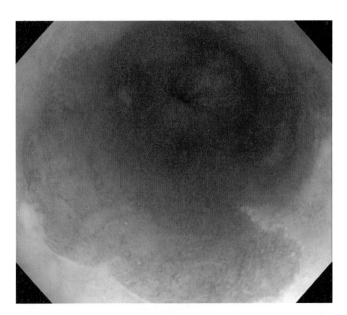

Figure 6–7. In this patient with long-segment Barrett's esophagus, the Z-line is relatively smooth.

a reddish color and coarse texture on endoscopic examination, whereas squamous epithelium has a pale, glossy appearance. The juxtaposition of these epithelia at the SCJ forms a visible line called the Z-line. As discussed, Western endoscopists generally identify the GEJ as the level of the most proximal extent of the gastric folds. The distal extent of the palisade vessels can also be used as a marker for the GEJ, but this level may differ from that of the proximal extent of the gastric folds. When the SCJ and GEJ coincide (Fig. 6–6), the entire esophagus is lined by squamous epithelium. When the SCJ is located proximal to the GEJ (see Fig. 6–2), there is a columnar-lined segment of esophagus. If the endoscopist takes biopsy specimens from that columnar-lined segment and histologic evaluation shows specialized intestinal metaplasia, the patient has Barrett's esophagus.

Several classification systems for Barrett's esophagus have been proposed on the basis of the extent of columnar-lined esophagus and the appearance of the Z-line. Perhaps the most widely used system classifies patients as having either "long-segment" or "short-segment" Barrett's esophagus.[15] Patients have long-segment Barrett's esophagus when the distance between the GEJ and the most proximal extent of the Z-line is 3 cm or more, and they have short-segment Barrett's esophagus when that distance is less than 3 cm. The cutoff value of 3 cm is arbitrary, and this classification has no clear implications regarding the pathogenesis of the condition or the clinical management of affected patients. Furthermore, there can be substantial variation in the appearance of the Z-line in patients with Barrett's esophagus (Figs. 6–7 to 6–9), and the short-long classification provides no specific information about that appearance.

In 2000, Wallner et al. proposed the ZAP (*Z*-line *AP*pearance) classification for evaluating the SCJ. The

ZAP classification has four categories[16]: grade 0—the Z-line is sharp and circular; grade I—the Z-line is irregular and there are tongue-like protrusions or islands of columnar epithelium (or both); grade II—there is a distinct, obvious tongue of columnar epithelium less than 3 cm in length; and grade III—there are distinct tongues of columnar epithelium greater than 3 cm in length, or the Z-line is displaced cephalad more than 3 cm. The likelihood of finding intestinal metaplasia (and hence having Barrett's esophagus) was shown to increase sig-

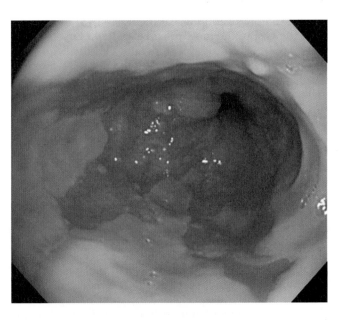

Figure 6–8. In this patient with short-segment Barrett's esophagus, the Z-line is jagged and eccentric.

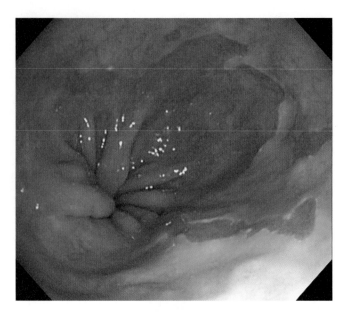

Figure 6–9. In this patient with short-segment Barrett's esophagus, the Z-line extends approximately 2 cm above the gastroesophageal junction (the tops of the gastric folds) on the right, but there is virtually no columnar-lined esophagus on the left.

nificantly with increasing ZAP grades, and the classification was found to have excellent reproducibility among endoscopists.[17] However, the clinical utility of the ZAP classification has not been established.

The International Working Group on the Classification of Oesophagitis is developing a "C and M" classification system for Barrett's esophagus that describes both the extent of circumferential metaplasia (C, measured from the GEJ to the most proximal extent of circumferential esophageal metaplasia) and the extent of the longest tongue of esophageal metaplasia (M, measured from the GEJ to the most proximal extent of esophageal metaplasia).[18] For example, a patient classified as C2M5 has columnar metaplasia involving the distal 2 cm of the esophagus in a circumferential fashion with a tongue of metaplasia that extends 5 cm above the GEJ. Presently, the advantages (if any) of this system over the others have not been established.

Some have argued that the term "Barrett's esophagus" itself is artificial and that the condition has been defined variably by investigators who have imposed arbitrary criteria that fit their personal perspectives.[19] In 1996, Spechler and Goyal proposed a simple classification system as follows: whenever columnar epithelium is seen in the esophagus, regardless of extent, the condition is called "columnar-lined esophagus." In these cases, biopsy specimens can be obtained from the esophageal columnar lining to seek specialized intestinal metaplasia. The condition can then be classified as either "columnar-lined esophagus with specialized intestinal metaplasia" or "columnar-lined esophagus without specialized intestinal metaplasia." Despite the simplicity and conceptual appeal of this system, the term Barrett's esophagus has

become so firmly entrenched among clinicians that it is unlikely to be abandoned.

SPECIALIZED ENDOSCOPIC TECHNIQUES FOR BARRETT'S ESOPHAGUS

A variety of specialized endoscopic techniques are available for the evaluation of Barrett's esophagus, including chromoendoscopy, magnification endoscopy, narrow-band imaging, endosonography, optical coherence tomography, and spectroscopy using reflectance, absorption, light-scattering, fluorescence, and Raman detection methods.[20-25] These techniques have been used to enhance the identification of both intestinal metaplasia in the esophagus and neoplasia in Barrett's esophagus. Only chromoendoscopy, magnification endoscopy, and narrow-band imaging will be discussed in this chapter.

In chromoendoscopy, the esophageal mucosa is painted either with dyes that stain the cells that absorb them or with dyes that accumulate in mucosal crevices to enhance the architectural features of the epithelium. When potassium iodide is absorbed by squamous epithelial cells, it binds to their glycogen and stains them brown. Application of this dye can help delineate the SCJ. For individuals who are at high risk for squamous cell cancer of the esophagus (e.g., patients who have had cancer of the head and neck, individuals living in high-incidence areas for squamous cell carcinoma such as northern China), potassium iodide staining has also been used to identify areas of early neoplasia in the squamous epithelium. Methylene blue dye is absorbed by intestinal-type cells, and this dye can be applied to identify areas of intestinal metaplasia in Barrett's esophagus. In addition, areas of dysplasia and early cancer in the specialized intestinal metaplasia of Barrett's esophagus can be identified by their failure to absorb methylene blue. One recent report has shown that application of methylene blue may cause DNA damage in Barrett's esophagus, and thus the use of this dye could conceivably be dangerous.[26] Indigo carmine is a chromoendoscopy dye that is not absorbed and is used to enhance architectural features. Cresyl violet dye stains the columnar cells that absorb it purple, and the dye also accumulates in crevices to enhance architectural features. Acetic acid, though not a dye, is often sprayed on the mucosa before chromoendoscopy as a mucolytic agent. Application of acetic acid also causes the columnar epithelium to swell, and this effect may enhance the evaluation of architectural features.

In magnification endoscopy, an optical zoom device is used to magnify the mucosa up to 150-fold. Magnification endoscopy is often combined with chromoendoscopy as just described. Investigators using this technique have identified a variety of "pit patterns" that might be typical of the intestinal metaplasia of Barrett's esophagus (Figs. 6–10 and 6–11).[27-29] Magnification endoscopy can also be combined with narrow-band imaging, which uses primarily blue light that penetrates

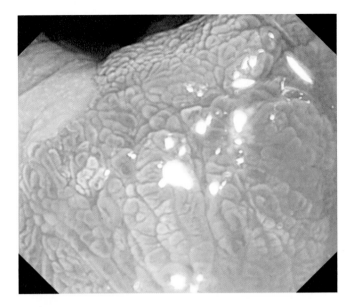

Figure 6–10. Magnification endoscopy of mucosa sprayed with acetic acid showing the pit pattern of columnar epithelium at the squamocolumnar junction. The relatively featureless squamous epithelium is seen adjacent to the columnar epithelium in the upper left corner of the slide.

only the superficial layers of the mucosa and is absorbed by hemoglobin (Fig. 6–12).

ENDOSCOPIC DIAGNOSIS OF REFLUX ESOPHAGITIS

Gastroesophageal reflux disease (GERD) is a condition in which gastric juice that refluxes into the esophagus

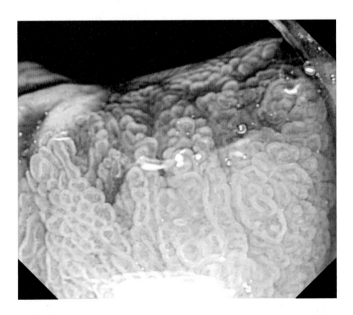

Figure 6–11. Magnification endoscopy of the region shown in Figure 6–10 after the application of indigo carmine dye.

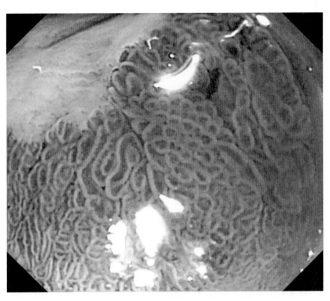

Figure 6–12. Magnification endoscopy of the region shown in Figure 6–10 combined with narrow-band imaging.

causes symptoms, tissue injury, or both.[30] Heartburn is the most common symptom of GERD, and tissue injury results when esophageal epithelial cells succumb to the caustic effects of the refluxed acid and pepsin. When these caustic agents cause macroscopic injury to the esophageal epithelium, the endoscopist can make a diagnosis of reflux esophagitis. However, more than 50% of patients who have typical GERD symptoms have normal endoscopic examinations.[31,32] Thus, it appears that GERD does not usually cause visible damage to the esophageal mucosa in most patients.

Mild changes of GERD that may be visible to the endoscopist include mucosal erythema, edema, hypervascularity, friability, and blurring of the SCJ. Identification of these changes is a subjective skill, however, and agreement among endoscopists regarding the presence of such minimal signs of reflux esophagitis can be very poor.[33,34] More severe GERD can result in esophageal erosions and ulcerations. Histologically, erosions are defined as superficial necrotic defects that do not penetrate the muscularis mucosae, whereas ulcerations are deeper defects that extend through the muscularis mucosae into the submucosa.[35] Endoscopically, these peptic esophageal lesions are identified on the basis of their gross features, and clinicians seldom have histologic confirmation that the lesions they call "esophageal ulcers" have in fact breached the muscularis mucosae. Thus, the distinction between esophageal ulceration and erosion is usually based on a subjective assessment of the depth of the necrotic lesion. One modern system for grading the severity of reflux esophagitis, the Los Angeles classification, avoids the problem of distinguishing erosions from ulcerations by referring to both as "mucosal breaks."[36]

More than 30 systems for the classification of reflux esophagitis have been proposed over the past few decades.[36] The endoscopic criteria for three of the most widely used systems are listed in Table 6–1.[34,36-38] All of the

Table 6–1 Classification Systems for Reflux Esophagitis

The Savary Miller Classification

Grade 0   Normal mucosa
Grade I   Discrete areas of erythema
Grade II   Noncircumferential erosions
Grade III Circumferential erosions
Grade IV   GERD complications (ulcers, strictures, Barrett's esophagus)

The MUSE (Metaplasia, Ulceration, Stricture, Erosion) Classification

	Metaplasia	Ulceration	Stricture	Erosion
Grade 0	M0 absent	U0 absent	S0 absent	E0 absent
Grade 1	M1 one	U1 one	S1 > 9 mm	E1 one
Grade 2	M2 circumferential	U2 ≥ 2	S2 ≤ 9	E2 circumferential

The Los Angeles Classification

Grade A   ≥1 Mucosal break <5 mm long that does not extend between the tops of 2 mucosal folds
Grade B   ≥1 Mucosal break >5 mm long that does not extend between the tops of 2 mucosal folds
Grade C   ≥1 Mucosal break that extends between tops of ≥2 mucosal folds involving <75% of the esophageal circumference
Grade D   ≥1 Mucosal break that involves ≥75% of the esophageal circumference

proposed systems have limitations, and no individual system has been shown to be clearly superior to another for establishing the diagnosis of GERD or for predicting the response to treatment. Arguably, the best validated and most widely used system is now the Los Angeles classification, which was proposed at the meeting of the World Congress of Gastroenterology in Los Angeles in 1994.[36] In this system, a mucosal break is defined as "an area of slough or erythema with a discrete line of demarcation from the adjacent, more normal-looking mucosa" (Fig. 6–13A and B). Esophagitis is graded on a scale of A to D, depending on the length and circumferential extent of the mucosal breaks (Fig. 6–14A and B; see also Fig. 6–13). Los Angeles grades C and D represent severe reflux esophagitis. Originally, grade D esophagitis was defined as a mucosal break that involved the entire circumference of the esophagus, but this was modified in 1999 to the criterion shown in Table 6–1 because it can be difficult to ascertain that a mucosal break is completely circumferential.[34]

ENDOSCOPIC EVALUATION OF PATIENTS WHO HAVE UNDERGONE ANTIREFLUX SURGERY

The two most commonly used fundoplication procedures (Nissen and Toupet) create characteristic folds in the proximal part of the stomach that are best appreci-

ated with the endoscope in the retroflexed position.[39] The folds of the fundoplication should be located just below the diaphragm (Fig. 6–15). If the folds are seen above the diaphragm, it is an indication that the fundoplication has herniated into the chest, which usually results from disruption of the crural repair. If there is a pouch of stomach proximal to the folds of the fundoplication, the condition is called a "slipped" fundoplication (e.g., a "slipped Nissen"). A slipped fundoplication can occur in two ways: (1) the fundoplication is fashioned in the correct location, but a portion of the stomach later herniates ("slips") through the fundoplication, or (2) the surgeon mistakes the proximal part of the stomach for the distal end of the esophagus and inadvertently fashions the fundoplication around the stomach. Although the latter situation represents an initial surgical error rather than later slippage (herniation), the condition is called a slipped fundoplication despite the misnomer. Finally, the absence of fundoplication folds suggests total disruption of the antireflux procedure (the "missin' Nissen"). Any of these abnormalities can render the antireflux surgery ineffective.

The folds of a properly constructed fundoplication should be oriented parallel to the diaphragm. An oblique orientation of the folds suggests twisting of the fundoplication or improper construction of the wrap involving the body rather than the fundus of the stomach (Fig. 6–16).[34] Either of these conditions can cause postoperative gastroesophageal reflux, dysphagia, or both. The folds should measure approximately 1 to 2 cm in

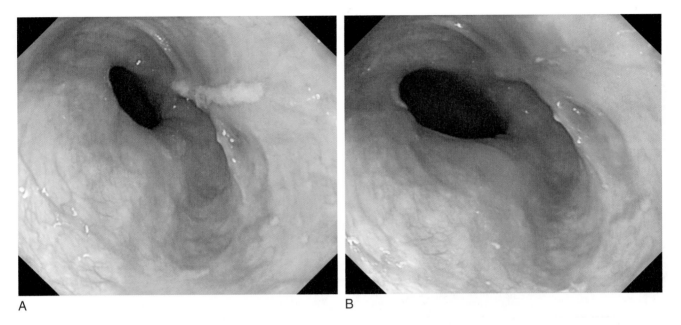

Figure 6–13. **A,** Endoscopic photograph of Los Angeles grade B esophagitis. There is a mucosal break defined as "an area of slough or erythema with a discrete line of demarcation from the adjacent, more normal-looking mucosa." Notice the whitish exudates covering the mucosal break, which is greater than 5 mm in length. In addition, scarring of the distal end of the esophagus is indicated by the fibrous strands that run perpendicular to the mucosal break at the 12- and 5-o'clock positions. **B,** Same area shown in **A** after the whitish exudates have been washed off. The mucosal break is still visible, but less prominent.

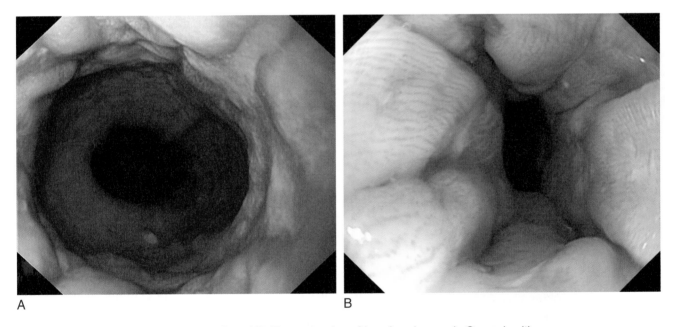

Figure 6–14. **A** and **B,** Two examples of Los Angeles grade C esophagitis.

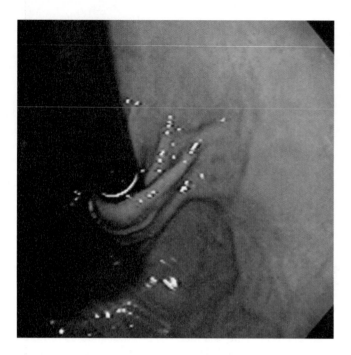

Figure 6–15. Endoscopic photograph of an anatomically correct Nissen fundoplication, retroflexed view. The fundoplication folds are located below the diaphragm and run parallel to the white distance line on the endoscope. (From Spechler SJ: The management of patients who have "failed" antireflux surgery. Am J Gastroenterol 99:552-561, 2004.)

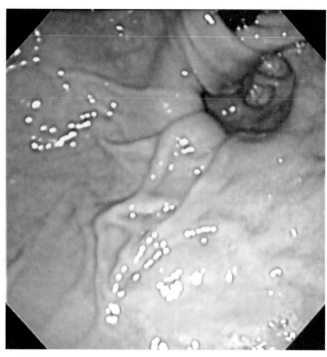

Figure 6–17. Endoscopic photograph of a paraesophageal hernia, retroflexed view. The herniated pouch of stomach is located next to the fundoplication folds. (From Spechler SJ: The management of patients who have "failed" antireflux surgery. Am J Gastroenterol 99:552-561, 2004.)

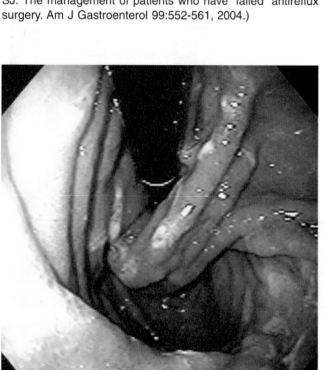

Figure 6–16. Endoscopic photograph of a slipped Nissen fundoplication, retroflexed view. The fundoplication folds are oriented obliquely to the white distance line on the endoscope, and there is a pouch of stomach proximal to the folds. (From Spechler SJ: The management of patients who have "failed" antireflux surgery. Am J Gastroenterol 99:552-561, 2004.)

span. A wider span indicates a too-generous fundoplication, which can cause dysphagia. A paraesophageal hernia can also cause dysphagia by pressing on the distal part of the esophagus (Fig. 6–17). The herniated portion of the stomach in these cases often originates from the fundoplication itself and may result from attempts to construct a "floppy" wrap.

ESOPHAGEAL CANCER

Esophageal cancers that are recognizable by conventional endoscopy appear as masses that protrude into the lumen of the esophagus. The masses are often nodular, irregular, and ulcerated, and the tumors may have a different color and texture than the surrounding normal mucosa. Squamous cell carcinoma and adenocarcinoma of the esophagus cannot be differentiated on the basis of endoscopic appearance, but the location of the tumor and its associated features may provide important clues regarding its histology. Tumors that involve the proximal and middle portions of the esophagus and that are separated from the stomach by a segment of squamous epithelium are very likely to be squamous cell carcinomas. Distal esophageal tumors can be either squamous cell carcinomas or adenocarcinomas. If there is associated Barrett's esophagus, the tumor is likely to be an adenocarcinoma (Figs. 6–18 and 6–19). However,

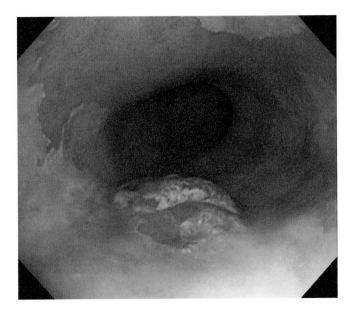

Figure 6–18.   Early cancer in Barrett's esophagus. Note the background of flat Barrett's epithelium with the nodular mass in the foreground.

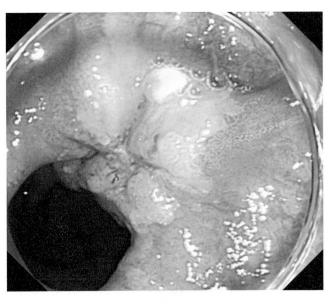

Figure 6–19.   Ulcerated cancer of the distal end of the esophagus.

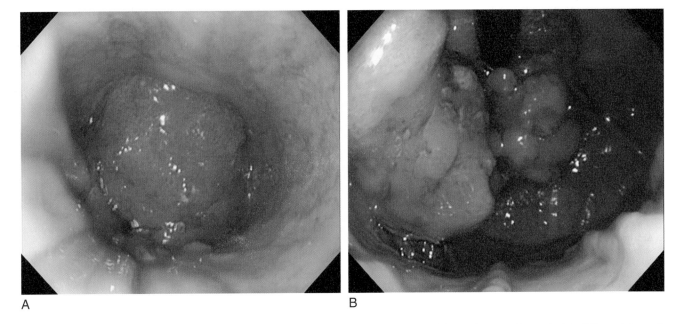

A   B

Figure 6–20.   Adenocarcinoma of the gastroesophageal junction photographed from the esophageal side **(A)** and from the gastric side **(B)**. If there is no Barrett's epithelium seen in the esophagus, it is not possible to determine whether such a tumor originated from the distal esophagus or from the gastric cardia.

adenocarcinomas that cause symptoms have often grown so large that they have obliterated any evidence of the Barrett's esophagus that spawned them. It can be especially difficult to determine the origin of an adenocarcinoma that straddles the GEJ (Fig. 6–20A and B). Such tumors can arise either from Barrett's esophagus or from the proximal part of the stomach. If no Barrett's esophagus is apparent, investigators have relied on the location of the tumor epicenter to classify the tumor as esophageal or "cardiac."

REFERENCES

1. Netter FH: Anatomy of the esophagus. In Oppenheimer E (ed): The CIBA Collection of Medical Illustrations, vol 3, Digestive System, Part I, Upper Digestive Tract. New York, CIBA Pharmaceutical Company, 1959, pp 34-46.
2. Goyal RK, Martin SB, Shapiro J, Spechler SJ: The role of cricopharyngeal muscle in pharyngoesophageal disorders. Dysphagia 8:252-258, 1993.
3. Mittal RK, Balaban DH: The esophagogastric junction. N Engl J Med 336:924-932, 1997.
4. Johnson LF, Moses FM: Endoscopic evaluation of esophageal disease. In Castell DO, Johnson LF (eds): Esophageal Function in Health and Disease. New York, Elsevier, 1983, pp 237-254.
5. Goyal RK, Bauer J, Spiro HM: The nature and location of the lower esophageal ring. N Engl J Med 284:1175-1180, 1971.
6. Ott DJ: Radiology of the oropharynx and esophagus. In Castell DO (ed): The Esophagus. Boston, Little, Brown, 1995, pp 41-91.
7. Paull A, Trier JS, Dalton MD, et al: The histologic spectrum of Barrett's esophagus. N Engl J Med 295:476-480, 1976.
8. Kim SL, Waring PJ, Spechler SJ, et al: Diagnostic inconsistencies in Barrett's esophagus. Department of Veterans Affairs Gastroesophageal Reflux Study Group. Gastroenterology 107:945-949, 1994.
9. Bozymski EM: Barrett's esophagus: Endoscopic characteristics. In Spechler SJ, Goyal RK (eds): Barrett's Esophagus: Pathophysiology, Diagnosis, and Management. New York, Elsevier, 1985, pp 113-120.
10. McClave SA, Boyce HW Jr, Gottfried MR: Early diagnosis of columnar-lined esophagus: A new endoscopic criterion. Gastrointest Endosc 33:413-416, 1987.
11. De Carvalho CA: Sur l'angio-architecture veineuse de la zone de transition esophago-gasgtrique et son interpretation fonctionnelle. Acta Anat 64:125-162, 1966.
12. Choi do W, Oh SN, Baek SJ, et al: Endoscopically observed lower esophageal capillary patterns. Korean J Intern Med 17:245-248, 2002.
13. Spechler SJ: The role of gastric carditis in metaplasia and neoplasia at the gastroesophageal junction. Gastroenterology 117:218-228, 1999.
14. Vianna A, Hayes PC, Moscoso G, et al: Normal venous circulation of the gastroesophageal junction. A route to understanding varices. Gastroenterology 93:876-889, 1987.
15. Sharma P, Morales TG, Sampliner RE: Short segment Barrett's esophagus. The need for standardization of the definition and of endoscopic criteria. Am J Gastroenterol 93:1033-1036, 1998.
16. Wallner B, Sylvan A, Stenling R, Janunger KG: The esophageal Z-line appearance correlates to the prevalence of intestinal metaplasia. Scand J Gastroenterol 35:17-22, 2000.
17. Wallner B, Sylvan A, Janunger KG: Endoscopic assessment of the "Z-line" (squamocolumnar junction) appearance: Reproducibility of the ZAP classification among endoscopists. Gastrointest Endosc 55:65-69, 2002.
18. Armstrong D: Review article: Towards consistency in the endoscopic diagnosis of Barrett's oesophagus and columnar metaplasia. Aliment Pharmacol Ther 20(Suppl 5):40-47, 2004.
19. Spechler SJ, Goyal RK: The columnar lined esophagus, intestinal metaplasia, and Norman Barrett. Gastroenterology 110:614-621, 1996.
20. Canto MIF, Setrakian S, Willis J, et al: Methylene blue–directed biopsies improve detection of intestinal metaplasia and dysplasia in Barrett's esophagus. Gastrointest Endosc 51:560-568, 2000.
21. Scotiniotis IA, Kochman ML, Lewis JD, et al: Accuracy of EUS in the evaluation of Barrett's esophagus and high-grade dysplasia or intramucosal carcinoma. Gastrointest Endosc 54:689-696, 2001.
22. Kobayashi K, Izatt JA, Kulkarni MD, et al: High-resolution cross-sectional imaging of the gastrointestinal tract using optical coherence tomography: Preliminary results. Gastrointest Endosc 47:515-523, 1998.
23. Georgakoudi I, Jacobson BC, Van Dam J, et al: Fluorescence, reflectance, and light-scattering spectroscopy for evaluating dysplasia in patients with Barrett's esophagus. Gastroenterology 120:1620-1629, 2001.
24. Kendall C, Stone N, Shepherd N, et al: Raman spectroscopy, a potential tool for the objective identification and classification of neoplasia in Barrett's oesophagus. J Pathol 200:602-609, 2003.
25. Bergman JJ, Tytgat GN: New developments in the endoscopic surveillance of Barrett's oesophagus. Gut 54(Suppl 1):i38-i42, 2005.
26. Olliver JR, Wild CP, Sahay P, et al: Chromoendoscopy with methylene blue and associated DNA damage in Barrett's oesophagus. Lancet 362:373-374, 2003.
27. Amano Y, Kushiyama Y, Ishihara S, et al: Crystal violet chromoendoscopy with mucosal pit pattern diagnosis is useful for surveillance of short-segment Barrett's esophagus. Am J Gastroenterol 100:21-26, 2005.
28. Toyoda H, Rubio C, Befrits R, et al: Detection of intestinal metaplasia in distal esophagus and esophagogastric junction by enhanced-magnification endoscopy. Gastrointest Endosc 59:15-21, 2004.
29. Endo T, Awakawa T, Takahashi H, et al: Classification of Barrett's epithelium by magnifying endoscopy. Gastrointest Endosc 55:641-647, 2002.
30. Spechler SJ: A 59-year-old woman with gastroesophageal reflux disease and Barrett esophagus. JAMA 289:466-475, 2003.
31. Armstrong D: Endoscopic evaluation of gastro-esophageal reflux disease. Yale J Biol Med 72:93-100, 1999.
32. Richter JE, Peura D, Benjamin SB, et al: Efficacy of omeprazole for the treatment of symptomatic acid reflux disease without esophagitis. Arch Intern Med 160:1810-1816, 2000.
33. Bytzer P, Havelund T, Hansen JM: Interobserver variation in the endoscopic diagnosis of reflux esophagitis. Scand J Gastroenterol 28:119-125, 1993.
34. Lundell LR, Dent J, Bennett JR, et al: Endoscopic assessment of oesophagitis: Clinical and functional correlates and further validation of the Los Angeles classification. Gut 45:172-180, 1999.
35. Grossman MI (ed): Peptic Ulcer: A Guide for the Practicing Physician. Chicago, Year Book, 1981.
36. Armstrong D, Bennett JR, Blum AL, et al: The endoscopic assessment of esophagitis: A progress report on observer agreement. Gastroenterology 111:85-92, 1996.
37. Savary M, Miller G: The Esophagus. Handbook and Atlas of Endoscopy. Solothurn, Switzerland, Verlag Gassman, 1978.
38. Armstrong D, Emde C, Inauen W, Blum AL: Diagnostic assessment of gastroesophageal reflux disease: What is possible vs. what is practical? Hepatogastroenterology 39(Suppl 1):3-13, 1992.
39. Spechler SJ: The management of patients who have "failed" antireflux surgery. Am J Gastroenterol 99:552-561, 2004.

7

Endoscopic Esophageal Ultrasonography

Thomas William Rice · Gregory Zuccaro, Jr.

Endoscopic esophageal ultrasonography (EUS) extended endoscopic examination of the esophagus beyond the mucosa into the esophageal wall and paraesophageal tissues. The diagnostic capabilities of surface ultrasound have been expanded by endoscopic placement of ultrasound transducers adjacent to the gastrointestinal mucosa. These transducers, operating at relatively high frequencies, provide detailed examination of the esophageal wall and surrounding tissues. EUS is the most significant advance in the diagnosis of esophageal disease since the introduction of flexible fiberoptic endoscopy. These intracorporeal examinations have proved beneficial in the diagnosis and treatment of both benign and malignant diseases of the esophagus and adjacent structures.

FUNDAMENTALS OF ULTRASONOGRAPHY

Sound is produced by vibration of a source within a medium. Vibration produces waves, cyclic compression, and rarefaction (expansion) of molecules in the medium, thus transmitting the sound wave through the medium. The number of cycles (compression and rarefaction) of a sound wave occurring in 1 second is the frequency and is measured in hertz. The frequency of sound waves audible to the human ear is between 20 and 20,000 Hz. Sound waves with frequencies higher than 20,000 Hz are ultrasound waves. Frequencies used in medical ultrasound imaging range from 1 to 20 million Hz (1 MHz to 20 MHz).

Ultrasound waves may be produced by electrical excitation of a piezoelectric crystal. The application of voltage across a crystal causes it to deform. Alternating electrical energy vibrates the crystal and produces sound waves. Conversely, if a sound wave deforms a crystal, electrical energy is produced. It is this ability to convert electrical energy into sound energy and, conversely, to convert sound energy into electrical energy that allows these crystals to function as both transmitters and receivers (i.e., as *transducers*). These transducers are responsive to a limited range of frequencies; hence, more than one transducer may be required for an ultrasound examination.

The speed of a sound wave within a medium (tissue) is defined by the following relationship: $V = (K/p)^{1/2}$. V is the velocity of the sound wave, K is the bulk modulus of the tissue (a measure of stiffness), and p is the density of the tissue.

The resistance to passage of a sound wave through tissue is called acoustic impedance (Z), which is defined by the following relationship: $Z = pV = (pK)^{1/2}$.

Sound waves travel best through dense or elastic tissue. Absorption of some of the energy of an ultrasound wave occurs as the wave passes through tissue. The amount of absorption is determined by tissue characteristics and the frequency of the sound wave. Higher-frequency waves have greater absorption.

Interactions occurring as a sound wave encounters different tissues are critical to the diagnostic capabilities of ultrasound. As a sound wave passes from one tissue to the next, a portion of the wave is transmitted and a portion is reflected. The reflected wave is received by the transducer, thereby providing the diagnostic information of ultrasound. The difference in acoustic impedance between the two tissues and the angle at which the sound wave enters the new medium (angle of incidence) determine the portion of the wave that is reflected and the portion that is transmitted. In tissue with similar acoustic impedance, most of the wave is transmitted. Soft tissue has excellent transmission qualities; the density and velocity vary only by 12% to 14% among different soft tissues. Because acoustic impedance is the product of velocity and density, the product of these small changes results in a 22% difference in acoustic impedance between fat and muscle.[1] Useless, bright echo images are obtained when an ultrasound wave encounters air or bone. Air is very compressible and of low density, whereas bone, although dense, has low compressibility and high reflectivity. These properties account for the poor transmission of ultrasound waves from tissue to air or tissue to bone. The amount of reflected sound is also related to the angle of incidence: as the angle of incidence increases, less sound is reflected. In addition, sound waves are bent as they travel from one tissue to the next. This process is termed *refraction*.

Absorption, reflection, and refraction are major sources of energy loss. Some ultrasound wave energy is also lost by scattering (diffusion), which occurs when a sound wave encounters heterogeneous tissue. Tiny particles within tissue (such as fat in muscle), smaller than the ultrasound wavelength, scatter the ultrasound wave. As a sound wave passes through tissue, a portion of its energy is lost; this is called *attenuation*. Attenuation increases as more tissues are encountered and as the wave travels farther from the source. If the returning ultrasound wave is not processed, the same tissue would be imaged differently, depending on its distance from the transducer. The intensity of the returning waves must be amplified (gain) to ensure that distant waves are correctly represented. Attenuation increases as ultrasound frequency increases.

Resolution is the ability to discriminate among different tissues with ultrasound waves. Depth or axial resolution is the ability to differentiate between two tissues along the path of the ultrasound wave. Lateral resolution is the ability to distinguish between adjacent tissues. Transducer characteristics and focus determine resolution. Higher frequencies allow better resolution but decreased tissue penetration.

Pulse-echo technique is used in EUS. Ultrasound waves are emitted for a brief period, followed by a subsequent listening period during which the reflected waves are received. The returning ultrasound waves are displayed such that the brightness is proportional to the amplitude of the returning ultrasound waves. This is known as *B-mode ultrasonography*. Because the amplitude is presented in a range from white to gray to black, the display is also termed *gray-scale ultrasound*. Individual scans are shown at a rate at which the eye cannot detect single images (12/sec). This fast-frame display is called *real-time ultrasound* and allows the ultrasonographer to study tissue temporally as well as spatially.

INSTRUMENTS AND TECHNIQUES

Because EUS does not provide adequate endoscopic inspection of the upper gastrointestinal tract, every ultrasound study should be preceded by a standard flexible endoscopic upper gastrointestinal examination. This provides precise location and mucosal definition (including biopsy) of the esophageal lesion and guides the ultrasound examiner. Intravenous administration of a narcotic, such as meperidine, and a benzodiazepine, such as midazolam, usually provides adequate sedation. The ultrasound endoscope is generally passed blindly through the oropharynx and hypopharynx. Care must be taken because the distal tip containing the transducer is

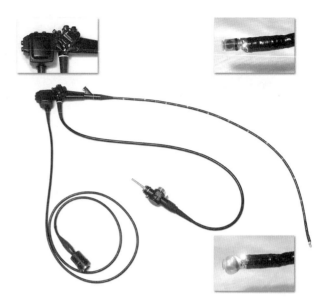

Figure 7–1. The Olympus GF-UM130 ultrasound endoscope. *Upper right inset*, The control section contains the deflection controls and air/water and suction valves similar to those on a standard endoscope. *Upper left inset*, The ultrasound transducer is housed in the tip of the endoscope. The forward oblique viewing endoscope and suction channel are proximal to the ultrasound transducer. *Lower left inset*, The distal tip of the ultrasound endoscope with the water-inflated contact balloon, which covers the ultrasound transducer.

rigid. For complete examination, the endoscope must be passed beyond the esophagus into the stomach.

The radial mechanical ultrasound endoscope (Fig. 7–1) is the principal instrument used for EUS. The ultrasound transducer is housed in the tip of the endoscope. It produces up to a 360-degree sector scan perpendicular to the transducer tip. Because the transducer is adjacent to tissues to be examined, higher frequencies than those used in extracorporeal ultrasound can be used. In the newest models a range of transducer frequencies from 5 to 20 MHz are available. These transducers allow adequate visualization of anatomic structures to a depth of 3 to 12 cm. An acceptable acoustic interface between the transducer and the tissue being examined must be obtained to ensure good-quality ultrasound images. This is most commonly accomplished by covering the tip of the endoscope with a latex balloon, which can be filled with water to provide an excellent acoustic interface (see Fig. 7–1). A less commonly used technique is rapid insufflation of the esophageal lumen with water. This provides an excellent, but transient acoustic interface without the tissue compression that may occur with the latex balloon. Current echoendoscopes also provide a video endoscopic image, albeit with a somewhat limited view in a forward oblique direction.

The control section contains the deflection controls and air/water and suction valves, similar to those on a standard endoscope (see Fig. 7–1). A water inflation/deflation system for the balloon is incorporated into the air/water and suction valve mechanisms. A direct-current

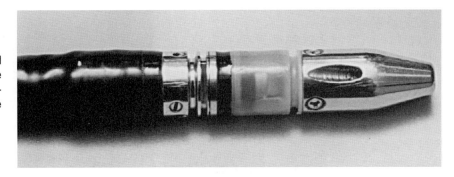

Figure 7–2. Radial mechanical blind probe. The tip is tapered to allow passage through tight strictures. The radial ultrasound transducer is positioned behind the tapered tip.

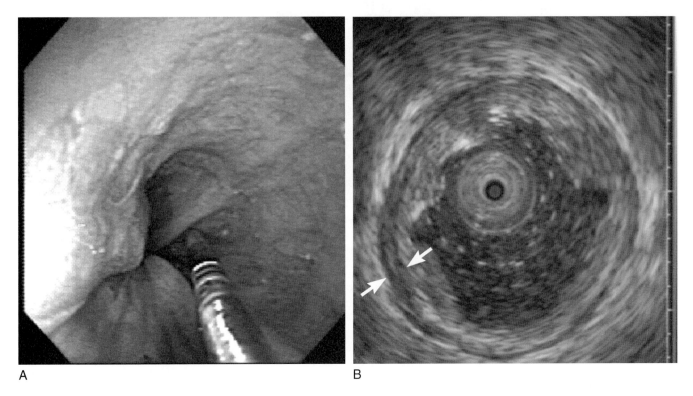

A   B

Figure 7–3. **A,** High-frequency (12 to 30 MHz) miniprobe passed through the operating channel of a standard endoscope. **B,** Miniprobe ultrasound image of a normal esophagus. The probe is not centered in the undistended esophageal lumen. The mucosa and submucosa are the inner hyperechoic layer. The muscularis propria (*arrows*) is the inner hypoechoic layer.

motor and drive mechanism that rotates the ultrasound transducer are housed in the control section. Current ultrasound endoscopes are totally immersible.

A radial mechanical blind probe (Fig. 7–2) is available for the evaluation of esophageal strictures. This echoendoscope provides images similar to those of larger-diameter radial mechanical echoendoscopes, but it has no endoscopic optical capabilities and is less than 8 mm in diameter. More commonly used in current practice are higher-frequency miniprobes passed through the operating channel of standard endoscopes (Fig. 7–3); these miniprobes provide radial images from 12 to 30 MHz.

These three instruments are used in conjunction with an image processor (Fig. 7–4). The image processor allows for adjustment of gain, contrast, and sensitivity

time control in order to regulate the strength of the returning echo at different depths. On-screen calibration and labeling can be done with the image processor. The image may be displayed on a video monitor or stored digitally or on videotape. The image processor has been refined and miniaturized with successive generations of endoscopic ultrasound equipment.

Newer electronic endoscopes are also available that have the advantage of providing color Doppler. They may be less susceptible to breakdown because moving parts are eliminated. In some cases, both radial and linear echoendoscopic examination may be possible with one power source and image processor system.

The curvilinear electronic echoendoscope (Fig. 7–5) also has also has video endoscopic capability and can produce up to a 180-degree oblique forward field. It

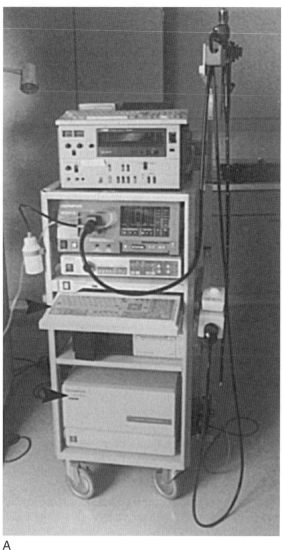

A

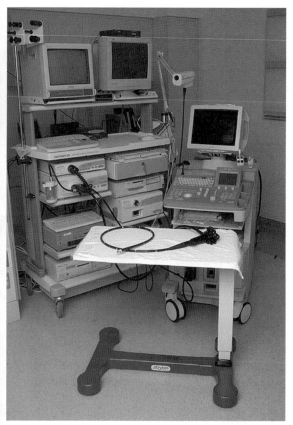

B

Figure 7–4. **A,** The Olympus EU-M20 image processor (*lower arrow*) is rack-mounted in a standard cart, which includes the other essential endoscopic equipment. The keyboard (*upper arrow*) can be used to measure and mark ultrasound findings. **B,** The complete system includes the light source rack, image processor, and ultrasound endoscope.

allows a range of scanning frequencies from 5 to 10 MHz with a depth of penetration of 4 cm or greater. This system can provide color Doppler examination and direct visualization of cytology needles passed into and beyond the esophageal wall.

Radial mechanical and electronic curvilinear scanners have increased the accuracy of EUS. However, the availability and use of two systems necessarily increase both the complexity and the cost of EUS examinations. For diagnostic purposes, the radial mechanical scanner is preferable because it allows a 360-degree view and is known as the "workhorse" of EUS. Because the radial mechanical scanner does not allow safe directed passage of a needle into the esophageal wall or adjacent tissue if a tissue sample is required for cytologic evaluation, the electronic curvilinear echoendoscope, powered by a separate system, is used. It is possible to perform both diagnosis and fine-needle aspiration (FNA) with the electronic linear echoendoscope alone, but the limitation in viewing field requires significant torque on the insertion tube to image the esophageal wall and adjacent tissues

for a 360-degree view. Comparable results, however, for staging examinations have been reported with the electronic curvilinear echoendoscope.[2] Both systems must be available for adequate EUS evaluation.

THE ESOPHAGEAL WALL AND ULTRASOUND ANATOMY

The esophageal wall is composed of three distinct layers: mucosa, submucosa, and muscularis propria (Fig. 7–6). The mucosa has three elements: epithelium, lamina propria, and muscularis mucosae. The innermost layer is stratified, nonkeratinizing squamous epithelium. It is separated and isolated from the remainder of the esophageal wall by a basement membrane. Immediately beneath is the lamina propria. This loose matrix of collagen and elastic fibers forms a superficial undulating layer; invaginations into the epithelium produce epithelial papillae. Lymphatic channels in the lamina propria are an anatomic feature unique to the esophagus. The

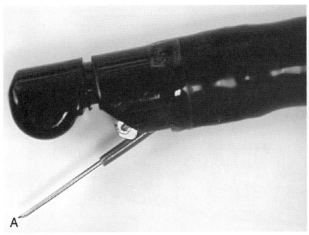

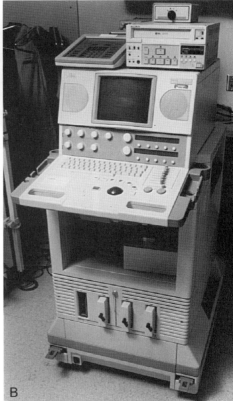

Figure 7–5. Curvilinear electronic endoscope **(A)** and image processor **(B)**. The optics and operating channel, through which a fine needle is passed, are positioned behind the linear ultrasound transducer. This echoendoscope requires a separate image processor.

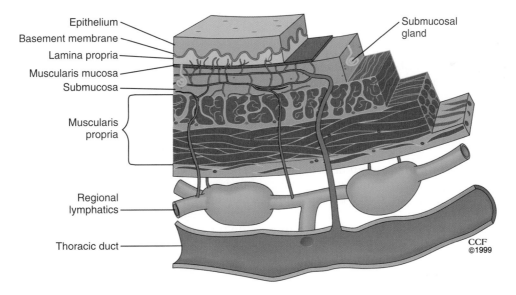

Figure 7–6. The esophageal wall is composed of mucosa, submucosa, and muscularis propria. The mucosa is composed of epithelium, lamina propria, and muscularis mucosae.

muscularis mucosae surrounds the lamina propria. This smooth muscle layer pleats the two inner layers of the mucosa into folds that disappear with distention of the lumen.

The submucosa is composed of connective tissues that contain a rich network of blood vessels and lymphatics. The dense submucosal lymphatic plexus facilitates early dissemination of esophageal malignancies. Elastic fibers and collagen combine to make this the strongest esophageal layer. Submucosal glands of mixed type are characteristic of the esophagus.

The muscularis propria is the muscular sleeve that provides the propulsive force necessary for swallowing. There are two layers of muscle: an inner circular layer

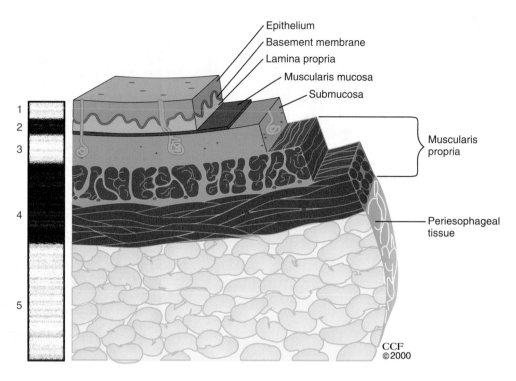

Figure 7–7. The esophageal wall is visualized as five alternating layers of differing echogenicity by esophageal ultrasound. The first layer, which is hyperechoic (white), represents the superficial mucosa (epithelium and lamina propria). The second layer, which is hypoechoic (black), represents the deep mucosa (muscularis mucosa). The third layer, which is hyperechoic (white), represents the submucosa. The fourth layer, which is hypoechoic (black), represents the muscularis propria. The fifth layer, which is hyperechoic (white) is the periesophageal tissue.

and an outer longitudinal layer. The upper cervical esophagus is composed entirely of striated muscle. There is a gradual transition from striated to smooth muscle within muscle bundles until the esophagus is entirely smooth muscle at the upper and midthird junction. Lymphatic channels pierce the muscularis propria and drain into regional lymphatics or directly into the thoracic duct.

The esophagus has no investing adventitia. The paraesophageal tissue is composed of fibrofatty tissue that lies directly against the outer fibers of the muscularis propria.

The normal esophagus is usually viewed as five discrete layers by EUS (Fig. 7–7). These layers are seen as alternating hyperechoic (white) and hypoechoic (black) rings. Studies have demonstrated that the five layers seen by EUS correspond to the balloon-mucosa interface, the mucosa deep to this interface, the submucosa and the acoustic interface between the submucosa and muscularis propria, the muscularis propria minus the acoustic interface between the submucosa and the muscularis propria, and the periesophageal tissue.[3,4] For clinical purposes, these layers represent the superficial mucosa, deep mucosa, submucosa, muscularis propria, and periesophageal tissue. In the upper part of the esophagus, with overdistention of the examining balloon or if the transducer is too close to the esophageal wall, only three layers of the esophageal wall may be apparent because the superficial mucosa, deep mucosa, and sub-

mucosa compose one hyperechoic layer. The thickness of each ultrasound layer is about equal and does not represent the thickness of the tissue layer but, instead, the time that it takes the ultrasound wave to traverse this layer.

ESOPHAGEAL CARCINOMA

The stage of an esophageal carcinoma, as defined by its anatomic extent, is the best predictor of outcome for patients with esophageal carcinoma. Recent refinements in the staging of esophageal carcinoma have resulted in the present staging system, which is based on the TNM classification (Box 7–1).[5] The primary tumor (T) is defined only by the depth of invasion; EUS is ideally suited for this determination. T1 tumors are confined to the submucosa or more superficial esophageal layers. T2 tumors invade into, but do not breach the muscularis propria. T3 tumors invade beyond the esophageal wall and into periesophageal tissue but do not invade adjacent structures. T4 tumors directly invade structures in the vicinity of the esophagus.

Lymph nodes in the area of the primary tumor, or regional lymph nodes (N), are characterized only by the presence (N1) or absence (N0) of metastases. Similarly, distant sites (M) are characterized by the presence (M1) or absence (M0) of metastases. The recent revision of the staging system for esophageal carcinoma subdivides distant metastatic carcinomas (M1) into M1a (distant,

Box 7–1 **TNM Classifications and Stage Groupings of Esophageal Carcinoma**

Classification

T: Primary Tumor

TX Tumor cannot be assessed
T0 No evidence of tumor
Tis High-grade dysplasia
T1 Tumor invades the lamina propria, muscularis mucosa, or submucosa. It does not breach the submucosa. Tumors may be subdivided into T1a (intramucosal) and T1b (submucosal)
T2 Tumor invades into and not beyond the muscularis propria
T3 Tumor invades the periesophageal tissue, but does not invade adjacent structures
T4 Tumor invades adjacent structures

N: Regional Lymph Nodes

NX Regional lymph nodes cannot be assessed
N0 No regional lymph node metastases
N1 Regional lymph node metastases

M: Distant Metastasis

MX Distant metastases cannot be assessed
M1a Upper thoracic esophagus metastatic to cervical lymph nodes
    Lower thoracic esophagus metastatic to celiac lymph nodes
M1b Upper thoracic esophagus metastatic to other nonregional lymph nodes or other distant sites
    Midthoracic esophagus metastatic to either nonregional lymph nodes or other distant sites
    Lower thoracic esophagus metastatic to other nonregional lymph nodes or other distant sites

Stage Grouping

Stage 0	Tis	N0	M0
Stage I	T1	N0	M0
Stage IIA	T2	N0	M0
	T3	N0	M0
Stage IIB	T1	N1	M0
	T2	N1	M0
Stage III	T3	N1	M0
	T4	Any N	M0
Stage IVA	Any T	Any N	M1a
Stage IVB	Any T	Any N	M1b

nonregional lymph node metastases) and M1b (other distant metastases).[5] M1a disease is further classified by tumor location: M1a tumors of the upper thoracic esophagus have metastasized to cervical nodes, and M1a tumors of the lower thoracic esophagus have metastasized to celiac lymph nodes. These TNM descriptors are grouped into stages with similar behavior and prognoses (see Box 7–1).

EUS may be used at two different periods in the course of esophageal carcinoma. The staging examination may be done before (clinical stage) or after (re-treatment stage) treatment.

Clinical Stage (cTNM)

Determination of cT Classification

Detailed images of the esophageal wall by EUS make it the most accurate modality available for determination of the depth of tumor invasion (T) before treatment (Figs. 7–8 to 7–11).[6-11] The same definition of the esophageal wall is not offered by computed tomography (CT). A thickened esophageal wall, the principal CT finding in esophageal carcinoma, is not specific for esophageal carcinoma and lacks the definition required to distinguish T1, T2, and T3 tumors.[12] In differentiation of T3 from T4 tumors, EUS is superior to CT. Evaluation of the fat planes is used to define local invasion at CT examination. The obliteration or lack of fat planes is not sensitive in predicting local invasion, but preservation of these planes is specific for the absence of T4 disease.[13-20] When compared with CT, EUS provides a more sensitive and reliable determination of vascular involvement.[21]

Experience with both examination technique and ultrasound interpretation is critical to accurately determine the clinical depth of tumor invasion. Seventy-five to 100 examinations are required before competence is obtained.[22,23] A review of 21 series reported an 84% accuracy of EUS for T classification.[24] Accuracy is not constant and varies with the T classification. In this meta-analysis, accuracy for T1 carcinomas was 83.5%, with 16.5% of tumors over-staged; accuracy for T2 was 73%, with 10% under-staged and 17% over-staged; accuracy for T3 was 89%, with 5% under-staged and 6% over-staged; and accuracy for T4 was 89%, with 11% under-staged.[24] A review of the literature shows variation in accuracy with T classification: 75% to 82% for T1, 64% to 85% for T2, 89% to 94% for T3, and 88% to 100% for T4.[24]

The greatest inaccuracy is reported for T2 tumors. EUS anatomy, in part, accounts for this problem. The muscularis propria is vital in defining T1, T2, and T3 tumors. For clinical assessment the fourth ultrasound layer is interpreted as the muscularis propria. This layer, however, does not include the interface between the submucosa and muscularis propria; it is contained in the third ultrasound layer. Thus, the border necessary to completely differentiate T1 from T2 tumors is contained in the third ultrasound layer. Since two boundaries must be assessed for determination of T2 and errors might occur at each, the inaccuracy is potentially twice that of T1 and T4 tumors.

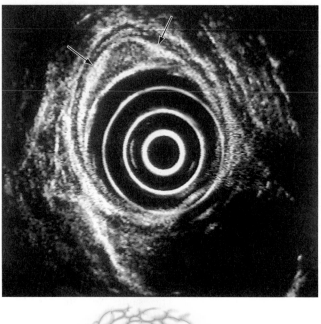

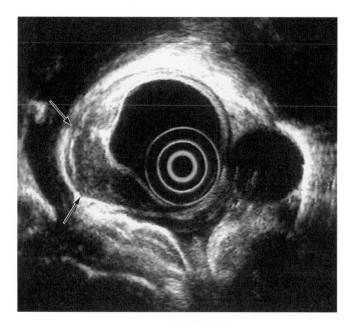

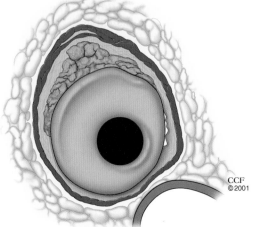

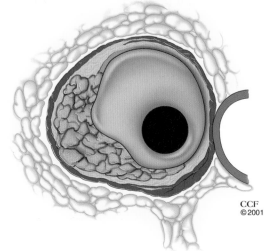

Figure 7–8. *Upper,* A T1 tumor as seen on esophageal ultrasound. The hypoechoic (black) tumor invades the hyperechoic (white) third ultrasound layer (submucosa) but does not breach the boundary between the third and fourth layers (*arrows*). *Lower,* A T1 tumor invades, but does not breach the submucosa.

Figure 7–9. *Upper,* A T2 tumor as seen on esophageal ultrasound. The hypoechoic (black) tumor invades the hypoechoic (black) fourth ultrasound layer but does not breach the boundary between the forth and fifth layers (*arrows*). *Lower,* A T2 tumor invades, but does not breach the muscularis propria.

Because invasion beyond the esophageal wall is important in determining therapy, some investigators have examined the accuracy of EUS in determining T classification dichotomously. When compared with T classification determined pathologically, EUS was 87% accurate, 82% sensitive, 91% specific, 89% positively predictive, and 86% negatively predictive of tumors confined to the esophageal wall (≤T2) or invading beyond the esophageal wall (>T2).[25] A systematic review of 13 studies also confirmed that EUS was highly effective in differentiating T1/T2 from T3/T4 tumors.[26]

EUS interpretation is not done in the absence of clinical information; patient history and preceding esophagoscopy and imaging are usually available. This fact was illustrated by Meining and colleagues, who reported that a blinded review of EUS studies was significantly less accurate than a retrospective review of EUS reports, 53% versus 73%, respectively.[27] When interpreters were unblinded and given endoscopy tapes, accuracy improved to 62%. Tumor length and luminal obstruction are known at the time of EUS and are predictive of the T classification.[28] In this report, tumor length greater than 5 cm had a sensitivity of 89% and specificity of 92% for diagnosing T3 tumors. Thirteen patients with luminal obstruction had at least T3 tumors. Clinically, EUS examinations are never interpreted in the absence of history and esophagoscopy.

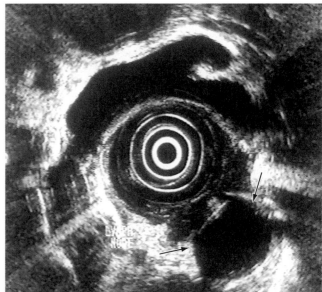

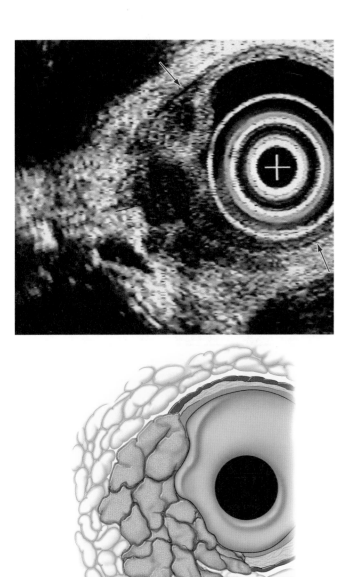

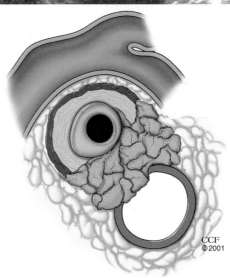

Figure 7–10. *Upper,* A T3 tumor as seen on esophageal ultrasound. The hypoechoic (black) tumor breaches the boundary between the fourth and fifth ultrasound layers (*arrows*) and invades the hyperechoic (white) fifth ultrasound layer (periesophageal tissue). *Lower,* A T3 tumor invades the periesophageal tissue but does not involve adjacent structures.

Figure 7–11. *Upper,* A T4 tumor as seen on esophageal ultrasound. The hypoechoic (black) tumor invades the aorta. The tumor breaches the boundary between periesophageal tissue and the aorta (*arrows*). *Lower,* A T4 tumor invades the aorta.

Esophageal obstruction caused by a malignant high-grade stricture prohibits staging in 19% to 63% of examinations.[11,29,30] Two studies have reported that EUS may be less reliable in nontraversable esophageal cancers.[10,31] Failure to pass an ultrasound probe beyond a malignant stricture has been found to be an accurate predictor of advanced stage. More than 90% of these patients have stage III or IV disease.[32] These discordant findings may be reconciled when viewed in the context of a study by Hordijk and colleagues[30] that assessed the severity of malignant strictures. In this study, the accuracy of T classification was 87% for nontraversable strictures, 46% for tight strictures that were difficult to pass, and 92% for easily traversable strictures. Options in the case of nontraversable strictures include limited examination of the proximal tumor margin, dilation and subsequent EUS examination, and the use of miniprobes. Limited examination of the tumor above the stricture has variable accuracy, but may be useful in staging if T3 or N1 disease is seen. Dilation of malignant strictures followed by EUS examination may be associated with an increased incidence of perforation.[32] However, it allows a complete examination in 42% to 95% of patients with high-grade strictures[33-35] and is not associated with perforation if careful stepwise dilation is performed. Careful dilation followed by EUS allowed Wallace and colleagues[35] to detect advanced disease in 19% of patients, mostly because of the detection of celiac lymph node metastases. This problem may be overcome by the use of miniature ultrasound catheter probes (see Fig. 7–4). Passed through the biopsy channel of the endoscope and advanced through the stricture, these probes accurately determined T classification in 85% to 90% of patients.[36-39] Because most of these data are uncontrolled, it is not clear whether the additional effort and cost provide staging benefits. These 20-MHz probes have limited depth of penetration, which may prevent full ultrasound assessment. Since most nontraversable tumors are at least T3, it is crucial to evaluate the outer boundary of the tumor and adjacent structures and regional lymph nodes, which may be outside the range of the miniprobe.

Conventional EUS does not image the mucosa well; however, EUS is useful in staging patients suspected of having high-grade dysplasia or intramucosal cancer by detecting unexpected submucosal invasion or regional lymph node metastases, or both.[40,41] High-resolution EUS has the ability to assess the mucosa and shows promise in staging superficial esophageal cancer.[42,43]

Determination of N and M (Nonregional Lymph Node) Classifications

In addition to size, EUS evaluates nodal shape, border, and internal echo characteristics in lymph node assessment (Fig. 7–12). Large (>1 cm in long axis), round, hypoechoic, nonhomogeneous, sharply bordered lymph nodes are more likely to be malignant; small, oval or angular, hyperechoic, homogeneous lymph nodes with indistinct borders are more likely to be benign.[44] In a retrospective review of 100 EUS examinations, EUS determination of N classification was 89% sensitive, 75% specific, and 84% accurate.[44] The positive predictive value of EUS for N1 cancer was 86%; the negative predictive value was 79%. A patient was 24 times more likely to have N1 cancer if EUS detected regional lymph nodes. The single most sensitive predictor in detecting N1 cancer was a hypoechoic internal echo pattern, followed by a sharp border, a round shape, and size greater than 1 cm. When all four factors are present, the accuracy of N1 detection is 80% to 100%.[44,45] Unfortunately, all four features are present in only 25% of N1 lymph nodes.[45] In a meta-analysis of 21 series, the overall accuracy of EUS determination of N status was 77%: 69% for N0 and 89% for N1.[24] The ability to use EUS to diagnose nodal metastases varies with the location. It is better in the assessment of celiac lymph nodes (accuracy, 95%; sensitivity, 83%; specificity, 98%; positive predictive value, 91%; negative predictive value, 97%) than in mediastinal lymph nodes (accuracy, 73%; sensitivity, 79%; specificity, 63%; positive predictive value, 79%; and negative predictive value, 63%).[46]

There are associations between the primary tumor and N classification. Close proximity of the regional node to the primary tumor is a predictor of N1 cancer.

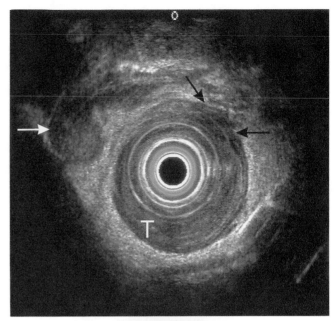

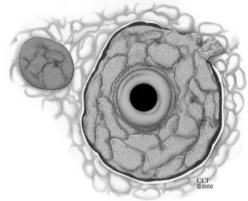

Figure 7–12. T3 N1 esophageal carcinoma. *Upper,* A T3 tumor (T) obliterates the ultrasound anatomy at this level. At 1 o'clock (*black arrows*), the tumor breaks through the fourth ultrasound layer and invades the fifth. An N1 regional lymph node (*white arrow*), close to the primary tumor, is large (2.2 cm in diameter), round, hypoechoic, and sharply demarcated. *Lower,* A T3 N1 tumor breaches the muscularis propria to invade periesophageal tissue and metastasizes to a regional lymph node.

Comparison of the echo characteristic of the tumor and regional lymph nodes is useful for EUS lymph node evaluation. The relationship of T classification to N1 must be considered during EUS examinations. The incidence of N1 cancer increases with deeper tumor invasion: for a patient with poorly differentiated adenocarcinoma, the probability of N1 is 17% for T1 tumors, 55% for T2, 83% for T3, and 88% for T4.[47] For T3 and T4 cancers, an EUS assessment of N0 does not ensure absence of N1 disease.

N classification accuracy and overall survival correlate with the number of lymph node metastases detected by EUS. Natsugoe and colleagues reported an accuracy of

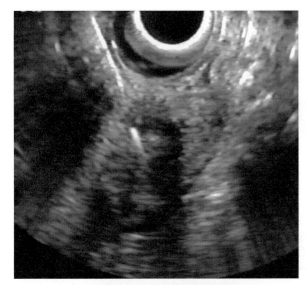

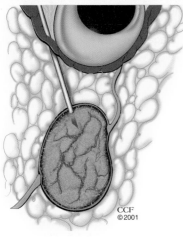

CCF
©2001

Figure 7–13.   Esophageal ultrasound fine-needle aspiration (FNA) of an N1 regional lymph node. *Upper,* Ultrasound image with a needle passed through the esophageal wall and into the N1 node. *Lower,* An N1 regional lymph node undergoing FNA under curvilinear electronic endoscopic examination.

84% with no N1 nodes, 60% with one to three, 43% with four to seven, and 96% with eight or more.[48] Five-year survival rates were 53%, 34%, 17%, and 0% for none, one to three, four to seven, and eight or more N1 lymph nodes, respectively.

Endosonography-directed fine-needle aspiration (EUS FNA) further refines clinical staging by adding tissue sampling to endosonography findings (Fig. 7–13).[49-53] In a multicenter study, 171 patients underwent EUS FNA of 192 lymph nodes.[54] Referent values for EUS FNA in determination of N classification were as follows: sensitivity, 92%; specificity, 93%; positive predictive value, 100%; and negative predictive value, 86%. Accuracy of N classification increased from 69% for EUS alone to 92% for EUS FNA. Two to three passes of the needle were made through each node. There was one nonfatal com-

plication: an esophageal perforation during dilation of an esophageal stricture before EUS FNA. Subsequent studies from Vazquez-Sequeiros and colleagues have confirmed and extended these findings.[52,53] In the most recent report, the first prospective, blinded study, EUS FNA was more accurate than EUS (87% versus 74%, respectively) as determined by histopathologic review of surgical specimens.[53] When compared with CT, EUS FNA changed the tumor stage in 38% of patients. Complications are extremely rare.[55] Unfortunately, some lymph nodes cannot be aspirated because of proximity to the primary tumor. Only nodes in which the needle path avoids the primary tumor are appropriate for EUS FNA because false-positive results might otherwise be obtained.

The combination of EUS and EUS FNA of celiac lymph nodes (M1a classification), deemed positive by EUS, had a sensitivity of 77%, specificity of 85%, positive predictive value of 89%, and negative predictive value of 71%.[56] EUS FNA confirmed a positive M1a classification in 94% of patients and was 98% accurate. EUS detection of M1a disease in the celiac axis and the avoidance of unnecessary surgery make EUS FNA the least costly staging strategy in patients with non-M1b esophageal cancer.[57]

For preoperative EUS examinations, N classification best predicts patient survival.[58] It is a superior predictor of patient survival than EUS determination of T and M1a classification. The use of EUS FNA is associated with improved recurrence-free and overall survival.[59] Therefore, careful EUS N classification with aggressive EUS FNA lymph node sampling is mandatory and critical to treatment planning and prognostication.

Determination of Non-nodal M1b Classification

EUS has limited value in screening for distant metastases (M1b). The distant organ must be in direct contact with the upper gastrointestinal tract for EUS to be useful. The left lateral segment of the liver and retroperitoneum are two such sites (Fig. 7–14).

Re-treatment Stage (yTNM)

After induction therapy, a subset of patients with esophageal cancer will be disease-free. Because significant morbidity and mortality are associated with surgery for esophageal cancer, the ability to detect patients who have no residual cancer (T0 N0) after induction therapy is theoretically desirable. Esophageal ultrasonography has been used in multiple clinical series for this purpose. Early series indicated that EUS was very accurate in determining T classification after chemotherapy. In these series, however, the presurgical therapy was largely ineffective in causing pathologic down-staging; therefore, EUS was accurate by merely indicating that no significant change had occurred.[60-62] In two series in which radiation therapy was provided along with chemotherapy, the accuracy of determination of T classification was again high (72% to 78%), but the prevalence of pathologic T0 disease was low or not

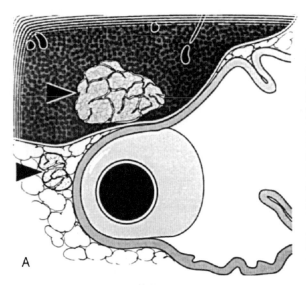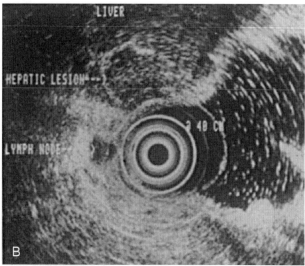

Figure 7–14. **A,** Hepatic metastasis (*upper arrow*) in the left lateral segment of the liver. A perigastric lymph node metastasis is shown (*lower arrow*). The esophageal ultrasound probe is seen in the gastric cardia. **B,** Hepatic metastasis (*upper arrow*) as seen from the gastric cardia by esophageal ultrasound. The metastasis was imaged only by esophageal ultrasound. A perigastric lymph node metastasis is shown (*lower arrow*). (From Rice TW, Boyce GA, Sivak MV, et al: Esophageal carcinoma: Esophageal ultrasound assessment of preoperative chemotherapy. Ann Thorac Surg 53:972, 1992.)

reported.[63,64] Accuracy of T classification can therefore be attributed primarily to a lack of tumor response to chemoradiotherapy.

Later series incorporate more aggressive regimens of chemoradiotherapy, with higher rates of significant down-staging of tumor and pathologic T0 N0 M0 cancer. In these series, up to 31% of patients had pathologic T0 N0 M0 stage grouping after chemoradiotherapy.[65] EUS was poor in accurately determining T classification, with reported rates of 27% to 47%.[65-69] The most common mistake made in determining T classification was overstaging because EUS is unable to distinguish tumor from inflammation and fibrosis produced by chemoradiotherapy. Similar difficulties in this differentiation have also been reported with EUS staging of rectal cancer.[70]

EUS accuracy for N classification after chemoradiotherapy has been reported in only four clinical series. The reported accuracy ranged from 49% to 71%.[65,67-69] The accuracy of N classification in patients who undergo chemoradiotherapy is lower than in patients not treated with chemoradiotherapy. Primary reasons for this inaccuracy are alterations in the ultrasound appearance of nodes after chemoradiotherapy such that established EUS criteria do not apply and residual foci of cancer within the nodes that are too small for detection by any modality other than pathologic analysis.

Change in maximal cross-sectional area before and after chemoradiotherapy appears to be a more useful means of assessing the response of esophageal cancer to preoperative therapy.[66,71] Chak and colleagues defined a response as a 50% or greater reduction in tumor area. Improved survival was reported in responders and responder subgroups who had surgery after chemoradiotherapy, adenocarcinoma, and T3 N1 M0 cancer before treatment.[71] Identification of persistent tumor in

lymph nodes by EUS FNA has been used to modify the treatment of patients receiving preoperative chemoradiotherapy.[72]

EUS has been useful in the diagnosis and restaging of patients with anastomotic recurrence that is not endoscopically visible.[73,74]

BENIGN ESOPHAGEAL DISEASES

Benign Esophageal Tumors

Detailed EUS examination of the esophageal wall has improved the diagnosis of benign esophageal tumors. EUS identification of intramural masses relies on both the layer from which the tumor arises (Table 7–1) and the ultrasound characteristics of the tumor. Homogeneous lesions that are anechoic, of intermediate echogenicity, or hyperechoic are almost exclusively benign.[75] A heterogeneous echo pattern may be seen in benign tumors, but this endosonographic finding, particularly in lesions greater than 3 cm to 4 cm in largest diameter, may be indicative of malignancy.

Tumors of the Mucosa

Fibrovascular polyps are collections of fibrous, vascular, and adipose tissue lined by normal squamous epithelium. Microscopically, fibrovascular polyps are expansions of the lamina propria.[76] These polyps usually arise in the cervical esophagus, extend into the esophageal lumen, and may reach into the stomach. Most patients eventually complain of dysphagia or respiratory symptoms, or both. Spectacular manifestations include regurgitation into the hypopharynx and mouth with subsequent aspiration and, occasionally, sudden death by

| Table 7–1 | Endoscopic Ultrasonographic Classification of Benign Esophageal Tumors |

EUS Layer	Esophageal Tumor
First/second (mucosa/deep mucosa)	Fibrovascular polyp
	Granular cell tumor
	Retention cyst
	Leiomyoma*
Third (submucosa)	Lipoma
	Fibroma
	Neurofibroma
	Granular cell tumor
Fourth (muscularis propria)	Leiomyoma*
	Cysts
Fifth	Cysts

*Leiomyomas may arise from the second or fourth ultrasound layer.

asphyxiation. Barium esophagography and CT best detect these lesions. Because fibrovascular polyps fill the esophageal lumen and have a composition similar to the mucosa, definition by esophagoscopy or EUS may be difficult or impossible.[77]

Granular cell tumors are the third most common benign esophageal tumor, and the esophagus is the most common gastrointestinal site of these tumors. Most are located in the distal end of the esophagus. Their origin is neural from the Schwann cell. Most patients with granular cell tumors are asymptomatic and rarely require surgery. At endoscopy, these lesions are yellow, firm nodules. Endoscopic biopsy is diagnostic in only 50% of patients.[78] EUS evaluation typically demonstrates a tumor less than 2 cm in diameter that has an intermediate or hypoechoic, mildly inhomogeneous solid pattern with smooth borders and rising from the inner two EUS layers.[78,79] Less than 5% originate from the submucosa. Malignant variants are rare and distinguished by size (>4 cm), nuclear pleomorphism, and mitotic activity.[80] Atypical EUS findings may predict the rare malignant granular cell tumors.

Tumors of the Submucosa

Esophageal stromal tumors are rare and include lipomas, fibromas, and hemangiomas. Lipomas are indirectly detected at esophagoscopy as a bulging of the overlying esophageal mucosa. They have a pale yellow appearance and soft texture when probed with an esophagoscope. Endoscopic biopsy usually produces normal overlying squamous epithelium because these samplings rarely penetrate the submucosa. EUS demonstrates a hyperechoic homogeneous lesion that originates in and is confined to the submucosal layer. Generally asymptomatic and most often found incidentally, lipomas require no EUS follow-up. Fibromas and neurofibromas are very

uncommon. At endoscopy, they are firm "to the touch." These lesions are less hyperechoic than lipomas. Symptomatic submucosal tumors are uncommon and the symptoms may be unrelated. These tumors are typically incidental findings of a "shotgun" investigation of atypical symptoms such as chest pain and cough. EUS is critical in diagnosis and, thus, in avoiding excision.

Hemangiomas may present with dysphagia and bleeding. Most hemangiomas are in the lower part of the esophagus and may be mistaken for esophageal varices. EUS examination reveals a hypoechoic mass with sharp margins arising from the second or third EUS layer.[81,82]

Tumors of the Muscularis Propria

Leiomyomas are benign smooth muscle tumors of the muscularis propria. Symptomatic tumors arising from the muscularis mucosae are rare, with the majority arising from the inner circular muscle layer in the distal and midthoracic esophagus.[83] EUS examinations reveal that the majority of esophageal leiomyomas are greater than 1 cm in diameter and are most frequently found in the muscularis mucosae.[84] Leiomyomas are the most common benign esophageal tumors and account for more than 70% of all benign tumors. There is no gender preponderance, and they typically occur in patients 20- to 50- years old, significantly younger than patients with esophageal carcinoma. Though frequently asymptomatic and discovered incidentally, leiomyomas can cause dysphagia, pain, or bleeding. Distal esophageal leiomyomas are often associated with symptoms of gastroesophageal reflux disease. Barium esophagography demonstrates smooth filling defects; esophagoscopy reveals a normal overlying mucosa. EUS displays a hypoechoic, sharply bordered tumor arising in the fourth ultrasound layer (Fig. 7–15). The diagnosis of small leiomyomas (<1 cm in diameter) may be enhanced with the use of miniature ultrasound probes.[84] Atypical EUS findings are a tumor larger than 4 cm, irregular margins, mixed internal echo characteristics, and associated regional lymphadenopathy. Endoscopic biopsies do not reach the muscularis propria. EUS FNA is unlikely to provide the cellular architectural characteristics necessary to differentiate leiomyomas from leiomyosarcomas, which are exceedingly rare. Malignant transformation of benign leiomyomas has been infrequently reported. Surgical resection, by minimally invasive techniques if possible, is indicated for symptomatic leiomyomas. In asymptomatic tumors with typical EUS features, expectant therapy plus EUS observation is indicated.

Miscellaneous Esophageal Diseases

Esophageal Cysts

Esophageal cysts, the second most common benign esophageal tumor, account for 20% of these lesions. The minority are acquired epithelial cysts arising in the lamina propria. Submucosal glandular inflammation is the suspected cause. The majority of esophageal cysts are congenital foregut cysts. They are lined with squamous,

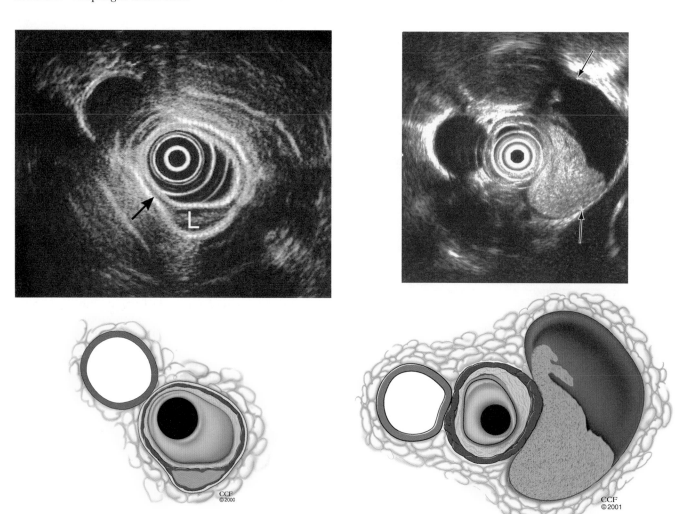

Figure 7–15. Esophageal leiomyoma. *Upper,* Endoscopic ultrasonography (EUS) of this most common benign tumor demonstrates a hypoechoic, homogeneous, well-demarcated tumor with no associated lymphadenopathy. EUS balloon overdistention blends the first three ultrasound layers into one hyperechoic layer. The tumor arises from and is confined to the fourth ultrasound layer (*arrow*). *Lower,* A benign leiomyoma arises from and is confined to the muscularis propria.

Figure 7–16. Foregut cyst. *Upper,* Endoscopic ultrasound demonstrates a mass (*arrows*) adjacent to the trachea and esophagus. The cyst has two components, one hyperechoic (white), representing proteinaceous material, and one hypoechoic (black), representing fluid. *Lower,* A foregut cyst in close proximity to the esophagus and trachea.

respiratory, or columnar epithelium and may contain smooth muscle, cartilage, or fat. Esophageal duplication is a subtype of foregut cyst; it is lined with squamous epithelium and its submucosal and muscularis elements interdigitate with the muscularis propria of the esophagus. EUS can clearly define the intramural or extraesophageal nature of these tumors and further determine their anechoic, cystic nature (Fig. 7–16).[85-88] Transesophageal EUS drainage of a foregut cyst has been reported, but drainage of the cyst without destruction of its lining may result in recurrence.[89]

Esophageal Varices

Esophageal varices have the typical appearance of blood vessels at EUS. Appearing as tubular, round, or serpigi-

nous echo-free structures, they may be visualized within the submucosa or in tissues adjacent to the esophagus (Fig. 7–17). These EUS patterns change after sclerosis.[90] Intravariceal sclerosis fills the varix with echogenic material representing thrombus. Paravariceal injection leads to obliteration of the varix with hypoechoic extravariceal thickening.

Achalasia

EUS findings in achalasia are controversial. Some authors have reported thickened esophageal wall in most patients examined.[91,92] This excessive thickening, however, may be artifactual. In a dilated and convoluted esophagus, the ultrasound transducer may orient at an angle oblique to the esophageal wall and give a false

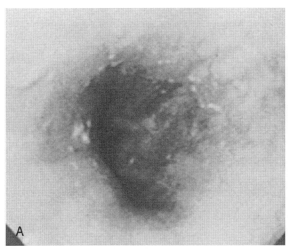
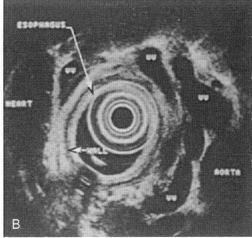

Figure 7–17.   Paraesophageal varices. **A,** At endoscopy, small varices are not visible. **B,** On esophageal ultrasound, the varices (VV) are prominent anechoic, tubular, and rounded structures outside the esophageal wall.

appearance of wall thickening.[93] The main role of EUS in achalasia is to exclude other mural abnormalities.[94-96]

PARAESOPHAGEAL DISEASES

EUS has been used to examine the mediastinal lymph nodes in patients with bronchogenic carcinoma.[97-99] In this setting, EUS has a reported positive predictive value of 77%, a negative predictive value of 93%, and an overall accuracy of 92% when using criteria similar to regional lymph node evaluation in esophageal carcinoma.[98] Anatomic constraints limit its usefulness for evaluation of lymph nodes in proximity to the airway. EUS FNA provides cytologic differentiation between benign and malignant lymphadenopathy[100] and has successfully diagnosed solid lesions of the mediastinum and lung.[75,101-103]

CONCLUSIONS

EUS and EUS FNA are essential in determining the clinical stage and directing treatment of esophageal cancer. The diagnosis of benign esophageal tumors requires EUS examination, which determines both the layer of origin in the esophageal wall and the ultrasound characteristics of the tumor. Because many of these tumors are asymptomatic, EUS affords simple follow-up and avoids unnecessary excision. EUS is a useful adjuvant for the diagnosis and treatment of paraesophageal disease.

REFERENCES

1. Kimmey MB, Martin RW: Fundamentals of endosonography. Gastrointest Endosc Clin N Am 2:557-573, 1992.
2. Vilmann P, Khattar S, Hancke S: Endoscopic ultrasound examination of the upper gastrointestinal tract using a curved-array transducer. A preliminary report. Surg Endosc 5:79-82, 1991.
3. Bolondi L, Casanova P, Santi V, et al: The sonographic appearance of the normal gastric wall: An in vitro study. Ultrasound Med Biol 12:991-998, 1986.
4. Kimmey MB, Martin RW, Haggitt RC, et al: Histologic correlates of gastrointestinal ultrasound images. Gastroenterology 96:433-441, 1989.
5. Greene FL, Page DL, Fleming ID, et al: AJCC Cancer Staging Manual. New York, Springer-Verlag, 2002.
6. Botet JF, Lightdale CJ, Zauber AG, et al: Preoperative staging of esophageal cancer: Comparison of endoscopic US and dynamic CT. Radiology 181:419-425, 1991.
7. Date H, Miyashita M, Sasajima K, et al: Assessment of adventitial involvement of esophageal carcinoma by endoscopic ultrasonography. Surg Endosc 4:195-197, 1990.
8. Heintz A, Hohne U, Schweden F, Junginger T: Preoperative detection of intrathoracic tumor spread of esophageal cancer: Endosonography versus computed tomography. Surg Endosc 5:75-78, 1991.
9. Tio TL, Cohen P, Coene PP, et al: Endosonography and computed tomography of esophageal carcinoma. Preoperative classification compared to the new (1987) TNM system. Gastroenterology 96:1478-1486, 1989.
10. Vilgrain V, Mompoint D, Palazzo L, et al: Staging of esophageal carcinoma: Comparison of results with endoscopic sonography and CT. AJR Am J Roentgenol 155:277-281, 1990.
11. Ziegler K, Sanft C, Zeitz M, et al: Evaluation of endosonography in TN staging of oesophageal cancer. Gut 32:16-20, 1991.
12. Reinig JW, Stanley JH, Schabel SI: CT evaluation of thickened esophageal walls. AJR Am J Roentgenol 140:931-934, 1983.
13. Consigliere D, Chua CL, Hui F, et al: Computed tomography for oesophageal carcinoma: Its value to the surgeon. J R Coll Surg Edinb 37:113-137, 1992.
14. Duignan JP, McEntee GP, O'Connell DJ, et al: The role of CT in the management of carcinoma of the oesophagus and cardia. Ann R Coll Surg Engl 69:286-288, 1987.
15. Kasbarian M, Fuentes P, Brichon PY: Usefulness of Computed Tomography in Assessing the Extension of Carcinoma of the Esophagus and Gastroesophageal Junction. Berlin, Springer-Verlag, 1988.
16. Kirk SJ, Moorehead RJ, McIlrath E, et al: Does preoperative computed tomography scanning aid assessment of esophageal carcinoma? Postgrad Med J 66:191-194, 1990.
17. Markland CG, Manhire A, Davies P, et al: The role of computed tomography in assessing the operability of oesophageal carcinoma. Eur J Cardiothorac Surg 3:33-36, 1989.
18. Rice TW, Boyce GA, Sivak MV: Esophageal ultrasound and the preoperative staging of carcinoma of the esophagus. J Thorac Cardiovasc Surg 101:536-543, discussion 543-544, 1991.
19. Ruol A, Rossi M, Ruffatto A: Reevaluation of Computed Tomography in Preoperative Staging of Esophageal and Cardial Cancers: A Prospective Study. New York, Springer-Verlag, 1987.

20. Sondenaa K, Skaane P, Nygaard K, Skjennald A: Value of computed tomography in preoperative evaluation of resectability and staging in oesophageal carcinoma. Eur J Surg 158:537-540, 1992.

21. Ginsberg GG, Al-Kawas EH, Nguyen CC: Endoscopic ultrasound evaluation of vascular involvement in esophageal cancer: A comparison with computed tomography [abstract]. Gastrointest Endosc 39:A276, 1993.

22. Fockens P, Van den Brande JH, van Dullemen HM, et al: Endosonographic T-staging of esophageal carcinoma: A learning curve. Gastrointest Endosc 44:58-62, 1996.

23. Schlick T, Heintz A, Junginger T: The examiner's learning effect and its influence on the quality of endoscopic ultrasonography in carcinoma of the esophagus and gastric cardia. Surg Endosc 13:894-898, 1999.

24. Rosch T: Endosonographic staging of esophageal cancer: A review of literature results. Gastrointest Endosc Clin N Am 5:537-547, 1995.

25. Rice TW, Blackstone EH, Adelstein DJ, et al: Role of clinically determined depth of tumor invasion in the treatment of esophageal carcinoma. J Thorac Cardiovasc Surg 125:1091-1102, 2003.

26. Kelly S, Harris KM, Berry E, et al: A systematic review of the staging performance of endoscopic ultrasound in gastro-oesophageal carcinoma. Gut 49:534-539, 2001.

27. Meining A, Dittler HJ, Wolf A, et al: You get what you expect? A critical appraisal of imaging methodology in endosonographic cancer staging. Gut 50:599-603, 2002.

28. Bhutani MS, Barde CJ, Markert RJ, Gopalswamy N: Length of esophageal cancer and degree of luminal stenosis during upper endoscopy predict T stage by endoscopic ultrasound. Endoscopy 34:461-463, 2002.

29. Dancygier H, Classen M: Endoscopic ultrasonography in esophageal diseases. Gastrointest Endosc 35:220-225, 1989.

30. Hordijk ML, Zander H, van Blankenstein M, Tilanus HW: Influence of tumor stenosis on the accuracy of endosonography in preoperative T staging of esophageal cancer. Endoscopy 25:171-175, 1993.

31. Catalano MF, Van Dam J, Sivak JMV: Malignant esophageal strictures: Staging accuracy of endoscopic ultrasonography. Gastrointest Endosc 41:535-539, 1995.

32. Van Dam J, Rice TW, Catalano MF, et al: High-grade malignant stricture is predictive of esophageal tumor stage: Risks of endosonographic evaluation. Cancer 71:2910-2917, 1993.

33. Kallemanis GE, Gupta PK, al-Kawas FH, et al: Endoscopic ultrasound for staging esophageal cancer, with and without dilation, is clinically important and safe. Gastrointest Endosc 41:540-546, 1995.

34. Pfau PR, Ginsberg GG, Lew RJ, et al: Esophageal dilation for endosonographic evaluation of malignant esophageal strictures is safe and effective. Am J Gastroenterol 95:2813-2815, 2000.

35. Wallace MB, Hawes RH, Sahai AV, et al: Dilation of malignant esophageal stenosis to allow EUS guided fine-needle aspiration: Safety and effect on patient management. Gastrointest Endosc 51:309-313, 2000.

36. Binmoeller KF, Seifert H, Seitz U, et al: Ultrasonic esophagoprobe for TNM staging of highly stenosing esophageal carcinoma. Gastrointest Endosc 41:547-552, 1995.

37. Hunerbein M, Ghadimi BM, Haensch W, Schlag PM: Transendoscopic ultrasound of esophageal and gastric cancer using miniaturized ultrasound catheter probes. Gastrointest Endosc 48:371-375, 1998.

38. McLoughlin RF, Cooperberg PL, Mathieson JR, et al: High resolution endoluminal ultrasonography in the staging of esophageal carcinoma. J Ultrasound Med 14:725-730, 1995.

39. Menzel J, Hoepffner N, Nottberg H, et al: Preoperative staging of esophageal carcinoma: Miniprobe sonography versus conventional endoscopic ultrasound in a prospective histopathologically verified study. Endoscopy 31:291-297, 1999.

40. Buskens CJ, Westerterp M, Lagarde SM, et al: Prediction of appropriateness of local endoscopic treatment for high-grade dysplasia and early adenocarcinoma by EUS and histopathologic features. Gastrointest Endosc 60:703-710, 2004.

41. Scotiniotis IA, Kochman ML, Lewis JD, et al: Accuracy of EUS in the evaluation of Barrett's esophagus and high-grade dysplasia or intramucosal carcinoma. Gastrointest Endosc 54:689-696, 2001.

42. May A, Gunter E, Roth F, et al: Accuracy of staging in early oesophageal cancer using high resolution endoscopy and high resolution endosonography: A comparative, prospective, and blinded trial. Gut 53:634-640, 2004.

43. Murata Y, Napoleon B, Odegaard S: High-frequency endoscopic ultrasonography in the evaluation of superficial esophageal cancer. Endoscopy 35:429-435, discussion 436, 2003.

44. Catalano MF, Sivak MV Jr, Rice T, et al: Endosonographic features predictive of lymph node metastasis. Gastrointest Endosc 40:442-446, 1994.

45. Bhutani MS, Hawes RH, Hoffman BJ: A comparison of the accuracy of echo features during endoscopic ultrasound (EUS) and EUS-guided fine-needle aspiration for diagnosis of malignant lymph node invasion. Gastrointest Endosc 45:474-479, 1997.

46. Catalano MF, Alcocer E, Chak A, et al: Evaluation of metastatic celiac axis lymph nodes in patients with esophageal carcinoma: Accuracy of EUS. Gastrointest Endosc 50:352-356, 1999.

47. Rice TW, Zuccaro G Jr, Adelstein DJ, et al: Esophageal carcinoma: Depth of tumor invasion is predictive of regional lymph node status. Ann Thorac Surg 65:787-792, 1998.

48. Natsugoe S, Yoshinaka H, Shimada M, et al: Number of lymph node metastases determined by presurgical ultrasound and endoscopic ultrasound is related to prognosis in patients with esophageal carcinoma. Ann Surg 234:613-618, 2001.

49. Wiersema MJ, Hawes RH, Tao LC, et al: Endoscopic ultrasonography as an adjunct to fine needle aspiration cytology of the upper and lower gastrointestinal tract. Gastrointest Endosc 38:35-39, 1992.

50. Wiersema MJ, Kochman ML, Chak A, et al: Real-time endoscopic ultrasound-guided fine-needle aspiration of a mediastinal lymph node. Gastrointest Endosc 39:429-431, 1993.

51. Mortensen MB, Pless T, Durup J, et al: Clinical impact of endoscopic ultrasound–guided fine needle aspiration biopsy in patients with upper gastrointestinal tract malignancies. A prospective study. Endoscopy 33:478-483, 2001.

52. Vazquez-Sequeiros E, Norton ID, Clain JE, et al: Impact of EUS-guided fine-needle aspiration on lymph node staging in patients with esophageal carcinoma. Gastrointest Endosc 53:751-757, 2001.

53. Vazquez-Sequeiros E, Wiersema MJ, Clain JE, et al: Impact of lymph node staging on therapy of esophageal carcinoma. Gastroenterology 125:1626-1635, 2003.

54. Wiersema MJ, Vilmann P, Giovannini M, et al: Endosonography-guided fine-needle aspiration biopsy: Diagnostic accuracy and complication assessment. Gastroenterology 112:1087-1095, 1997.

55. O'Toole D, Palazzo L, Arotcarena R, et al: Assessment of complications of EUS-guided fine-needle aspiration. Gastrointest Endosc 53:470-474, 2001.

56. Eloubeidi MA, Wallace MB, Reed CE, et al: The utility of EUS and EUS-guided fine needle aspiration in detecting celiac lymph node metastasis in patients with esophageal cancer: A single-center experience. Gastrointest Endosc 54:714-719, 2001.

57. Harewood GC, Wiersema MJ: A cost analysis of endoscopic ultrasound in the evaluation of esophageal cancer. Am J Gastroenterol 97:452-458, 2002.

58. Pfau PR, Ginsberg GG, Lew RJ, et al: EUS predictors of long-term survival in esophageal carcinoma. Gastrointest Endosc 53:463-469, 2001.

59. Harewood GC, Kumar KS: Assessment of clinical impact of endoscopic ultrasound on esophageal cancer. J Gastroenterol Hepatol 19:433-439, 2004.

60. Adelstein DJ, Rice TW, Boyce GA, et al: Adenocarcinoma of the esophagus and gastroesophageal junction. Clinical and pathologic assessment of response to induction chemotherapy. Am J Clin Oncol 17:14-18, 1994.

61. Hordijk ML, Kok TC, Wilson JH, Mulder AH: Assessment of response of esophageal carcinoma to induction chemotherapy. Endoscopy 25:592-596, 1993.

62. Roubein LD, DuBrow R, David C, et al: Endoscopic ultrasonography in the quantitative assessment of response to chemotherapy in patients with adenocarcinoma of the esophagus and esophagogastric junction. Endoscopy 25:587-591, 1993.

63. Dittler HJ, Fink U, Siewert GR: Response to chemotherapy in esophageal cancer. Endoscopy 26:769-771, 1994.

64. Giovannini M, Seitz JF, Thomas P, et al: Endoscopic ultrasonography for assessment of the response to combined radiation

therapy and chemotherapy in patients with esophageal cancer. Endoscopy 29:4-9, 1997.

65. Zuccaro G Jr, Rice TW, Goldblum J, et al: Endoscopic ultrasound cannot determine suitability for esophagectomy after aggressive chemoradiotherapy for esophageal cancer. Am J Gastroenterol 94:906-912, 1999.

66. Isenberg G, Chak A, Canto MI, et al: Endoscopic ultrasound in restaging of esophageal cancer after neoadjuvant chemoradiation. Gastrointest Endosc 48:158-163, 1998.

67. Laterza E, de Manzoni G, Guglielmi A, et al: Endoscopic ultrasonography in the staging of esophageal carcinoma after preoperative radiotherapy and chemotherapy. Ann Thorac Surg 67:1466-1469, 1999.

68. Kalha I, Kaw M, Fukami N, et al: The accuracy of endoscopic ultrasound for restaging esophageal carcinoma after chemoradiation therapy. Cancer 101:940-947, 2004.

69. Beseth BD, Bedford R, Isacoff WH, et al: Endoscopic ultrasound does not accurately assess pathologic stage of esophageal cancer after neoadjuvant chemoradiotherapy. Am Surg 66:827-831, 2000.

70. Fleshman JW, Myerson RJ, Fry RD, Kodner IJ: Accuracy of transrectal ultrasound in predicting pathologic stage of rectal cancer before and after preoperative radiation therapy. Dis Colon Rectum 35:823-829, 1992.

71. Chak A, Canto MI, Cooper GS, et al: Endosonographic assessment of multimodality therapy predicts survival of esophageal carcinoma patients. Cancer 88:1788-1795, 2000.

72. Agarwal B, Swisher S, Ajani J, et al: Endoscopic ultrasound after preoperative chemoradiation can help identify patients who benefit maximally after surgical esophageal resection. Am J Gastroenterol 99:1258-1266, 2004.

73. Catalano MF, Sivak MV Jr, Rice TW, Van Dam J: Postoperative screening for anastomotic recurrence of esophageal carcinoma by endoscopic ultrasonography. Gastrointest Endosc 42:540-544, 1995.

74. Lightdale CJ, Botet JF, Kelsen DP, et al: Diagnosis of recurrent upper gastrointestinal cancer at the surgical anastomosis by endoscopic ultrasound. Gastrointest Endosc 35:407-412, 1989.

75. Kawamoto K, Yamada Y, Utsunomiya T, et al: Gastrointestinal submucosal tumors: Evaluation with endoscopic US. Radiology 205:733-740, 1997.

76. Lewin KJ, Appelman HD: Mesenchymal tumors and tumor-like proliferations of the esophagus. In Rosai J, Sobin LH (eds): Tumors of the Esophagus and Stomach. Washington, DC, Armed Forces Institute of Pathology; 1996, pp 145-161. Atlas of Tumor Pathology; 3rd series, fascicle 18.

77. Schuhmacher C, Becker K, Dittler HJ, et al: Fibrovascular esophageal polyp as a diagnostic challenge. Dis Esophagus 13:324-327, 2000.

78. Palazzo L, Landi B, Cellier C, et al: Endosonographic features of esophageal granular cell tumors. Endoscopy 29:850-853, 1997.

79. Love MH, Glaser M, Edmunds SE, Mendelson RM: Granular cell tumour of the oesophagus: Endoscopic ultrasound appearances. Australas Radiol 43:253-255, 1999.

80. Goldblum JR, Rice TW, Zuccaro G, Richter JE: Granular cell tumors of the esophagus: A clinical and pathologic study of 13 cases. Ann Thorac Surg 62:860-865, 1996.

81. Araki K, Ohno S, Egashira A, et al: Esophageal hemangioma: A case report and review of the literature. Hepatogastroenterology 46:3148-3154, 1999.

82. Maluf-Filho F, Sakai P, Amico EC, Pinotti HW: Giant cavernous hemangioma of the esophagus: Endoscopic and echo-endoscopic appearance. Endoscopy 31:S32, 1999.

83. Takada N, Higashino M, Osugi H, et al: Utility of endoscopic ultrasonography in assessing the indications for endoscopic surgery of submucosal esophageal tumors. Surg Endosc 13:228-230, 1999.

84. Xu GM, Niu YL, Zou XP, et al: The diagnostic value of transendoscopic miniature ultrasonic probe for esophageal diseases. Endoscopy 30(Suppl 1):A28-A32, 1998.

85. Bhutani MS, Hoffman BJ, Reed C: Endosonographic diagnosis of an esophageal duplication cyst. Endoscopy 28:396-397, 1996.

86. Faigel DO, Burke A, Ginsberg GG, et al: The role of endoscopic ultrasound in the evaluation and management of foregut duplications. Gastrointest Endosc 45:99-103, 1997.

87. Lim LL, Ho KY, Goh PM: Preoperative diagnosis of a paraesophageal bronchogenic cyst using endosonography. Ann Thorac Surg 73:633-635, 2002.

88. Massari M, De Simone M, Cioffi U, et al: Endoscopic ultrasonography in the evaluation of leiomyoma and extramucosal cysts of the esophagus. Hepatogastroenterology 45:938-943, 1998.

89. Van Dam J, Rice TW, Sivak MV Jr: Endoscopic ultrasonography and endoscopically guided needle aspiration for the diagnosis of upper gastrointestinal tract foregut cysts. Am J Gastroenterol 87:762-765, 1992.

90. Yasuda K, Cho E, Nakajima M, Kawai K: Diagnosis of submucosal lesions of the upper gastrointestinal tract by endoscopic ultrasonography. Gastrointest Endosc 36(2 Suppl):S17-S20, 1990.

91. Bergami GL, Fruhwirth R, Di Mario M, Fasanelli S: Contribution of ultrasonography in the diagnosis of achalasia. J Pediatr Gastroenterol Nutr 14:92-96, 1992.

92. Deviere J, Dunham F, Rickaert F, et al: Endoscopic ultrasonography in achalasia. Gastroenterology 96:1210-1213, 1989.

93. Falk GW, Van Dam J, Sivak MV: Endoscopic ultrasonography (EUS) in achalasia. Gastrointest Endosc 37:241, 1991.

94. Barthet M, Mambrini P, Audibert P, et al: Relationships between endosonographic appearance and clinical or manometric features in patients with achalasia. Eur J Gastroenterol Hepatol 10:559-564, 1998.

95. Ponsot P, Chaussade S, Palazzo L, et al: Endoscopic ultrasonography in achalasia. Gastroenterology 98:253, 1990.

96. Ziegler K, Sanft C, Friedrich M, et al: Endosonographic appearance of the esophagus in achalasia. Endoscopy 22:1-4, 1990.

97. Kobayashi H, Danabara T, Sugama Y, et al: Observation of lymph nodes and great vessels in the mediastinum by endoscopic ultrasonography. Jpn J Med 26:353-359, 1987.

98. Kondo D, Imaizumi M, Abe T, et al: Endoscopic ultrasound examination for mediastinal lymph node metastases of lung cancer. Chest 98:586-593, 1990.

99. Potepan P, Meroni E, Spagnoli I, et al: Non–small-cell lung cancer: Detection of mediastinal lymph node metastases by endoscopic ultrasound and CT. Eur Radiol 6:19-24, 1996.

100. Mishra G, Sahai AV, Penman ID, et al: Endoscopic ultrasonography with fine-needle aspiration: An accurate and simple diagnostic modality for sarcoidosis. Endoscopy 31:377-382, 1999.

101. Fritscher-Ravens A, Petrasch S, Reinacher-Schick A, et al: Diagnostic value of endoscopic ultrasonography-guided fine-needle aspiration cytology of mediastinal masses in patients with intrapulmonary lesions and nondiagnostic bronchoscopy. Respiration 66:150-155, 1999.

102. Hunerbein M, Ghadimi BM, Haensch W, Schlag PM: Transesophageal biopsy of mediastinal and pulmonary tumors by means of endoscopic ultrasound guidance. J Thorac Cardiovasc Surg 116:554-559, 1998.

103. Pedersen BH, Vilmann P, Folke K, et al: Endoscopic ultrasonography and real-time guided fine-needle aspiration biopsy of solid lesions of the mediastinum suspected of malignancy. Chest 110:539-544, 1996.

8

Esophageal Motility

Rodney John Mason

The major function of the esophagus is to transport food from the mouth to the stomach. Secondary functions are to keep the esophagus empty, prevent regurgitation of gastric contents into the esophagus and trachea, and vent the stomach of excessive swallowed air. Functional disorders of the esophagus often give rise to symptoms before the development of injury recognizable by structural, histologic, or biochemical changes. They can exist for a period without causing morphologic changes while causing considerable symptoms. The symptoms typically associated with esophageal motility disorders are nonspecific and include dysphagia, regurgitation, and chest pain, which may be manifested as either a pressure-like sensation or retrosternal burning. Ascribing these symptoms to a specific esophageal abnormality in the absence of structural or histologic findings and without further investigation can lead to an error in diagnosis because a variety of gastric, duodenal, cardiac, and pulmonary disorders can cause symptomatology similar to esophageal abnormalities, thus making it difficult to differentiate and discriminate them from the latter. Furthermore, esophageal motility disorders can cause atypical symptoms, such as chest pain, chronic cough, or shortness of breath, that lead the investigator to suspect abnormalities of the heart or lung. Complicating matters even more, functional esophageal motility disorders can also occur concomitantly with gastroduodenal, cardiac, and pulmonary disease. Consequently, objective methods are required to confirm the presence of an esophageal motor abnormality and distinguish it from other conditions. Correct diagnosis of the abnormality and identification of the underlying cause are essential for the selection of appropriate therapy and to avoid failure or recurrence. This requires a sound understanding of normal esophageal physiology and the functional abnormalities that may result in tissue injury if allowed to persist.[1]

Esophageal motility disorders consist of a number of specifically identifiable disorders and a number of poorly characterized conditions that show a spectrum of esophageal motor abnormalities. The two best-characterized motility disorders, achalasia and diffuse esophageal spasm, represent only a small percentage of diagnosed motility disorders. The incidence of achalasia is 1 case per 100,000 population per year. As with any other chronic illness, prevalence exceeds incidence significantly. Familial clustering is observed, but a genetic relationship has not been established. Nutcracker esophagus is the most common motility disorder, but it is the most controversial in significance.

PHYSIOLOGIC ASPECTS OF ESOPHAGEAL MOTILITY

The esophagus is a muscular tube that traverses the neck and two body cavities—the chest and abdomen. The two body cavities have different pressure profiles, which is important for understanding esophageal motility. The intrapleural space that surrounds the esophagus in the chest cavity has a pressure that is essentially below atmospheric pressure during most of the respiratory cycle, whereas the distal esophagus in the abdominal cavity has a surrounding pressure that is always above atmospheric pressure. Striated muscle is found in the upper two thirds of the esophagus and nonstriated muscle is found in the lower third. In the upper quarter both layers are striated. In the second quarter of the esophagus, bundles of nonstriated muscle appear first on the internal aspect of the muscle and gradually replace the striated muscle more caudally. The act of alimentation requires the passage of food and drink from the mouth into the stomach. One third of this distance consists of the mouth and hypopharynx, and two thirds consist of the esophagus. To comprehend the mechanics of alimentation, it is useful to visualize the gullet as a mechanical model in which the tongue and pharynx function as a piston pump with three valves and the body of the esophagus and cardia function as a worm drive pump with a single valve. The three valves in the pharyngeal cylinder are the soft pallet, the epiglottis, and the cricopharyngeus. The valve of the esophageal pump is the lower esophageal sphincter (LES). Failure of the valves or the pumps leads to motility abnormalities manifested as difficulty in the

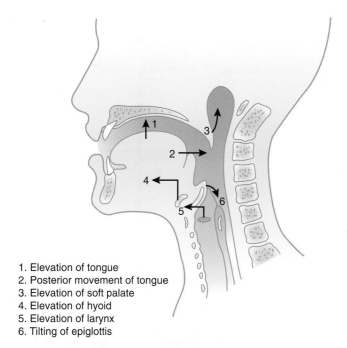

1. Elevation of tongue
2. Posterior movement of tongue
3. Elevation of soft palate
4. Elevation of hyoid
5. Elevation of larynx
6. Tilting of epiglottis

Figure 8–1. Sequence of events during the oropharyngeal phase of swallowing.

propulsion of food from the mouth to the stomach or regurgitation of gastric contents from the stomach into the pharynx.

Upper Esophageal Sphincter

The first phase of swallowing is the oral phase. Food is taken into the mouth in a variety of bite sizes, where it is broken up, mixed with saliva, and lubricated. When food is ready for swallowing, the tongue, acting like a piston, moves the bolus into the posterior oropharynx and forces it into the hypopharynx (Fig. 8–1). This marks the pharyngeal phase, and swallowing then passes out of conscious control and is entirely a reflex. Concomitant with posterior movement of the tongue, the soft palate is elevated, thereby closing the passage between the oropharynx and nasopharynx. This partitioning prevents pressure generated in the oropharynx from being dissipated through the nose. When the soft palate is paralyzed, as occurs after a cerebrovascular accident, food is commonly regurgitated into the nasopharynx. During swallowing, the hyoid bone moves upward and anteriorly to elevate the larynx and open the retrolaryngeal space. This action brings the epiglottis under the tongue (see Fig. 8–1). The backward tilt of the epiglottis covers the opening of the larynx to prevent aspiration. The entire pharyngeal portion of swallowing occurs within 1.5 seconds.

The pressure in the hypopharynx rises abruptly during swallowing to reach at least 60 mm Hg. A sizable pressure difference develops between the pharyngeal pressure and the less than atmospheric midesophageal or intrathoracic pressure (Fig. 8–2). This pressure gradient speeds the movement of food from the

hypopharynx into the esophagus when the cricopharyngeus or upper esophageal sphincter (UES) relaxes and opens and the cervical esophagus is appropriately compliant. The bolus is propelled through the open sphincter by the piston-like action of the tongue and the peristaltic contractions of the posterior laryngeal constrictors and is sucked into the thoracic esophagus by the pressure differential. Compliance of the striated muscle of the cervical esophagus is crucial for this phase of swallowing, and loss of compliance results in severe dysphagia. The UES closes within an additional 0.5 second, with the immediate closing pressure reaching approximately twice the resting level of 30 mm Hg. This postrelaxation contraction continues down the esophagus as a peristaltic wave (Fig. 8–3). The high closing pressure and initiation of the peristaltic wave prevent regurgitation of the bolus from the esophagus back into the pharynx. After the peristaltic wave has passed farther down the esophagus, the pressure in the UES returns to its resting level (see Fig. 8–3).

Swallowing can be started at will, or it can be reflexively elicited by stimulation of areas in the mouth and pharynx, including the anterior and posterior tonsillar pillars and the posterior lateral walls of the hypopharynx. The afferent nerves of the pharynx are the glossopharyngeal nerve and the superior laryngeal branches of the vagus. Once aroused by stimuli entering via these nerves, the swallowing center in the medulla coordinates the complete act of swallowing by discharging impulses through the 5th, 7th, 10th, 11th, and 12th cranial nerves, as well as the motor neurons of C1 to C3. Discharges through these nerves occur in a rather specific pattern and last for approximately 0.5 second. Little is known about the organization of the swallowing center except that it can trigger swallowing after a variety of different inputs, but the response is always a rigidly ordered pattern of outflow. After a cerebrovascular accident, this coordinated outflow may be altered and result in mild abnormalities of swallowing. In more severe injury, swallowing can be grossly disrupted and lead to repetitive aspiration.

The striated muscles of the cricopharyngeus and the upper third of the esophagus are activated by efferent fibers distributed through the vagus nerve and its recurrent laryngeal branches. Integrity of innervation is required for the cricopharyngeus to relax in coordination with the laryngohyoid elevation and pharyngeal contraction and resume its resting tone once a bolus has entered the upper part of the esophagus. Concomitantly, the striated muscle of the cervical esophagus must have the compliance to dilate and accept the swallowed bolus. Central nervous system damage from a variety of causes can interfere with innervation of the larynx, cricopharyngeus, and upper esophagus. The resulting loss of muscle function and compliance can predispose the patient to aspiration or dysphagia.

Esophageal Body

The pharyngeal activity in swallowing initiates the esophageal phase. Because of the helical arrangement of its circular muscles, the body of the esophagus functions

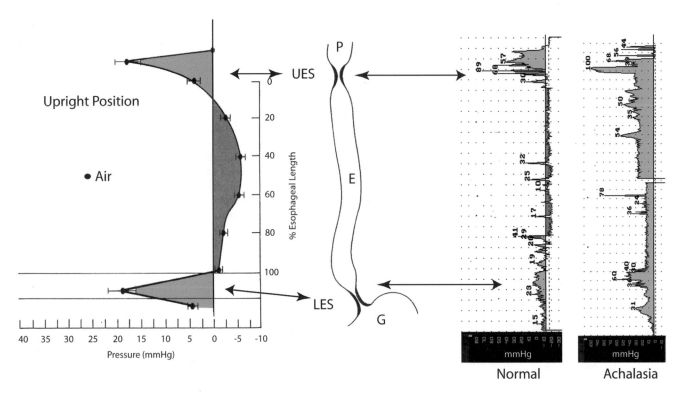

Figure 8–2. Resting pressure profile of the foregut showing the pressure differential between the atmospheric pharyngeal pressure (P), the less than atmospheric midesophageal pressure (E), and the greater than atmospheric intragastric pressure (G), with the interposed high-pressure zones of the upper esophageal sphincter (UES) and lower esophageal sphincter (LES). The necessity for coordinated relaxation of the UES and LES to move a bolus into the stomach is apparent. Esophageal work occurs when a bolus is pushed across the pressure gradient from the midesophageal area (E) into the stomach (G). A sample of a normal resting pressure profile is compared with the resting profile of a patient with achalasia. The patient with achalasia has a resting baseline pressure that is substantially above atmospheric pressure, a pattern of esophageal pressurization commonly seen in such patients.

as a worm drive propulsive pump and is responsible for transmitting a bolus of food from the distal end of the esophagus into the stomach. The esophageal phase of swallowing represents esophageal work performed during alimentation in that food is moved into the stomach from an intrathoracic pressure of −6 mm Hg to an average intra-abdominal pressure of +6 mm Hg, that is, a gradient of 12 mm Hg (see Fig. 8–2). Effective and coordinated smooth muscle function in the lower third of the esophagus is therefore important in pumping food into the stomach.

The act of pumping is termed peristalsis, which denotes a progressive sequential aboral contraction that traverses the entire esophagus. During this process the longitudinal muscle contracts and shortens, thereby providing a base for segmental contraction of the rings of the circular muscular fibers.[2] The circular muscle contractions can take the form of primary or secondary peristalsis or nonperistaltic tertiary contractions. Contraction of the striated esophageal muscle is dependent on sequential activation of neurons situated in the nucleus ambiguus. Peristalsis in the nonstriated muscle is mediated at the level of the dorsomotor nucleus of the vagus nerve at the level of the myenteric plexus.

Primary peristalsis is a biphasic response consisting of a wave of initial inhibition of the circular smooth muscle, followed by a wave of contraction.[3,4] Electrical stimulation, or the "on response," causes the circular muscle to relax. When the stimulus is removed (the off response), the muscle contracts. The latency of contraction is variable. The distal end of the esophagus shows greater inhibitory innervation than the proximal end does.[5] The shorter latency period in the proximal esophagus in conjunction with the longer latency in the distal esophagus results in the so-called latency gradient, which is thought to result in peristalsis down the esophagus (Fig. 8–4). The latency gradient appears to be mediated by nitric oxide. Blockage of nitric oxide reduces the latency between the onset of swallowing and esophageal contractions while increasing the velocity of the onset of propagation and thus converts a peristaltic contraction into a simultaneous contraction. The proximal esophagus is under greater cholinergic control than the distal esophagus, and an increase in cholinergic stimulation will delay the latency of contraction in the proximal esophagus and thereby result in the loss of peristalsis.[6] Longitudinal muscle contracts with stimulation and sustains contraction until the stimulus is removed.

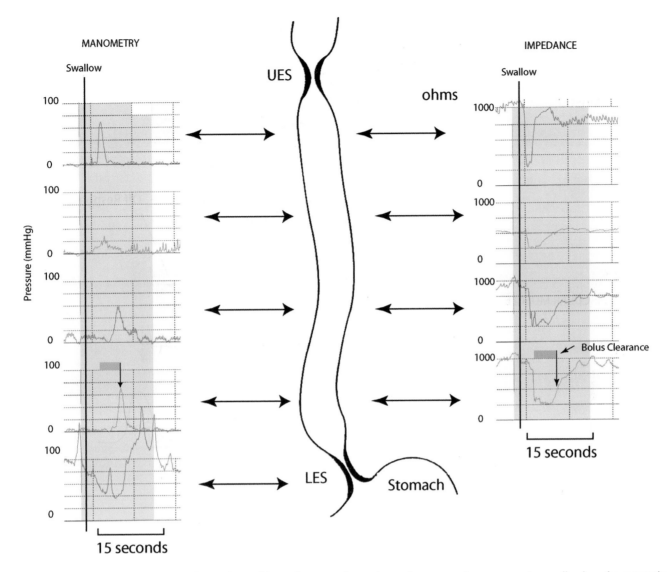

Figure 8–3. Combined intraluminal esophageal impedance and esophageal pressure in response to swallowing. An example of bolus transport is shown in channel 4. The duration of flow is depicted by the blue rectangle. The tail of the bolus corresponds to the maximum upstroke in the peristaltic contraction wave on the manometry tracing. The bolus clearance is antegrade and complete, and the manometry pressure wave is peristaltic. LES, lower esophageal sphincter; UES, upper esophageal sphincter.

The contraction wave appears manometrically as a bell-shaped curve and is seen to form when the circular muscle contracts around the pressure transducer on the manometry catheter. The peristaltic wave generates an occlusive pressure varying from 30 to 150 mm Hg (see Fig. 8–3). The wave rises to a peak in 1 second, lasts at the peak for about 0.5 second, and then subsides in about 1.5 seconds. The entire course of the rise and fall in occlusive pressure may occupy one point in the esophagus for 3 to 5 seconds. A small plateau is often seen before the sharp upstroke of the bell-shaped curve and represents the pressure within the swallowed bolus. The pressure is usually highest in the tail of the bolus. The peak of a primary peristaltic contraction initiated by a swallow moves down the esophagus at 2 to 4 cm/sec and reaches the distal esophagus about 9 seconds after

swallowing has been initiated (see Fig. 8–3). Consecutive swallows produce similar primary peristaltic waves, but when the act of swallowing is repeated rapidly, the amplitudes of the second and subsequent swallow fall within the refractory period of the first swallow and result in an esophagus that remains relaxed and refractory. The peristaltic wave occurs only after the last movement of the pharynx and forms the basis for the practice of spacing swallows at least 30 seconds apart.[7] This phenomenon is referred to as postdeglutitive inhibition.

Progress of the wave down the esophagus is caused by sequential activation of its muscles initiated by efferent vagal nerve fibers that arise in the swallowing center. Continuity of the esophageal muscle is not necessary if the nerves remain intact. If the muscles but not the nerves are cut, the pressure wave begins distally below

131

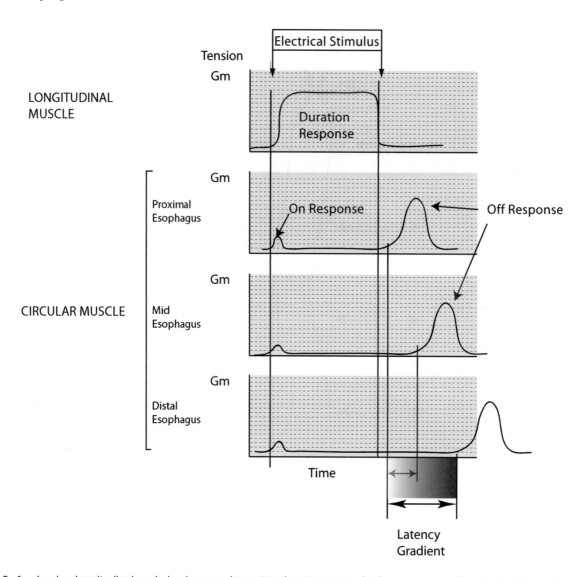

Figure 8–4. In vivo longitudinal and circular muscle contraction responses in the opossum after electrical stimulation. Longitudinal muscle shows a contraction response that is maintained throughout the duration of the stimulus (Duration Response). Circular muscle shows an initial brief contraction at the initiation of the stimulus (On Response), followed by a period of inhibition that is maintained throughout the duration of the stimulus. Once the stimulus is removed, there is a much greater contraction response (Off Response). The duration of inhibition increases while moving distally down the esophagus, the so-called latency gradient. This gradient results in propagation of a peristaltic contraction wave down the esophagus. Gm, contraction force in grams.

the cut because it dies out at the proximal end above the cut. This allows a sleeve resection of the esophagus to be performed without destroying its normal function. Afferent impulses from receptors within the esophageal wall are not essential for progress of the coordinated wave. However, afferent nerves do go to the swallowing center from the esophagus. If the esophagus is distended at any point, a contractual wave begins with forceful closure of the UES and sweeps down the esophagus. This secondary contraction occurs without any movement of the mouth or pharynx. Secondary contractions can occur as an independent local reflex to clear the esophagus of material left behind after passage of the primary wave, but they are less common than previously thought.

Despite the rather powerful occlusive pressure, the propulsive force of the esophagus is relatively feeble. If one attempts to swallow a bolus attached by a string to a counterweight, the maximum weight that one can overcome is 5 to 10 g. Orderly contractions of the muscular wall and anchoring of the esophagus at its inferior end are necessary for efficient and aboral propulsion to occur. Loss of the inferior anchor, as occurs with a large hiatal hernia, can lead to inefficient propulsion.

Lower Esophageal High-Pressure Zone

The esophagus passes through the right crus of the diaphragm at about the level of the 10th thoracic vertebra. The fascia on the inferior surface of the

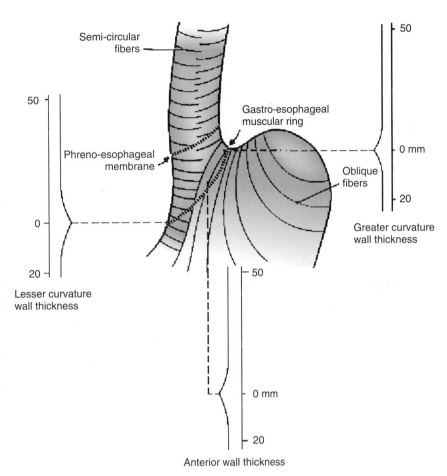

Figure 8–5. Schematic drawing showing wall thickness and orientation of fibers on microdissection of the cardia. At the junction of the esophageal tube and the gastric pouch, there is an oblique muscular ring composed of an increased muscle mass inside the inner muscular layer. On the lesser curve side of the cardia, the muscle fibers of the inner layer are oriented transversely and form semicircular muscle clasps that insert into the submucosal connective tissue. On the greater curve side of the cardia, these muscle fibers form long oblique loops that run parallel to the lesser curve of the stomach and encircle the distal end of the cardia and gastric fundus. (From DeMeester TR, Skinner DB: Evaluation of esophageal function and disease. In Glenn WWL [ed]: Thoracic and Cardiovascular Surgery, 4th ed. Norwalk, CT, Appleton-Century-Crofts, 1983, p 461, with permission.)

diaphragm is in continuity with the transversalis fascia, and fibroelastic fibers extend upward into the opening of the diaphragm in a cranial fashion to be attached to the wall of the esophagus about 2 cm above the gastroesophageal junction. Some of the elastic fibers penetrate to the mucosa of the esophagus and form the phrenoesophageal ligament. The esophagus below the phrenoesophageal ligament lies within the abdominal cavity and after a short distance of 2 to 3 cm enters into the stomach. A high-pressure zone can be identified in this area; it provides a pressure barrier between the esophagus and stomach and acts as the valve on the worm drive pump of the esophageal body. This barrier or high-pressure zone represents contributions made by the crus of the diaphragm,[8] the angle of His, and an intrinsic LES. Although an anatomically distinct LES has been difficult to identify, microdissection studies show that in humans, the sphincter-like function of this segment is related to the architecture of the muscle fibers at the junction of the esophageal tube and the gastric pouch[9] (Fig. 8–5). The lower esophageal muscle fibers are arranged as clasp and sling fibers. Clasp fibers have higher resting pressure and are less responsive to cholinergic stimulation.[10,11] This observation most probably accounts for the asymmetry of the sphincter, which shows more circularity on the left than on the right side and causes asymmetric LES pressure readings on manometric studies.[12] Nitric oxide causes LES relaxation, which is generated at the neuro-

muscular junction with some interaction by vasoactive intestinal polypeptide.[13] The sphincter actively remains closed to prevent reflux of gastric contents into the esophagus and opens via the relaxation that coincides with a pharyngeal swallow. LES pressure returns to its resting level after the peristaltic wave has passed through the esophagus (see Fig. 8–3). Consequently, any reflux of gastric juice that may occur through the open valve during a swallow is pumped back into the stomach. An important trigger for gastroesophageal reflux appears to be gastric distention, which results in shortening of the LES as it is taken up into the fundus of the expanding stomach. The progressive shortening of the sphincter reaches a point where the pressure in the remaining length gives way and the sphincter opens to allow reflux. Loss of sphincter barrier function also occurs if the pharyngeal swallow does not initiate a peristaltic contraction; in this case, coincident relaxation of the LES is unguarded, and reflux of gastric juice can occur. This appears to be the major cause of the so-called transient or spontaneous LES relaxations, thought by some to be a causative factor in gastroesophageal reflux disease (GERD).[14] In dogs, bilateral cervical parasympathetic blockade abolishes the LES relaxation that occurs with pharyngeal swallowing or distention of the esophagus.[15] This indicates that vagal function is important in maintaining LES barrier function and in coordinating LES relaxation with esophageal contraction. Rostral cells in motor neurons of the dorsal motor nucleus are involved in excitatory control of the LES, and caudal cells of the dorsal motor nucleus are involved in inhibition of the LES.[16,17]

The ability of the LES to protect the esophageal mucosa from excessive exposure to gastric juice depends on the resistance that it imposes to the flow of gastric juice from an environment above atmospheric pressure, the stomach, into an environment below atmospheric pressure, the esophagus (see Fig. 8–2). Clinical and in vitro studies have shown that this resistance is due to the integrated mechanical effect of sphincter pressure, overall length, and length exposed to the positive environmental pressure of the abdomen.[18-20]

PATHOPHYSIOLOGIC ASPECTS OF ESOPHAGEAL MOTILITY

In the normal situation, there is a coordinated interplay between the esophagus and its adjacent valves and compartments to propel food from the mouth to the stomach. Failure of the propulsive ability of a compartment hampers the forward movement of food and enhances regurgitation. Failure of the valve between two adjoining compartments results in exposure of the proximal compartment to the luminal contents of the distal compartment (i.e., gastroesophageal and esophagopharyngeal reflux).

Pharyngoesophageal Swallowing Disorders

Disorders of the pharyngoesophageal phase of swallowing result from dyscoordination of the neuromuscular events involved in chewing, initiation of swallowing, and propulsion of material from the oropharynx to the cervical esophagus. This results in dysphagia, nasal regurgitation, aspiration, and repetitive respiratory infections. The disorders can be categorized into one or a combination of the following: (1) inadequate oropharyngeal bolus transport, (2) inability to pressurize the pharynx,[21] (3) inability to elevate the larynx and open the UES, (4) impaired cricopharyngeal muscle relaxation and pharyngeal contraction, and (5) decreased compliance of the pharyngoesophageal segment and cervical esophagus secondary to restrictive myopathy.

Pharyngoesophageal swallowing disorders are usually an acquired condition that involves the central and peripheral nervous systems. Swallowing abnormalities caused by cricopharyngeal dysfunction are of increasing importance. The problem is associated with increasing age and carries high morbidity, mortality, and cost. Possible diseases and conditions include cerebrovascular accidents, brainstem tumors, poliomyelitis, multiple sclerosis, Parkinson's disease, pseudobulbar palsy, peripheral neuropathy, and operative damage to the cranial nerves involved in swallowing. Muscular diseases, such as radiation-induced myopathy, dermatomyositis, myotonic dystrophy, and myasthenia gravis, are less common. Occasionally, extrinsic compression as a result of thyromegaly, cervical lymphadenopathy, or hyperostosis of

the cervical spine can cause cervical dysphagia. It should be noted, however, that in our series, almost 40% of patients had no discernible underlying disease process that could be identified. The rapidity of the oropharyngeal phase of swallowing, movement of the gullet, and asymmetry of the cricopharyngeus account for the difficulty in assessing abnormalities of esophagopharyngeal swallowing disorders with manometry. Videocineroentgenography is the most objective test for evaluating oropharyngeal bolus movement, pharyngeal contraction, cricopharyngeal relaxation, and the dynamics of airway protection during swallowing.[22] Careful analysis of videocineroentgenographic studies and manometry with a specially designed catheter, ideally performed simultaneously (Fig. 8–6), can identify the cause of pharyngoesophageal dysfunction in most situations.[23] UES opening, UES relaxation, the concept of sphincter resistance, and compliance are key to understanding disorders related to the pharyngoesophageal segment. These factors are important for the clinician to keep in mind when distinguishing between frequently encountered radiologic abnormalities (e.g., cricopharyngeal bars) and clinically important disturbances in swallow function. A distinction must be made between two biomechanical events that are related but not synonymous, namely, UES relaxation and opening.

Characterization of pharyngoesophageal dysfunction and the associated mechanical abnormality of the swallow has potentially important clinical implications for the surgeon because the effect of a myotomy is mechanical. If a definite mechanical defect can be identified, myotomy may be of potential benefit to this subgroup of patients. The mechanical effects of a myotomy are to improve compliance, reduce resistance to transsphincteric flow, and improve the opening traction force on the UES. The efficacy of cricopharyngeal myotomy for some structural disorders of the UES (e.g., Zenker's diverticulum) is indisputable; however, the efficacy of procedures designed to reduce resistance to sphincteric flow in patients without Zenker's diverticulum is far less convincing and dependent on identification of some underlying mechanical abnormality of the UES. In patients with Zenker's diverticulum, it has been difficult to consistently demonstrate a motility abnormality of the pharyngeal phase of swallowing. The abnormality most apt to be present is loss of compliance in the pharyngoesophageal segment manifested by increased bolus pressure[24] (Fig. 8–7). Esophageal muscle biopsy results in patients with Zenker's diverticulum have shown histologic evidence of a restrictive myopathy correlating with decreased compliance of the upper esophagus on videocineradiographic and detailed manometric studies. These findings suggest that the diverticulum develops as a consequence of the repetitive stress of bolus transport through noncompliant muscle of the pharyngoesophageal segment. Other roentgenographic manifestations of a noncompliant segment in the proximal esophagus are a cricopharyngeal bar or more extended narrowing of the pharyngoesophageal segment. Dyscoordination of sphincter relaxation with pharyngeal contraction together with impaired sphincter opening is another cause of the development of Zenker's

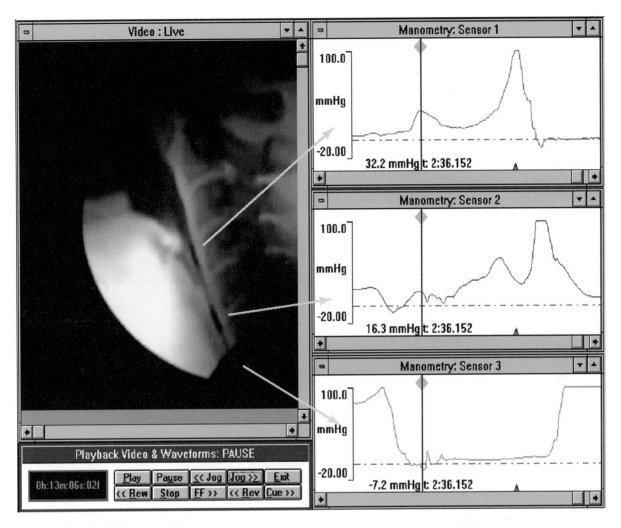

Figure 8–6. Combined manovideofluorography of the upper esophageal sphincter (UES) in a normal patient using a three-channel solid-state catheter with the distal transducer placed in the UES and the proximal two transducers in the pharynx. The UES is open and demonstrates a subatmospheric pressure drop before arrival of the bolus. The intrabolus pressure is depicted in the proximal channel of the manometry catheter. Manovideofluorography allows for optimal assessment of the dynamics involved in the pharyngeal swallow because manometric sphincter opening and bolus clearance can be accurately determined from the linked videoesophagogram and manometry tracing.

diverticulum. This may not occur throughout the full length of the sphincter and can easily be missed on manometric assessment because of movement of the cricopharyngeus on swallowing. Failure of the cricopharyngeal muscle to relax on swallowing, or so-called cervical achalasia, and failure of initiation of an esophageal contraction after a pharyngeal swallow have also been observed in patients with Zenker's diverticulum.[25]

Primary Motor Disorders of the Esophageal Body and Lower Esophageal Sphincter

Nonobstructive dysphagia (i.e., dysphagia in the absence of structural abnormalities) is the primary symptom of esophageal motor disorders. Its perception by the patient is a balance between the severity of the underlying cause that is producing the difficulty and the patient's

adjustment to that difficulty through alteration in eating habits. Consequently, any complaint of dysphagia requires a detailed assessment of the patient's dietary history in addition to a clear understanding of the physiologic abnormalities that may cause the patient's symptoms.[1]

Abnormalities that occur in the worm drive pump of the esophageal body or the LES can give rise to a number of disorders in the esophageal phase of swallowing. These disorders are due to primary abnormalities in the esophagus or result from a more generalized neural, muscular, or systemic disease (Box 8–1). With the introduction of standard esophageal manometry, a number of primary esophageal motility disorders have been reclassified from nonspecific to separate disease entities, including achalasia, diffuse esophageal spasm, the so-called nutcracker esophagus, and the hypertensive LES.[26] Classification of these disorders is usually based on

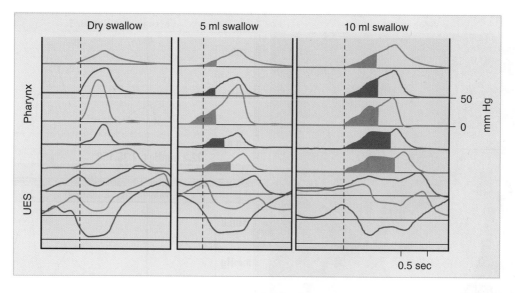

Figure 8–7. Manometric pharyngeal and upper esophageal sphincter (UES) tracings from a patient with a Zenker diverticulum. Tracings obtained during a dry, 5-ml, and 10-ml swallow are depicted. The intrabolus pressure wave (*shaded portion of tracing*) was above normal. With increasing bolus volumes there is a significant increase in intrabolus pressure, thus demonstrating loss of muscle compliance.

analysis of the manometric recordings of 10 wet swallows performed in a laboratory setting.[27] Recently, an updated classification of the primary esophageal motor disorders based on manometric abnormalities found in the LES and esophageal body has been proposed (Table 8–1).[28]

The pathogenesis of these primary abnormalities is either defective inhibition or defective excitatory innervation of the LES and esophagus. Achalasia is associated with loss of inhibitory innervation of the LES and loss of nitric oxide.[29,30] This unopposed excitatory innervation

leads to high LES pressure and defective or absent LES relaxation in patients with achalasia.

The technique of ambulatory 24-hour monitoring of esophageal motor activity multiplies the number of esophageal contractions available for analysis and provides an opportunity to assess esophageal motor function in a variety of physiologic situations. This increases the accuracy and dependability of the measurement.[31] The application of ambulatory 24-hour esophageal motility monitoring has shown that there are marked differences in the classification of esophageal motor disorders between standard manometry and ambulatory motility monitoring.[32] The degree of reclassification that occurs when analysis of esophageal motor function is conducted on the basis of ambulatory manometry indicates that the classic categories of esophageal motor disorders are inappropriate. This appears to be due to the intermittent expression of esophageal motor abnormalities that can be missed or overdiagnosed during the unphysiologic setting of standard manometry but are detected with a higher degree of reliability when motor activity is monitored over a 24-hour period under a variety of physiologic conditions. Based on these observations, esophageal motility disorders should be looked at as a spectrum of abnormalities that reflect various stages of deterioration of esophageal motor function rather than as separate entities.[1] This view is supported by the observation that the severity of esophageal motor disorders can progress or regress during the natural course of the disease.

Recently, we have seen the introduction of combined multichannel intraluminal impedance and esophageal manometry (Fig. 8–8). This technique allows for the simultaneous assessment of esophageal bolus transport together with esophageal manometry. With this technique, Tutuian and Castell[33] have shown that when

---

Box 8–1 **Esophageal Motility Disorders**

Primary

Achalasia, "vigorous" achalasia

Diffuse and segmental esophageal spasm

Nutcracker esophagus

Hypertensive lower esophageal sphincter

Nonspecific esophageal motility disorders

Secondary Esophageal Motility Disorders

Collagen vascular diseases: progressive systemic sclerosis, polymyositis and dermatomyositis, mixed connective tissue disease, systemic lupus erythematosus

Chronic idiopathic intestinal pseudo-obstruction

Neuromuscular diseases

Endocrine and metastatic disorders

Table 8–1   Manometric Classification of Primary Esophageal Motility Disorders

Manometric Classification	Motor Disorders	Manometric Findings
Inadequate LES relaxation	Achalasia	Elevated LES resting pressure
		Incomplete LES relaxation
		Elevated baseline esophageal pressure
		Absent distal esophageal peristalsis
	Atypical disorders of LES relaxation	
Uncoordinated motility	Diffuse esophageal spasm	Simultaneous esophageal contractions (>20%)
		Intermittent normal peristalsis
		Repetitive contractions (multipeaked waves >3)
		Prolonged contraction durations (>6 sec)
		Retrograde contractions
		Isolated incomplete LES relaxation
Hypercontracting esophagus	Nutcracker esophagus	Contraction amplitudes >180 mm Hg
		Increased contraction duration >6 sec
		Peristaltic contractions
	Hypertensive LES	Resting LES pressure >25 mm Hg
		May have partial LES relaxation
Hypocontracting esophagus	Ineffective esophageal motility	Increase nontransmitted peristalsis (>30%)
		Low distal peristaltic contraction amplitudes (<30 mm Hg)
	Hypotensive LES	Resting LES pressure <6 mm Hg

LES, lower esophageal sphincter.
Adapted from Spechler SJ, Castell DO: Classification of oesophageal motility abnormalities. Gut 49:145, 2001.

evaluating patients with motility disorders by combined multichannel intraluminal impedance and esophageal manometry, two distinct patterns emerge. Some patients have manometric pressure defects and associated defective bolus transit on impedance, whereas a second group of patients have pressure defects only (that is, normal bolus transit) (Table 8–2). Similar to the observations found when using ambulatory manometry, this study showed that manometry tends to overestimate the functional defect detected by impedance (Fig. 8–9). This most probably has important implications when assessing patients before antireflux surgery. Standard manometry appears to be too sensitive and should not be used alone to exclude or select patients for different surgical procedures. However, if normal esophageal function or isolated LES abnormalities are found on manometry, it is unlikely that impaired esophageal body peristalsis or clearance will be found with impedance. Isolated LES abnormalities impair bolus transit only when esophageal body contractions are defective. Of note is that there appears to be poor correlation between symptoms of dysphagia and abnormal bolus transport inasmuch as only

Table 8–2   Classification of the Primary Motor Disorders Based on Impedance Manometry

Impedance Classification	Manometric Findings	Prevalence of Normal Bolus Transport
Pressure defects *and* associated bolus transit abnormalities	Achalasia	0%
	Scleroderma	0%
	IEM	50%
	Diffuse esophageal spasm	5%
Pressure defects *only*	Nutcracker esophagus	97%
	Hypotensive LES	100%
	Hypertensive LES	96%
	Poor LES relaxation	100%

IEM, ineffective esophageal motility; LES, lower esophageal sphincter.
Adapted from Tutuian R, Castell DO: Combined multichannel intraluminal impedance and manometry clarifies esophageal function abnormalities: Study in 350 patients. Am J Gastroenterol 99:1011, 2004.

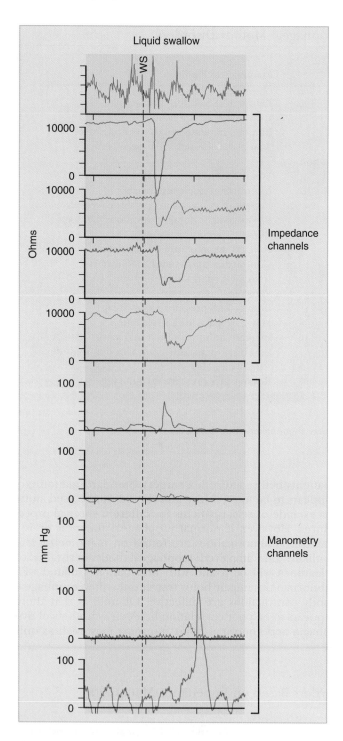

Figure 8–8 A sample tracing of a swallow using a combined multichannel impedance–manometry catheter. By linking the impedance tracing with the manometry tracing, the effectiveness of esophageal contraction pressure on bolus clearance can be evaluated.

50% of patients with dysphagia have abnormal bolus transit and about 30% of patients with no dysphagia have abnormal bolus transport (Fig. 8–10).

The symptom of dysphagia in patients without structural abnormalities of the esophagus can be caused by

distal obstruction from a nonrelaxing LES or by disorganized contractions of the esophageal body. In patients with a nonrelaxing sphincter, the function of the esophageal body deteriorates secondary to the distal obstruction and may recover if the obstruction is relieved early during the disease process. In patients with a primary motor disorder of the esophageal body, dysphagia appears to be due to an inability of the esophageal body to organize its motor activity into peristaltic contractions during meals. Ambulatory 24-hour monitoring of esophageal body function has shown that in normal asymptomatic volunteers, the prevalence of "effective contractions" (i.e., peristaltic contractions with sufficient amplitude to propel a bolus) increases with increasing states of consciousness (i.e., from sleep, to the upright position, to meal periods), probably because of a modulatory effect of the central nervous system on esophageal motor activity. Patients with nonobstructive dysphagia lack this ability to increase the prevalence of effective contractions with increasing states of consciousness.[34,35] Clinical studies using ambulatory esophageal motility have shown that the frequency of effective contractions increases during meal periods. Monitoring can be used to express the severity of esophageal body dysfunction on a linear scale. This can be related to the presence of nonobstructive dysphagia (Fig. 8–11), and it obviates the need for the current categories of esophageal motor disorders and permits objective assessment of the effect of medical or surgical therapy on esophageal body function.[35]

Esophageal contractions of an abnormally high amplitude or long duration have been suggested to be responsible for chest pain in patients with esophageal motor disorders.[36] Ambulatory 24-hour motility monitoring in these patients has, however, shown that the amplitude and duration of esophageal contractions associated with chest pain episodes are similar to those of asymptomatic contractions during the upright or supine recording. Esophageal chest pain episodes were preceded immediately by a markedly increased frequency of simultaneous and repetitive contractions.[32] Using simultaneous manometry, pH, and ultrasound imaging, Balaban et al.[37] have shown that these sustained esophageal contractions are related to the symptoms of chest pain and that the sustained contractions actually involve the longitudinal muscle of the esophagus and not the circular. The contractions may be confused with heartburn; however, it seems that the chest pain is on average about 25 seconds longer than that associated with a reflux event.[38] As in the heart, the esophageal blood supply may be interrupted during bursts of disorganized muscular contractions. Such interruption may become crucial in situations in which resting blood flow to the esophagus is already compromised, as has been shown for the hypertrophic esophageal muscle in patients with esophageal motor disorders. A burst of disorganized motor activity in this situation may give rise to ischemic pain. Consequently, chest pain caused by a burst of uncoordinated esophageal motor activity under ischemic conditions has been called *esophageal claudication*.[32] Studies using simultaneous manometry and high-frequency intraluminal ultrasound probes have shown an increase in muscle

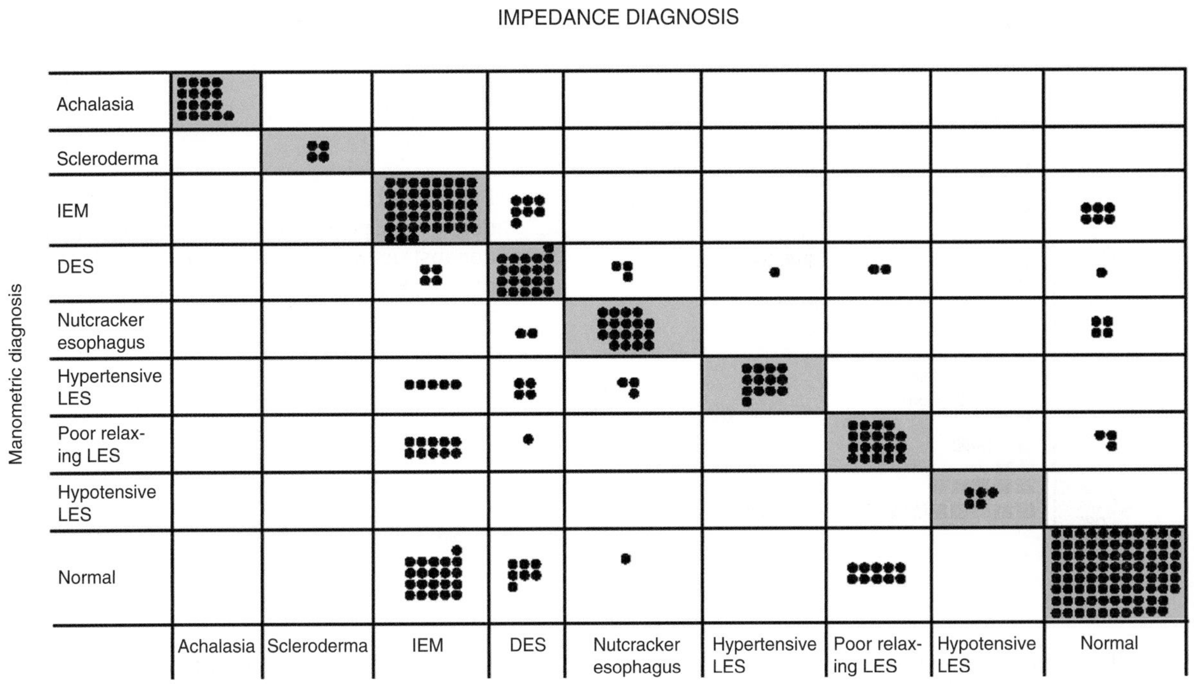

IMPEDANCE DIAGNOSIS

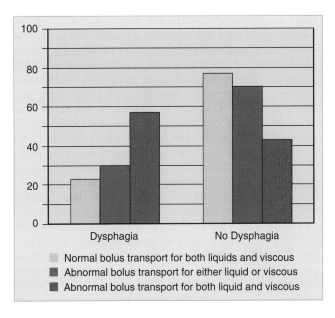

Manometric diagnosis	Achalasia	Scleroderma	IEM	DES	Nutcracker esophagus	Hypertensive LES	Poor relax-ing LES	Hypotensive LES	Normal
Achalasia	■■■								
Scleroderma		■■							
IEM			■■■	■■					■■
DES			■■	■■■	■	■	■■		■
Nutcracker esophagus				■■	■■■				■■
Hypertensive LES			■■	■■	■	■■			
Poor relax-ing LES			■■	■			■■		■
Hypotensive LES								■■	
Normal			■■	■■	■		■■		■■■

Figure 8–9. Classification of esophageal motor disorders in 350 patients with dysphagia or noncardiac chest pain according to findings on standard manometry or impedance. DES, diffuse esophageal spasm; IEM, ineffective esophageal motility; LES, lower esophageal sphincter. (Adapted from Tutuian R, Castell DO: Combined multichannel intraluminal impedance and manometry clarifies esophageal function abnormalities: Study in 350 patients. Am J Gastroenterol 99:1011, 2004.)

Figure 8–10. Prevalence of normal and abnormal bolus transport of liquids and viscous bolus material in patients with and without the symptom of dysphagia. Bolus transport was evaluated by combined multichannel intraluminal impedance and manometry. (Adapted from Tutuian R, Castell DO: Combined multichannel intraluminal impedance and manometry clarifies esophageal function abnormalities: Study in 350 patients. Am J Gastroenterol 99:1011, 2004.)

thickness and mass. When compared with normal subjects, patients with achalasia have the greatest increase in muscle thickness, followed by patients with diffuse esophageal spasm and those with nutcracker esophagus. It appears that the primary disorder is loss of this LES opening and relaxation and that the esophageal muscle hypertrophy is a secondary response to outflow obstruction at the level of the LES.[39]

Roentgenographic abnormalities in motility disorders such as segmental spasms with compartmentalization of the esophagus or the formation of a diverticulum are the anatomic results of disordered esophageal motor function. Detailed analysis will reveal that a motility disorder was usually present for years before documentation of these roentgenographic findings. The development of a diverticulum may temporarily alleviate the symptom of initial dysphagia during eating and replace it with the symptom of postprandial regurgitation of undigested food. In the few patients with a diverticulum in whom an abnormality of esophageal body or LES function cannot be identified manometrically, a traction or congenital cause of the diverticulum should be sought.

Diffuse esophageal spasm is relatively rare. There is evidence to support the fact that the dyscoordination usually seen in these patients is due to a deficiency of nitric oxide. Patients with higher contraction amplitudes have primarily chest pain and those with lower contraction amplitudes have primarily dysphagia. Although the pathophysiology is understood, the underlying cause of the loss in inhibitory nerves and degeneration of the

EFFECTIVE CONTRACTIONS DURING MEALS

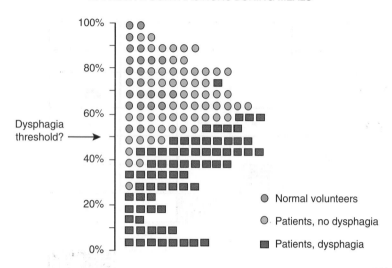

Figure 8–11. Prevalence of "effective contractions" during meal periods in normal volunteers, patients with nonobstructive dysphagia, and patients without dysphagia. Having less than 50% effective contractions during meals is associated with a high prevalence of nonobstructive dysphagia.

myenteric plexus is not known. GERD causes injury to the LES muscle. The inflammation somehow causes defective excitatory innervation that results in low contraction amplitudes or ineffective esophageal contractions. It is uncertain whether the monitor abnormality is primary or secondary to reflux damage.

Secondary Esophageal Motor Disorders

Esophageal motility disorders may also result from more generalized neural, muscular, or systemic metabolic abnormalities. The esophagus is particularly affected by almost any of the collagen vascular disorders; the most common are progressive systemic sclerosis, mixed connective tissue disease, polymyositis, and dermatomyositis (see Box 8–1).[40-42] Eighty percent of patients with progressive systemic sclerosis have an esophageal motor abnormality. In most cases, the disease follows a prolonged course and usually affects only the smooth muscle in the distal two thirds of the esophagus. In these patients the muscle fibers in the LES and esophagus are replaced by connective tissue.[43] Typical findings on esophageal manometry are normal peristalsis in the proximal striated esophagus and weak or absent peristalsis in the distal smooth muscle portion. LES pressure is progressively weakened as the disease advances, and this decline in pressure results in increased esophageal exposure to gastric juice because of a mechanically defective LES and poor clearance function of the esophageal body.[42]

In patients with polymyositis or dermatomyositis, the upper striated muscle portion is the major site of esophageal involvement, and such patients suffer from aspiration, nasopharyngeal regurgitation, and cervical dysphagia. Mixed connective tissue disease is associated with a mixture of the manometric findings of progressive systemic sclerosis and polymyositis. In patients with diabetes mellitus, an autonomic neuropathy is responsible for the findings of low contraction amplitude and double-peaked contraction waves. Infiltration of the

myenteric plexus of the LES in neoplastic disease and Chagas' disease is the cause of secondary achalasia. Patients with amyloidosis, alcoholism, and multiple sclerosis exhibit low-amplitude contractions in the distal esophagus.

Gastroesophageal Reflux Disease and Esophageal Motility Disorders

GERD is the most common foregut disorder in the Western world and accounts for approximately 75% of esophageal disorders. In about 50% of affected patients, it can lead to complications such as esophagitis, stricture, ulceration, Barrett's esophagus, repetitive pulmonary aspiration, recurrent pneumonia, and progressive pulmonary fibrosis.[44] Despite its prevalence, GERD can be one of the most challenging diagnostic problems in benign esophageal disease because the occurrence of specific symptoms or detection of endoscopic or histologic esophageal mucosal injury is unreliable in indicating the presence of the disease. With the introduction of 24-hour esophageal pH monitoring, the basic pathophysiologic abnormality of GERD (i.e., increased esophageal exposure to gastric juice) has been quantified.[45,46] This has provided an opportunity to conceptualize the pathophysiology of a complicated disease process, stimulated a rational stepwise approach to determine the cause of increased esophageal exposure to gastric juice, and led to the design of specific therapy to correct the underlying abnormalities. The problem is that there is no correlation between the majority of esophageal chest pain events and abnormal esophageal motor events or acid reflux events. Impedance testing has shown that there can, however, be non-acid reflux episodes and that the frequency of these non-acid reflux events in certain patients is high. Some of these patients demonstrate mechanical hypersensitivity to esophageal distention. Sarkar and colleagues have shown that in normal subjects and patients with symptoms, acid in the

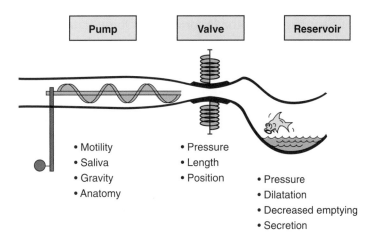

Figure 8–12. Mechanical model of the esophagus as a propulsive pump, the lower esophageal sphincter as a valve, and the stomach as a reservoir. Esophageal clearance of refluxed gastric juice is determined by esophageal motor activity, salivation, gravity, and the presence of an anatomic alteration such as a hiatal hernia. The competency of the lower esophageal sphincter depends on its pressure, overall length, and length exposed to abdominal pressure. Gastric function abnormalities causing gastroesophageal reflux include increased intragastric pressure, gastric dilatation, decreased emptying rate, and increased gastric acid secretion. (From DeMeester TR, Attwood SE: Gastroesophageal reflux disease, hiatus hernia, achalasia of the esophagus and spontaneous rupture. In Schwartz SI, Ellis H [eds]: Maingot's Abdominal Operations, 9th ed. Norwalk, CT, Appleton & Lange, 1989, with permission.)

esophagus induces a hypersensitivity that is mediated at the level of the spinal cord or higher.[47,48]

Three causes of increased esophageal exposure to gastric juice are known. The first is a mechanically defective LES, which accounts for about 60% to 70% of GERD and is due to inflammatory damage to the sphincter muscle.[20] Identification of this cause is important because antireflux surgery is the only therapy designed to correct the abnormality. The other two causes are inefficient esophageal clearance of refluxed gastric juice and abnormalities of the gastric reservoir that result in transient loss of the sphincter barrier because of progressive shortening of the sphincter with gastric distention. Conceptually, these three main causes of gastroesophageal reflux can be thought of as abnormalities of a pump, a valve, or a reservoir (Fig. 8–12). The relative contributions of each of these components of the antireflux mechanism to increased esophageal exposure to gastric juice should be determined before consideration of surgical therapy.

Failure of the LES can be caused by inadequate pressure, overall length, or intra-abdominal length (i.e., the portion of the sphincter exposed to the positive-pressure environment of the abdomen on manometry). Failure of one or two of the components of the sphincter may be compensated for by clearance of the esophageal body. Failure of all three sphincter components inevitably leads to increased esophageal exposure to gastric juice. The most common cause of a mechanically defective LES is inflammatory loss of myogenic function, which can result in loss of sphincter pressure, overall length, abdominal length, or a combination of these factors. Normal sphincter pressure can be nullified by an inadequate abdominal length or an abnormally short overall length of the sphincter.[20] Adequate abdominal length of the

sphincter is important in preventing reflux caused by increases in intra-abdominal pressure. Adequate overall length is important in preventing reflux caused by gastric distention, such as may occur with a meal.

The combined effects of sphincter pressure, overall length, and abdominal length can be determined by integrating the radial pressure exerted over the entire length of the sphincter. This can be done by calculating the volume of the three-dimensional sphincter pressure profile (i.e., the sphincter pressure vector volume).[19,49]

A second cause of increased esophageal exposure to gastric juice is inefficient esophageal clearance of refluxed material.[50] Because of failure to clear physiologic reflux, abnormal esophageal exposure to gastric juice can occur even in individuals who have a mechanically intact LES and normal gastric function. This situation is relatively rare, however, and ineffective clearance is more apt to be seen in association with a mechanically defective sphincter, where it augments the esophageal exposure to gastric juice by prolonging the duration of each reflux episode. The four factors important in esophageal clearance are gravity, esophageal motor activity, salivation, and anchoring of the distal esophagus in the abdomen. The bulk of refluxed gastric juice is cleared from the esophagus by a primary peristaltic wave initiated by a pharyngeal swallow. Secondary peristalsis initiated by either distention of the lower esophagus or a drop in intraesophageal pH is less important. Combined videocineradiographic and manometric studies have shown that failure of esophageal clearance can be caused by a nonperistaltic esophageal contraction waveform or contractions of low amplitude.[51] Salivation contributes to esophageal clearance by neutralizing the minute amount of acid that is left after a peristaltic wave. The presence of a hiatal hernia can also

Table 8–3	Prevalence of Esophageal Motor Disorders in Obese Patients

	Hong et al.[52] N = 61	Jaffin et al.[53] N = 111	Percentage
Hypotensive LES	10	28	22
Hypertensive LES	11		6
Achalasia		1	0.5
Diffuse esophageal spasm	2	8	6
Nutcracker esophagus	3	16	11
Ineffective esophageal motility	1		0.5
Nonspecific dysmotility	11	15	15

LES, lower esophageal sphincter.

cause increased acid exposure by reducing the efficiency of esophageal contractions through loss of its distal anchor.

Gastric abnormalities that increase esophageal exposure to gastric juice include gastric dilatation, increased intragastric pressure, a persistent gastric reservoir, and increased gastric acid secretion.[44] The effect of gastric dilatation is to shorten the overall length of the LES, which results in a decrease in sphincter resistance to reflux. Increased intragastric pressure occurs in patients with outlet obstruction caused by a scarred pylorus or duodenum, after vagotomy, or as a result of diabetic neuropathy. Persistence of the gastric reservoir results from delayed gastric emptying secondary to myogenic abnormalities, as seen in patients with advanced diabetes and diffuse neuromuscular disorders and after viral infections. Gastric hypersecretion can increase esophageal exposure to gastric juice by the physiologic reflux of the excessive volume of gastric juice of low pH that occurs in this condition.

Obesity and Esophageal Motility Disorders

Over recent years there has been a dramatic increase in the number of obese patients coming to the surgeon for surgical procedures designed to restrict eating and cause weight loss. This trend has resulted in a new group of patients with esophageal motility disorders. It appears that some of these obese patients have a preexisting motility disorder and that in others the surgery itself may cause a secondary esophageal motility disorder. This is particularly seen with operations that inherently produce a relative outflow resistance just below the gastroesophageal junction, such as the gastric banding procedure and Roux-en-Y gastric bypass. Various observational studies have shown that there appears to be an increase preoperatively in the manometric findings of a motility disorder in the obese population (Table 8–3). Although two studies have shown the prevalence of motility disorders to be high, namely, 54%[52] and 61%,[53] one study showed no increase in any esophageal dysmotility.[54] The correlation with symptoms is, however, only about 50%. Esophageal bolus transit determined by radionuclide

scintigraphy has also been shown to be significantly prolonged in patients with morbid obesity.[55,56] Part of the reason may be an increase in the esophageal-gastric pressure gradient. Body mass index has been shown to be positively related to intra-abdominal pressure,[57] and the increased pressure causes a relative outflow resistance and decreased flow from the esophagus to the stomach. The motility changes seen may also be related to altered gut neuropeptides inasmuch as it has been shown that neurotensin is significantly decreased and motilin is significantly increased in obese patients when compared with lean controls.[58] A small number of patients require reoperation and revision surgery after gastric banding because of esophageal dysmotility.[59-62] DeMaria et al.[59] reported that 71% of patients had a significant increase in esophageal diameter on barium studies that was associated with dysphagia, regurgitation, and vomiting. Weiss and associates[63] looked at esophageal manometry before and after gastric banding and showed significant deterioration in esophageal body function 6 months after surgery. This deterioration was mainly due to an increase in the number of simultaneous contractions and a significant decrease in contraction amplitude to less than 30 mm Hg. Some studies have, however, shown no deterioration in esophageal body function postoperatively. Theoretically, with weight loss there is normalization of gut hormones, a decrease in intra-abdominal pressure, and improvement in the esophageal-gastric pressure gradient. These factors would possibly be associated with an improvement in bolus transit and esophageal clearance of the esophagus, which has been demonstrated by Seymour et al.[56] Thus, the manometric findings may not be of clinical significance if there is no interference with bolus transit.

OBJECTIVE ASSESSMENT OF ESOPHAGEAL MOTILITY DISORDERS

A number of tests are available for the diagnosis and evaluation of esophageal motor disorders, but they vary greatly in reliability and appropriate application. When assessing patients with a suspected pharyngeal swallowing disorder, the gastrointestinal surgeon should ask seven key questions:

1. Does the patient aspirate?
2. Does the patient have a Zenker diverticulum?
3. Does the patient have some underlying disorder known to be associated with dysphagia (e.g., stroke, parkinsonism)?
4. In what swallowing phase does the abnormality occur (i.e., oral, preparatory, pharyngeal, or esophageal)?
5. Is the patient able to maintain adequate nutrition orally?
6. Is there manometric evidence of any swallowing dysfunction? Specifically, is their any manometric evidence of impaired sphincter opening or impairment to trans-sphincteric flow across the UES, and what is the state of the pharyngeal stripping wave?
7. Finally, if considering an operative procedure, has the upper esophageal high-pressure zone been localized manometrically?

Similarly, when assessing a patient with a suspected esophageal body or LES motor abnormality, the gastrointestinal surgeon should ask nine key questions:

1. Does the patient have pathologic acid gastroesophageal reflux?
2. Does the patient have a structural abnormality of the esophagus such as a diverticulum or hiatal hernia?
3. Does the patient have some underlying disorder known to be associated with an esophageal motor disorder (e.g., diabetes, alcoholism)?
4. Does the patient have a manometrically identifiable motor disorder of the esophageal body, such as achalasia?
5. Does the patient have defective esophageal bolus clearance, such as stasis, retrograde transport, or incomplete bolus transit?
6. Is the patient able to maintain adequate nutrition orally?
7. Is there impaired LES sphincter opening and resistance to bolus transport across the LES?
8. Is the LES mechanically defective?
9. Finally, if considering an operative procedure, are the manometric length of the esophagus, the esophageal contraction amplitudes, and the percentage of wet swallows that are considered effective known?

The answer to these questions can be determined only by performing additional tests on patients suspected of having an esophageal motility disorder. The diagnostic tests necessary may be divided into five broad groups: (1) tests to detect structural abnormalities of the esophagus, (2) tests to detect esophageal body contraction abnormalities, (3) tests to evaluate esophageal bolus clearance, (4) tests to provoke esophageal symptoms, and (5) tests to detect increased esophageal exposure to gastric and duodenal juice.

Tests to Detect Structural Abnormalities of the Esophagus

The first diagnostic evaluation in patients with suspected esophageal disease should be a contrast roentgenographic examination of the esophagus with full assessment of the stomach and duodenum, followed by upper gastrointestinal endoscopy with biopsy. Effective roentgenographic evaluation of the esophagus is dependent on the use of a combination of different examining techniques.

In any patient with dysphagia, endoscopy is indicated even in the face of a normal roentgenographic study. Regardless of the radiologist's interpretation of an abnormal finding, each structural abnormality of the esophagus should be confirmed visually and through biopsy. Endoscopy and biopsy are also necessary to assess for the presence of complications of GERD (i.e., esophagitis, stricture, and Barrett's esophagus). Fiberoptic endoscopic examination of swallowing is another valuable technique to assess pharyngeal sensitivity and swallowing. It provides a clear and direct view of the hypopharynx and larynx. Aspiration or evidence of aspiration can be directly observed. It allows for rapid clinical evaluation of patients in nursing homes, outpatient clinics, or intensive care units when videofluoroscopic examination is unavailable or unsuitable. It can evaluate vocal cord movement and the physical appearance of the pharyngeal and laryngeal structures.[64] The success of fiberoptic endoscopic examination of swallowing has led to the development of transnasal and transoral diagnostic endoscopy with narrow-diameter endoscopes (5.3 mm) in unsedated patients.[65]

The advance of endoscopic ultrasonography allows improved assessment of the esophageal wall. It is performed with a side-view endoscope that has a radial scanning ultrasound probe mounted at its tip. Contact with the esophageal wall is accomplished with a water-filled balloon over the ultrasound probe. This provides a circular ultrasound cross section of the esophageal wall that can be visualized on an image processor. On the ultrasound image, the wall of the esophagus consists of five layers that correspond to the acoustic reflections and the interfaces between them. With this technique, thickening of the wall in the distal end of the esophagus can easily be demonstrated in patients with achalasia and diffuse esophageal spasm. Fibrosis of the wall can be recognized in patients with scleroderma. Intramural tumors not seen on computed tomography or endoscopy can be detected and, in some situations, may be responsible for an observed motor disorder.[1]

Tests to Detect Esophageal Contraction Abnormalities

Many patients with symptoms of an esophageal motor disorder do not show a structural abnormality on standard roentgenographic and endoscopic evaluation. In these situations, esophageal function tests are necessary to identify a functional disorder. Tests to evaluate esophageal contraction abnormalities include stationary manometry of the pharyngoesophageal segment, esophageal body, and LES and ambulatory 24-hour esophageal motility monitoring.

Stationary Esophageal Manometry

Stationary esophageal manometry is a widely used technique to examine the motor function of the esophagus and its sphincters. It is indicated whenever a motor abnormality of the esophagus is suspected on the basis of complaints of dysphagia, odynophagia, or noncardiac chest pain and when the barium swallow or endoscopy does not show a clear structural abnormality.[1] Esophageal manometry is particularly necessary to confirm the diagnosis of specific primary esophageal motility disorders (i.e., achalasia, diffuse esophageal spasm, nutcracker esophagus, and hypertensive LES).[26] It also identifies nonspecific esophageal motility abnormalities and esophageal motor disorders secondary to systemic disease, such as scleroderma, dermatomyositis, polymyositis, and mixed connective tissue disease. Stationary manometry is the most accurate method for assessing LES function and has been the basis for identification and classification of the motor disorders of the esophageal body.[27] In patients with disorders of the pharyngoesophageal phase of swallowing, manometry is complementary to and should ideally be performed simultaneously with videocineroentgenography.[66,67] In patients with GERD, manometry of the esophageal body can identify a mechanically defective LES as the cause of increased esophageal acid exposure and evaluate the adequacy of esophageal clearance function.[44]

Esophageal manometry is performed with electronic pressure-sensitive transducers located within a catheter or water-perfused catheters with lateral side holes attached to transducers outside the body. The catheter usually consists of a train of five or more pressure transducers or water-perfused tubes bonded together with lateral openings placed at 5-cm intervals from the tip and oriented radially around the circumference. A special catheter assembly consisting of four or eight lateral openings at the same level, oriented radially at 90 or 45 degrees to each other, is useful when constructing a three-dimensional image of the LES. Other specially designed catheters are used to assess the UES. When water-filled catheters are used, the rate of water infusion must be adjusted to obtain reliable and reproducible pressure tracings. This is best achieved with a low-compliance pneumohydraulic capillary infusion system.[1]

The manometric catheter is passed through the nose and esophagus and into the stomach, and the gastric pressure pattern is confirmed. The catheter is withdrawn across the cardia to identify the high-pressure zone of the LES. Although some advocate steady, rapid withdrawal while patients hold their breath, we have found that stepwise withdrawal of the catheter at 0.5- or 1.0-cm intervals or slow motorized pullback at a speed of 1 mm/sec for 60 seconds provides reproducible and more quantitative information and allows patients to breathe normally during the procedure.[1,20] As the pressure-sensitive station is brought across the gastroesophageal junction, a rise in pressure off the gastric baseline identifies the beginning of the LES. The respiratory inversion point is identified when the positive excursions that occur with breathing in the abdominal cavity change to negative deflections in the thorax. The respiratory inversion point serves as the reference point at which the amplitude of LES pressure and the length of the sphincter exposed to abdominal pressure are measured. As the pressure-sensitive station is withdrawn into the body of the esophagus, the upper border of the LES is identified by the drop in pressure to the esophageal baseline. From these measurements, the resting pressure, abdominal length, and overall length of the sphincter are determined (Fig. 8–13). To account for the asymmetry of the sphincter, the pressure profile is repeated as each of the five radially oriented transducers is pulled through the sphincter, and sphincter pressure values above gastric baseline, overall sphincter length, and abdominal length of the sphincter are averaged. Alternatively, if the pressure-sensitive stations are radially oriented at the same level on the catheters, a single pull-through is all that is necessary.

Table 8–4 shows the values for these parameters in 50 normal volunteers without subjective or objective evidence of a foregut disorder. The level at which incompetence of the LES occurs was defined by comparing the frequency distribution of these values in the 50 healthy volunteers with the values for a population of similarly studied patients with symptoms of GERD.[20] The presence of increased esophageal exposure to gastric juice was documented by 24-hour esophageal pH monitoring. Based on these studies, a mechanically defective sphincter is identified by having one or more of the following characteristics: an average LES pressure of less than 6 mm Hg, an average length exposed to the positive-pressure environment in the abdomen of 1 cm or less, and an average overall sphincter length of 2 cm or less. When compared with the normal volunteers, these values are below the 2.5 percentile for sphincter pressure, overall length, and abdominal length.

If manometry of the LES is performed with four to eight radially oriented pressure transducers, a three-dimensional image of the sphincter can be constructed by plotting the pressure measured at each station of the pullback radially around an axis representing the gastric baseline.[19,49] For visual purposes, three-dimensional reconstruction of the sphincter pressure image can be enhanced by applying a cubic curve-smoothing interpolation that retains the original points while adding intermediate ones to give a smoother surface to the three-dimensional sphincter image and thus improve its readability. Commercially available computer programs enable the creation of three-dimensional sphincter images that can be rotated on a computer screen. This allows inspection of the sphincter image for asymmetry.

The volume circumscribed by the three-dimensional sphincter image integrates pressure exerted over the entire length and around the circumference of the sphincter into one value that represents sphincter resistance to reflux of gastric contents. This value has been termed the *sphincter pressure vector volume* and can be calculated with standard trigonometric formulas. Validation studies and application of this technique in a large

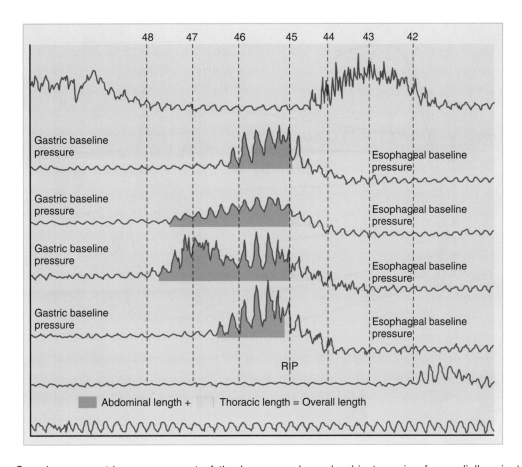

Figure 8–13. Sample manometric measurement of the lower esophageal sphincter using four radially orientated pressure transducers. The distances are measured from the nares. The asymmetry of the sphincter can be seen, as well as the portion of the sphincter exposed to abdominal pressure. RIP, respiratory inversion point.

number of patients with GERD have shown that calculation of the sphincter pressure vector volume is superior to standard techniques in assessing sphincter resistance to reflux of gastric juice,[19] particularly in patients with increased esophageal acid exposure but no mucosal injury and in those with borderline sphincter abnormalities.

To assess relaxation and postrelaxation contraction of the LES, a pressure transducer is positioned within the high-pressure zone, with a distal transducer located in

Table 8–4 Normal Manometric Values of the Lower Esophageal Sphincter (*N* = 50)

		Percentile	
	Median	**2.5**	**97.5**
Pressure (mm Hg)	13.0	5.8	27.7
Overall length (cm)	3.6	2.1	5.6
Abdominal length (cm)	2	.9	4.7
	Mean	**Mean − 2 SD**	**Mean + 2 SD**
Pressure (mm Hg)	13.8	4.6	23
Overall length (cm)	3.7	2.1	5.3
Abdominal length (cm)	2.2	.6	3.8

From DeMeester TR, Stein HJ: Gastroesophageal reflux disease. In Moody FG, Jones RS, Kelly KA, et al: Surgical Treatment of Digestive Disease, 2nd ed. Chicago, Year Book, 1989, p 65.

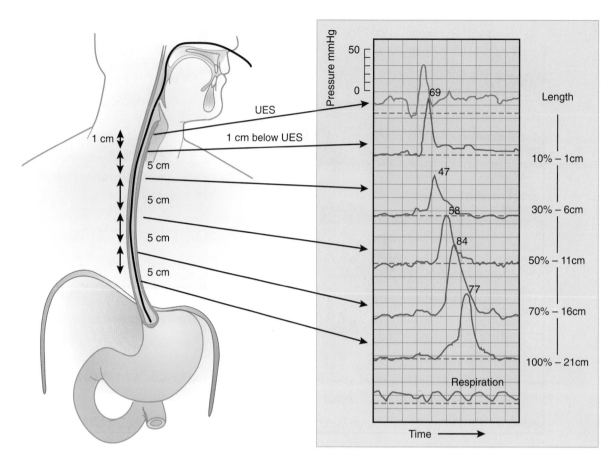

Figure 8–14. Schematic drawing combined with a sample manometric tracing showing placement of the transducers for standard manometry and the pressure response throughout the esophageal body during a swallow. UES, upper esophageal sphincter.

the stomach and the proximal transducer within the esophageal body. Ten wet swallows with 5 ml of water are performed. The pressure of the LES should drop to the level of gastric pressure during each wet swallow. The function of the esophageal body is assessed with three to five pressure transducers located at various levels in the esophagus. To standardize the procedure, the most proximal pressure transducer is placed 1 cm below the well-defined cricopharyngeal sphincter, with the distal orifices trailing at 5-cm intervals over the entire length of the esophagus. With this method, a pressure response throughout the whole esophagus can be obtained on swallowing (Fig. 8–14). The response to 10 wet swallows with 5 ml of room-temperature water is recorded. The amplitude, duration, and morphology of contractions (i.e., the number of peaks and repetitive activity) after each swallow are calculated at all recorded levels of the esophageal body. The delay between esophageal contractions at the various levels of the esophagus is used to calculate the speed of wave propagation and to classify contractions as peristaltic, simultaneous, or not transmitted. Based on this information, motor disorders of the esophagus are identified and classified (see Table 8–1). Typical manometric tracings of a patient with nutcracker esophagus, diffuse esophageal spasm, and achalasia are shown in Figures 8–15 through 8–17. Display of a

patient's values at the various levels of the esophagus against a background of normal values can make abnormalities more apparent (Fig. 8–18).

Because of the rapidity of events during the pharyngeal phase of swallowing, manometry in patients with suspected cricopharyngeal dysfunction should be performed with specially designed catheters. Both water-perfused and electronic systems have been used. Some advocate that electronic pressure-sensitive transducers are superior because they have a much higher frequency response than water-perfused catheters do and avoid the pharyngeal irritation that occurs with a water-perfused system.[66] The position, length, and pressure of the cricopharyngeal sphincter are assessed with a stationary pull-through technique. The manometry catheter is withdrawn in 0.5-cm intervals from the upper esophagus through the UES region into the pharynx.

To account for the anatomic asymmetry of the UES (Fig. 8–19), five measurements with the pressure transducers oriented in various directions are made, and an average is calculated. Localization of the upper and lower border of the UES can be determined manometrically during the station pull-through of the sphincter. Such localization may be helpful if an operative procedure is planned because a nasogastric tube can be marked at a

Text continued on p. 150

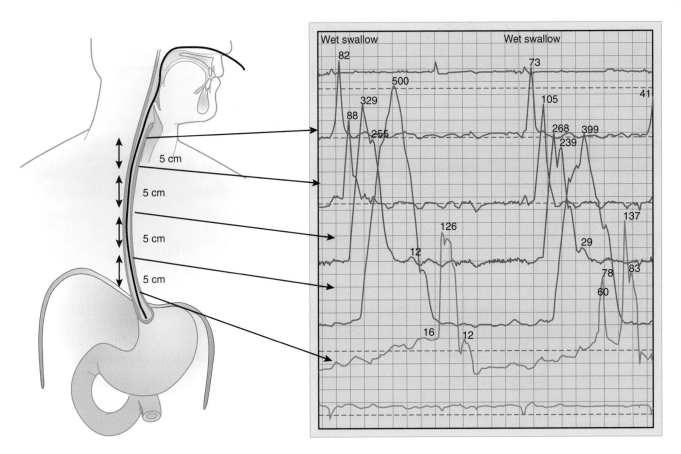

Figure 8–15. Manometric record from a patient with nutcracker esophagus showing distal esophageal peristaltic contractions of excessively high amplitude and long duration of contractions after wet swallows.

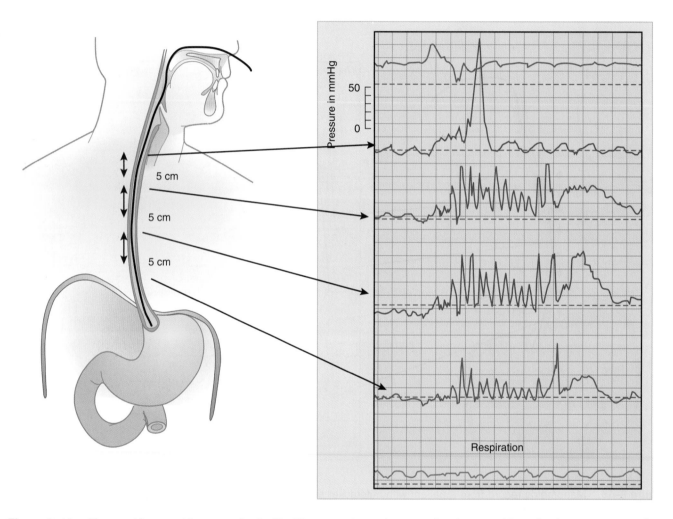

Figure 8–16.   Manometric record from a patient with diffuse esophageal spasm showing repetitive, simultaneous contractions in the distal esophageal body.

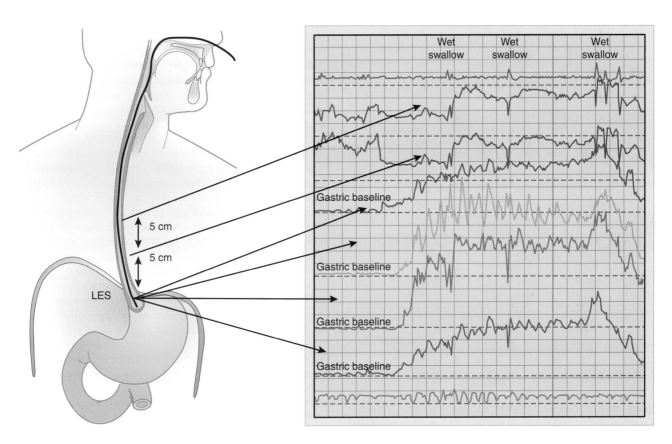

Figure 8–17.   Manometric record from a patient with achalasia showing failure of the lower esophageal sphincter (LES) to relax on swallowing. The esophageal body shows aperistalsis.

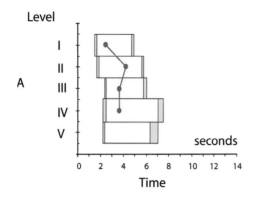

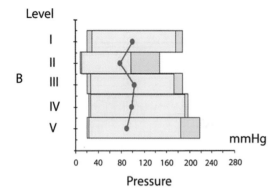

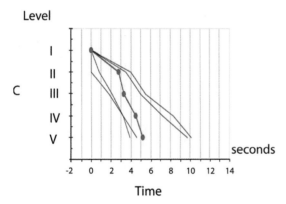

Figure 8–18. Graphic display of esophageal contraction characteristics at five levels of the esophagus (wet swallows). Patient values (*blue line*) are displayed against a background of normal values obtained in 60 asymptomatic volunteers (*solid lines*: 5th, 10th, 19th, and 95th percentiles). **A,** Duration of esophageal contractions. **B,** Amplitude of esophageal contractions. **C,** Wave progression.

site corresponding to the location of the patient's UES and placed in the patient's esophagus. During the operation the surgeon can then palpate the tip of the nasogastric tube, which will help guide the surgeon to the upper extent of the myotomy because failure to incorporate the proximal UES in the myotomy is one of the most frequent mistakes made. A dedicated water-perfused catheter consisting of eight lateral ports located at 0.5-cm intervals is of special use to evaluate abnormalities of sphincter opening and to detect

evidence of increased outflow resistance through the pharyngoesophageal segment. The opening of the UES is studied by placing one of the middle eight lateral pressure ports at the upper border of the cricopharyngeal sphincter while the other ports straddle the hypopharynx and upper esophagus (Fig. 8–20).[66] High-speed graphic recordings (50 mm/sec) are necessary to obtain an assessment of the coordination of cricopharyngeal relaxation with hypopharyngeal contraction.

The UES is opened by a traction force acting on the relaxed cricopharyngeus. This force is the consequence of the significant laryngohyoid elevation that occurs during the swallow. Normal swallowing and normal UES relaxation are associated manometrically with a subatmospheric pressure drop. The pressure at sphincter opening is determined by using a series of dry swallows. Atmospheric pressure is used as a baseline to determine whether the patient's opening pressure is subatmospheric. The pressure drop usually occurs early in the manometric tracing before any pharyngeal events can be seen (Fig. 8–21). An inability to achieve a subatmospheric pressure drop may be associated with impaired sphincter opening and relaxation (Fig. 8–22).

Normally, the sphincter is open and fully relaxed before the bolus arrives at this segment, and thus flow through the sphincter usually occurs with very little resistance. A measure of the resistance to flow through the sphincter can be determined by measuring the intrabolus pressure on the manometric tracing. Resistance to trans-sphincteric flow will occur if there is impaired sphincter opening, impaired relaxation, or decreased compliance of the upper esophageal musculature. Manometrically, this will be manifested by raised intrabolus pressure. Resistance to trans-sphincteric flow is determined by giving the patient a 5-ml bolus of water to swallow. This requires detection of the pressure at the bolus tail, which is most consistently and reliably determined by measuring the pressure just before the major upstroke of the pharyngeal stripping peristaltic contraction wave in the pharynx or just before the major upstroke of the UES postcontraction wave. Accurate determination of intrabolus pressure requires manovideofluorography (see Fig. 8–6); however, it is possible to get some indication of intrabolus pressure by routine manometry testing. Compliance of the pharyngoesophageal segment can also be determined by measuring intrabolus pressure during a series of swallows with an incremental increase in the swallowed volume. Compliance of the pharyngoesophageal segment is assessed by determining the rise in intrabolus pressure during a combination of 5-, 10-, and 15-ml swallows of water. There is usually only a slight increase in intrabolus pressure when going from a 5-ml to a 10-ml to a 15-ml swallow of water. A more steeply rising intrabolus pressure associated with an increase in swallow volume is indicative of decreased compliance of the pharyngoesophageal segment (see Fig. 8–7). Contraction amplitudes and wave progression of the pharyngeal stripping wave are assessed during the water swallows.

Carefully performed motility studies may demonstrate impaired sphincter opening, insufficient relaxation (Fig. 8–23) or premature contractions of the cricopharyngeus,

Figure 8–19. Three-dimensional pressure profile of the upper esophageal sphincter illustrating the short axial zone of maximal pressure and the marked radial asymmetry. UOSP, upper esophageal sphincter pressure. (From Welch RW, Luckmann K, Ricks PM, et al: Manometry of the normal upper esophageal sphincter and its alterations in laryngectomy. J Clin Invest 63:1039, 1979, with permission.)

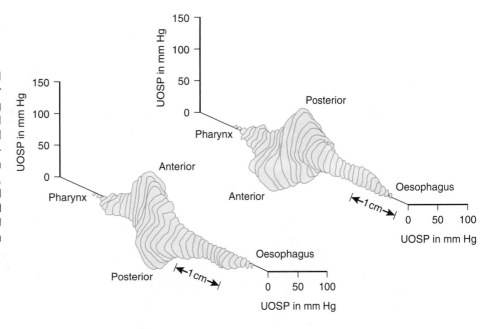

Figure 8–20. Record of a detailed manometric study of the pharyngoesophageal phase of swallowing showing the manometric correlates of pharyngeal peristalsis, elevation of the larynx, opening of the upper esophageal sphincter from proximal to distal, elevation of the cricoid, and the start of esophageal peristalsis.

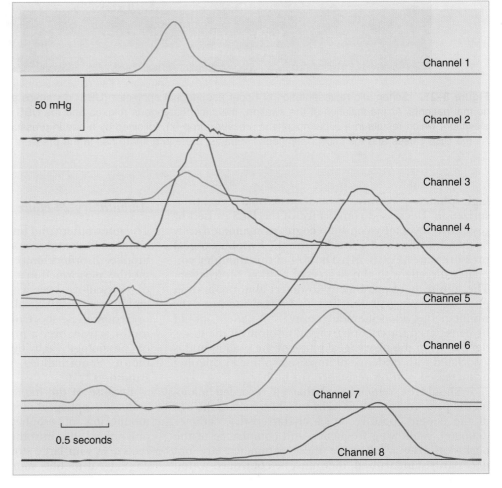

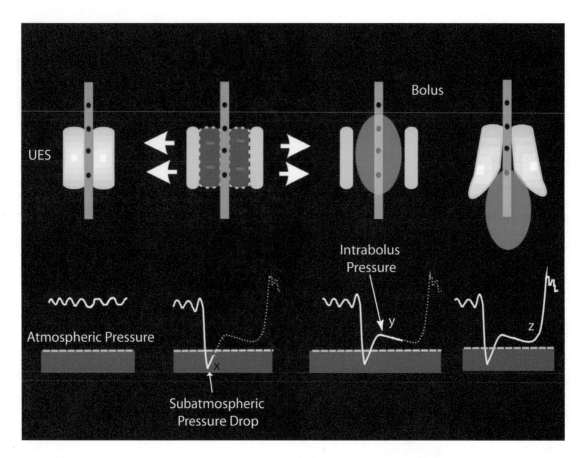

Figure 8–21. Schematic representation of upper esophageal sphincter (UES) dynamics and manometric correlates found in normal patients. At the initiation of the swallow, the cricopharyngeus relaxes and the UES is pulled open by the laryngohyoid elevation, which results in a subatmospheric pressure drop (x), followed by a rise in pressure as the bolus enters the UES (y). As the UES closes and the cricopharyngeus contracts, there is a sharp rise in the pressure tracing (z)

high sphincter pressure, or inadequate pharyngeal pressurization. Decreased compliance of the UES caused by restrictive myopathy can be recognized manometrically by the observation of a shoulder on the hypopharyngeal pressure wave (Fig. 8–24). The size of this shoulder correlates directly with the degree of outflow obstruction. The sensitivity of manometry to detect abnormalities in pharyngoesophageal function is further increased by simultaneous videocineradiography.[24,67] A patient should be considered for cricopharyngeal myotomy if the disorder occurs in the pharyngeal phase of the swallow and is associated with evidence of impaired sphincter opening or increased outflow resistance (or both).

It should be remembered that all recorded manometric pressures are affected by variables such as the age of the patient, posture, bolus characteristics, catheter diameter, swallowing frequency, and compliance of the perfusion system.[68] Because these parameters are not necessarily standardized, they must be controlled within an individual laboratory. Each laboratory should define normal values from volunteers who have no subjective or objective evidence of a foregut disorder; alternatively, one laboratory may adopt the normal values of another laboratory, provided that identical procedures and equipment are used.

Ambulatory 24-Hour Esophageal Manometry

The intermittent and unpredictable occurrence of motor abnormalities and symptoms in patients with esophageal motility disorders limits the diagnostic value of stationary motility performed in a laboratory setting and consisting of 10 swallows over a short period. The technique of ambulatory esophageal manometry was developed to overcome these shortcomings by monitoring esophageal motor activity over a prolonged period during a variety of physiologic activities and correlating esophageal motor abnormalities with spontaneously occurring symptoms.[31,69,70]

Because of the high sampling frequency required to evaluate esophageal motor activity, prolonged outpatient monitoring of esophageal motility became available only after the introduction of portable digital data recorders with large storage capacity. Today, ambulatory esophageal motility monitoring allows the evaluation of esophageal motor function based on more than 1000 contractions recorded over an entire circadian cycle under a variety of physiologic conditions (i.e., upright activity, eating, and sleeping). This technique provides a more than 100-fold larger database for the assessment of esophageal motor function than standard manometry does.[35]

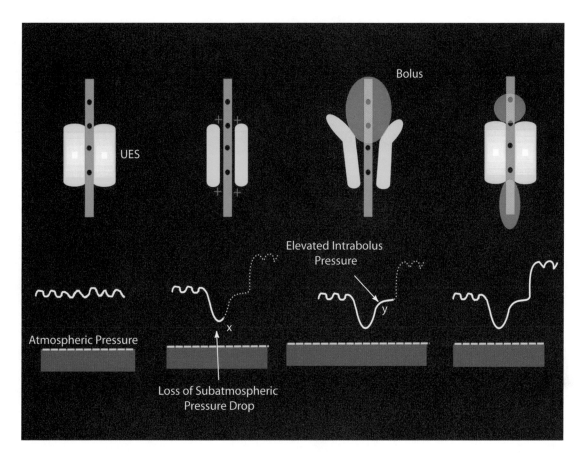

Figure 8–22. Schematic representation of upper esophageal sphincter (UES) dynamics and manometric correlates found in a patient with impaired sphincter opening and outflow resistance as a result of reduced compliance at the level of the UES. With impaired sphincter opening caused by either inadequate cricopharyngeus relaxation or impaired laryngohyoid elevation, there is loss of the normal subatmospheric pressure drop (x). With bolus entry into the UES, there is increased intrabolus pressure corresponding to the resistance to flow of the bolus through the UES (y).

Ambulatory esophageal motility monitoring is usually performed by placing a catheter with three or more electronic pressure transducers at 5-cm intervals above the upper border of the manometrically determined LES. The transducers are connected to a portable digital data recorder with sufficient memory to store pressure recordings from each channel over an entire circadian cycle. After placement of the transducers, the individuals are sent home and instructed to keep a diary for the next 24 hours in which they indicate when they retired for the night and awoke in the morning, when they ate their meals, and whenever a symptom occurred. The subjects are encouraged to perform normal daily activities during the study and to press an event marker when a spontaneous symptom occurs. After the 24-hour period, the subjects return to the laboratory, where the pressure transducers are removed and the data from the recorder are unloaded onto a personal computer. Data analysis is usually performed separately for the upright, supine, meal, and symptomatic periods with a computer program. This approach allows quantification of abnormal esophageal motor events and direct correlation of spontaneously occurring symptoms with motor abnormalities.

After its clinical introduction in 1985, ambulatory esophageal motility monitoring has been used primarily to identify esophageal motor abnormalities as the cause of noncardiac chest pain.[69,70] Recent studies in a larger number of unselected patients have found that many patients do not experience these typical symptoms during the 24-hour monitoring period.[32,71] Even when a spontaneous episode of chest pain occurred during the monitored period, motor abnormalities associated with the symptoms were rare and gastroesophageal reflux was found to be a far more frequent cause of noncardiac chest pain than esophageal motor disorders were. Consequently, ambulatory manometry in this situation should be performed simultaneously with esophageal pH monitoring and should be reserved for patients with daily symptoms.

Because of the enlarged database and the more physiologic conditions under which data are acquired, ambulatory manometry is superior to standard manometry for the evaluation of esophageal body function in patients with symptoms suggestive of a primary or secondary esophageal motor disorder.[35] The efficacy of esophageal motor activity can be determined by assessing the prevalence of peristaltic contractions with sufficient amplitude

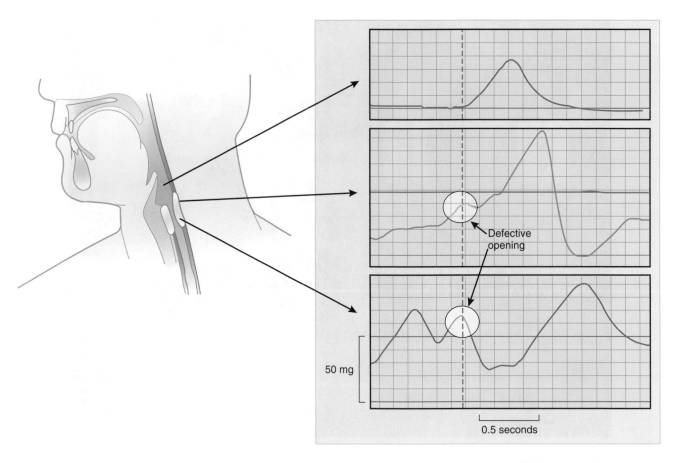

Figure 8–23. Manometric record showing defective and impaired upper esophageal sphincter (UES) opening. On initiation of the swallow, the UES should demonstrate a subatmospheric pressure drop. This record shows failure to achieve the drop.

to propel a bolus and clear refluxed gastric contents during the 24-hour monitoring period. Less than 50% of effective contractions during meals on ambulatory esophageal motility monitoring indicates the presence of a severe esophageal motor abnormality (see Fig. 8–11). Our experience with more than 300 ambulatory esophageal motility recordings in patients with esophageal motor disorders has shown that this approach allows quantification of the severity of a motor disorder and objective assessment of the effects of medical or surgical therapy.[35]

Tests to Evaluate Esophageal Bolus Clearance

Videocineroentgenography

High-speed cinerecording or videotaping of roentgenographic pharyngoesophageal contrast studies allows re-evaluation of individual swallows through review of the study at various speeds. The study is very useful for evaluation of the pharyngeal phase of swallowing. Observations that suggest oropharyngeal or cricopharyngeal dysfunction include misdirection of barium into the trachea or nasopharynx, prominence of the cricopharyngeal muscle (i.e., cricopharyngeal bar (Fig. 8–25), Zenker's diverticulum (Fig. 8–26), a narrow pharyngo-

esophageal segment, and stasis of contrast medium in the valleculae or hypopharyngeal recesses (Fig. 8–27).[72] These findings are not usually specific but are common manifestations of neuromuscular disorders that affect the pharyngoesophageal area. Studies using liquid barium, barium-impregnated solids, or radiopaque pills greatly aid in the evaluation of normal and abnormal motility in the esophageal body. Loss of the normal stripping wave or segmentation of the barium column with the patient in the recumbent position can be correlated with reduced contraction amplitude or abnormal waveforms in the esophageal body on manometry.[51,73] In addition, subtle structural abnormalities such as small diverticula, webs, and extrinsic impressions of the esophagus may be recognized only with motion-recording techniques.

Esophageal Transit Scintigraphy

Esophageal transit scintigraphy is another technique for the evaluation of esophageal function.[74] The esophageal transit of a 10-ml water bolus containing sulfur colloid is recorded with a gamma camera. Transit time is measured separately in the proximal and distal esophagus. With this technique, delayed bolus transit can be shown in patients with a variety of esophageal motor disorders,

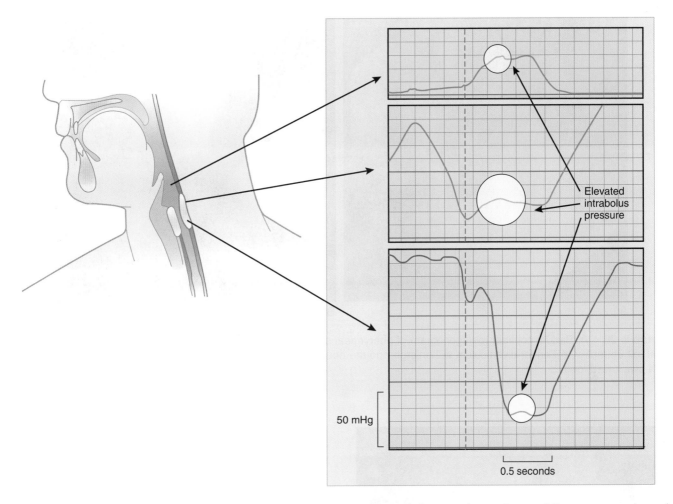

50 mHg

0.5 seconds

Figure 8–24.   Manometric record showing impaired sphincter opening and decreased compliance of the upper esophageal sphincter (UES) resulting in elevated intrabolus pressure on both the pharyngeal and UES manometric pressure waves.

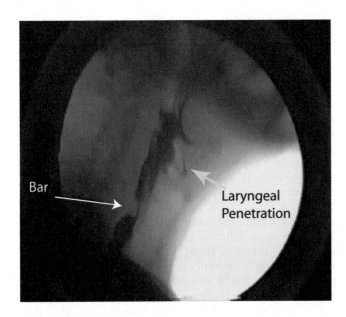

Bar

Laryngeal Penetration

Figure 8–25.   Barium contrast roentgenogram of pharyngeal swallowing activity showing a prominent cricopharyngeal indentation (*white arrow*) in a patient with dysphagia resulting from bulbar poliomyelitis. The patient also showed evidence of laryngeal penetration (*yellow arrow*).

including achalasia, scleroderma, diffuse esophageal spasm, nutcracker esophagus, and nonspecific motor disorders. It appears that transit scintigraphy is a reliable technique to quantify and document esophageal transit abnormalities.[21] However, the test lacks specificity because it cannot define the precise nature of a swallowing abnormality. Its best use is to quantify the effect of an esophageal motor abnormality by measuring esophageal emptying time.

Impedance

Impedance testing has recently been used to examine the clearance function of the esophagus and is indicated for all patients with suspected esophageal motility disorders. Impedance allows detection of all bolus movement in the esophagus without radiology. It is basically a measurement of opposition to electrical current flow. Esophageal impedance testing is performed with a specially designed catheter. The body of the catheter is electrically inert and has a series of ring electrodes spaced at various distances. The ring electrodes are essentially metallic conductors. An electrical current is sent to the individual electrodes with a current generator. The electrical conductivity between two ring electrodes

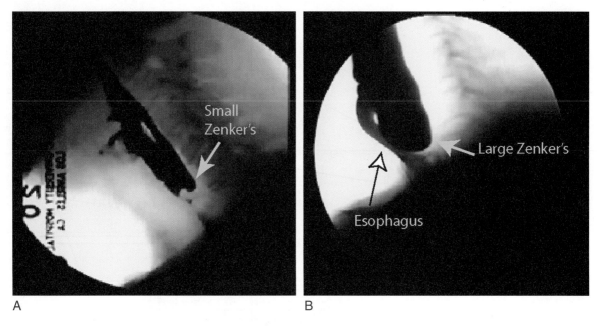

Figure 8–26. A, Barium contrast roentgenogram of pharyngeal swallowing activity showing a small early Zenker diverticulum. **B,** If left untreated, a Zenker diverticulum will enlarge and the pouch itself may cause obstruction of the esophagus when filled with swallowed food.

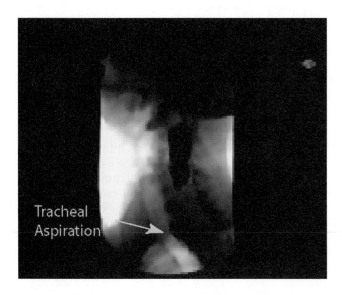

Figure 8–27. Barium contrast roentgenogram from a patient with cricopharyngeal achalasia and poor upper esophageal sphincter opening. There is significant retention of contrast medium at the level of the vallecula and piriform recesses, with no barium passing into the esophagus. The patient also shows significant aspiration of contrast into the trachea (*yellow arrow*).

can then be measured for this segment. A measure of the surrounding impedance can then be obtained and will reflect the background impedance of the esophageal wall. Any swallowed bolus, whether air, liquid, or solid, will have different impedance or conduct electricity differently. When a swallowed bolus spans two consecutive ring electrodes, electrical current flows between the two ring electrodes and the resistance can be measured. When no bolus is present, the impedance will be high. When the impedance falls, a bolus will be present between the two recording electrodes. A single impedance channel will detect bolus movement through the esophagus; however, if multiple impedance channels are used, it is possible to measure segmental changes and detect the direction of bolus movement and the propagation rate or clearance time (Figs. 8–28 and 8–29).

The impedance catheter is passed through the nose and esophagus into the stomach in much the same way as for esophageal manometry. The technique calls for obtaining baseline impedance for at least 5 seconds before a swallow. This baseline value represents the impedance of the surrounding esophageal mucosa and esophageal wall. Swallows consisting of normal saline and a viscous material that has a known standardized impedance value are then given. A liquid bolus is more electrically conductive than the esophageal lining. When a liquid bolus enters, impedance falls. Entry of the liquid bolus is depicted by a 50% drop in ohms from the pre-episode baseline impedance.[75] Bolus exit is depicted when the impedance returns to the 50% point on the impedance recovery slope of the curve. The difference yields the bolus clearance time. A gas bolus is less electrically conductive than the esophageal lining. When a gas bolus enters, impedance rises. Gas entry is defined by a 50% rise in impedance with a mean impedance of 3000 ohms or greater (Fig. 8–30).

The multichannel intraluminal impedance catheter has now been combined with a standard manometry catheter to create a unique way to examine esophageal function. Currently, the standard combined

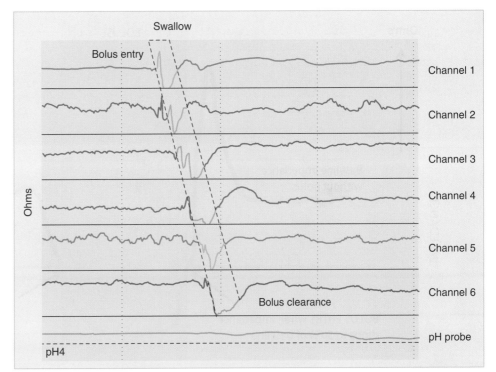

Figure 8–28. Impedance tracing depicting a normal liquid swallow. By using a multichannel catheter, the direction of bolus flow as well as the bolus clearance characteristics and propagation velocity can be calculated.

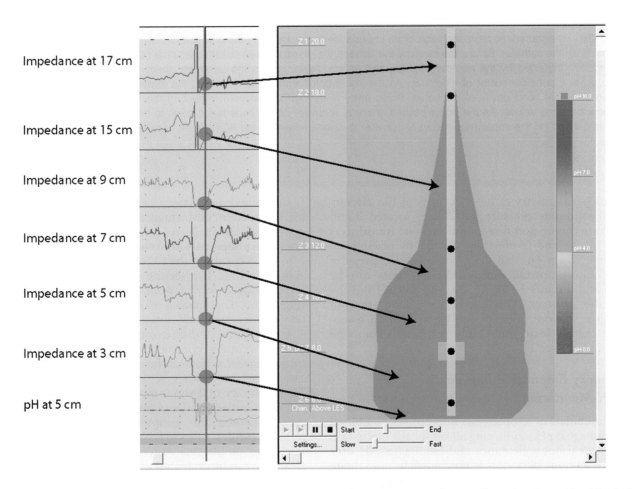

Figure 8–29. A sample tracing of an impedance record showing a software construct of a two-dimensional graphic of the bolus. A playback video of the bolus showing a two-dimensional moving waveform of the bolus as it traverses the esophagus can also be constructed. This can give further insight into bolus transit dynamics during a swallow.

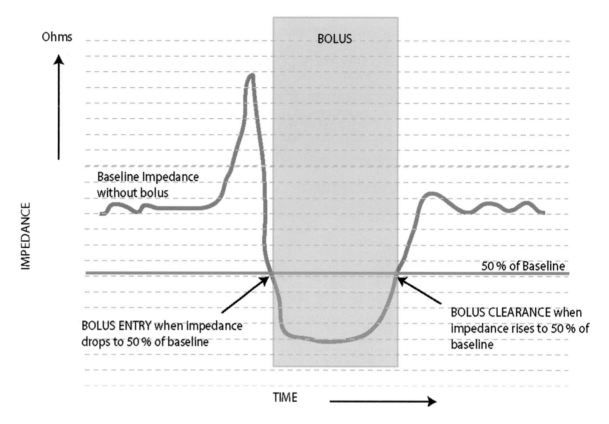

Figure 8–30. Diagrammatic representation of an impedance trace depicting the characteristics as the bolus enters the recording segment on the catheter. Before the swallow the impedance measured reflects the baseline conductivity of the segment and the impedance imparted by the esophageal wall and lumen. As air enters the segment, there is a sharp rise in impedance because air is a poor conductor of electricity. As the liquid bolus enters the segment, the impedance falls as a result of the increased electrical conductivity of the bolus. Bolus entry is defined by the point reflecting the 50% drop in impedance from preswallow baseline values. As the bolus passes, there is recovery of the impedance back to baseline values. The bolus exit position is defined on the impedance recovery curve at the point reflecting the 50% return to preswallow impedance.

impedance-manometry catheter consists of two circumferential solid-state pressure transducers located 5 and 10 cm from the tip and three unidirectional transducers spaced 15, 20, and 25 cm from the tip. By placing the impedance rings so that they straddle the pressure sensors, four impedance-measuring segments can be created at a distance of 10, 15, 20, and 25 cm from the tip of the catheter. This allows for quantization of esophageal squeeze pressure combined with an assessment of bolus velocity and clearance whether complete or incomplete (see Fig. 8–8).

Ambulatory Esophageal Impedance and pH Monitoring

Today, ambulatory esophageal impedance combined with esophageal pH monitoring allows for the evaluation of esophageal bolus clearance and esophageal pH over an entire 24-hour period. It is now possible to evaluate esophageal bolus clearance during eating, sleeping, and upright activity. The circadian motor pattern can be graphically displayed by showing the bolus clearance sequences (Fig. 8–31) during the monitored period.

Combined ambulatory pH and impedance monitoring is generally performed with a catheter that has six impedance channels and one to two pH electrodes. The impedance segments are usually positioned at 17, 15, 9, 7, 5, and 3 cm above the LES with the pH electrode 5 cm above the LES. If a second pH electrode is used, it is usually placed in the stomach to measure gastric pH (Fig. 8–32). This spacing allows for the optimum evaluation of retrograde and antegrade bolus movement.

It is possible to distinguish between primary and secondary peristaltic contractions. A determination of gastroesophageal reflux can be made, and it can further be categorized into either acid reflux or non-acid reflux. The advantage of 24-hour monitoring is that the patients can keep a diary of symptoms. Correlation can then be made between the symptoms and gastroesophageal reflux regardless of its pH. Noncardiac chest pain events related to esophageal distention and poor esophageal clearance can be evaluated with this new technique. Data analysis is usually performed with a computer program that specifically locates waveform areas with retrograde bolus movement. The program will also determine bolus entry and clearance points when reflux occurs and will

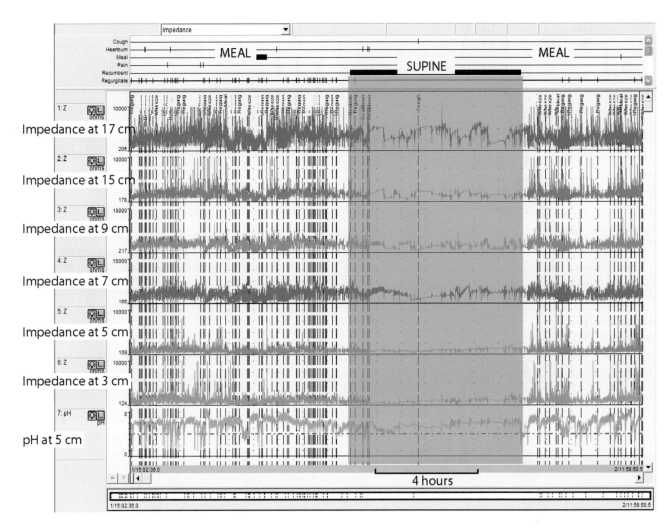

Figure 8–31. Condensed six-channel circadian esophageal combined impedance and pH motility tracing. Recording was started at 15:00 hours and terminated at 12:00 hours the next day. Time is shown on the x-axis. The six impedance segments were located 17 (*top tracing*), 15, 9, 7, 5, and 3 cm (*bottom tracing*) above the lower esophageal sphincter (LES). An electrode measuring pH was located 5 cm above the LES. Meal periods, the nighttime sleeping period, and reflux episodes are indicated at the bottom. The *dotted vertical lines* indicate the patient's symptoms during the recording period. Bolus movements and swallowing events in the esophagus are depicted by changes in impedance to give an indication of the motor activity occurring during the recording time. The circadian variability of esophageal motor activity can easily be recognized.

analyze the pH channel to determine drops below 4.0. In addition, the program will correlate the patient's specific symptoms with bolus movement and pH. In particular, the esophageal motor or clearance abnormalities associated with gastroesophageal reflux can be determined, and with a symptom index it is possible to ascertain whether the patient's symptoms are due to acid reflux or esophageal distention secondary to an esophageal clearance abnormality. The use of this tool in evaluating patients with esophageal motor disorders is still in its infancy, but it promises to yield further insight in these conditions. Currently, evaluation of antegrade swallows during a meal has to be reviewed manually. Although there are no reports on combined ambulatory multichannel intraluminal impedance and esophageal manometry, the technology exists to perform this acquisition.

Tests to Provoke Esophageal Symptoms

Acid Perfusion Test

Since its introduction in 1958 by Bernstein and Baker,[76] the esophageal acid perfusion test has been widely used to determine whether a patient's symptoms can be reproduced by infusion of acid into the esophagus. If positive, the test indicates that the esophagus is sensitive to acid and increased esophageal exposure to acid is assumed. In the original technique, the distal end of the esophagus was perfused with 0.1 N HCl at a rate of 6 to 8 ml/min with the patient sitting upright. Ideally, a placebo is also infused (i.e., acid is alternately perfused with physiologic saline without the patient knowing the identity of the perfusate). The patient is asked to report any symptom that develops during infusion. Consistent reproduction

COMBINED 6 SEGMENT IMPEDANCE
AND 2 CHANNEL pH CATHETER

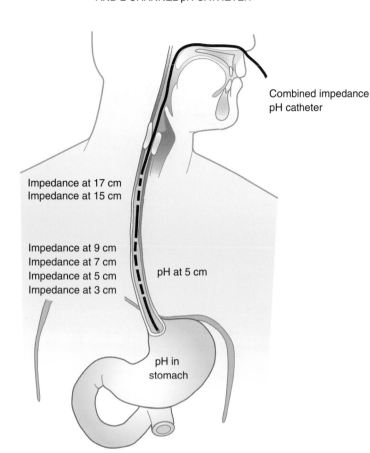

Combined impedance
pH catheter

Impedance at 17 cm
Impedance at 15 cm

Impedance at 9 cm
Impedance at 7 cm
Impedance at 5 cm
Impedance at 3 cm

pH at 5 cm

pH in
stomach

Figure 8–32. Placement of the catheter and location of the impedance segments and pH electrodes for combined ambulatory 24-hour esophageal impedance and pH monitoring.

of the patient's usual symptoms only during acid perfusion and rapid abatement during saline perfusion indicates a positive test. The development of symptoms during both the saline test and the acid perfusion test or the development of symptoms foreign to the patient's usual experience represents an equivocal test. Failure to develop any symptoms during a 30-minute acid perfusion indicates a normal test.

Various investigators have reported that 34% to 100% of patients with typical symptoms of GERD have a positive acid perfusion test. Failure to include certain components of gastric juice (e.g., pepsin, bile, pancreatic enzymes, food) in the perfusate may account for some of the normal results. A false-negative result can also occur in patients who have an insensitive esophagus. False-positive results are seen in 15% of symptomatic subjects. Of concern is that symptomatic subjects whose pain is not due to reflux may have a similar incidence of false-positive tests, thereby resulting in an erroneous diagnosis.

Edrophonium (Tensilon) Test

The edrophonium test has been introduced to identify chest pain of esophageal origin in patients in whom cardiac disease has been excluded.[77,78] The cholinesterase inhibitor edrophonium hydrochloride (Tensilon) is injected intravenously at a dose of 80 μg/kg. A syringe

with 1 mg of the antidote atropine should always be at hand when performing the test. The test is ideally placebo controlled. A positive test is defined as replication of chest pain similar to the pain that the patient experiences spontaneously after edrophonium injection but not placebo injection. The test is positive in 20% to 30% of patients with noncardiac chest pain but not in asymptomatic volunteers.[78] In both normal volunteers and symptomatic patients, edrophonium causes a marked increase in the amplitude and duration of esophageal contractions. Because reproduction of the patient's typical symptoms rather than a specific change in esophageal motility is considered the end point of the test, manometry does not have be performed. Disadvantages of the test are that its helpfulness is limited to only a small proportion of patients with chest pain, there is a risk of side effects, and it reproduces symptoms with an unphysiologic stimulus. The test should not be performed in patients with asthma, chronic obstructive airway disease, or cardiac arrhythmias. This test is rarely performed.

Esophageal Balloon Distention

Balloon distention of the esophagus was described in 1955 as a diagnostic test to distinguish esophageal from cardiac chest pain.[79] An inflatable balloon is positioned

10 cm above the LES and gradually inflated with air in 1-ml increments. Esophageal motility is simultaneously monitored. The test is considered positive when typical symptoms are reproduced with gradual distention of the balloon. Studies indicate that the procedure induces spastic esophageal motor activity and reproduces chest pain episodes in up to 50% of patients with noncardiac chest pain, but not in volunteers.[80] Although the test has greater diagnostic yield than drug provocative studies do, it is relatively invasive and provides no information on spontaneously occurring symptoms.

Tests to Detect Increased Esophageal Exposure to Gastric and Duodenal Juice

24-Hour Esophageal pH Monitoring

The most direct method of measuring increased esophageal exposure to gastric juice is 24-hour monitoring of esophageal luminal pH with an indwelling pH probe placed 5 cm above the upper border of the LES. It quantifies the actual time that the esophageal mucosa is exposed to acid gastric juice, measures the ability of the esophagus to clear refluxed acid, and correlates esophageal acid exposure to the patient's symptoms. A 24-hour monitoring period is necessary so that measurements are made over one complete circadian cycle. This allows for assessment of the effect of physiologic activity such as eating or sleeping on reflux of gastric juice into the esophagus. If a combined impedance-pH catheter is used, an assessment of all gastroesophageal reflux events, both acidic and nonacidic, can be made. The frequency of reflux episodes, their nature and duration, and the clearance time associated with the reflux event can be determined. Many patients with esophageal motor disorders have increased esophageal acid exposure that may be an important trigger for their symptoms or a secondary effect caused by poor esophageal clearance.

SUMMARY

Primary motor disorders of the esophagus affect neural as well as muscular elements of the UES, body of the esophagus, and LES. The cause of disorders of upper esophageal function is known in about 60% of patients, and the dysfunction is secondary to a variety of neurologic and muscular conditions. The cause in the remainder is uncertain. The cause of esophageal body and LES disorders is unknown; however, the hypertrophic myopathic state of the esophagus may be a consequence of LES dysfunction and the neural dysfunction may be secondary.[81]

SELECTED READINGS

Mason RJ, Bremner CG, DeMeester TR, et al: Pharyngeal swallowing disorders: Selection for and outcome after myotomy. Ann Surg 228:598, 1998.

Mittal RK, Bhalla V: Esophageal motor functions and its disorders. Gut 53:1536, 2004.

Nguyen HN, Silny J, Albers D, et al: Dynamics of esophageal bolus transport in healthy subjects studied using multiple intraluminal impedancometry. Am J Physiol 273:G958, 1997.

Spechler SJ, Castell DO: Classification of oesophageal motility abnormalities. Gut 49:145, 2001.

Tutuian R, Castell DO: Combined multichannel intraluminal impedance and manometry clarifies esophageal function abnormalities: Study in 350 patients. Am J Gastroenterol 99:1011, 2004.

REFERENCES

1. Stein HJ, DeMeester TR: Outpatient physiologic testing and surgical management of foregut motility disorders. Curr Probl Surg 29:413, 1992.
2. Bhalla V, Padda B, Puckett J: Longitudinal and circular muscle contract synchronously in the esophagus during peristalsis: A new way to look at the contraction of two muscle layers [abstract W1444]. Gastroenterology 126(Suppl 2):A-637, 2004.
3. Gidda JS, Goyal RK: Regional gradient of initial inhibition and refractoriness in esophageal smooth muscle. Gastroenterology 89:843, 1985.
4. Weisbrodt NW, Christensen J: Gradients of contractions in the opossum esophagus. Gastroenterology 626:1159, 1972.
5. Crist J, Gidda JS, Goyal RK: Characteristics of "on" and "off" contractions in esophageal circular muscle in vitro. Am J Physiol 246:G137, 1984.
6. Gidda JS, Buyniski JP: Swallow-evoked peristalsis in opossum esophagus: Role of cholinergic mechanisms. Am J Physiol 251:G779, 1986.
7. Meyer GW, Gerhardt DC, Castell DO: Human esophageal response to rapid swallowing: Muscle refractory period or neural inhibition? Am J Physiol 241:G129, 1981.
8. Mittal RK, Balaban DH:. The esophagogastric junction. N Engl J Med 336:924, 1997.
9. Liebermann-Meffert D, Allgower M, Schmid P, Blum AL: Muscular equivalent of the lower esophageal sphincter. Gastroenterology 76:31, 1979.
10. Muinuddin A, Xue S, Diamant NE: Regional differences in the response of feline esophageal smooth muscle to stretch and cholinergic stimulation. Am J Physiol Gastrointest Liver Physiol 281:G1460, 2001.
11. Preiksaitis HG, Diamant NE: Regional differences in cholinergic activity of muscle fibers from the human gastroesophageal junction. Am J Physiol 272:G1321, 1997.
12. Liu J, Parashar VK, Mittal RK: Asymmetry of lower esophageal sphincter pressure: Is it related to the muscle thickness or its shape? Am J Physiol 272:G1509, 1997.
13. Mashimo H, He XD, Huang PL, et al: Neuronal constitutive nitric oxide synthase is involved in murine enteric inhibitory neurotransmission. J Clin Invest 98:8, 1996.
14. Dent J, Holloway RH, Toouli J, et al: Mechanisms of lower oesophageal sphincter incompetence in patients with symptomatic gastrooesophageal reflux. Gut 29:1020, 1988.
15. Price LM, El-Sharkawy TY, Mui HY, et al: Effect of bilateral cervical vagotomy on balloon-induced lower esophageal sphincter relaxation in the dog. Gastroenterology 77:324, 1979.
16. Hyland NP, Abrahams TP, Fuchs K, et al: Organization and neurochemistry of vagal preganglionic neurons innervating the lower esophageal sphincter in ferrets. J Comp Neurol 430:222, 2001.
17. Rossiter CD, Norman WP, Jain M, et al: Control of lower esophageal sphincter pressure by two sites in dorsal motor nucleus of the vagus. Am J Physiol 259:G899, 1990.
18. Bonavina L, Evander A, DeMeester TR, et al: Length of the distal esophageal sphincter and competency of the cardia. Am J Surg 151:25, 1986.

19. Stein HJ, DeMeester TR, Naspetti R, et al: Three-dimensional imaging of the lower esophageal sphincter in gastroesophageal reflux disease. Ann Surg 214:374, 1991.

20. Zaninotto G, DeMeester TR, Schwizer W, et al: The lower esophageal sphincter in health and disease. Am J Surg 155:104, 1988.

21. Russell CO, Hill LD, Holmes ER 3rd, et al: Radionuclide transit: A sensitive screening test for esophageal dysfunction. Gastroenterology 80:887, 1981.

22. Kahrilas PJ, Dodds WJ, Dent J, et al: Upper esophageal sphincter function during deglutition. Gastroenterology 95:52, 1988.

23. Mason RJ, Bremner CG, DeMeester TR, et al: Pharyngeal swallowing disorders: Selection for and outcome after myotomy. Ann Surg 228:598, 1998.

24. Cook IJ, Gabb M, Panagopoulos V, et al: Pharyngeal (Zenker's) diverticulum is a disorder of upper esophageal sphincter opening. Gastroenterology 103:1229, 1992.

25. Bonavina L, Khan NA, DeMeester TR: Pharyngoesophageal dysfunctions. The role of cricopharyngeal myotomy. Arch Surg 120:541, 1985.

26. Vantrappen G, Janssens J, Hellemans J, et al: Achalasia, diffuse esophageal spasm, and related motility disorders. Gastroenterology 76:450, 1979.

27. Castell D, Richter J, Dalton C: Esophageal Motility Testing. Elsevier, New York, 1987.

28. Spechler SJ, Castell DO: Classification of oesophageal motility abnormalities. Gut 49:145, 2001.

29. Hirano I, Tatum RP, Shi G, et al: Manometric heterogeneity in patients with idiopathic achalasia. Gastroenterology 120:789, 2001.

30. Mearin F, Mourelle M, Guarner F, et al: Patients with achalasia lack nitric oxide synthase in the gastro-oesophageal junction. Eur J Clin Invest 23:724, 1993.

31. Eypasch EP, Stein HJ, DeMeester TR, et al: A new technique to define and clarify esophageal motor disorders. Am J Surg 159:144, 1990.

32. Stein HJ, DeMeester TR, Eypasch EP, et al: Ambulatory 24-hour esophageal manometry in the evaluation of esophageal motor disorders and noncardiac chest pain. Surgery 110:753, 1991.

33. Tutuian R, Castell DO: Combined multichannel intraluminal impedance and manometry clarifies esophageal function abnormalities: Study in 350 patients. Am J Gastroenterol 99:1011, 2004.

34. Singh S, Stein HJ, DeMeester TR, et al: Nonobstructive dysphagia in gastroesophageal reflux disease: A study with combined ambulatory pH and motility monitoring. Am J Gastroenterol 87:562, 1992.

35. Stein HJ, DeMeester TR: Indications, technique, and clinical use of ambulatory 24-hour esophageal motility monitoring in a surgical practice. Ann Surg 217:128, 1993.

36. Brand DL, Martin D, Pope CE 2nd: Esophageal manometrics in patients with angina-like chest pain. Am J Dig Dis 22:300, 1977.

37. Balaban DH, Yamamoto Y, Liu J, et al: Sustained esophageal contraction: A marker of esophageal chest pain identified by intraluminal ultrasonography. Gastroenterology 116:29, 1999.

38. Pehlivanov N, Liu J, Mittal RK: Sustained esophageal contraction: A motor correlate of heartburn symptom. Am J Physiol Gastrointest Liver Physiol 281:G743, 2001.

39. Tung HN, Schulze-Delrieu K, Shirazi S, et al: Hypertrophic smooth muscle in the partially obstructed opossum esophagus. The model: Histological and ultrastructural observations. Gastroenterology 100:853, 1991.

40. Marshall JB, Kretschmar JM, Gerhardt DC, et al: Gastrointestinal manifestations of mixed connective tissue disease. Gastroenterology 98:1232, 1990.

41. Stevens MB, Hookman P, Siegel CI, et al: Aperistalsis of the esophagus in patients with connective-tissue disorders and Raynaud's phenomenon. N Engl J Med 270:1218, 1964.

42. Zamost BJ, Hirschberg J, Ippoliti AF, et al: Esophagitis in scleroderma. Prevalence and risk factors. Gastroenterology 92:421, 1987.

43. Miller LS, Liu JB, Klenn PJ, et al: Endoluminal ultrasonography of the distal esophagus in systemic sclerosis. Gastroenterology 105:31, 1993.

44. DeMeester TR, Stein HJ: Gastroesophageal Reflux Disease, 2nd ed. Chicago, Year Book, 1989, p 65.

45. Demeester TR, Johnson LF, Joseph GJ, et al: Patterns of gastroesophageal reflux in health and disease. Ann Surg 184:459, 1976.

46. Johnson LF, Demeester TR: Twenty-four-hour pH monitoring of the distal esophagus. A quantitative measure of gastroesophageal reflux. Am J Gastroenterol 62:325, 1974.

47. Sarkar S, Aziz Q, Woolf CJ, et al: Contribution of central sensitisation to the development of non-cardiac chest pain. Lancet 356:1154, 2000.

48. Sarkar S, Hobson AR, Furlong PL, et al: Central neural mechanisms mediating human visceral hypersensitivity. Am J Physiol Gastrointest Liver Physiol 281:G1196, 2001.

49. Bombeck CT, Vaz O, DeSalvo J, et al: Computerized axial manometry of the esophagus. A new method for the assessment of antireflux operations. Ann Surg 206:465, 1987.

50. Helm JF, Dodds WJ, Riedel DR, et al: Determinants of esophageal acid clearance in normal subjects. Gastroenterology 85:607, 1983.

51. Kahrilas PJ, Dodds WJ, Hogan WJ: Effect of peristaltic dysfunction on esophageal volume clearance. Gastroenterology 94:73, 1988.

52. Hong D, Khajanchee YS, Pereira N, et al: Manometric abnormalities and gastroesophageal reflux disease in the morbidly obese. Obes Surg 14:744, 2004.

53. Jaffin BW, Knoepflmacher P, Greenstein R: High prevalence of asymptomatic esophageal motility disorders among morbidly obese patients. Obes Surg 9:390, 1999.

54. Korenkov M, Kohler L, Yucel N, et al: Esophageal motility and reflux symptoms before and after bariatric surgery. Obes Surg 12:72, 2002.

55. Mercer CD, Rue C, Hanelin L, et al: Effect of obesity on esophageal transit. Am J Surg 149:177, 1985.

56. Seymour K, Mackie A, McCauley E, et al: Changes in esophageal function after vertical banded gastroplasty as demonstrated by esophageal scintigraphy. Obes Surg 8:429, 1998.

57. Sanchez NC, Tenofsky PL, Dort JM et al: What is normal intra-abdominal pressure? Am Surg 67:243, 2001.

58. Weiss H, Labeck B, Klocker J, et al: Effects of adjustable gastric banding on altered gut neuropeptide levels in morbidly obese patients. Obes Surg 11:735, 2001.

59. DeMaria EJ, Sugerman HJ, Meador JG, et al: High failure rate after laparoscopic adjustable silicone gastric banding for treatment of morbid obesity. Ann Surg 233:809, 2001.

60. Greenstein RJ, Nissan A, Jaffin B: Esophageal anatomy and function in laparoscopic gastric restrictive bariatric surgery: Implications for patient selection. Obes Surg 8:199, 1998.

61. Peterli R, Donadini A, Peters T, et al: Re-operations following laparoscopic adjustable gastric banding. Obes Surg 12:851, 2002.

62. Weiss HG, Kirchmayr W, Klaus A, et al: Surgical revision after failure of laparoscopic adjustable gastric banding. Br J Surg 91:235, 2004.

63. Weiss HG, Nehoda H, Labeck B, et al: Treatment of morbid obesity with laparoscopic adjustable gastric banding affects esophageal motility. Am J Surg 180:479, 2000.

64. Langmore SE, Schatz K, Olsen N: Fiberoptic endoscopic examination of swallowing safety: A new procedure. Dysphagia 2:216, 1988.

65. Craig A, Hanlon J, Dent J, et al: A comparison of transnasal and transoral endoscopy with small-diameter endoscopes in unsedated patients. Gastrointest Endosc 49:292, 1999.

66. Castell JA, Dalton CB, Castell DO: Pharyngeal and upper esophageal sphincter manometry in humans. Am J Physiol 258:G173, 1990.

67. Kahrilas PJ, Logemann JA, Lin S, et al: Pharyngeal clearance during swallowing: A combined manometric and videofluoroscopic study. Gastroenterology 103:128, 1992.

68. Lydon SB, Dodds WJ, Hogan WJ, et al: The effect of manometric assembly diameter on intraluminal esophageal pressure recording. Am J Dig Dis 20:968, 1975.

69. Janssens J, Vantrappen G, Ghillebert G: 24-hour recording of esophageal pressure and pH in patients with noncardiac chest pain. Gastroenterology 90:1978, 1986.

70. Peters L, Maas L, Petty D, et al: Spontaneous noncardiac chest pain. Evaluation by 24-hour ambulatory esophageal motility and pH monitoring. Gastroenterology 94:878, 1988.

71. Soffer EE, Scalabrini P, Wingate DL: Spontaneous noncardiac chest pain: Value of ambulatory esophageal pH and motility monitoring. Dig Dis Sci 34:1651, 1989.

72. Ekberg O, Wahlgren L: Dysfunction of pharyngeal swallowing. A cineradiographic investigation in 854 dysphagia patients. Acta Radiol Diagn (Stockh) 26:389, 1985.

73. Massey BT, Dodds WJ, Hogan WJ, et al: Abnormal esophageal motility. An analysis of concurrent radiographic and manometric findings. Gastroenterology 101:344, 1991.

74. Tolin RD, Malmud LS, Reilley J, et al: Esophageal scintigraphy to quantitate esophageal transit (quantitation of esophageal transit). Gastroenterology 76:1402, 1979.

75. Nguyen HN, Silny J, Albers D, et al: Dynamics of esophageal bolus transport in healthy subjects studied using multiple intraluminal impedancometry. Am J Physiol 273:G958, 1997.

76. Bernstein LM, Baker LA: A clinical test for esophagitis. Gastroenterology 34:760, 1958.

77. Benjamin SB, Richter JE, Cordova CM, et al: Prospective manometric evaluation with pharmacologic provocation of patients with suspected esophageal motility dysfunction. Gastroenterology 84:893, 1983.

78. Richter JE, Hackshaw BT, Wu WC, et al: Edrophonium: A useful provocative test for esophageal chest pain. Ann Intern Med 103:14, 1985.

79. Kramer P, Hollander W: Comparison of experimental esophageal pain with clinical pain of angina pectoris and esophageal disease. Gastroenterology 29:719, 1955.

80. Barish CF, Castell DO, Richter JE: Graded esophageal balloon distention. A new provocative test for noncardiac chest pain. Dig Dis Sci 31:1292, 1986.

81. Mittal RK, Bhalla V: Esophageal motor functions and its disorders. Gut 53:1536, 2004.

9

pH and Bilirubin Monitoring

Leah M. Backhus • Ross M. Bremner

Gastroesophageal reflux (GER) is defined as excessive exposure of the esophageal lumen to refluxed gastric juice. Because gastric juice is characteristically acidic, recording intraluminal pH has become a convenient means of measuring this exposure. Similarly, knowing that gastric juice may contain duodenal contents refluxed from beyond the pylorus, measuring bilirubin in the refluxate has become a means by which duodenogastroesophageal reflux can be quantitated. This chapter discusses the relevance of pH and bilirubin monitoring as it pertains to foregut disorders, how these tests are accurately performed, and their applicability and limitations.

TESTS TO DETECT INCREASED ESOPHAGEAL EXPOSURE TO GASTRIC JUICE

To definitively make a diagnosis of gastroesophageal reflux disease (GERD), the presence of increased esophageal exposure to gastric juice has to be confirmed objectively. Historically, numerous methods have been used to characterize the extent of esophageal acid exposure, including symptom indices, esophagogastroduodenoscopy, videoesophagography, and scintigraphy. Each of these tests is limited in that they infer the presence of acid within the esophagus by indirect means and thus lack sensitivity. Consequently, a number of provocative tests have been designed to identify the esophagus as the cause of symptoms of GERD. Of these, the intraesophageal acid perfusion (Bernstein) test, the standard acid reflux test, and provocation maneuvers during barium esophagography are the most familiar. Common to all provocative tests is that they are dependent on the patient's perception and do not definitively prove an esophageal cause of a spontaneously occurring symptom. The sensitivity and specificity of various tests for GERD are listed in Table 9–1.

24-HOUR ESOPHAGEAL pH MONITORING

Extensive clinical experience has shown that 24-hour esophageal pH monitoring has the highest sensitivity and specificity for the detection of acid GERD. It is the most direct method of measuring increased esophageal exposure to gastric juice. It quantifies the actual time that the esophageal mucosa is exposed to acid gastric juice, measures the ability of the esophagus to clear refluxed acid, and correlates esophageal acid exposure to the patient's symptoms. It has been shown that a prolonged monitoring period is the most accurate means of detecting abnormal reflux because measurements are made over one complete circadian cycle.[1] The prolonged period allows for assessment of the effect of physiologic activity such as eating or sleeping on the reflux of gastric juice into the esophagus.

pH is a symbol for the logarithm of the reciprocal of the measure of hydrogen ion concentration and is mathematically described by the formula:

$$pH = -\log_{10}[H^+]$$

Because it is a logarithmic measurement, a solution with a pH of 1 contains 10 times the hydrogen ions of a solution with a pH of 2 and 1 million times (10^6) the activity of a solution with a pH of 7. A pH of 7 is considered neutral because at this pH the concentration of hydrogen ions equals the concentration of hydroxyl ions. The pH in the esophagus results from swallowed saliva and esophageal bicarbonate secretion and spans a range from 5 to 7. Because the esophagus normally has an intraluminal pH between 4 and 7 for 94% of the time, a pH of 4 has become the threshold that is used to detect increased esophageal acid exposure. Gastric acid secretion is responsible for a pH in the range of 1 to 2 and rarely more than 3, which is why a change in intraluminal esophageal pH to less than 4 quite reliably reflects reflux of gastric juice. The exception is patients taking antacids (especially proton pump inhibitors [PPIs]) or

Table 9–1	Sensitivity and Specificity of Tests for Gastroesophageal Reflux Disease		
Test		**Sensitivity (%)**	**Specificity (%)**
LES manometry (<10 mm Hg)		58	84
Esophagogastroduodenoscopy (>grade 1 esophagitis)		68	96
Mucosal biopsy		77	91
Gastroesophageal scintiscanning		61	95
Barium esophagography		40	85
Acid perfusion test (Bernstein)		79	82
Standard acid reflux test		84	83
Ambulatory 24-hour pH esophageal monitoring		96	96

LES, lower esophageal sphincter.

patients with achlorhydria. Exposure of the esophagus to higher concentrations of H^+ ions (i.e., lower pH) has also been correlated with the degree of mucosal injury.[2] Duodenal contents account for a pH environment of 6 to 8, which has given some investigators reason to interpret an esophageal pH greater than 7 as a reflection of reflux of duodenal contents into the esophagus.

HOW TO PERFORM A pH TEST

Instrumentation

pH Catheters/Probes Currently, two means of detecting pH in the esophagus are available. One is by means of a catheter-based electrode that is placed through the nose and situated 5 cm above the manometrically determined upper border of the lower esophageal sphincter (LES). This is the gold standard technique, and protocols regarding performance of the study are detailed later. Nasal and nasopharyngeal local anesthesia is recommended and is induced by asking the patient to sniff after 2% lidocaine jelly is squirted into the nose. Alternatively, cotton-tipped applicators with a topical anesthetic such as cocaine can be applied directly to the nasopharynx, but this is often uncomfortable for the patient.

A newer catheter-less technique is now also available. This technique is accomplished with a radiotelemetry device (Bravo probe) that is placed either at the time of endoscopy or via a transnasal catheter placement system and secured to the mucosa of the esophagus 6 cm above the visualized gastroesophageal junction. This technique is described briefly later.

Both systems rely on a pH detection probe located either at the end of the catheter or in the Bravo capsule. Different types of pH probes are available, with no single electrode being optimal (Fig. 9–1). Glass electrodes measure the electrical potential across a thin glass membrane set up by a concentration gradient of hydrogen ions; these electrodes have good reliability and sensitivity. The probes need to be soaked continuously in a saturated solution of KCl and have a relatively large diameter, which can potentially lead to more difficult insertion.[1,3] They are also comparatively expensive ($400 to $600). Antimony probes measure pH by virtue of a cor-

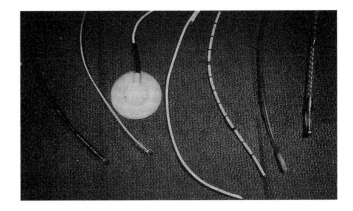

Figure 9–1. Types of pH probes.

rosion potential at the hydrogen ion and antimony surface. They are smaller, better tolerated, and cheaper than glass electrodes ($40 to $75). Values recorded by antimony probes are 2.1 ± 0.8 units higher in the alkaline range than those of glass electrodes and are therefore not useful for measuring alkaline GER.[4] Multiprobe catheters with proximal and distal electrodes are available and can be useful in evaluating patients with atypical symptoms and cervical esophageal acid exposure.[5]

Data-Recording Devices Solid-state data loggers are now lightweight, compact, and easily portable. They are usually worn on the patient's belt. The currently available data loggers record digital pH data every few seconds throughout the 24-hour period of study. These data loggers also have buttons (known as event markers) that allow the patient to record mealtimes, times of sleep, and any symptoms experienced during the study. The data recorded from the 24-hour study are uploaded to a personal computer at the end of the recording period for further analysis.

Software Analysis Various commercially available software programs are available to assist with the analysis. Once the data have been viewed in graphic format on the computer screen and the study periods of upright, supine, and meals have been validated, the software can provide an automated analysis of the entire 24-hour period of study and generate parameters of exposure as detailed later.

Protocols for Performing the Test

Catheter Systems Probes are always first calibrated in pH solutions with pH values of 1, 4, and 7 to ensure integrity of the probe. After calibration, the catheter is passed transnasally so that the tip of the electrode lies 5 cm above the upper border of the LES as measured previously with manometry. Studies have demonstrated that the LES moves cephalad a distance of up to 5 cm with swallowing.[6] Precise positioning is important because normal values for esophageal acid exposure vary with location of the probe. A probe too high will potentially miss reflux episodes and decrease sensitivity, whereas a probe positioned too low may drift into the stomach with swallowing and yield false-positive readings. Probes are recalibrated when the patient returns at the end of the 24-hour study period to rule out electrode failure or pH drift.

Preparation of the Patient Patients are instructed to not eat after midnight before a morning test. PPI use is stopped 2 weeks before the test, and H_2 receptor antagonists are discontinued 48 hours before the study.[7] Antacids may be used up until the night before. The probes are placed either transnasally (catheter based) or at the time of endoscopy (Bravo probe). Patients are allowed to go home and are encouraged to perform normal activities of daily living. Previous protocols have outlined dietary instructions that avoid acidic foods to limit false-positive results. Carbonated beverages have typically been forbidden because they have an acidic pH and may cause belching of gastric juice into the esophagus. Recently, however, the goal has been to minimize restrictions and encourage patients to record the foods that they have eaten along with their symptoms, which are analyzed together at the end of the study. In this way, the study period mimics their normal day (Box 9–1).

The Diary Patients are asked to keep an accurate diary during the 24 hours of the study or signal significant events by using the event marker buttons on the digital recording device. In particular, they are asked to document the start and end times of meals, the time when going to sleep and waking up, and the occurrence and nature of any symptoms experienced during the recording period. The latter has led to development of the symptom index, which is used by some investigators to correlate patient symptoms with esophageal pH changes. This index has been useful in patients with noncardiac chest pain and in those with other atypical symptoms such as cough or wheeze.[8]

Data Analysis At the end of the study, the data are downloaded from the data logger to a computer, which generates a pH tracing and data summary (Fig. 9–2). It is

---

Box 9–1 **Dietary Restrictions and Patient Instructions for 24-Hour Ambulatory Esophageal pH Testing**

pH Test Diet*

  Meat, fish, cheese, eggs
  Vegetables
  Noncitrus fruit
  Butter, margarine
  Bread, cereal
  Vanilla ice cream, candy
  Milk, water, coffee, tea

Avoid the Following

  Citrus fruits
  Grapefruit or other fruit juices
  Lemonade
  Alcohol
  Carbonated beverages
  Hard candy, lozenges, or chewing gum

*Smoking is allowed; however, note any/all cigarettes, cigars, pipe use, or chewing tobacco.

---

important to emphasize that 24-hour esophageal pH monitoring is not a test for reflux but rather a measurement of esophageal exposure to gastric juice. The measurement is expressed as the time that esophageal pH is below a given threshold during the 24-hour period. This single assessment, though concise, does not characterize the exposure. Consequently, two other assessments are necessary: the frequency of reflux episodes and their duration.

The units used to express esophageal exposure to gastric juice are (1) cumulative time that esophageal pH is below a chosen threshold (expressed as a percentage of the total, upright, and supine monitored time), (2) frequency of reflux episodes below a chosen threshold (expressed as the number of episodes per 24 hours), and (3) duration of the episodes (expressed as the number of episodes longer than 5 minutes per 24 hours and the time [in minutes] of the longest recorded episode).[9] Most centers use pH 4 as the threshold. With this threshold, it has been shown that there is a remarkable degree of uniformity of normal values for the six components throughout the world,[10] thus indicating that normal individuals have similar values for esophageal acid exposure despite nationality or dietary habits. Normal values obtained from 50 healthy volunteers are shown Table 9–2.[11]

To combine the result of the six components into one expression of overall esophageal acid exposure below a pH threshold, a pH score has been developed by

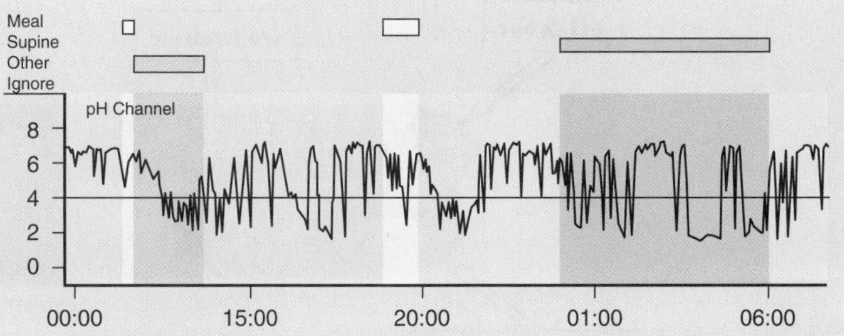

Figure 9–2. Display of a 24-hour esophageal pH monitoring study in a patient with increased esophageal acid exposure. DeMeester score (total): 92.5; DeMeester normal values: less than 14.72 (95th percentile).

Analysis results-pH channel
Acid period table

	Total	Uprigt	Supine	Meal	Postpr	Other
Duration of period	22:05	16:05	06:00	01:20	04:00	02:00
Number of refluxes	331	273	59	8	167	77
Number of long refluxes	6	1	5	0	0	0
Duration of longest reflux (min)	54	23	54	1	4	1
Time pH <4 (min)	228	105	124	2	46	17
Percent time pH <4 (%)	17.2	10.8	34.4	3.0	19.2	14.2
Minimum	0.5	0.5	1.3	2.3	1.7	2.1
Maximum	8.6	8.6	7.3	7.2	7.3	7.2
Mean	5.8	6.0	5.1	6.4	5.3	5.4
Median	6.6	6.7	6.4	6.6	5.4	5.7

Table 9–2 Normal Values of Six Components of the 24-Hour Record for 50 Healthy Volunteers

	Mean	95th Percentile
Total time pH <4 (%)	1.51	4.45
Upright time pH <4 (%)	2.34	8.42
Supine time pH <4 (%)	0.63	3.45
Number of episodes	19.00	46.9
Number of episodes ≥5 min	0.84	3.45
Longest episode	6.74	19.8

DeMeester et al. and is currently provided as an automatic option on most commercially available software products.[9] This score has been shown by receiver operating curves to be the most accurate means of assessing abnormal GER, although some centers still use the total time that the luminal esophagus has a pH below 4 as their predictor.[6,11] A composite score greater than 14.7 is considered pathologic.

The "Bravo" Probe

The Bravo (Medtronic, Shoreview, MN) pH system is a catheter-free esophageal pH monitoring system. It consists of an antimony pH electrode, a radio transmitter, and a battery contained in a capsule (Fig. 9–3). Capsule placement is accomplished with the aid of a delivery device and upper endoscopy or manometry. The delivery device is inserted through an anesthetized nostril and the probe positioned appropriately in the esophagus—5 cm above the manometrically determined proximal border of the LES. Alternatively, the probe can be positioned via the mouth, which is an easier procedure for the patient, but the accuracy of the method has not been defined. Those who are using the oral technique position the probe 6 cm above the endoscopically observed position of the squamocolumnar junction. A vacuum pump is attached to the port on the handle of the delivery device to draw a bleb of esophageal mucosa into the probe chamber. Once a steady vacuum has been achieved, the plunger on the handle of the delivery device is depressed to fire a locking pin through the bleb of mucosa, thus securing it to the esophagus. The vacuum is then released and the plunger rotated to detach the probe from the delivery device. The latter is subsequently removed from the patient. Proper capsule placement can be confirmed endoscopically while taking care to not dislodge the device. Esophageal pH is measured every 6 seconds, and two pH data points are transmitted every 12 seconds to the receiver unit over a 48-hour study period. The capsule is designed to dissolve in 3 to 7 days and pass through the gastrointestinal tract. There are reports of the probe remaining attached for longer periods, but without consequence.[12]

Studies using the Bravo catheter-free pH monitoring system are few; however, there are reports that claim the ability to obtain interpretable data 96% to 97% of the time.[12,13] The overall sensitivity and specificity in identifying patients with GERD vary with the length of the study period. Twenty-four-hour data yield a sensitivity and specificity of 67.5% and 89.7%. Using data from the worse of 2 days tested yields a sensitivity and specificity of 83.8% and 84.5%. Taking both days combined brings

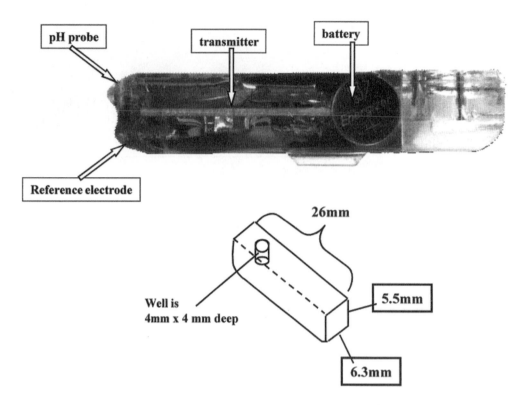

Figure 9–3.   Dimensions and electronics of the Bravo pH capsule. The capsule is oblong (6.3 × 5.5 × 26 mm). A well (diameter, 4 mm; depth, 4 mm) is located on the superior-lateral aspect of the probe. The well is connected to a custom-made vacuum unit capable of generating 600 mm Hg vacuum pressure to the well via the delivery system. An antimony pH electrode and reference electrode are located on the distal tip of the capsule, and an internal battery and transmitter are contained within the capsule.

those numbers to 64.9% and 94.8%.[12] The data highlight one advantage of the wireless system: patients may have less discomfort, which allows for a longer evaluation period and thus increases the sensitivity of the test. One disadvantage, however, is the price, which is approximately $225 versus $62 for a traditional pH probe.

24-HOUR AMBULATORY DETECTION OF ESOPHAGEAL BILIRUBIN EXPOSURE

Duodenogastroesophageal reflux (DGER) is defined as the pathologic regurgitation of duodenal contents into the stomach with subsequent reflux into the esophagus. Previous terms have been used to describe this process, including bile reflux and alkaline reflux. Neither is appropriate in that duodenal fluid consists of many substances besides bile and an esophageal pH higher than 7 does not necessarily coincide with reflux of duodenal contents.

DGER has been associated with complications of GERD, including stricture formation, complicated Barrett's esophagus, and adenocarcinoma. The mechanisms involved in the esophageal mucosal damage seen in DGER are not fully understood. Activated pancreatic enzymes can cause mucosal damage from direct exposure; however, bile acids are the predominant constituent

in DGER. Data from animal studies have shown that exposure of isolated esophageal mucosa to bile acids results in significant disruption of the mucosal barrier.[14,15] The extent of mucosal damage has been further linked to the conjugation state of the bile acids, as well as the pH of the refluxate. Conjugated bile acids and pepsin produce more injury at an acidic pH, whereas unconjugated bile acids and trypsin are more deleterious at a pH in the range of 5 to 8.[16] Twenty-four-hour gastric pH monitoring allows simultaneous evaluation of gastric acid secretion and an estimate of duodenogastric reflux and gastric emptying.

Bilitec Probe

Bechi et al. developed the apparatus known as the Bilitec probe (Medtronic), which indirectly measures bilirubin content in the stomach or esophagus, or in both.[17] In the absence of carotene and various lipids, the bilirubin concentration in a solution can be directly measured by spectrophotometry based on specific absorption at a wavelength of 453 nm. Surprisingly, reflux of alkaline components into the stomach is not completely neutralized by the gastric pH. Bile acids and lecithin are naturally present in the gastric environment, even at low pH values, and both taurine and glycine conjugated bile acids are present in the stomach at a pH of less than 2.

The apparatus used to measure the presence of bilirubin in the esophagus consists of a portable optoelectronic data logger weighing 1200 g that is strapped to the patient's side and a fiberoptic probe that is passed transnasally and positioned anywhere in the lumen of the foregut (Fig. 9–4). The spectrophotometric probes contain bonded optical fibers and are 3 mm in diameter and 140 cm in length. Two plugs connect 50% of the fibers to the light-emitting diodes and 50% to the receiving photodiode. The tip of the probe contains a 2-mm space for sampling. Fluids and blenderized solids can easily flow through the space and their bilirubin concentration measured. The probes are flexible, durable, easy to sterilize, and reusable.

The optoelectronic unit acts simultaneously as a light signal generator, a data processor, and a data storage device. The unit has two channels, thus allowing dual measurement with two probes if desired. The light source for each channel is provided by two light-emitting diodes that give off a 470-nm signal light (blue spectrum) and a 565-nm reference light (green spectrum). Optical signals reflected back from the probe are converted to electrical impulses by a photodiode. This electrical signal is then amplified and processed within the data logger (Minneapolis, Minnesota). Absorbance readings are averaged every two cycles. The system is capable of recording 225 individual absorbance values per hour and allows up to 30 hours of continuous monitoring. An in vivo validation study of the Bilitec fiberoptic system has shown that intraesophageal bilirubin absorbance correlates well with the presence of total bile acids and bilirubin.[18]

Performing the Test

For esophageal monitoring, the Bilitec probe is passed through an anesthetized nostril and positioned 5 cm above the upper border of the LES as previously determined by esophageal manometry. For intragastric monitoring, the probe is positioned 5 cm below the lower border of the LES. The test depends on patient avoidance of eating anything green or yellow or anything that may have green or yellow substances in it. As a result, patients are given a list of foods allowed during the study (Box 9–2). The probe is connected to a data logger and the patient allowed to go home and resume normal activities of daily living. As with pH monitoring, the patient returns at the end of the study period and data from the logger are uploaded to a computer and analyzed with commercially available software (Fig. 9–5).

Normal values for esophageal exposure to bilirubin from 35 healthy volunteers have shown a median percent time with absorbance greater than 0.2 of 0% and a 95th percentile of 1.7%. Consequently, abnormal esophageal exposure to bilirubin as measured by Bilitec monitoring is defined by absorbance above 0.2 greater than 1.7% of the total time of the study. In a study by Cuemo et al., the total bilirubin absorbance above 0.14 was 7.8 ± 2.2 (percentage of total study time) in patients without esophagitis, 11.7 ± 4.4 in patients with grade 1 to 2 esophagitis, and 17 ± 4.2 in those with grade 3 to 4

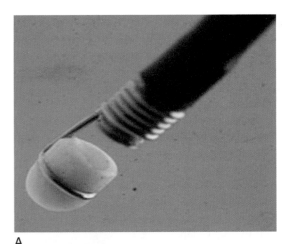

A

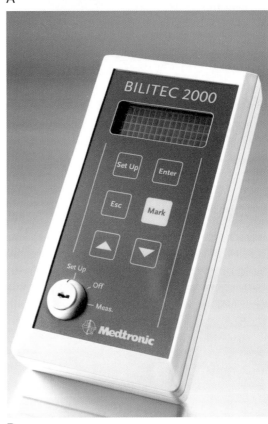

B

Figure 9–4.   Bilitec probe **(A)** and electronic data logger **(B)** for 24-hour esophageal bilirubin monitoring.

esophagitis.[19] Thus, esophageal bilirubin exposure correlates with the degree of esophageal mucosa damage.

CLINICAL USE OF AMBULATORY ESOPHAGEAL pH AND BILIRUBIN MONITORING

In the clinical setting, there are three main circumstances in which pH and bilirubin monitoring are useful in the day-to-day management of patients.

Box 9–2 **Dietary Restrictions and Patient Instructions for 24-Hour Ambulatory Bilirubin Monitoring**

Bilitec Test Diet

Bananas, apples

Saltine crackers

Cottage cheese

Chicken breast—skinless

Rice, pasta

Bread

Vanilla ice cream

Low-fat milk

Water

Avoid the Following

Carbonated beverages

Coffee

Tea

Alcohol

Butter, Margarine

Candy

Anything green or yellow or that might have green or yellow substances in it

Diagnosis of "Typical" Gastroesophageal Reflux Disease

GERD is such a common disorder that the acronym in now a household term. Who needs to be studied with 24-hour pH monitoring? It is obviously not feasible, nor necessary, to perform 24-hour pH testing on all patients with suspected reflux disease. The *American Journal of Gastroenterology* recently published guidelines regarding the diagnosis and evaluation of patients with suspected GERD.[20] Although it is recognized that symptoms may be a poor guide to the underlying disease, it is considered cost-effective in patients with "typical" symptoms (heartburn and acid regurgitation) to attempt a trial of PPIs. This acts as both a diagnostic and therapeutic approach, with further work-up being indicated in patients who do not appropriately respond.[21] Of course, this approach should not obviate education in terms of lifestyle changes that may help alleviate the degree of reflux, such as smoking cessation, moderation in alcohol consumption, and weight loss for those who are obese. The knee-jerk approach to prescribing PPIs for all patients with reflux symptoms will unfortunately subject many patients to unnecessary medication or miss patients with complicated reflux disease such as Barrett's esophagus or dysplasia. Physicians should be alerted to symptoms of dysphagia, odynophagia, anemia, or weight loss because they may be indicators of stricture, ulceration, Barrett's esophagus, or malignancy.

In patients with typical reflux symptoms (heartburn, regurgitation) *and* endoscopic findings of esophagitis (mucosal erosions), pH monitoring is probably unnecessary because this combination is about 97% specific for GERD, with infective esophagitis and pill-induced injury being nonreflux causes of mucosal damage.[22] Most patients, however, will have GERD without endoscopic evidence of mucosal injury (so-called endoscopically

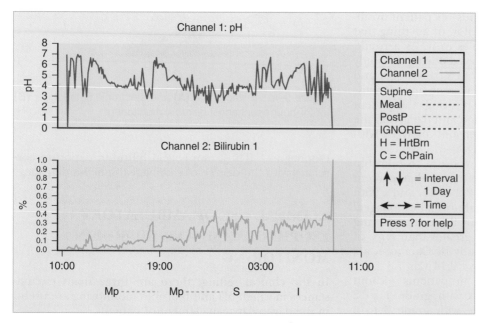

Figure 9–5. Display of a 24-hour esophageal pH and bilirubin monitoring system.

negative GERD), and to correctly document GERD as a source of the patients' symptoms, pH testing *is* necessary. Such an approach has also been shown to be cost-effective.[23] Certainly in endoscopically negative GERD, pH monitoring is considered essential before performing an antireflux operation so that a Nissen fundoplication is not performed on a patient without excessive esophageal exposure to gastric juice and an incompetent valve. It has been shown that the best surgical outcomes are achieved in patients with typical symptoms, abnormal pH scores, and a good response to acid-suppression therapy.[24] On the other hand, it is well documented that patients with achalasia may have symptoms suggestive of reflux disease, and performing an antireflux procedure in this situation has obvious consequences.

Some authors have also documented the value of increased exposure of the stomach and esophagus to bilirubin and have attempted to correlate such exposure with patient symptoms. There appears to be some valuable information regarding gastric symptoms; however, correlation with esophageal symptoms has been more difficult. Certainly, the most severe reflux patients have increased esophageal exposure to both acid and bile, as is the case in patients with Barrett's esophagus. Detection of increased bilirubin in the esophagus is a marker of more severe disease and possibly a marker of increased risk for complications of reflux, such as stricture, Barrett's esophagus, dysplasia, or adenocarcinoma.[25,26] Freedman et al. have noted that increased bilirubin exposure is also associated with less effective esophageal motility in patients with GERD.[27] Although useful in terms of understanding the pathophysiology of many of these diseases, bilirubin monitoring is not routinely carried out in the community during a work-up for GERD or esophageal symptoms, and usually these probes are found only in academic centers.

Diagnosis and Evaluation of Atypical Symptoms of Gastroesophageal Reflux Disease

GERD has been associated with so-called atypical symptoms such as cough, asthma, hoarseness, dental caries, chest pain, dysphagia, and globus sensation. It is recommended that pH testing be available in the diagnostic armamentarium of the physician diagnosing these disorders.

Asthma and Cough Alexander and colleagues noted that asthmatic patients have an increased prevalence of GERD symptoms and increased esophageal exposure to acid.[28] Schnatz and Castell also noted a high proportion (78%) of positive pH tests in patients with chronic cough or asthma.[29] Increased esophageal exposure to gastric juice in these patients is probably both cause and effect. Severe coughing plus wheezing increases intra-abdominal pressure and drives gastric juice into the negative-pressure environment of the chest, and esophageal acidification has been shown to result in a reflex bronchospastic response (Fig. 9–6). Furthermore, as noted later, chronic aspiration contributes to con-

tinued cough as well as progressive parenchymal fibrosis. Evidence of pharyngeal reflux on pH testing has been shown to assist in the identification of patients with respiratory symptoms who will benefit from an antireflux operation.[30]

Hoarseness and Dental Caries Reflux of gastric juice up to the laryngeal aditus or into the mouth has been associated with laryngeal symptoms and dental caries. In the work-up of patients suspected of having "high" reflux, catheters containing two or more probes have been used to assess reflux into the more proximal esophagus or even the pharynx.[31,32] Furthermore, the addition of impedance catheter monitoring has shown that reflux into the pharynx is more frequent than previously thought, even with pH monitoring. Kawamura et al. have shown that gaseous reflux with weak acidity is more common in patients with reflux-related laryngeal lesions.[33]

Noncardiac Chest Pain The esophagus has frequently been implicated as the cause of noncardiac chest pain. Twenty-four-hour pH monitoring has enabled us to understand this phenomenon, especially when combined with 24-hour ambulatory manometry. Chest pain that coincides with esophageal acidification during the study is evidence that the two may be related. Ambulatory manometry has shown that occasionally, esophageal acid exposure is associated with marked motor disturbances of the esophagus, although it has been difficult to show an association with pain exactly at the time of these abnormalities.[8,34] However, pH testing has been found to be predictive of a therapeutic response to omeprazole in severe refluxers with noncardiac chest pain.[35]

End-Stage Lung Disease and Lung Transplantation The role of GERD in patients with end-stage lung disease and in patients after lung transplantation has been underestimated in the past. A high proportion of patients with end-stage lung disease will have pathologic GERD, and it has been suggested that "silent" aspiration contributes to pulmonary injury in many of these patients. Similarly, the chronic cough associated with many end-stage lung diseases is thought to promote reflux because of the increased intra-abdominal pressure and trans-sphincteric gradient associated with coughing. One group found 35% of patients before lung transplantation to have GERD.[36] Recently, GERD has also been implicated as a significant adverse contributor to the development of bronchiolitis obliterans syndrome after lung transplantation.[37,38] Davis and colleagues have shown that 73% of patients after lung transplantation had GERD by pH monitoring.[37] This may in part be due to the significant number of patients with unrecognized GERD before transplantation, to vagal damage at the time of surgery, or to reflux-promoting side effects of the postoperative immunosuppressive medications. Nonetheless, this group has shown that fundoplication in lung transplant recipients with GERD is associated with significant improvement in lung function, particularly if performed before the late stages of bronchiolitis obliterans syn-

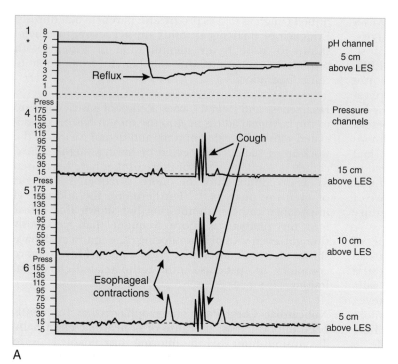

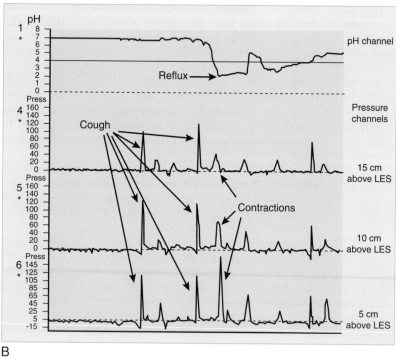

Figure 9–6. Cause-and-effect relationship between cough and esophageal acid exposure. **A,** Coughing precipitated by a reflux episode may be the result of occult aspiration of refluxed gastric juice or a reflex brought on by esophageal acidification. **B,** Conversely, increased intra-abdominal pressure as occurs with coughing may overcome antireflux mechanisms and result in a gastroesophageal reflux episode.

drome.[37] Furthermore, they have noted that many patients with progressive deterioration in lung function referred for transplantation have had stabilization of their pulmonary disease after fundoplication, again emphasizing the effect that GERD and silent aspiration have on pulmonary function. It is now believed essential to have a good understanding of a patient's reflux history before consideration of lung transplantation, and in our center all patients being considered will be evaluated for GERD by manometry, videoesophago-graphy, and 24-hour pH testing. Those with severe reflux and nonprohibitive risk for surgery will undergo fundo-plication before transplantation. Consideration is given to early post-transplant antireflux surgery in those who cannot undergo surgery before transplantation or in those in whom GERD develops after transplantation. pH monitoring has helped us understand the significance of GERD in this complex group of patients and continues to provide important information to direct therapy.

Evaluation of Patients Receiving Medical Therapy or After Surgery

As noted earlier, it is strongly recommended that pH testing, endoscopy, manometry, and videoesophagography be performed before contemplating antireflux surgery.[39] pH testing is also of value in evaluating patients after antireflux surgery and after initiation of medical therapy. Leite and colleagues noted that a significant number of patients are resistant to standard doses of omeprazole when studied with pH monitoring.[40] Katzka and associates studied patients while receiving PPI therapy with 24-hour pH testing. They showed that tolerance to standard PPI doses develops in a significant number of patients and they require ever-increasing doses of medication to control the acid secreted by the stomach and subsequent acid GER.[41] To evaluate the effect of the dose of PPIs in patients with recurrent or persistent symptoms, it is necessary to quantitate the esophageal acid exposure with 24-hour pH monitoring. Similarly, the 24-hour test is useful in evaluating patients with recurrent symptoms after laparoscopic fundoplication inasmuch as it has been shown that only about half these patients will have increased esophageal acid exposure.[42] Attributing the symptoms to failure of surgery without studying the patient via 24-hour pH testing may condemn a patient to an unnecessary redo operation.

pH monitoring has also been used to assess proximal esophageal acid exposure after esophagectomy and has shown that the acid secretory status of the stomach returns with time and that reflux of gastric juice into the proximal remaining esophagus does occur. Johansson and colleagues used this technique to compare the exposure of the cervical esophagus to acid after either transhiatal or Ivor-Lewis–type esophagectomy and have found that a cervical anastomosis is associated with higher acid exposure.[43]

INTEGRATED AMBULATORY FOREGUT MONITORING

The availability of portable digital recorders with large storage capacity now allows outpatient 24-hour monitoring of pharyngeal and esophageal motility simultaneously with esophageal and gastric pH.[44,45] Integrated evaluation of foregut motor and secretory function over an entire circadian cycle has thus become possible and has been found to be useful in many patients. In one study, integrated foregut monitoring established one or more functional or secretory abnormalities as the underlying cause of symptoms in 84% of the patients studied.[45] Prolonged ambulatory monitoring is the most physiologic way to assess foregut function and has the potential to replace the series of individual laboratory tests that have been necessary to thoroughly evaluate patients with complex foregut disorders. Ambulatory integrated foregut monitoring and computerized evaluation of the recorded data put into the physician's hand the ability to evaluate foregut motor and secretory abnormalities within the office. This will enable easier and more scientific evaluation of patients with symptoms possibly attributable to esophageal or gastric dysfunction.

SUGGESTED READINGS

Bremner RM, Bremner CG, DeMeester TR: Gastroesophageal reflux: The use of pH monitoring. Curr Probl Surg 32:429-558, 1995.

Bremner CG, DeMeester TR, Mason RJ, Bremner RM: Esophageal Motility Testing Made Easy. St Louis, Quality Medical, 2001.

Davis RD Jr, Lau CL, Eubanks S, et al: Improved lung allograft function after fundoplication in patients with gastroesophageal reflux disease undergoing lung transplantation. J Thorac Cardiovasc Surg 125:533-542, 2003.

DeMeester TR, Wang CI, Wernly JA, et al: Technique, indications, and clinical use of 24 hour esophageal pH monitoring. J Thorac Cardiovasc Surg 79:656-670, 1980.

Devault KR, Castell DO, American College of Gastroenterology: Updated guidelines for the diagnosis and treatment of gastroesophageal reflux disease. Am J Gastroenterol 100:190-200, 2005.

Johnson LF, DeMeester TR: Development of the 24-hour intraesophageal pH monitoring composite scoring system. J Clin Gastroenterol 8(Suppl 1):52-58, 1986.

Richter JE: Importance of bile reflux in Barrett's esophagus. Dig Dis 18:208-216, 2000.

Schnatz PF, Castell JA, Castell DO: Pulmonary symptoms associated with gastroesophageal reflux: Use of ambulatory pH monitoring to diagnose and to direct therapy. Am J Gastroenterol 91:1715-1718, 1996.

REFERENCES

1. Branicki FJ, Evans DF, Ogilvie AL, et al: Ambulatory monitoring of oesophageal pH in reflux oesophagitis using a portable radiotelemetry system. Gut 23:992-998, 1982.
2. Bremner RM, Crookes PF, DeMeester TR, et al: Concentration of refluxed acid and esophageal mucosal injury. Am J Surg 164:522-526, discussion 526-527, 1992.
3. de Caestecker JS, Heading RC: Esophageal pH monitoring. Gastroenterol Clin North Am 19:645-669, 1990.
4. Sjoberg F, Gustafsson U, Tibbling L: Alkaline oesophageal reflux—an artefact due to oxygen corrosion of antimony pH electrodes. Scand J Gastroenterol 27:1084-1088, 1992.
5. Jacob P, Kahrilas PJ, Herzon G: Proximal esophageal pH-metry in patients with 'reflux laryngitis.' Gastroenterology 100:305-310, 1991.
6. Jamieson JR, Stein HJ, DeMeester TR, et al: Ambulatory 24-h esophageal pH monitoring: Normal values, optimal thresholds, specificity, sensitivity, and reproducibility. Am J Gastroenterol 87:1102-1111, 1992.
7. Marks IM, Young GO, Winter T: Duration of acid inhibition after withdrawal of omeprazole in DU patients in remission. S Afr Med J 82:42A, 1992.
8. Dekel R, Martinez-Hawthorne SD, Guillen RJ, Fass R: Evaluation of symptom index in identifying gastroesophageal reflux disease–related noncardiac chest pain. J Clin Gastroenterol 38:24-29, 2004.
9. DeMeester TR, Wang CI, Wernly JA, et al: Technique, indications, and clinical use of 24 hour esophageal pH monitoring. J Thorac Cardiovasc Surg 79:656-670, 1980.

10. Emde C, Garner A, Blum AL: Technical aspects of intraluminal pH-metry in man: Current status and recommendations. Gut 28:1177-1188, 1987.

11. Johnson LF, DeMeester TR: Development of the 24-hour intra-esophageal pH monitoring composite scoring system. J Clin Gastroenterol 8(Suppl 1):52-58, 1986.

12. Pandolfino JE, Richter JE, Ours T, et al: Ambulatory esophageal pH monitoring using a wireless system. Am J Gastroenterol 98:740-749, 2003.

13. Ward EM, Devault KR, Bouras EP, et al: Successful oesophageal pH monitoring with a catheter-free system. Aliment Pharmacol Ther 19:449-454, 2004.

14. Johnson LF, Harmon JW: Experimental esophagitis in a rabbit model. Clinical relevance. J Clin Gastroenterol 8(Suppl 1):26-44, 1986.

15. Lillemoe KD, Johnson LF, Harmon JW: Alkaline esophagitis: A comparison of the ability of components of gastroduodenal contents to injure the rabbit esophagus. Gastroenterology 85:621-628, 1983.

16. Richter JE: Importance of bile reflux in Barrett's esophagus. Dig Dis 18:208-216, 2000.

17. Bechi P, Pucciani F, Baldini F, et al: Long-term ambulatory entero-gastric reflux monitoring. Validation of a new fiberoptic technique. Dig Dis Sci 38:1297-1306, 1993.

18. Barrett MW, Myers JC, Watson DI, et al: Detection of bile reflux: In vivo validation of the Bilitec fibreoptic system. Dis Esophagus 13:44-50, 2000.

19. Cuomo R, Koek G, Sifrim D, et al: Analysis of ambulatory duodeno-gastroesophageal reflux monitoring. Dig Dis Sci 45:2463-2469, 2000.

20. Devault KR, Castell DO, American College of Gastroenterology: Updated guidelines for the diagnosis and treatment of gastro-esophageal reflux disease. Am J Gastroenterol 100:190-200, 2005.

21. Juul-Hansen P, Rydning A: Endoscopy-negative reflux disease: What is the value of a proton-pump inhibitor test in everyday clinical practice? Scand J Gastroenterol 38:1200-1203, 2003.

22. Tefera L, Fein M, Ritter MP, et al: Can the combination of symptoms and endoscopy confirm the presence of gastroesophageal reflux disease? Am Surg 63:933-936, 1997.

23. Netzer P, Gut A, Heer R, et al: Five-year audit of ambulatory 24-hour esophageal pH-manometry in clinical practice. Scand J Gastroenterol 34:676-682, 1999.

24. Patti MG, Fisichella PM, Perretta S: Preoperative evaluation of patients with gastroesophageal reflux disease. J Laparoendosc Adv Surg Tech A 11:327-331, 2001.

25. Kauer WK, Peters JH, DeMeester TR, et al: Mixed reflux of gastric and duodenal juices is more harmful to the esophagus than gastric juice alone. The need for surgical therapy re-emphasized. Ann Surg 222:525-531, 1995.

26. Kauer WK, Burdiles P, Ireland AP, et al: Does duodenal juice reflux into the esophagus of patients with complicated GERD? Evaluation of a fiberoptic sensor for bilirubin. Am J Surg 169:98-103, 1995.

27. Freedman J, Lindqvist M, Hellstrom PM, et al: Presence of bile in the oesophagus is associated with less effective oesophageal motility. Digestion 66:42-48, 2002.

28. Alexander JA, Hunt LW, Patel AM: Prevalence, pathophysiology, and treatment of patients with asthma and gastroesophageal reflux disease. Mayo Clin Proc 75:1055-1063, 2000.

29. Schnatz PF, Castell JA, Castell DO: Pulmonary symptoms associated with gastroesophageal reflux: Use of ambulatory pH monitoring to diagnose and to direct therapy. Am J Gastroenterol 91:1715-1718, 1996.

30. Oelschlager BK, Eubanks TR, Oleynikov D, et al: Symptomatic and physiologic outcomes after operative treatment for extra-esophageal reflux. Surg Endosc 16:1032-1036, 2002.

31. Hanson DG, Conley D, Jiang J, et al: Role of esophageal pH recording in management of chronic laryngitis: An overview. Ann Otol Rhinol Laryngol Suppl 184:4-9, 2000.

32. Harrell S, Evans B, Goudy S, et al: Design and implementation of an ambulatory pH monitoring protocol in patients with suspected laryngopharyngeal reflux. Laryngoscope 115:89-92, 2005.

33. Kawamura O, Aslam M, Rittmann T, et al: Physical and pH properties of gastroesophagopharyngeal refluxate: A 24-hour simultaneous ambulatory impedance and pH monitoring study. Am J Gastroenterol 99:1000-1010, 2004.

34. Bremner CG, DeMeester TR, Mason RJ, Bremner RM: Esophageal Motility Testing Made Easy. St Louis, Quality Medical, 2001.

35. Fass R, Fennerty MB, Johnson C, et al: Correlation of ambulatory 24-hour esophageal pH monitoring results with symptom improvement in patients with noncardiac chest pain due to gastroesophageal reflux disease. J Clin Gastroenterol 28:36-39, 1999.

36. Young LR, Hadjiliadis D, Davis RD, et al: Lung transplantation exacerbates gastroesophageal reflux disease. Chest 124:1689-1693, 2003.

37. Davis RD Jr, Lau CL, Eubanks S, et al: Improved lung allograft function after fundoplication in patients with gastroesophageal reflux disease undergoing lung transplantation. J Thorac Cardiovasc Surg 125:533-542, 2003.

38. Verleden GM, Dupont LJ, Van Raemdonck DE: Is it bronchiolitis obliterans syndrome or is it chronic rejection: A reappraisal? Eur Respir J 25:221-224, 2005.

39. Patti MG, Diener U, Tamburini A, et al: Role of esophageal function tests in diagnosis of gastroesophageal reflux disease. Dig Dis Sci 46:597-602, 2001.

40. Leite LP, Johnston BT, Just RJ, et al: Persistent acid secretion during omeprazole therapy: A study of gastric acid profiles in patients demonstrating failure of omeprazole therapy. Am J Gastroenterol 91:1527-1531, 1996.

41. Katzka DA, Paoletti V, Leite L, et al: Prolonged ambulatory pH monitoring in patients with persistent gastroesophageal reflux disease symptoms: Testing while on therapy identifies the need for more aggressive anti-reflux therapy. Am J Gastroenterol 91:2110-2113, 1996.

42. Eubanks TR, Omelanczuk P, Richards C, et al: Outcomes of laparoscopic antireflux procedures. Am J Surg 179:391-395, 2000.

43. Johansson J, Johnsson F, Groshen S, et al: Pharyngeal reflux after gastric pull-up esophagectomy with neck and chest anastomoses. J Thorac Cardiovasc Surg 118:1078-1083, 1999.

44. Bremner RM, Hoeft SF, Constantini M, et al: Pharyngeal swallowing. The major factor in clearance of esophageal reflux episodes. Ann Surg 218:364-369, discussion 369-370, 1993.

45. Stein HJ, DeMeester TR: Integrated ambulatory foregut monitoring in patients with functional foregut disorders. Surg Annu 24:161-180, 1992.

Chapter

10

Multichannel Intraluminal Impedance

Radu Tutuian • Donald O. Castell

Multichannel intraluminal impedance (MII) is a relatively new technique for evaluating esophageal bolus transit during swallowing without the use of radiation and for monitoring gastroesophageal reflux (GER) independent of its pH. First described by Silny[1] in 1991, this technique has evolved over the years and is currently available for routine clinical use. The principles of MII are relatively simple, but important in understanding the advantages that MII has when combined with esophageal manometry (MII-EM) or pH (MII-pH).

PRINCIPLES OF MULTICHANNEL INTRALUMINAL IMPEDANCE

The principle for detecting the presence and movement of an intraesophageal bolus by MII is based on measuring differences in electrical conductivity determined by the presence of various materials within the esophagus. The basic components of the impedance circuit are two metal rings connected to an alternating current source. An isolator (i.e., body of the catheter) separates the rings so that the electrical circuit is closed by the electrical charges (i.e., ions) surrounding the catheter. Simply stated, impedance is a measure of electrical resistance in an alternating current circuit. While suspended in air, the impedance is very high. Once placed in the esophagus, the ions of the esophageal mucosa close the circuit and the system measures a relatively stable resistance of approximately 2000 to 3000 ohms. When a liquid bolus is present in the esophagus, the increased number of ions allows for better conductivity, thus decreasing the electrical impedance (Fig. 10–1). Based on differences in the electrical conductivity of air, esophageal mucosa, and liquids, intraluminal impedance can detect the entry and exit of boluses within the esophagus (Fig. 10–2).

The changes recorded by MII during bolus passage have been validated by simultaneous videofluoroscopy and impedance testing (Fig. 10–3).[2] Most recently,

Simren et al.[3] reported a strong correlation between fluoroscopy and impedance when measuring esophageal filling ($r^2 = .89$; $P < .0001$) and esophageal emptying ($r^2 = .79$; $P < .0001$) in a group of healthy volunteers. Imam et al.[4] have also reported on the correlation between MII and barium swallows in 13 healthy volunteers and indicated that barium and impedance bolus transit or stasis correlated in 97% (72/74) of swallows.

Mounting multiple impedance-measuring segments on a catheter allows determination of the direction of bolus movement based on the timing of changes in impedance at individual levels. A decline in impedance progressing proximally to distally indicates aboral (antegrade) bolus movement as seen during swallowing, whereas a rapid decline in impedance progressing distally to proximally is indicative of oral (retrograde) bolus movement as seen during reflux episodes (Fig. 10–4).

The ability of MII to assess bolus transit without the use of radiation offers a great opportunity to evaluate the functional implications of pressure measurements when combined with manometry (i.e., MII-EM). When combined with pH, MII expands the ability of reflux testing to evaluate the presence of refluxate independent of its pH, thereby allowing the detection of acid and non-acid GER.

COMBINED MULTICHANNEL INTRALUMINAL IMPEDANCE AND MANOMETRY

Combined MII-EM was approved by the U.S. Food and Drug administration as a diagnostic test for esophageal function in July 2002. Adding MII capability to the manometry catheter does not change the dimensions of the catheter. Therefore, from a patient perspective, combined MII-EM testing is no different from conventional esophageal manometry. Although impedance-measuring

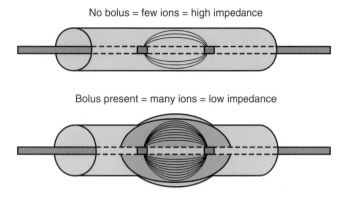

No bolus = few ions = high impedance

Bolus present = many ions = low impedance

Figure 10–1. Changes in intraluminal impedance are determined by an increased number of ions during the presence of a bolus.

segments can be added anywhere on the catheter, currently available designs place impedance rings around the pressure transducers so that pressure and bolus presence can be measured at the same level (Fig. 10–5).

Studies in our laboratory using normal volunteers have confirmed the ability of MII to characterize the transit of liquid, semisolid, and solid boluses through the esophagus.[5] In this study we found that liquid boluses of 1 to 10 ml produced the same changes in intraluminal impedance, thus indicating the high degree of sensitivity in identifying the presence of a bolus but the limited ability to estimate the volume of an intraesophageal bolus.

Normal values for this technique have been established by a multicenter study involving 43 healthy volunteers.[6] When MII changes during 10 saline and 10 viscous swallows were studied, it was found that more than 90% of these healthy volunteers cleared at least 80% of liquid swallows and at least 70% of viscous swallows, thus allowing us to establish normal values for esophageal bolus transit.

After studying 350 consecutive patients with various manometric abnormalities via combined MII-EM, we subsequently evaluated the ability of MII to characterize bolus transit abnormalities in different groups of patients.[7] All patients with achalasia and scleroderma of the esophagus were found to have abnormal liquid bolus transit (i.e., incomplete bolus transit for at least 30% of liquid swallows) and viscous bolus transit (i.e., incomplete bolus transit for at least 40% of viscous swallows). Normal liquid bolus transit was identified in at least 95% of patients with normal manometry, nutcracker esophagus, and isolated lower esophageal sphincter (LES) abnormalities (i.e., poorly relaxing LES, hypertensive and hypotensive LES). Approximately half the patients with ineffective esophageal motility (IEM) and distal esophageal spasm had normal liquid bolus transit (Fig. 10–6).

A more detailed study in 70 patients with IEM identified that there is no perfect (i.e., highly sensitive and highly specific) manometric cutoff that would predict complete bolus transit and that the current manometric criterion for diagnosing IEM (i.e., 30% or more manometrically verified ineffective swallows) is too sensitive and lacks the specificity for identifying patients with abnormal bolus transit. Normal bolus transit in the group of patients with IEM appeared to be dependent on distal esophageal amplitude (i.e., average amplitude at two distal esophageal sites 5 and 10 cm above the LES), the number of sites with low contraction amplitude, and the overall number of manometrically determined ineffective swallows (Fig. 10–7). Another important finding of this study (Fig. 10–8) was that approximately a third of patients with IEM had normal transit of liquid and viscous boluses (suggesting a mild functional defect), approximately a third had abnormal transit of either liquid or viscous boluses (i.e., moderate functional defect), and the remaining third of IEM patients had abnormal transit of both liquid and viscous boluses (i.e., severe functional defect).[8] Outcomes studies are warranted to evaluate whether grading of esophageal function defects in patients with manometrically verified IEM has the potential to identify patients at risk for postoperative dysphagia (i.e., those with a severe functional defect).

Combined MII-EM provides better information about bolus transit in patients with dysphagia after fundoplication.[9] Combined impedance-manometry and

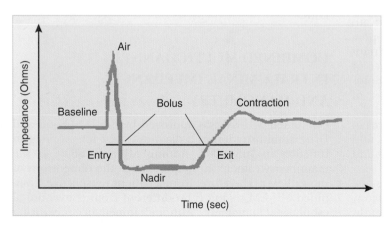

Figure 10–2. Impedance changes observed during bolus transit over a single pair of measurement rings separated by 2 cm. A rapid rise in resistance is noted when air traveling in front of the bolus head reaches the impedance-measuring segment, followed by a drop in impedance once the more conductive bolus material passes the measuring site. Bolus entry is considered to occur at the 50% drop in impedance from baseline relative to the nadir and bolus exit at the 50% recovery point from the nadir to the baseline. Lumen narrowing produced by the contraction transiently increases the impedance above baseline.

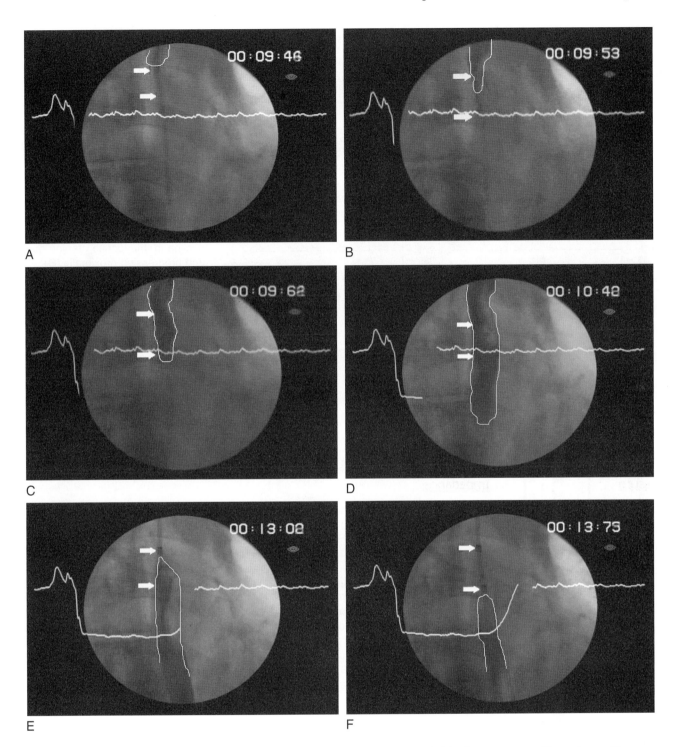

Figure 10–3.   Validation of impedance changes during bolus transit by combined videofluoroscopy and impedance. The *arrows* indicate the position of the impedance-measuring segment. The contour of the bolus is highlighted by drawing a margin in *white*. Before the bolus arrives in the impedance-measuring segment, the impedance has a relatively stable baseline value **(A)**. A bolus entering the segment will produce a rapid drop in impedance **(B)**, with a relatively stable nadir value reached once the liquid component of the bolus covers both segments **(C)**. The impedance will stay at these low values as long as the bolus is present between the rings **(D)**. Impedance starts rising once the tail of the bolus passes the proximal ring **(E)** and recovers to baseline once the tail of the bolus passes the second ring **(F)**. (Courtesy of Dr. J.H. Peters, University of Rochester, Rochester, NY.)

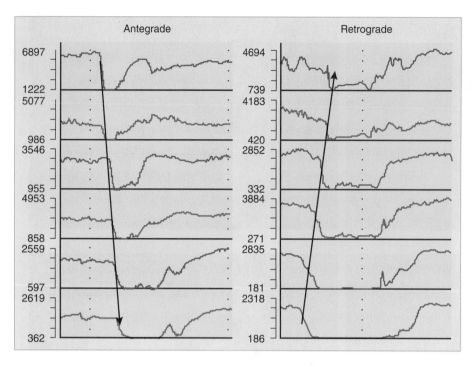

Figure 10–4. Bolus movement detected by multichannel intraluminal impedance. Swallowing is detected as antegrade bolus movement producing a decline in impedance starting proximally and progressing distally **(A)**, whereas reflux is detected as retrograde bolus movement producing a decline in impedance starting distally and progressing proximally **(B)**.

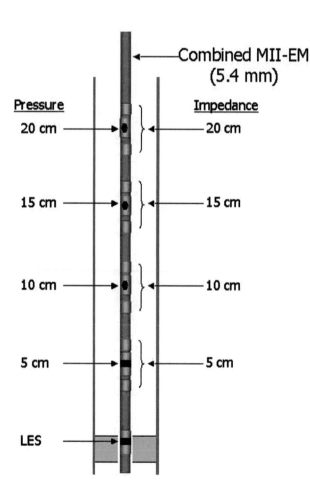

Figure 10–5. Nine-channel esophageal function catheter. Circumferential solid-state pressure sensors are located in the lower esophageal sphincter (LES) high-pressure zone (P5) and 5 cm above it (P4); unidirectional solid-state pressure sensors are located 10 cm (P3), 15 cm (P2), and 20 cm (P1) above the LES. Impedance-measuring segments are centered at 5 cm (Z4), 10 cm (Z3), 15 cm (Z2), and 20 cm (Z1) above the LES. MII-EM, multichannel intraluminal impedance with esophageal manometry.

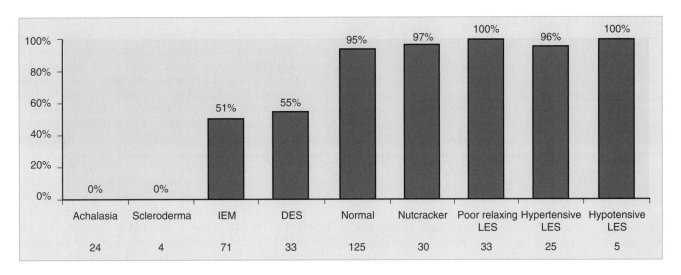

Figure 10–6. Percentage of 350 patients with normal liquid bolus transit based on manometric diagnoses. DES, distal esophageal spasm; IEM, ineffective esophageal motility; LES, lower esophageal sphincter.

Figure 10–7. Number of patients with normal/abnormal bolus transit depending on the number of manometrically verified ineffective swallows. A greater proportion of patients with less than five low-amplitude contractions had normal bolus transit as compared with those who had five or more low-amplitude contractions ($P < .05$).

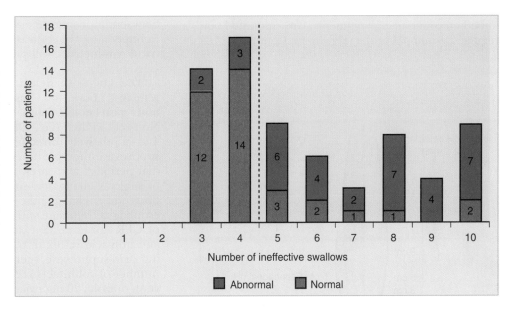

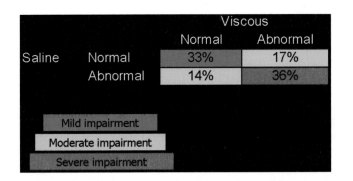

Figure 10–8. Degree of functional defect in patients with ineffective esophageal motility. Mild impairment, normal transit of both liquid and viscous boluses; moderate impairment, abnormal transit of liquid or viscous boluses; severe impairment, abnormal transit of both liquid and viscous boluses.

videofluoroscopy studies in patients with postfundoplication dysphagia indicate the ability of MII-EM to identify intraesophageal bolus pooling proximal to the fundoplication and retrograde escape of the bolus into the proximal esophagus after the completion of an otherwise normal peristaltic contraction. These studies underscore the potential of combined MII-EM to evaluate patients with esophageal symptoms after fundoplication.

Prospective studies evaluating the role of combined MII-EM in assisting in the selection of patients for antireflux surgery and in evaluating postoperative dysphagia are under way. The studies discussed earlier suggest that combined MII-EM, through its capability of assessing bolus transit during esophageal manometry without the use of radiation, has great potential to expand and refine the clinical diagnostic abilities of a modern esophageal testing laboratory.

COMBINED MULTICHANNEL INTRALUMINAL IMPEDANCE AND pH

For many years, the majority of clinicians and investigators considered esophageal pH monitoring the "gold standard" in diagnosing GERD, especially in the absence of endoscopically identified esophageal erosions. Esophageal pH monitoring quantifies the amount of distal esophageal acid exposure as the percentage of time when an intraesophageal pH less than 4 is recorded. This approach is very limited in detecting GER when the intraluminal pH does not go below 4.0. GER with a pH above 4.0 is difficult to detect by conventional pH monitoring, and different approaches (e.g., bilirubin monitoring, scintigraphy, manometry) have been proposed to overcome this limitation. Because impedance can detect the presence of refluxate in the esophagus independent of pH, bilirubin, and other factors and can be mounted on a regular pH catheter, MII has several advantages in monitoring GER. A recent consensus statement has identified combined MII-pH as the most sensitive test "to detect reflux of all types."[10]

For monitoring of GER via MII-pH, multiple impedance-measuring segments are mounted on a regular 2.1-mm pH probe (Fig. 10–9). Combined MII-pH

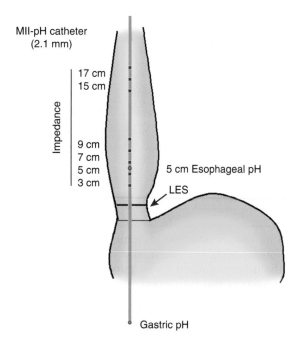

Figure 10–9. Combined multichannel intraluminal impedance (MII) and pH catheter. During reflux monitoring the esophageal sensor is located 5 cm above the proximal border of the lower esophageal sphincter (LES). Impedance-measuring segments are centered at 3, 5, 7, and 9 cm above the LES in the distal end of the esophagus and around 15 and 17 cm above the LES in the proximal end of the esophagus. This catheter also allows monitoring of gastric pH (10 cm below the LES).

represents a shift in the GERD testing paradigm. GER episodes are detected by retrograde (i.e., distal to proximal) declines in intraluminal impedance determined by increased conductivity of the liquid GER, whereas data from the esophageal pH sensor are simply used to categorize the GER into acid or non-acid (Fig. 10–10). Traditionally, GER with a pH above 4.0 is considered non-acid in order to underscore the difference in the acid reflux episodes detectable by conventional pH monitoring. In an attempt to comply with the chemical definition of acid and non-acid based on the chemical dissociation equation of water, a group of leading esophageal experts have proposed separating GER detected by MII into acid if the pH drops from above to below 4.0, weakly acidic if the pH is between 4.0 and 7.0, and non-acid if the intraesophageal pH during an MII-detected reflux episode remains above 7.0.[10]

In addition to the chemical properties of the gastroesophageal refluxate, MII has the ability to clarify some of its physical properties. MII can differentiate between liquid only, gas only, and mixed gas-liquid reflux episodes based on changes in intraluminal impedance. Gas or air has very poor electrical conductivity and, when present between impedance-measuring rings, will produce a rise in impedance; in contrast, liquid, which has better electrical conductivity, will produce a decline in impedance (Fig. 10–11).

The ability to detect GER episodes when the pH remains above 4.0 has important implications for both gastroenterologists and gastrointestinal surgeons. Non-acid reflux (i.e., GER episodes with a pH above 4.0) is relatively infrequent in subjects not taking acid-suppressive therapy; it occurs primarily in the postprandial periods[11] and rarely at night.[12] On the other hand, in subjects taking acid-suppressive therapy, the medications may change the composition of the gastroesophageal refluxate without affecting the total number of GER episodes.[13,14] Currently, normal values for acid and non-acid reflux in 60 healthy volunteers not receiving acid-suppressive therapy[12] and in a small ($N = 6$) number of volunteers receiving acid-suppressive therapy (omeprazole, 20 mg twice daily before meals) have been published.[14]

Non-acid reflux is not likely to cause esophageal lesions because esophageal mucosal healing rates of up to 90% have been documented in patients taking potent acid-suppressive therapy.[15] Quantifying non-acid reflux may be of interest in patients with supraesophageal (ear, nose, and throat and pulmonary) symptoms inasmuch as studies suggest that patients with pharyngeal lesions are more likely to have more gas-containing reflux episodes, a type of reflux episode detected primarily by impedance.[16] Although non-acid reflux may have a limited contribution to esophageal structural lesions, it appears to have a major role in causing persistent symptoms in patients taking acid-suppressive therapy. There is both direct evidence of postprandial symptoms being associated with non-acid reflux[13] and indirect data from a large PPI trial indicating that 35% to 40% of patients receiving acid-suppressive therapy continue to have symptoms.[15] Clarifying the relationship between reflux symptoms and ongoing GER (both acid and non-acid) is

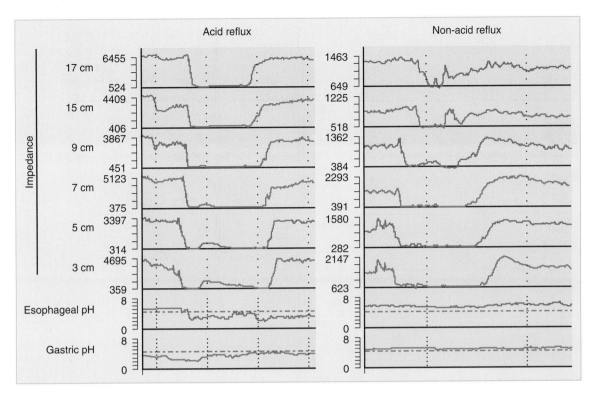

Figure 10–10.   Acid and non-acid reflux episodes detected by using combined multichannel intraluminal impedance (MII) and pH monitoring. Reflux episodes are detected by MII as a retrograde drop in impedance starting distally and moving proximally. Traditionally, a reflux episode is classified as acid if the esophageal pH drops below 4.0 or as non-acid if the pH remains above 4.0.

very important in clinical decision making because patients are more likely to be referred to gastroenterologists and gastrointestinal surgeons only after they have "failed" PPI trials.

Current clinical practice guidelines recommend empirical trials of PPIs instead of pH testing for patients complaining of reflux symptoms. The favorable side effect profile of PPIs has encouraged this initial step to be taken by primary care physicians, and patients are referred to specialists only if they have persistent symptoms with acid-suppressive therapy. In these circumstances esophageal pH testing is performed, but before testing, an important decision has to be made whether to test the patient while taking or while not taking PPIs. Esophageal pH testing without medication is more accurate, and a negative result (i.e., normal distal esophageal pH with negative symptom association) is very helpful in suggesting that the symptoms are not due to acid reflux. A positive esophageal pH test while not receiving therapy, on the other hand, does not necessarily explain why the patient is still having symptoms while taking PPIs. Esophageal pH testing during therapy is also helpful if the test result is abnormal (i.e., increased amount of distal esophageal acid exposure with therapy and a positive symptom association for acid reflux) because it suggests that the acid suppression may be insufficient. A negative esophageal pH test while receiving therapy cannot exclude non-acid reflux being associated with the residual symptoms. In our opinion, combined MII-pH has the potential to overcome this impasse. We propose the algorithm depicted in Figure 10–12 for evaluating patients with GERD symptoms.

In our experience[17] with MII-pH monitoring in more than 150 patients, less than 10% of patients with persistent symptoms during acid-suppressive therapy have symptoms associated with acid reflux (a group of patients who can potentially be detected by conventional pH alone). In the remaining 90% or more patients with symptoms while receiving twice-daily PPIs, combined MII-pH is of pivotal importance in separating those with persistent non-acid reflux associated with symptoms (about a third) from those with symptoms not associated with reflux (about two thirds). The type of reflux symptoms (typical versus atypical) plays a major role relative to whether they are associated with ongoing GER. In our experience, approximately half the patients with typical GERD symptoms had a positive symptom index for ongoing reflux, whereas more than 70% of patients with atypical symptoms had a negative symptom index with concurrent acid-suppressive therapy.

SUMMARY

MII is a valuable addition to both conventional manometry and pH testing. Combined MII-EM helps clarify the functional aspects of esophageal motility abnormalities

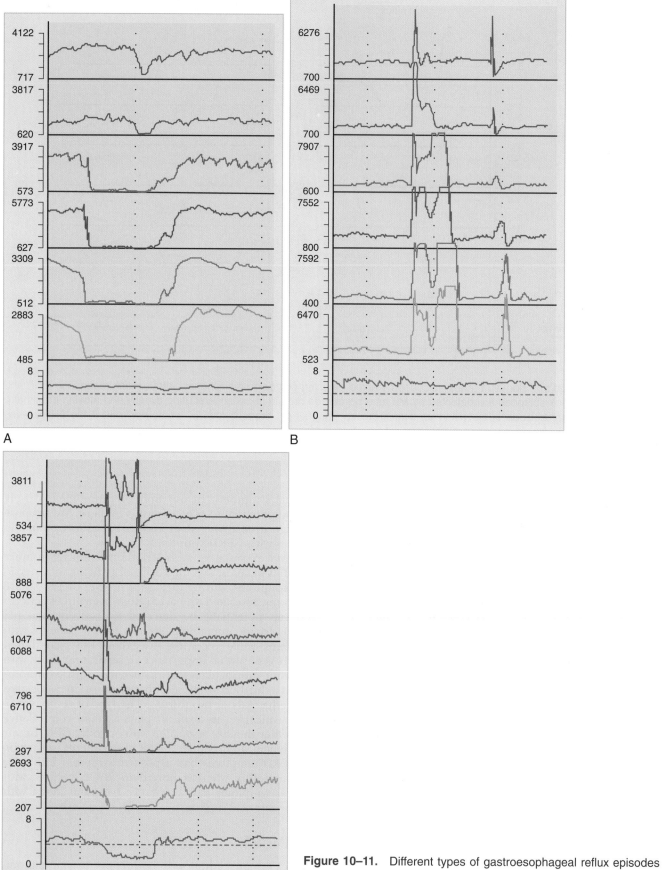

Figure 10–11.   Different types of gastroesophageal reflux episodes based on liquid-gas content: liquid only **(A)**, gas only **(B)**, and mixed gas and liquid **(C)**.

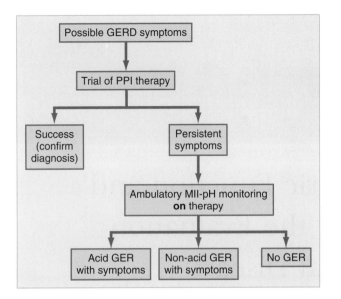

Figure 10–12. Suggested diagnostic gastroesophageal reflux disease (GERD) algorithm. GER, gastroesophageal reflux; MII-pH, combined multichannel intraluminal impedance and pH monitoring; PPI, proton pump inhibitor.

and has the potential to refine patient selection for antireflux procedures and to clarify the mechanisms of postfundoplication dysphagia. Combined MII-pH expands the ability to monitor for both acid and non-acid reflux and thus helps select patients who may benefit from antireflux procedures.

REFERENCES

1. Silny J: Intraluminal multiple electric impedance procedure for measurement of gastrointestinal motility. J Gastrointest Motil 3:151-162, 1991.
2. Blom D, Mason RJ, Balaji NS, et al: Esophageal bolus transport identified by simultaneous multichannel intraluminal impedance and manofluoroscopy. Gastroenterology 120:P103, 2001.
3. Simren M, Silny J, Holloway R, et al: Relevance of ineffective oesophageal motility during oesophageal acid clearance. Gut 52:784-790, 2003.
4. Imam H, Baker M, Shay SS: Concurrent video-esophagogram, impedance monitoring and manometry in the assessment of bolus transit in normal subject [abstract]. Gastroenterology 126(Suppl 2):A638, 2004.
5. Srinivasan R, Vela MF, Katz PO, et al: Esophageal function testing using multichannel intraluminal impedance. Am J Physiol 280:G457-G462, 2001.
6. Tutuian R, Vela MF, Balaji N, et al: Esophageal function testing using combined multichannel intraluminal impedance and manometry. Multicenter study of healthy volunteers. Clin Gastroenterol Hepatol 1:174-182, 2003.
7. Tutuian R, Castell DO: Combined multichannel intraluminal impedance and manometry clarifies esophageal function abnormalities. Study in 350 patients. Am J Gastroenterol 99:1011-1019, 2004.
8. Tutuian R, Castell DO: Clarification of the esophageal function defect in patients with manometric ineffective esophageal motility: Studies using combined impedance-manometry. Clin Gastroenterol Hepatol 2:230-236, 2004.
9. Imam H, Baker M, Shay S: Simultaneous barium esophagogram (Ba), impedance monitoring (Imp) and manometry (Ba-Imp-Manometry) in patients with dysphagia due to tight fundoplication [abstract]. Gastroenterology 126(Suppl 2):A-639, 2004.
10. Sifrim D, Castell D, Dent J, Kahrilas PJ: Gastro-oesophageal reflux monitoring: Review and consensus report on detection and definitions of acid, non-acid, and gas reflux. Gut 53:1024-1031, 2004.
11. Wildi SM, Tutuian R, Castell DO: The influence of rapid food intake on postprandial reflux: Studies in healthy volunteers. Am J Gastroenterol 99:1645-1651, 2004.
12. Shay S, Tutuian R, Sifrim D, et al: Twenty-four hour ambulatory simultaneous impedance and pH monitoring: A multicenter report of normal values from 60 healthy volunteers. Am J Gastroenterol 99:1037-1043, 2004.
13. Vela MF, Camacho-Lobato L, Srinivasan R, et al: Simultaneous intraesophageal impedance and pH measurement of acid and nonacid gastroesophageal reflux: Effect of omeprazole. Gastroenterology 120:1599-1606, 2001.
14. Tamhankar AP, Peters JH, Portale G, et al: Omeprazole does not reduce gastroesophageal reflux: New insights using multichannel intraluminal impedance technology. J Gastrointest Surg 8:888-896, 2004.
15. Castell DO, Kahrilas PJ, Richter JE, et al: Esomeprazole (40 mg) compared with lansoprazole (30 mg) in the treatment of erosive esophagitis. Am J Gastroenterol 97:575-583, 2002.
16. Kawamura O, Aslam M, Rittmann T, et al: Physical and pH properties of gastroesophagopharyngeal refluxate: A 24-hour simultaneous ambulatory impedance and pH monitoring study. Am J Gastroenterol 99:1000-1010, 2004.
17. Mainie I, Tutuian R, Agrawal A, et al: Symptoms on PPI therapy associated with non-acid reflux GERD. Am J Gastroenterol 99(Suppl):S14, 2004.

11

Tests of Gastric Function and Their Use in the Evaluation of Esophageal Disease

Karl-Hermann Fuchs

The pathophysiologic background of functional esophageal disorders is multifactorial.[1-3] The upper gastrointestinal tract is responsible for transport, reservoir function, and initiation of the digestion of food as an integrated system of different elements. Malfunction of only one of these constituents can have an impact on the whole process. The stomach and duodenum follow the esophagus and have special connections to the latter. The complex system of the antireflux barrier at the esophagogastric junction underlines the close relationship between the two organs. Malfunction or anatomic changes in the stomach and duodenum (or both) will have an influence on esophageal function and can be the background of esophageal disease.[1]

The clinical manifestation of esophageal functional disorders does not always allow for precise localization of the cause of the underlying problem.[4] Whereas heartburn and dysphagia are rather specific symptoms with a high probability of an esophageal origin, more nonspecific symptoms such as epigastric pain, nausea and vomiting, uncomfortable fullness and belching, hoarseness, and chronic cough lack this specificity. A number of other extraesophageal symptoms can occur in patients with gastroesophageal reflux disease (GERD), but they can also be present in other disorders or their presence can be a clue to concomitant disorders of the stomach, duodenum, or both.[1,3,5]

As a consequence, objective testing is needed to evaluate not only esophageal but also gastric and duodenal function, especially in patients in whom surgery is being considered. Even if classic esophageal functional testing such as 24-hour pH monitoring, as well as endoscopic or radiographic findings (or both), lead to a diagnosis, a work-up to evaluate function of the gastroduodenal segment should be completed before surgery because it can be involved in the process. It is important to evalu-

ate all involved functional defects along the upper gastrointestinal tract before changing one component by surgery since the remaining problems can lead to failure or new symptoms. Even if newly detected disorders will not lead to an alteration in the initial therapeutic plan, the information about a concomitant disorder is important for both the surgeon and patient because it could be the basis of a clinical problem in the future. Therefore, understanding of gastrointestinal pathophysiology and objective testing of gastric and duodenal function, as well as a focused history of symptoms regarding extraesophageal signs, are important in the management of esophageal disease.

PHYSIOLOGIC AND PATHOPHYSIOLOGIC ASPECTS OF THE STOMACH AND DUODENUM IN ESOPHAGEAL DISEASE

The physiologic tasks of the esophagus and stomach are transport, reservoir function, initiation of digestion by the secretion of acid and enzymes, and grinding of food. A major impairment is dysmotility causing obstruction and reflux.

Food is passed in small portions through the pharynx and esophagus into the stomach. In physiologic conditions this transportation process is well coordinated and usually occurs without any special mental effort. Once this process is disturbed by mechanical obstruction or malfunction of the esophagus and transport of the bolus is impaired, the person becomes aware of the swallowing process and realizes that such transport is difficult. Because of the physiologic connection between the gastric reservoir and the duodenum and esophagus, this phenomenon can also occur if gastric emptying is prohibited and the person feels that it is impossible to eat and swallow food. Any functional obstruction at the gastric level can cause or increase gastroesophageal reflux or inhibit transport.[1]

Duodenogastric reflux (DGR) has been known for years to influence esophageal exposure to gastric juice if duodenogastroesophageal reflux (DGER) occurs.[3,6,7] DGR is a physiologic phenomenon. If the amount of such reflux is excessive and exceeds a certain threshold, a mixture of duodenal juice and gastric acid can reach the esophageal lumen and cause damage.[6] Functional disorders of gastric acid secretion can have an impact on esophageal acid exposure.[8]

Two major functional disorders of the gastroduodenal segment are most relevant in esophageal disease: delayed gastric empting, and DGER. Both these disorders can occur as a primary dysfunction or be secondary to previous gastric surgery.

DELAYED GASTRIC EMPTYING

After the ingestion of fluids and solids, the gastric reservoir can be filled with several liters of volume. The stomach gradually dilates after a bolus enters as a result of relaxation, especially of the gastric fundus, where the storage of solids is accomplished. Dysfunction of accommodation of the gastric fundus can have an impact on functional disorders and the development of symptoms.[9,10] Motor activity is different in the fundic area, where relaxation, followed by low-amplitude tonic contractions, occurs to move solids more distal in the corpus. The gastric pacemaker is located in the upper part of the corpus and is responsible for orthograde motility from the corpus and antrum into the duodenum by creating a stimulus of approximately three contractions per minute. Fluids and small food particles leave the stomach earlier than solids do. When more than half the fluids are emptied, solids are moved by increasing fundic tonus toward the corpus in order to enter the antrum. The antral grinding mechanism will downsize the food particles for passage through the pylorus. If these particles are too large, they will be rejected back into the corpus via pyloric and antral motility to reenter the grinding process. Redistribution of food and fluids within the stomach can have a connection with the spectrum of symptoms.[11]

Gastric motor function includes, in addition to reception, storage, and grinding of food, mixing of food with acid and pepsin, discrimination between solids and fluids, recognition of the composition of food components such as fat and protein, and finally, advancement of chyme through the pylorus into the duodenum with the appropriate speed for further physiologic digestion. Duodenal motor activity is also involved in this process by varying duodenal resistance to the transpyloric flow of chyme.

Gastric and antroduodenal motility disorders may contribute to several foregut pathologies, such as gastroesophageal reflux, DGER, gastritis, and ulcerations, and are discussed as potential background for dyspep-

sia.[12-16] Delayed gastric emptying can be detected in patients with diabetes, neurologic disorders, and postoperative syndromes, as well as be a primary finding.[10] The classic clinical manifestation is early satiety, regurgitation and heartburn, uncomfortable fullness, nausea, vomiting, anorexia, and weight loss. The diagnostic workup consists of upper gastrointestinal endoscopy to verify mucosal damage, mechanical obstruction, or stenosis, as well as methods to evaluate gastric emptying, such as gastric emptying scintigraphy, the ^{13}C breathing test, antroduodenal manometry, gastric emptying ultrasound, barium sandwich emptying radiography, or any combination of these tests.

Gastric Emptying Scintigraphy

Scintigraphy, performed by ingesting a test meal with radioactive markers, is the most frequently used test for evaluation of gastric emptying.[17-19] It represents the optimal method, if performed by a validated protocol, because it allows for precise quantification. Solids as well as fluids can be marked with tracers, and emptying can be monitored with gamma cameras. It is important to use a posterior and anterior camera position in a sandwich technique to obtain representative data for calculation of geometric mean data.[19] Modern systems have dual-head gamma cameras. The most frequently used tracer is ^{99m}Tc, which has a short half-life of 6 hours. If fluid and solid emptying needs to be differentiated, ^{111}In is mixed, for example, with orange juice, and detected separately via the dual-isotope technique.

"Regions of interest" are marked in the upper abdominal quadrants such that the area of the stomach is covered, and initial and declining tracer activity is measured as food leaves the marked regions. Segments of the esophagus and stomach can also be differentiated to assess emptying of the proximal and distal parts of the stomach separately. Often, the time that it takes for 50% of the tracer to leave the "region of interest" is identified as the empting half-time. Alternatively, activity can be measured after 100 minutes or 2 hours (Figs. 11–1 and 11–2).

However, it must be emphasized that the results of gastric emptying scintigraphy have considerable interindividual and even intraindividual variability, which can be as high as 20% to 30%. This variability also depends on the food and tracer preparation. In clinical practice, it is convenient to mix the two components just before the test. However, fluids can wash the tracer off the solid food, which can lead to misinterpretation and therefore underestimation of the true emptying rate. More precise is a stronger bond between food and tracer, but tremendous logistic effort is required that cannot be realized in clinical practice.[18] It is important to follow a standardized protocol with a uniform meal and evaluation process.[17]

^{13}C Breathing Test

The advantage of this test is the absence of radiation problems because ^{13}C is a stabile isotope, and it is increasingly being used in clinical practice. The principle of this

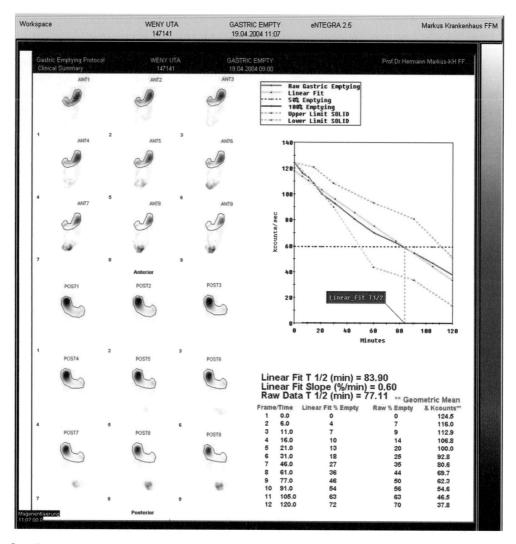

Figure 11–1. Gastric emptying scintigraphy with a dual-head gamma camera to evaluate emptying of solid food. The person investigated has normal emptying. (Investigation by M. Fobbe, Department of Radiology, Markus-Hospital, Frankfurt.)

method is based on emptying a combination of ^{13}C together with food (e.g., scrambled eggs) from the stomach to the duodenum. The tracer is mixed and fried together with the eggs to keep the marker on the semi-solid food when emptying occurs. In the small bowel, ^{13}C is oxidized to $[^{13}C]CO_2$, which is exhaled and measured. Breath tests are performed before and after ingestion for 2 or 4 hours. Several studies have shown the validity of this test.[21-22]

Antroduodenal Manometry

Antroduodenal manometry assesses gastric and duodenal motor activity, which can be altered in foregut disorders such as gastric emptying problems, non–ulcer-related dyspepsia, and GERD, as well as panmotility disorders associated with achalasia.[13,14,16,23-25] Functional obstruction by antroduodenal motility disorders can lead to gastric dilatation, widening of the lower esophageal sphincter, and gastroesophageal reflux, as well as retention of ingested gastric contents with stimulation of acid

secretion, thus increasing the potential for acid exposure in the esophagus.

Antroduodenal motility has been assessed by evaluating electrical activity or measuring the intraluminal mechanical activity of gastric and duodenal wall contractions by manometry. The latter is rather easy to manage in a clinical laboratory. Antroduodenal manometry can be performed with a perfusion manometry system in a gastrointestinal function laboratory or as a 24-hour monitoring test, depending on the equipment. Generally, a motility catheter is used with measuring points (openings on a perfusion catheter) or sensors (solid-state catheter) located a distance of 5 or 10 cm apart. Often, laboratories use catheters with a set of measuring points 1 cm apart at the pyloric region to record a representative image of this important segment. However, the choice of equipment depends on the particular patient, disorder, and questions that need to be answered with the test. Frequently, a six- or eight-channel system is used with 5-cm separation between the proximal three measuring points/sensors and 10-cm

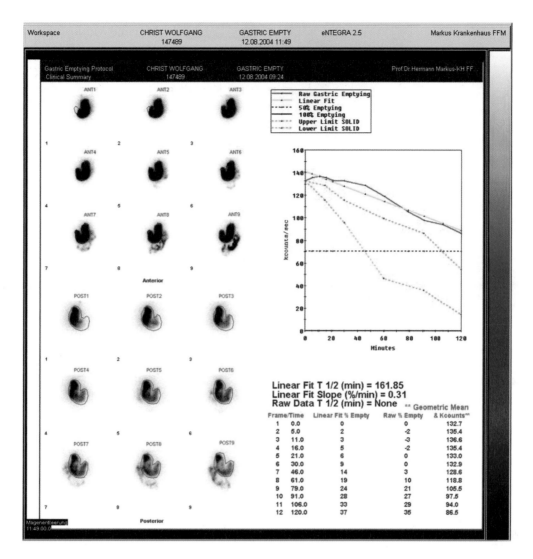

Figure 11–2.   Gastric emptying scintigraphy in a patient with gastroparesis showing delayed gastric emptying. (Investigation by M. Fobbe, Department of Radiology, Markus-Hospital, Frankfurt.)

separation between the distal two or three points. This setup enables valid assessment of both antral and duodenal motility without a special focus on the pyloric region.

Before the test, the patient has to discontinue taking all potentially motility-interfering drugs for at least for 48 hours. After 6 hours of fasting, the catheter is passed transnasally into the duodenum. Under fluoroscopic guidance or by endoscopic means, the final position of the catheter is achieved in the duodenum (Fig. 11–3). It is important that the two or three oral pressure sensors be located in the antrum 5 and 10 cm above the pylorus and the most distal two sensors be located in the distal part of the descending duodenum or even around the bend in the ascending part. Depending on the number of available recording channels or sensors, reliable data require two full recordings in the prepyloric antrum and two in the descending duodenum. During antroduodenal motor activity, the catheter will move considerably, in addition to movement of the pylorus and duodenum around the catheter. As a consequence, the channels or sensors in the pyloric region will sometimes record antral and sometimes record duodenal motility, depending on the position. This lead can be neglected in the final analysis, but it is a valuable parameter to be able to identify the pyloric region. If the purpose of the investigation is assessment of the pylorus, a special catheter is necessary that has many sensors positioned 1 cm apart over a distance of 5 to 10 cm to precisely register any movement and all contractions of the pylorus.

The protocol for the test depends on the equipment used, such as a solid-state sensor system or perfusion manometry. With the latter, the patient is connected to the perfusion pump and has to stay in the laboratory for the duration of the investigation. With the solid-state system, the patient should perform normal daily activities as much as possible. The patient should eat and drink at set meal times only and document this in the diary in order to provide data on both fasting and fed-state motility patterns. All special events and symptoms should be documented in the diary during the investigation.

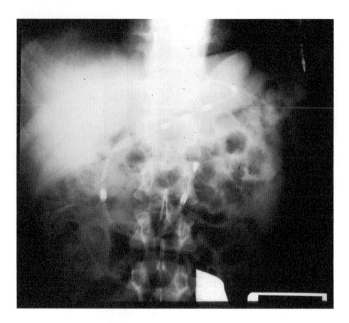

Figure 11–3. Fluoroscopic control after placement of an antroduodenal motility catheter for 24-hour antroduodenal manometry. It is important that the distal sensors be beyond the proximal duodenal bulb and be able to record duodenal motility in the descending and ascending portion of the duodenum.

Table 11–1	Normal Values of Antroduodenal Manometry in Healthy Volunteers	

Motility Criteria	Antrum	Duodenum
IMMC—phase duration (%)		
Phase I	15-30	10-25
Phase II	20-50	40-60
Phase III	3-5	3-5
Fed pattern	5-20	5-20
Antroduodenal linkage—orthograde migration	>80%	>80%
Contractions—phase II		
Frequency per minute	1-1.5	1.5-4.5
Mean duration (sec)	1.7-3.5	1.5-3.0
Mean amplitude (mm Hg)	10-25	10-20
Contractions—phase III		
Frequency per minute	2.5-4	7-14
Mean duration (sec)	1.5-4	1.3-3
Mean amplitude (mm Hg)	40-100	10-40
Contractions—fed pattern		
Frequency per minute	0.5-3	0.5-2.7
Mean duration (sec)	2-3.6	2-3.8
Mean amplitude (mm Hg)	15-35	13-28

IMMC, interdigestive migrating motor complex.
From Heimbucher J, Fuchs KH, Freys SM, Thiede A: Antroduodenal motility in patients with gastroesophageal reflux disease. Langenbecks Arch Surg Forum (Suppl I):89-93, 1998.

Usually, commercially available software will provide an analysis of the data. Normal data, generated from 30 normal healthy volunteers tested with the same standardized protocol as used for patients, are demonstrated in Table 11–1.

The recording system will analyze the contractions for each lead. The investigator identifies and, from the diary documentation, marks positions and activity patterns of the patient, such as mealtimes and upright and supine body positions, from which the fed pattern and phases I, II, and III of the interdigestive migrating motor complex (IMMC) can be deducted and separately analyzed (Figs. 11–4 and 11–5). Contraction frequency and morphology for phases II and III, as well as for the fed pattern, representative characteristics of the IMMC, and antroduodenal coordination are expressed. Depending on the purpose of the investigation, more parameters can be analyzed, but clinical experience has shown that contraction frequency and IMMC phase coordination, together with fed-pattern morphology, are the most sensitive in comparing data from healthy volunteers with data from patients with esophageal disorders.

Three major dysfunctions can be identified by antroduodenal manometry:

1. Antral hypomotility. Hypomotility is usually seen in patients with a decreased contraction amplitude and a decreased frequency of contractions. In some patients, this phenomenon is seen in the fasting as well as the postprandial state. A shortening or even absence of phase II and III and absence of a physiologic fed pattern is possible. Hypomotility during the fed state is regarded as the most severe problem.

2. Disturbance of phasic IMMC activity. When this problem is present, the physiologic sequence of phases from I to III does not occur on a regular basis or is absent. Instead, the phases are irregular in occurrence and duration. Antroduodenal coordination and linkage of phases can be absent. The percentage of orthograde migration of contraction patterns is decreased, as well as the number of complete IMMCs. This problem often occurs after previous upper gastrointestinal surgery, especially gastric surgery.

3. Focal dysfunction. Episodes of simultaneous contractions are recorded, followed by hypomotility segments. In addition, bursts of high-amplitude contractions may occur at only one level, so interpretation is difficult. This phenomenon can also be seen more frequently toward the oral side of an obstruction.

In patients with esophageal disorders, most often GERD, antroduodenal motility disorders can be associated with extraesophageal symptoms such as nausea, early satiety, uncomfortable fullness, and vomiting. Antral or antroduodenal hypomotility can be detected most frequently in these patients. Table 11–2 presents the results of a comparative study.[13] In these patients, the

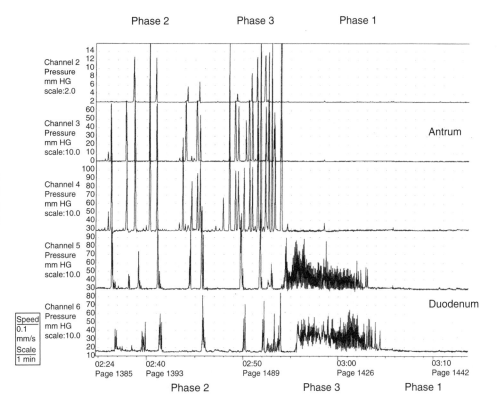

Figure 11–4. Example of a normal physiologic motility pattern of the interdigestive migrating motor complex as recorded by antroduodenal manometry.

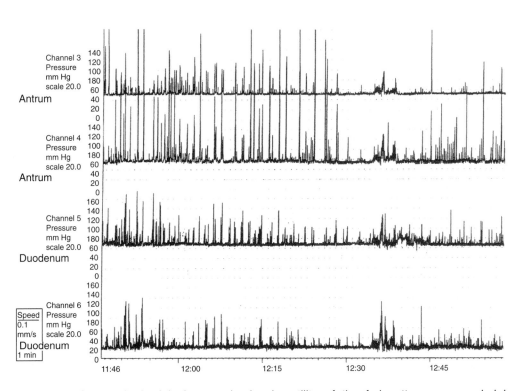

Figure 11–5. Example of normal physiologic antroduodenal motility of the fed pattern as recorded by antroduodenal manometry.

Table 11–2 Results of Antroduodenal Manometry in Patients with Gastroesophageal Reflux Disease Versus Healthy Volunteers

	Antrum			Duodenum		
	Control	**GERD**	**P**	**Control**	**GERD**	**P**
IMMC						
Number/24 hr	5	3	<.05	8	4	<.01
Duration (min)	120	122	NS	65	76	<.05
Frequency						
Total	1.1	0.8	<.01	1.8	1.9	NS
Upright	1.4	1.3	NS	2.1	1.9	NS
Supine	0.7	0.3	<.01	1.1	1.0	NS
Postprandial	1.7	1.0	<.05	4.7	3.2	<.01

IMMC, interdigestive migrating motor complex; NS, not significant.
From Heimbucher J, Fuchs KH, Freys SM, Thiede A: Antroduodenal motility in patients with gastroesophageal reflux disease. Langenbecks Arch Surg Forum (Suppl I):89-93, 1998.

number of IMMCs and hypomotility in both the antrum and duodenum can be the background for associated gastric symptoms. In patients with GERD, nonspecific symptoms such as nausea, epigastric pain, vomiting, and uncomfortable fullness are associated with the presence of antroduodenal dysmotility.

Additional Miscellaneous Gastric Emptying Tests

Assessment of the stomach and emptying of fluids or even standardized particles with real-time ultrasound has been shown to be helpful. Its high dependence on observer competence and its potential variability remain a problem. It is, however, a cheap and noninvasive procedure.

Radiographic barium burger studies to evaluate esophageal passage and gastric emptying can be performed in clinical practice in any radiology unit. Emptying is difficult to precisely quantify with this method, and radiation is invasive. Usually, the result is expressed as percent emptying after standardized time segments with respect to initial filling. It is helpful in clinical practice if no other more extensive evaluation is available.

Sophisticated technology such as the Barostat technique, single-photon emission computed tomography, and impedance epigastrography have been used, generally in research centers.[26,27] Further investigation will provide more insight into gastric physiology. There could be a simple alternative to assessment of gastric emptying in patients with gastroesophageal reflux, such as correlation of intraluminal pH values with gastric emptying data.[28-30]

DUODENOGASTROESOPHAGEAL REFLUX

DGR is a natural physiologic phenomenon.[30,31] It is part of the normal complex motility pattern of the upper gastrointestinal tract. The gastric mucosa is able to cope with a certain level of exposure to duodenal juice, including its various components, such as pancreatic enzymes and related agents, bile acids and bile salts, and varying amounts of bicarbonate. The constituents of duodenal juice have been demonstrated to have a tremendously damaging effect on gastric mucosa[32,33] and even more so on esophageal mucosa.[6,34] DGER is associated with two major clinical problems in gastrointestinal surgery: reflux problems after gastric surgery and Barrett's esophagus.[3,6,34,35]

In many patients with postgastrectomy syndromes and in some with postfundoplication problems, DGER is the major associated cause. As classic symptoms, Ritchie has defined epigastric pain, nausea, bile vomiting, and weight loss as indicating the possible presence of DGR.[33] In patients with mechanical and functional weakness of the lower esophageal sphincter, the combined problem will cause a mixed reflux. Accurate objective assessment of this pathologic process should include, in addition to endoscopic evaluation, 24-hour esophageal and gastric pH monitoring and 24-hour esophageal and gastric bilirubin monitoring.[31,34-38] Often, the problem can be corrected by surgical duodenal diversion procedures.

The association of Barrett's esophagus and its progression to cancer with DGER has been extensively investigated in the past. There is no doubt that DGER occurs significantly more frequently in GERD patients with Barrett's esophagus than in those without this condition.[6,34,35,39] Substantial experimental and clinical evidence is available to support the injurious effect of duodenal juice on esophageal mucosa.[39]

Evaluation of DGER has a long history and has involved several techniques, such as aspiration of intraesophageal fluid, scintigraphy, and pH monitoring in the esophagus and stomach. However, either the accuracy of the tests limited their diagnostic value or their invasive approach restricted their applicability in patients. Assessment by intraluminal probes connected to data loggers is currently still the most frequently used procedure. Objective assessment of DGER and its relationship to acid reflux is best evaluated by esophageal and gastric 24-hour pH and bilirubin monitoring.[31,40]

24-Hour Gastric pH Monitoring

After an 8-hour fasting period, pH probes are placed in the esophagus and stomach.[30,41] The gastric probe is positioned 5 cm below the lower boarder of the lower esophageal sphincter (Fig. 11–6). The probe is connected to a data logger and the data recorded over one circadian cycle of at least 20 hours. Both the pH probe and the bilirubin probe can be taped together if monitoring is performed as a combined test. During the test period, the diet is restricted to food with a pH between 5 and 7. Individuals are allowed to continue their daily activities exclusive of hard work or sports. If the test is performed in the hospital setting, the patients should move about, go for long walks, or sit in chairs and restrict their supine position to night hours. Body position and meal activities, as well as symptoms, should be documented in a diary. More important than in esophageal pH monitoring, in gastric pH monitoring mealtimes are standardized to three periods per day, and drinking must also be restricted to these periods and carefully documented.

Recorded pH data can be analyzed by a commercially available computer program (Medtronic GmbH, Düsseldorf, Germany). The analysis separates the 24-hour period into four different phases: upright, supine, mealtime, and postprandial periods. This is important because of the great influence of the meal on gastric intraluminal food and fluid (Fig. 11–7). The program provides data on intraluminal gastric pH, separated into the four different phases, as a frequency distribution of pH values from 0 to 1, 1 to 2, 2 to 3, 3 to 4, 4 to 5, 5 to 6, 6 to 7, and 7 to 8. Table 11–3 lists normal values of healthy volunteers.

Pathologic changes in this physiologic gastric pH spectrum can be determined. These changes can be identified as persistent gastric acidity when the percentage of pH distribution above pH 3 is less than 1% (Fig. 11–8). In contrast, a less acidic gastric pH environment can be detected if the intragastric pH profile is more frequently above pH 3 than the physiologic values are.[30,41] Figure 11–9 shows an example of a less acidic pH distribution

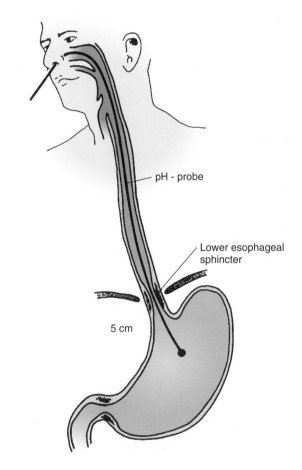

pH - probe

Lower esophageal sphincter

5 cm

Figure 11–6.   Positioning of the gastric pH probe and bilirubin monitoring probe in the proximal gastric lumen 5 cm below the lower border of the lower esophageal sphincter.

Figure 11–7. Physiologic 24-hour gastric pH monitoring record with a rather acidic gastric pH baseline interrupted by several rises in the pH value, mainly during meals consisting of food and drink with different pH values.

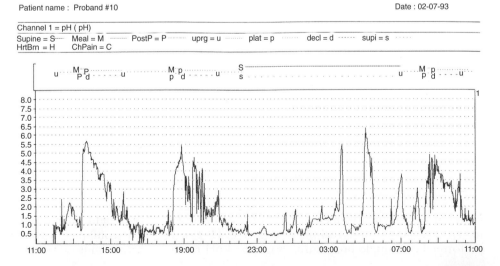

Patient name : Proband #10   Date : 02-07-93

Channel 1 = pH (pH)

Supine = S   Meal = M   PostP = P   uprg = u   plat = p   decl = d   supi = s
HrtBrn = H   ChPain = C

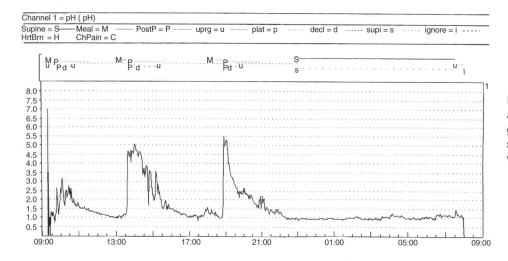

Figure 11–8. Persistent gastric acidity as measured by 24-hour gastric pH monitoring. The tracing shows hardly any changes in the very acidic gastric pH baseline.

Table 11–3 Normal Values for 24-Hour Gastric pH Monitoring in Healthy Volunteers: pH Value Distribution During a 24-Hour Circadian Cycle Exclusive of Mealtimes

Criteria	Body Position	5th Percentile	Median	95th Percentile
pH—mean	Upright	0.9	1.6	2.6
pH—mean	Supine	0.8	1.6	3.7
pH—intervals	Upright			
0-1		0	13.4	57.0
1-2		28	61.8	94.0
2-3		1.4	7.6	42.7
3-4		0	1.9	15.3
4-5		0	0.6	9.5
5-6		0	0.1	8.9
6-7		0	0	1.4
7-8		0	0	0.1
pH—intervals	Supine			
0-1		0	16.1	76.8
1-2		14	50.1	98.8
2-3		0	8.1	28.8
3-4		0	3.0	17.4
4-5		0	0.9	6.9
5-6		0	0	6.3
6-7		0	0	19.7
7-8		0	0	8.4

Data from Fuchs KH, DeMeester TR, Hinder RA, et al: Computerized identification of excessive duodenogastric reflux: Discriminant analysis of 24 hour gastric pH recording. Ann Surg 213:13-20, 1991; and Fuchs KH, Maroske J, Fein M, et al: Variability in the composition of duodenogastric reflux. J Gastrointest Surg 3:389-396, 1999.

in a patient with a high probability of reflux of duodenal juice with combined pH and bilirubin monitoring. It is clear that not all rises in pH in the recording are associated with reflux of bile and vice versa.[31]

An important application of 24-hour gastric pH monitoring in conjunction with esophageal pH monitoring is to verify negative esophageal pH testing (Fig. 11–10). If performed as a single procedure, esophageal pH moni-

toring in the event of a negative test does not tell the investigator whether acid in the gastric lumen influenced the refluxate. Combined esophageal and gastric pH monitoring will clarify the acidity in the stomach and the possible acid exposure in the esophagus, thereby shedding light on the competence of the antireflux barrier. The combined test can also be used to evaluate response in patients receiving proton pump inhibitor (PPI)

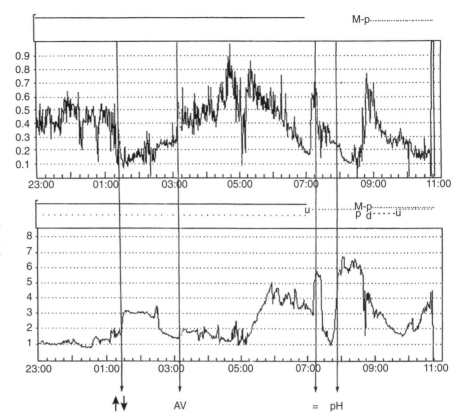

Figure 11–9. Example of a combined recording of 24-hour gastric pH monitoring and 24-hour gastric bilirubin monitoring showing changing acidity in the gastric lumen, as well as changing levels of absorption, indicating various levels of bile reflux. It is important to recognize that these changes do not occur simultaneously.

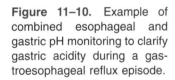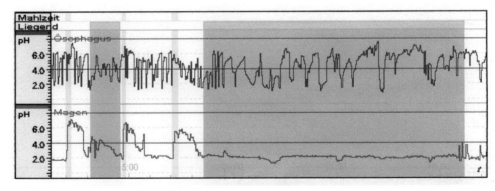

Figure 11–10. Example of combined esophageal and gastric pH monitoring to clarify gastric acidity during a gastroesophageal reflux episode.

therapy.[42-45] Persistent acidity of the gastric environment with PPI treatment enables the investigator to better interpret the therapeutic effect and allows for adjustment of dosage and timing.[46] Nightly acid breakthrough has been described as one of the causes of partial failure of PPI therapy in patients with GERD. In clinical practice, complex data analysis is often not even necessary. Visual control and evaluation of the 24-hour record will tell the investigator immediately the connection between the intraluminal gastric pH environment and esophageal acid exposure with regard to time during the circadian rhythm and duration of exposure. Accordingly, gastric pH testing is a valuable method in patients with esophageal disease that can help clarify pathophysiologic mechanisms, as well as control therapeutic activities.

24-Hour Bilirubin Monitoring

An indirect method to assess DGR or DGER is bilirubin monitoring by the Bilitec device. The system detects intraluminal bilirubin by spectrophotometric measurement. The spectophotometric probe contains optical fibers connected to light-emitting diodes and receiving photo diodes. This photoelectronic device can emit a 470-nm signal light and a 565-nm reference light. By reflection of signals from the probe, which is enveloped in esophageal and gastric fluids, the system can provide absorbance values that reflect intraluminal bilirubin concentrations. Several published validation studies have shown remarkable reliability of the system.[31,36-38,47] This test is valuable for the detection of bilirubin as an important marker of DGER.

The investigation is performed with a protocol similar to that for long-term pH monitoring. It is important to impose further dietary restrictions inasmuch as validation studies have shown that foods with a similar wavelength as bilirubin can cause severe artifacts.

Best is a diet consisting of food and drink with white or bright colors, such as chicken meat. Analysis of the recorded data provides absorption values distributed over the investigation period and subdivided into different phases, such as upright, supine, and meal periods. Table 11–4 presents normal data generated from healthy volunteers. Figure 11–11 illustrates pathologic bilirubin exposure in a patient with pathologic DGR and DGER.

Although DGR occurs physiologically, DGER has not been detected in normal healthy volunteers by bilirubin monitoring.[6,40] The role of DGER in Barrett's esophagus is well investigated and a documented fact.[35] Recent studies have shown that DGER and DGR can be associated with severe GERD.[40,48] The clinical application of such monitoring is limited to centers where the equipment is available. Because of the lack of a proven benefit or positive therapeutic effect in GERD patients with or without DGER, application of 24-hour bilirubin monitoring is limited. For precise determination of the severity of GERD, evaluation of DGER is necessary. Recently, a study in GERD patients has shown that the combination of esophageal pH and bilirubin monitoring is able to identify the reason for failure of PPI therapy.[48] Combined pH and Bilitec monitoring was superior to pH recording alone in detecting ongoing pathologic reflux in patients with poor clinical response to PPI treatment. In addition, gastric pH and bilirubin monitoring will provide the underlying basis for the intragastric acid and bile load. This information seems to also be helpful in surgical decision making. The documented presence of

Table 11–4   Normal Values of Esophageal and Gastric 24-Hour Bilirubin Monitoring in Healthy Volunteers

Percentage of Measured Time Above Threshold	25th Percentile	Median	95th Percentile
Esophagus—threshold absorption value >0.14			
Total time	0	0.5	11.8
Stomach—threshold absorption value >0.25			
Total time	0.35	1.45	28.2
Upright	0.08	0.85	15.4
Supine	0.07	0.75	37.7
Meal	0	0.1	14.5

Data from references 6, 31, 37.

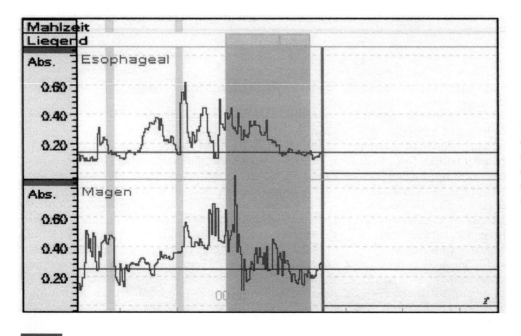

Figure 11–11. Example of combined esophageal and gastric bilirubin monitoring to clarify the level of gastric bile exposure during a gastroesophageal reflux episode.

pathologic esophageal and gastric acid and bilirubin exposure can make a stronger case for performing antireflux surgery, if all other indications are fulfilled.

Miscellaneous Gastric Functional Tests

Gastric acid secretion was studied for many years in clinical practice when gastroduodenal ulcer disease was still considered a problem of the secretory state.[8] This test was also used as a therapeutic control after surgery to reduce acid secretion, such as all forms of vagotomy. Because it is known that the majority of the ulcers develop from *Helicobacter pylori* infection or the use of nonsteroidal anti-inflammatory drugs, the clinical value of this test has diminished. Basal acid secretion was measured after overnight fasting by the instillation of a standardized saline solution and aspiration of the intragastric fluid with subsequent titration for determination of its hydrogen ion content. Basal acid secretion could vary between 0 and 5 mEq/hr. After stimulation with pentagastrin, the maximal secretory output of gastric acid can be determined and ranges between 10 and 15 mEq/hr. This test requires several hours of aspiration. Therefore, ambulatory 24-hour gastric pH monitoring is a better test for assessing intragastric acidity.

The Barostat test measures accommodation, gastric dilatation, and contractions, especially in the proximal part of the stomach.[26] Because it is a rather complex technology and requires testing in a laboratory, it is not used widely in clinical practice but remains a research tool in selected units. It can provide more insight into the relationship between esophageal function and gastric motility.[49]

Electrogastrography is technique that assesses gastric motility by monitoring electric activity. Initial experience with the cutaneous application of electrodes to record this activity has been achieved, but the clinical value of the recorded data is limited because of the need for investigation in a laboratory setting and a number of possible artifacts.

Measurement of impedance in the esophagus and gastroesophageal junction is increasingly gaining importance in assessing esophageal function.[50,51] Because the resistance of gastric mucosa is different from that of esophageal mucosa, however, application of impedance measurement to the gastric lumen is difficult.

ASSESSMENT OF GASTRIC FUNCTION IN ESOPHAGEAL DISEASE

The most important esophageal disorder that also involves the stomach is GERD. Gastric and duodenal dysfunction can have an influence on or even cause esophageal functional problems. As a consequence, assessment of gastric and duodenal function is important in both diagnosis and therapeutic decisions regarding esophageal disease. Such assessment is frequently necessary in patients with GERD, but it also relevant in patients with extensive gastrointestinal motility disorders such as achalasia associated with delayed gastric emptying or

panmotility problems with slow transit constipation, small bowel hypomotility, and delayed gastric emptying.

Especially in surgical patients, detailed evaluation of esophageal and gastric function is of utmost importance before surgery because postoperative failure can be caused by an underlying and undetected problem in gastric function.

REFERENCES

1. DeMeester TR: Definition, detection and pathophysiology of gastroesophageal reflux disease. In DeMeester TR, Matthews HR (eds): International Trends in General Thoracic Surgery, vol 3, Benign Esophageal Disease. St Louis, CV Mosby, 1987, pp 99-127.
2. Dent J, Brun J, Fendrick AM, et al: Geneva Workshop Group: An evidence-based appraisal of reflux disease management. Gut 44:1-16, 1999.
3. Fuchs KH, Freys SM, Heimbucher J, et al: Pathophysiologic spectrum in patients with gastroesophageal reflux disease in a surgical GI function laboratory. Dis Esophagus 8:211-217, 1995.
4. Costantini M, Crookes PF, Bremner RM, et al: Value of physiologic assessment of foregut symptoms in a surgical practice. Surgery 114:780-786, 1993.
5. Kahrilas PJ: Gastroesophageal reflux disease. JAMA 276:983-988, 1996.
6. Fein M, Ireland AP, Ritter MP, et al: Duodenogastric reflux potentiates the injurious effects of gastroesophageal reflux. J Gastrointest Surg 1:27-33, 1997.
7. Stein HJ, Barlow AP, DeMeester TR, Hinder RA: Complications of gastroesophageal reflux disease. Role of the lower esophageal sphincter, esophageal acid and acid/alkaline exposure, and duodenogastric reflux. Ann Surg 216:35-43, 1992.
8. Jenkins JX, Lanspa SJ: Acid secretory tests in the diagnosis of foregut surgical disease. Problems Gen Surg 9:92-103, 1992.
9. Bredenoord AJ, Chial HJ, Camilleri M, et al: Gastric accommodation and emptying in evaluation of patients with upper gastrointestinal symptoms. Clin Gastroenterol Hepatol 1:264-272, 2003.
10. McCallum RW, Chen JD, Lin Z, et al: Gastric pacing improves emptying and symptoms in patients with gastroparesis. Gastroenterology 114:598-601, 1998.
11. Piessevaux H, Tack J, Walrand S, et al: Intragastric distribution of a standardized meal in health and functional dyspepsia: Correlation with specific symptoms. Neurogastroenterol Motil 15:447-455, 2003.
12. Barlow AP, DeMeester TR, et al: The significance of the gastric secretory state in gastroesophageal reflux disease. Arch Surg 124:937-940, 1989.
13. Heimbucher J, Fuchs KH, Freys SM, Thiede A: [Antroduodenal motility in patients with gastroesophageal reflux disease.] Langenbecks Arch Chir Suppl Kongressbd 115(Suppl I):89-93, 1998.
14. Quigley EMM, Donovan JP, Lane MJ, Gallagher TF: Antroduodenal manometry: Usefulness and limitations as an outpatient study. Dig Dis Sci 37:20-28, 1992.
15. Schwizer W, Hinder RA, DeMeester TR: Does delayed gastric emptying contribute to gastroesophageal reflux disease? Am J Surg 157:74-81, 1987.
16. Stanghellini V, Ghidini C, Maccarini MR, et al: Fasting and postprandial gastrointestinal motility in ulcer and non-ulcer dyspepsia. Gut 33:184-190, 1992.
17. Buckles DC, Sarosiek I, McMillin C, McCallum RW: Delayed gastric emptying in gastroesophageal reflux disease: Reassessment with new methods and symptomatic correlations. Am J Med Sci 327:1-4, 2004.
18. Meyer JH, McGregor IL, Gueller R: ^{99m}Tc-tagged chicken liver as a marker of solid food in the human stomach. Dig Dis 21:296-304, 1976.
19. Ziessman HA, Fahey FH, Atkins FB, Tall J: Standardization and quantification of radionuclide solid gastric-emptying studies. J Nucl Med 45:760-764, 2004.
20. Bromer MQ, Kantor SB, Wagner DA, et al: Simultaneous measurement of gastric emptying with a simple muffin meal using [^{13}C]

octanoate breath test and scintigraphy in normal subjects and patients with dyspeptic symptoms. Dig Dis Sci 47:1657-1663, 2002.

21. Chew CG, Bartholomeusz FD, Bellon M, Chatterton BE: Simultaneous $^{13}C/^{14}C$ dual isotope breath test measurement of gastric emptying of solid and liquid in normal subjects and patients: Comparison with scintigraphy. Nucl Med Rev Cent East Eur 6:29-33, 2003.

22. Viramontes BE, Kim DY, Camilleri M, et al: Validation of a stable isotope gastric emptying test for normal, accelerated or delayed gastric emptying. Neurogastroenterol Motil 13:567-574, 2001.

23. Bortolotti M, Annese V, Coccia G: Twenty-four hour ambulatory antroduodenal manometry in normal subjects. Neurogastroenterol Motil 12:231-238, 2000.

24. Penning C, Gielkens HA, Hemelaar M, et al: Reproducibility of antroduodenal motility during prolonged ambulatory recording. Neurogastroenterol Motil 13:133-141, 2001.

25. Verhagen MA, Sambom M, Jebbink RJ, Smout AJ: Clinical relevance of antroduodenal manometry. Eur J Gastroenterol Hepatol 11:523-528, 1999.

26. Azpiroz F, Malagelada JR: Gastric tone measured by an electronic barostat in health and postsurgical gastroparesis. Gastroenterology 92:934-943, 1987.

27. Bennink RJ, van den Elzen BD, Kuiken SD, Boeckxstaens GE: Noninvasive measurement of gastric accommodation by means of pertechnetate SPECT: Limiting radiation dose without losing image quality. J Nucl Med 45:147-152, 2004.

28. Clark GWB, Jamieson JR, Hinder RA, et al: The relationship between gastric pH and the emptying of solids, semisolids and liquid meals. J Gastrointest Motil 5:273-279, 1993.

29. Estevao-Costa J, Dias JA, Campos M, et al: Can esophageal pH monitoring predict delayed gastric emptying? J Pediatr Surg 39:1537-1540, 2004.

30. Fuchs KH, DeMeester TR, Hinder RA, et al: Computerized identification of excessive duodenogastric reflux: Discriminant analysis of 24 hour gastric pH recording. Ann Surg 213:13-20, 1991.

31. Fuchs KH, Maroske J, Fein M, et al: Variability in the composition of duodenogastric reflux. J Gastrointest Surg 3:389-396, 1999.

32. Gowen GW: Spontaneous enterogastric reflux gastritis and esophagitis. Ann Surg 201:170-175, 1985.

33. Ritchie WP: Alkaline reflux gastritis: Late results on a controlled trial of diagnosis and treatment. Ann Surg 203:537-544, 1986.

34. Kauer WK, Peters JH, DeMeester TR, et al: Mixed reflux of gastric and duodenal juices is more harmful to the esophagus than gastric juice alone. The need for surgical therapy re-emphasized. Ann Surg 222:525-531, 1995.

35. Vaezi MF, Richter JE: Synergism of acid and duodenogastroesophageal reflux in complicated Barrett's esophagus. Surgery 117:699-704, 1995.

36. Bechi P, Pucciani F, Baldini F, et al: Long-term ambulatory enterogastric reflux monitoring. Validation of a new fiberoptic technique. Dig Dis Sci 38:1297-1306, 1993.

37. Fein M, Fuchs KH, Bohrer T, et al: Fiberoptic technique for 24-hour bile reflux monitoring—standard and normal values for gastric monitoring. Dig Dis Sci 41:216-225, 1996.

38. Vaezi MF, Lacamera RG, Richter JE: Validation studies of Bilitec 2000: An ambulatory duodenogastric reflux monitoring system. Am J Physiol 267:G1050-G1057, 1994.

39. DeMeester SR, DeMeester TR: Columnar mucosa and intestinal metaplasia of the esophagus: Fifty year controversy. Ann Surg 231:303-321, 2000.

40. Fein M, Maroske J, Fuchs KH: Where does bile in the esophagus come from? Importance of duodenogastric reflux in GERD. Br J Surg (in press).

41. Mela GS, Savarino V, Vigneri S, et al: Limitations of continuous 24-h intragastric pH monitoring in the diagnosis of duodenogastric reflux. Am J Gastroenterol 90:933-937, 1995.

42. Armstrong D: Review article: Gastric pH—the most relevant predictor of benefit in reflux disease? Aliment Pharmacol Ther 20(Suppl 5):19-26, 2004.

43. Frazzoni M, De Micheli E, Savarino V: Different patterns of oesophageal acid exposure distinguish complicated reflux disease from either erosive reflux oesophagitis or non-erosive reflux disease. Aliment Pharmacol Ther 18:1091-1098, 2003.

44. Gerson LB, Boparai V, Ullah N, Triadafilopoulos G: Oesophageal and gastric pH profiles in patients with gastro-oesophageal reflux disease and Barrett's oesophagus treated with proton pump inhibitors. Aliment Pharmacol Ther 20:637-643, 2004.

45. Kahrilas PJ: Review article: Is stringent control of gastric pH useful and practical in GERD? Aliment Pharmacol Ther 20(Suppl 5):89-94, discussion 95-96, 2004.

46. Katz PO, Hatlebakk JG, Castell DO: Gastric acidity and acid breakthrough with twice-daily omeprazole or lanzoprazole. Aliment Pharmacol Ther 14:709-714, 2000.

47. Romagnoli R, Collard JM, Bechi P, Salizzoni M: Gastric symptoms and duodenogastric reflux in patients referred for gastroesophageal reflux symptoms and endoscopic esophagitis. Surgery 125:480-486, 1999.

48. Tack J, Koek G, Demedts I, et al: Gastroesophageal reflux disease poorly responsive to single-dose proton pump inhibitors in patients without Barrett's esophagus: Acid reflux, bile reflux, or both? Am J Gastroenterol 99:981-988, 2004.

49. van den Elzen BD, Bennink RJ, Wieringa RE, et al: Fundic accommodation assessed by SPECT scanning: Comparison with the gastric barostat. Gut 52:1548-1554, 2003.

50. Balaji NS, Blom D, DeMeester TR, Peters JH: Redefining gastroesophageal reflux (GER). Surg Endosc 17:1380-1385, 2003.

51. Sifrim D, Castell D, Dent J, Kahrilas PJ: Gastro-oesophageal reflux monitoring: Review and consensus report on detection and definitions of acid, non-acid and gas reflux. Gut 53:1024-1031, 2004.

12

Epidemiology and Natural History of Gastroesophageal Reflux Disease

Alexander P. Nagle · Nathaniel J. Soper

The prevalence of gastroesophageal reflux disease (GERD) in the United States is high, with approximately 20% of the population experiencing weekly symptoms. Despite the fact that GERD is common, understanding the epidemiology and natural history of GERD is hampered by several factors, including an evolving definition of GERD, lack of a diagnostic gold standard, and a paucity of population-based data. Furthermore, there is an unclear demarcation between physiologic reflux and gastroesophageal reflux as a disease. Consequently, our understanding of the true epidemiology and natural history of GERD is limited.

EPIDEMIOLOGY OF GERD

Prevalence estimates of GERD primarily depend on the definition used in a given study. In general, GERD has been defined as a disorder in which gastric contents recurrently reflux into the esophagus and cause heartburn and other symptoms. GERD is typically classified into erosive and nonerosive disease based on endoscopic findings. In the absence of a gold standard for diagnosing GERD, various investigators have applied symptoms, endoscopic findings, 24-hour esophageal pH monitor-

ing, or even response to acid inhibitor therapy in an attempt to define GERD. The American College of Gastroenterology suggests the following definition of GERD: "chronic symptoms or mucosal damage produced by the abnormal reflux of gastric contents into the esophagus."[1] A group of experts at the Geneva Workshop on Reflux Management offered the following definition of patients with nonerosive reflux disease (NERD): "These are individuals who satisfy the definition of GERD but who do not have either Barrett's esophagus or definite endoscopic esophageal breaks."[2] A similar definition, proposed by Waring, cites "burning retrosternal discomfort for at least 3 months, but with normal esophageal mucosa on upper endoscopy."[3] Fass et al. proposed a different definition for NERD that underscores the close relationship between symptoms and reflux of gastric contents.[4] They defined NERD as the presence of typical symptoms of GERD caused by intraesophageal gastric contents in the absence of visible esophageal mucosal injury on endoscopy. However, there remains debate regarding when the frequency of symptoms denotes gastroesophageal reflux the disease versus occasional heartburn. The demarcation between "physiologic" and abnormal acid reflux remains undefined.

The prevalence of GERD differs, depending on the variable measured. Most studies have focused on symptoms (primarily heartburn) or endoscopic findings (i.e., esophagitis). Unfortunately, each approach has limitations. Questionnaire studies are limited by the poor correlation between symptoms and objective findings. In addition, questionnaires often do not recognize the myriad of extraesophageal symptoms associated with GERD. Alternatively, investigators have sought to define the prevalence of GERD in populations with the use of physiologic data, such as endoscopy and 24-hour pH monitoring. Although this approach has the strength of more objective criteria on which to base the diagnosis, it is invasive, time-consuming and expensive. Endoscopy misses the large group of GERD patients, approximately 50%, who suffer from nonerosive disease. Although 24-hour esophageal pH testing is useful in defining GERD, it is too resource intensive for assessing population-based prevalence.

Epidemiology of GERD Symptoms

When based on symptoms, GERD is common in Western countries (Table 12–1). In a nationwide population based study by the Gallup Organization in the United States, 44% of the population reported heartburn at least once a month.[6] Another survey of presumably healthy hospital employees demonstrated that 7% reported symptoms of heartburn daily and an additional 14% experienced it weekly.[5] More convincing data were obtained by Locke et al., who mailed out 2200 validated self-report questionnaires to a predominantly white population residing in Olmsted County Minnesota.[10] The prevalence of heartburn and acid regurgitation in the previous 12 months was noted to be 42% and 45%, respectively. Frequent symptoms occurring at least weekly were reported by 20% of respondents, with an equal gender distribution across all ages (Fig. 12–1). The majority reported that the heartburn was of moderate

---

Table 12–1 Studies Reporting GERD Symptoms by Questionnaire

Reference	Population	Symptoms Elicited	Frequency Reported	Percentage Affected
Nebel et al. (1976)[5]	U.S. hospital workers	Heartburn	Daily	7
Gallup Poll (1988)[6]	General U.S. sample	Heartburn	Monthly	44
			Weekly	14
			Yearly	42
		Acid regurgitation	Weekly	6
			Yearly	45
Jones et al. (1990)[7]	United Kingdom	Heartburn	Previous 6 months	18
Ruth et al. (1991)[8]	Sweden	Heartburn	Overall prevalence	21
		Regurgitation	Overall prevalence	20
Isolauri et al. (1995)[9]	Finland	Heartburn	That day	9
			Previous week	15
			Previous month	21
			Previous year	27
		Regurgitation	That day	5
			Previous week	15
			Previous month	29
			Previous year	45
Locke et al. (1997)[10]	Olmsted County, MN	Heartburn	Weekly	18
Norrelund and Pederson (1998)[11]	Norway	Heartburn	Previous 6 months	12
		Regurgitation	Previous 6 months	9
Valle et al. (1999)[12]	Italy	Heartburn	Daily	2.3
			Weekly	5.4
			Monthly	5.6
		Acid regurgitation	Daily	1.3
			Weekly	5.3
			Monthly	7
Frank et al. (2000)[13]	US and Canada	Heartburn	Weekly	6.2
			Previous 3 months	19.5
Louis et al. (2002)[14]	Belgium	Heartburn	Daily	6.3
			Weekly	11.3

Modified from Shaheen N, Provenzale D: The epidemiology of gastroesophageal reflux disease. Am J Med Sci 326:265, 2003.

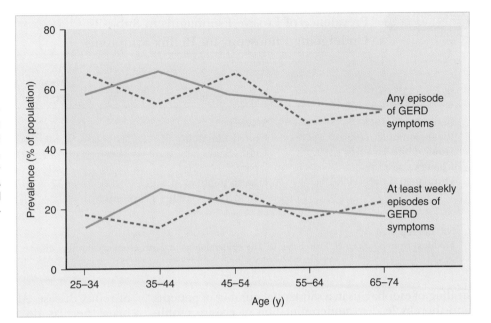

Figure 12–1. Prevalence of heartburn by age and sex in a random population sample. (Modified from Locke GR III, Talley NJ, Fett SL, et al: Prevalence and clinical spectrum of gastroesophageal reflux: A population-based study in Olmsted County, Minnesota. Gastroenterology 112:1448-1456, 1997.)

severity and had a duration of 5 years or longer, and only 5.4% reported a physician visit for reflux complaints within the previous year.

These data are similar to those of a recent Canadian study involving 1036 subjects in which the prevalence of heartburn in the previous 3 months was 43%; symptoms of moderate severity occurred at least once a week in 13%.[15] More variable prevalence rates for symptomatic GERD have been reported from Europe, with a range of 5% in Switzerland to 27% in Finland.[9] A Swedish study demonstrated a 21% cross-sectional prevalence of heartburn symptoms. Twenty percent also reported regurgitation and 12% reported noncardiac chest pain.[8] This population was evaluated 10 years later, and the prevalence of heartburn, acid regurgitation, and chest pain was essentially unchanged.[16] Louis et al. recently attempted to define the prevalence of heartburn in 2000 randomly selected Belgians.[14] They found that 6.3% of the population experienced daily substernal chest burning and 11.3% had weekly symptoms. Twenty-seven percent reported that they found their heartburn symptoms to interfere greatly with their daily activities. Similarly, Valle et al. recently reported on an Italian cohort of factory and hospital workers. They found that 21% described at least monthly symptoms of heartburn or regurgitation.[12]

As mentioned previously, prevalence estimates based on symptoms are limited by the poor correlation between symptoms and objective findings. This in part relates to the fact that GERD symptoms are not always caused by esophageal acid exposure. There are sufficient data to suggest that acid is not the only intraesophageal stimulus that can lead to a heartburn sensation. In fact, heartburn appears to be the "common pathway" of a variety of intraesophageal events, of which acid reflux is only one.

Epidemiology of GERD Based on Endoscopic Assessment

The prevalence of erosive esophagitis in the general population is difficult to ascertain in the absence of population-based studies. Estimates suggest that 7% of persons in the United States have erosive esophagitis.[17] Akdamar et al. reported that among 355 healthy volunteers undergoing upper endoscopy before inclusion in clinical trials, 13.8% had abnormal endoscopic findings and 8.5% had erosive esophagitis.[18] A study from China estimated a 5% rate of erosive esophagitis.[19] The prevalence of erosive esophagitis in those with reflux symptoms has also been extensively studied. There is a broad range in the reported prevalence of erosive esophagitis in those undergoing endoscopy in the literature, with rates ranging from 10% to 60% (Table 12–2). This range may represent underlying differences in the patients being studied, as well as differences in the availability of health services. In addition, many patients with GERD symptoms never seek medical attention. Voutilainen et al. performed upper endoscopy on 1128 Finnish patients with complaints of dyspepsia and reflux symptoms.[23] They found 25% of their population to have erosive esophagitis. In subjects complaining solely of reflux symptoms, 38% had esophagitis. Venables et al., in a multicenter study in the United Kingdom, studied the prevalence of esophagitis in patients in a general practice with heartburn as a predominant symptom.[24] Of the 944 patients studied, 32% were noted to have erosive esophagitis. One of the strengths of this study was the rapid access to endoscopy (within 14 days) from the time of the first evaluation in the primary care setting and the absence of antisecretory medications pending endoscopic evaluation. A considerable time lapse between clinical assessment and endoscopic evaluation may allow

Table 12–2 Prevalence of Erosive Esophagitis in Subjects Undergoing Endoscopy for Reflux Symptoms

Reference	Patient Population	Mean Age (yr)	Gender (% Female)	Erosive Esophagitis (%)
Behar et al. (1976)[20]	Sweden	52	64	35
Johansson et al. (1986)[21]	United Kingdom	NR	38	9.9
Howard and Heading (1992)[22]	Unites States	55.2	56	46
Chang et al. (1997)[19]	Japan	NR	38%	18.5
Voutilainen et al. (2000)[23]	Finnish population with dyspepsia or reflux symptoms	57	58	60

NR, not reported.

Modified from Shaheen N, Provenzale D: The epidemiology of gastroesophageal reflux disease. Am J Med Sci 326:269, 2003.

healing of esophagitis in a substantial number of patients and thereby lead to underestimation of erosive esophagitis. Achem et al. observed that the use of antisecretory medications may have accounted for the false-negative endoscopic results in up to 50% of patients with NERD.[25] Additionally, several groups have attempted to quantitate the amount of reflux in the normal population by 24-hour pH studies.[26,27] These studies have demonstrated considerable overlap between those with proven GERD and asymptomatic control subjects.[28,29] Thus, approximately a third to at most half of patients with GERD symptoms who seek medical help have erosive esophagitis. The amount of reflux experienced in the esophagus correlates only loosely with the signs and symptoms of reflux disease.

Population Risk Factors for GERD

Although GERD is ubiquitous, several risk factors have been suggested. The effect of age on the prevalence of reflux disease is inconsistent in the literature. Several groups have demonstrated that GERD symptoms are more common in older populations.[30,31] A Veterans Affairs study found evidence that more severe manifestations of reflux, such as strictures and ulcers, occur more commonly in elderly patients, probably as a result of cumulative acid injury to the esophagus over time. However, the finding of increasing prevalence of GERD symptoms with increasing age is not seen in all studies.[10] Some investigators have even found a negative association between GERD symptoms and age, with younger subjects suffering more severe symptoms than older persons.[7,32] Population-based studies also suggest a correlation between reflux symptoms and obesity. In morbidly obese patients, rates of both asymptomatic and symptomatic reflux have been reported to be high and directly correlate with weight.[33-36] The pathophysiology is most likely increased intra-abdominal pressure resulting in alterations in the gastroesophageal junction. Dietary factors, primarily high-fat diets, have been associated with a higher prevalence of GERD. The presence of a hiatal hernia has also been linked to more severe forms

of reflux disease. Although the majority of subjects with hiatal hernias do not have esophagitis, it has been demonstrated that most subjects with esophagitis do have a hiatal hernia.[37,38] Among those with esophagitis, the size of the hiatal hernia is also correlated with the severity of esophagitis, with those possessing the largest hernias having the most severe mucosal disease.[38,39] Additionally, Barrett's esophagus seems to be more common in those with a hiatal hernia.[40] Analysis of the gender ratio of patients with symptomatic GERD shows nearly equal proportions of men and women affected, but a male preponderance occurs with esophagitis (2 : 1 to 3 : 1) and Barrett's esophagus (10 : 1).[41-43] Pregnancy is associated with the highest incidence of symptomatic GERD; 48% to 79% of pregnant women complain of heartburn.[44] All forms of GERD affect whites more frequently than members of other races. There have been several case reports in the literature describing families with multiple members who have documented GERD. Jochem et al. described a family spanning three generations in which six cases of Barrett's esophagus were detected.[45] The acquisition of Barrett's esophagus was compatible with an autosomal form of inheritance. However, family members usually share other environmental risk factors for reflux besides genetic make-up. More research is needed regarding the genetic contribution to GERD.

The role of *Helicobacter pylori* with regard to the epidemiology of GERD remains unanswered. el-Serag and Sonnenberg observed opposing time trends in the prevalence of peptic ulcer disease and GERD in the United States: rates of peptic ulcer and gastric cancer fell between 1970 and 1995, whereas the prevalence of GERD and esophageal adenocarcinoma rose significantly (Fig. 12–2).[46] The authors speculated that the decreasing prevalence of *H. pylori* might play a contributory role to the increased prevalence of GERD. Data suggest that *H. pylori*–induced gastritis involves both the antrum and corpus and affects the parietal cell, thus reducing acid secretion and elevating gastric pH. Such infection may have a protective influence on the esophageal mucosa in patients susceptible to GERD. Furthermore, reversal of gastritis-associated hypochlorhydria renders individuals more susceptible to reflux of acid

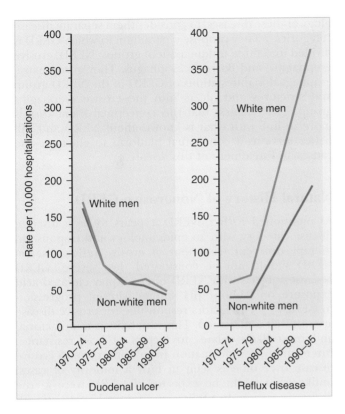

Figure 12–2. Opposing time trends in the rates of hospitalization for duodenal ulcer and gastroesophageal reflux disease. The computerized database of the U.S. Department of Veteran Affairs was used to analyze hospitalization rates. (Modified from El-Serag HB, Sonnenberg A: Opposing time trends of peptic ulcer and reflux disease. Gut 43:327-333, 1998.)

and the development of erosive esophagitis. Labenz et al. monitored patients with duodenal ulcer after antibiotic cure of *H. pylori* infection for 3 years.[47] The incidence of reflux esophagitis was 25.8% after eradication of *H. pylori* versus 12.9% in patients with persistent infection. Other groups have also observed higher rates of *H. pylori* infection in patients without than in those with severe forms of esophagitis characterized by erosions and Barrett's esophagus. Additional data suggest that *H. pylori* infection improves the efficacy of antisecretory therapy in healing esophagitis and maintaining remission.[48,49] These epidemiologic data have led some to believe that *H. pylori* should not be eradicated in patients with GERD. However, the fact that *H. pylori* is a risk factor for the development of peptic ulcer and gastric cancer has caused many practitioners to be uncomfortable with that recommendation. Long-term epidemiologic studies will be required to address this question more appropriately.

Finally, there is evidence that psychosocial factors promote health care seeking for GERD. Johnston et al. evaluated new patients with the primary complaint of heartburn and compared them with community controls with and without reflux symptoms.[50] They found that age and symptom severity were associated with seeking medical care. However, after controlling for these factors, they also found a higher incidence of phobia, obsessive disorder, and somatization in patients seeking medical care. Presumably, the interaction of heartburn with psychosocial factors is therefore relevant in promoting care seeking. Whether treatment of psychosocial distress assists in providing symptom relief has not been adequately explored.

Regional Variation in the Prevalence of GERD

Investigators internationally have attempted to describe the prevalence of reflux symptoms in their populations. The prevalence of GERD varies markedly between different populations. It seems that the prevalence of GERD symptoms and signs is greater in Western countries than in African or Asian cultures. Ho et al. recently described the prevalence of reflux symptoms in 696 randomly selected Chinese, Malays, and Indians living in Singapore.[51] They found that the prevalence of at least monthly heartburn among the Chinese, Malays, and Indians was 0.4%, 3.0%, and 5.3%, respectively. Corresponding percentages for at least monthly acid regurgitation among Chinese, Malays, and Indians were 0.4%, 2.1%, and 4.8%. These numbers are clearly lower than comparable percentages from Western populations. Chang et al. performed an endoscopic study of 2044 symptomatic Chinese patients.[19] They found that the incidence of erosive esophagitis in their cohort was 5%, much lower than that observed in Western cohorts. Of those who did have esophagitis, almost 90% had mild disease. Similarly, a recent publication reporting on the prevalence of GERD symptoms and complications in sub-Saharan Africa noted that "there are too few reports of GERD to allow analysis."[52] From these studies, it seems that the prevalence of GERD symptoms in non-Western cultures is significantly less than in the West. Possible reasons for the lower GERD prevalence include low dietary fat, lower body mass index, and lower maximal acid output related to infection with *H. pylori*.

Increasing Prevalence of GERD

One question of great importance, currently unanswered, is whether the prevalence of GERD is increasing. There is reason to believe that GERD may be becoming more common in the U.S. population. Hospitalization rates for erosive esophagitis, sometimes used as a surrogate for reflux disease, have increased severalfold over the past 3 decades.[53] Using the database of the Department of Veterans Affairs, el-Serag and Sonnenberg found that a discharge diagnosis of erosive esophagitis, esophageal ulcer, esophageal stricture, or hiatal hernia increased fourfold in nonwhites and sevenfold in whites between the periods 1970-1974 and 1990-1995.[46] Obesity, a putative risk factor for GERD, has been rising in epidemic proportions in the United States. In addition, esophageal adenocarcinoma, the cancer with which GERD is associated, has undergone a substantial increase in incidence over the last 30 years.[54] In the late 1970s, squamous cell carcinoma accounted for 70% of all esophageal tumors whereas adenocarcinoma accounted for only 17%. However, since then the prevalence of adenocarcinoma of the esophagus has continued to increase alarmingly; it now accounts for more than 50% of all esophageal cancers. Lagergren et al. have recently shown that adenocarcinoma of the esophagus was strongly associated with the presence of reflux disease (odds ratio, 44).[55] This association was found to be independent of the presence of Barrett's esophagus.

NATURAL HISTORY OF GERD

GERD is a chronic medical disorder, similar to arthritis or hypertension. Although reflux symptoms may appear to wax and wane, they probably do not disappear permanently in the majority of patients who seek medical care. Antisecretory medications, especially proton pump inhibitors, have made a tremendous impact on GERD and have resulted in significantly improved healing rates of erosive lesions and better symptom control. Consequently, erosive disease–related complications, such as esophageal strictures, have decreased significantly. Thus, medication use has probably modified the natural history of GERD. As a result, conducting studies in patients not exposed to medical therapy is now rare; it is ethically difficult to justify withholding therapy from patients with erosive esophagitis.

Traditionally, patients with erosive esophagitis were thought to have a more severe form of GERD and thus were at greater risk for complications such as stricture, ulcer, Barrett's esophagus, and even adenocarcinoma of the esophagus. The focus of esophageal mucosal injury as a step in disease progression was further reinforced by the concept that GERD is a "spectrum" of disease: on one end are patients with classic symptoms of GERD (heartburn and acid regurgitation) but without any evidence of mucosal injury, and on the other end are patients with erosive esophagitis and GERD complications. The "spectrum" hypothesis assumes that patients with GERD symptoms but no esophageal inflammation (NERD) represent only a milder form of the disease, a concept that resulted in a decade of therapeutic studies focused exclusively on GERD patients with erosive esophagitis. However, recent studies have demonstrated that patients with NERD are less likely to achieve complete symptomatic relief and need a longer time for symptom resolution during proton pump inhibitor therapy. Additionally, Fenton et al. reported that patients with NERD undergoing laparoscopic Nissen fundoplication are less likely to achieve symptom improvement or resolution, are more likely to experience postoperative dysphagia, and more commonly report dissatisfaction with surgery.[56] This unpredictable response to antireflux treatment in GERD patients without esophageal injury has perplexed many investigators. Consequently, much of the research interest in GERD in the last few years has shifted to further understanding of this disorder. Fass and Ofman have recently suggested that instead of looking at reflux disease as a continuum from nonerosive to erosive to stricture to Barrett's esophagus, it may be more appropriate, with regard to the epidemiology and pathophysiology of these diseases, to consider them separate disease categories.[57] They propose a paradigm in which GERD is divided into three unique patient groups: NERD, erosive esophagitis, and Barrett's esophagus. They group extra-esophageal manifestations of GERD in the NERD group and strictures and ulcers into the erosive esophagitis group. They suggest that this conceptual framework is more in line with what is known about NERD and will better serve as a conceptual platform to elucidate the causes and treatment of this disease.

Natural History of Nonerosive GERD

As mentioned earlier, NERD appears to be a discrete disease category, with an epidemiology and response to therapy different from that of erosive reflux disease. NERD should not be considered "less severe" GERD because subjects with NERD often display elevated acid exposure on 24-hour pH studies without progression to GERD.[58,59] The factors responsible for erosive disease are not well understood. This variability is multifactorial and most likely relates to factors of host resistance. Interestingly, transformation from nonerosive to erosive disease over time is seen in only a minority of cases, unlike what might be expected if GERD were a true disease spectrum. In a follow-up study of 17 patients with NERD over a 39-month period, McDougall et al. noted the development of new erosions in 24%.[53] At 6-month follow-up, Pace et al. observed new erosive changes in 15% of subjects with NERD treated with antacids or prokinetic drugs.[60] Unfortunately, both these studies are limited by small numbers, and further research is needed to truly understand the natural history of NERD. Currently, no data demonstrate an increased risk for Barrett's esophagus or esophageal adenocarcinoma in these patients over the long term.

Natural History of Erosive GERD

Although GERD symptoms may wax and wane over time, the data available suggest a more predictable course for those with erosive esophagitis. Since the early 1990s, proton pump inhibitors have been accepted as the mainstay of therapy for erosive GERD. Proton pump inhibitors not only have a greater success rate in healing than H_2 receptor antagonists do but also achieve healing faster. However, an important clinical question is whether ongoing medical therapy is required on a long-term basis after successful healing of esophageal erosions. Numerous studies have evaluated the course of erosive GERD patients with and without ongoing prophylactic therapy after the healing phase. Controlled studies have consistently showed that in the absence of ongoing maintenance therapy, a large number (up to 85%) of patients with erosive GERD will relapse within 6 months and the relapse rate is highest in those with the most severe grades of inflammation.

Most of the reported literature has focused on the short-term assessment of relapse, with only a few small case series reporting follow-up longer than 1 year. McDougall et al. conducted a postal questionnaire follow-up of 101 patients with erosive GERD 11 years after their initial diagnosis.[61] Only 15% of the patients remained asymptomatic without the use of medications. A further 26% reported infrequent symptoms, provided that they took regular antisecretory medications. However, the majority (51%) continued to have at least weekly symptoms of heartburn; half this group was taking regular antisecretory medication. The prevalence of endoscopically confirmed esophagitis in this study was unknown because the repeat endoscopy rate was only 8%. Based on this study, it appears that most patients with erosive GERD at index endoscopy will require chronic medical therapy. The long-term natural history of GERD in the absence of antisecretory therapy was retrospectively studied by Isolauri et al. in Finland.[62] Patients with symptomatic GERD were treated with lifestyle modification, antacids, prokinetic therapy, or any combination of these measures between 1973 and 1976. At initial assessment, 20 patients had erosions, but Barrett's esophagus was not found in any patient. After a median follow-up of 19 years, 14 patients continued to have erosions, but 6 new cases of long-segment Barrett's esophagus were detected. All cases of Barrett's esophagus developed in patients with previously documented erosive esophagitis. This suggests that suboptimal treatment of erosive esophagitis may have the potential to lead to the development of Barrett's esophagus. Furthermore, it has been shown that the degree of abnormal esophageal acid exposure directly correlates with the severity of esophagitis and is predictive of the development of stricture. An estimated 10% of patients who seek medical attention have strictures. However, up to a quarter of those with strictures do not have significant heartburn or regurgitation. In patients with Barrett's esophagus, strictures develop in 19% to 81%. Conversely, up to 50% of stricture are associated with Barrett's esophagus.

It is accepted that Barrett's esophagus results from chronic GERD. The prevalence of long-segment Barrett's metaplasia in patients who undergo upper gastrointestinal endoscopy is approximately 1% and increases with increasing severity of GERD.[63-65] In patients with GERD symptoms, the prevalence of Barrett's mucosa is 4.5% to 20%. In the United States, the average age of affected patients is 55 to 65 years, with a male-to-female ratio of 10:1 and a white-to-African American ratio of 10:1.[17,66] Although the annual incidence of adenocarcinoma in patients with long-segment Barrett's metaplasia has been reported to be as high as 1.5%,[67] an analysis in 2000 suggested that this risk is overestimated because of publication bias and that the actual incidence is probably closer to 0.5% per year.[68] Short-segment Barrett's metaplasia is clearly more prevalent than long-segment Barrett's metaplasia, but the precise incidence is difficult to define because published reports do not distinguish it from gastric cardia intestinal metaplasia. Although dysplasia and adenocarcinoma have been reported in patients with short-segment Barrett's metaplasia, the magnitude of this risk is unknown; reports attempting to quantify it concluded that the malignant potential of short-segment Barrett's metaplasia was much lower than that of long-segment Barrett's metaplasia.[69-72]

GERD would appear to be associated with a very low mortality rate. However, if one accepts that the development of Barrett's esophagus is part of the natural history of chronic GERD, death from adenocarcinoma should also be considered in the overall mortality figures for GERD.

CONCLUSION

Although GERD is widely reported to be one of the most prevalent clinical conditions afflicting the gastrointestinal tract, incidence and prevalence figures are based more on estimates than on actual data. This difficulty occurs partly because GERD and esophagitis cannot be differentiated by clinical history and partly because there is no gold standard for the recognition or exclusion of GERD. NERD is a relatively newly appreciated entity and may be more difficult to treat than classic erosive disease. Evidence is accumulating that these patients should be viewed as having a separate disease entity, not just a mild form of classic GERD. Large-scale, prospective data collection with standardized terminology and longitudinal follow-up will allow a clearer picture of the incidence, prevalence, natural history, and complications of GERD.

REFERENCES

1. DeVault KR, Castell DO: Updated guidelines for the diagnosis and treatment of gastroesophageal reflux disease. The Practice Parameters Committee of the American College of Gastroenterology. Am J Gastroenterol 94:1434-1442, 1999.
2. Dent J, Brun J, Fendrick AM, et al: An evidence-based appraisal of reflux management: The Geneva Workshop Report. Gut 44(Suppl 2):S1-S16, 1999.
3. Waring JP: Nonerosive reflux disease. Semin Gastrointest Dis 12:33-37, 2001.
4. Fass R, Fennerty MB, Vakil N: Nonerosive reflux disease—current concepts and dilemmas. Am J Gastroenterol 96:303-314, 2001.
5. Nebel OT, Fornes MF, Castell DO: Symptomatic gastroesophageal reflux: Incidence and precipitating factors. Am J Dig Dis 21:953-956, 1976.
6. A Gallup Organization national survey: Heartburn across America. Princeton, NJ, Gallup Organization, 1988.
7. Jones RH, Lydeard SE, Hobbs FD, et al: Dyspepsia in England and Scotland. Gut 31:401-405, 1990.
8. Ruth M, Mansson I, Sandberg N: The prevalence of symptoms suggestive of esophageal disorders. Scand J Gastroenterol 26:73-81, 1991.
9. Isolauri J, Laippala P: Prevalence of symptoms suggestive of gastro-oesophageal reflux disease in an adult population. Ann Med 27:67-70, 1995.
10. Locke GR III, Talley NJ, Fett SL, et al: Prevalence and clinical spectrum of gastroesophageal reflux: A population-based study in Olmsted County, Minnesota. Gastroenterology 112:1448-1456, 1997.
11. Norrelund N, Pederson PA: Prevalence of gastroesophageal reflux–like dyspepsia. Int Congr Gastroenterol 4:A10, 1998.
12. Valle C, Broglia F, Pistorio A, et al: Prevalence and impact of symptoms suggestive of gastroesophageal reflux disease. Dig Dis Sci 44:1848-1852, 1999.
13. Frank L, Kleinman L, Ganoczy D, et al: Upper gastrointestinal symptoms in North America: Prevalence and relationship to healthcare utilization and quality of life. Dig Dis Sci 45:809-818, 2000.
14. Louis E, DeLooze D, Deprez P, et al: Heartburn in Belgium: Prevalence, impact on daily life, and utilization of medical resources. Eur J Gastroenterol Hepatol 14:279-284, 2002.

15. Tougas G, Chen Y, Hwang P, et al: Prevalence and impact of upper gastrointestinal symptoms in the Canadian population: Findings from the DIGEST study. Am J Gastroenterol 94:2845-2854, 1999.

16. Ruth M, Mjornheim AC, Lundell L: Symptoms suggestive of esophageal disorders in a normal population—a 10 year follow-up study. Gastroenterology 112:A41, 1997.

17. Spechler SJ: Epidemiology and natural history of gastro-oesophageal reflux disease. Digestion 51(Suppl 1):24-29, 1992.

18. Akdamar K, Ertan A, Agrawal NM, et al: Upper gastrointestinal endoscopy in normal asymptomatic volunteers. Gastrointest Endosc 32:78-80, 1986.

19. Chang C-S, Poon S-K, Lien HC, et al: The incidence of reflux esophagitis among the Chinese. Am J Gastroenterol 92:668-671, 1997.

20. Behar J, Biancani P, Sheahan DG: Evaluation of esophageal tests in the diagnosis of reflux esophagitis. Gstroenterology 71:9-15, 1976.

21. Johansson KE, Ask P, Boeryd B, et al: Esophagitis, signs of reflux, and gastric acid secretion in patients with symptoms of gastroesophageal reflux disease. Scand J Gastroenterol 21:837-847, 1986.

22. Howard PJ, Heading RC: Epidemiology of gastroesophageal reflux disease. World J Surg 16:288-293, 1992.

23. Voutilainen M, Sipponen P, Mecklin JP, et al: Gastroesophageal reflux disease: Prevalence, clinical, endoscopic and histopathological findings in 1,128 consecutive patients referred for endoscopy due to dyspeptic and reflux symptoms. Digestion 61:6-13, 2000.

24. Venables TL, Newland RD, Patel AC, et al: Omeprazole 10 milligrams once daily, omeprazole 20 milligrams once daily, or ranitidine 150 milligrams twice daily, evaluated as initial therapy for relief of symptoms of gastro-esophageal reflux disease in general practice. Scand J Gastroenterol 32:965-973, 1997.

25. Achem SR, Malhi-Chowla N, David D, et al: The prevalence of endoscopic negative gastro-esophageal reflux at a tertiary care center. Gastroenterology 116:A107, 1997.

26. Katzka DA, Gideon RM, Castell DO: Normal patterns of acid exposure at the gastric cardia: A functional midpoint between the esophagus and stomach. Am J Gastroenterol 93:1236-1242, 1998.

27. Wiener GJ, Morgan TM, Copper JB, et al: Ambulatory 24-hour esophageal pH monitoring. Reproducibility and variability of pH parameters. Dig Dis Sci 33:1127-1133, 1988.

28. Weusten BL, Roelofs JM, Akkermans LM, et al: Objective determination of pH thresholds in the analysis of 24 h ambulatory oesophageal pH monitoring. Eur J Clin Invest 26:151-158, 1996.

29. Gastal OL, Castell JA, Castell DO: Frequency and site of gastroesophageal reflux in patients with chest symptoms. Studies using proximal and distal pH monitoring. Chest 106:1793-1796, 1994.

30. Wienbeck M, Barnert J: Epidemiology of reflux disease and reflux esophagitis. Scand J Gastroenterol Suppl 156:7-13, 1989.

31. Mold JW, Reed LE, Davis AB, et al: Prevalence of gastroesophageal reflux in elderly patients in a primary care setting. Am J Gastroenterol 86:965-970, 1991.

32. El Serag HB, Sonnenberg A: Associations between different forms of gastro-oesophageal reflux disease. Gut 41:594-599, 1997.

33. Fisher BL, Pennathur A, Mutnick JL, et al: Obesity correlates with gastroesophageal reflux. Dig Dis Sci 44:2290-2294, 1999.

34. Rigaud D, Merrouche M, Le Moel G, et al: Factors of gastroesophageal acid reflux in severe obesity. Gastroenterol Clin Biol 19:818-825, 1995.

35. Ruhl CE, Everhart JE: Overweight, but not high dietary fat intake, increases risk of gastroesophageal reflux disease hospitalization: The NHANES I Epidemiologic Followup Study. First National Health and Nutrition Examination Survey. Ann Epidemiol 9:424-435, 1999.

36. Locke GR III, Talley NJ, Fett SL, et al: Risk factors associated with symptoms of gastroesophageal reflux. Am J Med 106:642-649, 1999.

37. Berstad A, Weberg R, Froyshov Larsen I, et al: Relationship of hiatus hernia to reflux oesophagitis. A prospective study of coincidence, using endoscopy. Scand J Gastroenterol 21:55-58, 1986.

38. Petersen H, Johannessen T, Sandvik AK, et al: Relationship between endoscopic hiatus hernia and gastroesophageal reflux symptoms. Scand J Gastroenterol 26:921-926, 1991.

39. Jones MP, Sloan SS, Rabine JC, et al: Hiatal hernia size is the dominant determinant of esophagitis presence and severity in gastroesophageal reflux disease. Am J Gastroenterol 96:1711-1717, 2001.

40. Avidan B, Sonnenberg A, Schnell TG, et al: Hiatal hernia and acid reflux frequency predict presence and length of Barrett's esophagus. Dig Dis Sci 47:256-264, 2002.

41. Hirota WK, Loughney TM, Lazas DJ, et al: Specialized intestinal metaplasia, dysplasia, and cancer of the esophagus and esophagogastric junction: Prevalence and clinical data. Gastroenterology 116:277-285, 1999.

42. Reynolds JC, Rahimi P, Hirschl D: Barrett's esophagus: Clinical characteristics. Gastroenterol Clin North Am 31:441-460, 2002.

43. Avidan B, Sonnenberg A, Schnell TG, et al: Hiatal hernia size, Barrett's length, and severity of acid reflux are all risk factors for esophageal adenocarcinoma. Am J Gastroenterol 97:1930-1936, 2002.

44. Bainbridge ET, Temple JG, Nicholas SP, et al: Symptomatic gastro-oesophageal reflux in pregnancy: A comparative study of white Europeans and Asians in Birmingham. Br J Clin Pract 37:53-57, 1983.

45. Jochem VJ, Fuerst PA, Fromkes JJ: Barrett's esophagus associated with adenocarcinoma. Gastroenterology 102:1400-1402, 1992.

46. el-Serag HB, Sonnenberg A: Opposing time trends of peptic ulcer and reflux disease. Gut 43:327-333, 1998.

47. Labenz J, Blum AL, Bayerdorffer E, et al: Curing *Helicobacter pylori* infection in patients with duodenal ulcer may provoke reflux esophagitis. Gastroenterology 112:1442-1447, 1997.

48. Verdu EF, Armstrong D, Idstrom JP, et al: Effect of curing *Helicobacter pylori* infection on intragastric pH during treatment with omeprazole. Gut 37:743-748, 1995.

49. Labenz J, Tillenburg B, Peitz U, et al: *Helicobacter pylori* augments the pH-increasing effect of omeprazole in patients with duodenal ulcer. Gastroenterology 110:725-732, 1996.

50. Johnston BT, Gunning J, Lewis SA: Health care seeking by heartburn sufferers is associated with psychosocial factors. Am J Gastroenterol 12:2500-2504, 1996.

51. Ho KY, Kang JY, Seow A: Prevalence of gastrointestinal symptoms in a multiracial Asian population, with particular reference to reflux-type symptoms. Am J Gastroenterol 93:1816-1822, 1998.

52. Segal I: The gastro-oesophageal reflux disease complex in sub-Saharan Africa. Eur J Cancer Prev 10:209-212, 2001.

53. McDougall NI, Johnston BT, Collins JSA, et al: Disease progression in gastro-esophageal reflux disease as determined by repeat esophageal pH monitoring and endoscopy 3 to 4.5 years after diagnosis. Eur J Gastroenterol Hepatol 9:1161-1167, 1997.

54. Devesa SS, Blot WJ, Fraumeni JF Jr: Changing patterns in the incidence of esophageal and gastric carcinoma in the United States. Cancer 83:2049-2053, 1998.

55. Lagergren J, Bergstrom R, Lindgren A, Nyren O: Symptomatic gastroesophageal reflux as a risk factor for esophageal adenocarcinoma. N Engl J Med 340:825-831, 1999.

56. Fenton P, Terry ML, Galloway KD, et al: Is there a role for laparoscopic fundoplication in patients with non-erosive reflux disease (NERD)? Gastroenterology 118:A481, 2000.

57. Fass R, Ofman JJ: Gastroesophageal reflux disease—should we adopt a new conceptual framework? Am J Gastroenterol 97:1901-1909, 2002.

58. Lind T, Havelund T, Carlsson R, et al: Heartburn without oesophagitis: Efficacy of omeprazole therapy and features determining therapeutic response. Scand J Gastroenterol 32:974-979, 1997.

59. Juul-Hansen P, Rydning A, Jacobsen CD, et al: High-dose proton-pump inhibitors as a diagnostic test of gastro-oesophageal reflux disease in endoscopic-negative patients. Scand J Gastroenterol 36:806-810, 2001.

60. Pace F, Santalucia F, Bianchi PG: Natural history of gastro-oesophageal reflux disease without oesophagitis. Gut 32:845-848, 1991.

61. McDougall NI, Johnston BT, Collins JS, et al: Three- to 4.5-year prospective study of prognostic indicators in gastro-oesophageal reflux disease. Scand J Gastroenterol 33:1016-1022, 1998.

62. Isolauri J, Luostarinen M, Isolauri E, et al: Natural course of gastroesophageal reflux disease: 17-22 year follow-up of 60 patients. Am J Gastroenterol 92:37-41, 1997.

63. Cameron AJ, Zinsmeister AR, Ballard DJ, Carney JA: Prevalence of columnar-lined (Barrett's) esophagus: Comparison of population-based clinical and autopsy findings. Gastroenterology 99:918-922, 1990.

64. Spechler SJ, Zeroogian JM, Antonioli DA, et al: Prevalence of meta-plasia at the gastro-oesophageal junction. Lancet 344:1533-1536, 1994.

65. Winters C Jr, Spurling TJ, Chobanian SJ, et al: Barrett's esophagus: A prevalent, occult complication of gastroesophageal reflux disease. Gastroenterology 92:118-124, 1987.

66. Wienbeck M, Barnert J: Epidemiology of reflux disease and reflux esophagitis. Scand J Gastroenterol Suppl 156:7-13, 1989.

67. Drewitz DJ, Sampliner RE, Garewal HS: The incidence of adeno-carcinoma in Barrett's esophagus: A prospective study of 170 patients followed 4.8 years. Am J Gastroenterol 92:212-215, 1997.

68. Shaheen NJ, Crosby MA, Bozymski EM, Sandler RS: Is there pub-lication bias in the reporting of cancer risk in Barrett's esophagus? Gastroenterology 119:333-338, 2000.

69. Schnell TG, Sontag SJ, Chejfec G: Adenocarcinomas arising in tongues or short segments of Barrett's esophagus. Dig Dis Sci 37:137-143, 1992.

70. Sharma P, Morales TG, Sampliner RE: Short segment Barrett's esophagus—the need for standardization of the definition and of endoscopic criteria. Am J Gastroenterol 93:1033-1036, 1998.

71. Weston AP, Krmpotich PT, Cherian R, et al: Prospective long-term endoscopic and histological follow-up of short segment Barrett's esophagus: Comparison with traditional long segment Barrett's esophagus. Am J Gastroenterol 92:407-413, 1997.

72. Hirota WK, Loughney TM, Lazas DJ, et al: Specialized intestinal metaplasia, dysplasia, and cancer of the esophagus and esopha-gogastric junction: Prevalence and clinical data. Gastroenterology 116:277-285, 1999.

The Pathology of Gastroesophageal Reflux Disease

Parakrama Chandrasoma

Gastroesophageal reflux, which is defined as the entry of gastric contents into the esophagus, is an extremely common event that occurs sporadically in most people. Reflux is caused by failure of the normal lower esophageal sphincter mechanism. As Allison, in the first accurate description of reflux esophagitis in 1948,[1] stated: "A failure of this mechanism will allow acid to reach the esophagus, and in time this leads inevitably to inflammation and ulceration." At that time, ulceration and strictures were the dominant problems in patients with reflux disease. Since that time, other consequences of esophageal epithelial damage have been recognized: columnar-lined esophagus, first described by Allison and Johnstone in 1953[2] and correctly named by Barrett in 1957,[3] and adenocarcinoma of the esophagus. The last 3 decades have seen an alarming increase in the incidence of adenocarcinoma of the esophagus, which is now the most rapidly increasing cancer type in Western Europe and North America.[4,5] There is also a parallel, but less dramatic increase in the incidence of adenocarcinoma of the cardia.[6,7] Symptomatic gastroesophageal reflux is a risk factor for both esophageal and cardia adenocarcinoma, with odds ratios of 7.7 (confidence interval [CI], 5.3 to 11.4) and 2.0 (CI, 1.4 to 2.9), respectively, for those with symptoms and those without.[8] The risk increased with reflux severity; patients with long-standing and severe reflux symptoms had odds ratios of 43.5 for the development of esophageal adenocarcinoma and 4.4 for the development of adenocarcinoma of the cardia. The same study showed no increase in the incidence of squamous carcinoma of the esophagus in patients with reflux. This establishes that gastroesophageal reflux is very likely the cause of adenocarcinoma of the esophagus and cardia as defined in this study.

The amount of reflux into the esophagus can be assessed by determining the presence of some measurable component of the gastric refluxate, such as acid (the ambulatory 24-hour pH test)[9] or bilirubin (Bilitec test),[10] and by performing impedance studies, which detect the retrograde entry of fluid into the esophagus.[11] Studies using 24-hour pH testing have documented that symptoms associated with reflux occur when the pH is less than 4 for a period exceeding 4.5% of the 24-hour period.[12] It should be recognized that 4.5% of a 24-hour period is 64.8 minutes, which means that esophageal epithelium exposed to a pH less than 4 for less than 1 hour per day is not usually associated with symptoms. There is a probability that exposure not sufficient to cause symptoms may produce significant cellular pathologic changes in the esophagus; it is only when we develop the ability to recognize subclinical early disease that we will be able to begin making an effective impact on it. There is strong indirect evidence for subclinical reflux disease in that a significant number of patients with reflux-induced adenocarcinoma of the lower part of the esophagus have never had any symptoms of reflux.

The gastroesophageal refluxate contains many chemicals, including endogenous secretory products of the stomach such as acid and pepsin; duodenal contents such as the secretory products of the intestine, bile, and pancreatic juice, which frequently enter the stomach via duodenogastric reflux; and exogenous chemicals ingested as food. Correlation of esophageal damage with acid exposure by a 24-hour pH study does not necessarily indicate that the damage is caused by acid. The 24-hour pH study simply quantitates the amount of reflux; any injury-causing molecule in the refluxate that accompanies the acid will show a correlation with the 24-hour pH study abnormality. The 24-hour pH study is better than Bilitec for quantitating reflux because of the more constant presence of acid in the refluxate. This is not true, however, in patients who have atrophic gastritis and those taking acid-suppressive medications. Impedance studies have shown continuing reflux in patients taking acid-suppressive drugs, thus indicating that the esophageal epithelium continues to be subject to other molecules in the gastric refluxate after acid secretion has been suppressed.

Acid suppression has been the mainstay of treatment of reflux disease. In effect, this has been a human experiment over the past several decades that can be used to provide important conclusions. The manifestations of reflux disease that have declined in frequency, such as ulceration and stricture, are very likely directly caused by acid. Others such as Barrett's esophagus and adenocarcinoma, which have increased in prevalence, are very likely caused by unidentified molecules in the gastric refluxate other than acid.

There has been an unusual dichotomy in the minds of physicians treating patients with reflux, and this dichotomy persists to date. Reflux disease is seen as a squamous epithelial disease classified by symptoms as typical and atypical, classified by endoscopy as erosive and nonerosive, and graded by systems such as the Savary-Miller and Los Angeles systems by endoscopic changes in the squamous epithelium. Patients with reflux disease are treated by acid suppression, and the success of treatment is defined by relief of symptoms and healing of erosions.

Although everyone agrees that a columnar-lined esophagus is caused by reflux, physicians tend to regard it as a separate entity. When they see a columnar-lined esophagus, the intent is to make a diagnosis of Barrett's esophagus, which requires the presence of intestinal metaplasia in a biopsy specimen. This enters the patient into an endoscopic surveillance program to detect the occurrence of dysplasia and early adenocarcinoma. There is almost no recognition in practice that a columnar-lined esophagus is a manifestation of reflux disease and can be used to diagnose and classify reflux disease. The link that must exist between the pathology of reflux and Barrett's esophagus and adenocarcinoma is almost completely ignored.

DEFINITION OF NORMAL ENDOSCOPY AND HISTOLOGY

With most organs, normalcy is defined by autopsy examination of large numbers of patients of all ages who have never had symptoms related to that organ during life. When these are compared with the same organs that have had evidence of disease during life, differences between the normal and pathologic state can be determined. This usual method of establishing normalcy never occurred with regard to the epithelium of the esophagus. The new millennium dawned before the first autopsy study of the gastroesophageal junctional epithelium was published. The rapid postmortem autolysis that occurs in the columnar epithelium of the gastrointestinal tract after death is a serious deterrent to autopsy study. As a result, normalcy with regard to the esophagus was historically defined by the study of esophagectomy specimens and endoscopy, which are performed in

patients with the highest likelihood of esophageal disease. We must recognize that defining normalcy by studying an abnormal population is a potential source of serious error.

In 1961, Hayward defined normalcy for the anatomy and histology of the lower part of the esophagus.[13] Hayward did not cite any data for his conclusions but obviously drew from his experience with surgical specimens and endoscopy. According to Hayward, the distal 1 to 2 cm of the tubular esophagus was lined by columnar epithelium of cardiac (or junctional) type. This led to the general belief that persisted well into the 1990s that columnar lining in the distal tubular esophagus should be regarded as abnormal only if it exceeds 3 cm in length.

The recognition of short-segment Barrett's esophagus in the 1990s resulted in a change in the definition of normalcy.[14] As endoscopy became a common procedure, it was seen that squamous epithelium frequently extended to the end of the tubular esophagus. Endoscopic normalcy was therefore defined as the absence of any visible columnar lining in the esophagus (Box 13–1). The normal squamocolumnar junction was coincident with the proximal limit of the gastric rugal folds, which had become recognized as the best endoscopic indicator of the true gastroesophageal junction. This led to the recommendation that patients with any endoscopically visualized columnar epithelium in the esophagus undergo biopsy. When intestinal metaplasia is present in this biopsy tissue, a diagnosis of Barrett's esophagus is made; long- and short-segment disease is defined according to whether the endoscopic segment is greater or less than 2 cm (Figs. 13–1 and 13–2). Incredibly, when the biopsy specimen does not reveal intestinal metaplasia, the patient reverts to being classified as "normal," and the fact that there was an endoscopically visualized columnar-lined esophagus is largely ignored in practice (see Box 13–1).

Hayward also presented contradictory opinions in his paper about the distal extent of cardiac mucosa.[13] On the one hand he says that cardiac mucosa "extends a little way into the stomach" and has an illustration that clearly shows cardiac mucosa lining the proximal part of the stomach. On the other hand, Hayward states: "I suggest that junctional (cardiac) epithelium should be regarded as esophageal" and "the stomach should be described as lined by two sorts of epithelium, fundal and pyloric, except for a small area around the esophageal opening where esophageal junctional epithelium protrudes into it." Despite his stated belief that cardiac mucosa was esophageal, the effect of Hayward's paper was to establish a dogma that cardiac mucosa normally lined the proximal part of the stomach. This has no basis in fact, but exists to the present time.

When we performed our first autopsy study in the mid-1990s,[15] it was generally accepted that the distal 2 to 3 cm of the esophagus and an undefined part of the proximal stomach were normally lined by cardiac mucosa. Our autopsy study included 18 subjects who were prospectively studied by removing the gastroesophageal region and sectioning it vertically to examine the entire circumference microscopically. Astonishingly, 10 (56%)

Box 13–1   **Presently Accepted Endoscopic and Biopsy Definitions of Normal and Pathologic States**

1. **Endoscopic normalcy**: Coincidence of the squamocolumnar junction (Z-line) and the gastroesophageal junction (proximal limit of the rugal folds). There is no visible columnar lining in the esophagus, either as tongues of mucosa extending into the squamous epithelium or as a circumferential columnar-lined region in the tubular esophagus that separates the squamocolumnar junction from the proximal limit of the rugal folds.

2. Columnar-lined esophagus >3 cm (2 cm in some studies) with biopsy specimens showing intestinal metaplasia: **long-segment Barrett's esophagus.**

3. Columnar-lined esophagus >3 cm (2 cm in some studies) with biopsy specimens showing no intestinal metaplasia: **no conclusion.**

4. Columnar-lined esophagus <3 cm (2 cm in some studies) with biopsy specimens showing intestinal metaplasia: **short-segment Barrett's esophagus.**

5. Columnar-lined esophagus <3 cm (2 cm in some studies) with biopsy specimens showing no intestinal metaplasia: **normal or no conclusion.**

6. The practice guidelines of the American Gastroenterology Association recommend that patients who are endoscopically normal should not undergo biopsy. This recommendation is a statement that **ignorance is bliss.**

7. When there is no endoscopic abnormality and biopsy specimens show intestinal metaplasia, confusion reigns; some call this **"ultrashort-segment Barrett's esophagus"** and others call it **"intestinal metaplasia of the gastric cardia."**

8. When there is no endoscopic abnormality and biopsies show no intestinal metaplasia: **normal.**

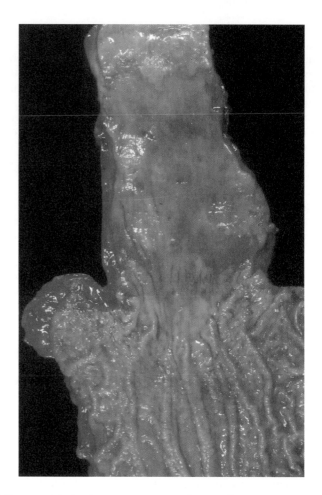

Figure 13–1. Long-segment columnar-lined esophagus characterized by flat columnar epithelium extending from the proximal limit of the rugal folds to the irregular squamocolumnar junction near the top of the picture. This is pathognomonic grossly and endoscopically for severe reflux disease. It is Barrett's esophagus only if intestinal metaplasia is demonstrated by biopsy.

subjects had no cardiac mucosa whatever, and those who did all had lengths of cardiac mucosa that were all less than 1 cm. The presence of cardiac mucosa in everyone was a myth when scientifically studied in an appropriate normal population for the first time (Figs. 13–3 and 13–4).

Jain et al.[16] confirmed the fact that cardiac mucosa is infrequently present at the junction in what is the only "normal" population studied. Many of these were patients who were undergoing upper endoscopic screening for nonesophageal diseases; many did not have clinical evidence of reflux, and the gastroesophageal region was endoscopically normal. Only 35% of these patients had cardiac mucosa in extensive sampling biopsies. Even studies in clinical endoscopy units with a bias toward patients with reflux show patients without cardiac mucosa, though much less frequently. Marsman et al.[17] found that pure cardiac mucosa was absent in 38% of patients in whom the actual squamocolumnar junction was present in the biopsy specimen. The data in these studies strongly suggest that cardiac mucosa is not universally present in the gastroesophageal junction and therefore highly unlikely to be normal epithelium.

If it is accepted that cardiac mucosa does not normally exist, the definition of histologic normalcy becomes feasible and in line with the endoscopic definition (Box 13–2). Normal histology can be defined as an esophagus that is completely lined by squamous epithelium (Fig. 13–5), ends normally at the squamocolumnar junction, and transitions at that point to gastric oxyntic mucosa (Fig. 13–6), which is characterized by rugal folds. Only two histologic zones exist normally: esophageal squamous epithelium and gastric oxyntic mucosa. The lower esophageal sphincter protects the

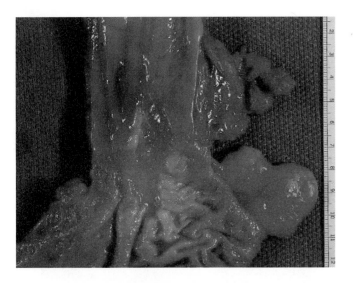

Figure 13–2. Short-segment columnar-lined esophagus characterized by flat columnar epithelium extending from the proximal limit of the rugal folds to the irregular squamocolumnar junction. This is pathognomonic of reflux disease of a lesser severity than in Figure 13–1. It is Barrett's esophagus only if intestinal metaplasia is demonstrated by biopsy.

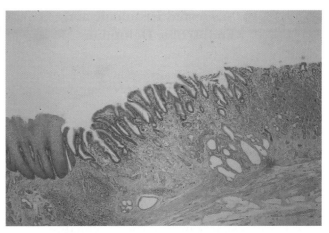

Figure 13–4. Squamocolumnar junction in a patient undergoing esophagectomy for squamous carcinoma of the midesophagus (hematoxylin-eosin stain). There is an approximately 0.6-cm length of cardiac mucosa interposed between the squamous epithelium (the Z-line) and gastric oxyntic mucosa (the gastroesophageal junction). This cardiac mucosa represents metaplastic columnar-lined esophagus, which is cellular evidence of reflux-induced damage.

squamous epithelium from gastric contents by normally preventing gastroesophageal reflux. A normal person has no acid-induced damage of the esophageal squamous epithelium. Endoscopy will be normal, the 24-hour pH study will be normal, and histology will reveal only squamous and gastric oxyntic mucosa.

We have proposed this concept of histologic normalcy for many years.[18] Although the trend is toward slow

acceptance, most people still continue to believe that a third histologic zone characterized by cardiac mucosa normally exists between esophageal squamous epithelium and gastric oxyntic mucosa. Authorities holding this belief agree that this zone is as small as 1 mm in some patients and almost always less than 5 mm. Marsman et al. hold this belief despite the fact that their own excellent study showed an absence of cardiac mucosa in 38% of patients.[17] Old dogmas die painfully, and the dogma that cardiac mucosa is found normally in the gastroesophageal junctional region is close to its demise. The problem is that until this dogma dies, there can be no histologic definition of normal. A biopsy sample showing cardiac mucosa can be considered "normal gastric

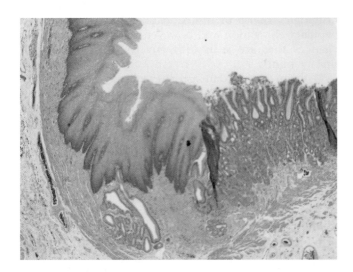

Figure 13–3. Squamocolumnar junction in a patient undergoing esophagectomy for squamous carcinoma of the midesophagus (hematoxylin-eosin stain). The squamous epithelium of the esophagus transitions directly to gastric oxyntic mucosa without intervening columnar-lined esophagus. This patient has no cellular evidence of reflux-induced damage.

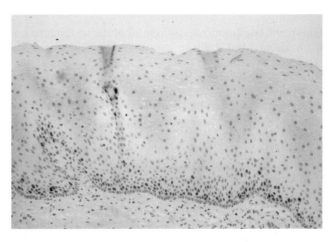

Figure 13–5. Normal squamous epithelium showing proliferative cells in the basal region (immunoperoxidase stain for Ki67).

Box 13–2 ## Suggested Histologic and Endoscopic Definitions

1. **Endoscopic normalcy:** coincidence of the squamocolumnar junction (Z-line) and the gastroesophageal junction (proximal limit of the rugal folds). There is no visible columnar lining in the esophagus.

2. **Histologic normalcy:** coincidence of the distal limit of the squamous epithelium and the proximal limit of gastric oxyntic mucosa. There is no microscopic esophageal metaplastic columnar epithelium between the two.

3. **Endoscopic columnar-lined esophagus:** the presence of any columnar epithelium between the squamocolumnar junction (Z-line) and the proximal limit of the gastric rugal folds, either as tongues of mucosa extending into the squamous epithelium or as a circumferential columnar-lined region that separates the squamocolumnar junction from the proximal limit of the rugal folds.

4. **Histologic columnar-lined esophagus:** the presence of any microscopic metaplastic esophageal columnar epithelium between the squamous epithelium and gastric oxyntic mucosa.

5. **Metaplastic esophageal columnar epithelium:** Cardiac mucosa with and without intestinal metaplasia and oxyntocardiac mucosa.

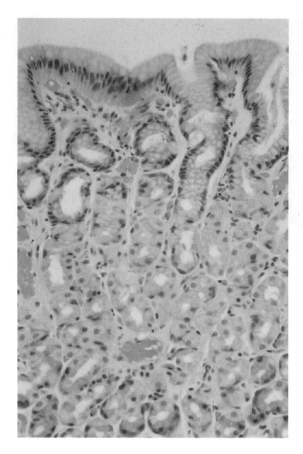

Figure 13–6.   Normal oxyntic mucosa of the stomach characterized by straight tubular glands composed of parietal and chief cells below the short foveolar pit (hematoxylin-eosin stain).

mucosa" or "normal esophageal epithelium" by those holding the belief that such mucosa is normal.

PATHOLOGY OF GASTROESOPHAGEAL REFLUX

Acid-Induced Damage

The stratified squamous epithelium of the esophagus has an unknown, but definite amount of resistance to acid exposure. Although reflux is an almost universal phenomenon, a majority of the adult population do not have symptoms of reflux. The structure of stratified squamous epithelium is designed to withstand injury; squamous cells have tight cell junctions that form an effective barrier to resist penetration by luminal molecules (see Fig. 13–5).

As the amount of acid exposure increases, the ability of squamous epithelium to resist injury is overwhelmed. The first change is most likely an increased rate of loss of surface cells, which stimulates a compensatory increase in the rate of proliferation of basal esophageal stem cells. Increased proliferative activity is manifested histologically by basal cell hyperplasia and elongation of the papillae of the epithelium. Expression of proliferative markers such as Ki67 is increased. These are the first

identifiable changes of reflux and are recognized as histologic criteria of reflux. Basal cell hyperplasia and papillary elongation are, however, relatively nonspecific changes that are seen with any cause of esophageal surface injury.

With increasing damage, the cell junctions between squamous cells separate, thereby resulting in dilated intercellular spaces. Tobey et al. showed by electron microscopic measurement that an increase in intercellular spaces results from exposure of esophageal squamous epithelium to acid.[19] Villanacci et al. have demonstrated that the severity of dilatation of intercellular spaces correlates with the severity of reflux.[20] This finding, which is equivalent to spongiosis of squamous epithelium, is a common finding in biopsy specimens from patients with reflux disease (Fig. 13–7).

Entry of acid into the epithelium produces direct cell damage that very likely results in the liberation of cytokines that stimulate sensory nerve endings in the epithelium, thereby causing heartburn. The fact that this symptom is effectively controlled by acid-suppressive drugs provides evidence that stimulation of nerve endings is an acid-dependent phenomenon.

The cell damage must also result in the release of cytokines that are chemotactic for eosinophil leukocytes.

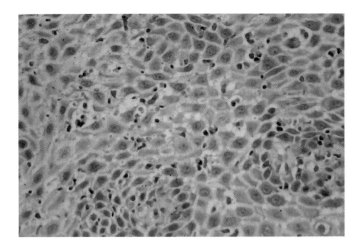

Figure 13–7. Reflux esophagitis showing squamous epithelium with intraepithelial eosinophils and separation of squamous cells (dilated intercellular spaces) (hematoxylin-eosin stain).

Intraepithelial eosinophils are a recognized criterion of reflux damage to squamous epithelium (see Fig. 13–7). The presence of intraepithelial eosinophils is nonspecific; eosinophils enter squamous epithelium in conditions other than reflux, such as eosinophilic esophagitis, which has an allergic basis.

With further cell damage, erosion and finally ulceration of the epithelium may occur. With ulceration, fibrosis of the submucosa and deeper layers may follow and lead to shortening of the esophagus and circumferential strictures. In the early days, the main clinical problem associated with reflux disease was the occurrence of ulcers and strictures. With the increasing efficacy and use of acid-suppressing agents in the treatment of reflux disease, complicated and nonhealing ulcers and complex strictures have become relatively uncommon. This suggests that acid is primarily responsible for the erosions and ulcerations that occur in squamous epithelium.

Separation of the tight junctions between squamous cells increases the permeability of squamous epithelium to luminal molecules. Tobey et al. have shown that in vitro exposure of squamous epithelium to acid permits the entry of small molecules up to 20 kD all the way down to the basal region of the epithelium.[21] Tobey and colleagues' studies are extremely valuable because the esophageal epithelium was exposed in vitro to acid alone and the damage described can therefore be directly attributed to acid. No other molecule in the refluxate has been shown to cause separation of squamous cells, and it is very likely that this is a unique injurious effect attributable to acid.

Acid is the key that opens the lock of the squamous epithelial barrier. Its action allows all the other molecular intruders in gastric refluxate to enter the squamous epithelium and interact with the proliferating stem cell population that is normally sequestered in the basal region.

Esophageal Squamous Epithelium Primed by Acid-Induced Damage

Whereas normal esophageal squamous epithelium has the capacity to resist the entry of luminal molecules, acid-damaged squamous epithelium permits the entry of such molecules. The degree of separation of squamous cells varies with the severity of acid-induced damage. With mild damage, only very small molecules enter the superficial region of the epithelium; as damage levels increase, the epithelium very likely becomes increasingly permeable to larger particles that penetrate a greater distance into the epithelium. With the maximum acid-induced damage, the squamous epithelium displays the characteristics of Tobey and colleagues' experimental model in which molecules up to a size of 20 kD penetrate the full thickness to reach the basal region of the squamous epithelium.[21]

Many patients with symptoms of reflux do not have erosive esophagitis. This condition has been termed nonerosive reflux disease (NERD). No histologic abnormality has been associated with NERD, largely because physicians perceive reflux disease as a purely squamous epithelial abnormality. These patients have intact and histologically normal esophageal squamous epithelium that, however, has been primed by acid-induced damage; light microscopy is not a sensitive method of detecting dilated intercellular spaces. Although it looks normal, the acid-primed squamous epithelium is like a sieve that permits the entry of small molecules.

Normal esophageal squamous epithelium is a dynamic structure that is multilayered and continually undergoing renewal. The renewal is directed by continuous proliferation of esophageal stem cells located in the basal layer of the epithelium (see Fig. 13–5). These stem cells are identical to the fetal foregut stem cells from which the esophagus developed. In the early fetal foregut, the esophageal stem cells were columnar in nature until the 20th week of gestation, when they acquired a genetic signal that directed squamous differentiation.[22,23] It should be recognized that the esophageal stem cell retains its multipotential capability to differentiate in any direction seen in the endoderm. The fact that it produces squamous epithelium means only that it expresses the genetic signal that directs squamous differentiation while genes that direct other types of differentiation are suppressed. The normal genetic signaling mechanism that directs squamous differentiation is yet unknown.

The esophageal stem cells proliferate during life to replace cells that are continuously lost at the surface. The first division of the stem cell in the basal zone produces a daughter cell that has been given the genetic signal to become squamous. This daughter cell divides a few times while differentiating into a keratinizing squamous cell and moves up the stratified epithelium to the surface. The average time for the daughter cell to be lost at the surface is 7.5 days.[24] By the time that it reaches the midregion of the stratified squamous epithelium, the cell has become terminally differentiated and incapable of mitotic division. This can be demonstrated by Ki67 staining. Ki67, which is an antigen expressed in cells that are in the mitotic cycle,[25] shows positive staining restricted to the basal two to three cell layers.

Epithelium that is primed by acid damage is different. Luminal molecules permeate through the epithelium and can reach the normally sequestered stem cells at the base of the epithelium. Interactions between these luminal molecules and surface receptors on the actively proliferating multipotential stem cells now become possible. These interactions must form the basis for the genetic changes that occur in these cells to drive the further evolution of this pathologic process.

Columnar Transformation—The First Genetic Switch

Columnar transformation has long been recognized as a complication of gastroesophageal reflux. Hayward, in 1961,[13] describes the process well: "When the normal sphincteric and valvular mechanism in the lower oesophagus and oesophago-gastric junction . . . fails, . . . reflux from the stomach occurs and acid and pepsin reach the squamous epithelium and begin to digest it. . . . In quiet periods some healing occurs, and in these periods the destroyed squamous epithelium may re-form, often with . . . junctional epithelium, usually not very healthy-looking. . . . Further reflux therefore attacks principally the squamous epithelium higher up. In the next remission it may be replaced by more junctional epithelium. . . . With repetition over a long period the metaplastic junctional epithelium may creep higher and higher. . . ."

Hayward, as did Barrett before him, believed that this process required erosion of the squamous mucosa.[3,13] It is now apparent that columnar transformation occurs without ulceration. Nonerosive acid-primed squamous epithelium, which has increased permeability, permits small molecules in the refluxate to enter the epithelium and, when the damage is severe, reach the basal region. These luminal molecules can interact with receptors on the surface of the proliferating stem cells. Such interactions can have many potential effects, but the one that is significant is columnar transformation of the epithelium. The exact mechanism by which this transformation takes place is not known, but it must involve a change in the genetic signal in the stem cell from squamous to columnar differentiation. This change can be either suppression of the normal squamous genetic signal, thereby permitting the epithelium to revert to its original fetal columnar state, or activation of a new genetic signal that directs columnar differentiation. The genetic basis for columnar metaplasia is not yet known, but its existence can be assumed by recognizing the phenotypic expression of the change, which is columnar transformation of the squamous epithelium.

The daughter cell of stem cell division that is given the genetic signal to differentiate into a columnar cell develops features of columnar cells, not squamous cells. One inevitable effect is the loss of normal cellular attachments, which results in loss of adhesion between the new columnar cell and its squamous neighbors and ultimately converts the area of epithelium involved into columnar epithelium. The area involved is short, possibly one cell,

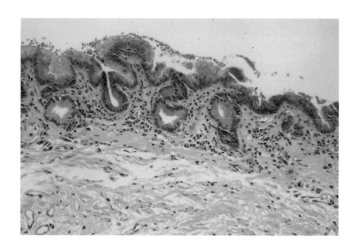

Figure 13–8. Newly formed metaplastic cardiac mucosa characterized by mucous cells lining the surface and a short foveolar pit (hematoxylin-eosin stain). Note the presence of chronic inflammatory cells in the lamina propria.

but as described by Hayward, the change is cumulative and results in a progressive increase in the amount of squamous epithelium that undergoes columnar transformation.[13]

The histologic product of the initial columnar metaplasia of esophageal epithelium is columnar epithelium devoid of specialized cells; these cells are recognized histologically as mucous cells, and the mucosa falls within the definition of cardiac mucosa (Fig. 13–8). The newly formed cardiac mucosa is interposed between the squamocolumnar junction and gastric oxyntic mucosa. In the earliest stages, the cardiac mucosa is so short that it is detectable only by histology; these patients have a normal appearance at endoscopy. When the columnar transformation reaches sufficient length, it becomes visible endoscopically as flat columnar epithelium interposed between the tops of the rugal folds and the squamocolumnar junction (see Fig. 13–2). This columnar epithelium may be seen as irregular tongues extending up into the squamous epithelium or as a circumferential segment.

Columnar transformation of the esophageal squamous epithelium to form cardiac mucosa is a change that is highly specific for reflux. It requires acid damage of the squamous epithelium to cause increased permeability, followed by a genetic switch resulting from an interaction between an unknown molecule in the refluxate and the esophageal stem cell. Although there is strong evidence that acid acts as the key to permitting access to the squamous epithelium, it is very likely that a molecule other than acid is responsible for the actual genetic switch that leads to columnar transformation in the stem cell. This is strongly suggested by the fact that columnar-lined esophagus has increased in prevalence in the past 3 decades despite increasingly effective acid suppression.

Cardiac Mucosa Is Reflux Carditis

The presence of cardiac mucosa between the squamous epithelium and gastric oxyntic mucosa has been incorrectly interpreted as normal gastric mucosa for nearly a century. The reason for this is surprising. Because autopsy studies were never performed, the original histologic data came from the study of esophagectomy specimens. The first successful thoracic esophagectomy was reported in 1913.[26] Between that time and 1953, when Allison and Johnstone first introduced the concept of columnar-lined esophagus,[2] the esophagus was thought to end at the squamocolumnar junction. Early histologists, studying abnormal esophagectomy specimens in the elderly, found cardiac mucosa distal to the squamous epithelium. In line with the definition of the time, they concluded that cardiac mucosa normally lined the proximal part of the stomach. This simple error led to great confusion. When Allison and Johnstone described the columnar-lined esophagus in 1953, they called it "oesophagus lined by gastric mucous membrane."[2] In 1957, Barrett disagreed with Allison's term and coined the more accurate term columnar-lined esophagus[3]; Barrett was stating the obvious: the esophagus is lined by esophageal epithelium, not gastric epithelium.

There has never been any evidence that cardiac mucosa is present in the true stomach. Allison and Johnstone, in their 1953 description of the columnar-lined esophagus, clearly showed that cardiac mucosa is restricted to the esophagus.[2] In a beautiful description of one of their esophagectomy specimens, Allison and Johnstone showed that the mucosa distal to the peritoneal reflection, which is the most accurate external marker for the gastroesophageal junction, is gastric oxyntic mucosa. Hayward,[13] to whom the dogma that cardiac mucosa lines the proximal part of the stomach is often attributed, also placed cardiac mucosa in the esophagus and not in the stomach, although his illustration shows cardiac mucosa extending into the proximal portion of the stomach, thus contradicting the ideas expressed in his own paper.

There is a great deal of evidence supporting the concept that columnar metaplasia of squamous epithelium to produce cardiac mucosa is a reflux-induced event. Oberg et al. showed that the presence of cardiac mucosa in a biopsy sample taken at the junctional region is associated with abnormal reflux.[27] In a study of 334 patients, the 246 with cardiac mucosa had a significantly greater likelihood of abnormality in a 24-hour pH study, as well as lower esophageal sphincter abnormality, than did the 88 patients who did not have cardiac mucosa. Glickman et al.,[28] in a study of pediatric patients with reflux disease, showed that patients who had greater than 1 mm of cardiac mucosa distal to the squamocolumnar junction had a greater likelihood of reflux symptoms than did patients with less than 1 mm of cardiac mucosa. This finding indicates that even a minute amount of cardiac mucosa (1 mm is about 30 cells, assuming that a mucous cell is 30 μm in diameter) is predictive of reflux.

When found, cardiac mucosa is always inflamed and shows reactive villiform change in the epithelium (Fig. 13–9).[2] Der et al.[29] showed that the amount of chronic

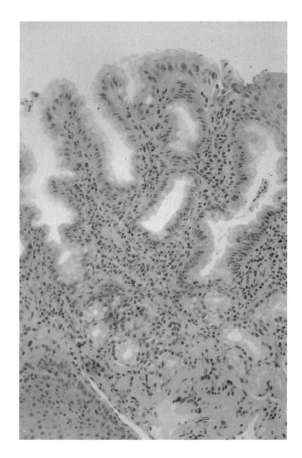

Figure 13–9. Well-formed cardiac mucosa showing only mucous cells (hematoxylin-eosin stain). There is evidence of damage indicated by severe chronic inflammation and by foveolar hyperplasia and serration, which has produced the villiform appearance typical of reflux carditis.

inflammation in cardiac mucosa correlates with 24-hour pH abnormality, thus making it likely that cardiac mucosa is damaged by the gastric refluxate. Because cardiac mucosa is always inflamed, its presence is equivalent to carditis. We believe there is adequate evidence that carditis is caused by reflux to use the term "reflux carditis." Because the generation of cardiac mucosa is a highly specific change that results from acid damage of esophageal squamous epithelium, followed by a genetic switch that causes the squamous stem cell to undergo cardiac metaplasia, we believe that reflux carditis is a highly specific histologic criterion of reflux disease. In fact, we use it to define reflux disease histologically.

There is controversy in the literature regarding the etiology of carditis. According to some authorities, carditis is a disease that can be produced by *Helicobacter pylori* infection, as well as by reflux.[30] Reports that show an association of carditis with *H. pylori* do not depend on histologic criteria to define carditis. Rather, they define carditis as the presence of inflammation in a biopsy sample taken distal to the anatomically defined gastroesophageal junction,[30] usually in patients with a normal endoscopic appearance. This definition is meaningless. In patients without reflux damage to squamous epithelium, a biopsy specimen immediately distal to the squamocolumnar junction will consist of gastric oxyntic mucosa, and inflammation therein is gastritis caused by *H. pylori* or autoimmunity. In patients who have microscopic reflux disease, a biopsy sample distal to the squamocolumnar junction contains reflux-induced cardiac mucosa; in these patients carditis will correlate with reflux. Cardiac mucosa is never generated from any change in gastric oxyntic mucosa; it is specific for acid-induced columnar metaplasia of the esophagus. Atrophy of gastric mucosa in chronic gastritis may result in loss of parietal cells in gastric mucosa and give rise to a flat mucosa composed of only mucous cells; this is atrophic gastritis, not carditis. No study in the literature that has defined carditis correctly by histologic criteria as inflamed cardiac mucosa has shown a relationship with anything other than reflux.[29,31,32]

Careful review of two papers shows that the lack of definition of terms plus failure to use histology is rife in the literature. A recent study in *Gastroenterology* by Rex et al.[33] in which screening biopsies of the region were evaluated for the prevalence of Barrett's esophagus shows the typical lack of histologic data. In 961 patients studied, visible columnar-lined esophagus was present in 176 patients, greater than 3 cm in 12 (all with intestinal metaplasia) and 0.5 to 3 cm in 164 (53 with intestinal metaplasia). There is no mention of histology apart from the presence or absence of intestinal metaplasia. A total of 940 patients in this study underwent biopsy of the cardia ("defined as the proximal edge of the gastric folds, just distal to the end of the tubular esophagus"); of these, "intestinal metaplasia (IM-cardia) was identified in 122 (12.9%)." There is no mention of any other histology except that seven of these patients had concomitant intestinal metaplasia in the tubular esophagus. Without knowledge of the histology in these cardiac specimens, it is impossible to know whether what the authors call IM-cardia is actually intestinal metaplasia in cardiac mucosa (which would be Barrett's esophagus because cardiac mucosa is esophageal metaplastic epithelium) or intestinal metaplasia in gastric oxyntic mucosa, which is atrophic gastritis. Lagergren and associates' highly influential report in the *New England Journal of Medicine* in 1999 uses the following definition in their methods section[8]:

> The distances between the gastroesophageal junction (defined as the point where the proximal longitudinal mucosal folds begin in the stomach) and the upper and lower borders of the tumor were measured. . . . For a case to be classified as a cancer of the gastric cardia, the tumor had to have its center within 2 cm proximal, or 3 cm distal, to the gastroesophageal junction,

According to these definitions, the *gastric cardia extends 2 cm proximal to the authors' own gastroesophageal junction!* Until reviewers of these most prestigious journals demand histologic data and standardize definitions, this subject will remain confused. The use of our suggested histologic definitions (see Box 13–2) is the only available answer to standardization because unlike clinical definitions, these histologic definitions are highly reproducible.[17,34,35]

We recommend using reflux carditis to define reflux disease at a cellular level. Its presence is a highly sensitive indicator of reflux. This definition converts reflux disease from a clinically defined entity to a histologically defined entity and forms a sound basis for scientific study. Patients with reflux carditis may or may not have symptoms; reflux carditis is the only method of identifying patients who have asymptomatic reflux. This is critical when one recognizes that the majority of patients with adenocarcinoma of the esophagus are asymptomatic. Patients with reflux carditis in a biopsy specimen may or may not have an abnormal 24-hour pH test. In our study, 39% of patients with reflux carditis had a pH test that was within the normal range.[29] It should not be surprising that levels of reflux insufficient to cause symptoms may cause cellular abnormalities. Reflux carditis is the histologic change seen in subclinical, asymptomatic reflux and in patients with symptoms who are presently classified as having NERD. Although the squamous epithelium is not eroded in these patients and although it may be histologically normal, it has undergone columnar transformation. Patients with NERD are histologically normal only because it is not recognized that their histologic abnormality is located in a place where it is not looked for; it is not in the squamous epithelium, but in the cardiac mucosa that is found immediately distal to the squamocolumnar junction.

The severity of reflux damage can be quantitated by the amount of squamous epithelium that has transformed into columnar epithelium. Csendes et al.[36] showed that the squamocolumnar junction moves proximally in a manner that correlated with the severity of reflux disease. We demonstrated that patients with greater than 2 cm of columnar transformation of the esophageal epithelium had highly significantly greater reflux by 24-hour pH study than did patients with less than 2-cm transformation.[37] Glickman et al.[28] showed that this correlation between reflux and the amount of cardiac mucosa present was significant at 1 mm, thus indicating that this is an exquisitely sensitive indicator of reflux disease.

The columnar transformation of squamous epithelium is a cumulative change. As Hayward described,[13] the amount of columnar metaplasia progressively increases with time. Because reflux is very common, the change is common. The number of people in the population who have cardiac mucosa is unknown but can be estimated as being between 35%, which was the number in Jain and colleagues' endoscopic study,[16] and 44%, which was the number in our autopsy study.[15] The prevalence is higher in clinical studies where there is an inevitable bias toward including patients with reflux. In our unit, 492 of 811 (60.5%) consecutive patients with less than 1 cm of columnar-lined esophagus had cardiac mucosa, with and without intestinal metaplasia.[38] In Marsman and associates' study, 62% of patients had cardiac mucosa.[17] Although the absence of cardiac mucosa is common in children, it becomes increasingly prevalent with increasing age.

We use these data to histologically grade reflux disease in a highly predictive manner as follows[27,37]: (1) *no evidence of reflux:* cardiac mucosa is absent in adequate biopsy samples taken from the junctional region in patients who are endoscopically normal; (2) *mild reflux:* cardiac mucosa is present in biopsy samples from patients without an endoscopically visible columnar-lined esophagus; (3) *moderate reflux:* cardiac mucosa is present in biopsy specimens from an endoscopically visible columnar-lined esophagus measuring less than 2 cm; and (4) *severe reflux:* cardiac mucosa present in biopsy specimens from an endoscopically visible columnar-lined esophagus measuring greater than 2 cm. This grading can be applied only if specimens are taken in a systematic manner at upper endoscopy, including specimens from patients who have no endoscopically visible abnormality. This practice is not presently recommended by the American Gastroenterology Association.

Evolution of Reflux Carditis

Hayward, in 1961, described cardiac mucosa as being an epithelium that was resistant to reflux.[13] Cardiac mucosa does not have any intraepithelial nerve endings and is probably less pain sensitive than squamous epithelium. However, there is much evidence that reflux damages cardiac mucosa. Cardiac mucosa invariably shows inflammation, with the number of eosinophils and plasma cells correlating with the severity of reflux, and it almost invariably displays reactive hyperplasia of the foveolar region, with elongation, serration, mucin distention of the cells, and smooth muscle proliferation (see Fig. 13–9).[29,39] In some cases, this hyperplastic cardiac mucosa produces small polypoid excrescences near the squamocolumnar junction.

The exact agents responsible for the damage to cardiac mucosa are unknown. These agents produce two effects on epithelial cells: (1) direct cell damage, which causes reactive hyperplasia, increased Ki67 expression, and chronic inflammation, and (2) molecular interactions at the cell surface that result in genetic changes. These genetic switches alter the differentiation model of cardiac mucosa and result in the development of specialized cells within the mucous cell–only cardiac mucosa. Many different types of specialized cells appear in metaplastic esophageal cardiac mucosa, including parietal cells, goblet cells, Paneth cells, pancreatic cells, and neuroendocrine cells. The appearance in cardiac mucosa of glands containing parietal cells is recognized as one of three main types of metaplastic esophageal epithelium (Fig. 13–10). Paull et al. called this fundic epithelium[35]; we call it oxyntocardiac mucosa because this epithelium is nowhere near the fundus of the stomach.[37] The appearance of goblet cells in cardiac mucosa results in intestinal metaplasia or the specialized columnar epithelium of Paull et al. (Fig. 13–11).[35,37]

Paull et al.,[35] in their classic study of the histology of columnar-lined esophagus, recognized that these three main epithelial types are seen in a very regular manner, and we have confirmed this finding.[40] When present, intestinal metaplasia was usually seen in the most proximal region of the segment of columnar-lined esophagus. The amount of intestinal metaplasia in any columnar-lined segment of esophagus varied from very short (one-gland Barrett's esophagus) to several centimeters.

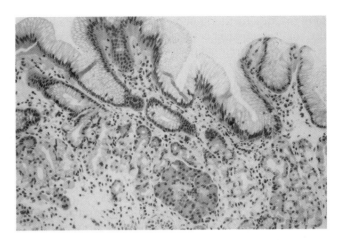

Figure 13–10. Oxyntocardiac mucosa showing lobulated glands containing parietal cells, mucous cells, and a focus of pancreatic metaplasia (hematoxylin-eosin stain). The chronic inflammation is mild.

In contrast, oxyntocardiac mucosa tends to be found in the more distal segment of the columnar-lined esophagus, a fact that was recognized even in Allison and Johnstone's original description of columnar-lined esophagus.[2] Cardiac mucosa was found proximal to oxyntocardiac mucosa and is frequently admixed with intestinal epithelium when the latter is present.

Intestinal Metaplasia—The Second Genetic Switch

Metaplastic cardiac mucosa in columnar-lined esophagus is an active epithelium. The proliferative stem cells are located in the basal region of the foveolar pit, where they multiply to renew the epithelium. The rate of proliferation depends on the rate of cell loss resulting from reflux-induced damage. Luminal molecules have access to the stem cells in cardiac mucosa and can interact with

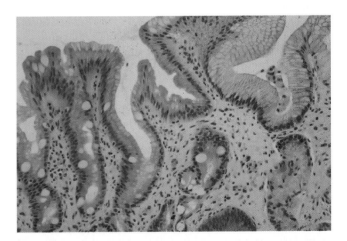

Figure 13–11. Intestinal metaplasia characterized by the presence of goblet cells (hematoxylin-eosin stain). Note the presence of residual nonintestinalized cardiac mucosa on the right side. Intestinal metaplasia defines Barrett's esophagus.

them to cause further genetic changes. Of these changes, intestinal metaplasia is the most important because it is necessary for carcinogenesis to progress.

There is good evidence that the genetic switch that causes intestinal differentiation in cardiac mucosa is activation of the *CDX* homeobox gene system, which includes CDX-1 and CDX-2.[41-43] These genes are suppressed in the normal esophagus and stomach. However, they are expressed in the normal small and large intestine and are believed to be the genes that drive differentiation in these sites.[41] CDX-2 is expressed in most cases of intestinal metaplasia of the esophagus.[42,43] In a quantitative study, we showed that CDX-2 expression was up-regulated in a stepwise manner from esophageal squamous epithelium (not expressed) to nonintestinalized cardiac mucosa (low level of expression) to intestinal metaplasia (highly significant expression). We interpreted these data to indicate that CDX-2 expression in the esophageal stem cell was the driving genetic signal causing intestinal metaplasia.

The pattern of CDX-2 expression in columnar epithelia of the esophagus also suggests that the metaplastic process is a multistep process: an intermediate columnar transformation to cardiac mucosa, followed by intestinal metaplasia in the cardiac mucosa. There is evidence from clinical observations to support such a two-step metaplastic process. Reflux-induced columnar-lined esophagus in children consists predominantly of cardiac mucosa without intestinal metaplasia.[44,45] After esophagectomy, cardiac mucosa develops in the esophagus above the anastomotic line in many patients. This progresses to intestinal metaplasia in some patients, often after many years.[46-48]

Recognition of this two-step process provides a potential method of preventing reflux-induced adenocarcinoma of the esophagus. Cardiac mucosa is easily identified by biopsy in the first phase of the metaplastic sequence, which can last many years before the development of intestinal metaplasia. Transformation of cardiac mucosa to intestinal metaplasia must occur as the result of an interaction of a luminal molecule and the stem cells in cardiac mucosa to cause CDX-2 activation. If this molecule can be identified and inactivated, CDX-2 activation and the resulting intestinal metaplasia in cardiac mucosa can be prevented. Because intestinal metaplasia is an essential precursor to reflux-induced carcinogenesis, prevention of CDX-2 activation will theoretically prevent the development of carcinoma.

Intestinal metaplasia does not occur randomly in the columnar-lined segment of the esophagus. Not only does intestinal metaplasia arise in the most proximal part of the columnar-lined segment, but there is also an increasing prevalence of intestinal metaplasia with increasing length of columnar-lined esophagus. In a study in which we mapped these epithelial types in columnar-lined esophagus,[38] almost 100% of patients with a columnar epithelium segment greater than 5 cm had intestinal metaplasia, as compared with 90% when the length was 3 to 4 cm, 70% when the length was 1 to 2 cm, and 15% when the length was less than 1 cm.

This distribution suggests that factors causing CDX-2 activation and intestinal metaplasia operate proximally in the esophagus much more than distally. Two reasons can be suggested for the proximal region of the esophagus providing a better milieu for intestinal metaplasia than the more distal region. First, it has been shown with the use of multiple-level pH electrodes that the pH tends to progressively increase more proximally in the esophagus. If the molecule that causes CDX-2 activation in cardiac mucosa is more active in an alkaline milieu, it could explain the distribution of intestinal metaplasia. Second, Fitzgerald et al.[49] have shown that pulse exposure to acid is associated with a greater proliferative rate in cells from columnar-lined esophagus than continuous exposure is. This suggests that pulse-type exposure is associated with a higher damage level than continuous exposure is. Pulse-type exposure is much more likely in the more proximal region of the esophagus, and the higher proliferative rate of the cells could also explain the higher likelihood of the genetic change required for intestinal metaplasia.

Oxyntocardiac Mucosa—The Benign Genetic Switch

Allison and Johnstone, in the original description of columnar-lined esophagus in 1953, recognized that the proximal region of the columnar-lined esophagus was lined by pure cardiac mucosa but that oxyntic (parietal) cells started appearing in the more distal region.[2] Paull et al., in their histologic classification of columnar-lined esophagus, recognized this mucosa, in which there are glands containing a mixture of parietal and mucous cells, as the third epithelial type; they called it "fundic" mucosa.[35] Because this has nothing to do with the gastric fundus, which is lined by pure gastric oxyntic mucosa, we prefer to use the term oxyntocardiac mucosa for this epithelium (see Fig. 13–10).[37]

Oxyntocardiac mucosa is an important epithelial type in the columnar-lined esophagus. As first reported by Paull et al. and confirmed by us, it is almost never associated with intestinal metaplasia.[35,38] As such, it is unlikely to progress to carcinogenesis; it is a benign epithelium.

Oxyntocardiac mucosa is formed when cardiac mucosa develops a genetic signal that causes its stem cells to differentiate into parietal cells and move downward into glands in the deeper part of the mucosa below the proliferative stem cell region in the base of the foveolar pit. Oxyntocardiac mucosa is very similar to gastric oxyntic mucosa, except for the presence of chronic inflammation, residual mucous cells in the glands, and frequent lobulation of the glands in contrast to the straight tubular glands of normal gastric mucosa (see Fig. 13–10). We postulate that oxyntocardiac mucosa develops when cardiac mucosa acquires a "gastric-type genetic signal" that results in the phenotypic expression of parietal cells that are highly specific for the stomach. The nature of this gastric-type genetic signal is unknown.

The distribution of oxyntocardiac mucosa in the columnar-lined esophagus is the exact opposite of intestinal metaplasia; it is present in the most distal segment.[2,35,40] It is the only epithelial type that is always present in the columnar-lined esophagus. In patients with very short (<1 cm) lengths of columnar-lined mucosa, oxyntocardiac mucosa represents the only metaplastic epithelium in about 20% of patients.[38] In our autopsy study, microscopic lengths of oxyntocardiac mucosa were present in some part of the squamocolumnar junction in all patients.[15] In these patients, all the cardiac mucosa had been transformed into oxyntocardiac mucosa.

The proliferative characteristics of oxyntocardiac mucosa show that it is less proliferative than cardiac and intestinal epithelia, thus indicating that it is associated with a low damage environment. The milieu in which oxyntocardiac mucosa occurs has damage factors that are opposite that in the proximal part of the esophagus (lower pH and continuous rather than pulse exposure to refluxate). The "gastric-type genetic signal" appears to be generated only in the low damage environment of the distal end of the esophagus.

Reversibility of Genetic Switches

We have suggested three genetic switches being responsible for the array of metaplasia that converts squamous epithelium to columnar. The first causes squamous epithelium to transform into undifferentiated cardiac mucosa composed of only mucous cells. Evolution of the columnar mucosa proceeds in one of two directions from cardiac mucosa. The development of a "gastric-type genetic signal" occurs in the low damage environment of the distal region and results in oxyntocardiac mucosa, which is characterized by the development of parietal cells. This is the benign pathway that is no longer susceptible to reflux-induced genetic transformations because it does not progress to intestinal metaplasia or adenocarcinoma. The second direction is the premalignant pathway. The development of intestinal-type genetic signals, probably the homeobox *CDX* genes, occurs in the high damage environment of the proximal end of the esophagus and results in the development of goblet cells, which defines intestinal (or Barrett-type) metaplasia. This is the only epithelium in columnar-lined esophagus that is at risk for the development of adenocarcinoma.

Genetic switches result from expression and suppression of normal genetic pathways in the cell as a result of cell surface interactions. They are reversible; removing or altering the surface interactions can drive these differentiation pathways in different directions. If this is true, intestinal metaplasia can revert back to cardiac mucosa if the *CDX* gene activation is reversed; cardiac mucosa can revert to squamous epithelium if it loses the first columnar genetic switch or becomes oxyntocardiac mucosa if it can be made to acquire the "gastric-type genetic signal." The ability to manipulate the columnar epithelia in the esophagus to move it away from intestinal metaplasia and toward squamous and oxyntocardiac mucosa is equivalent to preventing adenocarcinoma. We believe that the most beneficial reversion is the generation of oxyntocardiac mucosa because it is a full-thickness mucosal change. Squamous re-epithelialization of the surface is frequently associated with the presence of residual glandular elements below the epithelium, and these have been known to progress to adenocarcinoma.

The best method of manipulating these genetic shifts in columnar-lined esophagus is to characterize the nature of the interactions that cause the genetic changes and neutralize them. Until these specific interactions are characterized, however, the only logical method of achieving reversal is to alter the damage environment or abolish reflux completely. Acid-suppressive therapy is unlikely to achieve either of these goals; the reflux persists and may actually become even more alkaline, and the pulse effect does not change.[50] The fact that the prevalence of intestinal metaplasia and adenocarcinoma has risen even as acid suppression has improved is evidence that acid is a relatively minor factor in these genetic switches. On the other hand, successful antireflux surgery abolishes all reflux into the esophagus by creating a new valve. We have observed the phenotypic expression of some of these reversals; intestinal metaplasia accompanying short-segment Barrett's esophagus frequently reverses,[51] and we have observed an increased amount of oxyntocardiac mucosa in postfundoplication biopsy specimens as compared with preoperative specimens. Both these changes are highly beneficial and occur at a histologic level without any change in the endoscopic length of the columnar-lined esophagus. However, it is unlikely that fundoplication will have an impact on the incidence of adenocarcinoma of the esophagus, even if it is effective in preventing cancer in the individual patient, because of the high frequency of intestinal metaplasia and low frequency of adenocarcinoma.

The most promising point of attack in the attempt to prevent cancer is the stage of reflux disease before the development of intestinal metaplasia. The patients at risk in the future are those who have cardiac mucosa that is detectable by screening and biopsy. There is a long lag phase before cardiac mucosa progresses to intestinal metaplasia in most patients. Recognition of the molecular component in the refluxate that drives *CDX* activation and the "gastric-type genetic signal" can lead to the production of drugs that have an effect on these molecules and drive differentiation of cardiac mucosa away from intestinal metaplasia toward oxyntocardiac mucosa. This will theoretically prevent progression to adenocarcinoma. Of course, mass population screening is not cost-effective at the present time, but it may become so in the future if the incidence of adenocarcinoma continues its upward trend. In an individual patient undergoing endoscopy for any reason, taking a biopsy sample from the squamocolumnar junction is a screening opportunity.

Irreversible Genetic Mutations— Carcinogenesis in Intestinal Metaplasia

Once intestinal metaplasia develops in columnar-lined esophagus, the carcinogenetic pathway can begin. It probably occurs through a series of irreversible genetic mutations that are expressed phenotypically as low-grade dysplasia, high-grade dysplasia, and invasive adenocarcinoma. The exact molecular changes associated with these changes are unknown as yet.[52]

The frequency with which adenocarcinoma develops in patients with intestinal metaplasia is low. An individual who has intestinal metaplasia has a low risk for cancer; most patients do not progress. However, every patient with adenocarcinoma of the esophagus comes from the pool of patients who have esophageal intestinal metaplasia. There is no other pathway for adenocarcinoma of the esophagus. This set of data makes this disease very difficult to treat from a practical standpoint. Although it is impossible to ignore an individual patient with intestinal metaplasia because of the proven cancer risk, it stretches resources to keep all patients with intestinal metaplasia under surveillance, and the cost-effectiveness of such surveillance is questionable.

The development of adenocarcinoma in esophageal intestinal metaplasia is probably not related to its length. Although it was initially believed that only patients with long-segment Barrett's esophagus were at risk, there is convincing evidence now that short-segment Barrett's esophagus carries a similar risk.[14] The exact risk associated with very short segments of Barrett's esophagus is unknown because these patients remain undetected as a result of the standard of practice in gastroenterology that recommends that no biopsy be performed in patients without endoscopically visible columnar-lined esophagus. However, it is very likely that the junctional region adenocarcinomas that occur in asymptomatic patients are caused by a similar process as adenocarcinomas of the tubular esophagus. We have encountered patients who have had adenocarcinoma in extremely short lengths of columnar-lined esophagus.

The carcinogenic mechanism in reflux-induced adenocarcinoma is unique. Let us postulate that patients have different carcinogenic potential for reflux-induced adenocarcinoma of the esophagus resident in their gastric contents. Patients who have a high potential for carcinogenesis will remain without progression to cancer until intestinal metaplasia develops in the esophagus; at that time cancer can develop rapidly because of the high carcinogenic milieu irrespective of the amount of intestinal metaplasia that is present. In contrast, reflux-induced columnar metaplasia and intestinal metaplasia can develop in patients with a low carcinogenic milieu but not progress to dysplasia for long periods. If the major factor for development of adenocarcinoma in reflux disease is the carcinogenic potential of the refluxate, it is unlikely that present methods of surveillance will have an impact on the incidence of adenocarcinoma. Clinical experience supports such a hypothesis. Most patients in whom cancer is diagnosed do not have a long premalignant course, and most patients with long-segment Barrett's esophagus remain stable without progressing to cancer.

BARRETT'S ESOPHAGUS—DIAGNOSIS

The diagnosis of Barrett's esophagus at the present time is based on identification of goblet cells in a biopsy sample taken from an endoscopically visualized columnar-lined segment of esophagus (see Fig. 13–11). Goblet cells define intestinal metaplasia. There is

consensus that the goblet cells should be well defined and recognizable on routine hematoxylin-eosin–stained sections. Alcian blue staining at pH 2.5 is positive in goblet cells that contain acid mucin, in contrast to non-intestinalized columnar epithelium, which contains Alcian blue–negative neutral mucin. However, cardiac mucosa frequently shows Alcian blue positivity ("columnar blue cells") that is unrelated to intestinal metaplasia and probably represents a reactive phenomenon. As a result, if Alcian blue positivity is used to define intestinal metaplasia, there will be a significant overdiagnosis of Barrett's esophagus. Other types of mucin, sialomucin and sulfated mucin, can be demonstrated by high-iron diamine stain. This is not presently used in routine pathology practice or for defining intestinal metaplasia. The use of CDX-2 immunoperoxidase staining to define Barrett's intestinal metaplasia has been suggested but not accepted yet.[43]

Because most authorities follow the recommendations of the American Gastroenterology Association and avoid biopsy when endoscopic findings are normal, there is no attempt to diagnose the microscopic stage of Barrett's esophagus. It is obvious that a microscopic phase must precede the stage of the disease in which metaplastic epithelium is visible by endoscopy. If biopsies are performed in patients who are endoscopically normal, a significant percentage (probably 5% to 10%) of the population will have microscopic Barrett's intestinal metaplasia. This is easily recognized by histologic criteria as intestinal metaplasia occurring in cardiac (i.e., metaplastic esophageal) mucosa. It is distinguishable from chronic atrophic gastritis, which is the occurrence of gastric intestinal metaplasia in gastric oxyntic mucosa.

The most important practical function of the pathologist is to detect neoplastic change in Barrett's esophagus in patients undergoing either primary or surveillance biopsy. The neoplastic change progresses through low- and high-grade dysplasia to invasive adenocarcinoma (Figs. 13–12 to 13–14).

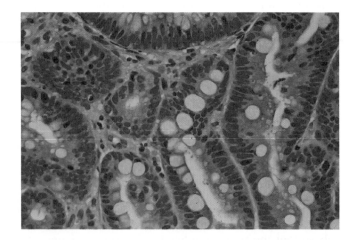

Figure 13–12. Intestinal metaplasia with low-grade dysplasia (hematoxylin-eosin stain). There is nuclear enlargement, stratification, and hyperchromasia. The glands are simple, and nuclear polarity is maintained. There is only minimal chronic inflammation.

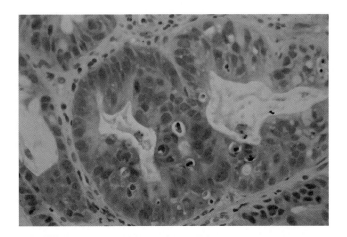

Figure 13–13. Intestinal metaplasia with high-grade dysplasia (hematoxylin-eosin stain). There is severe cytologic abnormality, complete loss of nuclear polarity, and early gland complexity.

The diagnosis of invasive adenocarcinoma and high-grade dysplasia is highly accurate and dependent on well-established criteria.[53] High-grade dysplasia (which includes the older terms severe dysplasia and carcinoma in situ) is characterized by a severe cytologic abnormality associated with complete loss of polarity of nuclei or the presence of gland complexity manifested by luminal bridging and cribriform architecture, or by both (see Fig. 13–13). Invasive carcinoma is characterized by the presence of irregularity of glands, often associated with microcystic change, and desmoplasia or the presence of single invasive cells in the lamina propria (see Fig. 13–14).

Differentiation of low-grade dysplasia from high-grade dysplasia is critical because high-grade dysplasia is an indication for esophagectomy in some centers. The fact that such differentiation is a problem should not be surprising; dysplasia is a continuous spectrum, and pathol-

ogists are drawing an artificial line separating low- from high-grade dysplasia. I tend to draw the line at a point where the specificity of the diagnosis of high-grade dysplasia is 100%; patients whom I consider to have high-grade dysplasia can proceed to esophagectomy. Increasing the specificity of the diagnosis of high-grade dysplasia necessarily decreases the sensitivity; I call borderline cases low-grade dysplasia, recommend a decreased surveillance interval, and defer the decision until future serial biopsies have been performed.

The diagnosis of low-grade dysplasia tends to have a greater degree of interobserver variation, even among experts.[53] Criteria for low-grade dysplasia are the presence of a cytologic abnormality that is significantly greater than normal with involvement of the surface epithelium to a similar extent as the foveolar region (see Fig. 13–12). When these strict criteria are used, low-grade dysplasia becomes an uncommon diagnosis in patients with Barrett's esophagus and justifies the decrease in surveillance interval that is recommended.

Most authorities recognize a category of "indefinite for dysplasia."[53] This category is used when cytologic changes are present but the criteria for low-grade dysplasia are not satisfied. I do not use the diagnosis "indefinite for dysplasia"; if there are no definite diagnostic criteria for low-grade dysplasia, it is negative for dysplasia. I use the term "reactive cytologic changes" for these cases. These patients simply stay at the regular surveillance interval for Barrett's esophagus that is recommended for nondysplastic Barrett's esophagus.

An important variable in the assessment of patients with columnar-lined esophagus is sampling. Harvesting biopsy specimens is a time-consuming activity for the endoscopist. It is not uncommon to see a sample with four to six biopsy specimens taken during surveillance endoscopy for long-segment Barrett esophagus. The chance of missing dysplasia in such a sample is significant. Patients under surveillance for Barrett's esophagus must undergo the four-quadrant biopsy per 2-cm segment protocol that is recommended. A correctly obtained surveillance biopsy sample from a 10-cm segment of Barrett's esophagus will have six separate levels with four specimens in each level.

HISTOLOGIC CLASSIFICATION OF REFLUX DISEASE

We recommend a histologic classification of reflux disease designed to predict cancer risk in patients, as well as histologically diagnose reflux disease and its severity (Box 13–3). This is highly controversial and not likely to be accepted, but we believe that there are more data to support it than any classification presently in use.

Any definition of reflux disease must recognize an end point. Present definitions use reversal of symptoms and healing of erosions and are helpful for the clinical management of patients with reflux. In the past 3 decades, however, the main life-threatening complication of reflux disease has become recognized as adenocarcinoma. Present definitions that use adenocarcinoma as an end point begin with Barrett's esophagus and not with

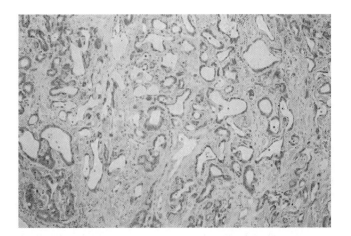

Figure 13–14. Invasive adenocarcinoma in Barrett's esophagus characterized by irregular malignant glands surrounded by desmoplasia (hematoxylin-eosin stain).

Box 13–3 Grading System for Reflux Disease

Grade 0: No Evidence of Reflux Disease (No Risk for Intestinal Metaplasia or Adenocarcinoma)

Definition: No cardiac mucosa or intestinal metaplasia at the junction

Features: These patients often have mild reflux by 24-hour pH test (within limits of normal or slightly abnormal) and are usually asymptomatic and endoscopically normal

Grade 0A: Normal: Only squamous epithelium and gastric oxyntic mucosa present

Grade 0B: Compensated reflux: Oxyntocardiac mucosa present in addition to squamous epithelium and gastric oxyntic mucosa

Grade 1: Reflux Disease (at Risk for Intestinal Metaplasia; No Risk for Adenocarcinoma)

Definition: Cardiac mucosa present at the junction; no intestinal metaplasia

Features: These patients often have an abnormal 24-hour pH test and may or may not be symptomatic and may or may not have endoscopically visible columnar-lined esophagus

Grade 1A: Mild reflux disease: 24-hour pH study often mildly abnormal, endoscopy normal, cardiac mucosa seen at microscopy

Grade 1B: Moderate reflux disease: Almost always have an abnormal 24-hour pH test; endoscopy shows a <2-cm short-segment columnar-lined esophagus

Grade 1C: Severe reflux disease: Severely abnormal 24-hour pH test; endoscopy shows >2-cm long-segment columnar-lined esophagus

Grade 2: Barrett's Esophagus (at Risk for Adenocarcinoma)

Definition: Intestinal metaplasia present

Features: Similar to those of reflux disease without intestinal metaplasia

Grade 2A: Microscopic Barrett's esophagus: Endoscopy normal; intestinal metaplasia in cardiac mucosa seen at microscopy

Grade 2B: Short-segment Barrett's esophagus: Almost always have an abnormal 24-hour pH test; endoscopy shows <2-cm short-segment columnar-lined esophagus

Grade 2C: Long-segment Barrett's esophagus: Severely abnormal 24-hour pH test; endoscopy shows >2-cm long-segment columnar-lined esophagus

Grade 3: Neoplastic Barrett's Esophagus

Definition: Histologic evidence of dysplasia/neoplasia present

Features: Similar to those of reflux disease and intestinal metaplasia

Grade 3A: Low-grade dysplasia

Grade 3B: High-grade dysplasia

Grade 3C: Invasive adenocarcinoma

reflux disease. The present classifications and grading systems seem to treat reflux disease and Barrett's esophagus as separate entities rather than different stages of one disease. The classification suggested here represents a unified concept that recognizes the entire reflux-adenocarcinoma sequence. The major grades in this system are designed to predict the risk for future adenocarcinoma. Subdivisions within each grade are designed to assess the amount of reflux-induced damage and are predictive of the severity of reflux-induced damage. Reflux-induced columnar transformation of squamous epithelium provides a far more accurate assessment of the severity of reflux than do changes in intact squamous epithelium. The length of columnar-lined esophagus has the greatest correlation with reflux when assessed by the 24-hour pH test. In many patients with a long-segment columnar-lined esophagus, who almost invariably have severe reflux, changes in squamous epithelium are frequently minimal. This is easy to understand; as the squamous epithelium moves proximally as a result of columnar transformation, it becomes removed from the point of reflux and separated from it by a buffer zone of columnar-lined esophagus.

The grading system recommended here recognizes the significance of the different genetic changes that occur in patients with reflux disease. Patients without reflux-induced genetic changes will have only normal squamous epithelium lining the esophagus. Patients enter grade 1 when cardiac mucosa develops as a result of columnar transformation. Cardiac mucosa remains as such or evolves by the development of specialized cells. If all the cardiac mucosa changes to oxyntocardiac mucosa, the patient moves out of the reflux-adenocarcinoma sequence and reverts back to grade 0. This is a very common circumstance in mild reflux disease; in patients with higher grades, conversion of columnar epithelium to oxyntocardiac mucosa essentially represents a histologic cure because oxyntocardiac mucosa does not progress to intestinal metaplasia and adenocarcinoma. When cardiac mucosa progresses in the direction of adenocarcinoma, intestinal metaplasia (grade 2) and increasing neoplastic change recognized morphologically as low-grade dysplasia, high-grade dysplasia, and adenocarcinoma (grade 3) develop. In the future, as molecular alterations specific for these changes are discovered, they can replace the morphologic criteria used at present to define these grades.

The most important element in this grading system is that it permits recognition of patients who are not at risk for adenocarcinoma or intestinal metaplasia. These patients are in grade 0 and probably represent about 50% to 60% of the general population and 35% to 40% of patients who undergo endoscopy for upper gastrointestinal symptoms and are endoscopically normal. If symptomatic, these patients can be confidently managed with acid suppression to heal and stabilize the squamous epithelium. Effective acid suppression in these patients is very likely to prevent the occurrence of columnar metaplasia because it reverses the squamous epithelial damage and removes exposure of the basally located stem cells to agents that cause genetic changes. Once cardiac metaplasia has occurred, however, the focus must shift to an attempt to convert it back to squamous epithelium or direct it to form oxyntocardiac mucosa. This grading system can form the basis for evaluating therapeutic measures that have an impact on esophageal columnar epithelium better than any other system in effect can.

REFERENCES

1. Allison PR: Peptic ulcer of the oesophagus. Thorax 3:20-42, 1948.
2. Allison PR, Johnstone AS: The oesophagus lined with gastric mucous membrane. Thorax 8:87-101, 1953.
3. Barrett NR: The lower esophagus lined by columnar epithelium. Surgery 41:881-894, 1957.
4. Blot WJ, Devesa SS, Kneller RW, Fraumeni JF Jr: Rising incidence of adenocarcinoma of the esophagus and gastric cardia. JAMA 265:1287-1289, 1991.
5. Pera M, Cameron AJ, Trastek VF, et al: Increasing incidence of adenocarcinoma of the esophagus and esophagogastric junction. Gastroenterology 104:510-513, 1993.
6. Powell J, McConkey CC: The rising trend in esophageal adenocarcinoma and gastric cardia. Eur J Cancer Prev 1:265-269, 1992.
7. Hansson LE, Sparen P, Nyren O: Increasing incidence of carcinoma of the gastric cardia in Sweden from 1970 to 1985. Int J Cancer 54:402-407, 1993.
8. Lagergren J, Bergstrom R, Lindgren A, Nyren O: Symptomatic gastroesophageal reflux as a risk factor for esophageal adenocarcinoma. N Engl J Med 340:825-831, 1999.
9. DeMeester TR, Wang CI, Wernly JA, et al: Technique, indications and clinical use of 24-hour esophageal pH monitoring. J Thorac Cardiovasc Surg 79:656-667, 1980.
10. Kauer WKH, Burdiles P, Ireland AP, et al: Does duodenal juice reflux into the esophagus of patients with complicated GERD? Evaluation of a fiberoptic sensor for bilirubin. Am J Surg 169:98-104, 1995.
11. Jamieson JR, Stein HJ, DeMeester TR, et al: Ambulatory 24-hour esophageal pH monitoring: Normal values, optimal thresholds, specificity, sensitivity, and reproducibility. Am J Gastroenterol 87:1102-1111, 1992.
12. Skopnik H, Silny J, Heiber O, et al: Gastroesophageal reflux in infants: Evaluation of the new intraluminal impedance technique. J Pediatr Gastroenterol Nutr 23:591-598, 1996.
13. Hayward J: The lower end of the oesophagus. Thorax 16:36-41, 1961.
14. Clark GW, Ireland A, Peters JH, et al: Short segment Barrett's esophagus: A prevalent complication of gastroesophageal reflux disease with malignant potential. J Gastrointest Surg 1:113-122, 1997.
15. Chandrasoma PT, Der R, Ma Y, et al: Histology of the gastroesophageal junction: An autopsy study. Am J Surg Pathol 24:402-409, 2000.
16. Jain R, Aquino D, Harford WV, et al: Cardiac epithelium is found infrequently in the gastric cardia [abstract]. Gastroenterology 114:A160, 1998.
17. Marsman WA, van Sandyck JW, Tytgat GNJ, et al: The presence and mucin histochemistry of cardiac type mucosa at the esophagogastric junction. Am J Gastroenterol 99:212-217, 2004.
18. Chandrasoma P: Pathophysiology of Barrett's esophagus. Semin Thorac Cardiovasc Surg 9:270-278, 1997.
19. Tobey NA, Carson JL, Alkiek RA, et al: Dilated intercellular spaces: A morphological feature of acid reflux–damaged human esophageal epithelium. Gastroenterology 111:1200-1205, 1996.
20. Villanacci V, Grigolato PG, Cestari R, et al: Dilated intercellular spaces as markers of reflux disease: Histology, semiquantitative score and morphometry upon light microscopy. Digestion 64:1-8, 2001.
21. Tobey NA, Hosseini SS, Argore CM, et al: Dilated intercellular spaces and shunt permeability in non-erosive acid-damaged esophageal epithelium. Am J Gastroenterol 99:13-22, 2004.
22. Johns BAE: Developmental changes in the oesophageal epithelium in man. J Anat 86:431-442, 1952.
23. Liebermann-Meffert D, Duranceau A, Stein HJ: Anatomy and Embryology. In Orringer MB, Heitmiller R (eds): The Esophagus, vol 1. In Zudeima GD, Yeo CJ (series eds): Shackelford's Surgery of the Alimentary Tract, 5th ed. Philadelphia, WB Saunders, 2002, pp 3-39.
24. Karam SM: Lineage commitment and maturation of epithelial cells in the gut. Front Biosci 4:286-298, 1999.
25. Gerdes J, Lemke H, Baisch H, et al: Cell cycle analysis of a cell proliferation–associated human nuclear antigen defined by the monoclonal antibody Ki-67. J Immunol 133:1710-1715, 1984.
26. Torek F: The first successful case of resection of the esophagus for carcinoma. Surg Gynecol Obstet 16:614-617, 1913.
27. Oberg S, Peters JH, DeMeester TR, et al: Inflammation and specialized intestinal metaplasia of cardiac mucosa is a manifestation of gastroesophageal reflux disease. Ann Surg 226:522-532, 1997.
28. Glickman JN, Fox V, Antonioli DA, et al: Morphology of the cardia and significance of carditis in pediatric patients. Am J Surg Pathol 26:1032-1039, 2002.
29. Der R, Tsao-Wei DD, DeMeester T, et al: Carditis: A manifestation of gastroesophageal reflux disease. Am J Surg Pathol 25:245-252, 2001.
30. Goldblum JR, Vicari JJ, Falk GW, et al: Inflammation and intestinal metaplasia of the gastric cardia: The role of gastroesophageal reflux and H. pylori infection. Gasteroenterology 114:633-639, 1998.
31. Bowery DJ, Clark GWB, Williams GT: Patterns of gastritis in patients with gastro-oesophageal reflux disease. Gut 45:798-803, 1999.
32. Lembo T, Ippoliti AF, Ramers C, Weinstein WM: Inflammation of the gastro-oesophageal junction (carditis) in patients with symptomatic gastro-oesophageal reflux disease: A prospective study. Gut 45:484-488, 1999.
33. Rex DK, Cummings OW, Shaw M, et al: Screening for Barrett's esophagus in colonoscopy patients with and without heartburn. Gastroenterology 125:1670-1677, 2003.
34. Sarbia M, Donner A, Gabbert HE: Histopathology of the gastroesophageal junction. A study on 36 operation specimens. Am J Surg Pathol 26:1207-1212, 2002.
35. Paull A, Trier JS, Dalton MD, et al: The histologic spectrum of Barrett's esophagus. N Engl J Med 295:476-480, 1976.
36. Csendes A, Maluenda F, Braghetto I, et al: Location of the lower esophageal sphincter and the squamocolumnar mucosal junction in 109 healthy controls and 778 patients with different degrees of endoscopic esophagitis. Gut 34:21-27, 1993.

37. Chandrasoma PT, Lokuhetty DM, DeMeester, TR, et al: Definition of histopathologic changes in gastroesophageal reflux disease. Am J Surg Pathol 24:344-351, 2000.

38. Chandrasoma PT, Der R, Ma Y, et al: Histologic classification of patients based on mapping biopsies of the gastroesophageal junction. Am J Surg Pathol 27:929-936, 2003.

39. Chandrasoma P: Non-neoplastic diseases of the esophagus. In Chandrasoma P (ed): Gastrointestinal Pathology. Stamford, CT, Appleton & Lange, 1999, pp 9-36.

40. Chandrasoma PT, Der R, Dalton P, et al: Distribution and significance of epithelial types in columnar lined esophagus. Am J Surg Pathol 25:1188-1193, 2001.

41. Silberg DG, Swain GP, Suh ER, Traber PG: Cdx1 and Cdx2 during intestinal development.. Gastroenterology 119:961-971, 2000.

42. Silberg DG, Furth EE, Taylor JK, et al: CDX1 protein expression in normal, metaplastic, and neoplastic human alimentary tract epithelium. Gastroenterology 113:478-486, 1997.

43. Phillips RW, Frierson HF, Moskaluk CA: Cdx2 as a marker of epithelial differentiation in the esophagus. Am J Surg Pathol 27:1442-1447, 2003.

44. Cooper JE, Spitz L, Wilkins BM: Barrett's esophagus in children: A histologic and histochemical study of 11 cases. J Pediatr Surg 22:191-196, 1987.

45. Qualman SJ, Murray RD, McClung HJ, Lucas J: Intestinal metaplasia is age related in Barrett's esophagus. Arch Pathol Lab Med 114:1236-1240, 1990.

46. Hamilton SR, Yardley JH: Regeneration of cardiac type mucosa and acquisition of Barrett mucosa after esophago-gastrectomy. Gastroenterology 72:669-675, 1977.

47. Oberg S, Johansson J, Wenner J, Walther B: Metaplastic columnar mucosa in the cervical esophagus after esophagectomy. Ann Surg 235:338-345, 2002.

48. Lord R, Wickramasinghe K, Johansson JJ, et al: Cardiac mucosa in the remnant esophagus after esophagectomy is an acquired epithelium with Barrett's-like features. Surgery 136:633-640, 2004.

49. Fitzgerald RC, Omary MB, Triadafilopoulos G: Dynamic effects of acid on Barrett's esophagus: An ex-vivo proliferation and differentiation model. J Clin Invest 98:2120-2128, 1996.

50. Vela MF, Camacho-Lobato L, Hatlebakk J, et al: Effect of omeprazole (PPI) on ratio of acid to nonacid gastroesophageal reflux. Studies using simultaneous intraesophageal impedance and pH (IE-IMP/pH). Gastroenterology 116:A209, 1999.

51. DeMeester SR, Campos GMR, DeMeester TR, et al: The impact of antireflux procedure on intestinal metaplasia of the cardia. Ann Surg 228:547-556, 1998.

52. Wijnhoven BPL, Tilanus HW, Dinjens WNM: Molecular biology of Barrett's adenocarcinoma. Ann Surg 233:322-337, 2001.

53. Montgomery E, Bronner MP, Goldblum JR, et al: Reproducibility of the diagnosis of dysplasia in Barrett esophagus: A reaffirmation. Hum Pathol 32:368-378, 2001.

14

The Gastroesophageal Barrier

Jeffrey H. Peters · Tom R. DeMeester

The gastrointestinal tract is a continuous hollow tube whose function is ingestion and digestion of food, absorption of chemical energy, and elimination of residue. These functions are performed separately in different compartments whose boundaries differ from our customary anatomic divisions of the gastrointestinal tract. Common to each compartment is a pumping mechanism to propel contents into the reservoir portion of the compartment, a sphincter to separate the pump from the reservoir, and the ability to maintain within the reservoir a distinct chemical, enzymatic, and pH environment appropriate to its function. In the most proximal compartment, the tongue and pharynx function as a pump; the upper esophageal sphincter, soft palate, and epiglottis function as valves; and the striated muscle portion of the upper esophagus functions as a receptacle. In the second compartment, the smooth muscle portion of the distal esophagus, characterized by peristaltic contractions of high amplitude, pumps food through a valve, the lower esophageal sphincter (LES), into the gastric fundus, which acts as a reservoir. In the third compartment, the antrum behaves as a pump to propel chyme through a valve, the pylorus, into a reservoir, the duodenum. Similarly, the small intestine pumps its contents through the ileocecal valve into a capacitance organ, the cecum. An important principle is that breakdown of function in one compartment of the gastrointestinal tract tends to produce secondary effects in the proximal compartments rather than in the distal compartments. Thus, problems originating in the stomach commonly cause symptoms in the esophagus or symptoms referable to the pharyngeal and laryngeal area. This concept of the gastrointestinal tract is important in understanding the pathophysiology of gastroesophageal reflux disease (GERD) and structuring a rational approach to its therapy.

The common denominator for virtually all episodes of gastroesophageal reflux, whether physiologic or pathologic, is loss of the normal gastroesophageal barrier and the resistance that it imposes to the flow of gastric juice from an environment of higher pressure, the stomach, to an environment of lower pressure, the esophagus. This barrier is composed of both anatomic (flap valve) and physiologic (sphincter) components that combined act to prevent reflux during stressed and unstressed conditions. Its key determinants include

1. The resting structural integrity of the LES
2. The frequency of swallow- and non–swallow-induced transient loss of sphincter competence
3. Anatomic configuration of the diaphragmatic crura and gastroesophageal flap valve represented by the angle of His

In severe GERD, reflux is usually due to a permanently nonexistent or reduced high-pressure zone. In early disease or normal subjects, it is usually due to a transient loss of the high-pressure zone.[1] The presence or absence of pathologic esophageal acid exposure (i.e., abnormal 24-hour pH studies) is influenced not only by the degree of barrier loss but also by the function of the esophagus and stomach, most importantly the effectiveness of esophageal peristalsis and clearance and any gastric motility abnormalities that affect gastric relaxation or distention (or both).

LOWER ESOPHAGEAL SPHINCTER

In humans, the primary physiologic barrier between the esophagus and stomach that confines the gastric fluid to the stomach is the lower esophageal "sphincter." The LES has few anatomic landmarks, but its presence can be identified by a rise in pressure over gastric baseline pressure as a pressure transducer is pulled from the stomach into the esophagus (Fig. 14–1). This high-pressure zone is normally present except in two situations: (1) after a swallow, when it is momentarily dissipated or relaxes to allow passage of food into the stomach (Fig. 14–2), and

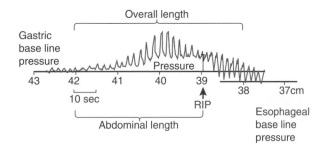

Figure 14–1. A pressure profile of the lower esophageal high-pressure zone or "sphincter" measured in a normal subject. The high-pressure zone has no anatomic landmarks, but is identified by a rise in pressure over the gastric baseline as the pressure transducer is pulled from the stomach into the esophagus. Note the long intra-abdominal portion identified by the positive respiratory excursions and the short intrathoracic portion identified by the negative respiratory excursions. The point where the respiratory excursions reverse is called the *respiratory inversion point*. The pressure scale is 3 mm Hg between *vertical dots*.

(2) during distention of the fundus with gas, when the high-pressure zone is eliminated to allow venting of the gas (a belch).

Three characteristics of the lower esophageal high-pressure zone, or "sphincter" as it is commonly referred to, maintain its resistance or "barrier" function to intra-gastric and intra-abdominal pressure challenges. Two of

these characteristics work together and are dependent on each other for proper sphincter function. They are its pressure, measured at the respiratory inversion point, and its overall length. The tonic resistance of the LES is a function of both its pressure and the length over which the pressure is exerted.[2,3] The shorter the overall length of the high-pressure zone, the higher the pressure must be to maintain sufficient resistance to remain competent (Fig. 14–3). Consequently, normal sphincter pressure can be nullified by a short overall sphincter length. Furthermore, as the stomach fills, the length of the sphincter decreases, rather like the neck of a balloon shortening as the balloon is inflated. If the overall length of the sphincter is abnormally short when the stomach is empty, with minimal gastric distention there will be insufficient sphincter length for the existing pressure to maintain sphincter competency, and reflux will occur. The integrated effects of radial pressure exerted over the entire length of the high-pressure zone can be measured to form a three-dimensional computerized image of the sphincter.[4] The volume of this image is a reflection of the sphincter's resistance and is called the sphincter pressure vector volume (Fig. 14–4). A calculated volume less than the 5th percentile in normal subjects is an indication of a permanently defective sphincter.

The third characteristic of the lower esophageal high-pressure zone, or "sphincter," is its position, and a portion of the overall length of the high-pressure zone should be exposed to positive intra-abdominal pressure. This portion of the high-pressure zone is commonly referred to as the abdominal length of the sphincter.

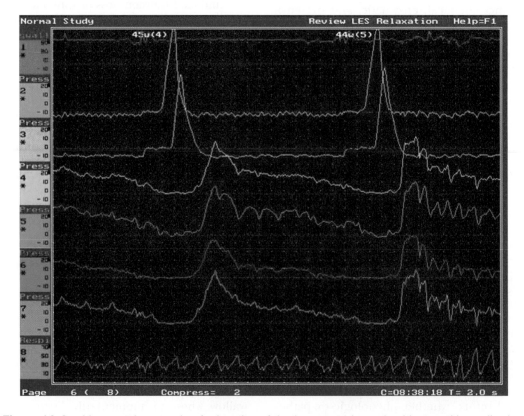

Figure 14–2. Manometric example of relaxation of the lower esophageal sphincter with swallowing.

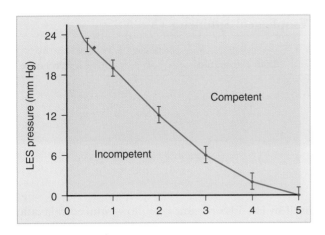

Figure 14–3. Relationship between the magnitude of pressure in the high-pressure zone measured at the respiratory inversion point and the overall length of the zone to the resistance to flow of fluid through the zone. Competent equals no flow. Incompetent equals flow of varied volume. Note that the shorter the overall length of the high-pressure zone, the higher the pressure must be to maintain sufficient resistance to remain competent. LES, lower esophageal sphincter.

During periods of increased intra-abdominal pressure, the resistance of the LES would be overcome if the abdominal pressure were not applied equally to the high-pressure zone and the stomach.[5-7] Think of sucking on a soft soda straw immersed in a bottle of Coke; the hydrostatic pressure of the fluid and the negative pressure inside the straw as a result of sucking cause the straw to collapse instead of allowing the liquid to flow up the straw in the direction of the negative pressure. If the abdominal length is inadequate, the sphincter cannot respond to an increase in applied intra-abdominal pressure by collapsing, and reflux is more liable to result.

If the high-pressure zone has an abnormally low pressure, a short overall length, or minimal exposure to the abdominal pressure environment in the fasting state, there is permanent loss of LES resistance and unhampered reflux of gastric contents into the esophagus throughout the circadian cycle. This is referred to as a permanently defective sphincter and is identified by one or more of the following characteristics: a high-pressure zone with an average pressure of less than 6 mm Hg, an average overall length of 2 cm or less, or an average length exposed to the positive-pressure environment of the abdomen of 1 cm or less.[8] When compared with normal subjects, these values are below the 2.5th percentile for each parameter (Table 14–1). The most common cause of a permanently defective sphincter is inadequate pressure, but the efficiency of a sphincter with normal pressure can be nullified by an inadequate abdominal length or an abnormally short overall length.

For the clinician, the finding of a permanently defective sphincter has several implications. Foremost, it is almost always associated with esophageal mucosal injury[9] and predicts that the patient's symptoms will be difficult to control with medical therapy.[10] It is a signal that surgical therapy is likely to be needed for consistent and long-term control of the patient's symptoms. It is now accepted that when the sphincter is permanently defective, it is irreversible, even when the associated esophagitis has healed.[11] The presence of a permanently defective sphincter is commonly associated with reduced esophageal body function, and if the disease is not brought under control, the progressive loss of effective esophageal clearance can lead to severe mucosal injury,

Figure 14–4. Computerized three-dimensional imaging of the lower esophageal sphincter. A catheter with four to eight radial side holes is withdrawn through the gastroesophageal junction. For each level of pullback, the radially measured pressure is plotted around an axis representing gastric baseline pressure. When a stepwise pullback technique is used, the respiratory inversion point (RIP) can be identified. (From Stein HJ, DeMeester TR, Naspetti R, et al: Three-dimensional imaging of the lower esophageal sphincter in gastroesophageal reflux disease. Ann Surg 214:374-384, 1991.)

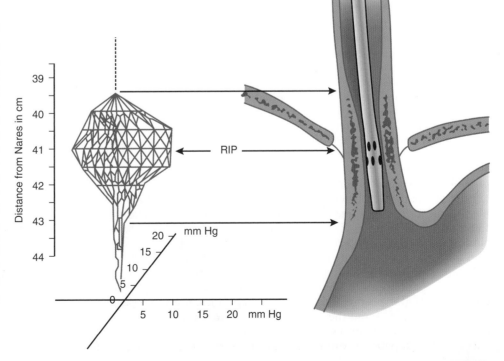

| Table 14–1 | Normal Manometric Values of the Distal Esophageal Sphincter ($N = 50$) |
| | |

Parameter	Median Value	2.5th Percentile	97.5th Percentile
Pressure (mm Hg)	13	5.8	27.7
Overall length (cm)	3.6	2.1	5.6
Abdominal length (cm)	2	0.9	4.7

repetitive regurgitation, aspiration, and pulmonary failure.[8,12,13]

TRANSIENT LOSS OF LOWER ESOPHAGEAL SPHINCTER COMPETENCE

Transient loss of the lower esophageal high-pressure zone occurs in association with swallowing and when the fundus is distended with gas, fluid, or food, which probably "unfolds" the sphincter. In 1980, Dent and Dodds reported that non-swallow–induced transient lower esophageal sphincter relaxation (tLESR) was a significant mechanism of gastroesophageal reflux in normal individuals and patients with GERD.[14] These spontaneous relaxations occurred without pharyngeal contraction, were prolonged (>10 seconds), and when reflux occurred, were associated with relaxation of the crural diaphragm. Indeed, Mittal et al. later showed that pharmacologic elimination of LES pressure to zero did not result in reflux unless crural diaphragmatic contraction was also absent.[15] Gastric distention, upright posture, and meals high in fat have all been shown to increase the frequency of tLESRs. These observations suggest that unfolding of the sphincter may be responsible for the loss of sphincter pressure.

As a result of these findings, tLESRs became commonly accepted as the major mechanism of gastroesophageal reflux regardless of the underlying severity of disease, despite evidence to the contrary. The fact that a hiatal hernia could be identified in more than 80% of patients with symptomatic gastroesophageal reflux and that most patients with erosive esophagitis and Barrett's esophagus had incompetent LES characteristics at rest were largely ignored. When these facts are taken into account, particularly in association with the known characteristics of tLESRs, it seems likely that they are (1) a physiologic response to gastric distention by food or gas, (2) the mechanism of belching, and (3) responsible for physiologic reflux episodes in individuals with normal LES and hiatal anatomy. Evidence supporting this conclusion was recently published by Van Herwaarden et al., who performed ambulatory esophageal manometry and pH studies on patients with and without hiatal hernia.[16] Although patients with hiatal hernia had greater esophageal acid exposure and more reflux episodes, the frequency of tLESRs and the proportion associated with reflux were similar in both groups. They concluded that excess reflux in patients with GERD and hiatal hernia is caused by low LES pressure, swallow-induced relaxation, and straining.

Transient loss of the high-pressure zone can also occur and is usually due to a functional problem of the gastric reservoir. Ingestion of excessive air or food can result in gastric dilatation and, if the active relaxation reflex has been lost, increased intragastric pressure. When the stomach is distended, the vectors produced by gastric wall tension pull on the gastroesophageal junction with a force that varies according to the geometry of the cardia; that is, the force is applied more directly when a hiatal hernia exists[5] than when a proper angle of His is present.[17,18] The force pulls on the terminal esophagus and causes it to be "taken up" into the stretched fundus, thereby reducing the length of the high-pressure zone, or "sphincter."[19] This process continues until a critical length is reached, usually about 1 to 2 cm, when the pressure drops precipitously and reflux occurs (Fig. 14–5). If

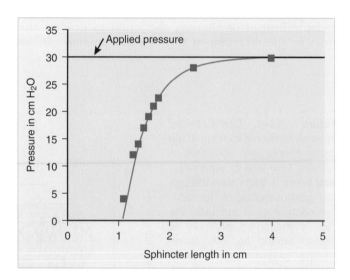

Figure 14–5. Relationship between resting sphincter pressure and sphincter length when applied pressure or "sphincter squeeze" is kept constant. Analysis was made with a model of the lower esophageal high-pressure zone. Note that as sphincter length decreased, the pressure recorded within the sphincter decreased only slightly until a length of 2 cm was reached, as which point sphincter pressure dropped precipitously and competency of the sphincter was lost. (From Pettersson GB, Bombeck CT, Nyhus LM: The lower esophageal sphincter: Mechanisms of opening and closure. Surgery 88:307-314, 1980.)

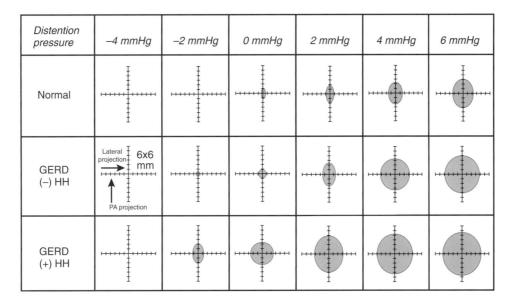

Figure 14–6. Radiographic measures of gastroesophageal junction opening size and shape under various clinical conditions for normal subjects, gastroesophageal reflux disease (GERD) patients without hiatal hernia (HH), and GERD patients with HH. Note the hiatal openings in patients with HH under conditions of minimal distention pressure. PA, posteroanterior. (Pandolfino JE, Shi G, Trueworthy B, Kahrilas PJ: Esophagogastric junction opening during relaxation distinguishes non-hernia reflux patients, hernia patients, and normal subjects. Gastroenterology 125:1018-1024, 2003.)

the pressure rather than the length of the high-pressure zone is measured, as with a Dent sleeve,[20] this event will appear as a spontaneous dissipation or "relaxation" of the high-pressure zone.

Gastric distention results in shortening of the length of the high-pressure zone along with a concomitant drop in LES pressure, which provides a mechanical explanation for "transient" relaxations of the LES without invoking a neuromuscular reflex. Rather than a "spontaneous" muscular relaxation, there is unfolding of the sphincter, secondary to progressive gastric distention, to the point at which it becomes incompetent. Consequently, non–swallow-induced relaxations of a normal high-pressure zone, or "sphincter," are inappropriately termed transient LES relaxations; rather, they should be called "transient sphincter shortenings." These "transient sphincter shortenings" occur in the initial stages of GERD and are the mechanisms for excessive postprandial reflux. After gastric venting, the length of the high-pressure zone is restored and competence returns, until distention again shortens it and encourages further venting and reflux. This sequence results in the common complaints of repetitive belching and bloating in patients with GERD. The increased swallowing frequency seen in patients with GERD aggravates gastric distention and is probably due to repetitive swallowing of saliva in an unconscious attempt to buffer acid refluxed into the esophagus.[21] Thus, the early pathogenesis of GERD may begin in the stomach, with gastric distention caused by overeating or the ingestion of fried foods, which delays gastric emptying, or subclinical gastric motility abnormalities.[22] Both characteristics are common in Western society and may explain the high prevalence of the disease in the Western world.

The mechanical forces set in play by gastric distention and their effect on sphincter unfolding are also influenced by the "geometry" of the gastroesophageal junction. The presence of a normal acute angle of His, in contrast to the abnormal dome architecture of a sliding hiatal hernia, markedly influences the ease with which the sphincter is pulled open (Fig. 14–6).[23] There is a close relationship between the degree of gastric distention necessary to overcome the high-pressure zone and the morphology of the cardia.[24] Greater gastric dilatation, as reflected by higher intragastric pressure, is necessary to "open" the sphincter in patients with an intact angle of His than in those with a hiatal hernia (Fig. 14–7). This is what would be expected if the high-pressure zone were shortened by mechanical forces and accounts for why a hiatal hernia is often associated with the presence of GERD.

In normal subjects, almost all reflux episodes are precipitated by belching. In patients with GERD, belching remains an important, but decreasing cause of reflux as the grade of esophagitis worsens.[25] Activities that produce a pressure gradient across the diaphragm, such as coughing, sniffing, or straining, become increasingly important in precipitating reflux as the degree of disease, graded according to the severity of esophagitis, becomes more severe. In patients with severe grades of esophagitis, episodes of acid reflux occur spontaneously, thus suggesting that the sphincter was permanently defective in its resting state and there is persistent loss of the barrier. Reflux episodes associated with belching are by inference due to gastric distention and are responsible for increased esophageal acid exposure in patients with early or less mucosal disease. In this situation there is a transient loss of the barrier. Mucosal damage caused

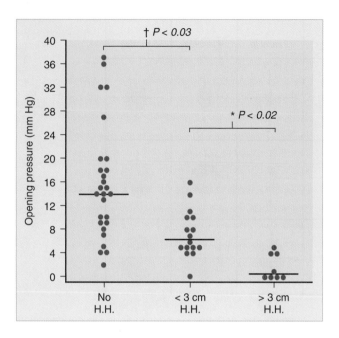

Figure 14–7. Intragastric pressure at which the lower esophagus endoscopically opened in response to gastric distention by air during endoscopy. Note that the dome architecture of a hiatal hernia (H.H.) influenced the ease with which the sphincter can be pulled open by gastric distention. (From Ismail T, Bancewicz J, Barlow J: Yield pressure, anatomy of the cardia and gastroesophageal reflux. Br J Surg 82:943-947, 1995.)

by repetitive exposure to gastric juice results in inflammatory injury to the underlying muscle.[26] Such injury leads to a permanently defective high-pressure zone, or "sphincter," that is initially due to the loss of abdominal length and eventually due to the loss of pressure and overall length. Subsequent inflammation in the esophagus results in the loss of its clearance ability and thereby leads to prolonged esophageal exposure to gastric juice.[27] This signals the presence of advanced disease and places the patient at risk for Barrett's metaplasia, stricture formation, and aspiration.

ANATOMIC ALTERATIONS

With the advent of clinical roentgenology, it became evident that a hiatal hernia was a relatively common abnormality, although not always accompanied by symptoms. Philip Allison in his classic treatise published in 1951 suggested that the manifestations of GERD were caused by the presence of a hiatal hernia.[28] For most of the next 2 decades, hiatal hernia was considered the primary pathophysiologic abnormality leading to GERD. Indeed, the Allison repair, among the first surgical attempts to treat GERD, was limited to reducing the hernia. Attention was slowly diverted away from hiatal hernia as the main pathophysiologic abnormality, however, as techniques of esophageal manometry developed in the late 1950s and 1960s allowed identification and study of the LES in subjects with and without reflux.

In 1971, Cohen and Harris published a study of the contributions of hiatal hernia to LES competence in 75 patients and concluded that hiatal hernia had no effect on gastroesophageal junction competence.[29] This paper, published in the *New England Journal of Medicine,* and the growing use of esophageal manometry shifted the emphasis away from hiatal hernia almost exclusively toward features of the LES as the primary abnormality in symptomatic GERD.

Perhaps serendipitously, studies of the phenomenon of tLESR identified the diaphragmatic crura as an important factor in preventing reflux during periods of loss of LES pressure. In normal subjects, even with absent LES pressure, reflux does not occur without relaxation of the crural diaphragm.[30] Coincidentally, Hill et al. stressed the importance of the physiologic flap valve created by the angle of His as a barrier to gastroesophageal reflux.[31] The endoscopic appearance of the flap valve can be correlated with abnormal esophageal acid exposure, thus emphasizing that the geometry of the gastroesophageal region is also important in barrier competence. Further evidence was provided by Ismail et al., who showed that the geometry of the gastroesophageal junction was an important factor in competency of the cardia regardless of sphincter status.[24] They reported a close relationship between the size of the hiatal hernia and the intragastric pressure required to open the sphincter, or the yield pressure. No relationship between yield pressure and LES resting pressure and length was found. Higher intragastric pressure was needed to open the sphincter in patients with an intact angle of His than in patients with a hiatal hernia. The presence of a hiatal hernia also disturbs esophageal clearance mechanisms, probably because of loss of anchorage of the esophagus in the abdomen. Kahrilas et al. have shown that complete esophageal emptying was achieved in 86% of swallows in control subjects without a hiatal hernia, in 66% of swallows in patients with a reducing hiatal hernia, and in only 32% of swallows in patients with a nonreducing hiatal hernia.[32] The impaired clearance in patients with nonreducing hiatal hernias suggests that the presence of a hiatal hernia contributes to the pathogenesis of GERD. Thus, present evidence is overwhelming that hiatal hernia does indeed play a significant, if not primary role in the pathophysiology of GERD.

INTEGRATED HYPOTHESIS OF THE PATHOPHYSIOLOGY OF GASTROESOPHAGEAL REFLUX DISEASE

The data support the likelihood that GERD begins in the stomach. Fundic distention occurs because of overeating and delayed gastric emptying secondary to the high-fat Western diet. The distention causes the sphincter to be "taken up" by the expanding fundus, thereby exposing the squamous epithelium within the high-pressure zone, which is the distal 3 cm of the esophagus, to gastric juice. Repeated exposure causes inflammation of the squamous epithelium, columnarization, and carditis. This is the initial step and explains why in early disease the esophagitis is mild and commonly limited to the very distal part of the esophagus. The patient compensates by increased swallowing, which allows saliva to bathe the injured mucosa and alleviate the discomfort induced by exposure to gastric acid. Increased swallowing results in aerophagia, bloating, and repetitive belching. The distention induced by aerophagia leads to further exposure and repetitive injury to the terminal squamous epithelium and the development of cardiac-type mucosa. This is an inflammatory process, commonly referred to as "carditis," and explains the complaint of epigastric pain so often registered by patients with early disease. The process can lead to a fibrotic mucosal ring at the squamo-columnar junction and explains the origin of a Schatzki ring. Extension of the inflammatory process into the muscularis propria causes progressive loss in length and pressure of the distal esophageal high-pressure zone, associated with increased esophageal exposure to gastric juice and the symptoms of heartburn and regurgitation. Loss of the barrier occurs in a distal-to-proximal direction and eventually results in permanent loss of LES resistance and explosion of the disease into the esophagus with all the clinical manifestations of severe esophagitis. This accounts for the observation that severe esophageal mucosal injury is almost always associated with a permanently defective sphincter. At any time during this process and under specific luminal conditions or stimuli, such as exposure time to a specific pH range, intestinalization of the cardiac-type mucosa can occur and set the stage for malignant degeneration.

REFERENCES

1. Mittal RK, Hollaway RH, Penagini R, et al: Transient lower esophageal sphincter relaxation. Gastroenterology 109:601-610, 1995.
2. Bonavina L, Evander A, DeMeester TR, et al: Length of the distal esophageal sphincter and competency of the cardia. Am J Surg 151:25-34, 1986.
3. DeMeester TR, Wernly JA, Bryant GH, et al: Clinical and in vitro analysis of gastroesophageal competence: A study of the principles of antireflux surgery. Am J Surg 137:39-46, 1979.
4. Stein HJ, DeMeester TR, Naspetti R, et al: Three-dimensional imaging of the lower esophageal sphincter in gastroesophageal reflux disease. Ann Surg 214:374-384, 1991.
5. Pellegrini CA, DeMeester TR, Skinner DB: Response of the distal esophageal sphincter to respiratory and positional maneuvers in humans. Surg Forum 27:380-382, 1976.
6. O'Sullivan GC, DeMeester TR, Joelsson BE, et al: The interaction of the lower esophageal sphincter pressure and length of sphincter in the abdomen as determinants of gastroesophageal competence. Am J Surg 143:40-47, 1982.
7. Johnson LF, Lin YC, Hong SK: Gastroesophageal dynamics during immersion in water to the neck. J Appl Physiol 38:449-454, 1975.
8. DeMeester TR, Johnson WE: Outcome of respiratory symptoms after surgical treatment of swallowing disorders. Semin Respir Crit Care Med 16:514-519, 1995.
9. Kuster E, Ros E, Toledo-Pimentel V, et al: Predictive factors of the long term outcome in gastro-oesophageal reflux disease: Six year follow up of 107 patients. Gut 35:8-14, 1994.
10. Lieberman DA: Medical therapy for chronic reflux esophagitis. Arch Intern Med 147:1717-1720, 1987.
11. Singh P, Adamopoulos A, Taylor RH, Colin-Jones DG: Oesophageal motor function before and after healing of oesophagitis. Gut 33:1590-1596, 1992.
12. Stein HJ, Eypasch EP, DeMeester TR, Smyrk TC: Circadian esophageal motor function in patients with gastroesophageal reflux disease. Surgery 108:769-778, 1990.
13. Tsai P, Peters J, Johnson W, et al: Laparoscopic fundoplication 1 month prior to lung transplantation. Surg Endosc 10:668-670, 1996.
14. Dent J, Dodds WJ, Friedman RH, et al: Mechanisms of gastroesophageal reflux in recumbent asymptomatic human subjects. J Clin Invest 65:256-267, 1980.
15. Mittal RK, Holloway R, Dent J: Effect of atropine on the frequency of reflux and transient lower esophageal sphincter relaxation in normal subjects. Gastroenterology 109:1547-1554, 1995.
16. Van Herwaarden MA, Samson M, Smout AJP: Excess gastroesophageal reflux in patients with hiatal hernia is caused by mechanisms other than transient LES relaxations. Gastroenterology 119:1439-1446, 2000.
17. Pettersson GB, Bombeck CT, Nyhus LM: The lower esophageal sphincter: Mechanisms of opening and closure. Surgery 88:307-314, 1980.
18. Marchand P: The gastro-oesophageal "sphincter" and the mechanism of regurgitation. Br J Surg 42:504-513, 1955.
19. Mason RJ, Lund RJ, DeMeester TR, et al: Nissen fundoplication prevents shortening of the sphincter during gastric distention. Arch Surg 132:719-726, 1997.
20. Dent J: A new technique for continuous sphincter pressure measurement. Gastroenterology 71:263-267, 1976.
21. Bremner RM, Hoeft SF, Costantini M, et al: Pharyngeal swallowing: The major factor in clearance of esophageal reflux episodes. Ann Surg 218:364-370, 1993.
22. Iwakiri K, Kobayashi M, Kotoyari M, et al: Relationship between postprandial esophageal acid exposure and meal volume and fat content. Dig Dis Sci 41:926-930, 1996.
23. Pandolfino JE, Shi G, Trueworthy B, Kahrilas PJ: Esophagogastric junction opening during relaxation distinguishes non-hernia reflux patients, hernia patients and normal subjects. Gastroenterology 125:1018-1024, 2003.
24. Ismail T, Bancewicz J, Barlow J: Yield pressure, anatomy of the cardia and gastroesophageal reflux. Br J Surg 82:943-947, 1995.
25. Barham CP, Gotley DC, Mills A, Alderson D: Precipitating causes of acid reflux episodes in ambulant patients with gastro-oesophageal reflux disease. Gut 36:505-510, 1995.
26. Zaninotto G, DeMeester TR, Bremner CG, et al: Esophageal function in patients with reflux-induced strictures and its relevance to surgical treatment. Ann Thorac Surg 47:362-370, 1989.
27. Rakic S, Stein HJ, DeMeester TR, Hinder RN: Role of esophageal body function in gastroesophageal reflux disease: Implications for surgical management. J Am Coll Surg 185:380-387, 1997.
28. Allison PR: Reflux esophagitis, sliding hiatal hernia and the anatomy of repair. Surg Gynecol Obstet 92:419-431, 1951.
29. Cohen S, Harris LD: Does hiatus hernia affect competence of the gastroesophageal sphincter? N Engl J Med 284:1053-1056, 1971.
30. Martin CJ, Dodds WJ, Liem HH, et al: Diaphragmatic contribution to gastroesophageal competence and reflux in dogs. Am J Physiol 263:G551-G557, 1992.
31. Hill LD, Kozarek RA, Kraemer SJM, et al: The gastroesophageal flap valve; in vitro and in vivo observations. Gastrointest Endosc 44:541-547, 1996.
32. Kahrilas PJ, Wu S, Lin S, Pouderoux P: Attenuation of esophageal shortening during peristalsis with hiatus hernia. Gastroenterology 109:1818-1825, 1995.

15

Esophageal Mucosal Injury and Duodenal Reflux

Hubert J. Stein ▪ Werner K. H. Kauer ▪ Dorothea Liebermann-Meffert

The existence of primary duodenogastroesophageal reflux disease, or excessive reflux of bile and pancreatic enzymes into the esophagus in patients with an intact stomach, has been questioned for years. Today, it is well established that both gastric juice and duodenal contents can reflux into the esophagus and contribute to esophageal mucosal injury, namely, inflammation, ulcerative esophagitis, intestinal metaplasia (so-called Barrett's esophagus), and esophageal adenocarcinoma.[1-4] Discoordination of antropyloroduodenal motility, frequently found after cholecystectomy, and defective barrier function of the lower esophageal sphincter are the underlying conditions predisposing to excessive reflux of duodenal contents through the stomach into the esophagus.[5] The individual and combined contributions of gastric juice and duodenal components to the development of esophageal mucosal damage have been studied extensively in vitro and in vivo.

ESOPHAGEAL MUCOSAL INJURY AND DUODENAL REFLUX IN ANIMAL STUDIES

Using a dog model, Bremner at al.[6] were the first to demonstrate that columnar epithelial metaplasia in the distal end of the esophagus could result from prolonged gastroesophageal reflux. This finding was confirmed by Gillen et al.,[7] who studied canine esophageal mucosa under basal conditions and in the presence of gastroesophageal reflux. Under normal conditions, mucosal defects in the esophagus are regenerated by squamous epithelium. In the presence of gastroesophageal reflux of acid or a combination of acid and bile, the mucosa is frequently regenerated by columnar epithelium.[8]

Lillimoe et al.[9] have shown that the reflux of bile and pancreatic enzymes into the stomach can protect or augment esophageal mucosal injury. In a rabbit whose gastric acid secretion maintains an acid environment, the presence of bile salts would attenuate the injurious effect of pepsin, and the acid gastric environment would inactivate trypsin. Such a rabbit would have bile-containing acid gastric juice that when refluxed into the esophagus would injure the mucosal barrier and the epithelium but would be less caustic than the reflux of acid gastric juice alone. In contrast, in a rabbit with significant duodenogastric reflux, a more alkaline intragastric pH environment may be present and encourage the solubility of bile salts.

This finding was supported in a study by Ireland et al.,[10] who manipulated rats so that the esophagus was exposed to reflux of gastric juice, duodenal juice, or a combination of both. In this rat model, the presence of gastric juice protected against the development of esophageal adenocarcinoma. The absence of gastric juice resulted in a threefold increase in the prevalence of adenocarcinoma. The protective effect of the stomach seems to be related to the secretion of acid because there was a progressive increase in the prevalence of esophageal adenocarcinoma as the amount of gastric acid that was permitted to reflux with duodenal juice into the esophagus was reduced. A recent study by Theisen et al.[11] using a similar rat model provided preliminary evidence of the mutagenic potential of bile reflux on esophageal epithelium. In rats suffering from duodenogastroesophageal reflux, specific mutations (*lacI* mutations) were markedly more frequent than would be expected and were similar to those found in the p53 mutations of human esophageal adenocarcinoma, thus providing a link to human esophageal cancer.

ESOPHAGEAL MUCOSAL INJURY AND DUODENAL REFLUX IN HUMAN STUDIES

Ambulatory 24-hour esophageal pH monitoring has become the gold standard for the diagnosis of gastroesophageal reflux disease.[12] In addition to significantly increased acid exposure, patients who suffer from gastroesophageal reflux disease can also have increased esophageal exposure to duodenal juice, especially when Barrett's esophagus is present on endoscopy and biopsy. On pH monitoring, this may be indicated by the time that the pH is greater than 7.[1,13] The alkaline component of the refluxed juice seems to result from contamination of the refluxed gastric contents with excessive duodenogastric refluxate.[14] Measurement of esophageal exposure to duodenal contents is, however, less dependable than measurement of esophageal acid exposure.[15]

A fiberoptic system (Bilitec) for circadian monitoring of duodenogastroesophageal reflux was proposed by Bechi et al.,[16] who used bilirubin as another indirect marker for reflux of duodenal juice. Major advantages of the system are that it allows prolonged simultaneous measurements at multiple sites in the foregut on an ambulatory basis and can be combined with pH monitoring. With the Bilitec system, it has been shown that patients who have reflux of acid gastric juice alone have less severe esophageal mucosal injury than do patients who have reflux of gastric juice contaminated with duodenal components.[17-19] Furthermore, reflux of duodenal juice into the esophagus is significantly more common in patients who have Barrett's esophagus than in patients who have erosive esophagitis or those with reflux who have no mucosal injury. In addition, the mean percentage of time that the esophagus is exposed to duodenal juice is markedly increased in patients who have Barrett's esophagus and is highest in the group of patients with high-grade dysplasia or early carcinoma in Barrett's esophagus.[17] Analysis of the circadian pattern of esophageal bilirubin exposure showed that bile reflux occurs primarily during the postprandial and supine periods.[17-19]

Simultaneous esophageal pH and bilirubin monitoring confirmed that esophageal exposure to duodenal juice occurs at all pH values.[20] In patients with gastroesophageal reflux, the presence of duodenal content within the esophagus could be demonstrated more than 15% of the time when the pH was less than 4, 19% of the time when the pH was between 4 and 7, and 6% of the time when the pH was higher than 7. Analysis of the cumulative period during which the esophagus was exposed to duodenal juice showed that the pH of the esophagus was between 4 and 7 more than 87% of the time. This pH is considered normal for the esophagus, and consequently such reflux goes undetected and unappreciated when analyzed by traditional pH criteria.

Only a few studies have measured reflux of duodenal juice into the esophagus directly. Via prolonged ambulatory aspiration in the distal end of the esophagus, it could be shown that patients who have reflux esophagitis and Barrett's esophagus have greater and more concentrated bile acid exposure to the esophageal mucosa than do normal subjects and reflux patients without mucosal injury.[13,18,20] This increased exposure occurs most commonly during the supine period while asleep and during the upright period after meals. Aspiration studies also delivered more details on the noxious effects of specific bile salts. Glycine conjugates of cholic, deoxycholic, and chenodeoxycholic acid have been identified as the predominant bile acids aspirated from the esophagus of patients with gastroesophageal reflux disease. This predominance is, as would be expected, due to the fact that glycine conjugates are three times more prevalent than taurine conjugates in normal human bile.

MECHANISM OF BILE ACID INJURY TO ESOPHAGEAL MUCOSA

In humans, a normal liver converts a daily average of 0.78 to 1.29 mmol of cholesterol into bile acids.[21-23] These primary bile acids, cholate and chenodeoxycholate, are synthesized from cholesterol by hepatocytes. Secondary bile acids, including deoxycholic and lithocholic acid, are formed as metabolic by-products of intestinal bacteria. Before secretion into the biliary tract, 98% of the bile acids are conjugated with taurine or glycine at a ratio of 3 : 1. Conjugation, especially with taurine, increases the solubility of bile acids by lowering their pK_a. Soluble bile acids can enter mucosal cells when they are in their non-ionized lipophilic form, specifically, at a pH between 2 and 5 for the conjugated bile acids. Because intracellular ionization results in entrapment, bile acids accumulate within intestinal cells. In vivo studies have shown that accumulation of bile acid in mucosal cells is driven by the pH gradient between the acidic lumen and the neutral cytosol; that is, intracellular accumulation is higher and occurs faster at a more acidic pH. The intracellular bile acid concentration can reach levels as high as eight times the luminal concentration.[24,25] Such excessive intracellular concentrations of bile acids result in increased mucosal permeability by dissolution of cell membranes and tight junctions and, eventually, cell death. This effect is related not only to the concentration of luminal bile acids but also to the time that the mucosa is exposed to bile acids. Depending on their conjugation status, bile acids, however, also precipitate irreversibly at an acidic pH. Precipitation occurs at a pH below 3 to 4 for unconjugated bile acids, whereas conjugated bile acids precipitate only at a pH below 1.5.[24] Because precipitated bile acids are innocuous, bile reflux into the stomach with an intact acid secretory capacity (i.e., a pH of about 1.2) does not cause any mucosal injury. At a pH between 2 and 4, conjugated bile acids are, however, both soluble and in an ionized form; that is, they are able to enter and accumulate in intestinal cells. Thus, the potentially injurious effect of bile reflux is not only related to the concentration of bile acids but also dependent on the pH.[26]

Recent studies have confirmed significant effects of bile acids on cellular physiology. Bile salts have been shown to activate protein kinase C and nuclear transcription factors.[27,28] Nuclear receptors for bile acids have been identified.[29] Parks et al. have shown that physiologic concentrations of free and conjugated chenodeoxycholic acid, lithocholic acid, and deoxycholic acid activate the farnesoid X receptor, a heretofore orphan nuclear receptor.[29] This provides evidence that bile acids may modulate nuclear activity. These findings, in concert with the strong link between gastroesophageal reflux and esophageal adenocarcinoma, suggest that bile salts may play a role in the pathogenesis of esophageal adenocarcinoma.[30]

Cyclooxygenase-2 (COX-2) has been shown to be involved in chronic inflammation and epithelial cell growth. The role of COX-2 in various stages of Barrett's esophageal metaplasia and in response to pulses of acid and bile salts in an ex vivo organ culture system was investigated by Shirvani and co-workers.[31] There was a progressive increase in expression of COX-2 with disease progression from Barrett's metaplasia to dysplasia and adenocarcinoma. This increase indicates that COX-2 overexpression is an early event in the neoplastic transformation process of Barrett's columnar metaplasia. Even more interesting, these studies showed that bile and acid could induce COX-2 expression in ex vivo human epithelial explants because COX-2 induction was increased significantly in the presence of acid and bile. The highest induction could be found when the explants were exposed to a 1-hour pulse of bile salts, which in part could be related to protein kinase C activation by bile salts.[32] Similar results were reported by Kawabe et al.,[33] who suggested that duodenogastroesophageal reflux may induce COX-2 expression and prostaglandin E2 production in esophageal epithelial cells and that COX-2–specific inhibitors may have a chemopreventive effect on esophageal carcinoma.

Thus, bile reflux into the esophagus may be linked to the development of adenocarcinoma arising in Barrett's esophagus.[34] The exact mechanism by which reflux of duodenal juice induces foregut cancer is unclear at the present time. Bile salts alone do not seem to be mutagenic, but they promote the mutagenicity of aromatic amines. Alternatively, bile acids and pancreatic enzymes may also facilitate the action of other endoluminal carcinogenic agents by disruption of the mucosal barrier and exposure of the proliferative epithelial compartment.[18]

SUMMARY

Gastric and bile acids are a particularly noxious combination when they interact with the mucosa of the esophagus. There is a critical pH range between 3 and 6 in which bile acids exist in their soluble, unionized form and can penetrate cell membranes and accumulate within mucosal cells. At a lower pH, bile acids are precipitated, and, at a higher pH, bile acids exist in their noninjurious, ionized form. Experimental and clinical studies have shown that increased esophageal exposure to bile in conjunction with acid predisposes to severe esophageal mucosal injury and is the key factor in the pathogenesis and malignant degeneration of Barrett's esophagus.

SUGGESTED READINGS

Guillem PG: How to make a Barrett esophagus: Pathophysiology of columnar metaplasia of the esophagus. Dig Dis Sci 50:415-424, 2005.

Stein HJ, Kauer WKH, Feussner H, et al: Bile acids as components of the duodenogastric refluxate. Hepatogastroenterology 46:66-67, 1999.

Triadafilopoulos G: Acid and bile reflux in Barrett's esophagus: A tale of two evils. Gastroenterology 121:1502-1506, 2001.

Vaezi MF, Singh S, Richter JE: Role of acid and duodenogastric reflux in esophageal injury: A review of animal and human studies. Gastroenterology 108:1897-1907, 1995.

REFERENCES

1. Stein HJ, Barlow AP, DeMeester TR, Hinder RA: Complications of gastroesophageal reflux disease: Role of the lower esophageal sphincter, esophageal acid/alkaline exposure, and duodenogastric reflux. Ann Surg 162:35-43, 1992.
2. Marshall REK, Anggiansah A, Owen JW: Bile in the esophagus. Clinical relevance and ambulatory detection. Br J Surg 84:21-28, 1997.
3. Vaezi MF, Singh S, Richter JE: Role of acid and duodenogastric reflux in esophageal injury: A review of animal and human studies. Gastroenterology 108:1897-1907, 1995.
4. Triadafilopoulos G: Acid and bile reflux in Barrett's esophagus: A tale of two evils. Gastroenterology 121:1502-1506, 2001.
5. Stein HJ, DeMeester TR: Outpatient physiological testing and surgical management of foregut motor disorders. Curr Probl Surg 24:415-555, 1992.
6. Bremner C, Lynch V, Ellis F: Barrett's esophagus: Congenital or acquired? An experimental study of esophageal mucosal regeneration in the dog. Surgery 68:209-216, 1970.
7. Gillen P, Keeling P, Byrne P, et al: Experimental columnar metaplasia in the canine esophagus. Br J Surg 98:2120-2128, 1988.
8. Guillem PG: How to make a Barrett esophagus: Pathophysiology of columnar metaplasia of the esophagus. Dig Dis Sci 50:415-424, 2005.
9. Lillimoe K, Johnson L, Harmon J: Alkaline esophagitis: A comparison of the ability of components of gastroesophageal contents to injure the rabbit esophagus. Gastroenterology 85:621-628, 1983.
10. Ireland A, Peters J, Smyrk T, et al: Gastric juice protects against the development of esophageal adenocarcinoma in the rat. Ann Surg 224:358-371, 1996.
11. Theisen J, Peters HJ, Fein M, et al: The mutagenic potential of duodenoesophageal reflux. Ann Surg 241:63-68, 2005.
12. Jamieson JR, Stein HJ, DeMeester TR, et al: Ambulatory 24-hour esophageal pH monitoring: Normal values, optimal thresholds, specificity and reproducibility. Am J Gastroenterol 87:1102-1111, 1992.
13. Stein HJ, Feussner H, Kauer WKH, et al: "Alkaline" gastroesophageal reflux: Assessment by ambulatory esophageal aspiration and pH monitoring. Am J Surg 167:163-168, 1994.
14. Attwood S, DeMeester TR, Bremner CG, et al: Alkaline gastroesophageal reflux: Implications in the development of complications in Barrett's columnar-lined lower esophagus. Surgery 106:764-770, 1989.
15. Stein HJ: Characterization of acid and alkaline reflux in patients with Barrett's esophagus. Dis Esophagus 105:107-111, 1993.
16. Bechi P, Pucciani F, Baldini F, et al: Long-term ambulatory enterogastric reflux monitoring. Validation of a new fiberoptic technique. Dig Dis Sci 38:1297-1306, 1993.
17. Stein HJ, Kauer WKH, Feussner H, et al: Bile reflux in benign and malignant Barrett's esophagus. Effect of medical acid suppression and fundoplication. J Gastrointest Surg 2:333-341, 1998.
18. Stein HJ, Kauer WKH, Feussner H, et al: Bile acids as components of the duodenogastric refluxate. Hepatogastroenterology 46:66-67, 1999.
19. Kauer WKH, Peters HJ, DeMeester TR, et al: Mixed reflux of gastric and duodenal juice is more harmful to the esophagus than gastric juice alone. Ann Surg 4:525-533, 1995.
20. Kauer WKH, Peter JH, DeMeester TR, et al: Composition and concentration of bile acid reflux into the esophagus of patients with gastroesophageal reflux disease. Surgery 122:874-881, 1997.

21. Schmid R: Bilirubin metabolism: State of the art. Gastroenterology 74:1307-1312, 1987.
22. Poland RL, Odell GB: Physiologic jaundice: The enterohepatic circulation of bilirubin. N Engl J Med 284:1-6, 1971.
23. Hofman AF: The enterohepatic circulation of bile acids in man. Clin Gastroenterol 6:3-24, 1977.
24. Schweitzer EJ, Bass BL, Batzri S, Harmon JW: Bile acid accumulation by rabbit esophageal mucosa. Dig Dis Sci 31:1105-1113, 1986.
25. Batzri BL, Harmon JW, Schweitzer EJ, et al: Bile acid accumulation in gastric mucosal cells. Proc Soc Exp Biol Med 197:393-399, 1991.
26. Barthlen W, Liebermann-Meffert D, Feussner H, Stein HJ: Effect of pH on bile acid concentration in human, pig, and commercial bile: Implications for measurement of 'alkaline' reflux. Dis Esophagus 7:127-130, 1994.
27. Beuers U, Throckmorton DC, Anderson MS, et al: Tauro-ursodeoxycholic acid activates protein kinase C in isolated rat hepatocytes. Gastroenterology 110:1553-1563, 1996.
28. Hirano F, Tanaka H, Makino Y, et al: Induction of the transcription factors AP-1 in cultured human colon adenocarcinoma cells following exposure to bile salts. Carcinogenesis 17:427-433, 1996.
29. Parks DJ, Blanchard SG, Bledsoe RK, et al: Bile acids; natural ligands for an orphan nuclear receptor. Science 284:1365-1368, 1999.
30. Lagergren J, Bergstrom R, Lindgren A, et al: Symptomatic gastroesophageal reflux as a risk factor for esophageal adenocarcinoma. N Engl J Med 340:825-831, 1999.
31. Shirvani V, Rodica O, Baljeet S, et al: Cyclooxygenase 2 expression in Barrett's esophagus and adenocarcinoma: Ex vivo induction of bile salts and acid exposure. Gastroenterology 118:487-496, 2000.
32. Fitzgerald R, Omary M, Triafilopoulos G: Dynamic effects of acid on Barrett's esophagus. J Clin Invest 98:2120-2128, 1996.
33. Kawabe A, Shimada Y, Soma T, et al: Production of prostaglandin E_2 via bile acid is enhanced by trypsin and acid in normal human esophageal epithelial cells. Life Sci 21:21-34, 2004.
34. Wilson K, Fu S, Ramajunam K, et al: Increased expression of inducible nitric oxide synthase and cyclooxygenase-2 in Barrett's esophagus and associated adenocarcinoma. Cancer Res 58:2929-2934, 1998.

16

Reflux Strictures and Short Esophagus

Allan Pickens · Mark B. Orringer

It has been estimated that 60% to 70% of all benign esophageal strictures in the United States are the consequence of reflux esophagitis.[1] Esophageal reflux strictures result from the inflammatory reaction that is induced in the esophagus by exposure to regurgitated gastric contents, both acid and alkaline.[2] It is unknown why strictures develop in certain patients with gastroesophageal reflux (GER). GER occurs independently of the presence or size of a hiatal hernia. Incompetence of the lower esophageal sphincter (LES) is the critical pathologic lesion. Reflux of gastric contents across the LES causes ulceration, submucosal edema, and inflammatory cell infiltration. Acute reflux esophagitis occurs in cycles and progresses to transmural fibrous infiltration. The inflammation may involve the muscular layers of the esophagus, as well as periesophageal soft tissues. Surrounding mediastinal edema and lymphadenopathy may be present. With healing, varying degrees of fibrosis occur. Contraction of collagen within the esophageal scar produces both circumferential narrowing and esophageal shortening.

Controversy regarding the concept of the "short esophagus" has existed for many years. Tileston reported patients with ulcerative reflux esophagitis and described associated esophageal stenosis.[3] As the term "reflux esophagitis" was popularized as a distinct clinical entity by Allison[4] and Barrett,[5] the occurrence of columnar epithelium distal to the stenosis in many of these patients began to be recognized. Although he was a pioneer in his efforts to define reflux esophagitis, Barrett unfortunately concluded that any portion of the swallowing passage that is lined by columnar epithelium is stomach.[5] Thus, the term "short esophagus" was coined because the columnar-lined esophagus distal to the stricture was regarded as stomach. With time, it became apparent that columnar lining of the lower part of the esophagus is an acquired lesion that results from reflux esophagitis.[6,7] Development of the techniques of esophageal manometry confirmed a definite, yet weak LES at the anatomic esophagogastric junction in patients with a columnar-lined lower esophagus. As a result, some investigators have disputed the very existence of a short esophagus and argue that the esophagogastric junction can always be reduced below the diaphragmatic hiatus for an antireflux operation.[8] Such thinking contradicts the preponderance of evidence from pathologic specimens, data from animal models, and the known response of tissue to burns. This is not the viewpoint of most esophageal surgeons, who recognize that fibrous contracture may occur in the esophagus just as it does at other sites in the body in response to a burn. Furthermore, it is apparent that acquired esophageal shortening in response to GER may occur even in patients who do not have esophageal fibrosis or stricture formation. Therefore, the term short esophagus can be applied appropriately to any patient who has an unacceptable degree of stretch of the distal esophagus once the esophagogastric junction is reduced below the diaphragm. This type of short esophagus may be found in association with hiatal hernia, Barrett's metaplasia, caustic ingestion, scleroderma, and Crohn's disease. It is reported that a shortened esophagus occurs in 10% to 15% of patients who undergo antireflux surgery.[9] Because the majority of antireflux operations are performed transabdominally, assessment of tension on the distal esophagus at completion of the repair is seldom possible. Furthermore, the elevation of the diaphragm caused by the pneumoperitoneum required for laparoscopy makes transabdominal assessment of esophageal tension less accurate. Consequently, esophageal shortening is grossly underestimated. Failure to recognize a short esophagus is thought to be responsible for 20% to 30% of surgical failures after open or laparoscopic fundoplication.[10] Reflux strictures and short esophagus have immediate and long-term implications for the success of antireflux operations.

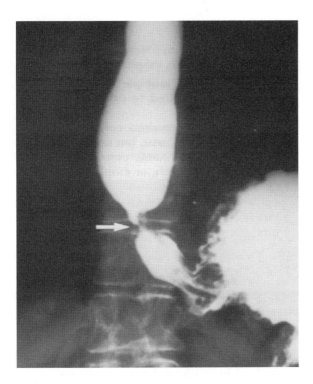

Figure 16–1. Barium esophagogram demonstrating the most frequent type of esophageal reflux stricture: a short stenosis *(arrow)* less than 2 cm occurring at the esophagogastric junction just proximal to a sliding hiatal hernia. (From Orringer MB: Short esophagus and peptic stricture. In Sabiston DC Jr, Spencer FC [eds]: Surgery of the Chest, 6th ed. Philadelphia, WB Saunders, 1995, p 1059.)

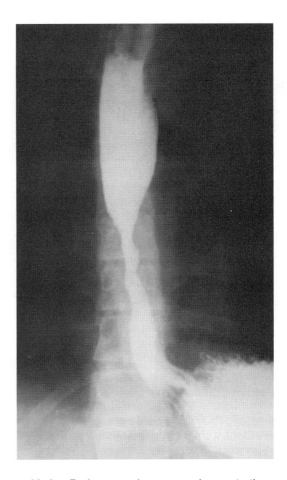

Figure 16–2. Barium esophagogram demonstrating an 8-cm-long esophageal reflux stricture that occurred after protracted vomiting. There is an associated sliding hiatal hernia. (From Orringer MB: Short esophagus and peptic stricture. In Sabiston DC Jr, Spencer FC [eds]: Surgery of the Chest, 6th ed. Philadelphia, WB Saunders, 1995, p 1060.)

ANATOMIC VARIATION AND EVALUATION

Esophageal reflux strictures occur in three general varieties. Most reflux strictures are 1 to 2 cm in length and are localized to the anatomic esophagogastric junction (Fig. 16–1). Less frequently, long strictures occur in the distal half or third of the esophagus in critically ill supine patients with nasogastric tubes (Fig. 16–2). Finally, short strictures form in the mid or upper thoracic esophagus at the squamocolumnar epithelial junction in patients with Barrett's esophagus (Fig. 16–3). The presence of a benign mid- or upper-esophageal stricture in a patient with GER should always alert the physician to the possibility of Barrett's esophagus. The stricture characteristically occurs at the squamocolumnar epithelial junction, and a sliding hiatal hernia is usually, but not always, present.

The presence of an esophageal reflux stricture is typically diagnosed by means of a barium esophagogram obtained in a patient who has dysphagia or reflux symptoms. There is debate regarding whether barium esophagography should be performed early in the evaluation of such esophageal symptoms or whether one should proceed directly to endoscopic evaluation. Endoscopy may be both diagnostic and therapeutic, but the barium esophagogram provides valuable anatomic information

about the esophagus that may help direct therapy and prevent endoscopic complications. The barium esophagogram provides information regarding the length, extent, and degree of narrowing of the stricture, which may be helpful in choosing the best method of dilatation. The barium esophagogram also appears to be more sensitive than endoscopy for the detection of subtle narrowing of the esophagus that is less than 10 mm in diameter.[11] Finally, the barium esophagogram provides an objective baseline record of the esophagus that can be used to assess the response to therapy or progression of disease.

Although it would obviously be desirable to treat GER before mural fibrosis occurs, early diagnosis of reflux esophagitis is hampered by the curious nature of this disease. A notoriously poor correlation between symptoms and the degree of esophagitis prevents physicians from relying on patient complaints as the primary indicator of the need for evaluation. The barium esophagogram provides no real information about the likelihood of successful stricture dilatation. The narrowing seen on a barium esophagogram in a patient with a

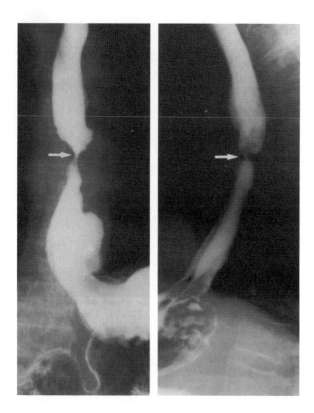

Figure 16–3. Posteroanterior *(left)* and lateral *(right)* views from an esophagogram demonstrating a short midesophageal stricture *(arrows)* in a patient with chronic reflux symptoms and dysphagia. This "high" stricture suggested Barrett's esophagus.

Grade I: distal esophageal mucosal erythema (which may obscure the esophagogastric squamocolumnar epithelial junction)

Grade II: mucosal erythema with superficial ulceration, typically linear and vertical and with an overlying fibrinous membranous exudate that is easily wiped away to leave a bleeding surface (which is often misinterpreted as "scope trauma" by an inexperienced endoscopist)

Grade III: mucosal erythema with superficial ulceration and associated mural fibrosis—a dilatable "early" stricture

Grade IV: extensive ulcerative and fibrous luminal stenosis, which may represent irreversible panmural fibrosis

In the Savary-Monnier classification,[13] there are five grades of reflux esophagitis:

Grade 1: single or multiple erosions (may be erythematous or covered by exudates) on a single mucosal fold

Grade 2: multiple erosions covering several mucosal folds (may be confluent, but not circumferential)

Grade 3: multiple circumferential erosions

Grade 4: ulcer, stenosis, or esophageal shortening

Grade 5: Barrett's epithelium (columnar mucosa re-epithelialization in the form of an island or strip or circumferential)

The Los Angeles classification of reflux esophagitis[14] similarly has five grades of esophagitis:

Grade 0: normal mucosa

Grade A: single erosion 5 mm or smaller on top of a fold

Grade B: single erosion greater than 5 mm on top of a fold

Grade C: confluent erosions 75% or less of the circumference

Grade D: confluent erosions greater than 75% of the circumference

Regardless of which endoscopic grading system is used, such objectivity in describing the pathologic changes seen endoscopically is preferable to the traditional designations of "mild," "moderate," or "severe" esophagitis, which have inherent wide variation and observer variability.

In addition to endoscopic grading of esophagitis, there is a need to classify reflux strictures according to the degree of resistance encountered during attempts at dilatation. The "hardness" of a reflux stricture reflects the degree of fibrosis present and has direct implications for successful treatment with conservative measures. The severity of a stricture can be classified on the basis of the degree of resistance encountered during dilatation. A *mild* stricture is defined as one in which minimal resistance is encountered as progressively larger dilators are passed through the stenosis. A *moderate* stricture requires some, but not excessive forceful dilatation. A *severe* stricture requires forceful dilatation and is inevitably associated with marked periesophageal inflammation

reflux stricture has two components: (1) edema and the cellular inflammatory reaction of acute reflux esophagitis and (2) varying degrees of fibrosis caused by previous reflux episodes. The ease with which progressively larger esophageal dilators can be passed through the radiographic narrowing (i.e., the "hardness" of the stricture) cannot be predicted from an esophagogram.

Endoscopic evaluation is recommended for most patients with dysphagia to establish a diagnosis, seek evidence of esophagitis, exclude malignancy, and implement appropriate therapy. Technologic advances in endoscopic optics and instruments have made the flexible esophagoscope the most common means of visualizing the esophageal lumen. Adequate esophageal biopsy and brushings for cytologic evaluation of the stricture should be performed at the initial endoscopic assessment of the stricture. The combination of esophageal biopsy and brushing establishes the diagnosis of carcinoma in more than 95% of patients with a malignant stricture. If there is no evidence of neoplasm with either of these studies, it is highly likely that the esophageal stenosis is benign.

A variety of classifications of esophageal inflammation have been proposed. Esophagitis is an endoscopic diagnosis, and several established classifications of reflux esophagitis may be applied to strictures. Skinner and Belsey[12] proposed four grades of esophagitis:

and mural thickening of the esophagus. Determination of the severity of a reflux stricture may not be possible with the flexible esophagoscope. Rigid esophagoscopy still has its place in the esophageal surgeon's armamentarium because it allows larger biopsy specimens to be harvested and permits direct assessment of stricture length and the degree of stenosis by direct gentle probing with a bougie. With a more severe stricture, it is dangerous to advance either the flexible or rigid esophagoscope. After the initial assessment and biopsy to exclude carcinoma, treatment of the esophageal reflux stenosis is addressed.

Preoperative assessment of the presence of a short esophagus is notoriously difficult. In a retrospective analysis of the preoperative predictability of a short esophagus in patients with stricture and paraesophageal hernia, an esophagogram had a sensitivity of 66% and a positive predictive value of 37%, whereas manometric length had a sensitivity of 43% and a positive predictive value of 25%.[15] Neither esophagography nor manometry was a reliable predictor of a short esophagus. Esophageal length is best evaluated in the operating room. It is helpful to think of a short esophagus as falling into two categories: (1) a truly nonreducible short esophagus in which the esophagogastric junction fails to reduce beneath the diaphragm and (2) a relatively short esophagus in which the esophagogastric junction fails to reduce beneath the diaphragm without undue tension. Perioperative endoscopic and radiologic studies document that both groups have an esophagogastric junction located at or above the hiatus. Both the truly nonreducible esophagus and the relatively short esophagus have sustained enough chronic damage to lead to actual intrinsic shortening. Some patients may have an apparently short esophagus that has a normal length accordioned into the mediastinum. The only absolute way to document esophageal shortening is direct assessment of the degree of tension remaining on the distal end of the esophagus after positioning of the esophagogastric junction below the diaphragm at the time of surgery.

TREATMENT

Nonoperative Management

Adequate treatment of esophagitis is critical to the prevention and management of esophageal stricture. Preventive treatment of esophageal reflux strictures is hampered by the fact that many patients remain relatively asymptomatic as their esophageal inflammation progresses through the initial pathologic and endoscopic stages of reflux esophagitis. In the era before proton pump inhibitors (PPIs), peptic strictures were widely regarded as fixed, fibrotic lesions that would respond only to dilatation or resection. Antireflux therapy was used to control symptoms of esophagitis and prevent progression of the stricture, but there was little expectation that elimination of reflux esophagitis would widen the established stenosis. Clinical trials comparing treatment with histamine receptor antagonists and placebo in

patients with peptic esophageal strictures supported this view.[16,17] These studies showed a significant decrease in reflux esophagitis in patients treated with histamine blockers, but no reduction in the need for stricture dilatation. It has been demonstrated that chronic, aggressive acid-suppression therapy with PPIs both improves dysphagia and decreases the need for subsequent esophageal dilatation.[18,19] In a study of 366 patients with peptic esophageal strictures who were randomly assigned to receive medical therapy with either omeprazole (20 mg daily) or ranitidine (150 mg twice daily) for 1 year after baseline stricture dilatation, repeat dilatation was required in 30% of patients in the omeprazole group versus 46% in the ranitidine group.[20]

The degree of esophagitis is believed to be as important as stricture diameter in causing dysphagia, and the esophagitis can be controlled with medical management. A good antireflux medical regimen includes compliant PPI use, true elevation of the head of the bed at night, regular use of antacids after meals, and refraining from eating for several hours before bedtime. Additional medications may be added as needed to help control reflux. Metoclopramide has been used because it enhances distal esophageal sphincter tone, increases gastric emptying, and relaxes the pyloric sphincter.[21] Sucralfate (aluminum sucrose sulfate) is used primarily in the intensive care setting to form a viscous fluid that binds protein exudates in areas of inflammation to function as a cytoprotective layer. For patients who remain symptomatic despite medical management, 24-hour esophageal pH monitoring can be used to document the adequacy of therapy in controlling acid reflux.

In addition to aggressive antireflux therapy, patients with benign esophageal strictures are usually treated with at least an initial dilatation. Up to 60% of patients require subsequent dilatation.[22] Many patients accept outpatient esophageal dilatation several times per year as a relatively minor price to pay for comfortable swallowing.

Some peptic strictures can be dilated initially with the flexible esophagoscope. The standard adult flexible esophagoscope is the size of a 32-French esophageal dilator, and a mild stricture can be dilated directly by advancing the instrument through the narrowing. Subsequently, blind passage of progressively larger tapered dilators is performed, beginning with a 32-French size and advancing to at least a 46-French size.

Four major types of esophageal dilating devices are commonly used: (1) mercury- or fiber-filled bougies that are passed blindly through the mouth (e.g., tapered Maloney dilators [Fig. 16–4] and blunt Hurst dilators); (2) gum-tipped dilators that are passed through the standard rigid esophagoscope (e.g., Jackson dilators [Fig. 16–5]); (3) polyvinyl bougies passed over a guidewire that is positioned within the stricture under endoscopic or fluoroscopic guidance (e.g., Savary dilators [Fig. 16–6]); and (4) balloon dilators that are passed over a guidewire or through the endoscope (e.g., TTS balloons). Esophageal dilators are sized by using the French gauge system, in which 1 French equals 3 mm (e.g., a 50-French dilator has a 1.5-cm diameter). Restoration of comfortable swallowing generally requires that at least a 46-French dilator be passed through the

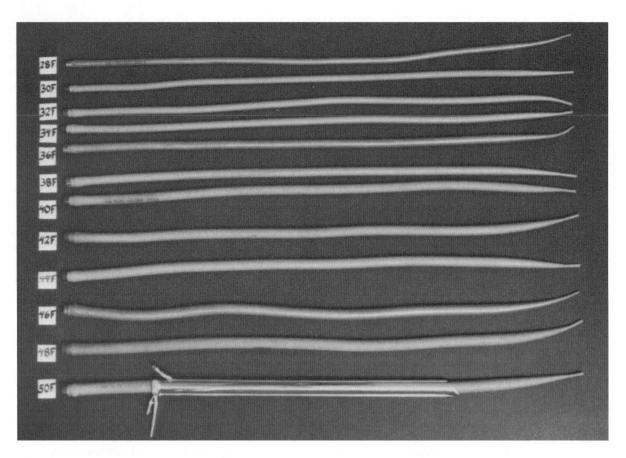

Figure 16–4.   Tapered Maloney esophageal dilators and Pilling 45-cm esophagoscope used to dilate dense, severe reflux strictures under direct vision.

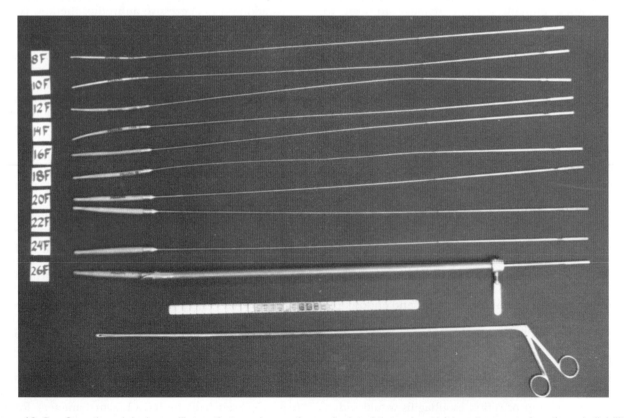

Figure 16–5.   Gum-tipped Jackson dilators that can be gently manipulated through a stricture to assess length and pliability of the obstruction. The 26 French is the largest dilator that will pass through a standard 45-cm rigid esophagoscope.

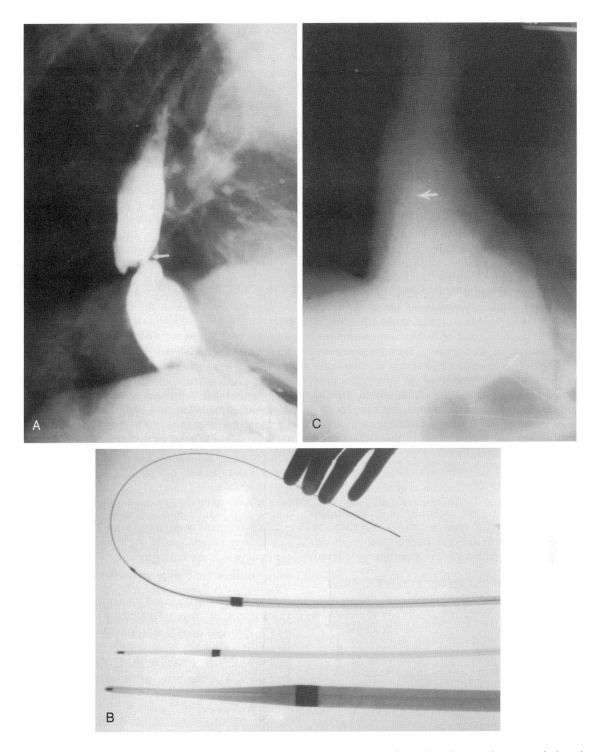

Figure 16–6.   A, Esophagogram showing an eccentric complex reflux stricture *(arrow)* at the esophagogastric junction proximal to a large sliding hiatal hernia. Because of the diverticulum-like configuration of the lumen in the region of the stricture, blind passage of a Maloney bougie was thought to be unsafe. **B,** Several sizes of polyvinyl Savary-Gillard dilators with a guidewire passed through the upper dilator. **C,** Radiographic confirmation of the proper course of the endoscopically placed Savary guidewire *(arrow)* through the esophageal stenosis and into the stomach (same patient as shown in **A**). Progressively larger Savary dilators up to 54 French were passed over the wire and through the stricture. Blind passage of Maloney dilators on an outpatient basis was then achieved without difficulty. (From Orringer MB: Short esophagus and peptic stricture. In Sabiston DC Jr, Spencer FC [eds]: Surgery of the Chest, 6th ed. Philadelphia, WB Saunders, 1995, p 1060.)

esophageal stricture; a larger size is preferable if it can be passed safely.

When dilating a stricture with bougies, the initial choice of dilator size is based on estimates from a barium esophagogram or endoscopic examination. A more physiologic approach to estimation of stricture diameter involves having the patient swallow barium spheres of known diameter, but this is seldom used in clinical practice and has not been found to improve dilatation results. The historic "rule of threes" is a clinical maxim that states that no more than three bougies of progressively increasing size should be passed at any one dilatation session to minimize the risk for esophageal perforation and hemorrhage.[23] Although this rule seems reasonable as a clinical guideline, no studies have verified that adherence to the rule improves dilatation efficacy or safety.[22] Furthermore, balloon dilatation routinely dilates strictures in one session to a diameter far greater than that achieved with three sequential bougies. Balloons are designed to burst if a certain pressure is exceeded during dilatation, but it is not clear that the burst pressure is less than that required to rupture a diseased esophagus. If one elects to dilate a stricture with tapered mercury-filled dilators rather than balloons, it seems a reasonable concession to the unvalidated rule of threes to pass bougies of progressively increasing diameter until resistance is first encountered and to pass no more than two subsequent bougies in the same session.[22] This may not be a reasonable approach when using polyvinyl (e.g., Savary) dilators passed over a guidewire because these dilators may not provide the operator with a meaningful tactile impression of stricture resistance. With polyvinyl dilators, the resistance to passage perceived by the operator may be more a function of friction produced by the guidewire than resistance created by the esophageal stenosis. In reality, there is no perfect predictor of impending complication from esophageal dilatation.

Mercury-filled bougies, or the fiber-filled bougies that have replaced them, are the dilator of choice for esophageal strictures with diameters larger than 10 to 12 mm.[24,25] These dilators are passed without a guidewire and frequently without fluoroscopic assistance. In addition, they can often be passed with minimal or no sedation. In fact, some patients can perform self-dilatation after proper instruction. The flexibility of fiber-filled dilators that contributes to their safety becomes a disadvantage when dilating complicated strictures that are long, tight, or tortuous. Fiber-filled dilators with diameters smaller than 10 mm (30 French) are so floppy that they may curl in the esophagus proximal to a tight stricture, thereby increasing the risk for perforation (Fig. 16–7). Complex strictures can be dilated under general anesthesia through a rigid esophagoscope with gum-tipped bougies that are passed through the stenosis under direct vision. Most standard rigid esophagoscopes will accommodate up to a 26-French bougie in this manner. After reaching this size, the rigid esophagoscope is removed and the dilatation is often continued blindly by passing a mercury-filled tapered dilator. Alternatively, a special-order rigid esophagoscope that accommodates up to a 50-French dilator may be passed to allow progressive

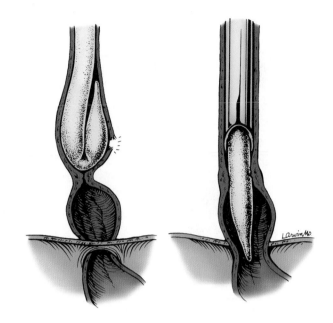

Figure 16–7. *Left,* Esophageal perforation caused by "curling" of an esophageal dilator passed blindly in an attempt to dilate a tight stricture. *Right,* A special-order, large rigid esophagoscope accommodates up to a 50-French dilator and permits dilatation of the stricture. (From Orringer MB: Complications of esophageal surgery and trauma. In Greenfield LJ [ed]: Complications in Surgery and Trauma, 2nd ed. Philadelphia, JB Lippincott, 1990, p 310.)

dilatation of the stricture under direct vision. With the decreasing popularity of rigid esophagoscopy, a Savary guidewire is passed through the flexible esophagoscope and across the stricture into the stomach. After removing the esophagoscope, progressively larger tapered Savary dilators are passed over the guidewire until there is an adequate lumen to permit endoscopic assessment along with biopsy and cytologic brushings. Alternatively, balloon dilatation over a guidewire or under endoscopic guidance has been shown to be effective.[26] Balloon dilators deliver only radial force, in contrast to pushed bougies, which deliver axial shear force as well as radial dilating force to the stricture. Despite the reported advantages of the isolated radial dilating force of the balloon, no studies have convincingly demonstrated that any dilator is superior.

The major complications of esophageal dilatation are perforation and bleeding. These two complications occur with approximately equal frequency. An American Society for Gastrointestinal Endoscopy survey found an average rate of perforation and bleeding of 0.2% with mercury-filled bougies and 2.5% with balloon dilatation.[27,28] The complication rate is highest with dilatation performed for strictures that are complex (i.e., long, tight, or tortuous). Endoscopic interventions such as a heater probe and injection can control most bleeding, but a contrast study is recommended if perforation is suspected. Although water-soluble contrast (e.g., diatrizoate meglumine [Gastrografin]) is commonly recommended for this study, such hypertonic agents can cause chemical pneumonitis if they are aspirated into the lungs. Consequently, these agents should not be used in sedated patients who have recently undergone an endoscopic procedure. Most patients experience pain and possibly pneumomediastinum after perforation. Dilute barium is recommended as the contrast agent of choice because it does not cause chemical pneumonitis and identifies small perforations with greater sensitivity. Perforations after stricture dilatation can be observed if contained or primarily repaired if not contained.

Stricture recurrence is common after initial dilatation. Neither the severity of the initial stenosis, the dilatation method, nor dilator size appears to have a major influence on the likelihood of stricture recurrence. Before PPIs became available, approximately 60% of patients would require multiple dilatations.[29,30] With PPI therapy, as few as 30% of patients may require repeat dilatation within 1 year.[19] There are reports that intralesional corticosteroid injection decreases the recurrence of refractory benign strictures and the need for subsequent endoscopic dilatation, but the exact mechanism is unknown.[31] It has been suggested that intralesional corticosteroids inhibit collagen synthesis and fibrosis, thereby reducing stricture severity. Self-expanding metal stents have also been used as an alternative treatment of refractory strictures.[32] The long-term potential consequences of such a foreign body in the esophagus are worrisome. Laser therapy has also been used for the treatment of refractory benign strictures.[33] This approach has not received widespread acceptance because of inability to assess the depth of penetration of the laser beam. Despite advances in technology, there is no reliable method to predict or totally eliminate the need for future dilatation of benign strictures. Dysphagia serves as the primary indicator of the need for additional treatment.

A patient who has a reflux stricture associated with Barrett's mucosa without endoscopic ulceration or histologic atypia may be treated effectively with a complete antireflux medical regimen, intermittent dilatation, and endoscopic surveillance at 1- or 2-year intervals to exclude dysplastic or neoplastic changes.

Once the esophageal stricture is dilated, gastric contents can again reflux into the esophagus and produce symptomatic GER. With the availability of highly effective antisecretory medications such as PPIs, concern about exacerbation of reflux symptoms should not be a major factor limiting the extent of dilatation. In fact, it has been suggested that esophageal dilatation in combination with antireflux medical therapy is the treatment of choice for virtually all patients with peptic esophageal strictures.[19] The poor operative results with long-term reflux control in patients treated with standard hiatal hernia repairs (e.g., Belsey, Nissen, or Hill operations) or the technical difficulty of esophageal resection with reconstruction has been used as a strong argument against the operative treatment of reflux strictures. Without question, the availability of PPI therapy has drastically reduced the need for operative intervention in patients with reflux strictures.

Surgical Treatment

Modern surgical advances have altered the traditional operative approach to reflux strictures. There is still a small, but definite population of patients with reflux strictures who are candidates for surgical intervention. These patients are debilitated by intractable reflux symptoms or dysphagia despite aggressive medical therapy and dilatation. There are two general approaches to the surgical treatment of esophageal strictures: (1) antireflux surgery with intraoperative stricture dilatation and (2) esophageal resection and reconstruction. Antireflux surgery combined with intraoperative dilatation produces success rates similar to those reported for nonsurgical dilatation therapy.[34-36] The major advantage is that successful surgery obviates the need for lifelong medical therapy with its attendant expense and inconvenience. However, there is no clear difference in the relief of dysphagia achieved with such surgery versus dilatation and medical therapy. There is a small operative mortality of less than 1% associated with fundoplication. The incidence of repeated dilatation after antireflux surgery for stricture ranges between 1% and 31%, which is still less than that reported for medical therapy and dilatation.[37] A thorough understanding of the "short esophagus" concept and the methods for addressing it is fundamental to obtaining good outcomes and avoiding complications such as "slipped" wraps and gastric herniation into the mediastinum.

Hayward first suggested that most reflux strictures could be treated successfully with operative dilatation in conjunction with an antireflux operation.[38] Hill et al. were the first in the United States to advocate this approach.[8] However, the presence of a peptic stricture with its inevitable esophageal shortening adversely affects long-term reflux control after standard antireflux operations. In a large retrospective review of the Belsey Mark IV operation, there was a 45% incidence of recurrent reflux or hernia in patients with esophagitis and stricture versus an 11% incidence of recurrent reflux or hernia in patients without esophagitis and stricture.[39] Based on these data, Belsey advocated distal esophagectomy and reconstruction with colon rather than a standard hiatal hernia repair in patients with a stricture and shortening. Mural inflammation, esophagitis, and esophageal shortening are characteristic of peptic esophageal strictures and prevent tension-free reduction of the 3 to 5 cm of distal esophagus below the diaphragm, which is a prerequisite for successful fundoplication. In addition, the Belsey repair requires placement of fundoplication sutures between the diaphragm, fundus, and inflamed distal esophagus. Any antireflux operation performed in the presence of mural inflammation or esophageal shortening jeopardizes the long-term success of the repair.

The most popular antireflux operations—the Belsey fundoplication[12] and the Nissen fundoplication[40]—advocate an intra-abdominal location of the gastroesophageal junction and require sutures in the distal end of the esophagus as part of the procedure. Despite the obvious undesirability of attempting to "drag" the esophagogastric junction of a shortened esophagus below the diaphragm, treatment of reflux strictures with a combi-

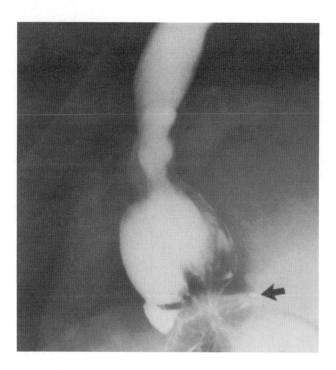

Figure 16–8. Esophagogram demonstrating a "slipped Nissen" fundoplication in an obese woman with esophageal shortening caused by reflux esophagitis. She had undergone an antireflux operation 9 months earlier. After initial control of reflux symptoms, regurgitation, pyrosis, and dysphagia developed. The stomach has "telescoped" through the fundoplication, the horizontal folds of which *(arrow)* can still be seen below the diaphragm. There is a recurrent hiatal hernia, and intermittent obstruction occurs.

nation of dilatation and a standard antireflux procedure has become common. The majority of standard antireflux operations are performed transabdominally, and the ability to assess the degree of esophageal shortening or tension on the distal esophagus after the completed fundoplication is limited. By elevating the diaphragm, the pneumoperitoneum required for laparoscopy further reduces the ability to assess distal esophageal tension. Attempting to pull down a shortened esophagus from an abdominal approach may produce elongation of the proximal part of the stomach, which is then inappropriately identified as the distal esophagus and wrapped by the fundoplication. The resultant "slipped Nissen" seen on subsequent barium esophagography is more a function of an improperly performed initial operation than disruption of the repair. A properly performed fundoplication that encircles the distal end of the esophagus but has been reduced beneath the diaphragm under tension is subject to dehiscence and slippage (Fig. 16–8). Any patient with a failed fundoplication should be evaluated with a barium swallow to delineate herniation and to define the anatomy, as well as upper endoscopy to assess the wrap and locate the esophagogastric junction. If symptoms indicate, an esophageal motility study should be performed to assess esophageal body function,

and a 24-hour pH study should be performed to evaluate acid reflux.[10] Reoperative surgery to correct such failure is known to have a higher rate of complications and less favorable long-term results.[41-44]

To circumvent the problem of trying to maintain the fundoplication below the diaphragm in a patient with esophageal shortening, some have advocated leaving the fundoplication within the thorax.[45,46] This approach creates an iatrogenic paraesophageal hiatal hernia with its potential for mechanical complications, including strangulation, perforation, ulceration, and bleeding. Such complications have been reported after intrathoracic fundoplication.[47,48] Although effective reflux control can be achieved whether the fundoplication is intra-abdominal or intrathoracic, there are obvious advantages when the reconstructed esophagogastric junction is intra-abdominal.

Combined Collis-Belsey Procedure

In 1971, Pearson and associates reported excellent reflux control in patients with strictures treated with the combination of esophagus-lengthening Collis gastroplasty[49] and Belsey repair.[50] The rationale for this approach followed the conclusions of the long-term Belsey study[39]: in a patient with a reflux stricture undergoing fundoplication, it should be possible to minimize recurrent reflux if additional distal esophageal length is made available, thereby minimizing tension on the repair and avoiding the need to suture the diseased esophagus. The combined Collis-Belsey operation is a transthoracic procedure performed through the sixth intercostal space (Fig. 16–9). After mobilizing the distal esophagus, the gastric fundus is delivered into the chest through the diaphragmatic hiatus. This involves routine ligation and division of several short gastric vessels along the high greater curvature of the stomach. With the surgeon's hand supporting the esophagogastric junction to reduce the risk for disruption, the anesthetist passes progressively larger Maloney tapered dilators per os, up to the 54- to 56-French range. With the dilator displaced against the lesser curvature of the stomach and the fundus retracted upward, the GIA stapler is applied to the stomach adjacent to the dilator and parallel to the lesser curvature. Use of the GIA stapler for construction of the gastroplasty tube keeps the operation closed. Advancement of the knife assembly creates a 5-cm-long tube extension of the esophagus. On rare occasion it may be necessary to apply the stapler a second time to gain an additional 2 to 3 cm of esophageal length. The staple line is oversewn, the dilator is removed, and the standard crural sutures are placed but left untied. A standard Belsey repair around the new distal esophagus (i.e., the gastroplasty tube) was recommended by Pearson and associates[51] (Fig. 16–10). After placing and tying two rows of three horizontal mattress sutures to secure the stomach below the diaphragm, the posterior crural sutures are tied. This creates a tension-free segment of intra-abdominal "esophagus" compressed by the partial fundoplication. The fundoplication sutures are placed into the healthy gastroplasty tube instead of the inflamed distal esophagus.

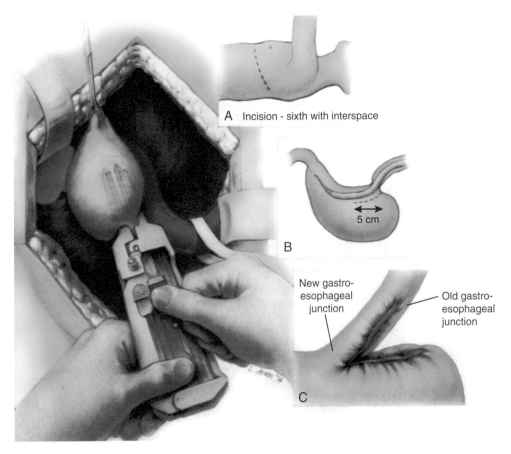

Figure 16–9. Construction of the Collis gastroplasty tube with the GIA surgical stapler. **A,** A sixth left interspace incision is used. **B,** The 54-French dilator inserted through the stricture is displaced against the lesser curvature of the stomach. The *dotted line* indicates the site of application of the stapler. The main illustration shows advancement of the knife assembly. **C,** The new functional distal esophagus is a 5-cm tube of healthy stomach. (From Orringer MB, Sloan H: An improved technique for the combined Collis-Belsey approach to dilatable esophageal strictures. J Thorac Cardiovasc Surg 68:298, 1974.)

Figure 16–10. Belsey reconstruction of the esophagogastric junction after construction of the Collis gastroplasty tube. *Main illustration,* Oversewing the staple suture line. **A,** Placement of the first row of three mattress sutures between the new distal "esophagus" and the gastric fundus. The posterior crural sutures have been placed but are left untied at this point. **B,** Placement of the second row of mattress sutures through the diaphragm, gastric fundus, and distal esophagus 2 cm proximal to the first row. **C,** The completed repair reduced beneath the diaphragm shows a 4-cm intra-abdominal distal esophageal segment (the gastroplasty tube) partially compressed by the Belsey fundoplication. The posterior crural sutures have been tied. (From Orringer MB, Sloan H: An improved technique for the combined Collis-Belsey approach to dilatable esophageal strictures. J Thorac Cardiovasc Surg 68:298, 1974.)

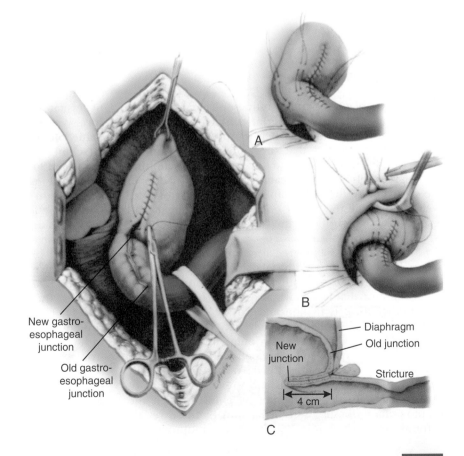

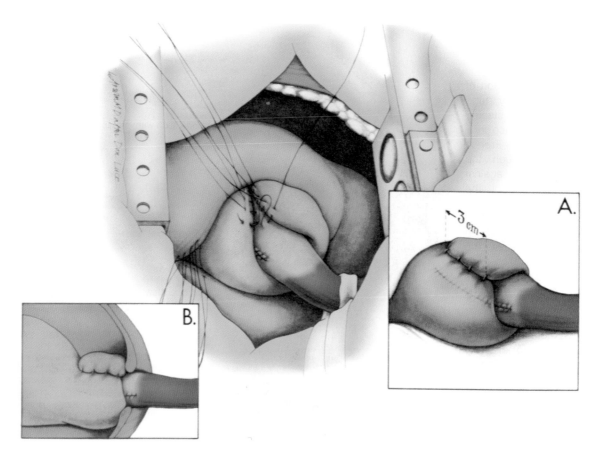

Figure 16–11. A 3-cm long fundoplication after Collis gastroplasty. Four seromuscular 2-0 silk sutures placed 1 cm apart *(main illustration)* result in a 3-cm-long fundoplication around the gastroplasty tube **(A),** not the proximal part of the stomach. **B,** The fundoplication reduced beneath the diaphragm. (From Stirling MC, Orringer MB: The combined Collis-Nissen operation for esophageal reflux strictures. Ann Thorac Surg 45:148, 1988.)

Collis-Nissen Procedure

With the use of postoperative intraesophageal pH monitoring, data emerged showing unsatisfactory long-term reflux control with the Collis-Belsey procedure. Orringer and Sloan[51] suggested that the amount of remaining gastric fundus was inadequate to perform a functioning 240-degree Belsey fundoplication after construction of the gastroplasty tube. To improve reflux control after performance of the Collis gastroplasty, Orringer and associates[52-54] described the use of a 360-degree Nissen-type fundoplication. The cut Collis gastroplasty combined with a 360-degree fundoplication has been successful in patients with dilatable reflux strictures that are amenable to an antireflux operation. Patients in whom initial endoscopic assessment has indicated that the stricture is benign and can be dilated with a 40-French bougie will most likely have a stenosis that can be dilated to the 56-French range at the time of a Collis-Nissen repair. In the combined Collis-Nissen operation, five or six short gastric vessels are routinely divided as the gastric fundus and greater curvature of the stomach are delivered into the chest through the diaphragmatic hiatus. Careful ligation of these vessels without undue tension is required to avoid injury to the

spleen and unrecognized intra-abdominal hemorrhage. Adhesions from previous operations at the hiatus may necessitate a diaphragmatic counterincision for exposure. When necessary, a 5- to 10-cm peripheral diaphragmatic incision is made 5 cm from the diaphragmatic attachment to the costal arch. Division of the costal arch is avoided to minimize postoperative incisional pain and chest wall instability. The reflux stricture is supported by the surgeon as the dilator is passed per os. The gastroplasty tube is constructed with the GIA stapler (see Fig. 16–9). To avoid narrowing of the "neo-esophagus," the gastroplasty and fundoplication are performed with either a 54-French dilator (in women) or a 56-French dilator (in men) within the esophagus.[54] The fundoplication is limited to 3 cm in length and is performed only around the gastroplasty tube (neo-esophagus) (Fig. 16–11). The fundoplication is fashioned with four interrupted seromuscular 2-0 silk sutures placed 1 cm apart, with each suture passing through the gastric fundus, gastroplasty tube, and gastric fundus again. The suture line is oversewn with a 4-0 running polypropylene Lembert seromuscular stitch. This is done prophylactically to prevent a fundoplication suture leak. The dilator is removed, and the fundoplication is reduced beneath the diaphragm. The fundoplication is secured to the undersurface of the diaphragm with three horizontal mattress sutures of 2-0 polypropylene suture placed between the fundoplication and the diaphragm around the circumference of the hiatus. The posterior crural sutures are tied to narrow the hiatus until it admits one finger comfortably alongside the esophagus. Silver clip markers are placed at the apex of the gastroplasty tube (the new gastroesophageal junction) before the fundoplication and at the edges of the diaphragmatic hiatus after the fundoplication has been reduced beneath the diaphragm. The distance between these two sets of silver clip markers on postoperative roentgenograms indicates the intra-abdominal segment of esophagus wrapped by the fundoplication (Fig. 16–12).

Although the severity of the stricture (i.e., the ease with which it can be dilated) cannot be predicted by its appearance radiographically or endoscopically, almost every reflux stricture can be dilated intraoperatively with the esophagus supported by the surgeon's hand as the dilator is passed. Stirling and Orringer found that 95% of esophageal reflux strictures could be dilated to a size compatible with comfortable swallowing (at least to 46 French but generally 54 or 56 French). Successful control of both reflux symptoms and dysphagia was accomplished in 77% of patients, but a 23% failure rate still leaves much to be desired. Occasionally, antegrade dilatation as described is not possible, and it may be necessary to pass a Hegar dilator retrograde through a high gastrotomy,[54] but this is rarely necessary.

When reflux disease has resulted in peptic stricture and shortening of the esophagus, long-term control of reflux with a standard antireflux operation is jeopardized.[39] The uncut Collis-Nissen gastroplasty is a technique designed to relieve distal esophageal obstruction and improve GER. Bingham[55] and Demos et al.[56] suggested retaining the benefits of a total fundoplication around a gastroplasty without transecting the gastric wall. Through a left thoracotomy, the anterior and posterior fundic walls are apposed over a bougie and stapled with a noncutting stapler. The remaining fundus is used to wrap the uncut gastroplasty. The fundoplication is secured with four sutures passed in front of the staple line. The fundoplication is reduced under the diaphragm and fixed in place by three sutures passing through the esophageal wall, apex of the fundoplication, and diaphragm. The procedure has the combined advantages of lengthening the distal esophagus while providing an "anchor" for the fundoplication to reduce the incidence of anatomic hernia recurrence or slipping of the esophagus out of the wrap.[57] Because mucosal apposition of the uncut gastroplasty tube may set the stage for recanalization, the uncut gastroplasty presents the potential for dehiscence of the gastroplasty. In a study of 80 patients who underwent this procedure, 1 patient required reoperation for a recurrent hernia.[58] In another review of 27 patients who underwent an uncut Collis-Nissen gastroplasty, 6 patients had slow esophageal emptying and 3 had occasional episodes of dysphagia. None required postoperative dilation. At least initially, ulcers and erosions healed in all 26 patients. It was concluded that the uncut Collis-Nissen procedure provides acceptable control of GER.[57]

More recently, several minimally invasive techniques have been developed to deal with an esophageal stricture in conjunction with a short esophagus. Decades of experience with the previously described open gastroplasty and fundoplications have established certain principles that are essential for successful outcomes in the treatment of this condition. These concepts include thorough preoperative testing, effective stricture dilatation, routine division of short gastric vessels, crural closure, and wraps performed without tension around 2.5 to 3 cm of tension-free intra-abdominal esophagus (the gastroplasty tube).[10] These principles are equally important in minimally invasive surgical treatment of esophageal strictures.

In the early years of laparoscopic fundoplication surgery, preoperative suspicion of a short esophagus was commonly listed as a contraindication to this approach, and the finding of esophageal shortening at surgery was an indication for conversion to an open procedure.[59] With rapidly evolving technology and increasing experience with minimally invasive approaches, an esophageal reflux stricture with an associated shortened esophagus can be treated while maintaining the benefits of a less invasive approach.

A standard setup for laparoscopic fundoplication is used despite the esophageal stricture or suspected shortened esophagus. Port placement is quite variable, but many surgeons use a midline port (camera), two subcostal retractor ports (liver retractor and assistant retractor), and two subcostal working ports (dissector, stapler, etc.). The phrenoesophageal ligament is dissected to access the distal 3 to 4 cm of esophagus. Care must be taken to preserve the vagi and avoid overly aggressive resection of the gastric fat pad, which can lead to perforation. Esophageal dilators are passed per os and their course in the stomach verified laparoscopically. Laparoscopic instruments are used to support the esophagus along its longitudinal axis during dilatation. Adequacy of the intra-abdominal length of the esophagus is assessed at this point. Assessment can be accomplished by holding the crura together with atraumatic graspers and releasing the stomach. There should be 2.5 to 3 cm of intra-abdominal esophagus without tension. If there is confusion about the location of the gastroesophageal junction, intraoperative endoscopy should be performed. Care must be taken to place the esophagus in position for measurement and avoid forcibly pulling it inferiorly (Fig. 16–13). Pulling the esophagus inferiorly, along with the diaphragmatic elevation created by the pneumoperitoneum, can cause misjudgment of adequate esophageal length. Excessive traction can elongate the proximal part of the stomach and cause it to resemble the esophagus. This can result in a misplaced wrap or a wrap under tension. If 2.5 cm of tension-free intra-abdominal esophagus cannot be obtained, the patient has a short esophagus and needs an esophageal lengthening procedure. Some suggest that extended transhiatal esophageal mobilization (>5 cm) will provide adequate esophageal length and reduce the incidence of fundoplication failure in patients with esophageal shortening.[60] Caution is advised when considering this extent of dissection from a transhiatal view because an esophageal

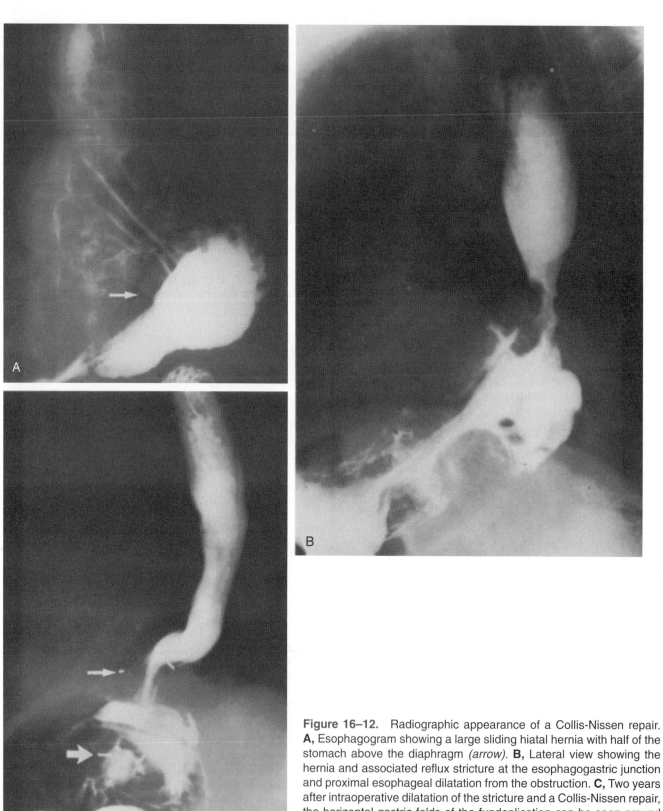

Figure 16–12.   Radiographic appearance of a Collis-Nissen repair. **A,** Esophagogram showing a large sliding hiatal hernia with half of the stomach above the diaphragm *(arrow)*. **B,** Lateral view showing the hernia and associated reflux stricture at the esophagogastric junction and proximal esophageal dilatation from the obstruction. **C,** Two years after intraoperative dilatation of the stricture and a Collis-Nissen repair, the horizontal gastric folds of the fundoplication can be seen around the gastroplasty tube. The *small arrow* indicates silver clips marking the diaphragmatic hiatus. The *large arrows* indicate clips at the new esophagogastric junction (the distal end of the gastroplasty tube). The esophageal stenosis has resolved, and there is now no proximal esophageal dilatation. (From Orringer MB: Short esophagus and peptic stricture. In Sabiston DC Jr, Spencer FC [eds]: Surgery of the Chest, 6th ed. Philadelphia, WB Saunders, 1995, p 1073.)

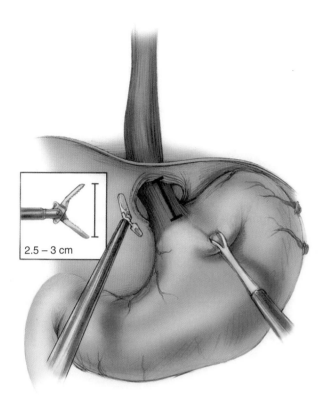

Figure 16–13. Intraoperative assessment of esophageal length. If there is confusion about the location of the gastroesophageal junction, intraoperative endoscopy should be performed. (From Horvath KD, Swanström LL, Jobe BA: The short esophagus: Pathophysiology, incidence, presentation, and treatment in the era of laparoscopic antireflux surgery. Ann Surg 232:630-640, 2000.)

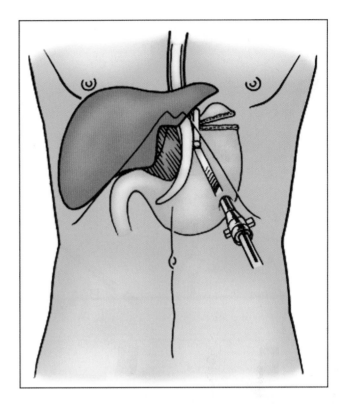

Figure 16–14. An endoscopic stapler is inserted and reticulated to make a horizontal staple line followed by a vertical staple line parallel to and abutting the dilator. A stapled wedge of stomach approximately 15 mL in volume is excised and removed. (From Terry ML, Vernon A, Hunter JG: Stapled-wedge Collis gastroplasty for the shortened esophagus. Am J Surg 188:258-294, 2004.)

lengthening procedure may be far wiser than risking severe hemorrhage, esophageal perforation, and vagus nerve injury.

Two laparoscopic Collis gastroplasty techniques have been described. They rely on laparoscopic esophageal and gastric mobilization, followed by creation of the gastroplasty tube and subsequent fundoplication. Swanström et al. described a totally laparoscopic version of the Collis gastroplasty with fundoplication.[37] With a standard setup for laparoscopic fundoplication, the initial description involved the use of an endoscopic circular stapler to create a window below the angle of His for the insertion of a linear stapler to create the neo-esophagus. This technique caused relative ischemia of the apex of the fundus. The minimally invasive Collis gastroplasty was revised to a stapled wedge gastroplasty.[61] The esophagus is mobilized and assessed for length. If there is less than 2.5 cm of tension-free intra-abdominal esophagus, the orogastric tube is removed and a 48-French dilator is advanced under vision with the laparoscope. A point approximately 3 cm inferior to the angle of His is marked with electrocautery. A left subcostal port is used to insert a reticulating endoscopic 45-mm linear cutting stapler that is maximally flexed. The assistant retracts the gastric fundus inferiorly, and the surgeon

maintains traction on the greater curve just below the angle of His as the stapler is advanced into position. The stapler is fired one to three times until the marked point inferior to the angle of His is reached. Once the transverse staple line is completed, a vertical staple line is created parallel to the esophagus and abutting the dilator (Fig. 16–14). The stapler is fired once or twice to produce a stapled wedge of stomach approximately 15 ml in volume, which is removed from the abdomen. This creates a tube, or neo-esophagus, that is 3 to 4 cm in length. The crura are closed, and a 360-degree tension-free fundoplication is performed around the neo-esophagus. The staple line is oriented so that it is apposed to the stomach wall. Swanström et al. described an alternative technique involving a combined laparoscopic and thoracoscopic Collis gastroplasty with fundoplication.[37] The essentials of this procedure involve placing an endoscopic stapler into the right chest (double-lumen intubation is not required), across the right mediastinal pleura, and transhiatally into the abdomen. This technique allows 3- to 4-cm stapling of the stomach parallel to the lesser curve. The resulting intra-abdominal neo-esophagus can subsequently be wrapped with the fundus (Fig. 16–15). After both minimally invasive Collis gastroplasty techniques, most patients undergo a contrast study

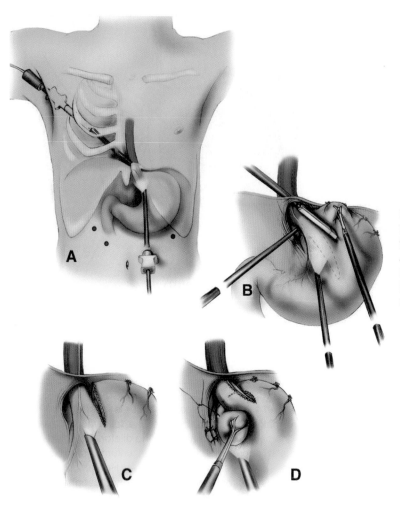

Figure 16–15.   A to **D,** After the neoesophagus has been created, a standard fundoplication is performed around it. (From Horvath KD, Swanström LL, Jobe BA: The short esophagus: Pathophysiology, incidence, presentation, and treatment in the era of laparoscopic antireflux surgery. Ann Surg 232:630-640, 2000.)

before discharge. The reported average length of hospital stay is 3 days, and most patients experience good results. Both techniques are reproducible and safe, but long-term follow-up is needed.

The Collis neo-esophagus typically lacks normal motility. This aperistaltic segment may theoretically be at risk during eventual dilatation or become a source of postoperative dysphagia. In any patient who continues to experience significant dysphagia after a Collis procedure, outpatient esophageal dilatations are performed liberally. A Collis gastroplasty also results in a small segment of gastric mucosa proximal to the newly constructed distal high-pressure zone. This "ectopic" gastric mucosa has been reported to secrete acid and cause localized esophagitis.[42,62] It is advisable to have all Collis gastroplasty patients closely monitored with objective testing. If esophageal acid exposure is documented, long-term medical therapy is indicated. Other complications from the gastroplasty procedure include leaks from the gastroplasty line and fistulas. Complications are reported to occur in up to 10% of open gastroplasty cases[10] and up to 22% of laparoscopic gastroplasty cases.[63] In our review of 240 patients who underwent primary transthoracic repair of paraesophageal hiatal hernias, with a Collis gastroplasty performed in 96% of cases, there was a 0.8% incidence of esophageal leak.[64]

Resection

In some situations a patient with an esophageal reflux stricture is best treated by esophageal resection. Such situations include extremely long nondilatable strictures, strictures with associated Barrett's mucosa with high-grade dysplasia, and strictures after multiple failed antireflux operations. Esophagectomy for nondilatable strictures was necessary in 22% of the patients with benign strictures from reflux disease reported by Bonavina et al.[65] A "nondilatable" stricture is generally defined as (1) one through which a dilator cannot be passed because of luminal narrowing or tortuosity, (2) one that causes persistent dysphagia despite dilatation, and (3) one with a previous perforation during dilatation. Complications of Barrett's esophagus were reported to be the indication for esophagectomy in 20% of patients undergoing resection for benign disease by Salamao et al.[66] Previous unsuccessful antireflux procedures constitute a common indication for esophagectomy for benign disease. Orringer reported a series in which 56% of resections for benign disease were performed for end-stage GER disease.[67] Repeated operations at the esophagogastric junction are associated with tissue damage, loss of function, and reduced blood supply leading to potential ischemic necrosis of either the distal esophagus or gastric fundus. Conserving a devitalized and dysfunctional esophagus invariably leads to poor outcomes. A number of reports have shown that after two previous antireflux procedures, the third antireflux operation is likely to fail in more than 50% of patients.[66,68]

The best conduit for esophageal reconstruction continues to be debated. Reconstruction for benign disease, such as a stricture, requires a substitute organ that is durable and associated with satisfactory long-term functional results. Important factors to consider when selecting the replacement conduit include absence of intrinsic disease, adequacy of blood supply, patient age, and the surgeon's own experience.[69] Proponents of gastric interposition emphasize the technical ease, single anastomosis, and faster return of normal alimentation.[66,70] Total thoracic esophagectomy with a cervical esophagogastric anastomosis is the authors' preferred approach in patients requiring esophageal resection for benign as well as malignant disease. Placing the esophageal anastomosis in the neck avoids the potential for mediastinitis associated with an intrathoracic anastomotic leak. The stomach is positioned in the posterior mediastinum in the original esophageal bed, and an end-to-side cervical esophagogastric anastomosis is constructed several centimeters from the apex of the gastric fundus. Clinically significant reflux is uncommon after a properly performed cervical esophagogastric anastomosis. In the largest series (>1500 patients) of transhiatal esophagectomy and cervical esophagogastric anastomosis, Orringer et al. reported anastomotic leak rates as low as 2.7%, clinically significant postoperative reflux in less than 10%, and good to excellent overall functional results in 70% of patients.[71,72] A cervical esophagogastric anastomotic leak after transhiatal esophagectomy is a predictor of subsequent unsatisfactory function; nearly half of such leaks result in an anastomotic stricture once healing of the fistula is complete. Dilatation of a cervical esophagogastric anastomosis is far safer than dilatation of an intrathoracic anastomosis. The stapled end-to-side cervical esophagogastric anastomotic technique described by Orringer and associates has been shown to decrease the incidence of anastomotic leaks and the need for anastomotic dilatation.[71]

An intrathoracic esophagogastric anastomosis is a poor choice for a patient who has reflux esophagitis with or without stricture. Resection of the lower esophageal sphincter and creation of an iatrogenic hiatal hernia with a portion of the stomach above and a portion below the diaphragm explain the reported 20% to 40% incidence of reflux esophagitis in the residual esophagus of patients undergoing an intrathoracic esophagogastric anastomosis.[73] The reflux that follows construction of an intrathoracic esophagogastric anastomosis may result in a recurrent peptic esophageal stenosis. Distal esophagectomy plus reconstruction with either a jejunal[45] or short-segment colonic interposition[74] is an excellent option in

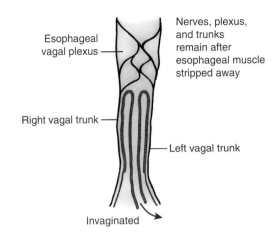

Figure 16–16. The esophagus is stripped out of the mediastinum with simultaneous mucosal inversion. The nerves are sheared off the muscularis propria with the esophageal plexus left intact (From Banki F, Mason RJ, DeMeester SR, et al: Vagal-sparing esophagectomy: A more physiologic alternative. Ann Surg 236:324-336, 2002.)

patients with reflux strictures requiring resection, and these procedures are associated with reasonable elimination of reflux symptoms. Both these reconstructions, however, are of considerable magnitude and are technically demanding. If an anastomotic stricture develops, dilatation of an intrathoracic esophagojejunal or esophagocolonic anastomosis is dangerous.

Vagal-sparing esophagectomy has been described as an ideal procedure for patients with end-stage benign esophageal disease.[75] This method of esophagectomy involves removal of the esophagus while preserving the vagal nerves and gastric reservoir. The esophagus is stripped out of the mediastinum and inverted in the process. This results in shearing the nerve fibers off the muscularis propria with the esophageal plexus left intact (Fig. 16–16). Colon is used as the replacement conduit. The preservation of gastric secretory, motor, and reservoir function reportedly allows normal alimentation, bowel regulation, and less weight loss. Vagal-sparing esophagectomy is reportedly associated with less postoperative dumping, diarrhea, and early satiety.[75]

One final method of indirect resectional therapy for esophagitis with stricture is partial gastrectomy and Roux-en-Y biliary diversion. Wangensteen and Levin were the first to report resolution of benign esophageal stenosis after partial gastrectomy for peptic ulcer disease.[76] The importance of bile in refluxed gastric contents in the development of severe esophagitis was then recognized both clinically and experimentally.[77,78] Consequently, some surgeons have treated reflux strictures with partial gastrectomy and Roux-loop gastrojejunostomy,[79] whereas others advocate antrectomy and Roux diversion in conjunction with resection.[80,81] In the opinion of the authors, it is difficult to rationalize leaving behind the inflamed, scarred, strictured esophagus, which may contain premalignant Barrett's epithelium, while sacrificing the healthy stomach, perhaps the best organ with which to replace the esophagus.

REFERENCES

1. Marks RD, Shukla M: Diagnosis and management of peptic esophageal strictures. Gastroenterologist 4:223-237, 1996.

2. Behar J, Ramsby G: Gastric emptying and antral motility in reflux esophagitis: Effect of oral metoclopramide. Gastroenterology 74:253-256, 1978.

3. Tileston W: Peptic ulcer of the esophagus. Am J Med Sci 132:240-265, 1906.

4. Allison PR: Peptic ulcer of the oesophagus. Thorax 3:20, 1948.

5. Barrett NR: Chronic peptic ulcer of the oesophagus and "oesophatitis." Br J Surg 38:175-182, 1950.

6. Allison PR, Johnston AS, Royce GB: Short esophagus with simple peptic ulceration. J Thorac Surg 12:432, 1943.

7. Mossberg SM: The columnar lined esophagus (Barrett's syndrome)—an acquired condition? Gastroenterology 50:671-676, 1966.

8. Hill LD, Gelfand M, Bauermeister D: Simplified management of reflux esophagitis with stricture. Ann Surg 172:638-651, 1970.

9. Waring JP: Surgical and endoscopic treatment of gastroesophageal reflux disease. Gastroenterol Clin North Am 31(4 Supp):S89-S109, 2002.

10. Horvath KD, Swanström LL, Jobe BA: The short esophagus: Pathophysiology, incidence, presentation, and treatment in the era of laparoscopic antireflux surgery. Ann Surg 232:630-640, 2000.

11. Ott DJ, Chen YM, Wu WC, et al: Radiographic and endoscopic sensitivity in detecting lower esophageal mucosal ring. AJR Am J Roentgenol 147:261-265, 1986.

12. Skinner DB, Belsey RH: Surgical management of esophageal reflux and hiatus hernia. Long-term results with 1,030 patients. J Thorac Cardiovasc Surg 53:33-54, 1967.

13. Ollyo JB, Fontolliet E, Brossard FL, et al: Savary's new endoscopic classification of reflux oesophagitis. Acta Endosc 22:307-320, 1992.

14. Armstrong D, Bennett JR, Blum AL, et al: The endoscopic assessment of esophagitis: A progress report on observer agreement. Gastroenterology 111:85-92, 1996.

15. Mittal SK, Awad ZT, Tasset M, et al: The preoperative predictability of the short esophagus in patients with stricture or paraesophageal hernia. Surg Endosc 14:464-468, 2000.

16. Ferguson R, Dronfield MW, Atkinson M: Cimetidine in treatment of reflux oesophagitis with peptic stricture. BMJ 2:472-474, 1979.

17. Starlinger M, Appel WH, Schemper M, Schiessel R: Long-term treatment of peptic esophageal stenosis with dilatation and cimetidine: Factors influencing clinical results. Eur Surg Res 17:207-214, 1985.

18. Koop H, Arnold R: Long-term maintenance treatment of reflux esophagitis with omeprazole: Prospective study in patients with H_2-blocker resistant esophagitis. Dig Dis Sci 36:552-557, 1991.

19. Marks RD, Richter JE, Rizzo H, et al: Omeprazole versus H_2-receptor antagonists in treating patients with peptic stricture and esophagitis. Gastroenterology 106:907-915, 1994.

20. Smith PM, Kerr GD, Cockel R, et al: A comparison of omeprazole and ranitidine in the prevention of recurrence of benign esophageal stricture. Gastroenterology 107:1312-1318, 1994.

21. Goldstein F, Thornton JJ 3rd, Abramson J, et al: Bile reflux gastritis and esophagitis in patients without prior gastric surgery, with pilot study of the therapeutic effects of metoclopramide. Am J Gastroenterol 76:407-411, 1981.

22. Spechler SJ: AGA technical review on treatment of patients with dysphagia caused by benign disorders of the distal esophagus. Gastroenterology 117:301-338, 1999.

23. Tulman AB, Boyce HW: Complications of esophageal dilatation and guidelines for their prevention. Gastrointest Endosc 27:229-234, 1981.

24. Marks RD, Richter JE: Peptic strictures of the esophagus. Am J Gastroenterol 8:1160-1173, 1993.

25. Nostrant TT: Esophageal dilatation. Dig Dis 13:337-355, 1995.

26. Saeed ZA, Ramirez FC, Hepps KS, et al: An objective end point for dilation improves outcomes of peptic esophageal strictures. Gastrointest Endosc 45:354-359, 1997.

27. Silvis SE, Nebel O, Rogers G, et al: Endoscopic complications. JAMA 235:928-930, 1976.

28. Kozarek RA: Hydrostatic balloon dilatation of gastrointestinal stenosis: A national survey. Gastrointest Endosc 32:15-19, 1986.

29. Ogilvie AL, Ferguson R, Atkinson M: Outlook with conservative treatment of peptic oesophageal stricture. Gut 21:23-25, 1980.

30. Benedict EB: Peptic stenosis of the esophagus. A study of 233 patients treated with bougienage, surgery, or both. Am J Dig Dis 11:761-770, 1966.

31. Kochhar R, Makharia GK: Usefulness of intralesional triamcinolone in treatment of benign esophageal strictures. Gastrointest Endosc 56:243-254, 2002.

32. Song HY, Jung HY, Park S, et al: Covered retrievable expandable nitinol stents in patients with benign esophageal strictures. Radiology 217:551-557, 2000.

33. Sanden R, Poesl H: Treatment of non-neoplastic stenoses with the neodymium-YAG laser—indications and limitations. Endoscopy 18:53-56, 1986.

34. Little AG, Naunheim KS, Ferguson MK, et al: Surgical management of esophageal strictures. Ann Thorac Surg 45:144-147, 1988.

35. Mercer CD, Hill LD: Surgical management of peptic esophageal stricture. Twenty-year experience. J Thorac Cardiovasc Surg 91:371-378, 1986.

36. Payne WS: Surgical management of reflux induced oesophageal stenosis: Results in 101 patients. Br J Surg 71:971-973, 1984.

37. Swanstrom LL, Marcus DR, Galloway GQ: Laparoscopic Collis gastroplasty is the treatment of choice for the shortened esophagus. Am J Surg 171:477-481, 1996.

38. Hayward J: The treatment of fibrous stricture of the oesophagus associated with hiatal hernia. Thorax 16:45-55, 1961.

39. Orringer MB, Skinner DB, Belsey RH: Long term results of the Mark IV operation for hiatal hernia and analyses of recurrences and their treatment. J Thorac Cardiovasc Surg 63:25-33, 1972.

40. Nissen R. Gastropexy and fundoplication in surgical treatment of hiatal hernia. Am J Dig Dis 6:954, 1961.

41. Ellis FH, Gibb SP, Heatley GJ: Reoperation after failed antireflux surgery: Review of 101 cases. Eur J Cardiothorac Surg 10:225-232, 1996.

42. Jobe BA, Harvath KD, Swanström LL: Postoperative function following laparoscopic Collis gastroplasty for the shortened esophagus. Arch Surg 133:867-874, 1998.

43. Stirling MC, Orringer MB: Surgical treatment after the failed antireflux operation. J Thorac Cardiovasc Surg 92:667-672, 1986.

44. Siewert JR, Isolauri J, Feussner H: Reoperation after failed fundoplication. World J Surg 13:791-797, 1989.

45. Moghissi I: Intrathoracic fundoplication for reflux stricture associated with short esophagus. Thorax 38:36-40, 1983.

46. Pennell T: Supradiaphragmatic correction of esophageal reflux strictures. Ann Surg 193:655, 1981.

47. Polk HC: Fundoplication for reflux esophagitis: Misadventure with the operation of choice. Ann Surg 183:645, 1976.

48. Richardson JD, Larson GM, Polk HC Jr: Intrathoracic fundoplication for shortened esophagus: A treacherous solution to a challenging problem. Am J Surg 143:29-35, 1982.

49. Collis JL: Gastroplasty. Thorax 16:197-206, 1961.

50. Pearson FG, Langer B, Henderson RD: Gastroplasty and Belsey hiatal hernia repair. An operation for the management of peptic stricture with acquired short esophagus. J Thorac Cardiovasc Surg 61:50-63, 1971.

51. Orringer MB, Sloan H: Complications and failings of the combined Collis-Belsey operation. Cardiovasc Surg 74:726-735, 1977.

52. Orringer MB, Orringer JS: The combined Collis-Nissen operation: Early assessment of reflux control. Ann Thorac Surg 33:534-539, 1982.

53. Orringer MB, Sloan H: Combined Collis-Nissen reconstruction of the esophagogastric junction. Ann Thorac Surg 25:16-21, 1978.

54. Stirling MC, Orringer MB. The combined Collis-Nissen operation for esophageal reflux strictures. Ann Thorac Surg 45:148-157, 1988.

55. Bingham JAW: Evolution and early results of constructing an antireflux valve in the stomach. Proc R Soc Med 67:4-8, 1974.

56. Demos NJ, Smith N, Williams D: New gastroplasty for strictured short esophagus. N Y State J Med 75:57-59, 1975.

57. Pera M, Deschamps C, Taillefer R, Duranceau A: Uncut Collis-Nissen gastroplasty: Early functional results. Ann Thorac Surg 60:915-921, 1995.

58. Allen MS, Trastek VF, Deschamps C, Pairolero PC: Intrathoracic stomach. Presentations and results of operation. J Thorac Cardiovasc Surg 105:253-259, 1993.

59. Peters JH, DeMeester TR: The lessons of failed antireflux repairs. In Peters JH, DeMeester TR (eds): Minimally Invasive Therapy of the Foregut. St Louis, Quality Medical, 1994, p 160.
60. Swanström LL, Hansen P: Laparoscopic total esophagectomy. Arch Surg 132:943-949, 1977.
61. Terry ML, Vernon A, Hunter JG: Stapled-wedge Collis gastroplasty for the shortened esophagus. Am J Surg 188:258-294, 2004.
62. Demos NJ: Stapled, uncut gastroplasty for hiatal hernia: 12 year follow-up. Ann Thorac Surg 38:393-399, 1984.
63. Awad ZT, Filipi CJ: The short esophagus: Pathogenesis, diagnosis, and current surgical options. Arch Surg 136:113-114, 2001.
64. Patel HJ, Tan BB, Yee J, et al: A 25-year experience with open primary transthoracic repair of paraesophageal hiatal hernia. J Thorac Cardiovasc Surg 127:843-849, 2004.
65. Bonavina L, Segalin A, Fumagilli U, et al: Surgical management of benign stricture from efflux oesophagitis. Ann Chir Gynaecol 84:175-178, 1995.
66. Salamao N, Gaboury L, Duranceau A: Esophagectomy for complications of gastroesophageal reflux disease. Probl Gen Surg 13:105-111, 1996.
67. Orringer MB: Resection of the esophagus. In Shields TW (ed): General Thoracic Surgery. Philadelphia, Lippincott Williams & Wilkins, 2000, pp 1697-1722.
68. Little AG, Ferguson MK, Skinner DB: Reoperation for failed antireflux operations. J Thorac Cardiovasc Surg 91:511-517, 1986.
69. Ferraro P, Duranceau A: Esophagectomy for benign disease. In Pearson FG, Cooper JD, Deslauriers J, et al: Esophageal Surgery, 2nd ed. Philadelphia, Churchill Livingstone, 2002, pp 453-463.
70. Orringer MB, Marshall B, Stirling MC: Transhiatal esophagectomy for benign and malignant disease. J Thorac Cardiovasc Surg 105:265-276, 1993.
71. Orringer MB, Marshall, Iannettoni MD: Transhiatal esophagectomy: Clinical experience and refinements. Ann Surg 230:392-400, discussion 400-403, 1999.
72. Orringer MB, Marshall B, Iannettoni MD: Eliminating the cervical esophagogastric anastomotic leak with a side-to-side stapled anastomosis. J Thorac Cardiovasc Surg 119:277-288, 2000.
73. Skinner DB, Belsey RH: Reconstruction with stomach. In Skinner DB, Belsey RH (eds): Management of Esophageal Disease. Philadelphia, WB Saunders, 1988, p 228.
74. Belsey RH: Reconstruction of the esophagus with left colon. J Thorac Cardiovasc Surg 49:33, 1965.
75. Banki F, Mason RJ, DeMeester SR, et al: Vagal-sparing esophagectomy: A more physiologic alternative. Ann Surg 236:324-336, 2002.
76. Wangensteen OH, Levin NL: Gastric resection for esophagitis and stricture of acid-peptic origin. Surg Gynecol Obstet 88:560, 1981.
77. Gillison EW, Capper WM, Airth GR, et al: Hiatus hernia and heartburn. Gut 10:609-613, 1969.
78. Safaie-Shirazi S, DenBesten L, Zike WL: Effects of bile salts on the ionic permeability of the esophageal mucosa and their role in the production of esophagitis. Gastroenterology 68:728-733, 1975.
79. Tanner NC, Westerholm P: Partial gastrectomy in the treatment of esophageal stricture after hiatal hernia. Am J Surg 115:449-453, 1968.
80. Holt CJ, Large AM: Surgical management of reflux esophagitis. Ann Surg 153:555-562, 1961.
81. Payne WS: Surgical treatment of reflux esophagitis and stricture associated with permanent incompetence of the cardia. Mayo Clin Proc 45:553, 1970.

17

Medical Therapy for Gastroesophageal Reflux Disease

Eugene Y. Chang · Blair A. Jobe

Although surgical antireflux procedures are indicated for complicated or medically refractory cases of gastroesophageal reflux disease (GERD), initial treatment relies primarily on medical therapy. Pharmacologic therapy for acid reflux has progressed from antacids to histamine H_2 receptor antagonists (H2RAs) and, most recently, to proton pump inhibitors (PPIs). An understanding of the proper use of these medications is important because a course of optimal medical management is generally warranted before considering surgery. Moreover, the limitations of therapy with H2RAs and PPIs should be recognized, particularly with regard to treatment and prevention of the complications of GERD. In this respect, it should be understood that GERD results from potentially three different pathophysiologic processes. First, the lower esophageal sphincter (LES) may be incompetent and allow the reflux of gastric contents into the esophagus. Second, the esophagus may have a motility disorder that results in impaired or delayed clearance of refluxate from the esophagus. Third, hypersecretion of acid in the stomach may contribute to increased esophageal exposure to acidity. In addition, delayed gastric emptying may impair the forward progression of stomach contents, thereby increasing the opportunity for reflux. It is important to distinguish among these processes when determining the most appropriate treatment for patients with GERD. Finally, a comprehensive understanding of the medical alternatives to surgery is necessary for proper counseling of a patient who wishes to make an informed decision regarding whether to undergo an antireflux operation.

LIFESTYLE MODIFICATIONS

Numerous studies have demonstrated physiologic factors that increase esophageal exposure to acid by decreasing LES pressure, prolonging acid clearance time, or both.

These factors include various foods, body position, and lifestyle variables.[1-6]

Foods

Certain foods have been shown to decrease LES pressure in human studies, including chocolate, peppermint, and spearmint[7] and foods rich in fat.[3,8,9] Other foods have been postulated to cause heartburn by direct irritation of the esophagus or by inducing the reflux of gastric contents. Chocolate and peppermint, for example, have been shown to increase esophageal reflux,[10] and a survey of individuals with and without symptoms of GERD identified chocolate as a food that precipitates heartburn.[11] Patients with esophagitis had a significant rise in esophageal exposure time to acid within 1 hour after eating chocolate.[12] Ingestion of onions has also been reported to increase esophageal exposure to acid.[13]

Beverages

Alcohol consumption has been associated with decreased LES pressure[14] and prolonged esophageal exposure to acid.[15] Although drinking coffee does not affect LES pressure, it has been shown to induce GERD symptoms, possibly by direct mucosal irritation and effects on acid production.[16] Similarly, beer, wine, and, to a lesser extent, tea and soft drinks have been associated with heartburn. This observation has been attributed to the osmolarity or acidity of these beverages.[17]

Body Position

Because patients typically report that symptoms are precipitated by reclining, practitioners naturally recommend that recumbent positions be avoided for 3 to 4 hours after a meal. When sleeping, patients have traditionally been advised to elevate the head of the bed. This is accomplished by resting on foam wedges or placing books underneath the legs of the bed to raise the head by 4 to 8 inches. In one study, patients with GERD reported a reduction in symptoms when sitting up or lying with the head of the bed elevated as opposed to lying flat. The same study showed reduced esophageal exposure to acid when the head of the bed was elevated by 28 cm versus lying flat.[1] In patients with GERD, placing 6-inch blocks under the head of the bed significantly improved acid clearance times and reduced esophageal exposure to acid.[2] These sleep positions, however, may not be acceptable to many patients because they may be uncomfortable and cause the sheets, the patient, and bedmate to slide toward the foot of the bed. Alternatively, patients may observe some improvement in symptoms in the left lateral decubitus position. This position has been reported to improve esophageal acid clearance and reduce the time with a pH less than 4 when compared with other positions.[18]

Obesity

GERD is more prevalent among morbidly obese patients,[19] and it is thought that this finding may be related to the persistently increased pressure gradient between the abdomen and thorax.[20] Similarly, tight-fitting clothing around the waist has also been inculpated as a contributor to heartburn.[20] Although obese patients with GERD are often given the classic recommendation to lose weight, clinical studies have failed to show any efficacy in treating GERD with this strategy. In one study, placing obese patients with erosive esophagitis on a 6-month weight loss program failed to produce any objective or subjective improvement despite demonstrable weight loss.[21]

Smoking Cessation

Cigarette smoking has been demonstrated to decrease LES pressure and prolong esophageal acid clearance in healthy individuals.[22-25] Although smoking cessation in individuals with GERD has been shown to reduce the number of upright reflux episodes, it failed to have any impact on total esophageal acid exposure time.[4] Furthermore, smoking did not appear to affect rates of healing in patients with esophagitis who were undergoing treatment with ranitidine or omeprazole.[26,27]

Recommendations for Lifestyle Modifications

Although the impact of lifestyle factors may be demonstrated on the basis of symptoms and esophageal acid exposure, it should be kept in mind that few prospective studies have been conducted to determine whether these measures are sufficiently efficacious as a treatment of GERD. However, lifestyle modifications often bring about benefits outside the gastrointestinal system and may augment pharmacologic therapy for GERD.

MEDICAL TREATMENT OF GERD SYMPTOMS

Antacids

Commonly used antacids include aluminum hydroxide and magnesium hydroxide, which exert their effects by neutralizing gastric acid. Because they are over-the-counter medications, antacids and acid suppressants have frequently been used as first-line therapeutic agents. These medications may produce mild short-term symptomatic relief of postprandial heartburn but are of very limited efficacy. A comparison of magnesium hydroxide and placebo in patients with esophagitis demonstrated that the antacid had only minimal effect on the frequency and severity of heartburn.[28] Furthermore, their use is limited by side effects, including diarrhea in the case of magnesium hydroxide and hypophosphatemia in patients taking aluminum hydroxide. Antacid foam tablets also failed to reduce esophageal acid exposure.[2] Sucralfate, a drug that reacts with gastric acid to produce a barrier coating the mucosa of the upper gastrointestinal tract, has demonstrated limited or no clinical efficacy in patients with GERD.

Promotility Agents

Cisapride, an agent that stimulates upper gastrointestinal motility through the indirect stimulation of acetylcholine release from the postganglionic nerve endings in the myenteric plexus, has been of value in the treatment of symptoms, thus underscoring the role of esophageal dysmotility and delayed gastric emptying in the pathogenesis of GERD. It reduces esophageal exposure to acid by increasing lower esophageal motility, reducing gastric emptying time, and increasing salivation.[29] It has typically been prescribed in a regimen of 10 mg four times a day. A study by Castell et al. demonstrated that when given at a dosage of 20 mg twice a day, it maintained the ability to reduce heartburn, regurgitation, eructation, and the use of antacids in comparison to placebo.[30] In this study, 67 of 188 patients reported a response in daytime heartburn, and 73 of 188 reported a response in nighttime heartburn. The most commonly reported adverse event was diarrhea, seen in 10% of patients. Because of a low incidence of cardiac arrhythmias, however, cisapride has been removed from the U.S. market and is issued only on a named-patient basis.

Other prokinetic agents that have been studied for GERD include metoclopramide, bethanechol, and domperidone. Unlike cisapride, however, none of these agents has consistently demonstrated clinical efficacy.[2,31] Furthermore, the side effects of metoclopramide (fatigue, restlessness, tremor, extrapyramidal movement disorders) further limit its usefulness. Domperidone is not available on the U.S. market. Tegaserod, a histamine 5-HT$_4$ receptor partial agonist, has been shown to have prokinetic effects and has demonstrated reduced esophageal exposure to acid at its lowest dose.[32] Whether this observation translates into an effect of therapeutic value remains to be seen.

Bethanechol, a cholinergic agent, was shown to decrease esophageal exposure time to acid in recumbent but not upright patients.[2] However, its use is limited by cholinergic adverse effects, including increased gastric acid secretion, bronchoconstriction, and increased bladder contraction.

H₂ Receptor Antagonists

The commonly used H2RAs, which include ranitidine and famotidine, are more efficacious than antacids and were once considered revolutionary in the treatment of GERD. These agents block the histamine receptor of the parietal cell, thus eliminating one of the pathways by which gastric acid secretion is promoted. The standard dosage of ranitidine is 150 mg twice a day; that of famotidine is 20 mg twice a day. H2RAs produce at least partial relief of symptoms in 50% to 70% of patients with GERD[33] and may be the most cost-effective approach to treating uncomplicated GERD in patients in whom symptomatic relief can be achieved. However, tolerance to an H2RA can develop within several weeks of starting therapy. Furthermore, in patients who have persistent symptoms despite treatment with an H2RA, escalation to a higher dose (ranitidine, 300 mg twice daily) has not been shown to improve symptoms significantly.[34] With the advent of more potent antisecretory agents, the role of H2RAs as primary therapy for GERD has largely been supplanted.

Proton Pump Inhibitors

PPIs include omeprazole, lansoprazole, pantoprazole, rabeprazole, and esomeprazole. They have become the mainstay of therapy and are often used as first-line treatment of GERD. Despite the widespread use of PPIs, an understanding of the optimal dosage schedule is lacking among nongastroenterologists.[35] This class of agents accumulates in the secretory canaliculi of active parietal cells and covalently binds to the proton-potassium ion exchange pump, irreversibly inhibiting it. Because the proton pump is maximally recruited to the secretory canaliculus after a period of fasting, the optimal time for once-daily dosing is 30 minutes before breakfast. For twice-daily dosing, a second dose is added before dinner.

In patients with GERD, omeprazole reduces heartburn, regurgitation, and the use of antacids.[36,37] In patients without esophagitis, omeprazole has been demonstrated to be superior to cisapride[38] and H2RAs in the short-term symptomatic control of GERD.[39] Maintenance of symptomatic remission generally requires continuous, lifelong therapy with PPIs. In patients with nonerosive GERD treated until symptomatic remission and then placed on a treatment strategy with a placebo, the majority taking the placebo become unwilling to continue the treatment strategy within 6 months.[40] In patients with esophagitis, symptomatic remission after 12 months of treatment with placebo fell to 34% versus 62% to 82% in patients who continued omeprazole therapy and 45% in patients treated with ranitidine.[41-43]

Alternatives to lifelong continuous therapy with PPIs have been studied and include strategies such as on-demand therapy. In contrast to scheduled dosing, on-demand therapy allows patients with infrequent symptoms to take the medication only when symptoms recur. Advantages of this regimen include the decreased use (and decreased cost) of medications. Proponents of this strategy also point out that patients told to take scheduled PPIs often take the medications on an on-demand basis despite the instructions given to them.[44] A major disadvantage, however, is that this strategy permits the recurrence of symptoms, which may take some time to resolve after resumption of the medication. When compared with placebo, on-demand therapy with omeprazole, 10 or 20 mg, or esomeprazole, 20 mg, in patients with nonerosive GERD was superior and well accepted by patients. In this study, 85% of patients taking the active medication were willing to continue the strategy at the end of 6 months of therapy.[40] Similar findings in studies using lansoprazole suggest that on-demand therapy with other PPIs may be feasible. Although on-demand therapy may be successful in patients with endoscopically negative GERD, its usefulness has not been demonstrated in those with GERD-related complications (such as erosive esophagitis)—these patients generally require lifelong continuous antisecretory agents. Another alternative to lifelong continuation of PPIs is a "step-down" strategy to less potent medications such as H2RAs or lower dosages of PPIs. In patients who have been rendered asymptomatic with PPIs or H2RAs, cisapride demonstrated no benefit over placebo in maintaining symptomatic remission, thus suggesting that it is not appropriate as a "step-down" agent.[45]

Response to a particular PPI varies among individuals, and this variation has been attributed to polymorphisms in the proton-potassium pump. Although numerous studies have been conducted to compare their efficacy in different situations,[46] there is generally little difference among PPIs with regard to their efficacy.[47]

Even though PPIs are generally well tolerated, they may be associated with side effects, with an overall incidence of 5%.[48] The most commonly reported side effects include headache, nausea, diarrhea, and abdominal pain.[49] In a study to assess the safety of omeprazole, 116 patients with Zollinger-Ellison syndrome were treated with dosages of omeprazole up to 60 mg twice daily for up to 114 months without any observed toxicity. In addition, no patients discontinued the medication secondary to drug-induced side effects.[50] Initial concerns that PPIs may lead to atrophic gastritis or gastric cancer have not been manifested.[48]

Acid suppression with antisecretory medications (including PPIs) has the major limitation that although these medications may eliminate the symptoms of esophageal reflux, they do not prevent the reflux of gastric contents into the esophagus. Simultaneous monitoring of intraesophageal impedance and pH (Fig. 17–1) can detect and discriminate between acid and non-acid reflux. Studies using impedance-pH monitors have demonstrated that PPIs shift the proportion of acid to non-acid reflux episodes, which dramatically reduces the number of acid reflux episodes but does not affect the

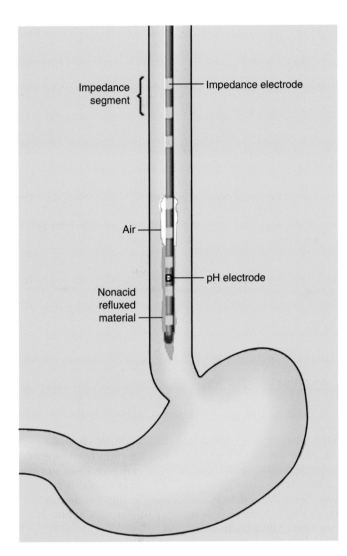

Figure 17–1. Simultaneous pH and impedance monitoring probe. Impedance is measured between electrodes along an intraesophageal catheter. One or more pH-sensing electrodes are also present. Whereas the pH probe detects esophageal acid exposure, impedance monitoring detects all forms of reflux irrespective of pH, including air (which raises the impedance between electrodes) and liquids (which decreases the impedance). Esophageal impedance also defines the proximity of the reflux episode in relation to the proximal end of the aerodigestive tract.

overall number of reflux episodes.[51] It has been suggested that persistence of non-acid reflux in the face of PPI therapy contributes to the pathogenesis of complications of Barrett's esophagus, such as stricture, ulceration, or carcinoma.[52] Furthermore, concern has been raised that acid-suppression therapy increases the risk for aspiration pneumonia because of loss of the antimicrobial effect of gastric acid. This possibility has been substantiated in a cohort study that demonstrated an increased risk for community-acquired pneumonia in patients taking PPIs and H2RAs.[53]

Nocturnal Acid Secretion

Despite therapy with PPIs, the stomach may not be rendered fully achlorhydric in some situations. Nocturnal gastric acid breakthrough is a phenomenon in which patients who are treated twice daily with PPIs have an intragastric pH less than 4 for at least 1 hour overnight. This has been reported in more than 70% of normal subjects and patients with GERD.[54,55] The mechanism by which it occurs is unclear, but explanations that have been put forth cite the limited duration of action of PPIs, the absence of food to buffer gastric acidity at night, and the possibility that the evening dose of PPI is less effective than the morning dose.[56] The addition of a nighttime H2RA has been shown to control nocturnal acid secretion.[56-58] However, recent studies suggest that nocturnal breakthrough returns after 1 week of therapy, which is probably due to the development of tolerance to the H2RA.[59] Nevertheless, the clinical significance of nocturnal acid breakthrough has not been well established, and it is recommended that in patients with difficult-to-manage GERD, the adequacy of acid suppression be determined by esophageal pH rather than intragastric pH.[59]

MEDICAL THERAPY FOR COMPLICATIONS OF GERD

Esophagitis

It is thought that esophagitis, a complication of GERD, requires more intensive therapy than nonerosive reflux does. Historically, H2RAs and promotility agents have been used to treat erosive esophagitis. Ranitidine,[60] cimetidine,[60] famotidine,[33] and nizatidine[61] have been shown to promote healing of esophagitis. After 12 weeks of therapy with standard doses, famotidine, ranitidine, and cimetidine produce healing in 68% to 74% of patients. Nizatidine, which has been given less attention, has demonstrated a 39% healing rate. Healing rates also vary with the grade of esophagitis; the probability of healing decreases with higher grades. Trials conducted with higher doses of H2RAs have demonstrated a slightly improved rate of endoscopically confirmed healing at approximately 77%.[60] Cisapride has also been shown to improve the healing of esophagitis, but it has very limited availability in the United States.[62]

PPIs are also effective in the treatment of esophagitis and have become the mainstay of therapy.[63] In a meta-analysis comparing H2RAs, PPIs, and placebo, esophagitis healed more quickly in patients treated with PPIs than in those treated with H2RAs.[64] This study demonstrated an overall 12-week healing rate of 79% to 88% with PPIs, 47% to 57% with H2RAs, and 19% to 37% with placebo.

Maintenance therapy for esophagitis requires lifelong continuation of PPI therapy. After successful treatment of esophagitis with omeprazole, only 14% of patients maintained on placebo remained in remission after 12 months as compared with 50% of patients who continued treatment with omeprazole, 10 mg, and 74% of

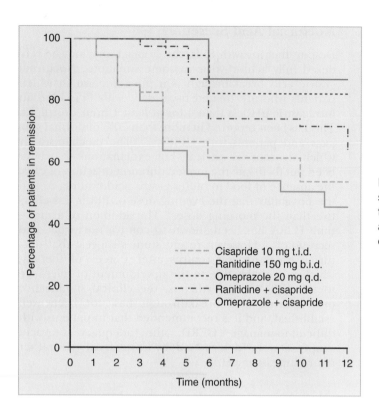

Figure 17–2. Percentage of patients remaining in remission from esophagitis while treated with various medications. (Adapted from Vigneri S, Termini R, Leandro G, et al: A comparison of five maintenance therapies for reflux esophagitis. N Engl J Med 333:1106-1110, 1995.)

those treated with omeprazole, 20 mg (Fig. 17–2).[42] Similar results have been noted for other PPIs.[65-67] When relapses occur, the vast majority take place within 12 months of therapy. Maintenance therapy with omeprazole continues to be effective at least 5 years after initiation of therapy.[68] The use of H2RAs as a step-down agent has been evaluated, but with disappointing results. In a study of 159 patients in which ranitidine, 150 mg twice daily, was compared with omeprazole, 20 mg taken daily, for the prevention of relapse of erosive esophagitis, 89% of patients in the omeprazole arm were free of esophagitis at the end of 12 weeks as compared with 25% in the ranitidine arm.[69] Another study of 392 patients showed a 72% 12-month remission rate in patients treated with omeprazole, 20 mg daily, versus 62% in those treated with omeprazole, 10 mg daily, and 45% in those treated with ranitidine, 150 mg twice daily.[42] These data argue against the use of H2RA as a step-down agent in the maintenance of remission.

Since the advent of PPIs, improvements in the success rate of treating esophagitis have been modest. Esomeprazole, an S-isomer of omeprazole, has shown some potential for improved results. Because it is undergoes less first-pass hepatic metabolism and has decreased plasma clearance, esomeprazole has higher bioavailability. In a study of 1960 patients, the pharmacodynamic advantages of this drug appear to translate into a small but statistically significant improvement over omeprazole. This study demonstrated a 94% healing rate after 8 weeks of treatment with esomeprazole, 40 mg daily, as compared with 87% in those treated with omeprazole, 20 mg daily.[70] Another potential improvement on treatment with omeprazole is the addition of a promotility agent. In a comparison of omeprazole and ranitidine with and without cisapride, the combination of omeprazole and cisapride produced higher remission rates than omeprazole alone did, although the difference did not appear to be statistically significant.[71] Progress with this strategy has been limited because cisapride has been removed from the U.S. market and other promotility agents have not been adequately evaluated.

Strictures

Peptic strictures of the esophagus are estimated to occur in 7% to 23% of patients with untreated reflux esophagitis.[72] The mainstay of therapy for esophageal strictures is mechanical dilation, which must be repeated if the stricture recurs. To date, there is no direct evidence that aggressive medical treatment of reflux prevents the *development* of esophageal strictures. Nonetheless, antisecretory therapy plays an important role in the management of esophageal strictures. An epidemiologic study has demonstrated a decline in the number of dilations performed in community hospitals as the use of PPIs has increased.[73] Aggressive therapy with PPIs (e.g., omeprazole, 20 to 40 mg/day) has been demonstrated to reduce the probability of needing redilatation when compared with H2RA therapy.[73,74] Despite improved healing rates for erosive esophagitis, H2RAs do not appear to reduce the need for dilation.[75] One report showed that the extent of dysphagia in patients with esophageal strictures depends not only on stricture diameter but also on the presence of esophagitis, thus suggesting a possible mechanism by which PPIs reduce the need for redilation.[76] Despite the higher cost of PPIs, the use of PPIs to treat patients with esophageal strictures appears to be more cost-effective than using H2RAs because of the decreased need for repeat endoscopy and dilation.[77]

Injection of triamcinolone into the stricture has also gained some interest. In a longitudinal study of 71 patients treated with four-quadrant injections of triamcinolone, it was found that the patients required dilation less frequently after starting treatment.[78] Potential adverse effects include esophageal candidiasis, although this was not observed in the study. No randomized, blinded studies to test the efficacy and safety of intralesional steroid injection have been performed.

Barrett's Esophagus

Evidence that adequate medical treatment of GERD prevents the development of Barrett's esophagus has largely been indirect.[79] Using a database of 2641 patients undergoing elective esophagogastroduodenoscopy, Lieberman et al. demonstrated that a longer duration of GERD symptoms was a significant risk factor for Barrett's disease, with an odds ratio rising steadily for patients with a longer history of symptoms. Patients who have had symptoms for longer than 10 years had an odds ratio of 6.4 for the development of Barrett's esophagus in comparison to those who have had symptoms for less than a year. In this study, Barrett's esophagus was 1.8 times more likely to develop in patients with a history of esophagitis, but this relationship did not reach statistical significance.[80]

It has long been thought that patients with GERD have a higher incidence of Barrett's disease, although evidence to support this notion is not entirely convincing, in part because of the unknown prevalence of GERD in the general population. Various studies have found that Barrett's disease has a prevalence of 3% to 15% in patients with GERD.[81,82] Most recently, a study of 378 consecutive veterans with a history of GERD who were undergoing a first upper endoscopy found that 13.2% of patients had biopsy-confirmed Barrett's disease.[83] Although the true prevalence of Barrett's disease in the general population is unknown, recent evidence suggests that it may be similar to the prevalence in patients with GERD. In a study enrolling 110 asymptomatic veterans undergoing screening colonoscopy, Barrett's disease was endoscopically visible in 25% of individuals, and an additional 16% with an endoscopically normal gastroesophageal junction had intestinal metaplasia on biopsy.[84] Such a high prevalence has not been confirmed in other studies, however. A larger study of 961 patients showed a 6.8% prevalence in all patients and a 5.6% prevalence in 556 patients who had never experienced heartburn.[85]

Controlled studies comparing the incidence of Barrett's esophagus in medically treated patients versus untreated patients are not available. In a cohort study comparing medical with surgical treatment of GERD, Barrett's esophagus developed in 12 of 83 patients treated with PPIs and cisapride over a follow-up period of 24 months, thus calling into question the ability of medical therapy to prevent Barrett's disease.[86] To date, no conclusive evidence has established that any therapy can prevent Barrett's disease.

Under the current recommendations of the American College of Gastroenterologists, Barrett's disease (intestinal metaplasia of the esophageal epithelium) should be treated to the end point of symptom control and maintenance of healed esophageal mucosa—the same treatment end points for GERD.[87] These recommendations are supported by a case-control study demonstrating that the risk for esophageal adenocarcinoma was strongly correlated with symptoms of heartburn or regurgitation. In this study, the strength of the association between symptoms and the development of adenocarcinoma was virtually identical in patients with Barrett's disease and those without, thus supporting the use of similar end points of treatment in both populations.[88]

Nonetheless, controversy exists over whether treatment should seek to accomplish more aggressive goals. In patients with Barrett's disease, treatment with PPIs to the point of eliminating the symptoms of reflux does not necessarily indicate that reflux into the esophagus has been eradicated. In one study of 30 patients with Barrett's esophagus whose symptoms had been completely eliminated with lansoprazole therapy, persistent pathologic acid reflux was demonstrated in 12 patients.[89] These findings have been confirmed in other studies[90] and are explained by the theory that patients with Barrett's disease may have a decreased visceral ability to sense acid reflux.[91] Furthermore, although the amount of bile reflux may be reduced by PPI therapy,[92] it persists in a substantial portion of Barrett's patients rendered asymptomatic with PPIs.[93] These findings raise the suggestion that PPI therapy in patients with Barrett's esophagus should be titrated according to pH monitoring rather than by symptomatic response, although no firm recommendation for pH monitoring is currently in place.

Because Barrett's disease is a significant risk factor for the development of esophageal adenocarcinoma, there has been considerable interest in the use of pharmacologic agents to prevent the progression to cancer. One form of chemoprevention is the use of acid-suppression mechanisms to normalize intraesophageal pH. Laboratory studies have offered theoretical evidence that effective control of intraesophageal pH may promote the regression of Barrett's esophagus or prevent progression to adenocarcinoma. In a prospective study of 42 patients, Ouatu-Lascar et al. demonstrated that patients with normalized intraesophageal pH have decreased proliferation cell nuclear antigen (PCNA) expression, which is a marker of cellular proliferation, and an increase in the expression of villin, a marker of differentiation.[94] It is unknown, however, whether these markers can reliably predict the likelihood of development of esophageal adenocarcinoma.

Clinical evidence to support this strategy has been inconsistent and suggests very modest benefits with medical therapy, at best. In one study, 68 patients with Barrett's esophagus were randomized to receive aggressive acid-suppression therapy (omeprazole, 40 mg twice a day) or standard therapy (ranitidine, 150 mg twice a day). Patients who received omeprazole showed significantly better normalization of intraesophageal pH and demonstrated a greater decrease in the area and length of Barrett's esophagus, with 8% demonstrating regression after 2 years.[95] An uncontrolled study of a cohort of 14 patients treated with omeprazole, 60 mg daily, showed a mean reduction in the length of Barrett's esophagus. Twelve patients in that study had complete normalization of intraesophageal pH. Several other studies of cohorts treated with H2RAs or PPIs have not demonstrated significant regression, but they may have been limited by their small sample size, short length of follow-up, or failure to normalize intraesophageal pH.[96,97] A finding that has been observed in multiple studies is the appearance of squamous islands of tissue within the field of intestinal metaplasia. Although it was hoped that the squamous islands were indicative of some form of regression, biopsies of these islands have demonstrated the presence of underlying columnar epithelium, thus suggesting that the islands represent overgrowth of squamous epithelium rather than true regression.[98] The prognostic significance of regression of the length or area of Barrett's metaplasia is unclear. A nonrandomized study demonstrated that patients with Barrett's disease in whom dysplasia did not develop were more likely to have been treated with PPIs and were treated for a longer duration than those in whom dysplasia did develop.[99]

Another potential approach to chemoprevention uses nonsteroidal anti-inflammatory drugs (NSAIDs). A large-scale case-control study using a national research database of patient records throughout the United Kingdom identified a lower odds ratio for the development of esophageal cancer in patients who were prescribed NSAIDs.[100] Another case-control study of 293 patients with esophageal adenocarcinoma demonstrated an odds ratio of 0.37 for the development of cancer in patients taking aspirin.[101] These results are supported by data from laboratory experiments, in which it was found that cyclooxygenase-2 (COX-2) inhibition is associated with antiproliferative and proapoptotic effects in Barrett's-associated esophageal adenocarcinoma cells in culture.[102] In a rat model of Barrett's esophagus, treatment with an NSAID or COX-2 inhibitor yielded lower rates of esophageal adenocarcinoma than did treatment with a placebo. Although Barrett's esophagus is associated with a 50- to 100-fold increase in the risk for adenocarcinoma in comparison to the general population, the absolute incidence is still small, as shown in a Mayo Clinic retrospective review in which adenocarcinoma developed in 2 of 104 patients observed an average of 8.5 years.[103] Consequently, the number of patients treated with a chemopreventive strategy to prevent a single case of esophageal adenocarcinoma would be very high. Such a strategy would therefore need to be safe, inexpensive, and readily available, thus making NSAIDs an appropriate candidate as a chemopreventive agent. Large-scale prospective trials to test chemoprevention strategies are needed.

EXTRAESOPHAGEAL MANIFESTATIONS OF REFLUX

Asthma

Several mechanisms have been demonstrated by which reflux induces the symptoms of asthma, including the microaspiration of gastric contents,[104-107] vagally mediated bronchoconstriction,[108,109] chest pain, and increased airway reactivity.[110,111] The cause-and-effect relationship between the two entities is not entirely clear because it has been postulated that asthma may contribute to GERD. Inspiratory airway obstruction may accentuate the negative thoracic pressure and alter the abdominal-thoracic pressure gradient, thus overcoming the valve mechanism of the gastroesophageal junction. Forced expiration in the presence of airway obstruction may cause the diaphragm to flatten and thereby compromise the anatomic antireflux mechanism.[112] Specific modalities to diagnose GERD-related asthma include sputum inspection for lipid-laden alveolar macrophages and scintigraphic technetium monitoring, but these tests are poorly sensitive for the condition and are rarely used in clinical practice. Dual-probe pH monitoring of the pharynx and distal esophagus is considered the standard for the diagnosis of GERD-related asthma and may document reflux of acidic material into the pharynx and correlate reflux events with respiratory symptoms. The temporal relationship between reflux events and respiratory symptoms is not entirely consistent. In a study of wheezing episodes in 48 patients, 10% of the episodes were preceded by reflux, 20% were followed by reflux, and 15% occurred concurrently.[113] Another study found that only 48% of cough or wheezing events correlated with reflux events.[114]

In practice, the diagnosis of reflux-induced asthma is made empirically on the basis of an improvement in pulmonary symptoms after treatment with antisecretory medications.[115] Although studies have sought to determine whether treatment of reflux improves respiratory symptoms in patients with GERD-related asthma, most are flawed by small sample size, short duration of treatment, and failure to demonstrate normalization of intraesophageal pH.[116-118] In a study performed by Harding et al., which evaluated PPI therapy in patients with GERD-related asthma, 30 patients were treated with 3 months of omeprazole.[119] The medication dosage was started at 20 mg daily and titrated according to 24-hour pH testing results until adequate acid suppression was achieved. Asthma symptom scores were assessed on monthly follow-up and demonstrated that 22 of the 30 patients showed at least 20% improvement in asthma symptom scores or peak expiratory flow. Among responders, asthma symptom scores decreased steadily from 1 month to the next over the 3-month period (Fig. 17–3). These findings suggest that the majority of patients with GERD-related asthma stand to benefit from treatment with PPIs and support treatment with a regimen of omeprazole for at least 3 months with monitoring of asthma symptoms, medication use, and peak expiratory flow. Patients who fail to improve with treatment should undergo 24-hour pH testing to assess the adequacy of acid suppression. In patients who do not respond to PPI therapy after pH probe–guided optimization, medical therapy is not likely to improve the symptoms (Fig. 17–4).

Chronic Cough

Patients with symptoms of cough persisting for at least 3 weeks in the absence of any known cause (confirmed by a normal chest radiograph) are considered to have

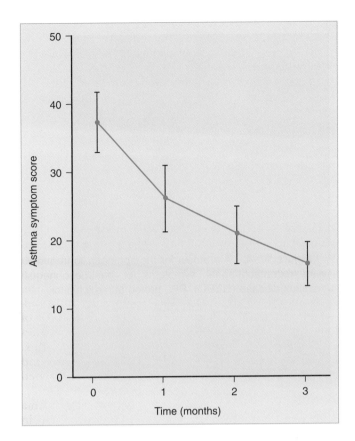

Figure 17–3. Time course of respiratory symptoms in patients with asthma and gastroesophageal reflux disease treated with acid suppression therapy. (Adapted from Harding SM, Richter JE, Guzzo MR, et al: Asthma and gastroesophageal reflux: Acid suppressive therapy improves asthma outcome. Am J Med 100:395-405, 1996.)

chronic cough. Among nonsmoking patients meeting these criteria, GERD is found to be the cause of the cough in 26% to 31% of cases.[120,121] As with asthma, the mechanism by which GERD leads to coughing may be multifactorial. Mechanisms include a vagally mediated esophagotracheobronchial reflex[122,123] and direct microaspiration of peptic contents into the airways.[124] Non-acid reflux may also play a role in contributing to chronic cough. Irwin et al. published the results of a cohort of eight patients with GERD-related cough confirmed by pH monitoring who failed acid-suppression therapy despite normalization of intraesophageal pH. After undergoing antireflux surgery, all patients had improvement in cough.[125] No studies have directly investigated the role of non-acid reflux in patients with chronic cough.

Chronic persistent cough attributable to GERD cannot be diagnosed on the basis of history alone because up to 75% of these patients may deny typical signs or symptoms of reflux.[123,126] The standard test for the diagnosis of GERD-related cough is dual-probe 24-hour esophageal pH monitoring. In addition to documenting reflux, pH testing may establish a temporal

relationship between reflux events and cough.[127] Because of the expense and discomfort posed by 24-hour pH monitoring, a trial of empirical PPI therapy is reasonable for patients with chronic cough and a history suggestive of GERD. However, in patients who lack any reflux symptoms and have a normal chest radiograph, ambulatory pH monitoring should be considered before initiating acid-suppression therapy.[112]

Aggressive antisecretory therapy may be successful in treating GERD-related cough. Poe and Kallay developed and tested a protocol in which patients with suspected GERD-related cough were initially treated with high-dose PPIs (e.g., omeprazole, 40 mg). If the patient had dysphagia or did not respond adequately to antisecretory therapy, a prokinetic agent (cisapride or metoclopramide) was added.[121] Among 54 patients with a history suggestive of GERD-related cough, 24 experienced resolution of the cough with PPI therapy. Eighteen required the addition of a promotility agent. After 6 weeks of therapy, resolution was achieved in 95% of responders. Patients who failed to respond to therapy after 2 months underwent a 24-hour pH test to assess for adequacy of acid suppression, and three patients were found to have normal DeMeester scores. This study supports the empirical use of high-dose PPIs for at least 6 weeks, with consideration for the addition of metoclopramide and 24-hour pH monitoring if symptoms do not improve.

Reflux Laryngitis

Among the otolaryngologic disorders associated with GERD, reflux laryngitis is perhaps the most common. Symptoms of reflux laryngitis include excessive throat mucus, chronic throat clearing, chronic cough, hoarseness, sore throat, halitosis, and a globus sensation. As with the other extraesophageal disorders, there is evidence to support more than one mechanism by which reflux leads to laryngitis, including direct exposure of the larynx to gastric acid refluxed through an esophageal-pharyngeal pathway.[128,129] Another postulated mechanism implicates a vagally stimulated chronic cough and throat clearing as a cause of laryngeal injury.[130]

In the diagnosis of reflux laryngitis, other causes of laryngitis should be considered and evaluated. Evaluation should include laryngoscopy (Fig. 17–5), which may show laryngeal edema and erythema, particularly in the posterior aspect of the larynx. Granulation or ulceration may also be seen.[131] Dual-probe pH testing, with one of the probes placed in the pharynx, may document the occurrence of esophagopharyngeal reflux. A high degree of suspicion for GERD should be maintained in patients with laryngitis because the majority of patients with pH-confirmed reflux laryngitis lack the typical symptoms of GERD.[132]

In practice, empirical therapy with antisecretory medication is considered reasonable, although placebo-controlled studies of the efficacy of PPI therapy in this context are few and give conflicting results. On the basis of currently available data, the optimal dose of PPI and optimal length of therapy are unknown.[133] A study by el-

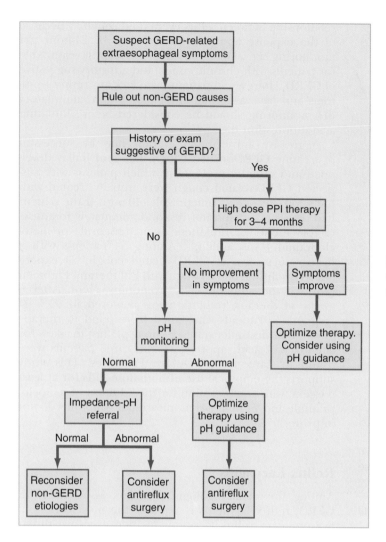

Figure 17–4. A protocol for the approach to treatment of extraesophageal symptoms of gastroesophageal reflux disease (GERD). PPI, proton pump inhibitor.

Serag et al. showed that in patients with reflux laryngitis treated with lansoprazole, 30 mg twice a day, 6 achieved a complete symptomatic response as compared with only 1 of 10 receiving a placebo.[134] A study conducted by Eherer et al. demonstrated similar results in patients given pantoprazole, 40 mg twice daily, but symptomatic improvement also occurred in patients given placebo, thus suggesting a role for watchful waiting in these patients.[135] Although the use of both cisapride and a PPI was associated with an improvement in symptoms in an uncontrolled trial,[136] no controlled studies have demonstrated the efficacy of adding promotility agents.

SUMMARY

Medical therapy for GERD includes both lifestyle modifications and pharmacologic interventions. Although a number of lifestyle modifications play a role in the education of patients with GERD, none of these strategies has been shown to be significantly efficacious when used alone for long-term treatment. Symptomatic relief from GERD can be reliably achieved with a number of agents, including PPIs, H2RAs, and promotility agents. Among the antisecretory therapies, PPIs are the most potent agents for reducing gastric acid production. To achieve the goal of long-term symptom control, lifelong therapy with PPIs may be needed, although various strategies can be used to step down to a less potent agent or reduce the frequency of dosing. In patients in whom erosive esophagitis develops, PPIs produce the highest and most durable remission rates, and lifetime therapy is generally required. Even though medical therapies have not been conclusively shown to prevent Barrett's esophagus and esophageal strictures, they play a significant role in treating underlying GERD symptoms in patients with these disorders. It is hoped that medical therapy may prevent the progression of Barrett's esophagus to dysplasia or adenocarcinoma, although studies have not conclusively demonstrated this effect. Extraesophageal manifestations of GERD include asthma, chronic cough, and laryngitis and continue to present a difficult set of disorders to treat. The diagnosis may not be straightforward because patients often have extraesophageal symptoms as the primary complaint, sometimes in the absence of typical GERD symptoms. Patients with extraesophageal symptoms of GERD generally require a long duration of high-dose acid-suppression therapy. Non-acid reflux may

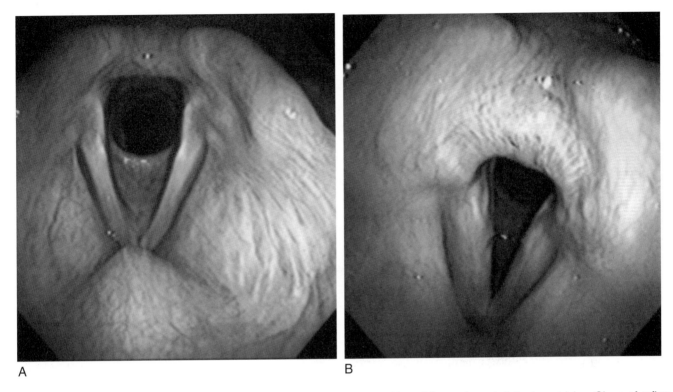

A   B

Figure 17–5.   Endoscopic images of the larynx. **A,** The normal larynx, with mobile cords and distinct ventricles. Signs of reflux laryngitis, such as granulation, erythema, edema, or posterior commissure hypertrophy, are not present. **B,** Vocal cord edema in a patient with reflux laryngitis.

also play a role in these disorders, which suggests that promotility agents may need to be added or antireflux surgery may be more appropriate. With the advent of impedance-pH monitoring, future studies are expected to refine the optimal therapy for extraesophageal symptoms.

REFERENCES

1. Stanciu C, Bennett JR: Effects of posture on gastro-oesophageal reflux. Digestion 15:104-1049, 1977.
2. Johnson LF, DeMeester TR: Evaluation of elevation of the head of the bed, bethanechol, and antacid form tablets on gastro-esophageal reflux. Dig Dis Sci 26:673-680, 1981.
3. Becker DJ, Sinclair J, Castell DO, Wu WC: A comparison of high and low fat meals on postprandial esophageal acid exposure. Am J Gastroenterol 84:782-786, 1989.
4. Waring JP, Eastwood TF, Austin JM, Sanowski RA: The immediate effects of cessation of cigarette smoking on gastroesophageal reflux. Am J Gastroenterol 84:1076-1078, 1989.
5. Meyers WF, Herbst JJ: Effectiveness of positioning therapy for gastroesophageal reflux. Pediatrics 69:768-772, 1982.
6. Castell DO, Richter JE:. The Esophagus. Philadelphia, Lippincott Williams & Wilkins, 2004.
7. Sigmund CJ, McNally EF: The action of a carminative on the lower esophageal sphincter. Gastroenterology 56:13-18, 1969.
8. Nebel OT, Castell DO: Lower esophageal sphincter pressure changes after food ingestion. Gastroenterology 63:778-783, 1972.
9. Price SF, Smithson KW, Castell DO: Food sensitivity in reflux esophagitis. Gastroenterology 75:240-243, 1978.
10. DeVault KR, Castell DO: Updated guidelines for the diagnosis and treatment of gastroesophageal reflux disease. The Practice Parameters Committee of the American College of Gastroenterology. Am J Gastroenterol 94:1434-1442, 1999.
11. Nebel OT, Fornes MF, Castell DO: Symptomatic gastroesophageal reflux: Incidence and precipitating factors. Am J Dig Dis 21:953-956, 1976.
12. Murphy DW, Castell DO: Chocolate and heartburn: Evidence of increased esophageal acid exposure after chocolate ingestion. Am J Gastroenterol 83:633-636, 1988.
13. Allen ML, Mellow MH, Robinson MG, Orr WC: The effect of raw onions on acid reflux and reflux symptoms. Am J Gastroenterol 85:377-380, 1990.
14. Hogan WJ, Viegas de Andrade SR, Winship DH: Ethanol-induced acute esophageal motor dysfunction. J Appl Physiol 32:755-760, 1972.
15. Vitale GC, Cheadle WG, Patel B, et al: The effect of alcohol on nocturnal gastroesophageal reflux. JAMA 258:2077-2079, 1987.
16. McArthur K, Hogan D, Isenberg JI: Relative stimulatory effects of commonly ingested beverages on gastric acid secretion in humans. Gastroenterology 83:199-203, 1982.
17. Feldman M, Barnett C: Relationships between the acidity and osmolality of popular beverages and reported postprandial heartburn. Gastroenterology 108:125-131, 1995.
18. Khoury RM, Camacho-Lobato L, Katz PO, et al: Influence of spontaneous sleep positions on nighttime recumbent reflux in patients with gastroesophageal reflux disease. Am J Gastroenterol 94:2069-2073, 1999.
19. Behar J, Sheahan DG, Biancani P, et al: Medical and surgical management of reflux esophagitis. A 38-month report of a prospective clinical trial. N Engl J Med 293:263-268, 1975.
20. Kitchin LI, Castell DO: Rationale and efficacy of conservative therapy for gastroesophageal reflux disease. Arch Intern Med 151:448-454, 1991.
21. Kjellin A, Ramel S, Rossner S, Thor K: Gastroesophageal reflux in obese patients is not reduced by weight reduction. Scand J Gastroenterol 31:1047-1051, 1996.
22. Chattopadhyay DK, Greaney MG, Irvin TT: Effect of cigarette smoking on the lower oesophageal sphincter. Gut 18:833-835, 1977.

23. Dennish GW, Castell DO: Inhibitory effect of smoking on the lower esophageal sphincter. N Engl J Med 284:1136-1137, 1971.

24. Kahrilas PJ, Gupta RR: Mechanisms of acid reflux associated with cigarette smoking. Gut 31:4-10, 1990.

25. Kjellen G, Tibbling L: Influence of body position, dry and water swallows, smoking, and alcohol on esophageal acid clearing. Scand J Gastroenterol 13:283-288, 1978.

26. Berenson MM, Sontag S, Robinson MG, McCallum RM: Effect of smoking in a controlled study of ranitidine treatment in gastroesophageal reflux disease. J Clin Gastroenterol 9:499-503, 1987.

27. Hetzel DJ, Dent J, Reed WD, et al: Healing and relapse of severe peptic esophagitis after treatment with omeprazole. Gastroenterology 95:903-912, 1988.

28. Graham DY, Patterson DJ: Double-blind comparison of liquid antacid and placebo in the treatment of symptomatic reflux esophagitis. Dig Dis Sci 28:559-563, 1983.

29. Patel R, Launspach J, Soffer E: Effects of cisapride on salivary production in normal subjects. Dig Dis Sci 41:480-484, 1996.

30. Castell DO, Sigmund C Jr, Patterson D, et al: Cisapride 20 mg b.i.d. provides symptomatic relief of heartburn and related symptoms of chronic mild to moderate gastroesophageal reflux disease. CIS-USA-52 Investigator Group. Am J Gastroenterol 93:547-552, 1998.

31. Ramirez B, Richter JE: Review article: Promotility drugs in the treatment of gastrooesophageal reflux disease. Aliment Pharmacol Ther 7:5-20, 1993.

32. Kahrilas PJ, Quigley EM, Castell DO, Spechler SJ: The effects of tegaserod (HTF 919) on oesophageal acid exposure in gastro-oesophageal reflux disease. Aliment Pharmacol Ther 14:1503-1509, 2000.

33. Sabesin SM, Berlin RG, Humphries TJ, et al: Famotidine relieves symptoms of gastroesophageal reflux disease and heals erosions and ulcerations. Results of a multicenter, placebo-controlled, dose-ranging study. USA Merck Gastroesophageal Reflux Disease Study Group. Arch Intern Med 151:2394-2400, 1991.

34. Kahrilas PJ, Fennerty MB, Joelsson B: High- versus standard-dose ranitidine for control of heartburn in poorly responsive acid reflux disease: A prospective, controlled trial. Am J Gastroenterol 94:92-97, 1999.

35. Barrison AF, Jarboe LA, Weinberg BM, et al: Patterns of proton pump inhibitor use in clinical practice. Am J Med 111:469-473, 2001.

36. Bate CM, Griffin SM, Keeling PW, et al: Reflux symptom relief with omeprazole in patients without unequivocal oesophagitis. Aliment Pharmacol Ther 10:547-555, 1996.

37. Lind T, Havelund T, Carlsson R, et al: Heartburn without oesophagitis: Efficacy of omeprazole therapy and features determining therapeutic response. Scand J Gastroenterol 32:974-979, 1997.

38. Galmiche JP, Barthelemy P, Hamelin B: Treating the symptoms of gastro-oesophageal reflux disease: A double-blind comparison of omeprazole and cisapride. Aliment Pharmacol Ther 11:765-773, 1997.

39. Venables TL, Newland RD, Patel AC, et al: Omeprazole 10 milligrams once daily, omeprazole 20 milligrams once daily, or ranitidine 150 milligrams twice daily, evaluated as initial therapy for the relief of symptoms of gastro-oesophageal reflux disease in general practice. Scand J Gastroenterol 32:965-973, 1997.

40. Talley NJ, Lauritsen K, Tunturi-Hihnala H, et al: Esomeprazole 20 mg maintains symptom control in endoscopy-negative gastro-oesophageal reflux disease: A controlled trial of "on-demand" therapy for 6 months. Aliment Pharmacol Ther 15:347-354, 2001.

41. Bate CM, Booth SN, Crowe JP, et al: Omeprazole 10 mg or 20 mg once daily in the prevention of recurrence of reflux oesophagitis. Solo Investigator Group. Gut 36:492-498, 1995.

42. Hallerback B, Unge P, Carling L, et al: Omeprazole or ranitidine in long-term treatment of reflux esophagitis. The Scandinavian Clinics for United Research Group. Gastroenterology 107:1305-1311, 1994.

43. Venables TL, Newland RD, Patel AC, et al: Maintenance treatment for gastro-oesophageal reflux disease. A placebo-controlled evaluation of 10 milligrams omeprazole once daily in general practice. Scand J Gastroenterol 32:627-632, 1997.

44. Schindlbeck NE, Klauser AG, Berghammer G, et al: Three year follow up of patients with gastrooesophageal reflux disease. Gut 33:1016-1019, 1992.

45. Hatlebakk JG, Johnsson F, Vilien M, et al: The effect of cisapride in maintaining symptomatic remission in patients with gastro-oesophageal reflux disease. Scand J Gastroenterol 32:1100-1106, 1997.

46. Frazzoni M, De Micheli E, Grisendi A, Savarino V: Lansoprazole vs. omeprazole for gastro-oesophageal reflux disease: A pH-metric comparison. Aliment Pharmacol Ther 16:35-39, 2002.

47. Wolfe MM, Sachs G: Acid suppression: Optimizing therapy for gastroduodenal ulcer healing, gastroesophageal reflux disease, and stress-related erosive syndrome. Gastroenterology 118(2 Suppl 1):S9-S31, 2000.

48. Reilly JP: Safety profile of the proton-pump inhibitors. Am J Health Syst Pharm 56(23 Suppl 4):S11-S17, 1999.

49. Richter JE, Kahrilas PJ, Hwang C, et al: Esomeprazole is superior to omeprazole for the healing of erosive esophagitis (EE) in GERD patients. Gastroenterology 118:A20, 2000.

50. Metz DC, Strader DB, Orbuch M, et al: Use of omeprazole in Zollinger-Ellison syndrome: A prospective nine-year study of efficacy and safety. Aliment Pharmacol Ther 7:597-610, 1993.

51. Vela MF, Camacho-Lobato L, Srinivasan R, et al: Simultaneous intraesophageal impedance and pH measurement of acid and nonacid gastroesophageal reflux: Effect of omeprazole. Gastroenterology 120:1599-1606, 2001.

52. Attwood SE, Ball CS, Barlow AP, et al: Role of intragastric and intraoesophageal alkalinisation in the genesis of complications in Barrett's columnar lined lower oesophagus. Gut 34:11-15, 1993.

53. Laheij RJ, Sturkenboom MC, Hassing RJ, et al: Risk of community-acquired pneumonia and use of gastric acid–suppressive drugs. JAMA 292:1955-1960, 2004.

54. Katz PO, Anderson C, Khoury R, Castell DO: Gastro-oesophageal reflux associated with nocturnal gastric acid breakthrough on proton pump inhibitors. Aliment Pharmacol Ther 12:1231-1234, 1998.

55. Castell DO: Medical, surgical, and endoscopic treatment of gastroesophageal reflux disease and Barrett's esophagus. J Clin Gastroenterol 33:262-266, 2001.

56. Peghini PL, Katz PO, Bracy NA, Castell DO: Nocturnal recovery of gastric acid secretion with twice-daily dosing of proton pump inhibitors. Am J Gastroenterol 93:763-767, 1998.

57. Peghini PL, Katz PO, Castell DO: Ranitidine controls nocturnal gastric acid breakthrough on omeprazole: A controlled study in normal subjects. Gastroenterology 115:1335-1339, 1998.

58. Katsube T, Adachi K, Kawamura A, et al: *Helicobacter pylori* infection influences nocturnal gastric acid breakthrough. Aliment Pharmacol Ther 14:1049-1056, 2000.

59. Fackler WK, Ours TM, Vaezi MF, Richter JE: Long-term effect of H2RA therapy on nocturnal gastric acid breakthrough. Gastroenterology 122:625-632, 2002.

60. McCarty-Dawson D, Sue SO, Morrill B, Murdock RH Jr: Ranitidine versus cimetidine in the healing of erosive esophagitis. Clin Ther 18:1150-1160, 1996.

61. Cloud ML, Offen WW, Robinson M: Nizatidine versus placebo in gastroesophageal reflux disease: A 12-week, multicenter, randomized, double-blind study. Am J Gastroenterol 86:1735-1742, 1991.

62. Lepoutre L, Van der Spek P, Vanderlinden I, et al: Healing of grade-II and III oesophagitis through motility stimulation with cisapride. Digestion 45:109-114, 1990.

63. Sontag SJ, Hirschowitz BI, Holt S, et al: Two doses of omeprazole versus placebo in symptomatic erosive esophagitis: The U.S. Multicenter Study. Gastroenterology 102:109-118, 1992.

64. Chiba N, De Gara CJ, Wilkinson JM, Hunt RH: Speed of healing and symptom relief in grade II to IV gastroesophageal reflux disease: A meta-analysis. Gastroenterology 112:1798-1810, 1997.

65. Robinson M, Lanza F, Avner D, Haber M: Effective maintenance treatment of reflux esophagitis with low-dose lansoprazole. A randomized, double-blind, placebo-controlled trial. Ann Intern Med 124:859-867, 1996.

66. Richter JE, Bochenek W: Oral pantoprazole for erosive esophagitis: A placebo-controlled, randomized clinical trial. Pantoprazole US GERD Study Group. Am J Gastroenterol 95:3071-3080, 2000.

67. Richter JE, Kahrilas PJ, Johanson J, et al: Efficacy and safety of esomeprazole compared with omeprazole in GERD patients with erosive esophagitis: A randomized controlled trial. Am J Gastroenterol 96:656-665, 2001.

68. Klinkenberg-Knol EC, Festen HP, Jansen JB, et al: Long-term treatment with omeprazole for refractory reflux esophagitis: Efficacy and safety. Ann Intern Med 121:161-167, 1994.

69. Dent J, Yeomans ND, Mackinnon M, et al: Omeprazole v ranitidine for prevention of relapse in reflux oesophagitis. A controlled double blind trial of their efficacy and safety. Gut 35:590-598, 1994.

70. Kahrilas PJ, Falk GW, Johnson DA, et al: Esomeprazole improves healing and symptom resolution as compared with omeprazole in reflux oesophagitis patients: A randomized controlled trial. The Esomeprazole Study Investigators. Aliment Pharmacol Ther 14:1249-1258, 2000.

71. Vigneri S, Termini R, Leandro G, et al: A comparison of five maintenance therapies for reflux esophagitis. N Engl J Med 333:1106-1110, 1995.

72. Richter JE: Peptic strictures of the esophagus. Gastroenterol Clin North Am 28:875-891, vi, 1999.

73. Guda NM, Vakil N: Proton pump inhibitors and the time trends for esophageal dilation. Am J Gastroenterol 99:797-800, 2004.

74. Smith PM, Kerr GD, Cockel R, et al: A comparison of omeprazole and ranitidine in the prevention of recurrence of benign esophageal stricture. Restore Investigator Group. Gastroenterology 107:1312-1318, 1994.

75. Ferguson R, Dronfield MW, Atkinson M: Cimetidine in treatment of reflux oesophagitis with peptic stricture. BMJ 2:472-474, 1979.

76. Dakkak M, Hoare RC, Maslin SC, Bennett JR: Oesophagitis is as important as oesophageal stricture diameter in determining dysphagia. Gut 34:152-155, 1993.

77. Marks RD, Richter JE, Rizzo J, et al: Omeprazole versus H_2-receptor antagonists in treating patients with peptic stricture and esophagitis. Gastroenterology 106:907-915, 1994.

78. Kochhar R, Makharia GK: Usefulness of intralesional triamcinolone in treatment of benign esophageal strictures. Gastrointest Endosc 56:829-834, 2002.

79. Fass R, Sampliner RE: Barrett's oesophagus: Optimal strategies for prevention and treatment. Drugs 63:555-564, 2003.

80. Lieberman DA, Oehlke M, Helfand M: Risk factors for Barrett's esophagus in community-based practice. GORGE consortium. Gastroenterology Outcomes Research Group in Endoscopy. Am J Gastroenterol 92:1293-1297, 1997.

81. Sharma P: Review article: Prevalence of Barrett's oesophagus and metaplasia at the gastro-oesophageal junction. Aliment Pharmacol Ther 20(Suppl 5):48-54, discussion 61-62, 2004.

82. Isolauri J, Luostarinen M, Isolauri E, et al: Natural course of gastroesophageal reflux disease: 17-22 year follow-up of 60 patients. Am J Gastroenterol 92:37-41, 1997.

83. Westhoff B, Brotze S, Weston A, et al: The frequency of Barrett's esophagus in high-risk patients with chronic GERD. Gastrointest Endosc 61:226-231, 2005.

84. Gerson LB, Shetler K, Triadafilopoulos G: Prevalence of Barrett's esophagus in asymptomatic individuals. Gastroenterology 123:461-467, 2002.

85. Rex DK, Cummings OW, Shaw M, et al: Screening for Barrett's esophagus in colonoscopy patients with and without heartburn. Gastroenterology 125:1670-1677, 2003.

86. Wetscher GJ, Gadenstaetter M, Klingler PJ, et al: Efficacy of medical therapy and antireflux surgery to prevent Barrett's metaplasia in patients with gastroesophageal reflux disease. Ann Surg 234:627-632, 2001.

87. Sampliner RE: Updated guidelines for the diagnosis, surveillance, and therapy of Barrett's esophagus. Am J Gastroenterol 97:1888-1895, 2002.

88. Lagergren J, Bergstrom R, Lindgren A, Nyren O: Symptomatic gastroesophageal reflux as a risk factor for esophageal adenocarcinoma. N Engl J Med 340:825-831, 1999.

89. Ouatu-Lascar R, Triadafilopoulos G: Complete elimination of reflux symptoms does not guarantee normalization of intrasophageal acid reflux in patients with Barrett's esophagus. Am J Gastroenterol 93:711-716, 1998.

90. Katzka DA, Castell DO: Successful elimination of reflux symptoms does not insure adequate control of acid reflux in patients with Barrett's esophagus. Am J Gastroenterol 89:989-991, 1994.

91. Trimble KC, Pryde A, Heading RC: Lowered oesophageal sensory thresholds in patients with symptomatic but not excess gastro-oesophageal reflux: Evidence for a spectrum of visceral sensitivity in GORD. Gut 37:7-12, 1995.

92. Menges M, Muller M, Zeitz M: Increased acid and bile reflux in Barrett's esophagus compared to reflux esophagitis, and effect of proton pump inhibitor therapy. Am J Gastroenterol 96:331-337, 2001.

93. Sarela AI, Hick DG, Verbeke CS, et al: Persistent acid and bile reflux in asymptomatic patients with Barrett esophagus receiving proton pump inhibitor therapy. Arch Surg 139:547-551, 2004.

94. Ouatu-Lascar R, Fitzgerald RC, Triadafilopoulos G: Differentiation and proliferation in Barrett's esophagus and the effects of acid suppression. Gastroenterology 117:327-335, 1999.

95. Peters FT, Ganesh S, Kuipers EJ, et al: Endoscopic regression of Barrett's oesophagus during omeprazole treatment; a randomised double blind study. Gut 45:489-494, 1999.

96. Cooper BT, Neumann CS, Cox MA, Iqbal TH: Continuous treatment with omeprazole 20 mg daily for up to 6 years in Barrett's oesophagus. Aliment Pharmacol Ther 12:893-897, 1998.

97. Sampliner RE: Effect of up to 3 years of high-dose lansoprazole on Barrett's esophagus. Am J Gastroenterol 89:1844-1848, 1994.

98. Sharma P, Morales TG, Bhattacharyya A, et al: Squamous islands in Barrett's esophagus: What lies underneath? Am J Gastroenterol 93:332-335, 1998.

99. El-Serag HB, Aguirre TV, Davis S, et al: Proton pump inhibitors are associated with reduced incidence of dysplasia in Barrett's esophagus. Am J Gastroenterol 99:1877-1883, 2004.

100. Farrow DC, Vaughan TL, Hansten PD, et al: Use of aspirin and other nonsteroidal anti-inflammatory drugs and risk of esophageal and gastric cancer. Cancer Epidemiol Biomarkers Prev 7:97-102, 1998.

101. Langman MJ, Cheng KK, Gilman EA, Lancashire RJ: Effect of anti-inflammatory drugs on overall risk of common cancer: Case-control study in general practice research database. BMJ 320:1642-1646, 2000.

102. Souza RF, Shewmake K, Beer DG, et al: Selective inhibition of cyclooxygenase-2 suppresses growth and induces apoptosis in human esophageal adenocarcinoma cells. Cancer Res 60:5767-5772, 2000.

103. Cameron AJ, Ott BJ, Payne WS: The incidence of adenocarcinoma in columnar-lined (Barrett's) esophagus. N Engl J Med 313:857-859, 1985.

104. Tuchman DN, Boyle JT, Pack AI, et al: Comparison of airway responses following tracheal or esophageal acidification in the cat. Gastroenterology 87:872-881, 1984.

105. Jack CI, Calverley PM, Donnelly RJ, et al: Simultaneous tracheal and oesophageal pH measurements in asthmatic patients with gastro-oesophageal reflux. Thorax 50:201-204, 1995.

106. Ruth M, Carlsson S, Mansson I, et al: Scintigraphic detection of gastro-pulmonary aspiration in patients with respiratory disorders. Clin Physiol 13:19-33, 1993.

107. Donnelly RJ, Berrisford RG, Jack CI, et al: Simultaneous tracheal and esophageal pH monitoring: Investigating reflux-associated asthma. Ann Thorac Surg 56:1029-1033, discussion 1034, 1993.

108. Wright RA, Miller SA, Corsello BF: Acid-induced esophagobronchial-cardiac reflexes in humans. Gastroenterology 99:71-73, 1990.

109. Schan CA, Harding SM, Haile JM, et al: Gastroesophageal reflux–induced bronchoconstriction. An intraesophageal acid infusion study using state-of-the-art technology. Chest 106:731-737, 1994.

110. Herve P, Denjean A, Jian R, et al: Intraesophageal perfusion of acid increases the bronchomotor response to methacholine and to isocapnic hyperventilation in asthmatic subjects. Am Rev Respir Dis 134:986-989, 1986.

111. Vincent D, Cohen-Jonathan AM, Leport J, et al: Gastro-oesophageal reflux prevalence and relationship with bronchial reactivity in asthma. Eur Respir J 10:2255-2259, 1997.

112. Harding SM, Richter JE: The role of gastroesophageal reflux in chronic cough and asthma. Chest 111:1389-1402, 1997.

113. Sontag S, O'Connell S, Khandelwal S: Does wheezing occur in association with an episode of gastroesophageal reflux [abstract]? Gastroenterology 96:482, 1989.

114. Avidan B, Sonnenberg A, Schnell TG, Sontag SJ: Temporal associations between coughing or wheezing and acid reflux in asthmatics. Gut 49:767-772, 2001.

115. Bowrey DJ, Peters JH, DeMeester TR: Gastroesophageal reflux disease in asthma: Effects of medical and surgical antireflux therapy on asthma control. Ann Surg 231:161-172, 2000.

116. Ekstrom T, Lindgren BR, Tibbling L: Effects of ranitidine treatment on patients with asthma and a history of gastro-oesophageal reflux: A double blind crossover study. Thorax 44: 19-23, 1989.

117. Ford GA, Oliver PS, Prior JS, et al: Omeprazole in the treatment of asthmatics with nocturnal symptoms and gastro-oesophageal reflux: A placebo-controlled crossover study. Postgrad Med J 70:350-354, 1994.

118. Meier JH, McNally PR, Punja M, et al: Does omeprazole (Prilosec) improve respiratory function in asthmatics with gastroesophageal reflux? A double-blind, placebo-controlled crossover study. Dig Dis Sci 39:2127-2133, 1994.

119. Harding SM, Richter JE, Guzzo MR, et al: Asthma and gastroesophageal reflux: Acid suppressive therapy improves asthma outcome. Am J Med 100:395-405, 1996.

120. Ours TM, Kavuru MS, Schilz RJ, Richter JE: A prospective evaluation of esophageal testing and a double-blind, randomized study of omeprazole in a diagnostic and therapeutic algorithm for chronic cough. Am J Gastroenterol 94:3131-3138, 1999.

121. Poe RH, Kallay MC: Chronic cough and gastroesophageal reflux disease: Experience with specific therapy for diagnosis and treatment. Chest 123:679-684, 2003.

122. Ing AJ, Ngu MC, Breslin AB: Pathogenesis of chronic persistent cough associated with gastroesophageal reflux. Am J Respir Crit Care Med 149:160-167, 1994.

123. Irwin RS, French CL, Curley FJ, et al: Chronic cough due to gastroesophageal reflux. Clinical, diagnostic, and pathogenetic aspects. Chest 104:1511-1517, 1993.

124. Benini L, Ferrari M, Sembenini C, et al: Cough threshold in reflux oesophagitis: Influence of acid and of laryngeal and oesophageal damage. Gut 46:762-767, 2000.

125. Irwin RS, Zawacki JK, Wilson MM, et al: Chronic cough due to gastroesophageal reflux disease: Failure to resolve despite total/near-total elimination of esophageal acid. Chest 121:1132-1140, 2002.

126. Irwin RS, Zawacki JK, Curley FJ, et al: Chronic cough as the sole presenting manifestation of gastroesophageal reflux. Am Rev Respir Dis 140:1294-1300, 1989.

127. Wunderlich AW, Murray JA: Temporal correlation between chronic cough and gastroesophageal reflux disease. Dig Dis Sci 48:1050-1056, 2003.

128. Shaker R, Milbrath M, Ren J, et al: Esophagopharyngeal distribution of refluxed gastric acid in patients with reflux laryngitis. Gastroenterology 109:1575-1582, 1995.

129. Jacob P, Kahrilas PJ, Herzon G: Proximal esophageal pH-metry in patients with "reflux laryngitis." Gastroenterology 100:305-310, 1991.

130. Ward PH, Berci G: Observations on the pathogenesis of chronic non-specific pharyngitis and laryngitis. Laryngoscope 92:1377-1382, 1982.

131. Koufman JA: The otolaryngologic manifestations of gastroesophageal reflux disease (GERD): A clinical investigation of 225 patients using ambulatory 24-hour pH monitoring and an experimental investigation of the role of acid and pepsin in the development of laryngeal injury. Laryngoscope 101(4 Pt 2 Suppl 53):1-78, 1991.

132. Wiener GJ, Koufman JA, Wu WC, et al: Chronic hoarseness secondary to gastroesophageal reflux disease: Documentation with 24-h ambulatory pH monitoring. Am J Gastroenterol 84:1503-1508, 1989.

133. Ormseth EJ, Wong RK: Reflux laryngitis: Pathophysiology, diagnosis, and management. Am J Gastroenterol 94:2812-2817, 1999.

134. El-Serag HB, Lee P, Buchner A, et al: Lansoprazole treatment of patients with chronic idiopathic laryngitis: A placebo-controlled trial. Am J Gastroenterol 96:979-983, 2001.

135. Eherer AJ, Habermann W, Hammer HF, et al: Effect of pantoprazole on the course of reflux-associated laryngitis: A placebo-controlled double-blind crossover study. Scand J Gastroenterol 38:462-467, 2003.

136. Hamdan AL, Sharara AI, Younes A, Fuleihan N: Effect of aggressive therapy on laryngeal symptoms and voice characteristics in patients with gastroesophageal reflux. Acta Otolaryngol 121:868-872, 2001.

18

Laparoscopic and Open Nissen Fundoplication

Swee H. Teh · Robert W. O'Rourke · John G. Hunter

Gastroesophageal reflux disease (GERD) is the most common disorder of the esophagus and gastroesophageal junction. With nearly half of Americans experiencing heartburn symptoms at least monthly, GERD is a serious health concern in the Western world. For the 6% to 10% of Americans who describe daily reflux symptoms, GERD increases the risk for esophageal stricture, Barrett's esophagus, and esophageal cancer and has a significant impact on work productivity.[1-3] The modern era of GERD therapy has brought advances in diagnosis and treatment and, subsequently, a better understanding of the pathophysiology of GERD. The single most important factor in the development of GERD is an incompetent lower esophageal sphincter.[4] Progressive dilation plus deterioration of the gastroesophageal valve mechanism results in loss of the antireflux barrier and allows for acid and bile reflux. The goal of antireflux surgery is to re-establish the competency of the lower esophageal sphincter while preserving the patient's normal swallowing capacity.[5]

Improved medical therapies in the form of H_2 receptor antagonists and proton pump inhibitors (PPIs) have brought both symptomatic relief and effective resolution of esophageal inflammation, which may help ameliorate some of the long-term sequelae of GERD, but medical therapy must be continued indefinitely and does not prevent bile reflux. Antireflux surgery provides a permanent anatomic and physiologic cure with symptomatic relief and prevents the adverse consequences of ongoing esophageal exposure to acid and bile refluxate.

The Nissen fundoplication is the gold standard for the operative treatment of GERD. This well-established procedure has proved to be both durable and safe over a period of more than 20 years. With introduction of the laparoscopic approach in the 1990s, the number of Nissen fundoplications performed annually has increased threefold.[6,7] Since Dr. Nissen's original fundo-

plication in 1937 to protect a gastroesophageal anastomosis, the Nissen fundoplication has undergone many modifications. The principles of modern Nissen fundoplication include secure crural closure and creation of a short (≤2 cm), 360-degree "floppy" fundoplication designed to most closely replicate the normal physiology of the gastroesophageal flap valve.[8]

This chapter discusses the technical aspects of laparoscopic and open abdominal Nissen fundoplication for GERD.

CLINICAL FEATURES

As with all operations, proper patient selection is essential for a successful outcome. A thorough history and physical examination, as well as appropriate laboratory tests, should be completed to establish a diagnosis of GERD and eliminate other potential causes of discomfort. Classic symptoms include heartburn, regurgitation, and dysphagia. The frequency and timing of reflux symptoms, the relationship to meals, symptom exacerbation in the supine or upright position, and difficulty swallowing should be noted. The response to medical therapy and the duration of medical therapy are also recorded.

In addition, patients may have atypical symptoms such as chronic cough, asthma, pulmonary disease, dysphagia, odynophagia, hoarseness, and chest pain. These patients should undergo cardiac evaluation, including a chest radiograph, electrocardiogram, and if indicated, pulmonary function tests, in addition to standard diagnostic evaluation for gastroesophageal reflux. Patients with atypical symptoms and those who fail to respond to medical therapy may show less improvement in symptoms after Nissen fundoplication than those with typical GERD symptoms.[9]

PREOPERATIVE EVALUATION

The preoperative evaluation of patients with GERD should be thorough. At a minimum, patients should undergo a barium swallow and esophagogastroduodenoscopy (EGD). Performance of an esophageal motility study (EMS) is currently a preoperative standard to detect esophageal motility disorders that may lead to troublesome postoperative dysphagia. Although it has been dogma that patients with ineffective esophageal motility (IEM) (mean distal peristaltic amplitude <30 mm Hg or >20% loss of peristalsis) should undergo a partial fundoplication to prevent postoperative dysphagia, recent studies have demonstrated that postoperative dysphagia after Nissen fundoplication is no greater with IEM than with normal esophageal motility.[10] We routinely perform a preoperative EMS because it also allows documentation of a motility "baseline" that may serve for comparison should postoperative dysphagia develop. Twenty-four-hour ambulatory pH monitoring is essential for the evaluation of patients with nonerosive reflux disease (NERD), supraesophageal symptoms, or lack of response to PPI therapy. Patients with typical reflux symptoms and erosive esophagitis (or Barrett's esophagus and peptic stricture) do not routinely need a pH study to prove the diagnosis of reflux preoperatively. In a multivariate analysis of factors predicting a good response to antireflux surgery, the best response to antireflux surgery (98% good to excellent results) occurred in patients who had symptom relief with PPIs, typical GERD symptoms, and a positive 24-hour pH study.[11]

Other new diagnostic devices that will play an increasingly important role in the diagnosis of GERD over the coming decade are the BRAVO pH probe (Medtronics, Minneapolis, MN) and multichannel intraluminal impedance (MII). The BRAVO probe monitors distal esophageal pH and transmits the data to a small external recorder worn on the belt for a duration of up to 48 hours. It has the advantage of being more comfortable than standard 24-hour pH probes. In addition, early data suggest that 48-hour BRAVO monitoring may have greater sensitivity for GERD than standard 24-hour monitoring does.[12] MII has similarly gained significant popularity for the detection of both acid and non-acid GERD. MII measures electrical resistance (impedance) between a series of electrodes on a catheter placed across the gastroesophageal junction and up the esophagus. Air within the esophageal lumen causes an increase in impedance, whereas the presence of liquid refluxate within the esophageal lumen causes a decrease in impedance. By determining the temporal sequence of impedance events, one can establish the directional flow of gas and liquid within the esophagus (i.e., distal flow: swallow; proximal flow: reflux event or belch). By coupling this technology with data from a standard pH probe, one can identify both acid and non-acid refluxate. In part because of lack of standardized analytic software, MII is currently considered a research tool only. However, this technology may become the best method to determine which patients will best respond to surgery. Those with significant symptoms and concomitant reflux events

(acid or non-acid) while taking acid-suppression therapy may be the ideal patients for surgical therapy.[13]

INDICATIONS FOR SURGERY

Although several innovative endoscopic methods for treating GERD have achieved modest popularity over the past 5 years, the indications for antireflux surgery have changed little and surgery remains the "gold standard" by which endoscopic procedures should be compared. Box 18–1 lists the primary indications for antireflux surgery.

There is rarely an indication for antireflux surgery in patients with uncomplicated GERD who are satisfied with medical therapy (single-dose or twice-daily PPI). Such patients are usually maintained on medical therapy as long as their symptoms are well controlled. In contrast, antireflux surgery should be seriously considered in patients with severe GERD and symptoms not controlled by medical therapy, patients who would like to avoid life-long antacid therapy, and those with severe complicated GERD (Barrett's esophagus, ulcer, stricture). In the latter group of patients, surgery may not be necessary if ulcer healing or a 24-hour pH probe while taking medications confirms the absence of acid reflux. However, because elimination of excessive reflux is difficult to achieve in these patients, who have the worst form of GERD, we generally believe that antireflux surgery should be considered. Preoperative endoscopic or medical treatment of esophageal stricture or peptic ulcer disease must be accomplished before surgery. In a patient with esophageal stricture, preoperative dilation to at least 16 mm (48 French) is advisable to minimize the chance that the customary postoperative dysphagia (a result of edema and early postoperative esophageal dysmotility) will be compounded by a tight stricture. If preoperative dilatation to 16 mm is successful—several sessions are sometimes necessary—it is usually possible to extend the

---

Box 18–1 **Primary Indications for Antireflux Surgery**

Patients with esophageal and/or extra-esophageal GERD symptoms that are responsive but not completely eliminated by PPIs

Patients with heartburn eliminated by PPIs but continued non-acid reflux

Patients with well-documented reflux events preceding symptoms such as chest pain, cough, or wheezing

Patients with GERD complications such as peptic stricture, Barrett's esophagus, or vocal cord injury while taking PPIs twice a day

Patients with well-documented GERD who desire to stop chronic PPI use despite excellent symptom control for any reason (e.g., side effects, lifestyle, expense)

dilation intraoperatively to 18 or 20 mm, the standard-size dilators used by surgeons for calibrating the fundoplication.

In certain subgroups of patients with severe GERD, antireflux surgery may not be indicated. Medically complicated, morbidly obese (body mass index >35 kg/m^2) patients with significant GERD should be treated by Roux-en-Y gastric bypass. Patients with Barrett's esophagus and high-grade dysplasia or adenocarcinoma should be treated by esophageal resection. Severe strictures that are not responsive to dilatation therapy should also be treated by esophageal resection. Patients with low-grade dysplasia should be treated with high-dose PPIs for 3 months, after which they should undergo repeat biopsy. Fundoplication may be considered in such patients if subsequent biopsy shows no progression to high-grade dysplasia or carcinoma. Finally, GERD patients with previous gastric surgery should be approached cautiously. GERD in patients after gastric bypass or vertical banded gastroplasty cannot be treated by fundoplication because the fundus has been anatomically disrupted by the previous surgery.

Once a decision is made to perform a surgical antireflux procedure on a patient with GERD, the next step is to decide which type of fundoplication to perform. Recent data support the concept that Nissen fundoplication is effective therapy for GERD and is not associated with significant long-term dysphagia, even in patients with IEM.[14] These data, combined with data suggesting that partial fundoplication is associated with high long-term failure rates,[15] have led to a significant decrease in the application of partial fundoplication in patients with GERD, regardless of esophageal peristaltic function. Currently, only patients with a "named" esophageal motility disorder, such as achalasia or scleroderma, should undergo partial fundoplication. Despite this recent trend toward complete (Nissen) fundoplication in most patients, emerging recent evidence suggests that long-term satisfactory results may be achieved with anterior partial fundoplication.[16] The debate regarding the role of partial fundoplication in the treatment of GERD therefore persists, although most experienced surgeons prefer to perform complete fundoplication in most patients.

PRINCIPLES OF NISSEN FUNDOPLICATION

Basic surgical principles guide the successful performance of Nissen fundoplication, regardless of the approach (laparoscopic or open). Box 18–2 lists the primary principles of Nissen fundoplication.

Open Versus Laparoscopic Nissen Fundoplication

Laparoscopic Nissen fundoplication was first reported by Dallemagne et al. in 1991.[17] Since then, several large clinical series of Nissen fundoplication have been reported, including longitudinal studies with long-term follow-up

---

Box 18–2 **Primary Principles of Nissen Fundoplication**

Circumferential crural dissection with preservation of the vagus nerves

Circumferential dissection of the esophagus at the gastroesophageal junction

Adequate mobilization of the esophagus (or Collis gastroplasty) to attain 2 to 3 cm of intra-abdominal esophagus without inferior traction

Crural closure with interrupted sutures

Gastric fundus mobilization and adequate short gastric vessel division

Creation of a short (<2 cm), floppy (loose around an 18- to 20-mm dilator) fundoplication anchored to the esophagus in several places

---

that demonstrate the results of both open and laparoscopic fundoplication to be equivalent.[18-20] Several randomized clinical trials published in the past decade have reached the same conclusion.[18,22-24] The laparoscopic approach is associated with shorter hospital stay, less postoperative pain, fewer wound-related complications, and earlier return to work. Despite these advantages, selection of the open versus the laparoscopic approach should depend on surgeon experience and the patient's previous surgical history. The intraoperative steps of surgical repair are relatively similar in both approaches. Laparoscopic Nissen fundoplication, however, requires that the surgeon possess advanced laparoscopic skills.

The approach to reoperative Nissen fundoplication is somewhat controversial. Some experts advocate that all reoperative surgery be performed through an open approach, but several large series have demonstrated equivalent results with laparoscopic and open reoperation.[25] Laparoscopic reoperation after open surgery, though feasible, may be tedious because the intra-abdominal adhesions associated with open surgery may be formidable.

LAPAROSCOPIC NISSEN FUNDOPLICATION

Position and Port Placement

After induction of general anesthesia, a Foley catheter and pneumatic calf compression devices are applied. The patient is placed in a split-leg position with both arms tucked and secured to the operating table. The surgeon stands between the patient's legs with the primary monitor over the patient's head. The first assistant stands to the patient's left, and the scrub technician stands to the patient's right. Pneumoperitoneum is achieved by inserting a Veress needle at the umbilicus.

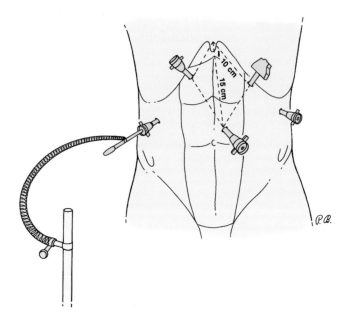

Figure 18–1. Preferred port site position for laparoscopic Nissen fundoplication.

A five-port (two 10-mm ports and three 5-mm ports) technique is used (Fig. 18–1). Additional ports may be placed as necessary. A 10-mm camera port is placed just superior and to the left of the umbilicus, approximately 15 cm below the xiphoid and medial to the inferior epigastric artery. A 45-degree laparoscope is placed through this port. The laparoscope camera may be managed by the first assistant or with a robotic camera holder. A thorough abdominal exploration with the laparoscope is routinely performed before initiating dissection. All secondary ports are placed under direct vision. With the patient in a steep reverse Trendelenburg position, a second port (10 mm) is next placed approximately 11 to 12 cm below the xiphoid process at the left costal margin. The third port (5 mm) is generally placed 8 to 10 cm farther down the left costal margin than the second port. This port should not be placed farther lateral than the anterior axillary line and may be limited by the reflection of the left colon. The fourth port, for liver retraction, is a 5-mm port placed on the right costal margin 12 to 15 cm from the sternal base (depending on the size of the liver). Alternatively, the liver can be retracted with a Nathanson retractor placed high in the subxiphisternal region. Finally, a 5-mm port is placed to the right of midline, at the level of the 10-mm dissecting port, so that it angles through the round ligament internally to lie immediately below the left edge of the liver.

Exposure

A 5-mm articulating liver retractor is placed through the right lateral port under laparoscopic visualization, and the left lobe of the liver is retracted anteriorly and superiorly to expose the hiatus. The right crus and caudate lobe of the liver should be clearly visible through the phrenoesophageal ligament if the liver retraction is adequate. The liver retractor is stabilized with an endoscopic instrument holder attached to the operating table. An atraumatic (Hunter type) grasper is placed through the left lateral port to assist in retraction of the stomach. The epiphrenic fat pad along the lesser curvature just below the esophagogastric junction is used for inferior retraction to minimize the risk of gastric or esophageal injury. The operating surgeon uses an atraumatic grasper in the left hand and a harmonic scalpel or electrosurgical dissecting scissors in the right hand.

Dissection

Lesser Curve

The pars flaccida of the gastrohepatic ligament is opened with the harmonic scalpel or scissors while taking care to preserve the hepatic branch of the vagus nerve, and the stomach is retracted to the patient's left and inferolaterally if possible. Preservation of this hepatic branch of the nerve may prevent impairment of gallbladder motility with subsequent cholelithiasis, although no data exist to support this theory. Nevertheless, some surgeons divide this structure routinely without significant adverse outcomes. In addition to the nerve, an aberrant left hepatic artery may be present in the pars flaccida in up to 13% of patients. If the gastrohepatic ligament is entered above the hepatic branch of the vagus nerve, the chance of encountering the aberrant left hepatic artery is minimal. Preservation of the aberrant left hepatic artery should be attempted if possible. On rare occasion, in the presence of an extremely large hiatal hernia it is necessary to divide the hepatic branch of the vagus or an aberrant left hepatic artery (or both) to reach the base of the right crus of the diaphragm. Clinically significant liver ischemia has not been reported in these circumstances.

Crus

Dissection of the lesser curve is extended superiorly, up to the esophagogastric junction, to reveal the caudate lobe below and expose the hiatus and the right crus of the diaphragm. The peritoneum overlying the right crus is incised, the medial border dissected, and the phrenoesophageal ligament divided along the apex of the hiatus (Fig. 18–2). Dissection is continued across the top of the crural arch until the left crus is exposed. The dissection is then carried down the border of the left crus until the angle of His and the gastric fundus limit further inferior dissection. The anterior vagus nerve crosses the esophagus in this region and should be identified and preserved. Periesophageal mediastinal dissection is initiated bluntly by introducing two round-nosed atraumatic graspers between the right crus and the esophagus and spreading horizontally (9- and 3-o'clock position) with the graspers closed (Fig. 18–3). This step is repeated to the left of the esophagus. The use of thermal devices is limited during mediastinal dissection to avoid undetected injury to the vagus nerves.

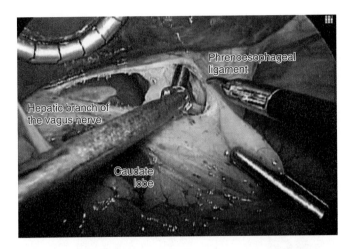

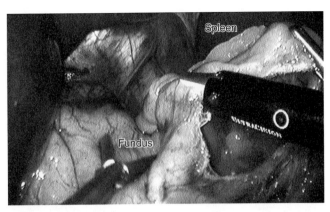

Figure 18–4. Taking down the greater curvature of the stomach by dividing the short gastric vessels.

Figure 18–2. Dissection of the lesser curve (extending superiorly) and the phrenoesophageal ligament along the apex of the hiatus.

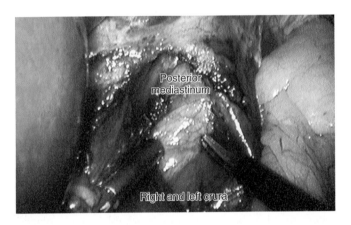

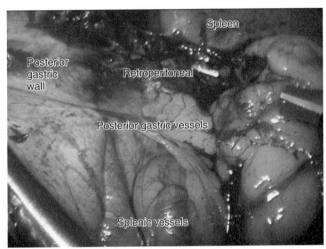

Figure 18–3. Horizontal (9- and 3-o'clock direction) spreading with closed graspers to open the posterior mediastinum.

Figure 18–5. Dissection of the retroperitoneal gastrophrenic fold. (Reproduced with permission from Jamie A. Koufman, MD, Voice Institute of New York.)

Fundus and Greater Curve

Dissection of the fundus of the stomach is begun by identifying the point on the greater curvature approximately a third of the distance from the angle of His to the antrum. A convenient landmark for this point is the inferior pole of the spleen or (occasionally visible) the left gastroepiploic artery. With the surgeon's left-hand instrument grasping the stomach adjacent to the greater curvature and retracting posteromedially and the first assistant retracting the greater omentum anterolaterally, the lesser sac is entered with the harmonic scalpel, approximately 5 to 10 mm away from the greater curve of the stomach (Fig. 18–4). The short gastric vessels are divided individually with the harmonic scalpel until the superior pole of the spleen is reached. As one proceeds superiorly, three strategies may help dissection in this area:

1. Expose the superior pole of the spleen with "triangular retraction." The three corners of retraction in the axial plane are the spleen tip, the surgeon's left-hand instrument retracting anteromedially on the anterior wall of the fundus, and the first assistant retracting posteromedially on the posterior wall of the stomach.

2. If the greater omentum obscures the superior pole of the spleen, it should be retracted inferiorly. This may be accomplished by introducing an additional port and grasper in the left flank or placing a "reefing" polypropylene suture in the greater omentum and retracting the omentum through the left lateral port with the two long ends of this suture.

3. Layer the dissection of the vascular structures at the superior pole of the spleen, starting with the visceral peritoneal reflection, then the short gastric vessels, and then the retroperitoneal gastrophrenic tissues. Dividing the pancreaticogastric peritoneal fold and the posterior gastric artery is necessary to fully mobilize the fundus and reach the base of the left crus posteriorly (Fig. 18–5).

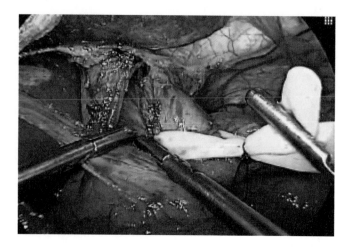

Figure 18–6. Penrose drain around the esophagus and secured with an Endoloop.

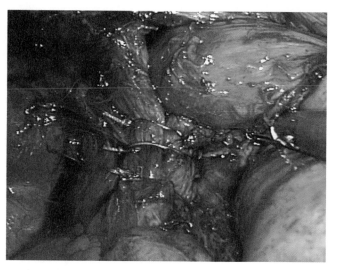

Figure 18–7. Crural closure with nonabsorbable suture starting posteriorly and working anteriorly.

Mediastinal and Posterior Esophagus

At the completion of gastric dissection, the base of the left crus is reached. If the earlier dissection reached the base of the right crus, the plane behind the esophagus is complete. Once this retroesophageal "tunnel" is made, a 4-inch-long, $\frac{1}{4}$-inch-wide Penrose drain is passed around the esophagus and secured with an Endoloop (Fig. 18–6). The first assistant places a toothed locking (gallbladder type) grasper on the secured Penrose drain and retracts inferiorly and to the patient's left. The esophagus is freed circumferentially within the mediastinum by blunt dissection. The posterior vagus is encountered adjacent to the esophagus and is generally retracted along with the esophagus. Dissection of the posterior vagus away from the esophagus exposes the vagus to injury later in the dissection. Although most of the mediastinal dissection can be done bluntly, an occasional aortoesophageal artery is encountered (usually high on the left) and should be controlled with the harmonic scalpel. The length of the mediastinal dissection depends on available intra-abdominal esophagus. In the presence of Barrett's esophagus, severe inflammation, stricture, giant hiatal hernia, or previous surgery, the esophagus is often foreshortened and will need extensive high mediastinal dissection or Collis gastroplasty, or both (see later).

To best assess intra-abdominal esophageal length, the Penrose drain is released and the distance from the gastroesophageal junction to the crural closure is measured. At least 2.5 cm of esophagus must be within the abdomen under no tension. If the maximal mediastinal dissection does not adequately reduce more than 2.5 cm of intra-abdominal esophagus, a Collis gastroplasty should be performed.

Repair

Crural Closure

The crura are closed from the right of the esophagus with interrupted nonabsorbable sutures placed 8 to 10 mm apart, 5 to 10 mm back from the crural edge. The peritoneal covering of the crura should be incorporated into the repair, and the sutures should be "staggered" in the anterior-posterior plane on the crura to avoid splitting the crural musculature along the length of the repair. The completed crural closure should be calibrated to the size of the esophagus containing a 56-French esophageal dilator (Fig. 18–7). One cannot close the crura with the dilator in place, but sutures can be added or cut out after the dilator has been used to properly size the crural aperture. To prevent reherniation, the crural closure is often performed with single 1-cm^2 Teflon felt patches, felt strips, or occasionally a piece of absorbable or nonabsorbable mesh placed across the crural closure. Several randomized trials have demonstrated a lower hernia recurrence rate when the closure is buttressed in this fashion.[26,27]

Fundoplication

The fundus is next passed posteriorly from left to right with atraumatic graspers to assess for adequate mobilization. The "shoeshine maneuver" involves sliding the fundoplication back and forth behind the esophagus to confirm good position (Fig. 18–8). One purpose of this maneuver is to confirm that no redundant fundus lies posterior to the esophagus after creation of the fundoplication. Grasping a point too low on the greater curvature may predispose to this error. The fundoplication should not retract significantly when the graspers are released. A 56- or 60-French esophageal dilator is then passed transorally into the stomach by the anesthesiologist under videoscopic vision by the surgeon. Good communication and slow advancement of the dilator are essential to minimize the risk of perforation at the esophagogastric junction. The dilator should pass without resistance. If resistance is encountered, the dilator is removed and a smaller dilator is passed. The size of the dilator is then increased until resistance is noted.

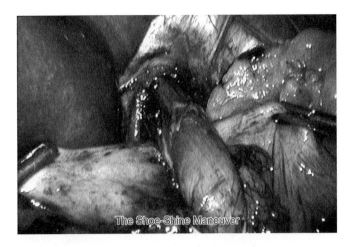

Figure 18–8. The "shoeshine maneuver" to ensure that the fundoplication is in good position without tension.

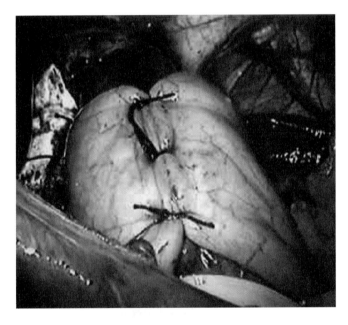

Figure 18–9. The completed Nissen fundoplication with three nonabsorbable sutures 1 cm apart.

After dilator placement, the most superior stitch of the fundoplication is placed 2 cm proximal to the esophagogastric junction with simple interrupted 2-0 nonabsorbable suture; full-thickness bites are taken through each side of the fundoplication and a partial-thickness esophageal bite in between. Two additional sutures are placed 1 cm above and 1 cm below the initial suture to create a 2-cm-long fundoplication that is secured to the esophagus just above the level of the esophagogastric junction (Fig. 18–9). Knots may be tied extracorporeally, but intracorporeal knotting decreases tissue trauma and optimizes knot tension and position. Some authors advocate infradiaphragm fixation of the fundoplication to the crura to prevent reherniation, but there is no evidence that this in any way decreases failure rates.

OPEN NISSEN FUNDOPLICATION

The principal steps in performing an open Nissen fundoplication are similar to the laparoscopic approach. Open Nissen fundoplication is indicated if surgeons do not have adequate laparoscopic experience or patients have dense adhesions because of previous upper gastrointestinal operations. Despite the improved tactile feedback with an open approach, it is important to note that exposure of the hiatus may be less easily achieved than with a laparoscopic approach. The techniques involved in open fundoplication are similar to those in laparoscopic fundoplication; the following sections therefore address only significant differences.

Exploration and Exposure

An upper midline incision with the use of a self-retaining retractor allows good exposure. A liver retractor placed close to the most posterior part of the left lateral lobe of the liver permits improved visualization. Optimal exposure is obtained when the diaphragm is seen to run vertically from the upper end of the incision directly posteriorly to the hiatus.

Lesser Curve

The thin gastrohepatic ligaments are incised, extended superiorly, and carried over the anterior surface of the esophagus as described earlier. Similarly, an aberrant left hepatic artery and hepatic branch of the vagus are protected if encountered in the pars flaccida. The anterior vagus is likewise identified and protected.

Crus

By retracting the lesser curve inferolaterally and to the right, the left crus is exposed. The right crus is dissected bluntly with the left fingers to create a retroesophageal space. A Penrose drain is passed around the lower part of the esophagus, excluding the posterior vagus nerve, and used as a retractor to provide better visualization of the retroesophageal space.

Mediastinal and Posterior Esophagus

With retraction on the Penrose drain, the esophagus can be dissected circumferentially. Similarly, the mediastinal dissection can be carried superiorly.

Fundus and Greater Curve

The loose attachments between the fundus and the left diaphragm are taken down. The short gastric vessels are ligated sequentially with the harmonic scalpel as described earlier or by serial division with clamps and suture.

Repair and Fundoplication

Crural repair and fundoplication are performed as described earlier. A "floppy" Nissen fundoplication requires that the fundic wrap admit the surgeon's index

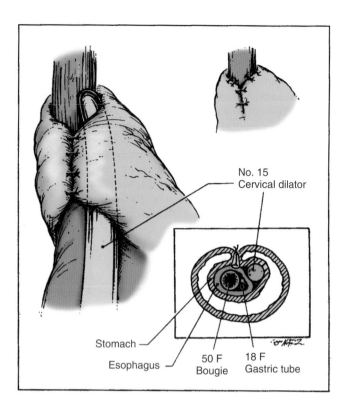

Figure 18–10. The original description of a "floppy" Nissen fundoplication by Donahue and Bombeck et al. in 1977.

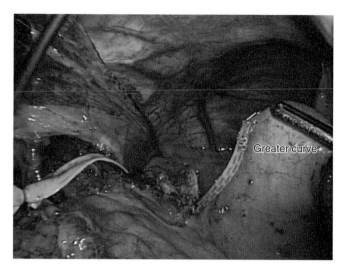

Figure 18–11. Laparoscopic stapling of the fundus from the greater curve toward the lesser curve.

finger between the wrap and the esophagus with the dilator in place (Fig. 18–10). Factors that influence the tightness of the wrap are the degree of mobilization of the fundus, the size of the esophageal dilator, and the sutures placed to create the fundoplication.

THE ACQUIRED SHORT ESOPHAGUS

The presence of a short esophagus increases the difficulty of laparoscopic Nissen fundoplication. Up to 20% of surgical failures with Nissen fundoplication are due to the lack of recognition of a short esophagus. A short esophagus is discovered more frequently in patients with esophageal stricture, Barrett's esophagus, and type III paraesophageal hernia. Esophageal foreshortening occurs as a result of recurrent acid peptic injury and subsequent fibrosis of the mediastinal esophagus. Given its pathogenesis, it is not surprising that esophageal stricture is often associated with esophageal foreshortening. Large hiatal hernias may also be associated with a short esophagus as a result of chronic cephalad displacement of the gastroesophageal junction. Preoperative results of barium swallow and EGD may provide an indication of a short esophagus, but no combination of preoperative clinical variables reliably predicts the presence of a short esophagus, and the diagnosis of this entity continues to be made definitively only in the operating room, where it is defined as failure to achieve 2.5 cm of intra-abdominal esophagus after standard mediastinal dissection techniques.

Collis gastroplasty achieves esophageal lengthening by using the gastric cardia to create a neo-esophagus. In open surgery, this can be performed easily by applying a cut staple on the left side and parallel to the esophagus with a 16-mm dilator in place. When a minimally invasive approach is used, the complexity of the procedure is increased. It can be accomplished either by a combined thoracoscopic-laparoscopic approach or by a totally laparoscopic approach.[28,29]

With the esophageal dilator in place, a thoracoscope is inserted through the third intercostal space in the anterior axillary line and passed through the chest until it meets the mediastinal pleura. This is visualized with a laparoscope in place in the abdomen. The thoracoscope is then removed, and a linear stapler is inserted through the same port until it meets the mediastinal pleura at the crura as seen with the laparoscope. Dissection from the abdomen allows for passage of the stapler into the abdomen, which is then applied to the stomach alongside the esophageal bougie at the gastroesophageal junction at the angle of His. Application of this stapler divides the upper part of the stomach from the angle of His distally, along the esophageal dilator, thus creating a neo-esophagus.

The totally laparoscopic approach to a short esophagus has evolved from a method using an EEA circular stapler to our current approach, which involves the use of a linear stapler and creation of a stapled wedge gastroplasty.[30] An esophageal dilator (16 mm) is placed to calibrate the width of the gastric tube. A mark is made 3 cm inferior to the angle of His adjacent to the dilator. The laparoscopic stapled wedge gastroplasty can be performed by applying the laparoscopic stapler horizontally from the greater curve toward the lesser curve with the esophageal dilator in place (Fig. 18–11). The gastroplasty is completed by firing a staple parallel to the dilator in the cranial direction and therefore lengthening the esophagus (Fig. 18–12). The superior portion of the body of the stomach is then used as the wrap. Elements of importance in fashioning the fundoplication include

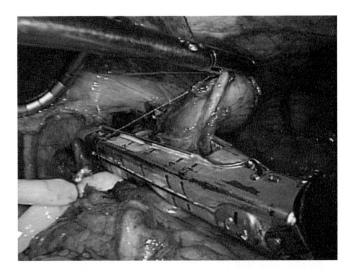

Figure 18–12. Lengthening of the esophagus by laparoscopic stapling parallel to the esophagus (with a dilator in place) in the cranial direction.

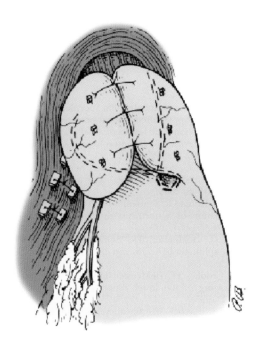

Figure 18–13. Final appearance of the fundoplication with the gastric portion of the staple line placed against the neo-esophagus.

placement of the initial suture of the fundoplication on the esophagus, immediately above the gastroesophageal junction, to ensure that acid-secreting (gastric) mucosa does not reside above the fundoplication. A second element that ensures safety and avoids wrap deformation is to place the gastric portion of the staple line against the neo-esophagus such that the tip of the gastric staple line sits adjacent to the middle suture of the fundoplication on the right side of the esophagus (Fig. 18–13). Before initiating a liquid diet we perform a water-soluble contrast study to ensure that no leak in the staple line is present.

POSTOPERATIVE CARE

A nasogastric tube is unnecessary after laparoscopic Nissen fundoplication. Patients are monitored on the regular floor and start clear liquids once they are awake and alert on the evening of surgery. The diet can be advanced to soft foods the following day. Patients may be dismissed home in 1 to 2 days. Although outpatient laparoscopic Nissen fundoplication has been performed, patient satisfaction is low, and management of pain and nausea may be difficult without parenteral access. Patients are advised to not eat large chunks of unchewed food for about 3 weeks, especially avoiding bread, meat, and raw vegetables. After the first 24 hours, postoperative pain can usually be managed with oral analgesia. We encourage 1-month follow-up; no studies are routine, but a barium swallow serves as an excellent screening test to evaluate postoperative dysphagia or reflux-like symptoms. In brief, if the fundoplication is intact and if a 12.5-mm barium tablet passes without difficulty, it is extremely unlikely that the symptoms are related to a technical deficiency of the repair.

SPECIFIC INTRAOPERATIVE AND POSTOPERATIVE COMPLICATIONS

Intraoperative complications include esophageal perforation, pneumothorax, splenic injury, bleeding, and missed visceral injury. Although these complications occur in less than 2% of all series,[30] the consequences can be grave.[31] Esophageal and gastric perforations occur in approximately 1.5% of cases and should be repaired primarily and buttressed with the fundoplication to minimize the risk for mediastinitis. We delay progression to a solid diet by 5 to 7 days when an esophageal repair has been performed.

Pneumothorax (1% to 5%) is usually self-limited but may cause immediate or delayed hemodynamic or respiratory consequences. When a pneumothorax is detected, we start by making the hole larger (to avoid a tension pneumothorax created by a one-way valve phenomenon). A red rubber catheter is inserted in the abdominal cavity with the tip placed through the rent in the pleura. At the completion of the operation, the wide end of the catheter is pulled out a trocar site and placed under water seal as the lung is re-expanded. A postoperative chest radiograph should be obtained and O_2 saturation monitored.

Splenic injury can take the form of infarction or bleeding. Superior pole infarction can occur with ligation of the short gastric arteries. Occasionally, some of these vessels enter the spleen directly without passing through the hilum and are end arteries to the upper pole. No further intervention is required if the tip of the spleen is infarcted. Rarely do patients have additional pain or fever under these conditions. Splenic bleeding, however, may require conversion to laparotomy and urgent splenectomy (0.5% to 1%). Incidental electrosurgery burns from arcing or inattention can result in delayed perforation and peritonitis. Meticulous dissection and gentle retraction can help prevent injury. An abdominal survey before closure can help identify any signs of bleeding.

Late complications can take many different forms. Even though Nissen fundoplication has greater than a 90% success rate in eliminating reflux symptoms, over time, new or recurrent foregut symptoms will develop in 2% to 17% of patients. Although some dysphagia, gas bloating, and mild residual esophagitis are not uncommon in the early postoperative period, these symptoms generally resolve by 3 to 6 months; severe or persistent symptoms may indicate failure. Two percent to 6% of patients undergoing antireflux surgery will eventually require a reoperation.[20,25] Reported causes of failure vary significantly between studies, but a slipped or misplaced fundoplication and dehiscence are each responsible in approximately 15% to 30% of patients, transthoracic herniation occurs in 10% to 60%, and tight fundoplication, missed motility disorders, and paraesophageal hernias account for other modes of antireflux surgery failure.

SHORT-TERM RESULTS

The overall short-term results in appropriately selected patients are excellent.[18,32] Minor self-limited symptoms may occur in the postoperative period in some patients. Up to 20% of patients will experience transient dysphagia, which is usually caused by postoperative edema secondary to surgical manipulation of the gastroesophageal junction. These symptoms typically improve without intervention within 6 weeks. EGD or barium swallow is indicated if symptoms persist. Dilatation may provide relief of persistent dysphagia, but reoperation may be indicated in patients who are not responsive to dilatation. The failure rate of Nissen fundoplication is approximately 1% per year.[25,33] Bloating is common in GERD patients, and the severity is not significantly different before or after surgery.[25] Other common symptoms after Nissen fundoplication are early satiety, nausea, and diarrhea. These symptoms are likely to improve with time and tend to respond to nonoperative therapy. Bilateral vagus nerve injury may result in gastroparesis.

LONG-TERM RESULTS

At 5 to 8 years' follow-up, more than 95% of patients report satisfaction with their laparoscopic Nissen fundoplication.[34,35] A minority of patients report persistent dysphagia and bloating. The cause of surgical failure is most often due to (1) complete disruption of the wrap, (2) a slipped Nissen fundoplication (in which part of the stomach lies above and part lies below the fundoplication), or (3) herniation of an intact wrap through the hiatus into the chest.[25,36] Surgical failures may require reoperation.[20,32] Patients should be cautioned that the results of reoperation for GERD are never as favorable as the results after a primary operation and that residual atypical symptoms may persist. Laparoscopic reoperative fundoplication is technically feasible by experienced surgeons.

CONCLUSION

Antireflux surgery is an excellent treatment option for patients with symptoms of GERD that are inadequately treated with medication, for patients who desire to avoid lifelong medical therapy, or for patients with significant complications from acid reflux. The impact of antireflux surgery on progression of Barrett's esophagus is not fully understood, and patients with Barrett's who undergo antireflux surgery still require routine endoscopic surveillance. The introduction of a laparoscopic approach to fundoplication should not alter the operative indications. Finally, to ensure successful surgical outcomes, an understanding of disease pathophysiology, preoperative diagnostic evaluation, appropriate patient selection, and complete familiarity with the various types of antireflux procedures available are essential.

By the time that this volume is in print, effective endoscopic therapies that approximate the outcomes of surgical fundoplication may be available. Regardless of these advances, surgical therapy for GERD will probably continue to play an important role in patients with complicated disease, such as those with large hiatal hernias or a shortened esophagus.

REFERENCES

1. Shaker R, Castell DO, Schoenfeld PS, Spechler SJ: Nighttime heartburn is an under-appreciated clinical problem that impacts sleep and daytime function: The results of a Gallup survey conducted on behalf of the American Gastroenterological Association. Am J Gastroenterol 98:1487-1493, 2003.
2. Wu AH, Tseng CC, Bernstein L: Hiatal hernia, reflux symptoms, body size, and risk of esophageal and gastric adenocarcinoma. Cancer 98:940-948, 2003.
3. Srinivasan R, Tutuian R, Schoenfeld P, et al: Profile of GERD in the adult population of a northeast urban community. J Clin Gastroenterol 38:651-657, 2004.
4. Zaninotto G, DeMeester TR, Schwizer W, et al: The lower esophageal sphincter in health and disease. Am J Surg 155:104-111, 1988.
5. Stein HJ, Crookes PF, DeMeester TR: Three-dimensional manometric imaging of the lower esophageal sphincter. Surg Annu 27:199-214, 1995.
6. Finlayson SR, Laycock WS, Birkmeyer JD: National trends in utilization and outcomes of antireflux surgery. Surg Endosc 17:864-867, 2003.
7. Fuchs KH, DeMeester TR, Albertucci M: Specificity and sensitivity of objective diagnosis of gastroesophageal reflux disease. Surgery 102:575-580, 1987.
8. Hunter JG, Trus TL, Branum GD, et al: A physiologic approach to laparoscopic fundoplication for gastroesophageal reflux disease. Ann Surg 223:673-685, discussion 685-687, 1996.
9. Farrell TM, Richardson WS, Trus TL, et al: Response of atypical symptoms of gastro-oesophageal reflux to antireflux surgery. Br J Surg 88:1649-1652, 2001.
10. Rydberg L, Ruth M, Abrahamsson H, Lundell L: Tailoring antireflux surgery: A randomized clinical trial. World J Surg 23:612-618, 1999.
11. Campos GM, Peters JH, DeMeester TR, et al: Multivariate analysis of factors predicting outcome after laparoscopic Nissen fundoplication. J Gastrointest Surg 3:292-300, 1999.
12. Tseng D, Rizvi AZ, Fennerty MB, et al: Forty-eight-hour pH monitoring increases sensitivity in detecting abnormal esophageal acid exposure. J Gastrointest Surg 9:1043-1051, discussion 1051-1052, 2005.
13. Castell DO, Vela M: Combined multichannel intraluminal impedance and pH-metry: An evolving technique to measure type and

proximal extent of gastroesophageal reflux. Am J Med 111(Suppl 8A):157S-159S, 2001.

14. Baigrie RJ, Watson DI, Myers JC, Jamieson GG: Outcome of laparoscopic Nissen fundoplication in patients with disordered preoperative peristalsis. Gut 40:381-385, 1997.

15. Horvath KD, Jobe BA, Herron DM, Swanstrom LL: Laparoscopic Toupet fundoplication is an inadequate procedure for patients with severe reflux disease. J Gastrointest Surg 3:583-591, 1999.

16. Watson DI, Jamieson GG, Lally C, et al: Multicenter, prospective, double-blind, randomized trial of laparoscopic Nissen vs anterior 90 degrees partial fundoplication. Arch Surg 139:1160-1167, 2004.

17. Dallemagne B, Weerts JM, Jehaes C, et al: Laparoscopic Nissen fundoplication: Preliminary report. Surg Laparosc Endosc 1:138-143, 1991.

18. Ackroyd R, Watson DI, Majeed AW, et al: Randomized clinical trial of laparoscopic versus open fundoplication for gastro-oesophageal reflux disease. Br J Surg 91:975-982, 2004.

19. Terry M, Smith CD, Branum GD, et al: Outcomes of laparoscopic fundoplication for gastroesophageal reflux disease and paraesophageal hernia. Surg Endosc 15:691-699, 2001.

20. Granderath FA, Kamolz T, Schweiger UM, et al: Long-term results of laparoscopic antireflux surgery. Surg Endosc 16:753-757, 2002.

21. Viljakka MT, Luostarinen ME, Isolauri JO: Complications of open and laparoscopic antireflux surgery: 32-year audit at a teaching hospital. J Am Coll Surg 185:446-450, 1997.

22. Lundell L, Dalenback J, Hattlebakk J, et al: Outcome of open antireflux surgery as assessed in a Nordic multicentre prospective clinical trial. Nordic GORD-Study Group. Eur J Surg 164:751-757, 1998. Erratum in Eur J Surg 165:1104, 1999.

23. Laine S, Rantala A, Gullichsen R, Ovaska J: Laparoscopic vs conventional Nissen fundoplication. A prospective randomized study. Surg Endosc 11:441-444, 1997.

24. Heikkinen TJ, Haukipuro K, Bringman S, et al: Comparison of laparoscopic and open Nissen fundoplication 2 years after operation. A prospective randomized trial. Surg Endosc 14:1019-1023, 2000.

25. Hunter JG, Smith CD, Branum GD, et al: Laparoscopic fundoplication failures: Patterns of failure and response to fundoplication revision. Ann Surg 230:595-604, discussion 604-606, 1999.

26. Granderath FA, Schweiger UM, Kamolz T, et al: Laparoscopic Nissen fundoplication with prosthetic hiatal closure reduces postoperative intrathoracic wrap herniation: Preliminary results of a prospective randomized functional and clinical study. Arch Surg 140:40-48, 2005.

27. Frantzides CT, Madan AK, Carlson MA, Stavropoulos GP: A prospective, randomized trial of laparoscopic polytetrafluoroethylene (PTFE) patch repair vs simple cruroplasty for large hiatal hernia. Arch Surg 137:649-652, 2002.

28. Swanstrom LL, Marcus DR, Galloway GQ: Laparoscopic Collis gastroplasty is the treatment of choice for the shortened esophagus. Am J Surg 171:477-481, 1996.

29. Johnson AB, Oddsdottir M, Hunter JG: Laparoscopic Collis gastroplasty and Nissen fundoplication. A new technique for the management of esophageal foreshortening. Surg Endosc 12:1055-1060, 1998.

30. Terry ML, Vernon A, Hunter JG: Stapled-wedge Collis gastroplasty for the shortened esophagus. Am J Surg 188:195-199, 2004.

31. Watson DI, Jamieson GG: Antireflux surgery in the laparoscopic era. Br J Surg 85:1173-1184, 1998.

32. Watson DI, Jamieson GG, Game PA, et al: Laparoscopic reoperation following failed antireflux surgery. Br J Surg 86:98-101, 1999.

33. Power C, Maguire D, McAnena O: Factors contributing to failure of laparoscopic Nissen fundoplication and the predictive value of preoperative assessment. Am J Surg 187:457-463, 2004.

34. Bammer T, Hinder RA, Klaus A, Klingler PJ: Five- to eight-year outcome of the first laparoscopic Nissen fundoplications. J Gastrointest Surg 5:42-48, 2001.

35. DeMeester TR, Bonavina L, Albertucci M: Nissen fundoplication for gastroesophageal reflux disease. Evaluation of primary repair in 100 consecutive patients. Ann Surg 204:9-20, 1986.

36. Hinder RA, Klingler PJ, Perdikis G, Smith SL: Management of the failed antireflux operation. Surg Clin North Am 77:1083-1098, 1997.

19

Partial Fundoplications

Lee L. Swanström

Subsequent to the incidental discovery of the efficacy of the 360-degree fundoplication as an effective antireflux procedure in the late 1950s, a proliferation of modifications were devised to either address specific physiologies or serve as a "more physiologic" alternative. For the most part, these were either modifications of Nissen's complete wrap that were designed to make it longer lasting or more physiologic or some sort of partial fundoplication. Partial fundoplications were proposed as a less "intense" or competent valve mechanism intended to minimize the common side effects of the original Nissen procedure—dysphagia, gas bloating, inability to vomit, and other complications.[1] Each of these repairs had schools of supporters, and many continue to be used today—particularly if they have made the transition to a laparoscopic application.

TYPES OF REPAIR

Belsey Mark IV Ronald Belsey began development of the repair associated with his name many years before the final publication of version "IV" in 1967.[2] Access for this repair is traditionally via a left thoracotomy, although thoracoscopic access has also been described. The Belsey repair involves mobilization of the distal end of the esophagus and proximal part of the stomach by opening up the hiatus from above and splitting the diaphragm if needed to bring sufficient stomach into the chest. Short gastric vessels are divided only enough to allow the fundus to be brought 270 degrees around the distal esophagus. The fundoplication is fashioned around a 54-French dilator. It is fixed with interrupted sutures to the wall of the esophagus. At completion, the wrapped gastroesophageal junction is reduced below the diaphragm and the crura repaired (Fig. 19–1).

Dor The Dor repair is a 180-degree anterior fundoplication performed via laparotomy or laparoscopy. It was initially described by Jacques Dor in 1962 as an alternative antireflux procedure to the Nissen fundoplication and remains widely used today as the most common antireflux adjunct after Heller myotomy for achalasia or distal diverticula (Fig. 19–2). The most common iteration of the Dor is to bring the greater curvature and anterior fundus up to the left crus and then across the anterior arc of the hiatus. It is frequently fixed to both the right crus and the right side of the esophagus to complete the "wrap."

Toupet Originally described as a more physiologic antireflux repair by its creator, the French surgeon Andre Toupet, this repair was initially a 180-degree posterior fundoplication (Fig. 19–3). It was subsequently modified to a 270-degree wrap for increased valve competency, and posterior crural repair is commonly added as well to minimize the high herniation rate seen in some laparoscopic series. Although this repair used to be little known in North America, the introduction of laparoscopic antireflux surgery has made it the most common repair after Nissen fundoplication.[3]

Watson David Watson and colleagues in Australia have published well-constructed comparative studies of a 90-degree partial fundoplication that seems to produce outcomes similar to those of other repairs.[4,5] This repair emphasizes an acute angle of His with the gastric fundus attached to the left side of the esophagus and the left crus only (Fig. 19–4).

Each type of partial repair, and all of their potential variations, have strong advocates and schools of practice. A very few places advocate partial fundoplication for all patients in an effort to minimize the undesirable side effects of a 360-degree wrap.[6] This school of thought was especially attractive in the early days of laparoscopic fundoplication because it was feared that patients who were undergoing a "minimally invasive" surgery would be particularly unhappy with even transient symptoms of dysphagia, gas bloating, inability to belch, and others.[7] This approach withered somewhat in the face of increasing reports of suboptimal long-term results with partial fundoplication, and today these repairs are used as one of the options for a "tailored" approach, with a Nissen repair being the standard treatment and a partial wrap

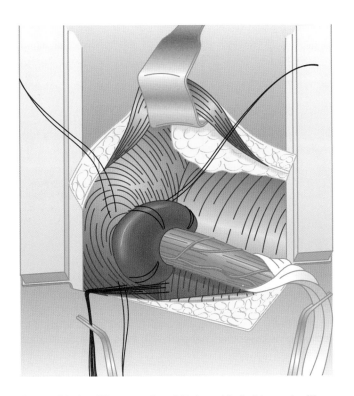

Figure 19–1. The completed Belsey Mark IV repair. (From Nyhus LM, Baker RJ, Fischer JE [eds]: Mastery of Surgery, 3rd ed. Boston, Little, Brown, 1997.)

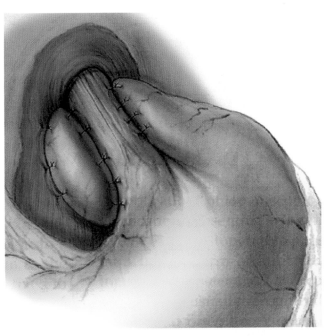

Figure 19–3. A completed 270-degree version of the Toupet fundoplication. (From Soper NJ, Swanström, LL, Eubanks WS [eds]. Mastery of Endoscopic and Laparoscopic Surgery, 2nd ed. Philadelphia, Lippincott Williams & Wilkins, 2004.)

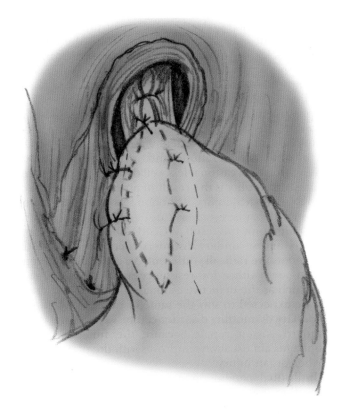

Figure 19–2. The finished Dor fundoplication as an adjunct to Heller myotomy.

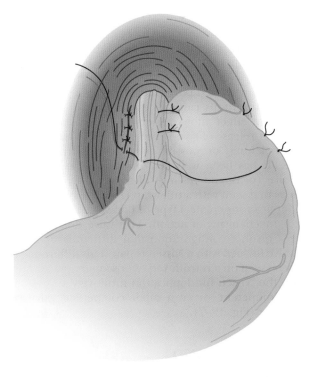

Figure 19–4. The 90-degree anterior fundoplication popularized by D.I. Watson. (From Eubanks WS, Swanström LL, Soper NJ [eds]: Mastery of Endoscopic and Laparoscopic Surgery. Philadelphia, Lippincott Williams & Wilkins, 2000.)

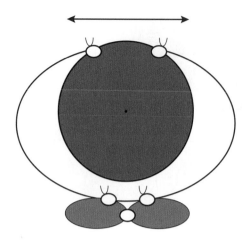

Figure 19–5. One of the differences between complete and partial fundoplications is the "hinge" effect of the exposed esophagus, which reduces the outflow and backflow characteristics of the repair.

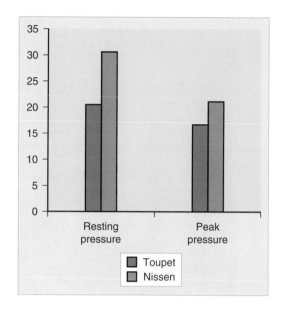

Figure 19–6. The resting and peak pressure of a Toupet fundoplication is lower than that seen with a Nissen fundoplication.

used for particular physiologic findings.[8] The description that follows is based on the use of partial fundoplication as one of the elements of a tailored approach.

MECHANISM

Partial fundoplications, like complete ones, function both by increasing outflow (and therefore "backflow") and resistance of the esophagus (augmentation of the resting pressure of the lower esophageal sphincter) and by restoring an anatomic "flap valve."[9] Outflow resistance, in turn, is a function of two phenomena. The first is the simple physics of resistance, in which the force of resistance to antegrade or retrograde bolus passage is equal to resting pressure times the length of the pressure zone. The second factor is, in effect, a hinge effect in which the uncovered portion of the esophagus common to all partial wraps can still expand easily (Fig. 19–5). This hinge effect allows easier passage of food boluses and easier release of gastric pressure, which can be good, as in belching, or possibly negative, as in continued reflux. It has been well demonstrated that the overall pressure (peak and resting) of a partial wrap is not as high as that seen with a full wrap (Fig. 19–6).[10] All partial fundoplications create a type of flap valve as one of their major mechanisms of action. This valve does, however, have a distinct configuration that distinguishes it from the valve formed with a Nissen repair. This difference can easily be seen on a retroflexed endoscopic view, and once again, the Nissen fundoplication intuitively appears as a more competent, or even super competent, valve configuration (Fig. 19–7).[9]

INDICATIONS AND CONTRAINDICATIONS

As previously discussed, a few centers perform a partial fundoplication for all patients with gastroesophageal reflux disease (GERD). This is, however, definitely a rare

approach. For the most part, partial wraps are used for very specific indications and, in most centers, performed in a small minority of reflux patients. As with any antireflux surgery, the patient should actually have gastroesophageal reflux. It must be well documented by history and a thorough work-up as described later. Specific indications for partial repairs include intrinsic physiologic abnormalities that make a Nissen repair unwise; idiosyncratic patient issues, which usually involve the absolute need to belch or vomit; psychological issues that make a Nissen repair ill advised; and intractable failure of a Nissen fundoplication (Table 19–1).

The most common indication for a partial wrap is for esophageal motility disorders (failed peristalsis). Motility disorders are commonly classified as either primary or secondary. Primary disorders have an intrinsic cause (myoneural degeneration) and include named disorders, as well as occasional less well defined disorders. Secondary dysmotility is the result of an extrinsic insult and direct esophageal injury. Although secondary dysmotility may include causes such as caustic ingestion, it is by far most commonly the result of GERD. Distinction between primary and secondary disorders is critical because the treatments are radically different. An intrinsic disorder is best treated with a low-resistance antireflux procedure inasmuch as the defective esophageal pump mechanism can be expected to stay the same or even deteriorate. A secondary dysmotility disorder can be well treated with a standard Nissen repair because the function of the esophagus almost always improves with the prevention of further organ injury.[10,11]

Individual patient physiology can represent a good indication for a partial fundoplication. An example includes patients whose initial complaint is significant dysphagia. If work-up reveals no treatable peptic stricture and GERD symptoms are trivial to the patient, partial

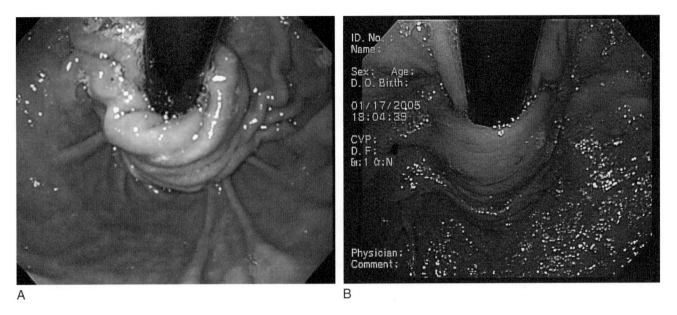

Figure 19–7.   A, Retroflexed endoscopic view of a Nissen valve. **B,** The same view after a Toupet fundoplication.

Table 19–1   Motility Disorders Treated by Fundoplication

Classification	Disorder	Manometric Characteristics
Primary	Achalasia	No peristalsis, nonrelaxing LES
	Vigorous achalasia	100% simultaneous contractions, nonrelaxing LES
	Diffuse esophageal spasm	High-amplitude, nonperistaltic contractions; normal or hypertensive LES
	Nutcracker esophagus	High-amplitude peristalsis (>180 mm Hg), normal or hypertensive LES
	Hypertensive LES	Normal body motility; high-pressure, possibly poorly relaxing LES
	Ineffective esophageal motility	Low-amplitude (<30 mm Hg) body contractions with all swallows and in all smooth muscle segments
	Nonspecific	Variable abnormal contractions throughout the entire smooth muscle of the esophagus
Secondary	Obstructive	Either low-pressure or high-pressure peristalsis in the distal esophagus
	Caustic ingestion	Decreased contractility throughout the affected segment
	GERD related	Progressively diminished amplitudes in the distal esophagus
	Pseudoachalasia (cancer infiltration)	Immotile esophagus in end-stage cases

GERD, gastroesophageal reflux disease; LES, lower esophageal sphincter.

fundoplication may be a wise choice. Another indication is severe aerophagia. This can be a result of gastroparesis, voluntary behavior such as air swallowing for postlaryngectomy esophageal speech, or unconscious adaptive (or maladaptive) behavior. The later is fairly common in the long-term GERD population but can still lead to crippling gas bloating after Nissen fundoplication if it is severe enough. Finally, some psychological conditions can make a partial wrap a preferred treatment. This category can include known eating disorders such as bulimia or simply the surgeon's analysis that an individual patient is psychologically unable to handle even the transient side effects (dysphagia, inability to belch,

gastric distention, and early satiety) common with a Nissen operation.

Contraindications include those common to any surgery—poor cardiac or pulmonary reserve and uncontrolled bleeding dyscrasias. All fundoplication patients should be carefully evaluated before surgery—even if laparoscopic surgery is planned. Conversion to an open procedure is always possible, and the surgery is still an esophageal procedure whether open or closed.

In addition, there are several relative contraindications related to the long-term function of these repairs. Because partial fundoplications offer somewhat less reflux protection, they should be used cautiously, if at all,

Table 19–2	Tests Ordered as Preoperative Evaluation for Reflux Disease	
Routine tesst	Upper endoscopy	Rule out malignancy
		Assess tissue damage
		Treat strictures
		Assess anatomy
	Esophageal manometry	Exclude primary esophageal motility problems
		Determine risk for dysphagia
		Assess LES status
		Aid in determination of esophageal length
	24-Hour pH test	Confirm the diagnosis of GERD
		Quantify the severity of reflux
		Correlate symptoms
		Establish a baseline for follow-up
Selective tests	Upper gastrointestinal radiographs	Measure transit time
		Assess anatomy
	Radionuclide gastric-emptying test	Quantify delayed gastric emptying
		Observe the gastric contribution to reflux
	Impedance manometry	Non-acid reflux
	Bilitec testing	Bile reflux (duodenal-gastric-esophageal reflux)
	Provocative testing (Bernstein, barostat)	Assess atypical symptoms

GERD, gastroesophageal reflux disease; LES, lower esophageal sphincter.

in patients with severe reflux, particularly those with normal esophageal motility. In a prospective study of the laparoscopic Toupet repair performed on 100 consecutive patients with reflux, it was noted that at 1-year follow-up, 50% of patients with preoperative DeMeester scores of 32 or higher had continued reflux versus 18% of those with scores lower than 32.[12] It is also a relative contraindication to perform a partial fundoplication in a patient with a relatively shortened esophagus because such shortening is typically a sign of chronic severe reflux (Barrett's esophagus, strictures, etc.) or is associated with a large hiatal hernia and shortening makes it difficult to carry out a technically adequate partial fundoplication, which requires at least 4 cm of intra-abdominal esophagus. The one exception is the Belsey repair, which benefits from the ability to extensively mobilize the thoracic esophagus. There are still some indications for an open approach as opposed to a laparoscopic one.[13] Such indications include multiple failed laparoscopic repairs, an extremely hostile abdomen or chest, and perhaps an associated giant paraesophageal hernia. As with any surgery, the approach and the technique should be tailored to the individual patient's physiology and psychology.

PREOPERATIVE EVALUATION

The preoperative evaluation of any reflux patient should be complete and thorough, particularly patients with abnormal physiology who are being considered for partial fundoplication. A structured gastrointestinal history, preferably with a standardized symptoms assessment tool, is extremely important and may help identify patients who should have a partial wrap because of psy-

chological or behavioral issues. Obviously, records of any previous gastrointestinal surgery should be reviewed, as well as copies of all previous foregut testing if at all possible. Not only should the reports of recent tests be reviewed, but the surgeon should also obtain and personally look at the actual physiology tests. Test reports done by nonsurgical investigators often neglect to comment on findings significant to the surgeon. This is particularly the case with upper endoscopy and motility testing, where determination of esophageal length, the size and type of hiatal hernia, and the anatomic appearance or grade of the valve have definite clinical meaning to the surgeon. All patients should undergo upper endoscopy to stage Barrett's esophagus, exclude cancer, grade the valve, assess gastric problems, and exclude findings that may make other studies dangerous, such as diverticula or strictures. Motility should likewise be evaluated in all cases to determine the type of motility disorder, state of the lower esophageal sphincter, and length of the esophagus. Twenty-four-hour pH testing as an absolute prerequisite to surgery is more controversial. We would argue that it should be done in all patients being considered for surgery to exclude those who have no reflux, determine the severity of their reflux, and serve as a baseline for follow-up should postoperative complaints arise. Other tests should be ordered as indicated by the patient's clinical findings or when standard tests fail to delineate the problem (Table 19–2).

SURGICAL TECHNIQUE

Laparoscopic abdominal procedures are typically performed with the patient in a split-leg position with arms outstretched. A basic five-port access pattern is used for

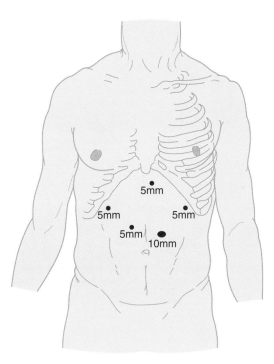

Figure 19–8. Laparoscopic trocar placement for partial fundoplication.

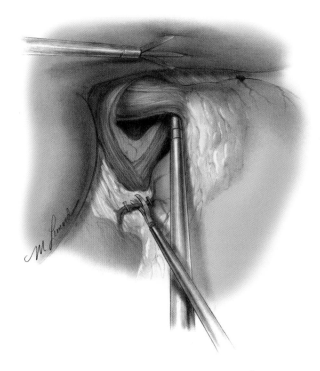

Figure 19–9. Using an angled laparoscope allows a retroesophageal window to be created under direct vision. (From Soper NJ, Swanström, LL, Eubanks WS [eds]: Mastery of Endoscopic and Laparoscopic Surgery, 2nd ed. Philadelphia. Lippincott Williams & Wilkins, 2004.)

any laparoscopic fundoplication (Fig. 19–8). Standard instruments required and some newer time-saving technologies are listed in Table 19–3. Monitors are positioned at the top of the table, and the operating surgeon stands either between the legs of the patient or on the patient's left. The assistant, who holds the laparoscope and retracts, stands on the patient's right or between the legs of the patient.

The left lobe of the liver is elevated without dividing the triangular ligament. The liver retractor is best fixed to a table-mounted retractor holder because secure retraction minimizes trauma to the liver. The assistant retracts the stomach downward and to the patient's left. The hepatogastric ligament is divided while preserving any significant anomalous liver arteries. The phreno-esophageal membrane is "nicked" at the apex of the esophageal hiatus, and blunt dissection is used to gain access to the lower mediastinum. The phrenoesophageal membrane can then be detached from the crura circumferentially with cautery or ultrasonic energy. Care should be taken to avoid stripping the peritoneal covering off of the crura because such stripping will compromise subsequent suture repair. Working from the right side and using the angled laparoscope, a window is created behind the esophagus (Fig. 19–9). The esophageal dissection is carried into the mediastinum via blunt and ultrasonic dissection as far as needed to bring the gastroesophageal junction at least 3 cm into the abdomen. The upper third of the gastric fundus is mobilized by dividing the short gastric vessels and the retrogastric attachments—a technical point that helps minimize tension on even partial fundoplications.

Table 19–3	Instruments for Laparoscopic Partial Fundoplication
Basic instruments	High-resolution laparoscopic camera
	Angled (45- or 30-degree) laparoscope
	Atraumatic liver retractor
	Table-mounted liver retractor holder
	Atraumatic graspers (Glassman)
	5-mm Babcock graspers
	Curved-tip needle holders
	Monopolar cautery scissors
	Multiple clip applier *or* ultrasonic coagulating shears
	Esophageal dilator
Advanced instruments	GIA staplers
	Flexible upper endoscope
	Bipolar scissors
	Clip applier
Optional labor-saving tools	Automatic suturing devices
	Ultrasonic coagulating shears

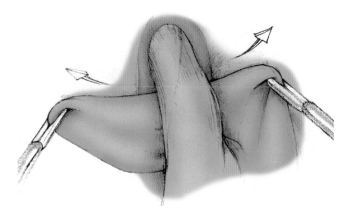

Figure 19–10. The "shoeshine" maneuver ensures that adequate fundus has been mobilized and the correct areas grasped.

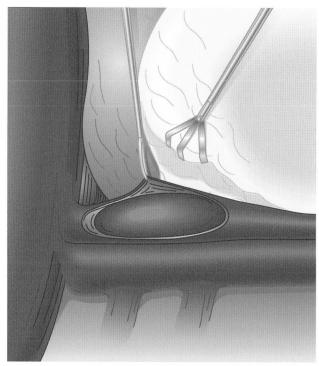

Figure 19–11. The left mediastinal pleura is opened longitudinally to expose the distal esophagus. (From Eubanks WS, Swanström LL, Soper NJ [eds]: Mastery of Endoscopic and Laparoscopic Surgery. Philadelphia, Lippincott Williams & Wilkins, 2000.)

Laparoscopic Toupet Procedure

The previously mobilized fundus is grasped from the right and brought behind the esophagus. The greater curvature is grasped on either side, and a "shoeshine" maneuver is performed to ensure that the correct portions of the stomach have been grasped and that the wrap is fully mobilized and loose enough (Fig. 19–10). The assistant then grasps the right side of the wrap and uses it to retract the esophagus to the patient's left. This maneuver exposes the posterior of the hiatus. A loose, nonobstructing hiatal closure is performed with interrupted posterior sutures of heavy woven polyester. Each of these posterior bites includes a slip of the posterior wrap. Additional sutures are placed from the greater curvature of both sides of the wrap to their corresponding crus. The repair is finished by passing a large dilator (54 to 58 French) and tacking the edges of the wrap to the esophagus at the 2- and 10-o'clock positions (see Fig. 19–3). The final result should be a tension-free, 270-degree fundoplication securely fixed to the diaphragm.[14]

Laparoscopic Dor Procedure

One advantage of the Dor anterior fundoplication is the possibility of preserving the posterior phrenoesophageal attachments. This is, of course, only possible if there is no esophageal shortening or hiatal hernia, which would require complete dissection and mobilization. Large hiatal hernias should be loosely closed, either posteriorly if a full dissection was performed or anteriorly if the posterior phrenoesophageal attachments were left intact. It is still preferable to divide the short gastric vessels to ensure the absence of tension on the repair. The Dor repair involves reconstruction of the angle of His by suturing the gastric fundus to the mid left crus. Subsequent sutures from the greater curve to the rim of the hiatus roll the fundus up and over the anterior gastroesophageal junction (see Fig. 19–2). The final result is a

180-degree anterior wrap that is securely fixed to the diaphragm.[15]

Transthoracic Belsey Mark IV Repair

The Belsey repair is generally performed via a left anterior-lateral thoracotomy, although occasional reports have surfaced of a similar repair done thoracoscopically.[16] Patients undergo general anesthesia with a double-lumen endotracheal tube and indicated monitoring lines. They are positioned in full right lateral decubitus position with care taken to adequately pad and protect dependent parts of the body. A muscle-sparing sixth intercostal incision is made and a self-retaining retractor is placed. The inferior pulmonary ligament is divided with cautery, and the mediastinum overlying the distal esophagus is opened longitudinally (Fig. 19–11). Blunt finger dissection is used to get around the esophagus, and a Penrose drain is placed to allow atraumatic retraction. Dissection is carried distally until the gastroesophageal junction is identified—it may be helpful to identify it via upper endoscopy at this point. The phrenoesophageal membrane is opened with cautery and the stomach is progressively mobilized into the chest by clipping and dividing the short gastric vessels. When adequate stomach wall is free, it is rolled up on the anterior of the esophagus and fixed in place with interrupted sutures (see Fig. 19–1). When tied, these sutures create a 180-degree partial fundoplication. The fundoplication is then reduced below the diaphragm while mobilizing the esophagus as far proximally as needed to avoid tension. The diaphragm is closed with interrupted non-absorbable sutures. A chest tube is placed, the thoracotomy is closed in standard manner, and an epidural catheter is placed at the end of surgery for optimal postoperative pain control.[15,17]

POSTOPERATIVE CARE

Patients generally stay in the hospital between 12 and 48 hours for laparoscopic surgery and 3 to 7 days for open surgery. A liquid diet can be started 6 hours after surgery in straightforward cases. In more complex cases (reoperative, myotomy, pyloroplasty, inadvertent gastrotomy, etc.), nothing is allowed orally until a water-soluble upper gastrointestinal radiograph is checked. Patients are advanced to a pureed diet and medications converted to liquid forms or crushed. Patients are instructed to remain on this diet for 2 weeks and then to slowly advance to solids. Care is taken to avoid postoperative nausea and vomiting because acute wrap herniation has been described in this scenario. It is our routine to bring all antireflux surgery patients back for physiology studies 6 to 8 months after surgery. At this visit a gastrointestinal symptoms assessment form is administered and 24-hour pH testing is performed. Upper endoscopy is performed if the patient has dysphagia or had Barrett's esophagus, strictures, or severe esophagitis preoperatively. In patients who had a motility disorder before surgery, an esophageal manometric examination is performed as well to assess the current state of their esophageal function.

RESULTS

A large amount of literature on outcomes has been published over the 40 years that partial fundoplications have been in use. The Belsey repair has lost a great deal of popularity both because of its relatively morbid access and because of outcomes showing lower efficacy than with other repairs (Table 19–4). The Dor repair has an excellent track record when used as an adjunct to Heller myotomy. In one of the larger series of the Dor repair in this capacity, Patti et al. reported an 11% incidence of reflux at 59 months' mean follow-up.[18] These results are typical of the outcomes achieved in most clinical reports of laparoscopic Heller/Dor procedures, which has resulted in it being the most commonly used adjunct to myotomy. Its use as primary antireflux surgery is so rare that there is no contemporary series reporting outcomes for the procedure. The Toupet procedure has become the most commonly used partial fundoplication. It is most often used as an alternative to a Nissen repair in cases of esophageal dysmotility, but there are also series and institutions describing its use as a standard antireflux procedure. Much like the Dor procedure, the Toupet repair works well for postmyotomy patients and for those with significant dysmotility. The results reported with its use as a primary antireflux procedure are conflicting. Several centers have long relied on the posterior partial wrap and report good results.[15,19,20] In addition, there have been three randomized prospective studies favorably comparing partial fundoplication with the "gold standard" Nissen. However, several North American reports have detailed a high rate of valve incompetence and wrap disruption with the Toupet procedure, particularly in patients more severe reflux disease (Table 19–5).[9,21-24]

CONCLUSION

Partial fundoplication has a long and controversial position in the history of antireflux surgery. The advent of laparoscopic approaches—with their increased volume and emphasis on postoperative quality of life—has created a resurgence of interest in partial fundoplication. Early results showing higher failure rates in at least some subsets of reflux patients dampened enthusiasm somewhat for these approaches, but there remain several indications and significant numbers of patients for whom partial wrap remains the best treatment of their reflux. All surgeons interested in an antireflux practice should be familiar with the indications and technical aspects of these procedures.

| Table 19–4 | Results of the Belsey Mark IV Repair |

Author	Study Type	No. Patients	Follow-up (yr)	Success Rate (%) Symptomatic/Objective
Dilling et al. (1977)	Review		4	64/53
Fenton et al. (1997)	Review	276	48.0	82/NA
Alexiou et al. (1999)	Review	90	11	71.9/NA
Champion (2003)*	Review	21	6.2	57/NA
Lerut et al. (1990)	Review	147	5	78/NA

*Thoracoscopic series.
NA, not available.

Table 19–5 Results of Laparoscopic Toupet Antireflux Surgery

Author	Study Type	No. Patients	Follow-up (mo)	Symptomatic/ Objective	Failure Rate Rate(%)
Erenoglu et al. (2003)	Retrospective	118 N	27.5	+/−	18 N
		26 T			16 T
Fernando et al. (2002)	Retrospective	163 N	19.7	+/−	7 N
		43 T			21 T
Zornig et al. (2002)	Prospective/randomized	100 N	4	+/+	12 N
		100 T			10 T
Jobe et al. (2004)	Prospective	100 T	24	+/+	48 T
Zugel et al. (2002)	Retrospective	40 N	19	+/−	12 N
		122 T			11 T
Farrell et al. (2001)	Retrospective	591 N	12	+/−	9 N
		78 T			21 T

N, Nissen; T, Toupet.

REFERENCES

1. Rydberg L, Ruth M, Lundell L: Mechanism of action of antireflux procedures. Br J Surg 86:405-410, 1999.
2. Skinner DB, Belsey RHR: Surgical management of esophageal reflux and hiatal hernia: Long-term results with 1,030 cases. J Thorac Cardiovasc Surg 53:33-54, 1967.
3. Carlson MA, Frantzides CT: Complications and results of primary minimally invasive antireflux procedures: A review of 10,735 reported cases. J Am Coll Surg 193:428-439, 2001.
4. Watson DI, Jamieson GG, Lally C, et al: Multicenter, prospective, double-blind, randomized trial of laparoscopic Nissen vs anterior 90 degrees partial fundoplication. Arch Surg 139:1160-1167, 2004.
5. Yau P, Watson DI, Ascott N, et al: Efficacy of a 90 degree anterior fundoplication vs a total fundoplication in an experimental model. Surg Endosc 14:830-833, 2000.
6. Holzinger F, Banz M, Tscharner GG, et al: [Laparoscopic Toupet partial fundoplication as general surgical therapy of gastroesophageal reflux. 1-year results of a 5-year prospective long-term study.] Chirurg 72:6-13, 2001.
7. Windsor JA, Yellapu S: Laparoscopic anti-reflux surgery in New Zealand: A trend towards partial fundoplication. Aust N Z J Surg 70:184-187, 2000.
8. Swanström LL: Partial fundoplications for gastroesophageal reflux disease: Indications and current status. J Clin Gastroenterol 29:127-132, 1999.
9. Jobe BA, Kahrilas PJ, Vernon AH, et al: Endoscopic appraisal of the gastroesophageal valve after antireflux surgery. Am J Gastroenterol 99:233-243, 2004.
10. Chrysos E, Athanasakis E, Pechlivanides G, et al: The effect of total and anterior partial fundoplication on antireflux mechanisms of the gastroesophageal junction. Am J Surg 188:39-44, 2004.
11. Heider TR, Behrns KE, Koruda MJ, et al: Fundoplication improves disordered esophageal motility. J Gastrointest Surg 7:159-163, 2003.
12. Jobe BA, Wallace J, Hansen PD, Swanström LL: Evaluation of laparoscopic Toupet fundoplication as a primary repair for all patients with medically resistant gastroesophageal reflux. Surg Endosc 11:1080-1083, 1997.
13. Migliore M, Arcerito M, Vagliasindi A, et al: The place of Belsey Mark IV fundoplication in the era of laparoscopic surgery. Eur J Cardiothorac Surg 24:625-630, 2003.
14. O'Keeffe T, Swanström LL: Laparoscopic partial fundoplications. In Soper NJ, Swanström LL, Eubanks S (eds): Mastery of Laparoscopic Surgery, 2nd ed. Boston, Little, Brown, 2004, pp 204-212.
15. Kneist W, Heintz A, Trinh TT, Junginger T: Anterior partial fundoplication for gastroesophageal reflux disease. Langenbecks Arch Surg 388:174-180, 2003.
16. Nguyen NT, Schauer PR, Hutson W, Landreneau R, Weigel T, Ferson PF, Keenan RJ, Luketich JD: Preliminary results of thoracoscopic Belsey Mark IV antireflux procedure. Surg Laparosc Endosc 8:185-188, 1998.
17. Baue AE: The Belsey Mark V procedure. Ann Thorac Surg 29:265-269, 1980.
18. Patti MG, Frisichella PM, Perretta S, et al: Impact of minimally invasive surgery on the treatment of esophageal achalasia: A decade of change. J Am Coll Surg 196:703-705, 2003.
19. Franzen T, Bostrom J, Tibbling GL, Johansson K: Prospective study of symptoms and gastro-oesophageal reflux 10 years after posterior partial fundoplication. Br J Surg 86:956-960, 1999.
20. Campbell AD, Ferrara BE: Toupet partial fundoplication. Correcting, preventing gastroesophageal reflux. AORN J 57:671-679, 1993.
21. Patti MG, Robinson T, Galvani C, et al: Total fundoplication is superior to partial fundoplication even when esophageal peristalsis is weak. J Am Coll Surg 198:863-869, 2004.
22. Oleynikov D, Eubanks TR, Oelschlager BK, Pellegrini CA: Total fundoplication is the operation of choice for patients with gastroesophageal reflux and defective peristalsis. Surg Endosc 16:909-913, 2002.
23. Bell RC, Hanna P, Mills MR, Bowrey D: Patterns of success and failure with laparoscopic Toupet fundoplication. Surg Endosc 13:1189-1194, 1999.
24. Horvath KD, Jobe BA, Herron DM, Swanstrom LL: Laparoscopic Toupet fundoplication is an inadequate procedure for patients with severe reflux disease. J Gastrointest Surg 3:583-591, 1999.

Esophageal Replacement for End-Stage Benign Esophageal Disease

Thomas J. Watson

The esophagus is a muscular pump bordered by two sphincters and responsible for only one essential task: the unidirectional movement of ingested food and saliva from the pharynx to the stomach. Prevention of reflux of gastric contents is inherent to this task. Unlike other portions of the gastrointestinal tract, the esophagus has no known endocrine, exocrine, immunologic, digestive, absorptive, or secretory roles. Despite the apparent simplicity of its responsibilities, the esophagus may exhibit derangements in function that can have a profound impact on an individual's overall health and quality of life. In most cases, the symptoms experienced by patients with esophageal disorders are minor, intermittent, and easily controllable with medications and subtle dietary or lifestyle modifications. In more advanced cases, patients may be referred for surgical therapy intended to improve foregut function or correct anatomic abnormalities. In a subset of patients, however, the severity of esophageal dysfunction and associated symptomatology is such that esophageal resection with replacement is the most appropriate option.

Patients who suffer the consequences of severe esophageal disorders or previously failed esophageal surgery are not uncommonly prescribed a myriad of ineffective or marginally beneficial medications in an effort to bring about symptomatic relief. These unfortunate individuals may seek input from multiple medical or surgical specialists in the process of evaluation and treatment. Considerable time and effort may be spent pursuing medical or minimally invasive therapies that despite being low risk, ultimately prove futile. Because previous surgery may have contributed to the problem or is perceived to have contributed, both patients and their treating physicians may be reluctant to consider referral for a repeat attempt at surgical remediation. In addition, complex reoperative esophageal surgery may be viewed as producing significant morbidity or mortal-

ity and resulting in marginal long-term functional success. Because of these factors, many patients have exhausted attempts at conservative management at the time of referral to a surgical specialist. The mere fact that the patient finally resorts to surgical evaluation frequently reflects the severity of the underlying pathology, even if a major surgical undertaking is the ultimate solution. Difficult foregut anatomic and functional problems, however, can rarely be successfully remediated through simple means and may require surgical reconstruction.

A major challenge facing esophageal surgeons is the decision whether to attempt fundoplication, myotomy, or other nonextirpative foregut procedure in the setting of advanced disease, especially in the reoperative setting, versus proceeding with the more invasive and potentially morbid option of resection and reconstruction. Despite the desire to avoid a large operation, the surgeon should understand that there are potential adverse consequences to repeat interventions around the esophagus, gastroesophageal junction (GEJ), or stomach that can have a negative impact on the ability to complete successful resection and reconstruction at a later date (Box 20–1). With regard to repeat fundoplication or myotomy, success is highly unlikely after two or three previous failures, depending on the circumstances. Repeated operations in the region of the GEJ can lead to local tissue ischemia and fibrosis, as well as risk iatrogenic vagal nerve injury with its sequelae. Preservation of a scarred and dysfunctional lower esophagus or upper stomach invariably leads to problems with dysphagia, weight loss, or pain. On the other hand, the patient's symptoms must be sufficiently severe to warrant a major extirpative procedure with its inherent risks. Because the functional outcome after esophageal replacement is never normal, the symptomatic result anticipated after esophageal replacement must be realistically assessed and compared

Box 20–1 Reasons to Abandon Attempts at Remedial Foregut Procedures

Additive morbidity/mortality

Further tissue damage with additional functional loss and increased adhesion formation

Loss of blood supply from repeat mobilization with risk of ischemic fibrosis/necrosis

Risk of iatrogenic vagal nerve injury with its sequelae

Compromise of potential esophageal replacement organ or organs

Table 20–1 Symptoms of End-Stage Esophageal Disease ($N = 104$)

Symptom	Percent
Dysphagia	90
Regurgitation	57
Heartburn	52
Weight loss	32
Chest pain	25
Epigastric pain	22
Vomiting	20
Cough	18
Nausea	18
Choking	9
Voice change	7
Diarrhea	3
Odynophagia	2
Anorexia	1
Bloating	1

From Watson TJ, DeMeester TR, Kauer WKH, et al: Esophageal replacement for end-stage benign esophageal disease. J Thorac Cardiovasc Surg 115:1241-1249, 1998.

Box 20–2 Mechanisms by Which Benign Esophageal Disease Can Lead to Esophageal Replacement

Inadequate nonoperative therapy

For gastroesophageal reflux disease

Inadequate acid suppression leading to stricture, bleeding, ulceration, perforation, or fistulization

Inadequate dilation of reflux-induced stricture

Necrosis of incarcerated paraesophageal hernia

For achalasia

Failed Botox injection

Failed pneumatic dilation

Inadequate surgery

For gastroesophageal reflux disease

Recurrent hiatal herniation

Improper fundoplication (e.g., malpositioned/"slipped," too tight, too long, angulated/twisted, excessive crural closure)

Improper Collis gastroplasty (e.g., too large, excess gastric mucosa above the fundoplication, leakage from the staple/suture line, persistent reflux)

Iatrogenic vagal nerve injury

For achalasia

Incomplete myotomy

Healing of myotomy

Complete fundoplication

Paraesophageal herniation

Iatrogenic vagal nerve injury

Other technical problems (e.g., angulation, tight hiatus)

Iatrogenic or traumatic injury to the esophagus, stomach, or vagus nerves

Endoscopic interventions

Mishaps during attempted endotracheal intubation

Operations on contiguous organs

Blunt or penetrating trauma

Caustic ingestion

Congenital abnormality

End-stage disease at initial evaluation

with the patient's preoperative status, and the magnitude of the anticipated improvements must be weighed against the potential surgical morbidity.

This chapter examines the characteristics of patient populations with end-stage, benign esophageal disease who are being considered for esophagectomy, the principles underlying successful reconstruction of the foregut, and data regarding safety and efficacy of the various reconstructive approaches.

CLINICAL MANIFESTATIONS OF END-STAGE BENIGN ESOPHAGEAL DISEASE

Symptoms in patients with end-stage esophageal disease can be quite variable (Table 20–1). The most common symptom driving the need for surgical intervention is dys-phagia, followed by regurgitation and heartburn. Other factors precipitating the need for esophagectomy can be acute hemorrhage, repetitive aspiration, or acute/subacute sepsis from ulceration, perforation, or fistulization (Box 20–2). Finally, foregut continuity may need to be re-established after previous esophageal exclusion/diversion or previously failed reconstruction.

Table 20–2	Nonmalignant Esophageal Conditions Leading to Esophageal Replacement

Diagnosis		No. Patients
End-stage gastroesophageal reflux disease		37
Undilatable stricture	25	
Other	12	
Advanced motility disorder		37
Traumatic or iatrogenic injury or spontaneous perforation		15
Corrosive injury		8
Congenital abnormality		6
Extensive leiomyoma		1

From Watson TJ, DeMeester TR, Kauer WKH, et al: Esophageal replacement for end-stage benign esophageal disease. J Thorac Cardiovasc Surg 115:1241-1249, 1998.

The most common nonmalignant conditions underlying the need for esophageal replacement are end-stage gastroesophageal reflux disease (GERD) and advanced motility disorders, in particular, achalasia (Table 20–2). In some cases, patients first seek medical attention while already manifesting end-stage disease. This fact underscores the ability of individuals to compensate for derangements in alimentary function through dietary, behavioral, and lifestyle modifications when symptoms are mild to moderate, thereby delaying evaluation for prolonged periods, even years. In some cases, disease progresses despite "appropriate" medical or surgical therapy. In other situations, inappropriate or poorly executed therapy can worsen foregut function by exacerbating existing symptoms or inducing new ones. Irreparable injury to the esophagus can occur from blunt or penetrating trauma or caustic ingestion. Iatrogenic injuries to the esophagus or stomach can occur as a result of endoscopic interventions, traumatic airway intubations, or operations on contiguous organs. In the latter case, the vagus nerves may be injured as well. Finally, some patients are initially seen in adulthood with the sequelae of congenital esophageal abnormalities after previous failed attempts at surgical correction.

PREOPERATIVE EVALUATION FOR FOREGUT RECONSTRUCTION

The functional and anatomic status of the foregut is assessed routinely before elective reconstruction by video barium upper gastrointestinal contrast studies, flexible esophagogastroduodenoscopy, and stationary esophageal manometry. Ambulatory esophageal pH monitoring with either a traditional transnasal pH catheter or an implantable Bravo probe (Medtronic, Minneapolis, MN) is performed when documentation of pathologic gastroesophageal reflux is critical to decision making. Other studies, such as radionuclide gastric emptying scans, multichannel intraluminal esophageal impedance tests, or bile monitoring, may be used on a selective basis.

Assessment of the patient's cardiopulmonary reserve is essential before any major surgical undertaking such as esophagectomy. A thorough history is obtained with specific concentration on respiratory difficulties at rest or with exertion, exercise tolerance, chest pain, and fatigability. Physical examination should concentrate on cardiopulmonary findings. When questions exist about coexistent cardiac or pulmonary disease based on the patient's age, comorbid conditions, physical signs, or symptoms, formal physiologic testing should be pursued. Pulmonary function testing, including expiratory flow, lung volumes, and diffusion capacity, can objectify the severity of concomitant obstructive or restrictive lung disease. Lung function should be optimized through smoking cessation, bronchodilators, expectorants, antibiotics, and pulmonary rehabilitation, as necessary. Cardiac imaging and stress testing can elicit subtle changes in cardiac function suggestive of ischemia, cardiomyopathy, or valvular heart disease. When coronary artery or valvular pathology is deemed significant, interventions such as angioplasty, coronary stenting, or even open heart surgery should be completed before elective esophageal surgery in an effort to minimize perioperative risk at the time of esophagectomy.

One advantage of esophagectomy in the setting of benign disease versus malignancy is that surgery can often be delayed pending optimization of cardiopulmonary issues, nutrition, or other comorbid diseases. Although the patient and treating physicians may feel a time pressure to treat an esophageal malignancy, end-stage esophageal disorders tend to be fairly long-standing problems that can be temporized while a thorough work-up is completed and risk factors addressed. Enteral or parenteral support may be pursued if a patient is unable to tolerate an adequate oral diet. Although no absolute thresholds exist for abandoning surgery because of pulmonary or cardiac compromise, such objective information can often assist the surgeon quite significantly in making a decision for or against esophageal reconstruction and in the type of operation chosen.

When the colon is being considered as a potential esophageal substitute, colonoscopy is performed to evaluate the status of the colonic mucosa. Mild diverticular disease is not generally a contraindication to the use of colon as an esophageal replacement, although extensive diverticulosis, frank diverticulitis, or inflammatory fibrosis may preclude colon interposition. Similarly, the presence of a few colonic polyps, whether hyperplastic or adenomatous, that can be removed before surgery does not preclude use of the colon. The presence of extensive polyposis or malignancy, however, is an absolute contraindication.

Some controversy exists regarding the necessity for routine preoperative mesenteric arteriography when colonic interposition is planned. Because the successful

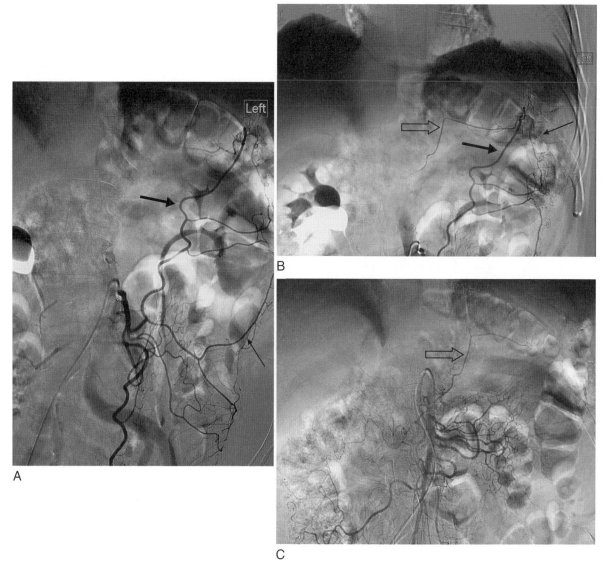

Figure 20–1. Mesenteric arteriogram in preparation for colon interposition. **A** and **B,** Selective injection of the inferior mesenteric artery. Note the ascending branch of the left colic artery *(broad arrows),* on which a left colon interposition is based, and the marginal artery of Drummond *(thin arrow).* **C,** Selective injection of the superior mesenteric artery in the same individual. Note the communication with the arcade from the inferior mesenteric artery *(hollow arrows).*

use of colon critically depends on adequate vasculature, the surgeon should have a low threshold to perform such studies. When arteriography is performed, selective injections of the celiac, superior mesenteric (SMA), and inferior mesenteric (IMA) arteries should be undertaken, including lateral views, with particular attention paid to any anatomic aberrancy. When the left colon is to be used for interposition, the most important angiographic finding is the status of the IMA, especially at its origin, which can be stenosed in elderly individuals or in those with peripheral vascular disease. Because the blood supply of a left colon interposition critically depends on adequate inflow from the IMA, significant stenosis of this vessel is a contraindication to use of the left colon for esophageal reconstruction.[1] A right colon interposition,

based on the middle colic branches of the SMA, can be used in this situation because it is not dependent on IMA inflow. Other angiographic features thought important to successful use of the left colon for interposition include a visible ascending branch of the left colic artery, a well-defined anastomosis between the left colic and middle colic systems (along the marginal artery of Drummond), and a single middle colic trunk before division into right and left branches (Fig. 20–1A-C). Because of its more reliable and predictable arterial inflow and venous outflow, not to mention its better size match to the native esophagus, the left colon is generally preferred over the right colon for esophageal replacement.

Because patients undergoing foregut reconstruction have not uncommonly undergone multiple previous

Box 20–3   **Features of the Ideal Esophageal Substitute**

Technically simple to construct

Minimal incisions

Minimal number of anastomoses

Adequate length to replace the excised esophageal segment

Reliable arterial and venous blood supply

Allows normal swallowing

Does not alter gastrointestinal function

Resistant to (or able to prevent) acid reflux

Durable with no long-term complications

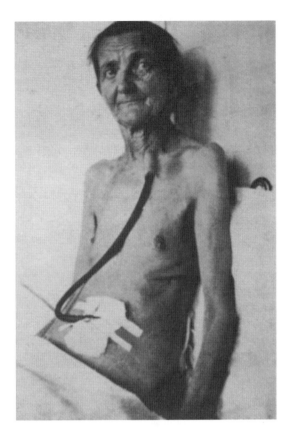

Figure 20–2. Franz Torek's first successful transthoracic esophagectomy patient (1913). An external rubber tube was used to establish continuity between a cervical esophagostomy and a gastrostomy.

abdominal operations, mesenteric arteriography can help define the resultant vascular anatomy and ascertain that vessels supplying planned esophageal substitutes are patent and not disrupted by previous surgeries. In particular, previous operations involving the greater curvature of the stomach may have disrupted the right gastroepiploic artery, critical to the blood supply of a planned gastric pull-up, or the middle colic artery and marginal artery of Drummond, critical to the blood supply of a planned colon interposition. Preoperative knowledge of such vascular abnormalities can help the surgeon plan surgery and save considerable time and effort during the procedure.

FEATURES OF THE IDEAL ESOPHAGEAL SUBSTITUTE

The goal of foregut reconstruction is return of normal alimentation in a durable fashion with a minimal risk for side effects, morbidity, and mortality. Because no esophageal replacement organ can perfectly replicate normal foregut function, a number of different conduits have been used, each with potential advantages and limitations. None of them fulfills all the criteria of an ideal esophageal substitute, and thus debate continues over which organ is best suited for this purpose (Box 20–3). It is noteworthy that as long ago as 1929, the observation was made that "Judging from the literature, it would seem that every method which ingenuity can invent has been practiced for the purpose of reestablishing the continuity of the esophagus after resection."[2] The field has advanced considerably since the first successful transthoracic esophagectomy performed by Torek in 1913,[3] in which an external rubber tube was placed between an end-esophagostomy and a gastrostomy (Fig. 20–2). Through trial and error with different esophageal replacement strategies and with accumulated experience, certain principles and controversies in foregut reconstruction have evolved.

CONTROVERSIES IN FOREGUT RECONSTRUCTION FOR BENIGN DISEASE

The debate surrounding foregut reconstruction for benign disease centers on several distinct, though interrelated controversies:

1. Long- versus short-segment esophagectomy
2. Operative approach to esophagectomy and reconstruction
3. Vagal-sparing versus standard esophagectomy
4. Esophageal replacement organ (stomach, jejunum, colon)
5. Esophagectomy as primary therapy for end-stage benign esophageal disease
6. Esophagectomy versus gastrectomy

Long- Versus Short-Segment Esophagectomy

In many cases of severe, end-stage esophageal disease, the significant anatomic or functional defect is localized to the region of the GEJ. Pertinent examples include a nondilatable distal esophageal stricture or failed fundoplication with recurrent hiatal herniation, slipped fundic wrap, and twisting or stenosis at the GEJ (Fig. 20–3).

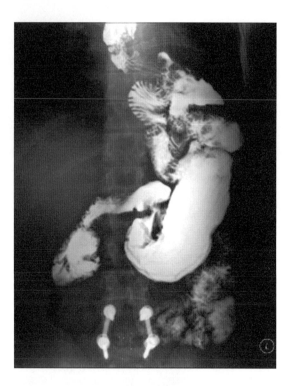

Figure 20–3. Distal esophagectomy and foregut reconstruction with colonic and jejunal interpositions. This patient underwent distal esophagectomy at the age of 7 for a nondilatable esophageal stricture. Reconstruction was initially performed with a colon interposition to the intact stomach. Bleeding from an ulcer within the distal interposed colon developed later, presumably from acid-induced injury, and led to segmental resection of the distal colon interposition and placement of a jejunal interposition between the proximal part of the colon and intact stomach. This barium upper gastrointestinal radiograph demonstrates the resultant reconstruction consisting of esophagus-colon-jejunum-stomach. Significant redundancy and tortuosity developed in the colonic and jejunal interpositions and led to dysphagia and regurgitation. The situation was eventually remediated at 38 years of age by excision of both the colonic and jejunal interpositions with primary esophagogastrostomy.

Another example is end-stage achalasia, with or without previous surgical myotomy or other intervention targeted at the lower esophageal sphincter (LES). In some circumstances, such as with underlying GERD, the esophageal body may demonstrate relatively normal peristalsis in response to swallowing. In other cases, such as with end-stage achalasia, the esophageal body may be relatively dilated and aperistaltic. Even in such cases, however, the esophageal body could be presumed to function no worse than a potential esophageal replacement conduit, which by nature may be similarly dilated and aperistaltic.

In many such cases of end-stage esophageal disease, resection could be limited to the region of the GEJ. Unlike esophageal resection for carcinoma, where the need for a wide resection margin generally mandates excision of a significant portion of the esophageal body, resection for benign disease can theoretically be much more limited. Certain advantages and disadvantages exist for limited esophageal resection versus the more commonly used strategy of resection of a much longer esophageal segment.

Pros of Short-Segment Esophageal Resection

The concept of leaving the majority of the esophagus in situ holds theoretical appeal. Less dissection is necessary to mobilize and resect only the GEJ versus the entirety of the esophagus, with less potential for hemorrhage, third-space fluid losses, or injury to surrounding structures such as the major thoracic blood vessels, thoracic duct, membranous airway, or recurrent laryngeal nerves. When compared with near-total esophagectomy plus cervical esophagogastrostomy, limited distal esophageal resection leaves a longer segment of normal squamous mucosa between the pharynx and stomach, which perhaps acts as a barrier against regurgitation of gastric contents into the pharynx, mouth, or airway. In addition, if the remaining esophagus is functionally normal, common sense would dictate that it is best to leave it intact if at all possible. Finally, limited resection may sometimes be accomplished through a laparotomy alone, thus obviating the need for an additional incision such as a thoracotomy or cervicotomy.

Cons of Short-Segment Esophageal Resection

Traditional teaching holds that limited resection of the GEJ, when reconstructed via primary esophagogastrostomy, is prone to significant gastroesophageal reflux. Low intrathoracic esophagogastric anastomoses (i.e., below approximately the level of the azygous vein) are thought best to be avoided because of this concern. The reason postulated for the increased incidence and severity of reflux in this setting is the high pressure differential between the positive pressure environment of the abdomen and the negative pressure environment of the thorax, exacerbated by loss of the LES barrier. This pressure differential drives gastric contents cephalad.

The extent to which significant gastroesophageal reflux actually occurs after short-segment esophagectomy is a matter of debate. In cases of palliative esophagectomy for advanced esophageal carcinoma, when the patient has a limited life expectancy, the importance of reflux over the ensuing months or few years of the patient's life may not be great. In cases of esophagectomy for benign disease, when life expectancy is measured in many years or decades, the potential adverse consequences of increased gastroesophageal reflux are much more worrisome. Reflux esophagitis, esophageal ulceration, stricture, or intestinal metaplasia may ensue and lead to disabling symptoms, anatomic derangements, or even esophageal carcinoma. In addition, regurgitation, aspiration, and pulmonary injury can lead to significant long-term morbidity. For these reasons, if a short segment of esophagus is resected for benign disease, reconstruction is best completed with a sufficiently long interposition of jejunum or colon between the remaining esophagus and stomach or with a primary Roux-en-Y esophagojejunostomy.

Table 20–3   Late Functional Results in 34 Patients Undergoing Short-Segment Intestinal Interposition of the Distal Esophagus

Grade	Symptoms	Colon	Jejunum
Excellent	Minimal or absent	9	7
Good	Slowed swallowing, occasional regurgitation, or both	4	6
Fair	Dysphagia with some solids, frequent regurgitation or intermittent dilation	3	2
Poor	Nutritional supplementation required	1	
Failure		2	

From Gaissert HA, Mathisen DJ, Grillo HC, et al: Short-segment intestinal interposition of the distal esophagus. J Thorac Cardiovasc Surg 106:860-867, 1993.

An additional issue relative to resection of short segments of the distal esophagus is that the subsequent esophageal anastomosis, whether it be to the stomach, small intestine, or colon, must frequently be intrathoracic in location. Only if there is sufficient length of abdominal esophagus can the subsequent anastomosis be placed in the abdominal compartment. Two potential problems relate to placement of the anastomosis within the thorax. The first is that a thoracotomy or thoracoabdominal incision is generally necessary, with its potential for significant pain, poor cosmetic or functional outcome, necessity for single-lung ventilation during surgery, and the additional time needed to open and close the incision and reposition the patient. Although a transhiatal anastomosis performed with a circular stapling device or thoracoscopic esophageal mobilization and anastomosis may obviate the need for a large thoracic incision, such techniques are not commonly feasible, especially in the setting of a reoperative procedure. The second potential problem is that the consequences of an intrathoracic leak may be more devastating than those resulting from a leak in the neck. Multiple surgical series have reported higher morbidity and mortality associated with intrathoracic esophageal leaks, which can lead to mediastinitis, empyema, and systemic sepsis, although these risks may be decreasing in recent years.[4] Relative to near-total esophagectomy with a cervical anastomosis, which can often be completed without a thoracic incision and places the anastomosis near the thoracic inlet, resection of a limited segment of the distal esophagus frequently carries with it the potential morbidity of both the thoracic incision and the intrathoracic anastomosis.

Clinical Experience with Short-Segment Esophageal Resection

The reported experience with resection of short segments of the distal esophagus for nonmalignant esophageal disease is quite limited. Gaissert et al. reported on 41 patients over a 20-year period at the Massachusetts General Hospital who underwent short-segment interposition of the esophagus with colon or jejunum, most for nonmalignant disease.[5] Colon was used in 22 patients and jejunum in 19. Seventy-six percent of the patients had previously undergone foregut surgical procedures, thus reflecting the severity and complexity of the underlying disease processes. As expected, all patients required a left thoracoabdominal incision or combined left thoracotomy and laparotomy. In the colon interposition group, the major complication rate was 45% with a median hospital stay of 17 days and a mortality of 4.5%. In the jejunal interposition group, the major complication rate was 31% with a median hospital stay of 21 days and a mortality of 10.5%. The overall mortality for the entire surgical series was 7.3%. Late follow-up was available on 34 patients at a mean of 87 months to assess long-term functional outcomes (Table 20–3). Most patients reported satisfactory long-term alimentation, although few claimed normal swallowing. Even though the number of patients was relatively small, the authors found little functional difference between jejunum and colon for the situations encountered, with both providing similar palliation of dysphagia and similar likelihood of regurgitation.

Operative Approach to Esophagectomy and Foregut Reconstruction

Mobilization of the esophagus can be accomplished successfully by open transthoracic, thoracoscopic, or transhiatal routes. In patients with end-stage nonmalignant esophageal disease, the esophagus may be relatively difficult to dissect because of the formation of periesophageal adhesions secondary to transmural fibrosis, previous surgery, or dilation of the esophageal body with neovascularization. Thus, a transthoracic route is often preferable to allow safe dissection under direct visualization.

Transhiatal esophagectomy (THE) has been well described for benign esophageal disease in selected patients. In the largest reported series from the University of Michigan, 1085 esophagectomies were attempted by the transhiatal route, 285 (26%) for benign disease.[6] THE was possible in 98.6% of patients in whom it was attempted, with only 15 patients (1.4%) requiring conversion to open thoracotomy. Reoperation for

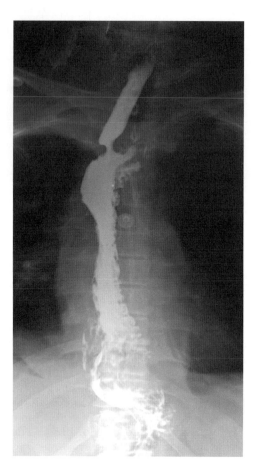

Figure 20–4. Cervical esophagogastric anastomotic stricture after esophagectomy and gastric pull-up.

mediastinal hemorrhage was necessary in five patients within 24 hours of surgery. Of course, such data are from a center with an extensive experience in resection via this approach. Extreme care and considerable judgment are necessary on the part of the operating surgeon to decide on suitable operative candidates. Similarly, the operating surgeon must have a low threshold for conversion to transthoracic resection should adhesions be dense, mobilization prove difficult, or significant bleeding ensue.

THE requires placement of the subsequent esophageal anastomosis in the neck or upper part of the thorax. Although the consequences of an intrathoracic leak are generally worse than those in the neck, the leak rate reported after cervical esophagogastrostomy is generally higher. The University of Michigan group reported a cervical anastomotic leak rate of 13%.[7] The incidence has fallen in recent years, however, with improvements in anastomotic techniques. In their hands, the clinically significant leak rate now falls in the range of 3%.[7]

Also of tremendous significance is the incidence of esophagogastric anastomotic strictures developing after cervical esophagogastrostomy (Fig. 20–4). The need for postoperative dilation has been reported to be as high as 77% after THE for benign disease, although it is rarely a disabling, long-term complication.[7] In view of the fact that many patients are referred for foregut reconstruc-

tion because of severe dysphagia, however, the persistence of dysphagia after surgery can be a significant adverse outcome.

An issue relevant to foregut reconstruction is the route of passage of the esophageal substitute. Most surgeons prefer to bring the conduit through the posterior mediastinum when it is available for this purpose. The native esophageal bed provides the straightest, shortest, and generally most convenient route for bringing an esophageal replacement conduit to the neck. Of course, this route may not be feasible when the esophagus has previously been resected and the esophageal bed is fibrosed. Another scenario that mandates the use of an alternative route is when the esophagus is bypassed rather than resected. An example of such a situation for benign esophageal disease occurs in the setting of a caustic injury, in which case extensive transmural esophageal inflammation and fibrosis may make esophagectomy hazardous (Fig. 20–5).

When the posterior mediastinum is not suitable for passage of the replacement conduit to the neck, the best available alternative is generally the substernal route. The stomach or colon can usually be brought to the cervical region through the substernal plane, although the jejunum will typically not reach this far when pedicled on its native mesenteric blood supply (Fig. 20–6). Of course, a free jejunal graft with microvascular anastomosis of the arterial inflow and venous outflow can be used to add length to a pedicled jejunal segment. Additionally, an interposed jejunal segment can be "supercharged" by microvascular anastomosis in the neck or upper part of the thorax.

As long as a previous sternotomy has not been performed, a sternotomy is not typically necessary to create an adequate substernal space. Technical details important to successful substernal transposition include a xiphoidectomy to prevent subsequent bony impingement of the conduit, direct dissection and mobilization of the diaphragmatic insertions to the lower part of the sternum to prevent compression in this region, and blunt hand dissection in the substernal plane to create adequate space. Most surgeons add a left hemimanubriectomy with resection of the head of the left clavicle and the head of the left first rib or, at a minimum, resection of the left sternoclavicular joint to create adequate space at the upper thoracic level (Fig. 20–7). Of course, in the setting of a previous sternotomy, a redo sternotomy, with its inherent risks, may be necessary to accomplish a substernal pull-up. Moreover, if a long length of proximal esophagus is available and the chosen esophageal replacement conduit is short, a sternotomy will allow a relatively low anastomosis in an intrathoracic, substernal position. Such an approach may permit a pedicled jejunal interposition or Roux limb of the jejunum to be used with a retrosternal esophagojejunal anastomosis if sufficient esophageal length remains.

Experience has shown that the anastomotic leak rate is higher for substernal conduits than for those brought through the posterior mediastinum. Among the 1030 surviving patients from the University of Michigan series in whom the stomach was positioned in the posterior mediastinum, anastomotic leaks developed in 13% versus

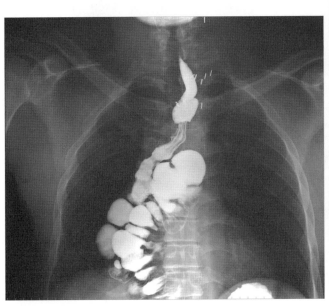

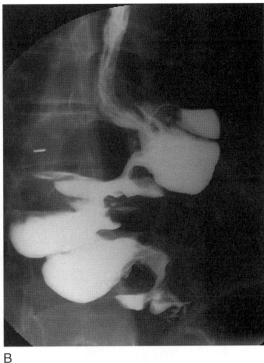

A

B

Figure 20–5. Substernal right colon interposition used to bypass a lye-induced esophageal stricture. **A,** Surgery was performed 22 years before this barium radiograph. **B,** Redundancy of the distal colon interposition developed over time.

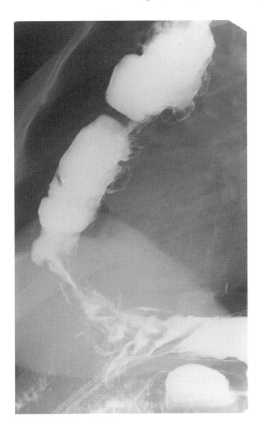

Figure 20–6. Substernal colon interposition. The substernal route was chosen because the patient had undergone resection of a previous gastric pull-up with an end-esophagostomy. The posterior mediastinum was not available for placement of the colon conduit.

an 86% leak rate in 7 patients reconstructed via retrosternal placement of the stomach.[6] Several mechanisms may explain the higher leak rate associated with a substernal conduit, including the relatively longer route of passage for the conduit plus the potential adverse effect on the blood supply, as well as the relative lack of surrounding soft tissue investment of the anastomosis, which may have a negative impact on wound healing. A substernally passed conduit places the cervical esophageal anastomosis essentially in a subcutaneous location, where it is unsupported during coughing or a Valsalva maneuver early in the postoperative period. On the contrary, when the conduit is placed in the native esophageal bed, the esophageal anastomosis is buttressed by the carotid sheath laterally, the prevertebral fascia posteriorly, and the membranous trachea anteriorly.

An option of last resort for bringing the colon or stomach to the neck is the subcutaneous route. Because of the obvious cosmetic and functional consequences, such a route should be used only when absolutely mandated and should virtually never be necessary. A technique was recently described for the use of tissue expanders to create an adequate subcutaneous space for passage of an esophageal replacement conduit after previous sternotomy.[8]

A final issue relative to colon and jejunal interpositions is whether they are positioned in an isoperistaltic or antiperistaltic fashion. A number of studies have confirmed that such interpositions typically empty by gravity and are not peristaltic.[5,9] Case reports, however, would suggest that over time, an antiperistaltic conduit may propel a food bolus in a retrograde fashion. Most

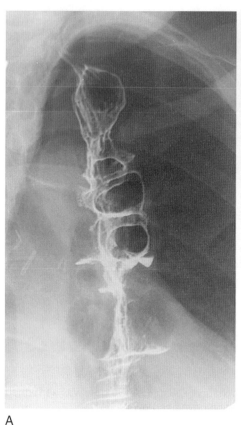

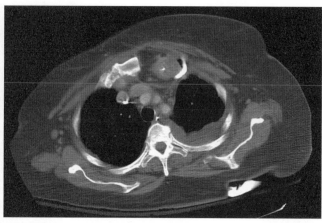

A

Figure 20–7. Substernal colon interposition. **A** and **B,** The left hemimanubrium and head of the left clavicle were resected to create adequate space for passage of the colon.

surgeons therefore prefer to place the esophageal replacement conduit in an isoperistaltic fashion.

Vagal-Sparing Versus Standard Esophagectomy

When esophagectomy is performed for malignancy, the vagus nerves are typically resected because of the potential for transmural spread of tumor and the desire to achieve a complete resection. For nonmalignant conditions leading to esophagectomy, the potential may exist to spare the vagus nerves at the time of resection. Such a vagal-sparing approach assumes, naturally, that the vagus nerves have not been disrupted by previous operative intervention such as myotomy or fundoplication and can be identified and preserved at the time of foregut reconstruction. Many of the side effects after esophagectomy probably relate to the associated vagotomy. By sparing the nerves, the potential exists for less alteration in gastrointestinal function after foregut reconstruction than is the case with a standard approach.

Vagal-sparing esophagectomy was initially reported by Denk in 1913,[10] who used a vein stripper and based the procedure on work performed on human cadavers. Akiyama et al. reintroduced the concept in 1994.[11] Either stomach or colon can be used as the esophageal substitute in this setting.

The technical details of the operation include the creation of a small anterior gastrotomy along the gastric cardia, mobilization and division of the cervical esopha-

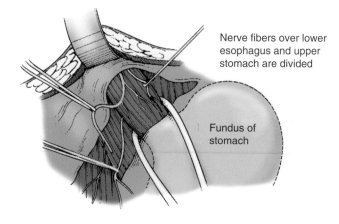

Nerve fibers over lower esophagus and upper stomach are divided

Fundus of stomach

Figure 20–8. Dissection of the abdominal vagal trunks for vagal-sparing transhiatal esophagectomy.

gus, passage of a vein stripper of suitable size through the gastrotomy proximally to the cervical esophagus, fixation of the cap of the vein stripper to the divided end of the esophagus by suture ligature, and eversion of the esophagus out of the stomach (Figs. 20–8 and 20–9). In the process the esophagus is stripped from its mediastinal divestments, with a layer of longitudinal esophageal muscle commonly left in situ. The dissection plane is typically quite easy to develop and does not offer much resistance on stripping. Umbilical tape is affixed to the

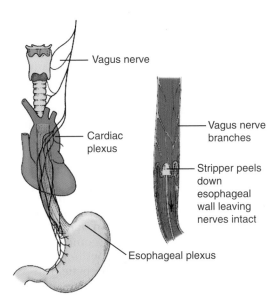

Figure 20–9. The technique of transhiatal vagal-sparing esophagectomy.

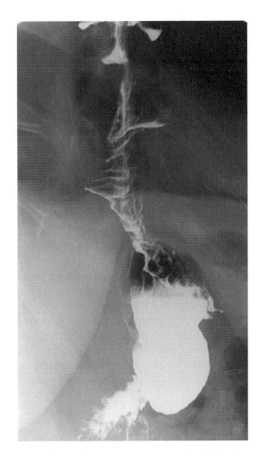

Figure 20–10. Colon interposition anastomosed to the gastric antrum. The proximal part of the stomach was resected to prevent problems with delayed gastric emptying, given that vagotomy was performed as part of a standard esophagectomy.

proximal tip of the esophagus being resected before eversion to allow passage of the tape though the mediastinum. The vagal plexus and main trunks are left intact. The esophagus is then divided near the GEJ. The resultant mediastinal tunnel must be dilated to allow adequate space for passage of the esophageal replacement conduit. Foley catheters with balloons inflated to progressively larger sizes (e.g., 30, 60, 90 ml) can be used for this purpose. The umbilical tape within the mediastinum denotes the proper plane for passage of the replacement organ among the vagal fibers, which can be somewhat web-like. The operation can be performed by open laparotomy or, in experienced hands, by a laparoscopic or hand-assisted technique.

If colon is used for interposition, the colon graft can be passed up through the posterior mediastinum along the path established by the umbilical tape. Anastomosis can then be performed proximally to the esophagus in the neck and distally to the intact stomach. Important differences between the techniques of colon interposition when performed with a vagal-sparing esophagectomy versus a standard esophagectomy are that a pyloroplasty is not necessary because pyloric innervation is preserved and the proximal part of the stomach is left intact. A common practice with colon interposition for malignancy is to resect the proximal two thirds of the stomach, either because of neoplastic involvement or because of the risk for gastroparesis and delayed gastric emptying should the denervated stomach be left intact (Fig. 20–10). By preserving vagal innervation, the stomach should function in normal fashion, thus allowing preservation of the normal gastric reservoir and antral pump.

If stomach is used for esophageal replacement, a highly selective vagotomy along the lesser gastric curvature is necessary to permit mobilization of the conduit. The left gastric artery is left intact in the process. A the-

oretical advantage of such a technique is better blood supply to the conduit than with a standard gastric pull-up, where the left gastric artery is divided, although this concept has not been proved in the laboratory or clinical settings. The stomach can then be brought to the neck via the posterior mediastinum, as for colon interposition.

Clinical experience with vagal-sparing esophagectomy is fairly limited. One study assessed physiologic parameters and clinical outcomes in patients undergoing vagal-sparing esophagectomy versus those undergoing esophagogastrectomy with colon interposition, standard esophagectomy with gastric pull-up, and asymptomatic normal volunteers.[12] Gastric acid production was assessed by Congo red staining. Vagal secretory function was quantitated by increases in gastric output and rises in serum pancreatic polypeptide levels in response to sham feeding. Vagal motor function was measured by gastric emptying scans and a questionnaire to evaluate dumping symptoms. Gastric reservoir function was estimated by meal capacities and postoperative changes in body mass index (BMI). The results showed that vagal-sparing esophagectomy preserved gastric acid secretion, gastric emptying, meal capacity, and BMI when compared with esophagogastrectomy plus colon interposition or standard esophagectomy with gastric pull-up. The incidence of dumping in patients undergoing vagal-sparing esophagectomy was 7% (1 of 15 patients), thus suggesting that the vagi were in fact preserved in most individuals. The only significant difference observed in patients who underwent vagal-sparing esophagectomy when compared with normal subjects was the speed with which they ate. This finding is intuitive if one considers that the main difference in operated individuals is the fact that they have a passive, nonperistaltic esophageal replacement conduit that would not be expected to transport food as rapidly as a normally peristaltic esophagus.

Several potential disadvantages of the vagal-sparing approach exist. The surgeon may be unable to ensure that the vagi are in fact preserved and that postoperative gastric emptying will not be an issue. Again, many surgeons would opt to resect the proximal part of the stomach or perform a pyloroplasty (or both) in cases in which the vagi are known to be compromised. The placement of acid-secreting gastric mucosa in juxtaposition to colonic mucosa can be problematic. Cases of colonic mucosal ulceration leading to pain or bleeding have been reported in this situation. Such ulceration would seem less likely when the proximal part of the stomach has been resected and the stomach is vagotomized. Finally, exposure of the hiatus to perform the operation may be technically challenging in obese patients. Whether the advantages of the vagal-sparing approach outweigh its disadvantages awaits further experience with longer follow-up on greater numbers of patients.

Choice of Esophageal Replacement Organ (Stomach, Colon, or Jejunum)

The preferred esophageal substitute is a widely discussed and debated issue. Because most esophagectomies are performed for carcinoma and the patient's life expectancy may be relatively short, the long-term functional outcome after esophageal replacement is often less of an issue in this scenario. In the case of foregut reconstruction for benign disease or early-stage malignancy, where life expectancy may be measured in many years or decades, the issue of the best functioning esophageal substitute is important and remains controversial.

The two organs most commonly used for esophageal replacement are the stomach and the colon. Each organ has been extensively evaluated, and each has its proponents. Closer analysis demonstrates that the stomach and colon possess several theoretical advantages and disadvantages in comparison to each other and to the jejunum.

Proponents of esophageal replacement via gastric pull-up tout the relative ease of gastric mobilization, the need for only a single (esophagogastric) anastomosis, and the relatively quick operative time and return of alimentation. In addition, where expertise exists, the operation can be completed through minimally invasive means, with laparoscopic gastric mobilization and cervical esophagogastrostomy or intrathoracic anastomosis accomplished via thoracoscopy.[13] The published experience with minimally invasive esophagectomy, however, has been predominantly for malignant or pre-malignant disease.

Disadvantages of use of the stomach include loss of the gastric reservoir with the potential for early satiety and dumping, as well as gastroesophageal reflux into the remaining esophageal remnant or pharynx. Placement of the stomach within the negative pressure environment of the thorax, coupled with loss of the normal GEJ antireflux barrier, predisposes the patient to reflux, regurgitation, and aspiration. Although there is general acceptance of the concept that a cervical esophagogastrostomy is less prone to reflux than an intrathoracic anastomosis is, particularly when placed low in the chest, reflux can occur in either scenario and may cause significant symptomatology or induce complications. Placement of gastric mucosa in juxtaposition to squamous esophageal mucosa predisposes the patient to proximal esophagitis, stricture, or Barrett's esophagus (BE) from chronic exposure of the remaining esophageal mucosa to gastric or duodenal content, or to both. A series from Japan demonstrated reflux esophagitis in 44% of patients and Barrett's metaplasia in 12% of patients monitored for more than 2 years after cervical esophagogastrostomy.[14] Another series from Öberg et al. demonstrated the development of metaplastic columnar mucosa within the cervical esophageal remnant in 15 of 32 patients (46.9%) after a gastric pull-up, 3 with intestinal metaplasia.[15] Of note, esophageal columnar metaplasia was more likely to occur in those with Barrett's mucosa resected at the time of esophagectomy than in those without, thus suggesting an underlying genetic predisposition to the development of metaplasia in susceptible individuals. The clinical significance of this metaplastic response, however, is uncertain in that the incidence of cancer in the esophageal remnant after esophagectomy and gastric pull-up is unknown and probably quite low. In contrast, the esophageal mucosa in patients undergoing colon interposition appears to undergo few histologic changes.

The blood supply to the proximal tip of the gastric conduit can be quite tenuous. The incidence of ischemic complications, such as esophagogastric anastomotic leaks or strictures, is relatively high as a result. The anastomotic leak rate after cervical esophagogastrostomy ranges between 3% and 20% in large surgical series.[6,13,16] Orringer and Stirling reported on 145 patients undergoing esophagectomy with gastric pull-up for benign disease.[17] Sixty-five percent of patients required immediate postoperative dilatation and 12% suffered from persistent dysphagia requiring regular anastomotic dilation or a home dilatation regimen. In a more recent publication from the same group, 77% of 251 patients undergoing THE and esophageal replacement with stomach for benign disease have required at least one postoperative anastomotic dilation, whereas only 4% have suffered from severe dysphagia requiring daily or weekly dilations.[6]

With regard to colon interposition (Fig. 20–11), several theoretical advantages have been suggested. The interposed colonic segment separates the remaining esophageal mucosa from acid-producing gastric

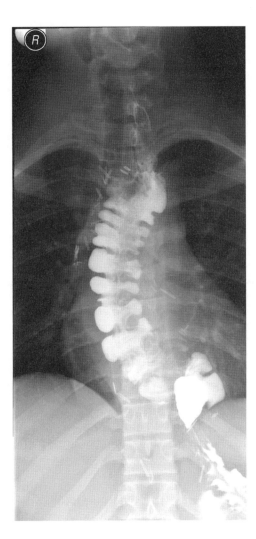

Figure 20–11. Colon interposition brought through the posterior mediastinum. A lye-induced esophageal stricture developed in this patient as a child and was initially treated by esophagectomy and reconstruction with a reversed gastric tube at the age of 6 years. Because the tube never emptied well, surgical remediation was undertaken 8 years later by excision of the gastric pull-up and left colon interposition to the intact gastric antrum.

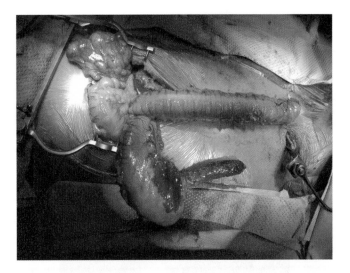

Figure 20–12. Operative photograph of an esophagus resected for a nondilatable lye stricture in a 3-year-old. Reconstruction was completed via a left colon interposition anastomosed distally to the gastric antrum.

mucosa and duodenal contents, as previously stated. The incidence of reflux-induced complications such as esophagitis, stricture, or BE is low. The blood supply to the colon, when mobilized appropriately, is generally quite robust. The incidence of ischemic complications at the esophageal anastomosis, such as leaks or strictures, is also quite low. In 85 patients undergoing colonic interposition for benign disease, Watson et al. reported an esophagocolonic leak rate of 3.5% and a need for postoperative anastomotic dilation in 5%.[16] Both these rates were much less than those after cervical esophagogastrostomy in their series, where anastomotic leaks occurred in 20% and the need for dilation in 30% of patients. Similarly, Briel et al. reported on 395 consecutive patients undergoing esophagectomy for both malignant and benign disease.[18] The development of either anastomotic leak or stricture was analyzed in patients undergoing gastric pull-up versus colonic interposition. Leaks and strictures were more common (14.3% versus 6.1%, $P = .013$; 31.3% versus 8.7%, $P < .0001$, respectively) and strictures were more severe after gastric pull-up.

The colon possesses a reservoir function that allows for a more normal meal capacity. The distal colonic segment and residual stomach remain in the positive pressure environment of the abdomen, thus helping guard against reflux (Figs. 20–12 and 20–13). In some individuals, the stomach is not suitable or available for use as an esophageal substitute. In such cases, the colon may serve the purpose quite well and can be anastomosed distally to a Roux limb of jejunum if the antrum has been resected or there is a significant gastric outlet obstruction. Finally, if the interposed colon becomes dilated or tortuous over the long term, it often can be successfully revised via a tailoring coloplasty or segmental resection.[16,19] A dilated, tortuous, or poorly emptying gastric pull-up, on the other hand, cannot be similarly remediated and requires replacement should significant dysfunction develop.

Disadvantages of the colon as an esophageal substitute are most apparent. The colon must be free of significant pathology, such as extensive diverticulosis, polyposis, or frank malignancy, and must be adequately evaluated and prepared for use, as for elective colon resection. Along with the need for three anastomoses (esophagocolonic, cologastric, and colocolonic), there is an inherently longer operative time with a greater extent of mobilization and dissection than with gastric pull-up. The operation may be technically challenging, especially in terms of preserving arterial inflow and venous drainage of the conduit. Seemingly minor mistakes in judgment or technique can have disastrous consequences with regard to maintenance of adequate vascularity. Leaks or strictures, or both, can occur at any of the anastomoses, and bowel obstruction can occur if the colonic mesentery is not adequately closed. Minimally invasive techniques for completion of the operation have yet to be mastered. The colon is generally thought to be slower to allow resumption of alimentation than the stomach is. Finally

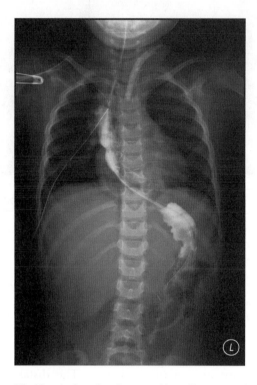

Figure 20–13. Left colon interposition. Postoperative contrast upper gastrointestinal radiograph of the patient in Figure 20–12 demonstrating the intact reconstruction.

and of great importance is the fact that colon interpositions are known to become dilated or tortuous (or both) when in place for many years. Such redundancy can lead to problems with dysphagia, regurgitation, or aspiration, although surgical remediation is often feasible, as stated earlier (Figs. 20–14 and 20–15).

Clinical experience with the jejunum as an esophageal substitute is much less than with either the stomach or colon (Fig. 20–16). This fact is largely due to the limited extent to which the jejunum can be brought into the thorax, either as a Roux limb or as a jejunal interposition, because of its short mesentery and tethered blood supply. Of course, a free jejunal interposition can be placed wherever there is suitable arterial inflow and venous outflow, although it is a technically more demanding procedure than the other options because of the need for microvascular anastomoses.

Extensive clinical experience has accumulated from a number of centers using different methods of esophageal reconstruction for end-stage nonmalignant esophageal disease. In the University of Michigan experience with THE for benign disease in 285 patients, the overall hospital mortality was 2.8%.[6] Follow-up data regarding long-term functional results were available in 242 of 251 hospital survivors (96%) at an average of 47 months. Results were considered excellent (completely asymptomatic) in 29%, good (mild symptoms requiring no treatment) in 39%, fair (symptoms requiring occasional treatment such as dilation or antidiarrheal medication) in 28%, and poor (symptoms requiring regular treatment) in 4%.

Curet-Scott et al. reported on the University of Chicago experience with colon interposition for benign disease.[20] Perioperative mortality was 3.8% in the 53

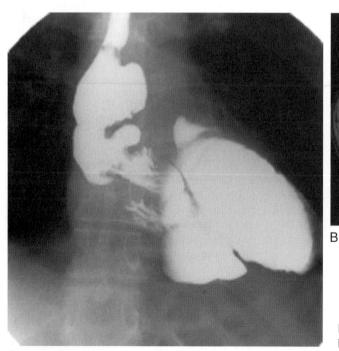

A

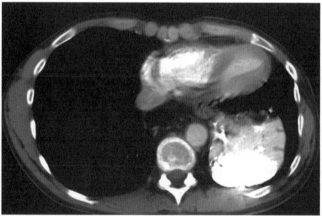

B

Figure 20–14. Dilated, redundant colon interposition. **A** and **B,** This situation can often be remediated via segmental resection with reanastomosis or a tailoring coloplasty (or both).

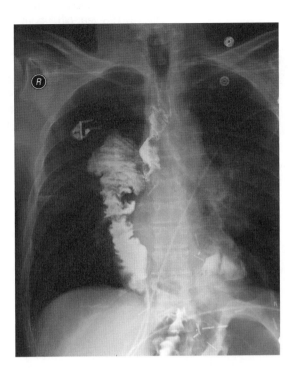

Figure 20–15. Right colon interposition brought through the posterior mediastinum. The intrathoracic portion of the colon is markedly redundant.

patients undergoing surgery, with a 26.4% major complication rate. Follow-up was complete in 83% of patients at an average of 5 years after reconstruction. Results were rated by patients and physicians, with 75% of the patients claiming good or excellent results and 72% classified as having good or excellent results by the physicians. There was, however, a 37% reoperative rate for treatment of delayed gastric emptying, anastomotic stricture, leak, or persistent symptoms. Despite the complication and reoperation rates, the authors stated that colon interposition remained their preferred technique for reconstruction after esophagectomy for benign disease.

At the University of Southern California, 104 patients with benign esophageal disease underwent esophageal reconstruction over a 21-year period.[16] For esophageal replacement, colon was used in 85 patients, stomach in 10, and jejunum in 9. Overall hospital mortality was 2% and the median hospital stay was 17 days. Forty-two patients who were at least 1 year after surgery answered a postoperative questionnaire concerning their long-term functional outcome. Ninety-eight percent of patients reported that the operation improved or cured the symptom driving surgery. Ninety-three percent were satisfied with the outcome of the operation. The number of patients undergoing esophageal reconstruction with stomach or jejunum, however, was too small to allow meaningful comparisons between the different types of reconstructions.

A report from the Mayo Clinic analyzed outcomes in 255 patients undergoing esophagectomy for benign disease between 1956 and 1997.[21] The esophageal substitute was stomach in 66%, colon in 27%, and small bowel in 7%. Perioperative mortality was 5% and morbidity was 56%. Median hospitalization was 14 days. Follow-up was available in 88.6% of patients at a median of 52 months after surgery. Improvement was noted in 77.4% of patients, with functional results classified as excellent in 31.8%, good in 10.2%, fair in 35.4%, and poor in 22.6%. The method of reconstruction did not appear to have an impact on late functional results.

The published reports on esophageal replacement for benign disease inherently reflect an institutional or surgeon-specific bias in terms of the types of reconstructions performed. Randomized trials comparing the different reconstructive options are lacking. Analysis of the published reports reveals that they suffer from a lack of uniform assessment of long-term symptomatic and functional outcomes. The long periods covered in the various reports also make results difficult to interpret in the setting of changing surgeons, refinements in operative technique, and advancements in perioperative care. Firm conclusions, therefore, regarding the optimal operative approach and esophageal replacement conduit for a given patient are lacking.

Esophagectomy as Primary Therapy for End-Stage Benign Esophageal Disease

Fortunately, the need for esophagectomy to treat end-stage motility disorders is rare. As mentioned previously, esophagectomy may be necessary after previous failed esophageal myotomy, fundoplication, or pneumatic dilatation or in patients with major complications such as perforation, ulceration, fistulization, or bleeding. On occasion, a patient is initially seen with an end-stage motility disorder, in the absence of previous interventions or complications, that cannot be remediated by a lesser procedure and requires an esophagectomy as primary therapy. The disease entity that stands as the model in such end-stage cases is achalasia. The largest body of literature, therefore, regarding esophagectomy as primary therapy for end-stage benign esophageal disease relates to achalasia.

Achalasia, though a relatively rare disease, is the most commonly treated of the primary motility disorders. Idiopathic achalasia occurs in approximately 0.5 to 1.0 per 100,000 population per year in the United States and Europe. It is characterized by esophageal body aperistalsis and propulsive failure with absent or incomplete LES relaxation in response to swallowing. The etiology and pathophysiology of achalasia are debated and not well understood but clearly relate to destruction of ganglion cells in the esophageal myenteric plexus of Auerbach, as well as abnormalities within the dorsal motor nucleus of the vagus. Clinically, achalasia is characterized by progressive dysphagia for solids and liquids, regurgitation, and sometimes chest pain or weight loss. Manometrically, achalasia is manifested as loss of LES relaxation in response to wet swallows, a hypertensive LES at rest, esophageal body aperistalsis, and esophageal body pressurization above atmospheric baseline.

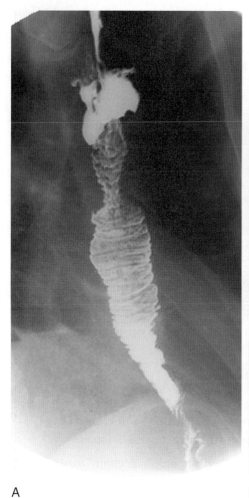

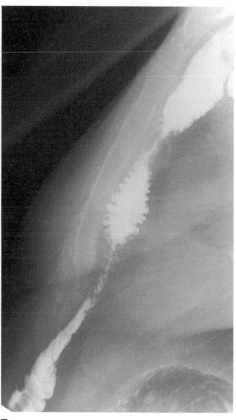

Figure 20–16A to **D.** Substernal jejunal interposition. The patient is a 53-year-old born with esophageal atresia. He underwent multiple esophageal operations during infancy, which culminated in a substernal jejunal interposition to the intact stomach approximately 50 years before this radiograph. Current complaints include dysphagia, regurgitation, and cough. Note the significant redundancy of the intra-abdominal segment of jejunum.

A

B

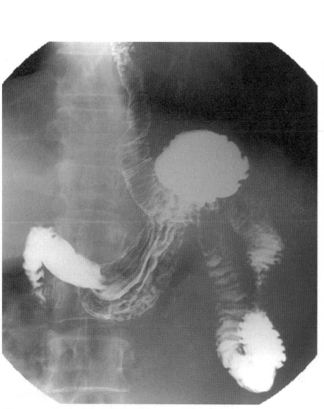

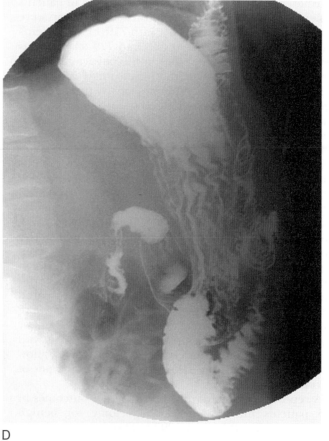

C

D

Box 20–4 **Hallmarks of End-Stage Achalasia**

Clinical: Severe dysphagia and/or regurgitation

Radiographic: Massive esophageal dilatation ("megaesophagus") and/or tortuosity ("sigmoid esophagus")

Pathologic: Reduction or absence of ganglion cells with fibrous replacement of the myenteric plexus

From Banbury MK, Rice TW, Goldblum JR, et al: Esophagectomy with gastric reconstruction for achalasia. J Thorac Cardiovasc Surg 117:1077-1084, 1999.

Box 20–5 **Mechanisms by Which Achalasia Can Lead to Esophageal Replacement**

Ulceration, bleeding, fistulization, perforation

Post-treatment reflux esophagitis/stricture

Development of carcinoma

Inadequate nonoperative therapy (Botox, dilatation)

Inadequate surgery
  Incomplete myotomy
  Healing of myotomy
  Complete fundoplication
  Paraesophageal herniation
  Other technical problems (e.g., angulation, tight hiatus)

End-stage disease at initial evaluation

The accepted therapies for achalasia are aimed at relieving the relative outflow obstruction at the LES and include smooth muscle relaxants, endoscopic botulinum toxin (Botox) injection, pneumatic dilation, and surgical myotomy. The latter can be performed in an open fashion, through the abdomen or thorax, or via minimally invasive approaches, either laparoscopic or thoracoscopic. Myotomy has been described with and without the addition of fundoplication, typically partial.

Therapy for achalasia is palliative, not curative in nature because treatment rarely returns normal function to an aperistaltic esophagus. Outcomes are therefore difficult to assess inasmuch as success is a relative term. In addition, objective outcome measures may not correlate with symptomatic findings.[22] Patients with achalasia typically learn to compensate for symptoms of dysphagia or regurgitation, or both, through a variety of dietary, behavioral, and lifestyle modifications, thus making symptomatic assessment of post-therapy outcome unreliable. Similarly, patients and their treating physicians may underestimate the severity of the physiologic derangements at the time of initial evaluation or after apparently successful intervention. Given these factors, it is no surprise that such patients not uncommonly have the manifestations of end-stage disease, which can be categorized by clinical, radiographic, and pathologic parameters (Box 20–4).

Achalasia may lead to the need for esophageal replacement through a number of mechanisms (Box 20–5). Esophageal stasis can lead to ulceration, bleeding, fistulization, or perforation of the esophageal body. GERD can result from therapy aimed at reducing the competency of the LES and can therefore lead not only to reflux symptoms but also to potential reflux-induced complications such as erosive esophagitis or stricture. Such complications are particularly difficult to correct in the setting of an aperistaltic esophagus. Successful treatment through nonextirpative remediation can be extremely unreliable. Achalasia is a known risk factor for the development of esophageal squamous cell carcinoma, presumably from the chronic esophageal mucosal inflammation associated with stasis esophagitis. Post-treatment gastroesophageal reflux can predispose to esophageal adenocarcinoma as well. Inadequate therapy, whether it is surgical or nonsurgical, can lead to gradual esophageal dilation or tortuosity (or to both), particularly if the patient is not closely monitored for the long term after intervention. As stated, patients tend to compensate for any difficulties encountered in eating and understate the severity of their ongoing symptomatology. For this reason, regular follow-up with the physician, including objective assessment of esophageal structure and function, is recommended indefinitely after therapy. Finally, patients may not be evaluated by the treating specialist until end-stage disease is already present. The fact that this continues to occur is testimony to the degree of compensation that patients can tolerate and the extent to which physiologic derangements can go underappreciated by the patient or primary physician.

With the availability of endoscopic or minimally invasive surgical therapies for achalasia, the question arises whether patients with end-stage achalasia at initial evaluation should ever be treated primarily with esophagectomy. Experience dictates that even significant megaesophagus can be treated with therapy aimed at the LES. As the degree of esophageal body tortuosity increases, however, the chance of success with such treatments diminishes because food must traverse a serpiginous route to reach the stomach. Botox injections in this setting will probably provide minimal, temporary palliation at best. Pneumatic dilation may be technically difficult to accomplish and risks perforation. Laparoscopic myotomy, though minimally invasive, risks potential compromise of the stomach for later use as an esophageal replacement organ and can place the vagus nerves amidst periesophageal fibrosis, thus making subsequent vagal-sparing esophagectomy difficult should the need arise. Primary esophagectomy should be considered when the anatomic and physiologic derangements are sufficiently severe, particularly in the setting of a tortuous or "sigmoid" esophagus. Such a decision requires considerable clinical experience and judgment, with the

Table 20–4   Esophageal Replacement for Achalasia

Institution	Year	No. Patients	Conduit	Mortality (%)	LOS (days)
USC[24]	1995	19	Colon	0	16
Mayo Clinic[25]	1995	37	Stomach: 26	5.4	12
			Colon: 6		
			Small bowel: 5		
Cleveland Clinic[26]	1999	32	Stomach	0	14
U. of Michigan[27]	2001	93	Stomach: 91	2	12.5
			Colon: 2		
Taiwan[28]	2003	9	Colon (short segment)	0	15

LOS, length of stay; USC, University of Southern California.

severity of the patient's symptoms, the anatomic and functional derangements, and associated comorbid conditions taken into account. Common sense would dictate that if any doubt remains about whether a less invasive therapy is indicated, conservative measures should be exhausted before proceeding with the more extensive and irreversible step of foregut resection and reconstruction.

Clinical experience regarding esophagectomy for end-stage achalasia comes from several sources. South American surgeons have extensive experience with primary esophagectomy for Chagas' disease, which has pathophysiologic and anatomic features similar to achalasia. Pinotti et al. reported on primary esophagectomy in 122 patients with Chagas' megaesophagus, with a 4.2% mortality rate and excellent/good functional outcomes in the vast majority.[23] Such experience demonstrates that esophagectomy can be performed safely on appropriately selected patients with end-stage benign megaesophagus.

Data regarding esophagectomy for achalasia come from several centers (Table 20–4). Operative approaches include a mix of transthoracic and transhiatal resections. Depending on institutional biases, patients had their foregut reconstructed with stomach, colon, or small intestine. A recent series from Taiwan reported on short-segment colon interposition for end-stage achalasia performed via a thoracoabdominal incision.[28] Mortality rates run acceptably low in these specialty centers, with lengths of stay consistent with esophagectomy for cancer. Outcomes in these series are reported with mean follow-up intervals of several years (Table 20–5). Given the nonuniformity in methods of assessing symptomatic responses, comparing outcomes across institutions and techniques is difficult. The data would suggest, however, that the vast majority of patients are symptomatically improved by esophageal replacement and are satisfied with the quality of their alimentation after surgery.

With regard to the safety of THE in the setting of megaesophagus, two reported series are noteworthy. Devaney et al. reported on 93 cases of attempted THE for achalasia.[27] Six operations were converted to a tho-

Table 20–5   Outcomes After Esophageal Replacement for Achalasia

Institution	Follow-up (yr)	Outcomes
USC[24]	6.0	93% cured/ improved/satisfied
Mayo Clinic[25]	6.3	91.4% excellent/good
Cleveland Clinic[26]	3.6	87% "felt better" than before
U. of Michigan[27]	3.2	93% "felt better" than before
Taiwan[28]	6.0	75% good/25% fair/25% worse

racotomy, and two patients required urgent thoracotomy for mediastinal hemorrhage within 24 hours of the initial operation. Banbury et al. reported on 32 esophagectomies for achalasia.[26] THE was attempted in 26 of these patients, with 5 converted intraoperatively to thoracotomy and no reoperations for bleeding. The take-home message from these series is that with experience and judgment, THE can be accomplished safely in the setting of megaesophagus, although the surgeon must exercise great care and be quick to convert to thoracotomy should transhiatal dissection prove difficult.

Proximal Gastrectomy or Gastric Bypass as a Remedial Operation for Benign Foregut Disease

The indications for esophageal replacement for nonmalignant conditions and the outcomes after esophagectomy are well studied and elucidated. A number of circumstances arise in which the pathology is localized to

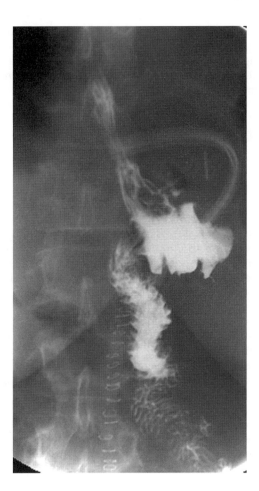

Figure 20–17.   Roux-en-Y gastric bypass used as remediation for multiple failed fundoplications.

which if normally functioning, allows propagation of a food bolus distally and acts as a barrier against the reflux of gastric or intestinal contents into the pharynx or airway. Because surgery is localized to the peritoneal cavity, the operation can typically be completed through a laparotomy alone, thus obviating the need for thoracotomy or cervicotomy. Not uncommonly, end-stage foregut disease is associated with gastric stasis or delayed gastric emptying, which can be addressed via a gastric operation. Finally, in this era of ever-increasing obesity, weight loss from gastric diversion can be a significant associated medical benefit, perhaps even outweighing the symptomatic benefit associated with foregut reconstruction.

An increasing body of literature is evolving regarding the control of GERD in patients undergoing RYGBP for morbid obesity.[29] Such an operation effectively diverts both acid and bile from the esophageal mucosa, with or without the addition of fundoplication or fundopexy. Controversy exists regarding whether fundoplication is more prone to failure in the setting of obesity. Recent reports demonstrate a higher rate of recurrent reflux in obese patients undergoing fundoplication than in overweight or normal-weight individuals.[30] Although other series have not been able to demonstrate such an association, these reports are limited in that they typically analyze results in obese (BMI >30) patients, with relatively few subjects falling in the morbidly obese (BMI >35 to 40) range. In a morbidly obese patient referred specifically for control of GERD, whether fundoplication or RYGBP is the procedure of choice remains unknown, although many surgeons at present are choosing the latter option when the patient so agrees. How best to handle a large hiatal hernia in the setting of morbid obesity and GERD is likewise a matter of debate.

A considerable body of literature also exists regarding distal gastrectomy with Roux-en-Y gastrojejunostomy for control of bile reflux gastritis. In this situation, a sizable proximal gastric remnant is typically left behind, whereas for control of GERD, little to no proximal gastric pouch should be left. Inherent to the success of using a Roux-en-Y bypass to control GERD is the need to eliminate as much acid-secreting mucosa as possible from the upper gastric remnant because the operation works by diversion of acid and bile from the esophageal mucosa rather than by augmentation of the antireflux barrier.

Csendes et al. reported on vagotomy and antrectomy with long-limb Roux-en-Y gastrojejunostomy as the preferred treatment option for patients with long-segment BE.[31] This choice of operation was based on the observations that fundoplication in the setting of BE is associated with a relatively high long-term failure rate and that dysplasia or carcinoma develops in a small proportion of patients with BE during follow-up. Because duodenogastric reflux is common in patients with BE and components of the duodenal refluxate are thought to be carcinogenic or injurious to the esophageal mucosa, antrectomy with Roux-en-Y diversion theoretically diverts the damaging components of the gastric refluxate from the esophageal mucosa. As a result of the added complexity and potential morbidity of such a reconstruction in comparison to fundoplication, especially when the

the GEJ or the upper part of the stomach (or to both), thus raising the question whether reconstruction would best be approached via partial proximal or total gastrectomy rather than esophagectomy. These situations differ from others, such as peptic ulcer disease or bile reflux gastritis, for which distal gastrectomy is an option.

The most notable example in which proximal gastrectomy or Roux-en-Y gastric bypass (RYGBP) is a consideration is in the setting of a failed fundoplication for GERD with or without associated gastroparesis (Fig. 20–17). The decision to attempt repeat fundoplication may be a difficult one in certain situations, particularly after two or more previous fundoplications or after a failed Collis gastroplasty, both of which can be difficult to remediate. In addition, the patient may be overweight or morbidly obese, perhaps contributing to breakdown of a previous operation or recurrence of reflux-related symptoms. The explosion in utilization of RYGBP or related operations for morbid obesity has contributed to the body of knowledge regarding the relative risks and benefits of gastric resection or bypass operations for benign disease.

When compared with esophagectomy, gastric resection or bypass is associated with a number of potential benefits. Obviously, the native esophagus is left intact, latter can be performed via a laparoscopic approach, the operation as proposed by Csendes et al. has not gained wide acceptance in the United States and Europe.

An issue of controversy is whether to resect the excluded distal gastric remnant after gastric bypass. Although such a resection is typically not performed in the setting of RYGBP for obesity, resection does appear to reduce or eliminate the potential risk for hemorrhage from the blind gastric pouch, the occurrence of gastrogastric fistulas, the development of marginal ulceration as a result of a retained antrum effect, bacterial overgrowth in the excluded pouch, and the development of a subsequent carcinoma that is not amenable to surveillance.[32] RYGBP with distal gastric resection is clearly more time-consuming and requires more extensive dissection than RYGBP without distal resection does. Whether the benefits of distal gastric resection outweigh the disadvantages merits further study and follow-up.

Little has been written about gastrectomy or RYGBP as a remedial antireflux operation after failed fundoplication in the obese. Raftopoulos et al. reported on seven morbidly obese individuals undergoing revision of an antireflux procedure to laparoscopic RYGBP.[33] The mean operative time was longer than 6 hours. Anastomotic strictures developed in five patients, and two were re-explored for gastric remnant herniation and intestinal obstruction. At a mean follow-up of 24 months, mean excess weight loss was 70.7%, and 70% of comorbid conditions were improved or resolved. In addition, GERD scores were significantly reduced. The authors concluded that laparoscopic RYGBP after failed antireflux surgery in the morbidly obese, though technically challenging, is a feasible and effective treatment of recurrent GERD and is associated with the additional advantages of weight loss and improvement of comorbid conditions.

At the University of Rochester, we have performed 12 RYGBP-type operations as remedial antireflux procedures after failed fundoplications in both normal-weight and obese individuals and have compared our results with those of a cohort of 25 individuals undergoing redo fundoplication.[34] The gastrectomy patients had a higher prevalence of preoperative endoscopic complications of GERD and multiple previous fundoplications than did those undergoing redo fundoplication. Mean symptom severity scores were improved significantly by both gastrectomy and redo fundoplication, but they were not significantly different from each other. Complete relief of the primary symptom was significantly greater after gastrectomy (89% versus 50%, $P = .044$). Overall patient satisfaction was similar in both groups. In-hospital morbidity was higher after gastrectomy than after redo fundoplication (67% versus 16%, $P = .003$), and new-onset dumping developed in two gastrectomy patients. Based on our findings, we concluded that in select patients with severe GERD and multiple previous fundoplications, the symptomatic outcome after gastrectomy is as good as or better than that after redo fundoplication. Gastrectomy is an acceptable treatment option for recurrent symptoms, particularly when another attempt at fundoplication is ill advised, such as in the setting of multiple previous fundoplications or failed Collis gastroplasty.

The indications for gastrectomy or RYGBP in the primary or reoperative settings, the pros and cons relative to esophagectomy, and situations in which a repeat attempt at fundoplication should be abandoned still require further elucidation.

CONCLUSIONS

End-stage benign esophageal disease is infrequently encountered in the general medical community. Most hospitals therefore lack the expertise to evaluate and treat patients suffering the manifestations of severe, end-stage esophageal disorders. In such patients, considerable judgment is necessary on the part of the surgeon in deciding when to continue further attempts at remediating foregut dysfunction through medical or surgical means and when to proceed with extirpation and reconstruction. Because the conditions that lead to reconstruction are often not immediately life-threatening, patients frequently remain inadequately treated for long periods before evaluation by a surgical specialist. On the other hand, the risks of a major surgical undertaking must be carefully weighed against the anticipated symptomatic benefit. When the severity of symptoms warrants further intervention and when the patient has been carefully assessed for comorbid disease and performance status, esophageal replacement should be considered. Because a volume-outcome relationship generally exists for esophagectomy, as for other major surgical procedures,[35] patients in need of esophageal replacement should be referred to a center with considerable experience in such types of surgery. Foregut reconstruction for end-stage nonmalignant esophageal disease can be performed safely in selected units with acceptable morbidity, low mortality, and excellent long-term alimentary function. The choice of operative approach and the type of foregut reconstruction should be tailored to the individual patient. With further experience and continued long-term assessment of outcomes, refinements in operative techniques and improvements in results will undoubtedly continue.

REFERENCES

1. Peters JH, Kronson J, Katz M, DeMeester TR: Arterial anatomic considerations in colon interposition for esophageal replacement. Arch Surg 130:858-862, 1995.
2. Saint JH: Surgery of the esophagus. Arch Surg 19:53-128, 1929.
3. Torek F: The first successful case of resection of the thoracic portion of the oesophagus for carcinoma. Surg Gynecol Obstet 16:614-617, 1913.
4. Martin LW, Swisher SG, Hofstetter W, et al: Intrathoracic leaks following esophagectomy are no longer associated with increased mortality. Ann Surg 242:392-399, 2005.
5. Gaissert HA, Mathisen DJ, Grillo HC, et al: Short-segment intestinal interposition of the distal esophagus. J Thorac Cardiovasc Surg 106:860-867, 1993.
6. Orringer MB, Marshall B, Iannettoni MD: Transhiatal esophagectomy for treatment of benign and malignant esophageal disease. World J Surg 25:196-203, 2001.
7. Orringer MB, Marshall B, Iannettoni MD: Transhiatal esophagectomy: Clinical experience and refinements. Ann Surg 230:392-403, 1999.

8. Kent MS, Gayle L, Hoffman L, Altorki NK: A new technique of subcutaneous colon interposition. Ann Thorac Surg 80:2384-2386, 2005.

9. Belsey R: Reconstruction of the esophagus with left colon. J Thorac Cardiovasc Surg 49:33-55, 1965.

10. Denk W: Zur radikaloperation des oesophaguskarzinoma. Zentralbl Chir 40:1065-1068, 1913.

11. Akiyama H, Tsurumaru M, Ono Y, et al: Esophagectomy without thoracotomy with vagal preservation. J Am Coll Surg 178:83-85, 1994.

12. Banki F, Mason RJ, DeMeester SR, et al: Vagal-sparing esophagectomy: A more physiologic alternative. Ann Surg 236:324-336, 2002.

13. Luketich JD, Alvelo-Rivera M, Buenaventura PO, et al: Minimally invasive esophagectomy: Outcomes in 222 patients. Ann Surg 238:486-494, 2003.

14. Ide H, Nakamura T, Okamoto F, et al: Reflux esophagitis after reconstruction of the esophagus using gastric tube: Factors for occurrence of reflux esophagitis and Barrett's epithelium. Paper presented at a conference of the International Society of Surgery, 1997, Acapulco, Mexico.

15. Öberg S, Johansson J, Wenner J, Walther B: Metaplastic columnar mucosa in the cervical esophagus after esophagectomy. Ann Surg 235:338-345, 2002.

16. Watson TJ, DeMeester TR, Kauer WKH, et al: Esophageal replacement for end-stage benign esophageal disease. J Thorac Cardiovasc Surg 115:1241-1249, 1998.

17. Orringer MB, Stirling MC: Transhiatal esophagectomy for benign and malignant disease. J Thorac Cardiovasc Surg 105:265-277, 1993.

18. Briel JW, Tamhankar AP, Hagen JA, et al: Prevalence and risk factors for ischemia, leak and stricture of esophageal anastomosis: Gastric pull-up versus colon interposition. J Am Coll Surg 198:536-542, 2004.

19. Schein M, Conlan AA, Hatchuel MD: Surgical management of the redundant transposed colon. Am J Surg 160:529-530, 1990.

20. Curet-Scott MJ, Ferguson MK, Little AG, Skinner DB: Colon interposition for benign esophageal disease. Surgery 102:568-574, 1987.

21. Young MM, Deschamps C, Trastek VF, et al: Esophageal reconstruction for benign disease: Early morbidity, mortality, and functional results. Ann Thorac Surg 70:1651-1655, 2000.

22. Vaezi MF, Baker ME, Achkar E, Richter JE: Timed barium oesophagram: Better predictor of long-term success after pneumatic dilation in achalasia than symptom assessment. Gut 50:765-770, 2002.

23. Pinotti HW, Cecconello I, da Rocha JM, Zilberstein B: Resection for achalasia of the esophagus. Hepatogastroenterology 38:470-473, 1991.

24. Peters JH, Kauer WK, Crookes PF, et al: Esophageal resection with colon interposition for end-stage achalasia. Arch Surg 130:632-636, 1995.

25. Miller DL, Allen MS, Trastek VF, et al: Esophageal resection for recurrent achalasia. Ann Thorac Surg 60:922-925, 1995.

26. Banbury MK, Rice TW, Goldblum JR, et al: Esophagectomy with gastric reconstruction for achalasia. J Thorac Cardiovasc Surg 117:1077-1084, 1999.

27. Devaney EJ, Iannettoni MD, Orringer MB, Marshall B: Esophagectomy for achalasia: Patient selection and clinical experience. Ann Thorac Surg 72:854-858, 2001.

28. Hsu H-S, Wang C-Y, Hsieh C-C, Huang M-H: Short-segment colon interposition for end-stage achalasia. Ann Thorac Surg 76:1706-1710, 2003.

29. Patterson EJ, Davis DG, Khajanchee Y, Swanstrom LL: Comparison of objective outcomes following laparoscopic Nissen fundoplication versus laparoscopic gastric bypass in the morbidly obese with heartburn. Surg Endosc 17:1561-1565, 2003.

30. Perez AR, Moncure AC, Rattner DW: Obesity adversely affects the outcome of antireflux operations. Surg Endosc 15:986-989, 2001.

31. Csendes A, Braghetto I, Burdiles P, Korn O: Roux-en-Y long limb diversion as the first option for patients who have Barrett's esophagus. Chest Surg Clin N Am 12:157-184, 2002.

32. Csendes A, Burdiles P, Papapietro K, et al: Results of gastric bypass plus resection of the distal excluded gastric segment in patients with morbid obesity. J Gastrointest Surg 9:121-131, 2005.

33. Raftopoulos I, Awais O, Courcoulas AP, Luketich JD: Laparoscopic gastric bypass after antireflux surgery for the treatment of gastroesophageal reflux in morbidly obese patients: Initial experience. Obes Surg 14:1373-1380, 2004.

34. Williams VA, Watson TJ, Gellerson O, et al: Gastrectomy as a remedial operation for failed fundoplication. Abstract presented at the 47th Annual Meeting of the Society for Surgery of the Alimentary Tract, May 20-24, 2006, Los Angeles.

35. Dimick JB, Pronovost PJ, Cowan JA, et al: Surgical volume and quality of care for esophageal resection: Do high-volume hospitals have fewer complications? Ann Thorac Surg 75:337-341, 2003.

21

Endoscopic Antireflux Repairs

Atif Iqbal · Charles J. Filipi · Henry Gale

Gastroesophageal reflux disease (GERD) affects millions of people worldwide. The prevalence of heartburn in a randomly selected adult population is approximately 20%. It is estimated that approximately a third of the adult population in the United States suffers from heartburn on a monthly basis and as many as 10% weekly.[1] Of these, approximately 7% have reflux esophagitis. Management of GERD has gained increasing attention during the past 2 decades because of a high prevalence in Western societies, a better understanding of the pathophysiology, new potent antisecretory drug therapies, the advent of minimally invasive surgery, and new transoral endoscopic therapies.[2] To understand the theoretical or probable mechanism of action of endoscopic antireflux procedures, the anatomy of the gastroesophageal junction (GEJ) and the pathophysiology of GERD as it is understood will be briefly reviewed.

REFLUX PATHOPHYSIOLOGY

Factors Opposing Reflux

The efficacy of the antireflux barrier at the GEJ is dependent on the "lower esophageal sphincter (LES) complex," the geometric profile of the cardia, and their changes as a result of gastric distention. Other factors such as gravity, intraperitoneal pressure, esophageal motility, and the mucosal barrier play a role in reflux prevention but will not be emphasized here.

The Lower Esophageal Sphincter Complex

Competence of the LES is maintained not just by the presence of a high-pressure zone but also by the length of the sphincter and its position relative to the diaphragmatic hiatus. It is known that resistance is directly proportional to the product of its pressure and length. A decrease in the pressure or overall length of the LES or just its abdominal segment predisposes to reflux because

it decreases the resistance imposed on the flow of gastric juice or bile from a higher-pressure cavity, the stomach, to a lower-pressure lumen, the esophagus. The most common cause of a permanently defective sphincter is inadequate pressure, but the efficiency of the sphincter can also be nullified by an inadequate abdominal length or an abnormally short overall length.[3]

Geometry of the Cardia and Its Role

The normal angle of His prevents the distending forces generated within the stomach to be transmitted to the LES, thus preventing its subsequent "unfolding."[3] As the normal geometry of the cardia disappears with increasing gastric distention, the gastric forces pull harder on the abdominal segment of the LES and cause it to be "taken up" into the stretching fundus. At a critical length of 1 to 2 cm, lower esophageal sphincter pressure (LESP) drops acutely and reflux occurs.[3] Figure 21–1 shows the circular muscle fiber thickening as proved by Liebermann et al.,[4] and the three circular muscle groups are demonstrated. Each muscle group improves LES tone by sustained contraction. The balance between the circular muscle groups and how they interact at their junctures is not understood; however, the vectors within which they work can be assumed to be in parallel with the fibers as demonstrated in Figure 21–1C and may be relevant to the force applied by the various endoscopic procedures.

Transient Lower Esophageal Sphincter Relaxation or Shortening?

In severe GERD, the LES, or the "high-pressure zone," is virtually nonexistent or greatly reduced. Reflux in this instance is understandable. However, the cause of reflux in milder disease with normal resting LESP is under considerable debate. It is believed that transient LES relaxations (tLESRs), or intermittent spontaneous

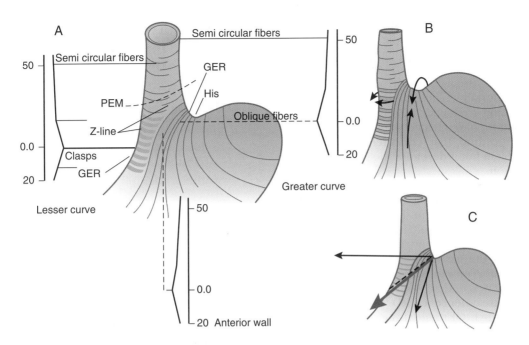

Figure 21–1.   Muscle groups of the gastroesophageal junction. **A,** Muscular orientation at the gastroesophageal junction, as described by Liebermann et al.[4] The *arrows* in **B** represent the direction of contraction of the underlying fibers. The *arrows* in **C** represent the vectors, with *black arrows* representing clasp and sling fiber vectors and the *blue arrow* the resultant vector. The length of the *arrows* correspond to the probable forces of contraction. The *dashed line* represents the gastroesophageal ring. GER, gastroesophageal reflux; PEM, phrenoesophageal membrane.

decreases in LESP, are responsible for reflux events.[5-8] Recent electrophysiologic data suggest that the relevant vagal afferent fibers terminate with specialized intraganglionic laminar endings. These deformity-sensitive transducers are lined in series with muscle fibers at the cardia and fundus and are believed to mediate both fundic receptive relaxation and elicitation of tLESRs.[9]

However, on a larger scale, the cause of tLESRs, the frequency of which increases with gastric distention,[4] can also be explained simply by oral intake. Mason et al. have shown that GERD is associated with shortening of LES length secondary to increasing gastric volumes, the so-called transient LES shortening (tLESS).[12] As further evidence, patients with early disease normally experience episodes of esophageal acid exposure shortly after meals. The increased swallowing frequency seen in GERD patients is an effort to neutralize the acid refluxed into their esophagus and is supportive evidence of intraprandial reflux in this population.[3] This, coupled with the ingestion of fatty foods, which delays gastric emptying, explains the rising incidence of GERD in the Western world.

Nissen fundoplication and endoluminal gastroplasty (ELGP)[2] have been shown to prevent LES shortening during gastric distention, thus minimizing GERD. In light of the aforementioned pathophysiologic factors, endoscopic therapies should prevent reflux in the following ways: (1) alter the compliance of the cardia and prevent transient LES shortening/relaxation, (2) increase baseline LES tone or, (3) increase baseline LES length.

Finally, none of the endoluminal therapies effectively reduces the distal end of the esophagus into the abdomen and effects a hiatal hernia repair. Hiatal hernias, even if small, alter the muscular vector force at the GEJ. Sling fibers and perhaps clasp fibers may be spread and stretched more by a hiatal hernia, especially with food intake and elevation of intragastric pressure secondary to Valsalva maneuvers. In addition, the angle of His is obliterated.

TRANSORAL ENDOSCOPIC PROCEDURE BACKGROUND

There has always been discussion and controversy among gastroenterologists and surgeons about treatment options for GERD. The majority of patients with GERD are best treated by proton pump inhibitors (PPIs). However, symptom relapse is common after cessation of treatment because PPIs suppress acid production without affecting the underlying disease mechanism. The rate of relapse reaches 100% in patients with low LESP,[10] and thus many patients must commit to lifelong therapy. Continuous PPI therapy also results in symptom relapse in up to 33% of patients, especially within the first 2 years. Moreover, 50% of patients continue to exhibit low intragastric pH and objective evidence of acid regurgitation despite complete symptomatic control with PPI therapy. Combined impedance-pH testing has highlighted the role of non-acid reflux in GERD. This leaves the patient prone to atypical manifestations of reflux disease, such as pulmonary symptoms, which are difficult to both diagnose and treat. Therefore, PPIs may not be an acceptable option for young patients facing lifelong medication use. There is good evidence that mechanical augmentation of the GEJ by fundoplication is a good treatment option for patients with severe progressive reflux disease.[3] However, laparoscopic antireflux surgery requires a general anesthetic, hospitalization, and postoperative lifestyle limitations for days to weeks; moreover, it is expensive and associated with postoperative morbidity and even mortality. These limitations, in conjunction with the rising frequency of reflux disease in the Western population, have created the need to develop a less invasive procedure that effectively addresses the underlying problem but is devoid of the shortcomings of the surgical option.

More than 10 years ago, the British gastroenterologist Paul Swain developed a sewing capsule attached to a flexible endoscope to perform limited surgical maneuvers in the gastrointestinal lumen. The idea of minimizing surgical trauma by performing operative procedures within the gastrointestinal tract provided a new perspective. As a consequence, in the past decade an entire spectrum of new endoscopic techniques have been developed for the treatment of GERD.[11] These procedures are listed in Box 21–1. Of these, three novel endoscopic therapies have been approved for use by the Food and Drug Administration. All procedures can be safely performed in an outpatient setting with conscious sedation.

SELECTION CRITERIA FOR ENDOSCOPIC THERAPY

The general selection criteria that have been used in most trials are shown in Figure 21–2. In addition, specific

---

Box 21–1 **Types of Endoluminal Therapy for Gastroesophageal Reflux Disease**

Endoscopic Suturing

Endoluminal gastroplasty (ELGP/EndoCinch)

Endoluminal full-thickness plicator (NDO plicator)

Syntheon ARD plicator

Radiofrequency Energy Delivery

Stretta procedure

Synthetic Implants/Injections

Implantable biopolymer (Enteryx)

Implantable prosthesis (Gatekeeper)

Implantable Plexiglas microspheres (PMMA)

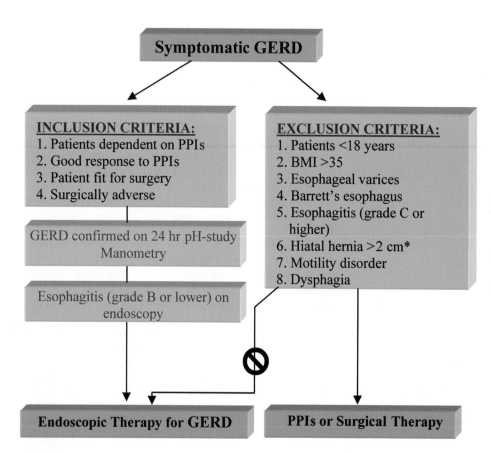

Figure 21–2. Inclusion/exclusion criteria for endoluminal therapies for gastroesophageal reflux disease (GERD). BMI, body mass index; PPIs, proton pump inhibitors. *Recently, some studies have included patients with a hiatal hernia >3 cm and Barrett's esophagus.

Symptomatic GERD

INCLUSION CRITERIA:
1. Patients dependent on PPIs
2. Good response to PPIs
3. Patient fit for surgery
4. Surgically adverse

GERD confirmed on 24 hr pH-study Manometry

Esophagitis (grade B or lower) on endoscopy

EXCLUSION CRITERIA:
1. Patients <18 years
2. BMI >35
3. Esophageal varices
4. Barrett's esophagus
5. Esophagitis (grade C or higher)
6. Hiatal hernia >2 cm*
7. Motility disorder
8. Dysphagia

Endoscopic Therapy for GERD

PPIs or Surgical Therapy

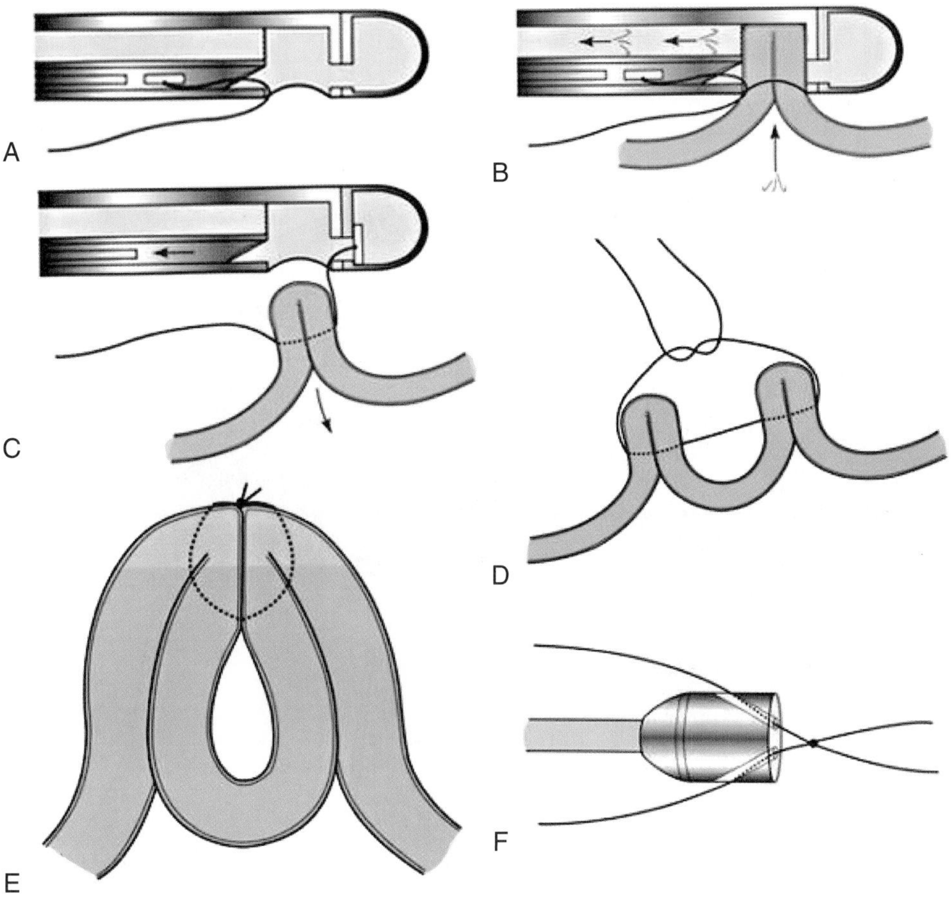

Figure 21–3. A, Drawing of a suturing device equipped with a vacuum chamber and a hollow needle in which a suture is attached to a tag. **B,** Tissue is drawn into the chamber by suction. The needle passes through the tissue, and the tag is captured in the distal chamber. **C,** The suction is then released. **D,** The procedure is repeated on an adjacent piece of tissue. **E,** On tightening the knot, the pieces of tissues are approximated. **F,** The suture is cut using a small device with internal knives.

patient selection criteria, if any, are mentioned in discussion of the respective procedures.

ENDOLUMINAL GASTROPLASTY

History

The first endoscopic approach to the GEJ involved the creation of an endoluminal valvuloplasty via a transgastric sewing technique. The valvuloplasty consisted of a full–wall thickness intussusception of the GEJ into the stomach to create a nipple-type valve; the configuration of the valve was maintained with eight staples, and stability was aided by an intramural injection of sodium morrhuate.[2] Safety, durability, and efficacy were tested in baboons.[12]

Swain et al. developed a mechanical aid that allowed passage of a needle and subsequent suture via the biopsy channel of an endoscope.[13] Later, the technique was modified to create plications endoscopically below and at the GEJ for the prevention of GERD.

Procedure

The endoluminal procedure requires a suturing capsule, suture tags, and an anchoring system that secures the suture and cuts the strands (Fig. 21–3). A short, 18-mm-outer-diameter overtube allows repeated intubations (approximately 12) while avoiding trauma to the esophageal mucosa. The choice of sedation depends on the patient's condition and general health. Usually, patients tolerate the procedure with conscious sedation. However, restless patients who have a class II airway require monitored anesthesia, and those with a class III or IV airway require a general anesthetic. Two to four plications are placed either longitudinally (one above the other), radially (next to each other), or spirally within the cardia. Each plication is formed by two stitches placed into the gastric submucosa, approximately 1 cm apart, and then pulled together. The procedure is performed via the following steps. After correct placement of the sewing capsule, suction is applied, the gastric wall is pulled into the hollow chamber of the capsule, and a straight needle loaded with nonabsorbable suture and a T tag is fired through the suctioned tissue. The system is reloaded and a second stitch is placed adjacent to the first. The two stitches are pulled together and cinched by a ceramic plug and ring via a second endoscope. Depending on the expertise of the operator and the number of plications intended, the procedure is completed within 40 to 60 minutes.

The application of cautery on opposing mucosal surfaces before plication may secure tissue apposition and promote long-term adherence. Its efficacy has been proved in pilot studies[14] but needs to be tested in a larger randomized controlled trial.

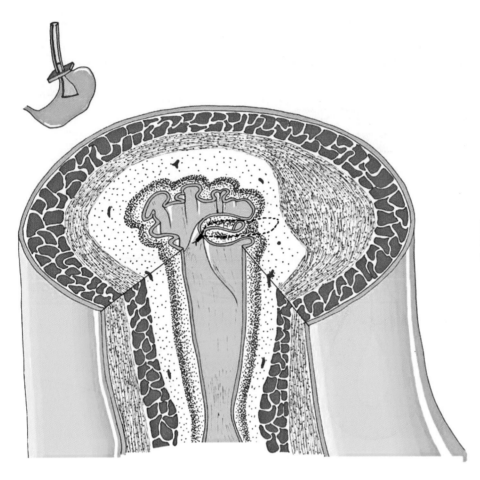

Figure 21–4. Cross-sectional illustration of changes seen with endoluminal gastroplication.

Histologic Changes

In animal models, the device has been shown to place the majority of stitches in the submucosal layer and is believed to do the same in humans. It has been found that everted intraluminal gastroplications do not result in fusion between mucosal folds, irrespective of suture depth. A flat scar is the final outcome and appears to be proportional to the amount of ischemia, foreign body reaction, and suture depth.[15] In a recent publication by Liu et al., ELGP was shown to cause muscular hypertrophy. Eight humans who had symptomatic relief with ELGP and pigs that underwent ELGP were examined by endoscopic ultrasound. The muscularis propria increased by 0.9 mm ($P < .01$) in humans and 2.6 mm by endoscopic ultrasonography and 2.1 mm by autopsy examination in the porcine model.[16] The changes observed with ELGP are shown in cross section in Figure 21–4.

Efficacy

The overall results with ELGP are tabulated in Table 21–1. The pooled data were obtained from 11 studies; however, an effort was made to avoid bias by including only studies that used off-PPI scoring as baseline and intent to treat.

Two multicenter trials are included in Table 21–1 and will be highlighted. In the first trial, 64 patients were ran-

domized to a circumferential or linear plication configuration.[17] All patients were dependent on antisecretory agents and had proven reflux by 24-hour pH monitoring. Manometry and endoscopy were performed to exclude patients with Barrett's esophagus, grade 3 or 4 esophagitis, large hiatal hernias, and an esophageal dysmotility disorder. No difference was found between the plication configuration groups, and postprocedure manometry and endoscopy showed no improvement in LESP or grade of esophagitis. A significant improvement in heartburn and regurgitation scores from baseline occurred, but the pH monitoring results, though significantly improved, showed only a 30% normalization rate.

In a second multicenter study, 85 symptomatic GERD patients not taking PPIs with proven reflux on 24-hour pH monitoring were included.[18] Upper endoscopy and manometry were also performed as baseline. Follow-up was scheduled at 3, 6, 12, and 24 months. Symptom scores and medication use were assessed at each follow-up, and pH-metry was performed at the 3-month follow-up. This study was different from others with respect to inclusion criteria inasmuch as it included patients with grade 3 esophagitis ($n = 10$), hiatal hernia larger than 2 cm ($n = 9$), Barrett's esophagus ($n = 4$), failed fundoplication ($n = 3$), and pulmonary symptoms ($n = 10$). The majority of patients had two plications performed (range, 1 to 3), and most had a circumferential plication (65%), with the remaining receiving a linear configuration (35%).

Table 21-1 Endoluminal Gastroplication: Pooled Results

Variable	≥1 mo	≥3 mo	≥6 mo	≥12 mo	≥24 mo
GERD-HRQL improvement	—	67% (56)	69% (110)	55% (15)	32% (31)
Heartburn improvement	89% (42)	79% (60)	75% (160)	74% (150)	54% (114)
Regurgitation improvement	78% (42)	72% (42)	61% (42)	55% (66)	—
Patients completely off PPIs	68% (22)	64% (22)	53% (57)	40% (414)	33% (105)
Patients with ≥50% reduction in PPI use	—	—	82% (59)	51% (113)	48% (105)
Improvement in quality-of-life scores SF-36 Physical	—	—	16% (66)	17% (15)	—
SF-36 Mental	—	—	9% (66)	NS (15)	—
QOLRAD	88% (22)	85% (22)	72% (22)	78% (22)	—
LESP improvement	—	NS* (194)	NS* (159)	NS* (21)	—
LES length improvement	—	NS* (194)	NS (130)	NS (21)	—
tLESR improvement	—	—	Yes (15)	—	—
Improvement in pH scores Total time pH <4	—	53% (170)	26% (62)	17%* (15)	—
Time upright pH <4	—	NS (53)	26% (68)	32% (21)	—
Time supine pH <4	—	NS (59)	NS (59)	NS (59)	—
Number of episodes	—	36% (121)	26% (29)	33% (21)	—
pH normalization	—	—	NS (15)	NS (15)	—
Healing of esophagitis	—	—	NS (108)	—	—
Residual plications	—	86% (26)	80% (15)	—	—
Re-treatment	—	—	11% (44)	15% (259)	—

The results expressed in the majority of studies are shown here. Numbers in parentheses are the numbers of patients studied to obtain the result.

*Signifies disagreement among studies.

GERD, gastroesophageal reflux disease; HRQL, health-related quality of life; LES, lower esophageal sphincter; LESP, LES pressure; NS, change not significant; PPI, proton pump inhibitor; QOLRAD, Quality of Life in Reflux and Dyspepsia questionnaire; SF-36, Short Form-36; tLESR, transient LES relaxation; —, data not available. Pooled data were obtained from references 17-27.

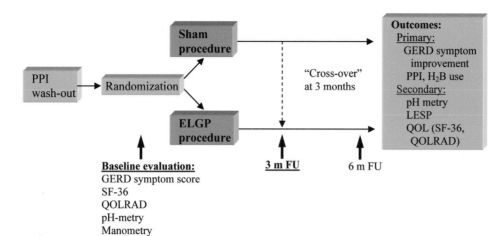

Figure 21–5. Endoluminal gastroplication (ELGP) sham study design. EGD, esophagogastroduodenoscopy; FU, follow-up; GERD, gastroesophageal reflux disease; LESP, lower esophageal sphincter pressure; PPI, proton pump inhibitor; QOL, quality of life; QOLRAD, Quality of Life in Reflux and Dyspepsia; SF-36, Short Form-36.

Twenty-four-month follow-up data demonstrated durable functional improvement and a sustained reduction in antisecretory medication use. Heartburn scores were reduced at both 1- (94%) and 2-year (78%) follow-up. Likewise, PPI use decreased, with 69% of patients using less than 50% of their baseline medication and 41% not taking any PPIs at 2-year follow-up. There was no change in LES length or pressure when measured at 3 months.

A sham-controlled, randomized, blinded single-institution study ($n = 34$) is under way, and 3-month follow-up is available.[28] The study design for the sham trial is shown in Figure 21–5. The study nurse and patients were blinded to the procedure performed. An overtube and two endoscopes were exchanged in all patients, and the conscious sedation dosing was similar. Four circumferential plications were placed when performing ELGP. At 3-month follow-up, heartburn frequency (69% versus 31%, $P = .03$) and severity (47% versus 17%, P = not significant) were improved in patients who underwent ELGP in comparison to those receiving the sham procedure. A significantly greater number of patients in the plication group discontinued their daily PPI/H_2B (75% versus 25%, $P = .03$). A significant reduction in the percentage of time that the pH was less than 4 was also observed; however, no difference was seen between groups regarding normalization of pH, median LESP, or quality of life. Limitations of this study include a probable type II error, a larger than expected sham effect, inadequate follow-up length, and lack of technique standardization. A randomized controlled trial of larger size with longer follow-up is needed for objective evidence of durable benefit.

Other studies of note have demonstrated a markedly improved quality of life at 1-year follow-up,[19] reduction of the rate of tLESRs by 37% at 6 months in a single-center study,[20] a significant increase in LES length in baboons,[29] and an increase in intra-abdominal but not total length of the LES after placement of three linear plications in dogs by Kadirkamanathan et al.[13]

Changes in Selection Criteria

A significant improvement in symptom scores and pH study results has been observed in 19 patients refractory to medications, although this improvement was less than that seen in other studies.[21] Short-term studies suggest that ELGP can be used as an effective salvage procedure for failed surgical fundoplication,[30,31] but this indication requires further study.

Effect of Plication Configuration and Number

The optimal configuration of plications is not known. In a small and unfortunately underpowered study by Davis et al., 22 patients with proven GERD were randomized to either a helical or a circumferential plication pattern. No difference in outcome was observed between configurations, although a trend in objective results favored the helical pattern.[22] It was proposed that the benefit of ELGP would be sustained at 18-month follow-up, but this was not substantiated, with no difference between groups and only 15% of patients being asymptomatic and not taking antisecretory medication. Raijman et al.[32] reported that the helical plication configuration demonstrated superior results at 6-month follow-up with regard to symptom control and medication use. The prevalence and persistence of these possible advantages are currently subject to investigation. Increasing the number of plications, when using the helical pattern, did not show a significant benefit at either 6- or 12-month follow-up.[22]

Complications

ELGP is generally safe over long-term follow-up and free of serious immediate side effects. The major and minor complications are shown in Table 21–7. Patients are instructed to take only oral fluids for the first 24 hours and to call their physician in the event of any chest pain or symptoms consistent with gastrointestinal bleeding.

Esophageal perforation can occur. Before the U.S. trials, Dr. Paul Swain encountered one patient who required open thoracotomy for a perforation of the esophagus, and in the initial multicenter trial a suture perforation occurred. This patient required 3 days of hospitalization and antibiotics and thereafter made an uneventful recovery. The perforation was thought to be secondary to a suture placed through the esophageal wall that allowed air to escape as evidenced by pneumomediastinum seen on computed tomography. A diatrizoate meglumine (Gastrografin) swallow followed by a barium study showed no extravasation.

Airway assessment is particularly important because hypoxemia and stridor may occur secondary to the overtube. Patients with class III and IV airways are at risk for these complications, whereas class I and II airways do not usually pose any serous problem unless there is a limitation in extension of the head or obesity. Patients who are obese, are combative during the preliminary endoscopy, or have a class IV airway should have either a general anesthetic or propofol sedation with careful monitoring. A dedicated anesthesiologist will improve procedure flow, thereby leading to a significant reduction in procedure time and possibly anesthesia-related complications.[33]

Recommended precautions include a training course for the entire team, preprocedure airway assessment, general anesthesia for combative patients and those with a class IV airway, and examination for active bleeding at the end of the procedure. To avoid a perforation, which is usually due to placement of a full-thickness suture within the esophageal wall, all stitches and plications should be placed below the squamocolumnar junction. If the suturing capsule needle does not retract after penetrating the tissue, the handle with the pusher rod should be disassembled rather than pulling the capsule away from the esophageal wall. Occasionally, the suture loops and locks at the tissue level as the second stitch is being placed. The needle literally goes through a loop and the suture will not slide through the tissue on removal of the endoscope. In this circumstance, the suture should be cut with endoscopic scissors; however, this can be difficult and pullout may be necessary. If tissue accompanies the knot, it should be sent to pathology for frozen section analysis. If the muscularis propria is included in the specimen, an esophagogram should be performed, followed by hospitalization.

Procedure Failure

Studies demonstrate that laparoscopic Nissen fundoplication (LNF) is feasible and effective after failed ELGP.[34,35] Patients should undergo upper gastrointestinal endoscopy before surgery, but suture removal is not necessary. No significant scarring or adhesions have been noted in the esophageal hiatus or inferior mediastinum at LNF, possibly because the stitches do not penetrate beyond the muscularis propria; penetration of the serosa has been shown to induce more scarring.[15] This in itself might contribute to the lack of durability in post-ELGP results. Although the technique is initially effective, long-term symptom control has yet to be established.

An interesting phenomenon that has been experienced by several investigators involved in the initial trials was diminishment of the patient's surgical adversity after ELGP. It appears that some patients, after taking an initial active step to rectify their reflux disorder, become more willing to find a definitive solution. This is potentially a positive effect of all intraluminal antireflux procedures and should be studied.

Alternatively, patients who experience recurrent GERD symptoms after ELGP may benefit from a second procedure. However, one study has demonstrated a significant trend toward earlier onset of recurrent symptoms after repeat ELGP.[23]

Advantages

Easy repeatability, short operative time, early discharge, no morbidity, and symptomatic improvement make ELGP an attractive option. Endoscopic gastroplication has proven short-term efficacy and has been demonstrated to be cost-effective for 1 to 2 years.[36]

Disadvantages

The absence of objective improvement after ELGP is disconcerting. No studies have shown improvement in LES pressure and the grade of esophagitis. pH monitoring results are mixed, but the rate of normalization is only 30% to 40% between studies. The lack of objective evidence of reflux control, in relation to improvement in symptoms, is best explained by a reduced volume of regurgitant confined to the less sensitive distal esophagus. This explanation does not, however, negate the deleterious effect of the acid within the distal esophagus and the chance for progression to complications such as stricture formation or even Barrett's esophagus.

Several studies have compared ELGP and LNF. Comparable improvement in symptom scores, PPI intake, and quality-of-life assessment has been seen. Patients who undergo LNF do have greater physiologic control of esophageal acid reflux, but at the expense of a higher incidence of postprocedure complications.[37] Chandalavada et al. compared 47 ELGP patients with 40 patients who had undergone laparoscopic antireflux surgery. Twelve-month follow-up demonstrated different results.[38] Surgical intervention offered a significantly greater reduction in medication use (87% versus 69%) and greater patient satisfaction (93% versus 66%). Similar patient satisfaction results (96% versus 78%) have also been reported by Velanovich et al.[39] Thus, surgery is superior to ELGP in patient satisfaction and objective improvement in reflux.

Summary

Endoscopic gastroplasty is a safe and moderately effective outpatient procedure that has been demonstrated to significantly improve symptoms and PPI requirements over at least a 1-year period.[19] Symptom relief is acceptable at 6 to 12 months, and the procedure is associated with minimal discomfort. These results support the use of ELGP in patients who are reluctant to undergo surgery or are at high surgical risk. Good symptomatic results are obtained in part by accuracy in placement of plications, but this seems to be highly operator dependent. Visualization is limited, and thus placement of stitches is difficult, especially after the first plication because of tissue distortion and accumulated blood. Finally standardization of technique has not been achieved. Further device modifications may be of assistance.

ENDOSCOPIC FULL-THICKNESS PLICATOR (NDO PLICATOR)

Current endoscopic suturing techniques usually involve submucosal suture placement, which may limit potential procedure-related complications but may also lead to early suture dehiscence and loss of long-term efficacy. This problem may theoretically be solved by full-thickness suturing or stapling devices that include the use of pledgets. Such an approach may, however, increase the risk for subsequent perforation. A novel technique of applying a full-thickness plication endoscopically has been developed and recently underwent clinical study in a U.S. multicenter trial. Selection criteria were similar to that shown in Figure 21–2.

Procedure

The NDO plicator (Fig. 21–6) is designed to apply a full-thickness pledget-reinforced U stitch near the GEJ with serosa-to-serosa apposition. The system consists of a reusable instrument and a single-use suture-based implant. Additionally, a proprietary endoscopic tissue retractor and a standard overtube are used to perform the procedure. A newer version of the instrument can be passed without an overtube and accepts a small transnasal gastroscope. The instrument passes two needles through tissue at the desired location to place the implant for tissue approximation, plication, and fixation. Controls on the instrument handle actuate the distal end of the device and provide for retroflexion of the distal end, opening and closing of the instrument arms, and delivery of the implant. The instrument contains two dedicated channels, one for insertion of the tissue retractor/plication device, the other for passage of the endoscope.[40] The tissue retractor is designed to engage the deep gastric wall, thereby allowing for creation of the serosa-to-serosa plication. The tissue retractor is configured in a helical fashion and includes a protective outer sheath to stabilize the gastric mucosa while engaging the wall. Typically, the retractor is inserted 1 cm distal to the GEJ, which allows the gastric wall to then be drawn into the arms of the instrument before deployment of the implant.

With the patient under conscious sedation, a gastroscope is passed into the stomach for endoscopic inspection and passage of a guidewire. The plication device is passed into the stomach after removal of the dilator and guidewire. The suture applicator is retroflexed and properly positioned under endoscopic vision. The endoscopic tissue retractor is then inserted to within 1 cm of the GEJ and advanced to the level of the muscularis, which is judged by visible tenting of the

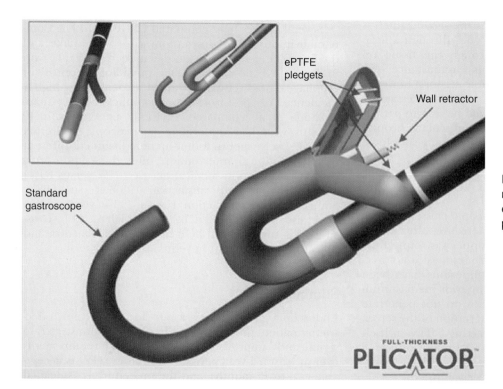

Figure 21–6. The NDO plicator mounted on a small-diameter endoscope. ePTFE, expanded polytetrafluoroethylene.

1. Plicator and gastroscope retroflexed

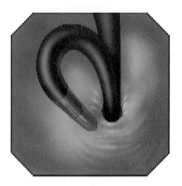

2. Arms opened, tissue retractor advanced to serosa

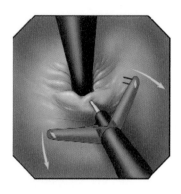

3. Gastric wall retracted, arms closed

4. Single pre-tied implant is deployed, securing serosa-to-serosa plication

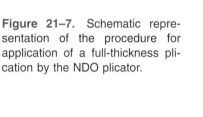

Figure 21–7. Schematic representation of the procedure for application of a full-thickness plication by the NDO plicator.

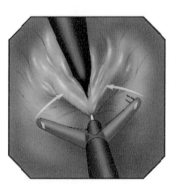

5. Full thickness plication restructures normal anti-reflux barrier

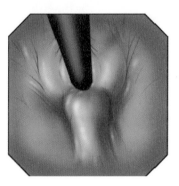

tissues around the entry point of the retractor. The gastric wall is next retracted and the instrument arms are closed on it. The pre-tied implant is deployed to secure a full-thickness plication. The tissue retractor is removed from the greater curvature side of the GEJ, the jaws are opened, and the entire assembly is removed from the stomach (Fig. 21–7). The approximate procedural time is 15 to 20 minutes.

Efficacy

Pooled results for the NDO plicator are shown in Table 21–2. A multicenter study enrolled 64 patients with symptomatic GERD who were dependent on antisecre-tory medication and showed evidence of esophageal acid exposure (pH-metry) without an underlying motility disorder. Follow-up was completed at 1, 3, and 6 months after the procedure and showed a significant reduction in GERD symptom scores, medication use, and esophageal acid exposure on 24-hour pH study that persisted at 1-year follow-up. No significant changes in esophageal manometry were noted.[41] At 6-month follow-up, there was a 63% improvement in symptom scores with elimination of PPI therapy in 74% and normalization of pH in 30% of patients. No patient required re-treatment during the 6-month follow-up. In this initial trial, one full-thickness plication was used. A pilot study involving seven patients also had similar results but failed

Table 21–2 NDO: Pooled Results

Variable		≥1 mo		≥3 mo		≥6 mo		≥12 mo		≥24 mo
GERD-HRQL improvement		42%	(7)	67%	(68)	63%	(68)	70%	(63)	—
Patients completely off PPIs		—		—		78%	(63)	75%	(58)	—
Improvement in quality-of-life scores	SF-36 Physical	28	(7)	6%	(61)	10%	(61)	31%	(7)	—
	SF-36 Mental	7%	(7)	7%	(61)	5%	(61)	10%	(7)	—
LESP improvement		—		NS	(61)			—		—
LES length improvement		—		NS	(61)			—		—
tLESR improvement						No				
Improvement in pH scores	Total time pH <4	—		—		29%	(43)	—		—
	Number of episodes	—		—		26%	(43)	—		—
	pH normalization	—		—		30%	(43)	—		—
Healing of esophagitis		—		—		NS	(7)	NS	(7)	—
Residual plications		—		—		100%	(7)	—		—
Re-treatment		—		—		0%	(64)	0%	(64)	—

All results displayed are significant. Numbers in parentheses show the number of patients studied to obtain the result.
GERD, gastroesophageal reflux disease; HRQL, health-related quality of life; LES, lower esophageal sphincter; LESP, LES pressure; NS, change not significant; PPI, proton pump inhibitor; SF-36, Short Form-36; tLESR, transient LES relaxation; —, data not available.
Pooled data were obtained from references 40-42.

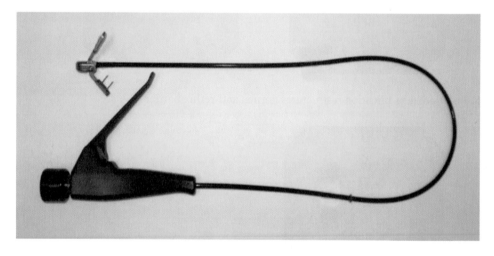

Figure 21–8. Syntheon plicator.

to show objective improvement of reflux.[42] Further studies with single versus multiple plications are anticipated. No sham-controlled trial has yet been completed, but one is being organized.

Complications

The most common complication was sore throat (spontaneously resolving within several days after the procedure). One gastric perforation did occur during the multicenter trial and was managed conservatively.

Summary

A single full-thickness plication placed at the GEJ is effective, reduces symptoms and medication use, and improves esophageal acid exposure. Further studies with longer follow-up will elucidate the safety of this procedure. A sham trial has just been completed. The initial appeal of a full-thickness plication is dampened by the results, but presumably with instrument and technique modification plus further experience, the results will improve.

SYNTHEON ARD PLICATOR

This promising new endoluminal suturing device has the capacity to place two stitches within the gastric wall at once, thus decreasing technical variability between operators (Fig. 21–8). The distance between the two stitches is predetermined. Withdrawal of the device is not necessary after each stitch, which may decrease procedure time and anesthesia-related complications. Results

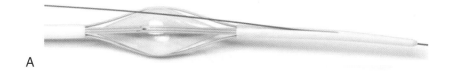

A

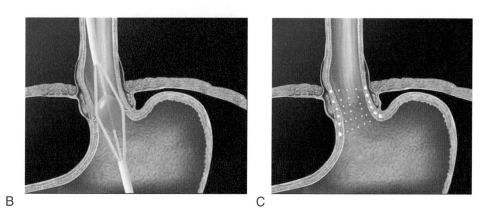

B   C

Figure 21–9. **A,** Stretta catheter with guidewire. **B,** Balloon assembly with struts and electrodes extending into the muscularis propria. **C,** A total of 56 lesions are applied as seen in this diagram.

with this device are not yet available, but a multicenter trial is planned. The device does have the ability to place sutures on the lesser curvature side of the GES.

STRETTA PROCEDURE

History

Radiofrequency (RF) energy has been used extensively in medicine since 1921 and is currently being used in the treatment of benign prostatic hypertrophy, cardiac arrhythmias, and metastatic liver lesions. The possibility of RF energy being used for GERD therapy was explored after successful treatment of snoring and sleep apnea. Endoscopic delivery of RF energy to the porcine GEJ was thus investigated and its effects assessed in a pilot study published in 2000.[43]

Patient Selection

RF augmentation of the LES has been widely used. More than 3500 procedures have been performed in the United States alone. Indications in the past have been confined to patients with early reflux disease. The Stretta procedure may have specific utility in morbidly obese patients, in those who have previously undergone gastric resection or a gastric bypass procedure, after a failed LNF,[44] or as an alternative to reoperation after disruption of fundoplication. In a porcine fundoplication disruption model, fluoroscopic guidance improved RF lesion accuracy, and therefore it has been suggested that fluoroscopic guidance be used to ensure probe placement.[45] Patients with failed antireflux surgery and subsequent RF therapy have experienced nonsignificant symptomatic improvement (decrease in heartburn score from 3.33 before the procedure to 2.75 after the procedure);

however, patient satisfaction scores are significantly improved.[46] The role of the Stretta procedure in postoperative fundoplication patients remains unclear.

Procedure

The Stretta catheter (Fig. 21–9A) is a flexible, hand-held, disposable, 20-French Savary-style dilator that is used in conjunction with the Curon (Sunnyvale, CA) control module. It is composed of a balloon basket assembly, four nickel titanium electrodes, and suction and irrigation capability. The balloon basket deploys four radially arranged electrodes into the smooth muscle of the GEJ. Tiny thermocouple temperature sensors within the electrodes provide temperature feedback to the RF generator. A target temperature is preselected and the power is automatically discontinued if the temperature exceeds the predetermined threshold. The needles also provide feedback on impedance, which allows the operator to know whether the needles are positioned correctly in the tissue.

The procedure is done under conscious sedation with upper endoscopy performed initially to evaluate the size of the hiatal hernia, if present, to determine the distance to the squamocolumnar junction and to place a guidewire as the endoscope is withdrawn. The catheter is placed over the guidewire into the stomach and withdrawn to the position of needle deployment. The guidewire is removed and suction and irrigation are connected. The balloon at the distal end of the catheter is inflated, the electrodes are deployed, and RF energy is applied for a specific period while monitoring the temperature and impedance levels (see Fig. 21–9B). Continuous cold water irrigation during the procedure prevents mucosal overheating and subsequent surface tissue injury. A first treatment ring of eight lesions is created by rotating the catheter 45 degrees and repeat-

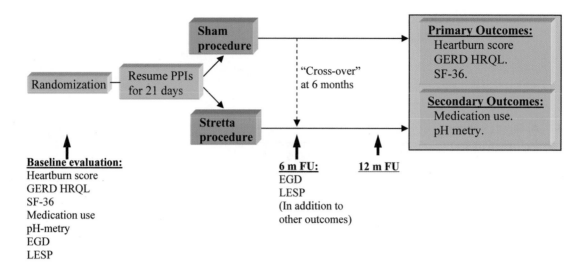

Figure 21–10.   The Stretta sham study design. EGD, esophagogastroduodenoscopy; FU, follow-up; GERD, gastroesophageal reflux disease; HRQL, health-related quality of life; LESP, lower esophageal sphincter pressure; PPI, proton pump inhibitor; SF-36, Short Form-36.

ing the same. Four such antegrade rings, each with eight lesions, are created at 0.5-cm intervals to a distance of 1 cm below the GEJ. Two further gastric "pull-back" rings, of 12 lesions each (three sets of deployment each), complete a set of thermal lesions (see Fig. 21–9C). Halfway through the procedure, an endoscope is reintroduced to verify the location of treatments, with subsequent adjustment distally or proximally to prevent superimposition of lesions. After recovery, patients continue their usual antireflux medication for 3 weeks.

It has been proposed that a modified technique be performed if variant anatomy such as a large hiatal hernia (>3 cm) or a failed Nissen fundoplication is present.[47] The modified technique creates six antero-grade treatment levels instead of four, beginning 1 cm above the squamocolumnar junction with 5 mm between levels; two sets of lesions are placed at each of the four proximal levels and three sets at the distal two levels.

Histologic Changes

Histologic assessment of porcine specimens has shown focal circular muscle thermal injury with normal mucosa, mild fibrosis, and no inflammation.[46] No randomized study has been completed to document the histologic changes in humans after the Stretta procedure, and the current animal studies suggest different findings. In a study involving 30 pigs, Utley et al. reported histologically normal muscle with occasional focal areas of collagen deposition at 8 weeks' follow-up,[43] whereas in a study involving 11 dogs, Kim et al. reported marked muscular hypertrophy as well as fibrosis within the muscle 7 months after the procedure when compared with control animals.[48] Measurements of the gastric cardia showed a significant (63%) increase in thickness. In animals, the procedure has also been demonstrated to increase LESP and mean muscular wall thickness.[48] Such results have not been proved in humans after the Stretta procedure.[49]

Efficacy

In the initial U.S. open-label trial,[50] 1-year follow-up showed a significant decrease in symptom scores. GERD-specific quality-of-life satisfaction scores and distal acid exposure were significantly improved over the baseline on-medication scores as well. However, normalization of pH monitoring scores did not occur in the majority of patients. In addition, LESP did not increase and esophagitis did not improve significantly at 6-month endoscopic follow-up.

The sham-controlled trial[51] study design is presented in (Fig. 21–10). The data showed significant improvement in symptom scores and quality of life at 6 and 12 months, but at 6 months there was no difference between groups in medication use. The grade of esophagitis did not show improvement, and in fact, grade 2 esophagitis increased in severity in both groups. Similarly, pH scores also failed to show significant improvement, unlike the previous uncontrolled studies.[50,52] The explanation for these findings may be altered sensitivity of the distal esophagus or unusual persistence of the sham effect.

In a registry series,[53] 558 patients underwent the Stretta procedure and experienced a significant improvement in GERD symptom control (from 50% to 90%) and patient satisfaction (from 23% to 86%) at a mean follow-up of 8 months. The onset of GERD relief occurred in less than 2 months in most patients (69%). The treatment effect was durable beyond 1 year, and most patients (51% at 1 year versus 96% before the procedure) were not taking any antisecretory drugs at follow-up. Most studies are limited to short-term follow-up (up to 12 months). For the first time, Torquati et al. reported long-term results in 41 patients, with 83% being highly satisfied at a mean follow-up of 27 months.[54] PPI use was discontinued in 56% of patients and was significantly reduced in 87%. Similarly, Reymunde and Santiage demonstrated significant and sustained improvement in antisecretory drug discontinuation (88%), GERD

Table 21–3   Stretta Procedure: Pooled Results

Variable		≥1 mo		≥3 mo		≥6 mo		≥12 mo		≥24 mo	
GERD-HRQL improvement		67%	(18)	67%	(16)	53%	(219)	65%	(113)	95%	(202)
Heartburn improvement		—		—		52%	(216)	61%	(163)	100%	(202)
Patients completely off PPIs		—		—		65%	(175)	55%	(163)	63%	(332)
Patients with ≥50% reduction in PPI use		—		—		67%	(141)	—		87%	(36)
Improvement in quality-of-life scores	SF-36 Physical	—		—		18%	(202)	20%	(113)	—	
	SF-36 Mental	—		—		14%	(171)	14%	(113)	—	
LESP improvement		—		—		NS*	(211)	—		—	
LES length improvement		—		—		NS	(18)	—		—	
tLESR improvement		—		NS	(36)	24%*	(20)	—		—	
Improvement in pH scores	Total time pH <4	—		53%	(170)	42%*	(180)	36%	(19)	8%	(36)
	Time upright pH <4	—		—		38%	(138)	—		—	
	Time supine pH <4	—		—		48%	(138)	—		—	
	Number of episodes	—		—		32%	(155)	—		—	
	pH normalization	—		—		36%	(22)	—		45%	(22)
Healing of esophagitis		—		—		—		NS	(85)	—	

The results expressed in the majority of studies are shown here. Numbers in parentheses are the numbers of patients studied to obtain the result.

*Signifies disagreement among studies.

GERD, gastroesophageal reflux disease; HRQL, health-related quality of life; LES, lower esophageal sphincter; LESP, LES pressure; NS, change not significant; PPI, proton pump inhibitor; SF-36, Short Form-36; tLESR, transient LES relaxation; —, data not available.

Pooled data were obtained from references 44, 46, 49-52, 54, 57, 58.

symptom scores (82%), and quality-of-life scores (44%) at more than 3 years of follow-up.[55] This encouraging evidence suggests that durability of results is the distinguishing attribute of the Stretta procedure.

Significant improvement in symptom scores and quality of life have also been observed in shorter-term studies.[49,50,53,56] Similarly, decreased PPI use and increased patient satisfaction have been seen consistently.[49,50,56] Most studies fail to demonstrate a beneficial effect of the Stretta procedure on esophagitis, but Triadafilopoulos et al.[52] showed an improvement in esophagitis grade, from 21% with grade 2 esophagitis to 9.3% after the procedure in 43 patients at 6 months. The role of the Stretta procedure in improving extraesophageal manifestations of GERD is still not clear; however, one study[44] suggests that respiratory benefit can be achieved if strict patient selection (abnormal pH study) is followed. Pooled results are shown in Table 21–3.

Complications

The major and minor complications are shown in Table 21–7. The five perforations and two deaths occurred during the learning curve and were due to poor patient selection and technical errors. No major complications were seen in the multicenter trial, and subsequent studies have not shown adverse effects on vagal nerve function or gastric emptying. The incidence and severity of complications observed with this procedure have steadily declined with the introduction of guidewire-

directed placement of the Stretta catheter, intense physician training, careful patient selection, provision and adherence to post-treatment guidelines, and standardized post-treatment discharge instructions (including a Stretta card with emergency contacts). The complication rate after the Stretta procedure has been less than 0.6% since introduction of the new technology and 0.13% in the last 12 months.

Recommended Precautions

Operators should check the position if abnormal impedance/temperatures are observed, use correct balloon pressures, control mucosal temperature carefully, minimize balloon pull-back pressure, and avoid nasogastric tube placement for 1 month after the procedure.

Alternatives After Treatment Failure

In the U.S. open-label trial, 5% of the patients elected to undergo fundoplication 6 to 12 months after the Stretta procedure because of an incomplete response or recurrent symptoms. In each case, there was no evidence of extraesophageal tissue abnormality, and the antireflux operation was performed in a normal manner and without difficulty. Richards et al.[44] compared the outcome of patients who underwent the Stretta procedure and those who underwent laparoscopic fundoplication at 6 months and found a comparable and significant improvement in Quality of Life in Reflux and Dyspepsia (QOLRAD) questionnaire, Short Form-12

(SF-12), and pH scores in both groups. However, medication use was significantly less in patients who had surgery (97% versus 58% not taking PPIs). Both groups were highly satisfied with their procedure. A repeat Stretta procedure is not recommended.

Summary

The Stretta procedure is a promising new endoscopic treatment of GERD. It significantly improves GERD symptoms and quality of life while eliminating the need for PPIs in the majority of patients. RF augmentation of the LES is probably safe, it is well tolerated, and symptom control at 6 to 12 months is acceptable. The future for the Stretta procedure will depend on its durability in long-term follow-up, continued and improved safety, third-party reimbursement, and determination of cost-effectiveness.

SYNTHETIC IMPLANTS/INJECTIONS

History

In the early 1980s, several groups studied the effectiveness of injected collagen or Teflon paste for the treatment of GERD. Most agents were first tested at the urinary bladder neck for female incontinence. Early investigations for the treatment of GERD provided proof of concept and healing of esophagitis in a small number of patients. However, the results were short-lived because of absorption of the collagen and recurrence of symptoms. In addition to these bulk-forming implants, injection therapy with sclerosing agents that induce focal necrosis and fibrosis have similarly been tried. Sodium morrhuate was used in 15 refractory GERD patients, but after a year of follow-up, the authors concluded that the therapy was ineffective.[59]

More recently, various injectable or implantable nonabsorbable biopolymers have been studied. These inert biocompatible substances are easy to place in an outpatient setting under conscious sedation and include Plexiglas spheres in bovine collagen, ethylene vinyl alcohol (Enteryx), and an expandable hydrogel prosthesis (Gatekeeper).

Properties of an Ideal Implant

1. The agent must be in a solution or suspension with viscosity low enough to easily traverse a needle.
2. It must undergo morphologic change, from liquid to a solid or semisolid state, when injected into the LES region. Such changes might be brought about by multiple mechanisms, such as collagen crosslinking as a result of body temperature, swelling of implants by imbibing body water, or an inflammatory response with subsequent collagen entrapment of the implant.
3. The implant and its effects must be durable.
4. It must be able to withstand the physical and chemical forces at the GEJ and resist both dissolution and migration.

5. It must be free of serious side effects and be cost-effective.
6. It must be noncarcinogenic and nonimmunogenic.
7. It must be sterile.
8. The optimal site for placement must be known. The implant commonly flows 1 to 2 cm cephalad or caudad from the injection site.
9. The optimal volume for long-term efficacy must be known. This varies between implants and is still not standardized.

ENTERYX

Enteryx consists of a biocompatible polymer (8% wt/vol ethylene vinyl alcohol polymer [EVOH] with a radiopaque contrast agent dissolved in the organic liquid carrier dimethyl sulfoxide [DMSO]). On contact with tissues or body fluids after injection, the solvent, DMSO, rapidly diffuses and induces precipitation of the polymer (EVOH) as a spongy mass. The low viscosity of Enteryx before dissipation of DMSO permits injection through a 23- to 25-gauge needle. It is not biodegradable and has no antigenic properties. Neither migration through blood vessels or lymphatics nor prosthetic contraction after injection has been observed.[60]

The three components of Enteryx—EVOH, DMSO, and tantalum—have previously been used together medically as a vascular embolization agent and as a membrane for hemodialysis and plasmapheresis. DMSO has been used as a solvent in medical applications since 1964 and is commercially available as the first treatment for interstitial cystitis. Tantalum-impregnated vascular stents have been available for some time.

Patient Selection

Enteryx is a treatment with promise but, like other endoluminal therapies, is lacking objective supportive data. Patients must understand that the procedure is irreversible.[61] Possible future indications for Enteryx include primary therapy for GERD in patients who respond to PPIs but prefer not to take medications daily, salvage therapy for PPI responders to reduce or eliminate daily medications, and salvage therapy for surgical failures.[61]

Enteryx therapy is clearly contraindicated in any individual who does not have physiologically documented GERD by pH study or endoscopic findings. It is also contraindicated in individuals who cannot undergo or tolerate endoscopy and those who have esophageal varices. There is no reported experience with this procedure in individuals with esophageal motility disorders, previous gastric or GERD surgery, scleroderma, Barrett's esophagus, hiatal hernias larger than 3 cm, or a body mass index greater than 35 or in patients who use anticoagulants other than aspirin.[62]

Procedure

The procedure is performed in an endoscopy suite equipped with fluoroscopy. Patients fast overnight and upper endoscopy is performed under conscious seda-

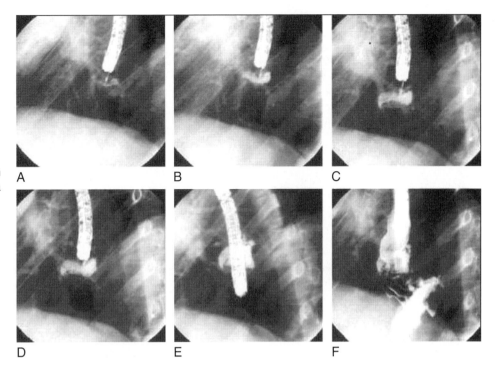

Figure 21–11. Enteryx injection under fluoroscopic control with a resultant prosthetic cuff.

tion. A long-needle catheter is filled with Enteryx after it has been flushed with DMSO to keep it liquefied as long as it stays within the catheter. The prepared injection needle is deployed and advanced into the muscularis propria at the appropriate level of the esophageal wall. The prosthesis is injected at a rate no greater than 1 ml/sec under combined fluoroscopic and endoscopic guidance (Fig. 21–11). The EVOH solidifies within the esophageal wall as the generated heat causes DMSO to dissipate. The injection is stopped if either submucosal or transmural injection is observed. Submucosal accumulation of material is seen endoscopically as a black bulge, and an extramural injection is demonstrated on fluoroscopy as either flow of material beyond the muscularis into the mediastinum or the abdominal cavity or lack of a visible deposit in the esophageal wall. If a circumlinear transverse path of material is visualized under fluoroscopy, the injection is completed at this site with a total of 1 to 2 ml. The procedure is considered satisfactory if 6 to 8 ml of Enteryx is delivered to the muscularis propria circumferentially without a submucosal or transmural injection. After the injection is complete at one site, the needle remains in place for 20 seconds to allow the material to stabilize and solidify and avoid leakage of the prosthesis into the esophageal lumen. Patients are usually discharged 2 to 4 hours after recovery.

Robert et al. reported Enteryx implantation in five pigs without the use of fluoroscopy. Enteryx was consistently deposited into the deep esophageal wall with a high degree of accuracy in a minimal amount of time. Placement was accurate in 85% and was transmural in just one instance. A human trial is under way to confirm these findings.[62]

Histologic Changes

Both gross and histologic examination in animals has shown that the implants persist as encapsulated, firm, smooth, slightly mobile ovoid masses several weeks after implantation. No evidence of pathologic inflammatory changes in the surrounding tissues has been observed.

Efficacy

Enteryx implantation significantly improves quality-of-life scores and medication use.[60,61] No change has been seen in the severity of esophagitis at endoscopy after Enteryx implantation. In general, the structural characteristics of the LES, including its length and pressure, are not altered significantly. Pooled results are shown in Table 21–4.

The 2-year follow-up results of the U.S. multicenter trial, which included 85 patients, were recently published[64] and showed PPI use to be eliminated in 74% of patients at 6-month follow-up. This effect was maintained in 64% of subjects at 2 years, whereas 74% were maintained on less than half their baseline PPI dosage. The improvement in symptom scores was 82% at 6 months and 70% at 2 years. Quality-of-life (SF-36) questionnaires demonstrated an improvement of 6% from baseline at 3 months and 3% at 12 months for the mental score, whereas the improvement in physical score was maintained at 12% at both 6- and 12-month follow-up. pH scores improved with 30% normalization, and there was a small but significant LES length augmentation (1 cm) after therapy.[65] No significant change in LESP was observed. The absence of change in LES resting pressure contrasts with findings from the pilot study, in which a

Table 21–4 Enteryx: Pooled Data

Variable		≥1 mo		≥3 mo		≥6 mo		≥12 mo		≥24 mo	
GERD-HRQL improvement		—		—		83%	(300)	70%	(300)	73%	(64)
Heartburn improvement		75%	(444)	81%	(441)	82%	(511)	71%	(583)	74%	(1985)
Regurgitation improvement		83%	(144)	91%	(141)	87%	(211)	77%	(283)	—	
Patients completely off PPIs		—		81%	(85)	76%	(412)	72%	(393)	65%	(106)
Patients with ≥50% reduction in PPI use		98%	(85)	91%	(141)	89%	(112)	80%	(93)	74%	(106)
Improvement in quality-of-life scores	SF-36 Physical	—		—		12%	(81)	12%	(74)	—	
	SF-36 Mental	—		—		6%	(81)	3%	(74)	—	
	QOLRAD	88%	(22)	85%	(15)	72%	(22)	—		—	
LESP improvement		—		—		NS	(81)	NS	(74)	—	
LES length improvement		—		—		33%	(81)	NS	(74)	—	
tLESR improvement		No									
Improvement in pH scores	Total time pH <4	—		—		27%	(101)	33%	(159)	—	
	Time upright pH <4	—		—		14%	(71)	37%	(261)	—	
	Time supine pH <4	—		—		NS	(71)	50%	(81)	—	
	Number of episodes	—		—		34%	(71)	31%	(160)	—	
	pH normalization	—		—		37%	(71)	38%	(195)	—	
Healing of esophagitis		—		—		—		—		—	
Residual implant volume		—		75%	(81)	—		—		—	
Re-treatment		—		18%	(44)	—		—		—	

All results displayed are significant. Numbers in parentheses are the numbers of patients studied to obtain the result.

GERD, gastroesophageal reflux disease; HRQL, health-related quality of life; LES, lower esophageal sphincter; LESP, LES pressure; NS, change not significant; PPI, proton pump inhibitor; QOLRAD, Quality of Life in Reflux and Dyspepsia questionnaire; SF-36, Short Form-36; tLESR, transient LES relaxation; —, data not available.

Pooled data were obtained from references 64-70.

significant increase in the LESP was observed at 6 months. This may have been due to the inclusion of patients with normal LESP at baseline or the smaller sample size in the pilot study. Importantly, most of the decline in treatment responders during follow-up occurred between 1 and 6 months. Between 6 and 12 months, the proportion of treatment responders remained stable. There was no evidence that the reduction in PPI use after the implant procedure was due to medication shifting.

The decline in residual implant volume seen after 1 month was attributable to sloughing of superficially implanted material until encapsulation was complete. There was no radiographic evidence of implant migration and after 3 months the residual volume remained stable ($P > .1$).[66] Twenty-two percent of patients were re-treated at the 3-month follow-up, 63% of whom improved at the 12-month follow-up, with 58% of patients not taking any PPIs and 5% reducing their PPI use by more than 50% of baseline.[65]

Multicenter randomized controlled sham trials with a "crossover" option starting at 3 months after randomization are currently under way in both Europe and the United States.[71] The European study design is shown in Figure 21–12. An interim report on 56 of the 64 total European patients has been announced with 3 months of follow-up. An improvement in GERD health-related quality of life (HQRL) was seen in 65% of patients in the

Enteryx arm versus 21% in the sham arm. The median change in symptom scores was 15 for the Enteryx group and 4 for the sham group. There was also a greater reduction in PPI use (64% versus 33%) and a lower crossover/re-treatment incidence (21% versus 71%) in the Enteryx group than in the sham group. Criteria for both crossover (for controls) and re-treatment (for the Enteryx group) were the same—an off-PPI HQRL score greater than 15.[71]

Johnson et al. reported that the likelihood of a successful clinical outcome is higher with more residual implant volume.[66] They showed that all patients who retained 5 ml of implant material eliminated or reduced PPI use by 50% and that the majority of subjects who retained more than 5 ml of Enteryx achieved a GERD-HRQL score of less than 15. Lehman et al. reported the procedure to be equally effective irrespective of the radiologic pattern evident at the time of implantation.[72] In a study evaluating predictors of outcome for Enteryx, Deviere et al.[73] showed that there was no statistically significant difference in PPI use or pH outcome by gender, but that GERD-HRQL symptom scores were significantly more likely to improve in males (86%; 57/66) than in females (67%; 32/48) ($P = .01$). Finally, Ganz et al. compared the endoscopic findings of patients from the multicenter study at 1-year follow-up with their baseline values (while taking PPIs) and reported that treatment with Enteryx provided improvement in esophagitis

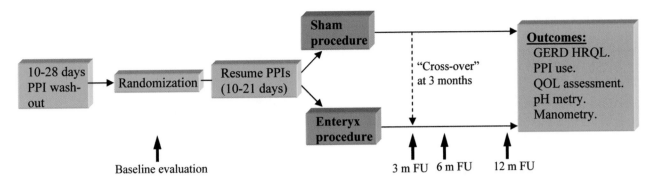

Figure 21–12. Enteryx sham study design. FU, follow-up; GERD, gastroesophageal reflux disease; HRQL, health-related quality of life; PPI, proton pump inhibitor; QOL, quality of life.

scores comparable to that provided by PPI medication.[74,75] This finding, however, has not been supported by other studies.

Complications

Complications are shown in Table 21–7. Recently, one death was reported in a patient as a result of inadvertent injection of Enteryx into the aorta. Further details are not yet available. Two patients experienced pericardial effusion after injection of the prosthesis and subsequently underwent a pericardial window procedure. A pleural effusion developed in two additional patients, but no other problems were recognized.

Recommended Precautions

All operators are required to receive hands-on laboratory training before clinical use. Injection techniques under fluoroscopic control are emphasized, and guidelines for prosthesis preparation are given. Most centers place patients on a liquid diet, followed by a soft diet the day of the procedure and then a normal diet the day after. Maintenance therapy with PPIs is continued for 10 to 14 days after implantation.

Summary

The procedure is uncomplicated and probably safe. Preliminary data are encouraging, although the pH normalization rate and LESP results are similar to those of other endoluminal procedures. Further follow-up is needed, but the present data suggest sustainable efficacy in patients requiring chronic maintenance therapy; however, re-treatment is often necessary. Subsequent to this writing, Boston Scientific withdrew the Enteryx procedure due to further procedural complications. Nevertheless, the lessons learned from this injection form of therapy remain valuable.

GATEKEEPER

Gatekeeper is a dehydrated hydrogel prosthesis implanted into the submucosa of the cardia/LES. It hydrates to 6 × 15-mm cylinder-shaped soft pliable cushions and is removable by endoscopy.[76]

Patient Selection

In addition to the general selection criteria already described, patients with esophageal varices, a peptic stricture, and morbid obesity were excluded from the trials for Gatekeeper.

Procedure

The Gatekeeper device consists of an overtube with separate channels for passage of an endoscope and a long delivery sheath. The overtube is inserted with the patient under conscious sedation. The injection capsule is placed through the overtube to straddle the squamocolumnar junction. A vacuum is created to stabilize the device and to draw the mucosa in. The injection needle is advanced into the submucosa, followed by the injection of 3 to 6 ml of sterile saline until blanching is observed. This is followed by removal of the injection needle and advancement of the needle assembly and delivery sheath into the mucosa, with the delivery sheath left in the submucosal plane. After the needle assembly has been retracted, the prosthesis is inserted into the proximal end of the delivery sheath and advanced to the submucosal level with a pushrod assembly. Up to six hydrogel implants are placed. The implants are small and "sliver"-like when introduced but swell to full size within 24 hours when hydrated. The procedure is shown in Figure 21–13.

Efficacy

In a limited number of patients, the Gatekeeper procedure has been shown to significantly decrease heartburn, improve quality of life and 24-hour pH-metry scores, and decrease medication use.[77] The success rate for implantation is 93%, whereas the procedural success rate was reported at 98.7%.[78] Pooled results for the Gatekeeper are shown in Table 21–5.

After completion of a 6-month pilot study[80] with favorable results, a European multicenter study was initiated.[79] Patients underwent manometry, endoscopy, 24-hour pH-metry, and symptom scoring before and after the proce-

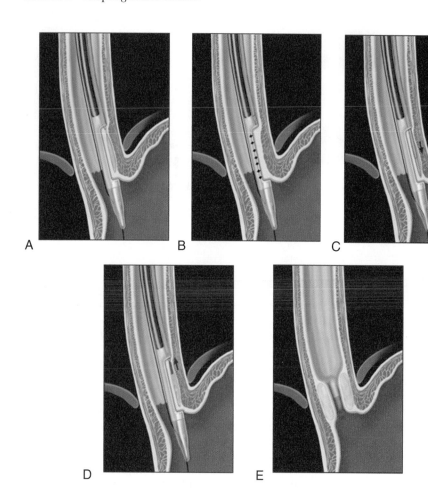

A   B   C

D   E

Figure 21–13.   A to **E,** Gatekeeper procedure.

Table 21–5   Gatekeeper: Pooled Results

Variable		≥1 mo		≥3 mo		≥6 mo	
GERD-HRQL improvement		65%	(55)	65%	(92)	74%	(91)
Regurgitation improvement		81%	(55)	94%	(49)	87%	(49)
Patients completely off PPIs		—		—		58%	(42)
Patients with ≥50% reduction in PPI use		—		—		54%	(67)
Improvement in quality-of-life scores	SF-36 Physical	16%	(61)	19%	(57)	17%	(57)
	SF-36 Mental	3%	(61)	8%	(57)	1%	(57)
LESP improvement		NS	(12)	16%	(78)	36%	(78)
LES length improvement		NS	(12)	—		NS	(78)
Improvement in pH scores	Total time pH <4	NS	(12)	10%*	(11)	32%*	(58)
	Time upright pH <4	—		NS	(27)	45%	(45)
	Time supine pH <4	—		NS	(27)	70%	(45)
	Number of episodes	—		42%	(27)	45%	(45)
	pH normalization	—		—		40%	(45)
Healing of esophagitis		58%	(62)	39%	(37)	45%	(53)
Residual plications		84%	(81)	73%	(69)	71%	(86)
Re-treatment		—		—		16%	(701)

The results expressed in the majority of studies are shown here. Numbers in parentheses are the numbers of patients studied to obtain the result.

*Signifies disagreement among studies.

GERD, gastroesophageal reflux disease; HRQL, health-related quality of life; LES, lower esophageal sphincter; LESP, LES pressure; NS, change not significant; PPI, proton pump inhibitor; SF-36, Short Form-36; —, data not available.

Pooled data were obtained from references 77-79.

dure. The average number of prostheses implanted was 4.3 (2 to 6). The final results showed significant improvement in symptom scores (HRQL score from 24 to 5), quality of life, pH parameters (percent time pH <4, 9.1% to 6.1%), and LESP (8.8 to 13.8 mm Hg) at 6 months.[78] The prosthesis retention rate was 70% at 6 months. Other studies with smaller numbers of patients have failed to demonstrate significant improvement in LESP; however, symptom scores and pH results show consistent improvement.[77,79]

An international, multicenter, randomized sham-controlled Gatekeeper trial has recently commenced.[81] Patients with symptomatic GERD requiring PPI therapy with evidence of GERD on 24-hour pH study and a symptom score greater than 20 while not taking medications are being included in the study. Up to eight implants will be placed circumferentially in the distal LES/cardia, with re-treatment offered to individuals if GERD symptoms persist. The initial 25 patients were lead-in–phase nonrandomized subjects, whereas the next 100 are to be randomized by sealed envelope at a ratio of 2 : 1 implant versus sham. Patients will take antisecretory medications on an as-needed basis.

Complications

The complications reported at 6-month follow-up are shown in Table 21–7.[78] In the largest multicenter study, severe complications developed in 2 of 40 patients (5%), including esophageal perforation caused by overtube placement and severe postprandial nausea (1 week after the procedure) leading to endoscopic removal of the prosthesis at 3 weeks.[78]

Advantages

The Gatekeeper prosthesis is removable by endoscopic means. A needle knife can be used to incise over the edge of the implant, which is then suctioned from its submucosal pocket.[76] Endoscopic ultrasound may be used for exact localization of the prosthesis. Of note, one of the two patients who had the prostheses removed did so 7 months after the procedure. All three prostheses were removed in the other patient 3 weeks after the procedure. No complication was encountered with either patient.

Summary

The Gatekeeper system is a safe and reversible procedure with acceptable to good prosthesis retention. Early results show efficacy on GERD-HRQL, SF-36, and pH monitoring. Many questions still remain unanswered, including its mechanism of action, durability, long-term safety, and placebo effect. A multicenter, randomized, sham-controlled study was initiated. However, the sponsoring company discontinued commercialization due to inefficacy.

PLEXIGLAS

A trial of gelatinous Plexiglas (polymethylmethacrylate [PMMA]) microsphere implants has been published by Feretis et al.[82] A mean volume of 32 ml was implanted submucosally, 1 to 2 cm proximal to the squamocolumnar junction, in 10 patients with a 21-gauge needle. Transient dysphagia was noted in one patient because of excessive implant volume. At a mean follow-up of 7.2 months, there was significant improvement in GERD-related symptoms and 24-hour pH studies (decreased from 24.5 to 7.2), but pH normalization was not seen. Ninety percent of patients were not taking any PPIs at 6-month follow-up. The procedure was found to be safe at short-term follow-up.

Minor and self-limited complications occurred in 4 of 10 patients (40%). Transient dysphagia and gas-bloating syndrome (10%) were thought to be due to excessive treatment with an implantation volume of 39 ml. Plexiglas injection was not associated with local or systemic complications and is not antigenic. PMMA is highly viscous, and therefore an endoscope with a larger biopsy channel that accommodates a large-caliber catheter was used for implantation. Longer follow-up studies are needed.[82] A multicenter study is currently being planned.

GENERAL OVERVIEW

The end points studied in most of the trials are GERD symptoms scores (HRQL), medication use, manometric findings, grade of esophagitis, and 24-hour pH study results. In general, the procedures are safe, with 3 deaths in 9000 to 10,000 cases. At present, the overall complication rates reported for ELGP, the Stretta procedure, Enteryx, and Gatekeeper are 11%, 6%, 6.7%, and 15%, respectively.[78] There is evidence of symptomatic relief with decreased medication use, but failure of an increase in LES length and pressure, healing of esophagitis, and improvement in pH scores. A cost analysis of PPI versus endotherapy for GERD is shown in Figure 21–14. A comparison of the results at 1-year follow-up for all procedures is shown in Table 21–6. An overview of the different endotherapies for GERD is shown in Table 21–7. A comparison of results in patients with EndoCinch, the Stretta procedure, and Enteryx at various follow-up intervals is also depicted in graphic format (Figs. 21–15 to 21–18).

Information on broader clinical applications, a possible spectrum of specific indications, and long-term results regarding the safety, endurance, and outcomes of these procedures has herein been reported. However, long-term efficacy, durability, and therapy-specific patient selection have yet to be elucidated inasmuch as the present literature consists of few publications, most of which are nonrandomized and have small numbers of patients, significant dropout rates, and lack of agreement on end points. To further confuse the issues, most of the larger studies are industry sponsored, and the results are often based on patients who underwent the procedure during the investigator's learning curve. The sham-controlled trials to date have been nonsupportive. The

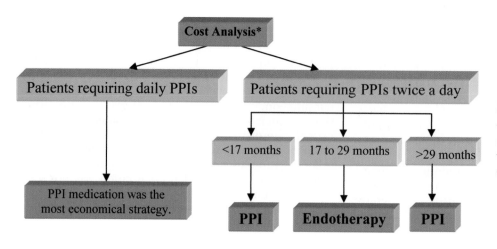

Figure 21–14. Cost analysis of proton pump inhibitor (PPI) therapy versus endotherapy in the treatment of gastroesophageal reflux disease. *Provided endotherapy failure rates remain greater than 20%.

Table 21–6   Endotherapy Result Comparisons: Pooled Data

Trial Results		ELGP	NDO Plicator	Stretta	Enteryx	Gatekeeper*
HDQRL improvement		55%	70%	65%	70%	74%*
Heartburn improvement		74%	—	61%	71%	—
Off PPIs	At 1 yr	40%	75%	55%	72%	58%*
	At >2 yr	33%	—	63%	65%	—
≥50% reduction in PPIs		51%	—	67%	80%	54%*
Quality-of-life improvement	SF-36 Physical	17%	31%	20%	12%	17%*
	SF-36 Mental	None	10%	14%	3%	1.4%*
Time pH <4: improvement		16%[†]	None	36%	33%	32%*
No. of reflux episode: improvement		33%[†]	—	None	31%	45%*
pH normalization		25%[†]	—	—	38%	40%*
LESP improvement		None	None	None[†]	None	None[†]
LES length improvement		None	None	None	None[†]	None
tLESR improvement		Yes	No	Yes	No	No
Healing of esophagitis		None	None	None	None	None
Sham trial		3-mo FU	Being planned	1-yr FU	Under way	Under way

All results are at 1-year follow-up except Gatekeeper. All results are statistically significant.
*Six-month follow-up data.
[†]Indicates controversy regarding results, but the results presented are the ones shown by the majority of studies.
ELGP, endoluminal gastroplication; FU, follow-up; HDRQL, Heartburn Dysphagic Regurgitation Quality of Life Score; LES, lower esophageal sphincter; LESP, LES pressure; None, change not statistically significant; PPI, proton pump inhibitor; SF-36, Short Form-36; tLESR, transient LES relaxation; —, not available.

Stretta sham trial provided unimpressive data, and the ELGP study was underpowered. Other sham trials are under way or in the planning stage.

PHYSIOLOGIC/ANATOMIC MECHANISMS OF ENDOLUMINAL THERAPIES

In the early stages of disease and in the absence of a hiatal hernia, the geometry and integrity of the cardia are normal. However, in the interprandial period and during periods of gastric stress, such as after meals, gastric distention alters the anatomy and makes the sphincter incompetent, probably because of sphincter shortening, which some term tLESS.[83] Such patients appear to be the ideal population for endoscopic antireflux procedures. LES dysfunction may also be caused by a loss of LES resistance that prevents it from serving as an effective reflux barrier, but this mechanism is seen only in more advanced GERD patients.

Most investigators believe that both the LES complex and the angle of His are crucial in the prevention of GERD. An understanding of the muscle fibers that form and maintain these structures anatomically might provide additional insight into the endoscopic treatment of GERD. Liebermann et al., in a carefully performed study, described the architecture of the GEJ musculature.[4] An oblique "ring" where muscular thickness is

| Table 21–7 | Procedure Characteristics and Complications: Pooled Data |

Variables		EndoCinch	NDO Plicator	Stretta	Enteryx	Gatekeeper
Procedure duration (mean)		68 min	20 min	69 min	33 min	35-60 min
Personnel required		1 physician and 2 assistants	1 physician and 2 assistants	1 physician and 2 assistants	1 physician and 2 assistants	1 physician and 2-3 assistants
Sedation required		Conscious sedation in 82%	NA	Conscious sedation in 100%	Conscious sedation in 100%	NA
Approximate no. of procedures performed		4000	200	4000	2600	225
Major complications	Perforation	0.075%	0.5%	0.125%	0%	0.4%
	Bleeding	0.05%	NA	0.05%	0%	0%
	Hypoxemia	0.075%	0%	0%	0%	0%
	Pleural effusion	0%	0%	0.025%	0.076%	0%
	Pericardial effusion	0%	0%	0%	0.076%	0%
	Aspiration pneumonia	0%	0%	0.05%	0%	0%
	Esophageal abscess	0%	0%	0%	0.038%	0%
	Ulceration over prostheses	0%	0%	0%	0%	0.4%
	Death	0%	0%	0.05%	0.038%	0%
Minor complications		Sore throat (0.35%) Chest soreness (0.17%) Abdominal pain (0.15%) Bloating (0.02%) Transient dysphagia (0.05%) Bronchospasm (0.01%)	NA	Superficial mucosal injury Burn at pad site (0.02%) Transient atrial fibrillation (0.02%) Bloating (0.02%) Gastroparesis and ulcerative esophagitis (0.02%) Low-grade fever Transient dysphagia Transient chest pain Topical anesthesia-related complications (e.g., allergy, hypotension)	Garlic odor for several hours (because of DMSO) Chest pain (82%) Transient dysphagia (13%) Belching/burping Bloating/flatulence Fever	Sore throat (15%) Chest pain (5%) Nausea/vomiting (0.8%) Erosive duodenitis (0.8%) Retrosternal pain (0.4%) Poor sleep (0.4%) Abdominal pain (0.4%) Rash (0.4%) Cough (0.4%)

Complications were obtained from pooled data.
DMSO, dimethyl sulfoxide; NA, not available.

maximal corresponds to the proximal most aspect of the gastric mucosal folds (see Fig. 21–1). This increase in thickness was attributed to an increase in the muscle mass of the inner circular muscle layer. On the lesser curvature side, these muscle bundles split to form semicircular short transverse "clasp" fibers above the gastroesophageal (GE) ring, whereas on the greater curvature side, they spread out as long oblique "sling" fibers. The direction of fibers suggests that the clasp fibers are more likely to contribute more to the barrier effect at the GEJ because the sling fibers are in fact almost parallel to the lesser curvature. As the GE ring is approached, both clasp and sling fibers increase in density and those in the outer coat remain unchanged. These site-specific changes in muscle density suggest that the inner circular ring plays a principal role in maintaining competence at

the GEJ whereas the outer layer may be suitable for a more generalized process such as gastric motility.

When the muscular contraction forces being exerted at the GEJ are represented by vectors, one vector is directed transversely from the angle of His toward the lesser curvature (clasp fiber vector) and the other is almost parallel to the lesser curvature (sling fiber vector). The resultant vector obtained is directed obliquely toward the lesser curvature and is parallel to the GE ring outlined by Liebermann et al. (see Fig. 21–1C). The GE ring appears to be the site of maximal resistance to the reflux of gastric contents inasmuch as the cross-sectional thickness of the muscle correlates with increased force of contraction/pressure generated within the lumen, assuming a solid pressure model. The GE ring is oblique, being higher on the greater curvature side, and is thickest posterolaterally.

Endoluminal Gastroplasty

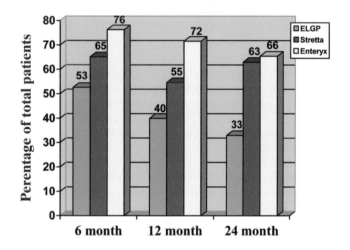

Figure 21–15. Percentage of total patients not taking proton pump inhibitors (PPIs) 6, 12, and 24 months after endoluminal gastroplication (ELGP), Stretta, and Enteryx procedures. All changes are significant when compared with baseline. Pooled data were obtained from references 18–24, 44, 46, 49, 50, 52, 54, 57, 65, 68, 70.

EndoCinch therapy has been shown to reduce distal esophageal acid exposure, but it does not eliminate it. The symptomatic improvement can be explained by a lower volume of refluxate reaching the more "sensitive" proximal esophagus. The decreased volume may correspond with a decreased frequency of tLESSs or tLESRs and failure to completely abolish them.

The mechanism by which ELGP improves competence of the GEJ remains unclear. Feitoza et al. demonstrated lack of fusion between the folds when sutures were placed intraluminally in the stomach of rabbits, irrespective of suture depth.[15] The degree of fibrosis, however, increases as the depth increases and is maximal with incorporation of the serosa. Endoscopic manipulation of mucosa before suture placement when performing electrocautery or mucosal resection has improved postoperative tissue healing.[84] ELGP may decrease tLESSs by scar formation.

Secondary scarring may impair the distensibility of the proximal stomach and may also affect neural pathways,

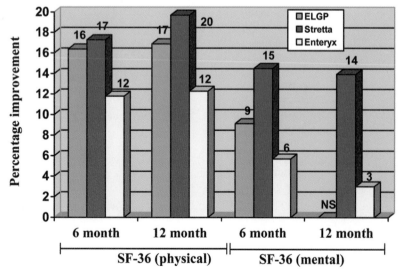

Figure 21–16. Improvement in quality-of-life scores (Short Form-36 [SF-36]), both physical and mental, at 6- and 12-month follow-up intervals after endoluminal gastroplication (ELGP), Stretta, and Enteryx procedures. NS, not significant. All other changes are significant when compared with baseline. Pooled data were obtained from references 17, 20, 50, 51, 52, 57, 65, 66.

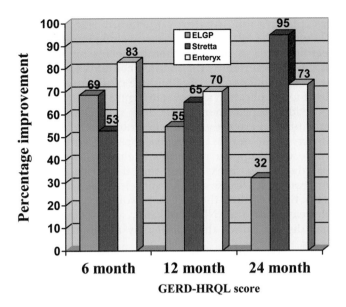

Figure 21–17. Degree of symptomatic improvement at 6-, 12-, and 24-month follow-up intervals after endoluminal gastroplication (ELGP), Stretta, and Enteryx procedures. All changes are significant when compared with baseline. GERD, gastroesophageal reflux disease; HRQL, health-related quality of life. Pooled data were obtained from references 17-22, 24, 25, 46, 50-52, 57, 58, 64, 65, 67-69.

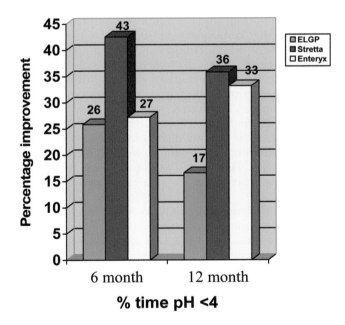

Figure 21–18. Improvement in the percentage of time that the pH is less than 4 at 6- and 12-month follow-up after endoluminal gastroplication (ELGP), Stretta, and Enteryx procedures. Only studies showing significant improvement in pH scores are considered. Pooled data were obtained from references 17, 20, 26, 44, 50, 52, 57, 65, 67, 69.

thereby reducing the rate of tLESRs and tLESSs. Such scar formation, when combined with the fact that ELGP has been shown to result in localized circular muscle hypertrophy in both humans and animals,[16] should lead to increased basal tensile strength and increased resistance to gastric distention.

ELGP increases smooth muscle thickness, but in an indirect fashion. Muscle inclusion within a plication has not been shown with ELGP; thus, muscularis propria gathering occurs rarely, if at all. Tissue apposition is initially realized secondary to mucosal/submucosal gathering, but it dissipates as a result of the lack of mucosal healing and the suture cheese wire effect (the suture seesawing with time through the tissue). The later is presumably caused by peristalsis and additional stressors such as food passage, belching, and vomiting. The scar formation and muscle hypertrophy seen with the current techniques and available devices are not durable and are therefore unable to reduce distal esophageal inflammatory changes and large-volume acid reflux. More strategically placed deeper plications may improve the results. Sling fiber gathering/hypertrophy is less likely to reduce GERD because the number of plications necessary is probably excessive for the technology available. Such may not be the case, however, for the lesser curvature and the underlying clasp fibers. Placement of plications on the GE ring will create hypertrophy apparently in the ideal location, but the exact location of the ring is not possible to identify endoscopically. To be sure of superimposition of plications on the ring, stitches should be applied along the lesser curvature because it is easily identified and close approximation of the capsule to the gastric wall is possible in this location. Placement of plications on the greater curvature is only technically possible 1 cm below the squamocolumnar junction. It is unsafe to go more proximally because suture perforation is more likely and the stomach flairs out more distally, thus making it impossible to place plications accurately since the endoscope with capsule will not work in the retroflexed position. More distally in the antegrade position, the capsule is placed remote from the target area in a partially distended stomach. With this remote position comes inaccuracy because it is impossible to reliably pull in a target area. Plications placed anteriorly or posteriorly are very often difficult to localize for the same reason and certainly do not easily correspond to the obliquity of the GE ring. In Figure 21–19A we propose plications that are more ideally placed to support (create hypertrophy of) the gastroesophageal ring, nature's anatomic point of apparent failure, and to reinforce the important clasp fibers. An additional linear row along the lesser curvature may make this approach the preferred endoscopic technique.

NDO Plicator

The degree of postprocedure inflammatory changes and fibrosis should be greater with a full-thickness plication. Feitoza et al.[15] showed maximal fibrosis with incorporation of serosa in the plication when compared with other depths of suture plication. The retention

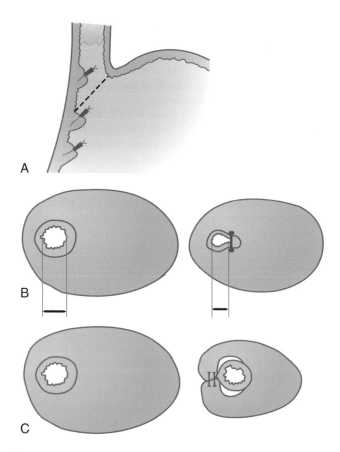

Figure 21–19. A, Anterior view of plications overlying the clasp fibers and reinforcing the gastroesophageal ring. **B,** Cross-sectional representation of the gastric lumen before and after the NDO plicator is applied. The plication may strangulate some of the sling fibers on the greater curvature side of the gastroesophageal junction but does decrease the esophageal lumen as indicated by the measurement lines. **C,** Schematic drawing of a Syntheon plication. The underlying clasp fibers may or may not be involved by the plication.

rate for sutures and thus the durability of results should also improve. Lengthening of the intra-abdominal segment of the LES[40] is expected with this technique.

It is our opinion that the full-thickness plication should be placed on the lesser curvature side of the GEJ. In this circumstance, the underlying clasp fiber forces would be reinforced rather than distracted (see Fig. 21–1) as when placing the plication on the greater curvature side of the GEJ. The bottom of the thickened LES and the angle of His are both augmented with the NDO plication, but the overall results of the procedure speak to either insufficient numbers of plications or anatomic/physiologic flaw. Further testing with more plications per patient appears to be in order. The new Syntheon plicator, which places the plication on the lesser curvature side, will also assist in further determining where the full-thickness plications should be applied. The NDO and Syntheon plicators are similar in that they both place a full-thickness U stitch, although the former places it on the greater curvature side of the GEJ and the Syntheon

can place it on the lesser curvature side (see Fig. 21–19C). The NDO plicator decreases the internal cross-sectional area of the GEJ, thereby decreasing the pressure being exerted by the luminal contents on the wall, but it may functionally disable some of the muscle fibers distal to the plication as shown in Figure 21–19B. Perhaps more ideal is placement of the deep suture on the lesser curvature, where presumably the anterior and posterior aspects of the fundus are opposed, as in Figure 21–19B. There would appear to be less likelihood of gathering and disrupting the GE ring, and if the inflammatory process is the cause of the muscle hypertrophy, the clasp fibers within the GE ring would be reinforced, whereas with the NDO plicator, the force applied may disrupt rather than ultimately augment the sling fibers.

Stretta Procedure

The unanticipated disparity between symptomatic improvement and acid exposure seen in the sham trial was surprising because acid exposure was expected to be less responsive to a sham effect than either symptom scores or medication use.[51] Previous multicenter studies have shown the contrary. This might be explained by the known poor correlation between GERD symptoms and 24-hour pH monitoring in so far as symptomatic improvement can occur with only slight variations in acid exposure. To explore this discrepancy, patients in the sham trial were divided into responders and nonresponders, depending on their symptomatic improvement. It was found that responders significantly improved their acid exposure when compared with nonresponders, which suggested that decreased acid exposure was accountable for at least part of the symptom improvement in the active treatment group. Alternative explanations proposed in the trial were a residual sham effect on symptoms or altered visceral sensitivity.[51] The later would explain the striking dichotomy between symptom relief and minimal to moderate improvement in acid reflux profiles. Diminished sensitivity may be due to destruction of chemosensitive or mechanosensitive nerve endings.[9]

The underlying mechanism of effect may be explained by multiple changes. First, mechanical alteration and thickening of the LES musculature probably lead to diminished reflux, as shown in the canine model.[48] Second, the progressive tissue remodeling and scar formation observed after the Stretta procedure may contribute to the decreased compliance and increased tensile strength of the GEJ, which also exerts its effect in decreasing tLESRs. This decrease in tLESRs has been shown in both animals and humans.[48,57]

Torquati et al. effectively addressed concerns about the durability of the procedure by reporting significant improvement in symptom scores, PPI use, and patient satisfaction at a mean follow-up of 27 months.[54] This study contradicts the contention that symptomatic improvement with the Stretta procedure is due to desensitization of the esophageal mucosa with a resultant decrease in PPI use but increased mucosal injury as a result of acid exposure. This was done by showing significant improvement in pH results at 27 months in patients who had responded to therapy. In light of this study, the durability of the procedure might be further increased by strict patient selection and inclusion of only patients who respond to PPIs before the procedure.

Although ablation of vagal afferent pathways of the reflex arc leading to decreased tLESRs has been proposed as a possible mechanism, studies of the pancreatic polypeptide response to sham feeding revealed normal responses, which suggests preservation of the vagal afferents.[49] Moreover, no microscopic or macroscopic evidence of damage to the vagus nerves has been demonstrated thus far except for a porcine model that showed destruction of enteric neural elements after treatment.[43] Delayed gastric emptying occurs in up to 25% of GERD patients and has been shown to improve after Nissen fundoplication. Recently, a study has suggested improvement in gastric emptying after the Stretta procedure, with 93% patients showing significant improvement and 83% complete normalization of gastric emptying.[85] This, in part, might contribute to the efficacy of the Stretta procedure.

Enteryx

Animal studies have shown a significant difference in yield pressure and yield volume with a raised threshold for transient relaxations after Enteryx injection.[86] Animal model findings verify this by showing that Enteryx undergoes fibrous encapsulation without a prolonged active inflammatory response.[86] The fibrous encapsulation may functionally lengthen the LES. The encapsulation/scarring is the probable mechanism of effect, but because the prostheses are placed high in the GEJ and scar formation is dependent on an unreliable distribution of the foreign body, this procedure requires further technical refinement.

The mechanism of action of Enteryx implantation in humans remains to be fully characterized. Enteryx injected circumferentially within and along the muscle layers of the LES incites a localized foreign body reaction and an acute inflammatory response leading to fibrous encapsulation of the Enteryx. Such encapsulation results in decreased LES compliance and distensibility during periods of gastric distention, thus preventing inappropriate LES relaxation/shortening. The "bulking" effect seen with some injectable treatments of urinary incontinence is not apparent for Enteryx because follow-up endoscopy has revealed no evidence of luminal narrowing.

Johnson et al. suggested that the main reasons for an inadequate clinical outcome and lack of durability were either insufficient material injected into the LES or loss of the implant because of sloughing of superficially injected material.[66] They showed that the clinical outcome was associated with the amount of residual implant. Patients with a residual volume of 5 ml had a better symptomatic outcome and greater improvement in medication use.

Gatekeeper

The reasons for failure and success are probably similar to those of the Enteryx procedure, with the exception of bulking and dispersion. The prosthesis does narrow the lumen, even at 6 months' follow-up endoscopy, and is self-contained. The maximum number of prostheses that can be safely applied requires investigation and perhaps manufacturing refinements.

CONCLUSION

Endoluminal therapy is an emerging field with continued prospects that may lead to substantial changes in patient care; however, the goal of such therapy needs to be healing of esophagitis. All studies to date allow the use of PPIs, and most gauge success by the number of patients decreasing their PPI dosage and symptomatic improvement. Meaningful conclusions cannot be made in this instance.

The scientific community needs to wait for industry-independent trials showing endoscopic and 24-hour pH monitoring follow-up data that establish long-term efficacy and prolonged symptomatic benefit. Cost-effectiveness and continued documentation of complications will better define the "true" role of these procedures in the management of GERD patients.

SELECTED READINGS

Corley DA, Katz P, Wo JM, et al: Improvement of gastroesophageal reflux symptoms after radiofrequency energy: A randomized, sham-controlled trial. Gastroenterology 125:668, 2003.

Filipi CJ, Lehman GA, Rothstein RI, et al: Transoral, flexible endoscopic suturing for treatment of GERD: A multicenter trial. Gastrointest Endosc 53:416, 2001.

Johnson DA, Ganz R, Aisenberg J, et al: Endoscopic implantation of enteryx for treatment of GERD: 12-month results of a prospective, multicenter trial. Am J Gastroenterol 98:1921, 2003.

Liebermann MD, Allgower M, Schmid P, et al: Muscular equivalent of the lower esophageal sphincter. Gastroenterology 76:31, 1979.

Triadafilopoulos G, DiBaise JK, Nostrant TT, et al: The Stretta procedure for the treatment of GERD: 6 and 12 month follow-up of the U.S. open label trial. Gastrointest Endosc 55:149, 2002.

REFERENCES

1. Locke GR, Talley NJ, Fell SL, et al: Prevalence and clinical spectrum of gastroesophageal reflux: A population-based study in Olmsted County, Minnesota. Gastroenterology 112:1448, 1997.
2. Peters JH: A current assessment of endoluminal approaches to the treatment of GERD. Personal communication.
3. DeMeester TR, Peters JH, Bremner CG, et al: Biology of gastroesophageal reflux disease: Pathophysiology relating to medical and surgical treatment. Annu Rev Med 50:469, 1999.

4. Liebermann MD, Allgower M, Schmid P, et al: Muscular equivalent of the lower esophageal sphincter. Gastroenterology 76:31, 1979.

5. Straathof JW, Ringers J, Lamers CB, et al: Provocation of transient lower esophageal sphincter relaxations by gastric distension with air. Am J Gastroenterol 96:2317, 2001.

6. Massey BT: Potential control of gastroesophageal reflux by local modulation of transient lower esophageal sphincter relaxations. Am J Med 3:186S, 2001.

7. Hirsch DP, Mathus-Vliegen EM, Dagli U, et al: Effect of prolonged gastric distention on lower esophageal sphincter function and gastroesophageal reflux. Am J Gastroenterol 98:1696, 2003.

8. Kahrilas PJ: GERD pathogenesis, pathophysiology and clinical manifestations. Cleve Clin J Med 70(Suppl):S4, 2003.

9. Kahrilas PJ: Radiofrequency therapy of the lower esophageal sphincter for the treatment of GERD. Gastrointest Endosc 57:723, 2003.

10. Liebermann DA: Medical therapy for chronic reflux esophagitis: A long-term follow-up. Arch Intern Med 147:1717, 1987.

11. Fuchs KH, Freys SM: Endoscopic antireflux therapy. Surg Endosc 17:1009, 2003.

12. Mason RJ, Filipi CJ, DeMeester TR, et al: A new intraluminal antigastroesophageal reflux procedure in baboons. Gastrointest Endosc 45:283, 1997.

13. Kadirkamanathan SS, Evans DF, Gong F, et al: Antireflux operations at flexible endoscopy using endoluminal switching techniques: An experimental study. Gastrointest Endosc 44:133, 1996.

14. Horatogis A, Hieston K, Lehman G: Evaluation of supplemental cautery during endoluminal gastroplication for treatment of gastroesophageal reflux disease [abstract]. Paper presented at Digestive Disease Week, Orlando, Fla, May 18-21, 2003.

15. Feitoza AB, Gostout CJ, Rajan E, et al: Understanding endoluminal gastroplications: A histopathologic analysis of intraluminal suture plications. Gastrointest Endosc 57:868, 2003.

16. Liu JJ, Glickman JN, Carr-Locke DL, et al: Gastroesophageal junction smooth muscle remodeling after endoluminal gastroplication. Am J Gastroenterol 99:1895, 2004.

17. Filipi CJ, Lehman GA, Rothstein RI, et al: Transoral, flexible endoscopic suturing for treatment of GERD: A multicenter trial. Gastrointest Endosc 53:416, 2001.

18. Chen YK, Raijman I, Ben-Menachem T, et al: Long-term experience with endoluminal gastroplication (ELGP): Clinical and economic outcomes of the US multicenter trial. Gastrointest Endosc 57:690, 2003.

19. Mahmood Z, McMahon BP, Arfin Q, et al: Endocinch therapy for gastro-oesophageal reflux disease: A one year prospective follow-up. Gut 52:34, 2003.

20. Tam WC, Holloway RH, Dent J, et al: Impact of endoscopic suturing of the gastroesophageal junction on lower esophageal sphincter function and gastroesophageal reflux in patients with reflux disease. Am J Gastroenterol 99:195, 2004.

21. Liu JL, Knapp R, Silk J, et al: Treatment of medication refractory gastroesophageal reflux disease with endoluminal gastroplication [abstract]. Gastrointest Endosc 55:AB257, 2002.

22. Davis R, Filipi CJ, Gerhardt J: Comparison of endoluminal gastroplication configuration techniques [abstract]. Am J Gastroenterol 97(9):30, 2002.

23. Menachem T, Chen Y, Raijman I, et al: Symptom recurrence after endoluminal gastroplication for GERD: Comparison of initial versus repeat ELGP [abstract]. Gastointest Endosc 57(5):130, 2003.

24. Liu JJ, Carr-Locke DL, Lee LS, et al: Endoluminal gastroplication for treatment of patients with classic gastroesophageal reflux symptoms and borderline 24-h pH studies [abstract]. Scand J Gastroenterol 39:615, 2004.

25. Rothstein RI, Filipi CJ: Endoscopic suturing for gastroesophageal reflux disease: Clinical outcome with the Bard EndoCinch. Gastrointest Endosc Clin N Am 13:89, 2003.

26. Caca K, Schiefke I, Söder H, et al: Endoluminal gastroplication for gastroesophageal reflux disease. Gastrointest Endosc 55(5):M1888, 2002.

27. Swain P, Park PO, Kjellin T, et al: Endoscopic gastroplasty for gastroesophageal reflux disease [abstract]. Gastrointest Endosc 51(4):AB4470, 2000.

28. Rothstein RI, Hynes ML, Grove MR, et al: Endoscopic gastric plication for GERD: A randomized, sham-controlled, blinded, single-center study [abstract]. Gastrointest Endosc 59:AB111, 2004.

29. Martinez-Serna T, Davis RE, Mason R, et al: Endoscopic valvuloplasty for GERD. Gastrointest Endosc 52:663, 2000.

30. Hong D, Swanstrom L: Endoscopic plication as salvage procedure for failed surgical fundoplications in select patients [abstract]. Surg Endosc 17(Suppl 1):S222, 2003.

31. Pazwash H, Gualtieri NM, Starpoli A: Failed surgical fundoplication: A possible new indication for endoluminal gastroplication [abstract 646]. Am J Gastroenterol 97:S212, 2002.

32. Raijman I, Walters R, Garza C, et al: Helical endoluminal gastroplication (ELGP) compared to standard ELGP in patients with gastroesophageal reflux disease [abstract]. Gastrointest Endosc 55:AB260, 2002.

33. Liu JJ, Knapp RM, Saltzman JR, et al: Impact of anesthesiologist on endoluminal gastroplication (ELGP) procedure [abstract]. Am J Gastroenterol 97:AB932, S2002.

34. Velanovich V, Ben Menachem T: Laparoscopic Nissen fundoplication after failed endoscopic gastroplication. J Laparoendosc Adv Surg Tech A 12:305, 2002.

35. Tierney BJ, Iqbal A, Filipi CJ: Effects of prior endoluminal gastroplication on subsequent laparoscopic Nissen fundoplication. Surg Endosc (in press).

36. Wiersema MJ, Levy MJ: Cost analysis of endoscopic antireflux procedures: Endoluminal plication vs. radiofrequency coagulation vs. treatment with a proton pump inhibitor. Gastrointest Endosc 59:749, 2004.

37. Mahmood Z, Byrne PJ, McCullouch J, et al: A comparison of Bard Endocinch transoesophageal endoscopic plication (BETEP) with laparoscopic Nissen fundoplication (LNF) for the treatment of gastroesophageal reflux disease (GORD). Gastrointest Endosc 55:463, 2002.

38. Chadalavada R, Lin E, Swafford V, et al: Comparative results of endoluminal gastroplasty and laparoscopic antireflux surgery for the treatment of GERD. Surg Endosc 18:261, 2004.

39. Velanovich V, Ben-Menachem T, Goel S: Case-control comparison of endoscopic gastroplication with laparoscopic fundoplication in the treatment of gastroesophageal reflux disease. Surg Laparosc Endosc Percutan Tech 12:219, 2002.

40. Pleskow D, Rothstein R, Lo S, et al: Endoscopic full-thickness plication for the treatment of GERD: A multicenter trial. Gastrointest Endosc 59:163, 2004.

41. Pleskow D, Rothstein R, Lo S, et al: Endoscopic full-thickness plication for GERD: 12-month multi-center study results. Am J Gastroenterol 98(9):18, 2003.

42. Chuttani R, Sud R, Sachdev G, et al: A novel endoscopic full-thickness plicator for the treatment of GERD: A pilot study. Gastrointest Endosc 58:770, 2003.

43. Utley DS, Kim MS, Vierra AM, et al: Augmentation of the lower esophageal sphincter pressure and gastric yield pressure after radiofrequency energy delivery to the lower esophageal sphincter muscle; a porcine model. Gastrointest Endosc 52:81, 2000.

44. Richards WO, Houston HL, Torquati A, et al: Paradigm shift in the management of gastroesophageal reflux disease. Ann Surg 237:638, 2003.

45. Mcclusky D, Khaitan L, Gonzalez R, et al: A comparison between standard technique and fluoroscopically guided radiofrequency energy delivery in the treatment of fundoplication disruption. Poster presented at the Society of American Gastrointestinal and Endoscopic Surgeons, Denver, March 31-April 3, 2004.

46. Go MR, Dundon JM, Karlowicz DJ, et al: Delivery of radio-frequency energy to the lower esophageal sphincter improves symptoms of gastroesophageal reflux. Surgery 136:786, 2004.

47. Noar M, Knight S, Bidlack D, et al: A modified technique for endoluminal delivery of radiofrequency energy for the treatment of GERD in patients with failed fundoplication or large hiatal hernia [abstract]. Gastrointest Endosc 55:258, 2002.

48. Kim MS, Holloway RH, Dent J, et al: Radiofrequency energy delivery to the gastric cardia inhibits triggering of transient lower esophageal sphincter relaxation and gastroesophageal reflux in dogs. Gastrointest Endosc 57:17, 2003.

49. DiBaise JK, Brand RE, Quigley EM: Endoluminal delivery of radiofrequency energy to the gastroesophageal junction in uncomplicated GERD: Efficacy and potential mechanism of action. Am J Gastroenterol 97:833, 2002.

50. Triadafilopoulos G, DiBaise JK, Nostrant TT, et al: The Stretta procedure for the treatment of GERD: 6 and 12 month

follow-up of the U.S. open label trial. Gastrointest Endosc 55:149, 2002.

51. Corley DA, Katz P, Wo JM, et al: Improvement of gastroesophageal reflux symptoms after radiofrequency energy: A randomized, sham-controlled trial. Gastroenterology 125:668, 2003.

52. Triadafilopoulos G, Dibaise JK, Nostrant TT, et al: Radiofrequency energy delivery to the gastroesophageal junction for the treatment of GERD. Gastrointest Endosc 53:407, 2001.

53. Wolfsen HC, Richards WO: The Stretta procedure for the treatment of GERD: A registry of 558 patients. J Laparoendosc Adv Surg Tech A 12:395, 2002.

54. Torquati A, Houston HL, Kaiser J, et al: Long term follow-up study of the Stretta procedure for the treatment of gastroesophageal reflux disease. Surg Endosc 18:1475, 2004.

55. Reymunde A, Santiage N: The Stretta procedure is effective at 3+ year follow-up for improving GERD symptoms and eliminating the requirement for anti-secretory drugs. Am J Gastroenterol 99(10):S29, 2004.

56. Houston H, Khaitan L, Holzman M, et al: First year experience of patients undergoing the Stretta procedure. Surg Endosc 17:401, 2003.

57. Tam WC, Schoeman MN, Zhang Q, et al: Delivery of radiofrequency energy to the lower oesophageal sphincter and gastric cardia inhibits transient lower oesophageal sphincter relaxations and gastro-oesophageal reflux in patients with reflux disease. Gut 52:479, 2003.

58. Noar M, Smith J: The Stretta procedure improves GERD symptoms and anti-secretory drug use at 2 years, while normalizing gastric emptying function in the majority of impaired subjects. Gastrointest Endosc 59(5):W1514, 2004.

59. Schlesinger PK, Donahue PE, Sluss K, et al: Endoscopic sclerosis of gastric cardia (ESGC) in severe reflux esophagitis: A human trial [abstract]. Gastrointest Endosc 40:33, 1994.

60. Deviere J, Pastorelli A, Louis H, et al: Endoscopic implantation of a biopolymer in the lower esophageal sphincter for gastroesophageal reflux: A pilot study. Gastrointest Endosc 55:335, 2002.

61. Edmundowicz SA: Injection therapy of the lower esophageal sphincter for the treatment of GERD. Gastrointest Endosc 59:545, 2004.

62. Ganz RA, Rydell M, Termin P: Accurate localization of Enteryx into the deep esophageal wall without fluoroscopy. Gastrointest Endosc 59:W1507, 2004.

63. Peters JH, Silverman DE, Stein A: Lower esophageal sphincter injection of a biocompatible polymer: Accuracy of implantation assessed by esophagectomy. Surg Endosc 17:547, 2003.

64. Cohen LB, Johnson DA, Ganz R, et al: Enteryx solution, a minimally invasive injectable treatment for GERD: Preliminary 24-month results of a multicenter trial [abstract]. Paper presented at the 68th Annual Scientific Meeting of the American College of Gastroenterology, Baltimore, Oct. 10-15, 2003.

65. Johnson DA, Ganz R, Aisenberg J, et al: Endoscopic, deep mural implantation of Enteryx for the treatment of GERD: 6-month follow-up of a multicenter trial. Am J Gastroenterol 98:250, 2003.

66. Johnson DA, Ganz R, Aisenberg J, et al: Endoscopic implantation of enteryx for treatment of GERD: 12-month results of a prospective, multicenter trial. Am J Gastroenterol 98:1921, 2003.

67. Johnson DA, Aisenberg J, Cohen LB, et al: Durability and long-term safety of Enteryx implantation for GERD: 24-month follow up of a prospective multicenter trial. Am J Gastroenterol 9(10):S296, 2004.

68. Aisenberg J, Al-Kawas F, Carr-Locke DL, et al: Enteryx FDA-mandated post-approval trial. Paper presented at the Physician

Dinner Symposium, Digestive Disease Week, New Orleans, May 16-20, 2004.

69. Lehman GA, Hieston KJ, Aisenberg J, et al: Enteryx solution, A minimally invasive injectable treatment for GERD: Current worldwide multicenter human trial results [abstract]. Gastrointest Endosc 57(5):AB96, 2003.

70. Neuhaus H, Schumacher B, Preiss C, et al: Enteryx solution, a minimally invasive injectable treatment for GERD: German multicenter experience [abstract]. Gastrointest Endosc 57:AB132, 2003.

71. Deviere J, Costamagna G, Neuhaus H, et al: Endoscopic implantation of Enteryx for the treatment of GERD: A randomized controlled trial Am J Gastroenterol 99(10):S296, 2004.

72. Lehman GA, Hieston K, Cohen LB, et al: Correlation between clinical outcome and Enteryx implant shape [abstract]. Gastrointest Endosc 59(5):AB149, 2004.

73. Deviere J, Cohen LB, Aisenberg J, et al: Predictors of Enteryx outcomes at 12 months [abstract]. Gastrointest Endosc 59(5):AB243, 2004.

74. Ganz R, Aisenberg J, Cohen L, et al: Enteryx solution, a minimally invasive injectable treatment for GERD: Analysis of endoscopy findings at 12 months. Gastrointest Endosc 57(5):M1743, 2003.

75. Puitt RE, Ganz RA, Brown M, et al: Treatment satisfaction and GERD symptoms among Enteryx patients. Am J Gastroenterol 99(10):S2, 2004.

76. Fockens P, Bruno M, Boeckxstaens G, et al: Endoscopic removal of the Gatekeeper system prosthesis. Gastrointest Endosc 55(5):260, 2002.

77. Fockens P, Bruno M, Hirsch D, et al: Endoscopic augmentation of the lower esophageal sphincter. Pilot study of the Gatekeeper reflux repair system in patients with GERD. Gastrointest Endosc 55(5):257, 2002.

78. Fockens P, Boeckxstaens G, Gabbrielli A, et al: Endoscopic augmentation of the lower esophageal sphincter for GERD: Final results of a European multicenter study of the Gatekeeper system [abstract]. Gastointest Endosc 59(5):AB242, 2003.

79. Fockens P, Costamagna G, Gabrielli A, et al: Endoscopic augmentation of the lower esophageal sphincter (LES) for the treatment of GERD: Multicenter study of the Gatekeeper reflux repair system [abstract]. Gastrointest Endosc 55(5):AB89, 2002.

80. Fockens P: Gatekeeper reflux repair system: Technique, preclinical and clinical experience. Gastrointest Endosc Clin N Am 13:179, 2003.

81. Lehman G, Watkins JL, Hieston K, et al: Endoscopic gastroesophageal reflux disease (GERD) therapy with Gatekeeper system. Initiation of a multicenter prospective randomized trial [abstract]. Gastrointest Endosc 55(5):W1597, 2002.

82. Feretis C, Benakis P, Dimopoulos C, et al: Endoscopic implantation of Plexiglas microspheres for the treatment of GERD. Gastrointest Endosc 53:423, 2001.

83. Mason RJ, Hughes M, Lehman GA, et al: Endoscopic augmentation of the cardia with a biocompatible injectable polymer (Enteryx) in a porcine model. Surg Endosc 16:386, 2002.

84. Felsher J, Farres H, Chand B, et al: Mucosal apposition in endoscopic suturing. Gastrointest Endosc 58:867, 2003.

85. Chuttani R, Sud R, Sachdev G, et al: Radiofrequency (RF) energy ablation of the cardia and esophagogastric junction corrects GERD-associated gastroparesis [abstract]. Gastrointest Endosc 57(5):AB675, 2003.

86. Mason RJ, Hughes M, Lehman GA, et al: Endoscopic augmentation of the cardia with a biocompatible injectable polymer in a porcine model [abstract]. Surg Endosc 14:S166, 2000.

History and Definition of Barrett's Esophagus

Reginald V. N. Lord

The current definition of Barrett's esophagus includes both macroscopic and microscopic criteria. *Macroscopically,* it requires the presence of any length of visible columnar mucosa in the tubular esophagus proximal to the gastroesophageal junction (GEJ). *Microscopically,* the definition requires that true goblet cells be seen, thus establishing the presence of intestinal metaplasia (IM, previously known as specialized epithelial type).[1-6] This definition seems straightforward, but the high frequency of misdiagnosis of Barrett's esophagus indicates the difficulty of accurately identifying it in all cases. Sources of difficulty include changes in the definition of Barrett's, the GEJ,[7] and the cardia, as well as varying terminology for IM that is seen only microscopically, conflicting reports regarding normal histology at the GEJ, and technical difficulties during endoscopy.

The macroscopic component of the diagnosis is usually assessed at endoscopy. The columnar mucosa appears as a homogeneous salmon-colored, reddish, or velvet mucosa distinct from the whiter normal squamous epithelial lining. The columnar mucosa is located proximal to the GEJ, which is defined as the proximal extent of the gastric rugal folds.[8] Columnar mucosa distal to the GEJ is gastric mucosa. IM distal to the GEJ is gastric IM, is associated with *Helicobacter pylori,* and is not related to reflux disease. The columnar mucosa may be either circumferential and project in one or more "tongues" or simply appear as a more irregular or "zigzag" squamocolumnar junction (Z-line) proximal to the GEJ.

It is important to define the GEJ as the proximal extent of the rugal folds rather than as the squamocolumnar junction because the squamocolumnar junction migrates proximally in patients who have gastroesophageal reflux disease, with the greatest cephalad displacement by definition occurring in those with Barrett's esophagus.[9] If the proximal margin of the rugal folds is not distinct, some deflation of the stomach may be needed because with overinflation the folds can flatten out. The endoscopist must make a particular effort to examine the GEJ and squamocolumnar junction in all patients. If there is any doubt about the presence of Barrett's esophagus, biopsy samples should be taken from this area, and the pathology request form should ideally state as accurately as possible the location of the biopsy in relation to the GEJ and squamocolumnar junction. The exact location of a biopsy in relation to the GEJ is sometimes uncertain because of technical difficulties in performing endoscopy. This problem is more likely in patients with a large hiatal hernia, esophagitis, or stricture. It can be helpful in these cases to take an additional specimen from the gastric antrum or body to establish whether gastric *H. pylori* colonization is present. If *H. pylori* is absent, any IM found in the region of the GEJ or squamocolumnar junction is most probably from an area proximal to the GEJ and related to reflux disease. If *H. pylori* is found in the gastric antrum or body, other features can help distinguish esophageal IM from gastric IM, including the presence of esophageal mucosal or submucosal glands or ducts,[10] the number of eosinophils, clinical features, and esophageal manometry and pH findings.[11,12]

The microscopic criterion for the definition of Barrett's esophagus requires detection of IM, which is defined by the presence of goblet cells. Goblet cells produce and contain mucin and are normally found in the small and large intestine, but not in the esophagus. They are identified on routine hematoxylin and eosin (H&E) staining by their round, weakly basophilic, cytoplasmic vacuole. H&E staining is sufficient to diagnose IM in most cases, but in equivocal cases, staining with alcian blue at pH 2.5 will help distinguish true goblet cells, which display strong positive blue vacuolar staining because of their acid mucin content, from "pseudogoblet" and "columnar blue" cells. Pseudogoblet cells are mucous cells lining the surface and foveolar regions and have cytoplasmic vacuoles containing neutral mucin. Although pseudogoblet cells are typically alcian blue negative, they may be weakly positive ("columnar blue" cells), in which case expert pathologic interpretation relying on cellular morphology will distinguish true goblet cells (IM) from non-IM mucosa. Some recommend selective, rather than routine use of alcian blue staining to confirm the presence of IM seen on H&E sections, thus limiting the likelihood of a false-positive diagnosis of IM because of the presence of alcian blue–positive pseudogoblet cells.[13]

If histopathology confirms the presence of IM, the length of Barrett's esophagus is defined as the distance from the GEJ to the most proximal extent of the macroscopic columnar-lined mucosa. The length of the Barrett's segment is thus not the length of IM. This distinction is important because of the zonation of epithelial types observed within the columnar mucosa.[2,3,5] When IM is present, it is situated most proximally within the columnar mucosa, immediately distal to the squamous mucosa. When IM and nonintestinalized columnar epithelium are both present, the IM is situated at this most cephalad zone, whereas the nonintestinalized epithelium is distal to the IM. Although a lack of zonation has been reported,[4,14] others with a large experience state that when present, IM is always found at the most proximal zone.[13] Consequently, the endoscopist should routinely biopsy this area in patients with suspected Barrett's esophagus.

The presence of Barrett's esophagus was previously defined according to the length of the columnar segment. The 3-cm rule stated that a 3-cm or greater length of macroscopic columnar mucosa was required to diagnose Barrett's esophagus. This rule was first suggested by Cedric Bremner at a 1983 conference in Chicago and was published shortly thereafter by Skinner et al.[15] and by Bremner.[16] Bremner recalls that "the reason why I suggested this was because of Hayward's paper [Hayward J: The lower end of the esophagus. Thorax 16:36-41, 1961]. [Hayward] stated that the normal esophagus could have a 2 cm length of columnar epithelium and so to avoid over-diagnosis of endoscopic Barrett's I suggested that we take 3 cm as the cut-off point" (Cedric Bremner, personal communication, 2005). Confusingly, a 2-cm rule was also used as an alternative to 3 cm.[8] Patients with columnar segments shorter than either of these lengths did not have Barrett's esophagus according to these older definitions.

The presence of IM was recognized as the critical factor for the definition of Barrett's esophagus after it was observed that goblet cells were not normally present in the esophagus and that the risk of malignant change was limited to those with IM.[5,15,17-19] Skinner wrote in 1989, "accordingly we now modify the definition of Barrett's esophagus to include all cases in which the metaplastic goblet cell–type of epithelium is found within the esophageal lumen at any level provided it is in continuity with gastric epithelium distally."[20] The length of the columnar segment is still used to define *long-segment Barrett's esophagus* (LSBE, also known as "traditional" Barrett's), in which the columnar segment is greater than 3 cm (or 2 cm) in length, and *short-segment Barrett's esophagus* (SSBE), in which the columnar segment is less than 3 cm (or 2 cm) in length. SSBE has been estimated as being 10 times more prevalent than LSBE.[21] Patients with LSBE have a greater likelihood of having more severe gastroesophageal reflux than patients with SSBE, as well as an incompetent lower esophageal sphincter,[22] but patients with SSBE are at risk for the development of Barrett's cancers.[23] The risk may be less than that in patients with LSBE, but a significant difference has not been shown.[24]

The term *ultrashort Barrett's esophagus* is a misnomer. It refers to the microscopic finding of IM in patients with no endoscopic columnar-lined esophagus. Because the macroscopic criterion for the definition of Barrett's is not met, these patients do not have Barrett's esophagus. Furthermore, the risk for malignant degeneration in these patients, though not accurately known, is very much less than in patients with Barrett's. A better term for these patients' condition is *cardiac mucosa with intestinal metaplasia* (CIM). This term does not include the words *Barrett's esophagus* and therefore does not have the potential for false alarm that the term *ultrashort-segment Barrett's esophagus* can have, particularly now that many patients research their diagnosis on the Internet.

Cardiac mucosa is a simple, mucinous columnar mucosa with foveolar hyperplasia, no parietal cells, and no goblet cells. It is found in the region of the GEJ in most adults in Western society. When present, it is almost invariably accompanied by an infiltrate of chronic or acute inflammatory cells and may thus be termed *carditis*.[25] In the past, it was believed that a length of cardiac mucosa was normally present in the most proximal section of the stomach, where it divides the gastric oxyntic mucosa from the esophageal squamous mucosa.[26] This prevailing view was challenged by a study suggesting that cardiac mucosa, rather than being a normally occurring mucosa, might be an acquired, metaplastic epithelium that develops in response to the reflux of gastric acid into the esophagus.[27] According to this hypothesis, the histology of a normal GEJ consists of squamous mucosa abutting gastric oxyntic mucosa, or the parietal cell–containing oxyntocardiac mucosa. Subsequent studies have confirmed that this histologic pattern—squamous epithelium directly abutting oxyntic or oxyntocardiac mucosa—does occur.[28,29] Several lines of evidence indicate that cardiac mucosa is, like Barrett's esophagus, an acquired epithelium that develops in response to gastroesophageal reflux.[30-33] These findings have led to the controversial hypothesis that cardiac mucosa and CIM, though not satisfying the criteria for the definition of Barrett's esophagus, may be early stages in the development of Barrett's esophagus.[34,35]

Using the current definition, the first definite report of Barrett's esophagus was published in 1951 by Lewis H. Bosher, Jr., and Frederick H. Taylor from Barnes Hospital, St. Louis, Missouri.[36] Bosher and Taylor reported a single case, that of an obese 63-year-old woman admitted with severe dysphagia as the primary symptom. Esophagoscopy showed a stricture 23 cm from the incisors, with "heterotopic gastric mucosa" lining the tubular esophagus below this, and the stomach within the abdomen. Esophagectomy was performed to resect the stricture and because it was thought that there was a risk for malignancy. Several photomicrographs are shown in which the "heterotopic gastric mucosa" is clearly IM. Furthermore, the microscopic description notes that the abnormal mucosa was "composed of glands which contained goblet cells. . . ." One photomicrograph shows the transition section where squamous mucosa is abruptly replaced by IM.[36] The authors distinguish their case, in which there was a small, easily reducible hiatal hernia, from "thoracic stomach associated with short esophagus."

Norman Barrett's article "Chronic Peptic Ulcer of the Oesophagus and 'Oesophagitis'" was published in 1950, 1 year before Bosher and Taylor's publication, and is often cited as the first report of Barrett's esophagus (Fig. 22–1).[37] In this article Barrett, who practiced principally at St. Thomas' Hospital, London, reviewed all published cases and contributed four new cases of "chronic peptic ulcer of the oesophagus." He concluded that these esophageal ulcers were chronic gastric ulcers in association with a congenital short esophagus, thereby adding considerably to the confusion regarding their cause.[37] Allison and Johnstone termed these ulcers *Barrett's ulcers*,[38] and the gastric-type epithelium surrounding them came to be known as Barrett's esophagus. The eponymous term *Barrett's esophagus* resulted through no effort of Barrett himself, who used the term *the lower esophagus lined by columnar epithelium* for the title of a 1957 publication in the journal *Surgery*.[39]

Were these ulcers in fact located within a segment of columnar-lined Barrett's esophagus? It is not possible to be certain now, but it is likely that Barrett's cases included some true cases of Barrett's esophagus and also some that were not Barrett's esophagus.[40] By attempting to explain both pathologies as a single entity, Barrett was led into misunderstanding. Two features of the 1950 publication suggest that there may have been at least some true cases of Barrett's esophagus. First, Barrett redefined the esophagus in this article as "that part of the foregut . . . which is lined by squamous epithelium," thus suggesting that he had to resort to redefinition to account for the columnar mucosa within a structure that might otherwise have been esophagus. Second, he stated that "in cases of congenital short oesophagus . . . the bare area is larger than

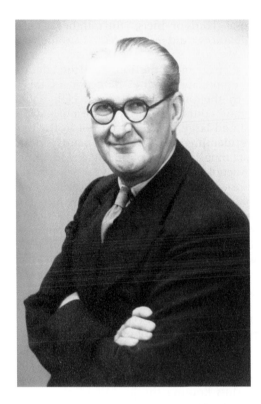

Figure 22–1.   Norman Barrett, senior surgeon at St. Thomas' Hospital, London, in 1958. (Courtesy of Julia Gough.)

usual."[37] With this comment Barrett seems to be attempting to explain the lack of a serosal surface on the columnar-lined gut above the diaphragm. Instead of the rather implausible suggestion that the absence of a serosal surface is due to an exceptionally large bare area of the stomach, it is reasonable to propose that there was no serosa because the columnar-lined intestine was esophagus. Although Barrett did not describe goblet cells within the "histologically gastric" mucosa, which would be expected in a long-segment columnar-lined esophagus, other publications, including the report by Bosher and Taylor, indicate that the pathologic nature of goblet cells in the stomach was not well appreciated at the time.[36] Barrett may thus not have thought it necessary to note the presence of goblet cells.

Other aspects of the publication indicate that at least some of the cases reported did not have Barrett's esophagus. Just as Barrett stated, these patients may have had a chronic peptic ulcer in an intrathoracic stomach, although the underlying abnormality was almost certainly herniation of the stomach through the esophageal hiatus rather than a congenital short esophagus. In support of this, Barrett stated that some cases of "congenital short oesophagus" had a partial covering of peritoneum above the crura (indicating that they were part of the stomach), and the case illustrated shows gastric rugal folds around the ulcer.[37] Finally, there is Barrett's reassessment of these ulcers and the columnar lining that surrounded them. Ten years after the initial report, when he had a greater understanding of esophageal mucosal disease, Barrett wrote, "ulcers that occur in the pouch of stomach that forms a sliding hiatal hernia are true gastric ulcers (Barrett, 1950) and have nothing to do with reflux."[41] In 1962 he wrote, "some years ago I pointed out that when a piece of stomach passes into a sliding hiatal or a paraesophageal hernia, it is not unusual for a typical peptic ulcer to develop in the abnormally placed segment of the stomach. Such an ulcer (Barrett's ulcer) has the character of a typical gastric ulcer. . . ."[42]

Barrett was thus probably unknowingly describing two different pathologic entities, only one of which was Barrett's esophagus. His other problem was that he erroneously considered that his cases had a congenital short esophagus. This conclusion was not so unreasonable at the time as it appears now because congenital short esophagus was an accepted condition at the time.[7,43-46] Indeed, as late as the 1978 second edition of *Surgery of the Alimentary Tract* by Shackelford there is a section titled "Brachyesophagus (Abnormally Short Esophagus)" with four pages devoted to congenital short esophagus.[47] One of the patients whom Barrett himself had seen was a 13-year-old boy "who had several other congenital deformities."[37] Columnar mucosa was found up to the level of the aortic arch, and the boy died of perforation into a pulmonary vein. Barrett later recognized his (and others') error regarding the congenital short esophagus theory and stated in 1960 that "it would have been better if the term [congenital short esophagus] had never been introduced. . . ."[41]

Allison and Johnstone clarified matters considerably in their 1953 publication "The Oesophagus Lined with Gastric Mucous Membrane."[38] They examined 115 patients with esophageal ulcers and stenosis and found 7 with columnar-lined esophagus, 1 of whom had certain IM. Noting that the columnar segments had no serosal layer but did have esophageal musculature, submucosal glands typical of the esophagus, islands of squamous epithelium, and an esophageal blood supply, they demonstrated the esophageal rather than gastric location of the columnar mucosa. Allison et al. had previously reported on 10 patients with esophageal ulcers, esophageal shortening, and "gastric" mucosa distal to a stricture, but it is not clear that these were cases of columnar-lined esophagus rather than hiatal hernia.[45]

Microscopic examination demonstrating esophageal muscle fibers had also confirmed the true anatomy of the columnar lining in studies conducted in Paris by Jean-Louis Lortat-Jacob and his wife M. Smith-Lortat-Jacob.[48-52] J.-L. Lortat-Jacob created the term *endobrachyesophagus* for the lower esophagus "lined by gastric mucosa."[50] Smith-Lortat-Jacob submitted her thesis on cases of columnar-lined esophagus in 1950, the same year as Barrett's initial publication.[48] "Inspired by his wife's doctoral thesis"[52] and after "a courteous and intelligent 'face à face' across the Channel"[52] with Barrett, J.-L. Lortat-Jacob published his findings in 1957.[49] Stein and Siewert note that the terms *endobrachyesophagus* and *Barrett's esophagus* are used synonymously in Europe.[53]

Is it possible that Barrett's esophagus is a disease that appeared only around the middle of the last century? This seems unlikely because in 1953 Allison and Johnstone found as many as 11 patients with "gastric"

mucosa in the esophagus among their 115 patients with esophageal ulcer and stenosis.[38] The prevalence of this disease in recent decades also argues against it being such a new disease. Autopsy studies estimate the prevalence to be 0.4% to 0.9% in the general population[54,55] and 3% to 12% in patients who undergo upper gastrointestinal endoscopy for the investigation of chronic reflux symptoms.[56-59] Endoscopy was not introduced until the late 1860s, but detailed autopsies were commonly performed in the 19th and early 20th centuries. All organs were examined at these autopsies and novel findings were reported regularly. It therefore seems likely that unless Barrett's esophagus was nonexistent or almost so, there should be some reports of columnar-lined esophagus before those of the 1950s. To investigate this hypothesis, some earlier publications that have been classified as early reports of columnar-lined esophagus are reviewed in the following text. These earlier descriptions all focus on esophageal ulcer and are reviewed only because they mention possible instances of columnar mucosa in the esophagus in association with the ulcers.

Alexander "Sandy" Lyall, from the Royal Infirmary and University in Glasgow, was a gifted investigator and physician who reported eight fatal cases of peptic ulcer of the esophagus in 1937.[60] The postmortem report on case 8, a Patrick C. aged 58 years who died of pneumonia but also had a large chronic distal esophageal ulcer, reads: "Closer examination of the mucous membrane in the region of the ulcer showed the presence of a remarkable state of affairs. The intact mucosa separating the lateral edges of the ulcer was found to be heterotopic gastric mucosa which extended as a tongue-shaped process of well-preserved tissue upwards from that of the fundus of the stomach." Microscopic examination showed that "the heterotopic gastric mucosa bore a resemblance to that found normally towards the pyloric end of the stomach, the glands being fairly short and wide. Oxyntic [parietal, HCl-secreting] cells were present, but were comparatively few in number."[60] This description of a tongue of columnar mucosa suggests that the patient had Barrett's esophagus, a possibility that is not excluded by the presence of a small number of parietal cells. Lyall cites articles by Fraenkel, Tileston, and Stewart and Hartfall as prior publications with heterotopic mucosa.

The case reported by Stewart and Hartfall in 1929, though sometimes listed as a report of Barrett's esophagus, is more likely to be one of only islet patches of columnar mucosa. The authors wrote that "a very interesting feature of the case here reported was the presence of two large patches of gastric mucous membrane in the upper oesophagus just below the level of the cricoid cartilage."[61] The illustration shows islets of columnar mucosa, the authors refer to islets, and they reference Schridde and Taylor, who also describe islet patches of columnar mucosa.[62,63] Whether nonislet (Barrett's) columnar-lined esophagus had been present inferior to these islets is unknown because the specimen had undergone extensive postmortem digestion in this region.[61]

In 1879 the great German physician Heinrich Irenaeus Quincke (Fig. 22–2) described three cases of esophageal ulceration with microscopic features

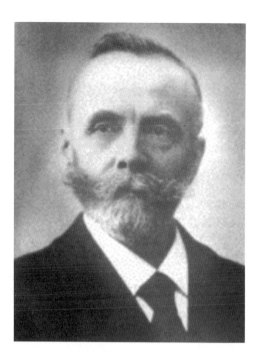

Figure 22–2. Heinrich Irenaeus Quincke, Geheimer Mediz-inalrath and chair of medicine at Bern and subsequently Kiel. Quincke's 1879 description of columnar mucosa in the esophagus may have been the first report of Barrett's esophagus.

"[usually only found in the stomach or small intestine]."[64,65] This report was perhaps the first of Barrett's esophagus and is also credited as being the first report of a Mallory-Weiss tear. It was one of many contributions by Quincke (1842-1922), whose teachers included Virchow, Heimholtz, and Wilms. Quincke was appointed to the chair in medicine at Bern, Switzerland, at the age of 31 and gave his name to seven medical eponyms. His greatest contribution is considered to be the introduction of lumbar puncture.

Wilder Tileston, from Boston, Massachusetts, reviewed the history of "ulcer of the oesophagus, resembling peptic ulcer of the stomach" in 1906 and noted that they were first described by Albers in 1839, their existence was supported by Rokitansky but denied by Zenker and Birch-Hirschfeld, and the matter was conclusively settled by Quincke's detailed report (1879) of three "clearly proved" cases.[64,66] Tileston excluded all cases reported before Quincke because of uncertainty of diagnosis but reviewed the 41 subsequently published cases and added 3 new cases of peptic ulcer of the esophagus. Microscopic examination was reported in only 14 of these 44 cases, but in 1 of these cases, reported by Fraenkel in 1899, there were "gastric glands present in oesophagus" with an ulcer at the cardioesophageal junction.[66,67] Tileston's first personal case might have had Barrett's esophagus. The patient had a large distal esophageal ulcer with perforation, and on microscopy, "near the edge of the ulcer, in the submucosa, [was] a large group of glands with columnar epithelium, resembling mucous glands in structure." The mucosa was absent because of postmortem digestion. Tileston's other two personal cases—

and almost all of the other published cases—are not suggestive of Barrett's esophagus but are seemingly reports of acute esophageal ulcer.[61]

It therefore seems likely, though admittedly uncertain, that Quinke in 1879, Fraenkel in 1899, Tileston in 1906, and Lyall in 1937 reported cases of Barrett's esophagus, and this condition has thus been occurring for more than 100 years. The focus of reports before the 1920s was on associated esophageal pathology, especially esophageal ulcer, lethal conditions were the primary interest, and autopsy was the predominant means of diagnosis. Large autopsy series with detailed examination of all organs were performed and reported. It seems reasonable to conclude that Barrett's esophagus must have been a rare disease before the second half of the 20th century. Lyall's 1 possible case, for example, was found in a series of 1500 postmortem examinations performed over the 4 years in which they "examined specially the oesophaguses."[60] Similarly, Stewart and Hartfall's case of an islet of columnar mucosa "is the first which we have encountered in over 10,000 autopsies performed during the last 18 years," thus suggesting that there were no true cases of Barrett's esophagus among this large number of postmortem examinations.[61] With the more widespread introduction of endoscopy and the consequent increased emphasis on more benign conditions, larger series of esophageal diseases were reported, but there were still very few reports of columnar mucosa in the esophagus, and the possibility that it was not "gastric heterotopia" was not realized until the 1950s. Reasons for the undoubtedly real increase in the incidence of both Barrett's esophagus and esophageal adenocarcinoma since the mid-20th century are beyond the scope of this chapter but discussed elsewhere.[68]

It is similarly difficult to be certain about the first report of Barrett's adenocarcinoma. Morson and Belcher's 1952 report of a case of esophageal adenocarcinoma arising above a columnar-lined esophagus, with the presence of IM noted, is usually credited as being the first definite report,[2] but there are several earlier reports of probable Barrett's-associated adenocarcinoma.[7,69-72] The development of esophageal cancer in association with a chronic "peptic" ulcer of the esophagus was described by Ortmann in 1901,[65] and Tileston wrote in 1906 that he had seen a similar specimen in Vienna.[61,66] Adler clarified the association between Barrett's esophagus and adenocarcinoma.[73]

ACKNOWLEDGMENT

The author gratefully acknowledges Julia Gough for permission to reproduce the photograph of her father (see Fig. 22–1).

REFERENCES

1. Trier JS: Morphology of the epithelium of the distal esophagus in patients with midesophageal peptic strictures. Gastroenterology 58:444-461, 1970.
2. Morson BC, Belcher JR: Adenocarcinoma of the oesophagus and ectopic gastric mucosa. Br J Cancer 6:127-130, 1952.

3. Abrams L, Heath D: Lower esophagus lined with intestinal and gastric epithelia. Thorax 20:66-72, 1965.

4. Mangla JC: Barrett's esophagus: An old entity rediscovered. J Clin Gastroenterol 3:347-356, 1981.

5. Paull A, Trier JS, Dalton MD, et al: The histologic spectrum of Barrett's esophagus. N Engl J Med 295:476-480, 1976.

6. Sampliner RE: Practice guidelines on the diagnosis, surveillance, and therapy of Barrett's esophagus. The Practice Parameters Committee of the American College of Gastroenterology. Am J Gastroenterol 93:1028-1032, 1998.

7. Goyal RK: Columnar cell–lined (Barrett's) esophagus. A historical perspective. In Spechler SJ, Goyal RK (eds): Barrett's Esophagus. Pathophysiology, Diagnosis, and Management. New York, Elsevier, 1985, pp 1-17.

8. McClave SA, Boyce HJ, Gottfried MR: Early diagnosis of columnar-lined esophagus: A new endoscopic diagnostic criterion. Gastrointest Endosc 33:413-416, 1987.

9. Csendes A, Maluenda F, Braghetto I, et al: Location of the lower oesophageal sphincter and the squamous columnar mucosal junction in 109 healthy controls and 778 patients with different degrees of endoscopic oesophagitis. Gut 34:21-27, 1993.

10. Ireland PE: Glands of the esophagus. Laryngoscope 43:351-368, 1933.

11. Hamilton SR: Reflux esophagitis and Barrett esophagus. In Goldman H, Appelman HD, Kaufman N (eds): Gastrointestinal Pathology. Baltimore, Williams & Wilkins, 1990, pp 11-68.

12. Odze RD: Unraveling the mystery of the gastroesophageal junction: A pathologist's perspective. Am J Gastroenterol 100:1853-1867, 2005.

13. Chandrasoma P: Non-neoplastic diseases of the esophagus. In Chandrasoma P (ed): Gastrointestinal Pathology. Stamford, CT, Appleton & Lange, 1999, pp 9-42.

14. Thompson JJ, Zinsser KR, Enterline HT: Barrett's metaplasia and adenocarcinoma of the esophagus and gastroesophageal junction. Hum Pathol 14:42-61, 1983.

15. Skinner DB, Walther BC, Riddell RH, et al: Barrett's esophagus. Comparison of benign and malignant cases. Ann Surg 198:554-565, 1983.

16. Bremner CG: Barrett's esophagus. Controversial aspects. In DeMeester TR, Skinner DB (eds): Esophageal Disorders. Pathophysiology and Therapy. New York, Raven Press, 1984, pp 233-240.

17. Haggitt RC, Tryzelaar J, Ellis FH, Colcher H: Adenocarcinoma complicating columnar epithelium–lined (Barrett's) esophagus. Am J Clin Pathol 70:1-5, 1978.

18. Reid BJ, Weinstein WM: Barrett's esophagus and adenocarcinoma. Annu Rev Med 38:477-492, 1987.

19. Weinstein WM, Ippoliti AF: The diagnosis of Barrett's esophagus: Goblets, goblets, goblets [editorial]. Gastrointest Endosc 44:91-95, 1996.

20. Skinner DB: What is the definition of Barrett's esophagus? In Guili R, McCallum RW (eds): Benign Lesions of the Esophagus and Cancer. Answers to 210 Questions. (O.E.S.O.). Berlin, Springer-Verlag, 1989, pp 620-621.

21. Spechler SJ, Zeroogian JM, Antonioli DA, et al: Prevalence of metaplasia at the gastro-oesophageal junction. Lancet 344:1533-1536, 1994.

22. Öberg S, DeMeester TR, Peters JH, et al: The extent of Barrett's esophagus depends on the status of the lower esophageal sphincter and the degree of esophageal acid exposure. J Thorac Cardiovasc Surg 117:572-580, 1999.

23. Clark GW, Ireland AP, Peters JH, et al: Short segment Barrett's esophagus: A prevalent complication of gastroesophageal reflux disease with malignant potential. J Gastrointest Surg 1:113-122, 1997.

24. Rudolph RE, Vaughan TL, Storer BE, et al: Effect of segment length on risk for neoplastic progression in patients with Barrett esophagus. Ann Intern Med 132:612-620, 2000.

25. Der R, Tsao-Wei DD, DeMeester T, et al: Carditis: A manifestation of gastroesophageal reflux disease. Am J Surg Pathol 25:245-252, 2001.

26. Hayward J: The lower end of the oesophagus. Thorax 16:36-55, 1961.

27. Öberg S, Peters JH, DeMeester TR, et al: Inflammation and specialized intestinal metaplasia of cardiac mucosa is a manifestation of gastroesophageal reflux disease. Ann Surg 226:522-530, 1997.

28. Chandrasoma PT, Der R, Ma Y, et al: Histology of the gastroesophageal junction: An autopsy study. Am J Surg Pathol 24:402-409, 2000.

29. Zhou H, Greco MA, Kahn E: Origin of cardiac mucosa. Ontogenic considerations. Mod Pathol 12:499A, 1999.

30. Öberg S, Peters JH, DeMeester TR, et al: Determinants of intestinal metaplasia within the columnar-lined esophagus. Arch Surg 135:651-655, 2000.

31. Öberg S, Johansson J, Wenner J, Walther B: Metaplastic columnar mucosa in the cervical esophagus after esophagectomy. Ann Surg 235:338-345, 2002.

32. Hamilton SR, Yardley JH: Regeneration of cardiac type mucosa and acquisition of Barrett mucosa after esophagogastrostomy. Gastroenterology 72:669-675, 1977.

33. Lord RV, Wickramasinghe K, Johansson JJ, et al: Cardiac mucosa in the remnant esophagus after esophagectomy is an acquired epithelium with Barrett's-like features. Surgery 136:633-640, 2004.

34. Chandrasoma P: Pathophysiology of Barrett's esophagus. Semin Thorac Cardiovasc Surg 9:270-278, 1997.

35. DeMeester SR, DeMeester TR: Columnar mucosa and intestinal metaplasia of the esophagus: Fifty years of controversy. Ann Surg 231:303-321, 2000.

36. Bosher LH Jr, Taylor FH: Heterotopic gastric mucosa in the esophagus with ulceration and stricture formation. J Thorac Surg 21:306-312, 1951.

37. Barrett NR: Chronic peptic ulcer of the esophagus and "oesophagitis." Br J Surg 38:175-182, 1950.

38. Allison PR, Johnstone AS: The oesophagus lined with gastric mucous membrane. Thorax 8:87-101, 1953.

39. Barrett NR: The lower esophagus lined by columnar epithelium. Surgery 41:881-894, 1957.

40. Lord RV: Norman Barrett, "doyen of esophageal surgery." Ann Surg 229:428-439, 1999.

41. Barrett NR: Hiatus hernia. BMJ 2:247-252, 1960.

42. Barrett NR: Benign stricture in the lower esophagus. J Thorac Cardiovasc Surg 43:703-715, 1962.

43. Keith A: On the origin and nature of hernia. Br J Surg 11:455-475, 1924.

44. Knaggs RL: On diaphragmatic hernia of the stomach and on torsion of the small omentum and volvulus of the stomach in association with it. Lancet 2:358-364, 1904.

45. Allison PR, Johnstone AS, Royce GB: Short esophagus with simple peptic ulceration. J Thorac Surg 12:432-457, 1943.

46. Frindlay L, Kelley AB: Congenital shortening of the oesophagus and the thoracic stomach results therefrom. Proc R Soc Med 24:1561-1578, 1931.

47. Shackelford RT: Esophageal strictures. In Shackelford RT (ed): Surgery of the Alimentary Tract. Philadelphia, WB Saunders, 1978, pp 215-356.

48. Smith-Lortat-Jacob M: Cinq Observations d'Ulcere Peptique de l'Oesophage [these pour le doctorat de medicine]. Paris, 1950.

49. Lortat-Jacob JL: L'endo-brachy-oesophage. Ann Chir 11:1247-1255, 1957.

50. Lortat-Jacob JL: What is the definition of Barrett's esophagus? In Guili R, McCallum RW (eds): Benign Lesions of the Esophagus and Cancer. Answers to 210 Questions. Berlin, Springer-Verlag, 1989, pp 619-620.

51. Guili R: The story of a modern disease. N. Barrett, J.L. Lortat-Jacob. Dis Esophagus 5:5-12, 1992.

52. Ribet ME: Surveillance of Barrett's esophagus [letter]. Ann Thorac Surg 55:1051-1052, 1993.

53. Stein HJ, Siewert JR: Barrett-Oesophagus—Endobrachyoesophagus: Norman Rupert Barrett und Jean-Louis Lortat-Jacob. Chirurg 65:110-111, 1994.

54. Cameron AJ, Zinsmeister AR, Ballard DJ, Carney JA: Prevalence of columnar-lined (Barrett's) esophagus. Comparison of population-based clinical and autopsy findings. Gastroenterology 99:918-922, 1990.

55. Ormsby AH, Kilgore SP, Goldblum JR, et al: The location and frequency of intestinal metaplasia at the esophagogastric junction in 223 consecutive autopsies: Implications for patient treatment and preventive strategies in Barrett's esophagus. Mod Pathol 13:614-620, 2000.

56. Barrett's esophagus: Epidemiological and clinical results of multicentric survey. Gruppo Operativo per lo Studio della Precancerosi dell'Esofago (GOSPE). Int J Cancer 48:364-368, 1991.

57. Winters CJ, Spurling TJ, Chobanian SJ, et al: Barrett's esophagus. A prevalent, occult complication of gastroesophageal reflux disease. Gastroenterology 92:118-124, 1987.

58. Cameron AJ, Ott BJ, Payne WS: The incidence of adenocarcinoma in columnar-lined (Barrett's) esophagus. N Engl J Med 313:857-859, 1985.

59. Lieberman DA, Oehlke M, Helfand M: Risk factors for Barrett's esophagus in community-based practice. GORGE consortium. Gastroenterology Outcomes Research Group in Endoscopy. Am J Gastroenterol 92:1293-1297, 1997.

60. Lyall A: Chronic peptic ulcer of the oesophagus: A report of eight cases. Br J Surg 24:534-547, 1937.

61. Stewart MJ, Hartfall SJ: Chronic peptic ulcer of the esophagus. J Pathol Bacteriol 32:9-14, 1929.

62. Schridde H: Über Magenschleimhaut-Inseln vom Bau der cardial-Drüsen Zone und fundus-Drüsen Region und den unteren, oesophagealen cardial-Drüsen gleichende Drüsen im obersten oesophagusabschnitt. Virchows Arch 175:1-14, 1904.

63. Taylor AL: The epithelial heterotopics of the alimentary tract. J Pathol Bacteriol 30:415-449, 1927.

64. Quincke H: Ulcus oesophagi ex digestione. Dtsch Arch Klin Med 24:72, 1879.

65. Ortmann K: Klinische Beiträge zur Erkrankung des Oesophagus durch Ulcus e Digestione. Munch Med Wochenschr 48:387, 1901.

66. Tileston W: Peptic ulcer of the oesophagus. Am J Med Sci 132:240-265, 1906.

67. Fraenkel A: Unknown. Wien Klin Wochenschr 12:1039, 1899.

68. Lagergren J: Adenocarcinoma of oesophagus: What exactly is the size of the problem and who is at risk? Gut 54(Suppl 1):i1-i5, 2005.

69. Smithers DW: Short oesophagus (thoracic stomach) and its association with peptic ulceration and cancer. Br J Radiol 18:199-208, 1945.

70. Mailer R: Carcinoma in a thoracic stomach (congenital short oesophagus). Br J Surg 35:426-428, 1948.

71. Dawson JL: Carcinoma in a herniated gastric cardia associated with short oesophagus. Br J Pediatr 23:270-273, 1950.

72. Eastwood GL, Bonnice CA: Barrett's esophagus—a special problem. In Castell DO, Wu WC, Ott DJ (eds): Gastroesophageal Reflux Disease: Pathogenesis, Diagnosis, Therapy. Mount Kisco, NY, Futura, 1985, pp 301-320.

73. Adler RH: The lower esophagus lined by columnar epithelium. Its association with hiatal hernia, ulcer, stricture, and tumor. J Thorac Cardiovasc Surg 45:13-34, 1963.

23

Pathophysiology of the Columnar-Lined Esophagus

Daniel S. Oh • Steven R. DeMeester

Gastroesophageal reflux disease (GERD) affects an estimated 20% of the population, and with direct and indirect costs exceeding $10 billion annually, it is the costliest gastrointestinal disorder in the United States.[1] Much of this extraordinary sum goes to pay for increasingly more potent and widely prescribed medications to suppress gastric acid production. Although these medications have been proved to relieve heartburn symptoms and heal esophagitis, they have failed to alter the malignant complications of reflux disease. The prevalence of Barrett's esophagus has been increasingly steadily in many Western countries, and in the United States the incidence of esophageal adenocarcinoma continues to increase faster than any other malignancy. Currently, it is outpacing the next closet cancer, melanoma, by a factor of 3.[2]

Because the esophagus is normally lined by squamous mucosa, it is clear that for adenocarcinoma to develop there must be a sequence of events that results in transformation of the normal squamous mucosa into columnar epithelium. This sequence begins with gastroesophageal reflux, and with continued injury, cardiac mucosa replaces the squamous mucosa in the distal esophagus. Subsequently, goblet cells indicative of intestinal metaplasia develop, and when there is a visible segment of columnar mucosa in the distal esophagus that shows intestinal metaplasia on biopsy, the criteria for Barrett's esophagus has been met. Barrett's esophagus is the precursor lesion for one of the most lethal malignancies that occurs in humans, esophageal adenocarcinoma.

DEFINITION

The definition of Barrett's esophagus has undergone many modifications and refinements as our understanding of the pathophysiology of this condition has evolved. In 1950 Dr. Norman Barrett described a columnar-lined foregut structure in the chest that he postulated to be a pouch of stomach that had herniated into the thorax secondary to either scarring or a congenitally shortened esophagus.[3] Shortly thereafter, however, Allison and Johnstone argued that the presence of esophageal submucosal glands indicated that this columnar-lined tubular structure was in fact esophagus.[4] In 1957 Barrett concurred and concluded that the normal squamous lining of the distal esophagus had been replaced by columnar mucosa in these patients.[5] Subsequently, a columnar-lined esophagus became known as Barrett's esophagus.

The first alteration in the definition of Barrett's esophagus came after John Hayward suggested that a junctional or buffer zone of columnar mucosa up to 2 cm in length was normally present at the gastroesophageal junction.[6] Despite the absence of supporting data or proof for this statement in his 1961 publication, Hayward's concept became widely accepted. This prompted concern regarding the potential for overdiagnosis of Barrett's esophagus given that up to 2 cm of columnar mucosa was considered normal, and by the 1980s it was necessary to have a minimum of 3 cm of columnar mucosa in the distal esophagus to make the diagnosis of Barrett's.[7]

Whereas all these modifications focused on the length of the columnar segment, Paull and colleagues introduced an entirely new concept by focusing on the histology of the columnar mucosa of Barrett's esophagus.[8] Using manometrically guided biopsies the authors reported that three types of columnar mucosa could be found in Barrett's esophagus: fundic, cardiac, and intestinal. Despite Paull and colleagues' detailed description, little significance was given to the histology of Barrett's until reports began surfacing in the 1980s that the intestinal type of Barrett's was the only one associated with the development of adenocarcinoma of the esophagus.[7,9,10] The critical importance of the histologic finding of goblet cells within a columnar-lined esophagus was thus established, and the *definition of Barrett's esophagus* now requires *both* an endoscopically visible segment of columnar lining in the distal esophagus *and* intestinal metaplasia on biopsy. A visible segment of columnar mucosa in the distal esophagus that does not have intestinal metaplasia on biopsy is not considered Barrett's esophagus and should be referred to simply as a columnar-lined esophagus. The premalignant significance of intestinal metaplasia on biopsy has relegated the length of the columnar segment to secondary importance. By current convention, *long-segment Barrett's* has intestinal metaplasia within a columnar-lined segment in the distal esophagus that is 3 cm or greater in length, whereas lengths less than 3 cm are called *short-segment Barrett's*. The finding of intestinal metaplasia within cardiac mucosa from an endoscopically normal-appearing gastroesophageal junction is not considered Barrett's esophagus and, instead, is called *intestinal metaplasia of the cardia (CIM)*.

EPIDEMIOLOGY

The prevalence of Barrett's esophagus appears to be increasing in the Western world. It has been debated whether this increase represents a true rise in incidence or is secondary to a heightened awareness of the dangers of reflux disease among practitioners and increased use of upper endoscopy to evaluate patients with reflux symptoms.[11] The most convincing epidemiologic evidence that the prevalence of Barrett's is actually increasing comes from a recent study in the Netherlands using their Integrated Primary Care Information database, which contains more than 500,000 computerized patient records. In this study there was a linear increase in the diagnosis of Barrett's that was even more pronounced if the increase was based on the number of upper endoscopies performed during the same period (from 19.8/1000 upper endoscopies in 1997 to 40.4/1000 upper endoscopies in 2002).[12] Epidemiologic studies in England have also demonstrated an age-specific increase in the prevalence of Barrett's per 100 upper endoscopies during the years 1982 to 1996.[13]

Thus, there is evidence that the prevalence of Barrett's is increasing, but it is clear that the true prevalence of Barrett's in the population is unknown and probably much higher than what would be expected based on clinical cases diagnosed by upper endoscopy. In one of the few autopsy studies that evaluated the prevalence of Barrett's, Cameron et al. found 376 cases per 100,000 people in Olmsted County, Minnesota.[14] This rate was approximately five times higher than the clinical prevalence of Barrett's in this same area (82.6 per 100,000). Further support for the concern about a large subclinical population of individuals with Barrett's comes from a study conducted in veterans by Gerson and colleagues.[15] They performed upper endoscopy in a group of patients undergoing routine sigmoidoscopy for colorectal cancer screening, none of whom had symptoms of reflux. Although there are obvious limitations to a study primarily involving older, white male military veterans, their finding that 25% of the patients had Barrett's is nonethe-

less concerning because on the basis of symptoms none of these patients would have been recommended to undergo upper endoscopy. These observations suggest that Barrett's goes undiagnosed in the majority of individuals, either because they ignore minor reflux symptoms or, as the study in veterans suggests, because they are truly asymptomatic.

RISK FACTORS FOR BARRETT'S ESOPHAGUS

Most studies of risk factors have focused on the more definitive end point of adenocarcinoma of the esophagus, and thus there are relatively few studies that specifically evaluate risk factors for Barrett's. However, because Barrett's is the leading risk factor for esophageal adenocarcinoma and both Barrett's and esophageal cancer are linked to gastroesophageal reflux, it is reasonable to extrapolate some of the risk factors defined for adenocarcinoma to Barrett's as well. The most significant risk factor for the development of Barrett's esophagus is longstanding GERD. Case-control studies have shown that individuals with the highest risk for Barrett's esophagus are those in whom reflux symptoms develop at an early age and thus have a long duration of symptoms.[16] Other risk factors for Barrett's esophagus include anatomic and physiologic abnormalities that predispose to severe gastroesophageal reflux, including the presence of a mechanically defective lower esophageal sphincter and a large hiatal hernia.[17] Most significantly, however, the factor that separates patients with reflux *and* Barrett's from those with reflux but *without* Barrett's is the composition of the refluxate, specifically, the presence of bile.[17,18]

Additional risk factors for Barrett's esophagus include age and gender. The prevalence of Barrett's increases in a linear fashion with age, starting at about 20 years old and peaking in the 70- to 79-year-old group.[13] The increase in females appears to start about 20 years later than in males, and the finding that females with Barrett's tend to be older than males with Barrett's has been shown in a number of studies.[13,18] Male gender is also a risk factor for Barrett's, but the explanation for this observation has not been clear until recently. We studied a large and carefully evaluated group of 796 patients with reflux symptoms, including 146 males and 63 females with Barrett's, and found that on average, females had less severe reflux disease than males did. Importantly, females with severe reflux were just as likely to have Barrett's as males with severe reflux, thus suggesting that it is the reduced prevalence of severe reflux rather than any protective effect of being a female that explains the significant sex difference in the prevalence of Barrett's.[18]

Ethnicity is another risk factor for Barrett's esophagus, with white individuals being at highest risk and Asians at the lowest.[19] However, these demographics are changing, perhaps as a result of the spread of fast food and a Western diet around the world. A recent study from Malaysia, where the population is composed equally of Malays, Chinese, and Indians, found an overall 6.2% prevalence of Barrett's, which is similar to that reported in many Western countries.[20] In another study, the prevalence of Barrett's in Hispanic Americans was found to be similar to that in white Americans.[21] Thus, it is becoming apparent that diet and lifestyle may play a more important role in reflux disease and Barrett's than do biologic differences between ethnic groups, although the lower frequency of Barrett's and esophageal adenocarcinoma in African Americans remains unexplained.[22,23]

The observation that the prevalence of Barrett's increases with advancing age is strong evidence that the condition is acquired. However, the possibility that there is a genetic risk factor for Barrett's esophagus and esophageal adenocarcinoma has emerged after the publication of case reports that describe finding Barrett's in multiple members of the same family and even in identical twins.[24-26] Further support for a genetic link comes from a cohort study by Chak and colleagues, where a positive family history of Barrett's esophagus or esophageal adenocarcinoma was significantly more common in white patients with Barrett's esophagus than in a GERD control group with a negative family history. In this study a positive family history increased the risk for Barrett's by 12-fold.[27] Others, though, have not confirmed this association. Romero et al. noted an increased prevalence of esophagitis in the relatives of Barrett's patients, but they found that increasing age and a longer duration of symptoms were stronger risk factors for Barrett's than a family history of Barrett's esophagus or esophageal adenocarcinoma.[28] Thus, a definitive genetic risk factor or "Barrett's gene" has not been proved to exist; instead, a predilection for severe GERD appears to run in families. There also seems to be individual variations in susceptibility to the development of Barrett's. Support for this concept comes from an intriguing finding by Oberg et al. in a study of the prevalence of cardiac mucosa and Barrett's after esophagectomy.[29] The authors evaluated the residual cervical esophagus above the anastomosis after esophagectomy and gastric pull-up. At the time of surgery the esophageal resection margins were pathologically shown to be squamous mucosa, and on follow-up upper endoscopy the authors found that columnar mucosa had developed in 47% of these patients. Interestingly, the likelihood of finding columnar mucosa above the anastomosis was higher in patients who underwent esophagectomy for adenocarcinoma than in those who underwent it for squamous carcinoma.

Other purported risk factors for reflux, Barrett's esophagus, or esophageal adenocarcinoma include obesity and dietary factors or medications that reduce the resting tone of the lower esophageal sphincter. The association between obesity and reflux disease is well established, but an association between obesity and Barrett's esophagus or esophageal adenocarcinoma has not been conclusively demonstrated.[17,30-33] These findings suggest that although obesity may predispose an individual to reflux disease, it does not appear to be an independent risk factor for Barrett's esophagus or esophageal adenocarcinoma. However, there is evidence linking medications that relax the lower esophageal sphincter with an increased risk for esophageal adenocarcinoma and, by inference, reflux disease and Barrett's.[34] Interestingly, the use of acid-suppression medications has also

been linked with a nearly threefold increase in the risk for esophageal adenocarcinoma, even when adjustments were made for the severity of reflux symptoms.[35] Thus, the widespread use of medications that affect gastric acidity and the function of the lower esophageal sphincter may be involved in the increasing prevalence of Barrett's esophagus and esophageal adenocarcinoma.

PATHOPHYSIOLOGY

The development of Barrett's is probably a two-step process. The first step involves the transformation of normal esophageal squamous mucosa to a simple columnar epithelium called cardiac mucosa. This conversion occurs in response to chronic injury produced by repetitive episodes of gastric juice refluxing onto the squamous mucosa. The change from squamous to cardiac mucosa probably occurs relatively quickly, within several years.[29] The second step in the pathophysiology of Barrett's is the development of goblet cells indicative of intestinal metaplasia within the columnar cardiac mucosa. There is evidence that this step proceeds over a period of 5 to 10 years.[29] Once present, Barrett's esophagus can progress to low- and high-grade dysplasia and ultimately to adenocarcinoma. This entire process is commonly described as the Barrett's metaplasia-dysplasia-carcinoma sequence.

Step 1: Metaplastic Columnarization with Cardiac Mucosa

To understand what constitutes a columnar-lined esophagus, an understanding of the anatomy and histology of the normal gastroesophageal junction is required. Unfortunately, the very definition of what is normal in this area remains controversial, with much debate centered on whether cardiac mucosa is normally present at the gastroesophageal junction. Although our understanding is gradually improving, Hayward's remark in 1961 that "the lower end of the oesophagus is a region where the pathology, the physiology, and even the anatomy are not quite clear" remains appropriate even today.[6] In one of the first reports describing the normal gastroesophageal junction, Hayward indicated that a junctional or buffer zone of columnar mucosa was normally interposed between the acid-secreting oxyntic gastric mucosa and the acid-sensitive squamous esophageal mucosa.[6] Though an appealing concept, Hayward provided no data in support of his theory and did not discuss the role of the lower esophageal sphincter, which had been demonstrated to exist before his publication. According to Hayward, this junctional mucosa was "normally" found in a length of up to 2 cm at the gastroesophageal junction. He also noted the following about this junctional mucosa: (1) it was histologically distinct from normal gastric fundic and pyloric epithelium, (2) it did not secrete acid or pepsin but was resistant to both, (3) it was not congenital but acquired, (4) it was mobile and varied in length—creeping progressively higher into the esophagus with continued gastroesophageal reflux, and (5) it was potentially reversible with correction of reflux. Furthermore, he pointed out that it was located in the esophagus and that it developed in association with gastroesophageal reflux.[6]

Now, over 40 years later, there is still dispute about the histology of the normal gastroesophageal junction. The preponderance of autopsy and clinical biopsy data suggest that in a normal individual, squamous esophageal mucosa transitions directly to oxyntic gastric mucosa at the gastroesophageal junction.[36,37] This situation is present in most children and adults younger than 20 years. However, in older adults, cardiac mucosa can be found in biopsy specimens from the gastroesophageal junction in approximately 50% of individuals, and the prevalence increases with age and the severity of reflux.[38,39] One center still disputes these findings and suggests instead that 1 to 4 mm of cardiac mucosa is a normal finding at the gastroesophageal junction. However, their definition of cardiac mucosa includes columnar cells with glands containing parietal cells, and this casts some doubt on their conclusions.[40,41] Nonetheless, it is clear that Hayward's concept is incorrect and that normally there is no cardiac mucosa or at most 4 mm of cardiac mucosa in the distal esophagus at the gastroesophageal junction. Longer lengths of cardiac mucosa are acquired secondary to chronic gastroesophageal reflux.

Supporting evidence for the concept that cardiac mucosa is acquired is derived from both clinical and experimental studies. Experimental evidence comes from a 1970 study by Bremner and colleagues in which a series of dogs underwent stripping of the distal esophageal squamous mucosa with or without cardioplasty to destroy the function of the lower esophageal sphincter. Squamous re-epithelialization occurred in animals without gastroesophageal reflux, whereas in animals with reflux after cardioplasty, the esophagus was re-epithelialized by a columnar epithelium that lacked submucosal glands and parietal cells—the equivalent of cardiac mucosa in humans.[42] There is also clinical evidence in humans that columnar mucosa can replace normal esophageal squamous epithelium in the setting of gastroesophageal reflux. After esophagectomy with gastric pull-up, reflux of gastric juice into the residual esophagus is common because there is no lower esophageal sphincter and a large hiatal hernia has been created. Postoperative endoscopy has revealed that in many of these patients columnar epithelium histologically identical to cardiac mucosa develops proximal to the anastomosis in the residual esophagus, in what had pathologically been proved to be squamous mucosa at the time of the operation. Several series have shown that this process is common and occurs in 50% or more of patients after esophagectomy with gastric pull-up. Furthermore, cardiac mucosa developed within 2 years of esophagectomy in many patients and was observed to increase in length with longer follow-up.[29,43-46] Importantly, the cardiac mucosa that develops in these patients proximal to the esophagogastric anastomosis has been shown to be biochemically similar to the cardiac mucosa found in unoperated patients at the native gastroesophageal junction.[43]

Additional support for the concept that cardiac mucosa is acquired comes from the fact that it is not found anywhere else in the gastrointestinal tract and, when present at the gastroesophageal junction, is always inflamed and demonstrates reactive changes unrelated to either *Helicobacter pylori* infection or mucosal disease elsewhere in the stomach.[47] This is atypical for normal epithelium. Moreover, the presence of cardiac mucosa can be correlated with objective markers of GERD, including an incompetent lower esophageal sphincter, increased esophageal acid exposure on 24-hour pH monitoring, a hiatal hernia, and erosive esophagitis.[39]

The earliest manifestation of GERD may in fact be the presence of microscopic foci of cardiac mucosa at the gastroesophageal junction. This leads to the question of why the finding of a microscopic length of cardiac mucosa at the gastroesophageal junction is so common, even in patients without the typical reflux symptoms of heartburn or regurgitation. Probably this is related to the pathophysiology of early reflux disease. Evidence is accumulating that reflux disease begins with gastric distention after large and particularly fatty meals. Gastric distention leads to effacement of the lower esophageal sphincter and exposure of the squamous mucosa at the distal extent of the sphincter to gastric juice. The pathophysiology of the gastroesophageal junction has best been studied by Fletcher et al. They noted that the gastric distention that occurs with eating can cause the lower esophageal sphincter to unfold by almost 2 cm in normal volunteers.[48] In addition, they identified an unbuffered acid pocket at the gastroesophageal junction after a meal, a phenomenon they attributed to gastric juice floating on a lipid layer after the ingestion of fatty food. By pulling back a pH catheter before and after a meal they were able to show that the pH step-up corresponding to the functioning lower esophageal sphincter moved proximally with gastric distention secondary to unfolding of the distal portion of the sphincter. By measuring acid exposure with a pH catheter positioned at the squamocolumnar junction and another located 5.5 cm proximal to the squamocolumnar junction, Fletcher et al. demonstrated significantly greater acid exposure at the squamocolumnar junction (median total percent time that the pH was less than 4, 11.7% versus 1.8% 5.5 cm proximal to the squamocolumnar junction).[49] This study confirmed the presence of significant acid exposure at the most distal intrasphincteric segment of the esophagus in patients with otherwise normal acid exposure 5.5 cm proximal to the squamocolumnar junction. These findings were subsequently extended when it was demonstrated that salivary nitrite is rapidly converted to nitric oxide when it comes in contact with gastric acid–containing physiologic levels of ascorbic acid, and this reaction was found to be maximal at the gastroesophageal junction.[50] The levels of nitric oxide generated at the gastroesophageal junction were potentially mutagenic and may play a role in the pathophysiology of this region.

It is likely that continued injury to the distal esophagus and lower esophageal sphincter leads to progressive loss of the abdominal length of the sphincter. What started as transient sphincter unfolding with gastric

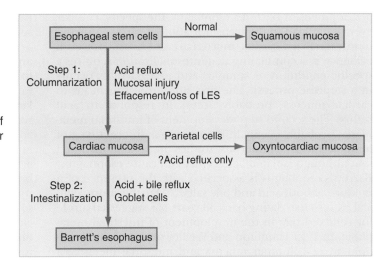

Figure 23–1. Hypothesis for the development of columnar mucosa in the esophagus. LES, lower esophageal sphincter.

distention gradually progresses to permanent sphincter destruction. With destruction of the sphincter, reflux disease is allowed to explode into the esophagus and can lead to an increase in the length of cardiac mucosa, either as tongues or as a circumferential replacement of the distal esophageal squamous mucosa. This leads to progressive migration of the squamocolumnar junction further proximally.[51,52] Confirmation of esophageal submucosal glands deep to areas lined by cardiac mucosa provides clear evidence that the development of cardiac mucosa is occurring in the esophagus in areas previously covered with squamous mucosa and not in the proximal part of the stomach.[52]

The precise details of the molecular mechanism by which squamous mucosa is transformed into cardiac mucosa remain unknown. However, there is probably a critical interaction between normally sequestered esophageal stem cells and an intraluminal stimulus that drives this metaplastic process. Tobey et al. demonstrated that exposure of esophageal squamous mucosa to gastric juice produces dilated intercellular spaces that allow molecules up to 20 kD in size to permeate down to the stem cells in the basal layer.[53] Perhaps the sensation of heartburn occurs as a result of stimulation of sensory afferent nerves by diffusion of hydrochloric acid through these intercellular spaces.[54] These ultrastructural changes occur before gross or microscopic changes become apparent. Thus, one possibility is that factors present in the refluxed juice that gain access to the basal layer stem cells via these dilated intercellular spaces induce a phenotypic transformation such that cardiac columnar mucosal cells rather than squamous cells are produced.

In summary, there is increasing evidence that at a normal gastroesophageal junction, squamous esophageal mucosa transitions directly with oxyntic mucosa of the stomach. Effacement of the lower esophageal sphincter occurs with gastric distention and leads to exposure of the distal esophageal squamous mucosa to acidic gastric juice. In combination perhaps with the generation of nitric oxide from salivary nitrite there is progressive injury to the lower esophageal sphincter, which in some patients leads to destruction of the

sphincter and escape of gastric juice proximally into the distal esophagus. The development of dilated intercellular spaces in the squamous epithelium in response to repetitive acid exposure may expose esophageal stem cells to components of the refluxate that stimulate a phenotypic change from squamous to columnar cardiac mucosa. Progression of reflux disease leads to a gradual migration of the squamocolumnar junction proximally and increasing lengths of cardiac mucosa in the distal esophagus.

Pathophysiology—Step 2: Intestinalization of Cardiac Mucosa

Cardiac mucosa is thought to be an unstable epithelium, in part because of the severe inflammatory and reactive changes noted on histologic examination. It is hypothesized that cardiac mucosa progress down one of two possible pathways based on a combination of environmental and genetic factors (Fig. 23–1). One pathway involves the expression of gastric genes and leads to the formation of parietal cells within cardiac mucosa. Gastric differentiation leads to a mucosa called oxyntocardiac mucosa, and this is thought to represent a regressive or favorable change because oxyntocardiac mucosa is not premalignant and appears to be protected from the development of intestinal metaplasia. In the second pathway, expression of intestinal genes causes the formation of goblet cells within cardiac mucosa. In contrast to gastric differentiation, intestinal differentiation represents a progressive or unfavorable change because this mucosa is premalignant. Both oxyntocardiac mucosa and Barrett's esophagus have less inflammation than cardiac mucosa does, which suggests that these mucosal types are more stable epithelia.[55]

The development of goblet cells marks the transformation of cardiac mucosa to intestinal metaplasia. When an endoscopically visible length of this mucosa is present in the esophagus, the definition of Barrett's esophagus has been met. Although gastroesophageal reflux is known to be the primary factor responsible for the development of Barrett's esophagus, the specific cellular events that lead to the transformation of cardiac mucosa to intestinalized cardiac mucosa are unknown. However, evidence is accumulating that intestinalization requires a specific condition or stimulus and that Barrett's occurs in a stepwise process. The first step, from squamous to cardiac mucosa, probably occurs in response to acid reflux. The second step, development of intestinal metaplasia, probably occurs in response to a different type of luminal insult. Numerous studies have demonstrated that although isolated acid reflux can cause esophagitis, Barrett's esophagus is associated with the presence of a mixture of both acid and bile salts.[56-58] Furthermore, clinical experience dating back 30 years has suggested a role for refluxed bile in the development of intestinal metaplasia. In 1977 Hamilton and Yardley observed the development of columnar mucosa and intestinal metaplasia above the esophagogastric anastomosis in a group of patients after esophagectomy. They noted that "severe symptoms of gastroesophageal reflux and bile staining of the refluxed material were documented only in the group with Barrett's. In addition, pyloroplasty had been performed more commonly in this group."[59] Recently, in two separate analyses of patients who had reflux with and without Barrett's, we found that the factor most associated with the presence of Barrett's esophagus in both males and females with GERD was abnormal bilirubin reflux as determined by Bilitec monitoring.[17,18] Interestingly, although all the patients in these studies had increased esophageal acid exposure by 24-hour pH monitoring, the necessity of acid in the refluxed material for Barrett's to develop is unclear. Scattered reports describing the development of Barrett's esophagus after total gastrectomy have circulated for a number of years, but a recent study clearly documents this process in eight patients at a median of 9 years postoperatively.[60] The authors noted that Barrett's was most likely to develop in patients with a reconstruction that permitted bile reflux into the esophagus. However, only one patient in this series had cardiac mucosa without intestinal metaplasia in the esophagus. This stands in stark contrast to the frequent development of cardiac mucosa in the residual esophagus after esophagectomy with gastric pull-up and supports the concept that cardiac mucosa develops in response to acidic reflux.[60,61]

Fitzgerald and colleagues reported several interesting observations on how the dynamics of mucosal exposure to luminal contents may affect columnar epithelial cell proliferation and differentiation. Using cultured human Barrett's biopsy specimens they demonstrated that continuous exposure to acidic media at pH 3.5 resulted in increased villin expression (a marker for epithelial cell differentiation) and reduced cell proliferation. Villin expression was not detected when the culture media was made more acidic (pH <2.5). In contrast, a dramatic increase in proliferation occurred when the Barrett's tissue was exposed to a short (1 hour) pulse of acidic media (pH 3.5) followed by a return to neutral pH.[62] Clinically, this same group has noted that effective acid suppression results in a shift of Barrett's epithelium away from proliferation toward differentiation.[63] However, the cellular consequences of duodenogastroesophageal reflux in the setting of gastric alkalization with acid-suppression medications were not addressed in this study.

It is hypothesized that the mechanism by which acid and bile interact to cause Barrett's esophagus is related to the ionized state of bile salts.[64] It appears that in a weakly acidic environment certain bile acids are particularly toxic. At a pH in the 3 to 6 range these bile salts are soluble and nonionized and can enter mucosal cells, accumulate, and cause direct cellular injury.[65] When the luminal pH is higher than their pK_a, these same bile acids are ionized and cannot cross the phospholipid membrane. Furthermore, when the luminal pH is lower, as it normally is in the stomach, bile acids precipitate out of solution and are harmless.[66] Thus, it is only at this critical pH range of 3 to 5 that certain bile acids become un-ionized and able to cross the cell membrane. Once inside the cell the pH is 7, and the bile acids become ionized and are trapped inside the cell, where they have been shown to result in mitochondrial injury, cellular toxicity, and mutagenesis.[67-70] Consequently, this midrange gastric pH of 3 to 5 is a danger zone for patients with duodenogastroesophageal reflux.

It remains uncertain whether the transformation of cardiac mucosa to intestinalized cardiac mucosa represents a phenotypic change secondary to the induction of genes or a mutational event within the columnar cells. Mendes de Almeida and colleagues have demonstrated biochemically that both cardiac mucosa and intestinal metaplasia express sucrase-isomaltase and crypt cell antigen—two small intestine marker proteins; however, in this study only three patients with cardiac mucosa were evaluated.[71] Kiron Das has developed a murine monoclonal antibody (DAS-1) that reacts specifically with normal colonic epithelial cells, and he subsequently found that it also reacts with an unknown epitope in Barrett's mucosa.[72] Griffel and colleagues reported that the DAS-1 antibody stained cardiac mucosa without intestinal metaplasia in seven patients and that histologic evidence of intestinalization on repeat biopsy samples later developed in six of the seven patients.[73] Likewise, we noted that the pattern of immunostaining with cytokeratins 7 and 20 was similar in cardiac mucosa and Barrett's.[74] These findings suggest that cardiac mucosa and intestinal metaplasia are biochemically similar and that cardiac mucosa is the precursor of intestinalized columnar epithelium, or Barrett's esophagus.

Currently, Barrett's esophagus is divided into short (<3 cm) and long (≥3 cm) segment types based on the endoscopically determined length of the columnar streak or column in the distal esophagus. Clinically, patients with long-segment Barrett's tend to have more severe reflux disease than do those with short-segment Barrett's. Patients with long-segment Barrett's have a higher prevalence of hiatal hernia, more commonly have a defective lower esophageal sphincter, and demonstrate greater esophageal acid and bilirubin exposure on 24-hour pH and Bilitec monitoring.[56,75] Despite the differences in length, there is evidence that short- and long-segment Barrett's are biochemically similar.[74,76] This finding is supported by the clinical observation that the risk for malignancy is similar in both short- and long-segment Barrett's esophagus.[77]

The presence of goblet cells is the sine qua non of Barrett's esophagus. The likelihood of finding intestinalization correlates with the length of the columnar segment, and once 4 cm of cardiac mucosa is present in the distal esophagus, nearly all patients will be found to have intestinal metaplasia on biopsy.[75,78] However, the location of goblet cells in a columnar-lined segment is not uniform, and often the entire length of columnar esophagus does not demonstrate intestinal metaplasia. Goblet cell density is greatest near the squamocolumnar junction and becomes more variable distally.[55] In other words, if intestinal metaplasia is present within a columnar-lined segment of the esophagus, it will always be present proximally at the squamocolumnar junction. Goblet cells may extend throughout the entire length of the columnar segment, but they might not. Interestingly, the length of Barrett's is determined by the endoscopic length of columnar mucosa and not by the length of mucosa showing intestinal metaplasia. In other words, a 6-cm segment of columnar mucosa with intestinal metaplasia only at the proximal 1 cm is still considered long-segment Barrett's esophagus, but the clinical behavior of this long-segment Barrett's may differ substantially from a 6-cm segment of columnar mucosa with intestinal metaplasia throughout the entire length. The current definition of Barrett's does not take this issue into account.

The time course for the development of goblet cells is uncertain, but it appears to take a minimum of 5 to 10 years.[64,79] Studies involving esophagectomy patients indicate that cardiac mucosa develops rapidly, often within 1 to 2 years. Intestinalization of the columnar segment in these patients occurs significantly later, typically after another 3 to 5 years.[44-46,59,61] These findings may reflect an accelerated course of events because these patients often have significantly greater reflux of acid and bile than the typical patient with GERD does. However, this clinically relevant human model does demonstrate the two-step process of Barrett's, starting with columnarization and subsequently followed by intestinalization in some patients.

The molecular mechanisms by which cardiac mucosa acquires goblet cells remain to be elucidated. However, there is increasing evidence that expression of the homeobox gene *Cdx2* plays a pivotal role. Expression of this gene increases with progression from squamous mucosa with esophagitis to cardiac mucosa and is maximal in the setting of intestinal metaplasia.[80-82] Experimental work suggests that *Cdx2* expression can be modulated by the pH of luminal material.[83] Furthermore, an individual's response to an inflammatory stimulus may also participate in the mucosal adaptation to reflux disease. Fitzgerald et al. have demonstrated that esophagitis and Barrett's esophagus have distinct cytokine profiles that reflect different inflammatory responses to reflux-induced injury.[84] Moreover, even within a given Barrett's segment, the inflammatory response is more severe at the proximal extent near the squamocolumnar junction, which may explain the greater tendency for intestinalization to occur at this location.[85] In addition, the specific cytokine polymorphism of a given individual may influence the development of Barrett's esophagus. Preliminary work from Gough and colleagues, for example, has demonstrated

that specific polymorphisms of interleukin-1 receptor antagonist and interleukin-10 are more common in patients with Barrett's than in those with esophagitis.[86] Thus, a genetically determined inflammatory response to reflux may influence the pathway of disease in each individual patient.

In summary, the second step in the formation of Barrett's esophagus involves the development of goblet cells within cardiac mucosa, a reflection of intestinalization of this columnar epithelium. The acquisition of goblet cells appears to be related to the composition of the refluxed material, particularly the presence of bile acids within the refluxed material. If present, goblet cells will always be found at the proximal portion of the columnar segment just distal to the squamocolumnar junction, with decreasing density distally. Goblet cells may or may not extend throughout the entire columnar segment, but identification of a single goblet cell is sufficient to diagnose Barrett's esophagus in the setting of a visible columnar segment in the distal esophagus. The specific genetic events that lead to the transformation of cardiac mucosa to intestinalized cardiac mucosa are unknown, but genes such as *Cdx2* probably participate, and the expression of these genes in response to reflux-induced mucosal injury may be variable in individuals and may influence the response of the mucosa to inflammatory injury.

DYSPLASIA AND MALIGNANT TRANSFORMATION

Barrett's esophagus is a premalignant mucosa and has an increased proliferation rate, decreased apoptosis, and an increased fraction of diploid and aneuploid cells in comparison to normal epithelium.[41,87] The combination of increased proliferation and decreased apoptosis allows genetic abnormalities to develop and accumulate and drives the development of dysplasia and malignant transformation in Barrett's.[88] Whereas nondysplastic Barrett's esophagus is a simple columnar epithelium with homogeneous nuclei arranged close to the basement membrane, dysplasia results in both cytologic and architectural abnormalities, including loss of nuclear polarity, a pleomorphic appearance, and the development of glandular distortion.[89] By convention, four broad categories are used by pathologists to describe the dysplastic process: (1) no dysplasia, (2) indefinite for dysplasia, (3) low-grade dysplasia, and (4) high-grade dysplasia. This classification system was adapted for use in Barrett's esophagus from that used in ulcerative colitis.[90,91] The most significant category, high-grade dysplasia, is characterized by carcinoma in situ with malignant cells that do not invade the lamina propria.

Grading of dysplasia has great clinical utility in stratifying the risk for subsequent cancer in patients with Barrett's, and to date it is the most important predictive marker for the development of invasive adenocarcinoma. However, the ability to grade dysplasia remains a subjective endeavor, particularly outside specialized centers and by those who are not expert gastrointestinal pathologists.[92] Even among focused gastrointestinal pathologists there is discordance, particularly with regard to the presence of low-grade dysplasia.[93] A new grading system called the Vienna classification has been proposed to reduce interobserver variation, but it has yet to be validated. This lack of precision inherent in histopathologic grading has stimulated efforts to identify more objective molecular and biochemical indicators of an increased risk for progression in patients with Barrett's. It has been demonstrated that in medically treated patients with Barrett's and low-grade dysplasia, the risk for progression is increased in patients with aneuploidy.[94] It is hoped that other molecular markers that are able to better predict which patients with Barrett's are at increased risk for progression will be identified in the future.

Investigating the molecular and genetic pathways by which Barrett's esophagus progresses to dysplasia and cancer not only increases our understanding of the pathophysiology of Barrett's esophagus but also aids in the identification of biomarkers for stratifying risk in an individual patient. It is hoped that ultimately, quantitative measurement of molecular changes will result in more objective end points for assessing the risk for dysplasia and cancer, as well as for assessing response to therapy. Perhaps not surprisingly, however, the genetic events associated with progression of Barrett's esophagus have been found to be diverse and varied. These events can be classified broadly as chromosomal events, characterized by loss or gain of chromosomal regions, molecular events, such as promotor hypermethylation, gene amplification or overexpression, and genetic mutations.[95] The specific changes that occur during progression to dysplasia and malignancy can be classified according to the general principles of carcinogenesis: (1) self-sufficiency and independence from external mitogenic growth signals, (2) insensitivity to antigrowth signals, (3) diminished apoptosis, (4) limitless replicative potential, (5) angiogenic capabilities, and (6) the ability to invade and metastasize.[88] A representative table of such changes studied to date in the Barrett's metaplasia-dysplasia-carcinoma sequence is shown in Table 23–1. Currently, there is no single unifying pathway that fully describes progression through this sequence of events similar to what has been done for sporadic colorectal cancer. Rather, there is increasing evidence that genetic and chromosomal abnormalities randomly accumulate and result in divergent clones of Barrett's mucosa that can progress to cancer. For malignant transformation to occur, it is hypothesized that at least 5 to 10 such genetic changes must accumulate within a given clone of cells.[96-98]

Despite being proposed by Virchow in 1863, the link between inflammation and cancer is only now becoming evident. One example of this link is the development of Barrett's esophagus and adenocarcinoma secondary to gastroesophageal reflux. Recent data indicate that a major mechanism by which reflux-induced inflammation can lead to carcinogenesis is via the nuclear factor-κB (NFκB) pathway, which has also been implicated in hepatocellular carcinoma secondary to hepatitis, cholangiocarcinoma secondary to ductal inflammation, squamous cell carcinoma of the skin, and colorectal carcinoma secondary to ulcerative colitis.[99,100] The NFκB pathway appears to be uniquely positioned to mediate this process because it has been shown to participate in the regulation of immune and inflammatory functions, as well as carcinogenesis. Stimulation of NFκB can occur through numerous factors, including cytokines, oxidants, and immune stimuli, which result in amplification of the inflammatory process. NFκB is responsible for downstream expression of many important and diverse proteins such as proinflammatory cytokines, chemokines, inflammatory enzymes, and adhesion molecules. One such downstream effector is cyclooxygenase-2 (COX-2), the rate-limiting enzyme in arachidonic acid conversion to prostaglandin.

Many investigators have focused on COX-2 in recent years because it appears to mediate the interaction between inflammation and carcinogenesis and has been implicated in multiple important carcinogenic mechanisms, including promotion of proliferation and angiogenesis, as well as inhibition of apoptosis.[101] COX-2 expression is usually undetectable in normal tissue, but it has been found to be up-regulated in Barrett's esophagus and increases in stepwise fashion during the progression to dysplasia and cancer.[102,103] It remains unclear at what point in the metaplasia-dysplasia-carcinoma sequence that COX-2 expression transitions from induced up-regulation secondary to inflammation and becomes permanent overexpression contributing to carcinogenesis. It is possible that COX-2 may play a significant role in the earliest stages of the metaplastic process, even before the development of Barrett's esophagus, because it is also expressed in the squamous epithelium of patients with reflux disease.[104] Recently, we have demonstrated that elevated COX-2 expression in patients with GERD is significantly reduced after antireflux surgery. In fact, it was normalized to levels expressed in control patients without reflux disease (manuscript submitted for publication). This observation demonstrates that increased COX-2 associated with gastroesophageal reflux is reversible. Furthermore, it is the first evidence that antireflux surgery alters gene expression in the esophagus and supports the controversial concept that antireflux surgery can have an impact on the natural history of reflux disease.

NATURAL HISTORY OF BARRETT'S ESOPHAGUS

Although widely accepted that Barrett's esophagus is a premalignant condition, the degree of risk remains uncertain. A meta-analysis by Shaheen et al. of 25 articles published between 1984 and 1998 concluded that the incidence of adenocarcinoma in patients with Barrett's was approximately 0.5% per patient-year, with a range of 0.2% to 2.9%.[105] However, these studies were performed in patients being treated for reflux, including those who underwent antireflux surgery, and thus these estimates may not reflect the true natural history of Barrett's progression. The incidence of low-grade dysplasia is reported to be approximately 4.3% per patient-year and that of high-grade dysplasia, 0.9% per patient-year.[106] Known risk factors for progression to dysplasia and

Table 23–1 Genetic Alterations in the Barrett's Metaplasia-Dysplasia-Carcinoma Sequence

Types of Alterations*	Comment
Abnormal Growth Signals	
Extracellular growth signals	
TGF-β_1	Overexpression, receptor alterations
aFGF, bFGF	Overexpression
TNF-α	Overexpression
TGF-α	Overexpression
Transcellular transducers	
EGFR (erbB-1)	Overexpression
HER2/neu (erbB-2)	Overexpression
Intracellular circuits	
Ras-Raf-MAPK pathway	Ras overexpression, mutations
APC	Inactivation (LOH, mutation, methylation)
Src	Overexpression
Loss of Antigrowth Signals	
Rb pathway	
Rb	Inactivation (LOH, mutation, methylation)
Cyclin D1, E	Overexpression
CDK	Loss of inhibitors
c-myc	Overexpression, aberrant localization
CDK inhibitors	
p16	Inactivation (LOH, mutation, methylation)
p15	Inactivation (LOH)
p27	Inactivation
p21	Inactivation
Loss of Apoptosis	
p53	Inactivation (LOH, mutation)
S-HODE	Reduced expression, proapoptotic
Fas	FasL overexpression, Fas sequestration
Decoy receptor 3	Overexpression, sequesters Fas
COX-2	Overexpression, blocks apoptosis
Bcl-2	Overexpression, inhibits apoptosis
Unlimited Replication	
Telomerase	Overexpression
Angiogenesis	
VEGF	Overexpression
COX-2	Overexpression, induces VEGF
Invasion and Metastasis	
E-cadherin	Reduced expression, aberrant localization
β-Catenin	Aberrant localization, overexpression
CD44	Isoform overexpression
DCC	Inactivation
Urokinase plasminogen activator	Overexpression
Cysteine protease cathepsin B (CTSB)	Overexpression
Src	Overexpression

*The six hallmarks of carcinogenesis. Adapted from Hanahan D, Weinberg RA: The hallmarks of cancer. Cell 100:57-70, 2000.
aFGF, acidic fibroblast growth factor; APC, antigen-presenting cell; bFGF, basic fibroblast growth factor; CDK, cyclin-dependent kinase; COX, cyclooxygenase; DCC, deleted in colon cancer; EGFR, endothelial growth factor receptor; LOH, loss of heterozygosity; MAPK, mitogen-activated protein kinase; Src, sarcoma; TGF, transforming growth factor; TNF, tumor necrosis factor; VEGF, vascular endothelial growth factor.

cancer include hiatal hernia size, the length of Barrett's esophagus, patient age, and the presence of cellular and molecular abnormalities, including abnormal ploidy status and p16 or p53 gene abnormalities.[94,107-110]

The natural history of dysplasia is not well characterized, but the risk for malignancy increases with the development of low- and high-grade dysplasia. The best data come from Reid and colleagues, and in a carefully monitored group of patients they reported that low-grade dysplasia progressed to cancer in 4% over a period of 5 years whereas high-grade dysplasia led to cancer in 61% at 5 years.[94] It is also clear that progression is variable, with some patients progressing at a steady pace over a period of several years and others having stable nondysplastic or low-grade dysplasia in Barrett's esophagus for many years and then rapidly progressing to high-grade dysplasia and cancer. Theisen et al. conducted a review of patients who received follow-up through the entire sequence of Barrett's esophagus, low-grade dysplasia, high-grade dysplasia, and adenocarcinoma to better understand the chronology of these events.[111] In a group of 28 patients with adenocarcinoma, a median of 24 months had passed from the initial diagnosis of Barrett's esophagus. Progression from low-grade to high-grade dysplasia occurred over a median of 11 months. Once high-grade dysplasia was diagnosed, the median time to diagnosis of cancer was 3 months. Although this timeline was variable for each individual, in this cohort of patients who had progression of Barrett's to cancer the process occurred within 3 years. However, because most Barrett's patients do not progress to dysplasia and cancer, the cohort in this retrospective study may not be applicable to all patients. Furthermore, since few of these patients had been in long-term Barrett's surveillance programs, it is not possible to separate prevalent from incident cancers in this group, and the actual month and year that Barrett's developed in each patient is also unknown. Thus, information on progression of Barrett's is largely anecdotal.

SCREENING AND SURVEILLANCE

There are currently no screening protocols for Barrett's esophagus in the United States. Although a history of chronic reflux symptoms in a white male older than 50 years was previously an indication for screening upper endoscopy, this recommendation was recently retracted by the American College of Gastroenterology.[112] The cost versus benefit of endoscopic screening continues to be debated, but perhaps as new technologies emerge such as the Pill-cam there will be lower-cost options that permit cost-effective screening to be performed. The other impediment has been the difficulty in determining appropriate candidates for screening because symptoms of reflux are not a reliable indicator for the presence or absence of reflux-related complications, including Barrett's. Thus, any screening strategy will have to be broadly applied independent of symptoms.

Endoscopic surveillance in patients with a diagnosis of Barrett's is less controversial, yet the cost-effectiveness and timing are debated, and in practice, surveillance in

patients is often sporadic.[113,114] The recommended biopsy protocol for surveillance of Barrett's esophagus is four-quadrant biopsies every 2 cm, with specimens taken at 1-cm intervals when high-grade dysplasia is present.[115,116] Occasionally, severe esophagitis may complicate the histologic differentiation of dysplasia versus cellular atypia secondary to inflammation, and repeat biopsy may be necessary after a period of aggressive acid-suppression therapy.

Recognizing the limitations of standard endoscopy, staining techniques have been used in an attempt to increase the sensitivity of diagnosing Barrett's esophagus and dysplasia. Among others, Lugol's iodine, toluene blue, indigo carmine, and methylene blue have been studied. Alternatively, new technologies, including high-magnification chromoendoscopes and a variety of light-scattering techniques, are also being investigated and may aid in recognition of abnormal mucosa and improve biopsy yield.[117] At this time, however, standard endoscopy with systematic four-quadrant biopsy of the columnar-lined esophagus remains the gold standard for the diagnosis and surveillance of Barrett's esophagus.

The recommended time interval for follow-up endoscopy is directly related to the presence or absence of dysplasia. The most recent practice parameters published by the American College of Gastroenterology suggest that when two consecutive endoscopies with biopsy confirm the absence of dysplasia, follow-up endoscopy can be done at 3-year intervals. The finding of low-grade dysplasia escalates follow-up to every 6 months for the first year, followed by annual endoscopy if low-grade dysplasia persists. High-grade dysplasia poses a special problem because of the difficulty with diagnosis and the risk of missing an occult cancer. Thus, the finding of high-grade dysplasia first requires (1) an immediate repeat endoscopy with biopsy every 1 cm to rule out cancer and (2) an expert pathologist consultation to confirm the diagnosis. Continued surveillance for high-grade dysplasia is controversial because it is associated with a significant risk for an occult carcinoma, particularly in long-segment Barrett's or when multifocal high-grade dysplasia is present.[118,119] If surveillance is chosen, it is recommended that it be undertaken every 3 months.[112] Any visible lesion or ulcerated area within a Barrett's segment must be carefully biopsied because of the high risk for associated cancer with these lesions.[118]

Determining appropriate recommendations for surveillance of Barrett's esophagus is difficult given our incomplete understanding of the natural history of this condition. The literature on surveillance and cancer incidence in Barrett's esophagus is compromised by heterogeneous patient groups and referral and publication bias.[105] Despite these uncertainties, surveillance of Barrett's patients has been shown to be beneficial. Patients in whom adenocarcinoma develops within a surveillance program tend to have earlier-stage disease and a better prognosis than do those who have de novo adenocarcinoma with symptoms from local tumor growth.[120-122] Furthermore, the cost of surveillance for Barrett's esophagus compares favorably with the widely accepted protocol of breast cancer detection with mammography. The cost per life-year saved is $4151 for esophageal adenocarcinoma versus $57,926 for breast cancer.[123]

An interesting dilemma arises in patients who have a columnar-lined segment of esophagus on endoscopy but do not have intestinal metaplasia on histology. This may simply represent a sampling error; however, even if a columnar segment is not intestinalized, there is a significant likelihood that it will become so in the future, particularly when the columnar segment approaches 3 cm in length.[78,124] Most agree that these patients should undergo follow-up endoscopy and biopsy, but consensus on the timing or frequency is lacking.

CONCLUSION

There is increasing evidence that at the normal gastroesophageal junction, esophageal squamous mucosa abuts oxyntic fundic mucosa of the stomach. With exposure to gastric juice the squamous mucosa is injured, and over time it becomes replaced by columnar cardiac mucosa. Deterioration of the lower esophageal sphincter allows reflux to extend up into the esophagus, and the squamocolumnar junction migrates proximally. Although it is likely that acidic gastric juice drives the transformation of squamous mucosa to cardiac mucosa, there is substantial evidence that other components of gastric juice, particularly bile acids, are essential for subsequent intestinalization of the cardiac mucosa to occur.

Barrett's esophagus is a premalignant mucosa, and the risk for malignant transformation is approximately 0.5% per patient-year. The finding of dysplasia is currently the most commonly used indicator of increased malignant risk, but it has high interobserver variability. It is expected that ultimately, molecular markers will prove more helpful than histology in Barrett's, and there are ongoing efforts to determine biomarkers that will better delineate an individual's risk for progression to cancer. Surveillance endoscopy in patients with Barrett's esophagus has proven efficacy, but it is time-consuming and haphazardly applied across the country. Currently, screening endoscopy is not recommended for Barrett's esophagus, but given the dramatic increase in the incidence of esophageal adenocarcinoma, new technologies that permit widespread and cost-effective screening are needed.

REFERENCES

1. Sandler RS, Everhart JE, Donowitz M, et al: The burden of selected digestive diseases in the United States. Gastroenterology 122:1500-1511, 2002.
2. Pohl H, Welch HG: The role of overdiagnosis and reclassification in the marked increase of esophageal adenocarcinoma incidence. J Natl Cancer Inst 97:142-146, 2005.
3. Barrett N: Chronic peptic ulcer of the oesophagus and 'oesophagitis.' Br J Surg 38:175-182, 1950.
4. Allison P, Johnstone A: The oesophagus lined with gastric mucous membrane. Thorax 8:87-101, 1953.
5. Barrett M: The lower esophagus lined by columnar epithelium. Surgery 41:881-894, 1957.
6. Hayward J: The lower end of the esophagus. Thorax 16:36-41, 1961.
7. Skinner DB, Walther BC, Riddell RH, et al: Barrett's esophagus. Comparison of benign and malignant cases. Ann Surg 198:554-565, 1983.
8. Paull A, Trier JS, Dalton MD, et al: The histologic spectrum of Barrett's esophagus. N Engl J Med 295:476-480, 1976.
9. Haggitt RC, Tryzelaar J, Ellis FH, Colcher H: Adenocarcinoma complicating columnar epithelium-lined (Barrett's) esophagus. Am J Clin Pathol 70:1-5, 1978.
10. Reid BJ, Weinstein WM: Barrett's esophagus and adenocarcinoma. Annu Rev Med 38:477-492, 1987.
11. Prach AT, MacDonald TA, Hopwood DA, Johnston DA: Increasing incidence of Barrett's oesophagus: Education, enthusiasm, or epidemiology [letter]? Lancet 350:933, 1997.
12. van Soest EM, Dieleman JP, Siersema PD, et al: Increasing incidence of Barrett's oesophagus in the general population. Gut 54:1062-1066, 2005.
13. van Blankenstein M, Looman C, Johnston B, Caygill CP: Age and sex distribution of the prevalence of Barrett's esophagus found in a primary referral endoscopy center. Am J Gastroenterol 100:568-576, 2005.
14. Cameron AJ, Zinsmeister AR, Ballard DJ, Carney JA: Prevalence of columnar-lined (Barrett's) esophagus. Comparison of population-based clinical and autopsy findings. Gastroenterology 99:918-922, 1990.
15. Gerson LB, Shetler K, Triadafilopoulos G: Prevalence of Barrett's esophagus in asymptomatic individuals. Gastroenterology 123:461-467, 2002.
16. Eisen GM, Sandler RS, Murray S, Gottfried M: The relationship between gastroesophageal reflux disease and its complications with Barrett's esophagus. Am J Gastroenterol 92:27-31, 1997.
17. Campos GM, DeMeester SR, Peters JH, et al: Predictive factors of Barrett esophagus: Multivariate analysis of 502 patients with gastroesophageal reflux disease. Arch Surg 136:1267-1273, 2001.
18. Banki F, Demeester SR, Mason RJ, et al: Barrett's esophagus in females: A comparative analysis of risk factors in females and males. Am J Gastroenterol 100:560-567, 2005.
19. Cameron AJ, Lomboy CT: Barrett's esophagus: Age, prevalence, and extent of columnar epithelium. Gastroenterology 103:1241-1245, 1992.
20. Rajendra S, Kutty K, Karim N: Ethnic differences in the prevalence of endoscopic esophagitis and Barrett's esophagus: The long and short of it all. Dig Dis Sci 49:237-242, 2004.
21. Bersentes K, Fass R, Padda S, et al: Prevalence of Barrett's esophagus in Hispanics is similar to Caucasians. Dig Dis Sci 43:1038-1041, 1998.
22. Kubo A, Corley DA: Marked multi-ethnic variation of esophageal and gastric cardia carcinomas within the United States. Am J Gastroenterol 99:582-588, 2004.
23. Rex D, Cummings O, Shaw M, et al: Screening for Barrett's esophagus in colonoscopy patients with and without heartburn. Gastroenterology 125:1670-1677, 2003.
24. Poynton AR, Walsh TN, O'Sullivan G, Hennessy TP: Carcinoma arising in familial Barrett's esophagus. Am J Gastroenterol 91:1855-1856, 1996.
25. Fahmy N, King JF: Barrett's esophagus: An acquired condition with genetic predisposition. Am J Gastroenterol 88:1262-1265, 1993.
26. Hassall E: Barrett's esophagus: Congenital or acquired? Am J Gastroenterol 88:819-824, 1993.
27. Chak A, Faulx A, Kinnard M, et al: Identification of Barrett's esophagus in relatives by endoscopic screening. Am J Gastroenterol 99:2107-2114, 2004.
28. Romero Y, Cameron AJ, Schaid DJ, et al: Barrett's esophagus: Prevalence in symptomatic relatives. Am J Gastroenterol 97:1127-1132, 2002.
29. Oberg S, Johansson J, Wenner J, Walther B: Metaplastic columnar mucosa in the cervical esophagus after esophagectomy. Ann Surg 235:338-345, 2002.
30. Nilsson M, Lagergren J: The relation between body mass and gastro-oesophageal reflux. Best Pract Res Clin Gastroenterol 18:1117-1123, 2004.
31. Lagergren J, Bergstrom R, Nyren O: No relation between body mass and gastro-oesophageal reflux symptoms in a Swedish population based study. Gut 47:26-29, 2000.

32. Lagergren J, Bergstrom R, Nyren O: Association between body mass and adenocarcinoma of the esophagus and gastric cardia. Ann Intern Med 130:883-890, 1999.

33. Gerson LB, Triadafilopoulos G: Screening for esophageal adenocarcinoma: An evidence-based approach. Am J Med 113:499-505, 2002.

34. Lagergren J, Bergstrom R, Adami HO, Nyren O: Association between medications that relax the lower esophageal sphincter and risk for esophageal adenocarcinoma. Ann Intern Med 133:165-175, 2000.

35. Lagergren J, Bergstrom R, Lindgren A, Nyren O: Symptomatic gastroesophageal reflux as a risk factor for esophageal adenocarcinoma. N Engl J Med 340:825-831, 1999.

36. Chandrasoma PT, Der R, Ma Y, et al: Histology of the gastroesophageal junction: An autopsy study. Am J Surg Pathol 24: 402-409, 2000.

37. Jain R, Aquino D, Harford W, et al: Cardiac epithelium is found infrequently in the gastric cardia. Gastroenterology 114:A160, 1998.

38. Chandrasoma PT, Der R, Ma Y, et al: Histologic classification of patients based on mapping biopsies of the gastroesophageal junction. Am J Surg Pathol 27:929-936, 2003.

39. Oberg S, Peters JH, DeMeester TR, et al: Inflammation and specialized intestinal metaplasia of cardiac mucosa is a manifestation of gastroesophageal reflux disease. Ann Surg 226:522-530, discussion 530-532, 1997.

40. Kilgore SP, Ormsby AH, Gramlich TL, et al: The gastric cardia: Fact or fiction? Am J Gastroenterol 95:921-924, 2000.

41. Chandrasoma P: Controversies of the cardiac mucosa and Barrett's oesophagus. Histopathology 46:361-373, 2005.

42. Bremner CG, Lynch VP, Ellis FH Jr: Barrett's esophagus: Congenital or acquired? An experimental study of esophageal mucosal regeneration in the dog. Surgery 68:209-216, 1970.

43. Lord RV, Wickramasinghe K, Johansson JJ, et al: Cardiac mucosa in the remnant esophagus after esophagectomy is an acquired epithelium with Barrett's-like features. Surgery 136:633-640, 2004.

44. Dresner SM, Griffin SM, Wayman J, et al: Human model of duodenogastro-oesophageal reflux in the development of Barrett's metaplasia. Br J Surg 90:1120-1128, 2003.

45. Lindahl H, Rintala R, Sariola H, Louhimo I: Cervical Barrett's esophagus: A common complication of gastric tube reconstruction. J Pediatr Surg 25:446-448, 1990.

46. O'Riordan JM, Tucker ON, Byrne PJ, et al: Factors influencing the development of Barrett's epithelium in the esophageal remnant postesophagectomy. Am J Gastroenterol 99:205-211, 2004.

47. Der R, Tsao-Wei DD, Demeester T, et al: Carditis: A manifestation of gastroesophageal reflux disease. Am J Surg Pathol 25:245-252, 2001.

48. Fletcher J, Wirz A, Young J, et al: Unbuffered highly acidic gastric juice exists at the gastroesophageal junction after a meal. Gastroenterology 121:775-783, 2001.

49. Fletcher J, Wirz A, Henry E, McColl KE: Studies of acid exposure immediately above the gastro-oesophageal squamocolumnar junction: Evidence of short segment reflux. Gut 53:168-173, 2004.

50. Iijima K, Henry E, Moriya A, et al: Dietary nitrate generates potentially mutagenic concentrations of nitric oxide at the gastroesophageal junction. Gastroenterology 122:1248-1257, 2002.

51. Csendes A, Maluenda F, Braghetto I, et al: Location of the lower oesophageal sphincter and the squamous columnar mucosal junction in 109 healthy controls and 778 patients with different degrees of endoscopic oesophagitis. Gut 34:21-27, 1993.

52. Chandrasoma PT, Lokuhetty DM, DeMeester TR, et al: Definition of histopathologic changes in gastroesophageal reflux disease. Am J Surg Pathol 24:344-351, 2000.

53. Tobey NA, Hosseini SS, Argote CM, et al: Dilated intercellular spaces and shunt permeability in nonerosive acid-damaged esophageal epithelium. Am J Gastroenterol 99:13-22, 2004.

54. Orlando RC: Pathogenesis of reflux esophagitis and Barrett's esophagus. Med Clin North Am 89:219-241, 2005.

55. Chandrasoma PT, Der R, Dalton P, et al: Distribution and significance of epithelial types in columnar-lined esophagus. Am J Surg Pathol 25:1188-1193, 2001.

56. Oberg S, Ritter MP, Crookes PF, et al: Gastroesophageal reflux disease and mucosal injury with emphasis on short-segment Barrett's esophagus and duodenogastroesophageal reflux. J Gastrointest Surg 2:547-553, discussion 553-554, 1998.

57. Fein M, Ireland AP, Ritter MP, et al: Duodenogastric reflux potentiates the injurious effects of gastroesophageal reflux. J Gastrointest Surg 1:27-33, 1997.

58. Kauer WK, Peters JH, DeMeester TR, et al: Mixed reflux of gastric and duodenal juices is more harmful to the esophagus than gastric juice alone. The need for surgical therapy re-emphasized. Ann Surg 222:525-531, discussion 531-533, 1995.

59. Hamilton SR, Yardley JH: Regeneration of cardiac type mucosa and acquisition of Barrett mucosa after esophagogastrostomy. Gastroenterology 72:669-675, 1977.

60. Peitz U, Vieth M, Ebert MH, et al: Small-bowel metaplasia arising in the remnant esophagus after esophagogastrostomy—a prospective study in patients with a history of total gastrectomy. Am J Gastroenterol 100:2062-2070, 2005.

61. Peitz U, Vieth M, Pross M, et al: Cardia-type metaplasia arising in the remnant esophagus after cardia resection. Gastrointest Endosc 59:810-817, 2004.

62. Fitzgerald RC, Omary MB, Triadafilopoulos G: Dynamic effects of acid on Barrett's esophagus. An ex vivo proliferation and differentiation model. J Clin Invest 98:2120-2128, 1996.

63. Ouatu-Lascar R, Fitzgerald RC, Triadafilopoulos G: Differentiation and proliferation in Barrett's esophagus and the effects of acid suppression. Gastroenterology 117:327-335, 1999.

64. DeMeester SR, Peters JH, DeMeester TR: Barrett's esophagus. Curr Probl Surg 38:558-640, 2001.

65. Schweitzer EJ, Bass BL, Batzri S, Harmon JW: Bile acid accumulation by rabbit esophageal mucosa. Dig Dis Sci 31:1105-1113, 1986.

66. DeMeester TR, Peters JH, Bremner CG, Chandrasoma P: Biology of gastroesophageal reflux disease: Pathophysiology relating to medical and surgical treatment. Annu Rev Med 50:469-506, 1999.

67. Schweitzer EJ, Bass BL, Batzri S, et al: Lipid solubilization during bile salt–induced esophageal mucosal barrier disruption in the rabbit. J Lab Clin Med 110:172-179, 1987.

68. Spivey JR, Bronk SF, Gores GJ: Glycochenodeoxycholate-induced lethal hepatocellular injury in rat hepatocytes. Role of ATP depletion and cytosolic free calcium. J Clin Invest 92:17-24, 1993.

69. Silverman SJ, Andrews AW: Bile acids: Co-mutagenic activity in the *Salmonella*-mammalian-microsome mutagenicity test: Brief communication. J Natl Cancer Inst 59:1557-1559, 1977.

70. Theisen J, Peters JH, Fein M, et al: The mutagenic potential of duodenoesophageal reflux. Ann Surg 241:63-68, 2005.

71. Mendes de Almeida JC, Chaves P, Pereira AD, Altorki NK: Is Barrett's esophagus the precursor of most adenocarcinomas of the esophagus and cardia? A biochemical study. Ann Surg 226: 725-733, discussion 733-735, 1997.

72. Das KM, Prasad I, Garla S, Amenta PS: Detection of a shared colon epithelial epitope on Barrett epithelium by a novel monoclonal antibody. Ann Intern Med 120:753-756, 1994.

73. Griffel LH, Amenta PS, Das KM: Use of a novel monoclonal antibody in diagnosis of Barrett's esophagus. Dig Dis Sci 45:40-48, 2000.

74. DeMeester SR, Wickramasinghe K, Lord RV, et al: Cytokeratin and DAS-1 immunostaining reveal similarities among cardiac mucosa, CIM, and Barrett's esophagus. Am J Gastroenterol 97:2514-2523, 2002.

75. Oberg S, DeMeester TR, Peters JH, et al: The extent of Barrett's esophagus depends on the status of the lower esophageal sphincter and the degree of esophageal acid exposure. J Thorac Cardiovasc Surg 117:572-580, 1999.

76. Ormsby AH, Vaezi MF, Richter JE, et al: Cytokeratin immunoreactivity patterns in the diagnosis of short-segment Barrett's esophagus. Gastroenterology 119:683-690, 2000.

77. Rudolph RE, Vaughan TL, Storer BE, et al: Effect of segment length on risk for neoplastic progression in patients with Barrett esophagus. Ann Intern Med 132:612-620, 2000.

78. Spechler S, Zeroogian J, Wand H, et al: The frequency of specialized intestinal metaplasia at the squamo-columnar junction varies with the extent of columnar epithelium lining the esophagus. Gastroenterology 108:A224, 1995.

79. DeMeester SR, DeMeester TR: Columnar mucosa and intestinal metaplasia of the esophagus: Fifty years of controversy. Ann Surg 231:303-321, 2000.

80. Eda A, Osawa H, Satoh K, et al: Aberrant expression of CDX2 in Barrett's epithelium and inflammatory esophageal mucosa. J Gastroenterol 38:14-22, 2003.

81. Phillips RW, Frierson HF Jr, Moskaluk CA: Cdx2 as a marker of epithelial intestinal differentiation in the esophagus. Am J Surg Pathol 27:1442-1447, 2003.

82. Marchetti M, Caliot E, Pringault E: Chronic acid exposure leads to activation of the cdx2 intestinal homeobox gene in a long-term culture of mouse esophageal keratinocytes. J Cell Sci 116:1429-1436, 2003.

83. Faller G, Dimmler A, Rau T, et al: Evidence for acid-induced loss of Cdx2 expression in duodenal gastric metaplasia. J Pathol 203:904-908, 2004.

84. Fitzgerald RC, Onwuegbusi BA, Bajaj-Elliott M, et al: Diversity in the oesophageal phenotypic response to gastro-oesophageal reflux: Immunological determinants. Gut 50:451-459, 2002.

85. Fitzgerald RC, Abdalla S, Onwuegbusi BA, et al: Inflammatory gradient in Barrett's oesophagus: Implications for disease complications. Gut 51:316-322, 2002.

86. Gough MD, Ackroyd R, Majeed AW, Bird NC: Prediction of malignant potential in reflux disease: Are cytokine polymorphisms important? Am J Gastroenterol 100:1012-1018, 2005.

87. Reid BJ, Sanchez CA, Blount PL, Levine DS: Barrett's esophagus: Cell cycle abnormalities in advancing stages of neoplastic progression. Gastroenterology 105:119-129, 1993.

88. Hanahan D, Weinberg RA: The hallmarks of cancer. Cell 100:57-70, 2000.

89. Flejou JF: Barrett's oesophagus: From metaplasia to dysplasia and cancer. Gut 54(Suppl 1):i6-i12, 2005.

90. Riddell RH, Goldman H, Ransohoff DF, et al: Dysplasia in inflammatory bowel disease: Standardized classification with provisional clinical applications. Hum Pathol 14:931-968, 1983.

91. Reid BJ, Haggitt RC, Rubin CE, et al: Observer variation in the diagnosis of dysplasia in Barrett's esophagus. Hum Pathol 19:166-178, 1988.

92. Alikhan M, Rex D, Khan A, et al: Variable pathologic interpretation of columnar lined esophagus by general pathologists in community practice. Gastrointest Endosc 50:23-26, 1999.

93. Skacel M, Petras RE, Gramlich TL, et al: The diagnosis of low-grade dysplasia in Barrett's esophagus and its implications for disease progression. Am J Gastroenterol 95:3383-3387, 2000.

94. Reid BJ, Levine DS, Longton G, et al: Predictors of progression to cancer in Barrett's esophagus: Baseline histology and flow cytometry identify low- and high-risk patient subsets. Am J Gastroenterol 95:1669-1676, 2000.

95. Jenkins GJ, Doak SH, Parry JM, et al: Genetic pathways involved in the progression of Barrett's metaplasia to adenocarcinoma. Br J Surg 89:824-837, 2002.

96. Fitzgerald RC: Genetics and prevention of oesophageal adenocarcinoma. Recent Results Cancer Res 166:35-46, 2005.

97. Walch AK, Zitzelsberger HF, Bruch J, et al: Chromosomal imbalances in Barrett's adenocarcinoma and the metaplasia-dysplasia-carcinoma sequence. Am J Pathol 156:555-566, 2000.

98. Wijnhoven BP, Tilanus HW, Dinjens WN: Molecular biology of Barrett's adenocarcinoma. Ann Surg 233:322-337, 2001.

99. Li Q, Withoff S, Verma IM: Inflammation-associated cancer: NF-kappaB is the lynchpin. Trends Immunol 26:318-325, 2005.

100. Ditsworth D, Zong WX: NF-kappaB: Key mediator of inflammation-associated cancer. Cancer Biol Ther 3:1214-1216, 2004.

101. McManus DT, Olaru A, Meltzer SJ: Biomarkers of esophageal adenocarcinoma and Barrett's esophagus. Cancer Res 64:1561-1569, 2004.

102. Kuramochi H, Vallbohmer D, Uchida K, et al: Quantitative, tissue-specific analysis of cyclooxygenase gene expression in the pathogenesis of Barrett's adenocarcinoma. J Gastrointest Surg 8:1007-1016, discussion 1016-1017, 2004.

103. Morris CD, Armstrong GR, Bigley G, et al: Cyclooxygenase-2 expression in the Barrett's metaplasia-dysplasia-adenocarcinoma sequence. Am J Gastroenterol 96:990-996, 2001.

104. Hamoui N, Peters JH, Schneider S, et al: Increased acid exposure in patients with gastroesophageal reflux disease influences cyclooxygenase-2 gene expression in the squamous epithelium of the lower esophagus. [erratum appears in Arch Surg. 2005 Mar140(3):249 Note: Valboehmer, Daniel (corrected to Vallbohmer, Daniel).] Arch Surg 139:712-716, discussion 716-717, 2004.

105. Shaheen NJ, Crosby MA, Bozymski EM, Sandler RS: Is there publication bias in the reporting of cancer risk in Barrett's esophagus? Gastroenterology 119:333-338, 2000.

106. Sharma P: Low-grade dysplasia in Barrett's esophagus. Gastroenterology 127:1233-1238, 2004.

107. Gopal DV, Lieberman DA, Magaret N, et al: Risk factors for dysplasia in patients with Barrett's esophagus (BE): Results from a multicenter consortium. Dig Dis Sci 48:1537-1541, 2003.

108. Weston AP, Banerjee SK, Sharma P, et al: p53 protein overexpression in low grade dysplasia (LGD) in Barrett's esophagus: Immunohistochemical marker predictive of progression. Am J Gastroenterol 96:1355-1362, 2001.

109. Weston AP, Badr AS, Hassanein RS: Prospective multivariate analysis of clinical, endoscopic, and histological factors predictive of the development of Barrett's multifocal high-grade dysplasia or adenocarcinoma. Am J Gastroenterol 94:3413-3419, 1999.

110. Reid BJ: p53 and neoplastic progression in Barrett's esophagus. Am J Gastroenterol 96:1321-1323, 2001.

111. Theisen J, Nigro JJ, DeMeester TR, et al: Chronology of the Barrett's metaplasia-dysplasia-carcinoma sequence. Dis Esophagus 17:67-70, 2004.

112. Sampliner RE: Practice Parameters Committee of the American College of Gastroenterology. Updated guidelines for the diagnosis, surveillance, and therapy of Barrett's esophagus. Am J Gastroenterol 97:1888-1895, 2002.

113. Falk GW, Ours TM, Richter JE: Practice patterns for surveillance of Barrett's esophagus in the United States. Gastrointest Endosc 52:197-203, 2000.

114. Cruz-Correa M, Gross CP, Canto MI, et al: The impact of practice guidelines in the management of Barrett esophagus: A national prospective cohort study of physicians. Arch Intern Med 161:2588-2595, 2001.

115. Levine DS, Haggitt RC, Blount PL, et al: An endoscopic biopsy protocol can differentiate high-grade dysplasia from early adenocarcinoma in Barrett's esophagus. Gastroenterology 105:40-50, 1993.

116. Reid BJ, Blount PL, Feng Z, Levine DS: Optimizing endoscopic biopsy detection of early cancers in Barrett's high-grade dysplasia. Am J Gastroenterol 95:3089-3096, 2000.

117. Sharma P: Review article: Emerging techniques for screening and surveillance in Barrett's oesophagus. Aliment Pharmacol Ther 20(Suppl 5):63-70, discussion 95-96, 2004.

118. Nigro JJ, Hagen JA, DeMeester TR, et al: Occult esophageal adenocarcinoma: Extent of disease and implications for effective therapy. Ann Surg 230:433-440, 1999.

119. Weston AP, Sharma P, Topalovski M, et al: Long-term follow-up of Barrett's high-grade dysplasia. Am J Gastroenterol 95:1888-1893, 2000.

120. Portale G, Peters JH, Hagen JA, et al: Comparison of the clinical and histological characteristics and survival of distal esophageal–gastroesophageal junction adenocarcinoma in patients with and without Barrett mucosa. Arch Surg 140:570-574, discussion 574-575, 2005.

121. Peters JH, Clark GW, Ireland AP, et al: Outcome of adenocarcinoma arising in Barrett's esophagus in endoscopically surveyed and nonsurveyed patients. J Thorac Cardiovasc Surg 108:813-821, discussion 821-822, 1994.

122. van Sandick JW, van Lanschot JJB, Kuiken BW, et al: Impact of endoscopic biopsy surveillance of Barrett's oesophagus on pathological stage and clinical outcome of Barrett's carcinoma. Gut 43:216-222, 1998.

123. Streitz JMJ, Ellis FHJ, Tilden RL, Erickson RV: Endoscopic surveillance of Barrett's esophagus: A cost-effectiveness comparison with mammographic surveillance for breast cancer. Am J Gastroenterol 93:911-915, 1998.

124. Oberg S, Peters JH, DeMeester TR, et al: Determinants of intestinal metaplasia within the columnar-lined esophagus. Arch Surg 135:651-655, discussion 655-656, 2000.

24

Surgical Treatment of Barrett's Esophagus

Jeffrey H. Peters

Norman Barrett described the condition that bears his name in 1950.[1] He believed that he was observing a congenitally short esophagus and an intrathoracic stomach.[2] Allison and Johnstone, with careful examination of seven esophagectomy specimens, showed conclusively in 1953 that it was indeed the tubular esophagus lined with columnar epithelium.[3] Despite its 50-year history, many aspects of Barrett's esophagus remain elusive and controversial, including the role of surgical treatment.[4,5] The uncertainty would be of little consequence were it not for the increasing number of, all too often, young men and women, many with few symptoms of gastroesophageal reflux, who have difficulty swallowing and are found to have esophageal adenocarcinoma.

There are five aims of therapy for patients with Barrett's esophagus. Ideally, they should be the same for both operative and nonoperative treatment and include

1. Providing long-term relief of symptoms
2. Allowing healing of reflux-induced esophageal mucosal injury, including stricture formation
3. Preventing progression to more advanced mucosal injury, dysplastic changes, or carcinoma
4. Inducing regression of dysplastic to nondysplastic Barrett's esophagus or intestinalized to nonintestinalized columnar epithelium
5. Completely eliminating and preventing any recurrence of high grade dysplasia

Achieving long-term success in the treatment of Barrett's esophagus can be difficult, particularly in those with long segments. This difficulty is due to the combination of several factors, including the fact that it represents severe gastroesophageal reflux disease (GERD), it is usually associated with large hiatal hernias, and it is a premalignant state. Acid-suppressive medication is increasingly being recognized to be inadequate, and ablative therapies remain difficult, complicated, and investigational. This leaves antireflux surgery as arguably the best treatment option, provided that long-term success can be shown.

RATIONALE FOR ANTIREFLUX SURGERY FOR BARRETT'S ESOPHAGUS

Relief of symptoms remains the primary force driving antireflux surgery in patients with nondysplastic Barrett's esophagus. Healing of esophageal mucosal injury and prevention of disease progression are important secondary goals. In this regard, patients with Barrett's esophagus are no different from the broader population of patients with gastroesophageal reflux. They should be considered for antireflux surgery when patient factors suggest severe disease or predict the need for long-term medical management, both of which are almost always the case in patients with Barrett's esophagus.

Several other factors are increasingly influencing the decision toward surgery, however. The first is the consideration that the ideal end point of treatment may not be simple symptomatic relief but rather elimination of pathologic esophageal acid exposure. This mindset is stimulated by the desire to prevent neoplastic development, together with the results of basic studies on the biology of Barrett's epithelium. These studies have shown disconcerting reflux-induced cellular changes in a Barrett's mucosa organ culture system.[6,7] Fitzgerald et al., for example, found that a dramatic increase in cellular proliferation resulted after Barrett's tissues were exposed to short pulses of acid at pH 3.5. Interestingly, continuous acid exposure had minimal effect. Cellular differentiation was also assessed by quantifying expression of the apical membrane cytoskeletal protein villin, which is important for brush border microvillus assembly. Increased villin expression was found with exposure to acid in a pH range of 3 to 5. Although these in vitro findings may not reflect the situation in vivo, the finding that short pulses of acid induce proliferation suggests that complete and continuous acid suppression is necessary to prevent these abnormal cellular biologic changes. Though theoretically possible with both medical and surgical treatment, complete esophageal acid control is more reliably provided by antireflux surgery.

Table 24–1   Clinical Features of Patients with Barrett's Esophagus and Gastroesophageal Reflux Disease and Esophagogastroduodenoscopy Controls

	Barrett's (n = 79)	GERD Controls (n = 94)	EGD Controls (n = 84)
Duration of symptoms (yr)*	16.4	11.8	13
Mean age at onset*	35.3	43.7	42.7
Esophagitis[†]	51 (65%)	33 (35%)	24 (29%)
Esophageal ulcer[†]	17 (22%)	7 (7%)	6 (7%)
Esophageal stricture[†]	21 (27%)	7 (7%)	5 (6%)
Hiatal hernia[†]	60 (76%)	41 (44%)	31 (37%)
Severe GERD[‡]	67 (85%)	55 (59%)	53 (63%)

*$P < .05$ for the Barrett's esophagus group versus either control group (Kruskal-Wallis test).

[†]Odds ratios for esophagitis, esophageal ulcer, esophageal stricture, and hiatal hernia greater than 3 cm for the Barrett's esophagus group versus either control group.

[‡]Severe GERD was defined as heartburn so painful that it awoke the patient or prevented sleeping.

Modified from Eisen GM, Sandler RS, Murray S, Gottfried M: The relationship between gastroesophageal reflux disease and its complications with Barrett's esophagus. Am J Gastroenterol 92:27-31, 1997.

Second, it is increasingly being recognized that normalization of esophageal acid exposure with medication is difficult in patients with Barrett's esophagus, even with proton pump inhibitors (PPIs). Sampliner et al. reported that a mean dose of 56 mg of omeprazole was necessary to normalize 24-hour esophageal pH studies after multipolar electrocoagulation.[8] Several studies have shown that nocturnal acid breakthrough resulting in supine GERD is common, even with 20 mg twice daily of PPI therapy.[9,10] Although this nocturnal acid breakthrough period can be reduced by taking a histamine H_2 receptor antagonist before sleep, short pulses of esophageal acid exposure still occur in some patients. Furthermore, once initiated, most patients with Barrett's esophagus will require lifelong treatment with PPIs both to relieve symptoms and to control any coexistent esophagitis or stricture.

Third is the recognition that Barrett's esophagus represents severe end-stage GERD, which will almost certainly require high-dose, lifetime drug therapy. The severity of the disease is demonstrated by clinical, physiologic, and basic biologic findings. A case-controlled epidemiologic study showed that patients with Barrett's esophagus have reflux symptoms at an earlier age and have more severe symptoms than age- and gender-matched GERD or upper endoscopy control patients do[11] (Table 24–1). Complications of reflux, including esophagitis, stricture, and ulceration, also occur more frequently in patients with Barrett's esophagus.[12] Physiologic studies reveal markedly abnormal esophageal acid exposure,[13] an incompetent lower esophageal sphincter,[14] and impaired esophageal body motility in a large majority of patients.[15] Both the frequency and the duration of reflux episodes are increased in comparison to patients with no intestinal metaplasia. Contractility of the esophageal body may be profoundly reduced in patients with Barrett's esophagus, thus resulting in prolonged contact times. The clinical and physiologic severity in

patients with short-segment Barrett's esophagus is generally intermediate between those with long-segment Barrett's and those with erosive esophagitis (Table 24–2).[16] Most patients with Barrett's esophagus have a hiatal hernia, which is often larger than in patients with reflux esophagitis without Barrett's.[17]

Studies of the constituents of the refluxate provide further indications that patients with Barrett's esophagus differ significantly from those with GERD without Barrett's esophagus. Patients with Barrett's esophagus are more likely to have mixed reflux of both gastric and duodenal contents into the esophagus.[18] Direct measurement of aspirated bile or measurement of esophageal bilirubin in the distal esophagus as a marker of duodenal juice has shown that duodenoesophageal reflux is significantly more frequent in those with Barrett's esophagus than in those with GERD without Barrett's.[19] A study of 100 patients with GERD found a significant association between the degree of mucosal injury and the presence of duodenogastroesophageal reflux rather than gastroesophageal reflux only.[18] Some animal model studies have indicated that duodenal reflux plays a significant role in esophageal tumor promotion.[20] It is likely that antireflux surgery results in more reproducible and reliable elimination of reflux of both acid and duodenal contents, although long-term outcome studies suggest that as many as 25% of post-Nissen patients will have persistent pathologic esophageal acid exposure confirmed by positive 24-hour pH studies.

OUTCOME OF ANTIREFLUX SURGERY IN PATIENTS WITH BARRETT'S ESOPHAGUS

Antireflux surgery is an excellent treatment option in most patients with Barrett's esophagus. It must be remembered, however, that patients with Barrett's esoph-

Table 24–2 Clinical and Anatomic Characteristics of Varying Degrees of Intestinal Metaplasia of the Esophagus and Gastroesophageal Junction

Characteristic	Total Population N (%)	GEJ-SIM N (%)	SSBE N (%)	LSBE N (%)	P Value
Sex (M/F)	394/344	25/22	45/19	35/5	.0001
White race	485 (66)	31 (66)	55 (86)	40 (100)	.0011
Hiatal hernia	252 (34)	19 (40)	39 (61)	32 (80)	.0001
Hernia size (cm)	2 (1-9)	2 (1-8)	3 (1-8)	4 (2-7)	.0001
Heartburn	343/550 (62)	20/34 (59)	33/40 (83)	10/16 (63)	.077
Duration of heartburn, yr (range)	2 (0.2-45)	3.5 (0.25-30)	3.5 (0.1-35)	20 (0.16-54)	.009
Esophagitis	110/549 (20)	7/34 (21)	10/40 (45)	3/16 (19)	.003
Dysplasia	0/720	2/47 (4.3)	4/50 (8)	2/13 (15)	
Cancer	0	1/47 (2.1)	1/50 (2)	2/13 (15.4)	
Dysplasia plus cancer	0	3/47 (6.4)	5/50 (10)	4/13 (31)	.043

GEJ-SIM, gastroesophageal junction—specialized intestinal metaplasia; LSBE, long-segment Barrett's esophagus; N, number of patients; SSBE, short-segment Barrett's esophagus.
Adapted from Hirota WK, Loughney TM, Lazas DJ, et al: Specialized intestinal metaplasia, dysplasia and cancer of the esophagus and esophagogastric junction; prevalence and clinical data. Gastroenterology 116:277-285, 1999.

agus generally have severe GERD, with its attendant sequelae such as a large hiatal hernia, stricture, shortened esophagus, and poor motility. These anatomic and physiologic features make successful antireflux surgery a particular challenge in this population. Indeed, recent data suggest that antireflux surgery in patients with Barrett's esophagus may not be as successful in the long term as in those without Barrett's. Once the decision for surgery is made, the most important features to identify before surgery are the presence of esophageal shortening, failed esophageal body motility, and dysplasia, each of which has significant bearing on the decision for surgical treatment, as well as the approach and type of antireflux procedure selected.

Choice of Operation

The antireflux procedure of choice is Nissen fundoplication. A laparoscopic approach will be appropriate for most patients, probably 80% to 85%. The remaining 15% to 20% of patients are best approached via open thoracotomy, which allows esophageal lengthening in the presence of a large hiatal hernia and esophageal shortening. Partial fundoplications should be used rarely, if at all in patients with Barrett's esophagus because most studies indicate that they provide inferior reflux control.[21,22] The superior reflux control provided by Nissen fundoplication probably justifies its use in patients with Barrett's esophagus even when disordered or low-amplitude peristalsis is present. The rationale for complete rather than partial fundoplication lies in the increasingly demonstrated importance of completely eliminating pathologic reflux and the prevention of disease progression in Barrett's patients.

Symptomatic Outcome

Studies focusing on the symptomatic outcome of antireflux surgery in patients with Barrett's esophagus document excellent to good results in 72% to 95% of patients 5 years after surgery.[23,24] Several have compared medical and surgical therapy. Attwood et al., in a prospective but nonrandomized study, reported on 45 patients undergoing either medical (26) or surgical (19) treatment of Barrett's esophagus.[25] The groups were similar in age, length of Barrett's segment, percent time with a pH less than 4, and length of follow-up. Mean symptom scores improved dramatically after antireflux surgery. Symptoms of heartburn, dysphagia, or both recurred in 88% of patients treated with medical therapy alone and in 21% after antireflux surgery. Reflux complications, largely the development of an esophageal stricture, occurred in 38% of the medically treated and 16% of the surgically treated patients ($P < .05$) over the 3-year follow-up period. Esophageal adenocarcinoma developed in one patient in each group. They concluded that antireflux surgery was superior to acid suppression for both control of symptoms and prevention of complications in patients with Barrett's esophagus.

Parilla and colleagues recently reported an update of a study originally published in the *British Journal of Surgery* in 1996.[26,27] One hundred one patients were enrolled over an 18-year period (1982 to 2000). Median follow-up was 6 years. Medical therapy consisted of 20 mg of omeprazole (PPI) twice daily since 1992 in all medically treated patients. Surgical therapy consisted of an open 1.5- to 3.0-cm Nissen fundoplication over a 48- to 50-French bougie with division of the short gastric arteries in 39% of patients and crural closure in all. Symptomatic outcomes in the two groups were nearly identical,

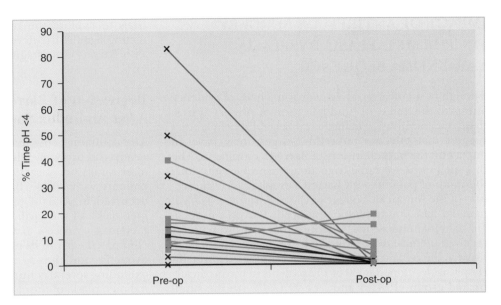

Figure 24–1. Twenty-four-hour distal esophageal pH results before and after Nissen fundoplication in 21 patients with Barrett's esophagus studied preoperatively and postoperatively. (From Hofstetter WA, Peters JH, DeMeester TR, et al: Long term outcome of antireflux surgery in patients with Barrett's esophagus. Ann Surg 234:532-539, 2001.)

although esophagitis, stricture, or both persisted in 20% of the medically treated patients versus only 3% to 7% of those after antireflux surgery. Fifteen percent of patients had abnormal acid exposure after surgery. Although pH data were not routinely collected in patients receiving PPI therapy, in the subgroup of 12 patients who did undergo 24-hour monitoring during treatment, 3 of 12 (25%) had persistently high esophageal acid exposure and most (75%) had persistently high bilirubin exposure.

In contrast, Csendes et al. have suggested that the long-term results of antireflux surgery in patients with Barrett's esophagus may not be as good as previously thought.[28] They reviewed their long-term results with "classic" antireflux surgery in 152 patients with both complicated and uncomplicated Barrett's esophagus. Fifty-four percent of those with uncomplicated Barrett's and 64% of those with Barrett's esophagus complicated by stricture or ulceration were classified as failures when symptoms were assessed 8 years postoperatively. Although this report challenges the long-term results of antireflux surgery in patients with Barrett's esophagus, it suffers from the fact that 85% of the patients were treated with a Hill repair, the results of which should not necessarily be extrapolated to patients undergoing Nissen fundoplication.

The outcome of laparoscopic Nissen fundoplication in patients with Barrett's esophagus has been assessed at 1 to 3 years after surgery. Hofstetter et al. reported the University of Southern California (USC) experience in 85 patients with Barrett's esophagus at a median of 5 years after surgery.[23] Fifty-nine had long-segment and 26 had short-segment Barrett's esophagus, and 50 were treated with a laparoscopic approach. Reflux symptoms were absent in 67 of 85 patients (79%). Recurrent symptoms developed in 18 (21%), and 4 resumed taking daily acid-suppressive medication. Seven patients underwent a secondary repair and were asymptomatic, thus raising the eventual successful outcome to 87%. Postoperative

24-hour pH levels were normal in 17 of 21 (81%) (Fig. 24–1). Ninety-nine percent of the patients considered themselves cured (77%) or improved (22%), and 97% were satisfied with the surgery.

Farrell and colleagues also reported symptomatic outcomes of laparoscopic Nissen fundoplication in 50 patients with both long- and short-segment Barrett's esophagus.[24] Mean scores for heartburn, regurgitation, and dysphagia all improved dramatically after Nissen fundoplication. Importantly, there was no significant decrement in symptom scores when 1-year results were compared with those 2 to 5 years postoperatively. They did find a higher prevalence of "anatomic" failure requiring reoperation in patients with Barrett's esophagus than in non-Barrett's patients with GERD. Others have reported similar results.[29,30]

Objective Measures of Reflux Control

Several studies have documented nearly complete elimination of both acid and alkaline reflux after fundoplication. Stein et al. showed that Nissen fundoplication provides normalization of both acid and bilirubin exposure in virtually all patients with Barrett's esophagus.[31] As mentioned earlier, normalization of duodenogastroesophageal reflux is not achieved with medical acid-suppression therapy. Csendes et al. reported extensive physiologic studies of Barrett's patients after combined fundoplication, highly selective vagotomy, and duodenal-switch bile diversion procedures.[32] Although these authors documented that the combined procedures abolished both acid and duodenogastroesophageal reflux, the extensive nature of the operation limits its appeal. Furthermore, as stated before, a properly performed Nissen fundoplication will prevent gastric juice of any nature from refluxing into the esophagus, thus making the additional procedures unnecessary.

IMPACT OF ANTIREFLUX SURGERY ON THE METAPLASIA-DYSPLASIA-CARCINOMA SEQUENCE

Though by no means proven, a growing body of evidence attests to the ability of fundoplication to protect against dysplasia and invasive malignancy. Several recent studies suggest that effective antireflux surgery may have an impact on the natural history of Barrett's esophagus. The first such evidence came from an analysis of longitudinal follow-up of patients with Barrett's esophagus in the registry of the American College of Gastroenterologists.[33] All patients had nondysplastic, quiescent Barrett's esophagus at initial endoscopy. One hundred fifty-two patients received medical treatment and 29 underwent antireflux surgery. Surveillance endoscopy was performed annually. Dysplasia developed in 30 of 152 patients in the medically treated group (19.7%) and 1 of 29 (3.4%) in the surgical group. A retrospective review of 118 patients with Barrett's esophagus who underwent antireflux surgery at the Mayo Clinic between 1960 and 1990 revealed three cancers occurring over an 18.5-year follow-up period.[34] All were found within the first 3 years after surgery. The fact that the development of adenocarcinoma was clustered in the early years after antireflux surgery and not randomly dispersed throughout the follow-up period strongly suggests that antireflux surgery altered the natural history of the disease, particularly given the fact that once dysplasia has developed, prospective studies show that carcinoma ensues in an average of 3 years. The occurrence of all observed cancers in the first few years suggests that the point of no return in the dysplasia-cancer sequence had already occurred before the time of surgery.

Further evidence that antireflux surgery may alter the natural history of Barrett's esophagus was reported by Katz et al.[35] This Veterans Affairs outcomes group retrospectively reviewed 102 patients undergoing annual surveillance for Barrett's esophagus from 1970 to 1994, for a total of 563 patient-years of follow-up. All specimens with any degree of dysplasia were blinded and re-reviewed. New-onset low-grade dysplasia developed in 19 patients, high-grade dysplasia in 4, and adenocarcinoma in 3. Antireflux surgery was associated with a significantly decreased risk for the development of dysplasia, the presence of which persisted in a multivariate analysis that took into account covariables such as age, sex, and smoking. Dysplasia did not develop in any of the 15 patients in this study after antireflux surgery. In the USC review noted earlier, no high-grade dysplasia or cancer developed in 410 patient-years of follow-up.[23] Finally, two prospective randomized studies found less adenocarcinoma in the surgically treated groups. Parilla et al. reported that although the incidence of dysplasia and adenocarcinoma was no different overall, significantly less dysplasia and no adenocarcinoma developed in the subgroup of surgical patients with normal postoperative pH studies.[27] Spechler and associates identified one adenocarcinoma 11 to 13 years after antireflux surgery versus four after medical treatment.[36] Most of these authors concluded that there is a critical need for future trials to explore the role of antireflux surgery in protecting against the development of dysplasia in patients with Barrett's esophagus.

Regression of Barrett's Esophagus After Antireflux Surgery

The common belief that Barrett's epithelium cannot be reversed is probably false. DeMeester et al. reported that after antireflux surgery, loss of intestinal metaplasia in patients with visible Barrett's esophagus was rare but occurred in 73% of patients with nonvisible intestinal metaplasia of the cardia.[37] This finding suggests that the metaplastic process may indeed be reversible if reflux is eliminated early in its process, that the cardiac mucosa is dynamic, and that as opposed to intestinal metaplasia extending several centimeters into the esophagus, intestinal metaplasia of the cardia is more likely to regress after antireflux surgery. Gurski et al. recently reviewed pretreatment and post-treatment endoscopic biopsy samples from 77 Barrett's patients treated surgically and 14 treated with PPIs.[38] Post-treatment histology was classified as having regressed if two consecutive specimens taken more than 6 months apart plus all subsequent specimens showed loss of intestinal metaplasia or loss of dysplasia. Histopathologic regression occurred in 28 of 77 (36.4%) patients after antireflux surgery and in 1 of 14 (7.1%) treated with PPIs alone ($P < .03$). After surgery, regression from low-grade dysplastic to nondysplastic Barrett's epithelium occurred in 17 of 25 (68%) patients and from intestinal metaplasia to no intestinal metaplasia in 11 of 52 (21.2%) (Fig. 24–2). Both types of regression were significantly more common in short-segment (<3 cm) than in long-segment (>3 cm) Barrett's esophagus: 19 of 33 (58%) and 9 of 44 (20%) patients, respectively ($P = .0016$). Eight patients progressed, five from intestinal metaplasia alone to low-grade dysplasia and three from low- to high-grade dysplasia. All those who progressed had long-segment Barrett's esophagus. On multivariable analysis, the presence of short-segment Barrett's esophagus and the type of treatment were significantly associated with regression; age, sex, surgical procedure, and preoperative lower esophageal sphincter and pH characteristics were not. The median time of biopsy-proven regression was 18.5 months after surgery, with 95% occurring within 5 years. Similar findings have been reported by the University of Washington group[39] and Hunter's group.[40] Although these studies do not conclusively prove the ability of antireflux surgery to reverse the changes of early Barrett's esophagus, they do provide encouragement that given early changes, the process may indeed be reversible.

Recent evidence suggests that the development of Barrett's esophagus may even be preventable. Despite being a very difficult hypothesis to study, Öberg et al. monitored a cohort of 69 patients with short-segment, nonintestinalized, columnar-lined esophagus over a median of 5 years of surveillance endoscopy.[14] Forty-nine of the patients were maintained on PPI therapy and 20 underwent antireflux surgery. Intestinal metaplasia was 10 times less likely to develop in these columnar-lined

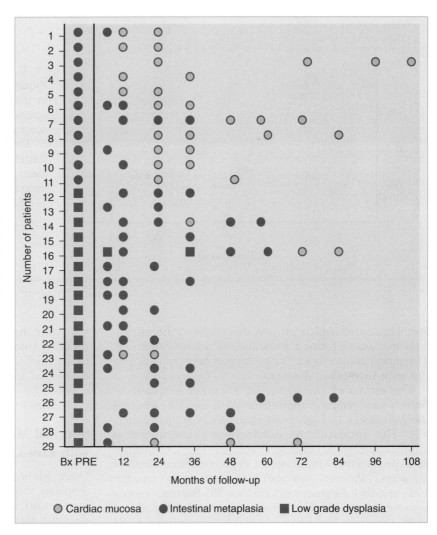

Figure 24–2. Schematic representation of histopathologic regression in 29 patients with Barrett's esophagus. (From Gurski RR, Peters JH, Hagen JA, et al: Barrett's esophagus can and does regress following antireflux surgery; a study of prevalence and predictive features. J Am Coll Surg 196:706-713, 2003.)

esophageal segments in patients treated with antireflux surgery over a follow-up span of nearly 15 years (Fig. 24–3) than in those treated with medical therapy. This rather remarkable observation supports the two-step hypothesis of the development of Barrett's esophagus (cardiac metaplasia followed by intestinal metaplasia) and suggests that the second step can be prevented if reflux disease is recognized and treated early and aggressively.

DYSPLASTIC BARRETT'S ESOPHAGUS

Dysplasia is defined as neoplastic epithelium that is confined within the basement membrane of the gland or epithelium within which it arose. The histopathologic classification of dysplasia in Barrett's epithelium relies on identification of cytologic and tissue architectural changes that were originally described in 1983 for ulcerative colitis[41] and subsequently modified for Barrett's esophagus.[42] Dysplasia is currently classified into four categories: (1) no dysplasia (intestinal metaplasia), (2) indefinite for dysplasia, (3) low-grade dysplasia, and (4) high-grade dysplasia. Before intervention, the diagnosis

of high-grade dysplasia should be confirmed by at least two expert pathologists. Unfortunately, there is considerable interobserver disagreement among even expert gastrointestinal pathologists,[43] particularly for the low-grade and indefinite categories. Repeat endoscopy with extensive biopsy should be performed if significant interobserver disagreement is encountered. Endoscopy with four-quadrant biopsy at 1-cm rather than 2-cm intervals within the visible columnar segment is recommended in the presence of dysplastic tissue (Table 24–3).[44] Even with this 1-cm protocol, it is not possible to be certain that cancer is not present in patients with known high-grade dysplasia. Emphasizing this fact is a study by Cameron and Carpenter in which they mapped esophagectomy specimens from 30 patients with high-grade dysplasia or early adenocarcinoma. The median surface area of the adenocarcinomas was 1.1 cm², and the three smallest cancers had surface areas of 0.02, 0.3, and 0.4 cm².[45]

It can be difficult to distinguish between high-grade dysplasia and well-differentiated intramucosal adenocarcinoma. Most use the term high-grade dysplasia for neoplastic changes involving the epithelium, but not extending into the lamina propria (i.e., superficial to the basement membrane).[46] Neoplastic disease involving the

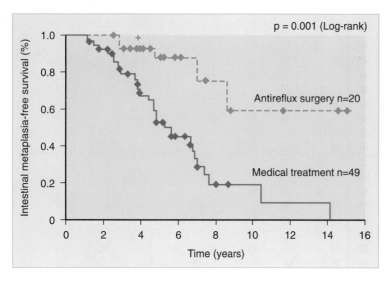

p = 0.001 (Log-rank)

Antireflux surgery n=20

Medical treatment n=49

Figure 24–3. Development of intestinal metaplasia in patients' nonintestinalized short segments of columnar-lined esophagus during medical and after surgical therapy for Barrett's esophagus. (From Öberg S, DeMeester TR, Peters JH, et al. The extent of Barrett's esophagus depends on the status of the lower esophageal sphincter and the degree of esophageal acid exposure. J Thorac Cardiovasc Surg 117:572-580, 1999.)

epithelium and lamina propria superficial to the muscularis mucosa is termed intramucosal adenocarcinoma. The term carcinoma in situ has largely been replaced by the term high-grade dysplasia.

The estimated prevalence of low-grade dysplasia in Barrett's esophagus ranges from 15% to 25%, whereas the prevalence of high-grade dysplasia is approximately 5%. The incidence of development of dysplasia is approximately 5% per year (Table 24–4).[47-50] O'Conner et al. prospectively monitored 136 patients for a mean of 4.2 years.[50] Patients with both long-segment (>3 cm, $n = 106$) and short-segment (<3 cm, $n = 30$) Barrett's esophagus were included. High-grade dysplasia developed in 4 (2.9%) patients and low-grade dysplasia developed in 24 (17.6%). The median time until the development of low-grade dysplasia was 3.0 years (range, 0.07 to 12.7 years). In another prospective investigation, Levine et al. studied 62 patients with Barrett's esophagus for a mean of 34 months.[51] The authors documented the development of

low-grade dysplasia in 10 of 39 patients with no dysplasia on entry into the study, one new case of high-grade dysplasia, and one invasive carcinoma. High-grade dysplasia developed in three patients with low-grade dysplasia at entry.

Surgical Management of Patients with Low-Grade Dysplasia

Once identified, Barrett's esophagus complicated by dysplasia should be treated aggressively with either PPI medication or fundoplication, preferably Nissen fundoplication. Deciding on the optimum treatment in patients with low-grade dysplasia or a persistent diagnosis of indefinite for dysplasia can be difficult. Because of the possibility of missing higher grades of dysplasia elsewhere in the esophagus as a result of sampling error, the uncertainty at the initial examination of the time from the development of low-grade dysplasia to the development of high-grade dysplasia, and the fact that antireflux surgery alters the anatomy of the gastroesophageal segment such that repeat biopsy may be more difficult, patients with low-grade dysplasia are best managed by continued surveillance for 6 to 12 months before the decision for surgery (Box 24–1). Three- to six-month endoscopic surveillance with four-quadrant biopsy at every 1 cm of the Barrett's segment is the optimal technique. If the dysplastic segment remains stable and no areas of high-grade dysplasia are detected during the surveillance period, antireflux surgery is a good option. If the dysplasia regresses after treatment, the surveillance interval can be extended to 1 year for the first 3 years and then to 2- or 3-year intervals if the regression persists. Surveillance endoscopy after antireflux surgery should be performed by an experienced endoscopist because of the difficulty of obtaining adequate biopsy samples within the fundoplication wrap.

Patients with low-grade dysplasia that persists after antireflux surgery may be the ideal group in which to perform Barrett's ablation or photodynamic therapy.

Table 24–3	Effect of Biopsy Protocol on Endoscopic Detection of Early Cancer in Barrett's Esophagus

Biopsy Protocol	Cancers Detected	% of Total
Visible lesions only	13/26	33
Every 2 cm without visible lesion	15/45	50
Every 2 cm and any visible lesion	32/45	71
Every 1 cm and any visible lesion	45/45	100

Adapted from Reid BJ, Blount PL, Feng Z, Levine DS: Optimizing endoscopic detection of early cancers in Barrett's high-grade dysplasia. Am J Gastroenterology 95:3089-3096, 2000.

| Table 24–4 | Prevalence of the Development of Dysplasia in Studies of Barrett's Esophagus |

Author	Barrett's Segment Length	No. of Patients	Mean Follow-up (yr)	No. of Patients Developing Dysplasia	% of Patients Developing Dysplasia/yr
Hameetemen et al.[47]	Long	50	5.2	10	3.8
McCallum et al.[33]	Long	152	4	30	4.9
Ortiz et al.[26]	Long	27	4	6	5.5
Sharma et al.[48]	Short	32	3	5	5.2
Weston[4] et al.[9]	Short	26	1.5	2	5.1
	Long	29	2	6	10.3
O'Conner et al.[50]	Short	30	4.2	4 (all lgd)	13.3
	Long	106	4.2	28 (4 hgd)	26

hgd, high-grade dysplasia; lgd, low-grade dysplasia.

Overholt et al. reported elimination of low-grade dysplasia in 13 of 14 patients with porfimer sodium (Photofrin) photodynamic therapy.[52] Ultrasonic ablation,[53] endoscopic mucosal resection,[54,55] and laser ablation or electrocoagulation[56,57] may also prove suitable treatment for patients with Barrett's low-grade dysplasia. It is worth noting that unsatisfactory results, including progression to malignancy, a high frequency of stricture formation, subsquamous Barrett's esophagus, and reappearance of Barrett's epithelium, have been reported after the use of these newer therapies. These techniques may thus be less suitable for the treatment of patients with high-grade dysplasia.

| Box 24–1 | **Management of Dysplasia** |

Indefinite for Dysplasia

Aggressive antireflux therapy (60 mg/day of a proton pump inhibitor plus a nocturnal H_2 blocker)

Rebiopsy in 3 months

Low-Grade Dysplasia

Aggressive antireflux therapy

Monthly surveillance for 6 to 12 months

Offer antireflux surgery if dysplasia is stable

High-Grade Dysplasia

Confirmation by two experienced pathologists

Esophagectomy (? extent)

Operative Management of High-Grade Dysplasia

There are three options for the management of patients with high-grade dysplasia; each has been advocated as the treatment of choice.

1. Endoscopic surveillance until carcinoma is identified
2. Mucosal ablation
3. Esophagectomy

The optimal treatment is controversial, in part because of the fact that the natural history of high-grade dysplasia is uncertain. Prospective studies documenting that a minority of patients progress to detectable adenocarcinoma support a conservative approach to the management of these patients. Watchful waiting, however, involves a time-consuming, labor-intensive, expensive protocol that is impractical in most practice settings. Large cohorts of patients with high-grade dysplasia have now been prospectively monitored at the University of Washington[51,58] and the University of Kansas[59] and retrospectively reviewed at the Hines Veterans Hospital in Chicago.[60] These data clearly show that cancer will be identified (*identified* is a more appropriate term than developed because many of these patients may have had carcinoma for some time before it is detected) in approximately 25% of patients at 1.5 years,[51] 50% at 3 years,[59] and up to 80% 8 years later.[58] The 80% figure should be interpreted in light of the fact that there is a 20% or so error rate in the pathologic diagnosis of high-grade dysplasia. Thus, the natural history of high-grade dysplasia is becoming clear. Most patients will have an invasive adenocarcinoma identified during a 5- to 10-year surveillance period, although a significant minority may not. Though far from perfect, these facts, particularly when viewed in association with p53 and cell cycle (flow cytometry) abnormalities, give the clinician significant information on which to base clinical decisions.

Underscoring these points, a decision analysis study that tested whether esophagectomy or continued surveillance is the optimal treatment for patients with high-grade dysplasia was recently reported in abstract form.[61] Seven strategies were tested, the first being immediate esophagectomy and the remaining six, surveillance for 3, 6, 12, 18, and 24 months and esophagectomy if cancer was identified and, finally, no cancer ever identified. The simulation continued until all patients died of cancer or other causes. A 5-year estimate of 20% to 50% for the development of cancer in patients with high-grade dysplasia was used (quite reasonable in view of the data presented earlier) and included operative mortality and both short- and long-term disability associated with esophagotomy. Immediate esophagectomy was the preferred treatment with all levels of cancer risk anywhere from 10% to 50%. Furthermore, immediate esophagectomy had the greatest gain in quality-adjusted life years. Esophagectomy remained the preferred treatment unless the cancer incidence fell below 3% at 5 years, the operative mortality rose to above 64%, or the quality-adjusted life years after esophagectomy declined to less than 0.5 (0 dead, 1 normal). These rather surprising data lend further credence to the decision for esophagectomy in patients with high-grade dysplasia.

Although efforts at effective ablation of dysplastic Barrett's esophagus have been ongoing for more than a decade, major obstacles remain.[62] Ablation of large segments of Barrett's epithelium is compromised by the fact that residual Barrett's epithelium remains in as many as half the patients and severe complications such as stricture or motility disturbances will develop in 25% to 30%. Effective ablation of small areas of dysplasia, whether by mucosal resection or thermal or photodynamic energy, requires accurate localization. Localization of a nonvisible area containing high-grade dysplasia is presently not possible, although technologies looming on the horizon such as optical coherence tomography may make this a clinical reality. Finally, investigators at the Mayo Clinic Rochester have found that despite the histologic absence of dysplasia after ablation, genetic abnormalities characterizing a premalignant epithelium remain.[63] Ablation is still an elusive goal.

Evidence supporting the performance of esophagectomy in patients with high-grade dysplasia comes from studies of esophagectomy specimens from patients with a preoperative diagnosis of high-grade dysplasia without carcinoma.[64] A report from the Cleveland Clinic that included the use of a jumbo forceps biopsy protocol found adenocarcinoma present in 10 of 28 patients who had a maximum preoperative diagnosis of high-grade dysplasia.[65] Despite the use of a surveillance protocol that entailed four-quadrant biopsy at 1- or 2-cm intervals within the Barrett's segment, the group at the University of California, San Francisco, recently reported that adenocarcinoma was present in the esophagectomy specimens of 4 of 11 patients with a maximum preoperative diagnosis of high-grade dysplasia.[66] Three of the cancer patients had disease not limited to the mucosa and died within 16 months of surgery. Overall, between a third and a half of patients with a maximum diagnosis of high-grade dysplasia will have occult adenocarcinoma. We

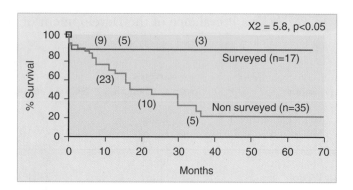

Figure 24–4. Kaplan-Meier survival curves for patients enrolled and not enrolled in an endoscopic surveillance program for Barrett's esophagus. (From Peters JH, Clark GWB, Ireland AP, et al: Outcome of adenocarcinoma arising in Barrett's esophagus in endoscopically surveyed and non-surveyed patients. J Thorac Cardiovasc Surg 108:813-822, 1994.)

believe that this fact justifies consideration of esophageal resection in all patients with a definite diagnosis of high-grade dysplasia. It is not possible with the present technology, including endoscopic ultrasound, to differentiate patients who do or do not harbor cancer. Importantly, the combination of regular surveillance and esophagectomy for patients with high-grade dysplasia has been shown to result in the detection of early-stage cancer and consequently high overall survival rates.[67,68] The 5-year survival rate approaches 90% in this setting (Fig. 24–4). When invasive cancer is found, most of these tumors will be limited to the wall of the esophagus, and few will have spread to the regional lymph nodes.

Extent of Resection for High-Grade Dysplasia

The standard surgical resection for patients with high-grade dysplasia includes total esophagectomy with removal of all Barrett's tissue and any potential associated adenocarcinoma. This is usually accomplished by transhiatal or transthoracic esophagectomy, with most expert centers favoring the transhiatal approach. Reconstruction generally requires a posterior mediastinal gastric "pull-up" procedure with placement of the anastomosis in the neck. Intrathoracic anastomoses are to be avoided because of the high prevalence of disabling reflux symptoms after an intrathoracic esophagogastrostomy. The mortality associated with this procedure should be less than 5% and is less than 1% in centers experienced in esophageal surgery. Functional recovery is good to excellent in the vast majority of patients.

Recently, we have used a transhiatal vagal-sparing esophageal stripping procedure, with colon interposition, as a more physiologic alternative to standard transhiatal esophagectomy in patients with high-grade dysplasia.[69] Sparing the vagal nerves improves the functional outcome by eliminating one of the major sources of postoperative alimentary morbidity after esophagectomy, namely, the postvagotomy effects of gastric atony and diarrhea. Its use is limited, however, to patients in whom there is little or no likelihood of lymph node metastases. Selecting such patients can be difficult. Recent data from our experience indicate that given careful endoscopic examination and biopsy, nodal disease is rare in the absence of a visible lesion.[70] The lymph node status of 10 patients with no endoscopically visible lesion and a biopsy diagnosis of high-grade dysplasia or intramucosal adenocarcinoma was retrospectively reviewed after en bloc esophagectomy. A total of 370 lymph nodes from these 10 patients were examined by both conventional histopathologic and immunohistopathologic methods. Only one lymph node contained metastatic disease. In contrast, 5 of 9 patients with an endoscopically visible lesion and a preoperative diagnosis of either high-grade dysplasia or intramucosal adenocarcinoma had metastasis to regional lymph nodes. If an endoscopically visible lesion is present, the frequency of submucosal disease is high. Because tumors that invade through the muscularis mucosa into the submucosa have a 60% or higher incidence of lymph node metastasis, it seems prudent to perform regional lymph node dissection with esophagectomy for the treatment of visible lesions, regardless of the histologic findings on biopsy (i.e., high-grade dysplasia or intramucosal carcinoma). Recent studies indicate, however, that in early adenocarcinoma in Barrett's esophagus, metastases do not appear to involve the splenic artery nodes and the spleen. Splenic artery dissection and splenectomy are therefore not necessary in this circumstance, nor is extended gastric resection.

Without question, removing the esophagus is a major undertaking often fraught with significant morbidity and mortality. What is often underestimated is the intensity of resources and emotional burden associated with the decision to pursue surveillance every 3 months. When given the option, many patients prefer to eliminate the possibility of development of esophageal adenocarcinoma, even if esophagectomy is the price to do so. Our challenge is to improve the state of the art such that this can be accomplished with as little morbidity as possible. After esophagectomy, average mortality has steadily decreased over the past 2 to 3 decades from higher than 25% to 2% to 4% in most centers. It approaches zero in large series of resection for benign disease[71] (in which patients with high-grade dysplasia can be included) and in units that have specifically focused on preventing death from esophageal resection, such as that in Hong Kong.[72] That being said, as the authors aptly point out, it is arguably the most sensitive surgical procedure to volume-outcome relationships.

REFERENCES

1. Lord RVN: Norman Barrett, "Doyen of esophageal surgery." Ann Surg 229:428-439, 1999.
2. Barrett NR: Chronic peptic ulcer of the esophagus and "oesophagitis." Br J Surg 38:175-182, 1950.
3. Allison P, Johnstone A: The oesophagus lined with gastric mucous membrane. Thorax 8:87-101, 1953.
4. DeMeester SR, DeMeester TR: Columnar lined mucosa and intestinal metaplasia of the esophagus; fifty years of controversy. Ann Surg 231:303-321, 2000.
5. Chandrasoma P: Norman Barrett: So close, yet 50 years from the truth. J Gastrointest Surg 3:7-14, 1999.
6. Fitzgerald RC, Omary MB, Triadafilopoulos G: Dynamic effects of acid on Barrett's esophagus. An ex vivo proliferation and differentiation model. J Clin Invest 98:2120-2128, 1996.
7. Fitzgerald RC, Omary MB, Triadafilopoulos G:. Altered sodium-hydrogen exchange activity is a mechanism for acid-induced hyperproliferation in Barrett's esophagus. Am J Physiol 275:G47-G55, 1998.
8. Sampliner RE, Fennerty B, Garewal HS: Reversal of Barrett's esophagus with acid suppression and multipolar electrocoagulation: Preliminary results. Gastrointest Endosc 44:532-535, 1996.
9. Katz PO, Anderson C, Khoury R, Castell DO: Gastro-oesophageal reflux associated with nocturnal gastric acid breakthrough on proton pump inhibitors. Aliment Pharmacol Ther 12:1231-1234, 1998.
10. Hatlebakk JG, Katz PO, Kuo B, Castell DO: Nocturnal gastric acidity and acid breakthrough on different regimens of omeprazole 40 mg daily. Aliment Pharmacol Ther 12:1235-1240, 1998.
11. Eisen GM, Sandler RS, Murray S, Gottfried M: The relationship between gastroesophageal reflux disease and its complications with Barrett's esophagus. Am J Gastroenterol 92:27-31, 1997.
12. Iascone C, DeMeester TR, Little AG, Skinner DB: Barrett's esophagus. Functional assessment, proposed pathogenesis, and surgical therapy. Arch Surg 118:543-549, 1983.
13. Gillen P, Keeling P, Byrne PJ, Hennessy TP: Barrett's oesophagus: pH profile. Br J Surg 74:774-776, 1987.
14. Öberg S, DeMeester TR, Peters JH, et al. The extent of Barrett's esophagus depends on the status of the lower esophageal sphincter and the degree of esophageal acid exposure. J Thorac Cardiovasc Surg 117:572-580, 1999.
15. Stein HJ, Hoeft S, DeMeester TR: Functional foregut abnormalities in Barrett's esophagus. J Thorac Cardiovasc Surg 105:107-111, 1993.
16. Hirota WK, Loughney TM, Lazas DJ, et al: Specialized intestinal metaplasia, dysplasia and cancer of the esophagus and esophagogastric junction; prevalence and clinical data. Gastroenterology 116:277-285, 1999.
17. Cameron AJ: Barrett's esophagus: Prevalence and size of hiatal hernia. Am J Gastroenterol 94:2054-2059, 1999.
18. Kauer WK, Peters JH, DeMeester TR, et al: Mixed reflux of gastric and duodenal juices is more harmful to the esophagus than gastric juice alone. The need for surgical therapy re-emphasized. Ann Surg 222:525-531, 1995.
19. Stein HJ, Feussner H, Kauer W, et al: Alkaline gastroesophageal reflux: Assessment by ambulatory esophageal aspiration and pH monitoring. Am J Surg 167:163-168, 1994.
20. Pera M, Cardesa A, Bombi JA, et al: Influence of esophagojejunostomy on the induction of adenocarcinoma of the distal esophagus in Sprague-Dawley rats by subcutaneous injection of 2,6-dimethylnitrosomorpholine. Cancer Res 49:6803-6808, 1989.
21. Horvath KD, Jobe BA, Herron DM, Swanstrom LL: Laparoscopic Toupet fundoplication is an inadequate procedure for patients with severe reflux disease. J Gastrointest Surg 3:583-591, 1999.
22. Jobe BA, Wallace J, Hansen PD, Swanstrom LL: Evaluation of laparoscopic Toupet fundoplication as a primary repair for all patients with medically resistant gastroesophageal reflux. Surg Endosc 11:1080-1083, 1997.
23. Hofstetter WA, Peters JH, DeMeester TR, et al: Long term outcome of antireflux surgery in patients with Barrett's esophagus. Ann Surg 234:532-539, 2001.
24. Farrell TM, Smith CD, Metreveli RE, et al: Fundoplication provides effective and durable symptom relief in patients with Barrett's esophagus. Am J Surg 178:18-21, 1999.
25. Attwood SEA, Barlow AP, Norris TL, Watson A: Barrett's oesophagus; effect of antireflux surgery on symptom control and development of complications. Br J Surg 79:1050-1053, 1992.
26. Ortiz A, Martinez de Haro LF, Parrilla P, et al: Conservative treatment versus antireflux surgery in Barrett's oesophagus; long term results of a prospective study. Br J Surg 83:274-278, 1996.

27. Parrilla P, Martinez de Haro LF, Ortiz A, et al: Long term results of a randomized prospective study comparing medical and surgical treatment in Barrett's esophagus. Ann Surg 237:291-298, 2003.

28. Csendes A, Braghetto I, Burdiles P, et al: Long term results of classic antireflux surgery in 152 patients with Barrett's esophagus; clinical radiologic, endoscopic, manometric, and acid reflux test analysis before and late after operation. Surgery 123:645-657, 1998.

29. Yau P, Watson DI, Devitt PG, et al: Laparoscopic antireflux surgery in the treatment of gastroesophageal reflux in patients with Barrett's esophagus. Arch Surg 135:801-805, 2000.

30. Patti MG, Arcerito M, Feo CV, et al: Barrett's esophagus: A surgical disease. J Gastrointest Surg 3:397-404, 1999.

31. Stein HJ, Kauer WK, Feussner H, Siewert JR: Bile reflux in benign and malignant Barrett's esophagus: Effect of medical acid suppression and Nissen fundoplication. J Gastrointest Surg 2:333-341, 1998.

32. Csendes A, Braghetto I, Burdiles P, et al: A new physiologic approach for the surgical treatment of patients with Barrett's esophagus: Technical considerations and results in 65 patients. Ann Surg 226:123-133, 1997.

33. McCallum RW, Plepalle S, Davenport K: Role of antireflux surgery against dysplasia in Barrett's esophagus [abstract]. Gastroenterology 100:A121, 1991.

34. McDonald ML, Trastek VF, Allen MS, et al: Barretts's esophagus: Does an antireflux procedure reduce the need for endoscopic surveillance? J Thorac Cardiovasc Surg 111:1135-1138, 1996.

35. Katz D, Rothstein R, Schned A, et al: The development of dysplasia and adenocarcinoma during endoscopic surveillance of Barrett's esophagus. Am J Gastroenterol 93:536-541, 1998.

36. Spechler SJ, Lee E, Ahmen D: Long term outcome of medical and surgical therapies for gastroesophageal reflux disease; follow-up of a randomized controlled trial. JAMA 285:2331-2338, 2001.

37. DeMeester SR, Campos GMR, DeMeester TR, et al: The impact of an antireflux procedure on intestinal metaplasia of the cardia. Ann Surg 228:547-556, 1998.

38. Gurski RR, Peters JH, Hagen JA, et al: Barrett's esophagus can and does regress following antireflux surgery; a study of prevalence and predictive features. J Am Coll Surg 196:706-713, 2003.

39. Low DE, Levine DS, Dail DH, Kozarek RA: Histological and anatomic changes in Barrett's esophagus after antireflux surgery. Am J Gastroenterol 94:80-85, 1999.

40. Bowers SP, Mattar SG, Smith CD, et al: Clinical and histologic outcome after antireflux surgery in Barrett's esophagus. J Gastrointest Surg 6:532-539, 2002.

41. Riddell RH, Goldman H, Ransohoff DF, et al: Dysplasia in inflammatory bowel disease: Standardized classification with provisional clinical applications. Hum Pathol 14:931-968, 1983.

42. Schmidt HG, Riddell RH, Walther B, et al: Dysplasia in Barrett's esophagus. J Cancer Res Clin Oncol 110:145-152, 1985.

43. Reid BJ, Haggitt RC, Rubin CE, et al: Observer variation in the diagnosis of dysplasia in Barrett's esophagus. Hum Pathol 19:166-178, 1988.

44. Levine DS, Haggitt RC, Blount PL, et al: An endoscopic biopsy protocol can differentiate high grade dysplasia from early adenocarcinoma in Barrett's esophagus. Gastroenterology 105:40-50, 1993.

45. Cameron AJ, Carpenter HA: Barrett's esophagus, high-grade dysplasia, and early adenocarcinoma: A pathological study. Am J Gastroenterol 92:586-591, 1997.

46. Haggitt RC: Pathology of Barrett's esophagus. J Gastrointest Surg 4:117-118, 2000.

47. Hameeteman W, Tytgat GNJ, Houthoff HJ, et al: Barrett's esophagus; development of dysplasia and adenocarcinoma. Gastroenterology 96:1249-1256, 1989.

48. Sharma P, Morales TG, Bhattacharyya A, et al: Dysplasia in short segment Barrett's esophagus; a prospective 3 year follow-up. Am J Gastroenterol 92:2012-2016, 1997.

49. Weston AP, Krmpotich PT, Cherian R, et al: Prospective long-term endoscopic and histological follow-up of short segment Barrett's esophagus; comparison with traditional long segment Barrett's esophagus. Am J Gastroenterol 92:407-413, 1997.

50. O'Connor JB, Falk GW, Richter JE: The incidence of adenocarcinoma and dysplasia in Barrett's esophagus; report on the Cleveland Clinic Barrett's Esophagus Registry. Am J Gastroenterol 94:2037-2042, 1999.

51. Levine DS, Haggitt RC, Blount PL, et al: An endoscopic biopsy protocol can differentiate high grade dysplasia from early adenocarcinoma in Barrett's esophagus. Gastroenterology 105:40-50, 1993.

52. Overholt BF, Panjehpour M, Haydek JM: Photodynamic therapy for Barrett's esophagus: Follow-up in 100 patients. Gastrointest Endosc 49:1-7, 1999.

53. Bremner RM, Mason RJ, Bremner CG, et al: Ultrasonic epithelial ablation of the lower esophagus without stricture formation. A new technique for Barrett's ablation. Surg Endosc 12:342-346, 1998.

54. Endo M: Endoscopic resection as local treatment of mucosal cancer. Endoscopy 25:672-674, 1993.

55. Inoue H, Takeshita K, Hori H, et al: Endoscopic mucosal resection with a cap-fitted panendoscope for esophagus, stomach, and colon mucosal lesions. Gastrointest Endosc 39:58-62, 1993.

56. Sampliner RE, Camargo E, Faigel D, et al: Efficacy and safety of reversal of Barrett's esophagus with high dose omeprazole and electrocoagulation [abstract]. Gastroenterology 116:A298, 1999.

57. Barham CP, Jones RL, Biddlestone LR, et al: Photothermal laser ablation of Barrett's oesophagus: Endoscopic and histological evidence of squamous re-epithelialisation. Gut 41:281-284, 1997.

58. Reid BJ, Levine DS, Longton G, et al: Predictors of progression to cancer in Barrett's esophagus; baseline histology and flow cytometry identify low and high risk subsets. Am J Gastroenterol 95:1669-1676, 2000.

59. Weston AP, Sharma P, Topalovski M, et al: Long term follow-up of Barrett's high grade dysplasia. An J Gastroenterol 95:1888-1893, 2000.

60. Schnell TG, Sontag SJ, Chejfec G, et al: Long term nonsurgical management of Barrett's esophagus with high grade dysplasia. Gastroenterology 120:1607-1619, 2001.

61. Provenzale D: Immediate esophagectomy or continued surveillance for Barrett's patients with high grade dysplasia?—a decision analysis [abstract]. Gastroenterology 120:A414, 2001.

62. Fennerty MB: Perspectives on endoscopic eradication of Barrett's esophagus; who are appropriate candidates and what is the best method. Gastrointest Endosc 49:S24-S28, 1999.

63. Krishnadath KK, Wang KK, Taniguchi K, et al: Persistent genetic abnormalities in Barrett's esophagus after photodynamic therapy. Gastroenterology 119:624-630, 2000.

64. Edwards MJ, Gable DR, Lentsch AB, Richardson JD: The rationale for esophagectomy as the optimal therapy for Barrett's esophagus with high-grade dysplasia. Ann Surg 223:585-589, 1996.

65. Falk GW, Rice TW, Goldblum JR, Richter JE: Jumbo biopsy forceps protocol still misses unsuspected cancer in Barrett's esophagus with high-grade dysplasia. Gastrointest Endosc 49:170-176, 1999.

66. Patti MG, Arcerito M, Feo CV, et al: Barrett's esophagus: A surgical disease. J Gastrointest Surg 3:397-404, 1999.

67. Peters JH, Clark GWB, Ireland AP, et al: Outcome of adenocarcinoma arising in Barrett's esophagus in endoscopically surveyed and non-surveyed patients. J Thorac Cardiovasc Surg 108:813-822, 1994.

68. Van Sandick JW, Lanschott JJ, Kuiken BW, et al: Impact of endoscopic biopsy surveillance of Barrett's esophagus on pathologic stage and clinical outcome of Barrett's carcinoma. Gut 43:216-222, 1998.

69. Banki F, Mason RJ, DeMeester SR, et al: Vagal sparing esophagectomy; a more physiologic alternative. Ann Surg 236:324-336, 2002.

70. Nigro JJ, Hagen JA, DeMeester TR, et al: Occult esophageal adenocarcinoma; the extent of disease and implications for effective therapy. Ann Surg 230:433-440, 1999.

71. Watson T, DeMeester TR, Kauer WKH, et al: Esophagectomy for end stage benign esophageal disease. J Thorac Cardiovasc Surg 115:1241-1249, 1998.

72. Patil NG, Wong J: Surgery in the "new" Hong Kong. Arch Surg 136:1415-1418, 2001.

Endoscopic Ablation of Barrett's Metaplasia and Dysplasia

Herbert C. Wolfsen · David Utley · Jeffrey H. Peters

BARRETT'S ESOPHAGUS

Barrett's esophagus develops as a result of chronic, pathologic reflux of gastroduodenal contents into the esophagus. The diagnosis is made initially by the endoscopic finding of salmon-colored epithelium in the distal esophagus, followed by histologic confirmation of specialized intestinal columnar epithelium (intestinal metaplasia [IM]) via biopsy.[1,2] Barrett's esophagus is classified by histology as either nondysplastic IM (hereafter IM), low-grade dysplasia (LGD), or high-grade dysplasia (HGD).

Barrett's esophagus is present in 1% to 2% of the adult U.S. population,[2-5] with recent reports suggesting a growing prevalence.[6,7] Rex et al. reported a 6.8% prevalence of IM in a general population of patients undergoing colonoscopy.[6] Among patients who reported symptoms of gastroesophageal reflux disease (GERD) in this study, the prevalence of IM, as might be expected, was even higher (8.6%). Gerson et al. reported a 25% prevalence of IM in a predominantly white, male, non-GERD population (>50 years of age) undergoing sigmoidoscopy.[7] The cause of this observed increase in the number of cases of Barrett's esophagus is unclear, but it may be related to the increase in the prevalence and awareness of GERD, more liberal use of endoscopy, and the broad use of antisecretory medications.

To assess the options available for the management of Barrett's esophagus, specifically, interventions intended to completely eradicate this lesion endoscopically before its progression to HGD or adenocarcinoma, the risk for progression of Barrett's esophagus must first be carefully considered.

RISK OF PROGRESSION TO DYSPLASIA AND ESOPHAGEAL ADENOCARCINOMA

The risk for a patient with nondysplastic Barrett's esophagus to progress to esophageal adenocarcinoma has been reported to be 0.4% to 1.0% per patient per year,[8-10] a risk 30 to 125 times higher than in the general population.[3,4,11] In 2005, according to the American Cancer Society, there were 14,520 new cases of esophageal cancer in the United States, the majority of which were adenocarcinoma, and 13,570 deaths associated with this disease.[12] This figure represents a 300% to 500% rise in U.S. esophageal cancer incidence over the last 30 years, an increase in incidence that surpasses that of all other cancers.[5]

Sharma et al. reported that on initial diagnosis of Barrett's esophagus in 1376 patients (Tables 25–1 and 25–2), LGD (7.3%), HGD (3.0%), or adenocarcinoma (6.0%) had *already* developed in a large number of patients.[8] Thereafter, 618 of the *nondysplastic* IM patients from this series underwent endoscopic surveillance for an average of 4 additional years. During this 4-year interval, a significant number of these previously nondysplastic IM patients progressed to LGD (16.1%), HGD (3.6%), or adenocarcinoma (2.0%). According to these data, the risk for a patient with nondysplastic IM to progress to either HGD or adenocarcinoma, diagnoses for which the standard of care is surgical esophagectomy, is *1.4% per patient per year*. Stated differently, 1 in 71 patients with nondysplastic Barrett's esophagus will have their esophagus removed every year because of the development of HGD or adenocarcinoma.

Table 25–1   Incidence of LGD, HGD, and Cancer at Primary Diagnosis of Barrett's Esophagus

New Case Diagnosis	Number	% of Cases
IM	1376	100
LGD	101	7.3
HGD	42	3.0
Cancer	91	6.7

HGD, high-grade dysplasia; IM, intestinal metaplasia; LGD, low-grade dysplasia.
Created from Sharma P, Reker D, Falok G, et al: Progression of Barrett's esophagus to high-grade dysplasia and cancer: Preliminary results of the BEST trial. Gastroenterology 120:A16, 2001.

Table 25–2   Incidence of LGD, HGD, and Cancer in Patients with Nondysplastic Barrett's Esophagus

Diagnosis	Total	% Risk in 4 Years	% Risk per Year
Total IM patients	618	NA	NA
New LGD	100	16.1	4.3
New HGD	22	3.6	0.9
Cancer	12	2.0	0.5

HGD, high-grade dysplasia; IM, intestinal metaplasia; LGD, low-grade dysplasia.
Created from Sharma P, Reker D, Falok G, et al: Progression of Barrett's esophagus to high-grade dysplasia and cancer: Preliminary results of the BEST trial. Gastroenterology 120:A16, 2001.

COLON POLYP/COLON AND RECTAL CARCINOMA VERSUS BARRETT'S ESOPHAGUS/ESOPHAGEAL ADENOCARCINOMA: A "PRECURSOR LESION" COMPARISON

According to the National Cancer Institute Surveillance, Epidemiology and End Results (SEER) database for 2005, the lifetime risk for the development of colon and rectal carcinoma (CRC) is 5.7%, whereas that for esophageal cancer is 0.5%.[13] In 2005 there were 145,290 new cases of CRC in the United States and 14,520 new cases of esophageal cancer. Although CRC has a much higher incidence than esophageal cancer (approximately a 10-fold difference), the age-adjusted death rate for CRC is 20.5 per 100,000 population versus 4.4 per 100,000 for esophageal cancer (less than a 5-fold difference). Furthermore, the death rate for CRC in males (all races) is 24.8 per 100,000 versus 7.7 per 100,000 for esophageal cancer (approximately a threefold difference). This dichotomy between the incidence and death

rate for CRC and esophageal cancer is due to the difference in 5-year survival rates for the two disease states: 64.1% for CRC versus 14.9% for esophageal cancer, with the latter being one of the lowest 5-year survival rates of any cancer diagnosis.

The risk for progression to CRC in a patient with polyps of the colon[14] and the risk for progression to esophageal adenocarcinoma in a patient with nondysplastic Barrett's esophagus[8-10] are identical—0.5% per patient per year. A patient with Barrett's esophagus, however, has an additional risk, that of HGD (0.9% per patient per year), which results in an aggregate risk of 1.4% per patient per year for the development of a disease state for which the standard of care is esophagectomy.[8]

The surgical intervention for most CRC stages is segmental colectomy or hemicolectomy, and that for most esophageal cancer stages and HGD is esophagectomy. The morbidity and mortality associated with removal of a segment of colon are relatively low, whereas esophagectomy carries a low, but real risk for longer-term complications and death. Mortality rates associated with esophagectomy for invasive cancer are typically 4% to 6%, but several recent reports suggest that in the setting of a patient with HGD it may be significantly lower (0% to 1%). Of note, evidence suggests a significant volume-outcome relationship for esophagectomy in that patients undergoing esophagectomy in small, low-volume hospitals incur a mortality rate as high as 25%.[15,16] A recent study evaluated the mortality associated with esophagectomy in 8657 patients in the United States from 1988 to 2000. Analysis of a random sample of 20% of these cases found that the overall in-hospital mortality rate was 11.3% but was lower in high-volume surgical centers (decreasing to 7.5%).[17] Additionally, several large studies have found that 30% to 50% of patients experienced at least one serious postoperative complication such as pneumonia, myocardial infarction, heart failure, or wound infection and that the average length of hospital stay was at least 2 weeks.[18] Anastomotic strictures requiring dilation occur in 30% to 50% of patients after gastric pull-up, and though a nuisance, they are rarely a significant problem for the patient.[19] Respiratory function may remain depressed for 6 months after esophagectomy.[20] Removal of the gastroesophageal junction and relocation of the stomach remnant into the chest may be associated with refractory gastroesophageal reflux, long-term pulmonary complications, and a risk for recurrence of Barrett's esophagus.[21,22] For these reasons most experts advocate a high intrathoracic or cervical anastomosis, which markedly diminishes these problems. Taken together, these observations suggest that referral to a high-volume center is probably in the patient's best interest.

PREVENTION OF COLON AND RECTAL CARCINOMA AND HIGH-GRADE DYSPLASIA/ADENOCARCINOMA

After the advent of barium radiography of the colon, it was hypothesized that the development of CRC was preceded by malignant transformation of adenomatous polyps, and subsequently the metaplasia-dysplasia-carcinoma sequence was proposed.[23] Surveillance studies with matched cohorts, such as the National Polyp Study, found that colon carcinoma was significantly less likely to develop in patients undergoing endoscopic removal of adenomatous polyps, a risk reduction that has approximated 80% to 90%.[14] Subsequently, the use of screening colonoscopy plus removal of colon polyps has been recognized as the most effective method for diagnosing and ultimately reducing the risk for development of CRC.[24] Therefore, the paradigm related to colon polyps and prevention of CRC is to (1) screen candidate patients for colon polyps (detect the precursor lesion for CRC) and (2) remove the precursor lesion, which has a 0.5% per patient per year risk for progression to CRC (prevent progression to CRC).

For Barrett's esophagus and prevention of esophageal adenocarcinoma, the current paradigm is clearly different: (1) do not screen patients, but rather detect Barrett's esophagus (precursor lesion for adenocarcinoma) incidentally on endoscopy indicated for GERD symptoms; (2) once detected, do not remove the precursor lesion, even though the lesion incurs a 1.4% per patient per year risk of progressing to HGD or adenocarcinoma; (3) survey patients with nondysplastic Barrett's esophagus every 3 years to detect progression to HGD or adenocarcinoma; and (4) remove the esophagus when HGD or adenocarcinoma is detected.

RATIONALE FOR ENDOSCOPIC REMOVAL OF BARRETT'S METAPLASIA AND DYSPLASIA

Given the elevated inherent risk for progression of nondysplastic Barrett's esophagus to HGD or adenocarcinoma, why then has a conservative "watch and wait" approach been the historic practice paradigm for these patients? The answer may lie in the fact that a technique for safe, effective (complete), and reproducible removal of all IM tissue in a given patient has been quite elusive. The endoluminal techniques that have been studied for removing Barrett's esophagus include circumferential balloon-based radiofrequency ablation,[25-30] photodynamic therapy (PDT),[31-47] endoscopic mucosal resection (EMR),[48-54] laser ablation,[3,55-61] argon plasma coagulation (APC),[3,55,62-73] multipolar electrocoagulation (MPEC),[3,55,74-78] and cryotherapy.[79-81]

There are multiple challenges inherent to achieving safe, effective, and reproducible removal of Barrett's esophagus, and each of these factors must be considered when evaluating a technique for managing this disease: (1) access (the targeted portion of the esophagus is approximately 30 to 40 cm from incisors); (2) the corrugated nature of the esophageal lumen (an uneven epithelial target); (3) mucous and gastric contents affecting the ablative effect of any energy source; (4) esophageal motility, which creates a moving ablation target; and (5) a very limited, tight margin between the ablation being "deep enough" (to the muscularis mucosae) and "too deep" (into the submucosa).

The ideal means to achieve safe, effective, and reproducible ablation of Barrett's esophagus should (1) be feasible for an endoscopist skilled in interventional techniques to perform; (2) be capable of removing all Barrett's epithelium; (3) result in no subsquamous IM (buried glands); (4) have a very low rate of complications, such as stricture formation, bleeding, and perforation; and (5) be well tolerated by the patient, thus enabling repeat therapy as needed for the lifetime of the patient for recurrent (new) or persistent disease, given the chronicity and GERD-related nature of Barrett's esophagus.

What depth of tissue ablation is required to effectively eliminate Barrett's esophagus? Ackroyd et al. reported that the thickness of nondysplastic IM ($500 \pm 4\,\mu m$; range, 390 to $590\,\mu m$) is very similar to that of normal squamous epithelium ($490 \pm 3\,\mu m$; range, 420 to $580\,\mu m$).[82] This narrow range and tight standard deviation for Barrett's thickness suggest that interpatient and intrapatient variability is very small. This information is promising in that if an ablation technique can be shown to repeatedly and uniformly penetrate at a minimum to the muscularis mucosae ($\approx 700\,\mu m$) and at a maximum to the top of the submucosa (≈ 1000 to $1500\,\mu m$), Barrett's epithelium can be reliably and safely removed. Proactive eradication of Barrett's esophagus, if safe and effective, could lead in the long-term to demonstration of a risk reduction for the development of adenocarcinoma.

Thus far we have reviewed the risk inherent for progression of nondysplastic Barrett's esophagus to HGD and adenocarcinoma, the comparison between the "precursor lesions" of colon polyps and nondysplastic Barrett's esophagus, and finally the rationale and ideal requirements for developing an endoprevention paradigm for proactively managing Barrett's esophagus. In the remainder of this chapter we review the presently available techniques for removing and ablating Barrett's esophagus.

CIRCUMFERENTIAL BALLOON-BASED RADIOFREQUENCY ABLATION

The most recently developed tool for ablation of Barrett's esophagus is a balloon-based electrode array (HALO^{360} system, BÂRRX Medical, Inc., Sunnyvale, CA) (Figs. 25–1 to 25–5). The balloon is used to dilate the targeted portion of the esophagus to a standardized pressure (0.5 atm), which transiently flattens the esophageal folds and submits the esophageal wall to a standardized tension or stretch. With the esophagus in a dilated state, a high-power, ultrashort ($\approx 300\,msec$) burst of ablative energy is applied to the epithelium to create a uniform depth of ablation of the muscularis mucosae ($\approx 1000\,\mu m$).[25]

The key features of this device that are intended to achieve a uniform ablation depth and wide-field removal of epithelium are (1) very high power (300 W), (2) ultrashort energy delivery time (<300 msec), (3) tightly spaced bipolar electrode array (<250 μm between electrodes), (4) standardized wall tension with balloon dilation, (5) standardized energy density (joules of energy

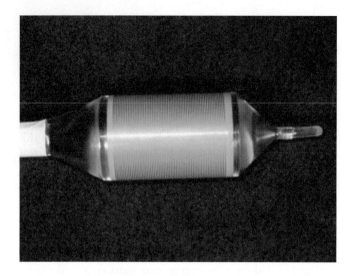

Figure 25–1. Balloon-based electrode (HALO[360] Ablation Catheter, BÂRRX Medical, Inc., Sunnyvale, CA). Three-centimeter length with 60 narrowly spaced circumferential electrode bands.

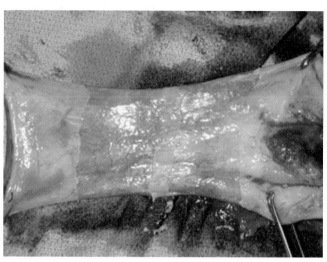

Figure 25–3. Resected human esophagus. Two separate ablation zones delivered via the HALO[360] system at 10 J/cm[2]. Squamous epithelium completely sloughed to the level of the muscularis mucosae.

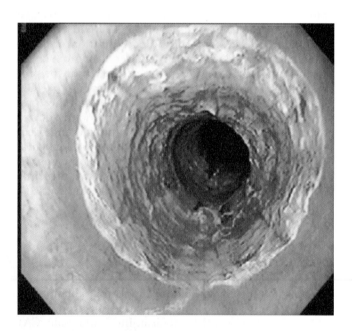

Figure 25–2. Endoscopic appearance after a single ablation with the HALO[360] system at 12 J/cm[2] in the human esophagus.

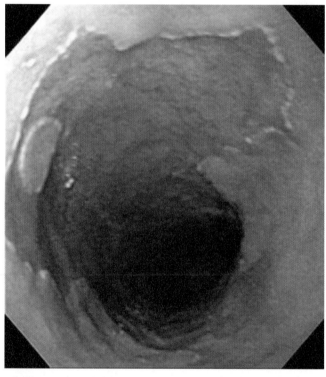

Figures 25–4. Human patient with low-grade dysplasia before ablation with the HALO[360] system.

delivered to each square centimeter of epithelium), and (6) large surface area of the electrode (>30 cm[2]).[25]

Why might each of these elements be important? High power (1) enables ultrashort energy delivery time (2), which mitigates the risk of thermal conduction deep into the esophageal wall and prevents injury to the submucosa. Submucosal injury would inevitably lead to stricture formation. Tight bipolar electrode array spacing (3), as assessed by finite element modeling and bench experimentation, further limits the depth of tissue heating. Finite element analysis is a technique to map electrical

field and heating characteristics. Changes in esophageal wall tension at the time of energy delivery could adversely affect the ablative effect, and it is therefore important to standardize the balloon inflation pressure (4) in order to control ablation depth. The endoscopist cannot be required to rely on visual evidence of heat-related changes in the epithelium as the end point for ablation. The ablation tool must therefore be automated and

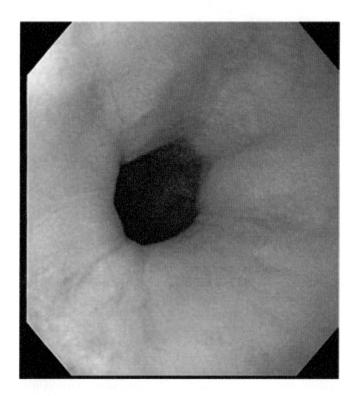

Figure 25–5. Human patient with low-grade dysplasia (LGD) 6 months after ablation with the HALO³⁶⁰ system at 12 J/cm² delivered twice. Baseline histology showed LGD, whereas all biopsy specimens from 6-month endoscopy showed normal squamous epithelium without subsquamous intestinal metaplasia.

capable of standardizing wall tension and delivering a precise amount of energy (5) to each surface area unit (J/cm²) to avoid undertreatment or unintended deep tissue injury. Finally, to ablate large areas of Barrett's esophagus, it is necessary to have a large electrode surface area (6), not just a small probe. This device ablates more than 30 cm² of epithelium in less than 1 second.

Ganz et al. reported on the use of this ablative device in a porcine model, as well as human esophagectomy patients.[25] Ablation depth was directly related to the energy density delivered, with 8 to 12 J/cm² resulting in complete removal of epithelium. There were no strictures and no significant submucosal injury within this energy density range. Deeper injury and subsequent stricture formation were evident at higher energy density settings (>20 J/cm²). A follow-on evaluation of this device in human subjects undergoing esophagectomy was included in this report. Ablation was performed 1 to 2 days before esophageal resection. Energy density settings of 10 and 12 J/cm² were used. Histologic examination revealed that removal of epithelium was complete in all areas of balloon electrode contact. The maximum depth of ablation was the muscularis mucosae, with no submucosal injury, thus corroborating the animal study findings in this energy density dose range.[25]

Dunkin et al. studied the effect of this device in a larger series of patients undergoing esophagectomy who received 10 or 12 J/cm² delivered once or twice. Complete removal of the esophageal epithelium without injury to the submucosa or muscularis propria was possible with the balloon-based electrode at 10 J/cm² (two overlapped applications in one treatment session) or 12 J/cm² (once or twice). A second application did not significantly increase ablation depth, and therefore overlapping ablations zones did not portend a significantly deeper injury.[28]

Sharma et al. reported on the use of this device in the multicenter dosimetry Ablation of Intestinal Metaplasia (AIM-I) trial in patients ($N = 32$) with nondysplastic IM. The procedure was performed with the use of conscious sedation on an outpatient basis. The median procedure time was 24 minutes. Energy densities evaluated were 8, 10, and 12 J/cm² (all delivered once). The procedure was well tolerated and there were no strictures or buried glands. Pathologic examination was performed by a centralized pathology service. After one application, most patients treated with 8 J/cm² had residual IM, whereas 10 and 12 J/cm² resulted in a respective 40% and 36% complete response (CR) rate (no histologic evidence of IM on four-quadrant biopsies). Given the equivalence of 10 and 12 J/cm², all patients were treated a second time with 10 J/cm², which resulted in a CR rate of 67% at 1 year.[26]

Fleischer et al. performed a larger follow-on study to AIM-I, deemed AIM-II, which included longer-segment (2 to 6 cm), nondysplastic IM. The median procedure time was 26 minutes. A single energy density setting was evaluated, 10 J/cm² (delivered twice). The procedure was well tolerated and there were no strictures or buried glands. At 12 months, the CR rate was 52%. Patients with persistent IM at 1 year typically exhibited focal disease only, in the form of small islands (the average clearance in the group with residual disease was 90%).[30]

Sharma et al. evaluated this device in patients with IM-LGD at 12 J/cm² (applied twice). They reported CR rates of 100% for LGD and 60% for IM at 1-year follow-up, with no strictures or buried glands.[27]

In a report by Smith et al., subjects underwent endoluminal ablation of one or two circumferential 3-cm segments of the esophagus that contained IM-HGD with the HALO³⁶⁰ system. Treatment settings were randomized to 10, 12, or 14 J/cm² and two to six applications. After esophagectomy, multiple sections from each ablation zone were evaluated by hematoxylin-eosin staining and microscopy. The maximum ablation depth was the lamina propria or muscularis mucosae in 10 of 11 specimens. One section treated at the highest energy (14 J/cm², four applications) had edema in the submucosa. In the well-overlapped areas of treatment, 91% (10/11) of specimens had no evidence of IM-HGD remaining. In one specimen the majority of IM-HGD was ablated, but small focal areas remained. In three specimens, IM-HGD was found at the edge of the treatment zones where overlap of the multiple energy applications was incomplete. They concluded that complete ablation of IM-HGD in 91% of treatment zones, without excessively deep injury, was possible with this device.[29] As a follow-on to these pilot dysplasia trials, a large, multicenter, randomized, sham-controlled trial is currently under way to compare ablation with the HALO[360] system plus esomeprazole with a sham ablation plus esomeprazole in patients with LGD or HGD.

PHOTODYNAMIC THERAPY

PDT involves the systemic administration of a photosensitizing pharmaceutical agent followed by the endoscopic delivery of light energy to the affected esophagus. Exposure to this drug-specific wavelength of laser light results in activation of the photosensitizer within esophageal epithelial cells and the subsequent formation of toxic intracellular oxygen metabolites that can result in cell death.[32] Although several photosensitizing agents (both oral and intravenous) have been evaluated for PDT, only porfimer sodium (PORPDT) has received regulatory approval to treat patients with Barrett's esophagus and HGD in the United States.[35]

There have been several published reports regarding the use of PORPDT for the treatment of patients with HGD.[31-43] In the most rigorous and comprehensive clinical trial, recently published by Overholt et al., 208 patients with HGD were randomized to receive either PORPDT plus omeprazole (OM) ($n = 138$) or OM alone ($n = 70$).[31] Average follow-up was 24.2 months. Most patients in the PORPDT group underwent more than one treatment session, with 47% receiving three sessions. There was a significant difference between PORPDT+OM and OM at 18 months for the primary end point (presence of HGD), with 75% of patients receiving PORPDT+OM and 36% of those receiving OM being free of HGD ($P < .0001$). Only 52% of patients receiving PORPDT+OM were free of all IM at any point in the follow-up, whereas 7% of those receiving OM were free of IM.

Patient tolerability was an issue for the PORPDT+OM group, including photosensitivity occurring up to 90 days after injection (69%), esophageal stricture (36%), vomiting (32%), noncardiac chest pain (20%), pyrexia (20%), dysphagia (19%), constipation (13%), dehydration (12%), nausea (11%), and hiccups (10%). No major adverse events occurred in the OM group. Within the PORPDT+OM group, 18 patients (13%) progressed to esophageal adenocarcinoma as compared with 20 patients (29%) in the OM group.

Mayo Clinic researchers have independently reported their experience with PDT in a total of 142 patients (69 patients treated with PORPDT at Jacksonville, FL, and 72 patients treated with either a hematoporphyrin derivative or PORPDT at Rochester, MN).[37,38] The 19- to 20-month follow-up was similar to that of Overholt et al. in that complete elimination of Barrett's mucosa was found in 52% and 35% of patients, respectively, and elimination of HGD in 100% and 88% of patients, respectively. These studies also included the adjunctive use of post-PDT thermal ablation with APC. Stricture rates were 22% and 27%, respectively, comparable to that of Overholt.

The paramount issues that continue to be associated with the use of PDT include patient toxicity (photosensitivity, postablation symptoms), safety (stricture forma-

tion, vomiting, pleural effusion, atrial fibrillation),[43] changes in motility after ablation,[44] persistent IM despite elimination of dysplasia in the majority of patients, and subsquamous IM reported in every PDT trial and as high as 51.5% in a recent study.[45]

Triadafilopoulos et al. found that PORPDT followed by surveillance was more cost-effective than esophagectomy for treating HGD despite incurring a greater lifetime cost ($47,310 versus $24,045), mainly because of a higher quality-adjusted length of life associated with PORPDT.[46]

ENDOSCOPIC MUCOSAL RESECTION

EMR techniques have been used to diagnose and treat HGD and carcinoma in selected patients with Barrett's esophagus. EMR is performed via a variety of techniques, such as an endoscopic cap with an internal snare device, a variceal ligation device, or a monofilament snare in conjunction with lifting the mucosa with biopsy forceps.[48] Generally, these resection techniques are performed after an injection into the submucosal layer separates the target mucosa from the deeper muscularis propria layer to mitigate against esophageal perforation. Once snared, coagulative energy is delivered to the snare wire as it is pulled into the cap to cut and coagulate the margins of the specimen. Mucosal resection creates a relatively large excisional mucosal biopsy specimen with a typical diameter of 15 to 20 mm, which allows detailed histologic analysis, including resection margins, provided that the excision specimen is intact and includes the entire lesion.

Ell et al. evaluated the role of EMR in 64 patients with Barrett's esophagus: 61 with early cancer and 3 with HGD.[52] After EMR, complete remission was achieved in 97% of patients who demonstrated the following baseline characteristics: lesion size less than 2 cm, histology showing moderately or well-differentiated adenocarcinoma or HGD, and lesion limited to the mucosa. The complete remission rate was lower (59%) in patients with more advanced baseline findings: lesion size larger than 2 cm and limited to the mucosa, poorly differentiated adenocarcinoma, or infiltration of the submucosa.

Although EMR may be a reasonable technique for primary diagnosis or selective treatment of localized lesions, such as HGD nodules, there are limitations to the extent of mucosa that can be safely resected before toxicity and stricture formation are incurred.[54] Furthermore, EMR is technically demanding for most endoscopists. When used for focal resection of suspicious areas such as nodules, focal nodules, plaques, and intramucosal carcinoma, the residual Barrett's mucosa must still be considered "at risk" for progression to HGD and adenocarcinoma, and subsequent wide-field treatment should be considered.

LASER ABLATION

Laser light sources (light amplification by stimulated emission of radiation) have been used for esophageal mucosal ablation and include neodymium:yttrium-aluminum-garnet (Nd-YAG, 1064 nm), potassium titanyl phosphate (KTP, 532 nm), and argon dye (514.5 nm). Mucosal depth of ablation and injury depend on the wavelength of the laser light energy used, treatment settings, and target tissue characteristics. Typically, Nd:YAG penetrates most deeply (up to 4 mm), whereas KTP is penetrates least deeply (≈1 mm).[3]

Reports of the use of laser ablation in Barrett's esophagus consist of small case series. In six of these reports,[56-61] complete ablation of all IM was achieved in 0% to 62% of cases after multiple treatment sessions. Buried glands were reported in some studies. Gossner et al. found that 20% of patients had subsquamous IM after laser ablation.[56]

The use of laser ablation has migrated away from primary therapy for Barrett's esophagus toward "spot ablation" salvage for wide-field ablation techniques, such as PDT, that experience high rates of residual focal nondysplastic IM.

ARGON PLASMA COAGULATION

APC is a system that delivers argon gas to the esophageal target epithelium via a through-the-scope catheter. As the gas exits the tip of the catheter, it is exposed to a monopolar electrode that ionizes the gas, which is carried to the tissue via the gas stream, thus returning to a common ground via a dispersive electrode.[3,62] As the energy passes through the epithelium, coagulation occurs. The depth of injury is dependent on the gas flow rate, power setting, duration of application, tissue hydration, and distance from the probe tip to the tissue.[3,62]

This technique has been used by several authors for the treatment of Barrett's esophagus with and without dysplasia.[63-73] Basu et al. reported that the best candidates for thermal ablation therapy are those with shorter segments of IM and good control of gastroesophageal reflux.[64] In this study, however, 44% of patients demonstrated subsquamous IM after treatment.

In 10 published cases series containing a diverse group of 221 patients with and without dysplasia,[63-72] CR rates for IM range widely from 0% to 99%. The observed inconsistency in results may be due to variability in technique, treatment settings, number of ablation sessions, ablation depth with APC, or any combination of these factors. Dulai et al. recently reported a comparison study between APC and MPEC.[73] This study was rigorously controlled with respect to treatment technique, treatment settings, number of treatment sessions, and follow-up, which may explain the more consistent results in comparison to other studies. They reported similar histologic CR rates for IM with APC (58%) and MPEC (65%), with 28 patients per group. The mean number of treatment sessions required to achieve these results was 3.8 (APC) and 2.9 (MPEC), with up to 6 sessions permitted. There was no subsquamous IM found in this study.

Complications related to APC for Barrett's esophagus that have been reported include pneumatosis, pneumoperitoneum, subcutaneous emphysema, pain, ulceration, stricture, bleeding, perforation, and even death.[63-72]

MULTIPOLAR ELECTROCOAGULATION

MPEC involves the delivery of radiofrequency energy to the tissue via a through-the-scope probe that delivers point coagulation to affected tissue. Energy travels between electrodes at the tip of the device and induces tissue coagulation. Like APC, laser ablation, and cryotherapy, the end point for treatment is visual coagulation.[3,55] In five case series,[74-78] 110 patients were treated with MPEC. The reported CR rate for IM ranged from 75% to 100%. Multiple sessions were required to achieve CR in all studies. All studies reported that adverse postablation symptoms were common; specifically, Kovacs et al. found that 41% of patients experienced dysphagia, odynophagia, or chest pain lasting up to 4 days.[76]

As with APC and laser therapy, MPEC is now most commonly used in the management of Barrett's esophagus for focal ablation of persistent IM after ablation with other modalities, such as PDT.

CRYOTHERAPY

Cryotherapy is not a new modality and has been used for tumor management in areas of the body other than the esophagus. More recently, cryotherapy has been studied in a limited manner for ablation of esophageal epithelium.[79,80] Liquid nitrogen is sprayed onto esophageal epithelium via a through-the-scope catheter. Previous attempts at using a "cold probe" were fraught with tissue sticking and ablation depth control. The mechanism of injury appears to include induced apoptosis and cryonecrosis.[81]

In a porcine model ($N = 20$), liquid nitrogen was sprayed onto squamous epithelium. Exposure time to the spray was varied between 10 and 60 seconds. The authors reported that 95% of the animals demonstrated complete ablation of the epithelium when sacrificed at 2 to 7 days. Stricture formation occurred in 15% of animals and aspiration pneumonia in 5%.[79]

CONCLUSION

Barrett's esophagus is caused by chronic pathologic exposure of the esophagus to gastroduodenal contents. The recurrent injury and resulting inflammation result in a metaplastic change in which the normal squamous lining of the esophagus is replaced by abnormal intestinalized columnar epithelium—a known precursor to esophageal adenocarcinoma. The prevalence of Barrett's esophagus is on the rise, but of much greater concern is the rapid rise in incidence of esophageal adenocarcinoma. For HGD and esophageal adenocarcinoma, surgical esophagectomy is the current standard of care. There is now a role for PDT in patients with HGD, and there are reports of the use of other ablation modalities and EMR for this diagnosis. A randomized sham-controlled trial is under way to evaluate the HALO[360] balloon-based ablation device for LGD and HGD in an attempt to demonstrate eradication of dysplasia without the associated morbidity of surgery or PDT.

In this chapter we presented data regarding a paradigm that should be considered and supported with continued clinical studies. This paradigm involves proactive endoprevention for Barrett's esophagus containing nondysplastic IM and LGD. Early eradication of this disease, before progression, is a reasonable approach if the technique is safe, reproducible, and effective at removing all diseased tissue.

REFERENCES

1. Spechler SJ: Barrett's esophagus. N Engl J Med 346:836-842, 2002.
2. Peters JH, Hagen JA, DeMeester SR: Barrett's esophagus. J Gastrointest Surg 8:1-17, 2004.
3. Eisen GM: Ablation therapy for Barrett's esophagus. Gastrointest Endosc 58:760-769, 2003.
4. Reid BJ: Barrett's esophagus and adenocarcinoma. Gastroenterol Clin North Am 20:817-834, 1991.
5. Shaheen N, Ransohoff DR: Gastroesophageal reflux, Barrett's esophagus and esophageal cancer. JAMA 287:1972-1981, 2002.
6. Rex DK, Cummings OW, Shaw M, et al: Screening for Barrett's esophagus in colonoscopy patients with and without heartburn. Gastroenterology 125:1670-1677, 2003.
7. Gerson LB, Shetler K, Triadafilopoulos G: Prevalence of Barrett's esophagus in asymptomatic individuals. Gastroenterology 123:636-639, 2002.
8. Sharma P, Reker D, Falok G, et al: Progression of Barrett's esophagus to high-grade dysplasia and cancer: Preliminary results of the BEST trial. Gastroenterology 120:A16, 2001.
9. O'Connor JB, Falk GW, Richter JE: The incidence of adenocarcinoma and dysplasia in Barrett's esophagus: Report on the Cleveland Clinic Barrett's Esophagus Registry. Am J Gastroenterol 94:2037-2042, 1999.
10. Drewitz DJ, Sampliner RE, Garewal HS: The incidence of adenocarcinoma in Barrett's esophagus: A prospective study of 170 patients followed 4.8 years. Am J Gastroenterol 92:212-215, 1997.
11. Provenzale D, Kemp JA, Arora S, Wong JB: A guide for surveillance of patients with Barrett's esophagus. Am J Gastroenterol 89:670-680, 1994.
12. American Cancer Society: Cancer Facts and Figures 2005. Atlanta, American Cancer Society, 2005.
13. Ries LAG, Eisner MP, Kosary CL, et al (eds): SEER Cancer Statistics Review, 1975-2002. Bethesda, MD, National Cancer Institute. http://seer.cancer.gov/csr/1975_2002/, based on November 2004 SEER data submission, posted to the SEER website 2005.
14. Winawer SJ, Zauber AG, Ho MN, et al: Prevention of colorectal cancer by polypectomy. The National Polyp Study Workgroup. N Engl J Med 329:1977-1981, 1993.
15. Urbach DR, Baxter NN: Does it matter what a hospital is "high-volume" for? Specificity of hospital volume-outcome associations for surgical procedures: Analysis of administrative data. BMJ 328:737-740, 2004.
16. Bartels H, Stein HJ, Siewert JR: Risk analysis in esophageal surgery. Recent Results Cancer Res 155:89-96, 2000.
17. Dimick JB, Wainess RM, Upchurch GR Jr, et al: National trends in outcomes for esophageal resection. Ann Thorac Surg 79:212-216, 2005.
18. Lerut TE, van Lanschot JJ: Chronic symptoms after subtotal or partial oesophagectomy: Diagnosis and treatment. Best Pract Res Clin Gastroenterol 18:901-915, 2004.
19. Orringer MB, Marshall B, Iannettoni MD: Eliminating the cervical esophagogastric anastomotic leak with a side-to-side stapled anastomosis. J Thorac Cardiovasc Surg 119:277-288, 2000.
20. Ikeguchi M, Maeta M, Kaibara N: Respiratory function after esophagectomy for patients with esophageal cancer. Hepatogastroenterology 49:1284-1286, 2002.
21. Shibuya S, Fukudo S, Shineha R, et al: High incidence of reflux esophagitis observed by routine endoscopic examination after gastric pull-up esophagectomy. World J Surg 27:580-583, 2003.
22. Wolfsen HC, Hemminger LL, DeVault KR: Recurrent Barrett's esophagus and adenocarcinoma after esophagectomy. BMC Gastroenterol 4:18, 2004.
23. Bond JH: Interference with the adenoma-carcinoma sequence. Eur J Cancer 31A:1115-1117, 1995.
24. Rex DK, Johnson DA, Lieberman DA, et al: Colorectal cancer prevention 2000: Screening recommendations of the American College of Gastroenterology. Am J Gastroenterol 95:868-877, 2000.
25. Ganz RA, Utley DS, Stern RA, et al: Complete ablation of esophageal epithelium with a balloon-based bipolar electrode: A phased evaluation in the porcine and in the human esophagus. Gastrointest Endosc 60:1002-1010, 2004.
26. Sharma VK, Overholt B, Wang KK, et al: A randomized multi-center evaluation of ablation of nondysplastic short segment Barrett's esophagus using BÂRRX Bipolar Balloon Device: Extended follow-up of the Ablation of Intestinal Metaplasia (AIM-I) Trial. Gastrointest Endosc 61:AB239, 2005.
27. Sharma VK, McLaughlin R, Dean P, et al: Successful ablation of Barrett's esophagus with low-grade dysplasia using BÂRRX bipolar balloon device: Preliminary results of the Ablation of Intestinal Metaplasia with LGD (AIM-LGD) Trial. Gastrointest Endosc 61:AB143, 2005.
28. Dunkin BJ, Martinez J, Bejarano PA, et al: Thin-layer ablation of human esophageal epithelium using a bipolar radiofrequency balloon device. Surg Endosc 20:125-130, 2006.
29. Smith CD, Dunkin BJ, Bejarano P, et al: Thin-layer ablation of intestinal metaplasia with high-grade dysplasia in esophagectomy patients using a bipolar radiofrequency balloon device (BÂRRX System). Gastroenterology 128:A809, 2005.
30. Fleischer DE, Sharma VK, Reymunde A, et al: A prospective multi-center evaluation of ablation of non-dysplastic Barrett's esophagus using the BÂRRX bipolar balloon device. Ablation of Intestinal Metaplasia Trial (AIM-II). Gastroenterology 128:A236, 2005.
31. Overholt BF, Lightdale CJ, Wang KK, et al: Photodynamic therapy with porfimer sodium for ablation of high-grade dysplasia in Barrett's esophagus: International, partially blinded, randomized phase III trial. Gastrointest Endosc 62:488-498, 2005.
32. Wang K: Photodynamic therapy made simple. Clin Perspect Gastroenterol March/April:90-100, 2001.
33. Webber J, Herman M, Kessel D, Fromm D: Current concepts in gastrointestinal photodynamic therapy. Ann Surg 230:12-23, 1999.
34. Kubba AK: Role of photodynamic therapy in the management of gastrointestinal cancer. Digestion 60:1-10, 1999.
35. Prosst RL, Wolfsen HC, Gahlen J: Photodynamic therapy for esophageal diseases: A clinical update. Endoscopy 35:1059-1068, 2003.
36. DeVault KR, Ward EM, Wolfsen HC, et al: Barrett's esophagus (BE) is common in older patients undergoing screening colonoscopy regardless of gastroesophageal reflux (GER) symptoms. Gastrointest Endosc 59:AB111, 2004.
37. Wolfsen HC, Hemminger LL: Photodynamic therapy for dysplastic Barrett's esophagus and mucosal adenocarcinoma. Gastrointest Endosc 59:AB251, 2004.
38. Wang KK, Wong Kee Song LM, Buttar NS, et al: Barrett's esophagus after photodynamic therapy: Risk of cancer development during long term follow up. Gastroenterology 126(Suppl 2):A-50, 2004.
39. Wang KK: Current status of photodynamic therapy of Barrett's esophagus. Gastrointest Endosc 49(3 Pt 2):S20-S23, 1999.
40. Wolfsen HC, Woodward TA, Raimondo M: Photodynamic therapy for dysplastic Barrett esophagus and early esophageal adenocarcinoma. Mayo Clin Proc 77:1176-1181, 2002.
41. Wang KK, Kim JY: Photodynamic therapy in Barrett's esophagus. Gastrointest Endosc Clin N Am 13:483-489, vii, 2003.
42. Wolfsen HC: Photodynamic therapy for mucosal esophageal adenocarcinoma and dysplastic Barrett's esophagus. Dig Dis 20:5-17, 2002.
43. Overholt BF, Panjehpour M, Haydek JM: Photodynamic therapy for Barrett's esophagus: Follow-up. Gastrointest Endosc 49:1-7, 1999.
44. Malhi-Chowla N, Wolfsen HC, DeVault KR: Esophageal dysmotility in patients undergoing photodynamic therapy. Mayo Clin Proc 76:987-989, 2001.
45. Ban S, Mino M, Nishioka NS, et al: Histopathologic aspects of photodynamic therapy for dysplasia and early adenocarcinoma arising in Barrett's esophagus. Am J Surg Pathol 28:1466-1473, 2004.
46. Rohini V, Triadafilopoulos G, Owens D, et al: Cost-effectiveness of photodynamic therapy for high-grade dysplasia in Barrett's esophagus. Gastrointest Endosc 60:739-756, 2004.

47. Nijhawan PK, Wang KK: Endoscopic mucosal resection of lesions with endoscopic features suggestive of malignancy or high grade dysplasia within Barrett's esophagus. Gastrointest Endosc 52:328-332, 2000.

48. Soetikno RM, Gotoda T, Nakanishi Y, Soehendra N: Endoscopic mucosal resection. Gastrointest Endosc 57:567-579, 2003.

49. Conio M, Cameron AJ, Chak A, et al: Endoscopic treatment of high-grade dysplasia and early cancer in Barrett's oesophagus. Lancet Oncol 6:311-321, 2005.

50. May A, Gossner L, Behrens A, et al: A prospective randomized trial of two different endoscopic resection techniques for early stage cancer of the esophagus. Gastrointest Endosc 58:167-175, 2003.

51. Rosch T, Sarbia M, Schumacher B, et al: Attempted endoscopic en bloc resection of mucosal and submucosal tumors using insulated-tip knives: A pilot series. Endoscopy 36:788-801, 2004.

52. Ell C, May A, Gossner L, et al: Endoscopic mucosal resection of early cancer and high-grade dysplasia in Barrett's esophagus. Gastroenterology 118:670-677, 2000.

53. Seewald S, Akaraviputh T, Seitz U, et al: Circumferential EMR and complete removal of Barrett's epithelium: A new approach to management of Barrett's esophagus containing high-grade intraepithelial neoplasia and intramucosal carcinoma. Gastrointest Endosc 57:854-859, 2003.

54. Rajan E, Gostout CJ, Feitoza AB, et al: Widespread EMR: A new technique for removal of large areas of mucosa. Gastrointest Endosc 60:623-627, 2004.

55. Haag S, Nandurkar S, Talley JJ: Regression of Barrett's esophagus: The role of acid suppression, surgery, and ablative methods. Gastrointest Endosc 50:229-240, 1999.

56. Gossner L, May A, Stolte M, et al: KTP laser destruction of dysplasia and early cancer in columnar-lined Barrett's esophagus. Gastrointest Endosc 49:8-12, 1999.

57. Salo JA, Salminen JT, Kiviluoto TA, et al: Treatment of Barrett's esophagus by endoscopic laser ablation and antireflux surgery. Ann Surg 227:621-623, 1998.

58. Bonavina L, Ceriani C, Carrazzone A, et al: Endoscopic laser ablation of nondysplastic Barrett's epithelium: Is it worthwhile? J Gastrointest Surg 3:194-199, 1999.

59. Barham CP, Jones RL, Biddlestone LR, et al: Photothermal laser ablation of Barrett's oesophagus: Endoscopic and histologic evidence of squamous re-epithelialisation. Gut 41:281-284, 1997.

60. Luman W, Lessels Am Palmer KR: Failure of Nd-YAG photocoagulation therapy as treatment for Barrett's esophagus: A pilot study. Eur J Gastroenterol Hepatol 8:627-630, 1996.

61. Weston AP, Sharma P: Neodymium:yttrium-aluminum garnet contact laser ablation of Barrett's high grade dysplasia and early adenocarcinoma. Am J Gastroenterol 97:2998-3006, 2002.

62. Ginsberg GG, Barkun AN, Bosco JJ, et al: The argon plasma coagulator. Gastrointest Endosc 55:807-810, 2002.

63. Tigges H, Fuchs KH, Maroske J, et al: Combination of endoscopic argon plasma coagulation and antireflux surgery for treatment of Barrett's esophagus. J Gastrointest Surg 5:251-259, 2001.

64. Basu KK, Pick B, Bale R, et al: Efficacy and one year follow-up of argon plasma coagulation therapy for ablation of Barrett's oesophagus: Factors determining persistence and recurrence of Barrett's epithelium. Gut 51:776-780, 2002.

65. Morino M, Rebecchi F, Giaccone C, et al: Endoscopic ablation of Barrett's esophagus using argon plasma coagulation (APC) following surgical laparoscopic fundoplication. Surg Endosc 17:539-542, 2003.

66. Schulz H, Miehlke S, Antos D, et al: Ablation of Barrett's epithelium by endoscopic argon plasma coagulation in combination with high dose omeprazole. Gastrointest Endosc 51:659-663, 2000.

67. Byrne JP, Armstrong GR, Attwood SE: Restoration of the normal squamous lining in Barrett's esophagus by argon beam plasma coagulation. Am J Gastroenterol 93:1810-1815, 1998.

68. Mork H, Barth T, Kreipe HH, et al: Reconstitution of squamous epithelium in Barrett's oesophagus with endoscopic argon plasma coagulation: A prospective study. Scand J Gastroenterol 33:1130-1134, 1998.

69. Van Laethem JL, Cremer M, Peny MO, et al: Eradication of Barrett's mucosa with argon plasma coagulation and acid suppression: Immediate and long-term results. Gut 43:747-751, 1998.

70. Pereira-Lima JC, Busnello JV, Saul C, et al: High power setting argon plasma coagulation for the eradication of Barrett's esophagus. Am J Gastroenterol 95:1661-1668, 2000.

71. Grade AJ, Shah IA, Medlin SM, Ramirez FC: The efficacy and safety of argon plasma coagulation therapy in Barrett's esophagus. Gastrointest Endosc 50:18-22, 1999.

72. Van Laethem JL, Jagodzinski R, Peny MO, et al: Argon plasma coagulation in the treatment of Barrett's high grade dysplasia and in situ adenocarcinoma. Endoscopy 33:257-261, 2001.

73. Dulai GS, Jensen DM, Cortina G, et al: Randomized trial of argon plasma coagulation vs. multipolar electrocoagulation for ablation of Barrett's esophagus. Gastrointest Endosc 61:232-240, 2005.

74. Montes CG, Brandalise NA, Deliza R, et al: Antireflux surgery followed by bipolar electrocoagulation in the treatment of Barrett's esophagus. Gastrointest Endosc 50:173-177, 1999.

75. Sharma P, Sampliner RE, Camargo E: Normalization of esophageal pH with high-dose proton pump inhibitor therapy does not result in regression of Barrett's esophagus. Am J Gastroenterol 92:582-585, 1997.

76. Kovacs BJ, Chen YK, Lewis TD, et al: Successful reversal of Barrett's esophagus with multipolar electrocoagulation despite inadequate acid suppression. Gastrointest Endosc 49:547-553, 1999.

77. Sampliner RE, Faigel D, Fennerty MB, et al: Effective and safe endoscopic reversal of nondysplastic Barrett's esophagus with thermal electrocoagulation combined with high-dose acid inhibition: A multicenter study. Gastrointest Endosc 53:554-558, 2001.

78. Fennerty MB, Corless CL, Sheppard B, et al: Pathologic documentation of complete elimination of Barrett's metaplasia following multipolar electrocoagulation therapy. Gut 49:142-144, 2001.

79. Johnston MH, Schoenfeld P, Mysore JV, Dubois A: Endoscopic spray cryotherapy: A new technique for mucosal ablation in the esophagus. Gastrointest Endosc 50:86-92, 1999.

80. Rodgers BM, McDonlad AP, Talbert JL, Donnelly WH: Morphologic and functional effects of esophageal cryotherapy. J Thorac Cardiovasc Surg 77:543-549, 1979.

81. Grana L, Ablin RJ, Goldman S, Milhouse E Jr: Freezing of the esophagus: Histologic changes and immunologic response. Int Surg 66:295-301, 1981.

82. Ackroyd R, Brown NJ, Stephenson TJ, et al: Ablation treatment for Barrett oesophagus: What depth of tissue destruction is needed? J Clin Pathol 52:509-512, 1999.

Chapter

26

Disorders of the Pharyngoesophageal Junction

André Duranceau

DEFINITION

Oropharyngeal dysphagia refers to difficulties in swallowing at the pharyngoesophageal level. This high or proximal dysphagia causes three categories of symptoms related to the fact that the oropharynx is involved in the function of swallowing, speech, and respiration. First, difficulty exists in propelling food or liquid from the oral cavity to the cervical esophagus. Regardless of whether the difficulty is initiating swallows, moving the bolus from the mouth to the pharynx, or food incarceration at the cricopharyngeus level, the result is difficulty swallowing. Second, when mechanical or functional obstruction impedes food or liquid transit, the bolus is misdirected back toward the mouth as pharyngo-oral regurgitation or through the nasopharynx as pharyngonasal regurgitation. The third category of symptoms relates to the larynx, with its role in phonation and respiration. Poor coordination plus hypopharyngeal stasis results in laryngeal and tracheal aspiration. The symptom complex of oropharyngeal dysphagia is for the most part associated with neurologic and neuromuscular disease. Idiopathic dysfunction of the upper esophageal sphincter (UES), with or without diverticulum formation, is also a frequent cause of oropharyngeal dysphagia. Previous treatment at the oropharyngeal level, either by surgery or by radiotherapy, may result in proximal dysphagia. Gastroesophageal reflux or transit abnormalities at the gastroesophageal junction may give rise to symptoms referred to the oropharyngeal level. The various causes of oropharyngeal dysphagia are classified in Box 26–1.

Patients with oropharyngeal dysphagia are difficult to assess. However, patients with these symptoms, when carefully selected, can be significantly improved by UES surgery.

The purpose of this chapter is to review the investigation of patients with oropharyngeal symptoms and clarify the role of surgery in managing these patients.

NORMAL FUNCTION

When a swallow is initiated, an organized sequence of events occurs that involves a sweeping action of the tongue, closing of the nasopharynx by the velopharyngeal muscles, and subsequent sequential contractions of the superior, medial, and inferior constrictor muscles. This sequence is difficult to evaluate because of the rapidity and variety of events that take place.

Tactile receptors in the pharynx elicit a series of reflex muscle activities that pull the pharynx up, elevate the hyoid bone, and bring the pharynx forward and upward.

Etiology of Pharyngoesophageal Dysfunction

Neurogenic
  Central
  Peripheral
Myogenic
  End-plate disease
  Muscular disease
Idiopathic dysfunction of the UES
  Isolated UES dysfunction
  UES dysfunction with a pharyngoesophageal diverticulum (Zenker's)
Iatrogenic
  Surgery
  Radiotherapy
Distal esophageal dysfunction
  Gastroesophageal reflux
  Motor disorders
  Esophageal obstruction
Mechanical
  Intrinsic
  Extrinsic
Psychogenic

Respiration ceases, the larynx is closed by the false and true vocal cords, and the epiglottis covers the laryngeal aditus. At the same time, the muscles of the upper middle and lower constrictors, which form a continuous sheet of muscle, are activated sequentially whereas the inferior constrictor remains inhibited during most pharyngeal muscle activity.[1,2]

Pharyngeal swallowing is divided into six phases:

1. When a bolus is present in the oral cavity, the soft palate is opposed to the posterior portion of the tongue, thereby closing the oropharynx.
2. Elevation of the soft palate and hyoid bone occurs while the entire pharynx is raised in a piston-like motion.
3. Active compression of the tongue on the bolus pushes it against and along the hard palate toward the entrance of the oropharynx. The soft palate elevates posteriorly and opposes the constrictor wall, thereby closing the nasopharynx. When the bolus passes the limits of the oropharynx, involuntary deglutition occurs, and the descending wave of peristalsis begins.
4. The hyoid bone reaches maximal elevation, and the larynx elevates to approach the hyoid. At this point the laryngeal vestibule closes, and the epiglottis tilts downward while pharyngeal peristalsis descends toward the hypopharynx.
5. With pharyngeal contraction, approximation of the pharyngeal wall, soft palate, and posterior of the tongue creates a closed chamber where the bolus is squeezed into the hypopharynx and through the open cricopharyngeal sphincter.
6. The pharyngeal airway reopens, and the soft palate, tongue, larynx, and hyoid bone return to their resting positions. The epiglottis springs back to a vertical position, and the laryngeal airway reopens when the pharyngoesophageal junction closes and resumes its elevated resting pressure.[1]

Sokol and associates[3] studied simultaneous cineradiographic and manometric activity of the pharynx and hypopharynx in asymptomatic subjects with the use of continuous perfusion techniques. At rest, the pressure in the pharyngeal cavity is equal to atmospheric pressure. In the hypopharynx, when the pharyngeal wall is collapsed and no air column exists, resting pressure increases progressively to a maximal pressure at the level of the cricopharyngeal muscle. On swallowing, pressure recordings show an initial double pressure peak corresponding to elevation of the laryngopharynx and simultaneous thrust of the tongue (E and I waves). Peak pharyngeal contraction follows these two initial waves; it is a peristaltic sequence starting radiologically as a stripping wave with closure of the velopharyngeal muscles, and it empties the pharyngeal contents into the hypopharynx. In the hypopharynx, the same small double peak is identified on swallowing and is attributed to upward laryngeal movement, tongue thrust, and progression of trapped air or the advancing bolus.

Accurate recording of pharyngeal motor events is not possible with a water-filled or a water-perfused system. For these reasons, Dodds and associates[4] studied human pharyngeal motor function in 12 recordings with an intraluminal strain gauge system. They observed that the pressure was highest in the hypopharynx, with amplitudes on contraction averaging 200 mm Hg. Peak contractions reached 600 mm Hg in one subject. Contraction pressure averaged 100 mm Hg in the oropharynx and 150 mm Hg in the nasopharynx. Wave duration decreased progressively from the nasopharynx to the hypopharynx, from 1.0 to 0.3 second, and peristaltic wave speed ranged between 9 and 25 cm/sec (Fig. 26–1). Observations by Kahrilas et al.[2,5,6] and Castell et al.[7,8] confirmed the difficulty of obtaining precise information on pharyngeal function.

The upper esophageal sphincter is a high-pressure zone 2.5 to 4.5 cm in length.[3] Within this zone is a shorter high-pressure zone, 1 cm long, of maximally elevated pressure that corresponds to the location of the cricopharyngeus muscle. This same pressure profile was described more recently by Kahrilas and Cook as reviewed by Sivarao and Goyal.[9] The cricopharyngeus is a muscle sling attached posteriorly to both laminae of the cricoid cartilage. It exerts its maximal pressure in an anteroposterior direction, at which point it closes the pharyngoesophageal junction and forms a crescentic slit seen at rigid esophagoscopy as the upper limit of the esophagus.

Winans[10] studied the pharyngoesophageal high-pressure zone of 18 human subjects with a special eight-lumen recording catheter that had recording orifices

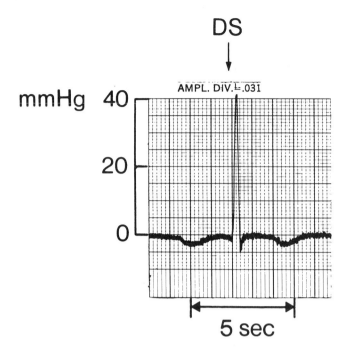

Figure 26–1. Pharyngeal contraction. A powerful single-peak contraction is produced with a duration of 0.4 second. This wave progresses at a speed of 9 to 25 cm/sec. DS, dry swallow.

spaced around its circumference. He observed significant pressure differences related to the position of the recording port, and this led to the concept of sphincter asymmetry (Fig. 26–2). In the UES, the greatest pressure (averaging 100 mm Hg) was recorded from the anterior and posterior orifices. Asoh and Goyal[11] showed that the UES is a high-pressure zone created mainly by the cricopharyngeus and inferior pharyngeal constrictor.

They observed that its asymmetry is not only radial but also axial. Pera and colleagues[12] documented a significant decrease in UES resting pressure in patients undergoing sequential surgical myotomy of the cricopharyngeus.

The high-pressure zone of the UES is attributable to continuous active muscle contraction and the elasticity of the surrounding structures. At rest, the cricopharyngeus is a striated muscle that receives its motor nerves from vagal nuclei through the vagi without synaptic interruption. The nerve endings come into direct contact with the motor end plates, and a continuous vagal discharge maintains the tonus of the sphincter at rest.[11,13]

On swallowing, a sequence of relaxations involving the pharyngoesophageal muscle groups is caused by the disappearance of action potentials in the muscle fibers (Fig. 26–3). Forward and upward displacement of the larynx is also involved in the opening mechanism of the sphincter. Although it is generally agreed that the cricopharyngeus is the major component of the UES, its wider pressure zone as observed by Sokol et al.,[3] Winans,[10] Welch et al.,[14] Goyal et al.,[15] and Sivarao and Goyal[9] must be explained by other factors. For instance, the passive elastic force may maintain a closed UES. If the nerve supply to the sphincter is removed, residual closing pressure remains. In addition, the circular muscle of the pharyngoesophageal junction may play a role.[16]

On swallowing, the UES high-pressure zone falls to resting atmospheric pressure and remains open to accommodate bolus transport through the sphincter area. This relaxation is brought about by cessation of vagal nerve stimulation and by vertical upward displacement of the larynx, which pulls the UES for about 2 cm. Full sphincter relaxation is observed for 0.5 to 1.2 seconds, and with passage of the hypopharyngeal contraction, the sphincter closes with a contraction that

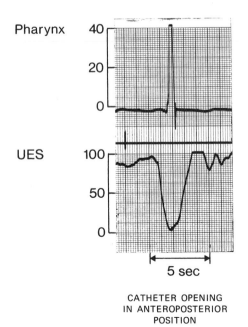

CATHETER OPENING
IN ANTEROPOSTERIOR
POSITION

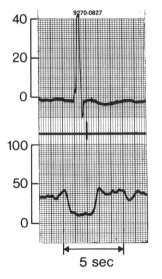

Figure 26–2. Asymmetry of the upper esophageal sphincter (UES). (From Winans CS: The pharyngoesophageal closure mechanism: A manometric study. Gastroenterology 63:768, 1972, with permission.)

CATHETER OPENING
IN LATERO LATERAL
POSITION

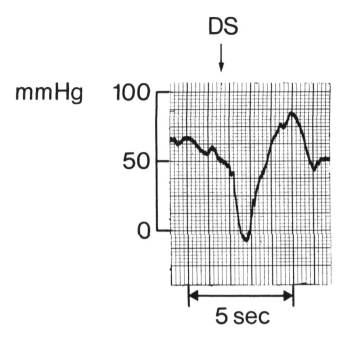

Figure 26–3. The high-pressure zone of the upper esophageal sphincter is caused by continuous active contraction of the cricopharyngeus muscle. DS, dry swallow.

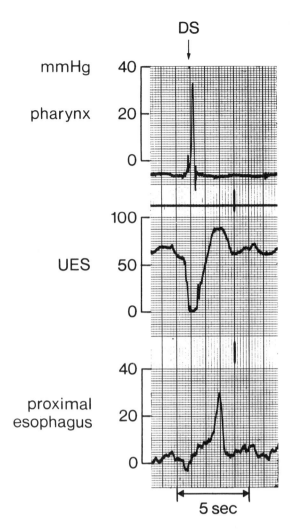

Figure 26–4. Pharynx, upper esophageal sphincter (UES), and cervical esophagus in action. During the rapid single contraction of the pharynx (13 cm), the high-pressure zone of the UES (18 cm) falls to ambient pressure. Passage of the contraction in the hypopharynx closes the sphincter, and the wave continues into the cervical esophagus (23 cm). DS, dry swallow.

creates a pressure that is often twice as high as the resting pressure in the sphincter (Fig. 26–4).

Physiologic evaluation of the UES is difficult because of recording issues. A single side-hole catheter recording must take into account the sphincter asymmetry. The eight-lumen circumferential recording catheter does not follow the upward movement of the sphincter on swallowing. Rapid pull-through techniques record a higher anteroposterior basal tone. A manometric recording device was proposed by Dent[17] and adapted to the UES by Kahrilas et al.[2]; it is a sleeve concept that is thought to record UES pressure behavior despite its movement during deglutition. However, evaluation of relaxation and coordination with pharyngeal contraction remains difficult. Castell and co-workers[7,8] proposed positioning the recording sensor above the high-pressure zone of the sphincter for that purpose, thereby allowing the opened sphincter, in its upward excursion, to be studied.

ASSESSMENT OF OROPHARYNGEAL DYSPHAGIA

Regardless of the cause, patients with oropharyngeal dysphagia must be assessed in a systematic fashion. Methods of investigation of the pharyngoesophageal junction have been reviewed by Cook and Kahrilas[18] and by Sivarao and Goyal.[9]

Clinical assessment of symptoms remains the most important step in classifying the disorder. Though subjective, it helps in obtaining the patient's medical history. The genealogy of transmitted disease can be clarified. For more objectivity, symptoms can be quantified in the

manner suggested for reflux disease.[19] This method is summarized in Table 26–1.[20]

Videofluoroscopic evaluation of swallowing is used to detect and analyze functional impairment of the pharyngoesophageal junction. It assesses the response of the oropharynx, palate, proximal airway, and proximal esophagus to swallows of varied volume and consistency and can identify the presence and mechanism of dysfunction. Videofluoroscopy can clarify an inability or delay in initiating swallows, the occurrence of bolus regurgitation or aspiration, or retention of the bolus in the pharynx. Conventional studies are inadequate because of the rapidity of events during the early phase of swallowing. The importance of this type of radiologic assessment is emphasized by the fact that the abnormal function is sometimes confined to one or two frames projected each second.[21] Delineation of specific muscle

| Table 26–1 | Symptom Score Applied to Oropharyngeal Dysphagia |

	1 Point	2 Points	3 Points	4 Points
Frequency	Occasional (<1/mo)	>1/mo, <1/wk	>1/wk, <daily	Daily
Duration	<6 mo	>6 mo, <24 mo	>24 mo, <60 mo	>60 mo
Severity	Mild: nuisance value	Moderate: spoils enjoyment of life	Marked: interferes with living normal life	Severe: terrible experience

For quantification of results: Add frequency and duration and then multiply by severity. Mild symptoms, 1 to 7; moderate symptoms, 8 to 15; marked symptoms, 16 to 23; severe symptoms, 24 to 32.

group abnormalities also requires the assistance of video technology.[22,23] Videofluoroscopic evaluation of swallowing with three-dimensional reconstruction was proposed, used, and perfected by Logemann and Kahrilas.[24]

Manometric evaluation of the entire esophagus must be performed. Assessment of the esophageal body and lower esophageal sphincter will rule out motor disorders and document the quality of lower esophageal sphincter tone. Specific manometric assessment of the UES quantifies the strength of pharyngeal contraction, the completeness of UES relaxation, and the timing of pharyngeal contraction relative to UES relaxation. However, precise recordings are limited in their depiction of events by a number of factors. The radial asymmetry of the sphincter requires multiple port recordings to sum the action of the sphincter[10] or a circumferential pressure-sensing transducer.[8,7] The Dent sleeve is a 6-cm perfused silicone membrane that also has the advantage of recording accurate resting pressure in the UES area.[2] It can record sphincter pressure at any level along the length of the membrane, even if movement displaces the sphincter. Assessment of sphincter relaxation and coordination with pharyngeal contraction is limited in accuracy by the upward movement of the larynx during the recording. Castell and associates[7,8] proposed positioning the recording sensor above the high-pressure zone of the sphincter for that purpose. Despite the sophistication of more recent manometric recordings, true abnormalities in function are undoubtedly underestimated in patients with pharyngoesophageal disorders. Integration of manometric data with fluoroscopic observation of the swallowing events was proposed and performed by Cook and colleagues.[25,26] The main advantage of this technique is detection and measurement of swallowing outcome and identification of subcategories of dysfunction, namely, impaired voluntary swallowing, impaired UES relaxation, and increased outflow resistance. The development of intrabolus pressure gradient recordings helped identify abnormal pathologic constriction in the UES during flow.[27]

Radionuclide pharyngoesophageal transit studies add quantitation to the symptoms. Boluses with different consistencies can be used to measure the poor emptying that results from oropharyngeal dysfunction. It adds to radiologic and manometric data by measuring the end result of any form of therapy that might be used in patients with transit abnormalities between the mouth, pharynx and proximal part of the esophagus.[28]

Endoscopic assessment of a patient with oropharyngeal dysphagia must be undertaken with great care. Anatomic abnormalities must be clearly delineated before any attempt at endoscopic evaluation. Flexible endoscopy can be used if no distortion is present. Any resistance to passage of the instrument should lead to assessment under general anesthesia. Examination under direct vision with a laryngoscope and short rigid esophagoscope should provide detailed visualization of the larynx, pharynx, hypopharynx, and esophageal inlet. No undue effort should be made to penetrate the cervical esophagus if resistance or abnormalities are encountered. Complete assessment of the esophageal body and cardia must be obtained in patients with oropharyngeal dysphagia. However, if any risk is entailed in the evaluation procedures, diagnosis and therapy for the proximal condition must prevail before completing the investigation of the remaining esophagus.

SURGICAL MANAGEMENT

Indications

Cricopharyngeal myotomy is a recognized treatment of patients with dysfunction of the pharyngoesophageal junction secondary to neurologic conditions. Intact voluntary swallowing and the absence of dysphonia are considered important prognostic factors for a successful outcome. In patients with oropharyngeal dysphagia caused by muscle disorders, cricopharyngeal myotomy is performed to remove the obstructive effect of the cricopharyngeus below a pharynx that is unable to mount a proper contraction to push the bolus into the cervical esophagus.

The only treatment available at present for idiopathic dysfunction of the UES and Zenker's diverticulum is surgery. The objective of the operation is to remove the effects of the restrictive myopathy affecting the UES. If the dysfunctional sphincter causes severe symptoms or if there is a symptomatic minute diverticulum present, extensive cricopharyngeal myotomy is completed over the pharyngoesophageal junction. When a diverticulum is present, cricopharyngeal myotomy remains the essen-

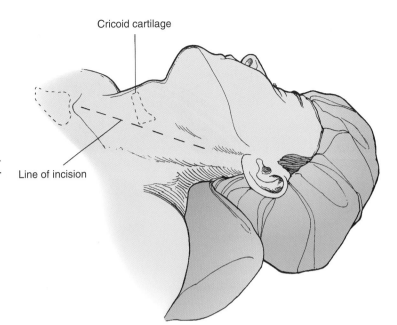

Cricoid cartilage

Line of incision

Figure 26–5. Position and incision for the operation. With a pillow under the shoulders, the head is in hyperextension and turned toward the right.

tial focus of treatment, and the diverticulum, seen as a complication of the dysfunction, is either suspended or resected.

Oropharyngeal dysphagia resulting from laryngectomy or from other extensive neck surgery may be encountered in patients so treated. Careful documentation of the UES dysfunction plus exclusion of any mechanical causes for the symptoms is important in these patients.

Operative Technique

Position and Incision

The patient lies in a supine position on the operating table. A pillow is placed under the shoulders to allow the head to be hyperextended and rotated toward the right. The anatomic reference point is the cricoid cartilage, into which the cricopharyngeus inserts. The incision follows the left interior border of the left sternomastoid muscle from the sternal notch to a point a few centimeters under the earlobe (Fig. 26–5).

Access to the Pharyngoesophageal Junction

The plane of access to the retropharyngeal area and to the superior mediastinum is between the large vessel sheath and the thyroid gland (Fig. 26–6A). Progressive division of the cervical tissue layers allows wide exposure of the pharyngoesophageal junction.

First, the subcutaneous tissues and platysma are divided. A branch of the cervical cutaneous nerve usually crosses the middle or proximal part of the incision; if low, the nerve must be divided, which can possibly result in some anesthesia or dysesthesia of the submandibular skin area. If the nerve is more proximal, it may be isolated and retracted for protection.

Next, the sternomastoid muscle is dissected free from the underlying prethyroid muscles and retracted laterally. The omohyoid muscle and both prethyroid muscles are then divided over the entire length of the incision to expose the thyroid gland and large vessels (see Fig. 26–6B).

At this point, the first surgical assistant exerts traction on the thyroid gland, and the middle thyroid vein, if present, is ligated and divided (see Fig. 26–6C). This allows the deep cervical fascia to be put under tension. It is opened proximally behind the pharynx, where the cellular plane between the pharyngeal wall and the prevertebral fascia is first identified. Progressive and careful opening of the fascia along the line of the incision is then completed to expose the interior thyroid artery, which is ligated laterally where it passes behind the carotid artery.

The assistant next retracts upward and contralaterally while exerting an eversion movement on the right side of the laryngeal and pharyngeal structures. The large vessels are retracted laterally to expose the entire posterior pharyngoesophageal junction. When a diverticulum is present and large enough, it can be recognized as a bulge at and below the pharyngoesophageal junction (Fig. 26–7). The recurrent laryngeal nerve is palpated and seen along the trachea just in front of the tracheoesophageal groove; it passes behind branches of the inferior thyroid artery.

Cricopharyngeal Myotomy

Extended cricopharyngeal myotomy of the pharyngoesophageal junction is the preferred technique when treating UES dysfunction of neurologic, muscular, idiopathic, or iatrogenic origin.[29,30]

Low-power diathermy is used on the superficial muscle layers of the posterior wall of the junction to trace

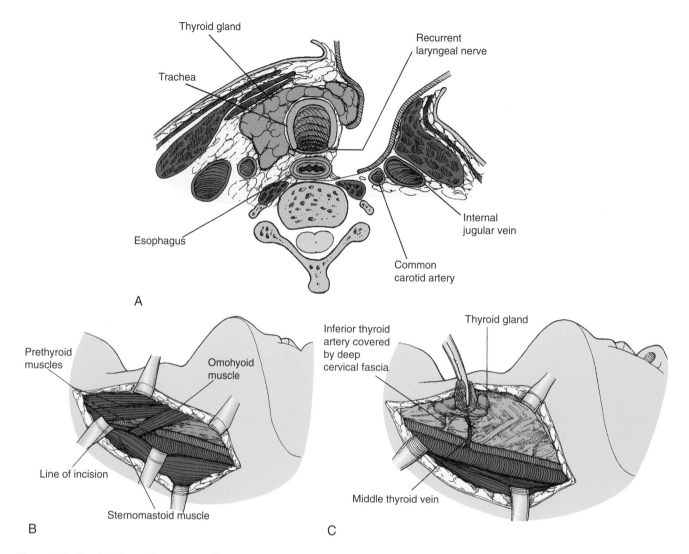

Figure 26–6.   A, Plane of access to the retropharyngeal space. **B,** The incision is oblique along the anterior border of the sternomastoid muscle. The omohyoid and prethyroid muscles are divided along the length of the incision. **C,** The middle thyroid vein is ligated, the thyroid is retracted toward the right, and the deep cervical fascia is put under tension to be opened proximally behind the pharynx. When the fascia is opened, the inferior thyroid artery is located and ligated.

the intended myotomy. The line of the myotomy is drawn along the right tracheoesophageal groove, which is everted toward the surgeon (Fig. 26–8A). A No. 36 Maloney bougie is passed into the esophagus and serves as a stent during the myotomy. The use of surgical loupes during this part of the operation permits better visualization of fine details while ensuring meticulous hemostasis. With a No. 15 scalpel blade, the myotomy is started on the cervical esophagus and progresses upward. Two to three centimeters of muscularis is divided on the esophagus. When the circular layer is divided, the esophageal mucosa is allowed to protrude between the divided muscle layers. Division of the muscle fibers of the pharyngoesophageal junction is then completed by extending the myotomy 2 cm more proximally.

The cricopharyngeus itself is not a well-identified structure. It corresponds to a thickening of the esophageal musculature at the point where it joins the

hypopharyngeal wall. The cricoid cartilage is the reference point for the posterior attachments of the cricopharyngeus. Once cut, the muscle retracts more readily toward the tracheoesophageal groove. An additional 2 cm of thickened muscle is transected on the hypopharynx, for a total myotomy of 6 cm.

After the cricopharyngeal myotomy has been completed, the muscularis is lifted from the underlying mucosa by dissecting a flap of muscle in the fine cellular plane between both layers. A transverse section of this flap is completed distally on the cervical esophagus and proximally at the pharyngeal level. Dissection of the muscularis from the mucosa is more difficult at the pharyngeal level than at the esophageal level because it is more adherent and the presence of a significant submucosal venous plexus may prove troublesome if torn or entered. The dissected flap of muscularis is resected for histologic examination (see Fig. 26–8B).

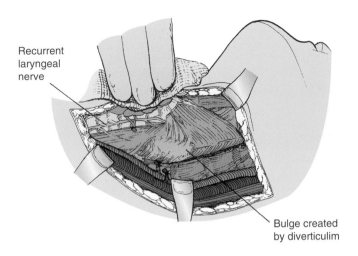

Recurrent laryngeal nerve

Bulge created by diverticulim

Figure 26–7. The pharyngoesophageal junction can be lifted and everted toward the surgeon. When there is a diverticulum present, it can be perceived as a bulge under adventitial tissues at the junction.

Cricopharyngeal Myotomy for a Pharyngoesophageal Diverticulum (Zenker's)

Minute Diverticula

A very small diverticulum, when symptomatic, is treated by an extended cricopharyngeal myotomy. Once the myotomy is completed, the small diverticulum disappears as part of the freed mucosa.

Established Diverticula (1 to 4 cm)

With the diverticulum freed and uplifted, the myotomy is started in the same manner on the cervical esophagus. The cervical esophageal mucosa is exposed. The cricopharyngeus muscle is then progressively transected (Fig. 26–9A). The muscle fibers are often seen to extend onto the body of the diverticulum itself, and division of these fibers is performed to free the entire collar of the sac. Lateral dissection to the left and right of the pouch allows proximal extension of the myotomy onto the hypopharyngeal wall. Two centimeters of hypopharyngeal muscle is transected with the same muscle flap created and resected for histologic analysis (see Fig. 26–9B).

The tip of the diverticulum left with thicker tissue is then uplifted. Fixation to the posterior pharyngeal wall is accomplished with four to five 3-0 silk sutures; these sutures anchor the thicker part of the diverticulum to the pharyngeal wall. Care is taken to not leave the collar of the sac in a dependent position. The lumen of the diverticulum should not be punctured by sutures to avoid contamination (see Fig. 26–9B).

Large Diverticula

If a pharyngoesophageal diverticulum is too large to uplift and place between the pharynx and prevertebral fascia, it must be resected. In this case, the myotomy is performed in the same way as already described.

With the Maloney bougie well secured in the esophageal lumen, a linear stapler is placed transversely 1 cm above the collar of the diverticulum (Fig. 26–10A). This may occasionally prove cumbersome if proper eversion of the posterior wall is difficult. An angulated linear stapler can be used for easier application. The diverticulum is then resected, with a 1-cm rim of collar tissue left distal to the stapled line. This tissue is uplifted and fixed to the transected muscle of the myotomy zone while leaving no portion of the collar in a dependent position. The myotomy area is left wide open to allow the suture line to heal in eversion and without the effect of a restrictive cricopharyngeus distal to it (see Fig. 26–10B).

Documenting the Integrity of the Mucosa

With the myotomy completed, accompanied by suspension or resection of the diverticulum, the mercury bougie is removed. A nasogastric tube is placed initially at the pharyngoesophageal junction, and 50 ml of air is injected through the tube while the myotomized zone is kept under saline to allow documentation of the integrity of the mucosa (Fig. 26–11).

Drainage and Closure

Nasogastric tube drainage with the tube directed toward the stomach is carried out after integrity of the myotomy site has been tested. The tube remains in place until normal peristalsis has resumed. There are two reasons for gastric drainage: to avoid blind passage of the nasogastric tube in the postoperative period if it should become necessary and to prevent gastric retention and possible regurgitation or vomiting in a patient whose UES has been removed.

We do not drain the operative site. Wound drainage may be open to discussion, especially if mucosal integrity has been documented. We used to place one Penrose drain at the thoracic inlet level and another behind the myotomized area. However, retrospective analysis of our results revealed a higher wound infection rate, mostly in patients with Zenker's diverticula. For these reasons we decided to not place drains anymore and instead use prophylactic antibiotics effective against aerobes and anaerobes. The wound is closed with a running stitch on the platysma and a resorbable subcuticular stitch on the skin.

Postoperative Care

Patients are mobilized immediately. The nasogastric tube is removed as soon as active peristalsis is documented. A liquid diet is started. Patients are discharged 72 hours after surgery with instructions for a pureed diet the first week and a soft diet during the second week. Normal food intake is then resumed.

Complications

Complications specific to this operation are recurrent laryngeal nerve trauma, hematoma formation, and infection with a salivary fistula. Meticulous technique should

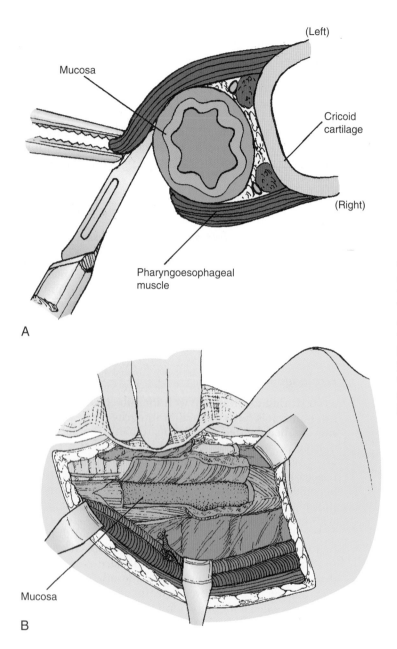

Figure 26–8. **A,** With the esophagus and pharynx everted toward the surgeon, the myotomy is started on the right side of the esophagus and the muscle is transected to the mucosal level. **B,** A sequential 6- to 7-cm myotomy is started on the cervical esophagus and then continued on the pharyngoesophageal junction, where the cricopharyngeus is located by identifying the cricoid cartilage. The thicker hypopharyngeal musculature is divided over a span of 2 to 3 cm. Transverse section of the muscle proximally and distally allows dissection of a muscle flap, which is resected for histologic analysis.

prevent all of these complications. Retropharyngeal hematoma, if it occurs, should be evacuated because of the prolonged resorption period in patients with poor swallowing function. When aspiration persists with absent phonation and disappearance of all protective mechanisms, sepsis from pulmonary infection is to be expected. In this extreme situation, we have resorted to permanent tracheostomy with laryngeal excision or exclusion (Fig. 26–12).

Results of Treatment

Neurologic dysphagia results from disruption of the swallowing mechanism in patients with central nervous system diseases or cranial nerve involvement. Stroke is the most frequent cause of this condition. Incoordina-

tion between pharyngeal contraction and sphincter relaxation is the pathologic result observed in these patients. It often results in misdirection of the swallowed bolus with pharyngeal and pharyngonasal regurgitation and frequent laryngotracheal aspiration. Complete absence of relaxation of the UES is seen mostly in these patients (Fig. 26–13A to C).

Oropharyngeal symptoms may be improved by myotomy, but they persist to a certain degree. The only significant improvement perceived by these patients is a reduction in aspiration episodes.[30]

When assessed radiologically, laryngeal penetration and tracheal aspiration are still observed frequently, even though the symptoms have improved. Radiologic signs of muscle group dysfunction as a result of the neurologic pathology, such as swallowing apraxia, pharyngeal and

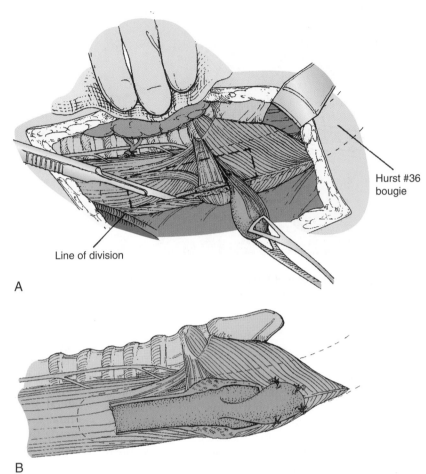

Figure 26–9. **A,** The diverticulum is freed and its tip uplifted and held in a small Duval clamp. A No. 36 bougie is passed into the esophagus and used as a stent. The myotomy is completed around the collar of the diverticulum, and the muscle to be analyzed is resected as described in Figure 26–8. **B,** This moderate-size diverticulum is uplifted and its tip fixed on the musculature of the posterior pharyngeal wall without leaving the collar of the sac in a dependent position.

Hurst #36 bougie

Line of division

A

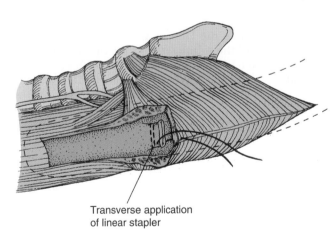

B

Figure 26–10. **A,** When a diverticulum is large, it is resected. An intraesophageal bougie protects the integrity of the lumen. A linear staple is applied to the collar of the diverticulum. The resection leaves a 1-cm rim of mucosa distal to the stapled line. **B,** The rim of the mucosa is uplifted and fixed on the muscularis of the transected hypopharyngeal wall. The myotomy is left open under the diverticulectomy site.

Transverse application of linear stapler

A

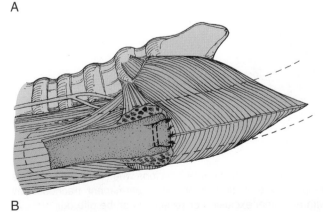

B

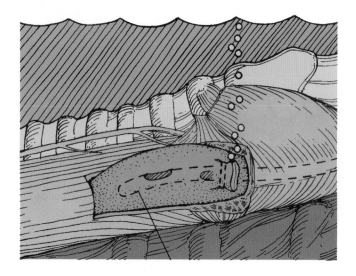

Figure 26–11. Air injected through a nasogastric tube into the submerged esophagus documents the integrity of the myotomized area.

epiglottic incoordination, hypopharyngeal stasis, and aspiration, all persist despite extensive cricopharyngeal myotomy. The functional obstruction and the imprint of the cricopharyngeus observed during the investigation are the only preoperative radiologic signs that are significantly reduced once the myotomy has been completed.

Manometry with specific assessment of the pharyngoesophageal junction shows a significant decrease in resting pressure in the UES, as well as a decrease in the opening time of the sphincter after the operation. These observations have been noted consistently after cricopharyngeal myotomy.[12,31,32] When a single liquid bolus of

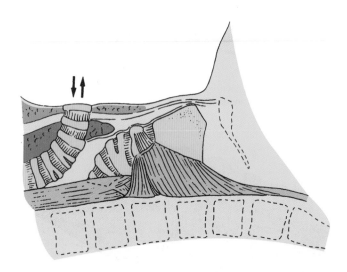

Figure 26–12. In extreme situations when aspiration persists despite an extended myotomy, a permanent tracheostomy with laryngeal exclusion or resection can be offered.

Box 26–2 **Prognostic Factors Affecting the Results of Cricopharyngeal Myotomy in Patients with Neurologic Diseases**

Intact voluntary deglutition

Adequate antepulsion and retropulsion of the tongue

Normal phonation

Absent dysarthria

10 ml is used for a radionuclide pharyngeal emptying study before and after myotomy, the dysfunction and the resulting emptying capacity are unchanged.

The clinical results of cricopharyngeal myotomy for neurologic dysphagia are influenced by the area of neurologic damage resulting from the stroke or the neurologic lesions. Lesions in the brainstem or from basilar artery thrombosis are associated with significant improvement. Lesions that are more diffuse show a poorer response. Patients with dysphagia from amyotrophic lateral sclerosis and motor neuron disease may have initial improvement, but since these conditions affect mostly the oral phase of deglutition, over time the cricopharyngeal myotomy does not help because the oral-phase abnormalities are untouched. Overall, the clinical improvement rate achieved by cricopharyngeal myotomy for neurologic dysphagia is influenced by the extent and location of damage in the nervous system. Approximately 80% of patients with a cerebrovascular accident are reportedly improved after the operation. When bulbar palsy and bulbar poliomyelitis are responsible for the dysphagia, the reported improvement is around 75%. Fifty percent of patients with amyotrophic lateral sclerosis and motor neuron disease are improved early, but over time the results are poor. Miscellaneous central lesions and bihemispheric damage result in more extensive difficulties that persist despite treatment.

The main prognostic factors for improvement of dysphagia in patients with neurologic disease are summarized in Box 26–2.

Myogenic Dysphagia

Oropharyngeal dysphagia of muscular origin is seen mostly in the oculopharyngeal form of muscular dystrophy. Williams et al.[33] have also studied the biomechanics and treatment outcome of patients with inflammatory myopathy. Oculopharyngeal muscular dystrophy has been investigated mostly in patients of French Canadian origin, in whom this myopathy has been transmitted in an autosomal dominant fashion over the last 12 generations.[34] Families affected by this condition are now found on all continents.

The dysphagia caused by muscular dystrophy is characterized by impaired function of the pharyngeal

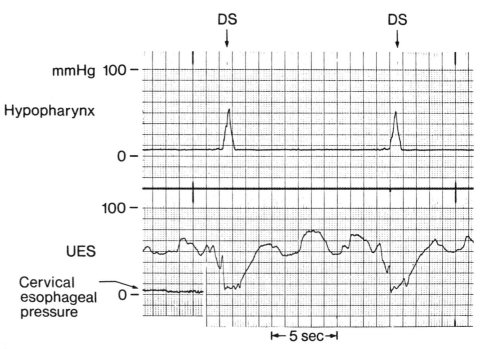

Figure 26–13. **A,** Hypopharyngeal contraction with normal relaxation to atmospheric pressure. DS, dry swallow; UES, upper esophageal sphincter. **B,** Achalasia of the UES in neurologic dysphagia.

Continued

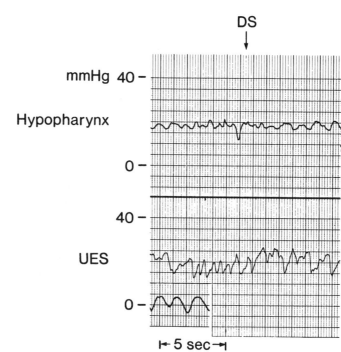

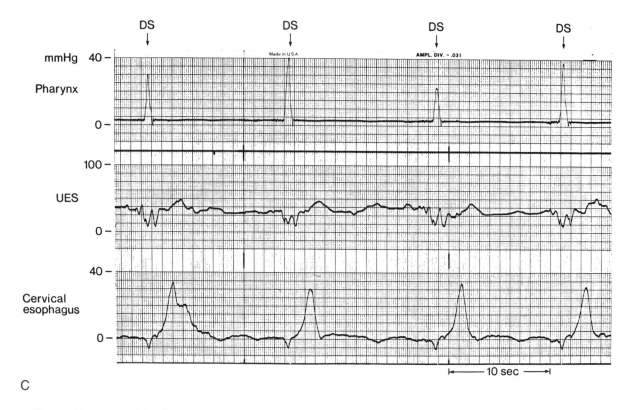

C

Figure 26–13, cont'd.   C, Incomplete relaxation of the UES in oropharyngeal dysphagia of neurologic origin.

muscles, which show weak and sluggish contractions. The severity of symptoms is paralleled by the severity of the dysfunction. These symptoms are esophageal and tracheobronchial in location. The dysphagia is identified at the sternal notch level and accompanied by frequent food incarceration at the upper sphincter level with resulting pharyngo-oral regurgitation. The velopharyngeal muscles are affected and incompetent, and pharyngonasal regurgitation results. Laryngeal penetration and tracheal aspiration are reported at mealtime. Saliva pooling in the hypopharynx and aspiration causing bronchorrhea occur during the night. Aspiration pneumonia is frequent. Peripheral muscle groups are affected, with bilateral ptosis usually being evident, as well as voice changes and limb weakness.

Radiologically, hypomotility of the pharynx with stasis of contrast material in the hypopharynx, valleculae, and piriform sinuses is observed frequently. The cricopharyngeus leaves a significant imprint on the radiopaque column on the lateral view in 80% of patients (Fig. 26–14). Aspiration episodes are recorded frequently. Radiologic observations correlate well with radionuclide emptying studies that document the delayed pharyngeal emptying capacity (Fig. 26–15A and B). When studied manometrically by intraluminal transducers, the pharyngoesophageal junction shows low pharyngeal pressure and weak pharyngeal contractions. The UES may have normal resting pressure but exhibits incoordination between a prolonged pharyngeal contraction and an abnormal and incomplete relaxation. Patients with

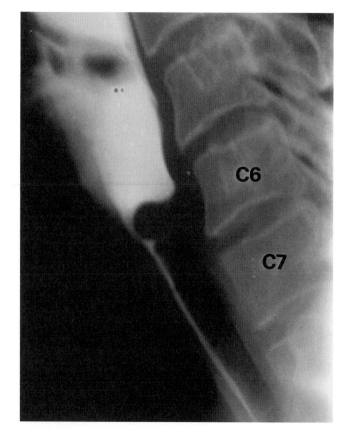

Figure 26–14. Prominent cricopharyngeus closing the esophageal mouth.

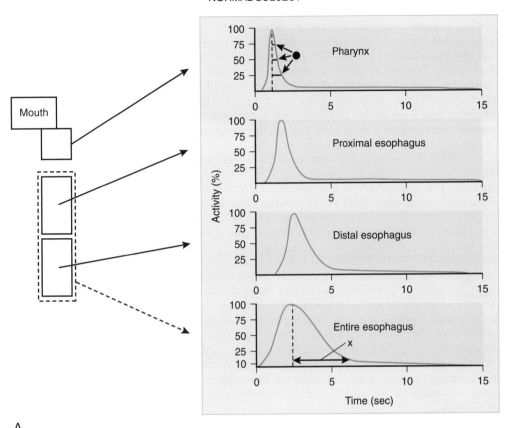

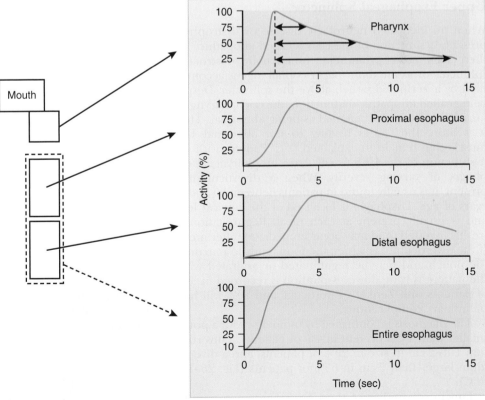

Figure 26–15. A, Radionuclide emptying capacity of the pharynx and esophagus in a normal individual. **B,** Radionuclide emptying study in a dystrophy patient. Prolonged retention of the bolus is quantified in the pharynx and esophageal body.

severe symptoms have more abnormalities in their manometric profile.[35]

The cricopharyngeal myotomy offered to these patients adheres to all the technical details described initially by Montgomery in his 1971 publication, the main goal of the operation being to maximally reduce the resistance caused by functional obstruction of the UES. As illustrated, the myotomy ends up as a myectomy involving 6 to 7 cm of the pharyngoesophageal junction because the posterior muscular wall of the junction is completely resected (see Fig. 26–8A and B).

The clinical results of the operation show significant improvement in swallowing comfort in 75% of operated patients. The improvement is appreciated more readily when swallowing solids than when voluntarily swallowing liquids. Tracheobronchial symptoms and nocturnal bronchorrhea improve as well. The stage of the disease and the extent of the muscular pathology and dysfunction affect the results. Patients with poor control of the laryngeal musculature and vocal cords show less improvement because of persistent aspiration. After cricopharyngeal myotomy, pharyngeal emptying scintigrams have documented improvement in clearing of a liquid bolus and in hypopharyngeal stasis.[32] The physiologic basis for improvement in symptoms is the significant reduction in resting pressure of the UES and the significant decrease in relaxation time for sphincter opening, thus suggesting reduced resistance to transit from the pharynx to the esophagus.[36]

Idiopathic Dysfunction of the Upper Esophageal Sphincter

When no identified neurologic disease or dystrophy is present, dysfunction of the UES is called idiopathic. It is then seen as a prominent, functionally obstructing sphincter or as an abnormal cricopharyngeus accompanied by a herniated pouch above the sphincter. Despite being called idiopathic dysfunction, the cricopharyngeus muscle has been documented as being abnormal. Thus, it is more the causes leading to this abnormal UES muscle that remain unexplained.[25,26,37] Patients with just dysfunction of the UES usually have oropharyngeal dysphagia of varying severity. When a diverticulum is present, it is usually found in patients between 60 and 70 years of age. Dysphagia is localized at the cervical level and is usually present at each meal. Regurgitation of freshly ingested food may occur immediately after meals. If the diverticulum is larger, the food tends to remain in the pouch and may be regurgitated or aspirated when the patient is lying down. Aspiration is recorded in 36% of patients with Zenker's diverticula, and 20% will have pulmonary complications.

The diagnosis is confirmed by radiology, with a pouch smaller than 1 cm present in 4% of patients, a diverticulum 1 to 2 cm in size in 20% of patients, and a diverticulum larger than 2 cm in 65% of patients (Fig. 26–16A to C).

Functional studies of the UES have demonstrated a sphincter pressure that was either normal, high, or low, with the type of recording method used having a definite influence on measurements. Incoordination between opening and closing of the cricopharyngeus against pharyngeal contraction was initially suggested.[38] However, sleeve recordings of the UES and measurement of intrabolus pressure in the hypopharynx when a diverticulum is present have been used by Cook et al.[25,26,39] to clarify the pathophysiology of the condition. In addition, they simultaneously observed the opening area of the sphincter on videoradiology. After identifying the restrictive pathology in the sphincter, they documented how the abnormal muscle restricted the opening surface of the esophageal mouth and caused incomplete opening of the sphincter during deglutition with resulting high hypopharyngeal intrabolus pressure. Thus, the progressive outpouching of the mucosa through the muscular wall of the hypopharynx just above the restrictive sphincter is a pulsion diverticulum and must be seen as a complication of the UES dysfunction.

The standard of care, when an established pharyngoesophageal diverticulum has been documented, is surgical.

Cricopharyngeal myotomy is the mainstay of treatment to correct an abnormal and restrictive UES. The diverticulum is seen as an anatomic complication of the dysfunctional sphincter, and it is treated according to its size. A simple cricopharyngeal myotomy will cause a minute diverticulum to disappear in the myotomized area (see Fig. 26–8B). Diverticula measuring up to 4 cm can be suspended and fixed on the posterior pharyngeal wall once the myotomy has been completed (see Fig. 26–9B). Diverticula larger than 4 cm usually need to be resected (see Fig. 26–10A and B).

Clinical and functional results are reported as excellent in 95% of treated patients.[37,38,40-42] Shaw and colleagues[43] documented the physiologic effects of the operation on the pharyngoesophageal junction. Myotomy of the junction with either resection or suspension of the diverticulum reduces intrabolus pressure in the hypopharynx to normal and returns the surface opening of the upper sphincter area to normal.

Endoscopic sphincterotomy with the use of a stapling device has been proposed. When performing the technique, the wall between the diverticulum and the esophageal lumen is divided. Use of this device is limited to large diverticula, and functional results have been shown to be acceptable on early follow-up. The remaining dependent pouch at the tip of the stapling line may explain persistent symptoms with this technique.

Oropharyngeal Dysphagia After Neck Surgery

Extensive neck surgery and laryngectomy may distort the muscular function as well as the innervation of the pharyngoesophageal junction. Laryngectomy has been documented to decrease UES resting pressure and reduce the asymmetry of the sphincter.[14,44] Up to 25% of laryngectomized patients may have a spastic sphincter, whereas dysphagia has been documented in nearly 40% of the operated population. Well-documented dysfunction of the UES after laryngectomy or extensive neck surgery may be improved by cricopharyngeal myotomy.

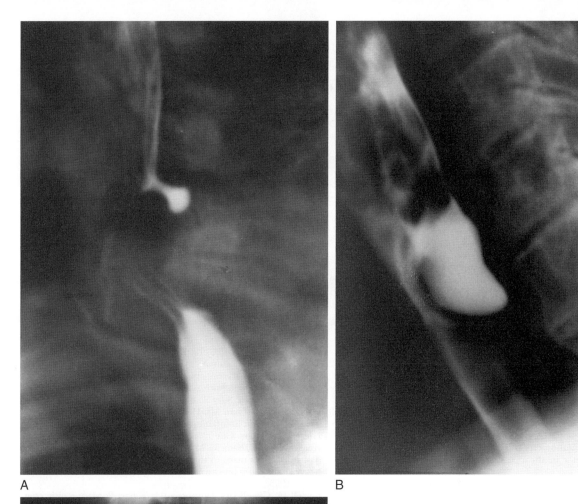

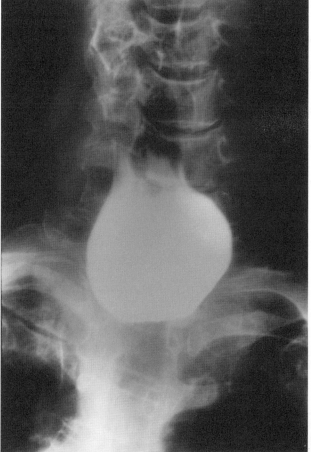

Figure 26–16. **A,** A symptomatic minute diverticulum is treated by extended cricopharyngeal myotomy. **B,** A moderate-size diverticulum is treated by cricopharyngeal myotomy, and the diverticulum is suspended and fixed on the posterior pharyngeal wall. **C,** A large diverticulum is usually resected once the cricopharyngeal myotomy has been completed.

Careful evaluation is required because the frequent use of radiotherapy in these patients may well be responsible for their symptoms.

REFERENCES

1. Donner MW, Bosma JF, Robertson DL: Neuromuscular disorders of the pharynx. Gastrointest Radiol 10:196, 1985.
2. Kahrilas PJ, Dent J, Dodds WJ, et al: A method for continuous monitoring of upper esophageal sphincter pressure. Dig Dis Sci 32:121, 1987.
3. Sokol EM, Hellmann P, Wolf BS, et al: Simultaneous cineradiographic and manometric study of the pharynx, hypopharynx, and cervical esophagus. Gastroenterology 51:960, 1966.
4. Dodds WJ, Hogan WJ, Lyndon SB, et al: Quantification of pharyngeal motor function in human subjects. J Appl Physiol 39:692, 1975.
5. Kahrilas PJ, Dodds WJ, Dent J: Upper esophageal sphincter function during deglutition. Gastroenterology 95:52, 1988.
6. Kahrilas PJ, Logeman JA, Lin S, Ergun GA: Pharyngeal clearance swallow: A combined manometric and video fluoroscopic study. Gastroenterology 103:128, 1992.
7. Castell JA, Dalton CB, Castell DO: Pharyngeal and upper esophageal sphincter manometry in humans. Am J Physiol 21:G73, 1990.
8. Castell JA, Dalton CB: Esophageal manometry. In Castell DO (ed): The Esophagus. Boston, Little, Brown, 1992, p 143.
9. Sivarao DV, Goyal RK: Functional anatomy and physiology of the upper esophageal sphincter. Am J Med 108:275, 2000.
10. Winans CS: The pharyngoesophageal closure mechanism: A manometric study. Gastroenterology 63:768, 1972.
11. Asoh R, Goyal RK: Manometry and electromyography of the upper esophageal sphincter in the opossum. Gastroenterology 74:514, 1978.
12. Pera M, Yamada A, Hiebert CA, Duranceau A: Sleeve recording of upper esophageal sphincter resting pressures during cricopharyngeal myotomy. Ann Surg 225:229, 1997.
13. Christensen J: The innervation and motility of the esophagus. Front Gastrointest Res 3:18, 1978.
14. Welch RW, Luckmann A, Richs PM, et al: Manometry of the normal upper esophageal sphincter and its alterations in laryngectomy. J Clin Invest 63:1036, 1979.
15. Goyal RK, Martin SB, Shapiro J, Spechler SJ : The role of cricopharyngeus muscle in pharyngoesophageal disorders. Dysphagia 8:252, 1993.
16. Zaino C, Jacobson HG, Lepow H, et al: The Pharyngoesophageal Sphincter. Springfield, IL, Charles C Thomas, 1970.
17. Dent J: A new technique for continuous sphincter pressure measurement. Gastroenterology 71:263, 1976.
18. Cook IJ, Kahrilas PJ: AGA technical review on management of oropharyngeal dysphagia. Gastroenterology 116:455, 1999.
19. De Dombal FT, Hall R: The evaluation of medical care from the clinician's point of view: What should we measure and can we trust our measurements? In Alperovitch A, De Dombal FT, Gremy F (eds): The Evaluation of the Efficacy of Medical Action. Amsterdam, Elsevier, 1979, p 13.
20. Duranceau A: Pharyngeal and cricopharyngeal disorders. In Pearson FG, Ginsberg RJ, Cooper JD, et al (eds): Esophageal Surgery, 2nd ed. New York, Churchill Livingstone, 2002, p 477.
21. Calceterra TC, Kadell BM, Ward PN: Dysphagia secondary to cricopharyngeal muscle dysfunction. Arch Otolaryngol 101:726, 1975.
22. Curtis DJ, Hudson T: Laryngotracheal aspiration: Analysis of specific neuromuscular factors. Radiology 149:517, 1983.
23. Curtis DJ, Cruess DF, Berg T: The cricopharyngeus muscle: A video recording review. Am J Radiol 142:497, 1984.
24. Logemann JA, Kahrilas PJ, Begelman J, et al: Interactive computer program for biomechanical analysis of video radiographic studies of swallowing. Am J Radiol 153:277, 1989.
25. Cook I, Blumbergs P, Cash K, et al: Structural abnormalities of the cricopharyngeal muscle in patients with pharyngeal (Zenker's) diverticulum. J Gastroenterol Hepatol 7:556, 1992.
26. Cook IJ, Gabb M, Panagopoulos V, et al: Pharyngeal (Zenker's) diverticulum is a disorder of upper esophageal sphincter. Gastroenterology 103:1229, 1992.
27. Anupam P, William RB, Cook IJ, Brasseur JG: Intrabolus pressure gradient identifies pathological constriction in the upper esophageal sphincter during flow. Am J Physiol Gastrointest Liver Physiol 285:G1037, 2003.
28. Taillefer R, Beauchamp G, Duranceau A: Radionuclide esophageal transit studies. In Van Nostrand D, Baum S (eds): Nuclear Medicine. Philadelphia, JB Lippincott, 1988, p 40.
29. Duranceau A, Jamieson GG, Beauchamp G: The technique of cricopharyngeal myotomy. Surg Clin North Am 63:833, 1983.
30. Duranceau A: The treatment of Zenker's diverticulum. Tech Gen Surg 4:1, 1994.
31. Poirier NC, Bonavena L, Taillefer R, et al: Cricopharyngeal myotomy for neurogenic oropharyngeal dysphagia. J Thorac Cardiovasc Surg 113:233, 1997.
32. Taillefer R, Duranceau A: Manometric and radionuclide assessment of pharyngeal emptying before and after the cricopharyngeal myotomy in patients with oculopharyngeal muscular dystrophy. J Thorac Cardiovasc Surg 95:868, 1988.
33. Williams RB, Grehan MJ, Hersch M, et al: Biomechanics diagnosis and treatment in inflammatory myopathy presenting as oropharyngeal dysphagia. Gut 52:471, 2003.
34. Brais B, Xie YG, Samson M, et al: The oculopharyngeal muscular dystrophy locus maps to the region of the cardia A and B myosin heavy chain genes on chromosome 14q 11.2-q 13. Hum Mol Genet 4:429, 1995.
35. Castell JA, Castell DO, Duranceau A, Topart P: Manometric characteristics of the pharynx, upper esophageal sphincter, esophagus, and lower esophageal sphincter in patients with oculopharyngeal muscular dystrophy. Dysphagia 10:22, 1995.
36. Duranceau A: Cricopharyngeal myotomy in the management of neurogenic and muscular dysphagia. Neuromusc Disord 7(Suppl 1):585, 1997.
37. Lerut T, VandeKerkhof J, Leman G, et al: Cricopharyngeal myotomy for pharyngoesophageal diverticula. Trends Gen Thorac Surg 3:351, 1987.
38. Ellis FN, Crozier RE: Cervical esophageal dysphagia: Indications for and results of cricopharyngeal myotomy. Ann Surg 194:279, 1969.
39. Cook IJ, Gabb M, Panagopoulos V, et al: Zenker's diverticulum: A defect in upper esophageal sphincter compliance? Gastroenterology 5:A98, 1989.
40. Orringer MB: Extended cervical esophagomyotomy for cricopharyngeal dysfunction. J Thorac Cardiovasc Surg 80:669, 1986.
41. Duranceau A: Oropharyngeal dysphagia. In Jamieson GG (ed): Surgery of the Esophagus. Edinburgh, Churchill Livingstone, 1988, p 434.
42. Sideris L, Chen LQ, Ferraro P, Duranceau A: The treatment of Zenker's diverticula: A review. Semin Thorac Cardiovasc Surg 11:337, 1999.
43. Shaw DW, Cook IJ, Jamieson GG, et al: Influence of surgery on deglutitive upper esophageal sphincter mechanics in Zenker's diverticulum. Gut 38:806, 1996.
44. Duranceau A, Jamieson GG, Hurwitz AL, et al: Alteration in esophageal motility after laryngectomy. Am J Surg 131:30, 1976.

Pathophysiology and Treatment of Zenker's Diverticulum

Toni Lerut · Willy Coosemans · Georges Decker ·
Paul De Leyn · Philippe Nafteux · Dirk Van Raemdonck

Pharyngoesophageal diverticulum was described for the first time as a pathologic entity by Ludlow in 1769.[1] However, it was Zenker who gave his name to this condition through a publication in 1877 in which he reported a series of 27 patients.[2] Already at that time Zenker presumed that the pouch is the consequence of "forces within the lumen acting against a restriction," a hypothesis that is indeed close to the modern understanding of its pathogenesis and remarkable because both endoscopy and radiology had yet to be invented. However, the mechanistic compression theory as a cause of symptoms would prevail until far into the 20th century and dominate therapeutic strategy as well (diverticulectomy). Only during the last decennia of the 20th century, thanks to new developments in imaging, endoscopy, manometry, and manofluorography, has better insight into the pathogenesis of Zenker's diverticulum (ZD) emerged and led to fundamental changes in the therapeutic strategy (myotomy of the cricopharyngeal muscle).

PHYSIOLOGY AND PHYSIOPATHOLOGY

ZD is defined as a blowout of the mucosa through a so-called locus minoris resistentiae on the posterior wall at the transition zone between the hypopharynx and the esophagus (Killian's triangle).[3] The proximal and lateral borders of this zone are the horizontal cricopharyngeal muscle distally and the oblique fibers of the thryropharyngeus muscle, which is part of the constrictor pharyngeus inferior muscle. At rest, the upper esophageal sphincter (UES) is closed because of tonic contraction. Within milliseconds after swallowing, a transient interruption of the muscle contraction relaxes the UES and allows passage of the bolus into the upper part of the esophagus. During this process the larynx moves forward and upward to facilitate opening of the relaxed sphincter.

At manometry it appears that UES pressure drops before its opening is visualized on simultaneous fluoroscopy. Conversely, manometric contraction precedes fluoroscopically visualized closure.

UES function also seems to be influenced by bolus volume. Kahrilas et al. showed that gradual bolus volumes modify movement and relaxation of the UES.[4] The larger the swallowed volume, the wider and longer the opening and the greater the oral motion of the UES.

The exact cause of the development of ZD remains unclear, and several hypotheses have been presented over time. For years the most widely accepted mechanism of development of ZD has been a functional disturbance of the pharyngoesophageal segment. Increased resting pressure of the sphincter, lack of complete relaxation, and in particular, incoordination between the hypopharynx and the sphincter have all been considered to play a role. The most frequently accepted hypothesis in this respect was that of premature relaxation and closure of the UES during swallowing as shown by Ellis and colleagues.[5] Cook et al.,[6] however, using a sleeve catheter for manometry and simultaneous videoradiography, found no difference between the timing of pharyngeal contraction and sphincter relaxation in patients with ZD and a control group. Nonetheless, they did find a significantly reduced sphincter opening in patients with greater intrabolus pressure. They concluded that ZD is a disorder of diminished UES opening, with increased hypopharyngeal pressure probably accounting for development of the diverticulum. Subsequent histologic examination of biopsy specimens taken at the time of surgery indicated

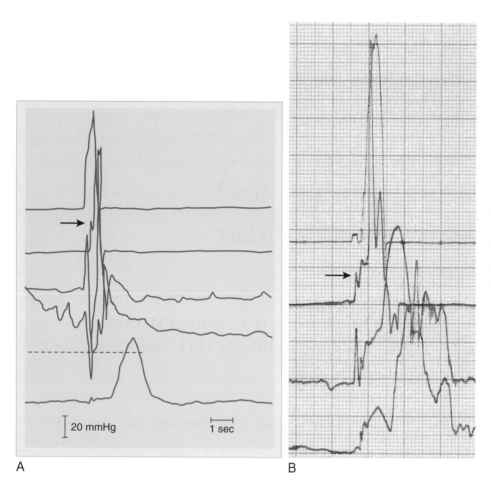

Figure 27–1. **A,** Manometric tracing of the upper esophageal sphincter (UES) in a healthy volunteer showing complete relaxation of the sphincter. The *arrow* indicates intrabolus pressure. **B,** Manometric tracing of the UES in a patient with Zenker's diverticulum indicating no relaxation of the sphincter. The *arrow* indicates the "shoulder" of increased intrabolus pressure. (Courtesy of E. Dejaeger.)

degenerative changes. They postulated that these degenerative muscle changes prevent the sphincter from opening completely because of lack of sufficient elasticity. The lack of compliance is reflected by the appearance of a "shoulder," or higher pressure, on manometric tracings when the bolus arrives (Fig. 27–1). This lack-of-compliance theory has been endorsed by our own studies on biopsy specimens harvested from a group of patients with ZD and a group of controls. Contractility, enzymohistochemistry, immunohistochemistry, and biochemistry studies were performed.[7]

Contractility Studies

Contractility studies showed a clear difference between diverticulum and control specimens (Table 27–1). In the diverticulum group, all the specimens had a slower and weaker contraction curve with a lower amplitude, a longer time to peak twitch, and a much longer relaxation half-time (Fig. 27–2). The values are statistically significant for the time to peak twitch, relaxation half-time, and increment in velocity of force, thus indicating reduced absolute force and slower contraction in patients with ZD.

The data obtained from pathologic, enzymohistochemical, and immunohistochemical analysis demonstrate an obvious disturbance of all analyzed parameters in ZD as compared with the control group (Table 27–2). In particular, atrophy, hypertrophy, size variation, necrosis, fibrosis, inflammation, and central nuclei were observed (Fig. 27–3). Ragged red fibers (abnormal accumulation of mitochondria) were seen frequently, and the presence of nemaline rods (abnormal densification of the Z-band) was occasionally noted. All changes were important enough to be considered pathologic. Only in two patients (5%) were all of the aforementioned normal. The distribution of fiber types was—with one exception—predominantly type I fiber, with an estimated 70% type I and 30% type II in the ZD group. In the control group, type II predominated in three specimens, whereas type II was predominant in some bundles in three other specimens (Fig. 27–4). Acetylcholinesterase and neurofilament staining showed a heterogeneous and weak pattern when compared with controls, at least in 75% of the 44 specimens. In most cases, more than 50% of the individual fibers did not stain (Fig. 27–5). In 10 patients, a biopsy specimen was taken from below the cricopharyngeal muscle at the level of the cervical esophageal muscle wall; in 8, it was combined with biopsy of the sternocleidomastoid muscle—all patients, of course, underwent cricopharyngeal muscle biopsy. The sternocleidomastoid biopsies were all strictly normal. Type II fiber clearly predominates (75% to

Table 27–1 Contractility Studies in 5 Controls and 5 Patients' with Zenker's Diverticulum

	TPT (msec)	½ RT (msec)	Amp (g)	DP/DT (g/msec)
Control	84	70	8.3	0.2
	72	70	1.4	0.05
	123	165	3	0.06
	61.5	123	6	0.08
	172	193	4.1	0.5
Total	102.5	124		0.32
	(±45.2)	(±55.4)		(±0.01)
ZD	324	188.0	0.9	0.006
	126	120	1.2	0.07
	490	312	0.7	0.01
	126	178	0.8	0.05
	72	193	0.5	0.01
Total	225	189		0.03
	(±156)	(±66)	(±0.001)	
	$P < .05$	$P < .05$	$P < .05$	

Amp, amplitude; DP/DT, force velocity increment; ½ RT, relaxation half-time; TPT, time to peak twitch; ZD, Zenker's diverticulum.

Table 27–2 Enzymohistochemical and Enzymoimmunologic Findings in 15 Control Specimens and 62 Zenker's Diverticulum Specimens

Dominant Fiber Type	Hypertrophy	Atrophy	Necrosis	Size Variation	Fibrosis	Central Nucleus	Inflammation	Nemaline Rods	Ragged Red Fibers	Acetylcholine-sterase	Neurofila-ments
Control											
I: 9	1/15	1/15	0/15	2/15	2/15	1/15		0/15	0/15	2/15	0/9
II: 3											
II: in some bundles: 3											
Zenker's Diverticulum											
I: 40	32/41	37/41	33/41	40/41	31/41	30/41	21/41	4/41	23/41	33/44	33/44

The denominator gives the number of patients in whom a given parameter was examined.

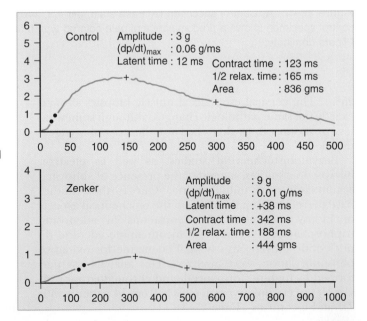

Figure 27–2. Contractility pattern of the cricopharyngeal muscle in a control specimen and Zenker's diverticulum.

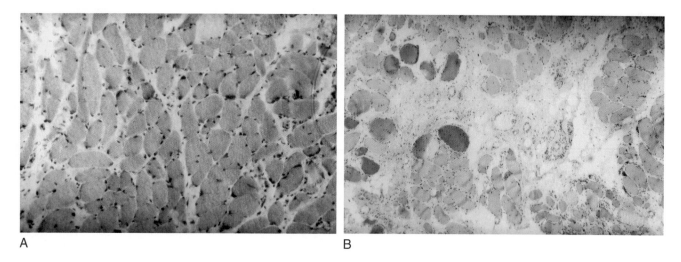

A   B

Figure 27–3. A, Control specimen (hematoxylin-eosin [H&E] stain, ×10). **B,** Diverticulum specimen (H&E, ×10). An irregular pattern of inflammation, increased fibrotic tissue, size variation, and necrosis is evident in the diverticulum specimen. Contrast with the regular-shaped organization of the muscle fibers without necrosis or inflammation in the control specimen.

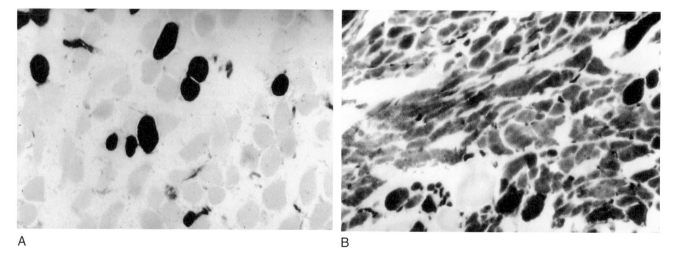

A   B

Figure 27–4. A, Control specimen (ATPase stain, pH 4.3, ×10). **B,** Diverticulum specimen (ATPase stain, pH 4.3, ×10). The control specimen shows a predominance of pale-colored type II fibers, whereas in the diverticulum specimen, dark-stained type I fibers dominate.

25%). The cervical esophageal muscle biopsies showed exactly the same pathologic changes, although somewhat less pronounced, as described for the cricopharyngeal muscle.

Enzymohistochemical studies, as well as electron microscopic studies, suggested the presence of abnormal accumulation of mitochondria. Our further studies have therefore been focusing on the biochemical aspects of biopsy specimens.[8] Concentrations of adenosine triphosphatase (ATPase) and nicotinamide adenine dinucleotide (NAD), an essential coenzyme for oxidative phosphorylation, were analyzed. This analysis was performed by high-performance liquid chromatography on samples of cricopharyngeal muscle from 14 patients with ZD and 6 controls (Table 27–3).

ATPase was found to be significantly reduced in the cricopharyngeal muscle of patients with ZD (5.8 μmol/g dry weight) when compared with the ATPase content of cricopharyngeal muscle from controls (10.4 μmol/g dry weight, $P = .0033$). NAD was equally significantly reduced in the cricopharyngeal muscle of patients with ZD (0.54 versus 0.903 μmol/g dry weight, $P = .0011$), thus suggesting deficient ATPase synthesis.

To exclude possible bias in values caused by the increase in fibrosis and subsequent decrease in the absolute amount of muscle fiber per gram dry weight, a study of creatine phosphokinase was performed. Creatine phosphokinase is an excellent measure of the absolute amount of muscle tissue present in a given biopsy specimen. There was no difference in creatine

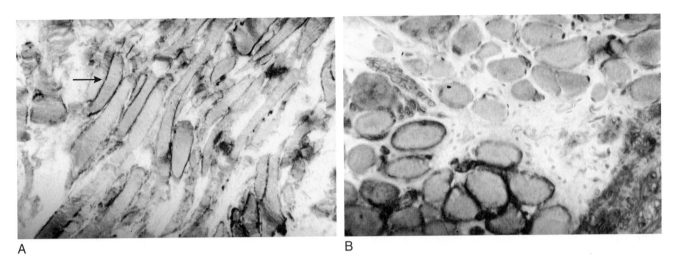

Figure 27–5. **A,** Control specimen (acetylcholinesterase stain, ×25). **B,** Diverticulum specimen (acetylcholinesterase stain, ×25). The dark-colored fibers represent the acetylcholinesterase staining. There is much more pronounced staining *(arrow)* in the control specimen **(A)** than in the diverticulum specimen **(B).**

Table 27–3 Biochemical Results

	n	ATPase, μmol/g Dry Weight	n	NAD, μmol/g Dry Weight	n	Creatine Phosphokinase, U/mg Dry Weight
Cricopharyngeus—ZD	14	5.8 (±2.9) (P = .033)	9	0.54 (P = .0011)	3	1.9 (±1)
Cricopharyngeus—control	6	10.4 (±2.2)	6	0.903	3	2 (±1.6)
Sternocleidomastoid—ZD	10	12.1 (±4.8)				
Sternocleidomastoid control	6	17 (±1.7)				

Standard deviations are in parentheses.
ATPase, adenosine triphosphatase; NAD, nicotinamide adenine dinucleotide; ZD, Zenker's diverticulum.

phosphokinase in cricopharyngeus muscle tissue from ZD patients and controls. These data strongly suggest that for the same amount of muscle tissue, ATPase and the energy charge are indeed deficient in the cricopharyngeal muscle of patients with ZD.

These studies seem to implicate both neurogenic and myogenic abnormalities as a potential underlying cause of the UES dysfunction. Further work performed by Venturi et al.[9] indicates a significantly higher collagen content in both the cricopharyngeal muscle and the muscularis propria of the esophagus below the cricopharyngeal muscle than in a control group. In the cricopharyngeal muscle, ratios of isodesmosine to desmosine and collagen to elastin were significantly higher in patients with ZD than in controls. These data, as well as our own data, indicate that both the cricopharyngeal muscle and the upper part of the striated cervical esophageal muscle are involved in the pathogenesis of ZD. These findings therefore support extension of the myotomy into the muscle of the proximal cervical esophagus below the cricopharyngeal muscle.

Most likely, no single pathogenic mechanism is solely responsible for the development of ZD. However, at this stage, poor UES compliance rather than cricopharyngeal incoordination appears to be the most plausible explanation. The increasing precision of imaging techniques, endoscopy, manometry, and manofluorography[10] has further endorsed the contention that ZD should be considered a pulsion diverticulum secondary to an underlying disturbance in function of the cricopharyngeal muscle and a so-called proximal UES. Gastroesophageal reflux has been implicated by some authors on the basis of a high prevalence of pathologic reflux in the ZD population. Chronic reflux of acidic gastric contents is thought to cause chronic damage to the cricopharyngeal muscle over time. However, this hypothesis has not been validated.[11] Dysfunction of the cricopharyngeal muscle is playing a premier role in the manifestation of symptoms, although the presence of the pouch, especially a larger one, is also contributing to the symptomatology.

Table 27–4	Zenker's Diverticulum: Clinical Features and Symptoms

Age (Mean, 68; Low, 38; High, 93)
50% >70 years
20% >80 years

Symptoms (Mean Duration, 37.4 Months)	
Dysphagia	80%
Regurgitation	58%
Choking	20%
Coughing	18%
Globus sensation	21%
Weight loss	23%
Others	14%
Associated Pathology	
Pulmonary infection	37%
Upper gastrointestinal pathology	60%
Documented reflux	44%
Other comorbid conditions	52%

These results are from our personal experience (*N* = 325).

SYMPTOMATOLOGY

The lack of compliance by the cricopharyngeal muscle and UES causes dysphagia (intrinsic dysphagia), the cardinal symptom, together with choking. Distention of the pouch by the incoming bolus and accumulation of food particles in the pouch may aggravate the sensation of dysphagia (extrinsic dysphagia). Regurgitation of undigested food particles, abnormal noise during swallowing, halitosis, the rare event of a visible swelling in the neck, and ear, nose, and throat symptoms are all manifestations of ZD (Table 27–4). Spontaneous evolution may result in life-threatening complications, in particular, cachexia or recurrent pulmonary infection and progression to end-stage respiratory insufficiency as a result of chronic aspiration. These complications are even more life-threatening inasmuch as ZD is a condition of the third age, with more than 50% of patients being older than 70 years and more than 20% being older than 80 years at the time of diagnosis.

One has to be aware that over 50% of patients have synchronous or metachronous complaints or documented pathologic changes of the upper gastrointestinal tract (or both). In particular, hiatal hernia and gastroesophageal reflux have to be looked for because of their high association with ZD. From our own material it appeared that 44% of the patients had pathologic reflux on 24-hour pH study or grade II or higher esophagitis at endoscopy.[7] These figures indicate that a full investigation of the upper gastrointestinal tract is mandatory in every patient with ZD, and if present, such associated pathologic change (e.g., gastroesophageal reflux) has to be treated "lege artis" (using the correct methods and procedures).

TREATMENT

Treatment is indicated for any symptomatic ZD. A variety of techniques are presently available and are discussed briefly.

Diverticulectomy and Diverticulopexy

Through a cervicotomy, preferably left sided, the diverticulum is identified and, after dissection of the pouch down to its neck, resected (diverticulectomy). The development of stapling devices that allow resection after staples have been fired has resulted in a clear decrease in the incidence of postoperative salivary fistula, the most important surgical complication. Nevertheless, data from the literature indicate an incidence of salivary fistula varying between 1% and 25%.[12,13] Moreover, because of a bare staple line on a fragile structure such as the mucosa, there is a tendency to wait somewhat longer before starting oral feeding. This delay will, of course, have a direct impact on the hospital stay, which in itself may increase the risk for comorbid conditions, especially in geriatric patients, and eventually result in an even longer hospital stay and possibly mortality.

To decrease the risk for postoperative leakage with a possibly fatal outcome, a technique has been developed by which the pouch is turned upside down after dissection and suspended on the prevertebral fascia of the cervical spine. This technique is called diverticulopexy.[14] Its main advantage is the fact that the esophageal lumen is not opened, thereby allowing patients to resume oral feeding the very same day or the day after the operation and thus resulting in a substantial decrease in hospital stay and a virtually nonexistent incidence of salivary fistula.

The Importance of Myotomy

Several authors have noticed recurrence of symptoms and pouch in a number of patients treated by simple diverticulectomy or diverticulopexy. Depending on the intensity of the follow-up and technical examinations applied, the recurrence rate after simple resection/diverticulopexy is reported to be between 2.5% and 20%.[13,14] It appears that recurrence is a slow process that requires several years. As a result, symptomatic recurrence will most likely not become apparent in very elderly patients.

In our own experience, it appeared that after simple diverticulectomy, which was the preferred method between 1953 and 1975, the incidence of symptomatic recurrence increased over time.[15] As a result of better understanding of the physiopathology, an increasing number of authors have underlined the importance of adding extramucosal myotomy of the cricopharyngeal muscle and proximal cervical striated muscle when performing either diverticulectomy or diverticulopexy (Figs. 27–6 and 27–7).[7,16] Although a randomized study has never been performed, there seems to be a consensus today that extramucosal myotomy is as an essential step in the treatment of ZD.

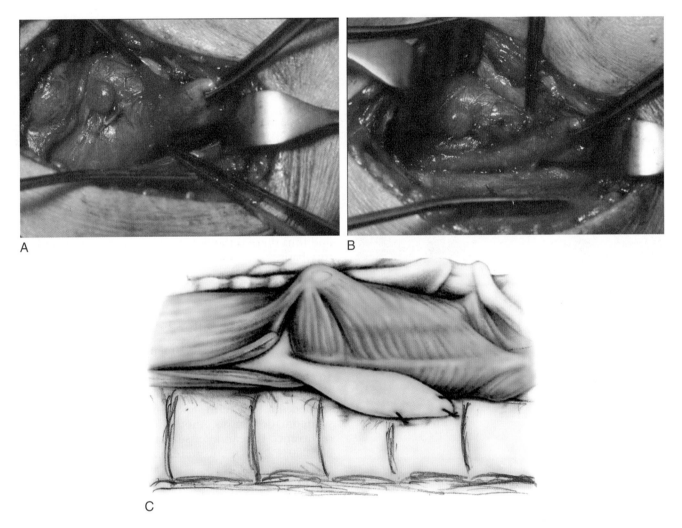

Figure 27–6. Myotomy and diverticulopexy in Zenker's diverticulum. **A,** The diverticulum is clearly visible. The forceps point toward the proximal border of the cricopharyngeal muscle. **B,** Same patient after performing a longitudinal extramucosal myotomy of the cricopharyngeal muscle and the proximal striated cervical muscle. **C,** Schema of the operation illustrating the diverticulopexy fixed to the prevertebral fascia.

With small diverticula (<2 cm), performance of solely extramucosal myotomy suffices to completely relieve the symptoms, which in itself seems to confirm the importance of the myotomy.

Endoscopic Techniques

The concept of an endoscopic approach dates back to the beginning of the 20th century. In 1917, Moscher described a technique by which the common wall between the esophagus and the pouch (the so-called cricopharyngeal bar) could be divided via an endoscopic approach.[17] Initially, the method resulted in high postoperative mortality. In 1960, Dohlman and Mattsson substantially improved this technique[18] by using a fixed rigid esophageal scope to allow better visualization of the cricopharyngeal bar and applying electrocoagulation. More recently, further refinement was obtained by replacing electrocoagulation with laser therapy and using magnifying devices.[19] The advantages of the endoscopic approach are evident: no open external approach and therefore less surgical trauma, shorter length of narcosis, and earlier resumption of feeding. The downside of the method is the fact that the cricopharyngeal bar can be incised only over a short distance because of the risk for perforation and subsequent mediastinitis. As a result, several sessions will be required in a substantial number of patients to eventually achieve complete symptomatic relief, but at the risk of higher morbidity.

However, with the introduction of videoscopic surgery, a method was developed by which a stapler is introduced through an endoscopic approach and an esophagodiverticulostomy is performed. After a sufficiently long myotomy of the cricopharyngeal bar and proximal cervical esophageal muscle, the anterior wall of the pouch and the posterior wall of the cervical esophagus are stapled along the line of transection (Fig. 27–8).[20-23] In addition to the myotomy, this method also enlarges the communication with the esophageal lumen of the pouch. This technique is clearly much more in alignment with the concept of a sufficiently long myotomy but without increasing the risk for a salivary fistula.

Negative aspects of the technique are the already documented risk for instrumental perforation and occasional leakage. Another disadvantage is that the pouch remains in its place and, despite enlargement of its basis, a so-called cul-de-sac persists. This may result in the accumulation of alimentary particles at the bottom of the

pouch and potentially cause regurgitation, coughing, or aspiration. Furthermore, it is evident that in a number of patients—10% to 15%—the method is not applicable, such as patients with ankylosis of the jaw, a prominent dental arch, and cervical kyphosis making hyperextension impossible. Finally, the procedure is difficult, if not impossible in patients with a diverticulum smaller than 3 cm because of the difficulty of introducing the stapler into the small pouch and the potential for an inadequate myotomy. Conversely, with a very large diverticula (>6 cm), several staples need to be fired, which might result in a too long a transection of the dorsal cervical esophageal wall and the eventual creation of a cloaca.

More recently, the endoscopic technique has been further refined to allow the use of flexible endoscopy, and thus there is the potential for treatment on ambulatory basis.[24,25]

RESULTS

Our Experience with 325 Patients

At our institution, the treatment of choice initially consisted of simple diverticulectomy. Between 1955 and 1975, 36 patients were treated in this manner. There was no postoperative mortality. Seven surviving patients were studied in long-term follow-up. One patient had a symptomatic stenosis. Another experienced symptomatic recurrence 16 years after surgery.[15] From 1975 to December 2003, 289 patients were operated on. Postoperative mortality was 0%.

The overall morbidity in this series is 8.5%, but it gradually decreased over the years to the point that it was 5.8% in 138 patients treated during the last 10 years. Overall in the series of 289 patients, three contained fistulas (0.1%) and three lesions of the recurrent nerve

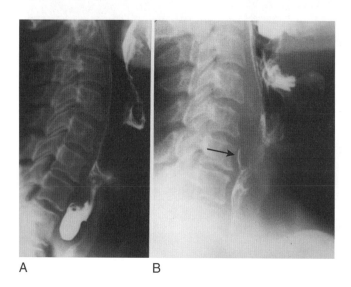

Figure 27–7.   **A,** Zenker's diverticulum: preoperative appearance with a contrast study. **B,** Same patient after extramucosal myotomy and diverticulopexy with free passage of the contrast material. The suspended diverticulum is visible as a small contrast line *(arrow).*

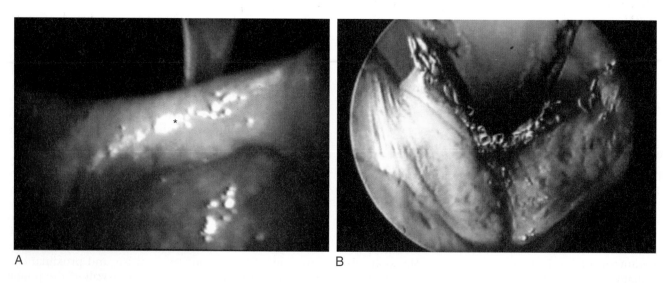

Figure 27–8.   Endoscopic approach. **A,** A cricopharyngeal bar *(asterisk)* is crossing the picture. The bottom of the picture shows the sac of the diverticulum. The upper part shows the entrance of the esophagus and the nasogastric tube in place in the esophagus. **B,** Same patient with an esophagodiverticulostomy after firing the endostapler. Note the V shape caused by retraction of the cricopharyngeal muscle.

(0.1%) with temporary vocal cord paralysis (Table 27–5) occurred. In addition, the mean hospital stay sharply decreased over the years from 8.3 days during the 1970s and mid-1980s to 2.6 days in the past 10 years. Typically, a contrast study is performed the day after surgery, and if no evidence of leakage is seen, normal oral alimentation is resumed and the patient is discharged.

The treatment of choice is extramucosal myotomy of the cricopharyngeal muscle and proximal cervical striated muscle combined with diverticulopexy. This type of operation has been performed in 265 patients; in 9 a simple myotomy was performed, the diverticulum itself being too small for diverticulopexy. In 4 patients, myotomy was combined with diverticulectomy, the reason being residual impaction of barium contrast material in the diverticulum. Finally, in 11 patients a videoendoscopic esophagodiverticulostomy was performed. An extended follow-up study was conducted twice over the years. The first analysis consisted of 178 patients in whom a myotomy plus diverticulopexy was performed between 1975 and 1996. Excellent to very good results were achieved in 90.6%. Eighty-five percent of the patients considered themselves totally asymptomatic. A fair to bad result was recorded in 3.4%. One patient had to undergo surgery again. In this patient a primary muscular disorder was considered the probable cause of the recurrent symptoms.

In these series a group of 28 patients who had been operated on more than 10 years previously were analyzed. Twenty-seven patients were completely asymptomatic. Between 1993 and August 2003, 138 patients were operated on and evaluated by means of a detailed questionnaire or outpatient clinic follow-up, or both. Excellent to very good results were obtained in 94% of the patients. Five patients (3.8%) had a fair result, three of them because of persistent symptoms of gastroesophageal reflux disease.

Of this group of 138 patients, 12 (8.7%) had been referred after previous endoscopic or open intervention. Redo interventions consisted of extramucosal myotomy and diverticulopexy in 11 and videoendoscopic esophagodiverticulostomy in 1. Excellent to very good results were achieved in 87% of this subgroup of patients.

In this series of 138 patients, 11 were treated by videoendoscopic esophagodiverticulostomy within the framework of a prospective study. There were no postoperative complications, but in further follow-up, recurrence of dysphagia and choking developed in two patients (Table 27–6). This appeared to be the consequence of a fibrotic tissue bar hampering passage of a solid bolus (Fig. 27–9). A redo intervention was performed, again via an endoscopic approach. Both patients remained asymptomatic afterward. As a result of these complications, the prospective study was interrupted and the treatment of choice today remains an open approach with myotomy and diverticulopexy because with both methods (open and endoscopic), resumption of oral alimentation can be started the day after surgery and the mean hospital stay is equally short. In other words, it appears that a videoendoscopic technique had no extra advantage with respect to resumption of oral alimentation and hospital stay.

Results from the Literature

Among many publications dealing with the treatment of ZD, a substantial number are providing only fragmentary results and also lack accurate information, such as the seriousness of complications and the improvement in preoperative symptoms. In addition, the definition of

| Table 27–5 | Zenker's Diverticulum: Postoperative Complications |

Complication	Number
Temporary speech symptoms	6
Infection/abscess	4
Pneumonia	3
Recurrent nerve paralysis	3
Hematoma	2
Fistula	3
Respiratory insufficiency	1
Thoracic duct leak	1
Other	3
Postoperative mortality	0

| Table 27–6 | Results of a Prospective Study to Evaluate Diverticuloesophagectomy |

Type of Procedure	No. of Preoperative Complications	No. of Postoperative Complications	Late Complications	Final Outcome
Open (n = 9)	—	Hematoma: 1	—	Excellent: 9
Endoscope (n = 11)	Subcutaneous emphysema: 1	Left vocal cord paresis: 1	Hematemesis: 1 Dysphagia Slight: 1 Moderate: 2	Excellent: 4 Good: 5 Fair: 2

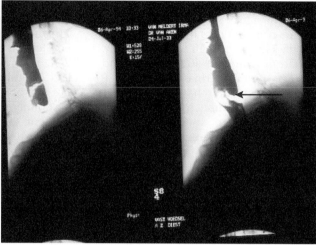

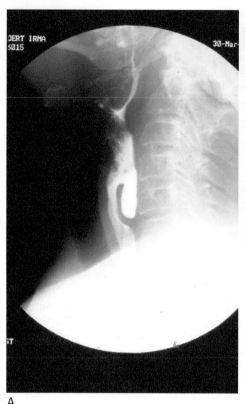

Figure 27–9. Endoscopic approach. **A,** Zenker's diverticulum preoperatively. **B,** Same patient postoperatively. A contrast study with a solid bolus indicates restriction of passage because of a fibrotic tissue indentation into the lumen *(arrow).*

recurrence when using the videoendoscopic approach lacks precision because the diverticulum by definition remains in place. Moreover, it is often unclear whether the redo surgery was incorporated as a recurrence in the results section when describing the final outcome. In analysis of the literature, one has to also take into consideration the date of publication, especially when studying the results of an open approach. Indeed, over the years, the progress of surgery in general and the improvement in perioperative management have undoubtedly resulted in a substantial decrease in surgical complications as reflected by more recent publications over the last decade. Tables 27–7 and 27–8 present an overview of the most relevant and larger series in the more recent literature dealing with ZD.[26-52]

The results of this overview indicate the consistent progress with regard to postoperative mortality during the last 2 decades. Mortality today is indeed very low. Morbidity seems to be similar for the different therapeutic approaches and is generally considered rather minor. It appears, however, that a videoendoscopic approach more frequently results in a need for reintervention and a clear and higher incidence of recurrence or insufficient control of symptoms. The incidence of total control of symptoms is clearly higher when using an open approach that includes myotomy than when using a videoendoscopic approach, in particular, endoscopic stapling, and this finding is also reflected in two comparative studies described in Table 27–9.[13,52]

WHICH TREATMENT?

Nowadays, ZD can be treated safely with a very low postoperative mortality rate irrespective of the type of treatment modality used. Equally irrespective of the treatment modality, oral alimentation can be started the day after (possibly the same day as) surgery with a very short mean hospital stay. In fact, the hospital stay is determined by the patient's comorbid conditions. This comorbidity can be serious and life-threatening inasmuch as ZD is indeed a condition of the third age. Precisely because of this fact, the goal of treatment of ZD is to provide a definitive solution with a single intervention for this often serious medical and social problem. Therefore, the treatment of choice is an approach or technique that in the long run offers the optimal guarantee for an excellent (i.e., totally asymptomatic) result.

Cosmetic considerations related to scar visibility are obsolete because in fact the scar is limited and barely visible after complete healing.

Data from the literature and in particular our own data seem to favor an open approach with extramucosal myotomy of the cricopharyngeal muscle and the proximal cervical striated muscle, combined with a diverticulopexy, as the technique of choice.

In occasional patients with contraindication to narcosis or open surgery, an endoscopic treatment modality may be the preferred method. Evidently, experience and mastery of the different techniques available are of paramount importance in determining the indication, type of treatment, and overall outcome.

Table 27-7 Open Approach

Author	Publication Year	Time Period	Method	N	Complications (%)	Mortality (%)	Results (%)		Recurrence
							Asymptomatic, Very Good	Partial Improvement	
Payne[26]	1992	1944-1978	D, DM, M	888	7.9	2	82	11	3.6
Laing[27]	1995	1979-1988	DM	67	16.4	NA	92.5	7.5	3
GEEMO multicenter report[8]	1996	1960-1982	D: 184	390	21		94		4.9
			DM: 121		10				4.9
			PM: 55		12.7	1.5			1.8
			M: 26		0				NA
			P: 4		0				7.6
Bonafede[28]	1997	1976-1993	M, DM, PM	87	24	3.5	78	13	NA
Zbaren[29]	1999	1987-1997	D, DM	66	15	1.5	77	11	6
Feussner[30]	1999	1982-1998	PM, DM	140	4.2	1	>90		0.8
Leporrier[31]	2001	1988-1998	DM, PM	40	17,5	0	92	8	0
Jougon[32]	2003	1987-2000	DM	73	4	0	99	1	0
Colombo-Benkmann[33]	2003	1985-1995	D, DM	79	15	0	76	19	2.5
Lerut	2004	1975-2003	PM, M, MD	289	8.5	0	94.2	3.8	0.03
Total				2119	10.5	1.4%			3.5%

D, diverticulectomy; GEEMO, Group Européen d'Etude des Maladies de l'Oesophage; M, myotomy; NA, not announced; P, diverticulopexy.

Table 27-8 Endoscopic Approach

Author	Publication Year	Time Period	Method	N	Complications (%)	Mortality (%)	Results (%)			Recurrence (%)
							Asymptomatic, Very Good	Partial Improvement		
Van Overbeek[19]	1994	1964-1992	Caut/CO_2L	545	6.7	1	90.6	8.6		NA
Ishioka[24]	1995	1982-1992	Caut	42	4.8	0	92.9	7.1		7.1
Von Doersten[34]	1997	1985-1994	Caut	40	25	0			92.5	0
Hashiba[35]	1999	Since 1978	Caut	47	14.9	0	96			4.3
Lippert[36]	2000	1984-1996	CO_2L	60	10	0	73	21		10
Nyrop[37]	2000	1989-1999	CO_2L	61	13.3	0	70	22		13
Mattinger[38]	2002	1974-1998	CO_2L	52	13.5	1			84.6	15.4
Krespi[39]	2002	1989-2001	CO_2L	83	4.8	0	85.5	11		7.5
Total				930	8.7	0.02				7.2
Peracchia[40]	1998	1992-1996	ESD	95	0	0	92.2	7.8		5.4
Van Eeden[41]	1999	1996-1997	ESD	18	5.9	0	53	35		NA
Cook[42]	2000	1995-1999	ESD	74	5	0	71	24		8.7
Luscher[43]	2000	1997-1998	ESD	23	4.3	0	76	14		4.3
Philippsen[44]	2000	1996-1996	ESD	14	0	0	57	21		NA
Sood[45]	2000	1992-1999	ESD	44	4.5	1	70	24		9
Jaramillo[46]	2001	1996-1999	ESD	32	3.7	0		80		7.4
Stoeckli[47]	2001	1997-2000	ESD	30	27	0		96		NA
Counter[48]	2002	1993-1997	ESD	31	9.7	0	50	44		22
Raut[49]	2002	1994-1998	ESD	25	8	0		48		32
Chang[50]	2003	1995-2001	ESD	150	12.7	0	73.3	22		11.8
Chiari[51]	2003	1997-2001	ESD	39	10	0	71	20		10.9
Total				575	7.8	0.02				10.9

Caut, electrocauterization; CO_2L, CO_2 laser; ESD, endoscopic stapler diverticulostomy.

Table 27-9 Comparative Studies of Long-Term Results

	Excellent Results		Excellent to Good Results	
	Open	**Endoscopic**	**Open**	**Endoscopic**
Gutschow, 2002[13] (1984-2002)	$n = 47$	$n = 28$	$n = 84$	$n = 79$
Diverticulum <3 cm	85%	25% $(P < .003)$	98%	57% $(P < .001)$
Diverticulum ≥3 cm	86%	56% $(P < .004)$	97%	88% $(P < .04)$
Zaninotto, 2003[52] (1993-2001)	$n = 34$	$n = 24$		
	100%	87.5% $(P < .05)$		

SUGGESTED READINGS

Belsey R: Functional diseases of the esophagus. J Thorac Cardiovasc Surg 52:164-188, 1966.

Chang C, Payyapilli R, Scher R: Endoscopic staple diverticulostomy for Zenker's diverticulum: Review of literature and experience in 159 consecutive cases. Laryngoscope 113:957-965, 2003.

Cook IJ, Gabb M, Panagopoulos V, et al: Pharyngeal (Zenker's) diverticulum is a disorder of upper esophageal sphincter opening. Gastroenterology 103:1229-1235, 1992.

Lerut T, Van Raemdonck D, Guelinckx P, et al: Zenker's diverticulum: Is a myotomy of the cricopharyngeus useful? How long should it be? Hepatogastroenterology 39:127-131, 1992.

Peracchia A, Bonavina L, Narne S, et al: Minimally invasive surgery for Zenker's diverticulum: Analysis of results in 95 consecutive patients. Arch Surg 133:695-700, 1998.

REFERENCES

1. Ludlow A: A case of obstructed deglution from a preternatural dilatation of, and bag formed in, the pharynx. Med Observ Inq 3:85-101, 1769.
2. Zenker F, von Ziemssen H: Krankheiten des Oesophagus. In Vogel FCW (ed): Handbuch der speciellen Pathologie und Therapie. Leipzig, Germany, Ziemssen, 1877, pp 1-87.
3. Killian G: The mouth of the esophagus. Laryngoscope 17:421-428, 1907.
4. Kahrilas P, Dodds W, Dent J, et al: Upper esophageal sphincter function during deglutition. Gastroenterology 95:52-62, 1988.
5. Ellis F, Schlegel I, Lynch V, Payne WS: Cricopharyngeal myotomy for pharyngoesophageal diverticulitis. Ann Surg 170:340-349, 1969.
6. Cook IJ, Gabb M, Panagopoulos V, et al: Pharyngeal (Zenker's) diverticulum is a disorder of upper esophageal sphincter opening. Gastroenterology 103:1229-1235, 1992.
7. Lerut T, Van Raemdonck D, Guelinckx P, et al: Zenker's diverticulum: Is a myotomy of the cricopharyngeus useful? How long should it be? Hepatogastroenterology 39:127-131, 1992.
8. Lerut T, Coosemans W, Cuypers P, et al: Cervical myotomy as therapeutic principle for pharyngoesophageal disorders. Dis Esophagus 9:22-32, 1996.
9. Venturi M, Bonavina L, Colombo L, et al: Biochemical markers in upper esophageal sphincter compliance in patients with Zenker's diverticulum. J Surg Res 70:46-48, 1997.
10. Dejaeger E, Pelemans W, Bibau G, et al: Manofluorographic analysis of swallowing in the elderly. Dysphagia 9:156-161, 1994.
11. Resouly A, Braat J, Jackson A, Evans H: Pharyngeal pouch: Link with reflux and oesophageal dysmotility. Clin Otolaryngol 19:241-242, 1994.
12. Sydow B, Levine M, Rubesin S, Laufer L: Radiographic findings and complications after surgical or endoscopic repair of Zenker's diverticulum in 16 patients. AJR Am J Roentgenol 177:1067-1071, 2001.
13. Gutschow C, Hamoir M, Rombaux P, et al: Management of pharyngoesophageal (Zenker's) diverticulum: Which technique? Am Thorac Surg 74:1677-1683, 2002.
14. Holinger P, Schild J: Zenker's (hypopharyngeal) diverticulum. Ann Otol Rhinol Laryngol 78:679-688, 1969.
15. Lerut T: Esophageal surgery at the end of the millennium. J Thorac Cardiovasc Surg 116:1-20, 1998.
16. Belsey R: Functional diseases of the esophagus. J Thorac Cardiovasc Surg 52:164-188, 1966.
17. Moscher H: Web and pouches of the esophagus: Their diagnosis and treatment. Surg Gynecol Obstet 25:175-187, 1917.
18. Dohlman G, Mattsson O: The endoscopic operation for hypopharyngeal diverticula: A roentgencinematographic study. AMA Arch Otolaryngol 71:744-752, 1960.
19. Van Overbeek J: Meditation on the pathogenesis of hypopharyngeal (Zenker's) diverticulum an a report of endoscopic treatment in 545 patients. Ann Otol Rhinol Laryngol 103:178-185, 1994.
20. Coosemans W, Lerut T, Van Raemdonck D: Thoracoscopic surgery: The Belgian experience. Ann Thorac Surg 56:721-730, 1993.
21. Hirsch D, Newbegin C: Autosuture GIA gun: A new application in the treatment of hypopharyngeal diverticula. J Laryngol Otol 107:723-725, 1993.
22. Collard J, Otte J, Kestens P: Endoscopic stapling technique of esophagodiverticulostomy for Zenker's diverticulum. Ann Thorac Surg 56:573-576, 1993.
23. Narne S, Bonavina L, Guido E, et al: Treatment of Zenker's diverticulum by endoscopic stapling. Endosurgery 1:118-120, 1993.
24. Ishioka S, Sakai P, Maluf F, et al: Endoscopic incision of Zenker's diverticula. Endoscopy 27:433-437, 1995.
25. Mulder C, den Hartog G, Robijn R, Thies J: Flexible endoscopic treatment of Zenker's diverticulum: A new approach. Endoscopy 27:438-442, 1995.
26. Payne W: The treatment of pharyngoesophageal diverticulum: The simple and complex. Hepatogastroenterology 39:109-114, 1992.
27. Laing M, Murthy P, Cockburn S: Surgery for pharyngeal pouch: Audit of management with short- and long-term follow up. J R Coll Surg Edinb 40:315-318, 1995.
28. Bonafede J, Lavertu P, Wood B, et al: Surgical outcome in 87 patients with Zenker's diverticulum. Laryngoscope 107:720-725, 1997.
29. Zbaren P, Schar P, Tschopp L, et al: Surgical treatment of Zenker's diverticulum: Transcutaneous diverticulectomy versus microendoscopic myotomy of the cricopharyngeal muscle with CO_2 laser. Otolaryngol Head Neck Surg 121:482-487, 1999.
30. Feussner H, Siewert J: Traditionelle extraluminale Operation des Zenker-Divertikels. Chirurg 70:753-756, 1999.
31. Leporrier J, Salamé E, Gignoux M, Ségol P: Diverticule de Zenker: Diverticulopexie contre diverticulectomie. Ann Chir 126:42-45, 2001.

32. Jougon J, Le Taillandier-de-Gabory L, Raux F, et al: Plaidoyer pour un abord externe par cervicotomie du diverticule de Zenker: À propos de 73 cas. Ann Chir 128:167-172, 2003.

33. Colombo-Benkmann M, Unruh V, Kriegelstein C, et al: Cricopharyngeal myotomy in the treatment of Zenker's diverticulum. J Am Coll Surg 196:370-378, 2003.

34. von Doersten P, Byl F: Endoscopic Zenker's diverticulotomy (Dohlman procedure): Forty cases reviewed. Otolaryngol Head Neck Surg 116:209-212, 1997.

35. Hashiba K, de Paula A, da Silva J, et al: Endoscopic treatment of Zenker's diverticulum. Gastrointest Endosc 49:93-97, 1999.

36. Lippert B, Folz B, Rudert H, et al: Management of Zenker's diverticulum and postlaryngectomy pseudodiverticulum with the CO_2 laser. Otolaryngol Head Neck Surg 121:809-814, 1999.

37. Nyrop M, Svendstrup F, Jorgensen K: Endoscopic CO_2 laser therapy of Zenker's diverticulum—experience from 61 patients. Acta Otolaryngol 543:232-234, 2000.

38. Mattinger C, Hormann K: Endoscopic diverticulotomy of Zenker's diverticulum: Management and complications. Dysphagia 17:34-39, 2002.

39. Krespi Y, Kacker A, Remacle M: Endoscopic treatment of Zenker's diverticulum using CO_2 laser. Otolaryngol Head Neck Surg 127:309-314, 2002.

40. Peracchia A, Bonavina L, Narne S, et al: Minimally invasive surgery for Zenker's diverticulum: Analysis of results in 95 consecutive patients. Arch Surg 133:695-700, 1998.

41. van Eeden S, Lloyd R, Tranter R: Comparison of the endoscopic stapling technique with more established procedures for pharyngeal pouches: Results and patient satisfaction survey. J Laryngol Otol 113:237-240, 1999.

42. Cook R, Huang P, Richstmeier W, et al: Endoscopic staple-assisted esophagodiverticulostomy: An excellent treatment choice for Zenker's diverticulum. Laryngoscope 110:2020-2025, 2000.

43. Luscher M, Johansen L: Zenker's diverticulum treated by the endoscopic stapling technique. Acta Otolaryngol Suppl 543:235-238, 2000.

44. Philippsen L, Weisberger E, Whiteman T, et al: Endoscopic stapled diverticulotomy: Treatment of choice for Zenker's diverticulum. Laryngoscope 110:1283-1286, 2000.

45. Sood S, Newbegin C: Endoscopic stapling of pharyngeal pouches in patients from the Yorkshire region. J Laryngol Otol 114:833-837, 2000.

46. Jaramillo M, McLay K, McAteer D: Long-term clinicoradiological assessment of pharyngeal pouch: A series of cases. J Laryngol Otol 115:462-466, 2001.

47. Stoeckli S, Schmid S: Endoscopic stapler-assisted diverticuloesophagostomy for Zenker's diverticulum: Patient satisfaction and subjective relief of symptoms. Surgery 131:158-162, 2002.

48. Counter P, Hilton M, Baldwin D: Long-term follow-up of endoscopic stapled diverticulotomy. Ann R Coll Surg Engl 84:89-92, 2002.

49. Raut V, Primrose W: Long-term results of endoscopic stapling diverticulotomy for pharyngeal pouches. Otolaryngol Head Neck Surg 127:225-229, 2002.

50. Chang C, Payyapilli R, Scher R: Endoscopic staple diverticulostomy for Zenker's diverticulum: Review of literature and experience in 159 consecutive cases. Laryngoscope 113:957-965, 2003.

51. Chiari C, Yeganehfar W, Scharitzer M, et al: Significant symptomatic relief after transoral endoscopic staple-assisted treatment of Zenker's diverticulum. Surg Endosc 17:596-600, 2003.

52. Zaninotto G, Narne S, Constantini M, et al: Tailored approach to Zenker's diverticula. Surg Endosc 17:129-133, 2003.

Epidemiology, Pathophysiology, and Clinical Features of Achalasia

Dan J. Raz ▪ Pietro Tedesco ▪ Marco G. Patti

Achalasia is a primary motility disorder of the esophagus characterized by aperistalsis and failure of the lower esophageal sphincter (LES) to relax appropriately in response to swallowing.[1] It is a chronic benign disease that is a common cause of dysphagia, yet its cause remains poorly understood. Sir Thomas Willis provided the first documented case report of achalasia in 1674, when he described his experience with esophageal dilation with a whalebone in a patient who had dysphagia and a dilated esophagus. To this day, the cornerstone of treatment of achalasia remains relief of the functional obstruction at the level of the gastroesophageal junction. In 1927, Hurst coined the term esophageal *achalasia,* meaning absence of relaxation, specifically, inadequate LES relaxation in the absence of mechanical obstruction.[2]

EPIDEMIOLOGY

The epidemiology of achalasia has not been thoroughly studied. The incidence of achalasia worldwide is estimated at 0.5 to 1 per 100,000 persons per year. It can occur at any age but has a peak incidence between the ages of 30 and 60 and is exceedingly rare in the first 2 decades of life.[3] In the University of California, San Francisco (UCSF), experience, the median age at diagnosis was 48 years (Fig. 28–1). Men and women are equally affected, with no ethnic predisposition to the disease.[4] There have been reports of "familial achalasia," but these cases represent less than 1% of cases in the literature and do not seem to follow any mendelian inheritance pattern.[5] The triple-A syndrome, or Allgrove's disease, is a rare condition consisting of achalasia, alacrima, and adrenocorticotropic hormone (ACTH)-resistant adrenal insufficiency. Severe skeletal and autonomic neuropathy, cerebellar dysfunction, and cognitive defects are also

part of the syndrome.[6] The disease almost always occurs in the first decade of life, and dysphagia is an early symptom. Most children have hypoglycemic or hypotensive episodes from adrenal insufficiency. Neurologic deterioration commonly occurs in the second or third decade of life. The syndrome follows an autosomal recessive inheritance pattern with variable penetrance. A genetic linkage analysis of families with triple-A syndrome has linked the disease to markers on 12q13, and recently, mutations have been localized to the *AAAS* gene.[6] Although achalasia significantly increases the risk for esophageal cancer, longitudinal studies indicate that achalasia does not affect life expectancy. The mean age of death of patients with achalasia in one series was 80 years, thus suggesting a relatively low frequency of esophageal cancer.[2]

PATHOGENESIS

The defining pathologic feature of achalasia is progressive inflammation and selective loss of the inhibitory myenteric neurons in Auerbach's plexus of the esophagus that normally secrete vasoactive intestinal polypeptide and nitric oxide. This results in failure of relaxation of the LES and aperistalsis of the esophageal body with subsequent functional obstruction at the level of the gastroesophageal junction and gradual dilatation of the esophagus.[7] Based on animal models and clinical observation, some authors have suggested that the primary event in achalasia is LES dysfunction with resulting outflow obstruction and secondary esophageal dilatation and loss of peristalsis.[2,7,8] According to this theory, relief of LES obstruction early in the disease would reverse the loss of peristalsis. Little et al. demonstrated that banding of the gastroesophageal junction in a feline model resulted in loss of peristalsis that was reversed with relief

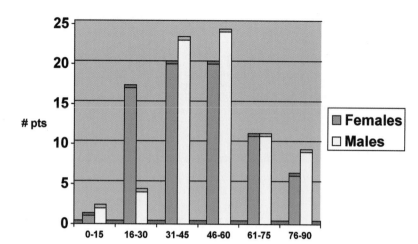

Figure 28–1. Age distribution in 148 untreated patients with achalasia.

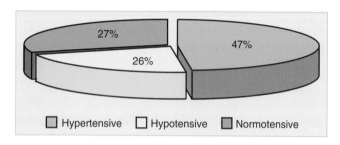

Figure 28–2. Lower esophageal sphincter pressure in untreated patients with esophageal achalasia.

of the obstruction.[9] Parilla described some return of peristalsis in patients after myotomy, which occurred more frequently in those who had a shorter duration of symptoms.[10] In our experience of 173 patients undergoing minimally invasive myotomy for achalasia, we found no return of peristalsis after treatment. Furthermore, the duration of symptoms at the time of myotomy had no effect on the outcome of the operation.[11] The theory of primary LES dysfunction is further flawed by the well-documented observation that less than 50% of patients with achalasia have a hypertensive LES. In fact, 25% of untreated patients with achalasia have a hypotensive LES (Fig. 28–2).[12] It is difficult to fathom that a hypotensive LES can produce a functional obstruction sufficient to cause aperistalsis.

The pathogenesis of achalasia remains elusive despite an understanding of the physiology of the disease. Overall, there is progressive esophageal dilation above the LES ranging from minimal dilation in early achalasia to an esophageal diameter of 10 to 14 cm in patients with long-standing disease. Mucosal changes, namely, ulceration and fibrotic thickening, can be present because of stasis of food and esophagitis. Histologically, neuritis and ganglionitis are seen early in the disease, with fibrosis gradually replacing the myenteric plexus in the esophageal body. Consequently, there is a marked decrease in intramuscular small nerve fibers and neurotransmitter-carrying vesicles in the remaining fibers.[7] Wallerian degenerative changes have been described in

the vagus nerve and dorsal motor nucleus of the vagus, and some investigators have reported impaired gastric acid secretion in patients with achalasia as a result.[13] Immunohistochemical studies show a marked inflammatory response mediated by cytotoxic T cells early in the disease, thus leading to the possibility of an infectious or autoimmune-mediated cause. The striking similarity of achalasia with Chagas' disease has further supported an infectious cause of primary achalasia. Although herpes simplex virus type 1 (HSV-1), HSV-2, polio, human papillomavirus, and measles have all been proposed as candidates in initiating the immune response, no infectious pathogens have been convincingly isolated from tissue samples either by electron microscopy or by polymerase chain reaction amplification.

HSV has been a prime candidate because of its neurotropic proclivity in other diseases such as trigeminal and facial neuritis. Recently, Castaglinolo et al. demonstrated that exposure of esophageal mononuclear cells isolated from the LES of patients with achalasia to HSV-1 antigens in vitro led to significantly elevated mononuclear cell proliferation and interferon-γ production when compared with controls. Based on this finding, they speculated that HSV-1 might initiate the inflammatory reaction leading to achalasia.[14] This result supports a causal relationship between HSV and achalasia, though not conclusively.

Certain class II major histocompatibility complex (MHC) antigens such as HLA-DQw1, HLA-DQB1, and HLA-DRB1 have been associated with achalasia.[15,16] A class II HLA association has been observed in autoimmune diseases such as rheumatoid arthritis and autoimmune endocrinopathies. Other postinfectious diseases, such as postgonococcal arthritis, have been linked to specific MHC antigens, although typically to class I alleles.[16] Also supporting an autoimmune cause is the presence of autoantibodies to myenteric plexus neurons in the serum of 39% to 64% of patients with achalasia versus 0% to 6% of healthy controls and patients with other esophageal disorders.[17,18]

Most consider the esophagopathy of achalasia and Chagas' disease to be clinically identical. Chagas' disease results from infection by the parasite *Trypanosoma cruzi* and is endemic to Central and South America, especially

Brazil, Venezuela, and northern Argentina. In chronic Chagas' disease there is progressive destruction of ganglion cells throughout the body, including the gastrointestinal tract. This neuropathy results in disturbed peristalsis leading to stasis and dilation predominantly in the esophagus, duodenum, and colon. Megaesophagus is present in 60% to 70% of patients with chronic Chagas' disease. The radiographic and manometric findings of patients with Chagas' disease are identical to those of patients with primary achalasia. Although primary achalasia and Chagas' disease are widely considered to be indistinguishable, some subtle differences between the two diseases do exist. In Chagas' disease there is denervation of both inhibitory and excitatory myenteric nerves, as opposed to the selective inhibitory neuronal loss seen in primary achalasia. Patients with Chagas' disease demonstrate hyposensitivity of the LES to gastrin, as opposed to hypersensitivity in primary achalasia. Finally, basal LES pressure is lower in Chagas' disease than in primary achalasia.[19] Because of more limited access to medical attention in developing nations where Chagas' disease is prevalent, there is typically a longer duration of symptoms and more pronounced esophageal dilation in these patients at the time of initial evaluation.[19]

CLINICAL FEATURES

The cardinal symptom of achalasia is dysphagia, which is present in almost all patients at the time of diagnosis. Most patients have had symptoms for more than 5 years before the diagnosis of achalasia is made and typically accommodate to their dysphagia by eating smaller quantities of food, avoiding solid food such as meat and bread, and drinking liquids with their meals. Often, patients are incorrectly given another diagnosis, most commonly gastroesophageal reflux disease (GERD), before eventually undergoing esophageal function tests that document achalasia. In our experience, 69% of untreated patients were taking acid-suppressing medications at the time of referral to our center.[4]

As the esophagus dilates, it becomes a reservoir of undigested food, and in severe cases it empties only when sufficient hydrostatic pressure is generated. Because of stasis in the esophagus, regurgitation occurs in 76% of patients, and 52% complain of heartburn.[4] Heartburn is due to stasis and fermentation of the food, and halitosis is a common complaint. Aspiration occurs usually at night when the patient is recumbent and can cause nocturnal cough, pneumonia, and pulmonary abscess.

Chest pain was present in 41% of patients referred to our center, even though it was never considered the main complaint.[4] The pain is probably due to esophageal wall distention, stasis esophagitis, or *Candida* esophagitis. Contrary to common belief, it is not related to younger age, shorter duration of symptoms, or the manometric finding of vigorous achalasia.[20]

Weight loss was present in 35% of patients with achalasia in the UCSF experience. It is usually due to an inability of the esophagus to empty and to *sitophobia,* or fear of eating. The average weight loss was 20 lb. Twenty percent of patients lost 1 to 15 lb, 7% lost 16 to 30 lb, and 8% lost more than 30 lb.[4] Severe weight loss over a short period in elderly patients should raise the suspicion of malignancy-induced or secondary achalasia.[2]

DIAGNOSTIC EVALUATION

Once the diagnosis of achalasia is suspected, a contrast esophagogram should be obtained. This test often shows distal esophageal narrowing (bird beak), an air-fluid level, slow emptying of the barium, and esophageal dilatation. Among our patients, the esophageal diameter was less than 4 cm in 30%, 4 to 6 cm in 50%, and greater than 6 cm in 16%. A sigmoid esophagus was present in 4% of patients and a hiatal hernia in 6%.[4]

The gold standard for the diagnosis of achalasia is esophageal manometry, which should be performed on all patients before initiating therapy. The defining manometric abnormality is lack of peristalsis of the esophageal body, as manifested by simultaneous, nonpropulsive contractions (Fig. 28–3). Impaired LES relaxation with swallowing is seen in 87% of patients. *Vigorous achalasia* is defined as the presence of nonpropulsive contractions with an amplitude greater than 37 mm Hg. Overall, there is no significant difference in age, sex, or duration of symptoms between patient with classic and vigorous achalasia or between patients with and without chest pain (Table 28–1).[20]

A hypertensive LES has been widely considered essential for the diagnosis of achalasia. However, many investigators have documented a hypertensive LES in only 50% of patients with achalasia. In our series of 145 untreated patients, only 43% of patients with achalasia had a hypertensive LES (>24 mm Hg), whereas 32% had a normotensive LES (14 to 24 mm Hg) and 25% had a hypotensive LES (<14 mm Hg) (see Fig. 28–2). In our experience, preoperative LES pressure did not affect the outcome of laparoscopic Heller myotomy.[12] In patients with a hypotensive LES and aperistalsis, it is important to differentiate achalasia from scleroderma. In contrast to patients with achalasia, those with scleroderma will frequently have a wide-open gastroesophageal junction on esophagography, a distal stricture or evidence of esophagitis on endoscopy, and evidence of GERD on pH monitoring.

Upper endoscopy should always be performed to exclude other disease such as cancer, peptic stricture, and scleroderma. In primary achalasia, the esophageal mucosa is usually normal, although there may be some esophagitis because of retained food. The endoscope should pass through the gastroesophageal junction without marked resistance. In previously treated patients, 24-hour esophageal pH monitoring differentiates heartburn secondary to real reflux from heartburn caused by stasis and fermentation of food in the distal esophagus.[21]

SECONDARY ACHALASIA

Secondary achalasia refers to esophageal motility abnormalities that are similar to achalasia but caused by other disease entities, most commonly malignancy and occa-

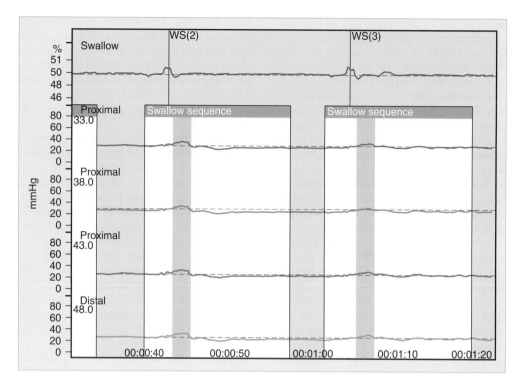

Figure 28–3.   Classic manometric findings in achalasia. Esophageal peristalsis is absent.

Table 28–1   Classic Versus Vigorous Achalasia

	Patients with Chest Pain (n = 117)	Patients Without Chest Pain (n = 94)	P Value
Age (yr)	49 ± 16	51 ± 14	NS
Sex (F/M)	56/61	41/53	NS
Duration of symptoms (mo)	71 ± 91	67 ± 67	NS
Dysphagia (score 0-4)	2.7 ± 1.4	2.6 ± 1.5	NS
Regurgitation (score 0-4)	1.8 ± 1.4	2.0 ± 1.5	NS
Esophageal diameter (cm)	4.5 ± 0.7	4.3 ± 0.8	NS
LES pressure (mm Hg)	15 ± 9	17 ± 11	NS
LES relaxation (% patients)	46	37	NS
Absent	44	52	NS
Partial	10	11	NS
Complete			
Vigorous achalasia	50	47	NS

From Perretta S, Fisichella PM, Galvani C, et al: Achalasia and chest pain: Effect of laparoscopic Heller myotomy. J Gastrointest Surg 7:595-598, 2003.

sionally intestinal pseudo-obstruction, postvagotomy states, amyloidosis, and sarcoidosis.

Malignancy-induced achalasia, often referred to as *pseudoachalasia,* accounts for up to 4% of patients with manometric findings of achalasia and is caused by adenocarcinoma of the gastric cardia in 75% of cases. The pathophysiology of pseudoachalasia involves direct tumor infiltration into the myenteric plexus causing denervation similar to that seen in primary

achalasia.[22] Malignant distal esophageal strictures caused by tumors involving the gastroesophageal junction and tumors involving the vagus nerve can similarly give rise to pseudoachalasia. Distant cancers such as prostate and pancreatic cancer have been reported to cause secondary achalasia via a paraneoplastic neuropathy. Age older than 60 years, duration of symptoms less than 1 year, and significant weight loss should raise suspicion of malignancy.[2] Endoscopic ultrasonography or computed tomography can help establish the diagnosis.

COMPLICATIONS OF ACHALASIA

Esophagitis is caused by irritation from stasis and by infection. Epiphrenic diverticula represent pulsion diverticula secondary to increased intraesophageal pressure. In addition, there is an association between achalasia and the development of squamous cell esophageal cancer, presumably because of chronic mucosal irritation. Achalasia patients in whom esophageal cancer develops typically complain of worsening dysphagia 15 to 30 years after their initial symptoms. The incidence of cancer varies widely in the literature from 0.3% to 20%.[2,7] In the most comprehensive prospective endoscopic surveillance study published to date, Meijssen et al. monitored 195 patients with achalasia by surveillance endoscopy for more than 10 years after endoscopic dilatation. Esophageal cancer developed in three patients, for a 1.5% incidence of cancer over the 10-year study, a 33-fold increased risk in comparison to historical controls.[23] Brucher et al. reported a 3.2% incidence of esophageal carcinoma in 124 patients with achalasia observed over a median of 5.6 years. The cancer developed 18 to 42 years after the patients experienced symptoms. Fifty percent of the cancers were early stage, and long-term survival was similar to that of esophageal cancer in patients without achalasia.[24] The effect of surgical myotomy or endoscopic therapies on decreasing the risk for cancer by decreasing the amount of esophageal stasis and mucosal irritation is unknown.

Surgical myotomy and endoscopic treatments of achalasia may also increase the risk for esophageal adenocarcinoma because of disruption of the LES with resulting gastroesophageal reflux and the development of Barrett's esophagus. GERD is documented by 24-hour pH monitoring in about a third of patients after endoscopic dilatation,[25] in 38% to 60% of patients after Heller myotomy without fundoplication,[21,25] but in only 8% to 15% with the addition of a partial fundoplication.[21,26] Overall, patients in whom Barrett's esophagus is diagnosed have an estimated 0.5% annual risk for esophageal cancer. The incidence of Barrett's esophagus and esophageal cancer is not well studied in patients undergoing surgical and endoscopic treatment of achalasia. In one series of 46 patients who underwent surgical myotomy without fundoplication, Barrett's esophagus developed in 9% on long-term follow-up.[27] Of the 30 patients in the literature with Barrett's esophagus and achalasia, adenocarcinoma developed in 25% after a mean follow-up of 22 years following treatment.[28] It is important to stress that this group of patients was not treated with laparoscopic Heller myotomy and fundoplication, the current surgical standard of care. Longer follow-up is necessary to accurately determine the incidence of Barrett's esophagus and esophageal adenocarcinoma after surgical myotomy with fundoplication for achalasia.

Patients who have previously been treated for achalasia and complain of recurrent dysphagia should undergo a complete evaluation, including barium swallow, upper endoscopy, esophageal manometry, and pH monitoring. Treatment should be tailored to the findings of these tests. For asymptomatic patients, the recommended frequency of surveillance endoscopy is debatable and not based on controlled studies.

REFERENCES

1. Patti MG, Fisichella PM, Perretta S, et al: Impact of minimally invasive surgery on the treatment of esophageal achalasia: A decade of change. J Am Coll Surg 196:698-703, 2003.
2. Reynolds J, Parkman H: Achalasia. Gastroenterol Clin North Am 18:223-255, 1989.
3. Podas T, Eaden J, Mayberry M, Mayberry J: Achalasia: A critical review of epidemiological studies. Am J Gastroenterol 93:2345-2347, 1998.
4. Raz D, Fogato L, Tedesco P, Patti MG: Clinical, radiological and manometric profile in patients with untreated esophageal achalasia. Dig Dis Sci (submitted for publication).
5. Zimmerman FH, Rosensweig NS: Achalasia in a father and son. Am J Gastroenterol 79:506-508, 1984.
6. Kimber J, McLean BN, Prevett M, Hammans SR: Allgrove or 4 "A" syndrome: An autosomal recessive syndrome causing multi-system neurological disease. J Neurol Neurosurg Psychiatry 74:654-657, 2003.
7. Wong RKH, Maydonovitch CL: Achalasia. In Castell DO, Richter JE (eds): The Esophagus, 3d ed. Philadelphia, Lippincott Williams & Wilkins, 1999, pp 185-213.
8. Vaezi MF, Richter JE: Diagnosis and management of achalasia. Am J Gastroenterol 94:3406-3412, 1999.
9. Little AG, Correnti FS, Calleja IJ, et al: Effect of incomplete obstruction on feline esophageal function with a clinical correlation. Surgery 100:430-436, 1986.
10. Parrilla P, Martinez de Haro LF, Ortiz A, et al: Factors involved in the return of peristalsis in patients with achalasia of the cardia after Heller's myotomy. Am J Gastroenterol 90:713-717, 1995.
11. Galvani C, Gorodner MV, Fogato L, Patti MG: Timing of surgical intervention does not influence return of esophageal peristalsis and outcome in patients with achalasia. Surg Endosc 19:1188-1192, 2005.
12. Gorodner MV, Galvani C, Fisichella PM, Patti MG: Preoperative lower esophageal sphincter pressure has little influence on the outcome of laparoscopic Heller myotomy for achalasia. Surg Endosc 18:774-778, 2004.
13. Dooley CP, Taylor IL, Valenzuela JE: Impaired acid secretion and pancreatic polypeptide release in some patients with achalasia. Gastroenterology 84:809-813, 1983.
14. Castaglinolo I, Brun P, Costantini M, et al: Esophageal achalasia: Is the herpes simplex virus really innocent? J Gastrointest Surg 8:24-30, 2004.
15. Verne GN, Hahn AB, Pineau BC, et al: Association of HLA-DR and DQ alleles with idiopathic achalasia. Gastroenterology 117:26-31, 1999.
16. Wong RKH, Maydonovitch CL, Metz SJ, Baker JR: Significant DQ w1 association in achalasia. Dig Dis Sci 34:349-352, 2004.
17. Storch WB, Eckardt VF, Wienbeck M, et al: Autoantibodies to Auerbach's plexus in achalasia. Cell Mol Biol (Noisy-le-grand) 41:1033-1038, 1995.
18. Verne GN, Eaker EY, Sallusito JE: Anti-myenteric neuronal antibodies in patients with achalasia. A prospective study. Dig Dis Sci 42:307-301, 1997.
19. Herbella FM, Oliveira DR, Del Grande JC: Are idiopathic and chagasic achalasia two different diseases? Dig Dis Sci 49:353-360, 2004.
20. Perretta S, Fisichella PM, Galvani C, et al: Achalasia and chest pain: Effect of laparoscopic Heller myotomy. J Gastrointest Surg 7:595-598, 2003.
21. Patti MG, Arcerito M, Tong J, et al: Importance of preoperative and postoperative pH monitoring in patients with esophageal achalasia. J Gastrointest Surg 1:505-510, 1997.

22. Moonka R, Patti MG, Feo CV, et al: Clinical presentation and evaluation of malignant pseudoachalasia. J Gastrointest Surg 3:456-461, 1999.

23. Meijssen MA, Tilanus HW, Van Blankenstein M: Achalasia complicated by oesphageal squamous cell carcinoma: A prospective study in 195 patients. Gut 33:155-158, 1992.

24. Brucher BL, Stein HJ, Bartels H, et al: Achalasia and esophageal cancer: Incidence, prevalence, and prognosis. World J Surg 25:745-749, 2001.

25. Shoenut JP, Duerksen D, Yaffe CS: A prospective assessment of gastroesophageal reflux before and after treatment of achalasia patients: Pneumatic dilation versus transthoracic limited myotomy. Am J Gastroenterol 92:1109-1112, 1997.

26. Richards WO, Torquati A, Holzman MD, et al: Heller myotomy versus Heller myotomy with Dor fundoplication for achalasia: A prospective randomized double-blind clinical trial. Ann Surg 240:405-412, 2004.

27. Jaakkola A, Reinikainen P, Ovaska J, Isolauri J: Barrett's esophagus after cardiomyotomy for esophageal achalasia. Am J Gastroenterol 89:165-169, 1994.

28. Guo JP, Gilman PB, Thomas RM, et al: Barrett's esophagus and achalasia. J Clin Gastroenterol 34:439-443, 2002.

29

Laparoscopic Esophageal Myotomy: Techniques and Results

Dave R. Lal ▪ Brant K. Oelschlager

Achalasia is a rare primary esophageal motor disorder characterized by ineffective relaxation of the lower esophageal sphincter (LES) and concomitant loss of esophageal peristalsis. The clinical manifestations of achalasia include progressive dysphagia and varying degrees of regurgitation, aspiration, chest pain, and weight loss. The reported incidence in the United States is 0.5 to 1 per 100,000. Although achalasia can occur at any age, a majority of patients are between the ages of 20 and 50 years. There is no gender preponderance.

Although the cause of achalasia is unknown, histologic examination of affected esophagi demonstrate myenteric inflammation with loss of ganglion cells and fibrosis of the myenteric plexus.[1] This destruction is probably autoimmune regulated because T lymphocytes predominate in the inflammatory infiltrate surrounding the myenteric plexus.[2] Additional research has shown achalasia patients to have decreased nitric oxide synthase in the myenteric plexus, which contributes to reduced nitric oxide production.[3] Nitric oxide is a key factor in gastrointestinal smooth muscle relaxation, including the LES.

Though first described more than 300 years ago, treatment of achalasia has evolved from dilatation with a whale bone to open and minimally invasive surgical myotomy, pneumatic dilatation, and botulinum toxin A (Botox) injection. This chapter discusses the medical and surgical management of achalasia.

DIAGNOSIS

Patients typically complain of a slow progression of dysphagia, first to solids and then to liquids. The dysphagia is usually accompanied by regurgitation, mild weight loss, and chest pain/discomfort associated with eating. Most patients relate a sensation of food getting stuck in their esophagus. Some adopt maneuvers, including standing and raising their arms above their heads, in an effort to use gravity to propel food into the stomach. Because of poor esophageal clearance, regurgitation of undigested food is common after meals and when lying supine. This regurgitation can lead to recurrent aspiration, pneumonia, and vocal hoarseness. Although patients complain of reflux, it is usually not due to gastric acid secretions but rather fermentation of undigested food that is pooled in the esophagus. Therefore, acid-suppressive medications provide little relief. In older patients (>55 years), those with a shorter duration of symptoms (<6 months), or those with more profound weight loss (>15 lb), it is crucial to rule out pseudoachalasia (presence of a distal esophageal tumor) as the cause of the symptoms.

The preferred initial diagnostic test for most patients with progressive dysphagia is a barium swallow. This inexpensive and readily available study reveals impaired peristalsis, a dilated esophagus, and the pathognomonic smooth tapering at the gastroesophageal (GE) junction commonly termed a "bird's beak" (Fig. 29–1A and B). In long-standing achalasia, the esophagus can become dilated and tortuous and has been termed sigmoid-shaped esophagus or megaesophagus (see Fig. 29–1C).

Manometry is required to diagnose achalasia. Manometric findings include failure of the LES to relax with deglutition and aperistalsis of the esophageal body. LES pressure is typically elevated (>40 mm Hg) but may be normal. Motor activity in the esophagus consists of low-amplitude (<40 mm Hg) simultaneous contractions. Occasionally, high-amplitude simultaneous contractions are seen, and these patients are classified as having vigorous achalasia.

Endoscopy is necessary to exclude pseudoachalasia and evaluate for atypical anatomy. Characteristic findings

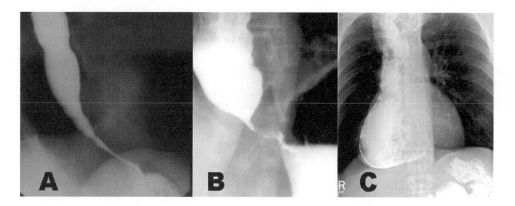

Figure 29–1.   Barium esophagograms of patients with varying stages of achalasia. All demonstrate the smooth tapering of the distal end of the esophagus termed a bird's beak. **A,** Early achalasia. Note the minimal esophageal dilatation. **B,** More typical esophagogram depicting a dilated esophagus in a patient with achalasia. **C,** Dilated and tortuous esophagus typically seen in patients with long-standing achalasia, termed megaesophagus or sigmoid-shaped esophagus. (Courtesy of Charles A. Rohrmann, Jr., M.D., University of Washington School of Medicine, Seattle.)

include a dilated esophagus with failure of the LES to open on insufflation and minimal resistance to passage of the scope through the GE junction. Retention of food and debris in the esophagus is common. Patients with achalasia have a 16-fold increased rate of esophageal cancer (typically squamous cell); thus, all mucosal abnormalities must be sampled by biopsy.[4] If concern for pseudoachalasia persists, computed tomography or endoscopic ultrasound (or both) should be added.

MEDICAL THERAPY

Pharmacologic Treatment

Nitrates and calcium channel blockers have been used with various degrees of success. Relief of symptoms is usually transient, limited to early or mild achalasia, and associated with side effects, including peripheral edema, dizziness, and headaches. Recently, sildenafil, a phosphodiesterase-5 inhibitor, has been shown to relax the LES.[5,6] The mechanism of action involves inhibition of phosphodiesterase-5, which results in increased nitric oxide and cyclic guanosine monophosphate within the LES. Like other pharmacologic treatments, sildenafil's effects last approximately 2 to 8 hours, and it may cause significant side effects. We occasionally prescribe pharmacologic therapy for short-term relief of severe symptoms in patients awaiting surgical myotomy.

Botulinum Toxin

Botox inhibits muscle contraction by blocking acetylcholine release from presynaptic nerve terminals. Treatments involve multiple injections around the GE junction via an endoscope. Although the initial success rate is high, long-term relief is not sustained. Zaninotto et al.[7] have published the only randomized controlled trial comparing Botox with surgical myotomy. In this

trial, patients randomized to receive Botox underwent two sessions of Botox injection within a 1-month period. Both techniques provided similar relief at 6 months. Prolonged follow-up at 2 years revealed that 87.5% of patients in the surgical group remained symptom-free whereas only 34% remained so in the Botox group ($P =$ .05). Previous Botox injections in patients undergoing surgical myotomy can lead to increased difficulty finding and dissecting the submucosal plane and a higher perforation rate.[8,9] Botox treatment should be reserved for patients unable to withstand surgery or unwilling to undergo an invasive procedure.

Pneumatic Dilatation

Pneumatic dilatation is performed under endoscopic or fluoroscopic guidance. The technique involves the inflation of polyethylene balloons, usually starting at 30 mm and progressing stepwise to 35 mm and occasionally to 40 mm. Inflation of the balloon and subsequent stretching of the distal esophagus result in fracture of the LES circular muscle. Patients typically undergo conscious sedation and have the procedure performed as an outpatient. Patients are observed after the procedure for approximately 6 hours to monitor for the reported 2% risk for esophageal perforation.[10] At 1 year, most authors have reported success rates around 70% for pneumatic dilatation. Dobrucali et al.[11] monitored their patients long-term and found that 54% continued to be symptom-free at 5 years. In comparison, Junginger et al.[12] reported on the long-term outcome in patients undergoing surgical myotomy. At a median of 88 months, 96% of the patients reported a very good or good outcome and 92% related no or very rare dysphagia. Similarly, Bonavina et al.[13] observed their Heller myotomy patients for a median of 64 months; 94% related their outcomes as excellent or good. In contrast to Botox injections, previous pneumatic dilatation does not hinder surgical myotomy.[8]

SURGICAL THERAPY

Approach

Before the introduction of minimal access surgery, Heller myotomies were routinely performed via a left thoracotomy. In the early 1990s, as minimally invasive techniques were developed, thoracoscopic cardiomyotomy was first described. The benefits of this minimally invasive technique were decreased postoperative pain and shorter hospital stay without compromise in relief of dysphagia.[14,15] Multiple factors in the mid-1990s led to the change in surgical approach from thoracoscopy to laparoscopy. First, surgeons were performing increased numbers of laparoscopic fundoplications and became more adept at operating on and around the esophagus and hiatus. Second, it became clear that extending the myotomy well onto the stomach was critical to consistent and durable relief of dysphagia.[16] Third, even with limited gastric myotomy, the incidence of postoperative reflux was high with the thoracoscopic approach. Additionally, laparoscopy avoided a double-lumen endotracheal tube and the need for single-lung ventilation and a postoperative chest tube. Multiple studies have affirmed the superiority of laparoscopic Heller myotomy by demonstrating shorter operative times and hospital stay with decreased postoperative dysphagia and reflux in comparison to the thoracoscopic approach.[16-18]

LAPAROSCOPIC HELLER MYOTOMY

Patient Positioning and Preparation

Patients are placed in a modified lithotomy position with a bean bag beneath them and both arms tucked at the sides. The bean bag overhangs the edge of the operative table to allow the formation of a saddle around the patient's perineum. This technique secures the positioning. The operative surgeon stands between the patient's legs with the assistant at the patient's left side. Monitors should be located ergonomically above the patient's head.

Port Placement

Initial access is obtained at the costal margin in the left upper quadrant. After establishing pneumoperitoneum with a Veress needle, a Visiport trocar (United States Surgical Corporation, Norwalk, CT) is inserted near the umbilicus. The abdomen is examined and four working ports are then placed under direct visualization, as shown in Figure 29–2. It is important to note that landmarks change with abdominal insufflation; therefore, port site markings should be performed after insufflation and visually checked intracorporeally to ensure proper reach and ergonomics. The camera port is placed approximately 10 to 12 cm inferior to the left upper quadrant port and 4 cm left of midline. The remaining ports include a 5-mm trocar in the right upper quadrant for the surgeon's left hand, a 10-mm trocar in the left lower quadrant for the assistant's right hand, and a 10-mm

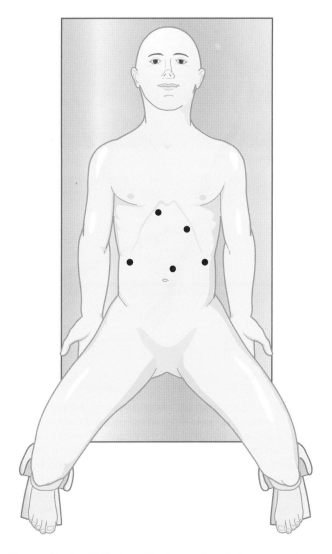

Figure 29–2. Patient positioning and port placement. (From Woltman TA, Oelschlager BK, Pellegrini CA: Achalasia. Surg Clin North Am 85:483-493, 2005, with permission.)

trocar in the right lateral quadrant for a liver retractor. After port placement, the patient is placed in steep reverse Trendelenburg positioning. Our preference for liver retraction is a paddle retractor that can be secured to the operative table with a Bookwalter retractor post and flexible arm (Codman, Raynham, MA). Alternatively, a 5-mm subxiphoid incision can be made and a Nathanson liver retractor (Cook, Bloomington, IN) used. A 10-mm 30-degree angled laparoscope provides superior visualization.

Operative Steps

Our initial approach involves dividing the left phrenoesophageal and phrenogastric ligaments to allow exposure of the left crus. Next, we mobilize the gastric fundus for later fundoplication. An ultrasonic dissector is used to divide the short gastric vessels, beginning at the inferior pole of the spleen and continuing superiorly to the

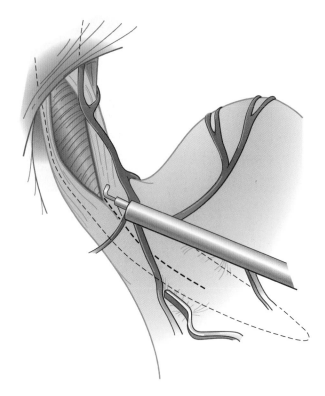

Figure 29–3. Laparoscopic Heller myotomy. A hook cautery is used to divide the outer longitudinal esophageal muscle for exposure of the underlying circular muscle. The *dashed line* in the background represents a lighted bougie in correct placement. A Babcock retractor is placed around the bougie and retracted caudally with slight tension on the esophageal muscle layers. (From Ali A, Pellegrini CA: Laparoscopic myotomy technique and efficacy in treating achalasia. Gastrointest Endosc Clin N Am 11:353, 2001, with permission.)

the esophagus caudally and laterally during hiatal and transmediastinal esophageal mobilization. Before the myotomy can be performed, a clear path must be made across the GE junction. We resect the cardioesophageal fat pad to the left of the anterior vagus nerve and at the same time mobilize the vagus off the esophagus. This allows a straight plane to perform the myotomy.

Essential to performing the myotomy is excellent visualization and exposure. A lighted 52-French bougie is placed in the body of the stomach; it serves to both illuminate the esophagus and muscle layers and provide a stable platform to perform the myotomy. A Babcock retractor is then draped over the bougie at the GE junction and retracted caudally. This motion exposes the anterior of the esophagus and myotomy path, and places the esophageal muscle fibers under slight tension, which aids in their identification and division. The myotomy is begun approximately 3 cm below the GE junction with an L-shaped hook electrocautery device. During the myotomy, electrocautery should be avoided unless absolutely necessary. Individual muscle fibers are divided by hooking them and applying gentle upward traction. Bleeding from the muscle or submucosa is controlled with pressure and time. These steps are important to avoid delayed perforation from unrecognized thermal mucosal injury. The longitudinal muscle fibers are divided first to expose the underlying circular muscle (Fig. 29–3). Once the circular muscles are divided, a mucosal plane is reached with smooth, white, bulging mucosa (Fig. 29–4). This plane is then carried cephalad onto the esophagus for a length of 6 to 8 cm. The entire myotomy therefore spans approximately 9 to 11 cm (3 cm below the GE junction to 6 to 8 cm above the GE junction). The most difficult dissection involves the 3-cm myotomy on the stomach. In this area, the plane of dissection becomes blurred with intervening sling muscular fibers, and the underlying gastric mucosa is thinner, thereby increasing the risk for perforation. Mucosal perforations are repaired with fine (4-0 or 5-0) absorbable monofilament suture and rarely require further intervention. Endoscopy can be used to evaluate the myotomy and check for a missed perforation.

After satisfactory cardioesophageal myotomy, we perform a Toupet fundoplication. The posterior fundus of the stomach is brought around the esophagus and secured to the right crus and the right cut edge of the myotomy. In a similar (in fact mirror image) fashion, the anterior fundus of the stomach is sutured to the left crus and left cut edge of the myotomy (Fig. 29–5). Rarely, patients with large hiatal hernias require curapexy closure of the hiatus. If we have an esophageal perforation, we perform an anterior (Dor) fundoplication to buttress the repair.

previously exposed left crus. The posterior attachments between the proximal part of the stomach and the retroperitoneum are also divided. Once the proximal stomach has been adequately mobilized to permit tension-free fundoplication, attention is turned to the gastrohepatic ligament. An avascular area close to the liver is incised and the incision carried craniad toward the esophageal hiatus to expose the right crus. Care is taken to preserve the nerves of Latarjet and aberrant vessels such as an accessory or replaced left hepatic artery. The anterior phrenoesophageal ligament and peritoneum overlying the anterior abdominal esophagus are divided while being cognizant of the underlying anterior vagus nerve. A posterior esophageal window is created to allow for a Toupet fundoplication. This is accomplished by dissecting to the base of the right crus under the esophagus and finding the confluence of the right and left crura. During this step the posterior vagus should be visualized and protected.

Adequate mediastinal esophageal mobilization is crucial for a long esophageal myotomy and tension-free fundoplication. If necessary, a Penrose drain may be placed around the GE junction and used to retract

Postoperative Management

Typically, patients receive liquids the evening of their operation. They are then advanced to a soft diet and discharged the following day. It is important to treat nausea aggressively with antiemetics. Patients are advised to avoid strenuous activity and heavy lifting for 4 to 6 weeks.

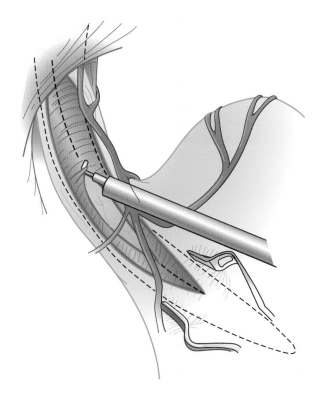

Figure 29–4. Laparoscopic Heller myotomy. Division of the inner circular muscle layer reveals the bulging underlying esophageal mucosa. Note the long length of the myotomy both distally onto the stomach and proximally on the esophagus. (From Ali A, Pellegrini CA: Laparoscopic myotomy technique and efficacy in treating achalasia. Gastrointest Endosc Clin N Am 11:353, 2001, with permission.)

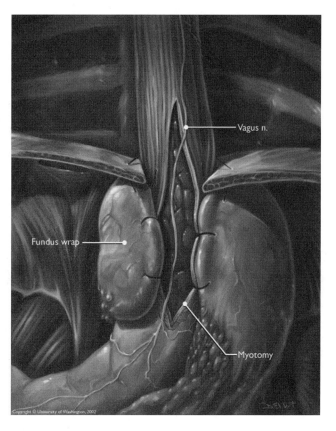

Figure 29–5. Completed laparoscopic Heller myotomy with posterior (Toupet) fundoplication. (Courtesy of the University of Washington, Seattle, with permission.)

A majority of patients resume normal activities within 1 to 2 weeks and a regular diet in 2 to 6 weeks.

CONTROVERSIES

Length of the Myotomy

The exact length and dimensions of the esophageal myotomy have been a source of debate. Multiple authors have shown a correlation between relief of dysphagia and length of myotomy carried onto the stomach. We first noted this association in our thoracoscopic group of patients in whom the myotomy extended 0.5 cm onto the gastric wall. The rate of persistent dysphagia was 27% as a result of the incomplete myotomy.[16] A critical flaw in the thoracoscopic approach is its inherent inability to perform an extended distal myotomy onto the stomach. Therefore, we switched our technique to a laparoscopic approach and incorporated a myotomy carried out 1 to 1.5 cm on the gastric wall. This additional length of myotomy distally decreased the postoperative dysphagia rate to 11%.[16] Similarly, Ramacciato et al.[19] compared outcomes in patients treated with thoracoscopic and laparoscopic Heller myotomy. In their study, myotomies

were carried onto the stomach for a distance of 1 cm in the thoracoscopic group and 2 cm in the laparoscopic group. They found that the thoracoscopic group had significantly more dysphagia than the laparoscopic group did (37.5% versus 5.8%, respectively, $P = .04$). Additionally, the median postoperative basal LES pressure was 15.5 mm Hg in the thoracoscopic group and 10.5 mm Hg in the laparoscopic group ($P = .0001$).

In 1998, our group hypothesized that postoperative dysphagia could be further decreased with an extended myotomy carried 3 cm distal to the GE junction. We compared outcomes in extended myotomy patients and those undergoing a short myotomy 1 to 1.5 cm onto the gastric wall. Our data clearly showed that an extended myotomy resulted in significantly less severity and frequency of postoperative dysphagia than a short myotomy did ($P = .001$ for both).[20] The frequency of postoperative heartburn, regurgitation, and chest pain was no different in patients with either an extended or short myotomy ($P = .36$, $P = .19$, $P = .71$, respectively). Additionally, postoperative 24-hour pH studies demonstrated no difference in proximal or distal esophageal acid exposure between extended and short myotomy ($P = .55$ and $P = .96$, respectively). These studies highlight the shortcomings of the thoracoscopic approach and importance of an extended distal myotomy.

Antireflux Procedure

Whether an antireflux procedure should be performed at the time of a Heller myotomy has been the most controversial surgical issue in the treatment of achalasia. Such is no longer the case; with few exceptions, an antireflux procedure should be performed. Performing a cardiomyotomy, in the vast majority of cases, renders the primary barrier to gastroesophageal reflux (GER) ineffective. Thus, a partial fundoplication that does not inhibit bolus transit from the aperistaltic esophagus into the stomach but diminishes GER would seem intuitive.

It has been shown that patients with achalasia have decreased esophageal chemoreceptors and therefore do not sense acid reflux as much as normal subjects do.[21] This is probably the reason for the low frequency of postoperative GER reported by patients treated with Heller myotomy and no antireflux procedure. Although the GER remains silent to the patient, continuous acid exposure of the esophagus can lead to peptic strictures, Barrett's esophagus, and esophageal cancer.[4] Proponents of cardiomyotomy without fundoplication cite their shorter operative times, diminished risk of causing dysphagia, and ease with which GER can be treated with modern acid-suppression medication.

We and others have long since said that an antireflux procedure was necessary to reduce the high rate of GER and could be done without increasing the rate of dysphagia.[12,13,16,18] Until recently, only meta-analysis and nonrandomized studies were available to base one's decisions. Richards et al.,[22] previous objectors to the need for an antireflux procedure, recently published the only prospective randomized double-blind study specifically addressing whether an antireflux procedure is necessary. In their study, 43 patients were randomized to undergo Heller myotomy alone or Heller myotomy plus Dor fundoplication. The addition of an antireflux procedure to Heller myotomy clearly decreased the incidence of GER (ninefold) without increasing the rate of dysphagia. In a comparison of the two groups, the incidence of pathologic GER was 47.6% in the Heller-only group and 9.1% in the Heller-plus-Dor group ($P = .005$). Distal esophageal acid exposure was significantly greater in the Heller group than in the Heller-plus-Dor group, 4.9% versus 0.4%, respectively ($P = .001$). The median postoperative LES pressure was 13.7 mm Hg in the Heller group and 13.9 mm Hg in the Heller-plus-Dor group. Subjectively, patients undergoing Heller-only and Heller-plus-Dor procedures reported similar decreases in the median dysphagia score (9 versus 8, $P = .79$). There are now few surgeons who do not perform an antireflux procedure after myotomy.

Fundoplication Technique

Because of the aperistaltic esophagus in achalasia patients, a complete 360-degree wrap is typically avoided. A majority of surgeons perform either an anterior (Dor) or a posterior (Toupet) 270-degree fundoplication. The advantage of the Dor fundoplication is its technical ease because it avoids extensive gastric mobilization and is able to buttress small mucosal perforations created during myotomy. A Toupet fundoplication inherently splays the myotomy edges apart, which theoretically prevents fibrosis between them and recurrent dysphagia. A small nonrandomized study showed that patients undergoing Toupet fundoplication had less postoperative reflux than did patients undergoing Dor fundoplication.[18] It is the authors' choice to perform a Toupet fundoplication for these advantages, although until a good randomized control trial comparing Dor with Toupet fundoplication is performed, this controversy will continue.

Sigmoid-Shaped Esophagus or Megaesophagus

Megaesophagus represents end-stage achalasia because the combination of an aperistaltic esophagus and failure of LES relaxation leads to progressive esophageal dilatation and lengthening with time (see Fig. 29–1C).[23] Previously, it was suggested that patients with megaesophagus be treated by esophagectomy rather than myotomy,[24-26] the rationale being that dilated, elongated, and often tortuous aperistaltic esophagi do not empty sufficiently to improve dysphagia, even when the LES is disrupted. As a result of the drastic decrease in morbidity with minimally invasive approaches, many surgeons have elected to attempt a myotomy first. Recently, two studies have demonstrated good postoperative results in patients with megaesophagus treated by Heller myotomy. The obvious advantage of a Heller myotomy is avoidance of the morbidity and mortality associated with esophagectomy. Patti et al.[27] performed laparoscopic Heller myotomy on patients who had a dilated esophagus (>6 cm) with a straight-axis configuration and a sigmoid-shaped configuration. They reported no increased difficulty in performing the surgery, no increase in complications, and excellent relief of dysphagia in both groups. Overall, 92% of patients in the study reported an excellent or good postoperative outcome. Likewise, Mineo and Pompeo[28] studied 14 patients with a sigmoid esophagus treated with a Heller myotomy. With a median follow-up of 85 months, excellent or good results were reported by 72%, and no patient required an esophagectomy. Postoperative dysphagia and regurgitation scores decreased significantly ($P = .002$ and $P = .001$, respectively) and were equivalent to postoperative scores from a nondilated esophagus group undergoing Heller myotomy. Health-related quality of life evaluated with a Short Form-36 questionnaire indicated statistically improved general health, social function, and mental health. Interestingly, esophageal width was found to narrow with time, on average 10 mm in 24 months.

COMPLICATIONS

Early complications are fortunately uncommon and include intraoperative esophageal perforation, pneumothorax, bleeding, intra-abdominal abscess, and wound infection. The esophageal perforation rate has been reported to be between 0% and 7% in most major studies.[22,29] Once identified, perforations are repaired by reapproximating the esophageal mucosa and buttressing the repair with an anterior (Dor) fundoplication. The Dor fundoplication is created by positioning the gastric fundus over (anterior to) the myotomy and perforation site. The fundus of the stomach is secured with sutures to the right and left crura, as well as the transected edges of the esophageal myotomy (Fig. 29–6).

Other complications occur in less than 3% of cases.[30] Pneumothorax typically develops when a rent is made in the pleura during mediastinal esophageal mobilization. If identified intraoperatively, the pleural defect may be primarily repaired with a suture or, if small, an endoclip. Rarely does the pneumothorax cause respiratory or circulatory embarrassment. If physiologic problems do occur, a majority resolve by decreasing the insufflation pressure to less than 10 mm Hg; if unsuccessful, a tube thoracostomy may be required. An asymptomatic pneumothorax discovered on a postoperative chest radiograph should be treated with oxygen supplementation via nasal cannula or face mask. These pneumothoraces resolve quickly because the carbon dioxide is rapidly absorbed by the body.

Late complications include recurrent dysphagia and GER. Postoperative dysphagia may be due to incomplete myotomy, perihiatal scarring, progressive dysmotility of the esophagus, peptic stricture, and obstructing tumor. Work-up of these patients should include esophagography, endoscopy, and repeat manometry. The most likely reason for recurrence of dysphagia is incomplete myotomy. As stated previously, we have found that extended myotomy significantly reduces postoperative dysphagia without increased GER.[20] Zaninotto et al.[31] reported on their experience with the development of dysphagia after laparoscopic Heller myotomy. Of 113 patients studied, 10 (8.8%) were considered surgical failures because of recurrent dysphagia or chest pain. Postoperative testing (performed on nine patients) identified that seven patients failed because of an incomplete myotomy distally, one for an incomplete myotomy proximally, and one as a result of megaesophagus, with the last cause being unknown. All patients underwent endoscopic pneumatic dilatation with 35- or 40-mm balloons inflated to a median of 6 psi for 1 minute. Seventy-eight percent of patients experienced complete resolution of their dysphagia or chest pain. The remainder underwent redo surgical myotomy. Likewise, Patti et al.[32] found that a majority of their postoperative failures were due to incomplete myotomy. These studies demonstrate that postoperative dysphagia is most likely due to incomplete myotomy and further support our group's advocacy of extended myotomy. Persistent dysphagia after surgery should first be approached with endoscopic dilatation and, if this fails, redo surgery.

As discussed earlier, symptomatic GER is rare in patients after Heller myotomy. However, if patients undergoing Heller myotomy without fundoplication are studied postoperatively, a significant amount will have pathologic acid reflux. Although it typically remains clinically silent, it does predispose the patient to Barrett's

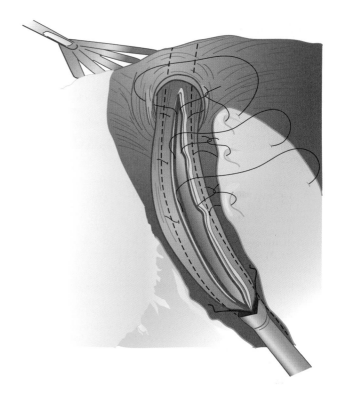

Figure 29–6. Laparoscopic Heller myotomy with anterior (Dor) fundoplication. The anterior fundus is sutured to the myotomy edges and both crura. (From Yim APC, Hazelrigg SR, Izzat MB, et al [eds]: Minimal Access Cardiothoracic Surgery. Philadelphia, WB Saunders, 2000, p 258.)

esophagus, peptic strictures, and cancer. It is therefore imperative that measures to minimize GER be implemented whether it is symptomatic or not. As discussed earlier, the most effective method of reducing GER is to perform a fundoplication in conjunction with myotomy. Six months after surgery, we study all patients with a 24-hour pH monitor to detect asymptomatic GER. Patients found to have abnormal esophageal acid exposure are placed on a regimen of proton pump inhibitors and monitored.

SUGGESTED READINGS

Oelschlager BK, Chang L, Pellegrini CA: Improved outcome after extended gastric myotomy for achalasia. Arch Surg 138:490-495, discussion 495-497, 2003.

Richards WO, Torquati A, Holzman MD, et al: Heller myotomy versus Heller myotomy with Dor fundoplication for achalasia: A prospective randomized double-blind clinical trial. Ann Surg 240:405-412, discussion 412-405, 2004.

Zaninotto G, Costantini M, Portale G, et al: Etiology, diagnosis, and treatment of failures after laparoscopic Heller myotomy for achalasia. Ann Surg 235:186-192, 2002.

REFERENCES

1. Goldblum JR, Rice TW, Richter JE: Histopathologic features in esophagomyotomy specimens from patients with achalasia. Gastroenterology 111:648-654, 1996.
2. Raymond L, Lach B, Shamji FM: Inflammatory aetiology of primary oesophageal achalasia: An immunohistochemical and ultrastructural study of Auerbach's plexus. Histopathology 35:445-453, 1999.
3. Mearin F, Mourelle M, Guarner F, et al: Patients with achalasia lack nitric oxide synthase in the gastro-oesophageal junction. Eur J Clin Invest 23:724-728, 1993.
4. Sandler RS, Nyren O, Ekbom A, et al: The risk of esophageal cancer in patients with achalasia. A population-based study. JAMA 274:1359-1362, 1995.
5. Bortolotti M, Mari C, Lopilato C, et al: Effects of sildenafil on esophageal motility of patients with idiopathic achalasia. Gastroenterology 118:253-257, 2000.
6. Eherer AJ, Schwetz I, Hammer HF, et al: Effect of sildenafil on oesophageal motor function in healthy subjects and patients with oesophageal motor disorders. Gut 50:758-764, 2002.
7. Zaninotto G, Annese V, Costantini M, et al: Randomized controlled trial of botulinum toxin versus laparoscopic Heller myotomy for esophageal achalasia. Ann Surg 239:364-370, 2004.
8. Patti MG, Feo CV, Arcerito M, et al: Effects of previous treatment on results of laparoscopic Heller myotomy for achalasia. Dig Dis Sci 44:2270-2276, 1999.
9. Horgan S, Hudda K, Eubanks T, et al: Does botulinum toxin injection make esophagomyotomy a more difficult operation? Surg Endosc 13:576-579, 1999.
10. Vaezi MF, Richter JE: Current therapies for achalasia: Comparison and efficacy. J Clin Gastroenterol 27:21-35, 1998.
11. Dobrucali A, Erzin Y, Tuncer M, Dirican A: Long-term results of graded pneumatic dilatation under endoscopic guidance in patients with primary esophageal achalasia. World J Gastroenterol 10:3322-3327, 2004.
12. Junginger T, Kneist W, Sultanov F, Eckardt VF: [Long-term outcome of myotomy and semi-fundoplication in achalasia.] Chirurg 73:704-709, 2002.
13. Bonavina L, Nosadini A, Bardini R, et al: Primary treatment of esophageal achalasia. Long-term results of myotomy and Dor fundoplication. Arch Surg 127:222-226, discussion 227, 1992.
14. Pellegrini CA, Leichter R, Patti M, et al: Thoracoscopic esophageal myotomy in the treatment of achalasia. Ann Thorac Surg 56:680-682, 1993.
15. Pellegrini CA: Esophageal surgery by the thoracoscopic approach. Semin Thorac Cardiovasc Surg 5:305-309, 1993.
16. Patti MG, Pellegrini CA, Horgan S, et al: Minimally invasive surgery for achalasia: An 8-year experience with 168 patients. Ann Surg 230:587-593, discussion 593-584, 1999.
17. Stewart KC, Finley RJ, Clifton JC, et al: Thoracoscopic versus laparoscopic modified Heller myotomy for achalasia: Efficacy and safety in 87 patients. J Am Coll Surg 189:164-169, discussion 169-170, 1999.
18. Raiser F, Perdikis G, Hinder RA, et al: Heller myotomy via minimal-access surgery. An evaluation of antireflux procedures. Arch Surg 131:593-597, discussion 597-598, 1996.
19. Ramacciato G, Mercantini P, Amodio PM, et al: The laparoscopic approach with antireflux surgery is superior to the thoracoscopic approach for the treatment of esophageal achalasia. Experience of a single surgical unit. Surg Endosc 16:1431-1437, 2002.
20. Oelschlager BK, Chang L, Pellegrini CA: Improved outcome after extended gastric myotomy for achalasia. Arch Surg 138:490-495, discussion 495-497, 2003.
21. Brackbill S, Shi G, Hirano I: Diminished mechanosensitivity and chemosensitivity in patients with achalasia. Am J Physiol Gastrointest Liver Physiol 285:G1198-G1203, 2003.
22. Richards WO, Torquati A, Holzman MD, et al: Heller myotomy versus Heller myotomy with Dor fundoplication for achalasia: A prospective randomized double-blind clinical trial. Ann Surg 240:405-412, discussion 412-405, 2004.
23. Shiino Y, Houghton SG, Filipi CJ, et al: Manometric and radiographic verification of esophageal body decompensation for patients with achalasia. J Am Coll Surg 189:158-163, 1999.
24. Devaney EJ, Lannettoni MD, Orringer MB, Marshall B: Esophagectomy for achalasia: Patient selection and clinical experience. Ann Thorac Surg 72:854-858, 2001.
25. Peters JH, Kauer WK, Crookes PF, et al: Esophageal resection with colon interposition for end-stage achalasia. Arch Surg 130:632-636, discussion 636-637, 1995.
26. Pinotti HW, Cecconello I, da Rocha JM, Zilberstein B: Resection for achalasia of the esophagus. Hepatogastroenterology 38:470-473, 1991.
27. Patti MG, Feo CV, Diener U, et al: Laparoscopic Heller myotomy relieves dysphagia in achalasia when the esophagus is dilated. Surg Endosc 13:843-847, 1999.
28. Mineo TC, Pompeo E: Long-term outcome of Heller myotomy in achalasic sigmoid esophagus. J Thorac Cardiovasc Surg 128:402-407, 2004.
29. Bloomston M, Durkin A, Boyce HW, et al: Early results of laparoscopic Heller myotomy do not necessarily predict long-term outcome. Am J Surg 187:403-407, 2004.
30. Martins P, Morais BB, Cunha-Melo JR: Postoperative complications in the treatment of chagasic megaesophagus. Int Surg 78:99-102, 1993.
31. Zaninotto G, Costantini M, Portale G, et al: Etiology, diagnosis, and treatment of failures after laparoscopic Heller myotomy for achalasia. Ann Surg 235:186-192, 2002.
32. Patti MG, Molena D, Fisichella PM, et al: Laparoscopic Heller myotomy and Dor fundoplication for achalasia: Analysis of successes and failures. Arch Surg 136:870-877, 2001.

Diffuse and Segmental Esophageal Spasm, Nutcracker Esophagus, and Hypertensive Lower Esophageal Sphincter

Tasha A. K. Gandamihardja · Cedric G. Bremner

This group of spastic conditions usually first comes to medical attention because of a history of chest pain, dysphagia, or both and often challenges the clinician with respect to making a correct diagnosis and initiating effective treatment. The cause and mechanism of the abnormalities remain unknown, but there has been progress in their management. Although radiologic investigation may suggest the diagnosis of a motility disorder, esophageal manometry, endoscopy, and pH testing are essential to give a precise appraisal of the problem.

DIFFUSE AND SEGMENTAL ESOPHAGEAL SPASM

Diffuse and segmental esophageal spasms are rare conditions. They are characterized by symptoms of substernal pain, dysphagia, or both; the radiographic appearance of localized, nonprogressive swallow responses (tertiary contractions); and an increased incidence of nonperistaltic contractions recorded on intraluminal manometry. The condition was first described by Osgood in 1889 as esophagismus.[1] In 1967, Fleshler described the syndrome of diffuse esophageal spasm (DES) as a clinical syndrome.[2] The chest pain or dysphagia may be precipitated by the ingestion of hot or cold foods, or it may occur spontaneously. Chest pain may be the predominant symptom and is sometimes indistinguishable from cardiac-type pain. Dysphagia may be less pronounced and intermittent in occurrence. This difference in symptomatology

separates esophageal spasm from achalasia, where dysphagia usually predominates.

The etiology of esophageal spasm is unclear. It has been suggested that the esophagus of patients with DES produces a hypersensitive response to cholinergic and hormonal stimulation, probably mediated by neural dysfunction.[3] A genetic link has also been proposed. The basic motor abnormality is a rapid progression of esophageal contractions down the esophagus without the normal latency gradient.

Investigations

Endoscopy Endoscopic examination is necessary to exclude an associated hiatal hernia or esophagitis.

Radiology Radiologic investigations may be normal in patients with DES and thus do not exclude the diagnosis. A variety of radiologic appearances have been described, such as "corkscrew" or rosary-bead esophagus (Fig. 30–1), segmental spasm, and pseudodiverticulosis, but in most cases the diagnosis is not obvious. Spasm may cause compartmentalization of the esophagus with resulting epiphrenic or midesophageal diverticula. Incomplete or absent primary peristalsis and mild to severe tertiary contractions have been described in about 70% of patients.[4] Impaired LES opening has also been reported.[5]

Manometry Manometry is essential for the diagnosis of esophageal spasm (Table 30–1). The criteria for

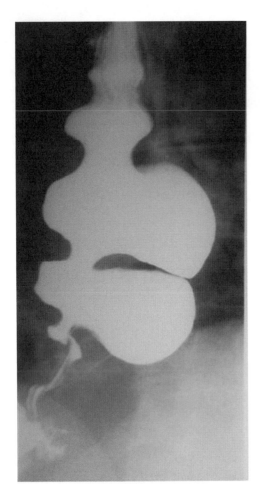

Figure 30–1. "Corkscrew esophagus" seen on a barium study of a patient who complained of dysphagia and chest pain.

diagnosis require that simultaneous swallow responses be present in at least three fifths of the esophageal body in 20% or more of wet swallows (Fig. 30–2).[6] It is important to appreciate that in esophageal spasm, the esophagus retains a degree of peristaltic contractions whereas in achalasia, there is no peristalsis. Because of this "misnomer," a plea has been made to describe the condition as "distal" esophageal spasm.[7] Furthermore, although DES has also been described as a motility disorder characterized by high-amplitude contractions, such contractions are not seen frequently. In one study, associated manometric features were repetitive (>3 peaks) contractions in 67% of subjects, high-amplitude contractions in 33%, spontaneous activity in 22%, prolonged duration of contractions in 11%, and LES abnormalities in 5%.[8] Other classic manometric findings include simultaneous multipeaked and repetitive responses to swallows (see Table 30–1).

Standard stationary esophageal manometry may, however, fail to detect the spasms, whereas ambulatory manometry may be more successful.[9]

Simultaneous contractions can occur in other diseases, such as achalasia, gastroesophageal reflux disease (GERD), diabetes, alcoholism, and connective tissue diseases. These conditions need to be ruled out before embarking on any possible surgical procedure.

pH Studies   Many patients with manometric findings of DES describe symptoms of gastroesophageal reflux. Some argue that the esophageal spasm in these patients is a consequence of acid exposure,[10] whereas others have argued that the aperistaltic nature of the esophagus causes poor clearance and hence retention of acid.[6] Reflux-induced and idiopathic DES cannot be differentiated on manometric features alone. Differentiation between GERD and DES may be based on the persistence of chest pain and dysphagia while the patients are taking acid-suppression therapy. Thus, in this group of patients, combined pH monitoring with simultaneous ambulatory

Table 30–1   Manometric Features of Primary Esophageal Motility Disorders

Disorder	Lower Esophageal Sphincter	Esophageal Body
Diffuse esophageal spasm	May be abnormal	>20% simultaneous contractions
		Other features may be present:
		Repetitive (>2 peaks) contractions
		Prolonged duration
		Spontaneous contractions
		High-amplitude contractions
		Intermittent normal peristalsis
Nutcracker esophagus	May be hypertensive	High-amplitude contractions (mean >180 mm Hg)
		Other features may be present:
		Prolonged duration (mean >6 sec)
		Normal peristaltic progression
Hypertensive lower esophageal sphincter	Baseline elevated (>27 mm Hg)	Normal peristaltic progression
	Normal relaxation or mild elevation of residual pressure	Ramp bolus pressure may be increased distally

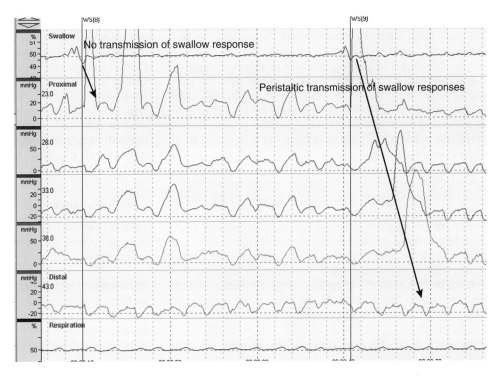

Figure 30–2. Manometric recording in a patient with diffuse esophageal spasm. The first swallow resulted in simultaneous swallow responses seen in the five channels, which are each 5 cm apart in the body of the esophagus. The second swallow, however, resulted in a normal peristaltic response. More than 20% simultaneous contractions with intermittent peristaltic contractions is required for the diagnosis of diffuse esophageal spasm.

24-hour esophageal motility studies may help differentiate the two conditions.

Treatment

Medical treatment of DES includes the use of muscle relaxants such as calcium channel blockers and nitrates. Psychosomatic treatment with antidepressants has been proposed as an effective mode of treatment because anxiety and depression have been found to be prevalent in this group of patients.[3] The use of endoscopically administered botulinum toxin provides initial symptom relief; however, repeated injections are usually necessary.[11] Medical treatment is generally geared toward symptom control, and the results are variable.

Surgery focuses on the mechanical dysfunction aspect of the condition, where bolus transit down the esophagus is restricted because of the presence of a functional obstruction resulting from simultaneous contractions as well as decreased muscle compliance.

Ambulatory motility studies performed during meals in patients with symptoms of dysphagia have shown that an association exists between increased simultaneous waveforms and decreased contraction amplitude of peristaltic waves. It has been shown that the presence of 75% or more simultaneous waveforms on ambulatory motility studies during meals is a good indication for surgical myotomy.[6] The presence of chest pain alone is not a sufficient indication for myotomy. Myotomy of the esophageal body relieves dysphagia by reducing the amplitude of esophageal contractions and the frequency of simultaneous, double-peaked and multipeaked, high-amplitude and long-duration contractions.[6]

The extent of the myotomy should be predetermined from the preoperative manometry study. The upper limit

of the myotomy is still a contentious issue among surgeons. To minimize outflow resistance, the lower limit usually extends distally across the lower esophageal sphincter (LES). This, however, eliminates the role of the sphincter as an antireflux barrier, and as a result an antireflux procedure needs to be performed to prevent reflux of stomach contents into the esophagus. A complete fundoplication will offer too much resistance (about 20 mm Hg) to esophageal emptying, and thus partial fundoplications have been preferred. A Dor or a modified Belsey procedure has been found to improve eating ability and significantly reduce the severity of chest pain, dysphagia, heartburn, and regurgitation.[6,12-14] In one study a Toupet fundoplication was reported to provide better relief from postoperative dysphagia.[15]

These procedures can now be carried out thoracoscopically or laparoscopically.

NUTCRACKER ESOPHAGUS

Nutcracker esophagus is a condition first described in 1979.[16] The majority of patients have chest pain, although dysphagia and symptoms of GERD may also be reported. The chest pain may be difficult to distinguish from cardiac pain, just as with DES. These patients are therefore often seen first by a cardiologist to rule out a cardiac cause before further referral. It is difficult to differentiate various esophageal motility disorders on the basis of symptoms alone, and thus further investigations are warranted.

The condition is characterized by high-amplitude peristaltic contractions in the distal end of the esophagus, with peak amplitudes greater than 2 SD above normal values recorded in individual laboratories (i.e., greater than 180 mm Hg), or a prolonged duration of contractions (or both).[17] The term "super squeezer" has also been used to describe the esophagus in this condition.

The etiology and pathogenesis of nutcracker esophagus is unclear. A few reports have documented the progression of nutcracker esophagus to achalasia, thus raising the question of whether it may be an abnormality occurring early in a spectrum of motility disorders that ends with achalasia.[18,19] Patients have been noted to have higher levels of somatization, anxiety, and depression, similar to those with esophageal spasm and irritable bowel syndrome. The similarities in symptoms suggest a possible generalized functional disorder in these patients.

Patients with nutcracker esophagus and chest pain have been found to have a low threshold for pain when their symptoms are reproduced by balloon distention. Furthermore, the esophageal reactivity to balloon distention is higher in these patients than in controls. The hypersensitivity and stiffness of the esophagus may play a role in the pathogenesis of chest pain in this condition.[20]

Recently, it has been suggested that gastroesophageal reflux may play an important role in the pathogenesis of nutcracker esophagus. A study found that 70% of patients with nutcracker esophagus had increased esophageal acid exposure with esophagitis and a positive symptom index.[21] The majority of patients with nutcracker esophagus and chest pain, however, did not have classic reflux symptoms. Among the patients who did suffer from GERD symptoms, 76% either improved after acid-suppression therapy or were symptom-free at an average of 10.7 months' follow-up. The authors concluded that patients with nutcracker esophagus may represent a subgroup of patients with acid reflux different from that in other reflux patients, given the lack of typical GERD symptoms. An important note, however, is that in this study nutcracker esophagus was defined as manometric contractions greater than 180 mm Hg at any level of the esophagus, rather than just the distal level used by the conventional definition.

Investigations

Endoscopy Endoscopic examination is necessary to rule out associated pathology such as hiatal hernia and esophagitis.

Radiology Barium studies are invariably normal. Occasionally, hiatal hernias are detected.

Manometry Manometry is essential for the diagnosis of nutcracker esophagus. Contraction amplitudes must exceed 2 SD above normal values determined for individual laboratories, be present in the two distal channels, and be peristaltic in waveform (Fig. 30–3). Other features seen in nutcracker esophagus include a prolonged duration of contractions (Fig. 30–4)[17] and a hypertensive sphincter, both of which are not required for the diagnosis.

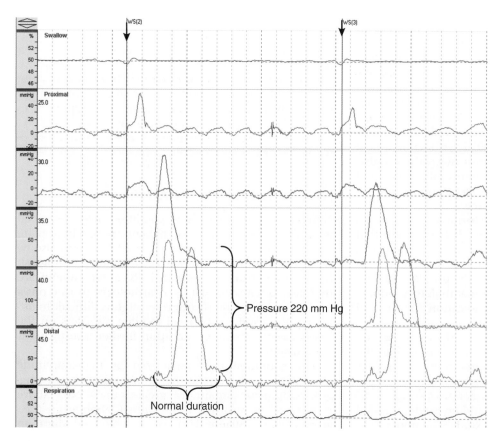

Figure 30–3. Manometric features of a nutcracker esophagus. High-amplitude, peristaltic responses to wet swallows were recorded in the distal three channels, which are each 5 cm apart. Contractions are of normal duration.

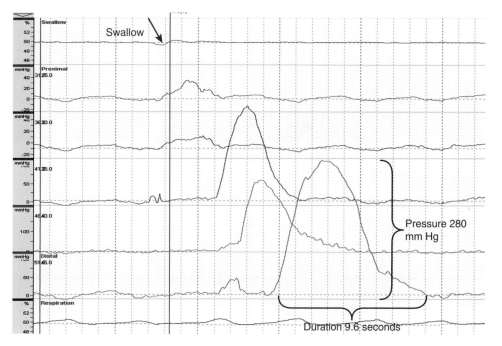

Figure 30–4. Nutcracker esophagus. On wet swallows, high-amplitude contractions are seen in the distal two channels (>180 mm Hg). The responses also have a prolonged duration (>6 seconds).

Of interest, when patients with nutcracker esophagus are monitored, changes in their manometric features may be seen. In one follow-up study, more than 50% of patients with nutcracker esophagus retained the initial manometric diagnosis and 33% had a change to segmental high-amplitude contractions.[17] Manometric changes to those typical of other esophageal motility disorders, such as DES and achalasia, and even to normal tracings have also been reported.[18,22-24]

Treatment

Medical treatment has produced variable results. The calcium channel blocker nifedipine has been shown to decrease esophageal contraction amplitude, but without associated improvement in symptoms,[25] whereas diltiazem has been shown to improve symptoms.[26]

Sildenafil, an inhibitor of phosphodiesterase type 5, has recently been shown to be a potential alternative treatment of nutcracker esophagus. It promotes guanosine 3′,5′-cyclic monophosphate accumulation, which then phosphorylates other intracellular signaling molecules to stimulate either smooth muscle relaxation or reduction in muscle excitability.[27] Sildenafil has been shown to decrease LES pressure and the amplitude of distal esophageal peristaltic pressure responses to swallows. However, the reduction in resting pressure was of short duration, which may limit the usefulness of this treatment.

Based on the high prevalence of GERD in patients with nutcracker esophagus, gastroesophageal reflux rather than an esophageal motility disorder has been suggested to be the cause of the chest pain experienced by patients. A recent double-blind, placebo-controlled, crossover study using the proton pump inhibitor lansoprazole as a means of acid-suppression therapy did not, however, produce significantly better pain relief than placebo did. Furthermore, no motility pattern change was seen during the study.[28] The role of acid in the pathogenesis of nutcracker esophagus needs further investigation.

Surgical treatment of nutcracker esophagus should therefore be undertaken with caution. A long myotomy performed because of the presence of chest pain and the finding of high-amplitude peristaltic contractions may aggravate the symptoms by rendering the esophagus aperistaltic. The chest pain may not be relieved, and dysphagia may result from the aperistalsis after the myotomy.

The observation that many patients improve with time has suggested a stress-related or psychological phenomenon playing a role in the pathogenesis of symptoms in these patients.

HYPERTENSIVE LOWER ESOPHAGEAL SPHINCTER

Hypertensive lower esophageal sphincter (HLES) is a primary motility disorder that was first described in 1960 by Code et al.[29] This condition is uncommon and, in order of frequency in our laboratory, is second to achalasia.

Typically, patients have symptoms of dysphagia (37% to 100%) and chest pain (33% to 100%).[30-36] These patients may also have the classic GERD symptoms of heartburn, regurgitation,[31,36] and epigastric pain.[30] In addition, it has been noted that patients with HLES have more of a nervous predisposition and display higher levels of anxiety and somatization.[1,35]

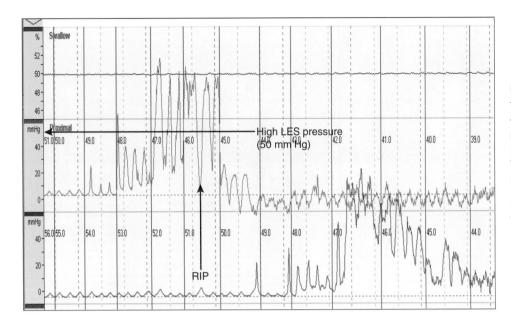

Figure 30–5. Manometric features of a hypertensive lower esophageal sphincter (LES). A pressure of 50 mm Hg was recorded in this stationary pull-through study of the LES. The pressure was measured at the midrespiratory phase at the respiratory inversion point (RIP). The upper limit of pressure at this point is 26 mm Hg.

Investigation

A thorough investigation is required to assist in the diagnosis of HLES.

Radiology Barium esophagography studies are either normal or demonstrate slight narrowing at the gastroesophageal junction.[35] Both upper gastrointestinal endoscopic studies and radionuclide solid esophageal emptying studies[37] are reported to be typically normal.

Manometry Esophageal manometry is essential for the diagnosis of this condition. HLES is characterized manometrically by the following:

- An elevated resting pressure in the LES that exceeds the upper limit of normal measured in a series of volunteers (Fig. 30–5). In Dr. DeMeester's laboratory at the University of Southern California, the upper limit of normal is 26 mm Hg, whereas in Dr. Castell's laboratory, it is 45 mm Hg.[38]
- Normal peristalsis of the esophageal body, thus distinguishing it from achalasia and DES.
- Incomplete LES relaxation (62% in our series),[31] although previously reported to be normal (Figs. 30–6 and 30–7).
- Increase in intrabolus pressure in the body of the esophagus. This, together with the presence of residual relaxation pressure (incomplete relaxation), suggests outflow obstruction.[31]

pH Studies Gastroesophageal reflux can occur in the presence of a hypertensive sphincter,[32,37] and approximately 25% of patients with HLES have been shown to have a positive 24-hour pH test. Transient LES relaxations are thought to be the cause of this paradoxical phenomenon.

The association between HLES and GERD is unclear, although fewer reflux episodes and a significantly lower total and supine percentage of time with the pH lower than 4 have been shown to occur in GERD patients with HLES than in those with symptoms of GERD alone.[30,37] Accordingly, the presence of HLES in patients with GERD may offer a protective barrier against refluxate and prevent the development of advanced grades of esophagitis.

Thus, to rule out GERD, pH studies are essential in patients with HLES.

Treatment

Treatment of HLES remains controversial. Previously, both medical and surgical options have focused mainly on reducing LES pressure. Medical drugs as the first line of symptomatic treatment have included the use of muscle relaxants such as calcium channel blockers, nitroglycerin, and nifedipine, with Botox injections and pneumatic dilatation reserved for resistant cases. However, the results of these treatment modalities are variable and often short-lived.

The recent demonstration of gastroesophageal acid reflux in patients with HLES has now challenged physicians to modify treatment modalities to suit individual needs. When HLES patients have GERD symptoms together with an abnormal ambulatory pH score, acid reflux therapy has been found to be effective therapy.[31,36] For the few nonresponders, an antireflux operation has been reported to result in a successful outcome. Nissen fundoplication performed in patients with HLES and GERD/type III hiatal hernia has been shown in one study to relieve symptoms of chest pain and dysphagia in all of the patients studied, with a good or excellent outcome in 81% of patients.[39]

On the other hand, when HLES is present without evidence of gastroesophageal reflux, LES myotomy with partial fundoplication has been shown to be effective

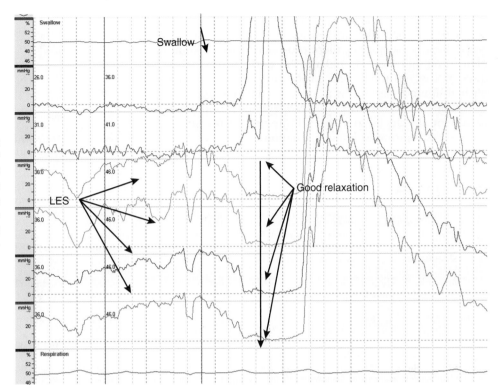

Figure 30–6. Swallow study in a lower esophageal sphincter (LES) that is hypertensive. LES pressure is recorded in channels 3 to 6, which are all at the same level in the sphincter. The sphincter relaxes to baseline during swallowing, thus confirming complete relaxation.

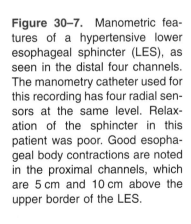
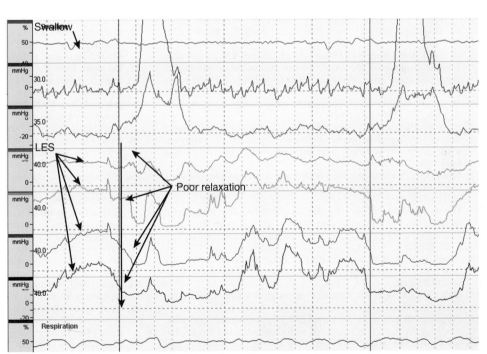

Figure 30–7. Manometric features of a hypertensive lower esophageal sphincter (LES), as seen in the distal four channels. The manometry catheter used for this recording has four radial sensors at the same level. Relaxation of the sphincter in this patient was poor. Good esophageal body contractions are noted in the proximal channels, which are 5 cm and 10 cm above the upper border of the LES.

therapy,[39,40] thus supporting a possible primary sphincter dysfunction. Because these patients have normal esophageal body motility, there is no reason why a complete fundoplication should not be performed at the time of the myotomy. This procedure is now accomplished in most patients by a laparoscopic approach.

Patients with HLES are a heterogeneous group, and treatment should be guided by both clinical investigations and symptoms at initial evaluation.

REFERENCES

1. Dalton CB, Castell DO, Hewson EG, et al: Diffuse esophageal spasm (DES): A rare motility disorder not characterized by high amplitude contractions. Dig Dis Sci 36:1025-1028, 1991.
2. Fleshler B: Diffuse esophageal spasm. Gastroenterology 52:559-564, 1967.
3. Clouse RE: Psychopharmacologic approaches to therapy for chest pain of presumed esophageal origin. Am J Med 92:106s-113s, 1992.
4. Chen YM, Oh DJ, Herson EG, et al: Diffuse esophageal spasm: Radiographic and manometric correlation. Radiology 170:807-810, 1989.
5. Prabhakar A, Levine MS, Rubesin S, et al: Relationship between diffuse esophageal spasm and lower esophageal sphincter dysfunction on barium studies and manometry in 14 patients. Am J Radiol 183:409-413, 2004.
6. Eypasch EP, DeMeester TR, Klingman RR, Stein HJ: Physiological assessment and surgical management of diffuse esophageal spasm. J Thorac Cardiovasc Surg 104:859-869, 1992.
7. Sperandino M, Tutuian R, Gideon RM, et al: Diffuse esophageal spasm: Not diffuse but distal esophageal spasm (DES). Dig Dis Sci 48:1380-1384, 2003.
8. Bassotti G, Pelli MA, Morelli A: Clinical and manometric aspects of diffuse esophageal spasm in a cohort of subjects evaluated for dysphagia and/or chest pain. Am J Med Sci 300:148-151, 1990.
9. Stein HJ, DeMeester TR, Eyspach EP, Klingman RR: Ambulatory 24-hour esophageal manometry in the evaluation of esophageal motor disorders and non-cardiac chest pain. Surgery 110:753-763, 1991.
10. Stuart RC, Hennesy TPJ: Primary disorders of esophageal motility. Br J Surg 76:1111-1120, 1989.
11. Storr M, Allescher HD, Rosch T, et al: Treatment of symptomatic diffuse esophageal spasm by endoscopic injections of botulinum toxin: A prospective study with long-term follow-up. Gastrointest Endosc 54:754-759, 2001.
12. Ellis FH Jr: Esophagomyotomy for non-cardiac chest pain resulting from diffuse esophageal spasm and related disorders Am J Med 92:129-131, 1992.
13. Henderson RD, Ryder D, Maryatt G: Extended esophageal myotomy and short total fundoplication hernia repair in diffuse esophageal spasm: Five-year review in 34 patients. Ann Thorac Surg 43:25-31, 1987.
14. Nastos D, Chen L-Q, Ferraro P, et al: Long myotomy with antireflux repair for esophageal spastic disorders. J Gastrointest Surg 6:713-722, 2002.
15. McBride PJ, Hinder RA, Filipi C, et al: Surgical treatment of spastic conditions of the esophagus. Int Surg 82:113-118, 1997.
16. Benjamin SB, Gerhardt DC, Castell DO: High amplitude, peristaltic esophageal contraction associated with chest pain and/or dysphagia. Gastroenterology 77:478-483, 1979.
17. Allen M, DiMarino AJ: Manometric diagnosis of diffuse esophageal spasm. Dig Dis Sci 41:1346-1349, 1996.
18. Anggiansah A, Bright NF, McCullagh M, Owen WJ: Transition from nutcracker esophagus to achalasia. Dig Dis Sci 35:1162-1166, 1990.
19. Paterson WG, Beck IT, Da Costa LR: Transition from nutcracker esophagus to achalasia: A case report. J Clin Gastroenterol 13:554-558, 1991.
20. Mujica VR, Mudipall RS, Rao SS: Pathophysiology of chest pain in patients with nutcracker esophagus. Am Gastroenterol 96:1371-1377, 2004.
21. Borjessen M, Pilhall M, Rolny P, Mannheimer C: Gastroesophageal acid reflux in patients with nutcracker esophagus. Scand J Gastroenterol 36:916-920, 2001.
22. Achem SR, Kolts BE, Burton L: Segmental versus diffuse nutcracker esophagus: An intermittent motility pattern. Am J Gastroenterol 88:847-851, 1993.
23. Narducci F, Bassotti G, Gaburri M, Morelli A: Transition from nutcracker esophagus to diffuse esophageal spasm. Am J Gastroenterol 80:242-244, 1985.
24. Traube M, Aaronson RM, McCallum RW, et al: Transition from peristaltic esophageal contractions to diffuse esophageal spasm. Arch Intern Med 146:1844-1846, 1986.
25. Richter J, Dalton CB, Bradely L, Castell DO: Oral nifedipine in the treatment of non-cardiac chest pain in patients with the nutcracker esophagus. Gastroenterology 93:21-28, 1987.
26. Richter JE, Spurling TJ, Cordova CM, et al: Effects of oral calcium blocker, diltiazem, on esophageal contractions. Studies in volunteers and patients with nutcracker esophagus. Dig Dis Sci 29:649-656, 1984.
27. Lee JI, Park H, Kim JH, et al: The effect of sildenafil on esophageal motor function in healthy subjects and patients with nutcracker esophagus. Neurogastroenterol Motil 15:617-623, 2003.
28. Borjessen M, Rolny P, Mannheimer C, Pilhall M: Nutcracker oesophagus: A double-blind, placebo-controlled, cross-over study of the effects of lansoprazole. Aliment Pharmacol Ther 18:1129-1135, 2003.
29. Code CF, Schlegel JF, Kelly ML, et al: Hypertensive gastroesophageal sphincter. Proc Mayo Clin 35:391-399, 1960.
30. Bassotti G, Alunni G, Cocchieri M, et al: Isolated hypertensive lower esophageal sphincter. Clinical and manometric aspects of an uncommon esophageal motor abnormality. J Clin Gastroenterol 14:285-287, 1992.
31. Gockel I, Lord RV, Bremner CG, et al: The hypertensive lower esophageal sphincter: A motility disorder with manometric features of outflow obstruction. J Gastrointest Surg 7:692-700, 2003.
32. Bremner CG: The hypertensive lower esophageal sphincter. In Stipa S, Belsey RHR, Moraldi A (eds): Medical and Surgical Problems of the Esophagus. No. 43 [Proceedings of the Sereno Symposium]. New York, Academic Press, 1981, pp 241-245.
33. Katada N, Hinder RA, Hinder PR, et al: The hypertensive lower esophageal sphincter. Am J Surg 172:439-442, 1996.
34. Pederson SA, Alstrup P: The hypertensive gastroesophageal sphincter. A manometric and clinical study. Scand J Gastroenterol 7:531-534, 1972.
35. Waterman DC, Dalton CB, Ott DJ, et al: Hypertensive lower esophageal sphincter: What does it mean? J Clin Gastroenterol 1:139-146, 1989.
36. Katzka DA, Sidhu M, Castell DO: Hypertensive lower esophageal sphincter pressures and gastroesophageal reflux: An apparent paradox that is not unusual. Am J Gastroenterol 90:280-284, 1995.
37. Sullivan SN: The supersensitive hypertensive lower esophageal sphincter. Precipitation of pain by small doses of intravenous pentagastrin. J Clin Gastroenterol 8:619-623, 1986.
38. Castell DO, Richter JE: The Esophagus, 3rd ed. Philadelphia, Lippincott Williams & Wilkins, 1999, p 216.
39. Tamhankar AP, Almogy G, Arain MA, et al: Surgical management of hypertensive lower esophageal sphincter with dysphagia or chest pain. J Gastrointest Surg 7:990-996, 2003.
40. Champion JK, Delisle N, Hunt T: Laparoscopic esophagomyotomy with posterior partial fundoplication for primary esophageal motor disorders. Surg Endosc 14:746-749, 2000.

Surgical Management of Esophageal Diverticula

Luigi Bonavina

Esophageal diverticula are epithelial-lined protrusions of the gut wall that remain in continuity with the lumen. They can occur at any level from the pharynx to the cardia and are generally acquired. An anatomic classification consisting of three categories (pharyngoesophageal, midesophageal, epiphrenic) is most commonly adopted, although the classic Rokitanski classification (pulsion and traction) still provides useful clues to the pathogenesis. Most esophageal diverticula are of the pulsion type and lack a muscular coat ("false" diverticula). Only midesophageal diverticula are of the traction type and have been considered "true" diverticula because they contain all layers of the esophageal wall. It has long been speculated that esophageal motor abnormalities are involved in the pathogenesis of diverticula, but the evidence remains inconclusive. Management of esophageal diverticula is dictated by the main clinical manifestations, most commonly dysphagia and regurgitation. Respiratory symptoms frequently occur in elderly patients, even in the absence of esophageal complaints, and require surgical therapy to prevent life-threatening episodes of aspiration.

PHARYNGOESOPHAGEAL (ZENKER'S) DIVERTICULUM

Pathophysiology

Toward the end of the 19th century, Zenker[1] formulated the hypothesis that a pharyngoesophageal diverticulum is caused by increased hypopharyngeal pressure producing herniation through an area of structural weakness, specifically, the junction of the inferior pharyngeal constrictor and the cricopharyngeus muscle, also known as Killian's triangle. Subsequent radiologic observations of a posterior indentation below the neck of the sac led to application of the term *cricopharyngeal achalasia*,[2] although manometric studies of patients with Zenker's diverticulum have often shown normal upper esophageal sphincter relaxation. Later, a reflex spasm of the cricopharyngeus muscle caused by presumed gastroesophageal reflux was implicated in the pathogenesis of the diverticulum.[3] An incoordination between pharyngeal and cricopharyngeal activity, with temporal premature contractions of the upper esophageal sphincter, was demonstrated by several investigators.[4-8] Other studies have focused on degeneration of the cricopharyngeal muscle,[9-12] with interstitial fibrosis being the main histologic finding.

Recent studies support the hypothesis that fibrosis of the cricopharyngeal muscle impairs upper esophageal sphincter opening by decreasing wall compliance. The reduced opening causes increased hypopharyngeal bolus pressure to compensate for the decreased cross-sectional area and maintain trans-sphincteric flow, and it can lead to the formation of a pulsion diverticulum through the weak Killian's triangle. Cook and colleagues[13] compared patients with Zenker's diverticulum and control subjects via simultaneous videoradiography and manometry. They were able to document significantly reduced sphincter opening and greater intrabolus pressure in patients with Zenker's diverticulum. They concluded that the primary abnormality in patients with Zenker's diverticulum is incomplete upper esophageal sphincter opening rather than abnormal coordination between pharyngeal contraction and upper esophageal sphincter relaxation or opening.

Thus, the act of swallowing in the presence of cricopharyngeal dysfunction, combined with the usual pressure phenomena during deglutition, is believed to generate sufficient transmural pressure to allow mucosal herniation (pulsion diverticulum) through an anatomically weak point in the posterior of the pharynx above the cricopharyngeus muscle. Because of the recurrent nature of the pressure involved and the constant distention of the sac with ingested material, the diverticulum progressively enlarges and descends toward the posterior and left lateral side of the neck.[14] Selective filling of the sac may compress and angulate the adjacent esophagus anteriorly. These anatomic changes obstruct swallowing. Moreover, because the neck of the diverticulum is above the cricopharyngeus, spontaneous emptying of the diverticulum is unimpeded and often associated with laryngotracheal aspiration, as well as pharyngo-oral regurgitation.

Symptoms and Diagnosis

Although a pharyngoesophageal diverticulum may be asymptomatic, symptoms develop early in the course of the disease in most patients. Once the pouch is established, it progresses in size (Figs. 31–1 and 31–2) and severity of symptoms and complications. Symptoms consist of cervical esophageal dysphagia, noisy deglutition, halitosis, and spontaneous regurgitation with or without coughing or choking episodes. The regurgitated food is characteristically undigested. If the condition is neglected, weight loss, hoarseness, asthma, respiratory insufficiency, and pulmonary infection leading to abscess are all potential complications. A gurgling mass may be appreciated in the left cervical region. The main complications of Zenker's diverticulum are nutritional and respiratory. Carcinoma arising in a pharyngoesophageal diverticulum is extremely uncommon.[15] Perforation of the diverticulum may occur after esophagoscopy, attempts at tracheal intubation, or accidental ingestion of a foreign body.

The diagnosis is confirmed by radiographic barium swallow with lateral views, which demonstrate posterior outpouching of the hypopharyngeal wall. Manometry is of little clinical value. Upper gastrointestinal endoscopy is useful to measure the longitudinal extension of the pouch and to exclude the presence of associated foregut disorders. However, the endoscopist should be warned of the possibility of a pharyngoesophageal diverticulum because of the risk for instrumental perforation. If passage of the endoscope under direct vision is unsuccessful, a guidewire can be inserted under fluoroscopic control through the esophageal inlet and the endoscope can be gently pushed over the instrument.

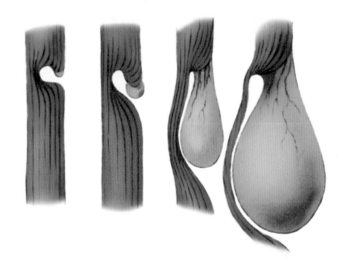

Figure 31–1.   Evolution of a pharyngoesophageal diverticulum from small to large. Note the prominence of the cricopharyngeus muscle within the spur between the esophagus and diverticulum.

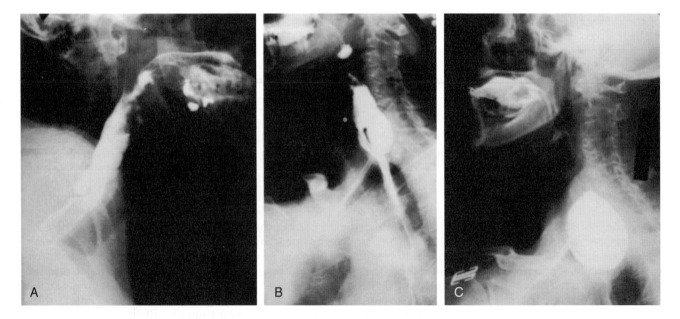

A   B   C

Figure 31–2.   Radiographic appearance of various sizes of pharyngoesophageal diverticula. **A,** Small. **B,** Moderate. **C,** Large. (**A** and **C** From Payne WS: Diverticula of the esophagus. In Payne WS, Olsen AM [eds]: The Esophagus. Philadelphia, Lea & Febiger, 1974; **B** from Payne WS, Clagett OT: Pharyngeal and esophageal diverticula. Curr Probl Surg 23:1-31, 1965.)

Treatment

Treatment of Zenker's diverticulum is indicated, regardless of its size, to relieve the disabling symptoms of oropharyngeal dysphagia and pharyngo-oral regurgitation and to prevent the life-threatening complication of aspiration pneumonia. The tendency of the pouch to progressively enlarge and the possible, though rare development of squamous cell carcinoma represent additional arguments in favor of early treatment.[15] Treatment is best done on an elective basis while the pouch is small or of moderate size and before complications have occurred. Advanced age is not a contraindication to surgical treatment. A recent review of patients 75 years or older who underwent surgical treatment of Zenker's diverticulum demonstrated an improvement rate of 94% with no operative death.[16] However, the nutritional status and respiratory condition of elderly patients with severe dysphagia and repetitive hypoxic episodes of aspiration are of special concern; in such circumstances, nutritional support and respiratory physiotherapy may be indicated before proceeding with surgical therapy. It has long been postulated that gastroesophageal reflux is common in patients with Zenker's diverticulum and that priority should be given to surgical correction of the reflux to prevent postoperative aspiration.[17] In most circumstances, medical treatment with proton pump inhibitors is effective for the treatment of mild degrees of gastroesophageal reflux, thus allowing the surgeon to proceed primarily with treatment of the diverticulum when the main complaint is obstructive dysphagia. If necessary, however, an antireflux repair can safely be performed during the same operative session.

Evolution of Current Management

Treatment of Zenker's diverticulum has evolved through a better understanding of the underlying pathophysiology of the disease. Surgical attempts to treat a disorder of the pharyngoesophageal junction date back to the past century, when Nicoladoni established a fistula to empty a Zenker diverticulum of its contents.[18] The first successful diverticulum resection was performed by Wheeler in 1885. This procedure was subsequently abandoned because of a high rate of leakage from the suture line and was replaced by a complicated two-stage operation to allow a more controlled salivary fistula. However, by the 1950s, almost all surgical therapy for Zenker's diverticulum used the one-stage technique of primary resection and closure.[19] Although the addition of cricopharyngeal myotomy to resection of the diverticulum had first been proposed by Aubin in 1936, it was not recognized until a few decades later that correction of the functional obstruction caused by the upper esophageal sphincter is an important component of the surgical procedure.[20] The objective documentation of increased intrabolus pressure resulting from inadequate sphincter opening[13] has strengthened the opinion of most esophageal surgeons that cricopharyngeal myotomy, alone or combined with resection or suspension of the diverticulum,[7] is an essential part of the surgical procedure irrespective of the presence of a manometric abnormality. Myotomy alone can be sufficient to treat small diverticula,[21] whereas myotomy combined with resection of the diverticulum has become the technique of choice for diverticula larger than 2 cm.[22]

An endoscopic approach to Zenker's diverticulum was first attempted almost a century ago by Mosher.[23] He divided the septum between the esophagus and the pouch with punch forceps, but this procedure was soon abandoned. The concept of endoscopically creating a common cavity between the esophagus and the pouch was restored to favor by Dohlman and Mattsson,[24] who introduced diathermy, and by van Overbeek,[25] who introduced laser treatment. Recent developments in minimally invasive surgery have led to the use of linear endoscopic stapling devices to suture and then divide the septum formed by the opposing walls of the esophagus and the diverticulum, a procedure that appears to be simpler and safer than electrocoagulation or laser therapy.[26,27]

Methods and Results of Surgical Therapy

The operation can be performed under general or locoregional anesthesia.[28] The patient is positioned supine on the operating table with a small pillow under the shoulders. The head is hyperextended and turned slightly to the right side. The neck is draped from the chin to below the clavicles. An oblique skin incision centered at the level of the cricoid cartilage is made along the anterior border of the left sternocleidomastoid muscle. The subcutaneous tissue and platysma are divided with cautery. The pharynx and cervical esophagus are exposed by retracting the sternocleidomastoid and carotid sheath laterally and the larynx and thyroid gland medially. Care is taken to not injure the recurrent laryngeal nerve, which runs in the tracheoesophageal groove. The diverticulum can be recognized as arising from the posterior wall of the pharynx at a point just above the level where the omohyoid muscle crosses the incision (Fig. 31–3). The pouch is grasped with Duval forceps and retracted cephalad. The loose connective tissue surrounding the diverticulum is carefully dissected to identify its neck on the posterior pharyngeal wall. The transverse fibers of the cricopharyngeal muscle can be identified just below the neck of the diverticulum. At this point, a right-angle forceps can be used to develop a dissection plane inferiorly between the muscularis and the mucosa, and the myotomy is performed with a No. 15 blade or curved scissors. Most sacs smaller than 2 cm simply disappear after the myotomy (Fig. 31–4). For diverticula between 2 and 4 cm, the myotomy is initiated at the neck of the diverticulum and extended inferiorly for about 4 cm (Fig. 31–5A). Simultaneously, a small peanut dissector is used to retract the muscle borders laterally. The diverticulum can be transected by the cut-and-sew technique and the mucosal defect closed with interrupted 4-0 PDS or Biosyn sutures. Larger diverticula should be resected with a TA stapling device, which improves the speed and safety of closure (see Fig. 31–5B and C). A 36-French bougie or an endoscope can be left

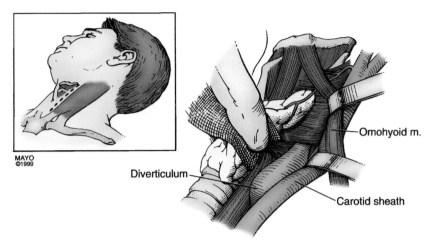

Figure 31–3. Surgical exposure of the retropharyngeal space is gained through an oblique left cervical incision oriented along the anterior border of the sternomastoid muscle *(inset)*. Retraction of the sternomastoid and carotid sheath laterally and the thyroid, pharynx, and larynx medially provides the necessary exposure of the diverticulum, which is located at a cervical level where the omohyoid crosses the surgical field. (Note that the omohyoid has been retracted cephalad to show the diverticulum.) (© Mayo Clinic, 1999.)

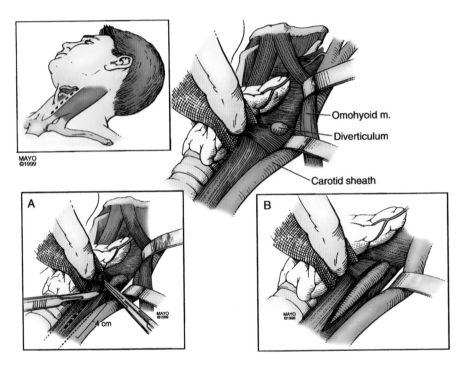

Figure 31–4. After connective tissue is dissected from the mucosal sac to identify the defect in the posterior pharyngeal wall, a posterior midline extramucosal myotomy is performed with a scalpel from the neck of the small sac inferiorly for a distance of 4 cm **(A)**. After retraction of the edges of the cut muscle with a peanut dissector, an almond-shaped diffuse bulge of mucosa through the myotomy is seen **(B)**. After the myotomy, the small diverticulum disappears. (© Mayo Clinic, 1999.)

in place to prevent narrowing of the lumen while the stapling device is applied. A the end of the operation, a standard nasogastric tube is applied, and a Penrose drain is placed in the retropharyngeal space.

A diatrizoate meglumine (Gastrografin) contrast study is performed the following day, and if satisfactory, the diet is resumed. The drain is removed 48 hours after the operation and the patient discharged home on the third postoperative day. If evidence of a mucosal leak is found on the radiographic study or if signs of excessive wound drainage develop, the drain is left in place, and the patient is fed nothing by mouth for 7 to 10 days. If repeat radiographs show persistent leakage, a central venous access is inserted and parenteral nutrition started to restore a positive nitrogen balance. Within 2 weeks it is usually possible, with either fistula sealing or a well-established drainage tract, to begin oral feeding. The

drain can be eventually removed with the expectation that the fistula will close spontaneously.

The results of the one-stage pharyngoesophageal diverticulectomy have been highly satisfactory. More than 800 patients were treated at the Mayo Clinic by this means, and the operative mortality rate was 1.4%.[19] The chief complications were recurrent nerve palsy (2.8%) and salivary fistula (2.5%). Generally, these complications clear spontaneously in a matter of days or weeks. In a 5- to 14-year follow-up of 164 patients, Welsh and Payne[29] found that 93% either were asymptomatic or had such rare and mild symptoms that they could be classified as having an excellent (82%) or a good (11%) result. Only 11 (7%) of the 164 had poor results, with or without anatomic recurrence, and required additional treatment. More recently, cricopharyngeal myotomy has been incorporated with equally satisfactory results. Late follow-up

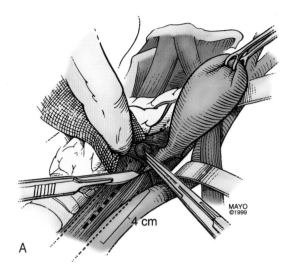

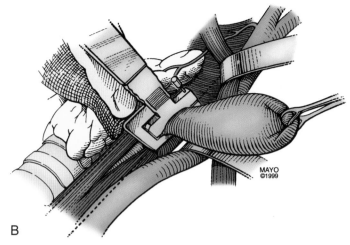

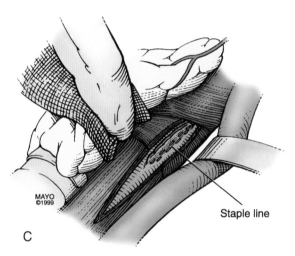

Figure 31–5. One-stage pharyngoesophageal diverticulectomy with myotomy. This procedure is used for the management of medium and large diverticula. **A,** A medium diverticulum is exposed through a left cervical incision as for a myotomy alone. Note that the omohyoid has been retracted cephalad and that a finger is used to retract the thyroid, rather than a metal instrument, to avoid injury to the recurrent nerve. The diverticulum has been dissected out to its neck, and its apex is held cephalad; with a 36-French catheter in the esophagus, an extra-mucosal myotomy is completed with the scalpel for a distance of 4 cm. **B,** Depending on the size of the diverticulum, a TA-15, TA-30, or TA-55 stapling device is selected. Most require a TA-30 with 4.8-mm staples. **C,** Note that the staple line is oriented along the long axis of the esophagus and that an indwelling 36-French esophageal catheter is used to prevent stenosis and minimize the length of any luminal narrowing. The mucosal closure is left uncovered. Drainage and closure are accomplished as for a myotomy alone. (© Mayo Clinic, 1999.)

results of Payne and Reynolds[30] show little change in the incidence of late pouch recurrence. Any radiographic recurrence was less likely to be symptomatic if the initial diverticulectomy was accompanied by myotomy. A similar outcome with no postoperative mortality, minimal morbidity, and very good to excellent results in 96% of patients has been reported in Europe.[22,31]

Two reviews on reoperation for recurrent pharyngoesophageal diverticula have clearly indicated an increased risk for early postoperative morbidity.[32,33] Reoperation on the upper esophageal sphincter can be a technical challenge because previous surgery often results in obliterated tissue planes and friable esophageal mucosa. The use of an indwelling bougie is particularly helpful, both as a landmark for the esophagus and as a stent over which the repair can be accomplished without fear of entering the esophageal lumen.[34]

Methods and Results of Endoscopic Therapy

The operation is routinely performed under general endotracheal anesthesia. The surgeon sits behind the

patient's head. The hypopharynx is entered with a modified Weerda diverticuloscope (Storz), which is gently pushed under vision behind the endotracheal tube. The instrument is held in place with a scope holder and a chest support (Fig. 31–6). A 5-mm wide-angle 0-degree telescope is inserted and connected to a cold-light source and to a videocamera to obtain a magnified view of the operative field on a television screen. The two self-retracting valves of the diverticuloscope, which can be approximated and angulated to fit the patient's hypopharyngeal anatomy, are then allowed to enter the diverticulum and the esophageal lumen, respectively. The septum between the esophagus and the diverticulum is therefore centered in the operative field. The longitudinal extension of the diverticulum can be checked with a graduated rod. This maneuver also allows the pouch to be straightened and the common wall to be elongated. A linear stapling device (ETS35, Ethicon Endo-Surgery) is used to divide the septum. The anvil is placed in the lumen of the diverticulum and the cartridge of staples in the lumen of the cervical esophagus. The instrument jaws are placed across the septum along the midline before firing (Fig. 31–7). With a single application of the endostapler, the

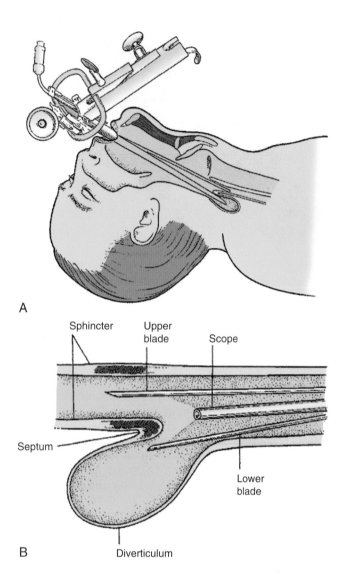

A

Sphincter   Upper blade   Scope

Septum

Lower blade

B   Diverticulum

Figure 31–6. **A,** Position of the Weerda diverticuloscope. **B,** Visualization of the septum interposed between the esophagus and diverticulum.

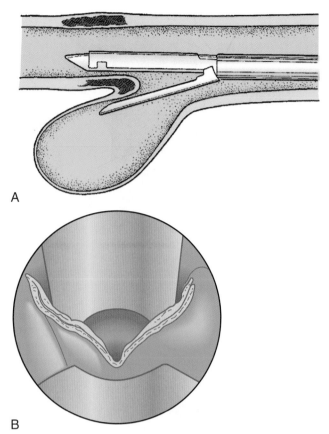

A

B

Figure 31–7. **A,** Suture and section of the septum with a linear endostapler. **B,** Frontal view of the divided septum. A common cavity has been created.

posterior esophageal wall is sutured to the wall of the diverticulum, and the tissue is transected between three rows of staples on each side. Multiple stapler applications may be necessary, depending on the size of the diverticulum. Coagulating endosurgical scissors may be used to complete the section at the distal end of the staple line. After removal of the stapler, the two wound edges retract laterally because of division of the cricopharyngeal muscle (see Fig. 31–7). Finally, the suture line is checked for hemostasis. The procedure requires a few minutes, and a nasogastric tube is not necessary. A Gastrografin swallow study is performed on the first postoperative day. The patient is then allowed to drink and eat and is discharged from the hospital 24 hours after surgery.

When compared with the conventional surgical operation, advantages of the endosurgical approach include absence of a skin incision, shorter operative time, minimal or absent postoperative pain, quicker resump-

tion of oral feeding, and shorter hospital stay. An additional advantage of this technique may be expected in patients who had undergone surgery in the left side of the neck or who have a recurrent diverticulum after a conventional operation.[35] In such circumstances, the conventional operation may pose a major technical challenge to the surgeon and is associated with a high risk for leakage or recurrent nerve palsy. On the other hand, the endoscopic approach may prove impossible in patients in whom neck hyperextension is limited and in those with reduced opening capacity of the mouth. Dental injury may occur as a result of difficult handling of the diverticuloscope in this setting. The best indication for the endosurgical technique is a medium-sized diverticulum 3 to 6 cm in length in which at least two staple cartridges can be applied and an adequate cricopharyngeal myotomy can be expected. A diverticulum smaller than 2 cm is a formal contraindication to the endosurgical approach because the common wall is too short to accommodate one cartridge of staples and allow complete division of the sphincter. This would result in an incomplete myotomy with persistent dysphagia.[36]

No prospective clinical trials have compared the endosurgical with the conventional surgical approach for the management of Zenker's diverticulum. Data from retrospective series or prospectively recorded case series consistently show that a satisfactory outcome is obtained in 96% of patients undergoing the endosurgical operation, with a 6% recurrence or persistence rate.[37] However, a retrospective comparison of endoscopic treatment with the stapler or laser against open surgery showed that only 75% of patients treated endoscopically were symptom-free at follow-up, as opposed to 97% of patients who underwent open surgery.[38]

EPIPHRENIC DIVERTICULUM

Pulsion diverticula can develop at any level of the esophageal body but have a predilection for the distal 10 cm. Epiphrenic diverticula generally project from the right posterior wall of the esophagus. The ratio of epiphrenic to pharyngoesophageal diverticula is 1 to 3.[39] However, the exact prevalence of this condition is unknown because asymptomatic cases are not usually discovered. Most epiphrenic diverticula are found in middle-aged or elderly patients, and male patients have a slight preponderance. Multiple diverticula can occur in up to 20% of cases.

Pathophysiology

With the advent of manometric studies, it has become evident that functional obstruction of the distal end of the esophagus may be not only the cause of the diverticulum but also a major cause of symptoms. Achalasia, diffuse esophageal spasm, hypertensive lower esophageal sphincter, and nonspecific motor abnormalities have all been seen in as many as two thirds of patients with epiphrenic diverticula.[40] It is inferred that increased motor activity and abnormal lower esophageal sphincter relaxation produce zones of increased intraluminal pressure through which outpouchings occur.[41-44] Therefore, the concept that epiphrenic diverticula are complications of esophageal motility disorders rather than primary anatomic abnormalities has gained widespread acceptance.

Symptoms and Diagnosis

The symptoms most commonly reported in patients with epiphrenic diverticula are dysphagia and regurgitation. Dysphagia is sometimes associated with esophageal obstruction. Regurgitation of indigested food is characteristically of large volume, frequently occurs at night, and is often precipitated by a change in position. Retrosternal pain or heartburn, or both, can be reported, and it may be difficult to determine whether these complaints are related to the motor disorder, the diverticulum itself, or coexisting gastroesophageal reflux disease. Pulmonary complications from aspiration occur in 24% to 45% of patients,[45,46] but this phenomenon is probably underestimated. Conversely, many patients with epiphrenic diverticula do not have definite symptoms. The diverticulum is often an incidental finding on barium swallow performed for unrelated reasons. Complications such as ulceration, bleeding, and spontaneous

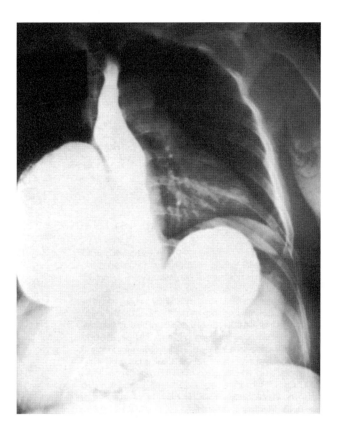

Figure 31–8.   Esophagus with a huge epiphrenic diverticulum occupying about half of the right thorax. Note the associated sliding esophageal hiatal hernia. (From Payne WS: Esophageal diverticula. In Shields TW [ed]: General Thoracic Surgery, 3rd ed. Philadelphia, Lea & Febiger, 1983, p 859.)

perforation are rare and may be due to caustic pills lodging in the pouch. Primary squamous cell carcinoma has been noted with epiphrenic diverticula, as have rare benign neoplasms, particularly leiomyoma.[39]

The diagnosis of epiphrenic diverticulum is established by a barium swallow study. The diverticulum appears as a round structure with a diameter of 1 to 5 cm (Fig. 31–8). Giant diverticula are rarely seen but can be larger than 10 cm. Patients with incapacitating symptoms should be further studied by esophagoscopy and esophageal manometry. Esophagoscopy allows evaluation of the mucosa for the presence of esophagitis and is also of value to detect associated lesions such as carcinoma, stricture, or hiatal hernia. In addition, the size and position of the diverticular neck can be precisely assessed, and this may be relevant if a laparoscopic surgical approach is planned. Esophageal manometry is crucial to assess the presence of an underlying motility disorder. The manometric findings may help determine the length of esophagomyotomy required to relieve the functional obstruction. Twenty-four-hour ambulatory motility testing can be helpful if the results of standard manometry are normal or indefinite.[45] If gastroesophageal reflux is suspected, a 24-hour pH study can also be performed to evaluate esophageal acid exposure. If not confirmed, the symptoms thought to be related to reflux may be caused by other conditions,

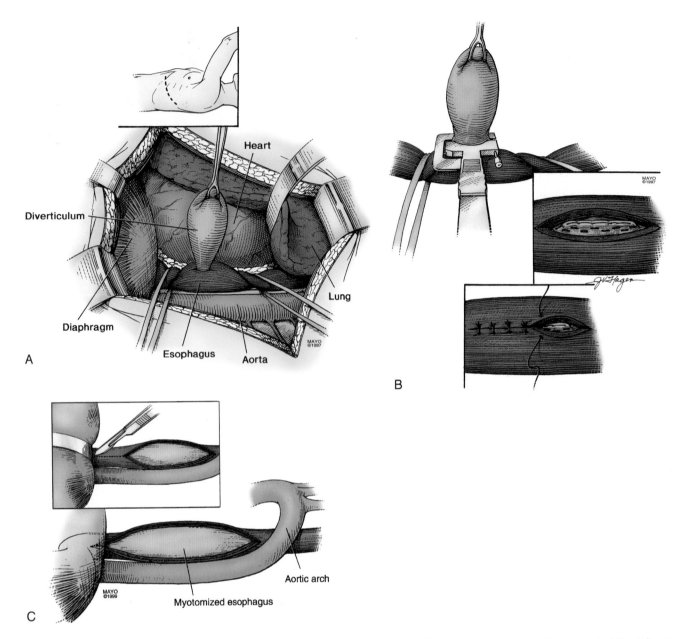

Figure 31–9. Surgical management of a pulsion diverticulum of the lower portion of the esophagus. Placement of the left posterolateral thoracotomy incision is shown in the *inset.* Exposure of the diverticulum is obtained when the chest is entered through the bed of the unresected left eighth rib. Note that the esophagus has been delivered from its mediastinal bed, tape has been passed around the esophagus, and the esophagus has been rotated to bring the diverticulum into view. The neck of the mucosal diverticulum has been dissected to identify the defect in the esophageal muscular wall **(A).** A TA stapling device is used to transect and close the diverticulum, followed by closure of the esophageal musculature over a mucosal suture line **(B).** The site of the diverticular incision has been rotated back to the right and is not visible. A long esophagomyotomy extending from the esophagogastric junction to the aortic arch has been performed. The musculature of the esophagus has been freed from about 50% of the circumference of the esophageal mucosal tube to allow the mucosa to bulge through the muscular incision **(C).** (© Mayo Clinic, 1999.)

such as abnormal motility or regurgitation of diverticular contents.

Treatment

Most patients with epiphrenic diverticula are asymptomatic and do not require treatment. Simple medical measures often provide good temporary control in mildly symptomatic patients. Benacci and associates,[47] reporting a series of 112 patients, described the natural history of the condition in a group of 47 asymptomatic individuals who did not undergo surgical therapy. Twenty of these patients were monitored for a median of 4 years (range, 1 to 17 years), and all remained symptom-free. Fifteen additional patients had mild symptoms without surgical intervention, and in none of them did incapac-

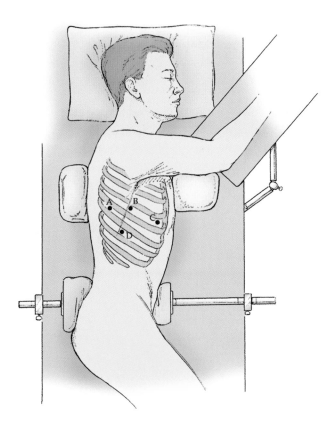

Figure 31–10. Port position for thoracoscopic resection of an esophageal diverticulum.

itating symptoms develop during follow-up (median, 11 years; range, 1 to 25 years). Although only half the patients with asymptomatic or mildly symptomatic disease had long-term follow-up available for review, progressive symptoms or complications did not develop in any of them. Therefore, patients with minimal symptoms should be managed conservatively and monitored at regular intervals. Neither size nor dependent location of the diverticulum usually correlates with symptoms. If symptoms are incapacitating or recurrent respiratory complications from aspiration are reported or suspected, surgical therapy is mandatory. Most esophageal surgeons agree that the ideal operation should include diverticulectomy, myotomy, and an antireflux repair. Streitz et al. have advocated selective use of myotomy in patients with documented motor abnormalities.[48]

Methods and Results of Surgical Therapy

The standard surgical technique consists of a diverticulectomy in conjunction with a long extramucosal esophagomyotomy, preferably through a left transthoracic approach (Fig. 31–9). The sac is mobilized and the diverticulectomy is performed longitudinally over an endoluminal bougie with a linear stapling device. The muscular wall is usually closed over the diverticular stump. An esophagomyotomy is performed not only to prevent suture line rupture and recurrence of the pouch

but also to relieve symptoms from the underlying motor disorder. The esophagomyotomy is performed opposite the site of the diverticulectomy and should be carried onto the stomach for a few millimeters. Controversy persists regarding whether all patients undergoing an esophagomyotomy should have a concomitant antireflux procedure. When preoperative gastroesophageal reflux or hiatal hernia is present, a modified Belsey Mark IV fundoplication should be performed.[49]

A reasonable alternative to the conventional operation is an epiphrenic diverticulectomy performed through either a thoracoscopic or a laparoscopic approach. The right thoracoscopic access has been chosen because the majority of pouches develop from the right side of the esophagus and are adherent to the right pleura or diaphragm, or both.[50,51] To overcome the difficulty of performing an esophagomyotomy from this side of the chest, it has also been suggested that pneumatic dilation of the lower esophageal sphincter be performed before the operation in patients with documented manometric abnormalities.[50] A double-lumen endotracheal tube is used to allow right lung retraction. The patient is placed in the left lateral decubitus position. Four ports are required: one for the camera, one for the lung retractor, and two for the operating devices (Fig. 31–10). Dissection is begun by taking down the inferior pulmonary ligament and freeing the right lower lobe to the level of the inferior pulmonary vein. The pleura overlying the esophagus is incised, and the right lateral aspect of the esophagus is dissected for a length of about 10 cm. Moderate insufflation and transillumination through an esophagoscope facilitate both dissection and resection of the diverticulum. The pouch can be grasped with a Babcock clamp and gentle traction applied to facilitate identification of the diverticular neck (Fig. 31–11). Once completely dissected, the diverticulum is excised with a reticulating linear endostapler (EndoGIA II) with a blue cartridge. The stapler must be oriented parallel to the longitudinal axis of the esophagus (see Fig. 31–11). If this step is unsatisfactory, a video-assisted approach can be used by performing a small thoracotomy and inserting a hand to assist in stapler orientation. One or two cartridges of staples are usually necessary. Endoscopic visualization is helpful to check placement of the stapler after closure of the jaws, as well to inspect the integrity of the suture line after resection. The muscle layer is closed over the mucosal suture with interrupted sutures of PDS or Biosyn. A standard chest tube is placed. A Gastrografin swallow study is performed on day 4, and the nasogastric tube is removed.

More recently, a laparoscopic approach has been advocated in an effort to simplify alignment of the stapler and facilitate performance of myotomy and fundoplication.[52] The patient is placed on the operating table in the lithotomy position with a 20-degree reverse Trendelenburg inclination. The surgeon stands between the legs. Pneumoperitoneum is established and five operating ports are placed in the upper part of the abdomen. After incision of the phrenoesophageal membrane, the dissection is begun on the right crus of the diaphragm. The esophagus is encircled with a Penrose drain for traction. Mediastinal dissection is performed bluntly close to the

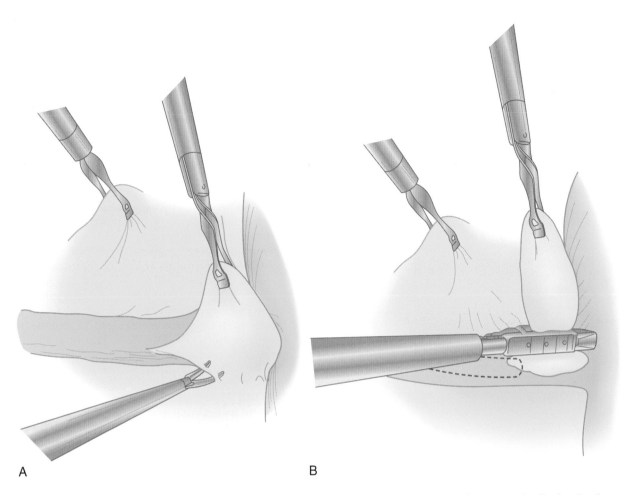

A   B

Figure 31–11. **A,** Dissection of an epiphrenic diverticulum through a right thoracoscopic approach. **B,** Application of the reticulating endostapler to the neck of the diverticulum.

esophageal wall until the diverticular pouch is reached. Moderate insufflation and transillumination through an endoluminal esophagoscope facilitate dissection of the diverticulum and identification of its neck. The pouch must be thoroughly cleaned of all adhesions. A reticulating linear endostapler (EndoGIA II) with a blue cartridge is introduced through the trocar in the left upper quadrant and applied parallel to the esophageal axis (Fig. 31–12). The stapler jaws are closed under endoscopic control. Further stapler application may be necessary to remove the diverticulum. The integrity of the suture line must be checked endoscopically, and then a few interrupted PDS or Biosyn sutures are placed to close the muscular wall. A Heller myotomy is performed on the opposite side of the esophageal wall with ultrasonic scissors. The myotomy is extended distally for about 2 cm on the gastric side with a sharpened hook (Fig. 31–13). A posterior hiatoplasty is performed with interrupted sutures. A Dor fundoplication is constructed by suturing the anterior fundic wall to the edges of the myotomy. The cranial sutures also attach the fundus to the anterior crura. A Penrose drain is placed in the subhepatic space. A Gastrografin swallow study is performed on postoperative day 4, and the nasogastric tube is removed.

Surgical treatment of an epiphrenic diverticulum results in resolution of symptoms in most patients.

However, the operative risks are significant. Among the 33 patients who underwent transthoracic resection of an epiphrenic diverticulum at the Mayo Clinic between 1975 and 1991, the mortality rate was 9%.[47] Death was caused by a clinically significant leak in two patients and by respiratory failure from aspiration during a Gastrografin swallow in the third individual. Six esophageal leaks occurred, four of which were benign and asymptomatic. Based on these data, operative intervention for asymptomatic or minimally symptomatic epiphrenic diverticula should be discouraged.[53] Although failure to perform myotomy in conjunction with diverticulectomy may be associated with suture line disruption and postoperative death, these sequelae are not inevitable results of its omission. Nevertheless, most esophageal surgeons agree that every effort should be made to correct associated esophageal disorders in order to minimize complications. Early radiographic examination of the esophagus before oral feeding is mandatory in the postoperative management of these patients. If leakage is documented, parenteral feeding should be continued for at least 3 weeks along with nasogastric aspiration, proton pump inhibitors, and antibiotics.

The long-term results of the operation are acceptable and durable. Patients are generally symptom-free if associated esophageal conditions have been adequately dealt

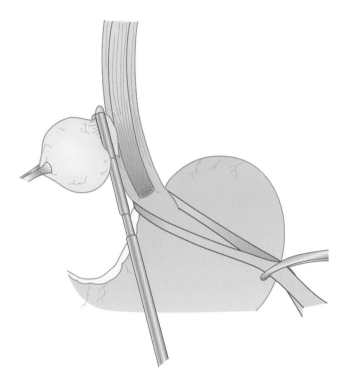

Figure 31–12.   Stapled resection of an epiphrenic diverticulum through a laparoscopic approach.

with during the operation. In the Mayo Clinic study,[47] the long-term follow-up ranged from 4 months to 15 years, with a median of 6.9 years. No recurrent diverticulum was observed. The overall results were good or excellent in 22 patients (76%), fair in 5 (17%), and poor in 2 (7%).

Sufficient data are not yet available to definitely recommend the minimally invasive surgical approach. Only small case series or case reports are found in the literature, and these procedures have been performed in just a few centers worldwide. Limitations of the right thoracoscopic approach include the fulcrum effect of thoracoports, difficult alignment of the stapler along the esophageal axis, and the impossibility of performing a distal myotomy from the right side of the chest. Theoretically, a video-assisted approach and patient repositioning for a laparoscopic myotomy and Dor fundoplication could overcome these limitations. The complete laparoscopic approach may represent the ideal procedure for patients with a truly distal epiphrenic diverticulum, but the short- and long-term results of this procedure are still awaited.[54,55]

MIDESOPHAGEAL DIVERTICULA

Midesophageal diverticula are traditionally thought to be caused by external "traction" in patients with mediastinal fibrosis or chronic lymphadenopathy from tuberculosis or histoplasmosis. In exceptional circumstances, mid-

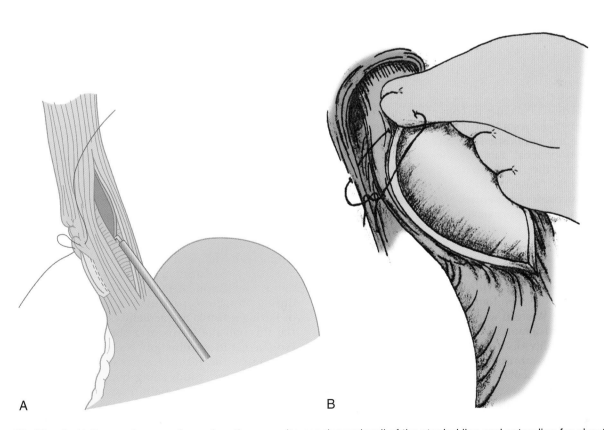

A   B

Figure 31–13.   A, Heller myotomy performed on the opposite esophageal wall of the stapled line and extending for about 2 cm on the gastric side. **B,** A Dor fundoplication is constructed by suturing the anterior fundic wall to the edges of the myotomy.

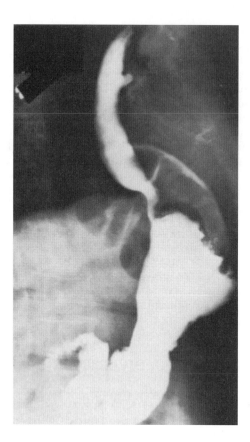

Figure 31–14. Esophagus with a traction diverticulum in the middle third of the thoracic portion in relation to the subcarinal lymph nodes. The patient was asymptomatic. (From Payne WS: Diverticula of the esophagus. In Payne WS, Olsen AM [eds]: The Esophagus. Philadelphia, Lea & Febiger, 1974, p 207.)

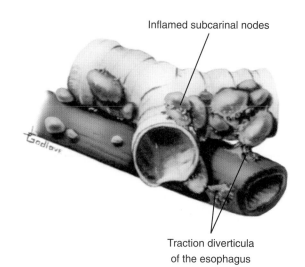

Inflamed subcarinal nodes

Traction diverticula of the esophagus

Figure 31–15. Traction diverticula of the esophagus occur most commonly in the middle third of the thoracic portion of the esophagus in relation to the granulomatous subcarinal lymph nodes. Note how the esophageal wall is tented by inflammatory lymph nodes. (From Payne WS, Clagett OT: Pharyngeal and esophageal diverticula. Curr Probl Surg 23:1-31, 1965.)

esophageal diverticula may be congenital and result from an abortive tracheoesophageal fistula or a foregut duplication that has established permanent communication with the esophageal lumen.[17] Because all layers are affected, these diverticula are considered to be "true" as opposed to the "false," pulsion-type diverticula in which only the mucosa is represented. Most traction diverticula arise within 4 to 5 cm proximal or distal to the carina and are associated with granulomatous diseases of the subcarinal lymph nodes (Figs. 31–14 and 31–15).[56] Inflamed nodes become anchored to the esophagus, and the contracting scar tissue tents up the esophageal wall to form a conical outpouching. With the progressive decline in the incidence of granulomatous disease of the mediastinum in the Western world, a pulsion theory became prominent and emphasized endoluminal forces secondary to motility disorders as the main pathogenetic mechanism of parabronchial diverticula,[57] analogous to epiphrenic diverticula. Nowadays, any pouch sited anywhere in the course of the esophageal body should be regarded as a pulsion diverticulum until proved otherwise.[44]

Occasionally, patients may complain of dysphagia, retrosternal discomfort, and regurgitation. However, the majority of midesophageal traction diverticula are totally asymptomatic and likely to remain so. In most circumstances, they appear to be incidental findings during esophageal radiography or endoscopy. It is thought that because of their wide-mouthed configuration and dependent drainage, they remain stable in size without causing symptoms. Carcinoma arising from a parabronchial diverticulum has rarely been reported.[58]

Complications of traction diverticula include bleeding and fistulas with the airways. Because of their rarity, precise diagnosis is often delayed or missed. Erosion of neighboring major blood vessels can produce massive upper gastrointestinal bleeding. More frequently, the hemorrhage is caused by friable granulation tissue or erosion of small bronchial or esophageal vessels.[59] Demonstration of a complication such as an acquired tracheobronchial esophageal fistula[60] may be delayed when the manifestation is recurrent pneumonia without the classic "swallow-cough" sequence. Esophageal radiography sometimes fails to define such a fistula unless the patient is in the prone position during examination. An alternative diagnostic technique consists of the simultaneous instillation of methylene blue in the esophagus during bronchoscopy. However, many patients suspected of having a fistula are actually aspirating ingested material through the larynx as a consequence of pharyngoesophageal incoordination. Surgical therapy consists of division of the fistula tract, closure of the esophagus in layers over an indwelling bougie, and closure of the airway (Fig. 31–16). A right thoracotomy is the approach of choice. Because of previously inflamed lymph nodes, extreme scarring is to be expected. Attention must be directed to correcting the distal esophageal obstruction if present. The risk for a recurrent fistula with the airways

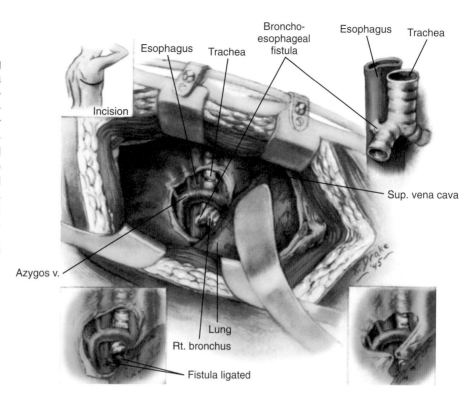

Figure 31–16. Technique for closing an acquired esophagobronchial fistula as a complication of a traction diverticulum of the esophagus. A right posterolateral thoracotomy incision *(upper left inset)* is made. For surgical exposure, the lung has been retracted anteriorly. Note the relationship of the esophagus, right main bronchus, and fistula to the neighboring sutures *(center).* The fistula before division and after division and ligation is seen in the *upper right* and *lower left insets.* The *lower right inset* shows the method of interposing pedicles of the mediastinal pleura between esophageal and bronchial closure. (From Payne WS, Clagett OT: Pharyngeal and esophageal diverticula. Curr Probl Surg 23: 1-31, 1965.)

is best minimized by the interposition of an intercostal muscle flap.

SUGGESTED READINGS

Benacci JC, Deschamps C, Trastek VF, et al: Epiphrenic diverticulum: Results of surgical treatment. Ann Thorac Surg 55:1109, 1993.

Bonavina L, Khan N, DeMeester TR: Pharyngoesophageal dysfunctions. The role of cricopharyngeal myotomy. Arch Surg 120:541, 1985.

Nehra D, Lord RV, DeMeester TR, et al: Physiologic basis for the treatment of epiphrenic diverticulum. Ann Surg 235:346, 2002.

Peracchia A, Bonavina L, Narne S, et al: Minimally invasive surgery for Zenker's diverticulum. Analysis of results in 95 consecutive patients. Arch Surg 133:695, 1998.

Rosati R, Fumagalli U, Bona S, et al: Diverticulectomy, myotomy and fundoplication through laparoscopy: A new option to treat epiphrenic esophageal diverticula? Ann Surg 227:174, 1998.

REFERENCES

1. Zenker FA, von Ziemssen H: Dilatations of the oesophagus. In Cyclopaedia of the Practice of Medicine, vol 3. London, Low, Marston, Searle & Rivington, 1878, p 46.
2. Sutherland HD: Cricopharyngeal achalasia. J Thorac Cardiovasc Surg 43:114, 1962.
3. Hunt PS, Connell AM, Smiley TB: The cricopharyngeal sphincter in gastric reflux. Gut 11:303, 1970.
4. Ellis FH Jr, Schlegel JF, Lynch VP, et al: Cricopharyngeal myotomy for pharyngo-esophageal diverticulum. Ann Surg 170:340, 1969.
5. Henderson RD, Marryatt G: Cricopharyngeal myotomy as a method of treating cricopharyngeal dysphagia secondary to gastro-esophageal reflux. J Thorac Cardiovasc Surg 74:721, 1977.
6. Lichter I: Motor disorder in pharyngoesophageal pouch. J Thorac Cardiovasc Surg 76:272, 1978.
7. Duranceau A., Rheault MJ, Jamieson GG: Physiologic response to cricopharyngeal myotomy and diverticulum suspension. Surgery 94:655, 1983.
8. Bonavina L, Khan N, DeMeester TR: Pharyngoesophageal dysfunctions. The role of cricopharyngeal myotomy. Arch Surg 120:541, 1985.
9. Cruse J, Edwards D, Smith J, Wyllie J: The pathology of cricopharyngeal dysphagia. Histopathology 3:223, 1979.
10. Skinner D, Belsey R: The pharynx, cricopharyngeus, and Zenker's diverticulum. Management of Esophageal Disease. Philadelphia, WB Saunders, 1988, p 409.
11. Lerut T, van Raemdonck D, Guelinckx P, et al: Pharyngo-oesophageal diverticulum (Zenker's): Clinical, therapeutic, and morphological aspects. Acta Gastroenterol Belg 53:330, 1990.
12. Venturi M, Bonavina L, Colombo L, et al: Biochemical markers of upper esophageal sphincter compliance in patients with Zenker's diverticulum. J Surg Res 70:46, 1997.
13. Cook JJ, Gabb M, Panagopoulos V, et al: Pharyngeal (Zenker's) diverticulum is a disorder of upper esophageal sphincter opening. Gastroenterology 103:1229, 1992.
14. Negus VE: Pharyngeal diverticula. Observations on their evolution and treatment. Br J Surg 38:129, 1950.
15. Huang B, Unni KK, Payne WS: Long-term survival following diverticulectomy for cancer in pharyngoesophageal (Zenker's) diverticulum. Ann Thorac Surg 38:207, 1984.
16. Crescenzo DG, Trastek VF, Allen MS, et al: Zenker's diverticulum in the elderly: Is operation justified? Ann Thorac Surg 66:347, 1998.
17. Belsey R: Functional disease of the esophagus. J Thorac Cardiovasc Surg 52:164, 1966.
18. Nicoladoni K: Behandlung der Oesophagusdivertikel. Wien Med Wochenschr 25:606, 1877.
19. Clagett O, Payne W: Surgical treatment of pulsion diverticula of the hypopharynx: One-stage resection in 478 cases. Dis Chest 37:257, 1960.

20. Ferguson M: Evolution of therapy for pharyngoesophageal (Zenker's) diverticulum. Ann Thorac Surg 51:848, 1991.
21. Ellis FH Jr, Crozier RE: Cervical esophageal dysphagia: Indications for and results of cricopharyngeal myotomy. Ann Surg 194:279, 1981.
22. Bonavina L, Bettineschi F, Fontebasso V, et al: Cricopharyngeal myotomy and stapling: Treatment of choice for Zenker's diverticulum. In Nabeya K, Hanaoka T, Nogami H (eds): Recent Advances in Diseases of the Esophagus, Tokyo, Springer-Verlag, 1993, p 207.
23. Mosher HP: Webs and pouches of the oesophagus, their diagnosis and treatment. Surg Gynecol Obstet 25:175, 1917.
24. Dohlman G, Mattsson O: The endoscopic operation for hypopharyngeal diverticula: A roentgencinematographic study. Arch Otolaryngol 71:744, 1960.
25. van Overbeek JJM: Meditation on the pathogenesis of hypopharyngeal (Zenker's) diverticulum and a report of endoscopic treatment in 545 patients. Ann Otol Rhinol Laryngol 103:178, 1994.
26. Collard JM, Otte JB, Kestens PJ: Endoscopic stapling technique of esophagodiverticulostomy for Zenker's diverticulum. Ann Thorac Surg 56:573, 1993.
27. Narne S, Bonavina L, Guido E, Peracchia A: Treatment of Zenker's diverticulum by endoscopic stapling. Endosurgery 1:118, 1993.
28. Hiebert CA: Surgery for cricopharyngeal dysfunction under local anesthesia. Am J Surg 131:423, 1976.
29. Welsh G, Payne WS: The present status of one-stage pharyngoesophageal diverticulectomy. Surg Clin North Am 53:953, 1973.
30. Payne WS, Reynolds RR: Surgical treatment of pharyngoesophageal diverticulum (Zenker's diverticulum). Surg Rounds 5:18, 1982.
31. Lerut T, van Raemdonck D, Guelincky P: Zenker's diverticulum: Is a myotomy of the cricopharyngeus useful? How long should it be? Hepatogastroenterology 39:127, 1992.
32. Huang B, Payne WS, Cameron AJ: Surgical management for recurrent pharyngoesophageal (Zenker's) diverticulum. Ann Thorac Surg 37:189, 1984.
33. Rocco G, Deschamps C, Martel E, et al: Results of reoperation on the upper esophageal sphincter. J Thorac Cardiovasc Surg 117:28, 1999.
34. Payne WS: The treatment of pharyngoesophageal diverticulum: The simple and complex. Hepatogastroenterology 39:109, 1992.
35. Narne S, Bonavina L, Antoniazzi L, et al: Safety and effectiveness of transoral stapling for recurrent Zenker diverticulum. In Pinotti H, et al (eds): Recent Advances in Diseases of the Esophagus, Bologna, Italy, Monduzzi Editore, 2001, p 701.
36. Peracchia A, Bonavina L, Narne S, et al: Minimally invasive surgery for Zenker's diverticulum. Analysis of results in 95 consecutive patients. Arch Surg 133:695, 1998.
37. Aly A, Devitt P, Jamieson G: Evolution of surgical treatment for pharyngeal pouch. Br J Surg 91:657, 2004.
38. Gutschow C, Hamoir M, Rombaux P, et al: Management of pharyngoesophageal (Zenker's) diverticulum: Which technique? Ann Thor Surg 74:1677, 2002.
39. Posthletwait RW: Diverticula of the esophagus. In Surgery of the Esophagus. Norwalk, CT, Appleton Century Crofts, 1986, p 129.
40. Allen TH, Clagett OT: Changing concepts in the surgical treatment of pulsion diverticula of the lower esophagus. J Thorac Cardiovasc Surg 50:455, 1965.
41. Dodds WJ, Stef JJ, Hogan WJ, et al: Distribution of esophageal peristaltic pressure in normal subjects and patients with esophageal diverticulum. Gastroenterology 69:584, 1975.
42. Debas HT, Payne WS, Cameron AJ, et al: Physiopathology of lower esophageal diverticulum and its implications for treatment. Surg Gynecol Obstet 151:593, 1980.
43. Bontempo I, Corazziari E, Mineo TC, et al: Esophageal motor activity in patients with esophageal diverticula. In DeMeester TR, Skinner DB (eds): Esophageal Disorders, Pathophysiology and Therapy. New York, Raven Press, 1985, p 427.
44. Evander A, Little AG, Ferguson MK, et al: Diverticula of the mid- and lower esophagus: Pathogenesis and surgical management. World J Surg 10:820, 1986.
45. Nehra D, Lord RV, DeMeester TR, et al: Physiologic basis for the treatment of epiphrenic diverticulum. Ann Surg 235:346, 2002.
46. Altorki NK, Sunagawa M, Skinner DB: Thoracic esophageal diverticula: Why is operation necessary? J Thorac Cardiovasc Surg 105:260, 1993.
47. Benacci JC, Deschamps C, Trastek VF, et al: Epiphrenic diverticulum: Results of surgical treatment. Ann Thorac Surg 55:1109, 1993.
48. Streitz J, Glick M, Ellis F: Selective use of myotomy for treatment of epiphrenic diverticula. Arch Surg 127:585, 1992.
49. Little AG, Soriano A, Ferguson MK, et al: Surgical treatment of achalasia: Results with esophagomyotomy and Belsey repair. Ann Thorac Surg 45:489, 1988.
50. Peracchia A, Bonavina L, Rosati R, Bona S: Thoracoscopic resection of epiphrenic esophageal diverticula. In Peters JH, Demeester TR (eds): Minimally Invasive Surgery of the Foregut. St. Louis, Quality Medical Publishing, 1995, p 110.
51. Peters JF, Bonavina L, Hagen JA: Thoracoscopic esophageal procedures. In Eubanks S, Swanstrom L, Soper N (eds): Mastery of Endoscopic and Laparoscopic Surgery. Philadelphia, Lippincott Williams & Wilkins, 2000, p 4878.
52. Rosati R, Fumagalli U, Bona S, et al: Diverticulectomy, myotomy and fundoplication through laparoscopy: A new option to treat epiphrenic esophageal diverticula? Ann Surg 227:174, 1998.
53. Orringer MB: Epiphrenic diverticula: Fact and fable [editorial]. Ann Thorac Surg 55:1067, 1993.
54. Stuart R, Wyman A, Chan A, et al: Thoracoscopic resection of oesophageal diverticulum: A case report. J R Coll Surg Edinb 41:118, 1996.
55. Anthuber M, Mayr M, Messmann H, Jauch K: A laparoscopic approach for the treatment of lower third esophageal diverticula. Langenbecks Arch Surg 386:582, 2002.
56. Dukes R, Strimian C, Dines D, et al: Esophageal involvement with mediastinal granuloma. JAMA 236:2313, 1976.
57. Kaye MD: Oesophageal motor dysfunction in patients with diverticula of the mid-thoracic oesophagus. Thorax 29:666, 1974.
58. Fujita H, Kakegawa T, Shima S, Kumagaya Y: Carcinoma within a middle esophageal (parabronchial) diverticulum: A case report and review of the literature. Jpn Surg 10:142, 1980.
59. Jonasson OM, Gunn LC: Midesophageal diverticulum with hemorrhage: Report of a case. Arch Surg 90:713, 1965.
60. Wychulis AR, Ellis FH Jr, Andersen HA: Acquired non-malignant esophagotracheobronchial fistula: Report of 36 cases. JAMA 196:117, 1966.

Chapter

32

Epidemiology, Risk Factors, and Clinical Manifestations of Esophageal Carcinoma

Daniel Vallböhmer ▪ Jan Brabender ▪
Paul M. Schneider ▪ Arnulf H. Hölscher

Esophageal cancer is one of the deadliest malignant tumors worldwide. During the last 30 years significant changes have occurred in the epidemiologic pattern of this disease, and recent studies have identified several risk factors for the development of esophageal cancer. These new findings serve as the focus of this chapter.

In 2005, esophageal cancer will be diagnosed in an estimated 14,520 people in the United States.[1] Of these, squamous cell carcinoma and adenocarcinoma are the most common types of primary esophageal malignancies.[2] Although esophageal cancer is uncommon, the incidence of esophageal adenocarcinoma in particular has increased dramatically over the last 25 years in the United States and large parts of Europe.[3-7]

Until the 1970s esophageal adenocarcinoma was a rare diagnosis worldwide. From 1926 to 1976, four large surgical series reported that only 0.8% to 3.7% of esophageal malignancies were adenocarcinoma and that squamous cell carcinoma overwhelmingly outnumbered adenocarcinoma.[5,7] Subsequently, the incidence of esophageal adenocarcinoma has increased rapidly in the Western world. In fact, the rate of increase in adenocarcinoma of the esophagus is greater than that of any other major malignancy in the United States (Fig. 32–1).[5] The absolute incidence increased approximately sixfold from 3.8 per million in 1973 to 1975 to 23.3 per million in 2001. For the same period (1975 to 2001), the incidence of squamous cell carcinoma of the esophagus fell from 31 to 19 per million (Fig. 32–2).[5]

Despite the fact that the incidence of esophageal adenocarcinoma has increased, it remains a relatively uncommon malignancy. The number of new cases per 100,000 white males in Western countries varies between 1 and 5, with the highest incidence in Great Britain, followed by Australia.[7] Other countries with relatively high-incidence populations are the United States and the Netherlands, whereas the incidence remains low in Eastern Europe and Scandinavia.[6]

MORTALITY/PROGNOSIS OF PATIENTS WITH ESOPHAGEAL CANCER

Esophageal cancer is expected to account for 13,570 cancer deaths in the United States in 2005.[1] Despite recent progress, esophageal cancer remains a highly lethal malignancy. The overall 5-year survival rate has increased from 4% in the 1970s to merely 14% currently.[8] With complete surgical removal of the tumor, the 5-year survival rate is 50% to 80% for stage I disease, 30% to

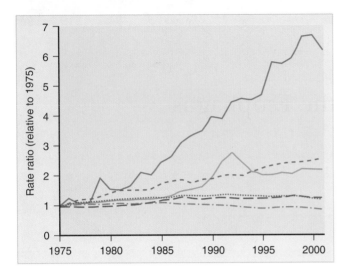

Figure 32–1. Relative change in incidence of esophageal adenocarcinoma and other malignancies (1975 to 2001). Data are from the National Cancer Institute's Surveillance, Epidemiology, and End Results program with age adjustment using the 2000 U.S. standard population. Baseline was the average incidence between 1973 and 1975. *Dark orange line,* esophageal adenocarcinoma; *purple short dashed line,* melanoma; *light orange line,* prostate cancer; *red dashed line,* breast cancer; *blue dotted line,* lung cancer; *green dashed and dotted line,* colorectal cancer. (From Pohl H, Welch HG: The role of overdiagnosis and reclassification in the marked increase of esophageal adenocarcinoma incidence. J Natl Cancer Inst 97:142-146, 2005.)

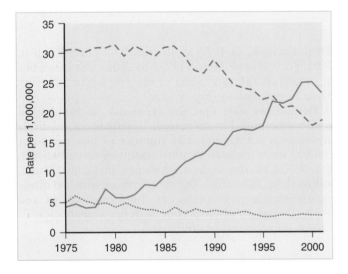

Figure 32–2. Histology and esophageal cancer incidence (1975 to 2001). Data are from the National Cancer Institute's Surveillance, Epidemiology, and End Results program with age adjustment using the 2000 U.S. standard population. *Dark orange line,* adenocarcinoma; *purple dashed line,* squamous cell carcinoma; *blue dotted line,* not otherwise specified. (From Pohl H, Welch HG: The role of overdiagnosis and reclassification in the marked increase of esophageal adenocarcinoma incidence. J Natl Cancer Inst 97:142-146, 2005.)

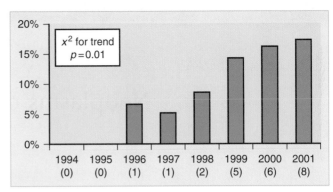

Figure 32–3. Incidence of esophageal adenocarcinoma in patients 50 years or younger at the University of Southern California. (From Portale G, Peters JH, Hsieh CC, et al: Esophageal adenocarcinoma in patients < or = 50 years old: Delayed diagnosis and advanced disease at presentation. Am Surg 70:954-958, 2004.)

40% for stage IIA disease, 10% to 30% for stage IIB disease, and 10% to 15% for stage III disease.[8]

AGE, SEX, AND RACE DISTRIBUTION

The incidence of esophageal adenocarcinoma increases with age, with a median age at diagnosis of 55 to 60 years and a striking male preponderance (7:1).[4,6] Interestingly, Portale et al. reported an increasing number of young patients with esophageal adenocarcinoma during the past decade at their institution (Fig. 32–3).[9] In this study consisting of 263 consecutive patients with resectable esophageal adenocarcinoma, 32 (12.2%) were 50 years or younger. It was found that these younger patients usually sought medical attention because of dysphagia, were symptomatic for a longer time before diagnosis, and had more advanced disease than older patients did. With appropriate aggressive treatment, survival was found to be similar, thus suggesting that liberal use of endoscopy and an aggressive diagnostic approach are paramount in young patients with dysphagia/symptoms of gastroesophageal reflux disease (GERD).

Esophageal adenocarcinoma incidence rates vary markedly by ethnicity. Kubo et al. recently analyzed the multiethnic and gender variability of the incidence of esophageal and cardia adenocarcinoma by using Surveillance, Epidemiology, and End Results cancer registry data between 1992 and 1998.[10] They demonstrated that white males' esophageal adenocarcinoma rate (4.2 per 100,000 population per year) was double that of Hispanics and fourfold higher than that of blacks, Asians, and Native Americans and that female rates were much lower than male rates for all ethnicities. Similar to esophageal adenocarcinoma, cardia adenocarcinoma rates were highest in white males (3.4 per 100,000 population per year). However, the ethnic differences were much less and female rates were comparable for almost all ethnicities, except Native Americans. In addition, it was found that the incidence rates of esophageal adeno-

Table 32–1	Risk Factors for Esophageal Adenocarcinoma and Squamous Cell Carcinoma	

	Esophageal Adenocarcinoma	Esophageal Squamous Cell Carcinoma
Age	↑	↑
Alcohol	0	↑
Caucasian race	↑	↓
Cholecystectomy	↑	0
Fruit and vegetables	↓	↓
Gastroesophageal reflux disease/Barrett's esophagus	↑	0
Helicobacter pylori infection	↓	?
Low socioeconomic status	↓	↑
Lower sphincter–relaxing medications	↑	0
Male sex	↑	↑
Nonsteroidal anti-inflammatory drugs	↓	↓
Obesity	↑	↓
Tobacco	↑	↑

↑, positive association; ↓, negative association; 0, no association.

carcinoma increased significantly only in whites and not in the other ethnic groups whereas cardia cancer rates did not increase for any ethnicity during this period. These findings suggest that cardia and esophageal adenocarcinomas are biologically distinct entities or that the incidence rate of cardia cancer represents a blending of gastric and esophageal carcinoma incidence rates. Current putative risk factors do not adequately explain this substantial variability.

Squamous cell cancer of the esophagus also has a male preponderance, with rates two to four times higher in males than in females.[4,6] In contrast to adenocarcinoma, squamous cell cancer incidence rates were highest in blacks (8.8 per 100,000 population per year) and Asians (3.9 per 100,000 population per year), and they were stable or declined for all ethnicities between 1992 and 1998, which could be influenced by the different socioeconomic variables existing between these ethnic groups.[10]

RISK FACTORS FOR SQUAMOUS CELL CANCER AND ADENOCARCINOMA

Obesity

Obesity is a risk factor for a number of gastrointestinal malignancies (Table 32–1). Calle et al. examined the relationship between body mass index (BMI) for men and women in 1982 and the risk for death from all cancers and from cancer at individual sites in a prospectively studied population of more than 900,000 U.S. adults (404,576 men and 495,477 women) who were free of cancer at enrollment.[11] They demonstrated that increased body weight was associated with increased death rates for all cancers combined and for cancers at multiple specific sites, including esophageal cancer (Fig. 32–4). In particular, those with the greatest BMI

(≥40) had death rates from all cancers combined that were 52% higher for men and 62% higher for women than for people of normal weight. In men, the relative risk for death was 1.52, and in women, the relative risk was 1.62. It is suggested that obesity, which increases the incidence of GERD, might result in an increase in the incidence of Barrett's esophagus, the most important risk factor for esophageal adenocarcinoma, thereby leading to a higher risk for the development of esophageal adenocarinoma.[3,12] In contrast, it is noted that esophageal squamous cell cancer decreases with increasing BMI.

Tobacco and Alcohol

Tobacco smoking and alcohol exposure have been identified as strong, independent risk factors for squamous cell cancer of the esophagus, but the risk depends mainly on the duration of smoking and the amount of alcohol consumed.[13,14] Cessation of smoking for 5 years reduces the risk by 50%, and abstinence from alcohol for at least 10 years reduces the risk to levels of nondrinkers.

For esophageal adenocarcinoma, smoking seems to be merely a moderate risk factor and alcohol consumption is not associated with an increased risk for this type of cancer.[15,16]

Diet and Nutrition

Squamous cell cancer and adenocarcinoma seem to be influenced by diet and nutrition in the same way. It has been shown that high intake of fruits and vegetables reduce the risk for both histologic types.[17-20] For example, Bollscheiler et al. demonstrated that low intake of vitamins C and E correlates significantly with the development of squamous cell carcinoma and adenocarcinoma.[20] Evidence suggests that in particular the

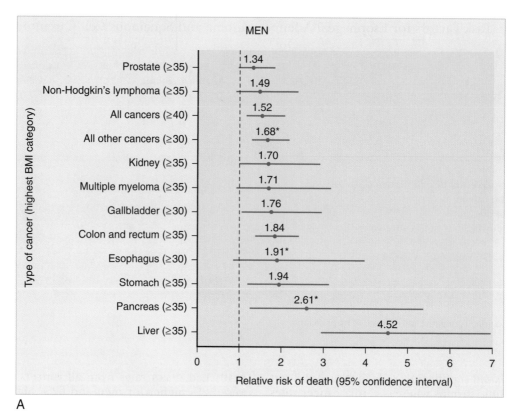

A

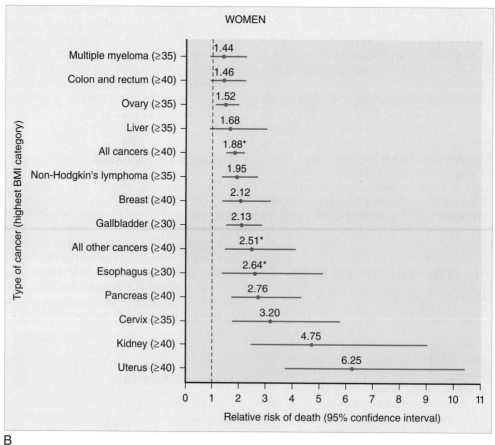

B

Figure 32–4. **A,** Summary of mortality from cancer according to body mass index for U.S. men in the Cancer Prevention Study II, 1982 through 1998. **B,** Summary of mortality from cancer according to body mass index for U.S. women in the Cancer Prevention Study II, 1982 through 1998. (From Calle EE, Rodriguez C, Walker-Thurmond K, Thun MJ: Overweight, obesity, and mortality from cancer in a prospectively studied cohort of U.S. adults. N Engl J Med 24;348:1625-1638, 2003.)

antioxidants in these dietary items seem to provide the protective effect.[21]

Nonsteroidal Anti-inflammatory Drugs

Cyclooxygenase-2 (COX-2) has been implicated as an important enzyme in the early development of several gastrointestinal cancers, including esophageal cancer.[22] COX-2 may contribute to cancer growth through several mechanisms, including increasing cells' longevity via inhibition of apoptosis and stimulation of angiogenesis.[23] Previous studies found an association between increased COX-2 expression and the development/progression of Barrett's esophagus, a premalignant condition of the esophagus strongly associated with esophageal adenocarcinoma.[24,25] Interestingly, epidemiologic studies suggest that the long-term use of nonsteroidal anti-inflammatory drugs (NSAIDs), which inhibit cyclooxygenases, are associated with a reduced risk for cancer, including both squamous cell cancer and adenocarcinoma of the esophagus.[26,27] Recently, Corley et al. performed a systematic review with a meta-analysis of nine observational studies consisting of 1813 cancer patients to evaluate the association of aspirin/NSAID use and esophageal cancer.[28] They described a significant protective association between the use of aspirin/NSAIDs and esophageal cancer and found that both intermittent and frequent medication use was protective. Therefore, aspirin/NSAIDs could protect against esophageal adenocarcinoma either by preventing the development of its primary precursor (i.e., Barrett's esophagus) or by diminishing the likelihood of Barrett's esophagus progressing to adenocarcinoma.

RISK FACTORS SPECIFIC TO ESOPHAGEAL ADENOCARCINOMA

Gastroesophageal Reflux Disease

GERD is a common disease that affects up to 30% of the Western population on a monthly basis. Its role in the development of esophageal adenocarcinoma has been investigated recently in several large epidemiologic studies. Lagergren et al. described a strong association between the risk for esophageal cancer and symptomatic GERD.[29] In this Swedish population-based, nationwide case-control study, 189 patients with esophageal adenocarcinoma and 820 control subjects were included. In persons with long-standing and severe symptoms of reflux, the odds ratio was 43.5 for esophageal adenocarcinoma. However, also in persons with recurrent symptoms of reflux occurring at least once per week, the risk for esophageal adenocarcinoma was increased eightfold. In a medical record–based case control-study by Chow et al. that included 196 patients with esophageal or cardia adenocarcinoma, a significantly twofold increased risk was found in persons with a recorded history of GERD, hiatal hernia, esophagitis/esophageal ulcer, or difficulty swallowing.[30] These results were validated in a case-control study of similar design in the United States.[31]

Finally, a Swedish cohort study of 65,000 male patients with a discharge diagnosis of heartburn, hiatal hernia, or esophagitis analyzed the relationship between GERD and esophageal adenocarcinoma.[32] The investigators reported a ninefold increased risk for esophageal adenocarcinoma in patients with endoscopic evidence of esophagitis.

Barrett's Esophagus

Barrett's esophagus is a condition in which the normal squamous epithelium of the distal end of the esophagus is replaced with metaplastic specialized intestinal-type epithelium as a sequela of chronic GERD.[33] This metaplastic condition is the most important risk factor for esophageal adenocarcinoma. In studies with a large sample size, the risk for development of esophageal adenocarcinoma was 30- to 60-fold higher in patients with Barrett's esophagus than in the general population.[6] Cameron et al. performed one of the earliest retrospective studies evaluating the malignant potential of Barrett's esophagus. In 18 of 122 patients, adenocarcinoma of the esophagus and Barrett's esophagus were found simultaneously, whereas in the remaining 104 patients, esophageal adenocarcinoma developed in 2 after a mean interval of 8.5 years.[34] In a Dutch prospective follow-up study by Hameeteman et al., 50 patients with Barrett's esophagus, without carcinoma at entrance to the study, were evaluated for a period of 1.5 to 14 years (mean, 5.2 years) to determine the dysplastic/malignant potential of Barrett's esophagus.[35] At the end of the observation period dysplasia had been found in 13 patients, in 10 scored as low grade and in 3 as high-grade, and adenocarcinoma had developed in another 5 patients. These data demonstrate that Barrett's esophagus is a premalignant condition that predisposes to the development of esophageal adenocarcinoma.

Lower Sphincter–Relaxing Medications

Several drugs are able to relax the lower esophageal sphincter and are thought to thereby increase the risk for development of esophageal adenocarcinoma because of an increase in the incidence of GERD. A Swedish case-control study tested the possible association between the use of sphincter-relaxing medications, such as nitroglycerin, anticholinergics, β-adrenergic agonists, aminophyllines, and benzodiazepines, and the risk for esophageal adenocarcinoma.[36] It was found that past use of sphincter-relaxing drugs was positively associated with risk for esophageal adenocarcinoma and that the association almost disappeared after adjustment for reflux symptoms, thus suggesting that promotion of reflux is the link between the use of sphincter-relaxing drugs and esophageal adenocarcinoma.

Helicobacter pylori Infection

Eradication of *H. pylori* is an effective strategy for chemoprevention of gastric cancer.[37] However, evidence suggests that such eradication is associated with a higher risk for esophageal adenocarcinoma. Two clinical studies, by Chow et al. and Simán et al., found that infection with *H. pylori* decreased the risk for esophageal cancer by 60% and by 50% to 80%, respectively.[38,39] The mechanism of this protective effect is still unclear. It is hypothesized that *H. pylori* infection induces atrophic gastritis and possibly increased intragastric ammonia production leading to protection against esophageal adenocarcinoma.[40]

WHY IS THE EPIDEMIOLOGY CHANGING?

Although the incidence of esophageal adenocarcinoma is rising dramatically, the reasons for this observation are still controversial. The increase may represent a true rise in disease burden; nevertheless, it may also be the result of overdiagnosis or reclassification. Pohl and Welch have recently examined the incidence, stage distribution, and disease-specific mortality of esophageal adenocarcinoma to determine whether the dramatic increase in incidence of this malignant disease represents merely overdiagnosis or reclassification or constitutes a real increase in disease burden.[5] They found that the distribution of esophageal cancer in general has changed and that the only location of disease manifestation with a rising incidence is the lower third of the esophagus, the typical location of adenocarcinoma, which suggests that reclassification of squamous cell cancer is unlikely to explain the change in epidemiology. In addition, they described an increased incidence of adjacent cardia cancer, thus demonstrating that even reclassification of cardia cancer is also unlikely to influence the rising incidence of esophageal adenocarcinoma. Finally, they excluded overdiagnosis as a factor influencing the rising incidence because in the last 30 years there has been just a minor change in the proportion of patients with localized disease and at the same time the mortality associated with esophageal adenocarcinoma has increased more than sevenfold. Therefore, they concluded that the increase in this cancer type represents a true increase in disease burden, thus suggesting that changes in the prevalence of known risk factors, specifically, GERD, obesity, or a decrease in *H. pylori* infection, might be possible explanations for the changing epidemiology. Nevertheless, if these risk factors contribute mainly to the increase in esophageal cancer, their incidence should also have risen in the last decades. Especially for GERD, thought to be one of the strongest risk factors, there is unfortunately a lack of data, so the future goal is to more carefully analyze the epidemiology of risk factors for esophageal cancer to ultimately prevent this disease in the future.

CLINICAL MANIFESTATIONS

Early symptoms in patients with esophageal cancer are normally absent. Therefore, at the time of diagnosis more than 50% of patients have an unresectable tumor or visible metastases.[8] The most common symptom in patients with this malignant tumor is dysphagia (74%). In addition, 57% of patients complain of weight loss and 17% of odynophagia (pain on swallowing food and liquids) at the time of diagnosis.[41] Other possible symptoms are cough, dyspnea, hoarseness, and pain (back, retrosternal, or abdominal). For patients with esophageal adenocarcinoma, Leers et al. recently confirmed that chronic GERD is a frequent factor in the clinical history of patients with this malignant disease.[42] Of the 117 patients included in this study, 86% reported having had heartburn or regurgitation at least several times in their lives. Moreover, 46% of the patients had reflux symptoms daily.

Usually, physical examination is unremarkable. However, if patients have metastatic disease, lymphadenopathy in the head and neck area, hepatomegaly, and pleural effusion can occur.

More recently, endoscopic surveillance of patients with Barrett's esophagus, the most important risk factor for esophageal adenocarcinoma, is becoming established. The rationale for this surveillance is twofold: to detect progression of disease to cancer and to allow early intervention while cure is still likely.[43] Peters et al. analyzed the clinical outcome of adenocarcinoma arising in Barrett's esophagus in endoscopically surveyed and nonsurveyed patients.[44] They reported that patients referred from surveillance programs for Barrett's esophagus have a better outcome and earlier stage than nonsurveyed patients do. Normally, these patients do not have the typical symptoms, such as dysphagia or weight loss, at the time of diagnosis but rather complain about typical reflux symptoms.

REFERENCES

1. Jemal A, Murray T, Ward E, et al: Cancer statistics, 2005. CA Cancer J Clin 55:10-30, 2005.
2. Klimstra DS: Pathologic prognostic factors in esophageal carcinoma. Semin Oncol 21:425-430, 1994.
3. Lukanich JM: Section I: Epidemiological review. Semin Thorac Cardiovasc Surg 15:158-166, 2003.
4. Crew KD, Neugut AI: Epidemiology of upper gastrointestinal malignancies. Semin Oncol 31:450-464, 2004.
5. Pohl H, Welch HG: The role of overdiagnosis and reclassification in the marked increase of esophageal adenocarcinoma incidence. J Natl Cancer Inst 97:142-146, 2005.
6. Lagergren J: Adenocarcinoma of oesophagus: What exactly is the size of the problem and who is at risk? Gut 54(Suppl 1):i1-i5, 2005.
7. Bollschweiler E, Wolfgarten E, Gutschow C, Hölscher AH: Demographic variations in the rising incidence of esophageal adenocarcinoma in white males. Cancer 92:549-555, 2001.
8. Enzinger PC, Mayer RJ: Esophageal cancer. N Engl J Med 349:2241-2252, 2003.
9. Portale G, Peters JH, Hsieh CC, et al: Esophageal adenocarcinoma in patients < or =50 years old: Delayed diagnosis and advanced disease at presentation. Am Surg 70:954-958, 2004.
10. Kubo A, Corley DA: Marked multi-ethnic variation of esophageal and gastric cardia carcinomas within the United States. Am J Gastroenterol 99:582-588, 2004.
11. Calle EE, Rodriguez C, Walker-Thurmond K, Thun MJ: Overweight, obesity, and mortality from cancer in a prospectively studied cohort of U.S. adults. N Engl J Med 348:1625-1638, 2003.
12. Lagergren J, Bergstrom R, Nyren O: Association between body mass and adenocarcinoma of the esophagus and gastric cardia. Ann Intern Med 130:883-890, 1999.

13. Castellsague X, Munoz N, De Stefani E, et al: Independent and joint effects of tobacco smoking and alcohol drinking on the risk of esophageal cancer in men and women. Int J Cancer 82:657-664, 1999.

14. Bosetti C, Franceschi S, Levi F, et al: Smoking and drinking cessation and the risk of oesophageal cancer. Br J Cancer 83:689-691, 2000.

15. Wu AH, Wan P, Bernstein L: A multiethnic population-based study of smoking, alcohol and body size and risk of adenocarcinomas of the stomach and esophagus (United States). Cancer Causes Control 12:721-732, 2001.

16. Gammon MD, Schoenberg JB, Ahsan H, et al: Tobacco, alcohol, and socioeconomic status and adenocarcinomas of the esophagus and gastric cardia. J Natl Cancer Inst 89:1277-1284, 1997.

17. Bosetti C, La Vecchia C, Talamini R, et al: Food groups and risk of squamous cell esophageal cancer in northern Italy. Int J Cancer 87:289-294, 2000.

18. Zhang ZF, Kurtz RC, Yu GP, et al: Adenocarcinomas of the esophagus and gastric cardia: The role of diet. Nutr Cancer 27:298-309, 1997.

19. Wolfgarten E, Rosendahl U, Nowroth T, et al: Coincidence of nutritional habits and esophageal cancer in Germany. Onkologie 24:546-551, 2001.

20. Bollschweiler E, Wolfgarten E, Nowroth T, et al: Vitamin intake and risk of subtypes of esophageal cancer in Germany. J Cancer Res Clin Oncol 128:575-580, 2002.

21. Mayne ST, Risch HA, Dubrow R, et al: Nutrient intake and risk of subtypes of esophageal and gastric cancer. Cancer Epidemiol Biomarkers Prev 10:1055-1062, 2001.

22. Wilson KT, Fu S, Ramanujam KS, et al: Increased expression of inducible nitric oxide synthase and cyclooxygenase-2 in Barrett's esophagus and associated adenocarcinomas. Cancer Res 58:2929-2934, 1998.

23. Fosslien E: Molecular pathology of cyclooxygenase-2 in neoplasia. Ann Clin Lab Sci 30:3-21, 2000.

24. Morris CD, Armstrong GR, Bigley G, et al: Cyclooxygenase-2 expression in the Barrett's metaplasia-dysplasia-adenocarcinoma sequence. Am J Gastroenterol 96:990-996, 2001.

25. Kuramochi H, Vallbohmer D, Uchida K, et al: Quantitative, tissue-specific analysis of cyclooxygenase gene expression in the pathogenesis of Barrett's adenocarcinoma. J Gastrointest Surg 8:1007-1017, 2004.

26. Thun MJ, Namboodiri MM, Calle EE, et al: Aspirin use and risk of fatal cancer. Cancer Res 53:1322-1327, 1993.

27. Funkhouser EM, Sharp GB: Aspirin and reduced risk of esophageal carcinoma. Cancer 76:1116-1119, 1995.

28. Corley DA, Kerlikowske K, Verma R, Buffler P: Protective association of aspirin/NSAIDs and esophageal cancer: A systematic review and meta-analysis. Gastroenterology 124:47-56, 2003.

29. Lagergren J, Bergstrom R, Lindgren A, Nyren O: Symptomatic gastroesophageal reflux as a risk factor for esophageal adenocarcinoma. N Engl J Med 340:825-831, 1999.

30. Chow WH, Finkle WD, McLaughlin JK, et al: The relation of gastroesophageal reflux disease and its treatment to adenocarcinomas of the esophagus and gastric cardia. JAMA 274:474-477, 1995.

31. Farrow DC, Vaughan TL, Sweeney C, et al: Gastroesophageal reflux disease, use of H$_2$ receptor antagonists, and risk of esophageal and gastric cancer. Cancer Causes Control 11:231-238, 2000.

32. Ye W, Chow WH, Lagergren J, et al: Risk of adenocarcinomas of the oesophagus and gastric cardia in patients with gastroesophageal reflux diseases and after antireflux surgery. Gastroenterology 121:1286-1293, 2001.

33. Peters JH, Hagen JA, DeMeester SR: Barrett's esophagus. J Gastrointest Surg 8:1-17, 2004.

34. Cameron AJ, Ott BJ, Payne WS: The incidence of adenocarcinoma in columnar-lined (Barrett's) esophagus. N Engl J Med 313:857-858, 1985.

35. Hameeteman W, Tytgat GNJ, Houthoff HJ, et al: Barrett's esophagus: Development of dysplasia and adenocarcinoma. Gastroenterology 96:1249-1256, 1989.

36. Lagergren J, Bergstrom R, Adami HO, Nyren O: Association between medications that relax the lower esophageal sphincter and risk for esophageal adenocarcinoma. Ann Intern Med 133:165-175, 2000.

37. Suerbaum S, Michetti P: *Helicobacter pylori* infection. N Engl J Med 347:1175-1186, 2002.

38. Chow WH, Blaser MJ, Blot WJ: An inverse relation between cagA+ strains of *Helicobacter pylori* infection and risk of esophageal and gastric cardia adenocarcinoma. Cancer Res 58:588-590, 1998.

39. Simán JH, Forsgren A, Berglund G, Florén CH: *Helicobacter pylori* infection is associated with a decreased risk of developing oesophageal neoplasms. Helicobacter 4:310-316, 2001.

40. Richter JE, Falk GW, Vaezi MF: *Helicobacter pylori* and gastroesophageal reflux disease: The bug may not be all bad. Am J Gastroenterol 93:1800-1802, 1998.

41. Daly JM, Fry WA, Little AG, et al: Esophageal cancer: Results of an American College of Surgeons Patient Care Evaluation Study. J Am Coll Surg 190:562-572, 2000.

42. Leers J, Bollschweiler E, Hölscher AH: Symptoms in patients with adenocarcinoma of the esophagus. Z Gastroenterol 43:275-280, 2005.

43. Provenzale D, Schmitt C, Wong JB: Barrett's esophagus: A new look at surveillance based on emerging estimates of cancer risk. Am J Gastroenterol 94:2043-2053, 1999.

44. Peters JH, Clark GW, Ireland AP, et al: Outcome of adenocarcinoma arising in Barrett's esophagus in endoscopically surveyed and nonsurveyed patients. J Thorac Cardiovasc Surg 108:813-821, 1994.

Esophageal Cancer: Current Staging Classifications and Techniques, Endoscopic Ultrasound, and Laparoscopic and Thoracoscopic Staging

Simon Law

Accurate staging serves three purposes: prognostication, source of information for stage-directed therapies, and quality control in clinical trials. Staging methods have evolved over the years, and there are now many staging techniques at our disposal, both invasive and noninvasive. Although these technologies undoubtedly have improved accuracy, the optimal methods remain controversial. Treatment strategies for esophageal cancer have also changed. A variety of endoscopic and surgical techniques and multimodality therapies are available to individual patients. Accurate staging assumes more importance for stage-directed therapy. This chapter details the current staging classifications and methods for esophageal cancer and highlights some of the difficulties and controversies.

STAGING SYSTEMS

Ideally, a staging system for cancer should be simple and easy to apply, provide sufficiently accurate and useful stratification of patients into different prognostic groups, and guide treatment. Unfortunately, no perfect system exists and constant modifications are required, depending on the knowledge gained. Currently, there are two main staging systems for esophageal cancer: the tumor-node-metastasis (TNM) system of the Union Internationale Contre le Cancer (UICC)[1] and the American Joint Committee on Cancer (AJCC),[2] which are uniform,

and the Guidelines for Clinical and Pathologic Studies on Carcinoma of the Esophagus advocated by the Japanese Society for Esophageal Diseases (JSED).[3]

Anatomic Subsites

Both systems divide the esophagus into anatomic segments for ease of classification (Fig. 33–1):

1. The cervical esophagus extends from the esophageal orifice (lower border of the cricoid cartilage) to the sternal notch (or thoracic inlet), which corresponds to approximately 18 cm from the upper incisor teeth.
2. The upper thoracic esophagus extends from the sternal notch to the tracheal bifurcation and measures approximately 24 cm from the upper incisor teeth.
3. The middle thoracic esophagus is the proximal half of the two equal portions between the tracheal bifurcation and the esophagogastric junction; it corresponds to roughly 32 cm measured from the upper incisor.
4. The lower thoracic esophagus is the thoracic part of the distal half of the two equal portions between the tracheal bifurcation and the esophagogastric junction.
5. The abdominal esophagus is the abdominal part of the distal half of the two equal portions between

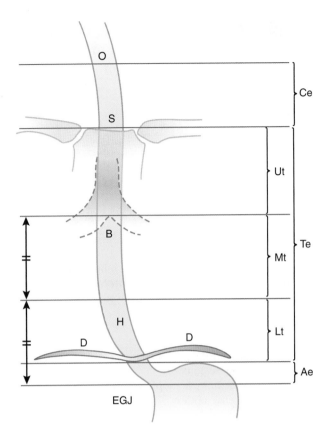

Figure 33-1. Description of the different levels of esophageal tumor. Ce, cervical esophagus; Te, thoracic esophagus; Ut, upper third; Mt, middle third; Lt, lower third; Ae, abdominal esophagus; EGJ, esophagogastric junction; O, esophagus; S, sternal notch; B, tracheal bifurcation; D, diaphragm; H, hiatus.

the tracheal bifurcation and the esophagogastric junction. The esophagogastric junction approximates 40 cm measured from the upper incisor.

Definitions of Depth of Tumor Infiltration (T Stage)

The depth of tumor infiltration classified by the Japanese system addresses the following:

1. TX: Depth of tumor invasion not able to be assessed
2. T0: No evidence of primary tumor
3. Tis: Carcinoma in situ (EP)
4. T1a: Invasion to the lamina propria mucosae (lpm) or up to but not beyond the muscularis mucosae (mm)
5. T1b: Invasion to but not beyond the submucosa (sm)
6. T2: Invasion to but not beyond the muscularis propria (mp)
7. T3: Invasion to the esophageal adventitia (Ad)
8. T4: Invasion to adjacent organs

In the current AJCC/UICC system, although T1 lesions are not subdivided into T1a and T1b officially, it is clear that T1a and T1b tumors are prognostically

Regional Lymph Nodes for Esophageal Cancer According to the American Joint Committee on Cancer TNM Classification

Cervical Esophagus

Scalene
Internal jugular
Upper and lower cervical
Periesophageal
Supraclavicular

Intrathoracic Esophagus (Upper, Middle, and Lower)

Upper periesophageal (above the azygous vein)
Subcarinal
Lower periesophageal (below the azygous vein)

Gastroesophageal Junction

Lower esophageal (below the azygous vein)
Diaphragmatic
Pericardial
Left gastric
Celiac

different in that T1b lesions are associated with a substantial chance of lymph node metastasis, so the nomenclature T1a and T1b is widely used. Studies on early cancer also indicate that subdivisions of mucosal and submucosal cancer are possible. Mucosal cancer is separated into intraepithelial cancer (m1), tumor involving the lamina propria (m2), and cancer penetrating the lamina muscularis mucosae (m3). Progressive depths of submucosal infiltration (sm1 to sm3) also indicate escalating chance of metastasis. This is increasingly of relevance, especially when high-frequency endoscopic ultrasound (EUS) and endoscopic mucosal resection techniques are used. In the Japanese system, "superficial cancers" are defined as carcinomas limited to the submucosal layer, whereas "early-stage cancers" are referred to as carcinomas with invasion into the mucosal layer but without metastasis (Tis N0 M0 and T1a N0 M0).

Nodal Metastases (N Stage)

The most controversial aspect in TNM staging is the classification of nodal metastases. Both the AJCC/UICC and the JSED systems use a topographic description of nodal metastases. The AJCC/UICC system is simpler and essentially regards periesophageal, mediastinal, and perigastric lymph node stations as "regional." For cervical esophageal cancer, only lymph nodes in the neck are regarded as regional (Box 33-1). For intrathoracic tumors, the celiac and cervical lymph nodes are classified as M1 disease, with subdivision into M1a and M1b depending on the site of the primary tumor. The latter also includes visceral organ metastases. The TNM stage groupings are shown in Table 33–1. A lymph node map that extends the nomenclature and numbering system used for the staging of non–small cell lung cancer has been suggested by the AJCC and is included in the staging manual (Fig. 33–2). In the Japanese system, lymph node stations are expanded in addition to that used for gastric cancer staging in Japan (Fig. 33–3 and Table 33–2). This system is substantially more complicated than that proposed by the AJCC. Lymph node stations are classified into N0 to N4, and just like gastric cancer, assignment of the N category depends on the location of the primary tumor (Table 33–3). Moreover, when pathologic information is available, the pN category is modified according to the number of lymph nodes found involved. For one to three metastatic nodes, no revision of the pN value is necessary; for four to seven nodal metastases, the pN value is modified upward by an increment of 1 (not beyond N4 cases); and when eight or more nodes are involved, a correction factor of 2 is used (not beyond N4). Thus, for example, in a patient found to have pN1 disease (by location), if eight nodes are found to be positive, the pN1 category is upgraded to pN3. Implicit within the staging system is that a minimum of four nodes need to be examined to allow this modification of the pN value. The final TNM combinations in different stages are shown in Figure 33–4. Lymph node stations are sometimes also classified according to a system proposed by Akiyama based on his extensive experience in three-field lymphadenectomy; it includes seven anatomic regions (Table 33–4). This system, however, has not been adopted by the JSED.

Cancer Around the Gastroesophageal Junction

For cancer around the gastroesophageal junction, a classification system proposed by Siewert and Stein is increasingly being used.[4] This system aims at subclassifying adenocarcinomas found within 5 cm proximal and distal to the anatomic gastroesophageal junction and is therefore of particular relevance in the West, where Barrett's esophagus and adenocarcinoma of the lower esophagus and gastric cardia are prevalent.[5,6] The system classifies tumors as type I to type III (esophageal, cardiac, and subcardiac), depending on the relative extent of involvement of either the esophagus or stomach (Fig. 33–5). The three types of cancers are different in patient demographics, possible cause, histopathologic features, and prognosis. Different treatment strategies are also advocated.[7] Further validation of this classification is needed to determine its reliability. In the East, where Barrett's esophagus and adenocarcinomas of the esophagus are uncommon, the system is perhaps less relevant[8]; lower esophageal cancers are mostly squamous, and there is no doubt about their cellular origin. Subcardiac cancers should probably be regarded as primarily gastric cancers. Classification and treatment of type II cancers centered on the gastroesophageal junction are most controversial,

and it is uncertain whether they should be staged as gastric or esophageal tumors.[9]

In the Japanese classification, depending on the relative extent of involvement of the esophagus and stomach, a simple descriptive method of EG, E = G, and GE is used. Realizing the problem of classification of junctional tumors, the assignment of nodal stations into N1 to N4

Table 33–1	Stage Groupings for Esophageal Cancer According to the AJCC TNM Classification

T: Primary tumor
- Tx   Tumor cannot be assessed
- Tis   In situ carcinoma
- T1   Tumor invades the lamina propria or submucosa; does not breach the submucosa
- T2   Tumor invades into but not beyond the muscularis propria
- T3   Tumor invades the adventitia but not the adjacent structure
- T4   Tumor invades the adjacent structure

N: Regional lymph nodes
- NX   Regional nodal status cannot be assessed
- N0   No regional lymph node involvement
- N1   Regional lymph node involved

M: Distant metastases
- MX   Distant metastases cannot be assessed
- M0   No distant metastasis
- M1a   Upper thoracic esophagus with metastases to the cervical nodes
        Lower thoracic esophagus with metastases to the celiac nodes
- M1b   Upper thoracic esophagus with metastases to other nonregional nodes or other distant sites
        Lower thoracic esophagus with metastases to other nonregional nodes or other distant sites
        Middle thoracic esophagus with metastases to the cervical, celiac, or other nonregional nodes or other distant sites

Stage Groupings

Stage	T	N	M
Stage 0	Tis	N0	M0
Stage I	T1	N0	M0
Stage IIa	T2	N0	M0
	T3	N0	M0
Stage IIb	T1	N1	M0
	T2	N1	M0
Stage III	T3	N1	M0
	T4	N0-N1	M0
Stage IVa	Any T	Any N	M1a
Stage IVb	Any T	Any N	M1b

From American Joint Committee on Cancer: AJCC Cancer Staging Manual. New York, Springer, 2002, pp 91-95.

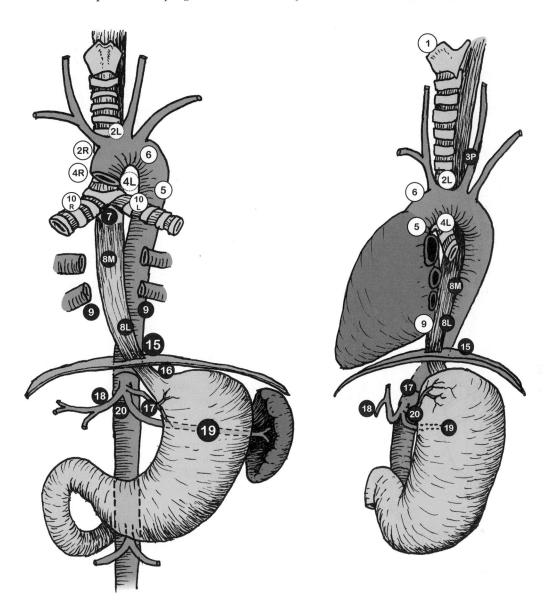

Figure 33–2.   Lymph node stations suggested by the American Joint Committee on Cancer manual. 1, Supraclavicular; 2R, right upper paratracheal nodes; 2L, left upper paratracheal nodes; 3P, posterior mediastinal nodes; 4R, right lower paratracheal nodes; 4L, left lower paratracheal nodes; 5, aortopulmonary nodes; 6, anterior mediastinal nodes; 7, subcarinal nodes; 8M, middle paraesophageal nodes; 8L, lower paraesophageal nodes; 9, pulmonary ligament nodes; 10R, right tracheobronchial nodes; 10L, left tracheobronchial nodes; 15, diaphragmatic nodes; 16, paracardial nodes; 17, left gastric nodes; 18, common hepatic nodes; 19, splenic nodes; 20, celiac nodes.

for these cancers is described as "tentative" by the JSED.[3] According to the Japanese Classification of Gastric Carcinoma endorsed by the Japanese Gastric Cancer Association, lymph node groupings also change when a cardia or proximal gastric cancer invades the esophagus.[10] To add to the confusion, the current Japanese gastric cancer nodal stations are classified from N0 to N3, whereas for esophageal cancer, the classification extends to N4. It is also observed that if the AJCC/UICC gastric cancer staging system is going to be used for type II or III cancers, assignment of nodal metastases changes from a topographic to a numerical one: N0 disease indicates no nodal disease, N1 is used for 1 to 6 involved regional

nodes, N2 for 7 to 15 nodes, and N3 for more than 15 involved nodes. The nomenclature of tumors around this area is therefore far from settled. Further work is urgently required to accurately reflect uniform and accurate staging of tumors around the gastroesophageal junction.

Which Staging System Should Be Used?

There is little disagreement with regard to T stage because it is reproducible and clear evidence of progressive metastatic potential and prognosis can be

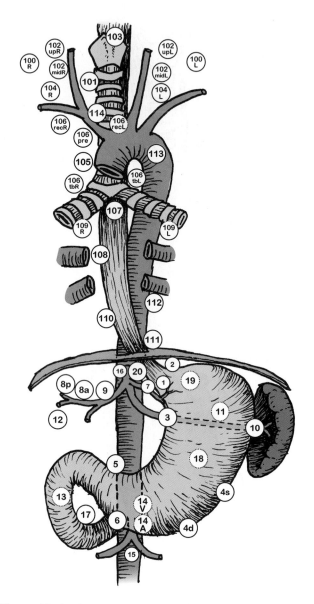

Figure 33–3. Lymph node stations according to the Japanese Society for Esophageal Diseases.

ogist's examination of the specimen together determine the number of lymph nodes retrieved; additional technique such as fat clearing also increases the yield.[11] At the author's institution, tissue at individual stations is dissected out and labeled for the pathologist to examine, but individual lymph nodes are not dissected out of the connective tissue and fat. This may be a practical compromise to ensure topographic accuracy without being too time-consuming for the surgeons.

The AJCC system is more widely used internationally. Assignment of nodal stations to simply N0 and N1 is perhaps oversimplified. The N1 versus M1a versus M1b descriptors also do not accurately identify prognostically different groups.[12] Currently, celiac lymph nodes are classified as M1a for lower thoracic esophageal tumors. Clearly, better survival can be achieved, with an approximately 10% or higher chance of cure at 5 years after surgical resection, as opposed to the more dismal prognosis with visceral metastases. Similarly, in patients with cervical nodal metastases, cervical lymphadenectomy can also result in long-term cure, especially when three-field lymphadenectomy is performed.[13]

The number of metastatic lymph nodes is recognized as an important prognostic factor. The TNM classification of gastric and colorectal cancer has already incorporated the number of lymph nodes in the pN classification category. Using the number of lymph nodes for staging implies a minimum number of retrieved nodes for histopathologic examination. The UICC recommends a minimum of 6 retrieved lymph nodes for an accurate nodal classification of esophageal cancer, 15 or more nodes for gastric cancer, and 12 or more for colorectal cancer.[1] Other authors have suggested a total of 12 for esophageal cancer.[14] The number of nodes resected is often used as a surrogate for quality control of lymphadenectomy. As already discussed, this reflects not only the extensiveness of the lymphadenectomy but also the manner in which the surgical specimens are handled and the conscientiousness of the pathologist. The Japanese style of specimen processing will invariably lead to more nodes examined, regardless of the extent of lymphadenectomy. This aside, various cutoff points of prognostic importance have been reported for the number of involved nodes: 0 or 1 versus 2 or more,[15] 0 versus 1 to 2 versus 3 or more,[12] 0 or 1 versus 2 to 7 versus 8 or more,[16] 1 to 4 versus 5 or more,[17-24] 0 versus 1 to 3 versus 4 or more,[25] 0 to 5 versus 6 or more,[26] and 1 to 7 versus 8 or more[27]; in addition, as used by the current Japanese system, cutoff points include 0 versus 1 to 3 versus 4 to 7 versus 8 or more.[3] The variety of combinations shows that although the number of involved nodes is recognized to be important, it is difficult to find a consensus. Other than the number of nodes, the lymph node ratio (number of positive nodes divided by the number sampled) was also found to have prognostic value.[28,29]

Modification of the current TNM staging system is clearly desirable, and various revisions have been suggested.[22-26] The AJCC task force for esophageal cancer strongly considered changing the TNM staging system for the latest version; however, it was thought that there were insufficient published data to support a proposal for a new system that would be widely accepted.[30]

demonstrated; accordingly, the AJCC/UICC and the Japanese system do not differ. How to classify nodal metastases and stage groupings is most controversial. Both systems use a topographic assignment for lymph node stations. The AJCC/UICC system is clearly simpler to apply. The problem with the Japanese method is that more detailed and meticulous handling of the surgical specimen is required. When a pathologic stage is assigned from esophagectomy specimens, close cooperation between the surgeon and pathologist is essential. In Japan, it is customary that individual lymph nodes be dissected from the surgical specimen by the operating surgeon before the specimen is sent to the pathologist, thereby ensuring topographic accuracy. In most Western practices this is not performed, and more reliance is placed on the pathologist. It is clear that the extent of lymphadenectomy and the thoroughness of the pathol-

Table 33–2   Lymph Node Stations According to the Japanese Society for Esophageal Diseases

Cervical and Mediastinal Lymph Nodes		Abdominal Lymph Nodes	
No.	Definition	No.	Definition
100	Superficial lymph nodes of the neck	1	Right cardial lymph nodes
101	Cervical paraesophageal lymph nodes	2	Left cardial lymph nodes
102	Deep cervical lymph nodes	3	Lymph nodes along the lesser curvature
103	Peripharyngeal lymph nodes	4	Lymph nodes along the greater curvature
104	Supraclavicular lymph nodes	5	Suprapyloric lymph nodes
105	Upper thoracic paraesophageal lymph nodes	6	Infrapyloric lymph nodes
106	Thoracic paratracheal lymph nodes	7	Lymph nodes along the left gastric artery
106-rec	Recurrent nerve lymph nodes	8	Lymph nodes along the common hepatic artery
106-rec L	Left recurrent nerve lymph nodes	9	Lymph nodes along the celiac artery
106-rec R	Right recurrent nerve lymph nodes	10	Lymph nodes at the splenic hilum
106-pre	Pretracheal lymph nodes	11	Lymph nodes along the splenic artery
106-tb	Tracheobronchial lymph nodes	12	Lymph nodes in the hepatoduodenal ligament
106-tb L	Left tracheobronchial lymph nodes	13	Lymph nodes on the posterior surface of the pancreatic head
106-tb R	Right tracheobronchial lymph nodes	14	Lymph nodes at the root of the mesentery
107	Subcarinal lymph nodes	14A	Lymph nodes along the superior mesenteric artery
108	Middle thoracic paraesophageal lymph nodes	14V	Lymph nodes along the superior mesenteric vein
109	Main bronchus lymph nodes (formerly: pulmonary hilar lymph nodes)	15	Lymph nodes along the middle colic artery
110	Lower thoracic paraesophageal lymph nodes	16	Lymph nodes around the abdominal aorta
111	Supradiaphragmatic lymph nodes (formerly: diaphragmatic lymph nodes)	17	Lymph nodes on the anterior surface of the pancreatic head
112	Posterior mediastinal lymph nodes	18	Lymph nodes along the inferior margin of the pancreas
113	Ligamentum arteriosum lymph nodes (Botallo's lymph nodes)	19	Infradiaphragmatic lymph nodes
114	Anterior mediastinal lymph nodes	20	Lymph nodes in the esophageal hiatus of the diaphragm

For more detailed subdivisions of individual lymph node groups, refer to the staging manual of the Japanese Society for Esophageal Diseases.

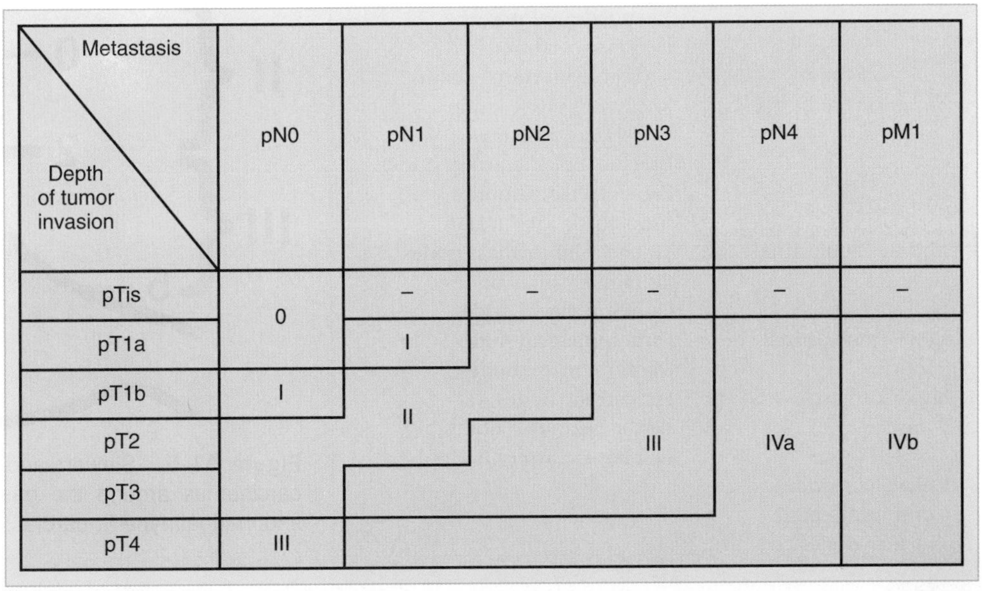

Figure 33–4. Stage groupings according to the Japanese Society for Esophageal Diseases.

Metastasis / Depth of tumor invasion	pN0	pN1	pN2	pN3	pN4	pM1
pTis	0	–	–	–	–	–
pT1a		I				
pT1b	I	II		III	IVa	IVb
pT2						
pT3						
pT4	III					

Table 33–3   Lymph Node Groups by Location of the Primary Tumor According to the Japanese Society for Esophageal Diseases

Tumor Location		N1	N2	N3	N4
Cervical esophagus (Ce)		101, 104	102, 106-rec	100, 103, 105, 106-tbL, 107, 108	106-pre, 106-tbR, 109, 110, 111, 112, 113, 114, 1, 2, 3, and others
Thoracic esophagus (Te)	Upper (Ut)	105, 101, 106-rec	104, 106-tbL, 107, 108, 109	102-mid, 106-pre, 106-tbR, 110, 111, 112, 1, 2, 3, 7	100, 102-up, 103, 113, 114, 4, 5, 6, 8, 9, 20, and others
	Middle (Mt)	108, 106-rec	101, 105, 106-tbL, 107, 109, 110, 1, 2, 3, 7	104, 111, 112, 20	100, 102, 103, 106-pre, 106-tbR, 113, 114, 4, 5, 6, 8, 9, and others
	Lower (Lt)	110, 1, 2	106-rec, 107, 108, 109, 111, 112, 3, 7, 20	101, 105, 106-tbL, 9, 19	101, 102, 103, 104, 106-pre, 106-tbR, 113, 114, 4, 5, 6, 8, 10, and others
Abdominal esophagus (Ae)		1, 2, 3, 20	110, 111, 7, 9, (4), (10), (11), 19	108, 5, 8, (112)	100, 101, 102, 103, 104, 105, 106, 107, 109, 113, 114, 6, and others
Esophagogastric junction*	EG E = G GE	1, 2, 3	7, 9, 10, 11, (110), (111), (4)	108, 5, 6, 8, (112), (12), (13), (14)	100, 101, 102, 103, 104, 105, 106, 107, 109, 15, 16, and others

For lymph nodes in parentheses, the D category is not affected by excision or nonexcision of these lymph nodes.
*Lymph node groups of the esophagogastric junction are tentative.

Table 33–4   Lymph Node Groups as Described by Akiyama

Anatomic Site	Lymph Node Group
Cervical nodes	Deep lateral nodes (spinal accessory chain)
	Deep external nodes
	Deep internal nodes (recurrent nerve chain)
Superior mediastinal nodes	Recurrent nerve chain
	Paratracheal nodes
	Brachiocephalic artery nodes
	Paraesophageal nodes
	Infra-aortic arch nodes
Middle mediastinal nodes	Tracheal bifurcation nodes
	Pulmonary hilar nodes
	Paraesophageal nodes
Lower mediastinal nodes	Paraesophageal nodes
	Diaphragmatic nodes
Superior gastric nodes nodes	Pericardiac nodes
	Lesser curvature nodes
	Left gastric artery nodes
Celiac axis nodes	
Common hepatic artery nodes	

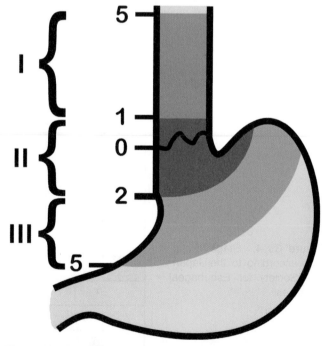

Figure 33–5. Siewert and Stein's classification of adenocarcinomas around the gastroesophageal junction. Type I, esophageal; type II, cardiac; type III, subcardiac.

The TNM system remains the most widely used, although the detailed topographic Japanese classification does have its merits. With the increasing amount of data accumulated, future changes in staging are inevitable. How best to integrate a topographic as well as a numerical component for nodal metastases remains to be determined. The minimal number and the stations of sampled lymph nodes required for adequate nodal staging, the optimal cutoff points for involved lymph nodes, the topographic locations of nodal stations that impart prognostic value, and whether the M1 category should be reserved for visceral metastases only are just some issues that need clarification. Because the incidence of lower esophageal and junctional adenocarcinoma is increasing while that of distal gastric cancer is decreasing, some concordance between staging of gastric, gastroesophageal junction, and lower esophageal adenocarcinoma is also desirable.

TNM Residual Tumor Classification

The R classification, an axillary classification within the TNM system, denotes the absence or presence of residual tumor after treatment and describes residual tumor as macroscopic or microscopic in amount.[31] The R category considers residual tumor at the primary tumor site, in the regional lymph nodes, and at distant sites. It may be used after surgical resection alone or after various combinations of nonoperative treatment. The R categories are defined as follows:

RX: The presence of residual tumor not able to be assessed
R0: No residual tumor
R1: Microscopic residual tumor
R2: Macroscopic residual tumor

R2 cases can be subdivided into R2a, in which there is no microscopic confirmation of residual tumor, and R2b, in which microscopic confirmation is available. The R1 category is reserved exclusively for cases in which residual tumor is found by histologic examination. This may apply to biopsy sampling of the regional tissue at the site of resection or a distant site at the time of surgery. It also applies to microscopic examination of the resection margins of the surgical resection specimen by the pathologist. In resected esophageal cancer specimens, the proximal and distal margins, as well as the lateral margins, should be examined pathologically for residual disease. Involvement of any margins despite gross macroscopic clearance at the time of surgery indicates an R1 resection. R1 should be used only if histologic examination reveals that the tumor is transected,[31] although some investigators have reported involvement of microscopic tumor within 1 mm or less of the resection margin as R1, and such cases are associated with a worse prognosis.[32] In tumor resection specimens from patients who have undergone lymphadenectomy, the "marginal" node is the one near the resection margin that is most distant from the primary tumor. Involvement of such a "marginal" or "apical" node, however, does not influence the R category. The R category naturally correlates with the stage of disease; the likelihood of palliative resection (R1-R2) migrates with advancing stage of disease, but R0 resections can also be performed for stage IV disease, provided that the metastatic lesion is resected as well.

Aside from stage, the R category is perhaps the strongest prognostic factor. It is also important with regard to quality assurance in oncologic treatment and facilitates comparison of treatment results if applied in a consistent manner. The need for additional treatment planning also depends heavily on the R category. This treatment-related variable should be carefully assessed and documented.

STAGING METHODS

Clinical staging requires a thorough physical examination and additional imaging methods. The physical sign indicative of metastatic disease that is most likely found is a palpable metastatic lymph node in the neck, particularly around the paratracheal region. Hoarseness of voice suggests recurrent laryngeal nerve palsy and thus signifies either direct tumor involvement or metastatic lymph nodes. Hepatomegaly with liver metastases is found only in very advanced disease. A simple chest radiograph may show metastases. Solitary lesions, however, may more likely indicate a primary pulmonary lesion.

Specific methods in clinical staging involve barium contrast studies, bronchoscopy, computed tomography (CT), percutaneous ultrasound of cervical lymph nodes with or without fine-needle aspiration (FNA) cytology, EUS with or without FNA, 2-[^{18}F]fluoro-2-deoxy-D-glucose (FDG) positron emission tomography (PET), and laparoscopy or thoracoscopy (or both).

Barium Contrast Study

Typical features on a barium contrast study include mucosal irregularity and shouldering, narrowing of the lumen, and proximal dilatation of the esophagus (Fig. 33–6). It gives a longitudinal graphic view of the tumor in relation to other mediastinal structures, especially the trachea and main bronchi. It is a useful guide to the endoscopist and the surgeon, and in addition, it is sensitive in depicting tracheal-airway fistulas. Tortuosity, angulation, axis deviation from the midline, sinus formation, and fistulation to the bronchial tree are signs indicative of advanced tumor that has traversed the adventitia and involved the neighboring fixed organs.[33]

Endoscopic Examination

A classification of the macroscopic endoscopic appearance of esophageal cancer is in use by the JSED.[3] Superficial tumors are classified into type 0-I (superficial and protruding), type 0-II (superficial and flat), and type 0-III (superficial and distinctly depressed). Advanced tumors are classified as type 1 (localized protruding), type 2 (ulcerative and localized), type 3 (ulcerative

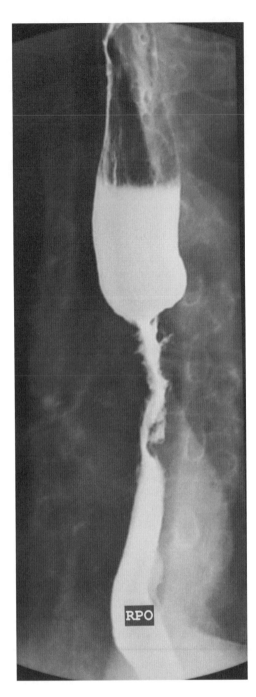

Figure 33–6. Barium contrast study showing a mid-esophageal tumor. Tumor stenosis with proximal dilatation of the esophagus is evident. The small sinuses are also suggestive of advanced infiltrative disease. RPO, right posterior oblique view.

specific (93%) in predicting the local extent of tumor (overall accuracy, 89%). Detailed analysis showed good sensitivity for type 0 (83%), which corresponds to T1 carcinoma, and for types 3 and 4 (82% and 83%), which represent T3 and T4 tumors. In endoscopic type 1 and type 2, the concordance with T stage (T2) was weak, with a sensitivity of 52%.[34]

Indirect information can be gained on the T stage and N stage by endoscopy alone. Esophageal tumors that are sufficiently large to cause luminal stenosis tend to be T3 and T4 lesions.[35] A tumor length greater than 5 cm is also predictive of T3 cancer with a sensitivity of 89%, specificity of 92%, positive predictive value (PPV) of 89%, and negative predictive value (NPV) of 92%.[36] Because advancing T stage correlates strongly with the presence of regional lymph node metastases, advanced-disease stage can often be inferred in patients with nontraversable tumors. In one study, 21 of 79 patients (26.6%) had high-grade malignant strictures precluding endosonographic examination without preceding esophageal dilatation. Nineteen of the 21 patients (90.5%) had stage III or IV disease by histopathologic examination of the surgical specimen.[37] Endoscopy alone, however, cannot distinguish T3 from T4 tumors, nor can distant metastases such as celiac lymph node or visceral metastases be predicted.

Endoscopic examination allows biopsy of the tumor, with or without brush cytology, to increase the diagnostic yield. In early tumors especially, Lugol's iodine chromoendoscopy is invaluable in localizing the extent of disease, in addition to directing biopsy at other dysplastic areas. Normal mucosa with its glycogen content should stain brown, with suspicious areas left unstained for directed biopsy. In patients with high-grade stenosis, endoscopically guided nasogastric tube insertion for tube feeding can be performed in the same setting.

Bronchoscopy

Use of the fiberoptic endoscope allows histologic confirmation of the cancer by biopsy or brush cytology. Flexible bronchoscopy is performed to assess tumor involvement of the tracheobronchial tree, especially tumors in the mid and upper portions of the esophagus. Signs of involvement include a widened carina, external compression, tumor infiltration, and fistulization. The last two signs contraindicate resection.[38] The gross macroscopic bronchoscopic appearance may not be accurate, and biopsy plus brush cytology is recommended. In one study involving patients with supracarinal cancer, endoluminal tumor mass, protrusion of the posterior tracheal wall, and signs of mucosal invasion were visible in 5.9%, 28.6%, and 4.1% of bronchoscopic examinations, respectively. However, in only 8.6% of 220 bronchoscopic examinations was cancer invasion proved by biopsy or cytology. Bronchoscopy excluded 18.1% of otherwise potentially operable patients from surgery because of airway invasion, with an overall accuracy of 93.3%.[39]

Bronchoscopic ultrasound has been investigated as a staging tool. The diagnosis of tracheobronchial invasion was based on an interruption in the most external hyper-

and infiltrative), type 4 (diffusely infiltrative), and type 5 (miscellaneous type). Types 0-I, 0-II, 1, 4, and 5 are further divided into subtypes. Corresponding barium contrast appearances are also included in the classification.

In a study of 209 patients correlating the UICC's T stage with the JSED's endoscopic categories, it was shown that endoscopic assessment was both sensitive (78%) and

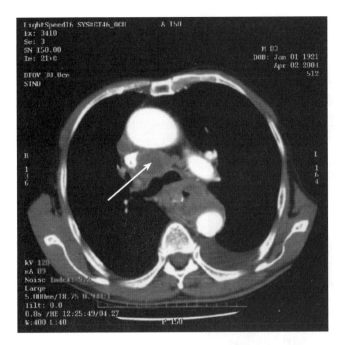

Figure 33–7. Computed tomography scan showing a midthoracic esophageal cancer with suspicious aortic infiltration, as well as a large precarinal lymph node *(arrow)*.

echoic layer of the tracheobronchus (corresponding to its adventitia). In one study, of 26 patients determined to be invasion-free by bronchoscopic ultrasound, only 2 had invasion, as compared with 7 of 22 patients who had invasion after CT scans had suggested that they did not. The examination had no complication.[40] The technique, however, is not commonly performed.

Computed Tomography

The main value of CT in staging esophageal cancer lies in its ability to detect distant disease, such as in the liver, lungs, bone, and kidneys. When a metastasis to the liver is larger than 2 cm, the sensitivity of diagnosis is 70% to 80%, although it drops to approximately 50% when it is less than 1 cm.[41] With adenocarcinoma of the gastroesophageal junction and gastric cardia, peritoneal metastases are more likely than with squamous cell cancer of the tubular esophagus. CT scanning is inferior to laparoscopy in detecting peritoneal metastases.[42] Solitary lung metastases are rare in patients with esophageal carcinoma[43] and, thus, when seen on CT, are more likely to be primary lung cancer or benign nodules and should be investigated as such.

CT cannot reliably distinguish the various T stages, and its use lies in the diagnosis of T4 disease (Fig. 33–7). One study showed that the sensitivity and specificity of CT in detecting T4 disease were 25% and 94%, respectively.[44] Obliteration of the fat plane between the esophagus and the aorta, trachea and bronchi, and pericardium is suggestive of invasion, but the paucity of fat in cachectic patients makes this criterion unreliable. Thickening or indentation of the normally flat membra-

nous trachea and left main bronchus is also suggestive of invasion, but it should always be confirmed by bronchoscopic examination. When the area of contact between the esophagus and the aorta extends for more than 90 degree of the circumference, an 80% accuracy of infiltration was reported,[45] but this is by no means absolute and the accuracy is inferior to that of EUS.

The sensitivity of detecting mediastinal and abdominal nodal involvement is suboptimal with CT because only size alone can be used as a diagnostic criterion. Intrathoracic and abdominal nodes greater than 1 cm are enlarged, and supraclavicular nodes with a short axis greater than 0.5 cm and retrocrural nodes greater than 0.6 cm are pathologic.[46] However, normal-sized lymph nodes may contain metastatic deposits, and enlargement of lymph nodes may be due to reactive and inflammatory hyperplasia. Recent studies using high-resolution helical CT scanning have demonstrated sensitivities of 11% to 77% and specificities of 71% to 95% for the detection of regional nodal disease.[47,48] CT is relatively insensitive in detecting celiac axis lymphadenopathy. Experience with magnetic resonance imaging (MRI) has shown limitations similar to those of CT, especially with respect to the low detection rate of mediastinal lymph nodes.[49]

Percutaneous and Endoscopic Ultrasound

Percutaneous ultrasound has a specific role in diagnosing cervical lymph node involvement, especially for squamous cell cancer, because the incidence of lymph node metastases in the neck is high, given the more proximal location of the tumor. Although lymph nodes are abundant in the neck (more than 300 in a normal adult), normal nodes are difficult to visualize because they are isoechoic to the surrounding fat. Sonographic examination of cervical lymph nodes usually begins with visualization of the common carotid artery and internal jugular vein at the base of the neck. Axial scans, transverse to the vessels, are performed in a cephalad direction. Nodes are viewed in relation to the carotid and jugular vein. Level IV, III, and II nodes are sequentially visualized anterior to and level V posterior to the vessels. Adenopathy can be a result of underlying inflammation in up to 50% of cases, whereas 20% to 40% of normal-sized nodes may harbor metastases; thus ultrasound-guided FNA is essential.

In a large study involving 519 patients, cervical lymph node metastasis was detected in 30.8% of patients (160/519). The sensitivity, specificity, and accuracy of ultrasound diagnosis in patients who underwent subsequent cervical lymphadenectomy were 74.5%, 94.1%, and 87.6%, respectively. In those who did not undergo neck dissection, the chance of cervical nodal recurrence was low at less than 5%.[50]

EUS is the only imaging modality able to distinguish the various layers of the esophageal wall, usually seen as five alternating hyperechoic and hypoecheoic layers (Fig. 33–8). Three general types of echoendoscopes can be used for staging: (1) a radial scanning endoscope, which provides a 360-degree view of the esophageal wall and surrounding tissues; it can operate at 5 to 20 MHz;

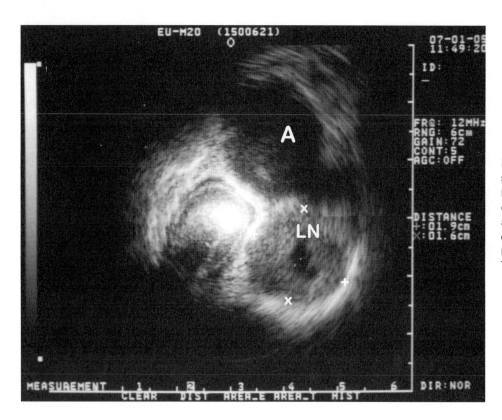

Figure 33–8. Endoscopic ultrasound image with a 12-MHz miniprobe placed at the gastroesophageal junction showing the aorta (A) and a large 2-cm adjacent lymph node (LN) with central necrosis. (Courtesy of K. E. Kwok, The University of Hong Kong.)

(2) EUS miniprobes, which can be passed through the accessory channel of the endoscope and provide 360-degree imaging at 12, 20, and 30 MHz; the high-frequency probes provide excellent resolution of the esophageal wall but have limited penetration and are best used for imaging superficial cancers; and (3) curved linear-array transducer endoscopes, which are primarily used for ultrasound guidance during FNA procedures such as sampling of the celiac lymph nodes; the lack of a 360-degree view makes it less user-friendly for T staging. The resolution and depth of penetration vary with the frequency of the ultrasound: at a frequency of 7.5 MHz, the depth of penetration is 9 cm with a resolution of 0.2 mm; the corresponding figures are 3 cm and 0.1 mm for 12 MHz.

The accuracy of EUS in locoregional staging is not questioned. The accuracy of EUS in T and N staging averages 85% and 75% versus 58% and 54% for CT.[51] Sensitivity and specificity tend to vary by T stage, with improved sensitivity as the T stage increases. In one series, the sensitivity was 58% for less than T2, 59% for T2, and 91% for greater than T2 disease.[52] A review of the literature shows variation in accuracy for T stage, as follows: 75% to 82% for T1, 64% to 82% for T2, 89% to 94% for T3, and 88% to 100% for T4.[53] One main limitation of EUS is an inability to pass the endoscope through the tumor stricture, which occurs in about a third of patients.[53-56] Although earlier studies suggested that dilatation would result in up to a 25% chance of perforation without much gain in diagnostic information,[35,37] more recent results show that dilatation can be performed safely, with the success rate of complete examination depending on the extent of dilatation: 36% for

11 to 12.8 mm and 87% for 14 to 16 mm.[57] An alternative is to use miniprobes; with a 6-French, 12.5-MHz miniprobe, overall accuracy in assessment of tumor infiltration depth and nodal disease is 90% and 78%, respectively.[58]

The use of higher-frequency echo-ultrasound allows fine distinction of early mucosal and submucosal esophageal cancer into intraepithelial cancer (m1), tumor involving the lamina propria (m2), tumor penetrating the lamina muscularis mucosae (m3), and various degree of submucosal infiltration (sm1 to sm3). The diagnostic accuracy was 80% when the muscularis mucosae was seen.[59] Such information is of particular importance when endoscopic mucosal resection is a treatment option for early cancer or for the detection of submucosal invasion, high-grade dysplasia, or carcinoma in situ in Barrett's esophagus.[60]

Ultrasonographic features of lymph nodes that suggest malignant involvement include echo-poor (hypoechoic) structure, sharply demarcated borders, rounded contour, and size greater than 10 mm, in increasing order of importance.[61] The four features just described, when each is present alone, may be inaccurate in diagnosing metastatic lymph nodes, but when all four are present, the accuracy reaches 80%. However, one study showed that all four features were present in only 25% of malignant nodes.[62] A collective review showed that the overall accuracy of staging nodal disease was 77%.[51]

Accuracy may differ for different lymph node locations. Its sensitivity is highest for the cervical and upper thoracic paraesophageal, infracarinal, left paratracheal, and recurrent laryngeal nodes. It is best with the para-

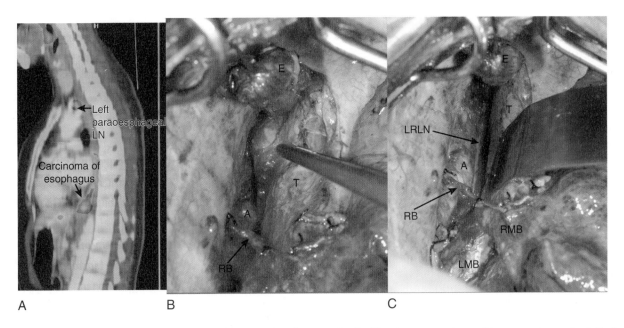

Figure 33–9. **A,** Positron emission tomography scan showing a patient with a lower esophageal tumor and a metastatic lymph node (LN) in the superior mediastinum. **B,** Operative photograph showing the lymph node identified in the left paratracheal area on the left recurrent laryngeal nerve. The forceps are pointing at the enlarged lymph node. A, aortic arch; E, esophageal stump; RB, right bronchial artery; T, trachea. **C,** Operative photograph showing the mediastinum after resection of the lymph node and mediastinal dissection. A, aortic arch; E, esophageal stump; LMB, left main bronchus; LRLN, left recurrent laryngeal nerve; RB, right bronchial artery; RMB, right main bronchus; T, trachea.

esophageal nodes and varies inversely with the axial distance of the nodes from the esophageal axis[63]; this is obviously related to the limited depth of penetration of EUS.

The availability of EUS-guided FNA increases the diagnostic accuracy of staging nodal disease because actual cytologic examination can be added to mere descriptive features (size, shape, border, and internal echo pattern). EUS-FNA is not ideal for detecting lymph nodes when the path of the needle may traverse through the primary tumor, in which case contamination by the primary tumor can lead to false-positive results. However, it is mostly distant nodes that are of importance, such as the celiac lymph nodes, for which even helical CT scanning is suboptimal in discerning.[44] EUS is better in identifying the celiac nodes, and EUS-guided FNA can help confirm the diagnosis. In a large series of 102 patients, the sensitivity of EUS in detecting celiac lymph nodes was 77%; specificity, 85%; NPV, 71%; and PPV, 89%.[64] In another report, when EUS-FNA was compared with CT, of 20 patients who satisfied the criteria for EUS-guided FNA directed toward the celiac nodes, 18 (90%) were positive for malignancy. CT was able to detect only 6 (30%) of the 20 cases of suspicious celiac lymph nodes, 5 (83%) of which were positive for malignancy by FNA.[65]

Combining cervical ultrasound and EUS can be highly accurate. In 329 patients who underwent esophagectomy, one-to-one comparisons between preoperative ultrasound, EUS, and histologic diagnosis were performed. The accuracy of combined ultrasound was 80.2% for regional lymph nodes, 91.5% for distant lymph nodes,

and 74.4% in overall stage groupings. When the number of metastatic nodes was classified into subdivisions of 0, 1 to 3, 4 to 7, and ≥8, accuracy rates were 83.8%, 59.7%, 43.3%, and 96%, respectively. More importantly, the preoperative combined ultrasound separation into the number of involved lymph node showed prognostic stratification close to the histologic diagnosis.[66] This type of examination of both the location and number of nodes with one-to-one comparisons with histologic findings does require experience and meticulous attention to detail, and such expertise may not be widely available.

FDG-PET Scans

The main limitations of CT in esophageal cancer staging are its insensitivity in diagnosing unresectability (T4 disease) and its inability to identify metastases in normal-sized lymph nodes. FDG-PET scans, by using the differential glucose metabolism of cancer, provide a functional assessment of lymph nodes even though they are not enlarged. PET scanning is gaining popularity in esophageal cancer staging,[67,68] and as more data have accumulated, the role of PET scanning is becoming clearer (Fig. 33–9).

For detection of a primary tumor, the sensitivity of PET ranges from 78% to 95%, with most false-negative tests occurring in patients with T1 or small T2 tumors,[47,69] thus suggesting limitations in spatial resolution of the PET imaging device, currently around 5 to 8 mm, as the cause of nonvisualization. Adenocarcinomas of the gastroesophageal junction and proximal part of the stomach sometimes show limited or absent FDG accumulation, regardless of tumor volume (FDG nonavidity). Some investigators have observed this phenomenon in as many as 20% of these patients, which seems to be related to the diffusely growing subtype and poorly differentiated tumors.[70]

PET does not provide enough definition of the esophageal wall and thus has no value in T staging. For locoregional nodal metastases, its spatial resolution is also insufficient to separate the primary tumor from juxtatumoral lymph nodes because of interference from the primary tumor, and thus most studies demonstrate poor sensitivity.[69,71] This is especially true for nodes in the middle and lower mediastinum, where most primary tumors are found. In one study, the sensitivity of PET for detecting cervical, upper thoracic, and abdominal nodes was 78%, 82%, and 60% respectively, but it was only 38% and 0%, respectively, for the mid and lower mediastinum.[47] The specificity of PET in detecting regional nodes is usually much better, with specificities of 95% to 100% reported.[69,71] The low rate of false-positive findings is important in preoperative staging.

The main utility of PET scanning seems to lie in its ability to detect distant metastases. Luketich and colleagues reported 69% sensitivity, 93.4% specificity, and 84% accuracy in detecting metastases with PET as compared with 46.1% sensitivity, 73.8% specificity, and 63% accuracy with CT.[68] Similar results were shown by others.[70]

A recent meta-analysis of 12 publications on the use of PET in esophageal cancer showed that the pooled sensitivity and specificity for the detection of locoregional metastases were 0.51 (95% confidence interval [CI], 0.34 to 0.69) and 0.84 (95% CI, 0.76 to 0.91), respectively. The PPV and NPV were 0.60 and 0.46, respectively. For distant metastases, the pooled sensitivity and specificity were 0.67 (95% CI, 0.58 to 0.76) and 0.97 (95% CI, 0.90 to 1.0), respectively. The corresponding PPV and NPV were 0.92 and 0.83. When 2 studies (out of 11) that had particularly low sensitivities for the detection of distant metastases were excluded (probably because they included more early tumors), the pooled sensitivity improved to 0.72 and the specificity to 0.95.[72] Specifically for the celiac nodes, the sensitivity, specificity, PPV, and NPV ranged from 53% to 98%, 77% to 100%, 79% to 100%, and 82% to 100%, respectively. This study highlights that the accuracy of PET in detecting locoregional nodes is only moderate. EUS-FNA may be better in this regard. PET is, however, more useful for picking up distant nodal and visceral metastases. Its specificity is especially high.

The diagnostic yield of PET for the detection of unsuspected metastases in early-stage disease (Tis, T1) may be low because the chance of lymph node metastases increases with increasing T stage. Cost-effectiveness in this setting is uncertain. It seems that PET should be performed in patients in whom standard staging methods (CT and EUS) demonstrate no distant metastatic disease. In such cases, PET may improve the detection of metastatic disease and thus change the management strategy.

Thoracoscopy and Laparoscopy

Thoracoscopy and laparoscopy have their advocates. Thoracoscopic staging usually involves a right-sided approach, with opening of the mediastinal pleura from below the subclavian vessels to the inferior pulmonary vein; lymph node sampling is then performed. Sometimes left-sided thoracoscopy is also performed to sample lymph nodes at the aortopulmonary window. Laparoscopic staging can include celiac lymph node biopsy, collection of peritoneal fluid for cytologic examination, and the use of laparoscopic ultrasound for detecting liver metastases. In a study of 53 patients whose staging included conventional CT and EUS, minimally invasive staging reassigned a lower stage in 10 patients and a more advanced stage in 7 patients (32.1%).[73] The multi-institutional study CALGB 9380 (Cancer and Leukemia Group B) reported on combined thoracoscopic and laparoscopic staging in 113 patients; the strategy was feasible in 73% of patients. Thoracoscopy and laparoscopy identified nodes or metastatic disease missed by CT in 50% of patients, by MRI in 40%, and by EUS in 30%. Although no deaths or major complications occurred, it did involve general anesthesia, one-lung anesthesia, a median operating time of 210 minutes, and a hospital stay of 3 days.[74]

The chance of metastases in the abdomen is considerably greater with adenocarcinoma of the lower esophagus and gastric cardia than with squamous cell cancer of the esophagus. Laparoscopy can be of use in diagnosing abdominal metastases such as peritoneal secondaries or identifying unsuspected cirrhosis, which is a relative contraindication to surgical resection for some investigators. Its value is minimal for more proximally located tumors.[75]

One recent study looked at the cost-effectiveness of different combinations of staging methods, including CT, EUS, PET, and thoracoscopy and laparoscopy. Although PET plus EUS-FNA was the most accurate staging combination, it was more expensive than CT plus EUS-FNA. Even though thoracoscopy and laparoscopy could identify some additional patients with advanced disease, the yield was small.[76] The study suggests that initial PET staging is indicated, and if no metastatic disease is identified, EUS with or without FNA should be performed. The limitations of these models include the selected patient population studied and assumptions regarding how patients with certain disease stages are treated. The controversies of M1a versus M1b disease and the significance of celiac node involvement have already been discussed. Given that PET scanning is still not widely available, it seems that CT and EUS should be the initial staging modalities, with PET indicated especially for patients found to have locally advanced tumor with no distant metastases. The invasiveness and cost of thoracoscopy and laparoscopy and the constantly improving noninvasive methods such as PET scanning make the use of minimally invasive staging less attractive. It should be reserved for patients in whom positive confirmation of metastatic disease not otherwise obtained is essential in deciding on treatment.

Therapy Monitoring

After nonsurgical treatment or neoadjuvant therapy, reassessment of tumor stage is unreliable because it is difficult to distinguish fibrosis, inflammation, and true histologic response. Often, epithelialization occurs despite residual tumor present in the wall of the esophagus. Biopsy of the mucosa will result in a false complete response. Neither CT nor EUS is accurate with regard to assessing response. EUS was only 27% to 48% and 38% to 71% accurate in assessing T stage and N stage, respectively.[77,78] In a study involving the use of CT scans, CT after chemoradiotherapy accurately staged the T classification in only 42%, over-staged 36% of patients, and under-staged 20%. CT had a sensitivity of 65%, a specificity of 33%, a PPV of 58%, and an NPV of 41% in evaluating the pathologic tumor response.[79]

Metabolic imaging with PET scanning holds promise. Brücher and colleagues reported PET after chemoradiation in patients with locally advanced squamous cell cancer.[80] Twenty-seven patients were assessed before and after chemoradiation. Responders were defined as having histologic findings of a complete response or 10% or less viable cells in the surgical specimen. In responders, FDG uptake decreased by 72%, whereas in nonresponders, it was reduced by 42%. A receiver operating characteristics analysis indicated that at a threshold of a 52% decrease in FDG uptake, the sensitivity in detecting a response was 100%, with a corresponding specificity of 55%. The PPV and NPV were 72% and 100%. These data imply that PET is excellent in identifying nonresponders. Nonresponders also had significantly worse survival after resection than responders did.

Flamens and colleagues also demonstrated the value of PET for evaluation of response. PET responders were defined as patients with complete or almost complete normalization of FDG uptake at the primary tumor site, together with complete normalization of all lymph node metastases seen on PET before chemoradiation. Serial PET had a predictive accuracy of 78% for a major response, with a sensitivity of 71% and a specificity of 82%.[81] False negativity (overestimation of response) is due to residual micrometastatic cancer foci falling below the detection threshold; thus, the sensitivity and PPV of a completely normal postinduction PET scan for the diagnosis of a complete pathologic response were only 67% and 50%, respectively. False positivity (underestimation of response) usually occurs at the primary tumor site, where inflammatory reactions may increase FDG uptake.

A recent comparative study using PET, CT, and EUS for the identification of pathologic responders after neoadjuvant therapy also showed that PET is more accurate for the prediction of response and survival than CT and EUS are. A postchemoradiation PET standard uptake value (SUV) of 4 or greater had the highest accuracy for pathologic response (76%). The inability to detect a complete histologic response, however, was again evident.[82]

Taking the potential use of PET further, it has been investigated as a means of predicting response early in the course of multimodal treatment. Weber and colleagues studied 40 patients with adenocarcinoma of the lower esophagus and gastric cardia (type I and II tumors). All patients had T3-4 Nx M0 disease. Chemotherapy was given, and PET was performed before and 14 days into treatment. Clinical response was assessed by a 50% or greater reduction in tumor length and wall thickness, and in those who underwent resection, histopathologic major response was also assessed. The reduction in tumor FDG uptake after 14 days of therapy was significantly different between responding (−54% ± 17%) and nonresponding tumors (−15% ± 21%). Optimal differentiation was achieved with a cutoff value of a 35% reduction in initial FDG uptake. Applying this cutoff value as a criterion for a metabolic response predicted clinical response with a sensitivity and specificity of 93% (14 of 15 patients) and 95% (21 of 22), respectively. Histopathologically complete or subtotal tumor regression was achieved in 53% (8 of 15) of the patients with a metabolic response but in only 5% (1 of 22) of those without a metabolic response. Patients without a metabolic response were also characterized by significantly shorter time to progression/recurrence and shorter overall survival.[83]

In a similar study by the same group, 38 patients with squamous cell cancer of the esophagus of stage cT3 cN0/+ cM0 were treated by chemoradiation. Patients underwent PET before therapy ($n = 38$), 2 weeks after initiation of therapy ($n = 27$), and preoperatively (3 to 4 weeks after chemoradiotherapy; $n = 38$). In histopathologic responders (<10% viable cells in the resected specimen), the decrease in SUV from baseline to day 14 was 44% ± 15%, whereas it was only 21% ± 14% in nonresponders ($P = .0055$). Metabolic changes at this time point were also correlated with patient survival ($P = .011$). The two studies described showed that changes in tumor metabolic activity after 14 days of preoperative treatment significantly correlated with tumor response and patient survival. PET might be used to identify nonresponders early during neoadjuvant treatment, thereby allowing for early modifications of the protocol. Thus, further cost and morbidity can be avoided in patients with little chance of a positive response.[84]

STAGE-DIRECTED THERAPY

The information derived from the staging methods described is useful only if a stage-directed therapy strategy is used. From the foregoing discussions, it seems clear that although the current stage segregation into stage I to IV has prognostic significance, further refinement is much needed. The separation of M1a and M1b, the significance of celiac or cervical lymph nodes, and the redefinitions of nodal disease are obvious controversies. Staging methods have improved accuracies, but the current techniques are unreliable in providing the precise number and location of nodal metastases. As a consequence, some surgeons even regard lymph node status (especially locoregional ones) as unimportant for deciding whether a primary resection should be performed because it cannot be predicted with sufficient accuracy preoperatively and, furthermore, regional nodes are resected routinely during esophagectomy.[85]

The assumption of benefit from stage-directed therapy is intuitive and reasonable and is obviously true for extreme cases such as T1a disease versus stage IV disease with visceral metastases. The finer distinction of patients into intermediate stages is difficult. It is even more controversial to consider the many options and combinations of treatments for each stage of disease, for which more studies are required to provide convincing evidence. Accurate staging is the prerequisite of quality control in clinical trials.

There is no doubt that staging methods will further improve and refinement of stage classification will evolve. As molecular techniques are coming of age, molecular classification may eventually be incorporated into tumor staging systems as well. The challenge is to constantly modify our treatment strategies according to new knowledge gained to give the best results to our patients.

SUGGESTED READINGS

Flamen P, Lerut T, Haustermans K, et al: Position of positron emission tomography and other imaging diagnostic modalities in esophageal cancer. Q J Nucl Med Mol Imaging 48: 96-108, 2004.

Korst RJ, Altorki NK: Imaging for esophageal tumors. Thorac Surg Clin 14:61-69, 2004.

Rice TW: Diagnosis and staging of esophageal carcinoma. In Pearson FG, Cooper JD, Deslauriers J, et al (eds): Esophageal Surgery, 2nd ed. Philadelphia, Churchill Livingstone, 2002.

Roöch T, Kassem AM: Endoscopic ultrasonography. In Classen M, Tytgat GNJ, Lightdale CJ (eds): Gastroenterological Endoscopy. New York, Georg Thieme, 2002, pp 199-220.

Wittekind C, Compton CC, Greene FL, Sobin LH: TNM residual tumor classification revisited. Cancer 94:2511-2516, 2002.

REFERENCES

1. Union Internationale Contre le Cancer: TNM Classification of Malignant Tumours. New York, Wiley-Liss, 2002.
2. American Joint Committee on Cancer: AJCC Cancer Staging Manual. New York, Springer, 2002, pp 91-95.
3. Japanese Society for Esophageal Diseases: Guidelines for Clinical and Pathologic Studies on Carcinoma of the Esophagus, 9th ed. Tokyo, Kanehara, 2001.
4. Siewert JR, Stein HJ: Classification of adenocarcinoma of the oesophagogastric junction. Br J Surg 85:1457-1459, 1998.
5. Ries LAG, Eisner MP, Kosary CL, et al (eds): SEER Cancer Statistics Review, 1975-2001. Bethesda, MD, National Cancer Institute, 2004.
6. Keighley MR: Gastrointestinal cancers in Europe. Aliment Pharmacol Ther 18(Suppl 3):7-30, 2003.
7. Siewert JR, Feith M, Werner M, Stein HJ: Adenocarcinoma of the esophagogastric junction: Results of surgical therapy based on anatomical/topographic classification in 1,002 consecutive patients. Ann Surg 232:353-361, 2000.
8. Goh KL, Chang CS, Fock KM, et al: Gastro-oesophageal reflux disease in Asia. J Gastroenterol Hepatol 15:230-238, 2000.
9. Steup WH, De Leyn P, Deneffe G, et al: Tumors of the esophagogastric junction. Long-term survival in relation to the pattern of lymph node metastasis and a critical analysis of the accuracy or inaccuracy of pTNM classification. J Thorac Cardiovasc Surg 111:85-94, 1996.
10. Japanese Gastric Cancer Association: Japanese Classification of Gastric Carcinoma, 2nd English ed, Gastric Cancer. Tokyo, Kanehara & Co. Ltd., 1998, pp 10-24.
11. Bunt AM, Hermans J, van de Velde CJ, et al: Lymph node retrieval in a randomized trial on western-type versus Japanese-type surgery in gastric cancer. J Clin Oncol 14:2289-2294, 1996.
12. Rice TW, Blackstone EH, Rybicki LA, et al: Refining esophageal cancer staging. J Thorac Cardiovasc Surg 125:1103-1113, 2003.
13. Tachibana M, Kinugasa S, Yoshimura H, et al: Extended esophagectomy with 3-field lymph node dissection for esophageal cancer. Arch Surg 138:1383-1389, 2003.
14. Dutkowski P, Hommel G, Bottger T, et al: How many lymph nodes are needed for an accurate pN classification in esophageal cancer? Evidence for a new threshold value. Hepatogastroenterology 49:176-180, 2002.
15. Tachibana M, Kinugasa S, Dhar DK, et al: Prognostic factors after extended esophagectomy for squamous cell carcinoma of the thoracic esophagus. J Surg Oncol 72:88-93, 1999.
16. Matsubara T, Ueda M, Yanagida O, et al: How extensive should lymph node dissection be for cancer of the thoracic esophagus? J Thorac Cardiovasc Surg 107:1073-1078, 1994.
17. Tabira Y, Yasunaga M, Tanaka M, et al: Recurrent nerve nodal involvement is associated with cervical nodal metastasis in thoracic esophageal carcinoma. J Am Coll Surg 191:232-237, 2000.
18. Tabira Y, Okuma T, Kondo K, Kitamura N: Indications for three-field dissection followed by esophagectomy for advanced carcinoma of the thoracic esophagus. J Thorac Cardiovasc Surg 117:239-245, 1999.
19. Nishimaki T, Suzuki T, Suzuki S, et al: Outcomes of extended radical esophagectomy for thoracic esophageal cancer. J Am Coll Surg 186:306-312, 1998.
20. Yano K, Okamura T, Yoshida Y, et al: The extent and number of metastatic lymph nodes limit the efficacy of lymphadenectomy in patients with oesophageal carcinoma. Surg Oncol 3:187-192, 1994.
21. Clark GW, Peters JH, Ireland AP, et al: Nodal metastasis and sites of recurrence after en bloc esophagectomy for adenocarcinoma. Ann Thorac Surg 58:646-653, 1994.
22. Skinner DB, Little AG, Ferguson MK, et al: Selection of operation for esophageal cancer based on staging. Ann Surg 204:391-401, 1986.
23. Ellis FH Jr, Heatley GJ, Krasna MJ, et al: Esophagogastrectomy for carcinoma of the esophagus and cardia: A comparison of findings and results after standard resection in three consecutive eight-year intervals with improved staging criteria. J Thorac Cardiovasc Surg 113:836-846, 1997.
24. Tachibana M, Kinugasa S, Dhar DK, et al: Dukes' classification as a useful staging system in resectable squamous cell carcinoma of the esophagus. Virchows Arch 438:350-356, 2001.
25. Korst RJ, Rusch VW, Venkatraman E, et al: Proposed revision of the staging classification for esophageal cancer. J Thorac Cardiovasc Surg 115:660-669, 1998.
26. Eloubeidi MA, Desmond R, Arguedas MR et al: Prognostic factors for the survival of patients with esophageal carcinoma in the U.S.: The importance of tumor length and lymph node status. Cancer 95:1434-1443, 2002.
27. Akiyama H, Tsurumaru M, Udagawa H, Kajiyama Y: Radical lymph node dissection for cancer of the thoracic esophagus. Ann Surg 220:364-372, 1994.
28. Roder JD, Busch R, Stein HJ, et al: Ratio of invaded to removed lymph nodes as a predictor of survival in squamous cell carcinoma of the oesophagus. Br J Surg 81:410-413, 1994.
29. Tachibana M, Dhar DK, Kinugasa S, et al: Esophageal cancer with distant lymph node metastasis: Prognostic significance of metastatic lymph node ratio. J Clin Gastroenterol 31:318-322, 2000.
30. Rusch VW: Should the esophageal cancer staging system be revised? J Thorac Cardiovasc Surg 125:992-993, 2003.
31. Wittekind C, Compton CC, Greene FL, Sobin LH: TNM residual tumor classification revisited. Cancer 94:2511-2516, 2002.
32. Dexter SP, Sue-Ling H, McMahon MJ, et al: Circumferential resection margin involvement: An independent predictor of survival following surgery for oesophageal cancer. Gut 48:667-670, 2001.

33. Akiyama H, Kogure T, Itai Y: The esophageal axis and its relationship to the resectability of carcinoma of the esophagus. Ann Surg 176:30-36, 1972.

34. Dittler HJ, Pesarini AC, Siewert JR: Endoscopic classification of esophageal cancer: Correlation with the T stage. Gastrointest Endosc 38:662-668, 1992.

35. Vickers J, Alderson D: Influence of luminal obstruction on oesophageal cancer staging using endoscopic ultrasonography. Br J Surg 85:999-1001, 1998.

36. Bhutani MS, Barde CJ, Markert RJ, Gopalswamy N: Length of esophageal cancer and degree of luminal stenosis during upper endoscopy predict T stage by endoscopic ultrasound. Endoscopy 34:461-463, 2002.

37. Van Dam J, Rice TW, Catalano MF, et al: High-grade malignant stricture is predictive of esophageal tumor stage. Risks of endosonographic evaluation. Cancer 71:2910-2917, 1993.

38. Cheung HC, Siu KF, Wong J: A comparison of flexible and rigid endoscopy in evaluating esophageal cancer patients for surgery. World J Surg 12:117-122, 1988.

39. Riedel M, Stein HJ, Mounyam L, et al: Extensive sampling improves preoperative bronchoscopic assessment of airway invasion by supracarinal esophageal cancer: A prospective study in 166 patients. Chest 119:1652-1660, 2001.

40. Osugi H, Nishimura Y, Takemura M, et al: Bronchoscopic ultrasonography for staging supracarinal esophageal squamous cell carcinoma: Impact on outcome. World J Surg 27:590-594, 2003.

41. Rice TW: Clinical staging of esophageal carcinoma. CT, EUS, and PET. Chest Surg Clin N Am 10:471-485, 2000.

42. Watt I, Stewart I, Anderson D, et al: Laparoscopy, ultrasound and computed tomography in cancer of the oesophagus and gastric cardia: A prospective comparison for detecting intra-abdominal metastases. Br J Surg 76:1036-1039, 1989.

43. Margolis ML, Howlett P, Bubanj R: Pulmonary nodules in patients with esophageal carcinoma. J Clin Gastroenterol 26:245-248, 1998.

44. Romagnuolo J, Scott J, Hawes RH, et al: Helical CT versus EUS with fine needle aspiration for celiac nodal assessment in patients with esophageal cancer. Gastrointest Endosc 55:648-654, 2002.

45. Picus D, Balfe DM, Koehler RE, et al: Computed tomography in the staging of esophageal carcinoma. Radiology 146:433-438, 1983.

46. van Overhagen H, Becker C: Diagnosis and staging of carcinoma of the esophagus and gastroesophageal junction, and detection of postoperative recurrence, by computed tomography. In Myers M (ed): Neoplasms of the Digestive Tract. Imaging, Staging and Management. Philadelphia, Lippincott-Raven, 1998, pp 31-48.

47. Kato H, Kuwano H, Nakajima M, et al: Comparison between positron emission tomography and computed tomography in the use of the assessment of esophageal carcinoma. Cancer 94:921-928, 2002.

48. Berger AC, Scott WJ: Noninvasive staging of esophageal carcinoma. J Surg Res 117:127-133, 2004.

49. Lehr L, Rupp N, Siewert JR: Assessment of resectability of esophageal cancer by computed tomography and magnetic resonance imaging. Surgery 103:344-350, 1988.

50. Natsugoe S, Yoshinaka H, Shimada M, et al: Assessment of cervical lymph node metastasis in esophageal carcinoma using ultrasonography. Ann Surg 229:62-66, 1999.

51. Rosch T: Endosonographic staging of esophageal cancer: A review of literature results. Gastrointest Endosc Clin N Am 5:537-547, 1995.

52. Rice TW, Blackstone EH, Adelstein DJ, et al: Role of clinically determined depth of tumor invasion in the treatment of esophageal carcinoma. J Thorac Cardiovasc Surg 125:1091-1102, 2003.

53. Saunders HS, Wolfman NT, Ott DJ: Esophageal cancer. Radiologic staging. Radiol Clin North Am 35:281-294, 1997.

54. Fok M, Cheng SW, Wong J: Endosonography in patient selection for surgical treatment of esophageal carcinoma. World J Surg 16:1098-1103, discussion 1103, 1992.

55. Bumm R: Staging and risk-analysis in esophageal carcinoma. Dis Esophagus 9(Suppl):20-29, 1996.

56. Bumm R, Wong J: Extent of lymphadenectomy in esophagectomy for squamous cell esophageal carcinoma: How much is necessary? Dis Esophagus 7:151-155, 1994.

57. Wallace MB, Hawes RH, Sahai AV, et al: Dilation of malignant esophageal stenosis to allow EUS guided fine-needle aspiration: Safety and effect on patient management. Gastrointest Endosc 51:309-313, 2000.

58. Hunerbein M, Ghadimi BM, Haensch W, Schlag PM: Transendoscopic ultrasound of esophageal and gastric cancer using miniaturized ultrasound catheter probes. Gastrointest Endosc 48:371-375, 1998.

59. Yanai H, Yoshida T, Harada T, et al: Endoscopic ultrasonography of superficial esophageal cancers using a thin ultrasound probe system equipped with switchable radial and linear scanning modes. Gastrointest Endosc 44:578-582, 1996.

60. Nijhawan PK, Wang KK: Endoscopic mucosal resection for lesions with endoscopic features suggestive of malignancy and high-grade dysplasia within Barrett's esophagus. Gastrointest Endosc 52:328-332, 2000.

61. Catalano MF, Sivak MV Jr, Rice T, et al: Endosonographic features predictive of lymph node metastasis. Gastrointest Endosc 40:442-446, 1994.

62. Bhutani MS, Hawes RH, Hoffman BJ: A comparison of the accuracy of echo features during endoscopic ultrasound (EUS) and EUS-guided fine-needle aspiration for diagnosis of malignant lymph node invasion. Gastrointest Endosc 45:474-479, 1997.

63. Chandawarkar RY, Kakegawa T, Fujita H, et al: Endosonography for preoperative staging of specific nodal groups associated with esophageal cancer. World J Surg 20:700-702, 1996.

64. Eloubeidi MA, Wallace MB, Reed CE, et al: The utility of EUS and EUS-guided fine needle aspiration in detecting celiac lymph node metastasis in patients with esophageal cancer: A single-center experience. Gastrointest Endosc 54:714-719, 2001.

65. Parmar KS, Zwischenberger JB, Reeves AL, Waxman I: Clinical impact of endoscopic ultrasound-guided fine needle aspiration of celiac axis lymph nodes (M1a disease) in esophageal cancer. Ann Thorac Surg 73:916-920, 2002.

66. Natsugoe S, Yoshinaka H, Shimada M, et al: Number of lymph node metastases determined by presurgical ultrasound and endoscopic ultrasound is related to prognosis in patients with esophageal carcinoma. Ann Surg 234:613-618, 2001.

67. Flanagan FL, Dehdashti F, Siegel BA, et al: Staging of esophageal cancer with 18F-fluorodeoxyglucose positron emission tomography. AJR Am J Roentgenol 168:417-424, 1997.

68. Luketich JD, Friedman DM, Weigel TL, et al: Evaluation of distant metastases in esophageal cancer: 100 consecutive positron emission tomography scans. Ann Thorac Surg 68:1133-1136, 1999.

69. Flamen P, Lerut A, Van Cutsem E, et al: Utility of positron emission tomography for the staging of patients with potentially operable esophageal carcinoma. J Clin Oncol 18:3202-3210, 2000.

70. Flamen P, Lerut T, Haustermans K, et al: Position of positron emission tomography and other imaging diagnostic modalities in esophageal cancer. Q J Nucl Med Mol Imaging 48:96-108, 2004.

71. Rasanen JV, Sihvo EI, Knuuti MJ, et al: Prospective analysis of accuracy of positron emission tomography, computed tomography, and endoscopic ultrasonography in staging of adenocarcinoma of the esophagus and the esophagogastric junction. Ann Surg Oncol 10:954-960, 2003.

72. van Westreenen HL, Westerterp M, Bossuyt PM, et al: Systematic review of the staging performance of 18F-fluorodeoxyglucose positron emission tomography in esophageal cancer. J Clin Oncol 22:3805-3812, 2004.

73. Luketich JD, Meehan M, Nguyen NT, et al: Minimally invasive surgical staging for esophageal cancer. Surg Endosc 14:700-702, 2000.

74. Krasna MJ, Reed CE, Nedzwiecki D, et al: CALGB 9380: A prospective trial of the feasibility of thoracoscopy/laparoscopy in staging esophageal cancer. Ann Thorac Surg 71:1073-1079, 2001.

75. Stein HJ, Kraemer SJ, Feussner H, et al: Clinical value of diagnostic laparoscopy with laparoscopic ultrasound in patients with cancer of the esophagus or cardia. J Gastrointest Surg 1:167-173, 1997.

76. Wallace MB, Nietert PJ, Earle C, et al: An analysis of multiple staging management strategies for carcinoma of the esophagus: Computed tomography, endoscopic ultrasound, positron emission tomography, and thoracoscopy/laparoscopy. Ann Thorac Surg 74:1026-1032, 2002.

77. Beseth BD, Bedford R, Isacoff WH, et al: Endoscopic ultrasound does not accurately assess pathologic stage of esophageal cancer after neoadjuvant chemoradiotherapy. Am Surg 66:827-831, 2000.

78. Zuccaro G, Rice TW, Goldblum J, et al: Endoscopic ultrasound cannot determine suitability for esophagectomy after aggressive chemoradiotherapy for esophageal cancer. Am J Gastroenterol 94:906-912, 1999.

79. Jones DR, Parker LAJ, Detterbeck FC, Egan TM: Inadequacy of computed tomography in assessing patients with esophageal carcinoma after induction chemoradiotherapy. Cancer 85:1026-1032, 1999.

80. Brücher BL, Weber W, Bauer M, et al: Neoadjuvant therapy of esophageal squamous cell carcinoma: Response evaluation by positron emission tomography. Ann Surg 233:300-309, 2001.

81. Flamen P, Van Cutsem E, Lerut A, et al: Positron emission tomography for assessment of the response to induction radio-chemotherapy in locally advanced oesophageal cancer. Ann Oncol 13:361-368, 2002.

82. Swisher SG, Maish M, Erasmus JJ, et al: Utility of PET, CT, and EUS to identify pathologic responders in esophageal cancer. Ann Thorac Surg 78:1152-1160, 2004.

83. Weber WA, Ott K, Becker K, et al: Prediction of response to preoperative chemotherapy in adenocarcinomas of the esophagogastric junction by metabolic imaging. J Clin Oncol 19:3058-3065, 2001.

84. Wieder HA, Brücher BL, Zimmermann F, et al: Time course of tumor metabolic activity during chemoradiotherapy of esophageal squamous cell carcinoma and response to treatment. J Clin Oncol 22:900-908, 2004.

85. Stein HJ, Brücher BL, Sendler A, Siewert JR: Esophageal cancer: Patient evaluation and pre-treatment staging. Surg Oncol 10:103-111, 2001.

Carcinoma of the Esophagus and Gastroesophageal Junction

Jeffrey A. Hagen • Brian E. Louie

Carcinoma of the esophagus and gastroesophageal junction (GEJ) remains one of the most difficult problems facing surgeons. Though relatively uncommon, these tumors are historically associated with a high mortality rate because of both the late stage of disease at initial evaluation and the many challenges associated with their treatment. Changes in the epidemiology of esophageal cancer have provided an opportunity for early detection, which together with the availability of new treatment modalities, has increased the number of patients who can be offered potentially curative surgical resection. At the same time, several controversies have arisen regarding the optimal treatment strategy. A number of new unproven therapeutic approaches have been advocated for patients with early cancer, such as mucosal ablation[1,2] and endoscopic mucosal resection.[3] For patients with more advanced-stage tumors, neoadjuvant chemoradiotherapy has been broadly applied despite the lack of clear evidence of benefit.[4-9] In some centers, the need for surgical resection at all has been questioned, with definitive chemoradiotherapy being offered instead. When surgery is performed, controversy persists regarding the extent of resection necessary,[10-14] and much of the debate has centered on the benefits of systematic lymph node dissection. This chapter reviews the current approach to the diagnosis and management of esophageal cancer, with an emphasis on improvements in clinical and pathologic staging. When combined with a better understanding of the natural history of disease, a logical and tailored treatment plan can be developed.

HISTORY

The history of surgery in the management of esophageal cancer is largely limited to the past century. Although tumors of the esophagus were recognized as early as the 12th century, attempts at surgical resection were not recorded until the late 19th century. The early experience was limited to resection of cervical esophageal cancer because of the risk for fatal pneumothorax associated with operations in the chest. After advancements in surgical and anesthetic techniques, most notably the availability of intratracheal administration of anesthetic gases, the first successful resection of an intrathoracic esophageal cancer was performed in the United States by Torek in 1913.[15] Gastrointestinal continuity was reestablished in this patient with the use of an extracorporeal tube. The first resection followed by reconstruction with esophagogastrostomy was performed in Japan by Ohsawa in 1932,[16] and it was popularized in the United States by Adams and Phemister at the University of Chicago in 1938.[17] Large series published in the mid-1940s detailed the risk associated with these early attempts at resection, with operative mortality rates as high as 60%.[18,19]

The history of radiation therapy for esophageal cancer is also relatively recent. First applied in the early 1920s, radiation therapy with crude delivery systems was associated with poor results and a high complication rate. In the latter half of the 20th century, the availability of more sophisticated equipment led to a rapid increase in the use of radiation therapy. At the same time, a variety of chemotherapeutic agents became available, which have increasingly been used alone or in combination with radiation therapy or surgery. To date, none of these combinations of therapies have been convincingly demonstrated to be superior to surgical resection alone, although the use of combined-modality therapy continues to increase.

EPIDEMIOLOGY

Esophageal cancer is the sixth leading cause of cancer death in the world,[20] although it remains relatively uncommon in North America. The most recent data available from the Surveillance, Epidemiology and End Results program of the National Cancer Institute indicate that 14,250 new esophageal cancers were diagnosed in the United States in the year 2004,[21] which represents 1% of all cancers and approximately 6% of gastrointestinal malignancies. Despite its relative rarity, the death rate remains high,[22] with an estimated 13,300 deaths attributed to esophageal cancer annually. This figure represents 2.4% of all cancer mortality and 10% of all deaths from gastrointestinal malignancy. It is four times more common in men than women, and in the United States it is three times more common in black than in white individuals.[23]

A dramatic change has occurred in the epidemiology of esophageal cancer over the past 2 decades.[24] The incidence of adenocarcinoma has risen faster than that of any other malignancy, and as a result it has replaced squamous cell carcinoma as the most common esophageal malignancy in most Western countries.[25] Although squamous cell carcinoma remains the most common type of esophageal cancer around the globe, particularly in developing areas such as the Caspian littoral region of Iran, northern China, and South Africa, the incidence of squamous cell cancer has fallen in the United States from 31 to 19 per million population between 1975 and 2001. During this same period, the incidence of adenocarcinoma has increased nearly 600% to 23.3 per million in 2001.[26]

There are clear differences in the epidemiologic profiles of patients with squamous cell carcinoma and adenocarcinoma of the esophagus. Esophageal adenocarcinoma is more common in white males and is strongly associated with a history of chronic gastroesophageal reflux disease (GERD). It also tends to occur at a younger age. In contrast, squamous cell carcinoma is more common in minority populations, including Asian and black Americans, and is more strongly associated with tobacco and alcohol consumption.

ETIOLOGY

The cause of esophageal cancer is unknown, but several clearly defined risk factors and associated medical conditions have been identified (Table 34–1).

Squamous Cell Carcinoma

Tobacco and alcohol consumption are the most well recognized risk factors for squamous cell carcinoma of

Table 34–1	Risk Factors Associated with Esophageal Carcinoma
Squamous cell carcinoma	Tobacco use Alcohol consumption History of head and neck cancer Achalasia Caustic injury Tylosis
Adenocarcinoma	Chronic gastrointestinal reflux disease Obesity Diet deficient in fruits and vegetables Diet high in animal protein and cholesterol

the esophagus. Case-control studies have shown that smoking is associated with a 2.3 to 15.5 relative risk for the development of squamous cell carcinoma, with regular consumption of alcohol bestowing a 2.5 to 19 relative risk. The effects of these agents appear to be synergistic.[27] Because these risk factors are associated with other aerodigestive malignancies, a patient with a history of previous lung or head and neck cancer carries an increased risk. The risk for a synchronous or metachronous esophageal cancer in a patient with a primary head and neck malignancy has been estimated to be between 3% and 9%.

Other conditions associated with chronic irritation of the esophagus that have been associated with an increased risk for squamous cell cancer of the esophagus include achalasia, caustic injury, and tylosis. Longstanding achalasia results in chronic stasis of food and saliva, which leads to fermentation and lowering of the pH of the esophagus to near gastric levels.[28] Over a period of 20 years or more such chronic irritation gives rise to the development of squamous cell carcinoma in approximately 5% to 10% of patients with achalasia.[29,30] Chronic irritation is also present in patients with a history of lye ingestion. Squamous cell carcinoma has been reported to occur in 1% to 5% of these individuals, usually 30 to 40 years after the episode of lye ingestion.[31,32] Irradiation of the esophagus has also been identified as a risk factor for squamous cell cancer of the esophagus, although the absolute risk appears to be small. Finally, tylosis (nonepidermolytic palmoplantar keratoderma), a rare, autosomal dominant disorder characterized by hyperkeratosis of the squamous epithelium of the palms and plantar surfaces of the feet, has been associated with an increased frequency of squamous cell carcinoma. Papillomas of the esophagus develop in these patients, and the risk for development of esophageal cancer has been estimated to be as high as 70%.[33]

Adenocarcinoma

The primary risk factor for esophageal adenocarcinoma is the presence of GERD. The best evidence of this relationship comes from a population-based study by Lagergren and associates.[34] Patients with reflux symptoms occurring more than three times a week had a 17-fold higher risk for adenocarcinoma, with a similarly increased risk in patients with higher reflux symptom scores and a duration of symptoms of more than 20 years. When combined, a patient with frequent severe reflux symptoms of prolonged duration had a nearly 44-fold higher risk for cancer. Other less well defined risk factors for esophageal adenocarcinoma include obesity and a diet deficient in fruits and vegetables. A diet rich in animal protein and cholesterol also appears to increase the risk for esophageal adenocarcinoma.[35,36]

Adenocarcinoma is unique among upper gastrointestinal malignancies in that a well-defined precursor lesion—Barrett's esophagus—has been identified. Barrett's esophagus is a condition associated with GERD in which there is a metaplastic transformation from the normal squamous epithelium in the distal esophagus to glandular epithelium with evidence of specialized intestinal metaplasia. It is a condition that was initially described in the late 1800s but has received heightened attention since the recognition by Hawe et al.[37] in 1973 that it was a precursor to the development of esophageal adenocarcinoma. Since then, the pathophysiologic mechanisms that lead to the development of Barrett's esophagus have been well defined. In addition, the histologic sequence of progression from reflux injury to cardiac metaplasia and reflux carditis, intestinal metaplasia, dysplasia, and ultimately, adenocarcinoma has been well described.[38] Recognition of this relationship between Barrett's esophagus (a known complication of GERD) and adenocarcinoma of the distal esophagus and GEJ has linked one of the most deadly malignancies known to humanity to the most common upper gastrointestinal disorder in Western civilization. Awareness of this relationship has resulted in another important recent change in the epidemiology of esophageal cancer—a documented increase in the number of esophageal cancers[39] detected at an early stage through early endoscopy in patients with reflux symptoms and the performance of surveillance endoscopy in those with Barrett's esophagus. The precise risk for the development of adenocarcinoma in patients with Barrett's esophagus is unknown, with recent estimates of 0.2% to 2.1% per year for patients without dysplasia, which translates into a lifetime risk for cancer that is 30 to 125 times greater than that of the general population.[40]

PATHOLOGY

The vast majority of esophageal neoplasms are malignant. Squamous cell carcinoma and adenocarcinoma account for over 90% of primary esophageal malignancies, with an assortment of other malignancies accounting for the remainder (Box 34–1). It has been estimated that metastatic lesions may actually outnumber primary esophageal malignancies, with metastatic melanoma,

---

Box 34–1 **Pathology of Esophageal Malignancies**

Squamous cell carcinoma
Adenocarcinoma
Leiomyosarcoma
Melanoma
Metastatic lesions

---

breast cancer, and lung cancer being the most common cell types.[41] Using autopsy data, Antler and associates[42] estimated that 4.5% of primary lung cancers had metastases to the esophagus that were not by direct extension. With more than 177,000 new lung cancers in 2004, this would amount to nearly 8000 patients with esophageal metastases from lung cancer alone, but most of these metastases are not clinically significant.

Squamous Cell Carcinoma

Grossly, squamous cell carcinoma usually appears as an exophytic lesion with a large fungating mass in the esophageal lumen, although a variant has been described that is manifested as an endophytic lesion with extensive submucosal spread and stricture formation. Multicentric tumors occur in 15% to 20% of cases. Whether they represent synchronous tumors or intramural metastases is controversial. Histologically, squamous cell cancers are composed of epithelial cells with characteristic intracellular bridges. Well-differentiated tumors have little nuclear pleomorphism and well-formed squamous pearls, whereas moderate to poorly differentiated tumors have considerable nuclear pleomorphism, and they may lack keratinization and intracellular bridges (Fig. 34–1).

Squamous cell cancers are distributed throughout the length of the esophagus. These tumors are located in the proximal third of the esophagus in 20% to 40%, the middle third in 50% to 60%, and the distal third in 10% to 20%. Tumors located in the proximal and middle thirds of the esophagus may involve the tracheobronchial tree by direct extension in up to 40%, with malignant tracheoesophageal fistula reported in 10% to 15%. In the confined space of the mediastinum, advanced proximal tumors may involve the recurrent laryngeal nerve, larynx, or thoracic duct. Middle third tumors can also invade the aorta and pericardium, whereas distal third tumors can involve the diaphragm, liver, and stomach.

Regional lymph node metastases are common in patients with squamous cell carcinoma, with the likelihood increasing as the tumor invades more deeply into the wall of the esophagus. For tumors confined to the mucosa, lymph node involvement is relatively rare (<5%), but with tumor invasion into the submucosa, node involvement is evident in 10% to 40% of patients.[43,44] The frequency of node involvement increases to 60% for tumors invading the muscularis

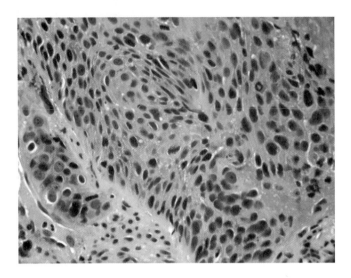

Figure 34–1. Photomicrograph of squamous cell carcinoma of the esophagus. (Courtesy of Dr. P. Chandrasoma, University of Southern California.)

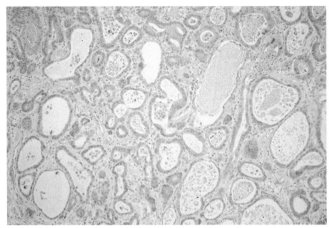

Figure 34–2. Photomicrograph of adenocarcinoma of the esophagus. (Courtesy of Dr. P. Chandrasoma, University of Southern California.)

propria and exceeds 80% in patients with transmural tumors.[45] The pattern of lymph node spread is not predictable because of the extensive lymphatic drainage system of the esophagus. Nodes far removed from the primary tumor may contain metastases, with abdominal lymph node involvement reported in up to 40% of patients with upper third tumors and a similar rate of cervical node involvement in patients with advanced tumors in the distal esophagus.[46]

Adenocarcinoma

Adenocarcinoma of the esophagus is most commonly manifested as a visible lesion grossly indistinguishable from the appearance of other types of tumors. They can be polypoid (5% to 10%), flat (10% to 15%), fungating (20% to 25%), or infiltrative (40% to 50%).[47] Upward of 40% to 60% of patients will have Barrett's mucosa identified in the resected esophagus, and it is believed that in the remainder Barrett's mucosa was present initially but was overgrown by the advancing tumor.[48] Histologically, these tumors are composed of irregularly shaped glands made up of cuboidal to columnar cells that infiltrate into the various layers of the esophageal wall. In the most poorly differentiated tumors, sheets of poorly formed glandular elements with signet ring cells can be found (Fig. 34–2).

The likelihood of lymph node spread in esophageal adenocarcinoma also depends on the depth of tumor invasion. The risk for node metastases is approximately 5% when the tumor is confined to the mucosa and 30% to 50% when it invades the submucosa.[49] Once the tumor penetrates the muscularis propria, more than 80% have at least one involved node.[50] The pattern of node dissemination is also not predictable, although involvement of the cervical nodes appears to be less frequent

than in patients with distal esophageal squamous cell cancer.

CLINICAL FEATURES

Esophageal cancer is typically initially detected in the sixth or seventh decade of life. Although dysphagia remains the most common initial symptom, heightened awareness of the relationship between reflux and esophageal adenocarcinoma has resulted in early diagnosis before the onset of dysphagia in an increasing number of patients. The reasons for evaluation in a consecutive series of 263 patients with esophageal adenocarcinoma are listed in Table 34–2.[51] Of note, more than half these patients had their cancer diagnosed at the time of endoscopy performed for indications other than dysphagia. In a third, endoscopy was performed for worsening foregut symptoms or for surveillance of known Barrett's esophagus. Occult bleeding and patient request accounted for another 18%. As might be expected, the symptom of dysphagia was associated with the presence of an advanced-stage tumor, whereas patients with other indications for endoscopy were more likely to have early tumors.

Weight loss is common in patients with esophageal cancer, and it is often more profound than in other types of cancer because of the combined systemic effects of malignancy and the obstructive effects of the tumor itself. Chest pain and odynophagia are also common, particularly in patients with bulkier tumors. These symptoms may arise from spasms occurring above an obstructing tumor or from ulceration of the esophagus. Ulceration of the tumor can also result in hematemesis, melena, or anemia. Less commonly, chest pain and odynophagia may arise from direct tumor extension into adjacent mediastinal structures. More advanced tumors may cause symptoms of hoarseness as a result of invasion of the recurrent laryngeal nerve, cough secondary to invasion of the airway, and aspiration pneumonia as a result of a malignant tracheoesophageal fistula.

Table 34–2   Comparison of Indication for Endoscopy and Pathologic Tumor Stage

Reason for Endoscopy:	N	Stage I (n = 97)	Stage II-IV (n = 166)	P Value
Dysphagia	129	20 (21)	109 (66)	<.0001
Barrett's surveillance	44	38 (39)	6 (4)	<.0001
Worsening of foregut symptoms	42	18 (19)	24 (14)	.39
Occult bleeding	32	12 (12)	20 (12)	1.0
Patient request	16	9 (9)	7 (4)	.11

Data are expressed as numbers of patients (%).

DIAGNOSIS

The diagnosis of esophageal cancer should be considered in any patient who complains of dysphagia. Evaluation should begin with a careful history and physical examination, followed by laboratory investigations, appropriate radiographic studies, and upper gastrointestinal endoscopy. The possibility of metastatic spread should be considered in a patient with profound weight loss or bone pain. Respiratory symptoms such as hoarseness, cough, or a history of aspiration pneumonia may indicate the presence of local tumor extension into adjacent mediastinal structures, which may preclude attempts at resection. Palpable cervical or supraclavicular adenopathy or a palpable nodular liver may indicate the presence of metastases. The history and physical examination should also focus on the patient's cardiopulmonary and nutritional status to anticipate the need for further preoperative functional assessment and nutritional supplementation.

Laboratory investigations should include a complete blood count because of the possibility of ulceration and bleeding. Liver function tests and measurement of the serum alkaline phosphatase level should also be performed to screen for metastatic disease to the liver or bone. In addition, the carcinoembryonic antigen (CEA) level should be measured in patients with adenocarcinoma. Though not diagnostic of esophageal adenocarcinoma, when elevated the CEA level can be useful in monitoring the results of therapy and the development of recurrence.[52]

EVALUATION

Chest Radiography

Chest radiography may be abnormal in as many as 50% of patients with locally advanced esophageal cancer, although the findings are generally nonspecific. An air-fluid level may be evident in patients with total or nearly total obstruction. Locoregionally advanced disease may also be evident by the presence of a soft tissue mass or bulky mediastinal adenopathy. In addition, a chest radiograph may reveal the presence of lung metastases or a pleural effusion.

Barium Esophagography

A contrast esophagogram provides useful information regarding the location of the tumor and an indication of the length of the primary tumor. The usual appearance of a lower third esophageal cancer is shown in Figure 34–3. The esophagogram typically reveals an irregular mucosal abnormality with dilatation of the proximal esophagus. By themselves, however, these findings are not diagnostic of cancer because benign strictures and esophageal dilatation in achalasia can have a similar appearance. Occasionally, a fistulous tract involving the tracheobronchial tree can be identified.

Upper Gastrointestinal Endoscopy

Evaluation of patients suspected of having esophageal cancer should always include endoscopy. In patients with dysphagia, the tumor is easily recognizable as a friable exophytic mass that is often ulcerated. Earlier-stage tumors may be more difficult to recognize, and biopsy should be performed on any abnormal-appearing mucosa. Careful attention should be paid to the possibility of synchronous lesions, especially in patients with squamous cell carcinoma.

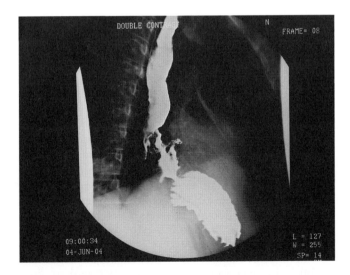

Figure 34–3. Esophagogram demonstrating a tumor at the gastroesophageal junction.

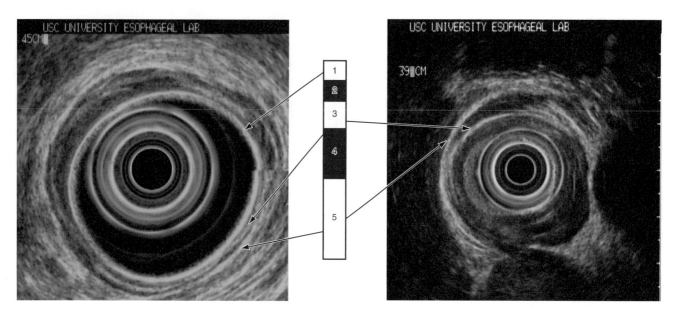

Figure 34–4. Endoscopic ultrasound appearance of a normal esophagus *(left)* and a T3 esophageal cancer *(right)*. The layers of the esophagus appear as alternating white (hyperechoic) and black (hypoechoic) rings. The first hyperechoic layer represents the mucosa (epithelium and lamina propria). The first hypoechoic or black ring represents the muscularis mucosa. The third layer is hyperechoic and represents the submucosa. The fourth layer is hypoechoic and identifies the muscularis propria. The last layer is hyperechoic and identifies periesophageal tissue. The tumor seen at 4 o'clock shows disruption of the third and fifth layers.

The endoscopic length of the tumor can provide useful information regarding the likelihood of lymph node involvement or systemic spread, or both. Tumors less than 5.0 cm in length are more likely to be T1 or T2 tumors, whereas tumors longer than 5 cm are more likely to be T3 or greater.[53] Patients found to have a high-grade luminal stenosis that precludes passage of an adult endoscope likewise have a greater likelihood of locally advanced tumor invasion.[54] Eloubeidi et al.[55] have shown that tumor length is also predictive of survival in the absence of nodal disease, with longer tumors associated with poorer survival.

Measurement of the distance between the tumor and the incisors provides useful information for treatment planning. The relationship between the tumor mass and important structures such as the cricopharyngeus, aortic arch, left main bronchus, and diaphragm can be determined. When the endoscope can be passed beyond the tumor, the stomach and duodenum should be examined. This evaluation should include a retroflexion maneuver to assess the fundus and cardia region of the stomach, which can be involved in a patient with a distal third cancer.

The diagnosis of esophageal cancer is usually made on the basis of biopsy samples obtained at the time of flexible endoscopy. The use of jumbo biopsy forceps increases the accuracy of endoscopic biopsy, but biopsy can be negative even when carefully performed, especially in patients with a tight stenosis. In these patients, careful dilatation before biopsy and brush cytology will usually establish the diagnosis. In a malnourished patient, consideration should be given to placement of a percutaneous gastrostomy tube at the time of endoscopy.

Endoscopic Ultrasound

Endoscopic ultrasound (EUS) is the best diagnostic tool available to assess the locoregional extent of disease. Introduced in the 1980s in Japan and the Netherlands for squamous cell carcinoma of the esophagus, it has recently grown in popularity in the United States for staging esophageal adenocarcinoma. The depth of tumor penetration of the esophageal wall and the presence of lymph node involvement can be assessed with an ultrasound probe attached to the tip of a flexible endoscope. The standard EUS probe uses ultrasound frequencies between 7.5 and 12 MHz. The typical appearance of a normal esophageal wall and the appearance of an invasive cancer are shown in Figure 34–4. Esophageal cancer appears as an irregular hypoechoic area of disruption of the normal esophageal wall architecture. Lymph nodes are categorized into three groups based on their appearance on EUS. Type 1 lymph nodes are poorly defined with diffuse homogeneous ultrasound echoes. These nodes are considered benign. Type 2 lymph nodes appear as well-defined structures with weak, relatively sonolucent echoes. Type 3 lymph nodes appear as well-defined structures with strong internal echoes and notching. Type 2 and 3 lymph nodes are considered malignant.

The accuracy of EUS in staging esophageal cancer has recently been reviewed.[56] EUS is 75% to 82% accurate in detecting T1 tumors, 64% to 85% accurate for T2 tumors, and 87% to 94% accurate for T3 disease. The accuracy of detecting invasion of adjacent structures approaches 100%. EUS is less accurate in assessing the depth of invasion for earlier-stage tumors because of difficulty distinguishing between intramucosal (T1a) and submucosal (T1b) invasion. This issue is of great importance inasmuch as alternatives to standard esophageal resection are increasingly being advocated, especially for patients with disease limited to the mucosa. In this setting, EUS has an accuracy of less than 20%.[57] It has been suggested that the use of higher-frequency ultrasound probes may increase the diagnostic accuracy of EUS in earlier-stage disease, but at present data are limited.[58,59] Endoscopic mucosal resection (EMR) may be a useful adjunct in staging these patients. Small mucosal abnormalities can be excised in their entirety via EMR so that a larger piece of tissue can be obtained for histologic evaluation to determine tumor depth. This approach has been shown to accurately predict tumor depth in all patients in a small series of patients who underwent EMR followed by esophagectomy.[60]

When locoregional nodes are assessed by EUS before esophagectomy and lymphadenectomy, the accuracy of identifying a malignant node ranges from 70% to 85%. The sensitivity of EUS in detecting node involvement ranges from 80% to 89%, but the specificity is only 50% to 75%. Fine-needle aspiration biopsy may improve these results. Given the relatively high false-positive rate of EUS assessment of lymph node involvement, caution should be exercised in basing important treatment decisions on the results of EUS.

Bronchoscopy

Bronchoscopic evaluation is mandatory for any patient with symptoms suggestive of airway invasion, such as cough or aspiration. In addition, all patients with a tumor located in proximity to the airway should undergo bronchoscopy. Bulky tumors in this location commonly cause a bulge in the membranous trachea or bronchus, although this finding does not always indicate invasion of the wall of the airway. Airway invasion should be suspected when the mucosa of the tracheobronchial tree is edematous or if it bleeds easily when contacted. Fixation of the mucosa on rigid bronchoscopy usually indicates invasion. Biopsy specimens should be obtained in this setting.

Computed Tomography of the Chest and Abdomen

Computed tomography (CT) remains a useful radiographic tool for evaluating a patient with esophageal cancer. It not only provides important information regarding the size of the primary tumor and the status of the mediastinal lymph nodes but also allows for assessment of the lungs, liver, and adrenal glands for metastases. The thickness of the tumor and its length can be estimated by CT. The normal esophageal wall is rarely more than 5 mm, and an asymmetric, thickened esophagus can be identified on CT in more than two thirds of patients with esophageal cancer.[61] However, the depth of invasion cannot be determined as accurately with CT as with EUS. Tumor depth is accurately predicted in only 30% to 50% in most series with a sensitivity of 43% to 73%

and a specificity of only 15% to 52%.[62] CT is generally better at distinguishing T4 from earlier-stage tumors. With the use of criteria such as obliteration of fat planes, thickening of adjacent tissue, and greater than 90 degrees of contact, direct invasion to an adjacent organ can be identified. Tracheobronchial invasion can be identified accurately in more than 85%, and aortic wall invasion can be detected in more than 80%. It has also been reported that performance of a CT scan in the prone position may enhance the accuracy of CT staging.[63] However, caution should still be exercised in precluding surgical resection based on radiologic criteria alone.

Computerized axial tomography is generally considered to be less accurate in determining lymph node involvement than other modalities such as EUS. Although many authors consider lymph nodes greater than 1 cm in size to be malignant, the actual size of the lymph node does not always correlate with pathologic review. In patients assessed with CT and the results compared with findings on esophagectomy and lymphadenectomy specimens, the overall accuracy was 65%, with a sensitivity of 60% and a specificity of 74%.[64]

Assessment for Metastases

The need for routine diagnostic tests to search for asymptomatic metastatic disease remains controversial. Scintigraphic studies such as a liver-spleen scan or a bone scan are rarely useful because they are relatively insensitive and seldom positive in patients without symptoms of metastases. In addition, benign abnormalities that can mimic metastases on bone scan are present in many patients, thus leading to additional and often costly investigations.

The broad availability of positron emission tomography (PET) has led to an improved ability to detect otherwise occult metastatic disease and can result in an alteration in clinical staging in as many as 20% of patients with esophageal cancer.[65,66] In a recent series of consecutive patients with esophageal cancer undergoing PET scanning, 12% were found to have otherwise unsuspected metastases, including metastases to nonregional lymph nodes and to other distant sites. As with other staging modalities, false-positive results can occur with PET, and therefore confirmatory biopsy specimens should always be obtained.

PET can also be used to identify regional lymph node involvement. In studies comparing CT, EUS, and PET scanning, PET appears to be more accurate in nodal staging than CT is, but it may be less accurate than EUS.[64] In studies in which PET findings were compared with lymph node histology after esophagectomy with formal lymphadenectomy, the accuracy of PET scanning was lower.[67] The major limitation in PET scan detection of mediastinal nodal involvement relates to the intense hypermetabolism present in the primary tumor, which tends to obscure activity in nodes in close proximity to the tumor mass. These are, of course, the nodes most likely to be involved. In addition, there are size limitations in the identification of lymph nodes with PET scanning, with an increasing false-negative rate for nodes smaller than 8 mm. The use of combined PET/CT appears to improve the accuracy of detecting node involvement, but false-positive and false-negative test results remain a problem.

Minimally Invasive Surgery for Staging Esophageal Cancer

Minimally invasive surgery using laparoscopy with or without thoracoscopy (MIS staging) has been proposed as an approach to staging esophageal cancer. The feasibility of this approach was recently evaluated in the Intergroup Trial CALGB 9380 (Cancer and Leukemia Group B).[68] In this trial, patients with esophageal carcinoma underwent comprehensive noninvasive staging with CT, EUS, and magnetic resonance imaging (MRI) and were then further staged with thoracoscopy and laparoscopy within 6 weeks of clinical staging. Overall, only 14% of patients had positive lymph nodes identified that were not detected by noninvasive testing. In addition, of the 13 patients identified as N0 on MIS staging, 3 (23%) had lymph node involvement at the time of resection, thus indicating that false-negative MIS staging may be quite common. The authors reported a median operating time of 210 minutes (40 to 865) and median length of stay of 3 days (1 to 35). No data on the complications or the ease or difficulty at the time of resection were reported. Although MIS staging may be feasible in as many as 73%, it does not appear to add much benefit over noninvasive testing, and the results do not appear to alter treatment in most patients. Many centers have abandoned MIS staging for these reasons and because of additional resource consumption.[69]

STAGING SYSTEM FOR ESOPHAGEAL CANCER

American Joint Committee on Cancer Staging System

Esophageal cancer is staged by using the tumor, nodal, and metastasis (TNM) system of categorization according to the American Joint Committee on Cancer (AJCC).[70] The goals of clinical staging are to determine the prognosis and allow selection of the most appropriate therapy. In the current staging system, the esophagus is divided into four regions. The cervical esophagus is defined as extending from the cricopharyngeus to the level of the thoracic inlet, which corresponds to a distance of approximately 18 cm from the incisors. The upper third of the thoracic esophagus is defined as extending from the thoracic inlet to the carina, which is located approximately 24 cm from the incisors. Middle third tumors are defined as those located between the carina and a point half the distance between the carina and the GEJ. The lower third of the esophagus extends from this point to the GEJ, located between 32 and 40 cm from the incisors.

Tumors are classified with the TNM system in accordance with the definitions listed in Table 34–3. T1 tumors

| Table 34–3 | TNM Descriptors |

Primary Tumor (T)

TX	Primary tumor cannot be assessed
T0	No evidence of primary tumor
Tis	Carcinoma in situ
T1	Tumor invades the lamina propria or submucosa
T2	Tumor invades the muscularis propria
T3	Tumor invades the adventitia
T4	Tumor invades adjacent structures

Regional Lymph Nodes (N)

NX	Regional lymph nodes cannot be assessed
N0	No regional lymph node metastases
N1	Regional lymph node metastases

Distant Metastases (M)

MX	Distant metastases cannot be assessed
M0	No distant metastases
M1	Distant metastases

invade into but not through the submucosa. These tumors are often subclassified as T1a and T1b for tumors limited to the lamina propria and submucosa, respectively, although this is not a component of the recognized staging system in use today. A tumor that invades into but not through the muscularis propria is designated a T2 lesion. Tumors that invade beyond the muscularis propria into the adjacent adventitia are classified as T3 tumors, whereas tumors that invade adjacent structures are classified as T4.

Lymph node status is classified according to the presence or absence of regional node involvement. Regional nodes are defined differently for tumors in different locations in the esophagus (Table 34–4). For tumors located in the cervical esophagus, the cervical, supraclavicular, and upper periesophageal lymph nodes are considered regional nodes. For tumors located in the GEJ, the periesophageal nodes below the azygos vein and the diaphragmatic, pericardial, left gastric, and celiac nodes are all considered to be regional nodes. The current staging system classifies involvement of any nonregional nodes as M1a disease. However, recent observations have questioned the validity of this practice, which has led to the suggestion that a category of N2 disease be added to better classify these tumors for prognostic purposes.

Combinations of TNM classifications are grouped into stages (Table 34–5). Stage 0 includes carcinoma in situ in the absence of node involvement or distant metastatic disease. Stage I tumors are limited to the lamina propria or submucosa in the absence of node involvement or distant metastases. T2 and T3 tumors without node involvement or distant metastases are classified as stage IIA. Tumors that are confined to the wall of the esophagus (i.e., T1 and T2 tumors) with regional node involvement are classified as stage IIB disease. Stage III includes T3 tumors with regional node involvement, as well as any

Table 34–4 Definitions of Regional and Nonregional Lymph Node Involvement by Tumor Location

Tumors of the Lower Thoracic Esophagus

Regional lymph nodes	Nonregional lymph nodes (M1a)
Upper periesophageal nodes (above the azygos vein)	Celiac nodes
Subcarinal nodes	
Lower periesophageal nodes (below the azygos vein)	

Tumors of the Midthoracic Esophagus

Regional lymph nodes	Nonregional lymph nodes (M1a)
Upper periesophageal nodes (above the azygos vein)	Not applicable
Subcarinal nodes	
Lower periesophageal nodes (below the azygos vein)	

Tumors of the Upper Thoracic Esophagus

Regional lymph nodes	Nonregional lymph nodes (M1a)
Upper periesophageal nodes (above the azygos vein)	Cervical nodes
Subcarinal nodes	
Lower periesophageal nodes (below the azygos vein)	

T4 tumor irrespective of node status. Stage IV tumors are classified in two groups: stage IVA for M1a tumors and stage IVB for M1b disease.

Inadequacies in the Current Staging System

The adequacy of the current staging system for esophageal cancer has been called into question for a number of reasons. First, it does not fully consider adenocarcinomas that arise at the GEJ. According to the current definitions, a tumor arising in the region of the GEJ that involves less than 2 cm of the esophagus is classified as a proximal gastric cancer without consideration

Table 34–5 Stage Groupings

Stage 0	Tis	N0	M0
Stage I	T1	N0	M0
Stage IIA	T2	N0	M0
	T3	N0	M0
Stage IIB	T1	N1	M0
	T2	N1	M0
Stage III	T3	N1	M0
	T4	Any N	M0
Stage IVA	Any T	Any N	M1a
Stage IVB	Any T	Any N	M1b

of the presence or absence of associated Barrett's epithelium, which most authorities consider a clear indication of the esophageal origin of these tumors. Second, it classifies "nonregional" lymph nodes in quite general terms while assigning tumors with metastases to these nodes as stage IV disease, which is considered unresectable. Third, the staging system does not consider the number of metastatic lymph nodes, a factor identified in several recent studies as being of prognostic importance. Finally, analysis of the performance of the current staging system in patients undergoing resection has shown that survival estimates do not differ significantly between several stage groups (i.e., the survival probabilities are not distinctive) and that TNM combinations included in the same stage grouping are dissimilar (i.e., the survival probabilities are not homogeneous).[45]

Clear epidemiologic evidence suggests that adenocarcinoma of the GEJ should be considered distinct from other types of gastric cancer. These so-called cardia cancers are increasing in frequency in Western countries at a time when other types of gastric cancer are clearly on the decline. In addition, identified risk factors and patient demographics more closely resemble those of esophageal than gastric cancer. Most importantly, a high percentage of these patients will have Barrett's-type intestinal epithelium in the distal esophagus, thus suggesting a common pathophysiology. Unless there is extensive gastric involvement, these tumors are approached the same from a therapeutic standpoint as well, with similar outcomes. All these facts suggest that tumors arising at or above the GEJ should be considered with adenocarcinomas arising higher in the tubular esophagus.

The classification of nonregional node involvement as metastatic disease stems from Japanese data limited to patients with squamous cell carcinoma. Although there is little doubt that survival in patients with involvement of nonregional nodes is worse than in patients with only regional nodes involved, it is also clear that survival in patients with nonregional node involvement is significantly better than the 4- to 6-month median survival reported in patients with visceral metastases.[71] Several recent publications have demonstrated 5-year survival rates as high as 17% in patients with squamous cell carcinoma when nonregional nodes are involved.[72,73] In a recent review of our experience with en bloc resections performed for distal esophageal adenocarcinoma,[74] 26 patients had distant node involvement, including 16 with involved celiac nodes. Survival rates at 5 years in these patients with stage IV disease according to the current staging system were 33% and 29%, respectively.

The current staging system also fails to account for the prognostic importance of the extent of lymph node involvement. Rather, lymph node status is considered to be a dichotomous variable despite reports from centers around the world documenting the importance of both the number of positive lymph nodes and the ratio of positive lymph nodes to the number of nodes removed. In 1982, Skinner and co-workers[14] first recognized the prognostic importance of the number of involved nodes and suggested a revised classification system in which limited node disease was defined by the presence of two or fewer node metastases. Skinner later revised this recommendation to a threshold of four or fewer node metastases based on subsequent analysis of additional patients undergoing en bloc resection.[75] Since that time, reports from several other investigators have reached similar conclusions.[71,74,76]

Classification according to the lymph node ratio (the number of nodes with metastases divided by the number of nodes removed) has also been proposed as being more accurate for prognostic purposes. Roder and colleagues[77] used a lymph node ratio of 20%, whereas more recent studies[55,78] would suggest that a lymph node ratio of 10% better stratifies patients with regard to survival. In our recently reported series of 100 en bloc resections for adenocarcinoma,[74] we found that the lymph node ratio appears to best stratify patients from the standpoint of 5-year survival. The 5-year survival rate was 92% for N0 disease versus only 18% in the setting of metastases to more than 10% of the nodes removed. Patients with node metastases and a lymph node ratio of less than 10% had an intermediate survival of 47%.

More recently, we have used immunohistochemistry (IHC) in an attempt to better classify patients with regard to lymph node involvement.[79] Twenty patients who had metastases to less than 10% of the nodes removed had IHC performed on all of the nodes removed. Overall, the 5-year survival rate in this group of patients was 55%. Additional node metastases were identified by IHC in 14 patients. When the number of IHC-detected node metastases was added to the number detected by hematoxylineosin staining and the lymph node ratio remained less than 10%, the survival rate was 77% at 5 years. In contrast, when the additional metastases detected by IHC resulted in a lymph node ratio of greater than 10%, the survival rate at 5 years was only 14%. Together, these observations have led to the suggestion that the lymph node staging system be revised such that patients with limited node involvement would be classified as N1 and patients with extensive nodal involvement as N2 disease.

The final inadequacy of the current staging system relates to the lack of distinctiveness and homogeneity of the stage groupings. This issue has been addressed in a recent review by Rice and colleagues[76] of their experience in 480 patients who underwent resection alone for esophageal cancer. They found a lack of homogeneity in the T1 classification and noted significant survival differences for tumors limited to the lamina propria (T1a) versus those that involved the submucosa (T1b). For reasons outlined in the preceding paragraph, they also noted a lack of homogeneity in patients with N1 disease, with a significant decrease in survival as the number of regional node metastases increased. In addition, these authors demonstrated a lack of distinctiveness between several of the stage groupings as currently defined. Although significant differences in survival were found between stages I, IIA, and III, they found no difference in survival between stage IIB, III, and IV disease. Based on these findings, they and others[71,76,80] have called for revision of the staging groupings in use for esophageal cancer (Table 34–6).

MANAGEMENT

Over the past 2 decades, management of esophageal cancer in Western countries has changed from the treatment of patients with advanced squamous cell carcinoma to those with earlier-stage esophageal adenocarcinoma occurring in the setting of Barrett's esophagus. The combination of increasing numbers of patients with very early-stage tumors along with the perceived high risk for mortality and morbidity associated with esophageal resection has spurred interest in a number of new and unproven therapeutic approaches, such as mucosal ablation and EMR. At the same time, patients with more advanced-stage tumors are increasingly being treated with combined-modality therapy (neoadjuvant chemoradiotherapy) despite a lack of clear evidence of the superiority of this approach. In some centers, the need for surgical resection is being questioned, with definitive chemoradiotherapy offered as primary therapy.[81] In addition, when surgery is performed, controversy persists in regard to the extent of resection necessary, with much of

Table 34–6		Proposed Revisions to the Staging Classification for Esophageal Cancer		

Stage	**Korst et al.[71]**	**Rice et al.[76]**	**Ellis et al.[80]**
0	T0 N0 M0, Tis N0 M0	N/A	T1 N0 M0
I	T1 N0 M0, T2 N0 M0	Tis, T1a N0 M0	T1 N1 M0, T2 N0 M0
IIA	T3 N0 M0 T1 N1 M0		T2 N1 M0, T3 N0 M0
IIB	T2 N1 M0 T3 N1 M0	T1b N0 M0, T1a N1 M0, T2 N0 M0	
III	T1-3 N2 M0	T3 N0 M0, T1b/T2 N1 M0, T3 N1 M0, T4 N0 M0	T3 N1 M0, Any T N2 M0
IV	T4 Any N M0 Any T Any N M1	T4 N1 M0, Any T N2 M0, Any T Any N M1	Any T Any N M1

the debate focused on the benefits of formal lymph node dissection.

Proponents of alternatives to primary resection cite as justification high surgical mortality rates of 10% to 15% and low 5-year survival rates of 20% to 25% after surgery. These statements, based largely on past experience with squamous cell cancer, give the perception that surgery is not curative in most patients with esophageal carcinoma and suggest that surgical therapy is no longer central in the treatment of these patients because the survival benefits are outweighed by the risks of resection. However, recent observations[51,82] suggest that the outcomes of surgical resection in the present era of improvements in perioperative care, which has resulted in increasing numbers of tumors being diagnosed at an earlier stage, are much better than commonly quoted, with overall survival rates after surgery approaching 50% and operative mortality rates of less than 5%.

Surgical Therapy

Surgical resection remains the primary mode of therapy for patients with cancer of the esophagus in the absence of systemic metastases. Surgery offers the highest likelihood of cure for patients with localized disease, and it can offer quality palliation for patients with more advanced disease. To obtain the best results, management of esophageal carcinoma should be individualized on the basis of a combination of factors, including the physiologic status of the patient, tumor location, and the stage of disease.

Patient Assessment

Esophageal cancer is a disease that occurs predominantly in the sixth and seventh decades of life. However, advanced age alone should not be considered a contraindication to esophageal resection. Although the risk for mortality is higher in patients older than 70 years, this increased risk is due to the higher frequency of comorbid medical conditions such as heart, liver, and kidney disease in the elderly population rather than age per se.[83] It is important to note that when operative mortality is excluded, long-term survival after resection in the elderly population is similar to that observed in younger patients. As a result, patients in their 80s and 90s can be considered candidates for potentially curative resection, but particular attention needs to be paid to the preoperative assessment of these patients.

The strong etiologic relationship between cancer of the esophagus and alcohol and tobacco use makes it imperative that patients be carefully screened for the presence of cardiovascular, pulmonary, and hepatic dysfunction regardless of their age. It has been estimated that between 20% and 30% of patients with esophageal cancer will have evidence of cardiovascular disease if carefully screened.[84] This evaluation should include noninvasive screening for coronary artery disease by either stress echocardiography or thallium imaging. In most patients, proper preoperative evaluation and perioperative management will allow the patient to undergo re-

section. The preoperative evaluation should also include pulmonary function testing and arterial blood gas analysis. Patients with significant impairment in the forced expiratory volume at 1 second (FEV_1 <1 L) and those with chronic bronchitis are at increased risk for respiratory complications after surgery.[85,86] The presence of hypercapnia ($PaCO_2$ >45 mm Hg) or hypoxemia (PaO_2 <55 mm Hg) is also associated with an increased risk for complications. Finally, cirrhosis of the liver is not uncommon in patients with esophageal cancer, particularly those with squamous cell carcinoma. Well-compensated cirrhosis (Child's classification A) alone is not a contraindication to resection of an otherwise curable cancer, but care should be exercised when considering resection in the setting of more advanced stages of cirrhosis.

Tumor location is also an important factor in selecting the most appropriate therapy for an individual patient. Tumors in the cervical esophagus and the upper third of the thoracic esophagus are less amenable to complete en bloc resection because of the comparatively close proximity of these tumors to the airway and important vascular structures. As a result, these tumors are preferentially treated by either definitive chemoradiotherapy or chemoradiation therapy followed by resection of any residual disease. For tumors of the lower esophagus and GEJ, selection of patients for surgical resection is based on the results of a complete clinical staging evaluation. A selective therapeutic approach that we have used is summarized in Figure 34–5.

Extent of Resection for Early Esophageal Adenocarcinoma

Because of the perceived high risk for morbidity and mortality associated with esophagectomy, a number of alternatives to resection have been proposed, particularly in patients with very early-stage tumors. Such alternatives include EMR, mucosal ablation via photodynamic therapy, and limited-resection techniques such as vagal-sparing esophagectomy (VSE). These treatments all focus on removal or destruction of the esophageal lesion only and do not include lymph node dissection. As a result, they are applicable only in situations in which the risk of lymph node involvement is very low. Patients with early-stage tumors, most often detected in the course of surveillance programs for Barrett's esophagus, are potential candidates for these alternative therapies. It has been shown that when a tumor is limited to the lamina propria (T1a tumors), the risk for lymph node metastases is very low. We have identified 2 patients, each with a single involved lymph node, out of 58 (3.4%) who underwent esophageal resection for a tumor limited to the lamina propria. In both patients, the involved node was located at the GEJ in immediate proximity to the tumor. When submucosal invasion is present, between 30% and 50% will have evidence of lymph node involvement,[74,87] which argues strongly for the need to perform a formal node dissection. As previously mentioned, it is difficult to reliably differentiate between these subgroups of T1 disease on clinical grounds. Even when EUS is performed, the accuracy of categorization between T1a and T1b disease

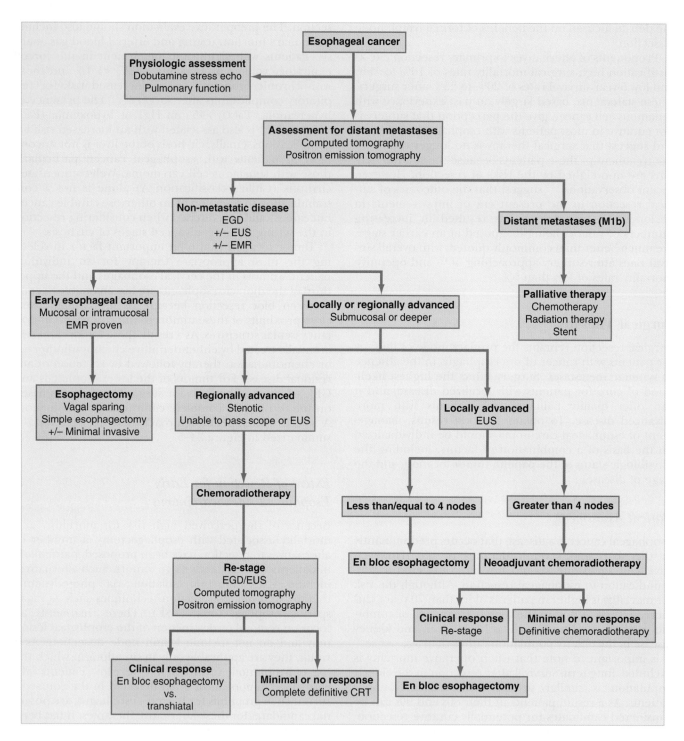

Figure 34–5. Therapeutic approach to esophageal cancer. CRT, chemoradiotherapy; EGD, esophagogastroduodenoscopy; EMR, endoscopic mucosal resection; EUS, endoscopic ultrasonography.

is no better than 20% to 30%.[56,88] We have recently described the utility of the endoscopic appearance of the Barrett's segment in differentiating between these early T1a and T1b tumors.[89] When no lesion is visible in the Barrett's mucosa and biopsy indicates the presence of intramucosal carcinoma, 80% have a tumor confined to the lamina propria. In contrast, when a lesion is visible, three quarters have a tumor that invades into the sub-

mucosa or beyond, and over half have node involvement. The former are potential candidates for more limited therapy, whereas the latter clearly need a formal cancer operation. More recently, we have performed EMR in patients with a visible lesion in an attempt to accurately determine the depth of invasion.[60] When EMR confirms the presence of a tumor limited to the lamina propria, treatment can be limited to removal of the esophagus

| Table 34–7 | Relationship between Tumor Depth and Lymph Node Status |

Tumor Depth	Prevalence of Node Metastases* (%)	Number of Involved Nodes† (Median [IQR])	Number with 1-4 Involved Nodes‡ (%)	Number with >4 Involved Nodes§ (%)
Intramucosal	1/16 (6.25)	2 (N/A)	1/16 (6.25)	0/16 (0)
Submucosal	5/16 (31.25)	1 (N/A)	4/16 (25)	1/16 (6.25)
Intramuscular	10/13 (76.92)	2 (1-4)	9/13 (69.23)	1/13 (7.69)
Transmural	47/55 (85.45)	5 (3-13.5)	22/55 (40)	25/55 (40)

*$\chi^2 = 42.0$, $P < .0001$ (chi-square test for trend).
†$\chi^2 = 11.02$, $P = 0.0116$ (Kruskal-Wallis); includes only patients with involved nodes.
‡$\chi^2 = 13.64$, $P = .0035$ (chi-square test for trend).
§$\chi^2 = 21.38$, $P < .0001$ (chi-square test for trend).
IQR, interquartile range.

without the need for formal lymph node dissection. In these patients, we advocate VSE.

Technique of Vagal-Sparing Esophagectomy The technique of VSE was developed to avoid the morbidity associated with division of the vagal nerves during standard esophagectomy.[90] The intent of the operation is to make esophagectomy more acceptable therapy to patients with end-stage benign disease and early malignant disease by avoiding some of the common gastrointestinal side effects of a standard esophagectomy.

VSE is performed through an upper midline abdominal incision and a second incision in the left side of the neck. The abdominal operation begins with identification of both the anterior and posterior vagus nerves. The nerves are encircled with tape for retraction purposes, and the nerve trunks are mobilized from the GEJ by a limited highly selective vagotomy. The proximal part of the stomach is transected with a linear stapling device above this point. When the stomach is to be used for reconstruction, the highly selective vagotomy is simply continued distally on the stomach to provide for greater mobility and creation of the gastric tube without injury to the vagus nerves.

The esophagus is then exposed in the neck and mobilized into the thoracic inlet where it can be divided as low as possible to preserve length for construction of the anastomosis. A gastrotomy is then made proximal to the point of gastric division, and a vein stripper is passed retrogradely up the esophagus. A stout ligature is applied around the esophagus and the vein stripper in the neck incision, and the esophagus is divided just above this point. The vein stripper is then used to remove the thoracic esophagus in an inverting fashion. After dilation of the esophageal bed with a 90-ml Foley catheter, the alimentary tract is reconstructed with either a colon interposition or a gastric pull-up.

We have compared the functional outcome of VSE with the results of standard transhiatal esophagectomy with gastric pull-up and esophagectomy with colon interposition.[91] Vagal secretory function was better preserved after VSE, as was vagal motor function. Gastric reservoir function was also more normal, and there was a significantly lower frequency of dumping and diarrhea after VSE. To date, experience with this technique in more than 100 patients with tumors confined to the lamina propria has confirmed the excellent quality of life after VSE, and in no patient has recurrent disease developed.

Extent of Resection for Localized Esophageal Cancer

Once the tumor has penetrated the submucosal layer, about half the patients will have node metastases. More than 80% of patients with invasion of the muscularis propria will have at least one involved lymph node.[49] In the event of transmural invasion, node involvement will be present in over 85%, and the median number of involved nodes and the proportion of patients with more than four involved nodes will increase (Table 34–7).[74] These patients, who have locoregionally advanced tumors, should be considered for resection based on the time-honored principles of surgical oncology, which emphasize the importance of complete resection. It is our preference to offer these patients en bloc resection.

Technique of En Bloc Esophagectomy The en bloc procedure is performed through an initial right thoracotomy followed by a midline laparotomy. The proximal anastomosis is performed through an incision made in the left side of the neck. The thoracic dissection includes removal of the azygos vein with its associated nodes, the thoracic duct, and the low paratracheal, subcarinal, paraesophageal, and parahiatal nodes in continuity with the resected esophagus. The block of tissue removed is bounded laterally on each side by the excised mediastinal pleura, anteriorly by the pericardium and membranous trachea, and posteriorly by the aorta and vertebral bodies.

The procedure begins with the patient in the left lateral decubitus position, and a posterolateral thoracotomy is performed with entry into the chest through the seventh or eighth intercostal space. The pleura overlying the lateral aspect of the vertebral bodies is incised from the level of the azygos arch to the diaphragm, and the intercostal veins are divided between ligatures as they enter the azygos vein. A dissection plane is then created by following each intercostal artery to reach the adventitial plane of the aorta. Blunt dissection continues across the anterior surface of the aorta until the left mediastinal pleura is reached. One or more hemiazygos communicating veins need to be ligated as they pass behind the aorta.

The anterior mediastinal dissection is performed along the posterior aspect of the pericardium, which is not removed unless the tumor is adherent. Once the left mediastinal pleura is reached, a vertical incision is made in the pleura just behind the pericardium and along the anterior aspect of the aorta at the limits of the previously created posterior dissection. The thoracic esophagus is then encircled with a Penrose drain for traction. The dissection plane along the anterior aspect of the aorta is then continued cephalad to a point just above the azygos arch, where the dissection is transitioned to the wall of the esophagus. In this transition, the right vagus nerve and the bronchial artery are divided. The anterior dissection is then continued cephalad along the pericardium until the subcarinal nodes are encountered. Careful dissection along the right main bronchus up to the carina and then distally along the left main bronchus allows removal of the entire subcarinal node packet in continuity with the resected esophagus. At this point, the anterior dissection is also transitioned to the wall of the esophagus by dividing the left vagus nerve. Blunt dissection from this point proximally should be performed as far as possible into the base of the neck to facilitate the later dissection.

As the en bloc dissection proceeds caudally, the thoracic surface of the diaphragm is reached. This should be incised with cautery to incorporate a portion of the esophageal hiatus with the specimen. The mediastinal tissue posteriorly just above the diaphragm includes the thoracic duct, which must be ligated carefully to prevent the development of chylothorax. A heavy silk ligature should be placed so that it incorporates all of the tissue anterior to the vertebral body and lateral to the aorta and esophagus. This ligature will also contain the azygos vein as it traverses the diaphragm, and the upper end of this vein is ligated flush with its confluence with the superior vena cava. The chest is closed after placement of a suction drain.

The abdominal portion of the operation begins at the porta hepatis, where all of the lymph node–bearing tissue overlying the hepatic arterial trunk and the portal vein is removed. This dissection is continued proximally along the hepatic artery to its origin from the celiac axis. The retroperitoneal tissue above the pancreas overlying the right crus of the diaphragm is dissected medially and superiorly so that it remains attached to the esophagectomy specimen. Attention is then turned to the greater curvature of the stomach, where the gastrocolic omentum is divided with preservation of the gastroepiploic arcade. This dissection should begin distally at the level of the pylorus and continue proximally to include division of the short gastric vessels. The use of a Har-

monic Scalpel (Ethicon Endo-Surgery, Cincinnati, OH) greatly facilitates this dissection. The short gastric vessels should be divided as close as possible to the spleen to preserve as many collateral vessels to the fundus as possible. The gastric fundus is rotated to the right to continue the dissection in the retroperitoneum, and all the node-bearing tissue above the splenic artery and overlying the left crus of the diaphragm is removed. The musculature of the diaphragmatic hiatus is then incised to meet the incision made in the diaphragm during the thoracic dissection. By retracting the stomach anteriorly, ample exposure of the celiac axis can be achieved to allow ligation of the coronary vein and the left gastric artery at its origin. A Kocher maneuver should be performed to allow maximum mobility of the stomach.

Exposure of the cervical esophagus is accomplished through an oblique left neck incision placed along the anterior border of the sternocleidomastoid muscle. This incision should extend from the sternal notch to a point half way to the ear lobe. The omohyoid, sternohyoid, and sternothyroid muscles are divided laterally. A dissection plane is then created between the contents of the carotid sheath and the trachea and esophagus to reach the prevertebral fascia. The inferior thyroid artery is divided between ligatures. Dissection is then continued posterior to the esophagus down into the thoracic inlet, where the dissection plane created during the thoracotomy is reached. The esophagus is encircled with a Penrose drain, and the upper thoracic esophagus is delivered up into the neck. A linear stapler is used to divide the esophagus as low as possible, and the specimen is removed through the abdomen.

Reconstruction is performed either by creation of a gastric tube after wide resection of the gastric cardia down to the fourth vein on the lesser curvature of the stomach or by using an isoperistaltic colon interposition based on the left colic artery. The gastric tube is created with a linear stapling device. This staple line should begin on the upper fundus at least 5 cm from the distal limit of the tumor and should continue to a point along the lesser curvature corresponding to the fourth or fifth branch of the left gastric artery. We prefer to oversew this staple line with a running absorbable suture to minimize the risk for a leak. A pyloromyotomy is then performed to aid in drainage from the vagotomized stomach. If an isoperistaltic colon interposition is used, the abdominal dissection also includes removal of the proximal two thirds of the stomach, the omentum, and the lymph nodes along the proximal two thirds of the greater curvature of the stomach.

Choice of Reconstruction   The choice of reconstruction by gastric pull-up or colon interposition is based on several factors. Generally, when the primary tumor is large or involves the proximal part of the stomach to a significant degree, a colon interposition should be performed to ensure adequate margins. However, in the setting of intrinsic colonic disease (polyps, diverticula, etc.) or variations in vascular supply that preclude use of the colon, a gastric pull-up or small intestinal interposition should be used.

In most patients undergoing resection for esophageal cancer, reconstruction is performed with a gastric conduit. The blood supply is very dependable, and only a single anastomosis is required. The major disadvantages of using the stomach include the complete lack of peristaltic activity and the tendency for persistent reflux into the remaining cervical esophagus that is directly connected to the acid-secreting stomach. In long-term survivors, this ongoing reflux can result in the development of recurrent Barrett's esophagus.[92] The need to preserve length may also result in more limited margins, especially for large or very distal tumors, which can result in local recurrence. As a result, with extensive involvement of the upper part of the stomach or in patients with a high expectation for long-term survival, we prefer to use an isoperistaltic left colon interposition.

The gastric pull-up is performed by wrapping the previously created gastric tube in a bowel bag to facilitate atraumatic passage to the neck. Care should be exercised to avoid excessive tension on the stomach or its gastroepiploic arcade during this maneuver, and twisting of the stomach must be avoided. The anastomosis is performed between the remaining cervical esophagus and the anterior wall of the gastric pull-up. We prefer to use a single-layer technique with placement of 4-0 monofilament absorbable sutures and tie the knots in the lumen. The last three or four sutures are placed in a modified Gambee fashion to achieve mucosal inversion. Gentle retraction on the gastric conduit from within the abdomen will remove redundancy in the gastric pull-up. Several nonabsorbable sutures should be placed between the stomach and the left diaphragmatic crus to prevent herniation of the stomach back into the thorax. A nasogastric tube is then carefully passed, a drain is placed in the neck, and the cervical wound is closed.

When a colon interposition is performed, the proximal part of the stomach is removed with the esophagectomy specimen by dividing the stomach at the level of the antrum. Leaving more denervated stomach can lead to gastric stasis and does not result in improved gastrointestinal function. The ascending colon and descending colon are mobilized completely. The segment of colon to be interposed derives its arterial supply from the ascending branch of the left colic artery and usually corresponds to the segment extending from the mid transverse colon to the proximal descending colon. This segment is mobilized by dissecting the middle colic artery back to its origin from the superior mesenteric artery, where it arises as a single trunk in most patients. After the middle colic artery and vein are temporarily occluded to ensure adequate collateral flow through the marginal artery, these vessels are ligated and divided.

The apex of the arc portended by the vascular pedicle is then marked with a suture, and the distance from this point to the neck is measured with umbilical tape. This tape is used to measure proximally from the first marking stitch to determine the point of transection of the proximal part of the colon. The divided colon is then passed through the bed of the resected esophagus wrapped in a bowel bag, and a single-layer monofilament anastomosis is performed to the remaining cervical esophagus.

Traction is gently applied to the colon from within the abdomen to eliminate redundancy, and the colon is secured to the left crus of the diaphragm with a nonabsorbable suture.

The colon is then divided with a linear stapler 5 to 10 cm below the point where it enters the abdomen. Care should be exercised to not leave too long an intraabdominal segment of colon because this will result in food retention. The mesentery should be divided immediately adjacent to the wall of the colon to avoid injury to the vascular pedicle. A two-layered anastomosis is then performed between the proximal divided colon and the antrum, and colon continuity is restored by a standard colocolostomy.

We routinely perform a catheter jejunostomy to provide for early postoperative feeding and to avoid the need for parenteral nutrition in the event of postoperative complications such as an anastomotic leak. The jejunostomy catheter is removed when the patient is able to maintain weight by oral feedings, usually 3 to 4 weeks postoperatively.

Transhiatal Esophagectomy Transhiatal esophagectomy has been advocated as an alternative to en bloc resection. Proponents cite lower morbidity and mortality rates associated with this approach, which eliminates the potentially debilitating thoracotomy incision.

Technique of Transhiatal Esophagectomy The procedure is performed through a midline laparotomy and an incision in the left side of the neck. Although an abdominal dissection similar to that described for the en bloc procedure can be performed, including the lymph nodes along the hepatic artery, the celiac trunk, and the left gastric artery and lesser curvature of the stomach, removal of the lower mediastinal lymph nodes is limited in this approach.

The operation begins with an abdominal lymph node dissection and gastric mobilization identical to that described for the en bloc procedure. After the stomach has been completely mobilized, the musculature of the esophageal hiatus is incised circumferentially. This not only ensures removal of any potentially involved parahiatal nodes but also enlarges the hiatal opening to facilitate the lower mediastinal dissection. The cervical esophagus is then exposed as described earlier.

Placement of appropriate retractors through the esophageal hiatus allows dissection of the lower thoracic esophagus under direct vision. This allows removal of many of the potentially involved periesophageal nodes from the lower mediastinum. When the limits of dissection under direct vision are reached, a hand is inserted into the mediastinum behind the esophagus. A relatively avascular plane can be developed that can reach the level of fingers of the opposite hand inserted in the neck incision behind the esophagus. A similar relatively avascular plane can then be developed anterior to the esophagus by working from both the abdomen and the neck. The lateral attachments on the left are dissected by reaching through the mediastinum posterior to the esophagus up into the neck incision. The index finger and thumb can then be used to bluntly dissect downward along the left side of the esophagus. In the lower mediastinum the vagal nerve trunks, which are separated from the esophagus by this maneuver, can be divided under direct vision after applying a large vascular clip. The right lateral attachments are mobilized in a similar manner by passing the right hand anterior to the esophagus and using the thumb and index finger to bluntly dissect the right lateral attachments. The upper thoracic esophagus is then delivered into the cervical wound, and it is divided with a linear stapling device as low as possible in the neck. The thoracic esophagus is then pulled down into the abdomen, the stomach is divided, and reconstruction is accomplished as described earlier.

Postoperative Care

Patients are routinely extubated at the completion of the operation, and they are admitted directly to the intensive care unit, where they are observed for 2 to 3 days after surgery. During the first 72 hours after surgery, patients are supported with a minimal amount of intravenous crystalloid and dextrose solutions. Continuous infusions of dopamine (3 µg/kg/min) and nitroglycerin (5 to 20 mg/min) are administered to aid graft perfusion. Albumin is used liberally to support blood pressure and urine output. A thoracic epidural catheter placed before the operation is used for postoperative pain management. This encourages early ambulation and assists in pulmonary toilet. Broad-spectrum antibiotics are continued for 24 hours after the operation.

After 72 hours, patients without complications are transferred to ward-level care. The infusions of dopamine and nitroglycerin are discontinued. Jejunal feedings are started at 15 ml/hr and increased by 15 ml daily until the target goal rate is achieved. Early mobilization and aggressive chest physiotherapy are continued on the ward. The nasogastric tube is removed when drainage is minimal and bowel function has returned. We routinely obtain a videoesophagogram 7 days after surgery to check for anastomotic leak and delayed conduit emptying. An oral diet, beginning with clear liquids and advanced to a soft diet over a period of 2 to 3 days, is gradually instituted with the patient sitting during and for 90 minutes after the meal. During this transition and after discharge, jejunal feedings are delivered at night to provide approximately 1000 calories until the patient is able to maintain hydration, weight, and nutrition with oral intake.

Complications

Despite recent improvements in perioperative management, postoperative morbidity and mortality after esophagectomy for cancer remain significant. These are large, technically demanding operations that are often performed on patients with compromised cardiopulmonary function. Nutritional disturbances are also common because of the combined effects of the cancer itself and the obstructing mass in the esophagus.

Complications occurring in a recent series of resections performed for esophageal adenocarcinoma are

| Table 34–8 | Perioperative Complications Occurring in 263 Consecutive Resections for Esophageal Adenocarcinoma |

Complication	*n*
Respiratory	61 (23%)
Pneumonia	25
Prolonged intubation	15
Empyema	5
Pleural effusion	16
Cardiovascular	44 (17%)
Arrhythmias	42
Myocardial infarction	2
Anastomotic	36 (14%)
Leak	31
Graft ischemia	5
Chylothorax	8 (3%)
Deep vein thrombosis/pulmonary embolism	9 (3%)
Gastrointestinal bleeding	1 (<1%)
Sepsis	4 (2%)
Urinary tract infection	3 (1%)
Wound infection	10 (4%)
Reoperation	30 (11%)
Abdominal bleeding	5
Anastomotic leak/graft necrosis	6
Sepsis/bowel infarction	3
Thoracic duct ligation	3
Empyema or continuous thoracic drainage	6
Fascial rupture/wound infection	7
Others	4 (2%)

summarized in Table 34–8.[51] Overall, 62% experienced at least one complication. Pulmonary complications, including pneumonia, acute respiratory distress syndrome requiring prolonged intubation, pleural effusion, and empyema, are among the most common complications and occurred in 23%. These complications can be minimized by early ambulation and careful attention to adequate pain control. Prevention of aspiration can be achieved by keeping the patient in the semi-upright position at all times and by meticulous attention to maintaining a functioning nasogastric tube. When necessary, a minitracheostomy can provide invaluable assistance in clearing retained secretions.

Cardiac complications occur in approximately 17% of patients, with the development of atrial fibrillation accounting for the majority of these complications. Though generally self-limited, they do require cardiac monitoring and treatment, which can prolong the intensive care unit stay. There is no evidence that prophylactic administration of antiarrhythmic drugs reduces the development of atrial fibrillation, although they are commonly used.

Anastomotic complications occur in 10% to 30% of patients, depending on the type of reconstruction performed. They appear to be more common after the use of neoadjuvant therapy, in patients with diabetes and hypertension, and in the obese.[93] Most of these leaks can be managed with local drainage and administration of antibiotics, as long as the vascular supply to the reconstruction is adequate. We recommend early endoscopy in any patient who is known or suspected to have a leak to exclude potentially life-threatening conduit ischemia, which can be present in as many as 14% of patients with an anastomotic leak.

Results

The goals of surgery in patients with esophageal cancer include elimination of dysphagia and improvement in long-term survival. Esophageal resection with reconstruction successfully achieves palliation of dysphagia in 80% to 90% of patients, but strictures do occur in 10% to 15% and may require intermittent dilatation. Weight loss, which is present in the vast majority of patients before surgery, is reversed in the majority, and most patients are able to return to work. Other potential complications of untreated esophageal cancer such as tumor pain, hemorrhage, and the development of an esophagorespiratory fistula can also be prevented.

Long-term survival after esophagectomy depends on a number of factors, such as the depth of tumor invasion, the number of involved lymph nodes, and the location of the tumor in the esophagus. The prognosis is better for tumors of the cervical esophagus and for those located at the GEJ than for tumors located in the thoracic esophagus. The impact of the type of resection performed on long-term survival remains a subject of debate. Although the results of single-institution series seem to indicate improved survival after en bloc resection, to date no prospective randomized trial has been reported with sufficient sample size to answer this question definitively.

We have recently reviewed our experience with 100 consecutive en bloc resections performed for esophageal adenocarcinoma.[74] Despite the fact that 55% had transmural invasion and node metastases were present in 63%, the overall survival rate at 5 years was 52%. Survival by AJCC stage is shown in Table 34–9. The survival rate after en bloc resection was higher than 94% for stage I disease, with an approximately 80% survival rate in patients with stage II disease. Even when stage III or IV disease was present, en bloc resection achieved long-term survival in approximately 25%. Similar results have been reported in several other relatively large single-institution series. Altorki and Skinner reported a 5-year survival rate of 40% in a series of 111 patients in which 60% had lymph node involvement and 59% had T3 or T4 disease.[94] The survival rate in patients with stage III disease was 39%. Collard and colleagues[95] have also reported a large experience with en bloc resection in a series of 235 patients, half of whom had N1 disease and more than 62% had T3 or T4 disease. The survival rate at 5 years was 49%, with 30% of the 98 patients with stage III disease surviving 5 years or more.

Table 34–9	Survival According to AJCC Stage Grouping
Stage (No. Patients)	Survival (%)
I (26)	94.4
IIa (9)	80.0*
IIb (11)	77.1†
III (32)	24.3‡
IV (16)	28.7

*P = NS for stage IIa versus stage IIb.
†P = .005 for stage IIb versus stage III.
‡P = NS for stage III versus stage IV.
AJCC, American Joint Committee on Cancer; NS, not significant.

A number of reports published recently have described the results of transhiatal esophagectomy. The overall 5-year survival rate has been reported at 18% to 27%,[96,97] with 10% to 15% survival rates in patients with stage III disease. Four recently published retrospective series compared survival after transhiatal and en bloc resection at a single institution.[13,97-99] Three of them reported improved survival after en bloc resection.

Proponents of transhiatal esophagectomy argue that the apparent benefit in overall survival associated with en bloc resection can be explained by the selection of patients with more favorable tumors for en bloc resection. They also explain the differences in survival by stage that have consistently been reported as being due to stage migration, which results from the more thorough lymph node sampling that undoubtedly occurs during an en bloc procedure. To address this question, Altorki et al.[13] reported outcomes after en bloc and transhiatal resection performed in patients with T3 N1 (stage III) disease. In this group of patients, stage migration cannot occur because all have locally advanced tumors with lymph node involvement. They reported a 4-year survival rate of 35% after en bloc resection, which was significantly better than the 11% survival rate observed after transhiatal esophagectomy. Ultimately, this debate can be resolved only by the completion of a large randomized controlled trial. To date, only one such trial has been reported, that by Hulscher and colleagues.[100] In this moderate-sized trial of 220 patients, the survival rate after en bloc resection was 39%, as opposed to a 27% survival rate after transhiatal esophagectomy. This difference, which amounted to a 44% improvement in survival after en bloc resection, was of borderline statistical significance (P = .08), thus suggesting that the study may have been underpowered.

There can be little doubt that the en bloc esophagectomy is a technically demanding operation that requires considerably more time to complete than standard esophagectomy does. A dedicated team of specialists is necessary to perform the procedure and to care for the patient after the operation to achieve acceptable morbidity and mortality rates. The technical expertise required to perform the surgery is demanding, and the learning curve is steep. Care after the operation is constant and complex for 10 to 14 days, but on occasion it can be much longer. In view of these issues, it is doubtful that the procedure will gain widespread acceptance until a prospective randomized trial is accomplished to show the benefit of the en bloc procedure. If such a study were to show the superiority of en bloc resection, it should be done in only a few select centers capable of organizing a team to perform the procedure and committed to providing care after the procedure.

The Role of Neoadjuvant Therapy

Increasingly, management of esophageal cancer has focused on multimodality therapy, with neoadjuvant chemoradiotherapy being administered to nearly all patients in many centers. This approach has made its way into the mainstream treatment of esophageal cancer despite the clear lack of convincing evidence of the superiority of this approach. The concept of neoadjuvant therapy in esophageal cancer was spurred by a general disappointment in the results of standard resections, which historically resulted in survival rates of 20% or less at 5 years. Rather than pursue more aggressive surgery, many centers chose to combine chemotherapy and radiation treatment with surgical resection in an attempt to increase the cure rate. Several phase II trials conducted in the early 1990s reported complete response rates of 10% to 20%, with improvement in survival in comparison to historical controls.[101-104]

This enthusiasm should have been tempered by awareness of the limitations of phase II trials. In particular, comparison with historical controls is known to introduce bias. The changes that have occurred in the epidemiology of esophageal cancer over the past several decades are well documented and have clearly resulted in detection of increasing numbers of cancers at an earlier, more curable stage. The results of surgical therapy also appear to be improving. The morbidity and mortality associated with surgery have declined, and our ability to deal with many side effects associated with treatment has also improved. For these and other reasons, the importance of the so-called historical control bias, which has been recognized since the 1950s, cannot be overemphasized.

As a result of these phase II trials, a number of randomized controlled trials have been conducted to assess the potential impact of combined-modality therapy for esophageal cancer. To date, the results of nine such trials have been reported. Of these, only one trial[9] was limited to patients with adenocarcinoma, whereas five trials included only patients with squamous cell cancer and three included tumors of both cell types. Only two of these trials have shown a benefit with routine administration of preoperative therapy. In each of these positive trials, a detailed review suggests several significant flaws.

The first randomized controlled trial to report improved survival with neoadjuvant therapy was published by Walsh et al. in 1996.[9] They reported the outcome in approximately 50 patients randomized to receive either preoperative 5-fluorouracil and cisplatin chemotherapy along with 40 cGy of external beam radiotherapy or surgical resection alone. They reported improved median survival (16 months versus 11 months) and better survival at 3 years after multimodality therapy. The major flaw in this study was the strikingly poor results achieved with surgery alone. They reported a 3-year survival rate of 6%, which is well below that reported in any recent surgical series. A detailed review of the manuscript reveals several possible explanations for the poor results reported for surgery alone. First, there was no standardization of surgical technique across the study centers, with at least five different operations being performed, depending on local preference. Second, the study also included proximal gastric cancers. Third, the prevalence of nodal metastases was nearly twofold higher in the surgery arm of the trial (82% versus 42%), thus suggesting that more advanced-staged tumors were randomized to surgical resection alone.

The only other randomized trial to report improved survival with neoadjuvant therapy was the Medical Research Council trial reported in 2002.[105] Approximately 400 patients were randomized to surgical resection alone or to 5-fluorouracil and cisplatin chemotherapy, followed by surgery. Radiation therapy was administered at the discretion of the study center. In this trial, 2-year survival was significantly better in the neoadjuvant therapy arm (43% versus 34%). Detailed review of the results of this trial raises several questions. First, the improved survival reported amounts to nine more patients surviving 2 years or more in the neoadjuvant therapy arm. However, there is evidence that the two groups may not have been comparable because the surgery-alone arm included 22 more patients with T4 tumors, 5 more patients with incomplete (R1) surgical resections, 22 more patients with lymph node involvement, and 18 more patients with distant lymph node involvement. Patients in the surgery-alone group were also more likely to have gross residual disease left behind (R2 resection), and in 13% of these patients no resection was performed. Combined, 26% of the surgery-alone group either had no resection or had incomplete resection as compared with a rate of only 14% in the neoadjuvant therapy arm. This difference in the extent of disease present may explain the difference in survival observed.

One consistent observation in nearly all reports of the outcome of neoadjuvant therapy has been the observation that patients who respond to neoadjuvant therapy have significantly better survival than nonresponders do. This observation has led to the use of response to therapy as a selection criterion in some centers for proceeding with surgical resection. Although it appears likely that neoadjuvant therapy does indeed benefit patients who respond, this implies that nonresponders fare correspondingly worse, particularly in the studies that report no difference in overall survival in comparison to surgery alone. There are at least two possible explanations for the reduced survival observed in patients who fail to respond to neoadjuvant therapy. First, it should be noted that the response rate to any particular chemotherapy regimen is at best 25% to 35%. In the remaining patients, the tumor is essentially left untreated during the 2 or 3 months that neoadjuvant therapy is given. During this period, the tumor may progress and these patients would probably have been better off if they had undergone resection initially. Administration of chemotherapy that has a significant impact on natural immunity without killing the patient's tumor cells may result in reduced protection from potential tumor metastases. The second possible explanation for reduced survival in nonresponders is that response to therapy may simply be a marker for tumors with less aggressive biologic behavior and therefore a better prognosis. If this is true, it is hardly an endorsement for the benefits of neoadjuvant therapy because it implies that the treatment itself was not of benefit. There are clinical data to suggest that such may be the case. In a randomized controlled trial involving 147 patients with squamous cell cancer, Law and co-workers[106] reported no difference in overall survival when neoadjuvant therapy was compared with surgical resection alone. As many others have shown, survival was better in patients who responded to neoadjuvant therapy than in those who did not. However, they also showed that patients who responded to neoadjuvant therapy had significantly smaller tumors on endoscopy at the time of randomization and had clinically earlier-stage tumors. In a report of the outcome of combined-modality therapy administered in a nonrandomized setting, Jiao et al.[107] showed that N status on MIS staging was the strongest predictor of response to neoadjuvant therapy, with a response rate of nearly 60% in patients with N0 disease versus only 15% when node metastases were present. Taken together, these observations suggest that response to therapy may be as much an indicator of a more favorable tumor as an indicator of a true benefit of the therapy administered.

Some evidence in the literature suggests that certain patients may be harmed by the routine administration of neoadjuvant therapy. Using a complicated statistical modeling approach, Rice and colleagues[108] have shown that survival in patients with clinical N1 disease that was down-staged to N0 disease after neoadjuvant therapy was similar to those staged N0 who had surgery alone, thus suggesting a benefit of combined-modality therapy in these patients. However, they also showed that survival was worse in patients with clinical N1 disease after neoadjuvant therapy if they failed to respond than in patients with similar clinical stage tumors that were treated by surgical resection alone. Using a similar statistical modeling approach in another publication,[109] the same group reported improved survival after neoadjuvant therapy in patients with clinical T3 N0 disease and in those with N1 disease if they responded to therapy. However, they concluded that survival was worse after neoadjuvant therapy in patients with clinical T1 or T2 tumors than would be expected had they undergone surgical resection alone.

SUMMARY

Changes in the diagnosis, evaluation, and treatment of carcinoma of the esophagus and GEJ have resulted in an improved prognosis for patients with this uncommon but deadly disease. Recent changes in epidemiology combined with a heightened awareness of the association between reflux, Barrett's metaplasia, and esophageal adenocarcinoma have allowed for earlier recognition and treatment. A more sophisticated approach to invasive and noninvasive preoperative staging with endoscopy, EUS, CT, and PET scanning has improved the selection of patients for a variety of treatment modalities. A tailored approach to the management of these patients can result in an overall 5-year survival rate greater than 50%, a dramatic improvement over the dismal results reported in the past.

SUGGESTED READINGS

DeMeester SR, DeMeester TR: Columnar mucosa and intestinal metaplasia of the esophagus: Fifty years of controversy. Ann Surg 231:303-321, 2000.

Hagen JA, DeMeester SR, Peters JH, et al: Curative resection for esophageal adenocarcinoma: Analysis of 100 en bloc esophagectomies. Ann Surg 234:520-530, discussion 530-531, 2001.

Nigro JJ, Hagen JA, DeMeester TR, et al: Prevalence and location of nodal metastases in distal esophageal adenocarcinoma confined to the wall: Implications for therapy. J Thorac Cardiovasc Surg 117:16-23, discussion 23-25, 1999.

Pohl H, Welch HG: The role of overdiagnosis and reclassification in the marked increase of esophageal adenocarcinoma incidence. J Natl Cancer Inst 97:142-146, 2005.

Rice TW, Blackstone EH, Adelstein DJ, et al: Role of clinically determined depth of tumor invasion in the treatment of esophageal carcinoma. J Thorac Cardiovasc Surg 125:1091-1102, 2003.

REFERENCES

1. Sabik JF, Rice TW, Goldblum JR, et al: Superficial esophageal carcinoma. Ann Thorac Surg 60:896-901, 1995.
2. Sampliner RE, Jaffe P: Malignant degeneration of Barrett's esophagus: The role of laser ablation and photodynamic therapy. Dis Esophagus 8:104-108, 1995.
3. Takeshita K, Tani M, Inoue H, et al: Endoscopic treatment of early oesophageal or gastric cancer. Gut 40:123-127, 1997.
4. Le Prise EL: [Cancer of the esophagus: Outcome of neoadjuvant therapy on surgical morbidity and mortality.] Cancer Radiother 2:763-770, 1998.
5. Bosset JF, Gignoux M, Triboulet JP, et al: Chemoradiotherapy followed by surgery compared with surgery alone in squamous-cell cancer of the esophagus. N Engl J Med 337:161-167, 1997.
6. Nygaard K, Hagen S, Hansen HS, et al: Pre-operative radiotherapy prolongs survival in operable esophageal carcinoma: A randomized, multicenter study of pre-operative radiotherapy and chemotherapy. The second Scandinavian trial in esophageal cancer. World J Surg 16:1104-1109, discussion 1110, 1992.
7. Apinop C, Puttisak P, Preecha N: A prospective study of combined therapy in esophageal cancer. Hepatogastroenterology 41:391-393, 1994.
8. Urba SG, Orringer MB, Turrisi A, et al: Randomized trial of preoperative chemoradiation versus surgery alone in patients with locoregional esophageal carcinoma. J Clin Oncol 19:305-331, 2001.
9. Walsh TN, Noonan N, Hollywood D, et al: A comparison of multimodal therapy and surgery for esophageal adenocarcinoma. N Engl J Med 15:462-467, 1996.

10. Orringer MB: Transhiatal esophagectomy without thoracotomy for carcinoma of the thoracic esophagus. Ann Surg 200:282-288, 1984.

11. Stark SP, Romberg MS, Pierce GE, et al: Transhiatal versus transthoracic esophagectomy for adenocarcinoma of the distal esophagus and cardia. Am J Surg 172:478-481, discussion 481-482, 1996.

12. Bumm R, Feussner H, Bartels H, et al: Radical transhiatal esophagectomy with two-field lymphadenectomy and endodissection for distal esophageal adenocarcinoma. World J Surg 21:822-831, 1997.

13. Altorki NK, Girardi L, Skinner DB: En bloc esophagectomy improves survival for stage III esophageal cancer. J Thorac Cardiovasc Surg 114:948-956, 1997.

14. Skinner DB, Dowlatshahi KD, DeMeester TR: Potentially curable cancer of the esophagus. Cancer 50(11 Suppl):2571-2575, 1982.

15. Torek F: The first successful case of resection of the thoracic portion of the esophagus for carcinoma. Surg Gynecol Obstet 16:614, 1913.

16. Ohsawa T: The surgery of the esophagus. Arch Jpn Chir 10:605, 1933.

17. Adams W, Phemister D: Carcinoma of the lower esophagus. J Thorac Surg 7:621, 1939.

18. Blalock A: Recent advances in surgery. N Engl J Med 231:261, 1944.

19. Sweet R: Surgical management of carcinoma of the mid esophagus. N Engl J Med 233:1, 1945.

20. Pisani P, Parkin DM, Bray F, Ferlay J: Estimates of the worldwide mortality from 25 cancers in 1990. [erratum appears in Int J Cancer 1999 Dec 10;83(6):870-3.] Int J Cancer 83:18-29, 1999.

21. Jemal A, Tiwari RC, Murray T, et al: Cancer statistics, 2004. CA Cancer J Clin 54:8-29, 2004.

22. Jemal A, Murray T, Ward E, et al: Cancer statistics, 2005. CA Cancer J Clin 55:10-30, 2005.

23. SEER Statistical Database. Esophageal cancer statistics. 2004.

24. Wang HH, Antonioli DA, Goldman H: Comparative features of esophageal and gastric adenocarcinomas: Recent changes in type and frequency. Hum Pathol 17:482-487, 1986.

25. Hesketh PJ, Clapp RW, Doos WG, Spechler SJ: The increasing frequency of adenocarcinoma of the esophagus. Cancer 64:526-530, 1989.

26. Pohl H, Welch HG: The role of overdiagnosis and reclassification in the marked increase of esophageal adenocarcinoma incidence. J Natl Cancer Inst 97:142-146, 2005.

27. Brown LM, Hoover R, Silverman D, et al: Excess incidence of squamous cell esophageal cancer among US black men: Role of social class and other risk factors. Am J Epidemiol 153:114-122, 2001.

28. Crookes PF, Corkill S, DeMeester TR: Gastroesophageal reflux in achalasia. When is reflux really reflux? Dig Dis Sci 42:1354-1361, 1997.

29. Meijssen MA, Tilanus HW, van Blankenstein M, et al: Achalasia complicated by oesophageal squamous cell carcinoma: A prospective study in 195 patients. Gut 33:155-158, 1992.

30. Peracchia A, Segalin A, Bardini R, et al: Esophageal carcinoma and achalasia: Prevalence, incidence and results of treatment. Hepatogastroenterology 38:514-516, 1991.

31. Appelqvist P, Salmo M: Lye corrosion carcinoma of the esophagus: A review of 63 cases. Cancer 45:2655-2658, 1980.

32. Hopkins RA, Postlethwait RW: Caustic burns and carcinoma of the esophagus. Ann Surg 194:146-148, 1981.

33. Harper PS, Harper RM, Howel-Evans AW: Carcinoma of the oesophagus with tylosis. Q J Med 39:317-333, 1970.

34. Lagergren J, Bergstrom R, Lindgren A, Nyren O: Symptomatic gastroesophageal reflux as a risk factor for esophageal adenocarcinoma. N Engl J Med 340:825-831, 1999.

35. Terry P, Lagergren J, Hansen H, et al: Fruit and vegetable consumption in the prevention of oesophageal and cardia cancers. Eur J Cancer Prev 10:365-369, 2001.

36. Mayne ST, Risch HA, Dubrow R, et al: Nutrient intake and risk of subtypes of esophageal and gastric cancer. Cancer Epidemiol Biomarkers Prev 10:1055-1062, 2001.

37. Hawe A, Payne WS, Weiland LH, Fontana RS: Adenocarcinoma in the columnar epithelial lined lower (Barrett) oesophagus. Thorax 28:511-514, 1973.

38. Chandrasoma PT, Lokuhetty DM, Demeester TR, et al: Definition of histopathologic changes in gastroesophageal reflux disease. Am J Surg Pathol 24:344-351, 2000.

39. Peters JH, Clark GW, Ireland AP: Outcome of adenocarcinoma arising in Barrett's esophagus in endoscopically surveyed and non-surveyed patients. J Thorac Cardiovasc Surg 108:813-822, 1994.

40. DeMeester SR, DeMeester TR: Columnar mucosa and intestinal metaplasia of the esophagus: Fifty years of controversy. Ann Surg 231:303-321, 2000.

41. Telerman A, Gerard B, Van den Heule B, Bleiberg H: Gastrointestinal metastases from extra-abdominal tumors. Endoscopy 17:99-101, 1985.

42. Antler AS, Ough Y, Pitchumoni CS, et al: Gastrointestinal metastases from malignant tumors of the lung. Cancer 49:170-172, 1982.

43. Endo M, Yoshino K, Kawano T, et al: Clinicopathologic analysis of lymph node metastasis in surgically resected superficial cancer of the thoracic esophagus. Dis Esophagus 13:125-129, 2000.

44. Araki K, Ohno S, Egashira A, et al: Pathologic features of superficial esophageal squamous cell carcinoma with lymph node and distal metastasis. Cancer 94:570-575, 2002.

45. Rice TW, Blackstone EH, Adelstein DJ, et al: Role of clinically determined depth of tumor invasion in the treatment of esophageal carcinoma. J Thorac Cardiovasc Surg 125:1091-1102, 2003.

46. Mandard AM, Chasle J, Marnay J, et al: Autopsy findings in 111 cases of esophageal cancer. Cancer 48:329-335, 1981.

47. Odze R, Goldblum J, Crawford J: Surgical Pathology of the GI Tract, Liver, Biliary Tract and Pancreas. Philadelphia, Elsevier, 2004.

48. Paraf F, Flejou JF, Pignon JP, et al: Surgical pathology of adenocarcinoma arising in Barrett's esophagus. Analysis of 67 cases. Am J Surg Pathol 19:183-191, 1995.

49. Nigro JJ, Hagen JA, DeMeester TR, et al: Prevalence and location of nodal metastases in distal esophageal adenocarcinoma confined to the wall: Implications for therapy. J Thorac Cardiovasc Surg 117:16-23, discussion 23-25, 1999.

50. Nigro JJ, DeMeester SR, Hagen JA, et al: Node status in transmural esophageal adenocarcinoma and outcome after en bloc esophagectomy. J Thorac Cardiovasc Surg 117:960-968, 1999.

51. Portale G, Hagen JA, Peters JH, et al: Modern 5-year survival in resectable esophageal adenocarcinoma: Single institution experience with 263 patients. J Am Coll Surg 202:588-596.

52. Clark GW, Ireland AP, Hagen JA, et al: Carcinoembryonic antigen measurements in the management of esophageal cancer: An indicator of subclinical recurrence. Am J Surg 170:597-600, discussion 600-601, 1995.

53. Bhutani MS, Barde CJ, Markert RJ, Gopalswamy N: Length of esophageal cancer and degree of luminal stenosis during upper endoscopy predict T stage by endoscopic ultrasound. Endoscopy 34:461-463, 2002.

54. Van Dam J, Rice TW, Catalano MF, et al: High-grade malignant stricture is predictive of esophageal tumor stage. Risks of endosonographic evaluation. Cancer 71:2910-2917, 1993.

55. Eloubeidi MA, Desmond R, Arguedas MR, et al: Prognostic factors for the survival of patients with esophageal carcinoma in the U.S.: The importance of tumor length and lymph node status. Cancer 95:1434-1443, 2002.

56. Kienle P, Buhl K, Kuntz C, et al: Prospective comparison of endoscopy, endosonography and computed tomography for staging of tumours of the oesophagus and gastric cardia. Digestion 66:230-236, 2002.

57. Hiele M, De Leyn P, Schurmans P, et al: Relation between endoscopic ultrasound findings and outcome of patients with tumors of the esophagus or esophagogastric junction. Gastrointest Endosc 45:381-386, 1997.

58. Kawano T, Ohshima M, Iwai T: Early esophageal carcinoma: Endoscopic ultrasonography using the Sonoprobe. Abdom Imaging 28:477-485, 2003.

59. Vazquez-Sequeiros E, Wiersema MJ: High-frequency US catheter-based staging of early esophageal tumors. Gastrointest Endosc 55:95-99, 2002.

60. Maish MS, DeMeester SR: Endoscopic mucosal resection as a staging technique to determine the depth of invasion of esophageal adenocarcinoma. Ann Thorac Surg 78:1777-1782, 2004.

61. Reinig JW, Stanley JH, Schabel SI: CT evaluation of thickened esophageal walls. AJR Am J Roentgenol 140:931-934, 1983.

62. Rasanen JV, Sihvo EI, Knuuti MJ, et al: Prospective analysis of accuracy of positron emission tomography, computed tomography, and endoscopic ultrasonography in staging of adenocarcinoma of the esophagus and the esophagogastric junction. Ann Surg Oncol 10:954-960, 2003.

63. Wayman J, Chakraverty S, Griffin SM, et al: Evaluation of local invasion by oesophageal carcinoma—a prospective study of prone computed tomography scanning. Postgrad Med J 77:181-184, 2001.

64. Kim K, Park SJ, Kim BT, et al: Evaluation of lymph node metastases in squamous cell carcinoma of the esophagus with positron emission tomography. Ann Thorac Surg 71:290-294, 2001.

65. Block MI, Patterson GA, Sundaresan RS, et al: Improvement in staging of esophageal cancer with the addition of positron emission tomography. Ann Thorac Surg 64:770-776, discussion 776-777, 1997.

66. Luketich JD, Schauer PR, Meltzer CC, et al: Role of positron emission tomography in staging esophageal cancer. Ann Thorac Surg 64:765-769, 1997.

67. Flamen P, Lerut A, Van Cutsem E, et al: Utility of positron emission tomography for the staging of patients with potentially operable esophageal carcinoma. J Clin Oncol 18:3202-3210, 2000.

68. Krasna MJ, Reed CE, Nedzwiecki D, et al: CALGB 9380: A prospective trial of the feasibility of thoracoscopy/laparoscopy in staging esophageal cancer. Ann Thorac Surg 71:1073-1079, 2001.

69. Wallace MB, Nietert PJ, Earle C, et al: An analysis of multiple staging management strategies for carcinoma of the esophagus: Computed tomography, endoscopic ultrasound, positron emission tomography, and thoracoscopy/laparoscopy. Ann Thorac Surg 74:1026-1032, 2002.

70. AJCC Cancer Staging Manual, 5th ed: Philadelphia, Lippincott-Raven, 1997, pp 65-69.

71. Korst RJ, Rusch VW, Venkatraman E, et al: Proposed revision of the staging classification for esophageal cancer. J Thorac Cardiovasc Surg 115:660-669, 1998.

72. A proposal for a new TNM classification of esophageal carcinoma. Japanese Committee for Registration of Esophageal Carcinoma. Jpn J Clin Oncol 15:625-636, 1985.

73. Iizuka T, Isono K, Kakegawa T, Watanabe H: Parameters linked to ten-year survival in Japan of resected esophageal carcinoma. Japanese Committee for Registration of Esophageal Carcinoma Cases. Chest 96:1005-1011, 1989.

74. Hagen JA, DeMeester SR, Peters JH, et al: Curative resection for esophageal adenocarcinoma: Analysis of 100 en bloc esophagectomies. Ann Surg 234:520-530, discussion 530-531, 2001.

75. Skinner DB: En bloc resection for neoplasms of the esophagus and cardia. J Thorac Cardiovasc Surg 85:59-71, 1983.

76. Rice TW, Blackstone EH, Rybicki LA, et al: Refining esophageal cancer staging. J Thorac Cardiovasc Surg 125:1103-1113, 2003.

77. Roder JD, Busch R, Stein HJ, et al: Ratio of invaded to removed lymph nodes as a predictor of survival in squamous cell carcinoma of the oesophagus. Br J Surg 81:410-413, 1994.

78. Chen JH, Wei GQ, Chen MY: [Prognostic evaluation of lymph node metastasis in thoracic esophageal cancer—an analysis of 212 cases.] Chung-Hua Chung Liu Tsa Chih [Chinese Journal of Oncology] 16:441-443, 1994.

79. Waterman TA, Hagen JA, Peters JH, et al: The prognostic importance of immunohistochemically detected node metastases in resected esophageal adenocarcinoma. Ann Thorac Surg 78:1161-1169, 2004.

80. Ellis FH, Watkins E, Krasna MJ, et al: Staging of carcinoma of the esophagus and cardia: A comparison of different staging criteria. J Surg Oncol 52:231-235, 1993.

81. Bedenne L, Michel P, Bouche D, et al: Randomized phase III trial in locally advanced esophageal cancer: Radiochemotherapy followed by surgery versus radiochemotherapy alone (FFCD 9102) [abstract]. Paper presented at a meeting of The American Society of Clinical Oncology, Orlando, Fla, 2002.

82. Stein HJ, Siewert JR: Improved prognosis of resected esophageal cancer. World J Surg 28:520-525, 2004.

83. Sugimachi K, Inokuchi K, Ueo H, et al: Surgical treatment for carcinoma of the esophagus in the elderly patient. Surg Gynecol Obstet 160:317-319, 1985.

84. Konder H: Analysis of cardiopulmonary function in esophageal cancer patients prior to surgery. Berlin, Springer-Verlag, 1988, p 249.

85. Giuli R, Sancho-Garnier H: Diagnostic, therapeutic, and prognostic features of cancers of the esophagus: Results of the international prospective study conducted by the OESO group (790 patients). Surgery 99:614-622, 1986.

86. Chan K, Wong J: Mortality after esophagectomy for carcinoma of the esophagus: An analysis of risk factors. Dis Esophagus 3:49, 1990.

87. Rice TW: Commentary: Esophageal carcinoma confined to the wall—the need for immediate definitive therapy. J Thorac Cardiovasc Surg 117:26-27, 1999.

88. Peters JH, Hoeft SF, Heimbucher J, et al: Selection of patients for curative or palliative resection of esophageal cancer based on preoperative endoscopic ultrasonography. Arch Surg 129:534-539, 1994.

89. Nigro JJ, Hagen JA, DeMeester TR, et al: Occult esophageal adenocarcinoma: Extent of disease and implications for effective therapy. Ann Surg 230:433-438, discussion 438-440, 1999.

90. Akiyama H, Tsurumaru M, Ono Y, et al: Esophagectomy without thoracotomy with vagal preservation. J Am Coll Surg 178:83-85, 1994.

91. Banki F, Mason RJ, DeMeester SR, et al: Vagal-sparing esophagectomy: A more physiologic alternative. Ann Surg 236:324-336, 2002.

92. Oberg S, Johansson J, Wenner J, Walther B: Metaplastic columnar mucosa in the cervical esophagus after esophagectomy. Ann Surg 235:338-345, 2002.

93. Briel JW, Tamhankar AP, Hagen JA, et al: Prevalence and risk factors for ischemia, leak, and stricture of esophageal anastomosis: Gastric pull-up versus colon interposition. J Am Coll Surg 198:536-541, discussion 541-542, 2004.

94. Altorki N, Skinner D: Should en bloc esophagectomy be the standard of care for esophageal carcinoma? Ann Surg 234:581-587, 2001.

95. Collard JM, Otte JB, Fiasse R, et al: Skeletonizing en bloc esophagectomy for cancer. Ann Surg 234:25-32, 2001.

96. Orringer MB, Marshall B, Stirling MC: Transhiatal esophagectomy for benign and malignant disease. J Thorac Cardiovasc Surg 105:265-276, discussion 276-277, 1993.

97. Horstmann O, Verreet PR, Becker H, et al: Transhiatal oesophagectomy compared with transthoracic resection and systematic lymphadenectomy for the treatment of oesophageal cancer. Eur J Surg 161:557-567, 1995.

98. Hagen JA, Peters JH, DeMeester TR: Superiority of extended en bloc esophagogastrectomy for carcinoma of the lower esophagus and cardia. J Thorac Cardiovasc Surg 106:850-859, 1993.

99. Putnam JB Jr, Suell DM, McMurtrey MJ, et al: Comparison of three techniques of esophagectomy within a residency training program. Ann Thorac Surg 57:319-325, 1994.

100. Hulscher JB, van Sandick JW, de Boer AG, et al: Extended transthoracic resection compared with limited transhiatal resection for adenocarcinoma of the esophagus. N Engl J Med 347:1662-1669, 2002.

101. Ajani JA, Roth JA, Ryan B, et al: Evaluation of pre- and postoperative chemotherapy for resectable adenocarcinoma of the esophagus or gastroesophageal junction. J Clin Oncol 8:1231-1238, 1990.

102. Forastiere AA, Orringer MB, Perez-Tamayo C, et al: Preoperative chemoradiation followed by transhiatal esophagectomy for carcinoma of the esophagus: Final report. J Clin Oncol 11:1118-1123, 1993.

103. Wolfe WG, Vaughn AL, Seigler HF, et al: Survival of patients with carcinoma of the esophagus treated with combined-modality therapy. J Thorac Cardiovasc Surg 105:749-755, discussion 755-756, 1993.

104. Stewart JR, Hoff SJ, Johnson DH, et al: Improved survival with neoadjuvant therapy and resection for adenocarcinoma of the esophagus. Ann Surg 218:571-576, discussion 576-578, 1993.

105. Medical Research Council Oesophageal Cancer Working Group: Surgical resection with or without preoperative chemotherapy in oesophageal cancer: A randomised controlled trial. Lancet 359:1727-1733, 2002.

106. Law S, Fok M, Chow S, et al: Preoperative chemotherapy versus surgical therapy alone for squamous cell carcinoma of the esophagus: A prospective randomized trial. J Thorac Cardiovasc Surg 114:210-217, 1997.

107. Jiao X, Krasna MJ, Sonett J, et al: Pretreatment surgical lymph node staging predicts results of trimodality therapy in esophageal cancer. Eur J Cardiothorac Surg 19:880-886, 2001.

108. Rice TW, Blackstone EH, Adelstein DJ, et al: N1 esophageal carcinoma: The importance of staging and downstaging. J Thorac Cardiovasc Surg 121:454-464, 2001.

109. Rice TW, Adelstein DJ, Chidel MA, et al: Benefit of postoperative adjuvant chemoradiotherapy in locoregionally advanced esophageal carcinoma. J Thorac Cardiovasc Surg 126:1590-1596, 2003.

35

Palliative Treatment of Carcinoma of the Esophagus

Thomas C. B. Dehn · Anthony S. Mee · Catherine Jephcott · Ruth Moxon

Despite advances in staging and in oncologic and surgical treatment of esophageal and junctional tumors, 5-year survival rates remain stubbornly between 10% and 15% at best. Thus, the majority of patients with these cancers will require some form of palliative treatment. As a result of unacceptably high postoperative mortality and morbidity, health commissioning bodies in both the United States and the United Kingdom have directed centralization of esophageal resection to centers performing a "high" volume of resectional surgery (in the United States, centers with more than 10 resections per annum; in the United Kingdom, units serving greater than 1 million population). It is enigmatic that no direction or resources have been allocated to the palliative treatment of such patients, who represent the majority of patients and for whom the appropriate choice of treatment is essential.

Patients requiring palliation fall into two groups: those who for reasons of metastatic disease, age, comorbid condition, or choice are unsuitable for radical surgery or chemoradiotherapy and those who have undergone treatment with curative intent but the disease recurs. The goals of palliative treatment are, first, to relieve the specific symptoms of dysphagia, mediastinal pain, and bleeding and, second, to delay death as a result of metastatic disease with minimal comorbidity. These goals must be accomplished within a few months inasmuch as 60% or more will have died within 6 months of diagnosis.[1]

Selection of palliative treatment must be individualized for each patient and be based on the physical characteristics and location of the tumor, the performance status and age of the patient, tumor burden, and expected survival. Other considerations are the availability of home support, traveling time between home and hospital, and finally, the local facilities and expertise at the hospital of treatment. These decisions can be difficult and should not be made by individual clinicians in isolation. In the United Kingdom National Health Service, all upper gastrointestinal cancer patients (whether undergoing curative or palliative treatment) are discussed at a weekly multidisciplinary team (MDT) meeting. The upper gastrointestinal MDT meeting is attended by upper gastrointestinal surgeons, gastroenterologists, radiologists, oncologists, histopathologists, and palliative care and cancer specialist nurses. The central figure in these meetings is the upper gastrointestinal cancer nurse specialist, who acts as the patient's advocate and the point of contact for the patient.

ASSESSMENT OF PATIENTS REQUIRING PALLIATIVE TREATMENT

The scope of clinical and laboratory investigations depends on the individual patient's circumstances. For example, an 80-year-old patient with ischemic heart disease, a 5-cm tumor causing grade IV dysphagia, and 5 hours' traveling time from the treatment center may best be served by a "one-off" treatment, such as a self-expanding stent or brachytherapy. Such a patient may require a full blood count and electrolyte assay to enable transfusion or rehydration to be delivered concurrently. Computed tomography (CT) and endoscopic ultrasound are superfluous and will not alter the management. A 50-year-old patient, however, with good performance status and celiac nodal or hepatic secondaries may require tumor staging by CT to further assess the metastatic load, as well as appropriate biochemistry evaluation to determine whether nephrotoxic chemotherapy may be administered.

Careful assessment must be made of the patient's dentition and ability to swallow. The site, length, and nature of the tumor (e.g., whether it crosses the cardia, is scirrhous or exophytic, and is single or multifocal) must be evaluated. This is best done endoscopically, although barium studies can assist when tumor growth precludes

Box 35–1   **Palliation of Malignant Dysphagia**

Endoscopically Delivered

Bougienage (dilatation)—can be rigid pulsion dilators such as the Savary-Gilliard or balloon dilators

Chemical—alcohol injection

Stents—self-expanding metal stents (SEMS). Stents can be covered/uncovered/impregnated with a chemotherapeutic agent

Thermal energy
 Nd-YAG laser
 Argon beam coagulation (ABC)
 Bipolar cautery (Bicap)
 Photodynamic therapy (PDT)

Oncologic Treatment

Radiotherapy
 External beam
 Brachytherapy

Chemotherapy
 Single agent
 Multiagent

Surgical

Palliative resection

Bypass surgery

Exclusion therapy and nutrition.

endoscopic assessment of the distal extent and dilatation is contraindicated.

Psychological support is paramount for patients with malignant dysphagia. This devastating symptom adversely affects quality of life and is embarrassing for both the patient and relatives in the social context of eating a meal.

The various methods available for palliation of malignant dysphagia are presented in Box 35–1. Table 35–1 lists the advantages and disadvantages of each method. Many of the treatments can be administered concurrently, with improved results—for example, external beam radiotherapy can enhance the effects of laser ablation of esophageal cancer.[2] The concept of one treatment being appropriate for all patients has been abandoned.

ENDOSCOPIC METHODS OF PALLIATION

Alcohol Sclerotherapy

Small (0.5 to 1 ml) aliquots of 98% ethanol can be injected sequentially into the tumor with an endoscopic varices needle. This method is cheap, readily available, and repeatable. Most patients experience some discomfort during and shortly after injection and require supportive analgesia. Randomized studies[3] have compared alcohol therapy with neodymium:yttrium-aluminum-garnet (Nd:YAG) laser ablation: both treatments produced similar improvement in dysphagia scores, but further treatments were required at the same time intervals (approximately 30 to 42 days). Return to feeding was achieved in similar proportion (laser, 88%; alcohol, 78%). The alcohol-treated group took a few days longer to begin normal feeding, probably because of the time needed to achieve tumor necrosis. Failure to relieve dysphagia—as indicated by stent insertion—was equivalent at around 12%.

Chemotherapeutic drugs (mitomycin C, bleomycin, cisplatin, and doxorubicin) have also been injected directly into esophageal tumors in the form of a gel matrix, but this technique has not gained widespread acceptance.

Bougienage

The first dilators were made of wax, hence the term "bougie" from the name of the Algerian town of Bougiyah, the medieval capital of the wax trade. The first description of their use took place 4 centuries ago. Mercury-filled dilators were introduced in 1915, but not until the development of fluoroscopically controlled, guidewire-assisted olive dilators in the 1950s (Eder-Puestow) was effective dilatation of neoplastic strictures possible. The subsequent development of hollow-core polyvinyl dilators (Savary-Gilliard) and through-the-scope (TTS) balloon dilators further refined these techniques.

The introduction of safe expansile metal prostheses has tended to supersede palliative esophageal dilatation for the relief of malignant dysphagia, although the latter remains a helpful initial approach in up to 90% of patients for whom a period of reasonable swallowing may be achieved.

Poiseuille's law and equation relate volume flow in a cylindrical tube model to the fourth power of the vessel's radius. Thus, a small decrease in the diameter of the esophagus by encroaching tumor can rapidly lead to worsening dysphagia and vice versa. A small improvement in luminal diameter may therefore be temporarily helpful. The technique of either bougienage or TTS balloon dilatation is simple and inexpensive and can easily be accomplished as a day (office) case, and the equipment is widely available. Although esophageal dilatation alone may effectively and safely palliate stenosis secondary to carcinoma, the effect is only temporary, particularly with carcinomas that are more scirrhous, for which the technique may need to be repeated every 10 to 14 days. Thus, even though up to 90% of patients will achieve palliation, the length of time before another dilatation is required is variable and unpredictable. Any initial savings over a prosthesis may therefore be lost by the need for repeat dilatation and, on rare occasion, by an inpatient stay after perforation. This complication may approach an incidence of 5% with neoplastic strictures and, though a major setback in any patient, is a

Table 35–1 Advantages and Disadvantages of Methods for Palliation of Malignant Dysphagia

Method	Advantages	Disadvantage
Bougienage	"Office" based Simple and inexpensive Readily available	Repeated treatments necessary Temporary relief of symptoms Risk of perforation
Stent	Short stay Simple Readily available "Treats" perforation/fistula Single treatment	Expensive May be painful Tumor overgrowth Stent slippage
Alcohol injection	"Office" based Inexpensive Readily available	Least reliable in efficacy Not beneficial for long tumors Repeated treatment necessary
Nd-YAG laser	Effective for exophytic, short tumors Office based	Expensive capital outlay Repeated treatments necessary Risk of post-treatment hemorrhage and perforation Not widely available
Argon beam coagulation	"Office" based Inexpensive Effective with short superficial tumors Less penetrative power than laser (less risk of perforation)	Repeated treatments Less effective with long, extensive tumors
Photodynamic therapy	"Office" based Prolonged length of effect Effective for long, tortuous tumors	Not readily available Photosensitivity
Radiotherapy *Brachytherapy*	Single treatment Successful with short tumors	Not widely available Esophageal lumen patency required No use with long tumors Time lag to efficacy
External beam	Reasonably effective	Wide effect Certain degree of patient fitness needed Repeated visits to hospital Time lag to efficacy
Chemotherapy	Effective with systemic disease	May require venous infusion and portable pump Toxic gastrointestinal and hematologic side effects Requires frequent monitoring

disaster for those in whom curative surgery is still a possibility because such patients can be rendered incurable by this complication. Preoperative dilatation in such potentially operable patients should either be avoided or be undertaken with particular caution.

Role of Esophageal Prostheses as Palliation for Obstructing Carcinoma

The alternative approach to dilatation, or placement of a per oral prosthesis, provides for more long-lasting palliation. Though originally placed surgically via a "pull-through" technique, the procedure was associated with high morbidity and mortality. The advent of fiberoptic endoscopy led to the development of pulsion techniques

of placing a plastic prosthesis over a guidewire under fluoroscopic control. A number of different prostheses became available, usually manufactured from radioresistant, radiopaque latex, rubber, or polyvinyl chloride that was reinforced with a nylon or metal coil to prevent kinking and included a proximal and distal flange to help prevent migration. These tubes were unpleasant and sometimes traumatic to place for both the patient and operator. The tumor frequently required maximal dilatation to 54 or 58 French before placement because a large "rammer" tube with an outside diameter of 30 mm was necessary to hold the endoprosthesis in place as the flanged wand was deployed to release the prosthesis in the required position. The procedure caused high morbidity in approximately 20% of patients with esophageal perforation rates of about 10%. Procedure-related mortality was usually less than 8% but could be as high as 25%. Despite these limitations, however, such plastic stents have provided effective palliation with relief of dysphagia for semisolid food in up to 90% of patients. Studies to determine whether combining modalities such as laser plus intubation were somewhat equivocal, with little advantage over each technique used singly.

The development of a new class of endoprostheses in the early 1990s was a major breakthrough. An expansile tube manufactured from metal mesh, compressed and restrained on a delivery device of small diameter, meant that maximal esophageal dilatation was no longer required before deployment. The ability of these self-expanding metal stents (SEMS) to expand to a large diameter also offered the prospect of rapid and effective palliation and other benefits with minimal morbidity and mortality. The high initial cost of these stents ($\approx$1250 Euros each) in comparison to plastic stents is more than compensated for by their ease of placement, reduced procedure time, reduction in morbidity and mortality, and decreased hospital stay, thus making them highly cost-effective.[4] One study showed that 4 weeks after insertion, the cost associated with SEMS and plastic endoprostheses was not significantly different.[5]

SEMS have been compared with other palliative modalities, including laser therapy and brachytherapy. A randomized trial of laser therapy alone versus uncovered stents seemed to favor uncovered stents for palliation of dysphagia.[6] However, a trial of single-dose brachytherapy seemed to give better long-term relief of dysphagia with fewer complications, although relief of dysphagia was more rapid with a stent.[7] Initial studies with stents impregnated with chemotherapeutic agents have, however, been disappointing.[8]

Stent designs vary. Although some original stents (e.g., Ultraflex) were bare mesh, which had the advantage of better anchoring properties,[9] there were problems with occasional rapid stent occlusion by tumor ingrowth. The use of covered stents has been shown to result in a reduction in the need for subsequent endoscopic procedures,[9,10] and their use is now standard practice. These stents have expanded flanges or flared ends to minimize migration, are simple to deploy, and are available in varying lengths. Studies comparing various types of covered stents in various locations indicate equal efficacy and complication rates for the different types of stents available.[11,12] Some authors have suggested that stenting for tumors of the distal esophagus and gastric cardia may be associated with a greater number of problems, particularly migration of the stent.[13,14] However, a randomized prospective comparison of the Flamingo Wallstent and Ultraflex for lower third tumors, including those across the gastroesophageal junction, failed to demonstrate any difference in efficacy or complication rates. There was, however, a suggestion that the lower end of the more flexible Ultraflex was less likely to impinge on the gastric wall and cause outlet obstruction.[12]

SEMS are effective not only for intrinsic esophageal neoplasms but also for extrinsic compression from mediastinal tumors and esophagobronchial fistulas. In this particular situation, nitinol-covered stents (e.g., Ultraflex) may be preferable to stainless steel–covered stents (e.g., Flamingo Wallstents) because they seemed to more frequently provide complete esophageal fistula sealing.[15]

Tumors of the cervical esophagus present a particular problem and can be difficult to manage.[16] Stents deployed too near the cricopharyngeus may cause odynophagia and a permanent foreign body sensation, and thus accurate placement is essential. Using stents that release proximally (e.g., Ultraflex) may be helpful in this situation. Similarly, with this proviso, stent placement after esophagectomy is also feasible.

Technique

Placement of SEMS is usually performed as a day case, either endoscopically with fluoroscopic control or radiologically. The patient is normally sedated with a benzodiazepine hypnotic, with or without throat spray and opioid analgesia, depending on the operator's preferences. The upper and lower margins of the tumor need to be demarcated, which is most conveniently accomplished by placing external skin markers under fluoroscopy. For endoscopic placement, impassable strictures may require gentle dilatation before passage of the endoscope and placement of a stiff guidewire into the distal antrum/proximal duodenum. The stent is advanced across the stricture, preferably leaving a covered margin of 1 cm distally and 2 cm proximally. Radiopaque markers on the stent release system allow accurate placement (Fig. 35–1). Releasing mechanisms vary in type and complexity. The Flamingo Wallstent has an outer constraining sheath that is retracted. This has the advantage of allowing resheathing and adjustment of prosthesis position, provided that not more than 50% of the stent has been deployed. The Ultraflex stent is constrained by a circumferential thread that is deployed by pulling on the suture ring. However, this stent is now available with a sheathing mechanism (Figs. 35–2 to 35–4). After release of the stent, the position can be checked with contrast or endoscopically (Fig. 35–5); in the absence of clinical indications of perforation, the patient is allowed to drink 2 hours later and to start a soft diet after 6 to 8 hours. Full expansion of the stent may take several hours, depending on the degree of stenosis and rigidity of the tumor.

Chest pain is common as the stent expands, but other than this, early complications are rare. If immediate perforation occurs, such as after initial dilatation, the operator should continue to deploy the stent to seal the perforation. In this case, a subsequent water-soluble contrast study to ensure that there is no continuing leak is necessary before allowing the patient anything by mouth.

The major disadvantages of the technique remain stent migration and tumor overgrowth at the proximal or distal ends of the prosthesis (Fig. 35–6). Stents that migrate into the stomach can usually be left in situ without complication or risk. If they do require removal, it is best achieved by passing a snare to the middle of the stent, compressing it, and pulling it upward in an inverted "V." If a stent has slipped, thereby allowing tumor to once again obstruct the lumen, or if tumor overgrowth occurs, a further stent can usually be

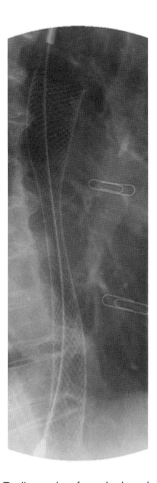

Figure 35–1. Radiograph of a deployed Flamingo stent crossing an esophageal tumor. The narrowing of the stent is at the area of the tumor. The paper clips are placed on the patient's skin and mark the proximal and distal extent of the tumor before stent deployment.

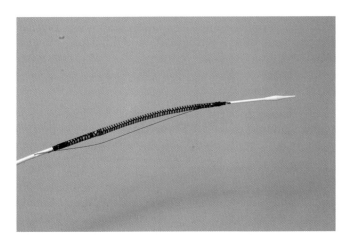

Figure 35–2. Ultraflex stent before deployment showing a retaining suture.

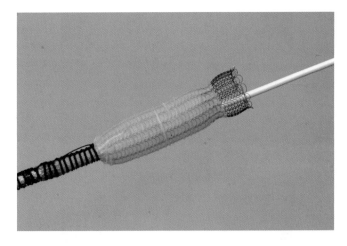

Figure 35–3. Ultraflex stent showing traction on the thread-releasing suture with stent release.

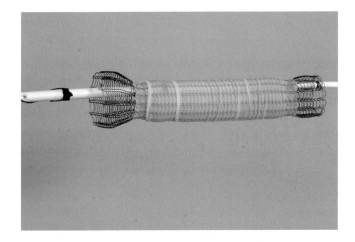

Figure 35–4. Ultraflex stent fully deployed.

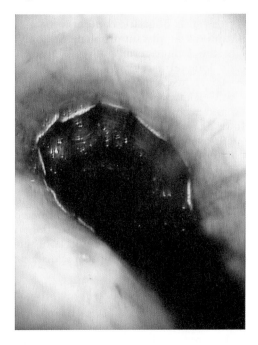

Figure 35–5. Endoscopic appearance of the proximal end of the stent after deployment.

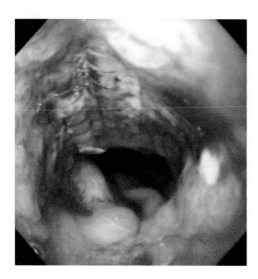

Figure 35–6. Endoscopic appearance of a tumor growing through an uncovered Ultraflex stent.

"piggy-backed" onto the original stent without difficulty. Laser, argon, or alcohol injection therapy can also be used for tumor overgrowth.

Special Considerations

Esophageal dilatation results in transient but significant bacteremia, and prophylactic antibiotics should be given to patients at moderate or high risk for endocarditis. Patients with friable tumors who are taking anticoagulants can bleed significantly after dilatation, and depending on the risks and circumstances, it may be appropriate to consider withdrawing or reversing oral anticoagulation before the procedure.

Stents placed across the gastroesophageal junction will allow free reflux of gastric contents into the esophagus. This can be a significant problem, not only initially but also in the longer term.[14] All patients should be placed on a long-term regimen of acid inhibition. To minimize such reflux, stents with antireflux mechanisms, usually a windsock-type valve at the lower end, have been developed and are reported to be effective in this situation.[17] However, a randomized trial has failed to demonstrate benefit over a standard open stent.[18]

Because stents do not usually allow completely normal swallowing of all solid food, it is essential that all patients with an esophageal stent have reasonable dentition to allow effective mastication. It is also useful to advise patients to disrupt food boluses with carbonated drinks every two to three mouthfuls to minimize the possibility of bolus impaction of the stent. Should bolus impaction fail to resolve spontaneously, endoscopic disimpaction is usually necessary.

Thermal Treatment

Heat can be used to destroy esophageal tumors. The three most common methods are argon beam coagulation (ABC), bipolar diathermy, and laser treatment.

Argon Beam Coagulation

ABC relies on the electrical ionization of argon gas, which is conducted down an argon coagulation probe passed through the endoscope instrument channel. A readily visible white/blue light is produced. The argon beam has a penetration depth of 2 to 3 mm, less than that of an Nd:YAG laser, and thus the risk for esophageal perforation is less but the number of treatments required may be more. The preferred method is to commence treatment distally; some patients may require prior esophageal dilatation. Heindorff et al.[19] from Denmark reported complete recannulation in one treatment session in 58% of 83 patients undergoing ABC; 26% required repeat treatments (average of six) at approximately 25- to 30-day intervals. Two thirds of patients maintained esophageal patency until the time of death, but in this study a third required stenting. Perforation can occur with ABC in approximately 2% of patient treatments.[20] Thus, ABC, perhaps unfairly, can be called a poor man's laser; when compared with the Nd:YAG laser, its advantages are relatively low capital and revenue costs and a slightly lower risk for esophageal perforation, but against these advantages must be weighed the increased number of treatment sessions required to maintain luminal patency.

Bipolar Electrocoagulation

Bipolar electrocoagulation uses olives of varying diameter mounted onto a semiflexible shaft that is passed over an endoscopic guidewire previously inserted into the stomach. An electric current is passed through the olive, which is placed at the level of the tumor. The applied current generates heat and produces tumor necrosis over a depth of 2 to 4 mm as the olive is pulled back through the tumor. This system is particularly suited to treat circumferential tumors because contact with normal esophageal tissue may result in perforation and fistulation. In a comparison of bipolar electrocoagulation and Nd:YAG laser treatment, approximately 85% of both groups experienced improvement in swallowing. Bipolar electrocoagulation is particularly suited for long circumferential tumors.

Nd:YAG Laser

The light energy of the laser is converted to heat by molecular agitation of tissue. The greater the absorption of light, the greater the molecular agitation and the greater the depth of tissue destruction. The usual depth of penetration of the Nd:YAG laser is up to 4 to 5 mm.

The preferred method of laser cannulization of esophageal tumors is retrograde therapy. Pretreatment lumen dilatation may be necessary in up to a third of patients to enable the endoscope to pass down the length of the tumor so that distal treatment can be performed first. In this manner the entire length of tumor can be treated in one session. Prograde treatment may result in an increased perforation rate.

Laser treatment is particularly indicated for short (<5 cm) exophytic tumors arising in the tubular esophagus. It has now become one of the standard treatments and may provide good palliation until death in up to 75% of patients.[21]

In a recent prospective study from Scotland of 948 patients undergoing palliative treatment of esophageal cancer, the laser was used in 117.[1] Trials comparing laser with stents and laser with bipolar coagulation have demonstrated similar efficacy, but morbidity and mortality were greater in patients in whom stents were used.

Complications of laser therapy include perforation (1% to 10%), although dilatation before laser treatment may be partially responsible for this. Perforation may be more common in those in whom laser treatment followed radiotherapy. Hemorrhage and tracheo-esophageal fistula have been reported, as has stricture formation, especially in patients with submucosal lesions. An analysis of 350 patients treated by laser alone showed that tumor length, histologic type, and site had no effect on either survival or relief of dysphagia; the worse the dysphagia score at initial evaluation, the poorer the survival.[22]

The effect of laser therapy can be enhanced by chemotherapy with epirubicin, cisplatin, and 5-fluorouracil (5-FU); this combination resulted in increased survival in comparison to laser alone and laser plus 5-FU/folic acid, in addition to no additional laser treatments being needed until the time of death.[22] The combination of external beam radiotherapy[2] or brachytherapy[23] and laser treatment can markedly reduce the requirement for further endoscopic therapy. Laser treatment may need to be repeated on average every 4 weeks, and tumor progression may require stent insertion (up to 27%).[22]

Lasers have been compared with SEMS in a randomized trial.[24] This study showed longer survival (125 days) in the laser group than in the stent group (68 days). The median hospital stay and cost of treatment (largely related to overnight hospital admission) for the laser group were twice that for the stent group. This study reported equally disappointing results in the relief of dysphagia 1 month after treatment in both the stent and laser groups but noted that pain was more prominent in the stent group.

Endoscopic Photodynamic Therapy

In photodynamic therapy (PDT) an exogenous synthetic photosensitizer is administered orally or intravenously, and after 2 to 3 days, during which time the photosensitizer accumulates in the malignant tissues (as well as normal tissues), light of appropriate wavelength is directed at the tumor by means of an endoscopic or a windowed balloon. The excited photosensitizer damages the mitochondrial and lysosome membranes and thereby induces cellular destruction. A randomized trial has shown PDT to be as effective as the Nd:YAG laser in the initial relief of dysphagia, but the effect was more long lasting in the PDT group[25] and may last up to 80 days.[26] Perforations were more common after laser treatment (7%) than after PDT (1%).

PDT is useful in patients with completely obstructed tumors, long and tortuous tumors, and high cervical

tumors in which it is difficult to use a laser probe. The depth of tumor destruction is very predictable after PDT therapy.

PDT is not widely available, thus limiting its potential for use. Moreover, natural light exposure may cause skin photosensitivity in up to 20%, but this problem can be reduced by the use of endogenous photosynthesizers. PDT application in selected patients may have dramatic results.

ONCOLOGIC MANAGEMENT

Options

Various treatment modalities can be implemented for the palliation of esophageal cancer, including radiotherapy (external beam and brachytherapy), chemoradiation, and chemotherapy. All have their place.

External beam radiotherapy and brachytherapy can be effective in palliating symptoms attributable to the primary disease, and in recent years chemoradiation has become an additional option. Locally advanced and disseminated disease can be helped by systemic chemotherapy. It can be given as a single agent or as combination therapy.

Patients who are not fit enough to tolerate active treatment can still benefit from best supportive care. Appropriate medications such as antiemetics, appetite stimulants, analgesics, and blood transfusions, given together with psychological and social support, can significantly improve the quality of life of terminally ill patients.

Radiotherapy

Patient Selection

Patients with predominantly local symptoms such as mediastinal pain, dysphagia, and local bleeding are likely to benefit most from local therapy. Radiation therapy is frequently the most appropriate choice in such circumstances.

Improvement in symptoms will often only occur over a number of weeks. Hence for patients with very severe dysphagia, stent insertion achieves a more immediate improvement in swallowing and is more appropriate. Radiotherapy may be offered subsequently should symptoms recur with the stent in situ.

Frail patients will frequently be offered relatively low-dose radiation schedules that may still provide meaningful palliation of symptoms for a period. Patients with good performance status but whose tumor is not suitable for radical therapy (usually because of the length and position of the tumor or regional or distant spread) can at times be offered higher-dose schedules, often with combined external beam radiotherapy and brachytherapy or sometimes combined with chemotherapy. These treatments may achieve more prolonged control of symptoms. The balance of risks and benefits with such interventions in the noncurative setting must be carefully weighed.

External Beam Radiotherapy

External beam therapy involves the application of radiation from an external source onto appropriate target areas within the patient. When used as a simple palliative treatment, it is relatively quick and easy to plan, verify, and deliver. All procedures are minimally invasive for the patient and involve a short visit to the simulator (either CT for virtual simulation where the tumor can be viewed directly on a planning CT scan or conventional simulation with real-time diagnostic x-ray image intensified screening and a barium swallow to visualize the tumor stricture), with a typical low-dose regimen consisting of 5 to 10 daily treatments. Each session takes approximately 10 to 15 minutes to set up and deliver.

This treatment is appropriate for patients with a bulky tumor (because the bulk of the disease can easily be encompassed in the irradiated volume), mediastinal pain, or a stricture that significantly interferes with the practicalities of administering brachytherapy. Disadvantages include the requirement for several visits to the radiotherapy department for treatment. In addition, adjacent noninvaded normal tissues may be irradiated and damaged. Modern radiotherapy technique includes shaping the radiation field to the shape of the tumor by excluding normal tissues with blocks or multileaf collimators. This is known as simple conformal radiotherapy. External beam radiotherapy has been shown to provide palliation of dysphagia in approximately 70% to 80% of patients and is effective until death in 50%. An increased dosage may achieve greater palliation by combining external beam therapy with local brachytherapy.

Brachytherapy

Intraluminal brachytherapy involves the insertion of a radioactive source into the lumen of the esophagus via an endoscope or nasogastric tube. Modern high-dose-rate (HDR) brachytherapy can deliver high doses of radiation over short periods, thereby allowing acceptable time for palliative treatment of patients. The usual isotope is iridium 192, and the dose is generally prescribed for treatment at a distance of 1 cm from the source. This treatment is practical and convenient for patients, who can often be treated in a single treatment session. Elderly patients (unless very frail) may prefer this. Moreover, since radiation is administered to the site of the tumor intraluminally, this treatment allows a high dose to be delivered to the tumor site with minimal irradiation of the surrounding normal tissues because of rapid falloff of the dose. This limits toxicity and is particularly suitable for patients with exophytic disease.

The major limitation of brachytherapy is the effective treatment distance. Treatment with ^{192}Ir is suboptimal at a distance greater than 1 cm; as a consequence, very thick tumors will be undertreated at their periphery.

Sources are usually introduced via a nasogastric tube. More frail patients can find the invasive nature of this treatment rather distressing. Furthermore, such treatment may not be technically feasible if the patient has a very tight stricture through which the introducing equipment cannot be passed; these patients require pretreatment dilation.

Homs et al.[27] reviewed 149 patients in a retrospective analysis. Patients were treated with HDR brachytherapy in one or two sessions at a median dose of 15 Gy. Six weeks after treatment, dysphagia scores had improved, although dysphagia had not improved in 51 patients. Procedure-related events occurred in 11 patients (7%), and late complications such as fistulas or retrosternal pain developed in 12 (8%). Procedure-related mortality occurred in 2%. At follow-up, 55 (37%) patients suffered recurrent dysphagia, and 34 (23%) required insertion of a stent.

A prospective randomized trial using HDR brachytherapy as the sole modality for palliation of advanced esophageal carcinoma was performed by the International Atomic Agency.[28] Two hundred thirty-two patients with inoperable squamous cell carcinoma of the esophagus were randomized to receive 18 Gy in three fractions or 16 Gy in two fractions on alternate days. The median overall dysphagia-free survival for the whole group was 7.1 months, and the median overall survival for the whole group was 7.9 months.

Combined Radiation Therapy

The combination of brachytherapy and external beam radiation therapy may offer effective palliation with acceptable complication rates.

Hujala et al.[29] reported on 40 patients with inoperable esophageal cancer treated with combined external (median dose, 40 Gy in 20 fractions) and intraluminal (median dose, 10 Gy in 4 fractions, on average 1 week after external beam radiotherapy) radiation therapy. Forty percent of patients attained immediate symptomatic relief, and no major complications were encountered.

Similarly, Sharma et al.[30] assessed 58 patients with advanced or recurrent esophageal carcinoma. Thirty-eight patients received intraluminal brachytherapy alone, and 20 received a combination of external beam radiotherapy and brachytherapy. Overall improvement in swallowing was seen in 22 patients (38%). The median dysphagia-free survival was 10 months. The overall complication rate was 30%. Strictures developed in 9 (16%) patients, ulceration in 6 (10%), and fistulas in 3 (5%).

Several trials have showed less favorable outcomes—particularly in the curative setting. The RTOG 92-07 trial[31] investigated 75 patients with carcinoma of the thoracic esophagus. Patients received a combined-modality regimen of 5-FU and cisplatin during weeks 1, 5, 8, and 11 concurrently with 50 Gy of external beam radiotherapy, followed by a boost during cycle 3 of chemotherapy with intraluminal brachytherapy—either at a low dose rate (19 patients not included in the final analysis because of low accrual) or at a high dose rate (56 patients, treatment given in weekly 5-Gy fractions during weeks 8, 9, and 10). The complete response rate was high at 73%, with a median follow-up of only 11 months. However, local failure occurred in 27% of patients. Acute toxicity was marked, with 58% having grade 3 toxicity and 26% grade 4, and treatment-related deaths occurred in 8%. In view of such toxicity, higher treatment doses are not suitable for palliation and can be considered in the curative setting only with considerable caution.

Chemoradiation

Chemoradiation combines radiation therapy with chemotherapy. It can offer the benefits available from both modalities and can increase the effectiveness of radiotherapy. Chemoradiation can have an important role in the management of unresectable esophageal cancer both for palliation of dysphagia and for longer-term disease control. This more aggressive approach verges toward giving radical regimens to incurable patients and is not considered appropriate by some authors. However, patients with good performance status, minimal comorbidity, and incurable disease may well benefit from a more intensive treatment regimen aimed at longer-term palliation than that achievable with the standard short-course palliative radiotherapy.

The practicalities of treatment planning and attendance over prolonged periods, together with probable toxicities (in the form of acute esophagitis, pneumonitis, and pericarditis with longer-term strictures and fistulas, as well as chemotherapy-induced toxicities), must be considered. Toleration of the side effects of treatment must be balanced against presumptive gain of symptom relief and longer-term benefit. All must be evaluated before undertaking complex treatments that may offer minimal improvement of symptoms over that derived from a simple and short treatment course. Modern radiotherapy techniques using conformal radiotherapy make this approach more appropriate for some patients.

Chemoradiation for suitable patients has been shown to be superior to external beam radiation alone. It is now standard practice to use 5-FU (by continuous infusion on days 1 to 4 and 29 to 33 and cisplatin on days 1 and 29), with concurrent external beam irradiation.

Two thirds of patients obtain palliation of dysphagia until death, but disadvantages of chemoradiation are the time taken to achieve palliation (up to 6 weeks) and discontinuation of chemotherapy as a result of toxicity (up to 25%).

Chemotherapy

Patient Selection

Chemotherapy is appropriate for patients who have symptoms from disseminated disease. The object in this situation is to palliate symptoms and improved quality of life rather than cure the disease. Local symptoms may also be palliated by chemotherapeutic agents, particularly if the tumor has become tolerant of radiation.

Therapy is chosen to suit the patient's fitness and tolerability of the toxicity profile. Different cytotoxic agents have differing toxicity profiles, and the physician and patient must together examine the risks and benefits of treatments. Side effects include general fatigue and malaise, myelosuppression with a risk for neutropenic sepsis, gastrointestinal problems (nausea, vomiting, and diarrhea), mucositis, hair loss, neurotoxicity, and renal toxicity among others.

Administration of cytotoxic drugs to patients with recurrent or metastatic carcinoma of the esophagus is often challenging. Such patients may be elderly with comorbid conditions. Their nutritional status is often poor, and their tumor burden is also frequently high. These factors together result in poor performance status and an impaired ability to tolerate treatment.

Each cycle of chemotherapy will consist of one or more drugs over a period of 3 or 4 weeks. Bolus administration of cytotoxic drugs will usually be given in a chemotherapy suite. Some regimens require continual administration as a protracted central infusion via an ambulatory device.

Regular review should be undertaken by the physician throughout the treatment period. Before each new cycle of chemotherapy the patient's toleration of treatment should be assessed.

Response to Treatment

Response is measured both subjectively and objectively. General well-being, pain control, level of fatigue, appetite, and swallowing ability are assessed. These subjective indices can be formalized by using quality-of life questionnaires, dysphagia scores, and pain scores and by analyzing analgesic requirements. Objective measurement of response is advisable midway through a course of treatment. CT images should be reviewed with the use of standard RECIST (response evaluation criteria in solid tumors) criteria. Direct visualization via endoscopy is helpful.

Ensuring an adequate response is essential. If one particular chemotherapeutic regimen is found to be ineffective, alternative regimens should be considered.

Over the last 25 years, many trials have investigated systemic therapy for esophageal cancer, but no regimen has evolved into the gold standard for patients with advanced disease. Several agents have shown modest activity when used alone, but in combination their activity is improved, with acceptable toxicity profiles.

Single-Agent Chemotherapy

Certain chemotherapeutic agents have been shown to be active against esophageal cancer when used alone, but response rates have been modest, with approximately 20% achieving brief symptomatic relief.

Combination Chemotherapy

Combination chemotherapy, though offering an improved response rate over single-agent treatment, may be limited in applicability.

Modern combination regimens include irinotecan and cisplatin. These agents were combined in view of their differing mechanisms of action and toxicity profiles. Ilson et al. used weekly cisplatin and irinotecan to treat 35 patients with advanced esophageal cancer and observed a 57% response rate.[32] The median duration of response was 4.2 months, the median survival was 14.6 months, and toxicity was acceptable; dysphagia and quality of life were improved in the majority of patients.

Several helpful chemotherapy regimens are available for patients with advanced esophageal cancer. Worthwhile benefits in quality of life, including relief of dysphagia in 60% to 80% of patients, can be achieved. Cisplatin-based therapy remains the most favored approach to treatment. The addition of newer drugs, such as irinotecan and paclitaxel, appears to achieve higher response rates, albeit with limited durations of response and increased toxicity.

New Agents

A most recent approach to cancer treatment lies in the production of agents that are designed to target specific molecules involved in potentially important oncologic processes, such as cell cycling, apoptosis, and angiogenesis. Such agents could theoretically produce greater disease responses without excessive toxicity. For example, bevacizumab, a recombinant humanized monoclonal antibody to vascular endothelial growth factor, which already has a place in the management of colorectal carcinoma, is currently being investigated in combination with radiotherapy for esophageal cancer and with irinotecan and cisplatin for gastric and gastroesophageal cancer.[33]

Similarly, the epidermal growth factor pathway is thought to be of importance in the pathogenesis of upper gastrointestinal malignancies.[34] Investigation of inhibitors of this pathway is ongoing.

Oncologic Treatment in Practice

Patients with Prominent Local Symptoms Such as Dysphagia, Pain, and Bleeding

Dysphagia can have a major impact on patient quality of life. Not only is nutritional status compromised with symptoms of general weakness and malaise, but social situations involving meals may also be difficult. Improvement of swallowing by localized therapy can have a major impact on the physical and psychological welfare of such patients.

A patient with a locally advanced esophageal tumor deemed unsuitable for more intensive radical therapy would be palliated with a simple course of palliative radiotherapy (either 20 Gy in 5 fractions or 30 Gy in 10 fractions). Radiotherapy can be planned in the conventional simulator, with patients in the supine position, their arms by their side, the use of a barium swallow, and the field edge placed to give a margin 5 cm superior and inferior and 2 cm lateral to the gross tumor volume, or a virtual simulation program using a CT planning scan to localize the tumor can be deployed (Fig. 35–7). This can allow slightly smaller fields to be used because it permits the physician to be more confident of the tumor position. The usual field arrangement is a parallel opposed pair with the dose directed at the midplane.

A patient with good performance status and minimal comorbidity but unsuitable for radical chemoradiation could be offered a treatment schedule consisting of external beam radiotherapy with or without a brachy-

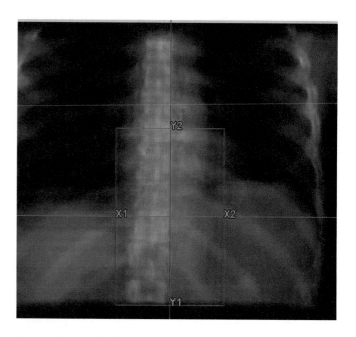

Figure 35–7. Palliative radiation field demonstrated on a digitally reconstructed radiograph. Field borders encompass the contoured volume of the tumor plus an appropriate margin. (Courtesy of Dr. R. Bulusu.)

therapy boost to the tumor bed. Such a regimen could be 30 Gy in 10 daily fractions or 40 Gy in 20 daily fractions, followed by a brachytherapy boost of 10 Gy at 1 cm 1 to 2 weeks later.

If the patient found traveling to the radiotherapy center troublesome and had an exophytic tumor such that brachytherapy could be appropriate for palliation, a single high-dose Selectron treatment could planned in the simulator with a barium swallow used for tumor localization. Radiotherapy would be delivered as a single HDR microSelectron treatment of 15 Gy at 1 cm.

If the patient was found to require rapid palliation within a few days because of severe dysphagia, radiotherapy may be considered less suitable than other approaches such as a stent or laser therapy, both of which would have a more immediate effect.

Patients with Systemic Symptoms

Patients with symptoms from disseminated disease such as nausea and malaise, respiratory symptoms from diffuse disease, or pain not amenable to focal irradiation should be offered systemic treatment in the form of chemotherapy. Performance status and comorbid conditions need to be considered when evaluating the tolerability of treatment. Diverse regimens with differing toxicities will be appropriate for various patients, and decisions must be made by both physicians and patients regarding the acceptability of toxicities as a result of treatment.

Best supportive care is appropriate for more frail patients with multiple existing comorbid conditions in whom the benefits of chemotherapy will be outweighed by the potential additional morbidity involved.

Surgical Therapy for Palliation

Before the development of endoscopic means of palliation, intraluminal esophageal stents were pulled through the esophagus into the stomach at laparotomy. Patients with esophageal obstruction were also treated by substernal or subcutaneous colonic interposition or, as a last desperate measure, by cervical esophagostomy and feeding gastrostomy.

The postoperative mortality and length of survival were such that these heroic and fruitless operations have no role in the 21st century when less invasive means of palliation are available.

On rare occasion it may be necessary to place an enteral feeding device to permit maintenance of nutrition when other palliation has failed or when the side effects of palliative treatment (e.g., radiation esophagitis) inhibit oral intake. This situation is most commonly encountered in younger patients who may wish to sustain nutrition for as long a period as possible.

Management of Terminal Patients

The terminal stages of locally advanced cancer of the esophagus are distressing for patients and caregivers. Patients may suffer intractable cough, aspiration, mediastinal pain, and an inability to swallow saliva. Management of the terminally ill is best undertaken by palliative care specialist doctors and nurses. Patients may need ambulatory opioid pumps, portable suction devices, and antisecretory medication. If oral intake is impossible, medication may need to be delivered by transdermal patch or per rectum.

SUMMARY

Palliation of esophageal cancer poses greater challenges than the management of potentially curable disease. It is as necessary to concentrate the care of these patients in centers that have a large range of treatments available and where sufficient experience may be gained as it is to centralize surgery in hospitals performing high volumes of resections.

ROLE OF THE UPPER GASTROINTESTINAL CLINICAL NURSE SPECIALIST

Patient Advocate/Support

The optimum time for the relationship between the clinical nurse specialist (CNS) and the patient to start is at diagnosis. Support at this time is crucial in enabling the patient and family to gain some control over the situation. Once an association is established, then acting as the patient advocate can become the focus. This is an important aspect of care because the majority of patients with upper gastrointestinal malignancy are elderly and tend to be very accepting of the treatment and advice given by the doctor. Patients who start a relationship at

this emotionally vulnerable time were found to value the relationship as being meaningful for themselves as well as their family because it developed at a significant life-changing event. A substantial part of the responsibility of a CNS is to support both the patient and the family through this disease, including nurturing the development and maintenance of hope. By achieving this, the nurse is able to bring about balance in the everyday changing life and enable a family to cope with the profound effect of the diagnosis of a terminal cancer.

The support of a health care professional empowers the patient to gain control by providing information to preserve a balance of knowledge, thereby letting patients hope for the best yet prepare for the worst. Doing so involves not only listening but also hearing what is not said in order to formulate a bigger picture of the individual and family. Individual knowledge of the patient's unique environment and culture is also necessary to achieve this goal. The specialist nurse can then use this knowledge to obtain resources that may be required, such as information, financial help, or psychological support. If this is realized, patients will be able to move forward with a positive attitude and visualize themselves as cancer survivors.

Planning is crucial after the diagnosis of a life-threatening illness, and it is the role of the health care team to be involved in this so that the plans made are realistic and in line with the patient's ability and life expectations.

Teacher/Educator

Once the initial shock of a cancer diagnosis is overcome, the majority of patients and caregivers require information, both about the disease and about the proposed treatment plan. Most patients and caregivers regard the CNS as the person with time to share and discuss the choice of treatment and the implications of this choice. Being part of the MDT enables the CNS to shape any treatment plan to a patient's requirement and inform the patient of the latest decision. The need for information continues throughout the cancer journey and emphasizes the importance of the nurse/patient relationship. Often, patients will contact the CNS after treatment to check progress or to receive advice. Written information to back up verbal discussion is always useful because it gives the patient something to reflect on and provokes questions. A patient who is distressed at the diagnosis and treatment can use the booklet to inform family and prevent seemingly endless repeated conversations. It is important that use of medical terminology be minimal and a low reading level be assumed.

Clinical Expert/Promoter of Quality Care

Someone with additional in-depth knowledge of a condition is in a prime position to influence the care that the patient and caregivers receive while undertaking treatment. This area of a CNS role can in some instances provide the key to the patient's cancer journey and enable it to be tailored where possible to individual needs. Gastrointestinal cancer has huge social implications for patients.[35] Living with cancer requires both physical and emotional strength. Use of nutritional supplements plus frequent meals is the key to weight maintenance and gain. The palliation achieved by stent use has enabled nutrition and hydration to continue in patients with severely advanced disease. This often simple measure goes some way to achieving calmness in both the patient and caregiver because most find the "starvation" aspect of this disease distressing.

Included within this area are the development and encouragement of patient support groups. These groups provide help to patients by patients. Every health care professional should reflect that "the true" expert of a condition is a person who has undergone a similar experience and can therefore fully empathize with the sufferer.

Researcher/Change Agent

Evidence-based practice is now recognized as the way to change clinical nursing practice. This may involve auditing a service (especially a newly developed one) to assess achievements and instigate changes to meet patient requirements.

REFERENCES

1. Thompson AM, Rapson T, Gilbert FJ, Park KGM: Endoscopic palliative treatment for esophageal and gastric cancer. Techniques, complications, and survival in a population-based cohort of 948 patients. Surg Endosc 18:1257-1262, 2004.
2. Sarjeant IR, Tobias JS, Blackman G, et al: Radiotherapy enhances laser palliation of malignant dysphagia: A randomised study. Gut 40:362-369, 1997.
3. Carazzone A, Bonavina L, Segalin A, et al: Endoscopic palliation of oesophageal cancer: Results of a prospective comparison of Nd-YAG laser and ethanol injection. Eur J Surg 165:351-356, 1999.
4. Ramirez FC, Dennert B, Zierer ST, Sanowski RA: Esophageal self-expandable metal stents—indications, practice, techniques and complications: Results of a national survey. Gastrointest Endosc 45:360-364, 1997.
5. O'Donnell CA, Fullarton GM, Watt E, et al: Randomised clinical trial comparing self-expandable metallic stents with plastic endoprosthesis and the palliation of oesophageal cancer. Br J Surg 89:985-992, 2002.
6. Adam A, Ellul J, Watkinson AF, et al: Palliation of inoperable esophageal carcinoma: A prospective randomised trial of laser therapy and stent placement. Radiology 202:344-348, 1997.
7. Homs MYV, Sterberg EW, Eijkenboom WMH, et al: Single-dose brachytherapy versus metal stent placement for the palliation of dysphagia from oesophageal cancer: Multi centre randomised trial. Lancet 364:1497-1504, 2004.
8. Manifold DK, Maynard ND, Cowling M, et al: Taxol coated stents in oesophageal adenocarcinoma [abstract]. Gastroenterology 114:A27, 1998.
9. Vakil N, Morris AI, Marcon N, et al: A prospective, randomised, controlled trial of covered expandable metal stents in the palliation of malignant esophageal obstruction at the gastro-esophageal junction. Am J Gastroenterol 96:1791-1796, 2001.
10. Hills KS, Chopra KB, Pal A, Westaby D: Self-expanding metal oesophageal endoprosthesis, covered and uncovered colon: A review of thirty cases. Eur J Gastroenterol. Hepatol 10:371-374, 1998.
11. Siersema PD, Hop WCJ, van Blankenstein M, et al: A comparison of three types of covered metal stents for the palliation of patients with dysphagia caused by esophagogastric carcinoma: A prospective, randomised study. Gastroendoscopy 54:145-153, 2001.
12. Sabharwal T, Hamady MS, Chui S, et al: A randomised prospective comparison of the Flamingo Wallstent and Ultraflex stent for palliation of dysphagia associated with lower third oesophageal carcinoma. Gut 52:922-926, 2003.
13. Siersema PD, Marcon N, Vakil N: Metal stents for tumours of the distal esophagus and gastric cardia. Endoscopy 35:79-85, 2003.
14. Laasch H, Lee S, Moss JG, et al: ROST—Registry of Oesophageal Stenting. First Report 2004. Published by the British Society of Interventional Radiology.
15. Dumonceau JM, Cremer M, Lalmand B, Deviere J: Esophageal fistula sealing: Choice of stent, practical management and cost. Gastrointest Endosc 49:70-78, 1999.
16. Conio M, Caroli-Bosc F, Demarquay JF, et al: Self-expanding metal stents in the palliation of neoplasms of the cervical oesophagus. Hepatogastroenterology 46:272-277, 1999.
17. Dua KS, Kozarek R, Kim J, et al: Self-expanding metal esophageal stent with anti-reflux mechanism. Gastrointest Endosc 53:603-613, 2001.
18. Homs MYV, Wahab PJ, Kuipers EJ, et al: Esophageal stents with antireflux valves, tumors of the distal esophagus and gastric cardia. A randomized trial. Gastrointest Endosc 60:695-702, 2004.
19. Heindorff H, Wojdemann M, Bisgaard T, Svendsen LB: Endoscopic palliation of inoperable cancer of the esophagus by argon electro-coagulation. Scand J Gastroenterol 33:21-23, 1998.
20. Eriksen JR: Palliation of non-resectable carcinoma of the cardia and oesophagus by argon beam coagulation. Dan Med Bull 49:346-349, 2002.
21. Bourke MJ, Hope RL, Chu G, et al: Laser palliation of inoperable malignant dysphagia: Initial and at death. Gastrointest Endosc 43:29-32, 1996.
22. Mason R: Palliation of malignant dysphagia: An alternative to surgery. Ann R Coll Surg Engl 78:457-462, 1996.
23. Spencer GM, Thorpe SM, Blackman GM, et al: Laser augmented by brachytherapy versus laser alone in the palliation of adenocarcinoma of the oesophagus and cardia: A randomised study. Gut 50:224-227, 2002.
24. Dalla HJ, Smith GD, Grieve DC, et al: A randomised trial of thermal ablative therapy versus expandable metal stents in the palliative treatment of patients with esophageal carcinoma. Gastrointest Endosc 54:549-557, 2001.
25. Lightdale CJ, Heier SK, Marcon NE, et al: Photodynamic therapy with porfimer sodium versus thermal ablation therapy with Nd-YAG laser for palliation of esophageal cancer: A multicentre randomised trial. Gastrointest Endosc 42:507-512, 1995.
26. Luketich JD, Christie NA, Buenaventura PO, et al: Endoscopic photodynamic therapy for obstructive esophageal cancer. Surg Endosc 14:633-637, 2000.
27. Homs MY, Eijkenboom WM, Coen VL, et al: High dose rate brachytherapy for the palliation of malignant dysphagia. Radiother Oncol 66:327-332, 2003.
28. Sur RK, Levin CV, Donde B, et al: Prospective randomised trial of HDR brachytherapy as a sole modality in palliation of advanced oesophageal cancer—an International Atomic Agency study. Int J Radiat Oncol Biol Phys 53:127-133, 2002.
29. Hujala K, Sipila J, Minn H, et al: Combined external and intraluminal radiotherapy in the treatment of advanced oesophageal cancer. Radiother Oncol 6:41-45, 2002.
30. Sharma V, Mahantshetty U, Dinshaw KA: Palliation of advanced/recurrent esophageal carcinoma with high dose rate brachytherapy. Int J Radiat Oncol Biol Phys 52:310-315, 2002.
31. Gaspar LE, Qain C, Kocha WI, et al: A phase I/II study of external beam, radiation, brachytherapy and concurrent chemotherapy in localized cancer of the oesophagus (RTOG 92-07): Preliminary toxicity report. Int J Radiat Oncol Biol Phys 37:593-599, 1997.
32. Ilson DH, Saltz L, Enzinger P, et al: Phase II trial of weekly irinotecan plus cisplatin in advanced esophageal cancer. J Clin Oncol 17:3270-3275, 1999.
33. Shah MA, Schwartz GK: Treatment of metastatic esophagus and gastric cancer. Semin Oncol 31:574-587, 2004.
34. Aloia TA, Harpole DH, Reed CE, et al: Tumour marker expression is predictive of survival in patients with oesophageal cancer. Ann Thorac Surg 72:859-866, 2001.
35. Bailey K: Management of dysphagia in patients with advanced oesophageal cancer. Gastrointestinal Nursing 2:18-22, 2004.

36

Multimodality Treatment of Esophageal Cancer

Waddah B. Al-Refaie · Wayne L. Hofstetter

Carcinoma of the esophagus is the fifth most common neoplasm of the digestive system, and it carries an alarmingly high fatality rate. According to recent data from the American Cancer Society, it is estimated that 14,520 new cases of esophageal carcinoma will be diagnosed in the United States in 2005, with estimated deaths of 13,570. In the last several decades treatment modalities and diagnostic imaging for esophageal carcinomas have undergone rapid transformation. Despite this progress, disease-free and overall survival has shown little improvement.[1] Adenocarcinoma is now considered the most common histologic type in North America and Europe, but squamous cell cancer of the esophagus still constitutes the majority of esophageal tumors in other parts of the world. Although controversy remains regarding the relative prognosis and efficacy of various treatment modalities for esophageal adenocarcinoma (EAC) and squamous cell carcinoma (SCC), most of the relevant studies in the past 20 years have either focused on SCC primarily or combined both histologies in the same study. To the extent that previous reports have described similar responses to therapy for both cell types and there have been no randomized studies that have proved such to be incorrect, we will discuss the treatment of esophageal cancer in general, with mention of the specific histology when available, the caveat to the reader being that the biologic activity of distal EAC and gastroesophageal junction tumor is quite possibly very distinct from that of proximal esophageal and mid-esophageal SCC.

RATIONALE FOR MULTIMODALITY TREATMENT

Historically, radiotherapy was the primary treatment of cancer of the esophagus, especially over the first 2 decades of the last century, but cure was considered a spurious event. The role of esophagectomy evolved in

the 1930s. Since then, with progress in anesthetic and surgical techniques, resection became the treatment of choice and relative gold standard for patients with localized disease. However, the more recent evolution in the understanding of cancer biology, en bloc resection techniques, and advances in critical care has failed to significantly improve the survival of patients with locally advanced disease over the past 30 years. It is known that most patients with esophageal cancer will have advanced disease at initial evaluation. Although patients would benefit from aggressive surgical therapy if their disease were detected at an early stage, we currently lack an effective screening modality for esophageal malignancy. Because of the modest results achieved with surgery alone, the lack of effective early detection strategies, and the fact that other treatment modalities have been shown to have efficacy to a certain extent, multimodality treatment became the focus of interest for several trials in an attempt to investigate the role and timing of each treatment method.

TREATMENT MODALITY

Radiation Therapy

Preoperative Radiation Therapy

At the turn of the last century, radiotherapy was considered the primary method of treatment of esophageal cancer. First applied as radium bougies and then as kilovoltage external beam therapy, radiation was shown to have the ability to down-stage tumors, achieve an occasional complete pathologic response, and sterilize areas outside the operative field. However, toxicity such as pulmonary fibrosis was a frequent complication of this treatment modality. Although radiation was originally applied as an alternative to esophagectomy, later treatment efforts sought to improve on the results of surgery with the use of preoperative or postoperative radiation treatment.

Table 36–1	Randomized Trials of Preoperative Radiation Therapy for Esophageal Cancer

Investigators	Year	Histology	Total Patients	Treatment	5-Year Survival (%)	P Value
Launois	1981	SCC	124	Surgery + XRT	9.5	NS
				(40 Gy) Surgery alone	11.5	NS
Gignoux (EORTC)	1987	SCC	208	Surgery + XRT	10	NS
				(30 Gy) Surgery alone	9	NS
Wang	1989	SCC	206	Surgery + XRT	35	NS
				(40 Gy) Surgery alone	30	NS
Arnott	1992	SCC/EAC	176	Surgery + XRT	9	NS
				(20 Gy) Surgery alone	17	NS

EAC, esophageal adenocarcinoma; EORTC, European Organization for Research and Treatment of Cancer; NS, not significant; SCC, squamous cell carcinomas; XRT, x-ray therapy.

Nonrandomized Trials of Preoperative Radiation Therapy Several nonrandomized trials have assessed preoperative radiation therapy, the earliest of which was conducted in 1970 by Akakura and colleagues and more recently by Liu in 1986.[2,3] These trials focused mainly on SCC, and the therapeutic approach ranged from hyperfractionated to hypofractionated radiation therapy in doses ranging from 20 to 64 Gy. Many of the uncontrolled trials showed significant improvement in resection rates and overall survival that was attributed to the additional radiation therapy. These studies were the basis for the subsequent randomized controlled trials that follow.

Randomized Trials of Preoperative Radiation Therapy The apparent success of the nonrandomized trials encouraged investigators to conduct several randomized prospective trials to establish whether preoperative radiotherapy (20 to 40 Gy) could have a role in decreasing local recurrence and improving survival in patients with esophageal cancer. These trials are summarized in Table 36–1.

Launois et al. (1981) randomized a total of 124 patients with SCC to preoperative radiation versus esophagectomy only.[4] The regimen involved 40 Gy of radiation over a period of 8 to 12 days, followed by surgery. This study resulted in no statistical significance in 5-year survival rates, which were 9.5% in the irradiated group versus 11.5% in the nonirradiated group. Moreover, the toxicity seen with the intense regimen of intermediate-dose radiotherapy resulted in a higher complication rate in the combined-therapy group.

In 1987, the European Organization for Research and Treatment of Cancer (EORTC, published by Gignoux et al.) randomized 208 patients with esophageal SCC to receive an intermediate dose of 33 Gy of preoperative radiation followed by surgery versus esophagectomy only.[5] The investigators found no differences in resectability between the groups, and postresectional pathologic analysis did not demonstrate convincing evidence of down-staging. At a mean follow-up of 3.6 years, this trial demonstrated no difference in overall survival:

49 weeks for the combined-treatment group and 48 weeks for surgery only (P = .943). A subset analysis revealed that patients without lymph node involvement who underwent complete resection also received no survival benefit from the addition of radiation (P = .846). The study did show benefit in patients with upper third neoplasms, whose mean survival was 161 weeks versus 97 weeks, thus favoring preoperative therapy (P = .04). In addition, a lower local failure rate was observed in patients randomized to the treatment arm (46%; P = .045), although attention should be focused on a very high local recurrence rate of 67% in the surgery-only arm of the study.

In a randomized trial from China, Wang et al. (1989) assigned a total of 206 patients to 40-Gy radiation and esophagectomy versus esophagectomy only.[6] The results showed a similar incidence of complete resection in both groups, and the overall 5-year survival rate was 35% in the radiation-plus-surgery arm versus 30% in the surgery-only arm. Despite the 5% trend, the improvement in survival was not significant. The authors noted that patients with a significant physiologic response to therapy (grade 3 to 4 esophagitis) had a higher survival rate in subgroup analysis and concluded that more effective radiation doses may be needed to confer an advantage.

From the United Kingdom, Arnott and colleagues (1992) performed a study involving 176 patients that also failed to demonstrate any survival benefit of low-dose preoperative radiotherapy.[7] Patients with SCC and EAC were randomized to receive 20 Gy of radiation followed by surgery versus esophageal resection alone. Five-year survival rates were 9% and 17%, respectively (P = NS), with a median survival of 8 months in both arms. The investigators identified by proportional hazard analysis that lymph node involvement, high tumor grade, and male sex were adverse prognostic features.

In 1998, Arnott et al. performed a summary meta-analysis that included 1147 patients, all of whom were enrolled in randomized trials and had adequate long-term follow-up.[8] They concluded that based on the existing trials, there was no clear evidence that preoperative radiation therapy could improve the survival of patients

Table 36–2   Randomized Trials of Postoperative Radiation Therapy (40-60 Gy) for Esophageal Cancer

Authors	Year	Histology	Total Patients	Treatment	Median Survival (mo)	3-Year Survival (%)	P Value
Teneiere	1991	SCC	221	Surgery + XRT	18	19*	NS
				Surgery alone	18	19*	
Fok	1993	SCC/EAC	130	Surgery + XRT	8.7	11	.02
				Surgery alone	15	22	
		Curative (subset)		Surgery + XRT	15	24	NS
				Surgery alone	21	28	
		Palliative (subset)		Surgery + XRT	7	0	.09
				Surgery alone	12	15	
Zieran	1995	SCC	68	Surgery + XRT	—	22	NS
				Surgery alone	—	20	
Xiao	2003	SCC/EAC	495	Surgery + XRT	—	43.5	NS
				Surgery alone	—	50.9	
		Stage III (subset analysis)	272	Surgery + XRT	—	35.1*	.0027
				Surgery alone	—	13.1*	

*Five-year survival rate.

EAC, esophageal adenocarcinoma; NS, not significant; SCC, squamous cell carcinomas; XRT, x-ray therapy.

with resectable esophageal carcinoma. Furthermore, there may be a modest improvement in survival of 3% to 4%, but a much larger trial or meta-analysis would need to be performed to confirm that this potential benefit would be statistically significant.

Despite the number of well-performed trials and inclusion of many patients, these trials have been noted to have several limiting factors. First, the inclusion of patients with differing histology and tumor location may have interfered with the outcomes. Second, although the use of low-dose radiation therapy as opposed to intermediate- or high-dose radiation in the preoperative setting may have resulted in fewer complications, the dose may not have been high enough to confer any significant biologic antitumor activity. Some investigators have argued that intermediate- to high-dose preoperative radiation therapy is necessary to observe a significant response in esophageal carcinomas, which may explain the lack of survival benefit seen when low-dose radiation therapy was used.

Postoperative Radiation Therapy

Temporal reports pointed to a high locoregional failure rate after esophagectomy with or without preoperative radiation. The toxicity of effective neoadjuvant radiation therapy and the apparent lack of locoregional control in patients with locally advanced disease who were treated with surgery alone led investigators to consider adjuvant radiotherapy. This modality of radiation therapy would be delivered at higher levels (40 to 60 Gy) in the postoperative period with less concern for the perioperative mortality that was previously thought to complicate the combination of intermediate- to high-dose radiation followed by esophagectomy. Postoperative radiation therapy was considered in the late 1960s, and a few small nonrandomized studies reported efficacy with this regimen. Because it had never been examined in a randomized controlled setting, beginning in the late 1980s several prospective trials were performed with the hypothesis that adjuvant radiation therapy could sterilize the mediastinum, achieve better local control, and therefore improve survival. These trials are summarized in Table 36–2.

In a large multicenter randomized adjuvant radiation trial reported by Teniere et al., 221 patients with squamous esophageal carcinomas were randomized to esophagectomy alone or esophagectomy with 45- to 55-Gy adjuvant radiation therapy.[9] At a follow-up of at least 3 years, the actuarial 5-year survival rate was similar at 19%, with a median survival of 18 months in both groups. Regional recurrence was significantly lower in patients receiving radiation therapy ($P < .02$); however, this difference occurred only in the subset of patients who were found to have no lymph node involvement. Patients with nodal disease spread showed no locoregional or survival benefit with intermediate-dose adjuvant radiation in this trial.

In 1993, Fok and co-workers from Hong Kong published a prospective, randomized trial involving 130 patients with SCC or adenocarcinoma of the esophagus in which the addition of adjuvant radiation therapy was compared with esophagectomy alone.[10] The two groups were subdivided into curative resection (CR) and palliative resection (PR). PR patients were defined as those who underwent R1 or R2 resection or whose pathologic examination revealed tumor infiltration beyond the esophagus or gross regional or distant lymph node involvement. In the curative arm (CR versus CR + radiation), no benefit in median survival was demonstrated. Actually, survival rates were lower in the postoperative radiation group, and this trend reached statistical significance when the whole study group was compared (CR and PR versus CR + radiation and PR + radiation;

$P = .02$). Local control was similar in the CR and CR + radiation patients, with a 10% versus 13% failure rate, respectively. In the PR versus PR + radiation group, the difference in the local recurrence rate reached statistical significance (46% versus 20%, $P = .04$). As one would expect, there were no differences in the incidence of distant failure found in the analyses. The investigators attributed the lower survival to the higher postoperative complication rates in the combination-treatment arm. This study established that radiotherapy may have some local control benefit in patients with locally advanced disease, but this benefit comes at the expense of high toxicity.

Zieren and colleagues published a study in 1995 on 68 patients with clinical stage II to IV SCC of the esophagus.[11] The treatment group underwent surgical resection followed by 56 Gy of adjuvant radiation therapy; the control group received surgical resection only. At a follow-up of at least 18 months, the 3-year survival rates were similar (22% versus 20% respectively). There were no differences in locoregional control, distant metastases, or elapsed time to failure between the two treatment groups. The authors concluded that adjuvant radiation was not justified in patients with "curative" surgery, although there could be a role for it in palliation.

In an ethically controversial trial, Xiao and co-workers (2003) demonstrated survival benefits with postoperative radiation therapy in patients with stage III esophageal cancer and positive lymph nodes.[12] In this large trial of 495 patients with SCC and EAC, 275 were randomized to surgery alone and 220 to surgery followed by 50- to 60-Gy radiation. The authors excluded 54 patients from the analysis who received lower-dose radiation treatment (<40 Gy) for several medical and social reasons, which later became a limitation of this trial.[12] The overall 5-year survival rates were 31.7% and 41.3%, respectively ($P = .45$). However, the 5-year survival rates of patients with lymph node involvement were 14.7% and 29.2%, respectively ($P = .0698$). Furthermore, the 5-year survival rates of subgroup stage III patients were 13.1% and 35.1%, respectively ($P = .0027$). Despite the significant findings, this trial generated a great deal of controversy because patients were not informed that they were part of a research study. In addition, this trial was criticized for the timing of randomization after resection, which introduced a significant selection bias in the study. The exclusion of 54 patients who received low-dose radiation (<40 Gy) further limits the conclusions that were reached in this trial.

Chemotherapy

There are several theoretical reasons to offer patients with esophageal cancer systemic chemotherapy. Distant failure is a common event leading to death in patients with esophageal cancer. Chemotherapy can potentially treat undetectable micrometastasis, and there is evidence that it can improve locoregional control. Neoadjuvant systemic chemotherapy has been shown to increase R0 resection rates and may down-stage unresectable (T4)

tumors, thus rendering patients potential candidates for resection. Combination chemotherapy has been found to have synergistic effects with radiation therapy. Finally, the response to preoperative systemic chemotherapy serves as a marker that can be used to influence later treatment.

Platinum-based chemotherapy has been the foundation for modern systemic treatment of esophageal carcinoma, hence its ubiquitous use in recent prospective randomized trials involving the use of chemotherapy. The results of many phase II studies using cisplatin and other agents in combination chemotherapy have been encouraging. In some experiences, chemotherapy has demonstrated clinical response in up to 50% of patients.[13] There have also been reports of complete pathologic response in up to 22% of patients who received chemotherapy alone.[14]

Randomized Trials of Preoperative Chemotherapy

Preoperative chemotherapy was compared with surgery alone in several prospective randomized trials that included patients with SCC and EAC. A summary of these trials is presented in Table 36–3.

In a small randomized trial, Roth et al. (1988) evaluated the role of perioperative cisplatin-based chemotherapy and esophagectomy versus surgery alone. Patients with mid-distal SCC (T4 and M1 patients excluded) were randomized to receive preoperative and postoperative systemic cisplatin, vinblastine, and bleomycin ($n = 19$) versus surgery only ($n = 20$).[15] With minimal dosage adjustment, all patients in the treatment arm tolerated the chemotherapy regimen. The frequency of complications and treatment-related mortality was similar in both groups. The complete resection rate was not statistically different between the treatment and control groups, although the trend favored the treatment group, which attained a higher percentage of patients with histologically negative resection margins (35% versus 21%). Despite a difference in the 3-year survival rate in the treatment and control groups (25% versus 5%, respectively; $P = .34$), median survival was 9 months for both groups; therefore no statistical difference was seen. The major contribution of this study was that the subset of patients who had a major or complete response to chemotherapy (47% and 5%, respectively) was shown to have a longer median survival than that of nonresponders (20 versus 6 months, $P = .008$). The responding patients also compared favorably with the surgery-only arm (8.6 months, $P = .05$). Despite the impact of response to chemotherapy, this study was limited by its small number of patients.

Likewise, Schlag (1992) assigned patients with SCC to cisplatin and 5-fluorouracil (5-FU) followed by surgery ($n = 29$) versus surgery only ($n = 40$). Although operative mortality was higher in the treatment arm than in the surgery-alone arm (21% versus 12%, respectively), there was no difference in overall median survival (8 versus 9 months, respectively).[16] Similar to Roth and colleagues' trial, this analysis demonstrated no survival benefit and was limited by the small number of patients.

Table 36–3 Randomized Trials of Preoperative Chemotherapy Versus Surgery Alone for Esophageal Cancer

Investigators	Year	Histology	Total Patients	Agent	3-Year Survival (%)	Median Survival (mo)	P Value
Roth	1988	SCC	39	Cisplatin, Vb, Bleo	25	9	NS
				None	5	9	
Schlag	1992	SCC	69	Cisplatin, 5-FU	—	8	NS
				None	—	9	
Law	1997	SCC	147	Cisplatin, 5-FU	44*	17	NS
				None	31*	13	
Kelsen	1998	SCC + EAC	440	Cisplatin, 5-FU	23	15	NS
				None	26	16	
Ancona	2001	SCC	96	Cisplatin, 5-FU	44	25	NS
				None	41	24	
MRCOCWP	2002	SCC + EAC + UD	802	Cisplatin, 5-FU	43*	16.8	<.005
				None	34*	13.3	

*Survival rates in the MRCOCWP trial were 2-year survival rates.
Bleo, bleomycin; EAC, esophageal adenocarcinoma; 5-FU, 5-fluorouracil; MRCOCWP, Medical Research Council Oesophageal Cancer Working Party; SCC, squamous cell carcinoma; UD, undifferentiated carcinoma; Vb, vinblastine.

In another trial using a similar regimen, Law et al. (1997) demonstrated no survival benefit with neoadjuvant chemotherapy.[17] In their trial, patients received cisplatin and 5-FU followed by esophagectomy ($n = 74$) versus esophagectomy alone ($n = 73$). Two-year survival rates were 44% in the treatment arm and 31% in the surgery-alone arm; median survival was 17 months and 13 months, respectively. Neither was statistically significant. A trial of 96 patients reported by Ancona et al. (2001) echoed these results. Equal numbers of patients received preoperative cisplatin and 5-FU and then esophagectomy ($n = 48$) or surgery alone ($n = 48$).[18] Three-year survival rates in the treatment arm versus surgery-alone arm were 44% and 41%, respectively, with a median survival of 25 and 24 months, respectively.

As part of the North America Intergroup Trial, Kelsen and colleagues (1998) conducted one of the largest trials (Trial 0113) on preoperative and postoperative chemotherapy in patients with SCC of the esophagus and EAC.[19] Of 440 treated patients, 227 underwent immediate esophagectomy and 213 were treated with 5-FU and cisplatin followed by esophagectomy. Endoscopic ultrasound was not uniformly used as a staging modality; therefore, response to chemotherapy in this trial was measured with barium contrast studies of the esophagus. Compliance was low: 66% completed the preoperative schedule and 38% were able to complete the postoperative regimen. Reported results showed that in both arms surgeons achieved a similar R0 resection rate (62% versus 59%, respectively). At a median follow-up of 55.4 months, the 3-year overall survival rate in the treatment group was 23% versus 26% in those who received surgery only ($P = .74$), and the median survival was 15 versus 16 months, respectively ($P = .53$). Disease-free survival was equivalent as well. Subset analyses revealed no difference in the survival of patients with SCC or EAC, and patients who were considered to have undergone curative procedures faired no differently with or without the addition of chemotherapy. The addition of chemotherapy also failed to achieve better local control in this trial. Locoregional failure rates were 32% and 31% ($P = $ NS) in the treatment and control arms of this trial, respectively. Distant failure was recorded in 41% versus 50% ($P = $ NS). The study is criticized for its relatively low compliance rate and the high locoregional failure rate seen in both arms of the study.

The only large phase III trial to show survival benefit with the addition of chemotherapy to surgery in patients with esophageal cancer was reported in the Medical Research Council (MRC) trial from the United Kingdom. In the largest trial addressing the role of preoperative chemotherapy, the MRC trial (2002) randomized 802 patients to receive preoperative chemotherapy followed by surgery versus esophagectomy only.[20] The chemotherapy regimen consisted of two cycles, 3 weeks apart, of cisplatin (80 mg/m^2) and continuous infusion of 5-FU (1000 mg/m^2). In contrast to many of the previous trials, patients in the chemotherapy arm tolerated their treatment well enough to achieve a compliance rate of 86%. The results showed a benefit in R0 resection rates for those who received preoperative chemotherapy (60% versus 54%; $P < .001$). At a median follow-up of 37 months, 2-year survival rates for the preoperative treatment group versus surgery alone were 43% and 34%, respectively ($P = .004$), with a median survival of 16.8 and 13.3 months, respectively. Although 9% of patients in each arm underwent preoperative external beam irradiation, this did not affect the differences seen in overall survival when reanalyzed with exclusion of these patients.

Overall, the two largest trials addressing the role of neoadjuvant chemotherapy in the treatment of

Table 36–4   Randomized Trials of Postoperative Chemotherapy for Esophageal Cancer

Investigators	Year	Histology	Total Patients	Treatment	5-Year Survival (%)	Median Survival (mo)	P Value
Pouliquen*	1996	SCC	120	Cisplatin + 5-FU	—	13	—
				Surgery alone	—	14	—
JCOG9204	2003	SCC	242	Cisplatin + 5-FU	52	—	0.13
				Surgery alone	61	—	
Armanios (phase II)	2004	EAC	59	Cisplatin and paclitaxel	60[†]	31	N/A

*Resections performed in this trial were for palliative purposes only.
[†]Two-year survival rate.
EAC, esophageal adenocarcinoma; 5-FU, 5-fluorouracil; JCOG, Japan Clinical Oncology Group; N/A, not applicable; SCC, squamous cell carcinoma.

potentially curative esophageal cancer have reported conflicting results, which does not fully support the use of this treatment modality.

The potential benefit of preoperative chemotherapy was evaluated in a meta-analysis of 1976 patients from 11 randomized clinical trials by Urschel et al. in 2003.[21] In this meta-analysis, neoadjuvant chemotherapy followed by esophagectomy did not achieve any survival benefit at up to 3 years. The authors offered two potential reasons for the failure of neoadjuvant chemotherapy to improve survival in patients with operable esophageal cancer. First, the current chemotherapeutic agents are not potent enough to treat micrometastasis. Second, treatment-related toxicities might hinder the effectiveness of preoperative chemotherapy. Although the rate of R0 resection was higher in patients treated with chemotherapy before surgery, the overall resection rate favored surgery alone (odds ratio, 1.71; 95% confidence interval [CI], 1.22 to 2.4; $P = .002$). This last finding is significant and is reiterated throughout many of the neoadjuvant trials.

Postoperative Chemotherapy

Despite the relative failure of preoperative and perioperative chemotherapy in previous trials, questions remained regarding the potential benefit of chemotherapy in the treatment of resectable esophageal cancer. Proponents of neoadjuvant therapy cite reasons mentioned in the previous text. Others argued that postoperative therapy could increase survival by allowing the selection of patients who were most likely to benefit from therapy while avoiding additional toxic therapy in those who had been shown to potentially derive the least amount of benefit. Table 36–4 summarizes the following studies.

Pouliquen et al. published the results of a multicenter, randomized study from France in 1996 that examined the role of additional chemotherapy after palliative surgical resection of esophageal SCC.[22] In this study, 120 patients who underwent esophagectomy and were found

to have pathologic N1 disease, incomplete resections (R1-2), or distant metastasis (M1) were randomized to receive postoperative chemotherapy with cisplatin and 5-FU to a maximum of eight cycles versus observation. In each group, patients were subdivided in the analysis into stratum I (N1) and stratum II (R1-2, M1). Compliance was considered excellent at 87%. The results showed no significant differences in survival. Median survival in the treated versus the untreated group was 13 and 14 months, respectively. Stratum I patients had a median survival of 20 months and an actuarial overall 5-year survival rate of 13%, with values similar in the treated and observed groups. Stratum II patients had a 0% 5-year survival rate, and there was no difference in the median survival in the treated and observed groups. The authors concluded that postoperative chemotherapy conferred no additional benefit to either subset of patients but did significantly decrease the treated patients' quality of life. There was 8% mortality attributed to adjuvant treatment in this study.

As part of the Japan Clinical Oncology Group study, Ando et al. (2003) reported a multicenter trial (JCOG9204) involving 242 patients with American Joint Committee on Cancer stage I to IV esophageal SCC.[23] In this randomized, phase III trial, 122 patients received surgery alone and 120 underwent surgery followed by two courses of cisplatin and 5-FU within 2 months of surgery. Full compliance with therapy was noted in 75% of patients, which was accomplished with limited treatment toxicity. Reported end points of the study after 63 months' median follow-up were 5-year disease-free survival, which was 45% for surgery versus 55% for esophagectomy plus adjuvant chemotherapy ($P = .037$), and 5-year overall survival, which was 52% versus 61%, respectively ($P = .13$). Subset analyses revealed that the disease-free benefit was observed only in the N1 group (38% versus 52%; $P = .04$) and not in the N0 patients (76% versus 70%; $P = .43$). This divergence between disease-free survival and overall survival may reflect a potential benefit of better local control achieved by the N1 population. Another explanation is that within this

| Table 36–5 | Studies Investigating Definitive Chemoradiation Therapy for Esophageal Cancer | | | | | | | |

Investigators	Year	Histology	Total Patients	Treatment	Median Survival (mo)	2-Year Survival (%)	P Value
RTOG 85-01	1992	SCC + EAC	121	Cisplatin + 5-FU + 50 Gy	12.5	38	.001
				64 Gy	8.9	10	
RTOG 90-12 (phase II)	1999	SCC	38	5-FU + cisplatin followed by 5-FU + cisplatin and 64 Gy	20*	20	—

*Five-year survival rate.

EAC, esophageal adenocarcinoma; 5-FU, 5-fluorouracil; RTOG, Radiation Oncology Therapy Group; SCC, squamous cell carcinoma.

multicenter trial, the extent of lymph node dissection differed significantly among participating institutions, which may have introduced a selection bias in the study via a stage migration effect.

A recent phase II trial reported by Armanios et al. in 2004 focused on adjuvant chemotherapy in patients with completely resected adenocarcinoma of the distal esophagus and gastroesophageal junction. In this multicenter trial, 59 patients with T2-4, N0-1, R0 disease were entered into the study, 89% (49/55) of whom had lymph node involvement.[24] Patients received intravenous cisplatin and paclitaxel every 21 days for four cycles. Compliance was noted at 84% for all four courses, and grade 3 or 4 toxicity developed in 54% (32/59) while on treatment. Median follow-up was 4 years with a 2-year overall survival rate of 60%. This was compared with historical controls and found to be significantly different (P = .0008). The pattern of first recurrence was at a distant site in 58% of patients and locoregional in 9%. In the light of the encouraging results of this study, the authors proposed validating these result in a randomized trial setting. In addition, they pointed out the disappointing systemic control offered by chemotherapy.

Chemoradiation

Definitive Therapy

Concern regarding the high morbidity and mortality rates associated with esophagectomy led investigators to consider chemoradiation therapy as definitive treatment of esophageal cancer. The synergistic antitumor effects and encouraging results seen with cervical esophageal SCC when using alternative therapies were valid reasons to apply this combined-treatment approach to other types of esophageal neoplasms.

Several nonrandomized trials investigating concurrent chemotherapy and radiation therapy demonstrated feasibility despite a high toxicity rate. Combination chemotherapy with concurrent radiation therapy was later found to achieve better survival in nonsurgical patients with esophageal SCC and EAC than chemotherapy or radiation alone was, and this finding forms the basis for modern combined-therapy trials. A summary of these trials is in presented in Table 36–5.

Herskovic and colleagues (1992) conducted an important prospective randomized Intergroup Trial (RTOG 85-01) comparing combined chemotherapy with concurrent radiation versus radiation therapy only. In this trial patients with SCC and EAC, T1-3, N0-1, M0 of the thoracic esophagus, were randomized to receive combined 5-FU (1000 mg/m^2) and cisplatin (75 mg/m^2) plus concurrent 50-Gy radiotherapy (n = 61) versus 64-Gy radiation therapy alone (n = 60). At a median follow-up of 17.9 months, significant survival advantages were demonstrated in the combination-treatment group. One-year and 2-year survival rates in the radiation-only group were 33% and 10%, respectively, versus 50% and 38%, respectively (P < .001), in the combined-therapy group. Median survival in both groups was 12.5 and 8.9 months, respectively. Despite high local recurrence rates in both groups, local and distant recurrent rates were significantly lower in the combination-treatment group.[25] The study was halted after accrual of 121 patients because of the obvious benefit of combined therapy over radiation alone. Not surprisingly, treatment-related toxicity was significantly higher in the combined-treatment arm (20% versus 3% rate of life-threatening toxicity). The authors concluded that the improvement seen in overall survival and local control comes at the cost of toxicity.

Long-term follow-up of RTOG 85-01 was published in 1999 by Cooper et al. After early termination of the accrual phase of the study, 73 more nonrandomized patients who received combined therapy were added.[14] At a minimum of 5 years of follow-up, 26% of the randomized and 14% of the nonrandomized patients in the combined modality group were alive versus 0% in the radiation-only arm (P < .001). Within the randomized patient group, 22% survived at least 8 years, and no deaths after 5 years were attributed to esophageal cancer. There was a trend toward longer survival in patients with SCC than in those with EAC (21% versus 13%), but this difference was not significant. Five-year survival rates in the randomized and nonrandomized patients receiving combined treatment were 26% and 14%, respectively; however, no patients survived 5 years in the radiation group. Toxicity, again, played a significant role in the delivery of treatment. Eight percent of the combined-treatment group had life-threatening side effects, and 2% died directly as a result of therapy, but there were no "late" toxic effects; patients who survived longer than 90 days had no more toxicity than the radiation-alone group did. This study showed that cure was possible without surgical intervention and that the incidence of cure rivaled the dismal results from surgery published in a review by Earlam and Cunha-Melo in 1980 (4% 5-year overall survival).[26]

To improve the local control results of the RTOG 85-01 trial, a proposal to intensify the dose of radiation and chemotherapy was made. Minsky et al. (1999), as part of Intergroup Trial 0122 (RTOG 90-12), published the results of a trial in which 45 patients were entered into a single-arm study, 38 of whom were eligible.[27] Patients with proximal to distal, T1-4, N0-1, M0 esophageal SCC were treated with three cycles of induction cisplatin (100 mg/m²/day) and 5-FU (1000 mg/m²/day), followed by an additional two cycles of 5-FU (1000 mg/m²/day) and cisplatin (75 mg/m²) with concurrent radiation treatment to a dose of 64 Gy. Treatment compliance was 69% for the induction phase, and 48% received the full radiation protocol. Reported complete response (radiographic) rates were 47%. After a median follow-up of 59 months, this trial failed to show an improvement in the locoregional failure rate seen in the original RTOG 85-01 trial. The actuarial 5-year survival rate was 20% with a median survival of 20 months. Shortcomings of the study included treatment-related mortality in 9% and the fact that 39% of the treated patients had T1-2 N0 disease. Despite any drawbacks, this study helped establish the basis of 50.4 Gy as an appropriate dose for definitive or neoadjuvant radiation therapy and re-emphasized the high complete response rate attainable with induction chemotherapy followed by concurrent chemoradiotherapy. This later became the platform for many trials involving surgery as well.

RTOG 92-07 was a study expanded from the 85-01 trial that was conducted to examine the role of additional brachytherapy in a phase I/II trial involving 49 patients with stage T1-2, Nx-1, M0 esophageal cancer that was limited to the thoracic esophagus. Adenocarcinoma was included in this trial (6%), although it was predominantly a study of esophageal SCC. Treatment consisted of concurrent radiotherapy to 50 Gy with two cycles of 5-FU and cisplatin. Two weeks after completion of external beam therapy, patients received an esophageal brachytherapy boost up to 15 or 20 Gy. Compliance with the concurrent chemoradiotherapy was excellent at 96% but dropped off to 69% (34/49) for the additional esophageal brachytherapy. The results showed no improvement over the RTOG 85-01 trial results in terms of tumor response, local control, or survival. There were, however, six cases (12% overall, 18% of treated patients) of treatment-related esophageal fistulas, which were ultimately fatal in three patients.

In a departure from the general direction that the field was moving, Sykes et al. (1998) published a manuscript on the use of definitive radiotherapy alone for the treatment of clinically localized esophageal SCC and EAC.[28] This was a descriptive cohort study of 101 patients who were treated definitively with radiation because they were medically unfit for resection or they chose radiation over surgery. A little over half the patients had disease localized to the mid to lower third of the esophagus, and 10% had adenocarcinoma. Radiotherapy was given over a period of 3 weeks to a total dose of 45 to 52.5 Gy, and treatment-related toxicity was considered tolerable. In this study the 5-year survival rate was 21% with a median survival of 15 months. Patients who lived longer than 3 years had significantly more involvement of the middle and lower esophagus than the upper. It appears that the results of this study have not been duplicated elsewhere.

Finally, a recent study in Germany published by Stahl and colleagues in 2005 sought to evaluate the additional benefit of surgery with chemoradiotherapy.[29] In a phase III trial, 172 patients were randomized to receive neoadjuvant induction chemotherapy, followed by concurrent chemoradiotherapy, followed by either observation or surgery. Inclusion was limited to patients with locally advanced (T3-4, N0-1, M0) upper to middle esophageal SCC. Their results showed that locoregional control was significantly better with the addition of surgery, but this failed to translate into a statistically significant survival advantage. Notable limitations of this study include the 66% eventual resection rate on an intent-to-treat basis of the patients randomized to the surgery arm, again emphasizing the lower overall resection rate of patients who undergo neoadjuvant therapy.

In summary, chemoradiation therapy without esophagectomy has a potential role in the treatment of locally advanced or metastatic disease. The standard of care for resectable esophageal cancer is still complete esophageal resection when possible, although the additional benefit of surgery in patients who have persistent locoregional disease or have had a complete response after induction therapy and concurrent chemoradiotherapy is also a study end-point of an ongoing multi-institutional phase II trial (RTOG 0246).

Preoperative Chemoradiation for Esophageal Cancer

Trials of definitive chemoradiation therapy demonstrated improved complete response rates and survival benefits over single-therapy modalities, but they continued to be hampered by high local recurrence. This led several investigators to use all three modalities in an attempt to improve survival through better local control. Mixed results were generated in the various nonrandomized trials. In almost all, cisplatin-based combination therapy was administered along with intermediate- to high-dose radiation therapy. Several international investigators have conducted prospective randomized trials consisting of chemoradiation therapy preceding esophageal resection, all of which except one have shown no survival benefit. A summary of these trials is presented in Table 36–6.

Nonrandomized Trials of Preoperative Chemoradiation for Esophageal Cancer In a nonrandomized trial, Donington et al. (2004) presented a single-institution

| Table 36–6 | | Randomized Trials of Preoperative Chemoradiation Therapy for Esophageal Cancer | | | | | |

Investigator	Year	Histology	Total Patients	Treatment	Median Survival (mo)	3-Year Survival (%)	P Value
Nygaard	1992	SCC	88	Surgery alone	7.5	9	NS
				Cisplatin/bleo + 35 Gy	7.5	17	
Le Prise	1994	SCC	86	Surgery alone	10	13.8	NS
				Cisplatin/5-FU + 20 Gy	10	19.2	
Apinop	1994	SCC	69	Surgery alone	7.4	10*	NS
				Cisplatin/5-FU + 40 Gy	9.7	24*	
Walsh	1996	EAC	113	Surgery alone	11	6	.01
				Cisplatin/5-FU + 40 Gy	16	32	
Bosset	1997	SCC	282	Surgery alone	18.6	37	NS
				Cisplatin + 37 Gy	18.6	39	
Urba	2001	SCC + EAC	100	Surgery alone	17.6	16	NS
				Cisplatin/Vb/5-FU + 45 Gy	16.9	30	
Burmeister	2002	SCC	256	Surgery alone	19	—	NS
				Cisplatin/5-FU + 35 Gy	22	—	

*Five-year survival rates
Bleo, bleomycin; EAC, adenocarcinoma; 5-FU, 5-fluoruracil; NS, not significant; SCC, squamous cell cancer; Vb, vinblastine.

study evaluating 75 patients with clinical stage III EAC.[30] Forty-seven patients received treatment with concurrent chemoradiation (50.4 Gy and two cycles of 5-FU plus cisplatin) followed by surgery, and 28 patients underwent esophageal resection only. Nineteen percent of patients who were treated with combined-modality therapy also underwent esophageal brachytherapy. The combined-treatment modality resulted in a 26% pathologic complete response rate. Positive margins were found more frequently in patients who did not undergo chemoradiotherapy (18% versus 4%), a finding mentioned in several other trials, but this trend was not statistically significant. At a median follow-up of 20 months, the authors concluded that there was no benefit to this trial of neoadjuvant chemoradiotherapy, citing 3-year disease-free survival rates in the combined-treatment and surgery-alone groups of 29% and 33%, respectively (P = .51). The 3-year overall survival rate was similar (42%) in both arms as well (P = .70).

Randomized Trials of Preoperative Chemoradiation for Esophageal Cancer Several randomized trials have been conducted to explore the role of chemoradiotherapy in resectable esophageal neoplasms. Only one of the numerous published randomized controlled trials has demonstrated a survival benefit with multimodality treatment. A summary of these trials is presented in Table 36–6.

Nygaard and colleagues conducted the first trial of this sort in Sweden in 1992 on 88 patients with esophageal SCC.[31] Forty-one patients underwent surgery only and 47 received chemotherapy consisting of cisplatin and bleomycin with radiation therapy followed by esophagectomy. R0 resection was accomplished in only

50% of cases in the treatment group. Although the mortality rate was higher in the neoadjuvant treatment group (24% versus 13%, respectively), median survival was similar at 7.5 months. The 3-year survival rate showed a trend favoring the neoadjuvant group (17% versus 9%, respectively), but it failed to reach statistical significance, and the trial therefore failed to demonstrate any survival benefit with the additional therapy. The question of whether to blame the study design and small patient numbers for the lack of significant findings or the lack of effective therapeutic alternatives was left to future studies.

Likewise, in 1994 Le Prise et al. published the results of a randomized trial in patients with SCC of the esophagus in which surgery alone was compared with preoperative chemoradiotherapy followed by surgery. In this trial, patients received *sequential* neoadjuvant chemoradiotherapy with 20-Gy radiation and cisplatin (100 mg/m^2)/5-FU (600 mg/m^2) followed by surgery (n = 41) versus surgery alone (n = 45).[32] In the combination-therapy arm, 95% of the patients completed their treatment course. There was a 10% complete response rate. At a short median follow-up of 16 months, the survival difference was not significant (3-year survival rates of 19.2% and 13.8%, respectively; P = .10). The limitations of this trial included small numbers of accrued patients, short follow-up, and a relatively low dose of preoperative radiation.

In the same year, Apinop et al. published the results of a similar trial involving 69 patients with locoregional, resectable, middle to distal esophageal SCC treated with preoperative cisplatin (100 mg/m^2) and 5-FU (1000 mg/m^2/day) plus 40 Gy of concurrent radiation therapy followed by esophagectomy in the treatment arm.[33] The 5-year survival rates in the combination group and surgery group were 24% and 10%, respectively, with a median survival of 9.7 and 7.4 months ($P = .4$). Again, a trend in survival was not demonstrated statistically in this small trial, and the overall survival in the surgery arm was low. However, subset analysis of this trial revealed that a partial or complete response to combined treatment had a favorable significant impact on survival ($P = .001$).

In 1997, Bosset et al. conducted a larger randomized trial that included 282 patients with esophageal SCC treated by esophagectomy alone ($n = 139$) versus esophagectomy after chemoradiotherapy ($n = 143$).[34] The preoperative treatment included cisplatin (80 mg/m^2) only with concurrent radiotherapy (37 Gy). At a median follow-up of 55 months, disease-free survival was found to be significantly longer in the combined-treatment group ($P = .003$); however, no overall survival benefit was demonstrated. In fact, both treatment groups shared similar median survival (18.6 months). Though not generally seen in other trials, the postoperative mortality rate in this trial was significantly higher in the combination-therapy group than in the surgery arm of this study (16.7% versus 5%; $P = .012$). The investigators proposed that higher doses of radiation (37 Gy), malnutrition (weight loss), and immunosuppression were potential reasons for the increased number of postoperative deaths.

Unlike the previously mentioned randomized trials that were mainly limited to esophageal SCC, there have been two randomized trials investigating the role of neoadjuvant chemoradiotherapy for both esophageal SCC and EAC. In 2001, Urba et al. from the University of Michigan published a randomized trial that included 100 patients with esophageal carcinoma (75% EAC/25% SCC) at all levels.[35] They compared concurrent chemoradiotherapy followed by transhiatal esophagectomy with surgery alone. The preoperative chemotherapy in this trial consisted of cisplatin ($20 \text{ mg/m}^2/\text{day}$), 5-FU ($300 \text{ mg/m}^2/\text{day}$), and vinblastine ($1 \text{ mg/m}^2/\text{day}$); the radiation was given to a dose of 45 Gy. At a substantial follow-up of 8.2 years the neoadjuvant treatment arm did not show any improvement in survival over surgery alone (median survival of 17 months in both groups). Although the 3-year overall survival rate in the chemoradiation group was superior by 14%, this was not statistically significant (30% versus 16%, respectively; $P = .15$). Disease-free survival echoed this trend. The local-regional failure rate, however, was significantly lower in the combination-therapy group (19% versus 42%; $P = .02$), but this had no bearing on the outcome. To put this in perspective, the concurrent incidence of distant disease relapse was similar for both groups, thus implying that although local control may have been improved by chemoradiotherapy, there was no effect on distant metastasis and overall survival. This randomized trial is unique for fair randomization in both arms in terms of patient histopathology; however, locoregional failure in the surgery arm is considered to be higher than that seen in previously published reports. Complicating this issue is the fact that locoregional failure is defined differently by different authors and is notoriously difficult information to obtain. The design of this trial may also have played a role in the negative findings of the study.

Several other small phase II trials tested a similar model of 5-FU, cisplatin, and concurrent radiotherapy. Some added induction chemotherapy before chemoradiotherapy, and this may improve locoregional control in locally advanced cases of esophageal cancer. All of them reported a relatively high incidence of compliance, R0 resection, and complete pathologic response, but they were also hampered by high locoregional or distant recurrence rates (or both). Although not all of them were designed to compare long-term survival, of those that were, none were able to show a significant benefit with the additional therapy.[36-41] The most notable finding in these trials was the improvement in survival seen in patients who demonstrate a complete or major response (no residual or microscopic disease seen on pathologic examination). Within the subset of patients who respond, survival in those with a down-staged post-treatment pathologic stage is similar to that of similarly staged patients treated with surgery alone.[42]

Walsh and colleagues (1996) from Ireland have been the only group to show a survival benefit for neoadjuvant chemoradiotherapy in patients with resectable EAC.[43] In this trial patients were randomized to receive preoperative 5-FU (15 mg/kg/day) and cisplatin (75 mg/m^2) with concurrent radiation (40 Gy) followed by surgery ($n = 58$) or surgery alone ($n = 55$). Patients randomized to the combined-treatment group had a favorable outcome when compared with patients who underwent esophagectomy only (3-year survival rate of 32% versus 6%, respectively; $P = .01$). However, this trial was heavily criticized for several aspects. First, the authors were inconsistent in their method of staging. Second, several patients included in the surgery-alone arm were stage IV. Third, the overall survival rate of patients randomized to the esophagectomy-only arm was 6% at 3 years, which is considered to be significantly lower than other reported experiences for esophageal resection. Fourth, there were statistical inconsistencies within the paper. Last, this trial had a relatively short median follow-up of 10 months.

In summary, randomized controlled trials using chemoradiation improved locoregional control and achieved a complete pathologic response in 26% to 47%, and in selected patients with an excellent response to neoadjuvant therapy, survival was more favorable. Overall, however, the results are conflicted regarding any potential survival benefit with this treatment modality, and there have been no definitive results to conclude that one modality is superior to the other.

META-ANALYSES

A comprehensive and well-presented series of meta-analyses was performed by Malthaner et al. (2004) to investigate the effect of surgery alone versus all other treatments in patients with resectable esophageal cancer.[44] In this publication, 34 randomized controlled trials and 6 meta-analyses were integrated into several basic treatment approaches. The authors referred to Arnott's meta-analysis (2000) of 1147 patients from five trials, which showed a hazard ratio for death of 0.89 (95% CI, 0.78 to 1.01; P = .062) for preoperative radiation therapy and esophagectomy versus esophagectomy only.[8] When postoperative radiation therapy plus surgery was compared with esophageal resection alone, there was no significant difference in survival at 1 year (overall risk ratio, 1.23; 95% CI, 0.95 to 1.59; P = .11). Of seven randomized trials examining preoperative chemotherapy and surgery versus surgery alone, the meta-analysis showed no difference in mortality risk at 1 year (relative risk ratio, 1.00; 95% CI, 0.83 to 1.19; P = .98). A separate meta-analysis investigating the utility of preoperative and postoperative chemotherapy plus surgery versus surgery alone did not detect any difference in mortality at 1 year (risk ratio, 0.99; 95% CI, 0.81 to 1.21; P = .93). Furthermore, no survival difference was noted at 3 years when the meta-analysis examined postoperative chemotherapy and surgery versus surgery alone (risk ratio, 0.94; 95% CI, 0.74 to 1.18; P = .59). Although the previous analyses of combined monotherapy and surgery demonstrated no survival benefit, a meta-analysis of trials investigating combined preoperative chemoradiation and surgery noted a decrease in 3-year mortality and better local control but a lower resection rate than with surgery alone (risk ratio, 0.87; 95% CI, 0.80 to 0.96; P = .004). These results were similar to those reported in meta-analyses performed by Fiorica et al. and Urschel et al. on neoadjuvant chemoradiotherapy.[21,45] However, the most recent meta-analysis, that by Greer et al. in 2005, weighted the observations of the individual studies according to their mean follow-up.[46] This analysis concluded that there may be a small survival benefit with neoadjuvant chemoradiation followed by surgery versus surgery alone, but this benefit did not reach statistical significance (risk ratio, 0.86; CI, 0.74 to 1.01; P = .07). The most interesting findings of this meta-analysis are that despite the fact that most of the randomized trials limited enrollment to clinically early disease, there was a lower overall rate of completion of therapy in the treatment arm (72% to 97%) than in the surgery-only arm (100%).

Postoperative Chemoradiation

Because one of the major drawbacks of chemoradiotherapy is toxicity, which may have led to the decrease in the overall resection rate in the previous studies, investigators attempted to focus additional therapy on a subgroup of patients who were thought to benefit most from the treatment. Ajani et al. from the University of Texas M.D. Anderson Cancer Center established the feasibility of this approach in a phase I/II study conducted on 35 patients with resectable adenocarcinoma of the esophagus and GE junction.[13] All patients received a total of six courses of chemotherapy (etoposide, 5-FU, and cisplatin) divided into two courses preoperatively and three to four courses postoperatively. Adjuvant radiation treatment was given if patients had positive margins or gross residual disease. There were no deaths related to esophagectomy, chemotherapy, or radiation treatment. The toxicities related to chemotherapy were moderate.

Several modern studies using this type of treatment protocol have been published; two have shown benefit with this treatment whereas other smaller studies have not. Rice et al. from the Cleveland Clinic randomized 83 patients with SCC or EAC to esophagectomy followed by adjuvant chemoradiation therapy versus esophagectomy only.[47] The stages were varied (pT1-4, pN0-1, pM0-1a). Of 83 patients, 31 patients with locoregionally advanced disease (pT1-4, pN0-1, pM0-1a) underwent esophageal resection and received postoperative cisplatin/5-FU and radiation, and 52 patients with advance disease (pT1-4, pN0-1, pM0-1b) received esophageal resection only. This trial demonstrated that patients with locoregionally advanced disease who received adjuvant chemoradiation had better median survival (28 versus 15 months, respectively; P = .05) and recurrence-free survival (22 versus 11 months, respectively; P = .04) than did those who underwent surgery alone. Another randomized study by Bédard et al. (2001) revealed in a multivariate model that adjuvant chemoradiotherapy was an independent predictor of survival and that overall median survival was improved (47.5 versus 14 months, respectively; P = .001).[48]

In summary, postoperative chemoradiotherapy remains a treatment option for patients who are at high risk for locoregional recurrence, and it may have benefit in a selected subgroup of patients. Difficulty with the administration of adjuvant therapy after undergoing esophagectomy may limit the overall efficacy of this modality.

NEW TREATMENT MODALITIES

Numerous trials have been performed to investigate the role and timing of esophagectomy, systemic chemotherapy, and radiation therapy. Combined-treatment modalities have resulted in improved 3-year mortality and complete resection rates in selected patient populations. On the other hand, the overall outcome of esophageal cancer remains dismal. This highlights the importance of considering new approaches to treatment, such as molecular-based targeted therapy. Evidence is evolving to demonstrate that biologic inhibitors can be potential adjuncts to our current armamentarium of treatment.

Cyclooxygenase-2 Inhibitors

Cyclooxygenase-2 (COX-2) is an inducible form of the COX enzyme that leads to the synthesis of prostaglandins. COX-2 is regulated by a variety of oncogenes and growth factors. An increasing body of evidence is supporting the fact that COX-2 contributes to the development of cancer, hence the utility of COX-2 inhibitors as a molecular target for the treatment and prevention of esophageal cancer. Two National Cancer Institute–sponsored trials are under way to evaluate the use of COX-2 inhibitors in reversing the dysplastic effect of Barrett's esophagus and its effect in a thermally ablated esophagus. Phase II trials (published in abstract form) using COX-2 inhibitors as part of the preoperative chemotherapy for locally advanced esophageal cancer have suggested a possible response to treatment. Unfortunately, recent reports of cardiac toxicity with COX-2 inhibitors may limit the ability to complete important ongoing trials. Diversion to inhibiting alternative pathways that ultimately lead to a common cascade are under way. It may be that derivative compounds such as dimethyl celecoxib could provide similar antitumor effect with a different safety profile.

Tumor Necrosis Factor

There is great interest in tumor necrosis factor-α (TNF-α) for its known immune response effect in causing severe tumor necrosis. Ongoing phase I/II protocols are taking place in which all patients will receive 5-FU, cisplatin, and 45-Gy external beam radiation therapy, followed by esophagectomy. A TNF-α–incorporated adenoviral vector will be injected in patients in a dose-escalating manner. Phase II will treat 50 patients in a single arm with preoperative chemoradiation therapy along with TNF-α biologic injection.

Epidermal Growth Factor Receptor

Epidermal growth factor receptors (EGFRs) are transmembrane glycoproteins with tyrosine kinase activity that play an important role in cell proliferation. Overexpression of EGFR has been found in several malignancies, including bladder, head and neck, breast, gastric, and colorectal carcinoma. In addition, several reports have identified EGFRs in normal esophagus, Barrett's esophagus, and poorly differentiated esophageal carcinoma. In an analysis of 38 patients with resectable esophageal carcinoma, Wilkinson and colleagues (2004) performed immunohistochemical analysis on paraffin-embedded tissue samples with the use of EGFR monoclonal antibodies.[49] In this interesting analysis, 13 of 23 patients with poorly differentiated esophageal cancer stained positive for EGFR ($P = .02$). Furthermore, it appears that EGFR correlates with outcome as evidenced by disease recurrence in 6 of 13 EGFR-positive patients ($P = .06$). Molecular target agents such as tyrosine kinase inhibitors are potential implications of this study for those who overexpress EGFR.

SUMMARY

A plethora of publications in the literature support or refute various modalities of treatment of SCC and adenocarcinoma of the esophagus. Surgery is the treatment of choice for early localized esophageal cancer. It appears that there is little role for combined perioperative monotherapy and surgery in patients with resectable lesions. Chemoradiotherapy may be beneficial in patients who have locally advanced disease, and the addition of surgical intervention in patients with locally advanced disease and a poor response to multimodality therapy should be considered palliative given the high incidence of regional and distant metastasis and poor overall outcome in that group. Limited current evidence shows some survival advantage to chemoradiation in the aftermath of esophagectomy, but this finding lacks the validation of a larger prospective randomized controlled trial.

As our understanding of esophageal cancer therapy evolves, the deficits remaining in esophageal cancer treatment modalities are becoming clearer. Careful staging, whether invasive or noninvasive, performed by contemporary investigators has helped us develop some understanding of the biology of this disease and has taught us that it is appropriate to approach the treatment of each patient with a stage-based algorithm.[50-52] Ultimately, the question remains whether current multimodality therapy is merely compensating for inadequate patient selection for surgery (a stage migration effect) or inadequate locoregional control (or both). If this were true, we may see improvement only in locoregional control with a marginal benefit on overall survival, and this is consistent with the trend of the relevant studies that we have reviewed. Certainly, future therapeutic effort needs to be directed at relatively chemoresistant and systemic disease. Further improvement in the overall treatment-related outcomes for esophageal cancer will depend on the innovation of novel molecular-based and biologic therapeutic agents and performance of statistically sound, well-constructed collaborative trials.

SUGGESTED READINGS

Ajani JA, Komaki R, Putnam JB, et al: A three-step strategy of induction chemotherapy then chemoradiation followed by surgery in patients with potentially resectable carcinoma of the esophagus or gastroesophageal junction. Cancer 92:279-286, 2001.

Bancewicz J, Clark PI, Smith DB, et al: Surgical resection with or without preoperative chemotherapy in oesophageal cancer: A randomised controlled trial. Lancet 359:1727-1733, 2002.

Cooper JS, Guo MD, Herskovic A, et al: Chemoradiotherapy of locally advanced esophageal cancer: Long-term follow-up of a prospective randomized trial (RTOG 85-01). Radiation Therapy Oncology Group. JAMA 281:1623-1627, 1999.

Kelsen DP, Ginsberg R, Pajak TF, et al: Chemotherapy followed by surgery compared with surgery alone for localized esophageal cancer. N Engl J Med 339:1979-1984, 1998.

Malthaner RA, Wong RK, Rumble RB, Zuraw L: Neoadjuvant or adjuvant therapy for resectable esophageal cancer: A systematic review and meta-analysis. BMC Med 2:35, 2004.

REFERENCES

1. Hofstetter W, Swisher SG, Hess K, et al: Treatment outcomes of resected esophageal cancer. Ann Surg 236:376-385, 2002.
2. Akakura I, Yoshizo N, Teruo K, et al: Surgery of carcinoma of the esophagus with preoperative radiation. Chest 57:47-57, 1970.
3. Liu G, Huang Z, Rong T, et al: Measures for improving therapeutic results of esophageal carcinoma in stage III: Preoperative radiotherapy. J Clin Oncol 32:248-255, 1986.

4. Launois B, Delarue D, Campion JP, Kerbaol M: Preoperative radiotherapy for carcinoma of the esophagus. Surg Gynecol Obstet 153:690-692, 1981.

5. Gignoux M, Roussel A, Paillot B, et al: The value of preoperative radiotherapy in esophageal cancer: Results of a study of the E.O.R.T.C. World J Surg 11:426-432, 1987.

6. Wang M, Gu XY, Yen WB, et al: Randomized clinical trial on the combination of preoperative irradiation and surgery in the treatment of esophageal carcinoma: Report on 206 patients. Int J Radiat Oncol Biol Phys 16:325-327, 1989.

7. Arnott SJ, Duncan W, Kerr GR, et al: Low dose preoperative radiotherapy for carcinoma of the oesophagus: Results of a randomized clinical trial. Radiother Oncol 24:108-113, 1992.

8. Arnott SJ, Duncan W, Gignoux M, et al: Preoperative radiotherapy in esophageal carcinoma: A meta-analysis using individual patient data (Oesophageal Cancer Collaborative Group). Int J Radiat Oncol Biol Phys 41:579-583, 1998.

9. Teniere P, Hay JM, Fingerhut A, et al: Postoperative radiation therapy does not increase survival after curative resection for squamous cell carcinoma of the middle and lower esophagus as shown by a multicenter controlled trial. Surg Gynecol Obstet 173:123-130, 1991.

10. Fok M, Sham JST, Choy D, et al: Postoperative radiotherapy for carcinoma of the esophagus: A prospective, randomized controlled study. Surgery 113:138-147, 1993.

11. Zieren HU, Muller JM, Jacobi CA, et al: Adjuvant postoperative radiation therapy after curative resection of squamous cell carcinoma of the thoracic esophagus: A prospective randomized study. World J Surg 19:444-449, 1995.

12. Xiao ZF, Yang ZY, Liang J, et al: Value of radiotherapy after radical surgery for esophageal carcinoma: A report of 495 patients. Ann Thorac Surg 75:331-336, 2003.

13. Ajani JA, Roth JA, Ryan B, et al: Evaluation of pre- and postoperative chemotherapy for resectable adenocarcinoma of the esophagus or gastroesophageal junction. J Clin Oncol 8:1231-1238, 1990.

14. Cooper JS, Guo MD, Herskovic A, et al: Chemoradiotherapy of locally advanced esophageal cancer: Long-term follow-up of a prospective randomized trial (RTOG 85-01). Radiation Therapy Oncology Group. JAMA 281:1623-1627, 1999.

15. Roth JA, Pass HI, Flanagan MM, et al: Randomized clinical trial of preoperative and postoperative adjuvant chemotherapy with cisplatin, vindesine, and bleomycin for carcinoma of the esophagus. J Thorac Cardiovasc Surg 96:242-248, 1988.

16. Schlag PM: Randomized trial of preoperative chemotherapy for squamous cell cancer of the esophagus. The Chirurgische Arbeitsgemeinschaft für Onkologie der Deutschen Gesellschaft für Chirurgie Study Group. Arch Surg 127:1446-1450, 1992.

17. Law S, Fok M, Chow S, et al: Preoperative chemotherapy versus surgical therapy alone for squamous cell carcinoma of the esophagus: A prospective randomized trial. J Thorac Cardiovasc Surg 114:210-217, 1997.

18. Ancona E, Ruol A, Santi S, et al: Only pathologic complete response to neoadjuvant chemotherapy improves significantly the long term survival of patients with resectable esophageal squamous cell carcinoma: Final report of a randomized, controlled trial of preoperative chemotherapy versus surgery alone. Cancer 91:2165-2174, 2001.

19. Kelsen DP, Ginsberg R, Pajak TF, et al: Chemotherapy followed by surgery compared with surgery alone for localized esophageal cancer. N Engl J Med 339:1979-1984, 1998.

20. Medical Research Council Oesophageal Cancer Working Group: Surgical resection with or without preoperative chemotherapy in oesophageal cancer. A randomised controlled trial. Lancet 359:1727-1733, 2002.

21. Urschel JD, Vasan H: A meta-analysis of randomized controlled trials that compared neoadjuvant chemoradiation and surgery to surgery alone for resectable esophageal cancer. Am J Surg 185:538-543, 2003.

22. Pouliquen X, Levard H, Hay JM, et al: 5-Fluorouracil and cisplatin therapy after palliative surgical resection of squamous cell carcinoma of the esophagus. A multicenter randomized trial. French Associations for Surgical Research. Ann Surg 223:127-133, 1996.

23. Ando N, Iizuka T, Ide H, et al: Surgery plus chemotherapy compared with surgery alone for localized squamous cell carcinoma of the thoracic esophagus: A Japan Clinical Oncology Group Study—JCOG9204. J Clin Oncol 21:4592-4596, 2003.

24. Armanios M, Xu R, Forastiere AA, et al: Adjuvant chemotherapy for resected adenocarcinoma of the esophagus, gastro-esophageal junction, and cardia: Phase II trial (E8296) of the Eastern Cooperative Oncology Group. J Clin Oncol 22:4495-4499, 2004.

25. Herskovic A, Martz K, Al-Sarraf M, et al: Combined chemotherapy and radiotherapy compared with radiotherapy alone in patients with cancer of the esophagus. N Engl J Med 326:1593-1598, 1992.

26. Earlam R, Cunha-Melo JR: Oesophageal squamous cell carcinoma: I. A critical review of surgery. Br J Surg 67:381-390, 1980.

27. Minsky BD, Neuberg D, Kelsen DP, et al: Final report of Intergroup Trial 0122 (ECOG PE-289, RTOG 90-12): Phase II trial of neoadjuvant chemotherapy plus concurrent chemotherapy and high-dose radiation for squamous cell carcinoma of the esophagus. Int J Radiat Oncol Biol Phys 43:517-523, 1999.

28. Sykes AJ, Burt PA, Slevin NJ, et al: Radical radiotherapy for carcinoma of the oesophagus: An effective alternative to surgery. Radiother Oncol 48:15-21, 1998.

29. Stahl M, Stuschke M, Lehmann N, et al: Chemoradiation with and without surgery in patients with locally advanced squamous cell carcinoma of the esophagus. J Clin Oncol 23:2310-2317, 2005.

30. Donington JS, Miller DL, Allen MS, et al: Preoperative chemoradiation therapy does not improve early survival after esophagectomy for patients with clinical stage III adenocarcinoma of the esophagus. Ann Thorac Surg 77:1193-1198, 2004.

31. Nygaard K, Hagen S, Hansen HS, et al: Pre-operative radiotherapy prolongs survival in operable esophageal carcinoma: A randomized, multicenter study of pre-operative radiotherapy and chemotherapy. The second Scandinavian Trial in Esophageal Cancer. World J Surg 16:1101-1110, 1992.

32. Le Prise E, Etienne PL, Meunier B, et al: A randomized study of chemotherapy, radiation therapy, and surgery versus surgery for localized squamous cell carcinoma of the esophagus. Cancer 73:1779-1784, 1994.

33. Apinop C, Puttisak P, Preecha N: A prospective study of combined therapy in esophageal cancer. Hepatogastroenterology 41:391-393, 1994.

34. Bosset JF, Gignoux M, Triboulet JP, et al: Chemoradiotherapy followed by surgery compared with surgery alone in squamous-cell cancer of the esophagus. N Engl J Med 337:161-167, 1997.

35. Urba SG, Orringer MB, Turrisi A, et al: Randomized trial of preoperative chemoradiation versus surgery alone in patients with locoregional esophageal carcinoma. J Clin Oncol 19:305-313, 2001.

36. Ajani JA, Komaki R, Putnam JB, et al: A three-step strategy of induction chemotherapy then chemoradiation followed by surgery in patients with potentially resectable carcinoma of the esophagus or gastroesophageal junction. Cancer 92:279-286, 2001.

37. Ajani JA, Walsh G, Komaki R, et al: Preoperative induction CPT-11 and cisplatin chemotherapy followed by concurrent chemoradiotherapy in patients with local-regional carcinoma of the esophagus or gastroesophageal junction. Cancer 100:2347-2354, 2004.

38. Burmeister BH, Denham JW, O'Brien M, et al: Combined modality therapy for esophageal carcinoma: Preliminary results from a large Australasian multicenter study. Int J Radiat Oncol Biol Phys 32:997-1006, 1995.

39. Entwistle JW III, Goldberg M: Multimodality therapy for resectable cancer of the thoracic esophagus. Ann Thorac Surg 73:1009-1015, 2002.

40. Ganem G, Dubray B, Raoul Y, et al: Concomitant chemoradiotherapy followed, where feasible, by surgery for cancer of the esophagus. J Clin Oncol 15:701-711, 1997.

41. Swisher SG, Ajani JA, Komaki R, et al: Long-term outcome of phase II trial evaluating chemotherapy, chemoradiotherapy, and surgery for locoregionally advanced esophageal cancer. Int J Radiat Oncol Biol Phys 57:120-127, 2003.

42. Swisher SG, Hofstetter W, Wu TT, et al: Proposed revision of the pathologic stage esophageal cancer staging system to accommodate pathologic response (pP) following preoperative chemoradiation (CRT). Ann Surg 241:810-820, 2005.

43. Walsh TN, Noonan N, Hollywood D, et al: A comparison of multimodal therapy and surgery for esophageal adenocarcinoma. N Engl J Med 335:462-467, 1996.

44. Malthaner RA, Wong RK, Rumble RB, et al: Neoadjuvant or adjuvant therapy for resectable esophageal cancer: A systematic review and meta-analysis. BMC Med 2:35, 2004.

45. Fiorica F, Di Bona D, Schepis F, et al: Preoperative chemoradiotherapy for oesophageal cancer: A systematic review and meta-analysis. Gut 53:925-930, 2004.

46. Greer SE, Goodney PP, Sutton JE, Birkmeyer JD: Neoadjuvant chemoradiotherapy for esophageal carcinoma: A meta-analysis. Surgery 137:172-177, 2005.

47. Rice TW, Adelstein DJ, Chidel MA, et al: Benefit of postoperative adjuvant chemoradiotherapy in locoregionally advanced esophageal carcinoma. J Thorac Cardiovasc Surg 126:1590-1596, 2003.

48. Bédard EL, Inculet RI, Malthaner RA, et al: The role of surgery and postoperative chemoradiation therapy in patients with lymph node positive esophageal carcinoma. Cancer 91:2423-2430, 2001.

49. Wilkinson NW, Black JD, Roukhadze E, et al: Epidermal growth factor receptor expression correlates with histologic grade in resected esophageal adenocarcinoma. J Gastrointest Surg 8:448-453, 2004.

50. Eloubeidi MA, Desmond R, Arguedas MR, et al: Prognostic factors for the survival of patients with esophageal carcinoma in the U.S.: The importance of tumor length and lymph node status. Cancer 95:1434-1443, 2002.

51. Hagen JA, DeMeester SR, Peters JH, et al: Curative resection for esophageal adenocarcinoma: Analysis of 100 en bloc esophagectomies. Ann Surg 234:520-530, 2001.

52. Nigro JJ, DeMeester SR, Hagen JA, et al: Node status in transmural esophageal adenocarcinoma and outcome after en bloc esophagectomy. J Thorac Cardiovasc Surg 117:960-968, 1999.

37

Benign Tumors and Cysts of the Esophagus

Richard F. Heitmiller · Molly M. Buzdon

Benign tumors and cysts of the esophagus are rare. A review of the literature does not indicate a change in their overall incidence or the distribution of specific types of tumors and cysts. No new classification schemes have been adopted. The majority of benign esophageal tumors and cysts continue to be small and produce no symptoms. Most are still found incidentally.

On the other hand, there have been dramatic advances in our ability to diagnose these lesions once they are identified. Historically, one of the most common indications for surgical resection was uncertainty of pathologic diagnosis. Such is no longer the case. Endoscopic esophageal ultrasound, transesophageal biopsy methods, and the digital imaging techniques of computed tomography (CT) and magnetic resonance imaging (MRI) with three-dimensional reconstruction result in a specific clinical diagnosis, often a pathologic diagnosis, with a high degree of confidence. Surgeons now have considerably more information available to determine which patients should undergo resection versus observation.

Another advancement in the management of patients with benign esophageal tumors and cysts is the introduction and refinement of endoscopic and minimally invasive methods to resect these lesions. Historically, surgical resection was accomplished by a standard thoracotomy approach that was safe and effective but a major surgical insult for a patient with a benign and generally asymptomatic lesion. Currently, increasing reports are documenting endoscopic resection of these lesions, especially those with a mucosal or intraluminal component. Intramural-extramucosal lesions can now frequently be resected with minimally invasive thoracoscopic and laparoscopic techniques.

Finally, pathologists have been able to study the molecular genetic profile of benign esophageal tumors to individually define tumor diagnosis and pathogenesis.

OVERVIEW

Incidence

Patterson[1] identified only 62 reported cases of benign esophageal tumors over the 215-year period 1717 to 1932. In separate autopsy series, Moersch and Harrington,[2] and Plachta[3] reported a prevalence of benign esophageal tumors and cysts of 0.59% (44/7459) and 0.45% (90/19,982), respectively. More recently, Attah and Hajdu identified only 26 benign esophageal tumors out of 15,454 autopsies over a 30-year review period.[4] The autopsy review by Plachta[3] best summarizes the overall characteristics of benign esophageal tumors and cysts. In that review, of the total 504 esophageal tumors identified at autopsy, 82% were malignant and 18% benign. Benign tumors were more common in males than females. The mean age of patients was 45 and 68 years for symptomatic and asymptomatic patients, respectively, although the age range was broad (22 to 92 years). Of the 90 benign esophageal tumors, the most common were leiomyomas in 49 (54%) patients, polyps in 23 (26%), cysts in 3 (3%), hemangiomas in 3 (3%), and papillomas in 2 (2%). There was a slightly increased prevalence of benign tumors involving the lower third of the esophagus.

Symptoms

Choong and Meyers[5] reported five clinical patterns in patients with benign esophageal tumors: asymptomatic, intraluminal obstruction, extramural extension with involvement of adjacent mediastinal structures, regurgitation of a pedunculated tumor, and mucosal ulceration with bleeding. Despite the fact that benign esophageal tumors may attain significant size, most patients are asymptomatic. Though uncommon, dysphagia is the second most common symptom. The reported incidence of dysphagia from benign esophageal tumors ranges from 0.075% to 0.14%.[2] Extraluminal compression of the adjacent airway results in cough and wheezing symptoms. Regurgitation of a pedunculated tumor is most commonly seen in patients with fibrovascular polyps. Bleeding is uncommon but has been reported in conjunction with esophageal hemangiomas.

Surgery

Ten percent (9 of 90) of patients with benign tumors required surgical treatment in Plachta's series.[3] More recent reports suggest that benign esophageal tumors and cysts are an infrequent indication for esophagectomy. Davis and Heitmiller[6] performed 45 esophagectomies for benign disease in which benign tumor was the indication in only 2 (4%) patients. The pathologic examination findings for these two cases were leiomyoma and melanotic schwannoma. Benign tumor was not an indication for transhiatal esophagectomy in any of the 166 cases reviewed by Orringer and Stirling.[7] In an operative series of 20 patients by Mansour et al.,[8] there were 13 leiomyomas, 4 cysts, 2 polyps, and 1 granular cell myoblastoma.

HISTORY

Sussius[9] is credited with the first description of a benign esophageal tumor, a leiomyoma, in 1559. Since that time there has been slowly accumulating experience with benign esophageal tumors and cysts, thus reflecting the infrequent occurrence of this pathologic condition. The first pathologic description of a leiomyoma is attributed to Virchow[10] in 1863. One of the earliest studies evaluating the prevalence of benign esophageal tumors was by Vinson et al.[11] from the Mayo Clinic in 1926. Of 4000 patients with dysphagia evaluated at the clinic, only 3 were found to have benign esophageal tumors as the cause of their symptoms. The infrequent occurrence was further established by Patterson[1] in 1932, who identified only 61 reported cases of benign esophageal tumor and cyst over the preceding 215 years. This fact is now a well-known characteristic of these tumors.

Although the majority of patients with benign esophageal tumors are asymptomatic, many of the early reports involved symptomatic patients. Arrowsmith[12] (1877) described a patient with a benign polypoid esophageal growth that resulted in such severe dysphagia that the patient died of malnutrition. Moersch and Harrington[2] (1944) noted that only 1 of 15 patients was asymptomatic. This undoubtedly reflects the fact that these reports antedated modern endoscopic and radiographic methods, which have since increased the probability of diagnosis of asymptomatic lesions.

One of the first reports of treatment was by Vater[13] in 1750, who described a patient whose esophageal polyp spontaneously separated and was regurgitated. In 1818, Dubois[14] successfully ligated a polypoid intraluminal esophageal neoplasm that later separated while the patient was sleeping and led to regurgitation, aspiration, and asphyxiation. Mackenzie[13] described two patients

whose tumor was removed with a probang, which is a long flexible rod with a sponge at one end. The first open surgical removal of a benign tumor is generally attributed to Oshawa[15] in 1933; however, Storey and Adams[16] identified a report 1 year earlier by Sauerbruch[17] of transpleural resection of a leiomyoma. The first successful surgery in the United States is attributed to Churchill[18] in 1937.

The most recent chapter in this historical review is still being written. The introduction of minimally invasive surgical methods approximately 25 years ago has challenged open surgical approaches for resecting benign esophageal tumors and cysts. Furthermore, as outlined in the beginning of the chapter, our ability to specifically diagnose these tumors and cysts, once they are identified, by endoscopic ultrasound (EUS), transesophageal endoscopic biopsy, and digital radiographic imaging methods has dramatically evolved. Finally, pathologists have been able to study the molecular genetic profile of benign esophageal tumors to determine their specific diagnosis and pathogenesis.

CLASSIFICATION

Three classification schemes have been proposed and are summarized in Box 37–1. The first classification system, advocated by both Sweet et al.[19] and Moersch and Harrington,[2] is based on both clinical and gross pathologic findings. They organized tumors according to the esophageal layer—mucosa, submucosa, and muscularis—from which they originated. The second is an anatomic classification attributed to Nemir et al.[20] in which esophageal tumors are organized by cell of origin into epithelial, nonepithelial, and heterotopic tumors. The third approach classifies benign tumors and cysts by location and clinical (radiographic and endoscopic) appearance. One example of this third approach, cited by Reed[21] and attributed to Herrera,[22] classifies tumors as intraluminal, intramural, and extramural. Another example, advocated by Avezzano et al.,[23] classifies tumors

---

Box 37–1 **Proposed Classification Schemes for Benign Esophageal Tumors**

Classification by esophageal layer of origin[2,19]
   Mucosal
   Submucosal
   Muscularis
Classification by anatomic site of origin[20]
   Epithelial
   Nonepithelial
   Heterotopic
Classification by location and clinical appearance[21-23]
   Intramural/extramucosal
   Intraluminal/mucosal
   Cysts and duplications

| Table 37–1 | Esophageal Mesenchymal Tumors | | |

Features	Schwannoma	Leiomyoma	GIST
Histology	Moderately cellular Peripheral lymphoid cuff	Eosinophilic cytoplasm	Highly cellular Spindle cells Basophilic appearance
Molecular genetic markers	+S-100, GFAP −CD117, CD34, SMA	+Desmin, SMA −CD117, CD34	+CD117, CD34
Gender ratio (M:F)	1:1	2:1	2:1
Mean age (yr)	54	35	63
Malignant potential	Lowest	Mixed	Highest

GFAP, glial fibrillary acidic protein; GIST, gastrointestinal stromal tumor; SMA, smooth muscle actin.
Data from references 22-29.

into two groups, intramural-extramucosal and mucosal-intraluminal. These two similar schemes are combined into the third classification based on clinical findings. The following description of specific benign tumors and cysts of the esophagus is organized according to this last classification scheme.

INTRAMURAL/EXTRAMUCOSAL

Mesenchymal Tumors

Previously, each benign esophageal tumor was thought to originate independently from precursor cells within the esophageal wall. For example, leiomyomas were thought to arise from smooth muscle cells of the muscularis mucosa, muscularis propria, vascular smooth muscle cells, or embryonic rest cells within the esophageal wall. However, increasing molecular genetic data indicate a common mesenchymal cell of origin for the three benign tumors *leiomyoma, gastrointestinal stromal tumor* (GIST), and *schwannoma*. Table 37–1 summarizes the histologic, immunohistochemical, and clinical characteristics of these three tumors.[22-29] Schwannomas are the least common of the three. They are positive for S-100 protein and glial fibrillary acidic protein (GFAP) but negative for CD117, smooth muscle actin (SMA), and CD34. Malignant potential is the lowest for the three mesenchymal tumors. Leiomyoma is the most common mesenchymal tumor. These tumors are positive for desmin and SMA but negative for CD117 and CD34. Malignant potential is closely related to tumor size. A large tumor, or documented growth, suggests a higher malignant potential. GIST is uncommon in the esophagus but more common than schwannoma. GIST is positive for CD117 and CD34. It has the highest malignant potential of mesenchymal tumors. The risk for malignancy, as with leiomyoma, increases with tumor size and with documented growth. However, even a smaller GIST with low mitotic activity can result in metastatic tumor recurrence, and reports indicate that a characteristic of all these tumors is expression of c-kit (CD117 antigen). The actual mesenchymal cell of origin is not known with

certainty, but resemblance to the interstitial cells of Cajal, which regulate gut peristalsis, suggests that they are the common cell of origin for these tumors. These cells retain the ability to grow and differentiate into smooth muscle cell (leiomyoma), stromal cell (GIST), and neural sheath (schwannoma) tumors. The terminology for these tumors remains confusing. Many still refer to each separately, whereas others call them *stromal tumors*. In this chapter they are grouped together as mesenchymal tumors in acknowledgment of their common mesenchymal cell of origin.

Leiomyoma

Leiomyoma accounts for approximately two thirds of all benign esophageal tumors. There have been many excellent reviews of the clinical and pathologic features of esophageal leiomyomas, including those by Storey and Adams,[16] Seremetis et al.,[10] Sweet et al.,[19] Posthlethwaite and Musser,[30] and Hatch et al.[31] The most recent comprehensive review, that by Lee et al.,[32] includes the time period 1900 to 2003. All these reviews present a picture of esophageal leiomyoma that is remarkably consistent.

Despite the fact that leiomyoma is the most common benign esophageal tumor, it is rare, with a reported incidence of 0.005% to 7.9% in autopsy series. Clinically, the prevalence is less because many tumors are small and remain undetected. Esophageal cancer is 50 times more common than leiomyoma. There is no evidence suggesting that the true, overall incidence is changing. The peak incidence at manifestation is between 30 and 50 years of age for both men and women (Fig. 37–1). The youngest and oldest reported patients are 9 and 83 years of age. Leiomyoma is more common in men than women with a ratio of 2 : 1.

Anatomically, leiomyomas are most commonly located in the lower two thirds of the esophagus. In the review by Hatch et al.,[31] the frequency of tumors in the upper, middle, and lower third of the esophagus was 8.5%, 38.2%, and 46.5%, respectively. An additional 6.8% of tumors involved both the lower third of the esophagus and the proximal part of the stomach. Leiomyomas most

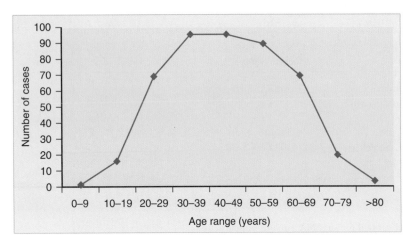

Figure 37–1. Leiomyoma: age at diagnosis.

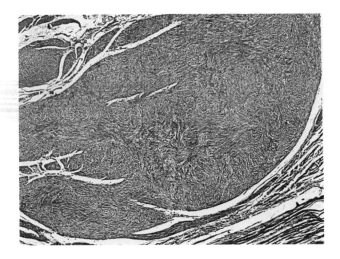

Figure 37–2. Photomicrograph of an intramural circumscribed leiomyoma demonstrating uniform spindle cells arranged in fascicles or whorls.

Table 37–2   Esophageal Leiomyoma: Major Symptoms

Symptom	Prevalence
Dysphagia	47.5%
Pain	45%
Pyrosis	40%
Weight loss	24%
Duration of symptoms	30% >5 yr
	30% >2 yr
	40% 11 mo*

*Average length of symptoms.
From Seremetis MG, Lyons WS, DeGuzman VC, Peabody JW: Leiomyomata of the esophagus. Cancer 38:2166-2177, 1976, with permission.

commonly occur as an extramucosal-intramural mass (72.4%), which is why they are included in this section; however, they may also be manifested as an extraluminal mass (19%) extending outside the esophagus into the mediastinum or as an intraluminal, polypoid mass (8.6%). Most tumors involve only a portion of the circumference of the esophageal wall, but 13% of leiomyomas are annular and involve the entire circumference of the bowel wall.

Leiomyomas are firm, rubbery, encapsulated masses that can assume many shapes—some uniform and others bizarre. Round, oval, spiral, horseshoe, and annular masses have been reported. Half these tumors are less than 5 cm in diameter, and 85% are less than 10 cm in diameter. Tumors ranging in size from several millimeters to 29 cm in diameter have been reported. Tumors exceeding 1000 g are termed giant. The histologic appearance demonstrates uniform spindle cells arranged in fascicles or whorls (Fig. 37–2). The vast majority of leiomyomas are solitary (97%). In some cases, the entire smooth muscle portion of the esophagus is filled with confluent small tumors, a condition termed leiomyomatosis.

Conditions that have historically been associated with esophageal leiomyoma include hiatal hernia, diverticulum, and achalasia. Amer et al.[33] documented esophageal motility disorders, distinct from achalasia, in four patients whose motility patterns normalized after removal of leiomyoma. The association of leiomyoma with esophageal motility disorders might be expected given that these tumors originate from the interstitial cells of Cajal, which are responsible for gastrointestinal motility. Other disorders that should be considered in the differential diagnosis of leiomyoma include esophageal cancer, other benign esophageal tumors or cysts, vascular anomalies, and lung and mediastinal tumors.

The symptoms related to leiomyoma, comprehensively reviewed by Seremetis et al.,[10] continue to be valid today and are listed in Table 37–2. Approximately half the patients with leiomyomas are asymptomatic. When symptoms are present, dysphagia and pain predominate. The pain is usually retrosternal or epigastric and is often described as a feeling of pressure. Unlike leiomyoma originating in the stomach, bleeding is rare. The patient's symptoms are of long duration. Sixty percent of patients reported symptoms for 2 years or longer. The remaining 40% of patients had symptoms for an average of 11 months. Storey and Adams[16] emphasized that in a symptomatic patient, multiple symptoms were the rule. They also noted that respiratory symptoms, including cough, dyspnea, or both, occurred in 10% of patients. Sweet et al.[19] identified tumor size as the single most important factor in determining the likelihood and severity of symptoms. In one report of a 13-year-old girl with hypertrophic osteoarthropathy and esophageal leiomyoma, the osteoarthropathy regressed rapidly after removal of the leiomyoma.[34]

There are no symptoms that specifically indicate that a patient has a leiomyoma. Fifty percent of patients with esophageal leiomyoma are asymptomatic. Often the symptoms, when present, are vague in their description and time of onset. Sometimes it is not even clear that the symptoms are related to the esophageal tumor. Therefore, diagnosis requires endoscopic or radiographic imaging.

Historically, most leiomyomas were identified as an incidental finding of an extramucosal, intramural esophageal mass on esophagoscopy. Even though a benign tumor was suspected, early surgical intervention was recommended because of the uncertainty in diagnosis. As mentioned in the beginning of the chapter, advances in diagnostic methods now result in the ability to diagnose the nature and extent of benign esophageal tumors with considerably greater confidence. As a result, patients can be appropriately triaged to surgical therapy versus observation.

Most esophageal leiomyomas cannot be visualized on plain chest films. Larger tumors, especially those that extend outside the esophageal wall, may be identified as a mediastinal mass.[35] On occasion, these tumors have been reported to contain focal areas of punctate calcification that could be identified in the posterior mediastinum on plain films.[36]

The characteristic features of leiomyomas on barium esophagography have been well described.[9,37-39] Oral contrast studies demonstrate a segmental lesion that focally impinges on the column of swallowed contrast (Fig. 37-3). This crescent-shaped tumor generally has half its mass in the esophageal wall and the rest extending into the lumen. The junction of the mass with the esophageal wall demonstrates sharp margins (approaching 90 degrees). There is little obstruction to flow of contrast. The mucosa overlying the mass is intact but smooth, as though it is stretched over the tumor. The mucosa on the opposite wall is intact. Proximal esophageal dilatation is unusual. Tumors near or involving the esophagogastric margin are often larger and angulate and flatten the esophageal lumen. Tumors near the esophagogastric junction may impair esophageal emptying, result in esophageal dilatation, and simulate achalasia. On CT most leiomyomas appear as eccentric, focal esophageal wall thickening. This finding has not been specific for leiomyoma, although radiologists are making progress in correlating CT findings with the specific pathologic diag-

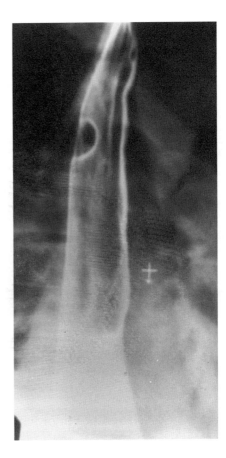

Figure 37–3. Contrast esophagogram demonstrating the characteristic findings of a leiomyoma.

nosis of benign esophageal tumors.[40] Administration of oral contrast helps in visualizing intramural esophageal leiomyomas. CT scanning is most helpful in evaluating larger tumors, especially those that extend outside the esophageal wall, to assess the interface between tumor and mediastinum.

The endoscopic characteristics of leiomyoma have also been well described[9,41] and include (1) a segmental tumor bulge into the lumen, (2) an intact overlying esophageal mucosa, (3) narrowing of the esophageal lumen without obstruction, and (4) a movable mass (Fig. 37–4). Ulceration of the mucosa overlying a benign esophageal leiomyoma is rare. In the past, endoscopic biopsy of extraluminal esophageal lesions was avoided for fear of bleeding or perforation. However, the safety of transendoscopic needle aspiration for cytologic evaluation is now well established. Often, a needle biopsy is performed in conjunction with EUS to more accurately establish the anatomy of the target lesion.

EUS has become instrumental in improving the diagnostic and staging accuracy of esophageal tumors. Rice[42] has classified benign esophageal tumors according to the five EUS esophageal layers. This classification is reproduced in Table 37–3. Leiomyomas are identified as arising from the fourth layer, or the muscularis propria. According to Rice, leiomyomas may arise from the muscularis mucosae in the second EUS layer, but they do so

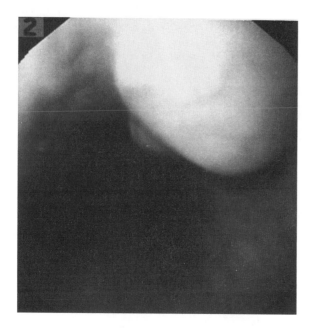

Figure 37–4. Endoscopic appearance of a leiomyoma illustrating the segmental tumor bulge, intact overlying mucosa, and luminal narrowing without obstruction.

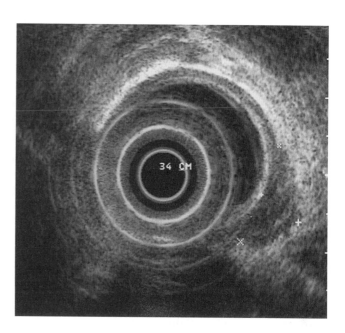

Figure 37–5. Endoscopic ultrasound of a leiomyoma demonstrating the size and location of the tumor. The tumor borders are marked by the three scan markers (*, x, +).

Table 37–3   Correlation of Endosonographic Layer and Pathology

Endoscopic Ultrasound Layer	Esophageal Tumor	Esophageal Cyst
First/second layer (mucosa and deep mucosa)	Squamous papilloma Fibrovascular polyp Granular cell tumor	Retention cyst
Third layer (submucosa)	Lipoma Fibroma Neurofibroma Granular cell tumor	
Fourth layer (muscularis propria)	Leiomyoma*	Cysts and duplications
Fifth		Cysts and duplications

*Leiomyomas most commonly arise as extraluminal/intramural masses. However, they may be manifested as intraluminal polypoid masses or with extraesophageal extension.

From Rice TW: Benign esophageal tumors: Esophagoscopy and endoscopic esophageal ultrasound. Semin Thorac Cardiovasc Surg 15:20-26, 2003.

only rarely. Therefore, EUS *location* of the tumor assists in the differential diagnosis. EUS can identify the size, shape, and extent of the tumor. It can identify lesions that would be too small to see by contrast esophagography or CT. In addition to location, the specific EUS *pattern* of leiomyoma is characteristic and includes a hypoechoic, homogeneous, well-demarcated mass with no associated lymphadenopathy (Fig. 37–5). EUS findings that are atypical for a benign leiomyoma include larger size (>4 cm), irregular margins, nonhomogeneous echoic pattern, and regional lymphadenopathy.

Historically, identification of an extraluminal-intramural esophageal mass was an indication for surgery because of the uncertainty of specific diagnosis and the inability to monitor the size of the lesion over time. Now, however, EUS and chest CT have increased the diagnostic accuracy and safety of nonoperative surveillance. Additionally, it is now well established that malignant degeneration of a benign leiomyoma is a very rare event generally heralded by a change in tumor size. Factors that need to be considered when selecting a patient for nonoperative management include tumor size, location, and patient symptoms. Leiomyomas that are small, extramucosal-intramural, without associated lymphadenopathy, and in asymptomatic patients may be observed without surgery. What size constitutes a "small" leiomyoma is not defined in the literature. Samphire et al.[43] consider small to be 2 cm or less. The principle of

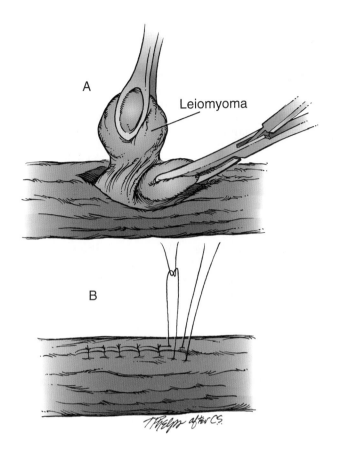

Figure 37–6. The technique of enucleation is illustrated. **A,** The esophageal muscular fibers are split and the leiomyoma is bluntly extracted from the esophageal wall. **B,** Once removed, the muscular defect is reapproximated.

nonoperative management is to monitor patients for the onset of symptoms or a change in size of the esophageal tumor. EUS, performed every 1 to 2 years, with or without chest CT, most accurately tracks tumor size.

Indications for resection include symptoms, uncertainty of diagnosis, larger size, mucosal erosion, regional lymph node enlargement, and tumor growth. Open resection has been the standard approach to resecting leiomyomas, but it is recently being challenged by minimally invasive and endoscopic methods. Lower third esophageal tumors are approached with a left thoracotomy. Tumors near the esophagogastric junction may be resected via laparotomy and a transhiatal approach. Leiomyomas proximal to the lower third are approach by right thoracotomy. In all cases, the tumor is localized visually and by palpation. The esophageal muscle is then split over the mass, which is then delivered from the muscular wall in a technique termed "enucleation" (Fig. 37–6). The mucosa is not generally involved, and intramural leiomyomas may be removed without entering the esophageal lumen. Once the mass is removed and the mucosa is inspected to ensure that it has not been inadvertently opened, the muscular fibers are reapproximated with interrupted sutures.

Resection of leiomyoma by the minimally invasive methods of thoracoscopy and laparoscopy is now well

established. The same technique as for open surgery is used to enucleate the tumor from the muscular wall. Samphire et al.[43] published an excellent description of thoracoscopic and laparoscopic enucleation of leiomyoma. More recently, Elli et al.[44] reported the successful use of robotic-assisted thoracoscopic resection of leiomyoma. Lee et al.[32] described an endoscopic-assisted method of enucleation called "combined endoluminal intracavitary thoracoscopic enucleation," or the "balloon push-out" method. At the time of thoracoscopy, an intraluminal balloon attached to an esophagoscope is inflated at the level of the leiomyoma and pushes the tumor outward toward the operating surgeon, thereby facilitating resection.

Several methods have been reported in which benign esophageal tumors are resected solely by endoscopic techniques. If an esophageal leiomyoma is intraluminal and polypoid, it may be removed via standard endoscopic polypectomy methods. Kinney and Waxman[45] reported their experience and reviewed the literature on a technique called endoscopic mucosal resection. In this method, a sclerotherapy needle is inserted into the esophageal wall under the submucosal tumor. Saline injection causes the tumor to protrude into the lumen in a polypoid fashion. The mass is then resected by standard polypectomy methods. Sun et al.[46] used suction on the submucosal tumor to pull it into the esophageal lumen, where it was "banded" at its base. Later, the tumor sloughed free into the gastrointestinal tract and the mucosal defect healed without further intervention. Park et al.[47] described an endoscopic, electrocautery method of resecting submucosal tumors. The technique results in successful but "piecemeal" resection of the tumor.

In some patients with diffuse esophageal leiomyomatosis or with particularly large tumors (>8 cm in size), esophagectomy is required. Esophagectomy is reported to be indicated in 10% of patients or less. Standard surgical techniques are used. Particular care should be taken to minimize the risk for postoperative gastroesophageal reflux.

In their collective review, Lee et al.[32] tabulated the results of resecting esophageal leiomyomas by thoracotomy, minimally invasive surgery, and endoscopic methods for the time period 1984 to 2001. With open thoracotomy, operative mortality for enucleation ranged from 0% to 1.3%. Complications were uncommon and minor, and 89% to 94% of patients were symptom-free 5 years after surgery. An earlier report by Rendina et al.[48] noted a mortality of 10.5% if esophagectomy was required. In one of the larger series reported to date by Bonavina et al.,[49] of 66 patients, 95.5% were managed by enucleation and 4.5% required esophagectomy. Enucleation was performed by thoracotomy in 50 (79%), laparotomy in 5 (8%), and videothoracoscopy in 8 (13%) patients. Indications for esophagectomy were either diffuse disease or large size. In their series there were no deaths. The number of cases reported in which leiomyomas are enucleated by thoracoscopy and laparoscopy is limited. However, it seems as though these approaches lower operative mortality in comparison to open methods, with similar favorable long-term outcomes. Whether the reduction in reported mortality is secondary to the minimally invasive methods or patient selection is not clear. The greatest danger with the use of minimally invasive methods is mucosal damage. When identified, it can be closed without conversion to an open approach. It is speculated that the application of robotic systems, with three-dimensional computer imaging, will further improve results. Endoscopic methods are new, and the number of reported cases and length of follow-up are limited. However, no deaths have been reported. Bleeding and symptoms from iatrogenic mucosal ulceration are the most prevalent problems encountered. Local recurrence, presumably from incomplete tumor resection, is the primary long-term concern. Overall, the data suggest a continued decline in operative mortality in the management of these tumors in adults.

Leiomyomas rarely develop in patients younger than 10 to 12 years.[21,50] In the pediatric age group, leiomyoma is more common in girls, and there is diffuse esophageal involvement in more than 91% of patients. Dysphagia is the most common initial symptom. Patients are often thought to have achalasia. Because of the diffuse nature of the disease in children, treatment requires esophagectomy in most patients. Operative mortality in pediatric patients is higher (21%), undoubtedly reflecting the greater percentage of esophagectomies required for these younger patients.[21,50]

Gastrointestinal Stromal Tumor

GISTs are mesenchymal tumors with specific molecular genetic features that differentiate them from leiomyomas and schwannomas.[25-29] These tumors most commonly develop in patients 40 years or older. They occur with equal frequency in both men and women. GISTs may occur anywhere along the gastrointestinal tract; however, they are most common in the stomach (60%). Less than 5% of GISTs are found in the esophagus. Benign tumors exceed malignant forms by a margin of 10:1. GISTs are firm, solid masses that on histologic examination demonstrate spindle cell morphology. Histologic differentiation between benign and malignant tumors is based on the presence and number of mitotic figures per high-power field (HPF). Tumors with 5 to 10 mitotic figures per HPF, or size greater than 10 cm in diameter, are considered to have high malignant potential. Even tumors with low mitotic counts per HPF are capable of generating metastatic disease.

Symptoms, diagnostic methods, and treatment options are the same as just discussed for leiomyoma.[40]

Tumor size is the best factor to determine whether to recommend surgery or observation. In general, tumor diameter greater than 5 cm, growth under observation, or symptoms are indications for surgical resection. Small GISTs can be enucleated by open or minimally invasive techniques as previously discussed. Larger GISTs, because of their adherence to the esophageal mucosa and their malignant potential, often require esophagectomy.

Schwannoma

Schwannomas are the least common of the esophageal mesenchymal tumors. The small number of reported cases makes it difficult to generalize about the patient characteristics of these tumors. The reported age range of patients is 47 to 62 years. No gender preponderance is noted. Grossly, schwannomas are tan masses that are firm and rubbery. Histologically, these tumors exhibit moderate cellularity and a characteristic peripheral rim of lymphoid cells. Some esophageal schwannomas have associated melanin pigmentation. Immunohistochemical studies demonstrate that these tumors are positive for S-100 protein and GFAP but negative for c-kit, CD34, and SMA.

Symptoms and diagnostic methods are similar to those for leiomyoma. Treatment options are to observe or resect these tumors. Resection options are the same as those described for leiomyoma. Of note, the majority of schwannomas are benign. Tumor size is the best predictor of malignant potential. The bigger the tumor, the greater the chance that it will be malignant. Post-treatment outcome is related to completeness of resection and whether the tumor is benign or malignant.[51-55]

Granular Cell Tumor

Granular cell tumor (GCT), also known as granular cell myoblastoma, is a rare submucosal tumor that infrequently involves the esophagus. Esophageal GCT and leiomyoma are both intramural submucosal tumors and share many clinical features, including initial symptoms, diagnostic work-up, and treatment options. Abrikossof is credited with the first description of an esophageal GCT in 1931.[9] GCT may occur in any organ system but is most commonly seen in the submucosa of the tongue (40%), skin (30%), breast (15%), and gastrointestinal tract (5%).[56-58] Most GCTs are benign; malignant GCTs account for only 2% to 3% of overall cases. Reports have documented both a male[59] and a female[56] preponderance of this tumor. More likely, GCT occurs equally in both sexes.[9] The average age at the time of diagnosis is 40 to 44 years. Despite accumulating experience with GCT, there is still controversy regarding its specific cell of origin, differentiation into benign and malignant tumor, and recommendations for optimal management.

The prevailing opinion is that GCT arises from neural cells within the esophageal wall. GCT cells have electron microscopic features similar to those of Schwann cells and stain for the neural proteins S-100 and neuron-specific enolase.[9,21] Only 1% to 2% of GCTs are found in the esophagus. Most GCTs, 50% to 63%, are located in the distal end of the esophagus. Multiple esophageal GCTs are reported in 20% of patients. When the esophagus is involved, it is the sole organ site in the majority of cases; however, in 5% to 14% of patients, GCT is identified in multiple organ sites.[56,60] Grossly, the tumor arises in the submucosa and protrudes into the esophageal lumen. GCTs have a characteristic pale yellow color. The overlying esophageal mucosa is intact, but it is often so translucent that it appears absent. Microscopically, tumor cells are pale staining with small nuclei and abundant cytoplasm that is characteristically granular in appearance (Fig. 37–7). The overlying mucosa shows pseudoepitheliomatous hyperplasia. There are no

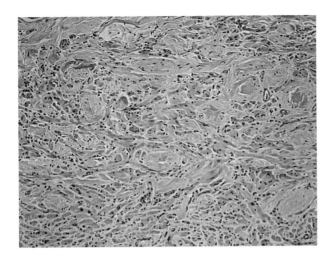

Figure 37–7. Photomicrograph of a granular cell tumor that has relatively uniform plump spindle cells containing coarsely granular eosinophilic cytoplasm.

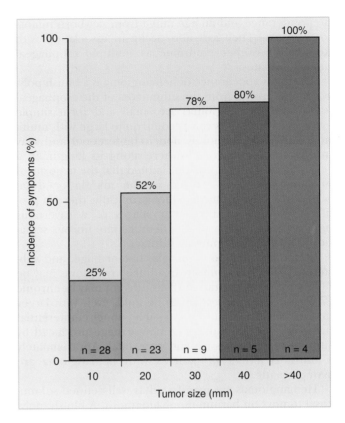

Figure 37–8. Incidence of symptoms as a function of granular cell tumor size. (From Coutinho DS, Soga J, Yoshikawa T, et al: Granular cell tumors of the esophagus: A report of two cases and review of the literature. Am J Gastroenterol 80:758-762, 1985, with permission.)

characteristic histologic findings defining malignant GCT. The diagnosis of benign versus malignant GCT is made on the basis of *both* clinical and histologic findings. Both local invasion and metastases have been reported with malignant GCT.

There are great similarities in the symptoms of esophageal GCT and leiomyoma. Symptoms include dysphagia, retrosternal pain or vague discomfort, and less frequently, nausea and vomiting. Fifty percent of patients with GCT are asymptomatic. Coutinho et al.[59] have demonstrated nicely that the frequency of symptoms is directly related to tumor size, as shown in Figure 37–8. In their series the frequency of symptoms in patients with tumors 10 mm or less, 11 to 20 mm, 21 to 30 mm, and 31 to 40 mm was 25%, 52.2%, 77.7%, and 80%, respectively. The differential diagnosis for patients with suspected GCT includes other benign esophageal tumors and malignant carcinoma.

As with patients with leiomyoma, the diagnosis is best made by contrast esophagography and endoscopy. A barium esophagogram demonstrates a smooth-walled filling defect impinging on the esophageal lumen. Smaller tumors are difficult to identify radiographically, whereas larger tumors may result in high-grade esophageal obstruction. Endoscopically, the tumor is visible as a yellowish "molar-shaped" polypoid lesion protruding into the lumen.[61] Endoscopic biopsy of these tumors is often nondiagnostic. EUS is helpful in defining the site of origin and the extent of these tumors. Tada et al.[61] described the EUS findings of esophageal GCT as hyperechoic solid masses surrounded by hypoechoic submucosa without continuity to the muscularis propria.

Management of patients with GCT remains controversial. Postlethwaite and Lowe[9] have argued that these tumors should be treated aggressively with surgical removal on diagnosis because of the inability to distinguish between benign and malignant tumors. Others have advocated conservative management with endoscopic follow-up for smaller, asymptomatic tumors.[62]

These authors site the low frequency of malignancy and availability of the tumor for endoscopic surveillance as justification for conservative management. This issue remains unresolved. There is agreement that symptomatic tumors or any tumor demonstrating rapid tumor growth is an indication for removal. Treatment in the past was limited to transthoracic excision; however, successful endoscopic mucosal resection has been described in several reports.[61,63-65] One report of endoscopic alcohol injection of a GCT under EUS guidance has been described,[66] as well as yttrium-aluminum-garnet (YAG) laser and argon plasma coagulation.[67,68]

Hemangioma

Hemangiomas are benign vascular tumors that originate from the esophageal submucosa. They are rare, with less than 100 reported cases in the literature. In Platcha's series,[3] hemangioma accounted for 3% of all benign esophageal tumors. Gentry et al.[69] found that only 11 of 261 (4.2%) gastrointestinal vascular tumors were located in the esophagus. The first description of an esophageal hemangioma, treated by radium application, is credited to Vinson et al.[70] in 1927. There are no data defining the demographics of patients with esophageal hemangioma. Riemenschneider and Klassen[71] noted a slight male preponderance and an age range from newborn infants to 72 years. They can also occur in association with Rendu-Osler-Weber syndrome as multiple esophageal hemangiomatosis.[72]

The gross appearance of hemangioma is a bluish polypoid mass arising from the submucosa of the esophageal wall. Some hemangiomas are small and form simple cystic masses. Others can become quite large with multinodularity. The tumor is noncircumferential and may involve the esophagus anywhere along its length. In a review of 58 patients, Govoni[73] noted that the majority of hemangiomas were located in the middle or distal portion of the esophagus. Microscopically, there is proliferation of benign vascular spaces of a cavernous nature. Multinodular masses demonstrate fibrous septation. The overlying mucosa is intact.

Symptoms include dysphagia, hemorrhage, and substernal pain or discomfort. In adults,[71] symptoms may be of relatively short duration (2 months) or may be chronic (7 years). Dysphagia tends to be mild, even with larger masses, because of the compressible, noncircumferential nature of these tumors. The hemorrhage produced by rupture may be massive and even fatal. Approximately a third to a half of patients with hemangioma are asymptomatic.

Hemangiomas are manifested as well-defined submucosal tumors on barium esophagography. A bluish, polypoid submucosal lesion is seen endoscopically. The mass is compressible endoscopically, and biopsy is not recommended.[74] EUS has been used to identify and "stage" these vascular tumors. In contrast to leiomyoma or GCT, CT is particularly helpful in making the diagnosis and planning treatment of hemangiomas.[75] MRI has also been described in the diagnosis of hemangioma, especially for larger tumors.

A wide variety of treatments have been proposed to manage esophageal hemangioma, including endoscopic resection,[76] YAG laser fulgaration,[77] sclerotherapy,[78] radiation therapy, and open or videothoracoscopic resection.[79] Surgical resection can usually be performed by either local resection or enucleation, although esophagectomy is occasionally required. The surgical procedures are safe with a mortality of approximately 2%.[9] There are no reports of recurrence after surgical resection. The results of endoscopic resection are limited to case reports but seem reasonable over a limited follow-up.

Other Intramural Tumors

All benign esophageal tumors are uncommon. The most common intramural tumors, leiomyoma, GCT, and hemangioma, have been separately discussed. Other rare intramural esophageal tumors have been reported. To be complete, they will be briefly covered in this section.

Rhabdomyomas are tumors of the striated skeletal muscle of the upper third of the esophagus. They are rare, and not enough patients have been identified to determine the clinical characteristics of these tumors. Lipomas and fibromas usually protrude into the esophageal lumen as a polyp, but they may form sub-

mucosal masses. Schwannomas share many pathologic and clinical features with leiomyoma. Both tumors arise from the interstitial stem cells of Cajal. Schwannomas produce the same symptoms as leiomyoma and are diagnosed in the same fashion. Recommended treatment is surgical enucleation. Endoscopic resection has been reported only once in the literature.[80]

Lipomas occur rarely as tumors of the submucosa and are usually found incidentally. They appear as a soft, pale yellow tumor with intact overlying mucosa. When evaluated by EUS, they are hyperechoic, homogeneous lesions that are confined to the submucosal layer. Biopsy samples are difficult to obtain because lipomas do not involve the mucosa. They do not require treatment or further follow-up because they have no malignant potential.[42]

Underlying submucosal inflammation can lead to inflammatory pseudotumors. These reactive pseudoneoplastic processes can occur throughout the body.[81] They may result from an underlying injury, such as perforation or the postoperative healing process, or can be secondary to an autoimmune disorder or subclinical infection. Epstein-Barr virus has also been implicated in the formation of these pseudotumors.[82-84] These tumors are composed of reactive blood vessels, fibroblasts, and polycellular inflammatory cells. Because they are submucosal lesions, biopsy may be inconclusive. Occasionally, they may cause ulceration of the overlying mucosa. Treatment strategies have included surgical excision or systemic corticosteroids, although the latter results in a high recurrence rate and is not without side effects.[85]

Congenital ectopic rests of pancreatic, thyroid, and parathyroid tissue have been reported in the esophageal wall.[9] In some cases this tissue has been hormonally active. In such cases, treatment is local resection or enucleation.

INTRALUMINAL/MUCOSAL

Fibrovascular Polyp

Fibrovascular polyps are the second most common benign esophageal tumor and the most common intraluminal tumor. Jang et al.[86] reported 56 cases in the literature in 1969. Fibrovascular polyp is a term that includes a broad range of specific intraluminal polyps, including fibromas, fibrolipomas, myomas, myxofibromas, pedunculated lipomas, and fibroepithelial polyps. The pathogenesis, clinical features, work-up, and treatment options are similar regardless of the specific histologic type of polyp. Though not proven, it is hypothesized that these polyps begin as a region of submucosal thickening that elongates into the esophageal lumen as a result of esophageal peristaltic action to form a polyp. Polyps most commonly originate from the proximal part of the esophagus just distal to the cricopharyngeus. They may achieve large size and result in esophageal dilatation or be long enough to reach into the stomach. The most dramatic clinical feature of fibrovascular polyps is their potential for regurgitation out through the oropharynx, where they may be reswallowed, severed by biting and expectorated, or aspirated.

Table 37–4	Age and Sex of 55 Patients with Fibrovascular Polyps	

Age (yr)	Men	Women
20-29	3	5
30-39	3	3
40-49	6	1
50-59	11	4
60-69	8	4
70-79	5	0
80-89	2	0

From Posthlethwaite RW, Lowe JE: Benign tumors and cysts of the esophagus. In Zuidema GD, Orringer MB (eds): Shackelford's Surgery of the Alimentary Tract, vol 1, 4th ed. Philadelphia, WB Saunders, 1996, pp 369-386.

Avezzano et al.[23] reported a male preponderance (75%) and a peak prevalence in the sixth and seventh decades. Posthlethwaite and Lowe[9] commented that polyps were seen in older men (average age, 54.7 years) and younger women (average age, 43.4). In their series, 69% of patients were men (Table 37–4).

Grossly, these polyps are cylindrical-shaped masses attached by a stalk to the esophageal wall, usually of the proximal esophagus. Polyps range in size from less than 1 cm to greater than 20 cm in length. The average size is 5 cm.[87] Polyps may be long enough that they extend into the stomach, where acid results in focal ulceration. A polyp's diameter may be wide enough that it results in esophageal dilatation. Multiple polyps have been reported. The site of origin within the esophagus is cervical, upper thoracic, middle, and lower esophageal in 80%, 2%, 8%, and 10%, respectively.[9] Histologically, these polyps are composed of mature fibrous tissue with varying amounts of vascularity and adipose tissue. Which of these three components is most prominent determines the specific name for the polyp (e.g., fibrolipoma, myxofibroma). Polyps are covered by intact, smooth mucosa. No malignant degeneration of these polyps has been reported, although at least one case of a coexisting squamous cell carcinoma has been identified.[87]

Aside from identifying a regurgitated polyp, no physical findings are characteristic of these tumors. Potential symptoms include intermittent dysphagia, regurgitation of the polyp, and respiratory symptoms. Polyps that extend into the stomach may ulcerate and bleed and thereby result in anemia and symptoms related to anemia. Levine et al.[88] reported that dysphagia (87%) and respiratory symptoms (25%) were most common. Regurgitation of the polyp into the mouth was noted in only 12% of patients. In their experience, the average duration of symptoms was 17 months; however, 44% of patients had symptoms for 6 months or less. Up to 30% of patients have been reported to be asymptomatic. Barium esophagography demonstrates a polypoid filling defect that may be seen to move within the esophageal lumen with a swallow. High-grade obstruction is uncommon. Larger polyps may cause esophageal dilatation

mimicking achalasia. Polyps may be missed on endoscopy because most originate in the proximal esophagus and are covered by normal mucosa. EUS demonstrates an echo-dense intraluminal polyp.[87] Findings on CT vary, depending on the amount of adipose and fibrovascular tissue. Polyps that contain a mixture of fibrovascular and adipose tissue appear as a heterogenous mass on CT, whereas those with a majority of adipose tissue appear as a fat-density lesion expanding the lumen of the esophagus, with a thin rim of contrast surrounding the polyp.[88] The differential diagnosis for a patient suspected of having a fibrovascular polyp includes polypoid schwannoma, leiomyoma, and hamartoma.

Treatment is resection of the polyp, including its point of origin and attachment. Historically, this has been accomplished by open surgical techniques in which the esophageal wall is opened, preferably 180 degrees opposite the base of the polyp, and the polyp and stalk excised along with a small cuff of mucosa. The mucosal defect is reapproximated and the esophagotomy closed. The procedure is performed via a cervical incision for proximal tumors and thoracotomy for more distal lesions. Endoscopic removal has been reported for polyps without excessive vascularity. Unless the polyp base is completely removed, however, local recurrence is possible. Treatment by either method is safe. No treatment-related deaths have been reported.[23]

Squamous Papilloma

Squamous papilloma is a rare, benign neoplastic disorder involving the esophageal mucosa. Autopsy series show a frequency of 0.01% to 0.04% of the general population.[89] Adler et al.[90] are credited with the first histologic description in 1959. Papillomas occur in males more frequently than females (2:1). Age at diagnosis ranges from 40 to 70 years. The etiology of papillomas is not known. Gastrointestinal reflux or other chronic mucosal irritation has been proposed as a potential cause. Human papillomavirus (HPV) is found in varying degrees in these tumors. Odze et al.[91] reported that 13 of 26 papillomas evaluated were positive for HPV, most commonly HPV type 16. Others[92-95] have found a more rare association of HPV with squamous papilloma, in the range of 0% to 4% of cases, even when tested by polymerase chain reaction. It is proposed that their etiology is multifactorial and may be a synergistic effect of mucosal irritation and HPV. There has been only one case report[96] of malignant degeneration associated with papillomavirus. Cases of progressive, fatal systemic dissemination have been reported.[97]

Papillomas are usually solitary, sessile lesions involving the distal end of the esophagus. Most lesions are small, less than 1 cm in diameter. Microscopically, papillomas are composed of a central core of connective tissue covered with hyperplastic squamous cells (Fig. 37–9).

The majority of patients with papillomas are asymptomatic, but some may complain of mild dysphagia. Because of an association of papillomas with gastroesophageal reflux and peptic ulcer disease,[90] some patients may initially be evaluated indirectly for

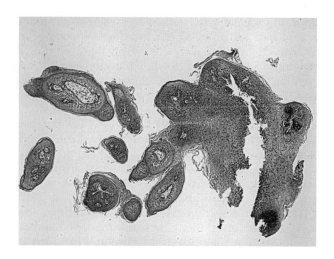

Figure 37–9. Photomicrograph of squamous papilloma showing no dysplastic squamous epithelium with a central core of connective tissue.

symptoms of these associated disorders. There are no characteristic findings on physical examination. Endoscopically, fleshy pink lesions, either sessile or pedunculated, are seen, usually in the distal end of the esophagus. Visually, the lesions may be mistaken for squamous carcinoma. The diagnosis is confirmed by biopsy. No further diagnostic or staging work-up has been advocated.

On the basis of published reports it is not clear whether these lesions should be observed or aggressively resected. Certainly, the diagnosis must first be confirmed and cancer ruled out by biopsy. If a lesion is localized and pedunculated, it should most likely be resected endoscopically and the patient monitored. Papillomas have been noted to recur and spread after treatment by laser fulguration, endoscopic resection, or surgical excision. Because of the risk of seeding, recurrence, or proliferation of disease, Politoske[92] concluded that papillomas should be removed with as little manipulation as possible.

CYSTS AND DUPLICATIONS

Cysts and duplications are included together because they share similar etiology, clinical and radiographic findings, and treatment options. Autopsy studies of the general population estimate the incidence of esophageal cysts to be 1 in 8200 patients.[98] Ten percent to 15% of all gastrointestinal duplications are esophageal in origin. Cysts are more commonly diagnosed in males than females and in children than adults. Cysts and duplications account for approximately 0.5% to 3.3% of all benign esophageal tumors. In children, however, duplications have been shown to account for 12% of mediastinal masses. It is estimated that only 25% to 30% of cysts occur in adults.[3,99,100] Posthlethwaite and Lowe[9] demonstrated a biphasic age distribution for patients with cysts. Forty-one percent of cases occurred in patients younger than 9 years, and 38% occurred in patients between the ages of 20 and 49 years. The first

Box 37–2 **Classification of Esophageal Cysts**

Congenital
  Duplication
    Bronchogenic
    Gastric
    Inclusion
  Other
    Neuroenteric
Acquired
  Retention (single or multiple)

Modified from Arbona JL, Fazzi GF, Mayoral J: Congenital esophageal cysts: Case report and review of the literature. Am J Gastroenterol 79:177-182, 1984.

description of a cyst is credited to Blassius in 1711, and the first surgical resection of a cyst was reported by Sauerbruch and Fick in 1931.[9] Arbona et al.[99] proposed a classification of esophageal cysts that is most commonly cited (Box 37–2).

Cysts and duplications are congenital in origin. One theory states that the early foregut is lined by ciliated columnar epithelium that grows and obliterates the lumen. Vacuoles are then secreted and subsequently coalesce, line up, and form the bowel lumen. It is postulated that single vacuoles become separated, remain within the esophageal wall, and develop into duplications or cysts.[21,99,101] Another theory has been advocated by Hutchison and Thomson.[100] Because the endodermal tube that is destined to form the gut is part of the yolk sac or archenteron, they propose that all developmental gastrointestinal cysts should be labeled "archenteric cysts." According to their theory, at an early stage in development, a *segment* of endoderm becomes separated and fails to become incorporated into the developing gut. This segment retains its endodermal competence and therefore directs the mesoderm to form surrounding muscular wall. However, because it is displaced, its histologic differentiation is less precise, thus accounting for the diversity of mucosal linings that these developmental cysts are noted to have.

Esophageal cysts are classified as duplications[21,99,101] if the cyst (1) is located within the esophageal wall, (2) is covered by two muscular layers, and (3) is lined by squamous epithelium or embryonic epithelium (columnar, pseudostratified, ciliated). Duplications are usually round, but they may be elongated tubular structures. The average diameter of spherical duplications is 4.5 cm. They are most frequently found in the lower part of the esophagus. In the collective series by Arbona et al.,[99] the location was the lower, middle, and upper esophagus in 60%, 17%, and 23%, respectively. A case of an esophageal duplication cyst manifested as an abdominal mass has been reported. Esophageal duplications can be associated with duplications elsewhere in the gastrointestinal tract. Duplication cysts are not linked to vertebral abnormalities. Malignancies arising in duplications are rare but have been reported in the literature.[102]

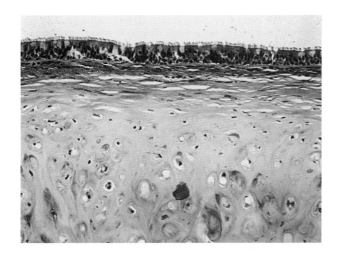

Figure 37–10. Photomicrograph of a bronchogenic cyst wall showing mature cartilage and respiratory-type pseudostratified ciliated columnar epithelium.

Bronchogenic cysts arising from the esophagus are rare.[99] These cysts are caused by an abnormality in lung bud separation from the primitive foregut. Cells from this evolving lung bud become sequestered within the esophageal wall and develop into a bronchogenic cyst. Pathologically, these cysts are located within the esophageal wall and contain cartilage (Fig. 37–10). Bronchogenic cysts are found within the middle and lower thirds of the esophagus and are not associated with vertebral anomalies. No neoplastic changes have been reported.

Gastric cysts are postulated to arise from cells that are destined to become stomach but fail to descend and remain within the esophageal wall. To be classified as a gastric cyst, it must be located within the esophageal wall, contain a muscular wall, and be lined with gastric mucosa.[99] Mucosal hydrochloric acid and enzyme production with ulceration and hemorrhage has been described.

Inclusion cysts are intramural cysts that contain respiratory or squamous epithelium, are not covered by muscle, and do not contain cartilage. They can therefore be differentiated from bronchogenic and duplication cysts. Arbona et al.[99] reported inclusion cyst location to be in the lower, middle, or upper esophagus in 66%, 24%, and 10% of patients, respectively. Cyst size ranged from 0.5 to 20 cm. They are not associated with vertebral abnormalities.

Neuroenteric cysts, also known as posterior mediastinal duplication cysts, arise during notochord separation from the foregut endoderm. At the time of separation, an endodermal diverticulum may form that remains fused to the esophagus or attached to it by a stalk and develops into a cyst. Neuroenteric cysts are found in the posterior mediastinum, are covered by muscle, and are lined by a variety of gastrointestinal mucosa.[99] Split notochord syndrome is described as a neuroenteric cyst associated with vertebral anomalies.[103] The vertebral anomalies may not be at the same level as the cyst.

The normal esophagus contains mucosal and submucosal glands that may coalesce to form acquired cysts. They may be single or multiple. If multiple, it is referred to as esophagitis cystica. These cysts range in size from a few millimeters to 3 cm in diameter and are located in the upper third of the esophagus.

No findings on physical examination are characteristic of cysts and duplications. Symptoms are related to size, location, and patient age. Respiratory symptoms, including cough and wheezing, are more common in children. Gastrointestinal symptoms, including dysphagia, epigastric and substernal pain, and anorexia and nausea, are more common in adults. The prevalence of gastroesophageal reflux seems to be increased in patients with cysts and duplications. According to Cioffi et al.,[104] 37% of patients are asymptomatic on initial evaluation. There has been one report of an acute rupture of an esophageal duplication cyst.[105] Findings on contrast esophagography and esophagoscopy are similar to those in patients with leiomyoma in which a smooth-walled submucosal mass is identified. EUS is helpful in defining the anatomy and establishing the diagnosis. CT is also helpful for both making the diagnosis and planning surgical therapy. MRI can likewise aid in diagnosis, with duplication cysts appearing as high–signal intensity structures on T2-weighted images.[106,107]

Management options include observation, aspiration, and surgical resection. Each option has advocates. Indications for resection include control of symptoms, increase in cyst size, and exclusion of malignancy. Surgically, cysts may be enucleated in a fashion similar to that used for leiomyoma. The procedure has been performed by open thoracotomy, video-assisted thoracoscopic, and laparoscopic techniques.[108]

REFERENCES

1. Patterson EJ: Benign neoplasms of the esophagus: Report of a case of myxofibroma. Ann Otol Rhinol Laryngol 41:942-950, 1932.
2. Moersch HJ, Harrington SW: Benign tumor of the esophagus. Ann Otol Rhinol Laryngol 53:800-817, 1944.
3. Plachta A: Benign tumors of the esophagus. Am J Gastroenterol 38:639-652, 1962.
4. Attah EB, Hajdu SI: Benign and malignant tumors of the esophagus at autopsy. J Thorac Cardiovasc Surg 55:396-404, 1968.
5. Choong CK, Meyers BF: Benign esophageal tumors: Introduction, incidence, and clinical features. Semin Thorac Cardiovasc Surg 15:3-8, 2003.
6. Davis EA, Heitmiller RF: Esophagectomy for benign disease: Trends in surgical results and management. Ann Thorac Surg 62:369-372, 1996.
7. Orringer MB, Stirling MC: Transhiatal esophagectomy for benign and malignant disease. J Thorac Cardiovasc Surg 105:265-277, 1993.
8. Mansour KA, Hatcher CR, Haun CL: Benign tumors of the esophagus: Experience with 20 cases. South Med J 70:461-464, 1977.
9. Posthlethwaite RW, Lowe JE: Benign tumors and cysts of the esophagus. In Zuidema GD, Orringer MB (eds): Shackelford's Surgery of the Alimentary Tract, vol 1, 4th ed. Philadelphia, WB Saunders, 1996, pp 369-386.
10. Seremetis MG, Lyons WS, DeGuzman VC, Peabody JW: Leiomyomata of the esophagus. Cancer 38:2166-2177, 1976.
11. Vinson PP, Moore AB, Bowing HH: Hemangioma of the esophagus. Am J Med Sci 172:416-418, 1926.
12. Arrowsmith R: Fatal case dysphagia produced by pylorus growth in the esophagus. Med Chir Trans 30:229-233, 1877.

13. Cited by MacKenzie M: Manual of Diseases of the Nose and Throat, vol 2. London, Churchill, 1884, p 1.

14. Dubois: Quoted by Mahoney JJ: Polypoid tumors of the esophagus: Report of two cases. Laryngoscope 50:1086-1091, 1940.

15. Oshawa T: Surgery of the esophagus. Arch F Jpn Chir 10:605, 1933.

16. Storey CF, Adams WC: Leiomyoma of the esophagus. Am J Surg 91:3-23, 1956.

17. Sauerbruch F: Presentations in the field of thoracic surgery. Arch F Klin Chir 173:457, 1932.

18. Churchill ED: Case records of the Massachusetts General Hospital, case no. 23491. N Engl J Med 217:955, 1937.

19. Sweet RH, Soutter L, Valenzuela CT: Muscle wall tumors of the esophagus. J Thorac Surg 27:13-31, 1954.

20. Nemir P Jr, Wallace HW, Fallahnejad M: Diagnosis and surgical management of benign disease of the esophagus. Curr Probl Surg 13:1-74, 1976.

21. Reed CE: Benign tumors of the esophagus. Chest Surg Clin North Am 4:769-783, 1994.

22. Herrera JL: Benign and metastatic tumors of the esophagus. Gastroenterol Clin North Am 20:775-789, 1991.

23. Avezzano EA, Fleischer DE, Merida MA, Anderson DL: Giant fibrovascular polyps of the esophagus. Am J Gastroenterol 85:299-302, 1990.

24. Went PT, Dirnhofer S, Bundi M, et al: Prevalence of KIT expression in human tumors. J Clin Oncol 15:4514-4522, 2004.

25. Miettinen M, Sarlomo-Rikala M, Sobin LH, Lasota J: Esophageal stromal tumors: A clinicopathologic, immunohistochemical, and molecular genetic study of 17 cases and comparison with esophageal leiomyomas and leiomyosarcomas. Am J Surg Pathol 24:211-222, 2000.

26. Miettinen M, Majidi M, Lasota J: Pathology and diagnostic criteria of gastrointestinal stromal tumors (GISTs): A review. Eur J Cancer 38(Suppl 5):S39-S51, 2002.

27. Miettinen M, Sarloma-Rikala M, Lasota J: Gastrointestinal stromal tumors: Recent advances in understanding of their biology. Hum Pathol 30:1213-1220, 1999.

28. Kwon MS, Lee SS, Ahn GH: Schwannomas of the gastrointestinal tract: Clinicopathological features of 12 cases including a case of esophageal tumor compared with those of gastrointestinal stromal tumors and leiomyomas of the gastrointestinal tract. Pathol Res Pract 198:605-613, 2002.

29. Miettinen M, Sarlomo-Rikala M, Lasota J: Gastrointestinal stromal tumours. Ann Chir Gynaecol 87:278-281, 1998.

30. Posthlethwaite RW, Musser AW: Changes in the esophagus in 1,000 autopsy specimens. J Thorac Cardiovasc Surg 68:953-956, 1974.

31. Hatch GF 3rd, Wertheimer-Hatch L, Hatch KF, et al: Tumors of the esophagus. World J Surg 24:401-411, 2000.

32. Lee LS, Singhal S, Brinster CJ, et al: Current management of esophageal leiomyoma. J Am Coll Surg 198:136-146, 2004.

33. Amer KM, Payne HR, Jeyasingham K: The relevance of abnormal motility patterns in intra-mural oesophageal leiomyomata. Eur J Cardiothorac Surg 10:634-640, 1996.

34. Massicot R, Aubert D, Mboyo A, et al: Localized esophageal leiomyoma and hypertrophic osteoarthropathy. J Pediatr Surg 32:646-647, 1997.

35. Griff LC, Cooper J: Leiomyoma of the esophagus presenting as a mediastinal mass. AJR Am J Roentgenol 101:472-481, 1967.

36. Gutman E: Posterior mediastinal calcification due to esophageal leiomyoma. Gastroenterology 63:665-666, 1972.

37. Harper RAK, Tiscenco E: Benign tumor of the oesophagus and its differential diagnosis. Br J Radiol 18:99, 1945.

38. Schatzki R, Hawes LE: The roentgenological appearance of extramucosal tumors of the esophagus. AJR Am J Roentgenol 43:1, 1942.

39. Glantz I, Grunebaum M: The radiological approach to leiomyoma of the esophagus with long-term follow-up. Clin Radiol 28:197-200, 1977.

40. Horton KM, Juluru K, Montgomery E, Fishman EK: Computed tomography imaging of gastrointestinal stromal tumors with pathology correlation. J Comput Assist Tomogr 28:811-817, 2004.

41. Lewis B, Maxfield RG: Leiomyoma of the esophagus. Case report and review of the literature. Int Abstr Surg 99:105, 1954.

42. Rice TW: Benign esophageal tumors: Esophagoscopy and endoscopic esophageal ultrasound. Semin Thorac Cardiovasc Surg 15:20-26, 2003.

43. Samphire J, Nafteux P, Luketich J: Minimally invasive techniques for resection of benign esophageal tumors. Semin Thorac Cardiovasc Surg 15:35-43, 2003.

44. Elli E, Espat NJ, Berger R, et al: Robotic-assisted thoracoscopic resection of esophageal leiomyoma. Surg Endosc 18:713-716, 2004.

45. Kinney T, Waxman I: Treatment of benign esophageal tumors by endoscopic techniques. Semin Thorac Cardiovasc Surg 15:27-34, 2003.

46. Sun S, Jin Y, Chang G, et al: Endoscopic band ligation without electrosurgery: A new technique for excision of small upper-GI leiomyoma. Gastrointest Endosc 60:218-222, 2004.

47. Park YS, Park SW, Kim TI, et al: Endoscopic enucleation of upper GI submucosal tumor by using an insulated-tip electrosurgical knife. Gastrointest Endosc 59:409-415, 2004.

48. Rendina EA, Venuta F, Pescarmona ED, et al: Leiomyoma of the esophagus. Scand J Thorac Cardiovasc Surg 24:79-82, 1990.

49. Bonavina L, Segalin A, Rosati R, et al: Surgical therapy of esophageal leiomyoma. J Am Coll Surg 181:257-262, 1995.

50. Bourque MD, Spigland N, Bensoussan AL, et al: Esophageal leiomyoma in children: Two case reports and review of the literature. J Pediatr Surg 24:1103-1107, 1989.

51. Kobayashi N, Kikuchi S, Shimao H, et al: Benign esophageal schwannoma: Report of a case. Surg Today 30:526-529, 2000.

52. Ngaage DL, Khan ZA, Cale AR: Esophageal melanotic schwannoma presenting with superior vena caval obstruction. Thorac Cardiovasc Surg 50:103-104, 2002.

53. Murase K, Hino A, Ozeki Y, et al: Malignant schwannoma of the esophagus with lymph node metastasis: Literature review of schwannoma of the esophagus. J Gastroenterol 36:772-777, 2001.

54. Manger T, Pross M, Haeckel C, Lippert H: Malignant peripheral nerve sheath tumor of the esophagus. Dig Surg 17:627-631, 2000.

55. Ohno M, Sugihara J, Miyamurea K, et al: Benign schwannoma of the esophagus removed by enucleation: Report of a case. Surg Today 30:59-62, 2000.

56. Giacobbe A, Facciorusso D, Conoscitore P, et al: Granular cell tumor of the esophagus. Am J Gastroenterol 83:1398-1400, 1988.

57. Sarma DP, Rodriguez FH, Deiparine EM, et al: Symptomatic granular cell tumor of the esophagus. J Surg Oncol 33:246-249, 1986.

58. Subramanyam K, Shannon CR, Patterson M: Granular cell myoblastoma of the esophagus. J Clin Gastroenterol 6:113-118, 1984.

59. Coutinho DS, Soga J, Yoshikawa T, et al: Granular cell tumors of the esophagus: A report of two cases and review of the literature. Am J Gastroenterol 80:758-762, 1985.

60. Maekawa H, Maekawa T, Yabuki K, et al: Multiple esophagogastric granular cell tumors. J Gastroenterol 38:776-780, 2003.

61. Tada M, Iida M, Yao T, et al: Granular cell tumor of the esophagus: Endoscopic ultrasonographic demonstration and endoscopic removal. Am J Gastroenterol 85:1507-1511, 1990.

62. Mineo TC, Biancari F, Francioni F, et al: Conservative approach to granular cell tumor of the oesophagus. Scand J Thorac Cardiovasc Surg 29:141-144, 1995.

63. Catalano F, Kind R, Rodella L, et al: Endoscopic treatment of esophageal granular cell tumors. Endoscopy 34:582-584, 2002.

64. Yasuda I, Tomita E, Nagura K, et al: Endoscopic removal of granular cell tumors. Gastrointest Endosc 41:163-167, 1995.

65. Esaki M, Aoyagi K, Hizawa K, et al: Multiple granular cell tumors of the esophagus removed endoscopically: A case report. Gastrointest Endosc 48:536-539, 1998.

66. Moreira LS, Dani R: Treatment of granular cell tumor of the esophagus by endoscopic injection of dehydrated alcohol. Am J Gastroenterol 87:659-661, 1992.

67. Norberto L, Urso E, Angriman I, et al: Yttrium-aluminum-garnet laser therapy of esophageal granular cell tumor. Surg Endosc 16:361-362, 2002.

68. Casetti T, Salzetta A, Michieletti G, et al: Endoscopic treatment of granular cell tumor of esophagus by argon plasma coagulation. Giorn Ital Endosc Dig 22:39-43, 1999.

69. Gentry RW, Dockerty MB, Clagett OT: Vascular malformations and vascular tumors of the gastrointestinal tract. Int Abstr Surg 88:281-323, 1949.

70. Vinson PP, Moore AB, Bowing HH: Hemangioma of the esophagus: Report of a case. Am J Med Sci 172:416, 1927.

71. Riemenschneider HW, Klassen KP: Cavernous esophageal hemangioma. Ann Thorac Surg 6:552-556, 1968.

72. Choong CK, Meyers MF: Benign esophageal tumors: Introduction, incidence, classification, and clinical features. Semin Thorac Cardiovasc Surg 15:3-8, 2003.

73. Govoni AF: Hemangiomas of the esophagus. Gastrointest Radiol 7:113-117, 1982.

74. Cantero D, Yoshida T, Ito T, et al: Esophageal hemangioma: Endoscopic diagnosis and treatment. Endoscopy 26:250-253, 1994.

75. Taylor FH, Fowler FC, Betsill WL Jr, Marroum MC: Hemangioma of the esophagus. Ann Thorac Surg 61:726-728, 1996.

76. Yoshikane H, Suzuki T, Yoshioka N, et al: Hemangioma of the esophagus: Endosonographic imaging and endoscopic resection. Endoscopy 27:267-269, 1995.

77. Shigemitsu K, Naomoto Y, Yamatsuji T, et al: Esophageal hemangioma successfully treated by fulguration using potassium titanyl phosphate/yttrium aluminum garnet (KTP/YAG) laser: A case report. Dis Esophagus 13:161-164, 2000.

78. Aoki T, Okagawa K, Uemura Y, et al: Successful treatment of an esophageal hemangioma by endoscopic injection sclerotherapy: Report of a case. Surg Today 27:450-452, 1997.

79. Ramo OJ, Salo JA, Baradini R, et al: Treatment of a submucosal hemangioma of the esophagus using simultaneous video-assisted thoracoscopy and esophagoscopy: Description of a new minimally invasive technique. Endoscopy 29:S27-S28, 1997.

80. Naus PJ, Tio FO, Gross GW: Esophageal schwannoma: First report of successful management by endoscopic removal. Gastrointest Endosc 54:520-522, 2001.

81. Saklani AP, Pramesh CS, Heroor AA, et al: Inflammatory pseudotumor of the esophagus. Dis Esophagus 14:274-277, 2001.

82. Arber DA, Weiss LM, Chang KL: Detection of Ebstein-Barr virus in inflammatory pseudotumor. Semin Diagn Pathol 15:155-160, 1998.

83. Arber DA, Van Kamel OW, et al: Frequent presence of Epstein-Barr virus in inflammatory pseudotumor. Hum Pathol 26:1093-1098, 1995.

84. Selves J, Meggetto F, Brousset P, et al: Inflammatory pseudotumor of the liver: Evidence for follicular dendritic reticulum cell proliferation associated with clonal Epstein-Barr virus. Am J Surg Pathol 20:747-753, 1996.

85. Mombaerts I, Schlingemann RO, Goldschmeding R, et al: Are systemic corticosteroids useful in the management of orbital pseudotumors? Ophthalmology 103:521-528, 1996.

86. Jang GC, Clouse ME, Fleischner FG: Fibrovascular polyp—a benign intraluminal tumor of the esophagus. Radiology 92:1196-1200, 1969.

87. Ming S: Tumors of the esophagus and stomach. In Firminger HI (ed): Atlas of Tumor Pathology, second series, fascicle 7. Washington, DC, Armed Forces Institute of Pathology, 1971, p 68.

88. Levine MS, Buck JL, Pantongrag-Brown L, et al: Fibrovascular polyps of the esophagus: Clinical, radiographic, and pathologic findings in 16 patients. AJR Am J Roentgenol 166:781-787, 1996.

89. Weitzner S, Hentel W: Squamous papilloma of esophagus. Am J Gastroenterol 50:391-396, 1968.

90. Adler RH, Carberry DM, Ross CA: Papilloma of the esophagus. J Thorac Cardiovasc Surg 37:625-635, 1959.

91. Odze R, Antonioli D, Shocket D, et al: Esophageal squamous papillomas. A clinicopathologic study of 38 lesions and analysis for human papillomavirus by the polymerase chain reaction. Am J Surg Pathol 17:803-812, 1993.

92. Politoske EJ: Squamous papilloma of the esophagus associated with the human papillomavirus. Gastroenterology 102:668-673, 1992.

93. Poljak M, Orlowska J, Cerar A: Human papillomavirus infection in esophageal squamous cell papillomas: A study of 29 lesions. Anticancer Res 15:965-969, 1995.

94. Carr NJ, Bratthauer GL, Lichy JH, et al: Squamous cell papillomas of the esophagus: A study of 23 lesions for human papillomavirus by in situ hybridization and the polymerase chain reaction. Hum Pathol 25:536-540, 1994.

95. Mosca S, Manes G, Monaco R, et al: Squamous papilloma of the esophagus: Long-term follow up. J. Gastroenterol Hepatol 16:857-861, 2001.

96. Van Cutsem E, Geboes K, Vantrappen G, et al: Malignant degeneration of esophageal squamous papilloma associated with the human papilloma virus. Gastroenterology 103:1119-1120, 1992.

97. Hording M, Hording U, Daugaard S, et al: Human papilloma virus type 11 in a fatal case of esophageal and bronchial papillomatosis. Scand J Infect Dis 21:229-231, 1989.

98. Whitaker J, Deffenbaugh L, Cooke A: Esophageal duplication cyst. Am J Gastroenterol 73:329-332, 1980.

99. Arbona JL, Fazzi GF, Mayoral J: Congenital esophageal cysts: Case report and review of the literature. Am J Gastroenterol 79:177-182, 1984.

100. Hutchinson J, Thomson JD: Congenital archenteric cysts. Br J Surg 41:15, 1953.

101. Kolomainen D, Hurley PR, Ebbs SR: Esophageal duplication cyst: Case report and review of the literature. Dis Esophagus 11:62-65, 1998.

102. Singh S, Lal P, Sikora SS, et al: Squamous cell carcinoma arising from a congenital duplication cyst of the esophagus in a young adult. Dis Esophagus 14:258-261, 2001.

103. Tarnay TJ, Chang CH, Migert RG, et al: Esophageal duplication (foregut cyst) with spinal malformation. J Thorac Cardiovasc Surg 59:293-298, 1970.

104. Cioffi U, Bonavina L, De Simone M, et al: Presentation and surgical management of bronchogenic and esophageal duplication cysts in adults. Chest 113:1492-1496, 1998.

105. Neo EL, Watson DI, Bessell JR: Acute ruptured esophageal duplication cyst. Dis Esophagus 17:109-111, 2004.

106. Bondestam S, Salo JA, Salonen OLM, et al: Imaging of congenital esophageal cysts in adults. Gastrointest Radiol 15:279-281, 1990.

107. Rafal RB, Markisz JA: Magnetic resonance imaging of an esophageal duplication cyst. Am J Gastroenterol 86:1809-1811, 1991.

108. Noguchi R, Hashimoto T, Takeno S, et al: Laparoscopic resection of esophageal duplication cyst in an adult. Dis Esophagus 16:148-150, 2003.

38

Perforation of the Esophagus

Dennis Blom

Perforation of the esophagus remains a highly lethal condition that constitutes a true surgical emergency. Successful management demands immediate diagnosis, sound clinical judgment, and institution of appropriate therapies.

The majority of perforations are iatrogenic and caused by instrumental rupture during diagnostic or therapeutic procedures. Spontaneous perforation, often referred to as Boerhaave's syndrome, is the etiologic cause in only 15% of such patients. Less common causes include penetration of the esophageal wall by a swallowed foreign body or trauma.[1] Pain is a striking and consistent symptom and strongly suggests that an esophageal rupture has occurred, particularly if located in the cervical area after instrumentation of the esophagus or in a substernal location in a patient with a history of recent vomiting. When subcutaneous emphysema is also present, the diagnosis is almost certain. The outcome of an esophageal perforation depends on four factors: (1) the cause and location of the perforation, (2) the underlying esophageal disorder, (3) the interval to diagnosis and treatment, and (4) patient comorbid conditions.

HISTORICAL BACKGROUND

In 1724, Hermann Boerhaave, a Dutch physician and one of Europe's leading physicians of the time, published the first description of spontaneous rupture of the esophagus after performing an autopsy on Barron van Wassenaer, the Grand Admiral of the Dutch navy. The admiral suffered from indigestion after large meals and often ingested emetics to induce vomiting for relief. The vivid description of his symptoms gives a lasting impression of the pain induced by spontaneous esophageal rupture: "But while he was sitting upon a chair trying to vomit, even though he did not feel any illness thus far, he suddenly gave forth a horrifying cry at which all the servants ran and they heard him complaining that something near the upper end of his stomach was ruptured, torn, or dislocated." He suggested that the pain was such that "in the most certain and vivid manner, death was coming and inevitable." He died within 24 hours. Boerhaave's autopsy demonstrated rupture of the lower third of the esophagus with free perforation into both pleural cavities. Boerhaave stated, "When it recurs again it can be recognized with the help of this description but cannot be remedied by the assistance from the medical profession." This statement was true for over 200 years, until the first successful repair of an esophageal perforation was reported separately by Barrett and by Olsen and Clagett in 1947.[2,3]

ETIOLOGY

The most common cause of esophageal perforation today is iatrogenic perforation secondary to medical instrumentation. In a comprehensive review of the literature, including 511 perforations, Jones and Ginsberg found that 43% were due to instrumentation of the esophagus, 19% were due to trauma, 16% were spontaneous, 8% were caused by operative injury, 7% were a result of foreign bodies, and 7% were due to tumors and other miscellaneous causes (Table 38–1).[1]

| Table 38–1 | Causes of Esophageal Perforation in 511 Patients in the Literature |

Cause	Percent
Instrumentation	43
Trauma	19
Spontaneous	16
Surgical	8
Foreign bodies	7
Tumor	4
Other	3

From Jones WG, Ginsberg R: Esophageal perforation: A continuing challenge. Ann Thorac Surg 53:534, 1992.

Diagnostic flexible esophagogastroduodenoscopy is a common procedure that is associated with low morbidity and mortality. A survey of more than 14,000 flexible endoscopies in England revealed a 0.05% incidence of perforation and a 0.008% mortality rate.[4] Rigid endoscopy carries a higher risk (0.8% to 1.1%).[5] An American Society of Gastrointestinal Endoscopy survey estimated an overall esophageal perforation rate after flexible upper endoscopy of 0.03% with an associated mortality of 0.001%.[6] The incidence increased to 0.4% after bougienage and 0.3% after pneumatic balloon dilatation. The incidence of perforation also increased to 4% when dilatation is performed for the treatment of achalasia and to 10% with dilatation of malignant strictures.[7,8] Endoscopic thermal therapy for gastrointestinal bleeding is associated with a 1% to 2% incidence of esophageal perforation, whereas palliative ablative procedures are associated with a 5% incidence and esophageal stents with a 5% to 25% incidence.[9,10] When perforation occurs secondary to diagnostic endoscopy, it is usually at the cricopharyngeus muscle; however, when therapeutic dilatation is performed, the location of the perforation is generally at or just proximal to the esophageal stenosis.

Spontaneous rupture, regardless of the cause (vomiting, weightlifting, excessive coughing, Heimlich maneuver, seizures, defecation, child birth), is secondary to the barotrauma associated with a sudden increase in intra-abdominal pressure.[11] If the upper esophageal sphincter fails to relax, this sudden increase in intra-abdominal pressure, frequently exceeding 200 mm Hg, can be completely transmitted into the thoracic esophagus, usually through a defective intrathoracic lower esophageal sphincter. Fifty percent of patients have concomitant gastroesophageal reflux disease, thus suggesting that decreased resistance to the transmission of abdominal pressure into the thoracic esophagus is a factor in the pathophysiology of the lesion. Because extragastric pressure remains almost equal to intragastric pressure, stretching of the gastric wall is minimal. The amount of pressure transmitted to the esophagus varies considerably, depending on the position of the gastroesophageal junction. When the gastroesophageal junction is in the abdomen and exposed to intra-abdominal pressure, the pressure transmitted to the esophagus is much less than when the junction is exposed to the negative thoracic pressure. In the latter situation, the lower esophageal pressure will frequently equal intragastric pressure if the glottis remains closed. Cadaver studies have shown that when this pressure exceeds 150 mm Hg, rupture of the esophagus is apt to occur. When a hiatal hernia is present and the sphincter remains exposed to abdominal pressure, the lesion produced is usually a Mallory-Weiss mucosal tear, and bleeding rather than perforation is the problem. This is due to stretching of the supradiaphragmatic portion of the gastric wall. In this situation the hernia sac represent an extension of the abdominal cavity, and the gastroesophageal junction remains exposed to abdominal pressure.

Trauma-related esophageal perforation is uncommon and may be categorized into blunt or penetrating injury. Perforation of the esophagus secondary to blunt trauma is rare (0.001%) and usually secondary to direct force or spinal fracture,[12] probably because of its posterior, well-protected location and the high lethality of these injuries when adjacent vital structures are also injured. Esophageal perforation as a result of blunt trauma most commonly occurs at the cervical esophagus and is often associated with other neck injuries.[13] Blunt trauma to the distal esophagus is exceedingly rare, with fewer than a dozen cases reported in the world literature.[14] Penetrating esophageal perforations caused by knife and missile injuries are more frequent than blunt perforation but are still relatively uncommon.[13] They too are almost always associated with other injuries and are often fatal.

Perforation of the esophagus can inadvertently occur during any esophageal, periesophageal, or gastric operation. Recently, laparoscopic foregut surgery has surged in popularity, and perforation during such surgery has been reported. Three mechanisms of injury accounted for a series of 17 gastric and esophageal laparoscopic perforations: improper retroesophageal dissection, passage of the bougie or nasogastric tube, and suture pull-through. Most injuries were repaired laparoscopically.[15]

Esophageal perforations secondary to the ingestion of foreign bodies most often occur at the normal acute angulations or physiologic narrowing of the esophagus, with the cricopharyngeus muscle being the most common location. Tumors, ingestion of caustic substances, retained pills, infections, severe peptic esophagitis, and Barrett's ulceration have all been reported as a cause of esophageal perforation.

CLINICAL FINDINGS

The clinical manifestation of esophageal perforation depends on three factors: (1) the location of the perforation, (2) the size of the perforation (i.e., the degree of surrounding contamination), and (3) the time elapsed since injury (i.e., the degree of surrounding inflammatory response, infection, and sepsis).

Patients with cervical esophageal perforation routinely complain of cervical pain, dysphagia, and odyno-

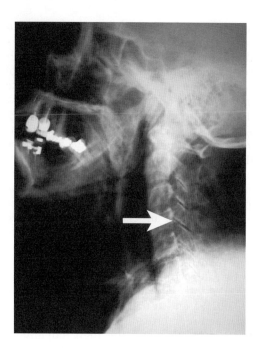

Figure 38–1. Chest roentgenogram showing air in the deep muscles of the neck after perforation of the esophagus *(arrow).* This is often the earliest sign of perforation and can be present without evidence of air in the mediastinum.

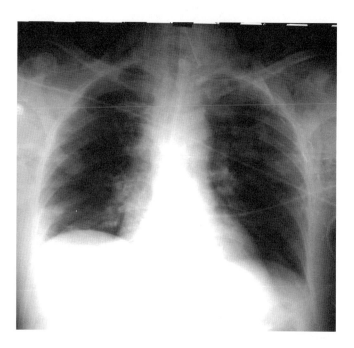

Figure 38–3. Chest radiograph of a patient with spontaneous thoracic esophageal perforation and subcutaneous emphysema.

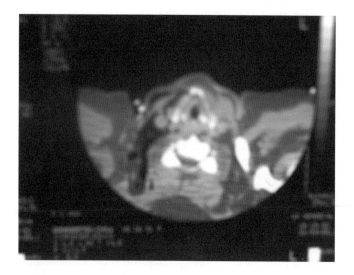

Figure 38–2. Computed tomography scan of a patient with a cervical perforation of the esophagus illustrating air in the deep muscle planes of the neck.

phagia. The pain is made worse by swallowing and movement, especially flexion of the neck. The neck is tender to examination, and crepitus is often noted. Fever usually develops early, and pleural effusions develop later, after 24 hours (Figs. 38–1 and 38–2).

Spontaneous rupture of the esophagus is often associated with a poor outcome and survival because of delay in recognition and treatment. Although there is gener-

ally a recent history of esophageal instrumentation, surgery, or vomiting, approximately 50% of patients have an atypical history, and in a small number of patients the injury occurs silently without any antecedent history. When the condition is visualized on a chest roentgenogram as air or an effusion in the pleural space, it is often misdiagnosed as pneumothorax or pancreatitis (Fig. 38–3). An elevated serum amylase level caused by extrusion of saliva through the perforation may fix the diagnosis of pancreatitis in the mind of an unwary physician. If the chest roentgenogram is normal, the diagnosis is often confused with myocardial infarction or a dissecting aneurysm.

Spontaneous rupture usually occurs on the left side of the distal esophagus into the left pleural cavity or just above the gastroesophageal junction. These patients are typically male (85%), 40 to 60 years of age, who have a history of recent emesis. Mackler's triad of thoracic pain, vomiting, and cervical subcutaneous emphysema is less reliable for the diagnosis of spontaneous esophageal perforation than once thought, and its absence should not exclude the diagnosis. Forty percent or more of patients will not exhibit this classic triad. Hematemesis is rare and, if present, is of small volume relative to the massive upper gastrointestinal bleeding associated with a Mallory-Weiss tear. Thoracic perforations cause substernal and epigastric pain. Mediastinal emphysema and pleural effusions are common, but early cervical subcutaneous emphysema is noted in only 20% or less of patients. Fever and sepsis develop with increasing contamination and inflammation of the mediastinum and pleural cavities. If left untreated, fulminant mediastinitis and hemorrhagic necrosis will develop and lead to an ever-increasing systemic inflammatory response, multiorgan failure, and cardiopulmonary collapse. Patients with an abdominal perforation have epigastric abdominal pain that is also often referred to the back and left shoulder; with time, signs of peritoneal irritation (rebound tenderness, muscle spasm, abdominal wall rigidity) and generalized peritonitis can develop.

DIAGNOSIS

Esophageal perforation, particularly spontaneous rupture of the esophagus, continues to be associated with poor survival because of the delay in recognition and treatment. The most important factor contributing to a delay in diagnosis is failure to consider esophageal perforation as a diagnostic possibility. All patients complaining of pain after endoscopy, especially if therapeutic dilatation was performed, should be suspected of having a perforation until proved otherwise. The diagnosis of Boerhaave's syndrome can be more elusive. The differential diagnosis includes perforated ulcer, acute pancreatitis, myocardial infarction, pneumonia, Mallory-Weiss tear, pneumothorax, dissecting aortic aneurysm, or incarcerated paraesophageal hernia. A careful history, physical examination, and appropriate laboratory tests should raise suspicion of esophageal perforation, exclude most of these incorrect diagnoses, and direct the clinician to the appropriate confirmatory radiologic studies.

Regardless of the cause, an urgent posteroanterior and lateral chest radiograph should be obtained. Abnormalities on the chest radiograph can be variable, depending on the time interval between the perforation and the roentgenographic examination, the site of the perforation, and the integrity of the mediastinal pleura (see Fig. 38–3). Mediastinal emphysema, a strong indicator of perforation, is present in only 40% of patients and usually takes at least 1 hour to develop. Mediastinal widening secondary to edema may not occur for several hours. Cervical emphysema is common with cervical perforation and mediastinal emphysema is rare; the converse is true for thoracic perforations. Frequently, air will be visible on a neck radiograph in the erector spinae muscles before it can be palpated or seen on a chest roentgenogram (see Fig. 38–1). The integrity of the mediastinal pleura influences the roentgenographic abnormality. Rupture of the pleura results in pneumothorax in 77% of patients. In approximately 70% of these patients the perforation is on the left side, 20% are right sided, and 10% are bilateral. If pleural integrity is maintained, mediastinal emphysema appears rapidly rather than pneumothorax. A pleural effusion secondary to inflammation of the mediastinum occurs late. In approximately 10% of patients the chest roentgenogram will remain normal.[16] The diagnosis is usually confirmed with a contrast esophagogram. This technique will demonstrate extravasation in 90% of patients (Fig. 38–4). The initial use of a water-soluble medium such as diatrizoate meglumine (Gastrografin) is preferred to prevent extravasation of barium into the mediastinum or pleura. If no leak is seen, a barium study should follow. Patients at high risk for aspiration should have a barium esopha-

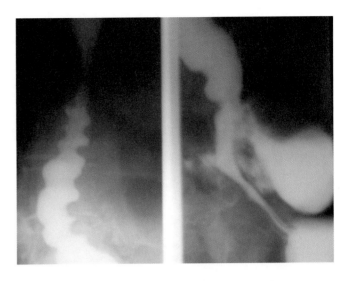

Figure 38–4. Roentgenographic study using water-soluble contrast material in a patient with a perforation of the esophagus. The patient is placed in the lateral decubitus position with the left side up to allow complete filling of the esophagus and demonstration of the defect.

gogram as their first study because of the risk for pulmonary edema from water-soluble contrast. Of concern is the reported 10% false-negative rate, which may be due to performing the roentgenographic study with the patient in the upright position. When upright, the passage of water-soluble contrast material can be too rapid to demonstrate a small perforation. The studies should be done with the patient in the right lateral decubitus position with water-soluble contrast followed by barium (see Fig. 38–4). In this position the contrast material fills the whole length of the esophagus, thereby allowing the site of perforation and its interconnecting cavities to be illustrated. One should not hesitate to repeat the radiographic evaluation if clinical suspicion remains high for perforation despite a negative work-up originally.

Computed tomography (CT) and esophagoscopy are also useful in complicated, equivocal cases or when an esophagogram is unavailable.[17]

CT is often the first imaging modality used in patients with severe chest pain. Subtle findings such as mediastinal gas or fluid, esophageal thickening, or small pleural effusions may suggest the diagnosis of esophageal perforation. CT scanning may be particularly useful to rule out other pathologic changes and causes of chest pain, and its sensitivity can be increased with the use of dilute oral contrast (Fig. 38–5).[17]

Flexible esophagoscopy is generally underused because of fear of extending the injury. It can provide important information about the location and extent of injury, the presence of coexisting disease, and the condition of surrounding tissues. Risks should be minimal if performed by an experienced surgeon prepared to definitively manage the esophageal perforation, either nonoperatively (Fig. 38–6) or surgically.

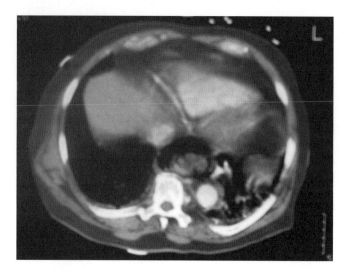

Figure 38–5. Abdominal computed tomography scan revealing mediastinal air and pneumothorax secondary to thoracic esophageal perforation.

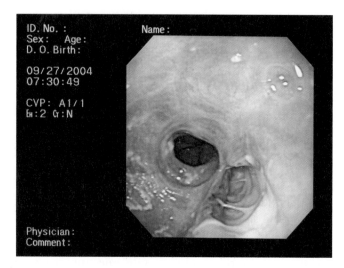

Figure 38–6. Esophagoscopy illustrating a large contained spontaneous esophageal perforation. The patient was successfully managed with nonoperative therapy.

MANAGEMENT OF ESOPHAGEAL PERFORATION

A tailored approach is critical to the successful management of esophageal perforation (Fig. 38–7). The outcome depends on the location of the perforation, the extent of tissue destruction, and the degree of inflammation and sepsis present, which is determined by the time interval between injury and initiation of treatment and the presence of underlying esophageal disorders. Treatment options include nonoperative therapy; periesophageal drainage alone; primary repair, with or without autologous tissue reinforcement;

esophageal resection; and exclusion and diversion in continuity.

Regardless of the treatment modality, the goals of treatment must include (1) prevention of continued contamination, (2) elimination and control of infection, (3) maintenance of the patient's nutritional status, and (4) restoration of the integrity and continuity of the alimentary tract.

Once esophageal perforation is suspected, immediate resuscitation should be initiated and consists of (1) discontinuation of all oral intake, (2) judicious placement of a nasogastric tube to decompress the stomach and decrease continued contamination, (3) aggressive intravenous volume support, and (4) broad-spectrum antibiotics with coverage of aerobic and anaerobic oral flora and fungi.

Nonoperative Therapy

Nonoperative management of esophageal perforation has been advocated and can be successful in select situations.[18-24] The choice of nonoperative therapy requires skillful and continuous clinical judgment and necessitates careful roentgenographic or endoscopic examination of the esophagus (or both).[10,11] This course of management usually follows a injury recognized during dilatation of esophageal strictures or pneumatic dilatation for achalasia or when there has been a significant delay in diagnosis with minimal symptoms and no signs of sepsis. Nonoperative management should not be used in patients who have free perforations into the pleural space or peritoneal cavity. Cameron and colleagues originally proposed criteria for nonoperative management of esophageal perforation in 1979, and they were updated by Altorjay et al. in 1997. These criteria include (1) intramural perforation; (2) transmural perforation that is not within the abdomen, is shown to be contained within the mediastinum, and drains well back into the esophagus; (3) perforation that is not associated with obstructive esophageal disease or malignancy; and (4) mild symptoms and minimal evidence of clinical sepsis.[18,19] If these conditions are met, it is reasonable to treat the patient with nothing by mouth, total parenteral nutrition, antibiotics, and intravenous proton pump inhibitors or H_2 receptor antagonists (or both) to inhibit acid secretion and diminish pepsin activity. Oral intake is resumed in 7 to 14 days, depending on subsequent roentgenographic findings. It is imperative that patients treated in this manner be continuously monitored and frequently reassessed for signs of physical deterioration. Operative intervention should be performed immediately if any of the criteria for continued nonoperative management are no longer met.[18,19]

Recently, the use of covered self-expandable stents has been reported for the conservative treatment of esophageal perforation in highly selected patients. Covered and self-expandable stents may be indicated and particularly useful in patients with extensive defects, in those with multiple comorbid conditions, and in the critically ill.[25-27]

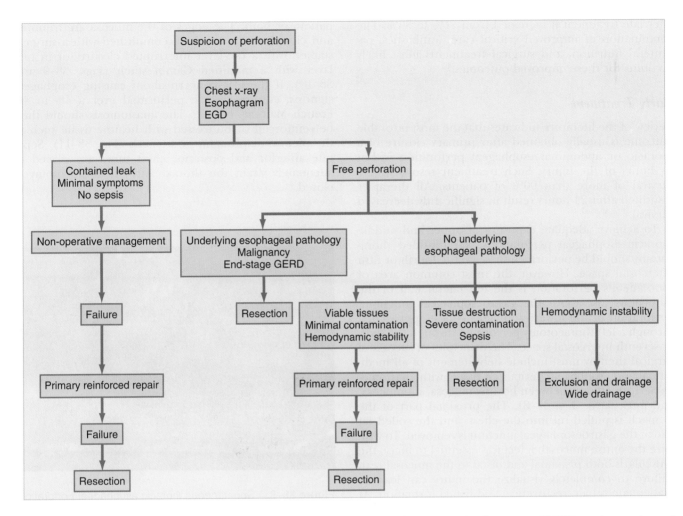

Figure 38–7.   Treatment algorithm for esophageal perforation. EGD, esophagogastroduodenoscopy; GERD, gastroesophageal reflux disease.

Surgical Management of Cervical Esophageal Perforation

Perforation of the cervical esophagus is seldom lethal. Most patients are candidates for cervical exploration and closure of the defect or drainage alone.[20,28-30] It is controversial whether closure offers any advantage over drainage alone.[1] In some instances, nonoperative approaches may suffice.[31]

Most cervical esophageal perforations can be surgically managed through a cervical approach using a longitudinal incision made along the anterior border of the left sternocleidomastoid muscle. The pharynx and cervical esophagus are exposed by retracting the sternocleidomastoid muscle and carotid sheath laterally and the thyroid and larynx medially. Routine division of the omohyoid, sternothyroid, and sternohyoid muscles gives ideal exposure. The middle thyroid vein and inferior thyroid arteries are identified and divided. The recurrent laryngeal nerve can be found as it courses in the tracheoesophageal groove, just anterior to the inferior thyroid artery. Retraction in this area is avoided. The esophagus is identified at the thoracic inlet as it overlies the spine

and is dissected circumferentially. The perforation is usually evident at this stage of the dissection. In the absence of severe inflammation, the perforation should be closed. A short myotomy is performed and the mucosal edges are trimmed. The mucosa is then approximated with interrupted sutures and the muscle layer closed separately. Placement of a closed suction drain and closure of the wound complete the procedure.

Surgical Management of Intrathoracic and Intra-abdominal Esophageal Perforations

The key to optimal management of a free thoracic or intra-abdominal esophageal perforation is not only early diagnosis but also immediate initiation of appropriate treatment. Recently, several investigators have documented a decline in mortality, both overall and in early and late treatment groups. Reeder et al. from the University of Chicago reported an overall survival rate of 91%, a 10% increase from the 81% reported a decade earlier from the same institution. The survival rate with early treatment improved from 91% to 95%, whereas after late treatment it increased from 71% to 86%. The combination of improved critical care, antibiotics, parenteral nutrition, and surgical treatments most likely accounts for these improved outcomes.[32]

Early Treatment

Review of the literature indicates that the most favorable outcome is usually obtained after primary closure of a thoracic or abdominal esophageal perforation within 24 hours of the injury. Such treatment results in the survival of more than 90% of patients. All therapies instituted after 24 hours result in significantly decreased survival.[20,28,30,33-37]

To achieve adequate exposure of upper and middle thoracic esophageal perforations, a right-sided thoracotomy should be performed through the fourth or fifth intercostal space. However, the most common area of spontaneous perforation is the left lateral wall of the esophagus just above the gastroesophageal junction.[1] Perforation of the lower esophagus is best approached through a left thoracotomy performed through the sixth or seventh intercostal space. The principles of successful surgical therapy must include débridement of all mediastinal and esophageal devitalized tissue, with anastomosis performed only between healthy mucosa, submucosa, and muscularis (Fig. 38–8). The proximal part of the stomach is pulled up into the chest, and the soiled fat pad at the gastroesophageal junction is removed. To visualize the entire mucosal defect it is essential to incise the muscularis both proximal and distal to the mucosal tear. Failure to completely visualize the injury can lead to inadequate repair, recurrence, and fistula formation. At this point, if nasogastric decompression has not been achieved, a tube can be placed under direct vision, pal-

pation, or both. The edges of the mucosa are trimmed and closed, which can be accomplished with a surgical stapler, with a two-layer interrupted closure, or in one layer with a modified Gambi stitch (Figs. 38–9 and 38–10). If there is concern about causing esophageal stenosis, closure can be performed over a 40- to 46-French Maloney bougie. The anastomosis should then be reinforced or buttressed with healthy tissue such as the pleura, diaphragm, or stomach (Fig. 38–11). Separate anterior and posterior chest tubes are placed to adequately drain the thorax, and the thoracotomy is closed.

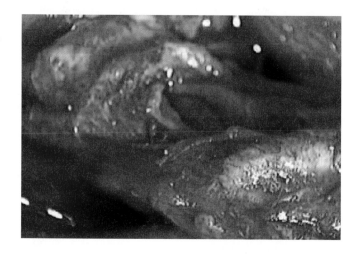

Figure 38–8. Spontaneous thoracic esophageal perforation. Notice the débridement to healthy tissue in preparation for closure.

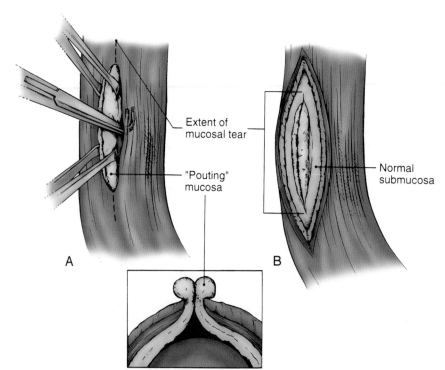

Extent of mucosal tear

"Pouting" mucosa

Normal submucosa

A

B

Figure 38–9. Primary repair of esophageal perforation illustrating exposure of the perforation. **A,** Extension of the muscular tear proximal and distal to the injury to allow complete exposure of the mucosal defect. The *inset* demonstrates the damaged pouting mucosa initially seen on inspection of the injury. **B,** Mobilization of the submucosa away from the muscular coat to allow exposure of the defect surrounded by normal submucosa and both the proximal and distal extent of the mucosal injury by extension of the muscular tear. (From Whyte RI, Iannettoni MD, Orringer MB: Intrathoracic esophageal perforation—the merit of primary repair. J Thorac Cardiovasc Surg 109:140, 1995.)

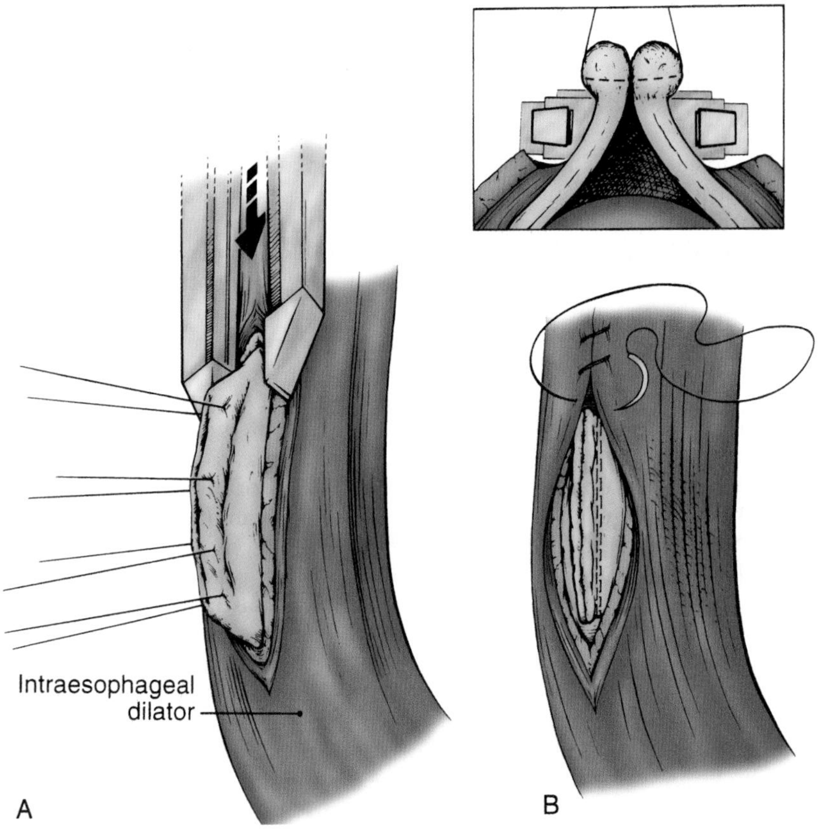

Figure 38–10.   Technique of primary repair of esophageal perforation illustrating **(A)** closure of the defect with a GIA surgical stapler after mobilization and exposure of the mucosal and submucosal tear beyond the muscular tear and **(B)** approximation of the muscular coat over the suture line with running absorbable suture. The stapler is applied over an intraesophageal bougie *(inset)* to healthy mucosa and submucosa, not to the inflamed edges of the defect. (From Whyte RI, Iannettoni MD, Orringer MB: Intrathoracic esophageal perforation—the merit of primary repair. J Thorac Cardiovasc Surg 109:140, 1995.)

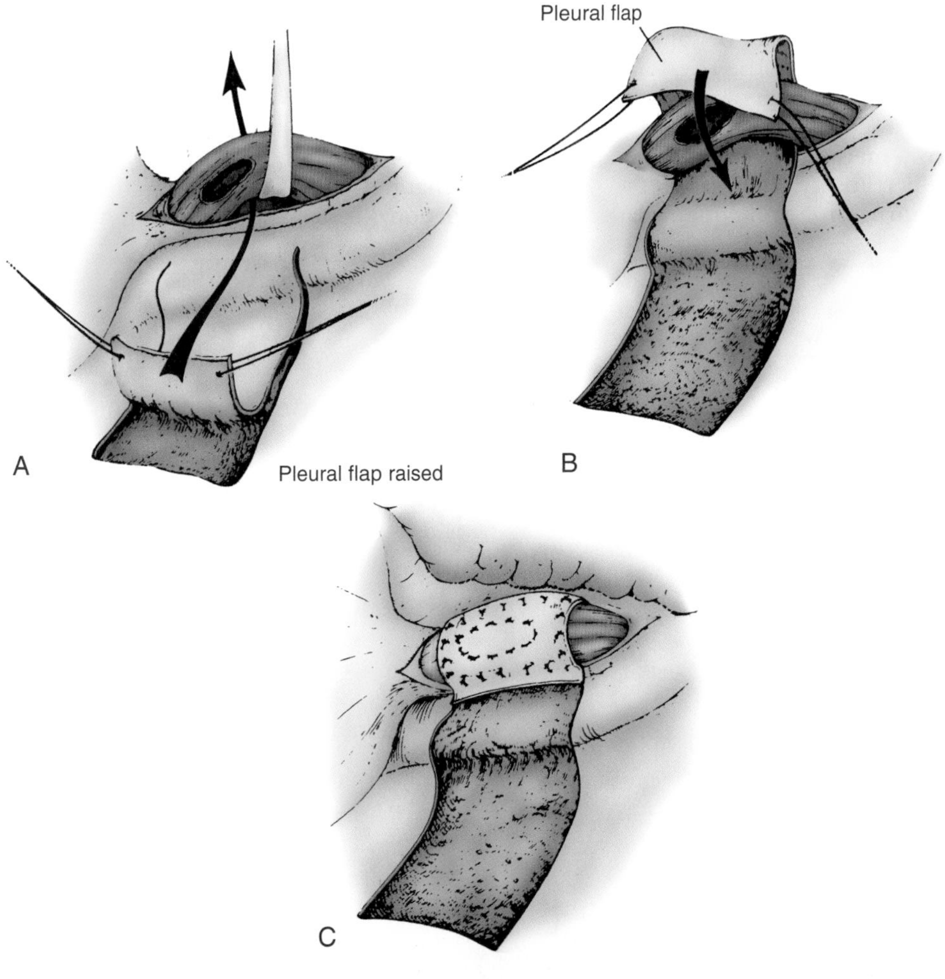

Intraesophageal dilator

A

B

Figure 38–11.   Pleural flap patch closure of a large esophageal defect. **A,** After mobilization of the esophagus, a pleural flap is raised. **B,** The flap is placed around the esophagus so that it covers the perforation. **C,** The flap is sutured to itself. Sutures are placed above and below at the margins of the flap as well as the perforation itself to tack the pleura firmly to the esophageal muscularis. (From Gricco HC, Wilkins FW: Esophageal repair following late diagnosis of intrathoracic perforation. Ann Thorac Cardiovasc Surg 20:337, 1975, by permission of The Society of Thoracic Surgeons.)

Pleural flap

Pleural flap raised

A

B

C

Late Treatment

Esophageal perforation with late or delayed diagnosis/ treatment results in increased mediastinal contamination, inflammation, tissue destruction, and hemodynamic instability. These factors make primary repair more difficult and prone to failure. A primary reinforced repair remains the procedure of choice, regardless of the time interval between injury and repair, if the principles previously described can be followed.[38] In the setting of extensive esophageal damage, mediastinitis, or severe underlying esophageal disease, esophagectomy is the best option.

Salo et al. reviewed 34 patients with esophageal perforations greater than 24 hours old. Nineteen of these patients underwent primary repair with drainage and 15 underwent primary esophagectomy. Hospital mortality was 68% in the group treated by closure and drainage and 13% in patients after esophagectomy. They concluded that esophagectomy is superior to primary repair in the setting of esophageal perforation with mediastinal sepsis.[39]

Esophagectomy can be accomplished through either a transhiatal or a transthoracic approach. The contaminated mediastinum is widely drained with closed suction drainage or chest tubes (or both). A gastrostomy and feeding jejunostomy are created for decompression and enteral nutrition. As much normal esophagus as possible should be saved before performing a cervical esophagostomy. In some situations the retained esophagus may be so long that it can be tunneled subcutaneously to exit on the anterior of the chest and saved for later reconstitution of alimentary tract continuity (Fig. 38–12). Recovery from sepsis is often immediate and dramatic as reflected by a marked change in the patient's course in 24 hours. On recovery from sepsis the patient is discharged and returns on a subsequent date for reconstruction with a substernal gastric or colonic interposition.[40] Failure to apply such aggressive therapy can result in mortality in excess of 50% in patients in whom the diagnosis has been delayed.[41]

In patients deemed unsuitable for resection because of hemodynamic instability and sepsis, an esophageal exclusion and diversion procedure with wide drainage of the mediastinum, stapled or ligated occlusion of the lower esophagus, and the formation of a cervical esophagostomy is preferred and can be performed quickly (Fig. 38–13). Gastrostomy and feeding jejunostomy may or may not be performed again, depending on the situation.[42-44]

In extreme cases, control of the esophageal fistula with a Silastic drain or T-tube and wide pleural drainage alone may be necessary.[45-46]

A free intra-abdominal esophageal perforation can lead to peritoneal contamination, peritonitis, and sepsis. However, if recognized early, abdominal perforation is associated with an excellent prognosis. The principles of repair are the same as for thoracic perforations, except that access may be gained through a celiotomy. The contaminated cavity (mediastinum, abdomen) is widely drained, and the injury is débrided, exposed, closed, and buttressed with a fundoplication or omental graft (Figs. 38–14 to 38–16). Enteral access by gastrostomy, tube jejunostomy, or both may also be performed.[47]

Esophageal perforation that occurs during laparoscopic foregut procedures and is recognized intraoperatively can be successfully repaired by primary closure and reinforcement with excellent outcomes. Schauer et al. reported 0% mortality, 0% postoperative leaks, and a mean hospital stay of 4.5 days in their patients who experienced a laparoscopic perforation recognized and repaired at the initial procedure. On short-term follow-up these patients reported no dysphagia or recurrence of their reflux symptoms. This outcome is in contrast to

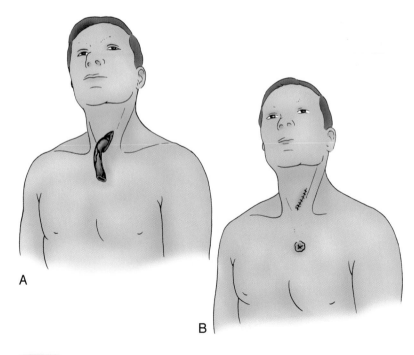

Figure 38–12. Construction of an anterior thoracic esophagostomy to preserve maximal length of esophagus. **A,** The mobilized thoracic esophagus is placed on the anterior chest wall to determine the location of the stoma. **B,** The esophagus is then tunneled subcutaneously and the esophagostomy is constructed. Stomal appliances are easily applied to the flat surface of the chest, and the additional esophageal length provided by the technique often facilitates later reconstruction. (From Orringer MB: Complications of esophageal surgery and trauma. In Greenfield LJ [ed]: Complications in Surgery and Trauma. Philadelphia, JB Lippincott, 1984, with permission.)

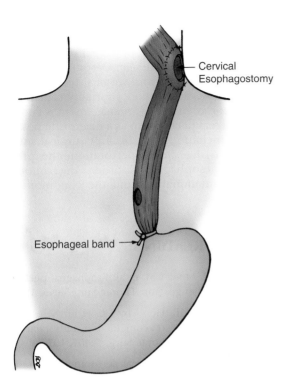

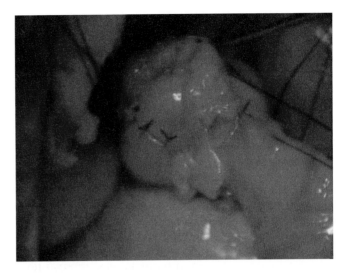

Figure 38–15. Perforation seen in Figure 38–14 after primary closure in two layers.

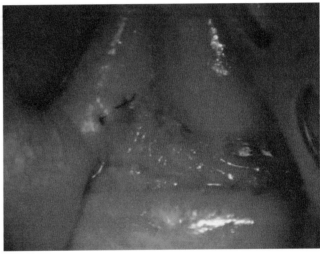

Figure 38–16. Repair of the perforation in Figure 38–14 after reinforcement of the closure with an omental graft.

Figure 38–13. Technique of esophageal exclusion. A side cervical esophagostomy diverts oral secretions. Reflux of gastric and biliary secretions is prevented by umbilical tape tied at the gastroesophageal junction. The tape is tied tightly enough to obstruct the lumen but not tight enough to cause mural ischemia. The vagus nerves are not included in the tie but lie superficial to it. (From Brewer LA III, Carter R, Mulder GA, Styles QR: Options in the management of perforations of the esophagus. Am J Surg 152:62, 1986.)

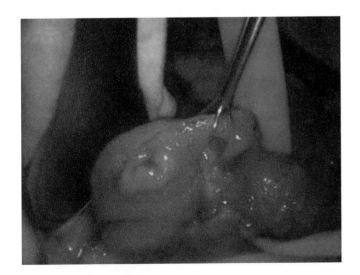

Figure 38–14. Perforation secondary to dilation, just below the gastroesophageal junction, in a patient with a hiatal hernia and esophageal stricture.

a 17% mortality in patients with a delayed diagnosis. Laparoscopic or thoracoscopic repair of these perforations can be achieved with good results, depending on the location of the perforation and the laparoscopic skill of the surgeon.[15] However, conversion to open repair is recommended in the majority of these cases, given the unforgiving nature of the esophageal wall, and should always be considered wise surgical judgment.

PERFORATION ASSOCIATED WITH ESOPHAGEAL DISEASE

Primary repair of an esophageal perforation in a patient with preexisting esophageal disease is often much more complex and can carry a much worse prognosis. Pathologic change that leads to distal esophageal obstruction will invariably lead to failure of a primary esophageal repair for perforation. It is therefore mandatory that the preexisting esophageal disorder be remedied at the same time as the perforation.[30,48,49]

Management of Esophageal Perforation After Dilation Therapy for Achalasia

Perforation of the esophagus after pneumatic dilatation for idiopathic motor disorders, specifically achalasia, requires special consideration, with treatment directed at both the perforation and the underlying esophageal disorder. For perforations that are contained within a localized region of the mediastinum and associated with minimal signs and symptoms, an initial course of non-operative therapy is warranted as previously discussed. Free perforations require prompt surgical intervention. Again, the surgical principles discussed in previous sections apply: (1) prevention of continued contamination, (2) elimination and control of infection, (3) maintenance of the patient's nutritional status, and (4) restoration of the integrity and continuity of the alimentary tract. The procedure is usually performed via a left thoracotomy. The mucosal edges are débrided and the mucosa closed with interrupted suture. Importantly, a myotomy that extends 2 to 3 cm distal to the gastro-esophageal junction on the gastric cardia and 3 to 4 cm proximal onto the body of the esophagus must be performed on the side opposite the perforation. The repair is then buttressed with a partial fundoplication such as a Dor, Thal patch, or Belsey Mark IV. Given prompt diagnosis and definitive treatment of the underlying esophageal motility disorder, the results of primary repair for esophageal perforation are excellent.

End-Stage Gastroesophageal Reflux, Intractable Strictures, Dysmotility, and Malignancy

In the situation of esophageal perforation associated with gastroesophageal reflux, intractable strictures, severe dysmotility (such as end-stage achalasia with esophageal tortuosity), caustic strictures, extensive devitalized tissue, or malignancy, esophageal resection is the procedure of choice. Primary repair, in this setting, often leads to decreased survival and increased subsequent morbidity when compared with primary resection.[28,36,48] Iannettoni et al. from the University of Michigan reported on the poor functional outcomes of 25 patients treated by primary repair for esophageal perforation in the presence of severe esophageal disease or strictures. Thirteen of these patients required at least one further operative treatment, and at least a third of the patients experienced chronic dysphagia requiring repeated dilatation or resection and reconstruction.[50] Esophageal resection can again be performed via a transthoracic or transhiatal approach. In a properly selected, stable patient, immediate reconstruction with a gastric graft and cervical esophagogastric anastomosis is possible and results in an excellent outcome.[51-53]

SUMMARY

Successful management of esophageal perforation continues to be a clinical challenge. Despite improvements in diagnostic, supportive, and surgical techniques since Boerhaave's classic description, mortality remains high. The most important aspect of management is consideration of esophageal perforation as a diagnostic possibility, aggressive resuscitation, and prompt surgical intervention tailored to the site of perforation, the presence of underlying esophageal disorder, the amount of surrounding contamination, and the condition of the patient.

SUGGESTED READINGS

Attar S, Hankins JR, Suter CM, et al: Esophageal perforation: A therapeutic challenge. Ann Thorac Surg 50:45, 1990.

Cameron JL, Kieffer HF, Hendrix TR, et al: Selective non-operative management of contained intrathoracic esophageal disruptions. Ann Thorac Surg 27:404, 1979.

Jones WG, Ginsberg R: Esophageal perforation: A continuing challenge. Ann Thorac Surg 53:534, 1992.

Reeder LB, Defilippi VJ, Ferguson MK: Current results of therapy for esophageal perforation. Am J Surg 169:615, 1995.

Salo JA, Isolauri JO, Heikkila LJ, et al: Management of delayed esophageal perforation with mediastinal sepsis—esophagectomy or primary repair? J Thorac Cardiovasc Surg 106:1088, 1993.

REFERENCES

1. Jones WG, Ginsberg R: Esophageal perforation: A continuing challenge. Ann Thorac Surg 53:534, 1992.
2. Barrett NR: Report of a case of spontaneous perforation of the esophagus successfully treated by operation. Br J Surg 35:216, 1947.
3. Olsen AM, Clagett OT: Spontaneous rupture of the esophagus: Report of a case with immediate diagnosis and successful surgical repair. Postgrad Med J 2:417, 1947.
4. Quine MA, Bell GD, McCloy RF, et al: Prospective audit of perforation rates following upper gastrointestinal endoscopy in two regions of England. Br J Surg 82:530, 1995.
5. Radmark T, Sandberg N, Pettersson G: Instrumental perforation of the oesophagus. A ten year study from two ENT clinics. J Laryngol Otol 100:461, 1986.
6. Silvis SE, Nebel O, Rogers G, et al: Endoscopic complications. Results of the 1974 American Society for Gastrointestinal Endoscopy Survey. JAMA 235:928, 1976.
7. Eckardt VF, Kanzler G, Westermeier T: Complications and their impact after pneumatic dilation for achalasia: Prospective long-term follow up study. Gastrointest Endosc 45:349, 1997.
8. Anderson PE, Cook A, Amery AH: A review of the practice of fiberoptic endoscopic dilatation of oesophageal stricture. Ann R Coll Surg Engl 71:124, 1989.
9. Jensen DM: Endoscopic control of nonvariceal upper gastrointestinal hemorrhage. In Yamada T, Alpers DH, Laine L, et al (eds): Textbook of Gastroenterology. Philadelphia, Lippincott Williams & Wilkins, 1999, p 2857.
10. Newcomer MK, Brazer SR: Complications of upper gastrointestinal endoscopy and their management. Gastrointest Endosc Clin N Am 4:551, 1994.
11. Tesler MA, Eisenberg MM: Spontaneous esophageal rupture. Int Abstr Surg 117:1, 1963.

12. Ketai L, Brandt MM, Schermer C: Nonaortic mediastinal injuries from blunt chest trauma. J Thorac Imaging 15:120, 2000.
13. Glatterer MS Jr, Toon RS, Ellestad C, et al: Management of blunt and penetrating external esophageal trauma. J Trauma 25:784, 1985.
14. Cordero JA, Kuehler DH, Fortune JB: Distal esophageal rupture after external blunt trauma: Report of two cases. J Trauma Injury Infect Crit Care 42:321, 1997.
15. Schauer PR, Meyers WC, Eubanks S, et al: Mechanisms of gastric and esophageal perforations during laparoscopic Nissen fundoplication. Ann Surg 223:43, 1996.
16. DeMeester TR: Perforation of the esophagus. Ann Thorac Surg 42:231, 1986.
17. Fadoo F, Ruiz DE, Dawn SK, et al: Helical CT esophagography for the evaluation of suspected esophageal perforation or rupture. AJR Am J Roentgenol 182:1177, 2004.
18. Cameron JL, Kieffer HF, Hendrix TR, et al: Selective non-operative management of contained intrathoracic esophageal disruptions. Ann Thorac Surg 27:404, 1979.
19. Altorjay A, Kiss J, Voros A, Bohak A: Nonoperative management of esophageal perforation—is it justified? Ann Surg 225:415, 1997.
20. Michel L, Grillo HC, Malt RA: Operative and nonoperative management of esophageal perforations. Ann Surg 194:57, 1981.
21. Lyons WS, Seremetis MG, deGuzman VC, et al: Ruptures and perforations of the esophagus: The case for conservative supportive management. Ann Thorac Surg 25:346, 1978.
22. Maroney TP, Ruiz EJ, Gordon RL, Pelligrini CA: Role of interventional radiology in the management of esophageal leaks. Radiology 170:1055, 1989.
23. Brown RH, Cohen PS: Nonsurgical management of spontaneous esophageal perforation. JAMA 240:140, 1978.
24. Mengold LR, Klassen KP: Conservative management of esophageal perforation. Arch Surg 91:232, 1965.
25. Gelbmann CM, Ratiu NL, Rath HC, et al: Use of self-expandable plastic stents for the treatment of esophageal perforations and symptomatic anastomotic leaks. Endoscopy 36:695, 2004.
26. White RE, Mungatana C, Topazian M: Expandable stents for iatrogenic perforation of esophageal malignancies. J Gastrointest Surg 7:715, 2003.
27. Mumtaz H, Barone GW, Beverly L, et al: Successful management of a nonmalignant esophageal perforation with a coated stent. Ann Thorac Surg 74:1233, 2002.
28. Brewer LA III, Carter R, Mulder GA, Styles QR: Options in the management of perforations of the esophagus. Am J Surg 152:62, 1986.
29. Loop FD, Groves LK: Esophageal perforations. Ann Thorac Surg 10:571, 1970.
30. Michel L, Grillo HC, Malt RA: Esophageal perforation. Ann Thorac Surg 33:203, 1982.
31. Tilanus HW, Bossuyt P, Schattenkerk ME, et al: Treatment of oesophageal perforation: A multivariate analysis Br J Surg 78:582, 1991.
32. Reeder LB, Defilippi VJ, Ferguson MK: Current results of therapy for esophageal perforation. Am J Surg 169:615, 1995.
33. Nesbitt JC, Sawyers JL: Surgical management of esophageal perforation. Am Surg 53:183, 1987.
34. Safavi A, Wang N, Razzouk A, et al: One-stage primary repair of distal esophageal perforation using fundic wrap. Am Surg 61:919, 1995.
35. Skinner DB, Little AG, DeMeester TR: Management of esophageal perforation. Am J Surg 139:760, 1980.
36. Ajalat GM, Mulder DG: Esophageal perforations: The need for an individualized approach. Arch Surg 119:1318, 1984.
37. Bladergroen MR, Lowe JE, Postlethwait RW: Diagnosis and recommended management of esophageal perforation and rupture. Am Thorac Surg 43:235, 1986.
38. Whyte RI, Iannettoni MD, Orringer MB: Intrathoracic esophageal perforation—the merit of primary repair. J Thorac Cardiovasc Surg 109:140, 1995.
39. Salo JA, Isolauri JO, Heikkila LJ, et al: Management of delayed esophageal perforation with mediastinal sepsis—esophagectomy or primary repair? J Thorac Cardiovasc Surg 106:1088, 1993.
40. Barkley C, Orringer MB, Iannettoni MD, Yee J: Challenges in reversing esophageal discontinuity operations. Ann Thorac Surg 76:989, 2003.
41. Attar S, Hankins JR, Suter CM, et al: Esophageal perforation: A therapeutic challenge. Ann Thorac Surg 50:45, 1990.
42. Urschel HC, Razzuk MA, Wood RE, et al: Improved management of esophageal perforation: Exclusion and diversion in continuity. Ann Surg 179:587, 1974.
43. Menguy R: Near-total exclusion by cervical esophagostomy and tube gastrostomy in the management of massive esophageal perforation. Report of a case. Ann Surg 173:613, 1971.
44. Laden DA, Dunnington GL, Rappaport WD: Stapled esophageal exclusion in acute esophageal rupture: A new technique. Contemp Surg 35:45, 1989.
45. Abbott OH, Mansour KA, Logan WD, et al: A traumatic so-called "spontaneous" rupture of the esophagus: A review of 47 personal cases with comments on a new method of surgical therapy. J Thorac Cardiovasc Surg 59:67, 1970.
46. Bufkin BL, Miller JI, Mansour KA: Esophageal perforation: Emphasis on management. Ann Thorac Surg 61:1447, 1996.
47. Berne CJ, Shader AE, Doty DB: Treatment of effort rupture of the esophagus by epigastric celiotomy. Surg Gynecol Obstet 129:277, 1969.
48. Larsson S, Pettersson G: Advisability of concomitant immediate surgery for perforations and underlying disease of the esophagus. Scand J Thorac Cardiovasc Surg 18:275, 1984.
49. Sarr MG, Pemberton JH, Payne WS: Management of instrumental perforations of the esophagus. J Thorac Cardiovasc Surg 84:211, 1982.
50. Iannettoni MD, Vlessis AA, Whyte RI, Orringer MB: Functional outcome after surgical treatment of esophageal perforation. Ann Thorac Surg 64:1606, 1997.
51. Altorjay A, Kiss J, Voros A, et al: The role of esophagectomy in the management of esophageal perforations. Ann Thorac Surg 65:1433, 1998.
52. Gupta NM: Emergency transhiatal oesophagectomy for instrumental perforation of an obstructed thoracic oesophagus. Br J Surg 83:1007, 1996.
53. Orringer MB, Stirling MC: Esophagectomy for esophageal disruption. Ann Thorac Surg 49:35, 1990.

Esophageal Caustic Injury

Peter F. Crookes

It was simple fire in a liquid form.

Mark Twain, *Tom Sawyer*, Chapter 12

HISTORY OF CAUSTIC INGESTION

Ingestion of poison either accidentally or with suicidal or homicidal intent has been known to humanity for thousands of years. The locally damaging effect of caustics or corrosives on the foregut has been also known for a long time.[1] Shakespeare records how Portia, the wife of Brutus, committed suicide by ingesting fire.[2] For the past 100 years two major subgroups of patients have continued to challenge health care agencies after caustic ingestion: children, who ingest caustic agents accidentally, and adults, who ingest them with suicidal intent. Accidental ingestion also occurs in adults and is more common in retarded or intoxicated individuals.

Children are at risk because cleaning materials, the most common toxic agents, are by convention kept in a cupboard beneath the kitchen sink. Toddlers who are unable to reach higher cupboards have easy access to these materials. It was a particular problem in the past because they were frequently kept in bottles resembling lemonade containers. The natural curiosity of children, combined with a proclivity to eat or drink anything in sight, made this a serious hazard. In the past 80 years, passionate lobbying has brought about federally mandated changes in the labeling and packaging of these materials by requiring them to be dispensed in characteristically shaped containers with childproof lids, as well as reducing their toxicity. However, the range of potentially injurious substances in a typical kitchen remains very large. The overall effect of these social changes has nevertheless been a significant reduction in the incidence and severity of accidental caustic ingestion in the United States, with the secondary consequence that most modern information now comes from countries where legislation is less restrictive, such as Turkey, India, France, and Eastern Europe.

Suicidal ingestion of caustic agents has also decreased in severity in the United States. As a mechanism of attempted suicide, caustic ingestion lags far behind ingestion of medications, gunshot wounds, leaping from a height, and hanging. However, in other cultures where firearms and pharmaceuticals are less readily available, caustic ingestion remains a significant social problem. The spectrum of ingested substances is a function of availability. In the Netherlands, for example, glacial acetic acid is commonly used by the Indonesian population. Within that community, suicidal ingestion of glacial acetic acid is frequent, with a high rate of complications and mortality.[3] In India, hydrochloric acid is widely used as a cheap toilet cleaner and is the agent most frequently swallowed in suicide attempts.[4] In the United States, glacial acetic acid and concentrated hydrochloric acid are not readily available, and cleaning agents are the most frequent caustic substances swallowed. The Toxic Exposure Surveillance System reported a total of 211,077 cleaning agent exposure incidents during 2003, of which exposure to hypochlorite (bleach) vastly outnumbered all other agents, with only one fatality reported in more than 52,000 exposures.[5]

PATHOPHYSIOLOGY

The injury inflicted by swallowed caustic substances is related to the nature of the agent and the amount swallowed. Accidental ingestion is associated with the consumption of lesser quantities because after the first gulp the patient will expectorate or try to dilute the agent, whereas in a deliberate suicide attempt, the initial revulsion and discomfort are ignored. Furthermore, in suicidal ingestions the patient may be socially isolated at the time and may delay seeking medical attention. In general, caustic alkali causes more profound injury than acid does because acid produces coagulative necrosis, which acts as a kind of barrier to limit deeper levels of injury, whereas alkali tends to cause liquefactive necrosis, thereby allowing deeper penetration.[6,7]

Phases of Injury

The initial contact with the toxic agent on the mucosa causes inflammation, which if severe leads to necrosis in the first 24 hours. Experimental studies have shown that severe transmural injury can develop after exposure to strong alkali (pH > 12) for even 1 second.[7-9] Thus, although the final outcome is very dependent on access to timely and expert medical treatment, the extent of injury is determined within a very short time of ingestion. Extensive thrombosis of submucosal vessels is observable at 48 hours, with inevitable necrosis of the mucosa. Although acid materials may produce an eschar that limits esophageal damage, they tend to induce pylorospasm and as a result lead to more severe gastric damage with the development of antropyloric strictures. Acid appears to be the causative agent in most cases of gastric stricture after caustic ingestion.

Purely esophageal damage is deeper with strong alkali agents. In the second and third week, granulation tissue begins to replace the necrotic slough, and the process of stricturing begins. It is in the period 4 to 14 days after injury when the esophagus is most likely to be perforated by endoscopy or dilation, and the traditional recommendation is therefore to avoid instrumentation of the esophagus at that time.

Spectrum of pH

The pH of the ingested material is a major factor in determining the extent of injury. The most severe damage is inflicted by strong alkalis such as sodium hydroxide. Lye is a nonspecific term used to describe any strong alkali used for making soap. It is found in drain cleaners such as Drano and Liquid-Plumr. The pH of these preparations is typically between 13 and 14. Floor stripper has a pH between 11 and 12, and household ammonia has a pH of 11. Most domestic cleaning products are much less alkaline, including Clorox (sodium hypochlorite) with a pH of 9, and cause correspondingly less damage. Strong acids are not commonly used in this country, but the concentrated hydrochloric acid used as a toilet cleaner in India has a pH of zero. Because the stomach physiologically contains hydrochloric acid in the pH range 1.2 to 1.5 and episodes of acid reflux in the pH range 2 to 3 are common in the esophagus, it may be wondered why concentrated hydrochloric acid is so damaging. It must be remembered that the household form is more than 10 times as concentrated as the physiologic form. In a normal stomach the presence of a low pH causes feedback inhibition of acid production. When a large quantity of concentrated HCl is ingested, pyloric spasm causes retention of the material in the antrum, where it overwhelms the normal defense mechanism.

Conceptually, the injury can be thought of in three categories:

1. Mild injuries, which involve only the mucosa and heal without sequelae
2. Moderate injuries, which heal with an esophageal stricture
3. Severe transmural injuries, which cause full-thickness damage leading to perforation acutely or dense, undilatable strictures in the recovery phase that require major foregut resection to restore the ability to eat

CLINICAL FEATURES

In the mildest form of injury, the patient goes to the emergency department (ED) with a history of caustic ingestion and reports only minor symptoms such as a sore throat or no symptoms at all. There may be normal mucosa or mild erythema in the oropharynx, but the voice is normal, patients can swallow their own saliva, and there is no systemic toxicity. This is commonly the situation with children.

With a substantial ingestion, the edema is more profound, and the patient is frequently drooling saliva, has a hoarse voice, is in severe distress with dysphagia, chest pain, and vomiting, and has tachycardia and leukocytosis. The oropharyngeal mucosa and lips may show ulceration or adherent sloughing. The more extensive the ingestion, the more likely that there will be full-thickness injury to the oropharynx, the tubular esophagus, and the stomach and surrounding organs. Hematemesis may indicate erosion into a major blood vessel. Abdominal tenderness is an ominous sign suggesting gastric necrosis.

Development of Strictures

With injury deeper than the mucosa, a stricture will develop in most patients in the recovery period. The location of the stricture depends on the rapidity with which the toxic material was transported down the esophagus. Damage tends to be maximal at areas of natural narrowing, such as the cricopharyngeal sphincter or the site of the left main bronchus. For reasons mentioned earlier, gastric stricture tends to be a consequence of concentrated acid consumption.[10]

PRINCIPLES OF MANAGEMENT

Management of caustic ingestion can be conveniently subdivided into three phases:

The *early phase*, which begins with arrival at the ED, deals with immediate assessment of the extent of injury, early resuscitation, and the disposition of the patient, whether to be discharged, admitted to the floor for observation, or sent to the intensive care unit (ICU) or directly to the operating room.

The *intermediate phase* involves managing the patient through the acute episode in the hospital by dealing with such issues as sepsis, aspiration, the need to maintain nutrition, and steering the patient though a potentially complicated postoperative course after resection of the esophagus, stomach, or both.

The *chronic phase* is aimed at restoring function once the patient has recovered from the acute attack and may involve elements such as psychosocial support and counseling and treatment of depression, nutritional support, repeated endoscopy for strictures, and major reconstructive surgery of the oropharynx and upper digestive tract.

EMERGENCY DEPARTMENT MANAGEMENT

Before any decision about disposition can be made, a basic clinical assessment must be carried out. Try to identify what and how much of the material the patient ingested. In children and ill or intoxicated adults, ask the accompanying family or friend. Assess the previous psychiatric background.

Examination follows the ABCs for any serious emergency. Check the airway. Stridor, coughing, drooling, and inability to speak are all signs of airway compromise, and the respiratory rate and the use of accessory muscles will give a warning of the need for intubation. Establish intravenous access in all symptomatic patients because they may sequester large amounts of extracellular fluid in the mediastinum and become hypotensive. Look at the oral mucosa, tongue, and pharynx for erythema and ulceration. More severe damage causes an adherent black or gray slough. Examine the neck for crepitus and tenderness and the abdomen for tenderness. Provide the patient with a suction catheter if drooling. Check routine chemistry and the blood count. These studies are useful as a baseline if the patient needs to be admitted. In all symptomatic cases it is wise to obtain immediate plain films of the chest and abdomen to look for signs of pneumothorax, pneumomediastinum, or pneumoperitoneum.

The results of this immediate clinical assessment will dictate whether the patient can be discharged home, whether endoscopy should be performed in the ED before the patient is either discharged or admitted, or whether the patient requires ICU admission or urgent surgery. The most severely ill patients with systemic signs (fever, tachycardia, leukocytosis, metabolic acidosis, and difficulty maintaining an airway) should be admitted to the ICU, resuscitated urgently, and have the endoscopic assessment performed under general anesthesia in the operating room.

Early Discharge

Prompt discharge with a follow-up appointment is appropriate only for a few patients who report no symptoms and have normal mental status. The patient should be afebrile and not have any tachycardia or abdominal tenderness on examination. Endoscopy is performed on all others. Patients with minimal systemic disturbance and no oral lesions on visual inspection may undergo endoscopy in the ED because if no damage is seen, it is reasonable to discharge them from the ED. The risk of any damage subsequently occurring is extremely low.

Follow-up of patients discharged early from the ED should involve social or psychiatric services. The parents of children who have ingested caustic agents are often plagued by guilt and may themselves need support. In others, neglect amounting to abuse may be responsible, and social services may need to assess the potential for other forms of abuse.[11]

Psychosocial support is also important for adult patients who may have fallen out with their families and whose social isolation may have led to the underlying depression that precipitated the ingestion episode.

Endoscopic Assessment

Endoscopy is the single most valuable diagnostic tool in planning the management of patients after caustic ingestion. It is indicated for all but the most trivial injuries. Significant esophageal damage can be present without any signs of oropharyngeal injury. Symptoms are important in identifying even trivial injuries, and several studies have clearly shown that a patient who is asymptomatic on initial evaluation will not have significant damage detected by endoscopy.[12] Thus, all symptomatic patients should be examined endoscopically. It used to be asserted that the endoscope should not be advanced past the first sign of injury, presumably because of a risk of worsening the damage, but this advice stemmed from the days of rigid endoscopy, and modern flexible narrow-caliber endoscopes passed with gentleness by a skilled operator do not increase the risk for perforation. The examination may be performed in the ED under sedation in patients with mild symptoms, but when the patient has mental status changes, is simultaneously intoxicated, or has drooling and difficulty swallowing, it is preferable to perform endoscopy under general anesthesia with airway protection in the operating room.

As a result of endoscopy, the injury can be classified into one of three major categories (Box 39–1). First-degree burns, or mere erythema, heal without incident. Second-degree burns tend to heal by stricturing. Third-degree burns are characterized by full-thickness necrosis and may require immediate esophagectomy if extensive.

Box 39–1   **Endoscopic Grading of Caustic Injury**

Grade 1: mucosal edema or hyperemia

Grade 2
  A: Friability, erosions, exudates
  B: As grade 2A plus deep or circumferential ulceration

Grade 3
  A: Scattered areas of necrosis with black or gray discoloration
  B: Extensive areas of necrosis

IN-PATIENT MANAGEMENT

Resuscitation

A patient with clinical or endoscopic signs of more severe injury will be admitted. Therapy is initially directed toward resuscitation and supportive management. Broad-spectrum antibiotics are generally recommended for moderate and severe injuries, but no controlled data are available because most workers report their own protocol. The oropharynx and esophagus are home to many virulent bacteria, and a damaged esophagus quickly becomes invaded, with the potential for systemic sepsis. Consequently, broad-spectrum antibiotics active against oral and intestinal flora are administered and should include gram-positive and anaerobic coverage, such as penicillin and metronidazole.

The patient should have nothing by mouth (NPO). Do not attempt to induce vomiting because any toxic material will cause damage on the way up, just as it did on the way down. Do not attempt to neutralize the material because thermal damage may be induced by the subsequent exothermic reaction.

Imaging Studies

Barium or contrast studies are of little value and may precipitate aspiration. Some recent work has rekindled interest in using a suspension of sucralfate labeled with technetium 99m to detect ulceration in the damaged esophagus. This method has good correlation with the endoscopic appearance because sucralfate adheres to ulcerated mucosa. It may be valuable in uncooperative children, in whom the risks associated with endoscopy and general anesthesia may be avoided.[13]

Steroids

The value of systemic steroids has been debated for years, but the general advice, based on a single randomized controlled trial in 1990, is that they confer no advantage.[14,15] Other recent nonrandomized series suggest that stenosis is reduced, but at the expense of a higher incidence of gastrointestinal hemorrhage.[16]

Acid Suppression

Acid suppression has been generally recommended to avoid exacerbation of the esophageal injury by superimposed gastroesophageal reflux (GER). Not only does the esophageal injury result in damage to the lower esophageal sphincter mechanism and lead to esophageal shortening, but GER can also be induced or aggravated by injury to the stomach as a result of pyloric stenosis.[17] Intravenous H_2 blockers are recommended for patients with NPO status. Thereafter, when oral liquids are tolerated, proton pump inhibitors are effective.

Stenting

Early dilation and stenting are sometimes recommended as a means to reduce the severity of future strictures. It seems intuitive that if contraction of collagen could be prevented in the first few weeks after injury, stricture severity could be reduced.[18] However, migration, bleeding, and tissue ingrowth sometimes requiring esophagectomy to remove the stent have all been reported, and the progression to stricture is likely to be determined by the initial injury rather than the treatment.

Early Stages of Recovery

Strictures begins within the first 2 to 3 weeks and may progress rapidly. Historically, dilation was associated with a high risk for perforation (Chevalier Jackson was fond of quoting the aphorism of Trousseau that "those who live by the bougie die by the bougie"), and a major advance in the management of severe caustic injuries in children was the introduction of Tucker's retrograde bougie technique.[19] This technique required the patient to swallow a string, which was retrieved at the time of creation of a gastrostomy. The gastrostomy was used for feeding, as well as for passing fusiform bougies over the string to dilate the stricture from below. Although passing retrograde bougies over a guide reduced the incidence of esophageal perforation, the large gastrostomy needed for passage of these bougies created troublesome skin problems. In recent times flexible endoscopy and through-the-scope balloon dilation have become the most common treatment, but passing Savary-type bougies over an endoscopically placed guidewire is also effective and considerably cheaper.

Maintenance of Nutrition

Throughout the patient's hospital course and early recovery period when numerous dilations are being performed, there is a serious risk for malnutrition as a result of the severe catabolic state and the fact that the priorities of the medical team are directed to immediately life-threatening considerations. Consequently, attention to nutrition is in danger of being overlooked. Patients may be fed via an indwelling nasogastric tube for fairly short periods, but long-term tolerance of this method is poor, and gastrostomy or jejunostomy is more commonly used. Gastrostomy may be performed endoscopically (percutaneous endoscopic gastrostomy [PEG]), but it should not be performed if the stomach is itself badly inflamed or if it is anticipated that the stomach is going to be used for eventual esophageal replacement. In this situation a feeding jejunostomy is superior, but bolus feeding by syringe is not tolerated in the jejunum, and instead, continuous infusion via a pump is required. A typical patient will need 30 kcal/kg/day, and because most enteral feeding formulas contain 1 kcal/ml, an average patient will require 2000 to 2500 ml/day, or 90 to 100 ml/hr over a 24-hour period. As the patient becomes more mobile, it is possible to cycle the tube feedings to deliver the same total amount over a shorter period, but rates above

160 ml/hr are often associated with discomfort and crampy abdominal pain. Total parenteral nutrition may be used but is associated with a risk for bacterial translocation, liver impairment, and acalculous cholecystitis, and thus the gastrointestinal tract should be used if possible.

Management of Severe Injuries

Patients with full-thickness injury to the foregut are at risk for serious systemic sepsis and extension of the injury to adjacent organs: the colon, pancreas, and duodenum in the abdomen and the tracheobronchial tree in the chest.[20,21] The combination of a systemic disturbance with hemodynamic instability (marked tachycardia or hypotension, oliguria, fever, and leukocytosis) and extensive injury on endoscopy is a strong indication to proceed to the operating room. One recent report of caustic ingestion injuries from Taiwan compared arterial blood gas data in patients who required surgery with those who did not. Acidosis was a prominent feature of the group requiring surgery (mean pH of 7.22, mean base excess of −12.0), but in the group treated conservatively, the mean pH was 7.38 with a mean base excess of −1.8. A marked acidosis therefore appeared to indicate a severe injury.[22] Some surgeons advocate laparoscopy because of the ease with which a rapid assessment of the stomach serosa can be made, and if no resection is required, a feeding jejunostomy is easily inserted. If the stomach shows signs of necrosis, the esophagus is also profoundly damaged and subtotal esophagectomy and total gastrectomy should be performed to prevent the spread of mediastinal or peritoneal sepsis.[23] The surgical details of esophagectomy are discussed elsewhere in this volume (Chapter 42). This might seem a radical step so early in the course of the illness, but it has the clear advantage of removing the major source of continued infection, and when performed early, it is a relatively easy and atraumatic operation. Although no level 1 evidence is available, several workers have noted that mortality and morbidity are reduced after the adoption of an aggressive surgical approach.[24] The stomach is mobilized in the abdomen and the distal esophagus mobilized though the hiatus by dividing the phrenoesophageal membrane and separating the distal esophagus from the right and left crura. The neck is then explored via an incision along the border of the left sternocleidomastoid muscle and the esophagus carefully mobilized away from the trachea. After dividing the omohyoid muscle and detaching the strap muscles close to their attachment to the manubrium and sternoclavicular joint, the esophagus is easily identified as the trachea and larynx are retracted medially and the carotid sheath laterally. As in all operations on the cervical esophagus, care must be taken to protect the recurrent laryngeal nerve, which lies in the sulcus between the trachea and esophagus and is at risk during mobilization of the anterior aspect of the esophagus. Once the cervical esophagus is safely encircled, a varicose vein stripper is inserted from the cardia up into the proximal end of the esophagus, the esophagus is transected in the neck, and the distal end is ligated

around the vein stripper. By careful and gentle traction, the esophagus can then be stripped out of the mediastinum with minimal blood loss and negligible mediastinal trauma. No attempt at reconstruction is made; the proximal end of the esophagus is brought out as a spit fistula, the duodenum is stapled off, and a feeding jejunostomy is inserted. The patient usually recovers quite quickly from this procedure, and subsequent definitive reconstruction is carried out electively many months later. Attention is paid to nutrition and psychological support in the interim. In time, the opening of the esophagostomy is likely to scar down. This process often continues for a year or more, and early reconstruction before the process is complete will risk the creation of a dense anastomotic stricture, which can be as difficult to manage as a typical corrosive stricture.

THE CHRONIC PHASE: RESTORATION OF FUNCTION

In patients who survive the initial crisis, the third phase of treatment involves either repetitive dilation of strictures in the preserved esophagus or surgical reconstruction.

Chronic Dilation

Several schemes have been devised to classify the severity and extent of caustic strictures, but in practice, the major distinction is between dilatable and nondilatable strictures. Some strictures are so severe that there is total luminal occlusion or they are so narrow and tortuous that dilation simply cannot be achieved with safety. In these patients, reconstruction is the only option. Milder strictures may be palliated by frequent dilation, but even these strictures have a higher incidence of perforation and require more frequent dilation than typical peptic strictures do. The study of Broor et al., in which the outcome of dilation was compared in 51 patients with caustic ingestion and 39 with peptic strictures, is instructive: of nine perforations in the series of dilations, eight occurred in the caustic group.[25] Another study from Korea using balloon dilation reported a 32% incidence of perforation. It is therefore clear that dilation is associated with significant morbidity in this population.[26] Many patients who survive the initial episode subsequently have severe strictures that can be physically dilated with some restoration of swallowing, but it is required so frequently, sometimes twice weekly, that recovery of normal life is impossible. Elective esophageal replacement may then be considered with expectation of good quality of life.

Intractable Esophageal Stricture

Resection or Bypass?

Unless the esophagus was resected at the time of the initial episode of ingestion, the surgeon has the option of simply bypassing the strictured esophagus and leaving it in situ. In most instances it is possible to bring up the esophageal substitute via a substernal route and perform the proximal anastomosis in the neck or pharynx. Esophageal bypass avoids the need to dissect out a densely scarred esophagus with the attendant risk of injury to the great vessels, thoracic duct, and the trachea or left main bronchus and the inevitable consequence of vagal injury. The disadvantage of bypass is that the remaining esophagus is prone to undergo cystic dilation, with occasional rupture.[27] It is inaccessible to endoscopic examination. If it is not disconnected from the stomach, it may be subject to severe acid reflux without the buffering effect of saliva. Finally, the esophagus has an increased risk for cancer after caustic injury. The magnitude of the risk is debated, but it is alleged that the risk is 1000 times that of the general population. It tends to occur many years after the injury, often more than 30 years later.[28,29] Many published reports do not distinguish between cancer in the portion of the esophagus in the food stream and cancer in the bypassed segment. It has been argued that the increased mortality as a consequence of attempted resection outweighs the theoretical advantage of reducing the cancer risk. Resection of the esophagus after transmural caustic injury can be a formidable undertaking. Thoracotomy is usually required because the dense periesophageal scarring, as a result of both the injury itself and possibly superimposed microperforations from numerous dilations, is difficult and dangerous to resect via the transhiatal route. Although the balance of evidence cannot be dogmatically determined, it can be confidently asserted that if esophagectomy is to be performed, it should be done in a high-volume center where experienced surgeons and intensive care is available.

Choice of Esophageal Substitute

There is an ongoing debate among esophageal surgeons about the relative merits of colon interposition versus gastric pull-up to replace a damaged esophagus. This debate is of most relevance to esophageal cancer, and the considerations are dealt with in detail elsewhere in this book. Gastric pull-up requires only one anastomosis, is generally quicker, and is increasingly being performed laparoscopically. However, the functional results tend to deteriorate over time with the development of symptomatic reflux, stricture, and columnar metaplasia above the anastomosis in the proximal esophageal remnant. In contrast, colon interposition is a more extensive procedure that requires three anastomoses, but the functional results remain stable or improve with time. We have recently shown in a long-term study of anastomotic stricture after esophagectomy that colon interposition is associated with a lower incidence of stricture than gastric pull-up.[30] When applied to caustic stricture, there are even stronger grounds for preferring colon interposition because the stomach has often been damaged by the caustic agent and is scarred and foreshortened.

Unusual cases occur in which both the stomach and the transverse colon have been damaged by the injury or resected before the ingestion episode. In such cases the right colon and terminal ileum may be available. If the colonic damage is extensive, recourse must then be made to the use of jejunum. The short mesentery of the jejunum generally precludes a jejunal limb from reaching to the cervical esophagus or pharynx. It is best to bring the limb of jejunum into the middle or upper mediastinum and then bridge the gap by harvesting a free flap of jejunum and anastomosing the artery and vein to the external carotid and jugular vein, respectively. The distal end may be anastomosed to the upper limit of the Roux limb of the jejunum, but it may be wise to let the free flap mature and the blood supply develop for several weeks before performing the proximal anastomosis in the pharynx.

One technique that was performed in the days before colon interposition or other gastrointestinal transposition procedures was the use of skin flaps. Early attempts with pedicled cervical skin flaps were associated with a very high failure rate because of leakage and stricture. A myocutaneous flap harvested from the pectoralis major muscle and based on the pectoral branch of the acromiothoracic artery may be tunneled under the clavicle and sutured into a pharyngeal defect, but this flap is too bulky to be used for a circumferential defect. As a general rule, these methods are of historical interest only and have been superseded because of the relative ease and reliability of reconstruction with the gastrointestinal tract.

Strictures in the Cervical Esophagus and Below

When the pharynx and laryngeal mechanism are spared and the esophageal stricture is located well below the cricopharyngeus, surgical treatment differs little from the standard principles of esophageal replacement for other more common diseases, with the caveat that a transthoracic rather than transhiatal approach is preferred (Fig. 39–1). The technique of colon interposition as described by DeMeester et al. in 1988 has never been bettered.[31] Certain important principles apply to the postoperative care of any patient after esophagectomy, including careful attention to fluid balance to avoid pulmonary overload, constant awareness of the high risk for aspiration, and vigilance to detect early signs of sepsis. Caustic ingestion is associated with an especially high risk for the development of an anastomotic stricture,[32] for several reasons. First, scarring in the proximal esophageal stump may continue to progress for more than 1 year after the initial insult. If there are strong clinical grounds for definitive surgical reconstruction during the first few months, care must be taken to resect well proximal to the strictured portion. Second, there may be tension on the anastomosis. Two techniques to reduce this tension are important: (1) a sufficiently long piece of colon should be mobilized by dividing the colon proximally so that it will reach high in the neck with ease, and (2) when using the substernal route, it is very helpful to excise the left half of the manubrium and the most distal portion of the left clavicle. This maneuver removes the risk of creating an anastomosis in a tight, crowded space.

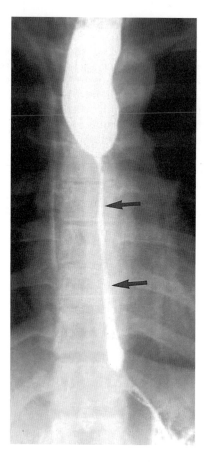

Figure 39–1. Stricture in the mid and distal portion of the esophagus, where conventional techniques of esophagectomy and reconstruction can bring about a good result.

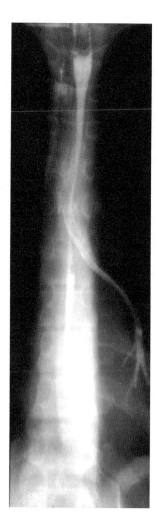

Figure 39–2. Stricture high in the cervical esophagus that was associated with an anastomotic stricture after colon interposition.

It is important to divide the clavicle medially, just lateral to the sternoclavicular joint, so that the costoclavicular ligament remains intact. This avoids the unsightly protrusion of the unattached clavicle.

One further technique to reduce the risk for anastomotic stricture is to perform it in two stages, as advocated by Ergun et al.[32] In this method the colon is generously mobilized and passed substernally up to the neck, where it is left in situ for 3 months, during which time it is claimed that the blood supply improves and thereby allows a safer definitive anastomosis in the neck. The authors report a stricture rate of 11%, which compares favorably with rates of 13% to 60% reported by other workers.

Oropharyngeal Stricture

Strictures high in the esophagus and pharynx are much harder to manage than those in the tubular esophagus or stomach (Fig. 39–2) because of the difficulty of restoring swallowing without creating intractable aspiration. A laryngeal or subglottic stricture is characterized by progressive dysphonia that eventually mandates tracheostomy. Injuries of this degree are easily recognized clinically by the presence of limited jaw opening and an inability to protrude the tongue as a consequence of fibrosis of the tongue base. Direct laryngoscopy shows that the epiglottis is scarred, deformed, and adherent to the pharyngeal wall. The vallecula and one or both piriform sinuses may be occluded by scarring. The epiglottis may be liberated by laser therapy, but scarring frequently redevelops. During this time the patient requires a tracheostomy. Most such patients are unable to phonate properly, and the voice is reduced to barely audible inarticulate squeaks. In this situation the chance of restoration of speech is so remote that the patient is better off with a primary laryngectomy and end tracheostomy. Once this key decision is made, a colon interposition or gastric pull-up can then be performed to the base of the tongue, and even the impaired pharyngeal apparatus that remains can generally be sufficient to permit the patient to have adequate swallowing for maintenance of nutrition without tube feeding. In the rehabilitation period the patient will need the services of a speech pathologist who specializes in laryngectomized patients, and some external mechanical larynx or the creation of a Bloom-Singer valve may be helpful in restoring the ability to communicate.

For patients with pharyngeal involvement but limited damage to the laryngeal mechanism, the ultimate goal of therapy is preservation of both swallowing and speech. The problem is not the physical provision of a conduit; it is the intractable aspiration that occurs. If both piriform sinuses are open, the prognosis for safe swallowing is relatively good. If one piriform sinus is preserved, it may still be possible to perform a safe anastomosis. When both are occluded by scarring, the larynx is also severely damaged. Many ingenious surgical solutions have been proposed, including anastomosis to the piriform sinus as advocated by Tran Ba Huy and Celerier[33] and pharyngocoloplasty as described by Popovici, a Romanian surgeon with a personal series of 253 esophageal reconstructions for caustic injury. Most of this extensive experience is available only in the French literature, but a summary is available in English.[34,35]

LONG-TERM CONSEQUENCES

The economic impact of serious caustic injuries is very significant. Young children with extensive injuries often remain in the hospital for several months and require numerous surgical and diagnostic procedures and anesthetics. The burden on their parents, who may have to move closer to a major referral center, is also very great. In adults with extensive injuries, prolonged ICU stay (averaging 58 days in the study by Cattan et al.) and the necessity for repeated interventions by surgeons, radiologists, and gastroenterologists are responsible for huge expenses that are rarely recouped by private institutions.[20]

In addition to the economic consequences, it has also been shown that there is an astonishingly high incidence, about 50%, of behavioral and educational problems in children who survive and that over a quarter of their families break up in the wake of the protracted period of stress.[36] In adults the risk for repeated suicide attempts is a real one, especially in the depressing situation in which a sequence of complications necessitates numerous additional surgeries. These considerations validate all the effort expended by lobbying groups to reduce the ease with which these devastating injuries occur.

REFERENCES

1. The Bible, II Kings 4:40.
2. Shakespeare W: Julius Caesar, Act IV, iii, 155.
3. Poley JW, Steyerberg EW, Kuipers EJ, et al: Ingestion of acid and alkaline agents: Outcome and prognostic value of early upper endoscopy. Gastrointest Endosc 60:372-377, 2004.
4. Lahoti D, Broor SL: Corrosive injury to upper gastrointestinal tract. Indian J Gastroenterol 12:135-141, 1993.
5. Watson WA, Litovitz TL, Klein-Schwartz W, et al: 2003 annual report of the American Association of Poison Control Centers Toxic Exposure Surveillance System. Am J Emerg Med 22:335-404, 2004.
6. Vancura EM, Clinton JE, Ruiz E, Krenzelok EP: Toxicity of alkaline solutions. Ann Emerg Med 9:118-122, 1980.
7. Gumaste VV, Dave PB: Ingestion of corrosive substances in adults. Am J Gastroenterol 87:1-5, 1992.
8. Baskerville JR, Nelson RE, Reynolds TL, Cohen M: Development of a standardized animal model for the study of alkali ingestion. Vet Hum Toxicol 44:45-47, 2002.
9. Yarington CT Jr: The experimental causticity of sodium hypochlorite in the esophagus. Ann Otorhinolaryngol 79:895-899, 1970.
10. Agarwal S, Sikora SS, Kumar A, et al: Surgical management of corrosive strictures of stomach. Indian J Gastroenterol 23:178-180, 2004.
11. Massa N, Ludemann JP: Pediatric caustic ingestion and parental cocaine abuse. Int J Pediatr Otorhinolaryngol 68:1513-1517, 2004.
12. Lamireau T, Rebouissoux L, Denis D, et al: Accidental caustic ingestion in children: Is endoscopy always mandatory? J Pediatr Gastroenterol Nutr 33:81-84, 2001.
13. Millar AJ, Numanoglu A, Mann M, et al: Detection of caustic oesophageal injury with technetium 99m–labelled sucralfate J Pediatr Surg 36:262-265, 2001.
14. Anderson KD, Rouse TM, Randolph JG: A controlled trial of corticosteroids in children with corrosive injury of the esophagus. N Engl J Med 323:637-640, 1990.
15. Ulman I, Mutaf O: A critique of systemic steroids in the management of caustic esophageal burns in children. Eur J Pediatr Surg 8:71-74, 1998.
16. Bautista A, Varela R, Villanueva A, et al: Effects of prednisolone and dexamethasone in children with alkali burns of the oesophagus. Eur J Pediatr Surg 6:198-203, 1996.
17. Mutaf O, Genç A, Herek O, et al: Gastroesophageal reflux: A determinant in the outcome of caustic esophageal burns. J Pediatr Surg 31:1494-1495, 1996.
18. Zhou J-H, Jiang Y-G, Wang R-W, et al: Management of corrosive esophageal burns in 149 cases. J Thorac Cardiovasc Surg 130:449-455, 2005.
19. Tucker JA, Turtz ML, Silberman HD, Tucker GF Jr: Tucker retrograde esophageal dilatation 1924-1974: A historical review. Ann Otol Rhinol Laryngol 83(Suppl 16):3-35, 1974.
20. Cattan P, Munoz-Bongrand N, Berney T, et al: Extensive abdominal surgery after caustic ingestion. Ann Surg 231:519-523, 2000.
21. Sarfati E, Jacob L, Servant JM, et al: Tracheobronchial necrosis after caustic ingestion. J Thorac Cardiovasc Surg 103:412-413, 1992.
22. Cheng YJ, Kao EL: Arterial blood gas analysis in caustic ingestion injuries. Surg Today 33:483-485, 2003.
23. Gossot D, Sarfati E, Celerier M: Early blunt esophagectomy in severe caustic burns of the upper digestive tract. Report of 29 cases. J Thorac Cardiovasc Surg 94:188-191, 1987.
24. Estrera A, Taylor W, Mills LJ, Platt MR: Corrosive burns of the esophagus and stomach: A recommendation for an aggressive surgical approach. Ann Thorac Surg 41:276-283, 1986.
25. Broor SL, Raju GS, Bose PP, et al: Long term results of endoscopic dilatation for corrosive oesophageal strictures. Gut 34:1498-1501, 1993.
26. Song HY, Han YM, Kim HN, et al: Corrosive esophageal stricture: Safety and effectiveness of balloon dilation. Radiology 184:373-378, 1992.
27. Kamath MV, Ellison RG, Rubin JW: Esophageal mucocele: A complication of blind loop esophagus. Ann Thorac Surg 43:263-269, 1987.
28. Tucker JA, Yarington CT Jr: The treatment of caustic ingestion. Otolaryngol Clin North Am 12:343-350, 1979.
29. Kim YT, Sung SW, Kim JH: Is it necessary to resect the disease esophagus in performing reconstruction for corrosive esophageal stricture? Eur J Cardiothorac Surg 20:1-6, 2001.
30. Briel JW, Tamhankar AP, Hagen JA, et al: Prevalence and risk factors for ischemia, leak, and stricture of esophageal anastomosis: Gastric pull-up versus colon interposition. J Am Coll Surg 198:536-541 2004.
31. DeMeester TR, Johansson KE, Franze I, et al: Indications, surgical technique, and long-term functional results of colon interposition or bypass. Ann Surg 208:460-474, 1988.
32. Ergun O, Celik A, Mutaf O: Two-stage coloesophagoplasty in children with caustic burns of the esophagus: Basis of delayed cervical anastomosis—theory and fact. J Pediatr Surg 39:545-548, 2004.
33. Tran ba Huy P, Celerier M: Management of severe caustic stenosis of the hypopharynx and esophagus by ileocolonic transposition via

suprahyoid or trans-epiglottic approach. Analysis of 18 cases. Ann Surg 207:439-445, 1988.

34. Popovici Z: Pharyngeal-oesophageal reconstruction with laryngeal preservation following severe caustic injury to the pharynx and oesophagus. In Hennessy TPJ, Cuschieri A (eds): Surgery of the Oesophagus. Oxford, Butterworth-Heinemann, 1992, p 32.

35. Popovici Z: Results of the surgical treatment of severe caustic pharyngo-esophageal stenosis. The value of complete reconstruction of the pharynx by transposition of the ileum and colon. Chirurgie 123:552-559, 1998.

36. deJong AL, Macdonald R, Ein S, et al: Corrosive esophagitis in children: A 30 year review. Int J Pediatr Otorhinolaryngol 57:203-211, 2001.

Paraesophageal and Other Complex Diaphragmatic Hernias

Matthew M. Hutter · David W. Rattner

Paraesophageal hernias (PEHs) merit consideration as a separate entity from the more common sliding hiatal hernia (HH) because they are associated with life-threatening complications such as strangulation, necrosis, and perforation of the stomach. As a result of the perceived high rate of complications and the high mortality of emergency surgery in this setting, surgical dogma has been to repair PEHs on diagnosis. Recent evidence, however, questions this dogma, and evidence-based guidelines recommend watchful waiting for elderly patients who are asymptomatic or minimally symptomatic. Only patients who are symptomatic require operative repair.

The principal components of surgery for PEH include reduction of the herniated stomach and other organs below the diaphragm, restoration of an intra-abdominal segment of esophagus, excision of the hernia sac, and repair of the defect in the diaphragm. Controversy exists regarding the best approach (laparoscopic versus transabdominal versus transthoracic), the need for routine fundoplication, the role of prosthetic mesh, the benefits of gastropexy, and the prevalence of the "short esophagus." These controversies are examined in this chapter.

Although this chapter focuses on PEH, it also discusses other complex hernias of the diaphragm, including

- Traumatic hernias
- Postoperative diaphragmatic hernias
- Parahiatal hernias
- Congenital diaphragmatic hernias in adults

CLASSIFICATION AND PATHOPHYSIOLOGY

All HHs are characterized by a portion—if not all—of the stomach protruding through an enlarged esophageal hiatus into the chest. HHs are thought to be caused by the combined forces of age, stress (negative intrathoracic pressure and positive intra-abdominal pressure), and degenerative processes on the diaphragm. HHs can be classified into four types, depending on the anatomic location of the gastroesophageal (GE) junction and the extent of herniated stomach or other organs (Fig. 40–1).

A *type I* hernia is known as a sliding HH and is characterized by upward displacement of the GE junction into the posterior mediastinum. The stomach remains in its usual longitudinal alignment (see Fig. 40–1). The development of an HH appears to be related to age and to structural deterioration of the phrenoesophageal membrane over time.[1] This deterioration is probably due to repetitive upward stretching of the phrenoesophageal membrane during swallowing, as well as the combined force of negative intrathoracic pressure and positive intra-abdominal pressure. This postulate is supported by the fact that power lifters, who develop high intra-abdominal pressure during weight training, have a higher incidence of sliding HH than do non-weightlifting age-matched controls.[2] A higher incidence of HH has also been found in people with inguinal hernias.[3] Although the majority of patients with HH are asymptomatic, the prevalence and size of the sliding HH correlate with increasing severity of reflux disease.[4]

Type II and *type III* hernias are known as paraesophageal hernias (see Fig. 40–1). Type II—a "true" PEH—is defined by a normally positioned intra-abdominal GE junction with upward herniation of the stomach alongside it. A type III hernia is known as a "mixed" hernia and is characterized by displacement of both the GE junction and a large portion of the stomach cephalad into the posterior mediastinum. The difference between a type I or sliding HH and a type III or mixed PEH is that with a type III hernia, a portion of the stomach lies cephalad to the GE junction.

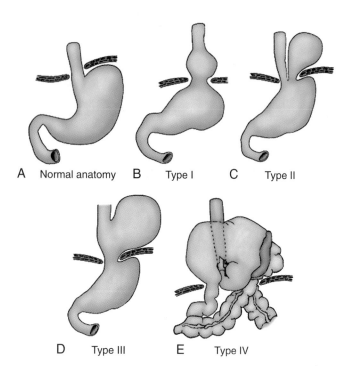

Figure 40–1. Types of hiatal hernia. **A,** Normal anatomy. **B,** Type I: sliding hiatal hernia. **C,** Type II: "true" parae-sophageal hernia. **D,** Type III: "mixed" paraesophageal hernia. **E,** Type IV: paraesophageal hernia containing other intra-abdominal organs. (From Duranceau A, Jamieson GG: Hiatal hernia and gastroesophageal reflux. In Sabiston DC Jr [ed]: Textbook of Surgery and the Biological Basis of Modern Surgical Practice, 15th ed. Philadelphia, WB Saunders, 1997, p 775.)

A PEH develops when there is a defect, possibly congenital, in the esophageal hiatus anterior to the esophagus.[5] Persistent posterior fixation of the GE junction is the essential difference between a PEH and a sliding HH. A type III or mixed hernia probably starts as a sliding HH, and over time as the hiatus enlarges, more and more of the fundus and body of the stomach herniate into the chest. Alternatively, a type III hernia could start as a type II hernia, with eventual migration of the GE junction cephalad.

In a *type IV* hernia, the esophageal hiatus has dilated to such an extent that the hernia sac also contains other organs such as the spleen, colon, or small bowel (see Fig. 40–1). Because of this altered anatomy, bowel obstruction and other complications may develop. PEHs initially develop on the left anterior aspect of the esophageal hiatus. The anterior gastric wall, or perhaps the epiphrenic fat pad itself, serves as a lead point, with the remainder of the stomach rolling up into the chest over time. The fundus must gain enough mobility from its intra-abdominal attachments to travel cephalad into the chest. This mobility is obtained by laxity in the gastrocolic and gastrosplenic ligaments, which normally help secure the stomach below the diaphragm. It is this laxity that allows volvulus to develop. Volvulus occurs when the stomach twists on itself, and this twisting leads to

obstruction of the stomach or esophagus and potentially perforation.

Two types of volvulus can occur: organoaxial and mesentericoaxial (Fig. 40–2). In organoaxial volvulus, the greater curvature of the stomach moves anterior to the lesser curve, along the axis of the organ. In mesentericoaxial volvulus, which is less common, the stomach rotates along its transverse axis. Gastric strangulation develops if the blood supply is compromised by distention of the herniated contents or a 360-degree twist of the stomach.

PREVALENCE

The actual prevalence of HH in the overall population is not known. Most patients are asymptomatic. Upper gastrointestinal (GI) barium studies in patients with GI complaints identify some type of HH in 15% of cases. The majority of hernias identified are incidental radiographic findings.

Greater than 95% of HHs are type I or sliding hernias. Less than 5% are PEHs. Of all PEHs, type III is the most common and is found more than 90% of the time,[6] type II is found 3.5% to 14% of the time, and type IV is the least common and occurs in only 2% to 5% of all PEHs.[4]

PEHs are four times more likely to develop in women than in men. The incidence of PEH increases with advancing age. Patients with PEH are on average significantly older than those with sliding HH: a mean of 61 years versus 48 years.[7] Familial cases of HH have been well documented and have an autosomal dominant mode of transmission.[8]

SYMPTOMS

Upward of 50% of patients with PEH are considered to be asymptomatic, although many of the symptoms are minor and may be overlooked. When patients are questioned carefully, 89% will actually have symptoms related to their hernia.[9] Symptoms include chest pain, epigastric pain, dysphagia, postprandial fullness, heartburn, regurgitation, vomiting, weight loss, anemia, and respiratory symptoms (Table 40–1).

When compared with a sliding HH, symptoms of dysphagia and postprandial fullness are more common with a PEH. The symptoms of heartburn and regurgitation that can be present with a sliding HH can also be present with a PEH and thus do not differentiate between the two.

Incarceration and Strangulation

The most serious complications of PEH are incarceration with obstruction of the stomach and gastric strangulation. Even mild dilation from incarceration with obstruction can lead to relative ischemia, ulceration, perforation, and ultimately sepsis. Borchardt's triad consists of chest pain, retching with an inability to vomit, and an inability to pass a nasogastric tube. This triad indicates an incarcerated intrathoracic stomach and is a true sur-

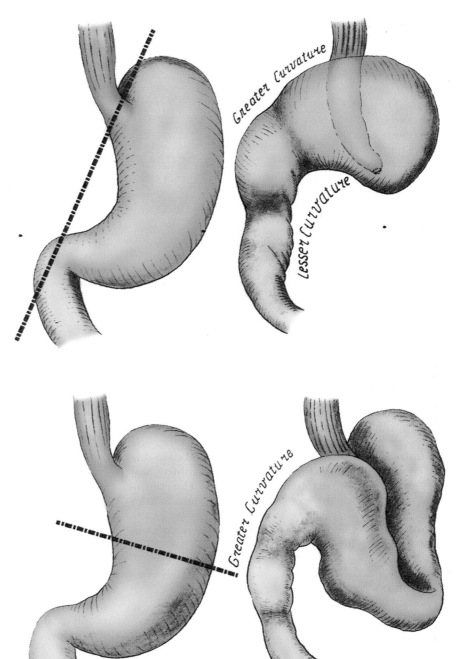

Figure 40–2. Gastric volvulus associated with paraesophageal hernias. *Top,* Organoaxial volvulus. Volvulus occurring along the longitudinal axis of the stomach leads to a true "upside down" stomach. The stomach becomes obstructed at both the cardia and the pyloroduodenal area. This type of gastric volvulus is the most common. *Bottom,* Mesentericoaxial volvulus. Folding of the stomach on itself along the transverse axis leads to pyloroantral obstruction. (From Menguy R: Surgical management of large paraesophageal hernia with complete intrathoracic stomach. World J Surg 12:416, 1988.)

gical emergency. It is often misdiagnosed as a myocardial infarction. Without timely surgical intervention, a life-threatening situation soon develops.

Compression of the Esophagus or Stomach

In a large PEH, symptoms are usually caused by the mechanical forces of the displaced stomach. In patients with organoaxial volvulus, or an "upside-down stomach," both the GE junction and the pylorus are relatively fixed

(see Fig. 40–2). Distention of a gastric volvulus is akin to wringing out a towel. The fluid trapped in the stomach leads to nausea, pain, and vomiting. As the stomach distends, the esophagus may be compressed and give rise to dysphagia or chest pain. Some patients complain of spitting up foamy fluid, or oral secretions that could not transit the obstructed GE junction. Interestingly, many patients with long-standing heartburn relate that their heartburn resolved at or about the same time that they began to complain of mechanically related symptoms such as postprandial "dry heaves" or chest pain. Vomit-

Table 40–1	Paraesophageal Hernias: Preoperative Symptoms and Findings

Typical heartburn	47%
Dysphagia	35%
Epigastric pain	26%
Vomiting	23%
Anemia	21%
Barrett's epithelium	13%
Aspiration	7%

Caveat: Many paraesophageal hernias are asymptomatic.
From Pierre AF, Luketich JD, Fernando HC, et al: Results of laparoscopic repair of giant paraesophageal hernias: 200 consecutive patients. Ann Thorac Surg 74:1909-1915, 2002.

ing is usually intermittent, but persistent vomiting suggests incarceration of the stomach.

Bleeding

Hematemesis or anemia is evident in about a third of patients with PEH. Bleeding can be caused by ischemia of the gastric mucosa or by "riding ulcers," otherwise known as "Cameron's ulcers." Cameron's ulcers are due to the constant abrasive force as the stomach rubs against or is pinched by the diaphragmatic hiatus.[10] The continuous movement of the stomach and esophagus as they travel up and down with respiration and swallowing compounds the problem. Anemia from a PEH resolves in 92% of patients after surgical repair.

Pulmonary Symptoms

Pulmonary symptoms associated with PEH include dyspnea because of the restrictive effects created by abdominal organs in the chest, pain with inspiration, or chronic cough. Recurrent aspiration from regurgitation can lead to pneumonia or a restrictive pulmonary disease.[11] With operative repair of the hernia, significant improvements in objective measurements of pulmonary function are usually achieved.[12]

DIAGNOSIS AND PREOPERATIVE EVALUATION

Although some patients have the symptoms just described, many are asymptomatic or minimally symptomatic. Physical examination can be remarkable for decreased breath sounds or dullness to percussion on the left side of the chest. Bowel sounds can often be auscultated in the chest in a person with a type IV HH. PEHs in asymptomatic or minimally symptomatic individuals are found during radiographic or endoscopic evaluations performed for other reasons.

Radiographic Studies

Chest radiographs often show opacity in the left side of the chest or an air-fluid level behind the cardiac silhouette. The lateral view usually demonstrates this opacity best (Fig. 40–3). A nasogastric tube that coils in the stomach can be used to demonstrate that this opacity is indeed an intrathoracic stomach. *Computed tomography* (CT) scans show these anatomic abnormalities with much more precision and can demonstrate whether other abdominal organs have migrated above the diaphragm as well. An *upper GI barium swallow* can be quite useful to assess anatomic detail, and it provides the diagnosis in almost all cases (Fig. 40–4). An upper GI study is also the best way to determine the location of the GE junction, which can help differentiate between a type II and type III hernia.

Endoscopy

Flexible fiberoptic endoscopy can be used to readily diagnose a PEH during retroflexed evaluation of the GE junction. Diagnostic findings of a type II PEH include a second orifice next to the GE junction and gastric rugal folds extending up into the opening. A type III PEH shows a gastric pouch extending above the diaphragm with the GE junction entering partway up the side of this pouch. Having the patient sniff can help identify the crura. Endoscopy can also be used to identify other intraluminal abnormalities, including ulcerations, gastritis, esophagitis, Barrett's esophagus, and mucosal-based neoplasms.

Manometry and 24-Hour pH Monitoring

Manometry and 24-hour pH monitoring are not very useful because the anatomic distortion of a PEH invariably makes the findings from these studies abnormal. We rely on fluoroscopic evaluation for a crude measure of esophageal motility. Because many patients are elderly, esophageal peristalsis is often abnormal, and thus symptomatology (presence or absence of dysphagia) is the best predictor of whether a patient will tolerate a full fundoplication. We recommend an antireflux procedure in most circumstances (see "Role of Fundoplication," later).

TREATMENT

Because PEH is an anatomic abnormality, no medical treatment can correct it. Although symptoms of gastroesophageal reflux disease (GERD) may be alleviated by acid suppression, the symptoms caused by mechanical forces such as ulceration, vomiting, and postprandial chest pain respond only to surgical restoration of normal anatomy. Endoscopic gastropexy has been described for use in the highest-risk patients; in this procedure the hernia is reduced with a gastroscope and fixed intraabdominally with a double percutaneous endoscopic gastrostomy (PEG) technique, with or without laparoscopic assistance.[13] However, surgical repair remains the mainstay of treatment of PEH.

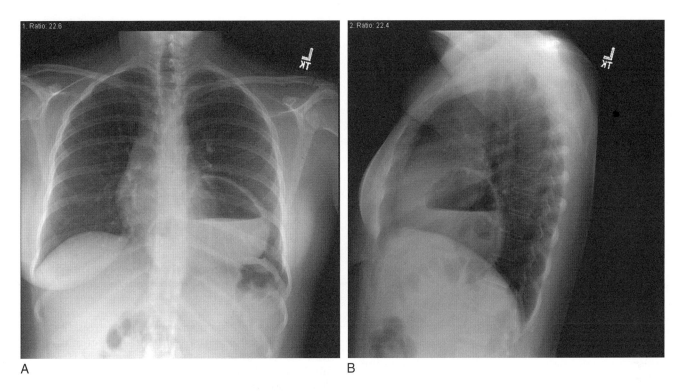

A B

Figure 40–3. Posteroanterior **(A)** and lateral **(B)** chest radiographs in a patient with a paraesophageal hernia. Notice the large air-fluid level behind the cardiac silhouette as a result of the intrathoracic stomach.

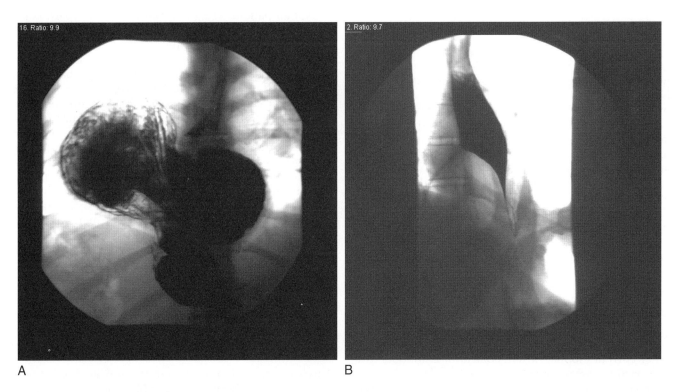

A B

Figure 40–4. Barium swallow in a patient with a paraesophageal hernia (same patient as in Fig. 40–3). **A,** Most of the stomach is in an intrathoracic position. **B,** Esophageal narrowing caused by compression from the intrathoracic portion of the stomach.

Indications

Traditional surgical teaching recommended operative reduction and repair of all PEHs once diagnosed, unless the patient was unfit for general anesthesia. The perceived need for prophylactic repair in all patients with a PEH is based on the theory that the mechanical complications leading to catastrophic life-threatening complications can occur without warning. This dogma was established in 1967 after publication of the classic report by Skinner and Belsey, who observed 21 patients without surgery.[14] Six of these 21 patients (29%) died of causes related to their PEH, including strangulation, perforation, bleeding, and acute dilation of the stomach. The authors concluded that elective surgery, with a 1% mortality rate, was preferable to the high mortality rate of emergency surgery.[14] This study, even though based on a small number of patients, was thought to characterize the natural history of PEH, as well as the morbidity and mortality associated with elective and emergency operations, and helped determine surgical practice for decades.

More recent evidence suggests that the risk of observing asymptomatic patients is much less, and therefore elective surgery should be reserved for symptomatic patients. In a 1993 article by Allen et al., 23 patients with a PEH who were asymptomatic were monitored for 20 years, and in only 4 of them did symptoms eventually develop.[15]

A recent study examined the outcomes of watchful waiting versus elective laparoscopic PEH repair in asymptomatic or minimally symptomatic patients.[16] This study used a Markov Monte Carlo decision analytic model based on pooled data from all published studies in this field and on nationwide, population-based data from the Nationwide Inpatient Sample. The authors found that published articles overestimated the mortality associated with emergency surgery when compared with the population-based data—17% versus 5.4%. Mortality with elective surgery was 1.4% in the population-based study. The annual probability of the development of acute symptoms requiring emergency surgery with the watchful waiting strategy was 1.1%. Using data for laparoscopic PEH repair as the benchmark for surgical treatment, this study concluded that routine elective repair would benefit only one in five patients. Furthermore, elective laparoscopic hernia repair in asymptomatic patients might actually decrease the quality-adjusted life expectancy for patients 65 years and older. Because progression of symptoms is slow and emergency surgery is seldom necessary, watchful waiting is the preferred approach for patients with large but relatively asymptomatic PEHs. Along with these landmark studies, multiple other current esophageal surgeons favor a nonoperative approach for asymptomatic patients.[9,15,17,18,19]

In contrast to asymptomatic patients, individuals who have either obstructive symptoms, bleeding, or complications of GERD associated with a PEH should undergo surgical repair. These patients are clearly the subgroup at risk for the development of life-threatening complications requiring emergency surgery. Elderly, high-risk patients who are symptomatic require specific consideration. Complex judgment is required to balance the risk associated with surgery, the type of surgical approach, and the extent of the procedure performed.

Surgical Approach

PEHs can be reduced and repaired from either a transthoracic or transabdominal approach. It would be optimal if the surgeon caring for patients with PEH were trained in all approaches and could truly individualize the approach to each patient's unique anatomy and risk profile. This, however, is rarely true in real-life practice. We do not believe that one operation is appropriate for all PEHs and use the following guidelines to select the approach. We preferentially repair PEH with a laparoscopic approach because of the high success rate and lower morbidity than with laparotomy or thoracotomy. This approach requires excellent advanced laparoscopic suturing and dissecting skills. In experienced hands, mobilization of the esophagus to the aortic arch can be routinely accomplished and a Collis gastroplasty added if necessary. In inexperienced hands, however, this is the most dangerous approach. Laparoscopic PEH repair is much more difficult than a routine laparoscopic antireflux operation and should probably not be attempted by the occasional laparoscopic surgeon. It is best if the operation is performed by an adequately trained surgeon so that the patient has the best chance for a safe and effective treatment.

Not all patients are good candidates for laparoscopic PEH repair. Those who have previously undergone open HH repair or laparoscopic PEH repair and obese patients are poor candidates for the laparoscopic approach. This group of patients is probably best approached transthoracically. Proponents of the transthoracic approach argue that it allows for complete esophageal mobilization and the best exposure for dissection of the hernia sac. A thoracotomy also provides easy exposure to perform a Collis gastroplasty. Disadvantages include the morbidity of a thoracotomy with incisional discomfort, pulmonary complications, and prolonged length of stay, as well as difficulty assessing the intra-abdominal organs. In our practice, open transabdominal approaches are reserved for patients being treated by gastropexy only. We believe that laparoscopic visualization is superior to that obtained via laparotomy—especially as one tries to work cephalad through the hiatus. Therefore, there is little advantage of laparotomy over laparoscopy in experienced hands if one chooses a transabdominal approach.

Laparoscopic Approach

Laparoscopic PEH repair confers the typical benefits of minimally invasive surgery—less blood loss and less third spacing of fluids, fewer pulmonary complications, and quicker recovery from surgery. This benefit is magnified in patients with PEHs, who tend to be elderly and debilitated and may not tolerate a thoracotomy or laparotomy well. The laparoscopic approach has additional unique advantages in that the view of the operative field is

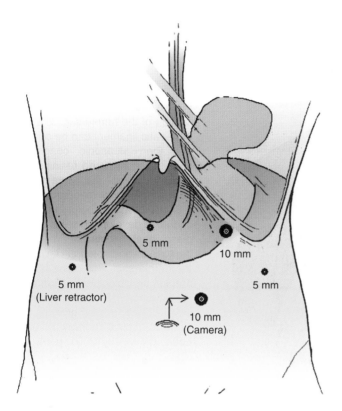

Figure 40–5. Trocar placement for laparoscopic paraesophageal hernia repair. A five-trocar technique is generally used, with two 10-mm trocars and three 5-mm trocars. (Adapted from Hutter MM, Mulvihill SJ: Laparoscopic management of pancreatic pseudocysts. In Zucker KA [ed]: Surgical Laparoscopy, 2nd ed. Philadelphia, JB Lippincott, 2001, p 647.)

magnified, thereby facilitating precise identification of tissue planes and vessels. Insufflation of CO_2 frequently establishes the correct dissection plane as one separates the peritoneal and pleural components of the hernia sac. The use of an angled scope also allows visualization of the mediastinum that cannot be obtained via laparotomy.

The disadvantages of a laparoscopic approach are the long learning curve and the need for advanced laparoscopic experience to perform this difficult operation safely and effectively. Some state that 30 to 50 laparoscopic fundoplications should be performed before attempting a laparoscopic PEH repair.[9] Such experience makes it easier to identify the anatomy, safely dissect the hernia sac from the mediastinum, and accurately place the crural sutures deep in the crura close to the aorta.

Laparoscopic Technique

The patient is placed supine, with the surgeon on the patient's right side. A five-port technique is used, with the initial 10-mm port placed via an open technique a few centimeters to the left of the midline and a few centimeters above the umbilicus (Fig. 40–5). Pneumoperi-

toneum is established, and a 10-mm 30-degree scope is used. A 10-mm port is placed in the left subcostal region, one or two fingerbreadths below the rib, a 5-mm trocar is placed inferior to this in the left anterior axillary line, a second 5-mm port is placed one hand's-breadth to the right of the camera port and a bit cephalad, and a third 5-mm port is placed on the right in the anterior axillary line for the liver retractor. Using atraumatic graspers, the stomach is grasped and traction is placed on it in an attempt to reduce it. The gastrohepatic ligament can be opened, and then ultrasonic coagulating shears can be used to incise the peritoneum at the anterolateral edge of the hiatus (Fig. 40–6). It is critical at this point in the procedure that the natural tissue plane that exists between the peritoneal and pleural layers of the hernia sac be developed. This plane is frequently areolar and bloodless. In patients who are highly symptomatic, however, inflammation can develop and make it more difficult to establish this plane. Once the plane is established, it can be carried circumferentially around the sac. Small vessels should be coagulated with the ultrasonic shears or cautery. At the cephalad margin one should identify the vagi and then roll the sac down into the abdomen. A laparoscopic peanut can be helpful for this blunt dissection (Fig. 40–7). Pneumothorax may develop during this dissection if the pleura itself is violated. Ordinarily, it is not of any consequence because the patient is being maintained on positive pressure ventilation. However, if the patient is hypovolemic or inadequately relaxed, tension pneumothorax can develop. Depressurizing the CO_2 in the abdomen will ameliorate this problem until volume status and anesthesia depth are corrected. Once complete dissection of the sac is performed, the sac is excised close to its attachment to the GE junction and removed so that it does not interfere with the subsequent repair. The anterior and posterior vagus nerves should be identified during the dissection and preserved during excision of the sac. If there is concern about the location of the vagus nerves or the sac is very thick and vascular, it is better to leave some excess sac than risk injury to the nerves or esophagus. It is, however, essential that the sac be completely detached from the crura and mediastinum. Residual attachments of the sac to the hiatus will lead to recurrence. With a rubber drain or tape around the esophagus, extensive mediastinal dissection with mobilization of the esophagus to the level of the aortic arch can be performed. The goal is to restore a suitable length (2.5 cm) of tension-free esophagus in the abdomen. The length should be measured with the esophagus unstretched and at the level where the crura are to be closed. The crura are then reapproximated with 0-Ethibond (Ethicon, Somerville, NJ) sutures tied over felt pledgets (Fig. 40–8). The left-handed grasper is placed on the left side of the aorta, and the needle is inserted through the base of the left crus. The needle can then be bounced off this grasper, which protects the aorta while ensuring that the suture gets a deep enough bite through the base of the crus. The sutures are placed starting caudally and tied, and additional pledgeted sutures are applied until only a 1-cm gap remains in the undistended esophageal hiatus. It is often helpful to lower the pressure of the

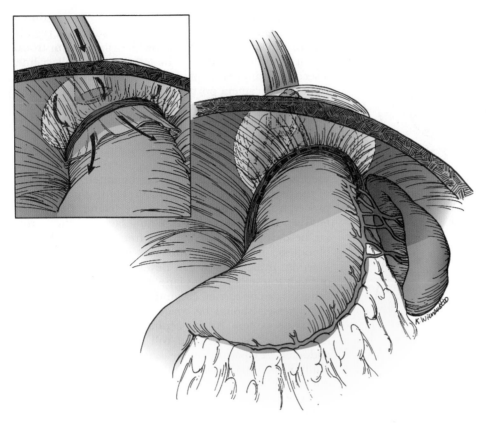

Figure 40–6. Laparoscopic dissection of the hernia sac. The gastrohepatic ligament can be opened, and then ultrasonic coagulating shears can be used to incise the peritoneum at the anterolateral edge of the hiatus (see *dotted line*). It is critical at this point in the procedure to develop the natural tissue plane that exists between the peritoneal and pleural layers of the hernia sac. This plane is often areolar and bloodless. (From Lee R, Donahue PE: Paraesophageal hiatal hernia. In Cameron JL [ed]: Current Surgical Therapy, 7th ed. St Louis, CV Mosby, 2001, p 44.)

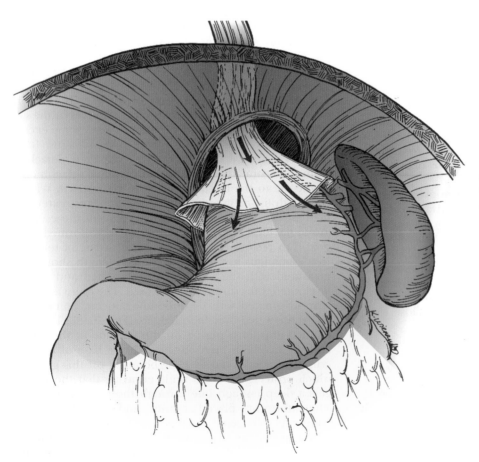

Figure 40–7. Laparoscopic dissection of the hernia sac (continued). The hernia sac is dissected circumferentially and seems to "tumble" down into the abdomen with gentle blunt dissection in the mediastinum with a laparoscopic peanut. (From Lee R, Donahue PE: Paraesophageal hiatal hernia. In Cameron JL [ed]: Current Surgical Therapy, 7th ed. St Louis, CV Mosby, 2001, p 45.)

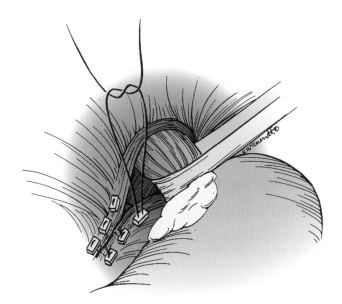

Figure 40–8. Crural closure. The crura are closed with simple interrupted pledgeted 0 braided polyester suture. Starting posteriorly, additional sutures are placed until there is a 1-cm space below the undistended esophagus. (From Lee R, Donahue PE: Paraesophageal hiatal hernia. In Cameron JL [ed]: Current Surgical Therapy, 7th ed. St Louis, CV Mosby, 2001, p 46.)

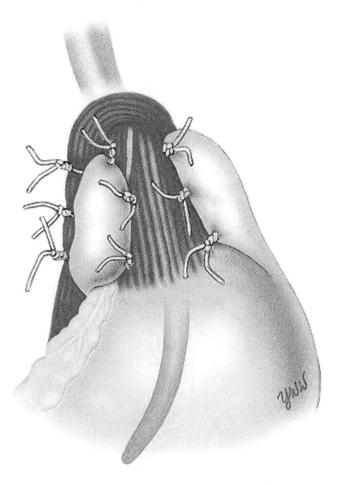

Figure 40–9. Completed Toupet fundoplication. Eight sutures are placed. Over a 54-French bougie, the top two sutures (one on the right, one on the left) include the esophagus, the fundus, and the edge of the crus. Two other sutures are placed on each side of the esophagus and include just the esophagus and fundus. One must be careful to avoid the anterior vagus nerve. Three crural sutures are seen toward the right on this diagram, and two sutures are placed posteriorly (not depicted) from the back of the wrap to the crural closure. In total, there are four points of fixation of the wrap to the crura. (From Champion JK, McKernan JB: Laparoscopic Toupet fundoplication. In Zucker KA [ed]: Surgical Laparoscopy, 2nd ed. Philadelphia, JB Lippincott, 2001, p 406.)

pneumoperitoneum to 8 to 10 mm Hg while closing the crura. The highest short gastric vessels are then divided, and either a 360-degree (Nissen) fundoplication or a 240-degree (Toupet) fundoplication is created (Fig. 40–9). In elderly patients or those with severe dysmotility seen on videoesophagograms, we prefer a partial fundoplication. The Toupet fundoplication also has the advantage of providing four points of fixation of the wrap to the crura. On completion of the repair, upper GI endoscopy can be useful if there is concern of esophageal injury or leak. We routinely perform an anterior gastropexy with two transfascial sutures of 2-0 Prolene (Ethicon, Somerville, NJ) at the conclusion of the repair.

A swallow study may be obtained on the first postoperative day to rule out leakage and reherniation if the dissection was difficult. Antiemetics should be given as part of the anesthetic and postoperative routine to prevent vomiting or retching. Clear liquids are started on the first postoperative day, and the patient is discharged home with instructions to start a full liquid diet on the second postoperative day and continue it for 1 week, at which time the diet is slowly advanced.

OUTCOMES

Outcomes of PEH repair reported in the literature are from a few high-volume, tertiary care centers that specialize in these procedures. Data from low-volume centers and population-based data are not available. The following results must therefore be interpreted with caution because they are not necessarily generalizable to all situations where these procedures are being performed.

Thoracic Approach The largest series using a thoracic approach was recently reported by Patel et al. from the University of Michigan.[20] A Collis gastroplasty was performed in 96% of their 240 cases. With a 42-month mean follow-up, the mortality rate was 1.7% and the complication rate was 8.5%, including three leaks. Nineteen (8%) anatomic recurrences were documented, 8 (3.3%) of which required reoperation. Maziach et al. from the University of Toronto reported a series of 94 cases, with 97% done transthoracically and 80% undergoing gastroplasty.[21] With a 94-month mean follow-up, the mortality rate was 2%, the major complication rate was 19%, including four leaks, and 2% required reoperation for recurrence.

Abdominal Approach In 2000, Geha et al. from the University of Illinois reported on 100 patients, 82 of whom were treated by an abdominal approach.[22] Two percent also required a Collis gastroplasty. There were two deaths in patients undergoing emergency operations and none in the elective group, with no recurrences. Williamson et al. from the Lahey Clinic reported on 119 patients with PEHs who underwent a transabdominal repair.[23] Follow-up in this study was for a median of 61.5 months, the mortality rate was 1.7%, and the complication rate was 11.8%. Eleven percent had symptomatic recurrences.

Laparoscopic Approach Pierre et al. from the University of Pittsburgh reported on 200 patients undergoing laparoscopic repair.[24] Fifty-six percent underwent a Collis gastroplasty, and 11% received polytetrafluoroethylene (PTFE) patches. With an 18-month median follow-up, the mortality rate was 0.5%, the complication rate was 28%, including six (3%) leaks, and 2.5% required reoperation for recurrence. Other laparoscopic series by Diaz et al. at Washington University ($N = 116$),[25] Andujar et al. from Allegheny Health System ($N = 166$),[26] and Mattar et al. from Emory ($N = 136$)[27] show similar mortality rates of 0% to 2.2% and complication rates of 4% to 10%. Gastroplasty was performed in less than 5% of these cases. Recurrence rates seen radiographically were as high as 22% to 33%; however, recurrences requiring reoperation occurred only at a rate of 2% to 3%. Many of the radiographically detected recurrences were small sliding HHs and were not thought to be clinically significant.

Laparoscopic Versus Open Repair Two single-institution studies retrospectively compared laparoscopic with open repair. Hashemi et al. at the University of Southern California (USC) looked at 54 patients: half underwent a laparoscopic procedure, a quarter underwent laparotomy, and a quarter underwent thoracotomy.[28] Although symptomatic outcomes were similar in both groups, 42% of the laparoscopic group had a recurrence on videoesophagography as compared with 15% in the open repair group. Schauer et al. at the University of Pittsburgh compared 95 consecutive cases, 70 performed laparoscopically and 25 performed with an open technique (19 transabdominal, 4 transthoracic).[29] The laparoscopic group had a significant reduction in blood loss, intensive care unit stay, ileus, hospital stay, and overall morbidity in comparison to the open group. Multiple studies also suggest that laparoscopic repair of PEH is successful and safe and leads to a shorter hospital stay with lower costs and greater patient satisfaction than with the open technique.[13,30-48]

The major concern about laparoscopic hernia repair is the recurrence rate. As mentioned earlier, the USC group reported a 42% reherniation rate in the laparoscopic group detected by videoesophagography as opposed to 15% in the open group.[28] The other laparoscopic series also show high anatomic recurrence rates

ranging from 22% to 30%. Despite this high radiographic recurrence rate, only 2% to 3% require operative repair for these recurrences, similar to the rate in the open studies. The high recurrence rates seen in the laparoscopic series may reflect the difficulty of placing sutures deeply into the crura or relaxed patient selection criteria such that patients who were considered unfit for thoracotomy were triaged to laparoscopic surgeons.

CONTROVERSIES

Role of Fundoplication

Controversy persists over whether to add an antireflux procedure to hiatal herniorrhaphy in patients with PEH.

There are many reasons to perform an antireflux procedure during PEH repair. First, an antireflux operation such as a Nissen, Toupet, Hill, or Belsey procedure can help hold the stomach in an intra-abdominal position. The bulky nature of the wrap or the suture fixation to the crura (or both) makes it more difficult for the stomach to reherniate into the chest. Second, it is very difficult to preoperatively assess which patients will have reflux symptoms once the hernia is reduced. Preoperative symptoms may be due to the distorted anatomy and poor esophageal clearance rather than reflux per se. Preoperative testing with pH probes and manometry in these patients does not provide much practical information because of the effects of their quite abnormal anatomy, as discussed earlier.

Third, the functionality of the GE junction is likely to be compromised by the operative dissection and reconstruction necessary to reduce the hernia sac and repair the hiatus. Even if function of GE junction were normal preoperatively, complete dissection of the hernia sac and mobilization of the esophagus mandate destruction of the posterior esophageal attachments, thereby predisposing to the development of reflux. Failure to perform an antireflux procedure can lead to symptomatic postoperative reflux in 20% to 40% of patients.[41]

The disadvantages of performing a fundoplication include additional time in the operating room and the added risk of complications specific to the fundoplication, such as dysphagia. However, because adequate dissection and crural closure have already been performed, we find that the addition of an antireflux procedure adds little time or morbidity. The risk of creating dysphagia or relative obstruction in a patient with inadequate esophageal motility is lessened by the liberal use of Toupet fundoplication. Furthermore, not all postoperative dysphagia is caused by the fundoplication—overly tight closure of the hiatus or severe postoperative fibrosis can also lead to dysphagia.

Prevalence of the "Short Esophagus"

Controversy persists over the need for an esophageal lengthening procedure in the repair of a PEH, mostly because of differing opinions about the prevalence of a "short esophagus." Most agree that a 2- to 3-cm segment of esophagus must be restored to the abdomen to perform an appropriate antireflux procedure. However, there is great controversy over how often this is encountered.

The prevalence of a "short esophagus" seems to be mostly related to the surgeon's perspective, the surgical approach, and how much effort the surgeon is willing to put forth in fully mobilizing the esophagus. The need for a Collis gastroplasty during PEH repair ranges from 0% in some series to as high as 96% in other series. Transthoracic series have the highest rates, whereas laparoscopic series have the lowest rates. Proponents of the liberal use of Collis gastroplasty point to the low recurrence rate of PEH attributable to decreased tension on the esophagus.

Patel et al., in their series of 240 patients undergoing transthoracic repair, performed an esophageal lengthening Collis gastroplasty in 96%.[20] In another large series of patients with large PEHs approached through the chest, the presence of a shortened esophagus requiring Collis gastroplasty was noted in 75 of 94 patients (80%).[21] One laparoscopic series has shown the need for Collis gastroplasty in 27% of cases.[31] Most series report that a shortened esophagus is present in approximately 10% of cases, although not all require gastroplasty.[48] In most laparoscopic series, gastroplasty is necessary in only 1% to 4% of cases.

There is no doubt that in certain circumstances a shortened esophagus does exist. Urbach et al. found that preoperative risk factors associated with finding a shortened esophagus requiring gastroplasty included the presence of a stricture, PEH, Barrett's esophagus, and redo antireflux surgery.[49] Repeated dilations or past perforations can also be risk factors.

Despite the added length of neo-esophagus created by the Collis gastroplasty, there are concerns about its liberal application, including the risk of placing gastric mucosa above the level of the newly created esophageal sphincter. There is also concern about leaks and bleeding from the staple line. Furthermore, when the short gastric vessels are divided, as is routine in laparoscopic approaches, the proximal end of the gastroplasty can become ischemic and result in a stricture or leak.

We have found that with adequate circumferential dissection of the hernia sac and extensive mediastinal dissection of the esophagus, the prevalence of a truly "short" esophagus is quite low. What appeared initially to be a short esophagus can usually be brought easily into the abdomen after adequate dissection and mobilization. Others have also shown that with such mediastinal dissection, highly selective rather than liberal use of Collis gastroplasty is appropriate.[50,51]

Need for Gastropexy or Gastrostomy

Gastrostomy and gastropexy have been suggested for patients who do not undergo an antireflux procedure, especially an elderly or debilitated patient who might not tolerate an extensive operation. Gastropexy helps keep the reduced stomach in an intra-abdominal position and can help reduce the chance of postoperative volvulus. It can be especially helpful as an adjunct to a repair with posterior fixation. Gastrostomy can do the same, but it can also allow for gastric decompression to permit a chronically incarcerated stomach time to regain its functionality. Because of the little risk and additional effort involved, anterior gastropexy should be added even if a fundoplication is performed.

Use of Prosthetic Mesh

It is tempting to draw on lessons learned from inguinal and ventral hernia repair and conclude that prosthetic mesh should be more widely used in repairing PEHs. However, the concern that the repetitive motions of swallowing and breathing will cause the mesh to erode into the GI tract over time, as happened with the Angelchik device,[52] should be taken seriously. Ideally, the crura should be closed under as little tension as possible. Prosthetic patches have been used to achieve a tension-free repair, but many surgeons are currently reluctant to use them near the GE junction. Although long-term results are not available, short- and medium-term results are extremely promising, with a recurrence rate close to zero when a prosthetic patch is used.

Multiple techniques have been described for patch placement, and both absorbable and nonabsorbable prostheses have been used.[53-65] A circular prosthesis that surrounds the esophagus with a keyhole cut out has been used with both polypropylene[56,57] and PTFE.[61] An A-shaped PTFE mesh patch that surrounds the crura has likewise been described.[59] Patches can also be used to buttress the crural repair without encircling the esophagus.

A randomized controlled trial of PTFE patch repair versus simple cruroplasty was conducted in patients undergoing laparoscopic Nissen fundoplication with a hiatal defect measuring 8 cm or greater, with 36 patients in each group.[65] A 3-cm keyhole was cut in a 13×10-cm PTFE patch for the esophagus to pass through, and the patch was secured to the diaphragm and crura with a straight hernia stapler. The study showed a marked decrease in recurrence rate in the prosthetic patch group—there were eight recurrences (22%) in the simple cruroplasty group and no recurrences in the PTFE patch group ($P < .006$).[65] At a mean follow-up of 3.3 years, there have been no erosions, strictures, or infections in the PTFE group.

Case series using polypropylene patches have reported no recurrences. Carlson et al. reported on 44 patients with large HHs and an intrathoracic stomach operated on through an open transabdominal approach using a keyholed polypropylene patch.[57] With a mean follow-up of 52 months, there were no clinical recurrences; however, one erosion was reported in a complicated patient. Granderath et al. from Austria used a polypropylene patch to buttress the crural closure rather than cutting a keyhole from the mesh via a laparoscopic approach performed on 24 patients undergoing redo laparoscopic antireflux procedures.[56] They found no recurrences with barium swallow at 1-year follow-up and no erosions or infections.

Overall, these series are quite encouraging regarding the application of prosthetic patches. The use of prosthetic patches to buttress PEH repairs is likely to evolve rapidly as longer-term data become available and newer studies report on the use of other prosthetic materials, including dual-sided expanded polytetrafluoroethylene (ePTFE), polypropylene coated with ePTFE or other nonadherent coating, and biodegradable patches. If erosion or other complications of the prosthetic patches do not develop over time, they should be used more liberally for large hiatal defects. Given the dynamic nature of the GE junction and the motion that occurs with swallowing and respiration, we remain concerned about keyhole mesh patches and the long-term potential complication of erosion—despite the fact that the short-term results as just described do not suggest erosion to be an issue. At this point we prefer to either make a relaxing incision in the diaphragm[17] or buttress the caudal extent of the crural closure as described by Granderath et al. to prevent the mesh from coming directly into contact with the esophagus.[56]

OTHER COMPLEX DIAPHRAGMATIC HERNIAS

Traumatic Hernias

Traumatic hernias can be caused by blunt force or penetrating objects, and management depends on whether they are identified acutely or in delayed fashion. Seventy-five percent of published traumatic hernias are due to blunt trauma, although the rate at a specific trauma center depends on the mix of penetrating versus blunt trauma in that specific geographic region.[66] Approximately 1% of patients admitted to the hospital after blunt trauma have a diaphragmatic injury: 69% are left-sided injuries, 24% are right sided, and 1.5% are bilateral. Fourteen percent are diagnosed in delayed fashion, and of the remaining cases, half are identified preoperatively and half during exploration. The mortality rate after an acute diagnosis is 3% to 17%, depending on the mechanism and associated injuries.[66,67]

In blunt trauma, rupture is usually due to increased intra-abdominal pressure related to falls or motor vehicle accidents. Diaphragmatic rupture generally occurs at the apex of the diaphragm in this situation.

Traumatic rupture of the diaphragm can be a diagnostic challenge. The diagnosis depends on a high index of suspicion, careful evaluation of the chest radiograph and CT scans, and meticulous inspection of the diaphragm when operating for concurrent injuries.[66] Although there have been advances in imaging the diaphragm,[68] no specific radiographic study can rule out a diaphragmatic injury, especially with penetrating trauma. The incidence of occult diaphragmatic injury with penetrating trauma to the lower left side of the chest is high, approximately 24%.[69] Delay in diagnosis with penetrating trauma increases mortality significantly—from 3% in the acute setting to 25% in the delayed group.[67] Therefore, some trauma surgeons recommend delayed laparoscopy in patients with left lower chest penetrating injuries if they do not otherwise have an indication for celiotomy.[69]

The surgical approach for repair of a diaphragmatic injury can be through either the abdomen or the chest. In the acute setting, most trauma surgeons use an abdominal approach because greater than 89% will have an associated abdominal injury.[66] Patients with a delayed diagnosis usually have significant adhesions to the intrathoracic organs, so a transthoracic approach should be considered. The surgical approach in a patient with a delayed diagnosis is controversial, but one must be prepared to operate on both sides of the diaphragm when undertaking such a case. Laparoscopic exploration and repair have also been undertaken in both the acute and chronic phases.[69-71] Creating a pneumoperitoneum when there is a diaphragmatic rupture can lead to a tension pneumothorax, so one must be prepared to decompress the chest urgently if necessary.

To fix the hernia defect, suture repair with interrupted, large nonabsorbable sutures is recommended. Direct suture repair is usually possible in the acute setting. In the chronic setting, a prosthetic patch is generally used. A chronic defect can be hard to close without a patch, and because the defect is not usually right at the GE junction, there is less concern about erosion by the patch.

Postoperative Diaphragmatic Hernias

Postoperative diaphragmatic hernias are due to alterations in the normal anatomy from surgical dissection of the hiatus. They may occur as a result of previous hernia repairs in this region, antireflux procedures, esophagomyotomy, partial gastrectomy, misguided chest tubes, or thoracoabdominal incisions in which the diaphragm is taken down.

After laparoscopic Nissen fundoplication, an iatrogenic PEH can develop in up to 6.3% of cases.[72] Early dysphagia after fundoplication can be caused by wrap herniation, which can readily be confirmed with a barium swallow. Symptomatic patients should undergo repair immediately. A laparoscopic repair is usually possible, although one must be prepared to perform an open procedure.[73]

Parahiatal Hernias

Parahiatal hernias are fleetingly rare, and some question their existence altogether in the absence of operative manipulation or trauma. A parahiatal hernia by definition arises lateral to the crural musculature, not through the esophageal hiatus itself. The clinical findings can be indistinguishable from those of a PEH.[74] Repair is similar to the repair of a PEH and can be performed laparoscopically or through an open approach.[74,75]

Congenital Diaphragmatic Hernias

Bochdalek hernias and Morgagni hernias occur as a result of incomplete embryologic development of the diaphragm. Most are repaired in children; however, 5% are found in adults.[76]

Bochdalek Hernias Bochdalek hernias, otherwise known as posterolateral hernias, account for 85% of congenital hernias. They occur on the left side 80% of the time. These hernias are diagnosed and repaired in children the majority of the time. Primary closure of small hernias can be performed with interrupted mattress sutures of nonabsorbable material, or larger defects can be repaired with a prosthetic patch. Both open and laparoscopic approaches have been described.[76]

Morgagni Hernias Foramen of Morgagni hernias, retrosternal hernias, and Larrey's hernias all describe the same entity and occur in the triangular space between the muscle fibers that make up the diaphragm; they extend from the xiphisternum and the costal margin to the central tendon of the diaphragm.[77] These hernias are thought to be due to congenital defects or absence of fusion of the muscle fibers in the diaphragm that is made worse by increased intra-abdominal pressure. Ninety percent are right sided because the pericardium itself prevents left-sided hernias.[78] Foramen of Morgagni hernias account for 3% to 4% of diaphragmatic hernias requiring surgery in both adults and children. Patients are usually asymptomatic, but anterior mediastinal masses are found incidentally on chest radiographs. Prompt surgical repair after diagnosis is prudent to avoid incarceration or strangulation of abdominal organs. A transabdominal route is the preferred choice. Although these hernias can be repaired laparoscopically, fixation of mesh and the use of tacks require skill and discretion to gain adequate fixation anteriorly and to not injure the pericardium and heart along the left margin of the defect. Prosthetic mesh is generally required to repair the defect.

SUGGESTED READINGS

Hashemi M, Sillin LF, Peters JH: Current concepts in the management of paraesophageal hiatal hernia. J Clin Gastroenterol 29:8-13, 1999.

Mattar SG, Bowers SP, Galloway KD, et al: Long-term outcome of laparoscopic repair of paraesophageal hernia. Surg Endosc 16:745-749, 2002.

Patel HJ, Tan BB, Yee J, et al: A 25-year experience with open primary transthoracic repair of paraesophageal hernia. J Thorac Cardiovasc Surg 127:843-849, 2004.

Pierre AF, Luketich JD, Fernando HC, et al: Results of laparoscopic repair of giant paraesophageal hernias: 200 consecutive patients. Ann Thorac Surg 74:1909-1915, 2002.

Stylopoulos N, Gazelle GS, Rattner DW: Paraesophageal hernias: Operation or observation? Ann Surg 236:492-501, 2002.

REFERENCES

1. Eliska O: Phreno-oesophageal membrane and its role in the development of hiatal hernia. Acta Anat 86:137-150, 1973.
2. Smith AB, Dickerman RD, McGuire CS, et al: Pressure-overload–induced sliding hiatal hernia in power athletes. J Clin Gastroenterol 28:352-354, 1999.
3. Deluca L, DiGiorgio P, Signoriello G, et al: Relationship between hiatal hernia and inguinal hernia. Dig Dis Sci 49:243-247, 2004.
4. Maish MS, DeMeester SR: Paraesophageal hernia. In Cameron JL (ed): Current Surgical Therapy, 8th ed. Philadelphia, CV Mosby, 2004.
5. Kleitsch WP: Embryology of congenital diaphragmatic hernia. I. Esophageal hiatus hernia. Arch Surg 76:868-873, 1958.
6. Hashemi M, Sillin LF, Peters JH: Current concepts in the management of paraesophageal hiatal hernia. J Clin Gastroenterol 29:8-13, 1999.
7. Peters JH, DeMeester TR: Gastroesophageal reflux and hiatal hernia. In Zinner MJ (ed): Maingot's Abdominal Operations, 10th ed. E Norwalk, CT, Appleton & Lange, 1997, p 834.
8. Carre IJ, Johnston BT, Thomas PS, Morrisson PJ: Familial hiatal hernia in a large five generation family confirming true autosomal dominant inheritance. Gut 45:649-652, 1999.
9. Floch NR: Paraesophageal hernias: Current concepts [editorial]. J Clin Gastroenterol 29:6-7, 1999.
10. Cameron AJ, Higgins JA: Linear gastric erosion. A lesion associated with large diaphragmatic hernia and chronic blood loss anemia. Gastroenterology 91:338-342, 1986.
11. Greub G, Liaudet L, Wiesel P, et al: Respiratory complications of gastroesophageal reflux associated with paraesophageal hiatal hernia. J Clin Gastroenterol 37:129-131, 2003.
12. Low DE, Simchuk EJ: Effect of paraesophageal hernia repair on pulmonary function. Ann Thorac Surg 74:333-337, 2002.
13. Kercher KW, Matthews BD, Ponsky JL, et al: Minimally invasive management of paraesophageal herniation in the high-risk patient. Am J Surg 182:510-514, 2001.
14. Skinner DB, Belsey RH: Surgical management of esophageal reflux and hiatus hernia. Long-term results with 1,030 patients. J Thorac Cardiovasc Surg 53:33-54, 1967.
15. Allen MS, Trastek VF, Deschamps C, Pairolero PC: Intrathoracic stomach. Presentation and results of operation. J Thorac Cardiovasc Surg 105:253-258, discussion 258-259, 1993.
16. Stylopoulos N, Gazelle GS, Rattner DW: Paraesophageal hernias: Operation or observation? Ann Surg 236:492-501, 2002.
17. Horgan S, Eubanks TR, Jacobsen G, et al: Repair of paraesophageal hernias. Am J Surg 177:354-358, 1999.
18. Dahlberg PS, Deschamps C, Miller DL, et al: Laparoscopic repair of large paraesophageal hiatal hernia. Ann Thorac Surg 72:1125-1129, 2001.
19. Treacy PJ, Jamieson GG: An approach to the management of para-oesophageal hiatus hernias. Aust N Z J Surg 57:813-817, 1987.
20. Patel HJ, Tan BB, Yee J, et al: A 25-year experience with open primary transthoracic repair of paraesophageal hernia. J Thorac Cardiovasc Surg 127:843-849, 2004.
21. Maziak DE, Todd TRJ, Pearson FG: Massive hiatus hernia: Evaluation and surgical management. J Thorac Cardiovasc Surg 114:53-62, 1998.
22. Geha AS, Massad MG, Snow NJ, Baue AE: A 32-year experience in 100 patients with giant paraesophageal hernia: The case for abdominal approach and selective antireflux repair. Surgery 128:623-630, 2000.
23. Williamson WA, Ellis FH Jr, Streitz JM Jr, Shahian DM: Paraesophageal hiatal hernia: Is an antireflux procedure necessary? Ann Thorac Surg 56:447-451, 1993.
24. Pierre AF, Luketich JD, Fernando HC, et al: Results of laparoscopic repair of giant paraesophageal hernias: 200 consecutive patients. Ann Thorac Surg 74:1909-1915, 2002.
25. Diaz S, Brunt LM, Klingensmith ME, et al: Laparoscopic paraesophageal hernia repair, a challenging operation: Medium-term outcome of 116 patients. J Gastrointest Surg 7:59-56, 2003.
26. Andujar JJ, Papasavas PK, Birdas T, et al: Laparoscopic repair of large paraesophageal hernia is associated with a low incidence of recurrence and reoperation. Surg Endosc 18:444-447, 2004.
27. Mattar SG, Bowers SP, Galloway KD, et al: Long-term outcome of laparoscopic repair of paraesophageal hernia. Surg Endosc 16:745-749, 2002.
28. Hashemi M, Peters JH, DeMeester TR, et al: Laparoscopic repair of large type III hiatal hernia: Objective follow-up reveals high recurrence rate. J Am Coll Surg 190:553-561, 2000.

29. Schauer PR, Ikramuddin S, McLaughlin RH, et al: Comparison of laparoscopic versus open repair of paraesophageal hernia. Am J Surg 176:659-665, 1998.

30. Oddsdottir M, Franco AL, Laycock WS, et al: Laparoscopic repair of paraesophageal hernia. New access, old technique. Surg Endosc 9:164-168, 1995.

31. Luketich JD, Raja S, Fernando HC, et al: Laparoscopic repair of giant paraesophageal hernia: 100 consecutive cases. Ann Surg 232:608-618, 2000.

32. Wiechmann RJ, Ferguson MK, Naunheim KS, et al: Laparoscopic management of giant paraesophageal herniation. Ann Thorac Surg 71:1080-1086, 2001.

33. Wu JS, Dunnegan DL, Soper NJ: Clinical and radiologic assessment of laparoscopic paraesophageal hernia repair. Surg Endosc 13:497-502, 1999.

34. Pitcher DE, Curet MJ, Martin DT, et al: Successful laparoscopic repair of paraesophageal hernia. Arch Surg 130:590-596, 1995.

35. Hawasli A, Zonca S: Laparoscopic repair of paraesophageal hiatal hernia. Am Surg 64:703-710, 1998.

36. Perdikis G, Hinder RA, Filipi CJ, et al: Laparoscopic para-esophageal hernia repair. Arch Surg 132:586-589, 1997.

37. Willekes CL, Edoga JK, Frezza EE: Laparoscopic repair of para-esophageal hernia. Ann Surg 225:31-38, 1997.

38. Gantert WA, Patti MG, Arcerito M, et al: Laparoscopic repair of paraesophageal hiatal hernias. J Am Coll Surg 186:428-432, 1998.

39. Horgan S, Eubanks TR, Jacobsen G, et al: Repair of paraesophageal hernias. Am J Surg 177:354-358, 1999.

40. van der Peet DL, Klinkenberg-Knol EC, Alonso Poza A, et al: Laparoscopic treatment of large paraesophageal hernias: Both excision of the sac and gastropexy are imperative for adequate surgical treatment. Surg Endosc 14:1015-1018, 2000.

41. Trus TL, Bax T, Richardson WS, et al: Complications of para-esophageal hernia repair. J Gastrointest Surg 1:221-228, 1997.

42. Behrns KE, Schlinkert RT: Laparoscopic management of para-esophageal hernia: Early results. J Laparoendosc Surg 6:311-317, 1996.

43. Huntington TR: Short-term outcome of laparoscopic para-esophageal hernia repair. A case series of 58 consecutive patients. Surg Endosc 11:894-898, 1997.

44. Krahenbuhl L, Schafer M, Farhadi J, et al: Laparoscopic treatment of large paraesophageal hernia with totally intrathoracic stomach. J Am Coll Surg 187:231-237, 1998.

45. Medina L, Peetz M, Ratzer E, Fenoglio M: Laparoscopic para-esophageal hernia repair. J Soc Laparoendosc Surg 2:269-272, 1998.

46. Edye MB, Canin-Endres J, Gattorno F, Salky BA: Durability of laparoscopic repair of paraesophageal hernia. Ann Surg 228:528-535, 1998.

47. Athanasakis H, Tzortzinis A, Tsiaoussis J, et al: Laparoscopic repair of paraesophageal hernia. Endoscopy 33:590-594, 2001.

48. Horvath KD, Swanstrom LL, Jobe BA: The short esophagus: Pathophysiology, incidence, presentation, and treatment in the era of laparoscopic antireflux surgery. Ann Surg 232:630-640, 2000.

49. Urbach DR, Khajanchee YS, Glasgow RE, et al: Preoperative determinants of an esophageal lengthening procedure in laparoscopic antireflux surgery. Surg Endosc 15:1408-1412, 2001.

50. O'Rourke RW, Khajanchee YS, Urbach DR, et al: Extended transmediastinal dissection: An alternative to gastroplasty for short esophagus. Arch Surg 138:735-740, 2003.

51. Madan AK, Frantzides CT, Patsavas KL: The myth of the short esophagus. Surg Endosc 18:31-34, 2004.

52. Varshney S, Kelly JJ, Branaan G, et al: Angelchik prosthesis revisited. World J Surg 26:129-133, 2002.

53. Scott JS: .www.lifecell.com/healthcare/procedures/abdominal/Scott.Hiatal%20Hernia.2004.Final.pdf.

54. Oelschlager BK, Barreca M, Chang L, Pellegrini CA: The use of small intestine submucosa in the repair of paraesophageal hernias: Initial observations of a new technique. Am J Surg 186:4-8, 2003.

55. Strange PS: Small intestine submucosa for laparoscopic repair of large paraesophageal hiatal hernias: A preliminary report. Surg Tech Int 11:141-143, 2003.

56. Granderath FA, Kamolz T, Schweiger UM, Pointner R: Laparoscopic refundoplication with prosthetic hiatal closure for recurrent hiatal hernia after failed antireflux surgery. Arch Surg 138:902-907, 2003.

57. Carlson MA, Condon RE, Ludwig KA, Schulte WJ: Management of intrathoracic stomach with polypropylene mesh prosthesis reinforced transabdominal hiatus hernia repair. J Am Coll Surg 187:227-230, 1998.

58. Champion JK, Rock D: Laparoscopic mesh cruroplasty for large paraesophageal hernias. Surg Endosc 17:551-553, 2003.

59. Casaccia M, Torelli P, Panaro F, et al: Laparoscopic physiological hiatoplasty for hiatal hernia: New composite "A"-shaped mesh. Physical and geometrical analysis and preliminary clinical results. Surg Endosc 16:1441-1445, 2002.

60. Edelman DS: Laparoscopic paraesophageal hernia repair with mesh. Surg Laparosc Endosc 5:32-37, 1995.

61. Frantzides CT, Richards CG, Carlson MA: Laparoscopic repair of large hiatal hernia with polytetrafluoroethylene. Surg Endosc 13:906-908, 1999.

62. Hui TT, Thoman DS, Spyrou M, et al: Mesh crural repair of large paraesophageal hiatal hernias. Am Surg 67:1170-1174, 2001.

63. Granderath FA, Schweiger UM, Kamolz T, et al: Laparoscopic antireflux surgery with routine mesh-hiatoplasty in the treatment of gastroesophageal reflux disease. J Gastrointest Surg 6:347-353, 2002.

64. Huntington TR: Laparoscopic mesh repair of the esophageal hiatus. J Am Coll Surg 184:399-400, 1997.

65. Frantzides CT, Madan AK, Carlson MA, Stavropoulos GP: A prospective, randomized trial of laparoscopic polytetrafluoroethylene (PTFE) patch repair vs simple cruroplasty for large hiatal hernia. Arch Surg 137:649-652, 2002.

66. Shah R, Sabanathan S, Mearns AJ, Choudhury AK: Traumatic rupture of diaphragm. Ann Thorac Surg 60:1444-1449, 1995.

67. Degiannis E, Levy RD, Sofianos C, et al: Diaphragmatic herniation after penetrating trauma. Br J Surg 83:88-91, 1996.

68. Iochum S, Ludig T, Walter F, et al: Imaging of diaphragmatic injury: A diagnostic challenge? Radiographics 22(Spec No):S103-S116, 2002.

69. Murray JA, Demetriades D, Asensio JA, et al: Occult injuries to the diaphragm: Prospective evaluation of laparoscopy in penetrating injuries to the left lower chest. J Am Coll Surg 187:626-630, 1998.

70. Meyer G, Huttl TP, Hatz RA, Schildberg FW: Laparoscopic repair of traumatic diaphragmatic hernias. Surg Endosc 14:1010-1014, 2000.

71. Frantzides CT, Madan AK, O'Leary PJ, Losurdo J: Laparoscopic repair of a recurrent chronic traumatic diaphragmatic hernia. Am Surg 69:160-162, 2003.

72. Watson DI, Jamieson GG, Devitt PG, et al: Paraoesophageal hiatus hernia: An important complication of laparoscopic Nissen fundoplication. Br J Surg 82:521-523, 1995.

73. Seelig MH, Hinder RA, Klingler PJ, et al: Paraesophageal herniation as a complication following laparoscopic antireflux surgery. J Gastrointest Surg 3:95-99, 1999.

74. Scheidler MG, Keenan RJ, Maley RH, et al: "True" parahiatal hernia: A rare entity radiologic presentation and clinical management. Ann Thorac Surg 73:416-419, 2002.

75. Rodefeld MD, Soper NJ: Parahiatal hernia with volvulus and incarceration: Laparoscopic repair of a rare defect. J Gastrointest Surg 2:193-197, 1998.

76. Richardson WS, Bolton JS: Laparoscopic repair of congenital diaphragmatic hernias. J Laparoendosc Adv Surg Tech A 12:277-280, 2002.

77. Minneci PC, Deans KJ, Kim P, Mathisen DJ: Foramen of Morgagni hernia: Changes in diagnosis and treatment. Ann Thorac Surg 77:1956-1959, 2004.

78. Comer TP, Clagett OT: Surgical treatment of hernia of the foramen of Morgagni. J Thorac Cardiovasc Surg 52:461-468, 1966.

41

Congenital Disorders of the Esophagus

R. Cartland Burns

The purpose of this chapter is to familiarize surgeons with common congenital problems of the esophagus, to understand the embryologic events leading to formation of the defect, and to understand the surgical principles of caring for children with these anomalies. The primary congenital disorders of the esophagus are those that result from failure of formation (esophageal atresia [EA]), incomplete separation of the aerodigestive tract (tracheoesophageal fistula [TEF] and cleft), duplication, stenosis, and external compression (vascular ring).

EMBRYOLOGY AND ANATOMIC CONSIDERATIONS

Comprehension of the embryologic development of the esophagus serves to improve understanding of the congenital diseases that affect the esophagus, in addition to providing a framework to understand the essential anatomic considerations that have a bearing on important surgical principles useful for the treatment of these disorders. This topic is covered in detail elsewhere and is only briefly mentioned here.

The median ventral diverticulum (eventually forming the trachea) begins to form during the third week after conception (day 22 to 23), and the stomach forms sequentially in a posterior position. The esophagus develops from the endodermal tissue between these two structures. The trachea and esophagus elongate during the next 10 days, and separation of the two structures proceeds in a cranial direction to complete division of the esophagus and trachea by day 34 to 36. The esophagus has attained its full length by day 49 and continues to grow rapidly during the first postnatal years (Fig. 41–1).[1]

During the course of development the lumen of the esophagus becomes nearly filled with epithelial cells by the eighth week. A single lumen is restored by the process of vacuolization, perhaps mediated by regulated apoptosis as is suspected in other portions of the gastrointestinal tract.[2-4]

Sympathetic innervation is derived from mediastinal branches of the thoracic sympathetic trunk and from the celiac plexus. Parasympathetic innervation arises from the vagus nerve.[4] Vascular supply in the upper esophagus is derived from branches arising from the inferior thyroid artery, and the lower esophagus is supplied by segmental branches arising directly from the aorta.

ESOPHAGEAL ATRESIA AND TRACHEOESOPHAGEAL FISTULA

Historical Points

Esophageal and tracheoesophageal atresia has captured the fascination of the medical community since it was first described in 1670, when Durston described pure EA.[5,6] Proximal EA with distal TEF was subsequently described by Thomas Gibson in 1697.[7] Despite knowledge of the anomaly, no surgical treatment was effective until 1939, when Ladd and Leven, working independently, performed a staged approach to feeding via gastrostomy, division of the fistula, and eventual reconstruction with a skin tube created on the anterior chest wall.[5,8] Before this time, all reported attempts at correction were met with uniform mortality.[9] Subsequent work by Cameron Haight in 1941 resulted in the first successful primary repair accomplished by thoracotomy. He later modified the approach to the extrapleural route, which remains the most popular approach even today.[10,11] Recently, reports are demonstrating the feasibility of the thoracoscopic approach for the surgical management of EA-TEF.[12,13]

Development

Developmental understanding of the malformation is largely limited to animal models demonstrating the

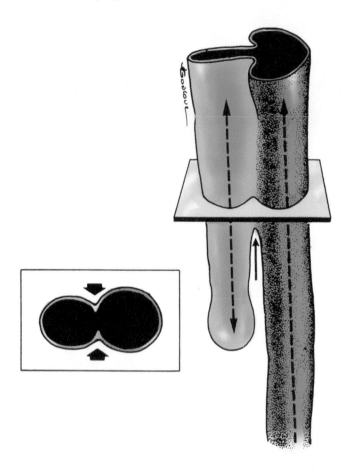

Figure 41–1. The trachea *(red)* forms as a diverticulum from the primitive foregut, and both structures elongate. Two cellular ridges form *(inset)* and divide the two structures into the trachea *(red)* and esophagus *(pink)*. This process begins at the caudal end and proceeds in a cranial direction *(arrow)*. (From Skandalakis J, Gray S: Embryology for Surgeons. 2nd ed. Baltimore, Williams & Wilkins, 1994, p 65.)

lesion. These malformations are primarily induced by exposure to the teratogen doxorubicin (Adriamycin),[14,15] and EA and foregut duplications develop in the embryo in a dose-related manner. The effect of the anthracycline antibiotic on apoptosis seems relevant to the restoration of a continuous lumen in this animal model.[16] Various candidate genes regulating these processes appear to be the HOX D group and the SHH and GLI signaling pathway, which have also been linked to anomalies in the VACTERL constellation (vertebral, anorectal, cardiac, tracheoesophageal, renal, and limb anomalies).[11]

Classification

EA and TEF occur in a predictable pattern and are categorized by anatomic variation as described by Gross in his classic textbook.[17] In this volume, Gross described six anatomic variations of the esophageal anomaly, demonstrated in Figure 41–2. Type C, proximal EA and

distal TEF, is the most common and represents 85% of cases. Pure atresia (type A), though less common (6%), may present a greater surgical challenge because of inadequate esophageal length for repair. The upper pouch fistulas in types B and D may be overlooked because of attention focused on the atretic esophagus. They will subsequently be found when persistent coughing and symptoms of aspiration prompt investigation. Similarly, TEF without atresia (type E) is characterized by symptoms of gastroesophageal reflux (GER) and choking spells with feeding. Type F congenital esophageal stenosis arises from various embryologic errors and is discussed in detail later.

Associated Abnormalities

As many as 50% of children with EA or TEF (or both) will have other important anomalies.[18-24] In many cases the associated anomalies will have a greater impact on the overall prognosis for the child than the foregut anomaly. Accordingly, it is important to conduct a thorough investigation for such abnormalities. Anomalies associated with EA include those found in the VACTERL constellation of anomalies,[25,26] as well as several other less common deformities.

Holder[27] and subsequently Dunn et al.[28] reported that associated anomalies were most common in pure EA without fistula and least common in cases of H-type TEF without atresia. These anomalies involve, in order of frequency, the cardiovascular (ventricular septal defect most common), gastrointestinal (imperforate anus, duodenal and other atresia, malrotation), and genitourinary systems (hypospadias, cryptorchidism, renal malformation, urinary obstruction and exstrophies).

The CHARGE association is seen in 2% of patients with EA[29] and includes coloboma, heart defects, choanal atresia, mental retardation, genital hypoplasia, and ear anomalies.

Esophageal anomalies may be seen in patients with Down's syndrome, and in these cases one must investigate for evidence of duodenal atresia, cardiac defects, and Hirschsprung's disease.

Tracheomalacia is common in children with EA and may be mild with insignificant clinical findings or may be severe enough to result in respiratory compromise. The upper part of the trachea is the most commonly involved area and corresponds to the area adjacent to the obstructed upper pouch of the esophagus. The commonly accepted mechanism is pressure-induced malacia from the dilated upper pouch, and it is associated with a deficiency of tracheal cartilage. The tracheomalacia will typically improve in time after correction of the atresia, but it may be problematic, with stridor requiring treatment. Usual management includes careful attention to feeding, avoidance of aspiration, and evaluation for GER, which will exacerbate the condition. Tracheal suspension (aortopexy) is occasionally needed in severe cases and improves the tracheal obstruction by lifting the aorta and its attachments to the trachea anteriorly. This maneuver creates an external "stent" that relieves the obstructive symptoms.

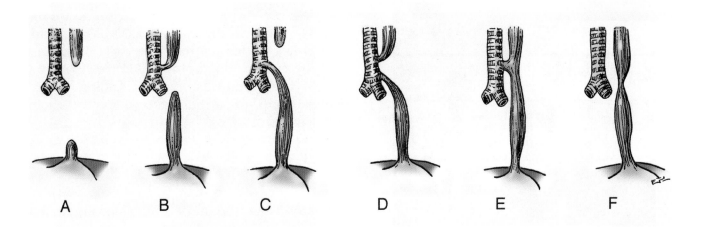

Figure 41–2.   Classic stratification of the most common varieties of esophageal atresia and tracheoesophageal fistula as outlined by Robert Gross in 1953. **A,** Pure esophageal atresia without fistula, also called "long-gap" atresia. **B,** Esophageal atresia with a proximal tracheoesophageal fistula. **C,** The most common anatomic relationship of esophageal atresia and distal tracheoesophageal fistula. **D,** Esophageal atresia with both proximal and distal tracheoesophageal fistulas. This variety may be more common than once reported, and an upper pouch fistula is always suspected. **E,** Tracheoesophageal fistula without atresia. Also known as an H-type fistula, this lesion is usually high in the trachea and generally approachable through a cervical incision. **F,** Congenital esophageal stenosis. (From Gross RE: Atresia of the esophagus. In Gross RE [ed]: The Surgery of Infancy and Childhood. Philadelphia, WB Saunders, 1953, p 76.)

Clinical Findings and Diagnostic Evaluation

Prenatal diagnosis is becoming more common and more accurate.[30-32] The ultrasound findings of a dilated upper esophagus, small stomach, and polyhydramnios are all suggestive of EA. When EA is suspected in the antenatal period, it is desirable to offer the family counseling by a pediatric surgeon, neonatologist, and geneticist. These parents may wish to consider amniocentesis or chorionic villus sampling. At the very least, they can be educated about the diagnosis, associated anomalies, and treatment options and possibilities before the delivery, when the diagnosis of anomalies can be overwhelming.

The newborn's clinical symptoms are related to the anatomic findings. EA results in failure to swallow saliva, apparent marked salivation, and drooling. Attempts at feeding are accompanied by coughing, choking, and regurgitation of undigested milk or formula. These events are usually followed by the attempted passage of nasogastric or orogastric tubes, which are met with resistance and are seen to be coiled in the upper pouch on chest radiographs. Radiographs will demonstrate a gasless abdomen in patients with pure EA (Fig. 41–3) or air in the abdomen in those with atresia and TEF (Fig. 41–4). Abdominal distention may be present in children with TEF, but not with pure atresia. In patients with distal intestinal atresia (duodenal atresia, small bowel atresia, imperforate anus), the abdominal distention may be marked and can cause respiratory compromise. Isolated TEF is associated with coughing, choking, and apparent aspiration episodes with every feeding.

Diagnostic evaluation should give consideration to confirmation of the presence of EA, which may be as simple as an inability to pass an orogastric tube with the tip coiled in the upper pouch. A plain radiograph will confirm this location, demonstrate the presence or absence of air in the intestine, and identify vertebral anomalies. Barium may be instilled into the upper pouch (diluted, 1 ml) to confirm the diagnosis, but it is not frequently necessary. This study may demonstrate an upper pouch fistula, although it has been shown to have a significant rate of inaccuracy, and a great deal of care is required to avoid aspiration through the larynx and resultant soiling of the lungs. Because associated anomalies are common, preoperative studies should include a thorough physical examination, echocardiogram, and renal ultrasound. Chromosome analysis may be considered if not completed in the prenatal period.

Management Considerations

The presence of EA or TEF is not a surgical emergency, but it does require diligence in protection of the infant's lungs because tracheobronchial aspiration is common and can contribute to significant pulmonary complications, including pneumonitis. Aspiration of saliva can occur via the larynx or aspiration of gastric contents via the distal TEF. The upper pouch saliva is suctioned with an orogastric sump tube to clear secretions. The oral route is preferred because infants are obligate nasal breathers and the nasal route risks compromising the airway. Gastric reflux through the distal TEF is reduced by maintaining the infant in an upright, preferably prone position. Spontaneous ventilation is preferred to prevent continuous gaseous distention of the stomach. On occasions when intubation and mechanical ventilation are required, low inspiratory pressures are preferred. These and all surgical neonates require 10% dextrose solutions to prevent hypoglycemia, as well as careful attention to

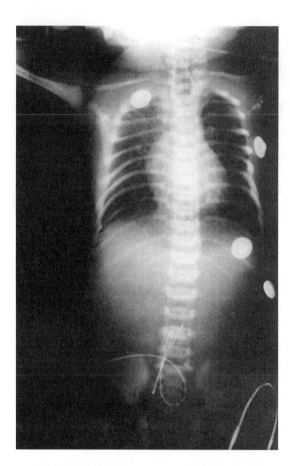

Figure 41–3. Typical radiograph in an infant with esophageal atresia demonstrating the orogastric tube coiled in the atretic proximal esophagus without a patent tracheoesophageal fistula as shown by the gasless abdomen. (From Ashcraft KW, Murphy JP, Sharp RJ, et al [eds]: Pediatric Surgery, 3rd ed. Philadelphia, WB Saunders, 2000, p 353.)

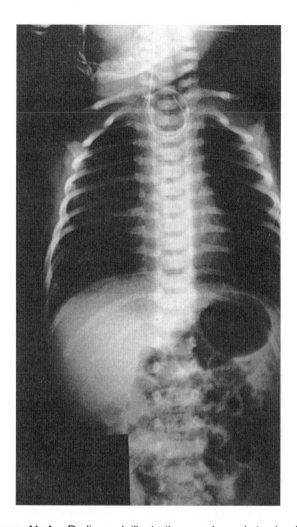

Figure 41–4. Radiograph illustrating esophageal atresia with the orogastric tube coiled in the atretic upper esophageal pouch. Air in the bowel indicates a distal tracheoesophageal fistula. This radiograph does not exclude the presence of the upper pouch fistula seen in type B. (From Ashcraft KW, Murphy JP, Sharp RJ, et al [eds]: Pediatric Surgery, 3rd ed. Philadelphia, WB Saunders, 2000, p 353.)

maintenance of electrolyte balance. Perioperative broad-spectrum antibiotics are instituted as well. In some instances, children with long-gap atresia have been allowed to be cared for at home before definitive repair, which may be delayed for months after birth.[33-35]

Preoperative evaluation will allow identification of pertinent associated anomalies, some of which will adversely affect the outcome of an infant with EA. Historically, Waterston's criteria were used to separate infants into risk groups based on prematurity and associated anomalies.[36] This classification scheme was highly relevant when it was developed; however, modern surgical and neonatal care has shifted focus to alternative considerations in perioperative planning. Several recent studies have shown that physiologic status, specifically respiratory status and life-threatening anomalies, are the primary prognostic factors in the current treatment of EA and TEF.[37-39] With these guidelines, current success rates in children without life-threatening associated anomalies and with good respiratory function approach 100% with primary division of TEF and repair of EA. In children with associated cardiac anomalies and low birth weight (<1500 g), perioperative risk is much greater, with only a 22% survival rate.[40]

Operative Management

Proximal EA with distal TEF is usually managed by primary division of the fistula and repair of the atretic esophagus. Division of the TEF allows more controlled ventilation and prevents further soiling of the tracheobronchial tree, whereas repair of the EA reconstitutes gastrointestinal tract continuity. Many surgeons prefer rigid bronchoscopy at the outset of the proposed repair of the anomaly to assess for the presence of a proximal pouch fistula. The operative strategy is coordinated with the anesthesiologist, and a right thoracotomy is preferred in the usual case of a left-sided aortic arch. Either left main stem intubation or low-volume ventilation is helpful for posterior mediastinal exposure. The child is placed in the decubitus position, and a muscle-sparing thoracotomy is performed in the fourth or fifth intercostal space. The latissimus dorsi and serratus anterior muscles are mobilized off the chest wall, and the intercostal space is identified. The intercostal muscle is

Figure 41–5. After dividing the intercostal muscles, the parietal pleura is encountered and protected. By gentle dissection, the parietal pleura is separated from the chest wall and a retropleural plane is developed. The retropleural plane allows easy control of the ipsilateral lung during dissection and prevents intrapleural soiling in the event of an anastomotic leak.

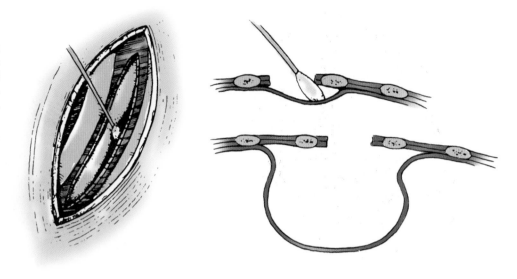

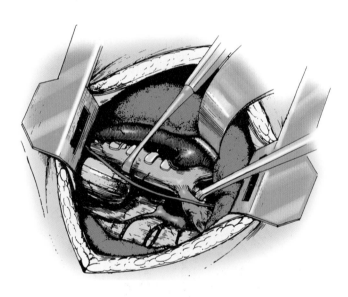

Figure 41–6. The azygos vein is identified and divided near its junction with the superior vena cava. The location of the azygos vein directs the surgeon to the region of the tracheal carina, where a distal tracheoesophageal fistula is usually found. The tracheal anatomy is carefully confirmed to avoid erroneous division of a bronchus.

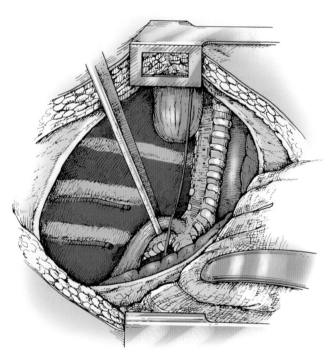

Figure 41–7. The tracheoesophageal fistula is dissected to allow control of the fistula near the trachea. A vessel loop allows traction on the fistula, which will immediately improve ventilation. The vagus nerve (if found) is carefully preserved. (From Ashcraft KW: Atlas of Pediatric Surgery. Philadelphia, WB Saunders, 1994, p 40.)

divided with care to avoid pleural violation. A retropleural dissection is conducted carefully to mobilize nearly the entire lateral and posterior aspect of the chest (Fig. 41–5). The azygos vein is encountered and divided between ligatures (Fig. 41–6). The distal TEF can be identified at this point and is usually distended with air at each inspiration. The distal portion of the esophagus is dissected circumferentially at the level of the fistula and encircled with a vessel loop (Fig. 41–7). At this point the surgeon can occlude the fistula and the anesthesiologist will confirm adequate (usually improved) ventilation. The fistula is divided with absorbable monofilament sutures on the trachea while taking care to not deprive

the trachea of an adequate lumen nor retain an esophageal remnant as a tracheal diverticulum (Fig. 41–8). The distal esophagus is controlled with a fine suture, and attention is turned to locating and mobilizing the proximal esophagus. The proximal esophagus is mobilized as widely as possible to allow a tension-free anastomosis (Fig. 41–9). Mobilization of the distal esophagus has traditionally been discouraged, although recent

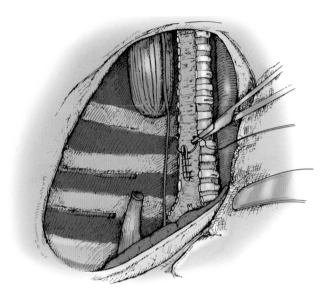

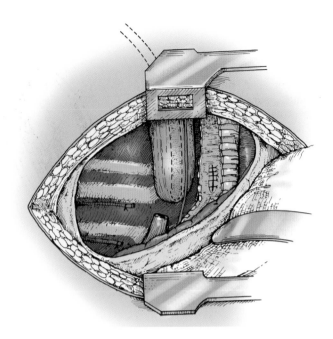

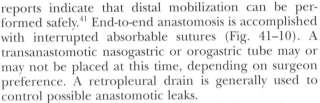

Figure 41–8. The tracheoesophageal fistula is divided at the junction with the trachea by sequential transection and suture repair of the trachea. This is performed sequentially to avoid the development of a large air leak complicating ventilation. The trachea is repaired with absorbable monofilament sutures to avoid narrowing the trachea or preserving a tracheal diverticulum. (From Ashcraft KW: Atlas of Pediatric Surgery. Philadelphia, WB Saunders, 1994, p 41.)

Figure 41–9. The upper pouch is mobilized with the assistance of the anesthesiologist by placing an orogastric tube into the upper pouch and distending the upper part of the esophagus. The two ends of the esophagus are assessed for feasibility of primary anastomosis. (From Ashcraft KW: Atlas of Pediatric Surgery. Philadelphia, WB Saunders, 1994, p 41.)

reports indicate that distal mobilization can be performed safely.[41] End-to-end anastomosis is accomplished with interrupted absorbable sutures (Fig. 41–10). A transanastomotic nasogastric or orogastric tube may or may not be placed at this time, depending on surgeon preference. A retropleural drain is generally used to control possible anastomotic leaks.

Primary repair of both deformities is ideal; however, in children with significant risk factors, division of the fistula may be undertaken as a primary procedure and gastrostomy performed for access to the distal gastrointestinal tract for nutritional management. In this case, the distal esophagus is secured to the prevertebral fascia to prevent retraction and to aid in identifying this structure at subsequent reconstruction.

Pure EA is frequently associated with a long gap between the proximal and distal atretic segments. The gap may prohibit primary repair of the deformity, and such children are usually managed with an initial gastrostomy for enteral feeding access.[42] Delayed repair is then planned, with consideration for mobilization of both the proximal and distal segments. The literature is replete with descriptions of innovative techniques and operative strategies for the management of patients with long-gap EA, thus bearing witness to the fact that it presents a true surgical challenge. Several techniques have been proposed for increasing the length of the proximal esophagus, such as bougienage[43] or intraoperative myotomy of either the upper pouch, the lower pouch, or both.[44-49] Some authors have reported success with creation of a fistula between the proximal and distal

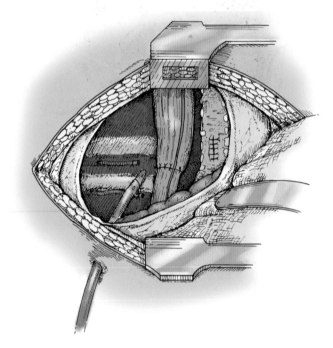

Figure 41–10. A primary repair is achieved with an accurate single-layer anastomosis created with interrupted, absorbable sutures. The posterior row of sutures is preplaced and then tied with the assistant holding traction to release tension from the anastomosis. The anterior row of sutures is then placed and tied. A tube thoracostomy is placed near the anastomosis to control a possible anastomotic leak. Some prefer to suture the tube in place with fast-absorbing suture. (From Ashcraft KW: Atlas of Pediatric Surgery. Philadelphia, WB Saunders, 1994, p 43.)

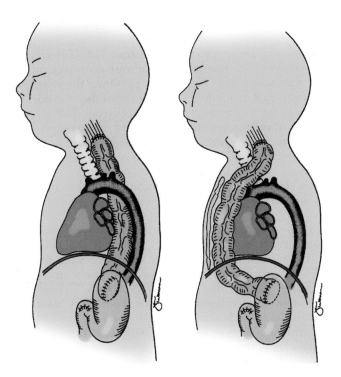

Figure 41–11. Colonic interposition has been used successfully as a replacement esophageal conduit and is shown in the substernal position, as well as in the preferred native esophageal position in the posterior mediastinum. (From Dillon PA: Esophagus. In Oldham KT, Colombani PM, Foglia RP, et al [eds]: Principles and Practice of Pediatric Surgery, vol 2. Philadelphia, Lippincott, Williams, & Wilkins, 2005, p 1034.)

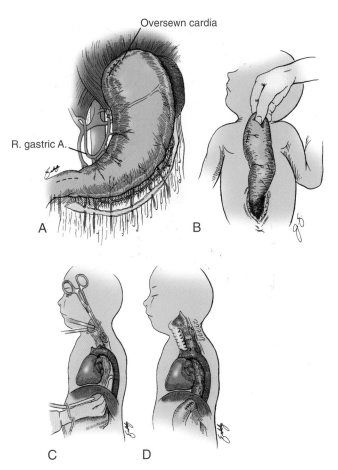

Figure 41–12. **A** to **D,** Gastric transposition has been used to replace the missing esophagus and, with extensive mobilization, will reach into the neck. The vagus nerves are sacrificed, thus necessitating pyloroplasty. (From Dillon PA: Esophagus. In Oldham KT, Colombani PM, Foglia RP, et al [eds]: Principles and Practice of Pediatric Surgery, vol 2. Philadelphia, Lippincott, Williams, & Wilkins, 2005, p 1035.)

ends of the esophagus and subsequently dilating the tract.[50] Recently, several reports have demonstrated success with the technique of mobilizing the proximal and distal esophagus, followed by placement of external sutures tethering the ends to a button. The button is subsequently tightened to produce tension on the esophagus and stretch the atretic segments into proximity, followed by primary anastomosis.[51-54] Still other authors have promoted primary repair of the atretic segments regardless of the amount of tension on the anastomosis.[55,56] The multiplicity of techniques and reports supports the conventional wisdom that the native esophagus remains the preferred conduit for the thoracic gastrointestinal tract; however, the occasion does arise in which replacement is required. In such cases the literature describes acceptable outcomes with the interposition of colon (Fig. 41–11), small bowel, or gastric conduit (Figs. 41–12 and 41–13).[57-64]

Recent reports have described thoracoscopic repair of EA and TEF.[12,13,65] The procedure has been proved to be safe and effective, but it requires a specialized unit with a dedicated endoscopic surgical team. The occasional laparoscopist will find the procedure tedious and will probably not reproduce the current excellent outcomes offered by the open procedure.

Complications

Complications associated with repair of EA and TEF can be considered to be either perioperative or late in nature. Perioperative complications are limited primarily to anastomotic leak or disruption. This complication occurs in approximately 15% of patients and usually responds (95%) to simple drainage, which is generally established at the time of anastomosis.[66-68] The development of an anastomotic leak is usually due to inaccurate surgical technique, poor perfusion, or excessive tension on the anastomosis. These factors can generally be avoided, but in some cases they are inevitable and a leak will occur. An anastomotic leak is diagnosed by detecting the presence of pneumothorax or pleural effusion in the first 24 to 48 hours postoperatively or by a leak on an esophagogram performed routinely at 5 to 7 days postoperatively before instituting enteral feeding. The principles of management of an anastomotic leak include adequate drainage and nutritional repletion with parenteral nutrition. These children are maintained

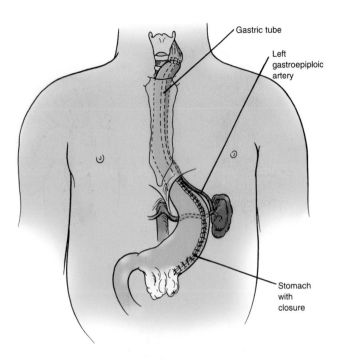

Figure 41–13. The reversed gastric tube can be fashioned from the greater curvature of the stomach and may be mobilized to reach the upper pouch in the neck. (From Dillon PA: Esophagus. In Oldham KT, Colombani PM, Foglia RP, et al [eds]: Principles and Practice of Pediatric Surgery, vol 2. Philadelphia, Lippincott, Williams, & Wilkins, 2005, p 1036.)

on antibiotics for the duration of the leak. Even large leaks are successfully managed with conservative techniques and rarely require a reoperation.

Later complications include anastomotic stricture, which in many cases is a secondary complication after an anastomotic leak. Stricture may also occur as a result of GER, and a stricture that does not respond rapidly to treatment should alert the surgeon to consider treatment of GER by fundoplication.[69] The incidence of stricture is reported to be as high as 40%.[70] An anastomotic stricture is suspected when there is impaction of food, feeding intolerance, or dysphagia. The diagnosis is confirmed by either esophagography or esophagoscopy, which may also be therapeutic. Treatment consists of dilation, and the type of dilator is based on surgeon preference. Dilators include those passed antegrade, such as a Maloney- or Savary-type bougie. Pneumatic dilation is also available and may offer the advantage of fluoroscopic guidance; when the balloon is filled with contrast material, it provides a dynamic view of the stricture and dilation.[70] If dilation is unsuccessful, the surgeon should consider the possibility of GER being a contributing factor, and contrast studies and pH monitoring should be performed before considering local resection and anastomosis.

Recurrent TEF usually occurs in association with an anastomotic leak (approximately 10%)[71-73] and is probably related to local inflammation and poor healing of the primary lesion. A high index of suspicion is needed to identify a recurrent TEF because the symptoms may be nonspecific. These children generally have symptoms of coughing, choking, and feeding intolerance. Recurrent pneumonia is also seen with recurrent TEF. If suspected, the diagnosis is pursued by contrast esophagography, esophagoscopy, and bronchoscopy. Once the diagnosis is confirmed, treatment options must be considered. Options for the management of recurrent TEF include repeat thoracotomy for very early recurrence. The operative management of this lesion should include repeat division of the fistula, repair of the esophagus and trachea, and placement of tissue between the two structures. The choice of tissue is variable and has included an intercostal muscle flap, pleural flap, pericardium, and azygos vein. Recent innovative techniques have been described and include cauterization, fibrin glue, and histoacryl glue.[72,74-79]

Tracheomalacia is commonly associated with EA and TEF and may result in respiratory symptoms, including expiratory stridor or a barking-type cough.[80] These children may have symptoms ranging from noisy breathing to apneic spells leading to life-threatening events. The trachea lacks its normal rigidity because of one of several causes, and this allows the trachea to collapse under the positive pressure of expiration or straining. The traditional wisdom regarding tracheomalacia associated with EA and TEF holds that the dilated upper pouch of the esophagus exerts pressure on the posterior wall of the trachea and causes the trachea to be easily deformable.[81,82] Further information has found a high incidence of primary tracheal defects in patients with EA/TEF and thus raises support for consideration of tracheomalacia as a primary airway defect.[83] Suspicion of tracheomalacia can be confirmed by bronchoscopy with spontaneous ventilation (Fig. 41–14) or by radiographic means.[84-87] Although most children with tracheomalacia will improve with time, those with severe manifestations require intervention. The primary form of treatment is aortopexy to achieve elevation of the vascular structures anteriorly for relief of pressure on the trachea. This can be accomplished by direct suturing (Figs. 41–15 and 41–16), a pericardial sling, or more recently, thoracoscopic techniques.[88-92] Occasionally, a child will fail to respond to vascular suspension and will require a tracheostomy, and tracheal stenting has been used with limited success.[93-95]

ESOPHAGEAL DUPLICATION

Esophageal duplication cysts represent anomalous structures arising from the primitive foregut and are frequently described as dorsal enteric remnants.[96] These remnants arise from the foregut early during development and may be found as cystic structures in the superior mediastinum or more commonly in the posterior mediastinum. The cyst may be lined with any type of epithelium found in the foregut structures, including ciliated respiratory epithelium and enteric (commonly gastric) mucosa.[97-100] The gastric mucosal remnants may secrete acid and cause the cyst to erode into adjacent structures. Most commonly, these cysts do not communicate with the lumen of the esophagus, although mus-

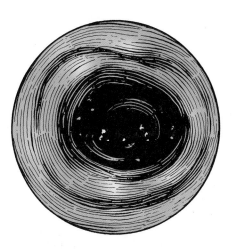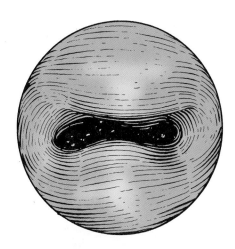

Figure 41–14. Bronchoscopic evaluation of a patient with tracheomalacia reveals a compromised lumen; this is demonstrated during spontaneous ventilation as positive pressure holds the lumen in a distended position and may lead to error in diagnosis. Insufficient tracheal rings may be identified as well. Some prefer to complete the aortopexy under bronchoscopic guidance to confirm correction of the compression. (From Rob and Smith's Operative Surgery: Pediatric Surgery, 4th ed. Boston, Butterworth, 1988, p 126.)

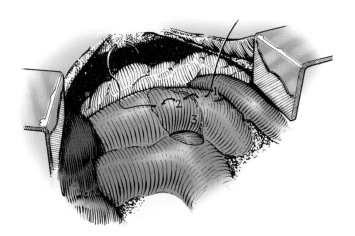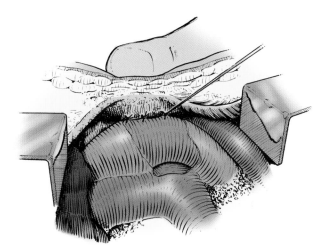

Figure 41–15. The aorta is mobilized anteriorly through the pericardium, and usually three sutures are placed partial thickness into the aorta. Care is taken to avoid dissection of the tissues between the vascular structures and the trachea because these fibrous attachments are necessary to create the lift or external stenting of the trachea. (From Rob and Smith's Operative Surgery: Pediatric Surgery, 4th ed. Boston, Butterworth, 1988, p 129.)

Figure 41–16. The sutures are tied to complete the aortopexy. The aorta is approximated to the posterior of the sternum. This is usually accomplished while the assistant is depressing the sternum to avoid excessive traction on any of the aortic sutures. (From Rob and Smith's Operative Surgery: Pediatric Surgery, 4th ed. Boston, Butterworth, 1988, p 129.)

cularis mucosae may be shared. A cleavage plane usually exists between the two structures.

These abnormalities are associated with vertebral anomalies in as many as 50% of cases, and there is nearly a 50% incidence of associated additional intestinal duplications. In some cases the lesion will cross the diaphragm, and a cyst manifested as a thoracic duplication will be originating from below the diaphragm.[101] Additionally, the cyst may be associated with a vertebral anomaly, with extension into the spinal canal, and it is then termed a neurenteric cyst.[102] Because the preoperative evaluation usually focuses on the chest, the surgeon

must remain vigilant about the possibility of transdiaphragm extension.[96,97,102]

Symptoms attributed to these lesions depend on the size of the cyst and the pressure of the mass on surrounding structures.[103] Such symptoms usually include airway irritation (cough, dyspnea), failure to thrive, or esophageal symptoms (dysphagia, chest pain). Cysts containing gastric mucosa may give rise to hemorrhage or perforation as a result of ulceration. Occasionally, the gastric mucosa will cause erosions into the lung, bronchi, or esophagus. In these cases, pulmonary hemorrhage or hematemesis may develop.[104]

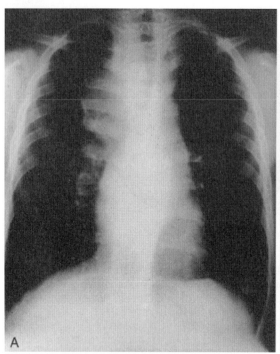
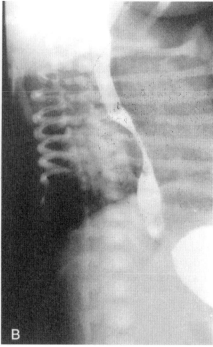

Figure 41–17. A child with vague respiratory symptoms or solid food dysphagia is found to have a mediastinal mass on a plain chest radiograph **(A).** The esophagus is deformed by the mass as seen on the contrast study **(B).** (From Ashcraft KW, Murphy JP, Sharp RJ, et al [eds]: Pediatric Surgery, 3rd ed. Philadelphia, WB Saunders, 2000, p 320.)

Evaluation

Duplication cysts are generally found on plain radiographs as part of the evaluation for vague respiratory or esophageal symptoms. Physical examination findings are rarely specific, and radiographs show a clearly defined spherical or ovoid mass in the mediastinum. Esophagography is usually performed and reveals a deformation of the esophagus caused by the cyst in proximity to the esophagus (Fig. 41–17). Computed tomography or magnetic resonance imaging further defines the lesion and allows preoperative planning.[105-111]

Treatment

The preferred management of thoracic enteric duplications is excision (Fig. 41–18). The approach is usually transpleural and can be safely accomplished by thoracotomy, as described for the treatment of EA, or by thoracoscopic techniques for surgeons accustomed to advanced thoracoscopy.[106,112] The principles of surgical therapy for these cysts demand complete excision to avoid the complication of retained gastric mucosa leading to further erosion. When the muscularis is inseparable from the esophagus, it may be allowed to remain; however, the entire mucosa must be excised. During dissection, one may find that erosion is present and the mass may be densely adherent or eroded into surrounding lung parenchyma or bronchial structures. Rarely, this will necessitate pulmonary lobectomy to complete the resection. As mentioned earlier, lesions with transdiaphragm extension are usually amputated in the chest, and the abdominal portion is dealt with separately.

CONGENITAL ESOPHAGEAL STENOSIS

Congenital esophageal stenosis (CES) caused by a developmental defect is a rare disorder and occurs in only 1 per 25,000 to 50,000 live births. The deformity is associated with other anomalies in nearly a quarter of patients, including primarily EA or TEF, anorectal malformations, hypospadias, and craniofacial malformations.[113,114]

True CES is not associated with GER and is a developmental defect categorized into one of three types.[115]

A *tracheobronchial remnant* (TBR) is the most common type of CES and results from errors in separation of the enteric and respiratory foregut structures during early fetal development (fourth week of gestation).[116] Respiratory remnants are retained in the esophagus and are usually manifested as a cartilaginous rest causing obstruction of the esophagus. These lesions are most commonly found in the distal third of the esophagus and result in dysphagia or feeding intolerance. The occurrence of TBR in association with EA is well described, and such remnants are usually found in the distal end of the esophagus.[117,118]

Idiopathic fibromuscular hypertrophy (FMH) or *stenosis* is nearly as common as TBR and develops as a result of hypertrophy of submucosal muscle and fibrous tissue. The overlying mucosa is normal. The cause of FMH is unclear, and it has been compared with the findings associated with pyloric stenosis, although there is no clear relationship. This lesion usually occurs in the middle third of the esophagus and again is characterized by dysphagia and feeding intolerance. FMH may involve a short segment of stenosis or may extend as long as 4 cm and result in an hourglass shape on contrast esophagography.

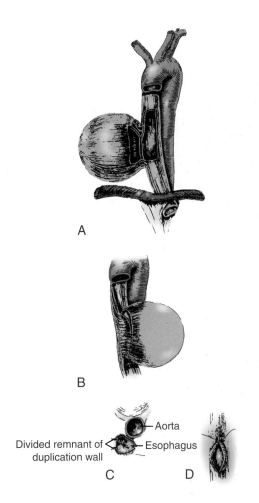

Figure 41–18. A duplication cyst arises from the muscular wall of the esophagus and rarely communicates with the lumen of the esophagus **(A)**. The cyst is mobilized from the esophagus, with the esophageal mucosa left intact. If necessary, only the mucosal lining of the cyst is removed to avoid entry into the lumen of the esophagus **(B and C)**. The muscular remnants are closed over the esophageal defect to prevent perforation or the development of a diverticulum **(D)**. (From Raffensperger JG, ed: Swenson's Pediatric Surgery, 5th ed. Norwalk, CT, Appleton & Lange, 1990.)

A *congenital membranous web (CMW) or diaphragm* occurs less frequently and may represent an incomplete form of EA. This lesion occurs in the middle third of the esophagus and appears as a short segment of incomplete obstruction. The web is generally found when children begin to take solid foods at approximately 6 months of age because the web usually allows the passage of liquids.

Diagnostic evaluation of CES is important because the three varieties of this anomaly require different forms of therapy. A child with feeding intolerance should undergo contrast esophagography, which will demonstrate narrowing of the esophagus. The character of the narrowing is helpful in determining the type of obstruction. Both FMH and CMW usually occur in the middle third of the esophagus, and TBR is most common in the distal third. FMH may be a longer narrowing with an hourglass impression, whereas CMW is narrow with a small opening in the web that is usually eccentric. TBR will be seen as a short-segment stenosis in the lower esophagus. If esophagoscopy is performed, the TBR will be found to be an unyielding distal obstruction, whereas FMH will usually permit passage of the esophagoscope. CMW will be seen as a mucosal-lined obstruction with a small pinhole opening.[113,119,120] Recently, ultrasound has been used for the evaluation of CES and may provide some useful information in differentiating the type of CES.[121]

Treatment options usually begin with attempts at dilation with either bougie dilators or pneumatic dilators, depending on surgeon preference. Several reports have demonstrated successful results with dilation alone for FMH, and this is generally the therapy of choice. The risk of perforation appears low, and although dilation may be repeated on several occasions, the outcome is usually good. CMW has been treated with dilation as well; however, resection or division of the web is much more likely to be needed to achieve good functional results. The web may be divided or ablated endoscopically, thus avoiding thoracotomy. TBR does not respond well to dilation, and although it is safe to attempt dilation, this course of treatment is rarely successful. Because TBR is usually a short-segment obstruction, it is generally amenable to resection and anastomosis, although there are reports of enucleation of the cartilaginous bar without esophageal resection. TBR may be located very near the lower esophageal sphincter, and resection may therefore interfere with its function. In these cases, consideration should be given to antireflux procedures.[113,122-124]

The outcome of CES is generally very good, although associated anomalies have an impact, as do chromosomal defects.

VASCULAR COMPRESSION

Compression of the esophagus can be caused by aberrant vascular structures commonly referred to as vascular rings. These anomalies are usually related to a double aortic arch encircling both the trachea and esophagus (Fig. 41–19), a right aortic arch and ligamentum arteriosum encircling both the trachea and esophagus, or an aberrant right subclavian artery arising from the left and passing behind either the trachea or esophagus (Fig. 41–20). In each anomaly, the aberrant vascular structure compresses the esophagus and thereby results in dysphagia.[125-127]

The diagnosis is based on historical factors and imaging studies. The symptoms are primarily related to dysphagia, especially when starting solid foods, or they may be associated with tracheal compression manifested by inspiratory stridor or recurrent pneumonia. The site of compression is at the level of the aortic arch, and contrast esophagography shows a winding or steeply angled compression in the case of an aberrant subclavian artery. This lesion can be differentiated from CES by contrast esophagography, echocardiography, or more recently, magnetic resonance angiography.[128-130]

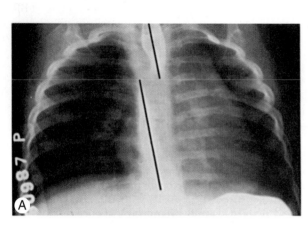

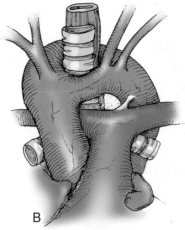

Figure 41–19. Vascular compression of the esophagus is seen on a contrast esophagogram as an angulated obstruction **(A).** The anatomic relationships of the double aortic arch depict the cause of esophageal obstruction, as seen in **B.** (From Ashcraft KW, Murphy JP, Sharp RJ, et al [eds]: Pediatric Surgery, 3rd ed. Philadelphia, WB Saunders, 2000, p 343.)

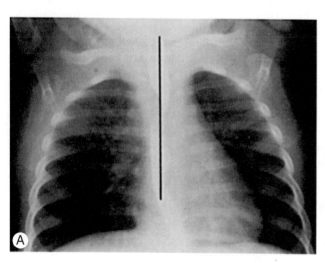

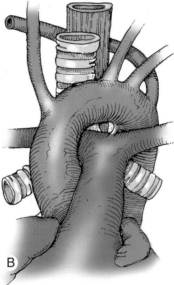

Figure 41–20. A and **B,** The anatomic relationships of an aberrant subclavian artery demonstrate the mechanism of esophageal compression resulting in solid food dysphagia. (From Ashcraft KW, Murphy JP, Sharp RJ, et al [eds]: Pediatric Surgery, 3rd ed. Philadelphia, WB Saunders, 2000, p 343.)

Treatment

Vascular compression of the esophagus is treated by division of the offending vessel through an anterolateral thoracotomy. Each anomaly is evaluated individually; however, the usual approach is to divide the smallest vessel or the aberrant vessel. In cases of double aortic arch, when the left (anterior) arch is small, the left arch is divided distal to the left subclavian artery; alternatively, in patients with a smaller right (posterior) arch, it is divided near the junction with the descending aorta. In those with equal-sized arches, the right (posterior) arch is divided. In either case the operation includes division of the ligamentum arteriosum or ductus arteriosus and lysis of the fibrous tissue between the trachea and esophagus to release the constriction around the esophagus.

In cases of persistent right aortic arch with left ligamentum arteriosum, the approach includes division of the ligamentum arteriosum and lysis of the fibrous tissue surrounding the esophagus and trachea.

An aberrant right subclavian artery causing symptoms of dysphagia should be divided at its origin from the aorta, and it can usually be approached through a posterolateral thoracotomy, unlike the previous lesions.[125,130-134]

REFERENCES

1. Skandalakis J, Gray S: Embryology for Surgeons, 2nd ed. Baltimore, Williams & Wilkins, 1994.
2. Fairbanks TJ, Kanard RC, De Langhe SP, et al: A genetic mechanism for cecal atresia: The role of the Fgf10 signaling pathway. J Surg Res 120:201-209, 2004.
3. Fairbanks TJ, Kanard R, Del Moral PM, et al: Fibroblast growth factor receptor 2 IIIb invalidation—a potential cause of familial duodenal atresia. J Pediatr Surg 39:872-874, 2004.
4. Hillemeier AC: Development of the esophagus. In Lebenthal E (ed): Human Gastrointestinal Development. New York, Raven Press, 1989, p 242.
5. Ladd WE: The surgical treatment of esophageal atresia and tracheo-esophageal fistulas. N Engl J Med 230:625-637, 1944.

6. Durston W: Philosophical transaction of the Royal Society. Trans R Soc 1670.

7. Gibson T: Anatomy of Humane Bodies Epitomized, 5th ed. Awnsham & Churchill, 1697.

8. Leven NL: Congenital atresia of the esophagus with tracheo-esophageal fistula. J Thorac Surg 10:648-657, 1941.

9. Lanman TH: Congenital atresia of the esophagus: A study of thirty two cases. Arch Surg 41:1060-1083, 1940.

10. Haight C: Congenital atresia of the esophagus with tracheo-esophageal fistula. In Mustard WT (ed): Pediatric Surgery. Chicago, Year Book, 1969, p 357.

11. Spitz L: Esophageal atresia: Past, present, and future. J Pediatr Surg 31:19-25, 1996.

12. Bax KM, van Der Zee DC: Feasibility of thoracoscopic repair of esophageal atresia with distal fistula. J Pediatr Surg 37:192-196, 2002.

13. Rothenberg SS: Thoracoscopic repair of tracheoesophageal fistula in newborns. J Pediatr Surg 37:869-872, 2002.

14. Diez-Pardo JA, Baoquan O, Navarro C, Tovar JA: A new rodent experimental model of esophageal atresia and tracheoesophageal fistula: Preliminary report. J Pediatr Surg 31:498-502, 1996.

15. Qi BQ, Beasley SW, Williams AK: Evidence of a common pathogenesis for foregut duplications and esophageal atresia with tracheo-esophageal fistula. Anat Rec 264:93-100, 2001.

16. Williams AK, Qi BQ, Beasley SW: Temporospatial aberrations of apoptosis in the rat embryo developing esophageal atresia. J Pediatr Surg 35:1617-1620, 2000.

17. Gross RE: Atresia of the esophagus. In Gross RE (ed): The Surgery of Infancy and Childhood. Philadelphia, WB Saunders, 1953, pp 75-102.

18. Beasley SW: Influence of associated anomalies on the management of oesophageal atresia. Indian J Pediatr 63:743-749, 1996.

19. Chittmittrapap S, Spitz L, Kiely EM, Brereton RJ: Oesophageal atresia and associated anomalies. Arch Dis Child 64:364-368, 1989.

20. Ein SH, Shandling B, Wesson D, Filler RM: Esophageal atresia with distal tracheoesophageal fistula: Associated anomalies and prognosis in the 1980s. J Pediatr Surg 24:1055-1059, 1989.

21. Engum SA, Grosfeld JL, West KW, et al: Analysis of morbidity and mortality in 227 cases of esophageal atresia and/or tracheoesophageal fistula over two decades. Arch Surg 130:502-508, 1995.

22. German JC, Mahour GH, Woolley MM: Esophageal atresia and associated anomalies. J Pediatr Surg 11:299-306, 1976.

23. Kimble RM, Harding J, Kolbe A: Additional congenital anomalies in babies with gut atresia or stenosis: When to investigate, and which investigation. Pediatr Surg Int 12:565-570, 1997.

24. Rejjal A: Congenital anomalies associated with esophageal atresia: Saudi experience. Am J Perinatol 16:239-244, 1999.

25. Bauman W, et al: VATER oder ACTERL syndrom. Klin Pediatr 188:328, 1976.

26. Quan L, Smith DW: The VATER association: Vertebral defects, Anal atresia, T-E fistula with esophageal atresia, Radial and Renal dysplasia: A spectrum of associated defects. J Pediatr 82:104-107, 1973.

27. Holder TM, Cloud DT, Lewis JE Jr, Pilling GP IV: Esophageal atresia and tracheoesophageal fistula: A survey of its members by the surgical section of the American Academy of Pediatrics. Pediatrics 34:542-549, 1964.

28. Dunn JC, Fonkalsrud EW, Atkinson JB: Simplifying the Waterston's stratification of infants with tracheoesophageal fistula. Am Surg 65:908-910, 1999.

29. Tellier AL, Cormier-Daire V, Abadie V, et al: CHARGE syndrome: Report of 47 cases and review. Am J Med Genet 76:402-409, 1998.

30. Malinger G, Levine A, Rotmensch S: The fetal esophagus: Anatomical and physiological ultrasonographic characterization using a high-resolution linear transducer. Ultrasound Obstet Gynecol 24:500-505, 2004.

31. Matsuoka S, Takeuchi K, Yamanaka Y, et al: Comparison of magnetic resonance imaging and ultrasonography in the prenatal diagnosis of congenital thoracic abnormalities. Fetal Diagn Ther 18:447-453, 2003.

32. Shulman A, Mazkereth R, Zolel Y, et al: Prenatal identification of esophageal atresia: The role of ultrasonography for evaluation of functional anatomy. Prenat Diagn 22:669-674, 2002.

33. Aziz D, Schiller D, Gerstle JT, et al: Can "long-gap" esophageal atresia be safely managed at home while awaiting anastomosis? J Pediatr Surg 38:705-708, 2003.

34. Bass J: A technique to facilitate nursing care in patients with long-gap esophageal atresia. Pediatr Surg Int 18:749-750, 2002.

35. Hollands CM, Lankau CA Jr, Burnweit CA: Preoperative home care for esophageal atresia—a survey. J Pediatr Surg 35:279-281, 2000.

36. Waterston DJ, Bonham Carter RE, Aberdeen E: Oesophageal atresia: Tracheo-oesophageal fistula. Lancet 1:819-822, 1962.

37. Deurloo JA, de Vos R, Ekkelkamp S, et al: Prognostic factors for mortality of oesophageal atresia patients: Waterston revived. Eur J Pediatr 163:624-625, 2004.

38. Choudhury SR, Ashcraft KW, Sharp RJ, et al: Survival of patients with esophageal atresia: Influence of birth weight, cardiac anomaly, and late respiratory complications. J Pediatr Surg 34:70-73, discussion 74, 1999.

39. Filston HC, Rankin JS, Grimm JK: Esophageal atresia. Prognostic factors and contribution of preoperative telescopic endoscopy. Ann Surg 199:532-537, 1984.

40. Spitz L, Kiely EM, Morecroft JA, Drake DP: Oesophageal atresia: At-risk groups for the 1990s. J Pediatr Surg 29:723-825, 1994.

41. Auldist AW, Beasley SW, Myers NA: Long-gap oesophageal atresia. Pediatr Surg Int 12:620, 1997.

42. Beasley SW: A practical approach to the investigation and management of long gap oesophageal atresia. Indian J Pediatr 63:737-742, 1996.

43. de Lorimier AA, Harrison MR: Long gap esophageal atresia: Primary anastomosis after esophageal elongation by bougienage and esophagomyotomy. J Thorac Cardiovasc Surg 79:138-141, 1980.

44. Tannuri U, Teodoro WR, de Santana Witzel S, et al: Livaditis' circular myotomy does not decrease anastomotic leak rates and induces deleterious changes in anastomotic healing. Eur J Pediatr Surg 13:224-230, 2003.

45. Giacomoni MA, Tresoldi M, Zamana C, Giacomoni A: Circular myotomy of the distal esophageal stump for long gap esophageal atresia. J Pediatr Surg 36:855-857, 2001.

46. Lessin MS, Wesselhoeft CW, Luks FI, DeLuca FG: Primary repair of long-gap esophageal atresia by mobilization of the distal esophagus. Eur J Pediatr Surg 9:369-372, 1999.

47. Davison P, Poenaru D, Kamal I: Esophageal atresia: Primary repair of a rare long gap variant involving distal pouch mobilization. J Pediatr Surg 34:1881-1883, 1999.

48. Schneeberger AL, Scott RB, Rubin SZ, Machida H: Esophageal function following Livaditis repair of long gap esophageal atresia. J Pediatr Surg 22:779-783, 1987.

49. Schwartz MZ: An improved technique for circular myotomy in long-gap esophageal atresia. J Pediatr Surg 18:833-834, 1983.

50. Sigge W, Wurtenberger H, Franz A, Albrecht M: Bridging a gap in oesophageal atresia using Rehbein's technique: Dilatation of a thread canal. Z Kinderchir 41:5-9, 1986.

51. Lopes MF, Reis A, Coutinho S, Pires A: Very long gap esophageal atresia successfully treated by esophageal lengthening using external traction sutures. J Pediatr Surg 39:1286-1287, 2004.

52. Al-Qahtani AR, Yazbeck S, Rosen NG, et al: Lengthening technique for long gap esophageal atresia and early anastomosis. J Pediatr Surg 38:737-739, 2003.

53. Gaglione G, Tramontano A, Capobianco A, Mazzei S: Foker's technique in oesophageal atresia with double fistula: A case report. Eur J Pediatr Surg 13:50-53, 2003.

54. Foker JE, Linden BC, Boyle EM Jr, Marquardt C: Development of a true primary repair for the full spectrum of esophageal atresia. Ann Surg 226:533-541, 1997.

55. Bagolan P, Iacobelli Bd B, De Angelis P, et al: Long gap esophageal atresia and esophageal replacement: Moving toward a separation? J Pediatr Surg 39:1084-1090, 2004.

56. Hagberg S, Rubenson A, Sillen U, Werkmaster K: Management of long-gap esophagus: Experience with end-to-end anastomosis under maximal tension. Prog Pediatr Surg 19:88-92, 1986.

57. Shokrollahi K, Barham P, Blazeby JM, Alderson D: Surgical revision of dysfunctional colonic interposition after esophagoplasty. Ann Thorac Surg 74:1708-1711, 2002.

58. Spitz L, Kiely E, Pierro A: Gastric transposition in children—a 21-year experience. J Pediatr Surg 39:276-281, 2004.

59. Ludman L, Spitz L: Quality of life after gastric transposition for oesophageal atresia. J Pediatr Surg 38:53-57, 2003.

60. Spitz L: Gastric transposition for esophageal substitution in children. J Pediatr Surg 27:252-257, 1992.

61. Anderson KD, Noblett H, Belsey R, Randolph JG: Long-term follow-up of children with colon and gastric tube interposition for esophageal atresia. Surgery 111:131-136, 1992.

62. Halsband H: Esophagus replacement by free, autologous jejunal mucosa transplantation in long-gap esophageal atresia. Prog Pediatr Surg 19:22-36, 1986.

63. Pineschi A, Pini M, Torre G, Levi N: Gastric tube oesophagoplasty for oesophageal atresia: A follow-up study. Part II: Radiologic, endoscopic and histologic controls. Z Kinderchir 40:16-20, 1985.

64. Pineschi A, Torre G, Levi N: Gastric tube oesophagoplasty for oesophageal atresia: A follow-up study. Part I: Clinical controls. Z Kinderchir 40:13-15, 1985.

65. Holcomb GW III, Rothenberg SS, Bax KM, et al: Thoracoscopic repair of esophageal atresia and tracheoesophageal fistula: A multi-institutional analysis. Ann Surg 242:422-428, discussion 428-430, 2005.

66. Calisti A, Oriolo L, Nanni L, et al: Mortality and long term morbidity in esophageal atresia: The reduced impact of low birth weight and maturity on surgical outcome. J Perinat Med 32:171-175, 2004.

67. Kay S, Shaw K: Revisiting the role of routine retropleural drainage after repair of esophageal atresia with distal tracheoesophageal fistula. J Pediatr Surg 34:1082-1085, 1999.

68. McKinnon LJ, Kosloske AM: Prediction and prevention of anastomotic complications of esophageal atresia and tracheoesophageal fistula. J Pediatr Surg 25:778-781, 1990.

69. Wheatley MJ, Coran AG, Wesley JR: Efficacy of the Nissen fundoplication in the management of gastroesophageal reflux following esophageal atresia repair. J Pediatr Surg 28:53-55, 1993.

70. Allmendinger N, Hallisey MJ, Markowitz SK, et al: Balloon dilation of esophageal strictures in children. J Pediatr Surg 31:334-336, 1996.

71. Rickham PP, Stauffer UG, Cheng SK: Oesophageal atresia: Triumph and tragedy. Aust N Z J Surg 47:138-143, 1977.

72. Ghandour KE, Spitz L, Brereton RJ, Kiely EM: Recurrent tracheo-oesophageal fistula: Experience with 24 patients. J Paediatr Child Health 26:89-91, 1990.

73. Goh DW, Brereton RJ: Success and failure with neonatal tracheo-oesophageal anomalies. Br J Surg 78:834-837, 1991.

74. Holder TM, Ashcraft KW, Sharp RJ, Amoury RA: Care of infants with esophageal atresia, tracheoesophageal fistula, and associated anomalies. J Thorac Cardiovasc Surg 94:828-835, 1987.

75. Tzifa KT, Maxwell EL, Chait P, et al: Endoscopic treatment of congenital H-type and recurrent tracheoesophageal fistula with electrocautery and histoacryl glue. Int J Pediatr Otorhinolaryngol Nov 29, 2005.

76. Lopes MF, Pires J, Nogueira Brandao A, et al: Endoscopic obliteration of a recurrent tracheoesophageal fistula with enbucrilate and polidocanol in a child. Surg Endosc 17:657, 2003.

77. Delarue A, Paut O, Simeoni J, et al: Costal cartilage grafting for repair of a recurrent tracheoesophageal fistula in a 1.6-kg baby with esophageal atresia. Pediatr Surg Int 18:162-164, 2002.

78. Hoelzer DJ, Luft JD: Successful long-term endoscopic closure of a recurrent tracheoesophageal fistula with fibrin glue in a child. Int J Pediatr Otorhinolaryngol 48:259-263, 1999.

79. Wiseman NE: Endoscopic closure of recurrent tracheoesophageal fistula using Tisseel. J Pediatr Surg 30:1236-1237, 1995.

80. Nasr A, Ein SH, Gerstle JT: Infants with repaired esophageal atresia and distal tracheoesophageal fistula with severe respiratory distress: Is it tracheomalacia, reflux, or both? J Pediatr Surg 40:901-903, 2005.

81. Messineo A, Filler RM: Tracheomalacia. Semin Pediatr Surg 3:253-258, 1994.

82. Filler RM, de Fraga JC: Tracheomalacia. Semin Thorac Cardiovasc Surg 6:211-215, 1994.

83. Usui N, Kamata S, Ishikawa S, et al: Anomalies of the tracheobronchial tree in patients with esophageal atresia. J Pediatr Surg 31:258-262, 1996.

84. Briganti V, Oriolo L, Buffa V, et al: Tracheomalacia in oesophageal atresia: Morphological considerations by endoscopic and CT study. Eur J Cardiothorac Surg 28:11-15, 2005.

85. Inoue K, Yanagihara J, Ono S, et al: Utility of helical CT for diagnosis and operative planning in tracheomalacia after repair of esophageal atresia. Eur J Pediatr Surg 8:355-357, 1998.

86. Lindahl H, Rintala R, Malinen L, et al: Bronchoscopy during the first month of life. J Pediatr Surg 27:548-550, 1992.

87. Kao SC, Smith WL, Sato Y, et al: Ultrafast CT of laryngeal and tracheobronchial obstruction in symptomatic postoperative infants with esophageal atresia and tracheoesophageal fistula. AJR Am J Roentgenol 154:345-350, 1990.

88. van der Zee DC, Bax KM: Thoracoscopic repair of esophageal atresia with distal fistula. Surg Endosc 17:1065-1067, 2003.

89. Weber TR, Keller MS, Fiore A: Aortic suspension (aortopexy) for severe tracheomalacia in infants and children. Am J Surg 184:573-577, 2002.

90. Schaarschmidt K, Kolberg-Schwerdt A, Bunke K, Strauss J: A technique for thoracoscopic aortopericardiosternopexy. Surg Endosc 16:1639, 2002.

91. Filler RM, Messineo A, Vinograd I: Severe tracheomalacia associated with esophageal atresia: Results of surgical treatment. J Pediatr Surg 27:1136-1140, 1992.

92. Applebaum H, Woolley MM: Pericardial flap aortopexy for tracheomalacia. J Pediatr Surg 25:30-31, 1990.

93. Tazuke Y, Kawahara H, Yagi M, et al: Use of a Palmaz stent for tracheomalacia: Case report of an infant with esophageal atresia. J Pediatr Surg 34:1291-1293, 1999.

94. Blair GK, Cohen R, Filler RM: Treatment of tracheomalacia: Eight years' experience. J Pediatr Surg 21:781-785, 1986.

95. Martin WM, Shapiro RS: Long custom-made plastic tracheostomy tube in severe tracheomalacia. Laryngoscope 91:355-362, 1981.

96. Smith JR: Accessory enteric formations: Classification and nomenclature. Arch Dis Child 35:87-89, 1960.

97. Ware GW, Conrad HA: Thoracic duplication of alimentary tract. Am J Surg 86:264-272, 1953.

98. Takeda S, Miyoshi S, Minami M, et al: Clinical spectrum of mediastinal cysts. Chest 124:125-132, 2003.

99. Yasufuku M, Hatakeyama T, Maeda K, et al: Bronchopulmonary foregut malformation: A large bronchogenic cyst communicating with an esophageal duplication cyst. J Pediatr Surg 38(2):e2, 2003.

100. Prasad A, Sarin YK, Ramji S, et al: Mediastinal enteric duplication cyst containing aberrant pancreas. Indian J Pediatr 69:961-962, 2002.

101. Knight J, Garvin PJ, Lewis E Jr: Gastric duplication presenting as a double esophagus. J Pediatr Surg 18:300-301, 1983.

102. Wakisaka M, Nakada K, Kitagawa H, et al: Giant transdiaphragmatic duodenal duplication with an intraspinal neurenteric cyst as part of the split notochord syndrome: Report of a case. Surg Today 34:459-462, 2004.

103. Haller JA, Shermeta DW, Donahoo JS, White JJ: Life-threatening respiratory distress from mediastinal masses in infants. Ann Thorac Surg 19:365-370, 1975.

104. Macpherson RI, Reed MH, Ferguson CC: Intrathoracic gastrogenic cysts: A cause of lethal pulmonary hemorrhage in infants. J Can Assoc Radiol 24:362-369, 1973.

105. Weiss LM, Fagelman D, Warhit JM: CT demonstration of an esophageal duplication cyst. J Comput Assist Tomogr 7:716-718, 1983.

106. Koizumi K, Haraguchi S, Hirata T, et al: Thoracoscopic surgery in children. J Nippon Med Sch 72:34-42, 2005.

107. Kawahara H, Kamata S, Nose K, et al: Congenital mediastinal cystic abnormalities detected in utero: Report of two cases. J Pediatr Gastroenterol Nutr 33:202-205, 2001.

108. Al-Sadoon H, Wiseman N, Chernick V: Recurrent thoracic duplication cyst with associated mediastinal gas. Can Respir J 5:149-151, 1998.

109. Daldrup HE, Link TM, Wortler K, et al: MR imaging of thoracic tumors in pediatric patients. AJR Am J Roentgenol 170:1639-1644, 1998.

110. Rizalar R, Demirbilek S, Bernay F, Gurses N: A case of a mediastinal neurenteric cyst demonstrated by prenatal ultrasound. Eur J Pediatr Surg 5:177-179, 1995.

111. Siegel MJ, Sagel SS, Reed K: The value of computed tomography in the diagnosis and management of pediatric mediastinal abnormalities. Radiology 142:149-155, 1982.

112. Michel JL, Revillon Y, Montupet P, et al: Thoracoscopic treatment of mediastinal cysts in children. J Pediatr Surg 33:1745-1748, 1998.

113. Amae S, Nio M, Kamiyama T, et al: Clinical characteristics and management of congenital esophageal stenosis: A report on 14 cases. J Pediatr Surg 38:565-570, 2003.

114. Bonilla KB, Bowers WF: Congenital esophageal stenosis; pathologic studies following resection. Am J Surg 97:772-776, 1959.

115. Ramesh JC, Ramanujam TM, Jayaram G: Congenital esophageal stenosis: Report of three cases, literature review, and a proposed classification. Pediatr Surg Int 17:188-192, 2001.

116. Zhao LL, Hsieh WS, Hsu WM: Congenital esophageal stenosis owing to ectopic tracheobronchial remnants. J Pediatr Surg 39:1183-1187, 2004.

117. Yeung CK, Spitz L, Brereton RJ, et al: Congenital esophageal stenosis due to tracheobronchial remnants: A rare but important association with esophageal atresia. J Pediatr Surg 27:852-855, 1992.

118. Mahour GH, et al: Congenital esophageal stenosis distal to esophageal atresia. Surgery 69:936-939, 1971.

119. Setty SP, Harrison MW: Congenital esophageal stenosis: A case report and review of the literature. Eur J Pediatr Surg 14:283-286, 2004.

120. Luedtke P, Levine MS, Rubesin SE, et al: Radiologic diagnosis of benign esophageal strictures: A pattern approach. Radiographics 23:897-909, 2003.

121. Usui N, Kamata S, Kawahara H, et al: Usefulness of endoscopic ultrasonography in the diagnosis of congenital esophageal stenosis. J Pediatr Surg 37:1744-1746, 2002.

122. Vasudevan SA, Kerendi F, Lee H, Ricketts RR: Management of congenital esophageal stenosis. J Pediatr Surg 37:1024-1026, 2002.

123. Takamizawa S, Tsugawa C, Mouri N, et al: Congenital esophageal stenosis: Therapeutic strategy based on etiology. J Pediatr Surg 37:197-201, 2002.

124. Segnitz RH: Treatment of a five-pound infant with congenital esophageal stenosis. Wisc Med J 55:447-451, 1956.

125. Backer CL, Ilbawa MN, Idriss FS, DeLeon SY: Vascular anomalies causing tracheoesophageal compression. Review of experience in children. J Thorac Cardiovasc Surg 97:725-731, 1989.

126. Tucker BL, Meyer BW, Lindesmith GG, et al: Congenital aortic vascular ring. Arch Surg 99:521-523, 1969.

127. Levine S, Serfas LS: Dysphagia lusoria secondary to complete vascular ring. Am J Surg 113:435-438, 1967.

128. van Son JA, Julsrud PR, Hagler OJ, et al: Surgical treatment of vascular rings: The Mayo Clinic experience. Mayo Clin Proc 68:1056-1063, 1993.

129. Lillehei CW, Colan S: Echocardiography in the preoperative evaluation of vascular rings. J Pediatr Surg 27:1118-1120, 1992.

130. Chun K, Colombani PM, Dudgeon DL, Haller JA Jr: Diagnosis and management of congenital vascular rings: A 22-year experience. Ann Thorac Surg 53:597-602, 1992.

131. Mihaljevic T, Cannon JW, del Nido PJ: Robotically assisted division of a vascular ring in children. J Thorac Cardiovasc Surg 125:1163-1164, 2003.

132. Bove T, Demanet H, Casimir G, et al: Tracheobronchial compression of vascular origin. Review of experience in infants and children. J Cardiovasc Surg (Torino) 42:663-666, 2001.

133. Sebening C, Jakob H, Tochtermann U, et al: Vascular tracheobronchial compression syndromes—experience in surgical treatment and literature review. Thorac Cardiovasc Surg 48:164-174, 2000.

134. van Son JA, Bossert T, Mohr FW: Surgical treatment of vascular ring including right cervical aortic arch. J Card Surg 14:98-102, 1999.

42

Techniques of Esophageal Reconstruction

Christopher R. Morse • Douglas J. Mathisen

Esophageal resection and reconstruction remain a major therapeutic challenge for surgeons involved in the care of patients with benign and malignant disease of the esophagus. Despite major advances in postoperative care, operative mortality rates worldwide remain unacceptably high. Much of the operative mortality is related to the complications of anastomotic leak. "Acceptable" leak rates of 8% to 10% are still reported today. With whatever conduit is chosen, the operation requires careful planning and preparation of the patient, strict attention to technical details of the operation, and dedicated postoperative care. Resection and reconstruction are inevitable for malignant disease, but every attempt should be made to preserve the native esophagus in patients with benign disease because no esophageal substitute achieves "normal" swallowing comparable to that of the esophagus.

In the final analysis, a general thoracic surgeon must be thoroughly familiar not only with the technical aspects of various visceral esophageal substitutes but also with the appropriate selection of a particular conduit under specific circumstances. Accordingly, this chapter is intended to provide both details of surgical technique and the physiologic concepts that constitute the basis for selection of a particular organ for creation of a replacement "esophagus" (esophagoplasty).

HISTORICAL BACKGROUND

The first successful resection of the cervical esophagus was reported by Czerny in 1877.[1] Torek is credited with the first resection of the thoracic esophagus in 1913.[2] Successful resection plus intrathoracic reconstruction of the esophagus was reported by Oshawa in 1933.[3] Sweet and Churchill in 1942 reported a three-layer technique of anastomosis that gave results superior to those of many contemporary reports today.[4] Sweet's series in 1954 of 141 patients with an operative mortality rate of 15% and a leak rate of 1.4% was remarkable for its time and is still

acceptable by today's standards.[5] In 1946, Ivor Lewis popularized the laparotomy and right thoracotomy approach for tumors of the middle third of the esophagus—an approach that still bears his name.[6] Mahoney and Sherman published their results of colon replacement after total esophagectomy in 1954.[7] Replacement of the distal esophagus with a short-segment colon interposition was reported in 1965 by Belsey[8] and with jejunum by Brain in 1967.[9] As recently as 1990, Muller et al. in another collective review reported that the overall operative mortality for curative and palliative resection of the esophagus was 11% and 19%, respectively.[10] Mathisen and associates reported an operative mortality rate of 2.9% and no leaks at the Massachusetts General Hospital.[11] Others have reported similar excellent results from single institutions, but it is obvious that the challenge still remains.

OPTIONS IN REPLACING THE ESOPHAGUS

Surgeons involved in the care of patients with esophageal disease should be familiar with all the conduits available for esophageal replacement. Individual circumstances may dictate the choice of substitute, or unexpected operative findings may cause a change in plan. The surgeon should be flexible enough to tailor the choice of substitute to suit the patient and the underlying disease process. Many factors dictate which option is chosen: benign or malignant disease, availability of conduit, comorbid conditions such as chronic obstructive pulmonary disease or vascular occlusive disease, steroid-dependent conditions, previous irradiation, and ultimately, the surgeon's preference. Some methods of reconstruction, such as antethoracic skin tubes or prosthetic replacements, are primarily of historical significance but should be remembered for the rare patient for whom no other option is available. Other methods, such as the reversed gastric tube, are suitable alternatives but have never gained popularity.

The three standard visceral substitutes used for replacing the esophagus, in the order of both frequency and preference, are the stomach, colon, and jejunum.

Stomach

The liberal blood supply of the stomach makes it the most reliable organ for use in intrathoracic replacement of the esophagus. Of its five feeding arterial sources, the left gastric artery, the left gastroepiploic artery, and the short gastric arteries may be divided, with the right gastric and right gastroepiploic arteries left to supply the entire transpositioned stomach. Division of these arteries is possible because of the presence of extensive intrinsic collaterals within the gastric wall. A second reason for the reliability of the stomach in replacement of the esophagus is its size and contour, which after total division of the greater and lesser omenta and lateral peritoneal liberation of the duodenal sweep (Kocher's maneuver), permit the stomach to be brought to the neck. When maximum length is required, the true fundus of the stomach should be used for anastomosis rather than the gastroesophageal junction. Skeletonizing the lesser curve also gives added length with little ischemic risk. Moreover, use of the stomach for esophageal replacement requires only a single anastomosis, either in the chest or in the neck. Use of the stomach also allows for a portion of the omentum to be used to wrap the anastomosis. The stomach can be transposed by either the posterior mediastinal route in the bed of the native esophagus or the substernal route. The posterior mediastinal route is the preferred route in most patients.

Colon

The colon may be used for extended lengths of esophageal replacement or for bypass (i.e., when it is necessary to reach to the neck). When the left colon is selected and placed in an isoperistaltic direction, it derives its blood supply from the inferior mesenteric artery through the left colic artery. If the antiperistaltic direction is used, the midcolic artery becomes the feeding source. When shorter segments of colon are required, the transverse colon based on the middle colic artery and the splenic flexure supplied by the left colic artery are the primary options. Although the right colon can be used in some circumstances, the lack of a reliable marginal artery and its limited mobility make it an option only when others have been exhausted.

Jejunum

The jejunum is most frequently used as a short segment replacing the distal esophagus, more often in benign disease and particularly for reflux acid-peptic stricture. In these cases, the proximal jejunum is used as a short interposition graft with a segment beginning just distal to the first jejunal arterial branch from the superior mesenteric artery. In asthenic patients with a long jejunal mesentery, the jejunum may be brought to a level above the aortic arch, and in young children particularly, it may even reach all the way to the cervical level. More often, however, when such length is mandated by the lack of other available options, arterial and venous augmentation may be necessary, such as an internal mammary artery–to–jejunal artery anastomosis. For short-segment replacement of the cervical esophagus, a free *autograft* of small intestine may be used; arterial and venous anastomoses are accomplished by conventional microvascular techniques to, for example, the superior thyroid artery and the anterior facial vein.

Specific factors ultimately come into play in selection of the viscus used to replace the esophagus, including (1) availability, related to previous surgical resections; (2) anomalous anatomic variants, particularly in blood supply; (3) possible pathologic processes in the viscus under consideration; (4) technical reliability of the vascular supply necessary for appropriate anastomotic healing; and (5) always, the experience of the operating surgeon.

Throughout this discussion, emphasis is placed repeatedly on blood supply. *The first and foremost requisite for successful replacement of the esophagus is adequate circulation, both arterial input and venous drainage, in the substituting organ.* An anastomosis cannot heal by primary intention in the absence of reliable circulation in both ends to be joined.

TECHNICAL VARIABLES

In addition to selection of the viscus to be used for esophageal replacement, the surgeon has three other choices to consider when planning the ideal technical operation: (1) the surgical approach, (2) the route for replacement of the new "esophagus," and (3) the level of the anastomosis.

Placement of Incision

For distal partial esophagectomy and anastomosis below the aortic arch, there is almost general agreement on use of a left transthoracic or thoracoabdominal incision. With upward paravertebral extension and Sweet's double-rib resection (or double intercostal incisions), the left-sided approach can be extended to any level of the intrathoracic esophagus if necessary, although dissection of large carcinomas at the level of the aortic arch may pose technical challenges.

For midesophageal carcinomas, the conventional approach is use of the double incisions of Lewis: a midline laparotomy for gastric mobilization and a high right-sided posterolateral thoracotomy for esophageal dissection and execution of a high intrathoracic anastomosis. This operative approach may be extended to include a third, cervical incision to allow resection of a greater length of proximal esophageus and a cervical anastomosis as described by McKeown.[12]

Yet another surgical approach is the transhiatal esophagectomy of Orringer, in which a high midline

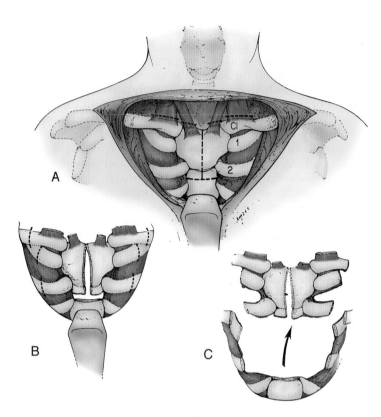

Figure 42–1. **A,** The anterior cervical skin and platysma are elevated inferiorly over the pectoral fascia, especially in the midline. The sternocleidomastoid muscle is detached from the sternal and clavicular attachments. **B** and **C,** Resection of a plate of sternum, clavicle, and the first and second ribs. Usually, the left half is all that is required to enlarge the thoracic inlet, but both sides may be needed in special circumstances.

laparotomy and transhiatal dissection are combined with a cervical incision to allow proximal esophageal dissection and performance of the anastomosis.[13] Extensive division of the hiatus allows greater visualization of the distal esophagus. Partial resection of the manubrium and the first and second ribs (Fig. 42–1) permits better visualization and dissection of the cervicothoracic esophagus in some patients. Both these techniques allow esophagectomy to be performed under direct visualization in most patients.

Finally, the rapidly advancing technology of laparoscopy has been applied to esophageal disease. Both a transhiatal technique and a method involving thoracoscopic mobilization of the esophagus have been described.[14,15] Both involve a cervical anastomosis. Initial reports have demonstrated minimally invasive esophagectomy to have outcomes similar to those of most open procedures and potentially shorter hospital stay with better quality of life. With improving instruments and advancing robotic technology, minimally invasive esophagectomy may come to occupy a more prominent role in the management of esophageal carcinoma.

Route of Replacement

Four options are available when choosing the route of replacement: (1) posterior mediastinal through the bed of the resected esophagus; (2) anterior mediastinal in the retrosternal position; (3) lateral transpleural, usually behind the lung root; and (4) the antethoracic or presternal subcutaneous route. The fourth choice has never achieved universal popularity, primarily because of cosmetic considerations.

The orthotopic posterior mediastinal route for placement of the conduit is the most widely used if the esophagus has been removed. It is the shortest and most direct route and does not require dissection and preparation of the second port of access.

The retrosternal route is used most commonly for bypass of the esophagus when it has been decided, because of tumor unresectability, condition of the patient, or staging, to not resect the esophagus. This choice may require enlarging the thoracic inlet by resecting the head of the clavicle and the anterior end of the first rib to ensure adequacy of room for the replacement and to be certain that there is no compression of the essential vascular supply (see Fig. 42–1). The retrosternal route is noted to be longer than posterior mediastinal positioning by 2 to 3 cm.

The transpleural route is seldom used but may be necessary if the usual anterior mediastinal route has been transgressed by a previous median sternotomy, particularly for an open cardiac surgical operation.

Level of Anastomosis

If the transhiatal approach to esophagectomy is used, there is no option; the anastomosis is always performed at the cervical level. Likewise, the three-incision technique for near-total removal of the esophagus uses a cervical anastomosis. However, if distal esophagectomy is planned, a decision regarding the level of anastomosis is paramount. A level must be chosen that permits complete removal of the tumor with a negative resection margin. It must also allow construction of a secure anastomosis with full visual exposure. Because of these considerations, intrathoracic anastomoses at the middle to high level are better accomplished from the right-sided thoracic approach.

The most important aspect of a successful esophagectomy and replacement (at least in terms of postoperative recovery) is performance of a safe, intact anastomosis. *The technical goal of all esophageal surgeons is a zero anastomotic leakage rate.*

GUIDELINES IN MAKING THE CHOICE

For malignant disease in particular, the stomach is the most reliable replacement for the esophagus. Its intrinsic blood supply is the most extensive and the stomach's pliability allows it to reach any necessary level. It has stood the test of time and has now been in general use since the 1938 report of Adams and Phemister.[16] The principal drawback in using the stomach is the development of reflux esophagitis resulting in stricture at or above the anastomosis. Although pyloric drainage procedures and anastomosis-wrapping techniques are used to minimize the possibility of damaging reflux, practice has shown that the higher the anastomosis is placed, the less likely the development of esophagitis.

In patients with a nondilatable peptic stricture of the distal esophagus, interposition of a segment of intestine is the preferred method of replacement after esophageal resection. The choice between colon and jejunum is mainly one of the surgeon's preference and experience. Either organ can provide a satisfactory physiologic "barrier" against ongoing gastroesophageal reflux while maintaining the entire stomach in its normal abdominal anatomic location. An esophagogastric anastomosis, particularly at the distal esophageal level for reflux peptic disease, is fraught with a high incidence of postoperative esophagitis and the danger of possible life-threatening nocturnal tracheobronchial aspiration. On the other hand, in elderly or medically compromised patients, the esophagogastric distal anastomosis may be used because of the expedience of the procedure and the reliability of the circulation.

For a long esophageal replacement in patients with benign disease (i.e., usually stricture, either peptic or corrosive), the colon is given first consideration. Its reliable marginal arterial circulation, especially between the left branch of the middle colic and the left colic arteries, permits isoperistaltic replacement of the left colon all the way through the posterior mediastinal esophageal bed to the level of the neck. An alternative route, even after resection, is placement through a retrosternal tunnel.

For esophageal bypass without resection, the colon is also the viscus of choice. It is placed behind the sternum unless obliteration of the anterior mediastinum by previous surgery, mediastinal irradiation, or malignant disease requires transpleural replacement. The side and position (in front of or behind the root of the lung) are the surgeon's choice. Bypass rather than esophageal resection may be selected because of either the extent of an invasive carcinoma or the physiologic status of the patient, both of which may prevent successful transpleural resection. In addition, some general thoracic surgeons prefer to stage a procedure in the event of corrosive destruction of the esophagus by first performing a looping esophageal bypass and, later, esophageal resection.

STUDIES USEFUL IN THE DECISION-MAKING PROCESS

A viscus cannot be used to replace the esophagus unless it is intrinsically healthy (i.e., free of its own disease) and has an adequate arterial supply and venous return. The three methods used to assess these characteristics are (1) endoscopy, (2) arteriography, and (3) barium contrast radiology.

Endoscopy

Endoscopy provides the greatest amount of information when it can be applied appropriately. For instance, if the fiberoptic esophagogastroscope can be negotiated through an esophageal carcinoma or stricture, it provides information about (1) the presence or absence of a second carcinoma, (2) the presence or absence of peptic ulceration or gastritis, and (3) the adequacy of the pyloric channel. In evaluating the colon for use as replacement of the esophagus, colonoscopy is essential. It provides the opportunity for total inspection and thus eliminates the possibility of the presence of a polyp, small carcinoma, or other unsuspected lesion in either the substitute viscus or the residual colon that does not participate in the replacement. It may not provide information about diverticulitis unless it is extensive or actually obstructive.

Arteriography

There is room for a difference of opinion about the need for arteriography. The arterial supply of the stomach is abundant because of its five primary vessels, and its intrinsic network of interconnecting communications is so extensive that arteriography is not necessary. Anomalies in arterial supply are neither too common nor sufficiently severe to cause concern, even with the necessary disconnection from the adjacent omentum, spleen, colon, and celiac axis. For the colon, however, the situation is quite the opposite. The adequacy of the segmental arterial supply is inconstant. First, atherosclerotic involvement of the colonic vessels is common, particularly in the older population so frequently affected by esophageal carcinoma. The origin of the inferior mesenteric artery is a particular site of atherosclerotic narrowing. Second, the variety and frequency of anomalies in colonic blood supply require clarification before a decision can be made about (1) the utility of the colon as a replacement of the esophagus and (2) which portion to use. Numerous variants have been identified by careful anatomic dissection, and anomalies have been found in more than 10% of patients studied by mesenteric arteriography as reported by Sonneland and colleagues.[17] The

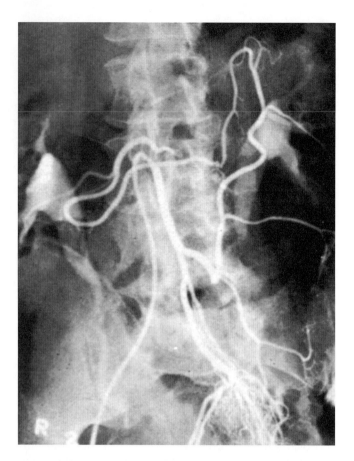

Figure 42–2. This inferior mesenteric arteriogram demonstrates filling of the left colic artery around the splenic flexure, through the anastomotic branch to the middle colic artery, and even (overlying the right renal pelvis) to the right branch of the middle colic artery and the hepatic flexure. This anatomy ensures successful use of the left hemicolon for esophagocoloplasty.

point of strategic interest is the marginal communication between the left branch of the middle colic artery and the ascending portion of the left colic artery (Fig. 42–2). Successful use of the left colon depends on this critical marginal artery. The distribution of the right colic artery is inconsistent, and an unreliable communication with the right branch of the middle colic artery or the ileocolic artery makes selection of the right colon sometimes risky. The true benefit of colonic arteriography lies in the fact that it provides a clear anatomic "road map" *preoperatively* to eliminate any surprise or confusion in the operating room. The most common useful arteriographic findings are stenosis at the origin of the inferior mesenteric artery, inadequacy of the marginal artery, failure of communication of the right and left branches of the middle colic artery, and a short trunk of the middle colic artery precluding access and division. Knowledge of these findings before surgery saves considerable time intraoperatively. A complete study includes transfemoral retrograde catheter opacification of the inferior mesenteric artery, the superior mesenteric artery, *and* the celiac axis. Complications of such a study in experienced radiographic hands are uncommon.

Barium Contrast Radiography

The contrast barium esophagogram still provides a good "road map" for the surgeon to assess the length of tumor involvement, proximity of the tumor to the aortic arch, and involvement of the lesser curve of the stomach. It is especially helpful in making a decision between the thoracoabdominal approach and the Ivor Lewis approach. A contrast barium enema is helpful to rule out neoplasms and extensive diverticulosis when considering use of the colon.

A concluding point in this section on diagnostic studies is that none of the three studies is actually applicable to the jejunum. The jejunum has a consistent blood supply and is always long enough, at least for short esophageal replacement. It is not accessible to endoscopy. The detail provided by a small bowel barium follow-through examination is marginal. For these reasons, indeed, many surgeons give the jejunum preference as the viscus for replacement of the esophagus.

ESOPHAGOGASTROSTOMY

The surgical technique for esophageal replacement by the stomach is best considered by reducing it to its component steps: (1) mobilization of the stomach, (2) lengthening of the stomach, (3) drainage of the stomach, (4) transposition of the stomach, and (5) anastomosis. Each step is described here with a preferred method of performance and the reason why it is performed in this manner. The actual esophageal dissection is described elsewhere.

Mobilization of the Stomach

Detaching the stomach from its complicated intraabdominal anatomic relationships requires full operative exposure, which is best achieved by performing a standard upper midline laparotomy (used for combined incisions, including the abdominal–right thoracic and the transhiatal-cervical) or a left thoracoabdominal incision (used for distal esophageal resections). Although the stomach may be detached for distal esophagectomy via a strictly transthoracic, transdiaphragmatic approach, this method does not provide optimal exposure.

The initial step in mobilizing the stomach is division of the greater omentum outside the gastroepiploic arcade, which is formed by the right gastroepiploic artery from the gastroduodenal artery at the pyloric end of the stomach and the left gastroepiploic artery from the splenic artery toward the proximal end of the stomach. This division is facilitated by grasping the transverse colon, lifting it out of the incision distally, and entering the lesser omental sac at a point where the omentum is thinnest and most transparent, usually at the midpoint of the stomach or slightly to its left. The dissection is carried all the way to the level of the pylorus, with division of the small omental branches of the epiploic arcade. These vessels may be coagulated, clipped, or tied. The use of fine ligatures is preferred to avoid any retrograde coagulum, which might compromise the integrity of the gastroepiploic arcade, and to avoid metal clips, which might compromise the clarity of detail of any subsequent computed tomography scan. The dissection is then directed toward the spleen, where the left gastroepiploic artery is ligated at the upper end of the arcade above the segmental artery to the stomach.

The short gastric (gastrolienal) arteries are divided carefully between hemostatic clamps and ligated securely. The more proximal of these vessels may be quite short and require the application of suture ligatures. Ligatures on the stomach must be tied securely because there have been instances in which these ties slipped off when the stomach later became distended in the thorax. Finally, there is a posterior branch from the splenic artery to the posterior aspect of the cardia that is very constant; division of this branch completes the liberation of the greater curvature.

The reflection of peritoneum at the esophagogastric junction is divided, and blunt finger or right-angled clamp dissection permits the surgeon to encircle the abdominal esophagus. Circumferential passage of an empty Penrose rubber drain allows upward traction on this end of the stomach during dissection of the lesser curvature. If the entire stomach is to be used to replace the esophagus, the vagus nerves are divided at this point. If the proximal part of the stomach itself is to be resected, the branches of the vagus nerves are included when the stomach is transected. The rather avascular, thin gastrohepatic omentum is entered low on the stomach, and a second Penrose drain is passed around the stomach at about the level of the incisura to permit downward traction during dissection of the lesser curvature.

Attention is directed toward exposing the origin of the left gastric artery at the trifurcation of the celiac axis. This structure is approached most easily from the posterior aspect of the stomach, which is elevated to the right by the assistant applying traction on the two Penrose drains. It is necessary to divide the filmy, avascular adhesions between the back of the stomach and the retroperitoneum that extend from the pylorus to the superior edge of the pancreas. At this point, the celiac axis and its three branches can be identified by palpation as the left thumb and forefinger encircle what is left of the lesser curvature attachments. The left gastric artery is exposed by sharp dissection. It is doubly ligated at its origin with heavy nonabsorbable suture material, such as No. 0 silk. The first ligature is placed and tied firmly before the artery is actually divided so that should the ligature break during tying, a freely spurting major artery is avoided. Two hemostatic clamps are then applied distal to this first ligature, and the artery is divided between them. A stitch is placed on the left gastric artery 5 mm distal to the first tie. The artery on the gastric side is managed best with a secure stitch ligature. The left gastric vein is usually identified separate from the artery and is handled in similar fashion. The tissue remaining now includes branches of the vagus nerves and the sympathetic chains, which extend upward to the Penrose tape previously placed to encircle the esophagogastric junction; this tissue is divided between clamps and suture-ligated because vessels frequently arise from the undersurface of the liver to the highest point on the lesser curvature.

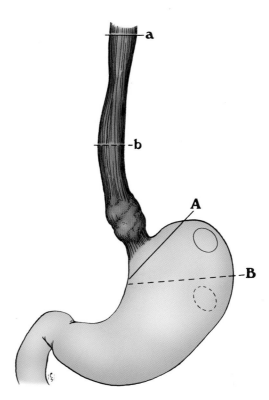

Figure 42–3.   The gastric fundus should be preserved (A) to maximize gastric length, which will permit extension of the gastric tube to the neck (a) if necessary. For a distal lesion where only a portion of the esophagus need be resected (b), it is important not to assume adequate gastric length and prematurely amputate the gastric fundus (B). A complete *circle* indicates the proposed esophagogastric site.

The stomach is now free except for the duodenum with the right gastric and right gastroepiploic arteries and the esophagus with its two vagus nerves. Depending on the procedure, the stomach is now handled in one of two ways:

1. If the primary operation is a distal esophagogastrectomy, the nodes along the left gastric artery and celiac axis have been dissected carefully so that they remain in continuity with the stomach. The stomach is transected *from* a point on the greater curvature opposite the level of emergence of the left gastroepiploic artery *to* a point on the lesser curvature below the lowest branch of the left gastric artery with the GIA or TA90 stapler (Fig. 42–3). The lesser curvature point of transection may actually be carried distally to a point below the incisura. The stapled gastric margin is turned in with interrupted No. 4-0 silk Lembert sutures.

2. If the operation planned is a more proximal esophagectomy of the Ivor Lewis type, nothing further need be done at this point. Transection of the stomach at the cardia is carried out once the stomach is drawn through an enlarged hiatus into the right hemithorax after the right thoracic esophageal dissection. This method allows less

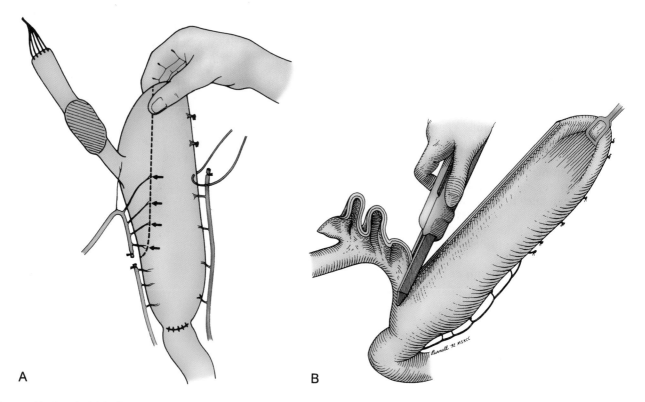

A   **B**

Figure 42–4. **A,** This illustration demonstrates both removal of the lesser curvature of the stomach and elongation of the stomach by traction on the greater curvature. The subsequent esophagogastric anastomosis will be made to a point toward the greater curvature from the surgeon's thumb. (From Akiyama H: Surgery for carcinoma of the esophagus. Curr Probl Surg 17:56, 1980.) **B,** Multiple applications of the GIA-60 stapler are used to "unfold" the lesser curvature and achieve maximal length of the gastric tube. (From Shriver CD, Spiro RH, Burt M: A new technique of gastric pull-through. Surg Gynecol Obstet 177:519, 1993.)

opportunity for possible torsion of the stomach as it is drawn upward. The operator must be careful to not pull the stomach too tightly when mobilizing it into the chest, which could result in compression by the hiatus or in redundancy of the stomach in the chest with resultant poor emptying.

Lengthening of the Stomach

After completion of the dissection just described, lengthening of the stomach is achieved by right lateral peritoneal pancreaticoduodenal mobilization, the so-called Kocher maneuver. It is begun distal to the pylorus along the second portion of the duodenum, with particular care taken to preserve the right gastric artery and to remain anterior to the common bile duct. The peritoneum alone is divided, and the dissection is carried around the C curve of the duodenum along the inferior margin of its third portion. The duodenum can then be dissected free posteriorly by blunt dissection behind the pancreas and in front of the inferior vena cava. The Kocher maneuver permits the duodenum to assume an almost vertical axis as the stomach is drawn up into the thorax. This allows the stomach to reach the cervical level with the pylorus then lying at the level of the diaphragmatic hiatus.

Akiyama has described resection of the lesser curvature of the stomach to gain additional length (Fig.

42–4A).[18] This maneuver may be needed to remove a lymphatic drainage siphon, but aside from dividing both anterior and posterior branches of the left gastric artery individually, excision of the lesser curvature is not usually necessary to gain length. This procedure can be accomplished by use of the linear stapler (see Fig. 42–4B).

Because of the peculiar shape of the stomach, maximal length is obtained by applying upward traction on a point high on the greater curvature of the stomach, actually the highest point of the fundus (see Fig. 42–4A). The location of this point is determined by moving the right thumb and forefinger along on the greater curvature while applying upward traction to find the point providing maximal length.

Drainage of the Stomach

Opinion regarding the necessity for a pyloric drainage procedure after esophagectomy is varied. Actual practice is largely the result of personal experience. There are staunch supporters of routine pyloric drainage and those who favor it only when pyloric obstruction is encountered.

Huang and colleagues, in a prospective study of pyloroplasty versus no pyloroplasty after esophagectomy, showed no difference in gastric emptying time.[19] If gastric outlet obstruction at the level of the pylorus per-

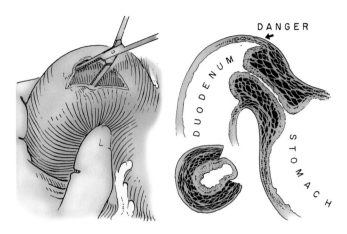

Figure 42–5. Pyloromyotomy. The 3-cm incision across the pylorus provides complete exposure of the sphincter muscle for division down to the mucosal layer. Fine hemostatic forceps are helpful in this dissection. The principal risk of entry into the duodenum is shown in the cross section at the *right,* where the duodenal mucosa covers the undersurface of the pyloric muscle at the duodenal aspect.

sists, surgical intervention is invariably required. This can be difficult in a patient after esophagogastrectomy, especially if an Ivor Lewis or transhiatal approach has been used, because the pylorus is usually located at or near the hiatus, thus making exposure difficult. Balloon dilation may be successful in patients who have undergone a pyloromyotomy and failed conservative measures for correction of gastric outlet obstruction.

From a physiologic standpoint, a gastric drainage procedure makes sense. In the early clinical experience with vagotomy for peptic ulcer disease, it became clear that obstructive symptoms were encountered frequently when vagotomy was performed without a drainage procedure. After esophagectomy, gastric stasis may be observed when the anastomosis is examined radiologically at the initial postoperative study. Because gastroesophageal reflux is common after an intrathoracic anastomosis of the esophagus and stomach and peptic stricture is always a possibility, most experienced general thoracic surgeons now perform a drainage procedure.

A pyloromyotomy is preferred by most. It does not detract from the length of the stomach when the stomach must be brought to the neck, and the pylorus retains some of its barrier capacity against the reflux of bile and pancreatic juice into the stomach (Fig. 42–5). Performance of a complete pyloromyotomy is not always an easy technical task. The best teachers of the proper technique are pediatric surgeons, who gain considerable experience from the Ramstedt-Fredet operation for hypertrophic pyloric stenosis.

The myotomy is limited to 3 cm. Transfixion sutures of silk around the pyloric vein on either side of the myotomy site facilitate exposure by reducing bleeding and permitting lateral traction. With the left hand placed behind the gastroduodenal junction and lifting the pyloric channel forward, the incision is begun directly over the easily palpable pyloric muscle with an unused No. 15 Bard-Parker blade. The surgeon's thumb retracts

the muscle downward as it is divided while the assistant provides countertraction upward. When the submucosal plane is reached, the myotomy incision is carried onto the first portion of the duodenum, which presents the only real danger of entry into the lumen. The last muscle fibers are often best separated with good exposure and light and the use of fine, vertically cutting scissors.

If entry into the duodenum does occur, the safest course of action is to convert the procedure to a pyloroplasty. The Heineke-Mikulicz method of closure suffices, again limiting the length of the incision to no more than 2 to 3 cm. Continuous fine inverting chromic catgut or polyglycolic acid sutures are used for closure of the inner layer, and interrupted Lembert sutures of fine silk are used for the reinforcing, outer layer. A single-layer closure is also acceptable. Tacking a portion of adjacent residual omentum over the pyloromyotomy or pyloroplasty provides an additional safety measure against subsequent leakage.

Transposition of the Stomach

If the esophagus has been removed, the stomach is placed in the posterior mediastinal or orthotopic position. If a bypassing conduit is planned, a retrosternal tunnel must be constructed to allow anterior mediastinal transposition of the stomach.[20] Of the various placement options for the stomach, the orthotopic position is the shortest. Ngan and Wong measured the distances of the various positions used for gastric replacement of the esophagus.[21] The orthotopic route was an average of 2 cm less than the retrosternal route; the latter was an additional 2 cm less than the presternal subcutaneous route of passage.

The Ivor Lewis right-sided thoracotomy approach to esophageal dissection permits the mobilized stomach to be drawn gently through the hiatus into the orthotopic position. Then after confirming that torsion of the stomach has not occurred, the cardia or more distal part of the stomach is transected with a GIA or TA90 stapler, and the staple line is inverted with interrupted fine silk Lembert sutures.

If the retrosternal route is chosen, the diaphragmatic attachments to the back of the sternum are sharply divided, and this avascular opening is gradually dilated from the width of two fingers to a size that permits upward passage of the entire hand (Fig. 42–6). With the palm upward, the areolar tissue and pleural membrane are swept gently from the midline to the patient's left until the plane of dissection developed through a left oblique cervical incision is encountered. The left pleural membrane does not approach as close to the midline as the right does, and therefore blunt dissection to the left is less likely to result in entering the pleura. Hemodynamics must be monitored carefully to watch for hypotension or arrhythmia. If symptoms develop, the hand must immediately be withdrawn and blunt dissection continued only when the changes resolve. If either pleural space is entered, placement of a thoracostomy tube (No. 28 Argyle) is required. A portable chest radiograph is always taken before the patient is moved from the operating table because an unsuspected pneumothorax can be managed easily in the operating room.

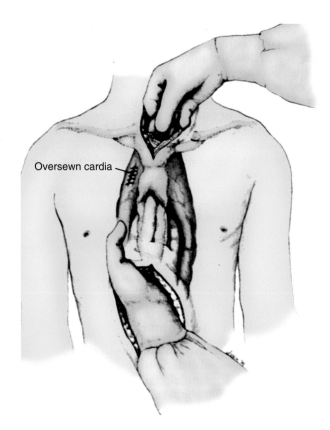

Oversewn cardia

Figure 42–6. The retrosternal tunnel has been bluntly dissected with the finger so that the entire hand can be extended upward in the anterior mediastinum. This figure illustrates passage of the stomach through this tunnel to the thoracic inlet and the cervical incision. Note that the thoracic inlet has been enlarged by resection of the inner end of the clavicle and a portion of the manubrium. (From Orringer MB, Sloan H: Substomal gastric bypass of the excluded thoracic esophagus for palliation of esophageal carcinoma. J Thorac Cardiovasc Surg 70:836, 1975.)

Anastomosis

In patients undergoing esophageal resection, the anastomosis may be placed below the aortic arch (as in a left-sided thoracoabdominal approach for carcinoma of the cardia or very distal esophagus), at the apex of the right hemithorax (as in the conventional Ivor Lewis approach), or in the neck for subtotal esophagectomy. If an anterior mediastinal approach is used, the anastomosis must be placed in the neck. This procedure may actually be the most critical part of the operation. In our experience at Massachusetts General Hospital, the esophagogastric anastomosis is sufficiently secure that placing it in the mediastinum is not a concern. Thus, placement of the anastomosis in the neck is dictated *solely* by the extent of disease, not by fear of possible leakage at the anastomotic suture line.

For more than 50 years we have used a two-layer anastomosis of interrupted fine (4-0) silk. Meticulous attention to detail is required in this technique. No clamps of any sort are permitted on the edges of the anastomotic tissue. The cutting cautery is not used to transect the

esophagus; only a new sharp scalpel blade is used. There must be no tension on the respective edges of the esophagus and stomach. Placement of a given stitch is guided by gentle traction on the preceding one, and the edges are handled as little as possible with forceps. The interrupted technique prevents purse-stringing of the anastomosis and allows patent capillaries to extend to the precise edges of the anastomosed structures.

The details of the anastomosis have previously been described by Wilkins[22] and by Mathisen and colleagues.[11] It is an end-to-side (esophagus-to-stomach) technique. A point on the stomach is selected on its anterior aspect at least 2 cm from the gastric transection line in what was the fundus of the stomach and toward the greater curvature. A small circle (the size of a nickel) is scored in the gastric serosa with a scalpel. This maneuver exposes the intramural plexus of vessels, which are then individually suture-ligated with fine silk, thus minimizing ooze and preserving a bloodless field for suture placement (Fig. 42–7). With the specimen still attached to the esophagus at this point, the esophagus is reflected proximally to expose the area of planned transection. A long right-angled occluding clamp is placed just distal to the planned anastomotic line (i.e., toward the specimen). The clamp assists in providing exact exposure of the anastomosis and at the same time prevents spillage of gastric contents or tumor cells from the specimen.

1. The first row of 4-0 silk sutures is an outer posterior row placed in horizontal mattress fashion between the muscularis of the esophagus and the seromuscular layer of the stomach (see Fig. 42–7A). Four to six of these sutures are placed first and then tied carefully, always drawing the stomach upward to the esophagus by positioning the tying left forefinger above the point of actual approximation. The esophagus is a fixed structure that cannot be brought down distally, and its muscular coats are fragile and do not hold sutures as well as those of the stomach. The outer posterior row of sutures covers only about a third of the circumference to allow better exposure when placing the next layer. The corner ties are left long and marked with hemostats.

2. The esophagus is then opened with a scalpel 4 to 5 mm distal to the initial row of stitches, and the incision is extended around each corner. The mucosal layer of stomach is incised, and the scored button is removed. The pinkish gray esophageal mucosa is exposed carefully (it tends to retract) by spreading (not grasping) the opening in the esophagus. The inner posterior stitches, also 4-0 silk, are placed and tied as one proceeds (see Fig. 42–7B). Each stitch is placed about 5 mm back from the cut edge on either structure. The needle must be pulled through each edge separately because trying to include both edges in one pass of the needle causes tearing. The use of atraumatic grasping forceps is necessary to place the first stitch, but subsequent grasping of mucosa is usually unnecessary. Elevation of the previous stitch guides placement of the next. The entire posterior mucosal row is

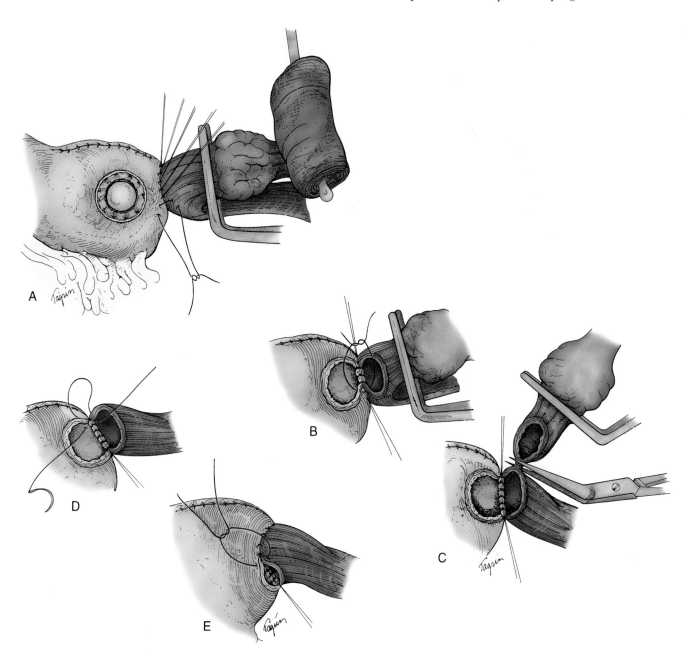

Figure 42–7.   A, The first step in the Sweet anastomosis developed at the Massachusetts General Hospital. An end-to-side anastomosis is being initiated with excision of a button of gastric wall. This button must not be placed too close to the gastric turn-in. The button can actually be placed quite close to the greater curvature, often between the last two branches of the gastroepiploic arcade. The outer posterior row of the anastomosis is being performed with interrupted mattress sutures of fine silk placed across the longitudinal muscle fibers of the esophagus. Our preference is to place all these sutures before tying. **B,** The gastric button has been excised. With the specimen still attached and excluded with the right-angle clamp, the mucosae of the esophagus and stomach are approximated with interrupted fine silk sutures. **C,** Completion of the posterior inner row and excision of the specimen. **D,** The corner of the anastomosis is being turned to begin the anterior row of sutures. These are placed, again in interrupted fashion, with the knots tied on the inside. **E,** Completion of the anastomosis with mattress sutures of interrupted silk in the outer anterior row. Each suture approximates the muscularis of the esophagus to the seromuscular layer of the stomach. These sutures are placed in horizontal mattress fashion (not as actually shown) so that there is less risk of cutting through. (From Mathisen DJ, Grillo HC, Wilkins EW Jr, et al: Transthoracic esophagectomy: A safe approach to carcinoma of the esophagus. Ann Thorac Surg 45:137, 1988.)

completed, with the corner sutures left uncut. Transection of the esophagus is now completed, and the specimen is removed (see Fig. 42–7C). The nasogastric tube is directed downward through the anastomosis to the level of the gastric antrum and is fixed by the anesthetist to the patient's nose.

3. The anterior inner row is continued in interrupted fashion, with the stitches placed so that the knots are always tied within the lumen (see Fig. 42–7D). The assistant holds the previous tie down and away as each subsequent stitch is secured. This method allows complete inversion of the mucosal layer. The previous suture is then cut after tying each subsequent stitch. This row of sutures is tied from either end toward the middle so that a final horizontal mattress suture can be placed to complete the anterior mucosal row.

4. The outer anterior row is placed in horizontal mattress fashion over what is left, which is about two thirds of the circumference (see Fig. 42–7E). The serosa of the stomach is brought as much as 1 cm above the inner mucosal layer. Because the anastomosis has been placed 2 cm or more down the apex of the stomach posteriorly and the stomach has been folded upward anteriorly, a valve-like luminal orifice has been created that helps minimize the possibility of gastroesophageal reflux. The stomach is suspended by a series of nonabsorbable sutures to the fascia overlying the thoracic spine. This minimizes the possibility of downward drag of a potentially full stomach on the fragile anastomosis.

Whether the esophagogastrectomy is performed as a replacement of the esophagus or as a bypass of it, it may be accompanied by placement of a feeding jejunostomy. The jejunostomy is used for feeding purposes if there is any difficulty with the anastomosis or delay in postoperative gastric emptying. It also provides access for immediate postoperative substantive caloric feeding, obviates the need for total intravenous parenteral nutrition, and promotes healing at the anastomotic sites by providing a catabolic state for the patient.

One week after surgery, barium swallow is used to evaluate the esophagogastric anastomosis and gastric emptying. If there are no issues, the patient is allowed small amounts of clear liquids. Gastric dilatation must be evaluated by chest radiography as oral intake commences. If delayed gastric emptying is identified, oral intake should be stopped and nasogastric decompression instituted. A prokinetic agent such as metoclopramide (Reglan) should be started. A second trial of oral liquids should be attempted several days later. If the patient fails again, balloon dilatation of the pylorus should be considered. The jejunostomy tube is usually removed at the first postoperative visit (1 month).

Functional Results

Despite the vast experience with the stomach as an esophageal substitute, little information is available on long-term functional results. Orringer and associates have reported the early and late results of transhiatal esophagectomy in patients with benign and malignant disease.[23] As they note, functional results are better demonstrated in patients undergoing surgery for benign disease because of longer survival data. Among patients with benign disease who underwent esophagectomy, data have been accumulated on 242 patients over an average of 47 months. The overall functional result in patients with benign disease was reported as excellent in 29% (asymptomatic), good in 39% (mild symptoms requiring no intervention), fair in 28% (occasional episodes of dumping or requiring occasional dilatation), and poor in 4% (requiring regular treatment).

Orringer et al. also reported on 721 patients at an average of 29 months after transhiatal esophagectomy for esophageal cancer.[23] The overall functional results were reported as excellent, or asymptomatic, in 54% of patients. The results were reported as good in 28%, fair in 15%, and poor in 3% of patients.

ESOPHAGOCOLOPLASTY

The term *esophagocoloplasty* is used arbitrarily in this section to denote either replacement or bypass of the esophagus by colon. As clearly described already, the stomach is the first choice for replacing the esophagus. However, when the stomach has previously been removed, even partially, the colon is the viscus of choice. In addition, when bypass of an unresectable esophageal carcinoma is required, the colon offers the best possibility of providing successful palliation. An advantage to colon grafts is the length available, but colon interposition can cause significant morbidity and is a technically complex procedure. The specific indications for esophagocoloplasty are presented in Box 42–1.

Box 42–1 **Indications for Esophagocoloplasty**

Malignant Tumors

Replacement of esophagus after gastrectomy

Bypass of unresectable carcinoma

Palliation of esophagotracheal or bronchial fistula

Staged complex esophageal resections

Benign Conditions

Staged bypass of caustic esophageal stricture

Esophageal atresia (congenital) when primary anastomosis is not feasible

Bypass of a long peptic esophageal stricture in a physiologically impaired patient

Preoperative Preparation

Emphasis has already been placed on evaluating the colon by colonoscopy, mesenteric arteriography, and barium enema. Of these, evaluation of the colon's arterial blood supply by arteriography is the most vital because it provides important detail on the variable colic arteries. In older patients, the presence of atherosclerotic plaque is also identified by these studies. Any of a number of major mesenteric arterial anomalies may be identified. Although in most cases the details of this anatomy can be worked out by intraoperative transillumination of the colonic mesentery, arteriographic study saves both time and confusion during the actual conduct of the operation.

Adequate colon preparation is essential to primary healing of the esophagocolic anastomosis in the neck, where spillage of residual fecal contents must be avoided. Mechanical cleansing of the colon is accomplished with polyethylene glycol (GoLYTELY), and enemas are rarely required and should not be administered within 12 to 18 hours before surgery. Oral antibiotics are favored by some, with 1 g of neomycin and 1 g of erythromycin every 4 hours for three doses being the most common regimen. Broad-spectrum antibiotics are initiated parenterally on call to the operating theater, and maintenance doses are continued in bolus intravenous fashion during the procedure and 48 hours after.

The route of reconstruction must be considered. The posterior mediastinal route for placement of the conduit is often available after esophageal resection. However, when it has been decided, because of tumor unresectability or the condition of the patient, to not resect the esophagus, a retrosternal approach may be taken (described in the next section). In addition, the subcutaneous route may be necessary if the usual anterior mediastinal route has been transgressed by a previous median sternotomy, particularly for an open cardiac surgical operation. This approach requires a mandatory ventral hernia to allow the colon to enter the subcutaneous tissue of the chest. Finally, a transpleural route may be used with the colon passing through the esophageal hiatus and pleural space.

Operative Technique

Retrosternal positioning of the colonic bypass is ideally suited to a two-team approach, an abdominal team and a cervical team. The cervical team should delay incision until the exploratory findings in the abdomen are clearly favorable: (1) absence of major intra-abdominal metastatic disease and (2) the presence of a suitable length of colon with a proper arterial blood supply and venous drainage. The abdominal mobilization of the colon described subsequently is the same for any of the routes or reconstructions.

Standard endotracheal anesthesia is used and the patient is placed supine on the operating table with the head turned to the right. Hyperextension of the neck is achieved with elevation of the shoulders by a thyroid bag. The operative field is prepared from the left mastoid process to the symphysis pubis. A nasogastric tube is passed to the point of esophageal obstruction or into the stomach.

Abdominal Team

A long midline or left paramedian laparotomy incision is used that extends from the xiphoid process to below the umbilicus. Careful exploration is needed to search for hepatic metastases, left gastric artery–celiac axis node metastases, peritoneal or omental implants of tumor, a possible second gastric carcinoma, or other unsuspected intra-abdominal processes.

The colon is then mobilized from the ascending to the sigmoid level. Freeing the colon from the omentum and from the right and left peritoneal reflections is not difficult but must be accomplished carefully. The general surgical background of the thoracic surgeon is a helpful attribute. Important points in this dissection are, in order of approach, (1) total detachment of the omentum from the colon, leaving it attached to the stomach but preserving the midcolic vessels as the posterior leaf of the omentum is peeled off the transverse mesocolon; (2) mobilization of the splenic flexure without injury to the spleen, a process that is more easily accomplished after the left peritoneal reflection has been incised, thereby permitting downward traction on both the transverse and descending colon; and (3) freeing of the hepatic flexure from the duodenum and retroperitoneal structures in the right upper quadrant.

This subtotal freeing of the colon now permits it to be elevated for appropriate transillumination and visualization of all colic vessels. The left hemicolon is preferred for use as the bypassing conduit because of its more reliable blood supply and an advantageous size match. The marginal artery between the left branch of the midcolic artery and the ascending portion of the left colic artery is critical, and its presence and adequacy on the preoperative arteriogram must be verified (see Fig. 42–2). The midcolic artery is no less critical. Because the length of the necessary colon bypass takes one to the hepatic fixture, a bifurcation of the midcolic artery well out from its superior mesenteric arterial source is required; a bifid origin of the right and left branches of the midcolic artery does not permit retrograde blood flow all the way from the left colic artery to the hepatic flexure. *Isoperistaltic placement of the colon segment is preferred* (Fig. 42–8).

To use the left colic artery as the source of blood supply, the midcolic vessels are now divided at their origin from the superior mesenteric vessels and doubly ligated (Fig. 42–9). For complete mobility of the hepatic flexure, the right colic vessels must also often be divided. The distance from the point where the colon is tethered by the left colic artery is measured to the level of the midneck. The distance is then measured around the colon toward the hepatic flexure, and the appropriate transection point is carefully identified. The colon is divided with the GIA stapler both at this point and at the juncture of the descending and sigmoid colon. The colon can then be passed behind the stomach through a wide aperture made in the avascular gastrohepatic omentum. This maneuver allows the left colic artery and

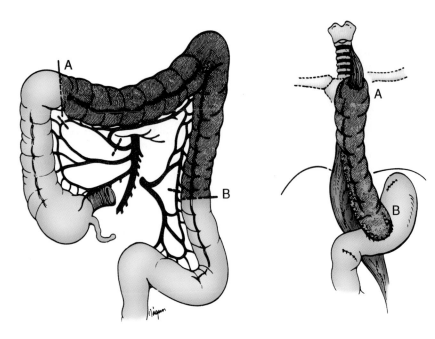

Figure 42–8. Schematic illustration showing use of the left colon to replace the esophagus. Points A and B are determined by the length of colon necessary to reach the neck. The left colic artery provides the blood supply. The middle colic artery is divided. The colon is placed, always, in isoperistaltic fashion such that the segment near the hepatic flexure is anastomosed to the esophagus in the neck and the end near the sigmoid colon is attached to the antrum of the stomach in the abdomen.

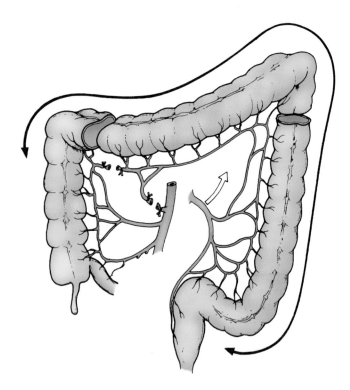

Figure 42–9. The long line with *arrows* at both ends illustrates the extent of colon to be freed for left colon replacement of the esophagus. Blood supply is provided through the inferior mesenteric artery, the left colic artery, and the anastomotic branch connecting the middle colic artery. The middle colic artery has been divided near its origin from the superior mesenteric artery.

vein to extend the shortest distance and prevents angulation or potential compression by a dependent full stomach.

The mobilized residual abdominal colon can now be reanastomosed. Our preference has been to use an end-to-end, two-layer, inverting anastomosis of interrupted fine silk and running catgut suture. An important detail is closure of the colon mesentery to minimize the likelihood of internal herniation of small intestine. This closure usually lies slightly caudad to the ligament of Treitz and often requires approximation of the mesentery to the posterior peritoneum.

With a viable colon segment, the second team can begin the cervical incision and the abdominal team can start to bluntly develop the retrosternal tunnel. Particular attention is paid to the thoracic inlet portion of this tunnel, and it should be big enough to admit four fingers. The inlet can be enlarged if necessary as described earlier (see Fig. 42–1). The colon segment is then gently drawn upward by means of a guiding heavy silk thread, with care taken to keep its mesentery on the right without any twisting. An impediment in venous return may result in subsequent venous thrombosis and failure of the colon bypass. Viability of the upper end of the segment must be verified not only by visual inspection of its color but also by palpable observation of arterial pulsation, by the application of a Doppler probe, or by incisional demonstration of arterial blood flow.

The cologastric anastomosis is carried out in end-to-side fashion to the anterior aspect of the midportion of the stomach with an inner layer of running 4-0 catgut and an outer layer of interrupted 4-0 silk suture.

The pylorus is palpated to determine the need for a pyloric drainage procedure (an opportunity is available at the time of cologastric anastomosis to palpate the pylorus from within). In general, pyloric drainage is required only if the esophagus is being removed and the vagus nerves divided; a simple bypass does not compromise gastric innervation, and stasis is not likely to be an issue.

Gastric decompression is provided by a Stamm gastrostomy placed proximal to the cologastric anastomosis. A No. 18 Foley catheter works effectively and is brought out through a stab incision placed laterally in the left upper quadrant. The stomach is secured to the anterior peritoneum in four quadrants around the tube with 3-0 silk sutures.

Cervical Team

A left-sided oblique cervical incision is a useful approach to the cervical esophagus. It requires dividing the omohyoid muscle, retracting the sternocleidomastoid muscle laterally, dividing the inferior thyroid artery and often the middle thyroid vein, detaching the sternal insertions of the peritracheal muscles, and entering the avascular prevertebral plane. The esophagus is readily apparent by palpation of its inlaying nasogastric tube.

The esophagus is encircled, with care taken to not damage the membranous portion of the trachea or the recurrent laryngeal nerves. Even unilateral vocal cord palsy enhances the possibility of postoperative aspiration. The mobilized esophagus is transected 2 to 3 cm distal to the cricopharyngeus and its proximal end marked with silk sutures at the corners and left open without clamping. The distal end is turned in with two layers, one stapled and the second with inverting 4-0 interrupted silk sutures.

The critical esophagocolic anastomosis is carried out in end-to-end fashion with two layers of inverting, interrupted 4-0 silk. The actual suture material is not as important as the two-layer, interrupted technique. Use of the left colon minimizes the size discrepancy between the two lumens, and proper interval spacing of the sutures or the addition of a short vertical incision at the end of the esophagus permits an anastomosis with no redundant tissue. The nasogastric tube, withdrawn to transect the esophagus, is replaced distally into the colon bypass before completing the anterior row of sutures: It provides evacuation of colonic air, monitors postoperative bleeding, and minimizes the potential for tracheal aspiration. The nasogastric tube is routinely left in overnight and removed on postoperative day 1.

The neck is closed without drains unless there is persistent oozing or contamination (the abdominal incision has now been closed by the abdominal team). A portable chest radiograph is obtained before the endotracheal tube is removed, and pneumothorax is decompressed by means of a thoracostomy tube.

Postoperative Care

The most important consideration in postoperative management is viability of the colon bypass segment. An extremely reliable indicator that the segment may be compromised is a persistently high fever. Endoscopy is hazardous because of the fresh anastomosis, and the appearance of the mucosa is not always a consistent indi-

| Table 42–1 | Indications for Colon Esophageal Bypass |

Diagnosis	No. of Patients
Neoplastic	88
Esophageal cancer	78
Proximal gastric cancer	3
Laryngeal cancer	3
Thyroid cancer	3
Malignant carcinoid	1
Non-neoplastic	48
Stricture	35
Caustic	16
Peptic	14
Radiation	5
Congenital atresia	10
Motility disorder	3

From Wain JC: Long segment colon interposition. Semin Thorac Cardiovasc Surg 4:336, 1992.

cator of viability. The best method of assessing the colon conduit is a second-look operation. The neck incision can be opened easily under local anesthesia, and the upper end of the colon segment can be inspected directly. If the segment is nonviable, the entire colon bypass must be immediately removed from its retrosternal location. A necrotic colon persisting in the anterior mediastinum is a source of possible death. In one case of failed colon bypass in our experience, the residual viable colon was brought up subcutaneously, and the resultant gap was ultimately bridged with a free jejunal autograft.

Feedings are begun by gastrostomy on the second day with the patient fed in a semierect position to minimize possible gastrocolic reflux. A barium esophagogram is carried out on the seventh postoperative day. Oral feeding is then begun gradually if the anastomosis proves to be intact.

Results

Wain reported our results with long-segment colon substitution of the esophagus in 136 patients.[24] Indications were neoplasms in 88 and non-neoplastic disorders in 48 (Table 24–1). The left colon was used in 100 of 136 (74%) and the right colon in 36 of 136 (26%). Major acute complications included graft ischemia (4 of 100 with the left colon, 8 of 36 with the right colon) and cervical anastomotic leak (Table 24–2). Thirty-day operative mortality rates were 16% in the neoplastic group and 0% in the non-neoplastic group (Table 24–3). The differences in operative mortality between benign and malignant disease were corroborated in a review by Postlethwait (Table 24–4).[25] Late complications included proximal anastomotic stenosis (eight), graft redundancy (four), bile reflux (two), and esophageal mucocele (one). Among operative survivors, excellent function (no dysphagia, stable weight) was obtained in 88% (107 of 122), good function (mild dysphagia, stable weight) in 10% (12 of 122), and poor results in only 2.5% (3 of 122).

Wain and colleagues further analyzed 52 patients who had undergone long-segment colon interposition for

Table 42–2   Acute Complications of Colon Esophageal Bypass

Diagnosis	No. of Patients
Technical	
Graft ischemia	12
Left colon	4
Right colon	8
Cervical anastomotic leak	8
Vocal cord paresis	3
Acute nonvascular perforation	1
Sternal necrosis	1
Other	
Pneumonia	15
Wound infection	9
Small bowel obstruction	4
Pulmonary embolism	2
Cholecystitis	1

From Wain JC: Long segment colon interposition. Semin Thorac Cardiovasc Surg 4:336, 1992.

Table 42–3   Cause of Operative Mortality in Long-Segment Colon Bypass for Neoplasm

Cause	No. of Patients
Colon necrosis	7
Respiratory failure	5
Metastatic disease	1
Sudden cardiac death	1

From Wain JC: Long segment colon interposition. Semin Thorac Cardiovasc Surg 4:336, 1992.

acquired disease.[26] Pneumonia was the most frequent complication, and it occurred in 24 patients. Graft ischemia was noted in 5 patient (3 of 46 with left colon interposition and 2 of 6 patients with right colon interposition), and late complications included anastomotic strictures in 24 patients, all managed with dilatation. Episodes of aspiration pneumonia were noted in three patients more than 6 months after the procedure. Median survival was 11.5 years, and 11 of 50 patients maintained their weight. A modified diet for aspiration or moderate dysphagia was necessary in 33 of 50 patients. Five patients required continuous enteral feeding to maintain weight.

Redundancy of the colon in the chest or abdomen is a potentially serious complication. In a group of 69 long-segment colon interpositions, Jeyasingham et al. noted a 25% incidence of colonic redundancy.[27] Of the group of patients, supra-aortic redundancy developed in 4, supra-diaphragmatic redundancy in 11, and subdiaphragmatic redundancy in 7. The authors hypothesized that as a thin-walled structure the colon dilated in response to negative intrathoracic pressure above potentially obstructing landmarks. Of the patients in whom redundancy developed, 15 required operative intervention.

Colon bypass requires precise attention to technical detail for a successful outcome. The major complications and causes of operative mortality are often related to technical failure. When successful, the colon has proved to be an effective conduit with which to replace the esophagus.

ESOPHAGOJEJUNOPLASTY

Jejunum represents the third alternative for esophageal replacement. As a replacement, it can be used in one of three ways: (1) as an interposition graft retaining its vascular supply with branches from the superior mesenteric artery and vein, (2) as a Roux-en-Y limb, or (3) as an autograft. Jejunum is most frequently used as a short-segment interposition graft after resection of a distal esophageal stricture, although it may also be used to restore continuity after distal esophagectomy for carcinoma when the stomach has previously been removed. The anatomy of its mesentery makes long-segment interposition difficult, although in children, a Roux-en-Y loop readily reaches the neck. As an autograft, it is used for resection of short

Table 42–4   Colon Interposition Operative Mortality

	Benign		Malignant	
	No. of Patients	Deaths (%)	No. of Patients	Deaths (%)
Through 1961	54	11.1	78	21.8
Through 1971	655	7.5	245	24.5
Through 1981	474	4.9	367	16.6
Total	1183	6.8	690	20.0

From Postlethwait RW: Surgery of the Esophagus, 2nd ed. Norwalk, CT, Appleton-Century-Crofts, 1986, p 505.

cervical esophageal segments containing carcinoma, after extensive cervical trauma involving damage to the esophagus, or for augmentation of a failed colonic esophageal bypass.

Interposition

The short jejunal interposition for distal esophageal resections is described here because it is the most common application of esophagojejunoplasty. A left-sided thoracoabdominal incision provides the exposure necessary for both the esophageal procedure and preparation of the jejunum. The proximal part of the jejunum is identified and lifted out of the abdomen for transillumination of its mesentery (Fig. 42–10). The first jejunal artery is identified and preserved to maintain vascular integrity of the 10 to 12 cm of jejunum adjacent to the ligament of Treitz. After determining the length of jejunum needed, the upper three or four jejunal arteries to this measured segment are exposed. With the help of the transilluminating light, these arteries are isolated and occluded sequentially with atraumatic bulldog clamps to test the reliability of one jejunal artery to provide circulation to this segment. The peritoneum is reflected carefully from either side of the mesentery outward to the primary anastomotic arcade, the tissue intervening between the jejunal arteries is incised, and the necessary jejunal arteries and veins are divided and securely ligated with 2-0 silk. For longer reaches of the jejunal segment, one or two points on the secondary anastomotic arcade may require division (Fig. 42–11).

The jejunal segment is now separated from normal intestinal continuity by proximal and distal applications of the GIA stapler. The pedicled segment to be interposed is then brought through the transverse mesocolon. Because the segment has a proclivity to retain its curved

axis, the stapled proximal end of the segment is turned in with interrupted 3-0 silk Lembert sutures. The distal end of the jejunal segment is anastomosed first to the posterior aspect of the fundus of the stomach with a two-layer technique of interrupted 4-0 silk and continuous 4-0 chromic catgut. The esophagojejunal anastomosis is carried out in end-to-side fashion at a point 2 cm away from the jejunal turn-in on its antimesenteric border (Fig. 42–12). This is done with the same technique of two inverting layers of interrupted silk suture as

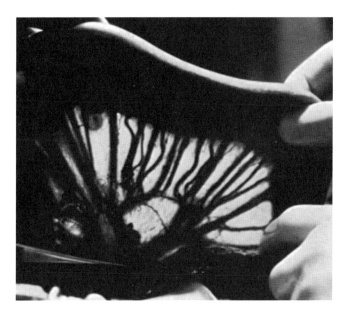

Figure 42–10. Transillumination of the jejunum demonstrates the jejunal branches of the superior mesenteric artery and permits selection of an appropriate one for reliable blood supply to the segment to be used in esophagojejunoplasty.

Figure 42–11. **A** and **B,** Diagrammatic illustration of (1) preservation of the highest jejunal artery, (2) division of the next three jejunal arteries, and (3) two points of division of a secondary arcade in **B.** Particular care must be taken that an arcade exists from the feeding arterial source (in this case, the fourth jejunal artery) all the way to the transected margin. (From Ring WS, Varco RL, L'Heureux PR, et al: Esophageal replacement with jejunum in children: An 18 to 33 year follow-up. J Thorac Cardiovasc Surg 83:918, 1982.)

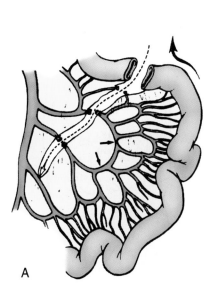

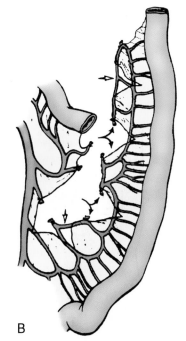

A

B

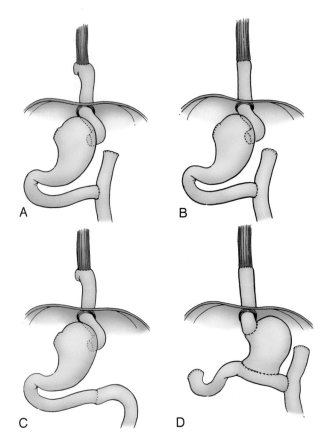

Figure 42–12. A-D, Methods of reconstruction using jejunum. (From Postlethwait RW: Surgery of the Esophagus, 2nd ed. Norwalk, CT, Appleton-Century-Crofts, 1986, p 500, with permission.)

described in the section on esophagogastrostomy. An end-to-end anastomosis constructed with an outer layer of silk and an inner running catgut suture restores jejunal continuity.

Roux-en-Y Limb

When there is no stomach for jejunal interposition, a Roux-en-Y jejunal limb may be used. This procedure involves only two anastomoses—esophagojejunal and an end-to-side jejunojejunal—instead of the three needed for an interposed segment. The higher the jejunum must reach in the chest or even to the neck, the more jejunal arteries that must be divided to provide adequate length of the Roux-en-Y limb. Unfortunately, this requirement increases the possibility of vascular failure at the tip of the jejunal segment and explains why jejunum is generally considered the third choice for esophageal replacement. Ring and associates state that jejunum is the first choice in children, but their illustrations (Fig. 42–13) show a process of staging the esophagojejunal anastomosis with an unanastomosed jejunal stoma in the neck in the first stage, presumably planned to be certain of its viability, and subsequent esophagojejunal anastomosis.[28]

In cervical esophagojejunoplasty, there is always the option of vascular enhancement by microvascular anastomosis of the internal mammary artery or a branch of a carotid artery to the jejunal mesentery arterial arcade. A suitable draining vein must also be identified and anastomosed under these circumstances. Payne and Fisher described a unique experience with "free jejunal transfer circulatory augmentation of pedicled intestinal inter-

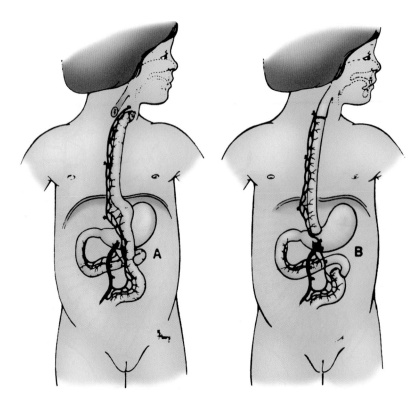

Figure 42–13. Use of the jejunum to replace the esophagus in a child. The jejunum readily reaches the neck. **A,** The proximal end of the jejunum is brought out as a cervical stoma to permit secondary performance of the esophagojejunal anastomosis. **B,** The distal end of the jejunum has been divided and anastomosed to the antrum of the stomach and the cervical anastomosis completed. (From Ring WS, Varco RL, L'Heureux PR, et al: Esophageal replacement with jejunum in children: An 18 to 33 year follow-up. J Thorac Cardiovasc Surg 83:918, 1982.)

Figure 42–14. Reconstruction of the cervical esophagus with a free jejunal graft according to the technique described by Hester et al. (1980). **A,** Tumor extirpation and neck dissection are completed. **B,** After abdominal exploration, a suitable segment of proximal jejunum is isolated on its pedicle, and the bowel is divided proximally and distally while ensuring that the only blood supply to the segment is through the pedicle. **C,** The artery and vein of the chosen segment are cleaned of adventitia with use of the operating microscope. **D,** The proximal bowel anastomosis is completed with interrupted 3-0 Vicryl sutures. **E,** The arterial and venous anastomoses to the chosen donor vessels are done. **F,** The distal bowel anastomosis is completed with interrupted 3-0 Vicryl sutures. **G,** A small window of dimethicone (Silastic) sheeting is left over the jejunum to allow close postoperative observation of the replant. (From Skinner DB, Belsey RHR: Management of Esophageal Disease. Philadelphia, WB Saunders, 1988.)

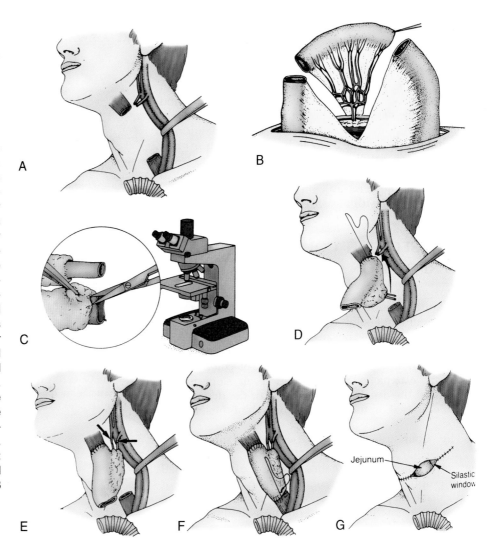

positions using microvascular surgery," in which the details of a number of variants of esophagojejunoplasty are described to solve unusual problems of cervical esophageal replacement.[29] When contemplating the use of jejunum for a long-segment replacement of the esophagus, such as to the cervical level, a thoracic surgeon he would be well advised to consult a microvascular surgical practitioner to prepare for the possible need for circulatory augmentation.

Free Transfer

Two teams accomplish the free transfer procedure most expeditiously. Attention in this discussion is focused on the abdominal procurement ("harvesting") team. Through a routine laparotomy, a suitable segment of jejunum is selected, preferably at least 40 cm distal to the ligament of Treitz (Fig. 42–14B). The principal issue in selecting the site is obtaining an appropriate length of a jejunal artery and vein for later vascular anastomosis. The character of the bowel itself is an additional consideration in that it must have adequate caliber and be free of intrinsic disease. Once the length of jejunum needed is

determined, it is transected proximally and distally with a GIA stapler. The mesentery is divided in a V fashion to the origin of the perfusing vessels. The isolated segment is now allowed to perfuse until the cervical team is prepared to carry out the actual transfer (see Fig. 42–14A). Meanwhile, jejunal continuity is re-established by end-to-end anastomosis as described in the preceding section.

The jejunal autograft, with the artery and vein carefully occluded by noncrushing bulldog clamps, is moved to the cervical incision. The segment is placed in the cervical esophageal bed in an isoperistaltic fashion. The proximal jejunal anastomosis is performed first to the cervical esophagus or hypopharynx with two layers of inverting interrupted 4-0 silk as described for esophagogastrostomy (see Fig. 42–14D). This provides enough fixation and stability to allow performance of the two microvascular anastomoses without concern for tension or torsion. A suitable neck artery (the inferior thyroid, transverse cervical, or common carotid artery itself) is used for the vascular anastomosis, which is performed with 10-0 nylon monofilament sutures under the operating microscope (see Fig. 42–14E). The microvascular bulldog clamps are released, and the jejunal autograft is allowed to perfuse. A two-layer anastomosis of the distal jejunum to the esophagus is then completed, again using inverting, interrupted fine silk sutures (see Fig. 42–14F). Finally, venous anastomosis to the facial vein, the middle thyroid vein, or one of the jugular veins is carried out.

The cervical incision is usually closed without drainage. A thermistor probe has been used as a method of monitoring viability of the jejunal graft. Alternatively, a Silastic "window" can be used for direct observation of the jejunal segment for 24 to 48 hours and then primarily closed once viability is ascertained (see Fig. 42–14G). It is preferred that a nasogastric tube not be allowed to pass through the cervical jejunum; gastric drainage can be accomplished with a gastrostomy tube.

SHORT-SEGMENT COLON INTERPOSITION

Short-segment colon interposition is an alternative to jejunal interposition of the distal esophagus. Preparation of the patient and colon is as described for long-segment colon interposition. Because extensive length is not required, more options exist, and arteriography is not as critical. The most popular segment of colon to use for distal esophageal replacement is an isoperistaltic segment of the distal transverse colon or the descending left colon based on the ascending branch of the left colic artery.

The operation is usually performed through an extended left thoracoabdominal incision to allow mobilization of the colon segment, resection of the diseased distal esophagus, and anastomosis of the colon segment to the distal esophagus and posterior wall of the stomach. Left colon segments are based on the ascending branch of the left colic artery. Transverse colon segments are based on the middle colic artery. The colon segment should be isoperistaltic. In our experience, the left colon was used more commonly ($n = 19$) than the transverse colon ($n = 3$).[6] The length of colon segment needed is mobilized, and the vascular pedicle is identified but not skeletonized. The bowel is divided with staplers and the colon segment placed in a posterior mediastinal position while avoiding tension or torsion of the vascular pedicle. The proximal anastomosis is end to end with a two-layered closure of interrupted 4-0 silk. The distal anastomosis is end to side, most commonly to the posterior gastric wall. This allows the colon to be positioned in a more direct, straight path than an anastomosis to the anterior gastric wall does. At least 12 cm of colon is desirable to prevent reflux. A nasogastric tube through the colonic segment is used initially, and gastrostomy or jejunostomy is performed when indicated. The hiatus is carefully tacked to the colon to prevent herniation of abdominal contents. A gastric drainage procedure is always performed.

Results of Short-Segment Colon and Jejunal Interposition

Jurkiewicz and Paletta recounted their experience with 130 free jejunal interpositions and reported a graft sur-

Table 42–5	Indications for Short-Segment Intestinal Interposition of the Distal Esophagus

Diagnosis	No. of Patients
Gastroesophageal reflux disease	34
Failed antireflux repair	21
Nondilatable stricture	9
Complication of treatment of chalasia	2
Complication of myotomy for motility disorder	1
Complication of intrathoracic esophagogastrostomy	1
Esophageal moniliasis with stricture	2
Barrett's esophagus with carcinoma in situ	2
Leak from esophagotomy	1
Carcinoma of the esophagus	1
Leiomyosarcoma of the esophagus	1

From Gaissert HA, Mathisen DJ, Grillo HC, et al: Short segment intestinal interposition of the distal esophagus. J Thorac Cardiovasc Surg 106:860, 1993.

Table 42–6	Major Complications After Intestinal Interposition

Complication	No. of Patients
Colon	
Pneumonia/acute respiratory distress syndrome	4*
Graft perforation	1
Colon perforation, subphrenic abscess	1
Chylothorax	1
Pulmonary edema	1
Pulmonary embolus	1
Deep vein thrombosis	1
Jejunum	
Pneumonia	3
Graft necrosis	1*
Gastric perforation	1
Paraparesis, aortoenteric erosion	1
Transient recurrent nerve injury	1
Myocardial infarction	1*

*Cause of operative mortality.
From Gaissert HA, Mathisen DJ, Grillo HC, et al: Short segment intestinal interposition of the distal esophagus. J Thorac Cardiovasc Surg 106:860, 1993.

vival rate of 92%.[30] The operative mortality rate was 5%. The main cause of graft failure is often arterial or venous insufficiency, and if graft failure does occurs, a second attempt with another free jejunal graft should be made, with success rates of 50% to 75% being attained. A pharyngocutaneous fistula is a common postoperative complication that was reported in 33 of 101 patients in Jurkiewicz and Paletta's series. Twenty-four of these fistulas closed spontaneously; the others were managed by a second graft or simple drainage.

Gaissert and associates published our results with jejunal (19 patients) and short-segment colon (22 patients) interposition of the distal esophagus.[31] Indications for intestinal interposition are listed in Table 42–5. Multiple previous operations were common and had occurred in more than 75% of patients. Major complications developed in 45% of patients (10 of 22) after colon interposition, and the hospital mortality rate was 4.5% (Table 42–6). Major complications after jejunal interposition occurred in 31% of patients, and the hospital mortality rate was 10.9%. Late functional results in 32 patients with a mean follow-up of 87 months were excellent in 26, fair in 5, and poor in 1.

Intestinal interposition is a technically demanding procedure that requires strict attention to detail to avoid catastrophic complications and ensure the greatest chance for success.

REFERENCES

1. Czerny V: Neue Operationen. Zbl Chir 4:443, 1877.
2. Torek F: The first successful case of resection of the thoracic portion of the esophagus for carcinoma. Surg Gynecol Obstet 16:614, 1913.
3. Oshawa T: Surgery of the esophagus. Arch Jpn Surg 10:605, 1933.
4. Sweet RH, Churchill ED: Transthoracic resection of tumors of the esophagus and stomach. Ann Surg 116:566, 1942.
5. Sweet RH: Thoracic Surgery, 2nd ed. Philadelphia, WB Saunders, 1954, p 309.
6. Lewis IL: The surgical treatment of carcinoma of the oesophagus. With special reference to a new operation for growths of the middle third. Br J Surg 34:18, 1946.
7. Mahoney EB, Sherman CD Jr: Total esophagoplasty using intrathoracic right colon. Surgery 35:937, 1954.
8. Belsey R: Reconstruction of the esophagus with left colon. J Thorac Cardiovasc Surg 49:33, 1965.
9. Brain RHF: The place of jejunal transplantation in the treatment of simple strictures of the esophagus. Ann R Coll Surg Engl 40:100, 1967.
10. Muller JM, Erasmi H, Stelzner M, et al: Surgical therapy of oesophageal carcinoma. Br J Surg 77:845, 1990.
11. Mathisen DJ, Grillo HC, Wilkins EW Jr, et al: Transthoracic esophagectomy: A safe approach to carcinoma of the esophagus. Ann Thorac Surg 45:137, 1988.
12. McKeown KC: Total three-stage oesophagectomy for cancer of the oesophagus. Br J Surg 63:259, 1976.
13. Orringer MB, Orringer JS: Esophagectomy without thoracotomy: A dangerous operation? J Thorac Cardiovasc Surg 85:72, 1983.
14. Luketich JD, Alvelo-Rivera M, Buenaventura PO, et al: Minimally invasive esophagectomy: Outcomes in 222 patients. Ann Surg 238:486, 2003.
15. Luketich JD, Nguyen NT, Schauer PR: Laparoscopic transhiatal esophagectomy for Barrett's esophagus with high-grade dysplasia. JSLS 2:75, 1998.
16. Adams WE, Phemister DB: Carcinoma of lower thoracic esophagus: Report of successful resection and esophagogastrostomy. J Thorac Surg 7:621, 1938.
17. Sonneland J, Anson BJ, Beaton LE: Surgical anatomy of the arterial supply to the colon from the superior mesenteric artery based upon a study of 600 specimens. Surg Gynecol Obstet 106:385, 1958.
18. Akiyama H: Surgery for carcinoma of the esophagus. Curr Probl Surg 17:56, 1980.
19. Huang GJ, Zhang DC, Zhang DW: A comparative study of resection of carcinoma of the esophagus with and without pyloroplasty. In DeMeester TR, Skinner DB (eds): Esophageal Disorders: Pathophysiology and Therapy. New York, Raven Press, 1985, p 383.
20. Ong GB: The Kirschner operation—a forgotten procedure. Br J Surg 60:221, 1973.
21. Ngan SYK, Wong J: Lengths of different routes for oesophageal replacement. J Thorac Cardiovasc Surg 91:790, 1986.
22. Wilkins EW Jr: Esophageal anastomotic techniques: The esophagogastric anastomosis. In Wu Y, Peters R (eds): International Practice in Cardiothoracic Surgery. Beijing, Science Press, 1985, p 590.
23. Orringer MB, Marshall B, Iannettoni MD: Transhiatal esophagectomy for treatment of benign and malignant esophageal disease. World J Surg 25:196, 2001.
24. Wain JC: Long segment colon interposition. Semin Thorac Cardiovasc Surg 4:336, 1992.
25. Postlethwait RW: Surgery of the Esophagus, 2nd ed. Norwalk, CT, Appleton-Century-Crofts, 1986, p 505.
26. Wain JC, Wright CD, Kuo EY, et al: Long-segment colon interposition for acquired esophageal disease. Ann Thorac Surg 67:313, 1999.
27. Jeyasingham K, Lerut T, Belsey RH: Functional and mechanical sequelae of colon interposition for benign oesophageal disease. Eur J Cardiothorac Surg 15:327, 1999.
28. Ring WS, Varco RL, L'Heureux PR, et al: Esophageal replacement with jejunum in children: An 18 to 33 year follow-up. J Thorac Cardiovasc Surg 83:918, 1982.
29. Payne WS, Fisher J: Esophageal reconstruction: Free jejunal transfer or circulatory augmentation of pedicled interpositions using microvascular surgery. In Delarue NC, Wilkins EW Jr, Wong J (eds): International Trends in General Thoracic Surgery, vol IV, Esophageal Cancer. St Louis, CV Mosby, 1988.
30. Jurkiewicz MJ, Paletta CEL: Free jejunal graft. In Current Therapy in Cardiothoracic Surgery. Philadelphia, BC Decker, 1989, p 206.
31. Gaissert HA, Mathisen DJ, Grillo HC, et al: Short segment intestinal interposition of the distal esophagus. J Thorac Cardiovasc Surg 106:860, 1993.

43

Complications of Esophageal Surgery

Andrew C. Chang ▪ Mark B. Orringer

ANATOMIC AND PHYSIOLOGIC CONSIDERATIONS

Many of the complications of esophageal surgery are directly related to specific features of esophageal anatomy and physiology. Detailed knowledge and thorough understanding of these characteristics by the surgeon are essential to identify potential pitfalls of esophageal surgery and avert complications before they occur. When performing esophagoscopy, for example, one must bear in mind the three naturally occurring sites of esophageal narrowing: the upper esophageal introitus, or the cricopharyngeal sphincter; the level of the aortic arch and left main stem bronchus; and the esophagogastric junction (Fig. 43–1). The rigid esophagoscope must be manipulated appropriately through these points of narrowing to minimize the risk for injury during esophagoscopy. One distinct feature of esophageal anatomy is its unusually fatty submucosa, which allows greater mobility of the overlying squamous mucosa. When performing an esophageal anastomosis manually, meticulous technique is essential to ensure such that every suture transfixes the mucosal edge, which at times may retract more than 1 cm from the cut esophageal margin (Fig. 43–2). The esophagus is also unique in the gastrointestinal tract because it lacks a serosal layer. The soft and often tenuous muscle holds sutures poorly and cannot be relied on to maintain a fundoplication, for example, unless the associated submucosa is transfixed by the esophageal stitch.

The esophagus is nourished by four to six paired aortic esophageal arteries, as well as collateral circulation from the inferior thyroid, intercostal and bronchial, inferior phrenic, and left gastric arteries. The segmental "poor" blood supply of the esophagus has frequently been incriminated as the cause of anastomotic disruption. However, the submucosal collateral circulation of the esophagus is extensive, and even after the cardia has been divided and the intrathoracic esophagus mobilized completely out of the chest, the distal end of the esophagus maintains good arterial bleeding as long as the inferior thyroid arteries remain intact. Poor technique, not poor blood supply, is the more likely explanation for the complication of esophageal anastomotic disruption. Finally, the parasympathetic innervation of the esophagus is supplied by the vagus nerves, and the recurrent laryngeal nerve supplies the upper portion of the esophagus. Recurrent laryngeal nerve injury during esophageal surgery may result in one of the most devastating complications, cricopharyngeal muscle dysfunction with subsequent incapacitating cervical dysphagia and aspiration pneumonia.[1] Similarly, injury to the vagal nerve trunks during distal esophageal operations may produce neurogenic dysphagia or gastric atony and pylorospasm, which are very troublesome complications after esophageal surgery.

Physiologic considerations influence other complications of surgery on the esophagus. The pathophysiology of gastroesophageal reflux and secondary reflux esophagitis directly influences the results of antireflux surgery and hence the complication of recurrent reflux. For example, it has been demonstrated that the incidence of recurrent reflux in patients undergoing the standard Belsey Mark IV transthoracic hiatal hernia repair in the presence of esophagitis or stricture is between 25% and 75%.[2,3] In patients with intramural inflammation and esophageal shortening secondary to reflux esophagitis, the esophageal sutures of the Belsey repair may not be reliable, and tension on the repair to reduce the requisite 3 to 5 cm of distal esophagus below the diaphragm sets the stage for recurrence of the hernia (Fig. 43–3). These same considerations apply to the Nissen fundoplication and the Hill posterior gastropexy, which also aim to restore an intra-abdominal segment of distal esophagus and require esophageal or periesophageal sutures (Fig. 43–4). To avert the complication of disruption of the repair as a consequence of (1) the

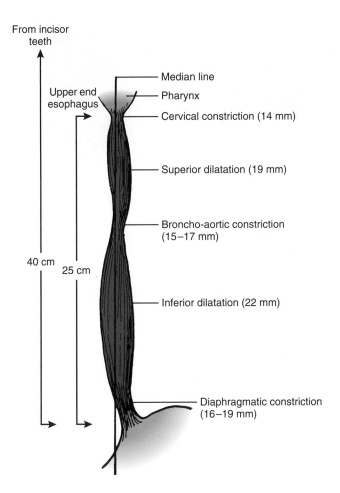

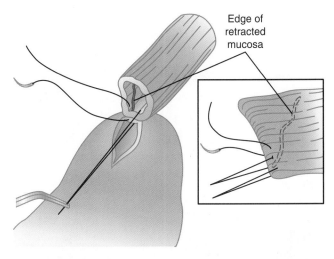

Figure 43–2. Failure of an esophageal anastomotic suture to transfix the mucosa is a function of the fatty submucosa, which permits mobility of the overlying mucosa and allows it to retract. The mucosa must be identified and deliberately transfixed with each suture placed to achieve mucosal apposition and avoid an anastomotic leak. (From Orringer MB: Complications of esophageal surgery and trauma. In Greenfield LJ [ed]: Complications in Surgery and Trauma, 2nd ed. Philadelphia, JB Lippincott, 1990, p 303.)

Figure 43–1. Normal esophageal constrictions, dilatations, and measurements. (From Shackelford RT [ed]: Surgery of the Alimentary Tract, vol 1, 2nd ed. Philadelphia, WB Saunders, 1978.)

need to suture an inflamed esophagus and (2) tension on the repair, the esophagus-lengthening Collis gastroplasty can be combined with fundoplication.[4-6] The gastroplasty tube functions as a new distal esophagus and provides healthy, resilient tissue (i.e., the gastric wall) around which to perform the fundoplication. Furthermore, the additional "esophageal length" provided by the gastroplasty tube reduces tension on the repair. The presence of reflux esophagitis and a peptic stricture also complicates an antireflux procedure if the stricture is perforated during attempted dilation.

An intrathoracic esophagogastric anastomotic leak, perhaps the most dreaded complication of esophageal surgery, in part owes its morbidity to associated gastroesophageal reflux. An intrathoracic esophagogastric anastomosis is almost invariably associated with the development of reflux esophagitis, in contrast to a cervical esophagogastric anastomosis, which is rarely associated with clinically significant reflux. Although it has been argued that with appropriate attention to detail, an intrathoracic esophagogastric anastomosis can be performed reliably and with an exceedingly low morbidity

rate,[7] the potential for an anastomotic leak and secondary mediastinitis cannot be eliminated totally, and this fact perhaps more than anything else has influenced our current "defensive posture" that the best esophagogastric anastomosis is a cervical anastomosis because the consequence of a leak is a salivary fistula and not life-threatening mediastinitis and sepsis.

Gastroesophageal reflux after esophageal resection and esophagogastric anastomosis may be responsible for life-threatening aspiration of gastric contents into the tracheobronchial tree in the early postoperative period. For this reason, initial decompression of the intrathoracic stomach with a nasogastric tube and placement of the patient in a 45-degree head-up position are important. Similarly, because of the potential for regurgitation and aspiration after eating, patients who have a fresh esophagogastric anastomosis should not be permitted to undergo postural drainage as part of their postoperative pulmonary physiotherapy within 1 to 2 hours of mealtime.

The potential pulmonary complications, primarily aspiration pneumonia, resulting from esophageal obstruction secondary to a variety of causes cannot be overestimated. Particularly in a patient with megaesophagus as a result of advanced achalasia, the risk for massive regurgitation and aspiration on induction of general anesthesia is enormous. Awareness of this possibility dictates the need for esophageal decompression and emptying by nasogastric tube in these patients before rapid-sequence induction of general anesthesia and endotracheal intubation.

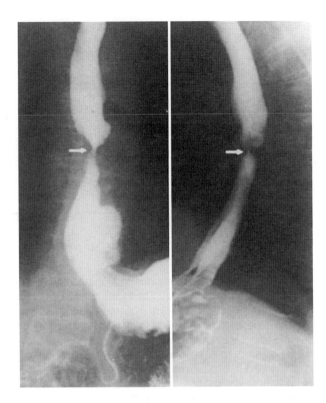

Figure 43–3. Posteroanterior *(left)* and lateral *(right)* views from a barium swallow examination showing a sliding hiatal hernia with a midesophageal stricture *(arrow)* at the squamocolumnar junction in a patient with Barrett's esophagus. Standard antireflux operations (Hill, Belsey, or Nissen) require reduction below the diaphragm of not only the esophagogastric junction but also the distal 3 to 5 cm of esophagus. The esophageal shortening and periesophageal fibrosis secondary to reflux esophagitis in this patient prevented a tension-free standard repair.

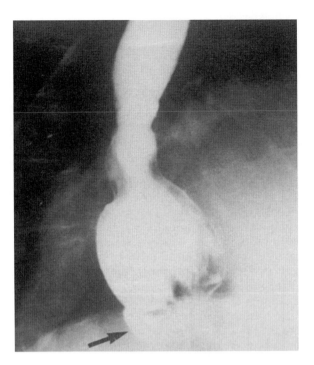

Figure 43–4. Slipped Nissen fundoplication in a patient who was operated on for reflux complicated by a short esophagus and stricture. Tension on the repair resulted in subsequent disruption of it. The proximal part of the stomach has herniated through the fundoplication *(arrow)* and is seen above the level of the diaphragm.

ESOPHAGEAL PERFORATION

Perforation of the thoracic esophagus, with resultant mediastinitis, poses a devastating threat. Regardless of the cause of perforation (Box 43–1), delay in recognition and definitive management increases concomitant mortality and morbidity. Repair of an acute esophageal tear in an otherwise normal esophagus within 6 to 8 hours carries a risk of morbidity that is essentially the same as that imposed by elective esophagotomy and primary esophageal closure. If operative intervention is delayed beyond this early period, local inflammation greatly jeopardizes primary healing of the esophageal tear and mortality rises dramatically.[8-10]

Esophageal instrumentation accounts for the large majority of iatrogenic perforations, with the cricopharyngeal area most commonly injured (Fig. 43–5). Perforation of the mid and distal esophageal segments is most likely to occur after biopsy or dilatation. Spontaneous perforation usually occurs after straining (Boerhaave's syndrome), with rupture involving the left posterior aspect of the distal esophagus.[11]

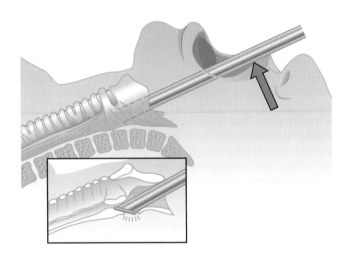

Figure 43–5. Mechanism of endoscopic cervical esophageal perforation. In performing rigid esophagoscopy, it is essential that a gentle, steady lifting force *(arrow)* be exerted to displace the larynx and cricoid cartilage forward. Failure to overcome the natural pull of the upper esophageal sphincter against the cricoid cartilage results in a typical posterior perforation *(inset)* (From Orringer MB: Complications of esophageal surgery and trauma. In Greenfield LJ [ed]: Complications in Surgery and Trauma, 2nd ed. Philadelphia, JB Lippincott, 1990, p 309.)

Box 43–1   Causes of Esophageal Perforation

Instrumental

Endoscopy
    Direct injury
    Injury occurring during removal of a foreign
      body

Dilatation

Intubation (esophageal, endotracheal)

Noninstrumental

Barogenic trauma
    Postemetic
    Blunt chest or abdominal trauma
    Other (e.g., labor, convulsion, defecation)

Penetrating neck, chest, or abdominal trauma

Postoperative
    Anastomotic disruption
    Devascularization after pulmonary resection,
      vagotomy, or repair of hiatal hernia

Injury after ingestion of a caustic agent

Erosion by adjacent infection with a resultant
    fistula involving the tracheobronchial tree,
    pericardium, pleural cavity, or aorta

Pathologic
    Severe reflux esophagitis
    Candidal, herpetic, and opportunistic
      infection

Diagnosis

Patients with esophageal perforation typically have pain directly referred from the site of injury. The presence of mediastinal air or hydropneumothorax on a chest radiograph in a patient suspected of having a perforation is confirmatory. However, a normal chest radiograph does not exclude the possibility of esophageal perforation. Not every esophageal tear is a full-thickness disruption. For example, pneumatic dilatation of the esophagus for achalasia may result in a tear of the distal esophageal mucosa and submucosa. Air insufflation through a flexible esophagoscope may result in mediastinal, cervical, or subcutaneous air, thereby exaggerating the extent of injury. After esophagoscopy or an esophageal operation, postoperative pain or fever should be considered to be caused by esophageal perforation until proved otherwise. Contrast esophagography should be performed immediately to limit any further delay in establishing proper drainage or definitive repair, or both. Water-soluble contrast esophagography, followed by dilute barium, best identifies the site of perforation (Fig. 43–6) and establishes whether the perforation is communicating with either the pleural or peritoneal cavities or is confined to the mediastinum.

Treatment

Once the diagnosis of esophageal perforation is established, oral intake by the patient should cease. Aggressive intravenous fluid resuscitation, facilitated by using either a central venous pressure catheter or a pulmonary artery catheter, is indicated if there is hypovolemia associated with an intrathoracic perforation. Broad-spectrum antibiotic coverage is initiated. The presence of carious teeth increases the risk for morbidity in patients with esophageal injury because of the virulence of swallowed oral bacteria. Thus, oral hygiene should not be neglected in a patient with an esophageal perforation.

There is controversy about the best method of treatment of patients with esophageal perforations. Nonoperative "conservative" therapy is successful in some patients with esophageal perforation, primarily those with preexisting periesophageal and mediastinal fibrosis that contains the injury. Thus, for an esophageal disruption in which contrast material extends only a few millimeters from the esophageal lumen and the patient is doing well clinically, antibiotic therapy, chest tube drainage as indicated, and observation may suffice.[12-14] More frequently, however, a successful outcome after esophageal perforation requires surgical intervention (Fig. 43–7).

Perforation of the cervical and upper thoracic esophagus is approached through an oblique cervical incision that parallels the anterior border of the left sternocleidomastoid muscle (Fig. 43–8). The sternocleidomastoid muscle and carotid sheath are retracted laterally and the trachea and thyroid gland medially. If the perforation can be identified, it is closed with absorbable polyglycolic acid sutures. If the injury cannot be visualized adequately for repair, the retroesophageal prevertebral space is dissected bluntly with the finger and the superior mediastinum is drained with two 1-inch Penrose drains brought out through the neck wound. Esophageal perforations at the level of the tracheal bifurcation can generally be treated successfully with such a cervical approach. Midthoracic esophageal perforations must be approached through a right thoracotomy, and those of the distal third of the esophagus are approached through a left thoracotomy.

Traditional surgical dogma teaches that esophageal perforations beyond 6 to 12 hours in duration are virtually impossible to repair primarily because the pouting inflamed mucosa at the edge of the tear holds sutures poorly. Isolated reports, however, have emphasized that even after a marked delay in repair, successful closure of the esophageal injury may be possible.[8,15] Several groups have found that the majority of esophageal tears can in fact be repaired successfully with meticulous surgical technique that includes identification of adjacent submucosa by dissecting away the overlying muscle, definition of the limits of the mucosal tear (Fig. 43–9), reapproximation of the disrupted mucosa and submucosa with a surgical stapler (Auto Suture Endo GIA II Stapler, U.S. Surgical Corporation, Auto Suture Company Division, Norwalk, CT),[16] and reapproximation of the muscle over the staple suture line (Fig. 43–10). Limited esophagomyotomy performed 180

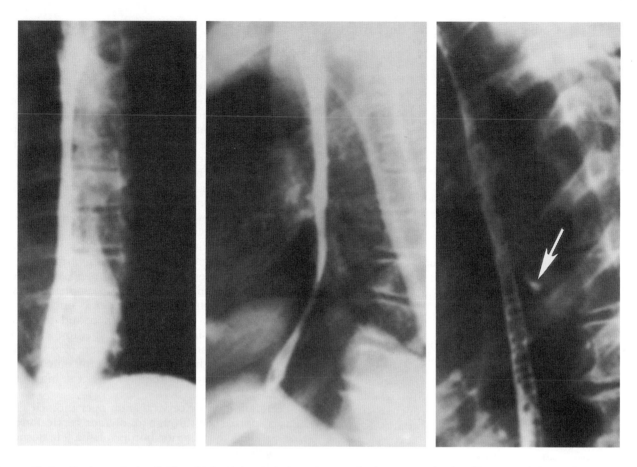

Figure 43–6.   Posteroanterior *(left)* and lateral *(center)* views from a diatrizoate meglumine (Gastrografin) esophagogram in a patient with acute caustic injury that was incorrectly dilated prematurely within 10 days of caustic ingestion. There was still acute inflammation in this esophagus, and the patient had fever and chest pain after dilation. Despite the negative Gastrografin swallow, dilute barium was administered *(right),* and a perforation *(arrow)* of the midesophagus was demonstrated. (From Orringer MB: Complications of esophageal surgery and trauma. In Greenfield LJ [ed]: Complications in Surgery and Trauma, 2nd ed. Philadelphia, JB Lippincott, 1990, p 312.)

degrees opposite the site of injury may permit enough advancement of adjacent esophageal wall for adequate repair of the perforation.[17] In patients with chronic mediastinitis and pleural reaction, the adjacent mediastinal pleura is thickened and provides an excellent flap with which to reinforce the esophageal suture line. Alternatively, if insufficient parietal pleural thickening is available to provide adequate support for the suture line, reinforcement with a pedicled intercostal muscle flap, omentum, pericardium, visceral pleura, or diaphragm can be carried out.[18,19] The mediastinal pleura must be opened from the apex of the chest to the diaphragm to permit wide drainage of the mediastinum. After copious irrigation of the mediastinum and pleural cavity and decortication of any acute fibrinous exudate that may have formed over the lung, a large-bore chest tube is left near the esophageal suture line so that if disruption occurs, the result will be an esophagopleural cutaneous fistula.

When treating an esophageal perforation, associated esophageal disease cannot be ignored. Thus, a perforation proximal to a carcinoma or a caustic or reflux stricture may necessitate emergency esophagectomy with either primary or delayed esophageal reconstruction. In

patients with an esophageal perforation and a long-standing history of reflux stricture, postoperative dysphagia requiring repeated esophageal dilatation is more likely to develop. In this subset of patients, consideration should be given to primary esophagectomy if their physiologic status at the time of surgery permits.[20] Alternatively, if it is possible to dilate a benign stricture intraoperatively to relieve the distal obstruction, closure of a proximal esophageal perforation may be successful. A subsequent disruption of the esophageal closure may still eventually heal if dilatation of the associated stricture is continued. A perforated pulsion diverticulum of the esophagus may be resected within several hours of the injury. The associated obstruction must be dealt with and the esophageal neuromotor dysfunction responsible for formation of the pouch relieved by performing a concomitant esophagomyotomy.

PROCEDURAL COMPLICATIONS

Esophagoscopy

Technologic advances in the development of flexible fiberoptic instruments have greatly facilitated the

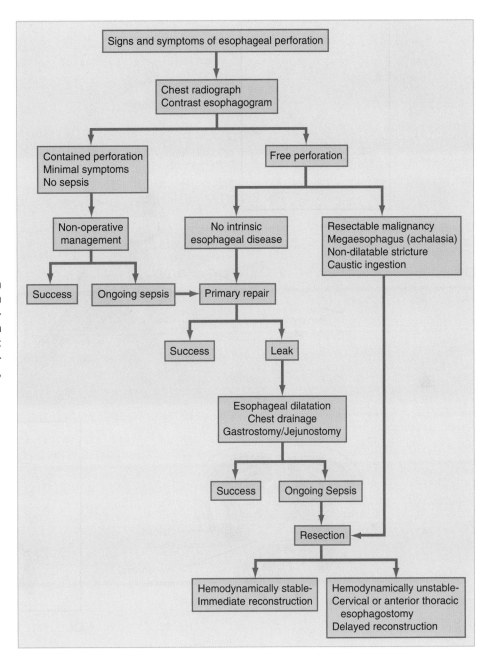

Figure 43–7. Treatment algorithm for esophageal perforation. (From Chang AC, Iannettoni MD: Complications of esophageal surgery. In Mulholland MW, Doherty GA [eds]: Complications in Surgery. Philadelphia, Lippincott Williams & Wilkins, 2006.)

performance of esophagogastroscopy, particularly with the advent of endoscopic ultrasound. Furthermore, there has been a concomitant increase in the number of these studies being performed on an outpatient basis. The consequences of esophageal disruption, however, have not changed. Perforation occurs in 0.8% of all patients during flexible upper endoscopy, with rates as high as 4% in patients undergoing esophageal dilatation.[21] Perforation after rigid esophagoscopy can occur in as many as 5% of patients after therapeutic procedures (e.g., biopsy, dilatation, or removal of a foreign body) and in up to 1.5% of patients after rigid esophagoscopy alone.[22] To avoid perforation during esophagoscopy, certain basic principles must be acknowledged:

1. Adequate preoperative and intraoperative sedation and anesthesia are mandatory. In some cases, general anesthesia is the only means of creating acceptable conditions for performing esophagoscopy for both the patient and the surgeon.
2. Esophagoscopy should not be carried out unless a barium esophagogram has been performed and reviewed by the endoscopist. The barium swallow provides information about preexisting disease and its expected location (Fig. 43–11). For example, a Zenker diverticulum identified on a contrast esophagogram should be expected to be encountered at the level of the upper esophageal sphincter, approximately 15 cm from the upper

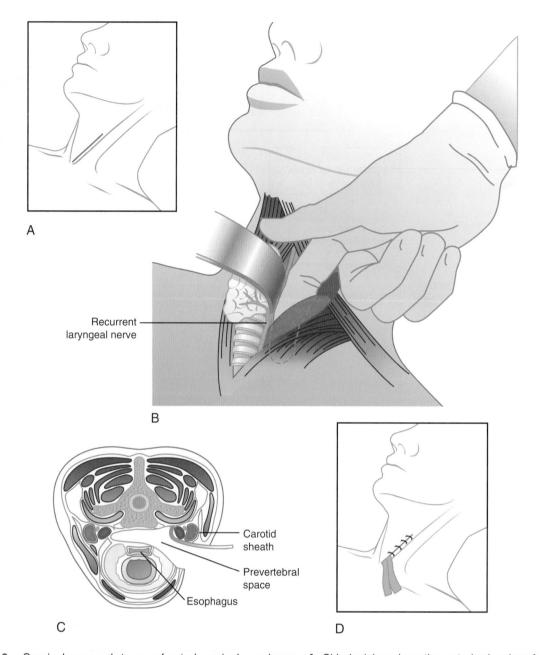

A

Recurrent
laryngeal nerve

B

Carotid
sheath

Prevertebral
space

Esophagus

C

D

Figure 43–8.   Surgical approach to a perforated cervical esophagus. **A,** Skin incision along the anterior border of the left sternocleidomastoid muscle from the level of the cricoid cartilage to the sternal notch. **B,** Blunt dissection into the superior mediastinum along the prevertebral fascia medial to the sternocleidomastoid muscle and carotid sheath. Injury to the recurrent laryngeal nerve in the tracheoesophageal groove must be avoided. **C,** Schematic view of the prevertebral space to be drained. **D,** Placement of two 1-inch rubber drains to allow establishment of an esophagocutaneous fistula. (From Orringer MB: The mediastinum. In Nora PF [ed]: Nora's Operative Surgery, 3rd ed. Philadelphia, WB Saunders, 1990, p 374.)

incisors. A midesophageal carcinoma at the level of the tracheal bifurcation is encountered approximately 25 cm from the upper incisors. An epiphrenic diverticulum is encountered before the esophagoscope reaches the esophagogastric junction at a point 40 cm from the upper incisors. Perforation of a cervical esophageal diverticulum or a midesophageal stricture cannot be justified because the endoscopist was unaware of these lesions as a result of neither obtaining nor personally reviewing a barium swallow examination beforehand.

3. Failure to introduce the rigid esophagoscope properly through the upper esophageal sphincter may result in a perforation. The cricopharyngeus muscle originates from the cricoid cartilage, and the natural "pull" of this muscle against the cartilage will result in a posterior perforation unless the larynx is "lifted" anteriorly as the esophagoscope is advanced.

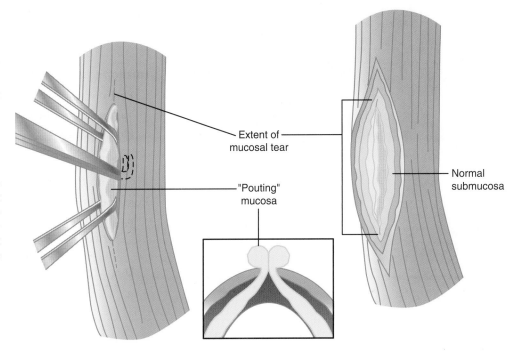

Figure 43–9. Technique of primary repair of an esophageal perforation. Mucosa at the site of the tear *(inset)* is grasped with Allis clamps **(A),** and the adjacent esophageal muscle is mobilized around the entire tear until 1 cm of normal submucosa is exposed around the defect **(B).** (From Whyte RI, Iannettoni MD, Orringer MB: Intrathoracic perforation: The merit of primary repair. J Thorac Cardiovasc Surg 109:140, 1995.)

Extent of mucosal tear

Normal submucosa

"Pouting" mucosa

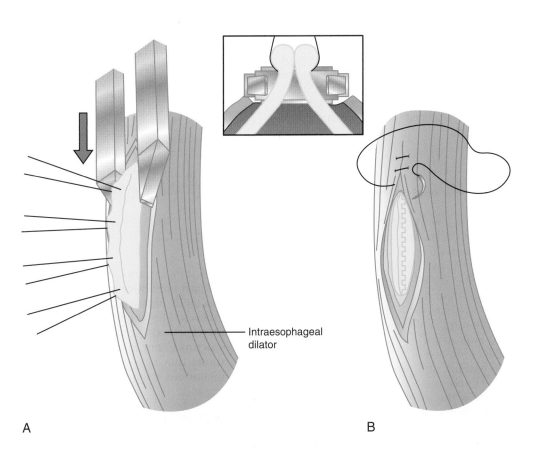

Intraesophageal dilator

A   B

Figure 43–10. Technique of primary repair of an esophageal perforation (continuation of Fig. 43-9). Traction sutures placed along the inflamed mucosal edge of the tear elevate the submucosa so that an Endo GIA II cartridge (3.5-mm staples) can be applied and deployed. The esophageal lumen is maintained by passage of an intraesophageal dilator (**A** and *inset*). The staple line is covered by approximating the adjacent muscle with running absorbable suture (**B**). (From Whyte RI, Iannettoni MD, Orringer MB: Intrathoracic perforation: The merit of primary repair. J Thorac Cardiovasc Surg, 109:140, 1995.)

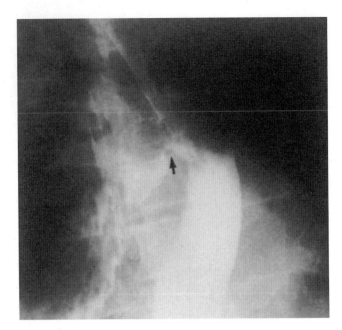

Figure 43–11. Gastrografin swallow showing a midesophageal perforation *(arrow)* after rigid esophagoscopy in a patient who had dysphagia. An outside "normal" barium swallow report had been accepted, and esophagoscopy was performed without the endoscopist seeing the contrast study. In this patient, a large subcarinal mass of lymph nodes secondary to sarcoidosis was displacing the esophagus to the left, as is evident in this posteroanterior view. Without knowledge of this abnormal course of the esophagus in this patient, the esophagoscope was advanced, and a perforation occurred. The surgeon performing esophagoscopy is responsible for seeing the barium swallow examination in the patient before passing the esophagoscope.

4. The esophagoscope should not be advanced unless the lumen is visible.
5. As the esophagoscope is advanced, adjustment must be made for the natural course of the esophagus. Because the distal esophagus courses anteriorly and to the left as it joins the stomach, the instrument must be angled toward the right side of the patient's mouth and the occiput of the head lowered as the esophagoscope is advanced into the distal end of the esophagus, particularly when performing rigid endoscopy.
6. The initial dilatation of a tight esophageal stricture is frequently painful, and adequate sedation and anesthesia are important to minimize patient discomfort and allow the surgeon to concentrate on the visual field. When a rigid esophagoscope is used for this initial evaluation, flexible gum-tipped Jackson bougies are inserted through the stricture under direct vision, and the pliability and extent of the stenosis are assessed. With a mild "soft" stenosis, dilatation by advancing the esophagoscope through the stenosis might be possible. With firmer, high-grade strictures, it is safer to pass progressively larger dilators through the narrowing.

Box 43–2 Complications of Hiatal Herniorrhaphy

Intraoperative Complications

Perforation

Vagus nerve injury

Hemorrhage
　Splenic laceration
　Short gastric vessel

Postoperative Complications

Perforation
　Stricture
　Suture placement
Dysphagia
　Mechanical
　　Tight hiatal closure
　　Excessive fundoplication
　　Inadequate gastroplasty
　Edema
　Gastric atony, pylorospasm
Early anatomic recurrence
　Crural repair disruption
Functional
　Postvagotomy diarrhea
　Ileus
Cardiac tamponade
Chylothorax
Pleural effusion
Incisional pain

Modified from Patel HJ, Tan BT, Yee J, et al: A twenty-five year experience with open primary transthoracic repair of paraesophageal hiatal hernia. J Thorac Cardiovasc Surg 127:843, 2004.

This can be accomplished by using the Savary-Gilliard guidewire and dilating system, under fluoroscopic guidance, or Maloney tapered esophageal dilators. The latter instruments are our preference for repeated outpatient dilatations of esophageal strictures; they do not require the sedation or anesthesia that is necessary when endoscopic balloon dilatations are performed.

Hiatal Hernia Repair

Hiatal herniorrhaphy, though conceptually quite simple, can result in a number of serious complications (Box 43–2). Acute esophageal perforation can occur when concomitant esophagoscopy is performed during an antireflux operation or when a distal esophageal stricture is disrupted during intraoperative dilatation. A delayed perforation, usually within 1 week of surgery, may occur

Figure 43–12. A, Barium swallow examination in a 49-year-old man who was treated for a gunshot wound in the esophagus and trachea 23 years earlier. At that operation, the tracheal and esophageal holes were débrided and repaired, and the esophagus was incorrectly wrapped circumferentially with a mobilized intercostal muscle pedicle. Subsequent regeneration of cartilage from the perichondrium of the intercostal pedicle resulted in severe dysphagia and the high-grade upper esophageal stenosis with proximal esophageal dilation that is shown. **B,** Postoperative barium swallow after a repeat right thoracotomy and partial resection of the encircling cartilaginous and muscle ring. The lumen was greatly improved, and the dysphagia was relieved.

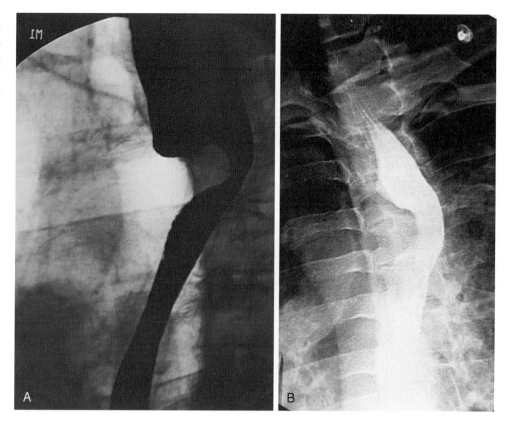

when esophageal sutures placed too deeply during the repair result in local mural necrosis.

Acute esophageal tears recognized intraoperatively should be approached transthoracically and repaired and the esophageal suture line reinforced either with the fundoplication if the tear is in the distal esophagus or with pedicled anterior mediastinal fat or a pedicled intercostal muscle flap if the tear is higher. When an intercostal muscle pedicle is used to reinforce an esophageal suture line, it should be sutured to the esophagus as an onlay patch, not placed circumferentially around the esophagus; otherwise, regeneration of bone or cartilage from the perichondrium or periosteum mobilized with the flap may result in a late obstructing ring around the esophagus (Fig. 43–12). When a reflux stricture is perforated during attempted dilation at the time of a planned antireflux operation, unless the involved tissues are relatively healthy and amenable to repair, resectional therapy is generally a better option. Although most reflux strictures can be dilated and many regress after an antireflux procedure has been carried out, disruption of a stricture during attempted dilation is one of the definitions of an "undilatable" stricture that justifies esophageal resection. Our preference in this situation is to proceed with transthoracic esophagectomy and then reposition the patient supine and carry out a cervical esophagogastric anastomosis. Several additional options for the treatment of a disrupted distal stricture are available. Unfortunately, none is without its associated morbidity. The Thal fundic patch esophagoplasty uses adjacent gastric fundus to "patch" the opened narrowed esophagus. This procedure not only relies on healing of

the opened, inflamed distal esophagus to which the stomach is sutured but also requires the addition of an intrathoracic fundoplication (Thal-Woodward procedure) to control gastroesophageal reflux, in effect, creating an iatrogenic paraesophageal hiatal hernia. The high incidence of suture line disruption and mechanical complications associated with this operation condemns its use. For the same reason, we oppose the use of an intrathoracic fundoplication (without a Thal procedure) to control reflux (Fig. 43–13). The complications of such an approach outweigh its benefits.

Gastric ulceration may complicate 3% to 10% of fundoplications and may occur with both supradiaphragmatic fundic wraps and intra-abdominal fundoplications. In the former, one is dealing with a complication of an iatrogenic paraesophageal hiatal hernia, and operative repair is generally indicated. In the latter, ulceration may be due to relative ischemia in the wrap, and treatment with H_2 receptor blockers, proton pump inhibitors, or cytoprotective agents may suffice.

The development of fever, chest pain, or respiratory distress during the first week after a hiatal hernia operation mandates a contrast study, and if a distal esophageal perforation is diagnosed, treatment usually involves reoperation. The site of the perforation is identified intraoperatively, at times by insufflating air through a nasogastric tube. A leak from an intra-abdominal fundoplication suture may be closed and reinforced with adjacent omentum. If the leak is in the chest, pedicled anterior mediastinal fat, intercostal muscle, or pleura is used to reinforce the closure through a transthoracic approach. A jejunostomy feeding tube should be placed

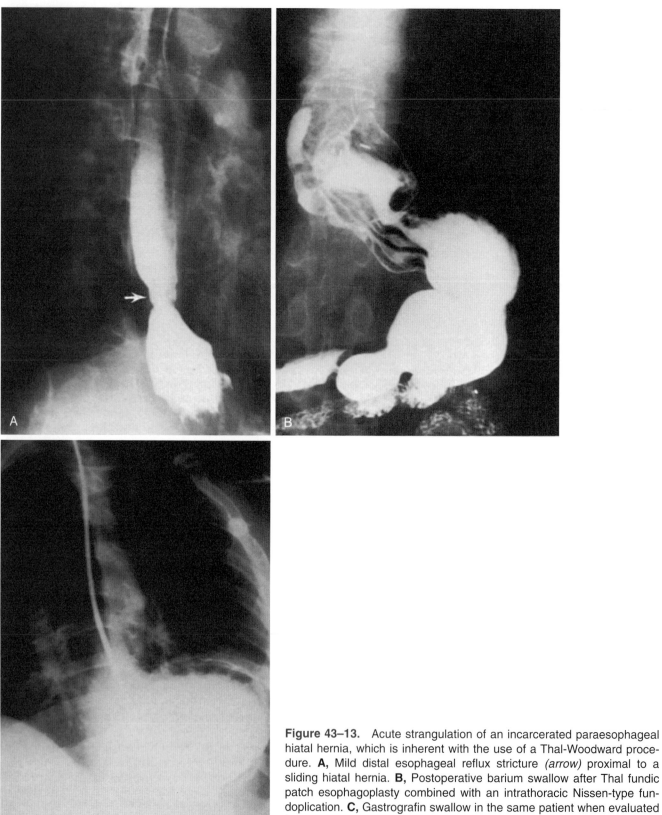

Figure 43–13.   Acute strangulation of an incarcerated paraesophageal hiatal hernia, which is inherent with the use of a Thal-Woodward procedure. **A,** Mild distal esophageal reflux stricture *(arrow)* proximal to a sliding hiatal hernia. **B,** Postoperative barium swallow after Thal fundic patch esophagoplasty combined with an intrathoracic Nissen-type fundoplication. **C,** Gastrografin swallow in the same patient when evaluated for acute chest pain and shortness of breath. There was gross dilation of the incarcerated intrathoracic stomach. Nasogastric decompression was required, and the patient was subsequently treated by distal esophagectomy and short-segment colonic interposition.

to allow nutritional support and unimpeded ambulation in case the repair is unsuccessful and an esophageal fistula ensues. Either a large-bore chest tube should be left near the thoracic esophageal repair or a drain should be placed near the transabdominally repaired fundoplication to ensure external drainage of a recurrent fistula. There have been recent reports suggesting the use of self-expanding Silastic-covered esophageal stents for the treatment of postoperative esophageal leaks because of the touted ability to remove or reposition such devices once healing is complete. However, long-term follow-up is not readily available. In a normal-caliber esophagus, such devices appear to be more prone to distal migration into the stomach. Furthermore, the radial force exerted by these stents when placed in a pathologically narrowed esophagus may result in relative ischemia with possible extension of the esophageal injury and enlargement of the esophageal leak. The use of such devices should therefore be undertaken with caution and reserved for patients who are otherwise not suitable candidates for surgery.[23]

Low retrosternal dysphagia after an antireflux operation may have one of several causes: (1) distal esophageal edema after intraoperative manipulation, (2) distal esophageal motor dysfunction as a result of manipulation of the vagus nerves, (3) obstruction caused by too tight a fundoplication, (4) or obstruction from excessive closure of the hiatus. Performance of the fundoplication over at least a 54-French intraesophageal dilator minimizes the likelihood of this latter complication. Dysphagia after truncal vagotomy has been recognized for more than 40 years, and it is apparent that esophageal neuromotor dysfunction may follow manipulation of the vagus nerves at the level of the distal esophagus. This complication after antireflux surgery is more likely with a transthoracic than with a transabdominal repair because both exposure and displacement of the main vagal trunks are more frequent with the former approach. Such patients have dysphagia immediately after the antireflux procedure. On barium swallow examination, the distal esophagus is tapered and empties poorly, similar to the picture of achalasia or esophageal spasm. Reassurance plus maintenance of a soft diet for several days is usually adequate therapy, although passage of an esophageal dilator is at times required for relief. This problem typically subsides spontaneously, but occasionally reoperation, takedown of the repair, and at times even esophageal resection may be needed.

Another complication of intraoperative vagus nerve injury occurring during hiatal hernia repair is impaired gastric motility or pylorospasm resulting in delayed gastric emptying and secondary gastric dilation. This complication has direct implications for the long-term success of hiatal hernia repair because sustained gastric dilation in conjunction with a competent distal esophageal sphincter mechanism may eventually result in disruption of the esophageal sutures used to construct the fundoplication and failure of the repair. When gastric dilation develops immediately after surgery in a patient who has undergone an antireflux operation, a 7- to 10-day trial of gastric decompression with a nasogastric tube is indicated. At times, an anticholinergic (e.g., atropine,

0.4 mg either per os or intramuscularly every 4 to 6 hours) may relieve the associated pylorospasm. However, this problem should not be permitted to persist indefinitely, and it is best to perform an early gastric drainage procedure (pyloromyotomy or pyloroplasty) than to risk recurrent gastroesophageal reflux. Finally, vagal nerve injury may result in varying degrees of "dumping syndrome" (i.e., postprandial diarrhea, cramping, abdominal pain, nausea, diaphoresis, palpitations). This problem generally subsides within a few months, but at times long-term management with antidiarrheal medication and dietary restriction may be required.

Chylothorax after an antireflux procedure may result from injury to the thoracic duct, which passes from the abdomen through the aortic hiatus and then courses in the lower part of the chest anterior to the spine between the esophagus and the aorta. Injury may occur during mobilization of the cardia or during placement of the crural sutures. This complication is heralded by prolonged chest tube drainage after a transthoracic repair, and the true cause of this serosanguineous drainage may not become apparent until the patient's diet is liberalized and its fat content increases. If chylothorax is present, the oral administration of 60 to 90 ml of cream for 4 to 6 hours will result in chest tube drainage of opalescent and milky chyle. The diagnosis can also be established by staining the fluid with Sudan R, which stains the globules of fat. Determination of cholesterol and triglyceride levels in the fluid is not usually necessary. A cholesterol-triglyceride ratio of less than 1 is characteristic of a chylous effusion, whereas nonchylous effusions have a ratio of greater than 1. In most cases, chylothorax after hiatal hernia repair can be managed nonoperatively by administering a low-residue elemental diet and maintaining prolonged chest tube suction. If the output of chyle remains significant (>400 to 600 ml per consecutive 8-hour periods) after 7 to 10 days of this treatment, reoperation with identification and ligation of the injured thoracic duct is indicated.

Acute postoperative hemorrhage after an antireflux operation is most often the result of bleeding from an unsecured divided short gastric vessel along the high greater curvature of the stomach. This possibility should always be borne in mind as the short gastric vessels are divided and ligated before performing a fundoplication. Hemorrhage from these vessels may be a particularly treacherous complication after transthoracic hiatal hernia repair because the resulting hypovolemic shock may be attributed to other causes (e.g., myocardial infarction) when there is minimal chest tube drainage and the chest roentgenogram shows no hemothorax. The proper course of therapy is abdominal exploration, evacuation of the blood, and ligation of the bleeding vessel. Splenic injury also occurs in a small percentage of patients undergoing antireflux surgery, particularly during reoperations. The incidence of splenic injury is slightly higher with transabdominal than with transthoracic antireflux operations, particularly in obese patients. Rarely, postoperative hemorrhage is manifested as a pericardial effusion causing tamponade and cardiopulmonary collapse. This complication may arise from avulsion of an epicardial vessel, disruption of pericardial adhesions during esophageal mobilization for repair of a large hiatal hernia, or inadvertent injury to the myocardium during placement of diaphragmatic crural sutures. Rapid diagnosis by surface echocardiography followed by sternotomy, relief of tamponade, and repair of the bleeding vessel is indicated.[24]

Before the patient is discharged from the hospital after an antireflux operation, a barium swallow examination should be routinely performed to document the postoperative appearance of the reconstructed esophagogastric junction. At times, this contrast study may reveal a "silent" localized extravasation of contrast material at the site of one of the fundoplication sutures that was placed too deeply. If the patient is asymptomatic and the "leak" is very small, no therapy may be required because the supporting fundoplication has prevented a more major disruption. A far more disconcerting radiographic finding on a "routine" postoperative barium swallow obtained before discharge is asymptomatic migration of the fundoplication or gastric fundus into the chest as a result of disruption of the posterior crural repair (Fig. 43–14). This iatrogenic paraesophageal hiatal hernia is subject to the same mechanical complications of paraesophageal herniation as in a patient who has had no surgery. Reoperation is necessary to reduce the fundoplication back into the abdomen and to replace the posterior crural sutures if they have pulled through the crural muscle (or to narrow the hiatus further if they have not) before postoperative adhesions form between the herniated stomach and adjacent tissues and make any subsequent repair more complicated. It may be difficult to tell an asymptomatic patient recovering from an antireflux operation that a reoperation is necessary, but conservative management of this problem is ill advised.

Controversy remains regarding the role of surgical therapy in patients with complications of gastroesophageal reflux disease, particularly Barrett's esophagus. Both symptoms and the requirement for antisecretory medications decrease significantly after an antireflux operation.[25] However, no long-term data are available regarding regression of Barrett's esophagus, regarded as a precursor lesion to esophageal adenocarcinoma. Currently, patients with Barrett's esophagus who are undergoing hiatal herniorrhaphy should continue to be monitored by routine surveillance esophagoscopy with biopsy to screen for progression from metaplasia to dysplasia and esophageal adenocarcinoma.[26]

Laparoscopic Antireflux/ Hiatal Hernia Surgery

Since 1991, when the first reports of laparoscopic antireflux surgery were published, minimally invasive surgical approaches to the diaphragmatic esophageal hiatus have been used with increasing frequency. Although mortality rates for laparoscopic fundoplication have been low (0% to 1.4%), early morbidity rates are acceptable, and conversion rates to an open procedure range from 0% to 14%, the learning curve for this operation is substantial.[27]

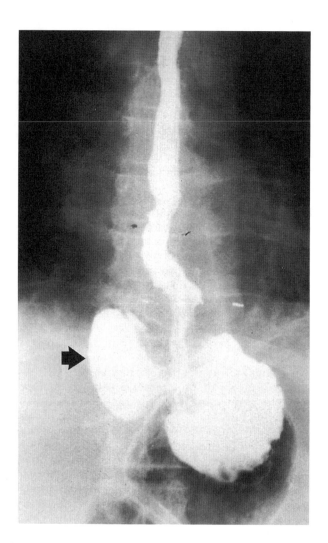

Figure 43–14. Asymptomatic partial migration of the fundoplication into the chest through the diaphragmatic hiatus 1 week after a Collis-Nissen hiatal hernia repair (the *arrow* indicates the portion of fundoplication above the diaphragm). Although asymptomatic, this patient underwent a reoperation, with the fundoplication reduced and secured below the diaphragm and the hiatus narrowed further to prevent later potential complications of this paraesophageal hernia. (From Orringer MB: Complications of esophageal surgery and trauma. In Greenfield, LJ [ed]: Complications in Surgery and Trauma. Philadelphia, JB Lippincott, 1984, p 275.)

In obese patients, in those with intra-abdominal adhesions from previous surgery, or in those with an unusually large left hepatic lobe, visualization of the operative field may be so difficult that persistence in performing the "closed" operation may be frankly dangerous. The latter factors remain indications for open transthoracic hiatal hernia repair. Perforations of the distal esophagus or gastric fundus have been reported during laparoscopic fundoplication. Blind dissection posterior to the esophagus should be avoided to prevent this complication. When recognized at the time of or soon after surgery, laparoscopic repair is feasible, but conversion to an open procedure may be the best option.

Early postoperative dysphagia may result from an overly tight fundoplication, which is more likely to occur with minimally invasive procedures because tactile sensation cannot be used to assess the tightness of the wrap. Performance of the fundoplication over at least a size 54-French Maloney dilator minimizes the likelihood of this complication. Postoperative dysphagia as a result of fibrotic stenosis of the muscular esophageal hiatus, attributed to diathermy injury during esophageal dissection, has also been reported and treated with laparoscopic hiatal division. Persistent dysphagia after a laparoscopic fundoplication that is refractory to dilatation therapy may necessitate reoperation, takedown of the wrap, and construction of a looser fundoplication. The authors' approach for such reoperative procedures is transthoracic, generally with a combined esophageal-lengthening Collis gastroplasty and Nissen fundoplication. Additional complications of laparoscopic fundoplication include pneumothorax or pneumomediastinum from CO_2 tracking into the chest during the operation, incisional hernia at a port site, and herniation of the fundoplication through the diaphragmatic hiatus (particularly when the crura were not approximated well or at all at the time of the original operation).

As enthusiasm for laparoscopic fundoplication has grown, this approach has also been used to repair large paraesophageal hiatal hernias, which are often associated with an attenuated, abnormally wide esophageal hiatus in an obese patient. In 1983, Pearson and associates emphasized that esophageal shortening is common in these patients, most of whom have combined sliding and paraesophageal hiatus hernias, and they used the combined Collis gastroplasty–fundoplication operation liberally in this group.[28,29] With the laparoscopic approach one cannot assess the degree of tension on the distal esophagus that results from reduction of the esophagogastric junction below the diaphragm because, again, direct manual palpation of the esophagus is not possible. Furthermore, with the diaphragms pushed abnormally upward by CO_2 insufflation into the abdomen during the operation, a false sense of ease of reduction of the esophagogastric junction into the abdomen may occur. Although several groups have developed minimally invasive techniques for combined Collis gastroplasty and fundoplication with acceptable short-term results,[30,31] our group believes that most large combined sliding and paraesophageal hiatal hernias should be approached through the chest with an open operation, generally a combined Collis gastroplasty and Nissen fundoplication. The increasing number of fundoplications that have "slipped" through the hiatus into the chest after laparoscopic repair probably reflect, at least in part, a lack of recognition by the original surgeon that there was unacceptable tension on the repair. Recurrent herniation of an intact or a partially disrupted fundoplication is the most common reason for failure of laparoscopic fundoplication. Body habitus is another important but often overlooked factor in recurrence after laparoscopic (or any) antireflux operations; obesity is present in a significant number of patients who experience disruption of repairs.

Another laparoscopic technique for the repair of paraesophageal hiatal hernias involves the use of mesh to close the diaphragmatic defect. This is an ill-conceived operation because the constant diaphragmatic motion against the adjacent esophagus at the hiatus may result in esophageal or gastric erosion and perforation. This approach is mentioned only to condemn its use.

Esophageal Resection and Visceral Esophageal Substitution

In almost every large series of patients undergoing a traditional esophageal resection and substitution with either stomach or intestine, the leading causes of death are (1) respiratory insufficiency associated with the physiologic insult of a combined thoracic and abdominal operation and (2) sepsis from mediastinitis secondary to disruption of an intrathoracic anastomosis. As a result, our group has adopted a general policy of performing no intrathoracic esophageal anastomoses and prefers a cervical esophagogastric anastomosis instead. A cervical esophagogastric anastomotic leak generally represents little more acute morbidity than a salivary fistula, and spontaneous closure with local wound care is the rule. Our group has reported a dramatic reduction in the incidence of postoperative cervical esophagogastric anastomotic leak to less than 3% with a side-to-side stapled cervical esophagogastric anastomosis[32] constructed with the Auto Suture Endo GIA II Stapler. The authors have also found that a transhiatal esophagectomy without thoracotomy plus a cervical esophagogastric anastomosis is applicable in most patients requiring esophageal resection and reconstruction for both benign and malignant disease. This procedure minimizes the operative insult to the patient by avoiding a thoracotomy. The incidence of postoperative pulmonary complications is thereby reduced, and the possibility of mediastinitis resulting from an intrathoracic leak is virtually eliminated.

The authors recommend the use of a 14-French rubber catheter feeding jejunostomy tube secured in place with a Witzel maneuver, not a "needle catheter" jejunostomy, in every patient undergoing esophagectomy and esophageal reconstruction. The jejunostomy tube is regarded as an "insurance policy" in case anastomotic disruption necessitates an alternative means of nourishment. If use of the tube is not required postoperatively, it is removed after several weeks. Alternatively, if an anastomotic leak occurs, a feeding jejunostomy tube is safer and more effective in providing calories than intravenous hyperalimentation.

Anastomotic Leak

After completion of a cervical esophageal anastomosis, the neck wound is closed loosely with only four or five 4-0 sutures over a $\frac{1}{4}$-inch Penrose drain placed adjacent to the anastomosis. If an anastomotic leak does occur, the neck wound is opened at the bedside in its entirety, and the wound is gently packed with gauze. The size of the leak can be estimated by having the patient drink water and evaluating the amount that escapes from the neck wound with a disposable bedside suction catheter. Generally, within several days of opening the wound, the drainage diminishes considerably, and the patient may resume oral intake while maintaining steady gentle pressure over the wound to occlude the fistula. Passage of tapered Maloney dilators (generally 40 and 46 French) at the bedside during the first week after drainage of the cervical fistula ensures that no element of obstruction from either local edema or spasm contributes to continued drainage of the fistula.[33] More than 98% of cervical esophagogastric anastomotic leaks are small and respond to the open drainage and packing as described. A small proportion, however, are associated with catastrophic complications: major gastric tip necrosis necessitating takedown of the anastomosis, construction of a cervical esophagostomy, and resection of nonviable stomach; vertebral body osteomyelitis; epidural abscess with resultant paraplegia; pulmonary microabscesses from an internal jugular vein abscess; and tracheoesophagogastric anastomotic fistula.[34]

Early disruption of an intrathoracic esophageal anastomosis occurring within the first 10 critical days after surgery is characterized by the signs and symptoms of mediastinitis: fever, chest pain, tachycardia, tachypnea, respiratory distress, peripheral cyanosis, vasoconstriction, hypotension, and shock. When coupled with a chest roentgenogram that demonstrates hydrothorax or pneumothorax, there is little question about the diagnosis. The diagnosis should nonetheless be confirmed with a contrast study. In an otherwise asymptomatic patient found to have a small (<1 cm) contained anastomotic leak on a routine postoperative barium swallow, observation alone may be sufficient. In most cases, however, anastomotic disruption warrants urgent re-exploration, irrigation of the chest and mediastinum, repair of the fistula if possible, and chest tube drainage. A localized anastomotic leak with viable adjacent tissue may be amenable to direct suture repair. A pedicled flap of anterior mediastinal fat, an intercostal muscle flap, pleura, or omentum should be mobilized to reinforce the repair. Decompression of the esophageal substitute with a nasogastric tube, placement of a jejunostomy tube for nutritional support, and appropriate antibiotics complete the therapy. After removal of the chest tubes, a barium swallow examination should be performed 10 days after the reoperation to be certain that healing has occurred. If disruption of the anastomosis recurs, a controlled esophagopleural cutaneous fistula should be established. Rib resection with placement of a large-bore drainage tube adjacent to the fistula may be required to ensure that all drainage from the esophageal leak can flow freely out of the chest. Gastric contents that are aspirated through the nasogastric tube can be returned to the alimentary tract through the jejunostomy tube to minimize electrolyte imbalance and to simplify fluid and electrolyte replacement.

During re-exploration of the chest for a disrupted esophageal anastomosis, extensive local necrosis of the tissue with a major anastomotic dehiscence mandates takedown of the anastomosis, resection of nonviable stomach, and replacement of the remaining stomach into the abdomen. Only nonviable distal esophagus

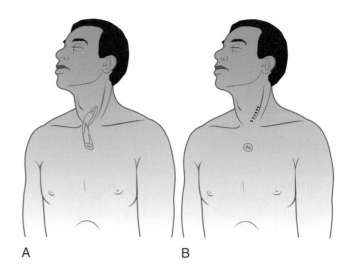

A   **B**

Figure 43–15. Construction of an anterior thoracic esophagostomy instead of a traditional end cervical esophagostomy. **A,** The mobilized thoracic esophagus is placed on the anterior chest wall so that the location of the stoma can be determined. **B,** All viable remaining esophagus is preserved and tunneled subcutaneously, and an end anterior thoracic esophagostomy is constructed. Stomal appliances are readily applied to the flat anterior surface of the chest, and when performing a later colon interposition, 7 to 12 cm of esophagus is available for the reconstruction. (From Orringer MB: Complications of esophageal surgery and trauma. In Greenfield LJ [ed]: Complications in Surgery and Trauma, 2nd ed. Philadelphia, JB Lippincott, 1990, p 317.)

should be resected. However, a diverting lateral cervical esophagostomy with oversewing of the divided proximal intrathoracic esophagus should not be attempted. Not only is disruption of the intrathoracic esophageal suture line likely, but if subsequent reconstruction is possible, management of the remaining segment of intrathoracic esophagus also presents a considerable technical problem. The best alternative is to mobilize the esophagus circumferentially well into the neck through the thoracic incision. After the thoracotomy is closed, an end esophagostomy, with the patient returned to the supine position, should be performed. As indicated earlier, the submucosal collateral circulation of the esophagus is excellent, and most of the length of the thoracic esophagus will remain viable as long as at least one inferior thyroid artery remains intact. Therefore, after delivering the divided thoracic esophagus out of the neck incision, the maximum length of remaining esophagus should be preserved to facilitate later reconstruction. This is achieved by developing a subcutaneous tunnel anteriorly to the left clavicle onto the chest wall and constructing an anterior thoracic esophagostomy. An esophagostomy stoma placed on the relatively flat upper anterior chest wall is much more easily cared for by the patient because a stomal appliance is more readily adapted to this location than to the usual site of a standard cervical esophagostomy (Fig. 43–15). A feeding jejunostomy is, of course, required until later esophageal reconstruction can be performed.

When colon or jejunum has been used to replace the esophagus and necrosis of the graft is documented at re-exploration for an anastomotic leak, there is similarly little recourse but to remove the nonviable graft and insert a feeding tube. If the patient survives the sequelae of the mediastinal sepsis, later reconstruction can be considered.

Anastomotic Stricture

Although the management of a cervical anastomotic leak is generally straightforward and seldom associated with death, the long-term sequelae of a cervical leak are far from inconsequential. As many as 50% of cervical esophagogastric anastomotic leaks result in an anastomotic stricture as healing occurs, which is an unsatisfactory outcome of an operation that is intended to provide comfortable swallowing. The implications are similar in patients who survive an intrathoracic esophageal anastomotic leak. Our group has previously reported an anastomotic leak rate averaging 13% in nearly 1100 transhiatal esophagectomy patients at the University of Michigan, with subsequent anastomotic strictures developing in nearly half of these patients,[35] consistent with reports in the literature for the incidence of both anastomotic leak (5% to 26%) and stenosis (10% to 31%).[36-38] Without question, prevention of an anastomotic leak is the key to a successful functional outcome in these patients. In our initial experience with the side-to-side stapled cervical esophagogastric anastomosis, which has been associated with an anastomotic leak rate of less than 3%, we observed a dramatic reduction in the need for late postoperative anastomotic dilatations.[32]

In a patient who has experienced an esophageal anastomotic leak, early passage of a 46-French or larger dilator within 1 week of drainage is carried out to maintain a satisfactory lumen and prevent late high-grade stenosis. A cervical fistula generally heals within 7 to 10 days of external drainage. When the patient returns for follow-up within 2 weeks of discharge, a 46-French or larger Maloney dilator is passed through the anastomosis. If the patient has no dysphagia and there is no resistance to passage of the dilator, the need for subsequent dilatations is dictated by the return of cervical dysphagia. In patients with anastomotic narrowing that prevents the free passage of a 46-French or larger Maloney dilator, a more aggressive program of esophageal dilatation is undertaken. With an early program of weekly dilatations, anastomotic healing in a patent configuration is often achieved. Patients whose anastomotic stricture produces resistance as the dilator is passed may need more frequent dilatations. In this situation, the patient is taught over a period of several weeks to pass a 46- or 48-French dilator with the assistance of a family member or friend. Once facility with passage of the dilator is achieved, the patient is issued a dilator with instructions to pass it daily for 1 week, then every other day for 1 week, and then at increasingly longer intervals until the longest duration between dilatations without recurrence of dysphagia can be established. With this aggressive initial program of dilatation, long-term comfortable swallowing with little or no need for subsequent dilatations is generally achieved. Few patients require anastomotic revision. Occasionally, endoscopic injection of steroids into a refractory anastomotic scar facilitates the management of this problem.[39,40]

Pulmonary Complications

Respiratory insufficiency after esophageal resection and reconstruction is exceedingly common and is associated with a mortality rate of up to 40%.[41,42] Patients with esophageal squamous cell cancer, particularly those treated with preoperative chemoradiation, may have a greater risk for postoperative pulmonary morbidity, including pleural effusion, pneumonia, and respiratory insufficiency after esophagectomy.[43] A vital part of minimizing postoperative pulmonary complications after esophageal resection and reconstruction is rigorous preoperative pulmonary physiotherapy. The authors insist on total abstinence from cigarette smoking for a minimum of 3 weeks before esophagectomy. Home use of an incentive inspirometer and instruction in deep-breathing exercises are also begun 3 weeks preoperatively. This investment of time and energy in improving the patient's preoperative respiratory status is repeatedly rewarded by a lower incidence of postoperative pulmonary complications after esophageal resection and reconstruction. Postoperatively, patients are extubated immediately after surgery and resume pulmonary physiotherapy as early as possible. Adequate postoperative analgesia, particularly epidural anesthesia, is of great value in minimizing postoperative pulmonary problems.

One of the most disastrous complications after esophageal resection is the development of a fistula between the tracheobronchial tree and either the esophagus or the esophageal substitute, generally at the anastomotic site. Among 207 patients with malignant esophagorespiratory fistulas treated at the Memorial Sloan-Kettering Cancer Center in New York, Burt and associates reported 13 patients in whom fistulas developed after resection for esophageal carcinoma.[44] Once a fistula between the airway and adjacent alimentary tract develops, there is little option other than to prevent continued contamination of the respiratory tree by identifying and dividing the fistula and repairing the airway, generally a major undertaking in a desperately ill patient.

Gastric Outlet Obstruction

The need for a routine gastric drainage procedure after the vagotomy that inevitably accompanies esophagectomy has been debated. It has been shown, for example, that most patients who undergo esophagectomy and esophagogastric anastomosis without a concomitant drainage procedure do not have difficulty with gastric outlet obstruction.[45,46] However, in a prospective trial in which 200 patients undergoing esophageal resection were randomized to receive either pyloroplasty or no gastric drainage procedure, gastric emptying was found to be four times longer in those who did not have a pyloroplasty.[47] Adverse postprandial symptoms were less frequent in those who had a drainage procedure, and there was no morbidity from the pyloroplasty. For the

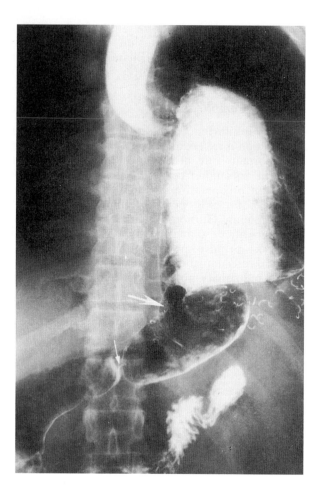

Figure 43–16. Barium study in a patient with regurgitation and dilatation of the intrathoracic stomach after esophagectomy for distal-third carcinoma. This complication was the result of two technical errors: failure to enlarge the diaphragmatic hiatus sufficiently, with resultant relative obstruction at the diaphragmatic hiatus *(large arrow),* and failure to perform a gastric drainage procedure, with resultant pyloric obstruction *(small arrow).* (From Orringer MB: Complications of esophageal surgery and trauma. In Greenfield LJ [ed]: Complications in Surgery and Trauma, 2nd ed. Philadelphia, JB Lippincott, 1990, p 318.)

occasional patient in whom significant gastric outlet obstruction does develop after esophageal resection (Fig. 43–16), the outcome may be disastrous: aspiration pneumonia and impaired nutrition because of an inability to eat. Furthermore, a reoperation to perform a drainage procedure may be very difficult after the stomach has been mobilized into the chest. For these reasons, the authors advocate performance of a gastric drainage procedure in every patient undergoing esophagectomy and esophageal reconstruction; our preference is a Ramstedt-type extramucosal pyloromyotomy, which avoids the intra-abdominal suture line of a pyloroplasty. After performing the pyloromyotomy, silver clip markers placed at the level of the pylorus aid in interpreting the subsequent radiologic studies used to evaluate gastric emptying. In more than 1500 such pyloromyotomies

performed during esophageal bypass or replacement with stomach, our group has experienced one leak postoperatively. This leak resulted in fatal peritonitis. Intrathoracic gastric outlet obstruction may also result from failure to enlarge the diaphragmatic hiatus adequately before mobilizing the stomach into the chest. The diaphragmatic hiatus should accommodate at least three fingers comfortably alongside the mobilized stomach to prevent this complication.

Diaphragmatic Hiatal Obstruction or Herniation

Not only must the hiatus be enlarged sufficiently to prevent the esophageal substitute from becoming obstructed at the level of the diaphragm, but the esophageal replacement, whether stomach or intestine, should also be carefully sutured to the edge of the diaphragmatic hiatus to prevent subsequent herniation of abdominal viscera through the hiatus and into the chest (Fig. 43–17). As our group and others have observed, this complication may occur acutely within the first several days after surgery or years after the esophagectomy.[48,49] Such a hernia may be an asymptomatic finding on a postoperative chest roentgenogram on which intestinal gas is seen above the level of the hiatus, or the patient may have vague left upper quadrant abdominal or lower thoracic discomfort, nausea, and vomiting, as is the case with chronic traumatic diaphragmatic hernias. Because the risk for incarceration and strangulation of the herniated viscera is substantial, reduction of the hernia is advised. Herniation of intestine through the diaphragmatic hiatus after esophagectomy can generally be repaired transabdominally. In the case of chronic traumatic diaphragmatic hernias, the opening in the diaphragm is relatively small, and the herniated viscera may become adherent to adjacent intrathoracic structures and require a transthoracic approach for reduction. The majority of herniations of intestine alongside the intrathoracic stomach, on the other hand, occur through a relatively patulous hiatus. Reduction of the hernia and narrowing of the hiatus are readily achieved through the abdomen. As is the case with other complications that follow esophageal surgery, this situation can also generally be prevented. When the esophageal substitute has been brought through the diaphragmatic hiatus and the anastomosis has been completed, several heavy diaphragmatic crural sutures should be used to narrow the hiatus so that it admits three fingers alongside the stomach or colon. Then a few interrupted sutures should be placed between the edge of the diaphragmatic hiatus and the visceral esophageal substitute to limit the migration of other intra-abdominal viscera through the hiatus into the chest. Finally, the divided triangular ligament of the mobilized liver should be sutured to the edge of the hiatus to provide one additional barrier to herniation at this site.

Chylothorax

Because of the proximity of the thoracic duct and the esophagus, chylothorax after esophagectomy is a recognized complication. Ligation of the divided

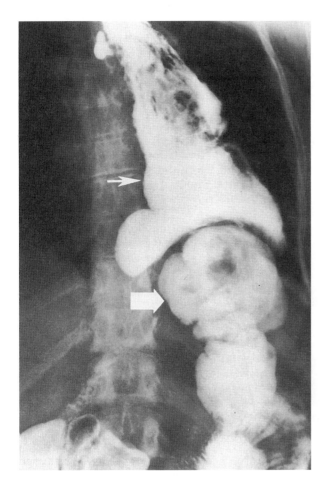

Figure 43–17. Herniation of the splenic flexure of the colon *(large arrow)* through the diaphragmatic hiatus after esophageal replacement with stomach for a caustic stricture. No sutures had been placed between the intrathoracic stomach *(small arrow)* and the edge of the diaphragmatic hiatus to prevent this complication. (From Orringer MB: Complications of esophageal surgery and trauma. In Greenfield LJ [ed]: Complications in Surgery and Trauma, 2nd ed. Philadelphia, JB Lippincott, 1990, p 318.)

periesophageal tissues at the time of esophagectomy minimizes this complication. When compared with the relatively healthy patient who sustains a chylothorax after aortic surgery, however, this complication in a debilitated patient with esophageal obstruction is not well tolerated, with reported mortality as high as 50%.[50,51] Patients with chronic esophageal obstruction are already nutritionally depleted. Further loss of protein-rich chyle is not well tolerated. Only a few days should be expended in trying to treat this complication nonoperatively. With aggressive operative intervention and direct ligation of the point of thoracic duct injury, patient salvage is the rule.[52] Thoracic duct ligation at the point where the thoracic duct emerges through the diaphragmatic hiatus can be accomplished by either right posterolateral thoracotomy or video-assisted thoracoscopic surgery.

Pancreatitis

Postoperative pancreatitis may occur after esophagectomy as a result of pancreatic injury during performance of either the Kocher maneuver or gastric mobilization. The possibility should be suspected in patients in whom unexplained fever, respiratory distress, or prolonged ileus develops after esophagectomy. The diagnosis is confirmed by determining serum amylase and lipase levels. Standard treatment of pancreatitis with nasogastric tube decompression of the gastrointestinal tract and administration of intravenous fluids is usually sufficient, although progression to fatal hemorrhagic pancreatitis may ensue.

Splenic Injury

Injury to the spleen may occur during esophagectomy, particularly during mobilization of the stomach for esophageal replacement. Careful avoidance of undue traction on the short gastric vessels during gastric mobilization and early division of adhesions between the stomach and the spleen on opening the abdomen minimize this complication. Routine splenectomy as part of the "cancer operation" for esophageal carcinoma is not advocated because splenectomy is associated with a well-documented increased morbidity of its own.

Peripheral Atheroembolism

Thromboembolic sequelae after transhiatal esophagectomy have been reported in two patients and attributed to inadvertent dislodgement of debris from the diseased aorta in the process of mobilizing the esophagus through the diaphragmatic hiatus.[53] This complication has not been encountered by our group in a combined experience totaling more than 1500 transhiatal esophagectomies.

Complications of Substernal Esophageal Replacement

Several unique complications of esophageal replacement are related to retrosternal placement of the esophageal substitute. The most obvious is potential obstruction at the level of the retrosternal neohiatus because of failure to create an adequate opening (Fig. 43–18). When creating a retrosternal tunnel, it is our practice to dilate this space until the entire hand and forearm can be inserted retrosternally to ensure sufficient room for either the stomach or the colon. Compression along with obstruction of the retrosternal esophageal substitute at the superior opening into the anterior mediastinum is a function of the posterior prominence of the clavicular head, which narrows the anterior thoracic inlet. For this reason, when performing a retrosternal interposition of stomach or colon, which requires relocation of the cervical esophagus anteriorly from its usual position to the left and posterior to the trachea, the medial third of the left clavicle, the adjacent manubrium, and usually the medial first left rib as well should be resected to ensure an adequate opening into the anterior mediastinum.

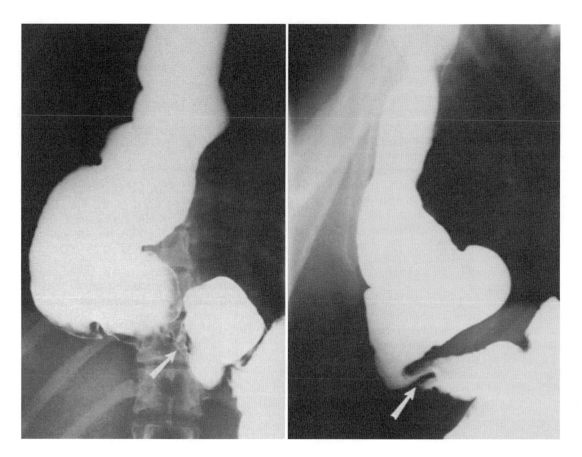

Figure 43–18.   Posteroanterior *(left)* and lateral *(right)* views from a barium swallow showing early postoperative obstruction of a retrosternal colonic interposition at the level of the diaphragm *(arrows)* as a result of failure to create an adequate opening in the diaphragm.

Complications of Bypassing or Excluding the Native Esophagus

Management of the diseased native esophagus is controversial when performing retrosternal replacement of the esophagus. An esophagus that is severely strictured from a caustic injury, for example, may simply be left in the posterior mediastinum and bypassed with a retrosternal colon. The potential complications arising from the residual diseased esophagus, however, mandate that it be removed whenever possible. The small but definite increased risk for late development of carcinoma in the caustic strictured esophagus is a less compelling reason to resect it than the potential for subsequent reflux esophagitis. A caustic injury may destroy the lower esophageal sphincter mechanism as a result of subsequent fibrosis, and reflux symptoms and severe esophagitis in the native esophagus may develop in such a patient undergoing substernal colon interposition (Fig. 43–19).

Although substernal bypass of the excluded esophagus with either stomach or colon has been used for the treatment of both benign and malignant disease, the complications from such an approach are appreciable. The excluded esophagus may become a giant posterior mediastinal mucocele that causes respiratory distress as

a result of tracheobronchial compression (Fig. 43–20). Of more immediate concern in the postoperative period is the incidence of disruption of the distal end of the excluded esophagus with a resultant left subphrenic abscess. When esophageal replacement is necessary for benign disease, the authors advocate resection of the esophagus. It is always preferable to place the esophageal substitute in the posterior mediastinum in the original esophageal bed because (1) this is the shortest distance between the neck and the abdominal cavity; (2) if subsequent anastomotic dilation is required, it is far safer and more direct to perform it when one does not have to negotiate the anterior angulation of a cervical esophagus that has been anastomosed to a retrosternal graft; and (3) the incidence of postoperative cervical anastomotic leak is lower. In the original esophageal bed in the neck, the anastomosis is buttressed by adjacent tissues: the spine posteriorly, the carotid sheath laterally, the trachea medially, and the strap muscles anteriorly. An esophageal anastomosis to a retrosternal colon or stomach is basically subcutaneous in the neck and is relatively unsupported. Coughing or a Valsalva maneuver against a closed upper esophageal sphincter results in distention of the retrosternal esophageal substitute with increased pressure on the anastomosis and a higher anastomotic leak rate. If esophageal bypass is performed in

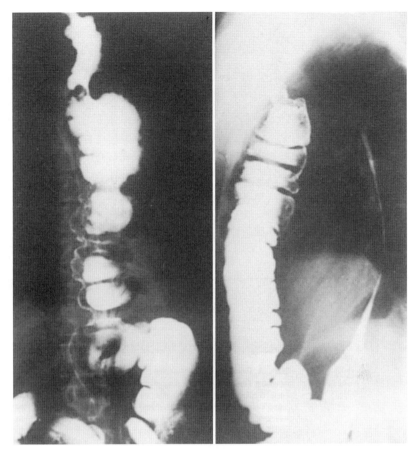

Figure 43–19. Posteroanterior *(left)* and lateral *(right)* views from a barium swallow performed in a patient who had undergone a retrosternal colonic bypass for a caustic esophageal stricture 4 years earlier. This patient had experienced severe reflux symptoms for 2 years before being evaluated for upper gastrointestinal bleeding secondary to reflux esophagitis. The lateral film shows simultaneous opacification of both the colon graft and the native esophagus, which filled as a result of a grossly incompetent lower esophageal sphincter. Resection of the native esophagus was required to relieve the severe reflux esophagitis.

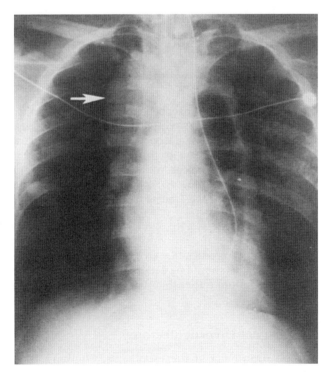

Figure 43–20. Posteroanterior chest roentgenogram in a 27-year-old man being evaluated for acute respiratory distress 2 years after undergoing substernal gastric bypass of the excluded thoracic esophagus for a caustic stricture. The patient had compression of the tracheobronchial tree by a huge posterior mediastinal mucocele *(arrow)* that had formed in the excluded esophagus. An endotracheal tube was required to relieve the airway obstruction. A nasogastric tube is seen in the retrosternally placed stomach. A right-sided thoracotomy and resection of the dilated esophagus were carried out.

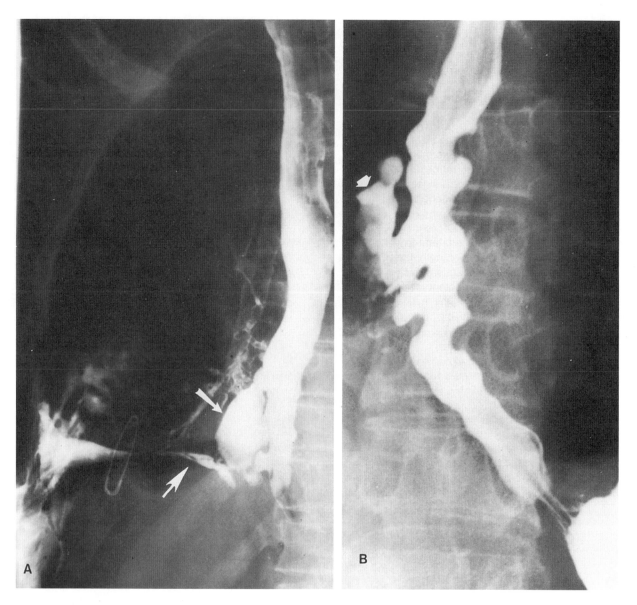

Figure 43–21. **A,** This esophagogram shows an esophagopleural cutaneous fistula *(large arrow)* and a recurrent esophageal diverticulum *(small arrow)* in a patient who had previously undergone resection of the diverticulum without esophagomyotomy. **B,** The patient's underlying esophageal neuromotor problem is evident in this view from the same study, which shows a typical corkscrew esophagus. The relative obstruction secondary to intermittent spasm distal to the esophageal suture line had not been relieved when the diverticulum was resected; hence disruption of the suture line with fistula formation and recurrence of the diverticulum *(arrow)* followed. (From Orringer MB: Complications of esophageal surgery and trauma. In Greenfield LJ [ed]: Complications in Surgery and Trauma, 2nd ed. Philadelphia, JB Lippincott, 1990, p 320.)

patients with unresectable esophageal carcinoma, the distal esophagus should be decompressed into a Roux-en-Y limb or jejunum rather than excluded.[54,55]

Esophageal Diverticulectomy

Pulsion diverticula of the esophagus, whether oropharyngeal (Zenker's diverticulum) or intrathoracic, result from associated distal esophageal obstruction, most often neuromotor dysfunction. Thus, if the underlying neuromotor abnormality responsible for formation of the

diverticulum is not addressed at the time of diverticulectomy, failure to relieve the distal obstruction may result in disruption of the suture line (Figs. 43–21 and 43–22). After resection of a diverticulum, the esophagus should be insufflated with air through an indwelling nasogastric tube positioned within the esophagus, and an air leak should be looked for by immersing the pouting esophageal submucosa in saline solution (Fig. 43–23). The most opportune time to treat such a pinhole leak is at the time of surgery, and a single 5-0 monofilament stitch may avert a great deal of postoperative morbidity. Alternatively, if a cervical esophageal leak occurs after

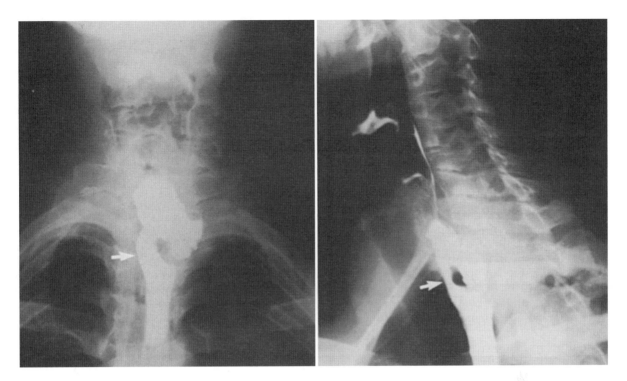

Figure 43–22.   Posteroanterior *(left)* and lateral *(right)* views of a barium swallow in a patient with a recurrent Zenker diverticulum after two previous diverticulectomies, each one complicated by disruption of the suture line and an esophagocutaneous fistula. The undivided cricopharyngeus muscle *(arrow)* causing the obstruction distal to the pouch is evident. An esophagomyotomy to relieve this neuromotor dysfunction causing the obstruction had not been performed. A third diverticulectomy, this time combined with esophagomyotomy, resulted in relief of dysphagia. The diverticulum has not recurred after 10 years of follow-up.

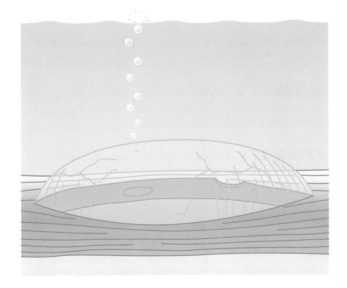

Figure 43–23.   Testing for inadvertent esophageal perforation after esophagomyotomy. The esophageal mucosa is distended by insufflating air down an intraesophageal nasogastric tube. Air bubbles escaping from the esophagus submerged under saline indicate a perforation. (From Orringer MB: Complications of esophageal surgery and trauma. In Greenfield LJ [ed]: Complications in Surgery and Trauma, 2nd ed. Philadelphia, JB Lippincott, 1990, p 322.)

diverticulectomy and esophagomyotomy, the neck wound must be opened, irrigated, and drained, as described earlier for the treatment of cervical anastomotic disruption. Nutrition may be maintained with either nasogastric feedings or total parenteral support. Broad-spectrum antibiotics are administered. With an adequate esophagomyotomy that has relieved the distal obstruction, the incidence of leak from a diverticulectomy suture line should be exceedingly low. If a cervical salivary fistula does occur, however, spontaneous closure within 7 to 10 days should be expected. If an intrathoracic esophageal suture line leak occurs within several days of diverticulectomy, immediate re-exploration of the chest with closure of the fistula and reinforcement with anterior mediastinal fat, adjacent pleura, intercostal muscle, or omentum is indicated.

Esophagomyotomy for Achalasia or Esophageal Spasm

The megaesophagus of achalasia may contain 1 to 2 L of stagnant intraesophageal contents. Induction of general anesthesia in such a patient represents the most dangerous part of the operation. Because a nasogastric tube interferes with deep breathing and adequate clearing of pulmonary secretions, one should not use an intraesophageal nasogastric tube for several days preoperatively to decompress the dilated esophagus. Rather, the patient is restricted to a clear liquid diet for 2 days before the operation, and then immediately before induction of general anesthesia, with the patient in a sitting position, a nasogastric tube is passed, and the esophagus is aspirated and evacuated. Rapid-sequence induction of anesthesia is then carried out while constant pressure is maintained on the cricoid cartilage to prevent regurgitation of esophageal contents into the pharynx until the endotracheal tube balloon is inflated. Once the airway is protected, rigid esophagoscopy is carried out, and the esophagus is evacuated and irrigated.

After completion of the esophagomyotomy, integrity of the esophageal mucosa is documented by insufflating air into the esophagus through an indwelling intraesophageal nasogastric tube. As described earlier, identification plus closure of an inadvertent esophageal injury at this point is far simpler than when the perforation is detected hours to days after surgery. Patients with achalasia are frequently referred for surgery after failed pneumatic dilatation or, more recently, unsuccessful intrasphincteric injection of botulinum toxin. These previous endoscopic interventions may increase the difficulty of identifying tissue planes at the time of subsequent esophagomyotomy. In particular, patients who have previously undergone botulinum toxin injection and obtained some relief of achalasia symptoms are more likely to have periesophageal fibrosis and, consequently, a greater risk, as high as 50%, for esophageal perforation during esophagomyotomy and less palliation of their symptoms after surgery. Periesophageal fibrosis was less prevalent in patients who had previously been treated by pneumatic dilatation, and it did not appear to affect surgical outcomes after esophagomyotomy.[56,57]

Regardless of the approach used, potential complications exist and may require reoperation in 10% to 15% of patients after esophagomyotomy. If a complete distal esophagomyotomy is not performed and the obstruction relieved, dysphagia and regurgitation will continue in the immediate postoperative period and a reoperation may be necessary.[58] Alternatively, if the esophagomyotomy is carried onto the stomach to ensure adequate relief of the esophageal obstruction, the uncoordinated lower esophageal sphincter may be converted to an incompetent one, with ensuing long-term complications of reflux esophagitis. Furthermore, a "long" esophagomyotomy, greater than 5 cm with extension onto the stomach, has been associated with "diverticularization" of the mucosa in long-term follow-up.[59,60]

Controversy exists about the need for a concomitant antireflux procedure with the distal esophagomyotomy, which may render the lower esophageal sphincter incompetent.[61-63] With a few notable exceptions, the majority of esophageal surgeons now advocate partial fundoplication to prevent the subsequent development of gastroesophageal reflux after esophagomyotomy for achalasia.[64] A Belsey-type partial fundoplication has been recommended when esophagomyotomy is approached transthoracically, whereas Toupet (posterior) or Dor (anterior) fundoplasty is typically recommended after transabdominal esophagomyotomy. When performing a fundoplication to ensure lower esophageal sphincter

competence in an atonic esophagus, care must be exercised to avoid subsequent obstruction as a result of overaggressive fundoplication.

Among the more difficult problems of surgery for achalasia is the development of recurrent dysphagia and regurgitation secondary to esophageal obstruction occurring 1 or more years after a previous esophagomyotomy. Although esophagomyotomy has become the standard surgical approach to patients with achalasia, in those with a tortuous megaesophagus and a supradiaphragmatic pouch of esophagus, delayed esophageal emptying may occur even after a satisfactory esophagomyotomy. Furthermore, a patient who has undergone a previous esophagomyotomy and has recurrent symptoms has only a 40% to 70% chance of experiencing a good result from a "redo" esophagomyotomy.[65,66] Finally, esophagomyotomy remains a palliative operation for patients with esophageal motor disorders involving the body of the esophagus and lower esophageal sphincter. Patients with achalasia remain at risk for the development of esophageal squamous cell carcinoma and should undergo routine surveillance upper endoscopy after esophagomyotomy. In patients with either recurrent or persistent symptoms of achalasia, with or without associated reflux esophagitis, esophagectomy may provide the best option by eliminating the esophageal obstruction as well as the potential for the late development of carcinoma.[67]

SUGGESTED READINGS

Luketich JD, Grondin SC, Pearson FG: Minimally invasive approaches to acquired shortening of the esophagus: Laparoscopic Collis-Nissen gastroplasty. Semin Thorac Cardiovasc Surg 12:173, 2000.

Patti MG, Feo CV, Arcerito M, et al: Effects of previous treatment on results of laparoscopic Heller myotomy for achalasia. Dig Dis Sci 44:2270, 1999.

Zwischenberger JB, Savage C, Bidani A: Surgical aspects of esophageal disease: Perforation and caustic injury. Am J Respir Crit Care Med 165:1037, 2002.

REFERENCES

1. Henderson RD, Boszko A, VanNostrand AW, et al: Pharyngoesophageal dysphagia and recurrent laryngeal nerve palsy. J Thorac Cardiovasc Surg 68:507, 1974.
2. Salama FD, Lamont G: Long-term results of the Belsey Mark IV antireflux operation in relation to the severity of esophagitis. J Thorac Cardiovasc Surg 100:517, 1990.
3. Orringer MB, Skinner DB, Belsey RH: Long-term results of the Mark IV operation for hiatal hernia and analyses of recurrences and their treatment. J Thorac Cardiovasc Surg 63:25, 1972.
4. Pearson FG, Langer B, Henderson RD: Gastroplasty and Belsey hiatus hernia repair. An operation for the management of peptic stricture with acquired short esophagus. J Thorac Cardiovasc Surg 61:50, 1971.
5. Orringer MB, Orringer JS, Dabich L, et al: Combined Collis gastroplasty–fundoplication operations for scleroderma reflux esophagitis. Surgery 90:624, 1981.
6. Pearson FG: Hiatus hernia and gastroesophageal reflux: Indications for surgery and selection of operation. Semin Thorac Cardiovasc Surg 9:163, 1997.

7. Lam TC, Fok M, Cheng SW, et al: Anastomotic complications after esophagectomy for cancer. A comparison of neck and chest anastomoses. J Thorac Cardiovasc Surg 104:395, 1992.

8. Michel L, Grillo HC, Malt RA: Esophageal perforation. Ann Thorac Surg 33:203, 1982.

9. White RK, Morris DM: Diagnosis and management of esophageal perforations. Am Surg 58:112, 1992.

10. Bufkin BL, Miller JI Jr, Mansour KA: Esophageal perforation: Emphasis on management. Ann Thorac Surg 61:1447, 1996.

11. Zwischenberger JB, Savage C, Bidani A: Surgical aspects of esophageal disease: Perforation and caustic injury. Am J Respir Crit Care Med 165:1037, 2002.

12. Cameron JL, Kieffer RF, Hendrix TR, et al: Selective nonoperative management of contained intrathoracic esophageal disruptions. Ann Thorac Surg 27:404, 1979.

13. Andersen OS, Giustra PE: Nonoperative management of contained esophageal perforation. Arch Surg 116:1214, 1981.

14. Michel L, Grillo HC, Malt RA: Operative and nonoperative management of esophageal perforations. Ann Surg 194:57, 1981.

15. Flynn AE, Verrier ED, Way LW, et al: Esophageal perforation. Arch Surg 124:1211, 1989.

16. Whyte RI, Iannettoni MD, Orringer MB: Intrathoracic esophageal perforation: The merit of primary repair. J Thorac Cardiovasc Surg 109:140, 1995.

17. Orringer MB: Complications of esophageal surgery and trauma. In Greenfield LJ (ed): Complications in Surgery and Trauma, 2nd ed. Philadelphia, JB Lippincott, 1990, p 313.

18. Gouge TH, Depan HJ, Spencer FC: Experience with the Grillo pleural wrap procedure in 18 patients with perforation of the thoracic esophagus. Ann Surg 209:612, 1989.

19. Wright CD, Mathisen DJ, Wain JC, et al: Reinforced primary repair of thoracic esophageal perforation. Ann Thorac Surg 60:245, 1995.

20. Iannettoni MD, Vlessis AA, Whyte RI, et al: Functional outcome after surgical treatment of esophageal perforation. Ann Thorac Surg 64:1606, 1997.

21. Hernandez L, Jacobson J, Harris M: Comparison among the perforation rates of Maloney, balloon, and Savary dilation of esophageal strictures. Gastrointest Endosc 51:460, 2000.

22. Kubba H, Spinou E, Brown D: Is same-day discharge suitable following rigid esophagoscopy? Findings in a series of 655 cases. Ear Nose Throat J 82:33, 2003.

23. Langer FB, Wenzl E, Prager G, et al: Management of postoperative esophageal leaks with the Polyflex self-expanding covered plastic stent. Ann Thorac Surg 79:398, 2005.

24. Patel HJ, Tan BB, Yee J, et al: A twenty-five year experience with open primary transthoracic repair of paraesophageal hiatal hernia. J Thorac Cardiovasc Surg 127:843, 2004.

25. Khaitan L, Ray WA, Holzman MD, et al: Health care utilization after medical and surgical therapy for gastroesophageal reflux disease: A population-based study, 1996 to 2000. Arch Surg 138:1356, 2003.

26. Bowers SP, Mattar SG, Smith CD, et al: Clinical and histologic follow-up after antireflux surgery for Barrett's esophagus. J Gastrointest Surg 6:532, 2002.

27. Watson DI, Baigrie RJ, Jamieson GG: A learning curve for laparoscopic fundoplication. Definable, avoidable, or a waste of time? Ann Surg 224:198, 1996.

28. Pearson FG, Cooper JD, Ilves R, et al: Massive hiatal hernia with incarceration: A report of 53 cases. Ann Thorac Surg 35:45, 1983.

29. Maziak DE, Todd TR, Pearson FG: Massive hiatus hernia: Evaluation and surgical management. J Thorac Cardiovasc Surg 115:53, 1998.

30. Johnson AB, Oddsdottir M, Hunter JG: Laparoscopic Collis gastroplasty and Nissen fundoplication. A new technique for the management of esophageal foreshortening. Surg Endosc 12:1055, 1998.

31. Luketich JD, Grondin SC, Pearson FG: Minimally invasive approaches to acquired shortening of the esophagus: Laparoscopic Collis-Nissen gastroplasty. Semin Thorac Cardiovasc Surg 12:173, 2000.

32. Orringer MB, Marshall B, Iannettoni MD: Eliminating the cervical esophagogastric anastomotic leak with a side-to-side stapled anastomosis. J Thorac Cardiovasc Surg 119:277, 2000.

33. Orringer M, Lemmer J: Early dilation in the treatment of esophageal disruption. Ann Thorac Surg 42:536, 1986.

34. Iannettoni MD, Whyte RI, Orringer MB: Catastrophic complications of the cervical esophagogastric anastomosis. J Thorac Cardiovasc Surg 110:1493, 1995.

35. Orringer MB, Marshall B, Iannettoni MD: Transhiatal esophagectomy: Clinical experience and refinements. Ann Surg 230:392, 1999.

36. Dewar L, Gelfand G, Finley RJ, et al: Factors affecting cervical anastomotic leak and stricture formation following esophagogastrectomy and gastric tube interposition. Am J Surg 163:484, 1992.

37. Vigneswaran WT, Trastek VF, Pairolero PC, et al: Transhiatal esophagectomy for carcinoma of the esophagus. Ann Thorac Surg 56:838, 1993.

38. Gandhi SK, Naunheim KS: Complications of transhiatal esophagectomy. Chest Surg Clin N Am 7:601, 1997.

39. Kirsch M, Blue M, Desai RK, et al: Intralesional steroid injections for peptic esophageal strictures. Gastrointest Endosc 37:180, 1991.

40. Lee M, Kubik C, Polhamus C, et al: Preliminary experience with endoscopic intralesional steroid injection therapy for refractory upper gastrointestinal strictures. Gastrointest Endosc 41:598, 1995.

41. Law SY, Fok M, Cheng SW, et al: A comparison of outcome after resection for squamous cell carcinomas and adenocarcinomas of the esophagus and cardia. Surg Gynecol Obstet 175:107, 1992.

42. Gillinov AM, Heitmiller RF: Strategies to reduce pulmonary complications after transhiatal esophagectomy. Dis Esophagus 11:43, 1998.

43. Doty JR, Salazar JD, Forastiere AA, et al: Postesophagectomy morbidity, mortality, and length of hospital stay after preoperative chemoradiation therapy. Ann Thorac Surg 74:227, 2002.

44. Burt M, Diehl W, Martini N, et al: Malignant esophagorespiratory fistula: Management options and survival. Ann Thorac Surg 52:1222, 1991.

45. Urschel JD, Blewett CJ, Young JE, et al: Pyloric drainage (pyloroplasty) or no drainage in gastric reconstruction after esophagectomy: A meta-analysis of randomized controlled trials. Dig Surg 19:160, 2002.

46. Ludwig DJ, Thirlby RC, Low DE: A prospective evaluation of dietary status and symptoms after near-total esophagectomy without gastric emptying procedure. Am J Surg 181:454, 2001.

47. Fok M, Cheng SW, Wong J: Pyloroplasty versus no drainage in gastric replacement of the esophagus. Am J Surg 162:447, 1991.

48. Katariya K, Harvey JC, Pina E, et al: Complications of transhiatal esophagectomy. J Surg Oncol 57:157, 1994.

49. Heitmiller RF, Gillinov AM, Jones B: Transhiatal herniation of colon after esophagectomy and gastric pull-up. Ann Thorac Surg 63:554, 1997.

50. Merigliano S, Molena D, Ruol A, et al: Chylothorax complicating esophagectomy for cancer: A plea for early thoracic duct ligation. J Thorac Cardiovasc Surg 119:453, 2000.

51. Wemyss-Holden SA, Launois B, Maddern GJ: Management of thoracic duct injuries after oesophagectomy. Br J Surg 88:1442, 2001.

52. Orringer MB, Bluett M, Deeb GM: Aggressive treatment of chylothorax complicating transhiatal esophagectomy without thoracotomy. Surgery 104:720, 1988.

53. Magee MJ, Landreneau RJ, Keenan RJ, et al: Peripheral atheroembolism from the aorta complicating transhiatal esophagectomy. Am J Surg 60:634, 1994.

54. Kirschner M: Ein neues Verfahren der oesophagus plastik. Arch Klin Chir 114:606, 1920.

55. Meunier B, Stasik C, Raoul J-L, et al: Gastric bypass for malignant esophagotracheal fistula: A series of 21 cases. Eur J Cardiothorac Surg 13:184, 1998.

56. Patti MG, Feo CV, Arcerito M, et al: Effects of previous treatment on results of laparoscopic Heller myotomy for achalasia. Dig Dis Sci 44:2270, 1999.

57. Wiechmann RJ, Ferguson MK, Naunheim KS, et al: Video-assisted surgical management of achalasia of the esophagus. J Thorac Cardiovasc Surg 118:916, 1999.

58. Patti MG, Molena D, Fisichella PM, et al: Laparoscopic Heller myotomy and Dor fundoplication for achalasia: Analysis of successes and failures. Arch Surg 136:870, 2001.

59. Chen L-Q, Chughtai T, Sideris L, et al: Long-term effects of myotomy and partial fundoplication for esophageal achalasia. Dis Esophagus 15:171, 2002.

60. Ellis FH Jr: Failure after esophagomyotomy for esophageal motor disorders. Causes, prevention, and management. Chest Surg Clin N Am 7:477, 1997.

61. Richards WO, Sharp KW, Holzman MD: An antireflux procedure should not routinely be added to a Heller myotomy. J Gastroint Surg 5:13, 2001.

62. Peters JH: An antireflux procedure is critical to the long-term outcome of esophageal myotomy for achalasia. J Gastrointest Surg 5:17, 2001.

63. Lyass S, Thoman D, Steiner JP, et al: Current status of an antireflux procedure in laparoscopic Heller myotomy: Outcomes of laparoscopic fundoplication for gastroesophageal reflux disease and paraesophageal hernia. Surg Endosc 17:554, 2003.

64. Ellis FH Jr, Watkins E Jr, Gibb SP, et al: Ten to 20-year clinical results after short esophagomyotomy without an antireflux procedure (modified Heller operation) for esophageal achalasia. Eur J Cardiothorac Surg 6:86, 1992.

65. Gorecki PJ, Hinder RA, Libbey JS, et al: Redo laparoscopic surgery for achalasia. Surg Endosc 16:772, 2002.

66. Ellis FH Jr, Crozier RE, Gibb SP: Reoperative achalasia surgery. J Thorac Cardiovasc Surg 92:859, 1986.

67. Devaney EJ, Iannettoni MD, Orringer MB, et al: Esophagectomy for achalasia: Patient selection and clinical experience. Ann Thorac Surg 72:854, 2001.

Femoral Hernia

Daniel E. Swartz · Edward L. Felix

A femoral hernia (Greek *hernios*, offshoot or bud) is a protrusion of preperitoneal fat, bladder, or peritoneal sac with or without intraperitoneal contents through the femoral ring. It becomes clinically evident once the exit of the femoral canal, or the femoral orifice, is breached. Accounting for 2% to 8% of adult groin hernias, a femoral hernia is three to five times more common in women than men, rarely occurs in children, and is most commonly seen in patients between the ages of 40 and 70 years, with a peak incidence during the sixth decade. Since the laparoscopic era, the reported incidence of femoral hernia has increased to 11% of groin hernias.[1,2] Approximately 27,000 femoral herniorrhaphies are performed annually in the United States.

ANATOMY

The femoral canal is an elliptically shaped inverted cone measuring approximately 2 cm in length that extends from the femoral ring superomedially to the femoral orifice inferolaterally (Fig. 44–1A and B). Located just medial to the femoral vessels, it is lined by the transversalis fascia and normally contains lymphatics, adipose tissue, and commonly the lymph node of Cloquet (Fig. 44–2). The femoral ring, or entrance to the canal, is lined by the iliopubic tract anterosuperiorly after it crosses anterior to the femoral vessels. The fibers of the iliopubic tract spread out in a fan-shaped manner, the superior fibers of which curve posteriorly, insert into the superior ramus, and form the medial margin of the ring. The inferior fibers of the iliopubic tract descend vertically to join the fascia lata and form the medial wall of the femoral canal. The femoral ring, furthermore, is bordered inferoposteriorly by Cooper's ligament and laterally by the femoral sheath. The femoral canal is enveloped by the fascia lata, with the superficial layer forming the anterior wall and the deep layer forming the posterior wall. The medial wall of the canal is composed of the descending fibers of the iliopubic tract and fascia lata, which are supported by the lacunar (Gimbernat's) ligament. The femoral canal normally ends blindly; however, when a femoral hernia is present, an opening known as the femoral orifice is created. The femoral orifice is bounded posteriorly by the pectineal fascia, laterally by the femoral sheath, anteriorly by the superior cornu of the fascia lata, and medially by the fan-shaped fibers of the iliopubic tract.[3,4]

HISTORY

Femoral hernia was first distinguished from inguinal hernia by Guy de Chauliac in 1363 in his text *Chirugia Magna*.[5] It was further described by Barbette in 1687, but the first detailed account of femoral canal anatomy was not recorded until 1817 by Cloquet.[6] There are three classic approaches to a femoral hernia: femoral, inguinal, and preperitoneal. The femoral approach was first described by Socin in 1879. He performed high ligation of the sac alone and noted a high recurrence rate. Bassini, in 1885, used a femoral approach to close the femoral ring with suture. He sutured the inguinal ligament to the pectineal fascia and lacunar ligament. Marcy,

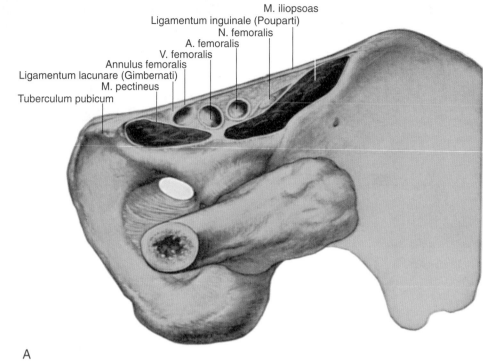

M. iliopsoas
Ligamentum inguinale (Pouparti)
N. femoralis
A. femoralis
V. femoralis
Annulus femoralis
Ligamentum lacunare (Gimbernati)
M. pectineus
Tuberculum pubicum

A

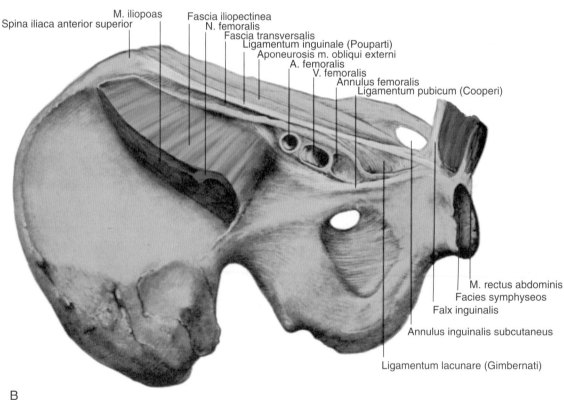

M. iliopoas
Spina iliaca anterior superior
Fascia iliopectinea
N. femoralis
Fascia transversalis
Ligamentum inguinale (Pouparti)
Aponeurosis m. obliqui externi
A. femoralis
V. femoralis
Annulus femoralis
Ligamentum pubicum (Cooperi)

M. rectus abdominis
Facies symphyseos
Falx inguinalis

Annulus inguinalis subcutaneus

Ligamentum lacunare (Gimbernati)

B

Figure 44–1. Bone and ligamentous anatomy of the femoral canal and related structures as viewed from the thigh **(A)** and from the pelvis **(B)**.

in 1892, used a purse-string suture to close the femoral ring.[7] It was not until 1974 that a tension-free repair with a cylindrical roll of polypropylene mesh to plug the femoral canal was described by Lichtenstein and Shore.[12] This approach was subsequently modified by

others, including Gilbert, Rutkow and Robbins, and Bendavid.[4,8,9]

The inguinal approach to a femoral hernia was first described by Annandale in 1876.[10] His repair consisted of high ligation of the sac. The first repair approximating

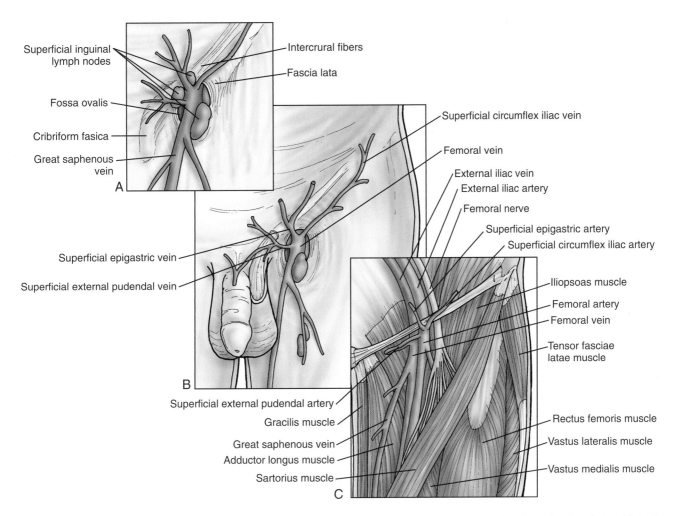

Figure 44–2. Superficial inguinofemoral dissection. **A,** Relationship of the fossa ovalis to the deep fascia of the thigh, the inguinal ligament, and the superficial vessels. **B,** The fossa ovalis cleared of the lymphatic contents and the cribriform fascia. **C,** Exposure of the contents of the femoral trigone (of Scarpa) after all superficial structures and the deep fascia have been removed.

Cooper's ligament to the inguinal ligament was described by Ruggi in 1892. Later, Moschowicz included an inguinal floor repair to reduce the potential for recurrence of an inguinal hernia.[11] Lotheissen first described using Cooper's ligament to repair a ruptured inguinal ligament during inguinal herniorrhaphy in 1898, and this technique was later popularized by McVay and Anson in 1942 as an anatomic repair of femoral and direct inguinal hernias. They astutely noted that the transversus abdominis muscle and transversalis fascia inserted onto Cooper's ligament and not the inguinal ligament. This repair became widely accepted and more recently has included placement of prosthetic mesh plugs via the femoral ring to obliterate the canal.[4,8,9,12]

The preperitoneal approach was first described by Annandale in 1876 and further advanced by Cheatle[13] (1920) and later Henry[14] (1936) through a low midline incision. The linea alba was carefully divided with the peritoneum left intact, and the plane of dissection was bluntly created by separating the peritoneum from the bladder and pelvic brim. McEvedy used an oblique incision over the lateral border of the rectus sheath to access this plane and sutured the conjoined tendon to Cooper's ligament in 1950. Nyhus et al. (1960) advanced this procedure by using a transverse incision cephalad to the superior border of the pubis to expose the femoral ring. The hernia was reduced, the sac ligated, and the repair performed by approximating Cooper's ligament to the iliopubic tract. They later modified the technique by buttressing the repair with polypropylene mesh and reduced the recurrence rate to less than 1%.[15] In 1973, Stoppa et al. used a posterior midline approach to place a large sheet of polyester mesh bilaterally.[16] A unilateral preperitoneal hernia repair using ring-supported mesh inserted through a small 2- to 3-cm incision was subsequently popularized by Kugel.[17]

The first laparoscopic transabdominal preperitoneal (TAPP) inguinal hernia repair using a mesh plug and polypropylene buttress was reported by Schultz et al. in 1990.[18] By 1993, Felix and others demonstrated that the plug was unnecessary with a laparoscopic approach and that a large sheet of mesh covering all potential hernia sites was the key to the repair.[19] The preperitoneal approach, whether open or laparoscopic, is different from the inguinal or femoral approaches in that it repairs the entire posterior floor, including the femoral defect, in all patients. In 1993, McKernan and Laws reported the first laparoscopic totally extraperitoneal (TEP) approach mimicking the open technique of Stoppa.[20] A laparoscopic intraperitoneal onlay mesh was described around the same time but was quickly abandoned because of intra-abdominal adhesions and a high recurrence rate.[5]

ETIOLOGY

A femoral hernia was initially thought to be of congenital origin with a preformed peritoneal sac. Careful anatomic studies by Keith in 1923, however, led to abandonment of this theory.[21] The acquired theory is now the most widely accepted. It proposes elevated intra-abdominal pressure as the causative factor, such as during pregnancy, constipation, and bronchitis. Preperitoneal fat is displaced through the femoral ring and may pull peritoneum with it and thereby create a sac. The normally closed femoral orifice is then opened. Femoral hernias may also be produced iatrogenically when a conventional Bassini repair under tension distorts and opens the femoral ring.

DIAGNOSIS

The classic manifestation is pain or a lump in the groin, or both. Physical examination often reveals a small nonreducible mass below the inguinal ligament. The differential diagnosis includes inguinal hernia, lymphadenopathy, lipoma, and pseudohernia. A femoral pseudohernia is a nonpathologic entity seen in extremely thin patients with bilateral masses below the inguinal ligament and medial to the femoral vessels that resolve on recumbency. The cause is accentuation of a normal fat pad and Cloquet's lymph node, which normally reside in the femoral canal, and no treatment is necessary.[6]

The presence of an incarcerated hernia in the groin should immediately raise suspicion that it is a femoral hernia because incarcerated femoral hernias outnumber all other incarcerated abdominal wall hernias combined.[4] Differentiating between a femoral and an inguinal hernia, although difficult at times, is important. The likelihood of strangulation at 3 and 21 months is 20% and 45% for femoral and only 3% and 4.5% for inguinal hernias, respectively,[22] and strangulation is associated with a mortality rate of 6% to 23%.[4] The sensitivity and positive predictive value of physical examination by surgeons have been shown to be only 50% and 37.5%, respectively.[22] There have been reports of the use of contrast herniography, color Doppler ultrasound, and computed tomography to diagnose femoral hernias, but no rigorous study has been performed to determine their accuracy.[23-26] Physical examination therefore remains the mainstay of preoperative diagnosis.

Nyhus described two ways to differentiate femoral from inguinal hernias: first, the pubic tubercle will be felt superior and medial to a femoral hernia; in contrast, it will be felt inferior and lateral to an inguinal hernia. Second, with the hernia reduced, the examiner places a finger at the medial end of the inguinal ligament and has the patient cough. A femoral hernia will appear below the finger, whereas an inguinal hernia will appear above it.[27] Another method is to follow the adductor longus tendon caudally from the inguinal ligament and place fingers lateral to the tendon (one fingerbreadth medial to the femoral artery) and have the patient cough. The presence of a bulge suggests that it is an inguinal hernia because a femoral hernia should stay reduced.[22]

TREATMENT

As previously discussed, there are three basic approaches to treatment: femoral, inguinal, and preperitoneal, the latter of which includes open and laparoscopic approaches. Suture, mesh, or both may be used in all three approaches. Each technique has advantages and disadvantages, but in the hands of skilled and experienced surgeons, each has been shown to have low complication and recurrence rates. With a nonincarcerated, nonstrangulated femoral hernia, any of the techniques may be applied; with incarceration or strangulation, however, the femoral and laparoscopic TEP repairs should be avoided. Although a majority of surgeons have espoused the open inguinal approach in the presence of incarceration and strangulation, the authors prefer a laparoscopic TAPP approach. In the presence of strangulation, bowel resection will be required and prosthetic mesh should be avoided. Franklin et al. have recently reported using a biologic mesh composed of porcine small intestinal submucosa (Surgisis, Cook Surgical, Bloomington, IN) intraperitoneally to repair strangulated inguinal and incisional hernias. Even with gross contamination, the authors reported no mesh-related complications or recurrences in 58 hernia repairs with a 19-month follow-up.[28] Further studies are needed before advocating the routine use of mesh for strangulated or contaminated hernias.

The femoral approach is the simplest, requires the least dissection, and may be performed with local anesthesia (Fig. 44–3). This approach is most appropriate for a nonincarcerated, nonstrangulated femoral hernia and for high-risk surgical patients. Incarcerated hernias have been treated in this manner, although it can be difficult because visualization of femoral ring anatomy is poor. After making an inguinal or subinguinal incision, the subcutaneous fascia is divided to reveal the intact external oblique aponeurosis. The hernia sac, located just inferior to the aponeurosis, is dissected, opened, and emptied. If the hernia is incarcerated, it may be released by incising the lacunar (Gimbernat's) ligament medially and, failing that, the inguinal ligament. With the femoral approach this is often a blind maneuver and a counteringuinal incision may be required for better visualization. Once the hernia is free, the sac is opened, the contents are inspected and returned to the abdominal cavity, and the sac is ligated. The femoral canal is obliterated either with sutures or with a cylindrical polypropy-

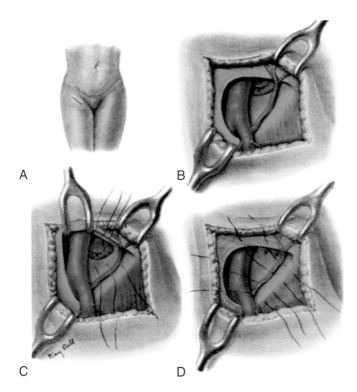

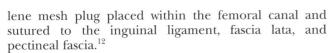

Figure 44–3. The femoral approach to repair of a right femoral hernia with suture. **A,** Incision. **B,** Dissection of the femoral orifice and canal. **C,** Placement of nonabsorbable sutures between the inguinal ligament, fascia lata, and pectineal fascia. **D,** View of the completed repair.

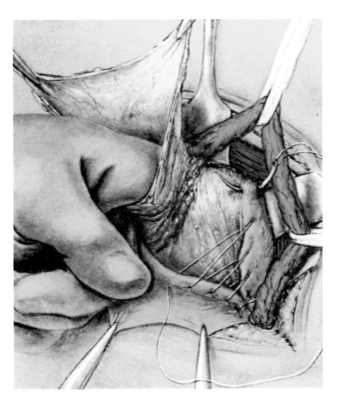

Figure 44–4. Examination for a concomitant femoral hernia during inguinal hernia repair. Examination for a concomitant inguinal hernia during repair of a femoral hernia should similarly be performed.

lene mesh plug placed within the femoral canal and sutured to the inguinal ligament, fascia lata, and pectineal fascia.[12]

The excellent exposure of the femoral ring provided by the classic inguinal approach facilitates release of the incarcerated hernia, as well as the opportunity to resect gangrenous intestine. An inguinal incision is made in the skin and carried down through the subcutaneous layers. The external oblique aponeurosis is opened in the line of its fibers from the cephalad aspect of the external ring medially until the internal ring is exposed laterally. The external oblique aponeurosis is cleared of the cremasteric muscle attachments, and the cord structures are mobilized. Careful examination of the cord and inguinal floor is necessary to exclude the presence of a concomitant inguinal hernia (Fig. 44–4). The floor of the inguinal canal (transversalis fascia) is opened and the femoral hernia sac exposed. If necessary, an aberrant obturator artery may be ligated at this point. In the event of an incarcerated hernia, the contents of the sac must be examined for viability after the hernia is reduced. An incarceration is released by dividing the fibers of the iliopubic tract and lacunar ligament at the medial edge of the femoral ring. In rare cases the inguinal ligament must be divided, but this should be avoided if possible because of the increased likelihood of recurrence. Once the contents of the hernia sac are examined and returned to the abdominal cavity, the sac is ligated at the level of the peritoneal cavity and the repair is performed.

It can be done either by suture approximation of the iliopubic tract to Cooper's ligament (Fig. 44–5) or, preferably, in the absence of strangulation, by polypropylene mesh repair to obliterate the femoral ring and canal. This may be achieved with several shapes of plugs, including cylindrical,[12] umbrella,[5] or dart with a base[29] fashioned to the inguinal ligament and iliopubic tract anteriorly, Cooper's ligament posteriorly, the femoral sheath laterally, and the iliopubic tract and lacunar ligament medially with nonabsorbable suture. Inguinal herniorrhaphy should be included to prevent an iatrogenic hernia.[11] Because of reports of chronic pain after the use of mesh plug repairs,[30] Amid at the Lichtenstein Hernia Institute has abandoned the use of plugs in favor of a polypropylene mesh sheet that covers the femoral ring in addition to the inguinal floor.[31]

The open, preperitoneal approach remains popular[13-16] because it permits excellent exposure, it allows for rapid intraperitoneal access to control any strangulated viscera, and mesh permits repair of all three potential hernia sites, including a femoral hernia (Fig. 44–6). Access is through a transverse lower abdominal incision 3 cm cephalad to the typical inguinal incision. The subcutaneous fascia is dissected to expose the anterior rectus sheath and external oblique aponeurosis. The anterior rectus sheath is divided cephalad to the internal ring, and the rectus abdominis is retracted medially to expose the posterior inguinal wall. The sac is carefully reduced while maintaining control of the contents for

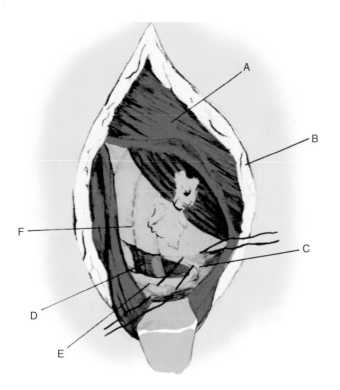

Figure 44–5. Inguinal approach to repair of a femoral hernia using suture approximation of the iliopubic tract to Cooper's ligament. Closure of the peritoneum (sac excision and ligation) has already been performed.

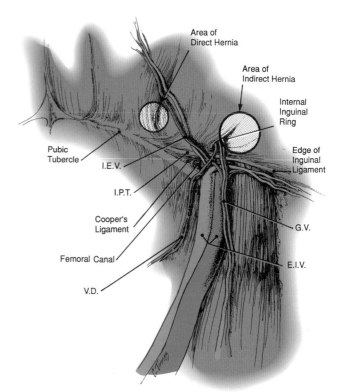

Figure 44–6. Schematic view of the extraperitoneal anatomy as seen from the open or laparoscopic preperitoneal approach. Direct and indirect hernia spaces, as well as the femoral canal, are shown. E.I.V., external iliac vein; I.E.V., inferior epigastric vessel; I.P.T., iliopubic tract.

examination. If the hernia is incarcerated, an incision through the iliopubic tract where the fibers insert onto Cooper's ligament at the medial border of the femoral ring should release it. Once strangulation is excluded by opening the sac and examining its contents, the peritoneum is closed. Small primary femoral hernias (Nyhus type IIIC) can be repaired with three to five nonabsorbable sutures approximating the iliopubic tract to Cooper's ligament. Large, recurrent, or complex femoral hernias (Nyhus type IV) can be repaired in the same manner but usually require a mesh buttress. Alternatively, they may be repaired with mesh without suture approximation of the femoral ring. Polypropylene mesh is placed as a sheet that covers the femoral ring and the direct and indirect spaces with a 2- to 3-cm overlap.

The Kugel repair is the newest modification of the preperitoneal approach. A ring-reinforced double layer of polypropylene mesh (Davol, Cranston, RI) is placed in the preperitoneal space through a small 3-cm oblique incision by blunt finger dissection.[17] Today, mesh repairs are preferred by most surgeons, but in the presence of contamination or strangulation, prosthetic material should be avoided.

The laparoscopic approach to hernia repair has become increasingly popular with advanced laparoscopic surgeons. The technique combines the benefits of laparoscopic procedures (reduced postoperative pain and early return to activities) and the preperitoneal approach (excellent exposure, easy intraperitoneal access for visceral examination or resection, and cover-

age of all three potential groin hernia sites with a single sheet of mesh). There are two accepted techniques: TAPP and TEP (Fig. 44–7). Many surgeons favor the TEP technique for elective repairs because it avoids potential intraperitoneal complications, but the TAPP technique is equally acceptable.[2] Most surgeons perform TAPP repairs for hernias with incarceration or strangulation because of improved visibility and control of incarcerated viscera, but Ferzli et al. have suggested that the TEP technique can also be used.[32] If necessary, bowel resection may be performed either laparoscopically or with conventional laparotomy, depending on the experience of the surgeon.

The TEP technique involves dissection of the preperitoneal space and the cord structures beyond the separation of the vas deferens and testicular vessels, as well as any hernia within the indirect, direct, or femoral spaces.[19] The peritoneum must be dissected back so that it lies completely posterior to the inferior edge of the mesh. When a TAPP technique is used, the peritoneum is opened 2 cm superior to the internal ring and is dissected down to expose all three potential groin hernia sites. After completing the hernia repair, a TAPP technique requires careful reapproximation of the peritoneum. Whether a TAPP or TEP technique is used, incarcerated femoral hernias are released by dividing the superomedial aspect of the femoral ring where the

Table 44–1   Recurrence Rates After Primary Femoral Hernia Repair

Author	Year	N	Approach	Follow-up	Recurrence (%)
Amid[3]	1994	200	Femoral, mesh plug	1-15 yr	0.5
Bendavid[4]	1994	329	Inguinal, mesh plug	—	1.8
Felix[2]	1997	85	TAPP, TEP	2 yr (median)	0
Glassow[36]	1985	1138	Femoral, suture	—	1.9
Hachisuka[7]	2003	67	Femoral, mesh	—	1.5
Hernandez[37]	2000	51	TAPP	1 yr	0
Kapiris[38]	2001	19	TAPP	3.75 yr	0
Swarnkar[39]	2003	43	Femoral, mesh plug	2 yr (median)	0
Trabucco[29]	1994	40	Femoral, mesh dart	1-4 yr	2.5

TAPP, transabdominal preperitoneal; TEP, totally extraperitoneal.

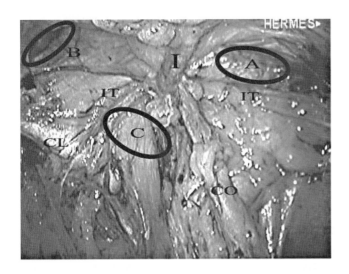

Figure 44–7. View of the extraperitoneal anatomy during a laparoscopic totally extraperitoneal technique. A, direct hernia; B, indirect space; C, femoral space; CL, Cooper's ligament; CO, spermatic cord structures; I, inferior epigastric vessels; IT, iliopubic tract medial and lateral to the inferior epigastric vessels.

iliopubic tract inserts into Cooper's ligament. Once all the dissection is completed, a polypropylene mesh is placed over the entire floor. The mesh may be fixed in place with anchors or placed without fixation. The authors' preferred technique is the use of preformed mesh (Bard 3-D Max) that conforms to the pelvis and does not require fixation.[33,34]

RESULTS

A comprehensive list of primary femoral hernia repair studies and their outcomes is presented in Table 44–1. Swarnkar et al. reported no recurrences to a median 2-year follow-up in 43 femoral hernias repaired via a femoral approach with a polypropylene mesh plug.[35] Trabucco reported a single recurrence (2.5%) with a 1- to

4-year follow-up in 40 femoral hernias repaired via dart-shaped polypropylene mesh plugs through an inguinal approach.[29] Bendavid fashions an umbrella-shaped polypropylene mesh placed via an inguinal approach and has reported a 1.8% recurrence rate in 329 repairs.[4] Glassow has reported repair of 1138 primary femoral hernias by suture via a femoral approach, with 21 recurrences (1.9%).[36]

Hernandez-Richter and colleagues reported no recurrences in a 12-month follow-up of 51 femoral hernias repaired by a laparoscopic TAPP technique.[37] Kapiris et al. retrospectively reported the outcomes of laparoscopic TAPP repairs in 3017 patients over a 7-year period, including 16 femoral hernia repairs. The authors reported 22 recurrences for a rate of 0.72%, but only 5 recurrences in the last 3205 patients when a larger (10 × 15 cm) sheet of mesh was used.[38] Felix and associates reported using both TEP and TAPP techniques to repair 1173 groin hernias, 16 of were pure femoral hernias and 69 had a femoral component to an inguinal hernia. Of these 85 femoral hernias, there were no recurrences over a 2-year median follow-up.[2] In another series of 90 recurrent inguinal hernias repaired laparoscopically with TAPP and TEP techniques, 8 hernias had a femoral component, and no re-recurrences were discovered during a median 14-month follow-up.[39]

COMMENTARY

The incidence of femoral hernias is relatively rare when compared with that of inguinal hernias. Femoral hernias account for 2% to 8% of all groin hernias. Differentiating femoral from inguinal hernias preoperatively is an inexact science, and definitive diagnosis requires surgical examination. Crawford et al. found that a preoperative diagnosis of groin hernia was incorrect 56% of the time in 253 patients, with ipsilateral femoral hernias and contralateral inguinal and femoral hernias frequently being missed.[1] Unlike the unnecessary attempt to distinguish indirect from direct inguinal hernias preoperatively because both spaces are examined and repaired with an anterior approach, unsuspected femoral hernias may be missed with an anterior approach and lead to a "femoral" recurrence of the groin hernia repair. Mikkelsen et al. reviewed the Danish surgical database of 34,849 groin hernias repaired over a 3-year period and noted that the incidence of "recurrent" femoral hernia after inguinal herniorrhaphy was 15 times higher than the rate of primary femoral hernias found in that population.[40] The main advantage of the preperitoneal approach, open or laparoscopic, is the ability of the surgeon to accurately examine for and repair all groin hernias at the same time, hence potentially eliminating all missed hernias.

Surgeons at our center routinely perform laparoscopic repair of all groin hernias unless there is a contraindication such as anesthetic risk or obliteration of the preperitoneal space as a result of previous surgery or irradiation. Routine use of the laparoscope has led to the discovery of unsuspected femoral hernias in up to 11% of patients undergoing inguinal herniorrhaphy,[1,2] which suggests that the commonly touted femoral hernia rate of 2% to 8% underestimates its true incidence. Laparoscopic groin hernia repair requires extensive experience on the part of the surgeon in both TAPP and TEP techniques and has a significant learning curve.[41,42] Previous studies have found that severe complications, though rare, occur more frequently with laparoscopic than with open repair.[41,43-45] However, other series reported by experienced surgeons demonstrate low complication rates and recurrence rates of 0% to 2%, comparable to those in the open literature.[46-48] The preperitoneal approach, whether open or laparoscopic, is the preferred approach for recurrent femoral hernias because the femoral approach is associated with a 10% recurrence rate.[35] The approach that each surgeon uses should be based on the clinical situation, as well as the surgeon's experience and results. The aim of this chapter has been to provide a review of the commonly used repairs and a framework with which to select the most appropriate one.

SUGGESTED READINGS

Amid PK: Lichtenstein tension-free hernioplasty: Its inception, evolution and principles. Hernia 8:1, 2004.

Felix EL: Laparoscopic extraperitoneal inguinal hernia repair. In Eubanks WS, Swanstrom LS, Soper NJ (eds): Mastery of Endoscopic and Laparoscopic Surgery, 2nd ed. Philadelphia, Lippincott Williams & Wilkins (in press).

Hachisuka T: Femoral hernia repair. Surg Clin North Am 83:1189, 2003.

REFERENCES

1. Crawford DL, Hiatt JR, Phillips EH: Laparoscopy identifies unexpected groin hernias. Am Surg 64:976, 1998.
2. Felix EL, Michas CA, Gonzalez MH Jr: Laparoscopic hernioplasty: Why does it work? Surg Endosc 11:36, 1997.
3. Amid PK, Shulmann AG, Lichtenstein IL: Femoral hernia (Part I): Anatomy of the femoral canal. In Bendavid R (ed): Prostheses and Abdominal Wall Hernias. Boca Raton, FL, CRC Press, 1994, p 408.
4. Bendavid R: Femoral hernia (Part III): An "umbrella" for femoral hernia repair. In Bendavid R (ed): Prostheses and Abdominal Wall Hernias. Boca Raton, FL, CRC Press, 1994, p 413.
5. Lau WY: History of treatment of groin hernia. World J Surg 26:748, 2002.
6. Bendavid R: Femoral pseudo-hernias. Hernia 6:141, 2002.
7. Hachisuka T: Femoral hernia repair. Surg Clin North Am 83:1189, 2003.
8. Gilbert AI: Sutureless repair of inguinal hernia. Am J Surg 163:331, 1992.
9. Rutkow IM, Robbins AW: "Tension-free" inguinal herniorrhaphy: A preliminary report on the "mesh plug" technique. Surgery 114:3, 1993.
10. Read RC: British contributions to modern herniology of the groin. Hernia 9:6, 2005.
11. Moschowitz AV: Femoral hernia; a new operation for radical cure. N Y J Med 21:1087, 1907.
12. Lichtenstein IL, Shore JM: Simplified repair of femoral and recurrent inguinal hernias by a "plug" technique. Am J Surg 128:439, 1974.
13. Cheatle G: An operation for the radical cure of inguinal and femoral hernia. BMJ 2:68, 1920.
14. Henry AK: Operation for a femoral hernia: My midline extraperitoneal approach. Lancet 1:531, 1936.
15. Nyhus LM, Condon RE, Harkins HN: Clinical experiences with preperitoneal hernia repair for all types of hernia of the groin. Am J Surg 100:234, 1960.
16. Stoppa R, Petit J, Abourachid H, et al: Procede original de plastie des hernia de l'aine: L'Interposition sous fixation d'une prothese en tulle de Dacron par voie mediane sous-peritoneale. Chirurgie 99:199, 1973.
17. Kugel RD: The Kugel repair for groin hernias. Surg Clin North Am 83:1119, 2003.
18. Schultz LS, Graber JN, Peritrafitta J, Hickok DF: Laser laparoscopic herniorrhaphy: A clinical trial preliminary results. J Laparoendosc Surg 1:41, 1990.
19. Felix EL: Laparoscopic extraperitoneal inguinal hernia repair. In Eubanks WS, Swanstrom LS, Soper NJ (eds): Mastery of Endoscopic and Laparoscopic Surgery, 2nd ed. Philadelphia, Lippincott Williams & Wilkins (in press).
20. McKernan JB, Laws HL: Laparoscopic repair of inguinal hernias using a totally extraperitoneal prosthetic approach. Surg Endosc 7:26, 1993.
21. Keith A: On the origin and nature of hernia. Br J Surg 11:455, 1924-5.
22. Hair A, Paterson C, O'Dwyer PJ: Diagnosis of a femoral hernia in the elective setting. J R Coll Surg Edinb 46:117, 2001.
23. Bergenfeldt M, Ekberg O, Kesek P, Lasson A: Femoral hernia: Clinical significance of radiologic diagnosis. Eur J Radiol 10:177, 1990.
24. Stabile Ianora AA, Midiri M, Vinci R, et al: Abdominal wall hernias: Imaging with spiral CT. Eur Radiol 10:914, 2000.
25. Weng TI, Wang HP, Chen WJ, et al: Ultrasound diagnosis of occult femoral hernia presenting with intestinal obstruction. Am J Emerg Med 19:333, 2001.
26. Zhang GQ, Sugiyama M, Hagi H, et al: Groin hernias in adults: Value of color Doppler sonography in their classification. J Clin Ultrasound 29:429, 2001.
27. Nyhus LM: The preperitoneal approach and iliopubic tract repair of inguinal hernias. In Nyhus LM, Condon RE (eds): Hernia, 4th ed. Philadelphia, JB Lippincott, 1995, p 153.
28. Franklin ME Jr, Gonzalez JJ, Glass JL: Use of porcine small intestinal submucosa as a prosthetic device for laparoscopic repair of hernias in contaminated fields: 2-year follow-up. Hernia 8:186, 2004.
29. Trabucco E: Femoral hernia (Part II): Femoral plug hernioplasty. In Bendavid R (ed): Prostheses and Abdominal Wall Hernias. Boca Raton, FL, CRC Press, 1994, p 411.
30. Amid PK: Personal communication, 2004.
31. Amid PK: Lichtenstein tension-free hernioplasty: Its inception, evolution and principles. Hernia 8:1, 2004.
32. Ferzli G, Shapiro K, Chaudry G, Patel S: Laparoscopic extraperitoneal approach to acutely incarcerated inguinal hernia. Surg Endosc 18:228, 2004.
33. Bell R, Price J: Laparoscopic inguinal hernia repair using an anatomically contoured three-dimensional mesh. Surg Endosc 17:1784, 2003.

34. Felix EL, Swartz DE: Laparoscopic hernioplasty without fixation. Paper presented at a meeting of the Society of American Gastrointestinal Endoscopic Surgeons, 2003, Los Angeles.

35. Swarnkar K, Hopper N, Nelson M, et al: Sutureless mesh-plug hernioplasty. Am J Surg 186:201, 2003.

36. Glassow F: Femoral hernia: Review of 2105 repairs in a 17 year period. Am J Surg 150:353, 1985.

37. Hernandez-Richter T, Schardey HM, Rau HG, et al: The femoral hernia: An ideal approach for the transabdominal preperitoneal technique (TAPP). Surg Endosc 14:736, 2000.

38. Kapiris SA, Brough WA, Royston MS, et al: Laparoscopic transabdominal preperitoneal (TAPP) hernia repair: A 7-year two-center experience in 3017 patients. Surg Endosc 15:972, 2001.

39. Felix EL, Michas CA, McKnight RL: Laparoscopic repair of recurrent hernias. Surg Endosc 9:135, 1995.

40. Mikkelsen T, Bay-Nielsen M, Kehlet H: Risk of femoral hernia after inguinal herniorrhaphy. Br J Surg 89:486, 2002.

41. Neumayer L, Giobbie-Hurder A, Jonasson O, et al: Open mesh versus laparoscopic mesh repair of inguinal hernia. N Engl J Med 350:1819, 2004.

42. Wright D, O'Dwyer P: The learning curve for laparoscopic hernia repair. Semin Laparosc Surg 5:227, 1998.

43. Hair A, Duffy K, McLean J, et al: Groin hernia repair in Scotland. Br J Surg 87:1722, 2000.

44. McCormack K, Scott NW, Go PMNYH, et al on behalf of the EU Hernia Trialists Collaboration: Laparoscopic techniques versus open techniques for inguinal hernia repair (Cochrane Review). In The Cochrane Library. Chichester, UK, John Wiley & Sons, 1:CD001785, 2003.

45. Tetik C, Arregui ME, Dulcuq JL, et al: Complications and recurrences associated with laparoscopic repair of groin hernias. A multi-institutional analysis. Surg Endosc 8:1316, 1994.

46. Felix E, Scott S, Crafton B, et al: Causes of recurrence after laparoscopic hernioplasty. Surg Endosc 12:226, 1998.

47. Phillips EH, Arregui M, Carrol J, et al: Incidence of complications following laparoscopic hernioplasty. Surg Endosc 9:16, 1995.

48. Tschudi J, Wagner M, Klaiber C, et al: Controlled multicenter trial of laparoscopic transabdominal preperitoneal hernioplasty vs Shouldice herniorrhaphy. Surg Endosc 10:845, 1996.

45

Basic Features of Groin Hernia and Its Repair

Sathyaprasad C. Burjonrappa · Samuel Cemaj ·
Robert J. Fitzgibbons, Jr.

HISTORY

The earliest written records dealing with inguinal hernias (*hernios* in Greek = budding) date back to approximately 1500 BC. Early operations involved ligation of the sac and cord at the level of the external ring with excision of the sac, cord, and testis. Celsus (3 to 64 AD) is credited with bringing the more advanced Greek medicine to Rome (Greco-Roman Era, 460 BC to 467 AD). Notable figures such as Herophilus, Erasistratus, Heliodorus, and Galen, influenced by Hippocrates, "the father of medicine," and Aristotle, "the philosopher," performed and wrote about hernia surgery with a scientific understanding of anatomy and the use of anesthesia and hemostasis by ligature. During medieval times—the "Dark Ages" (Middle Ages, 476 AD to the 15th century)—the technical advances of Alexandrian and Greco-Roman surgery were largely lost. Surgery was usually performed by barbers, most of whom were ignorant and often illiterate. Hot cautery devices were commonly used to destroy tissue and control bleeding as the art of tying off a bleeding vessel disappeared. The use of any type of anesthesia was absent, and mutilation of the testicle and castration were thought to be necessary to cure a hernia. Needless to say, complications from these brutal methods were numerous.

The Renaissance (15th through mid-17th centuries) heralded many improvements for society, and surgery was no exception. Ambroise Pare is considered by many to be the father of modern surgery. Among many contributions was his understanding of the importance of ligating vessels to control bleeding instead of hot oil or cautery. The use of anesthesia was reinstated for inguinal hernia surgery, and preserving the testicle became an essential part of the operation as described by Casper Stromayr in 1559. The 18th century surgeon/anatomists

were the first to publish treatises with illustrations based on detailed anatomic dissections. Sir Percivall Pott's *Treatise on Ruptures* refuted the older theories concerning the cause of hernias and methods of treatment (Fig. 45–1). While being the first to describe congenital hernias, he also gave a detailed description of the operative repair of incarcerated and strangulated hernias. Richter, a German surgeon, described the partial enterocele strangulation that still bears his name in *Abhandlung von den Bruchen*, one of the best-written hernia treatises of that time. A French contemporary, Alexis Littre, described herniation of a Meckel diverticulum. Jean Louis Petit recommended surgical repair of strangulated hernias only and described an external herniotomy without entering the sac, an operation that is eponymously linked to him. He also described the inferior lumbar triangle formed by the latissimus dorsi muscle, external oblique muscle, and iliac crest. It was John Hunter who renamed the lacunar ligament as Gimbernat's ligament after the Spanish anatomist described his technique of incision of the lacunar ligament for reduction of femoral hernia contents. Camper, a physician and philosopher, was the first to describe the processus vaginalis and the superficial fascia laying over the subcutaneous tissue in his *Icones Herniarum*.[1]

By the first decade of the 19th century, giants such as Astley Cooper, Franz Hesselbach, and Antonio Scarpa produced high-quality anatomy atlases that facilitated the development of modern hernia repairs. Marcy, an American surgeon and pupil of Lister, was the first to recognize the importance of the transversalis fascia and closing the internal ring when repairing an inguinal hernia. Furthermore, he emphasized the need for antisepsis. Edoardo Bassini, another pupil of Lister, described his technique of dissecting and ligating the sac high in the retroperitoneal space after dividing the transversalis fascia and emphasized the importance of including the transversalis fascia in his posterior wall buttress, which

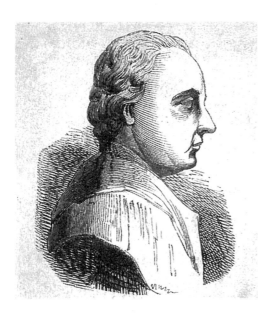

Figure 45–1. Percivall Pott (1714-1788) gave a detailed description of the operative repair of incarcerated and strangulated hernias, among many other contributions to the field. (From Rutkow IM: A selective history of hernia surgery in the late eighteenth century: The treatises of Percivall Pott, Jean Louis Petit, D. August Gottlieb Richter, Don Antonio de Gimbernat, and Pieter Camper. Surg Clin North Am 83:1021-1044, 2003.)

involved suturing the internal oblique and transversus abdominis with the upper layer of the transversalis fascia in one layer (Bassini's famous triple layer!) to the lower leaf of the transversalis fascia and the inguinal ligament with interrupted silk sutures.[2] His final results published in 1894, with a 100% follow-up at 5 years, revealed 8 recurrences in 206 operations with no operative mortality.[3] These phenomenal results have earned him the title of Father of Modern Herniorrhaphy.

Unfortunately, the results achieved by Bassini were not reproduced when his operation was adopted by the general surgical community. Protégés of Bassini have pointed out that modifications in the technique decreased its effectiveness. Perhaps most notable was omission of division of the transversalis fascia in favor of blindly grasping tissue beneath the internal oblique muscle and sewing it to the inguinal ligament. The basis of this modification was fear of bladder or neurologic injury, or both, caused by entering the preperitoneal space. This "good stuff to good stuff" approach did not result in an entirely reproducible procedure because of the variability of what was actually grasped by the Allis forceps. The only Bassini modification that offered consistently comparable results was the multilayered Shouldice repair, reported by surgeons at the Shouldice Clinic in Toronto. However, this operation was hard to teach because of difficulty understanding what was really being sewn to what. Unless specifically trained at the Shouldice Clinic with an opportunity to work with the surgeons there, the various layers in the medial flap are not reliably identified by surgeons to develop the multiple suture lines.

Proponents of prosthetic material began to express the opinion that these materials might be the solution for achieving the holy grail of a "tension-free" repair as early as the 1950s. However, the vast majority of surgeons were disinclined to use foreign material for an inguinal hernia repair because of fear of infection, erosion into surrounding structures, rejection, cost, and even carcinogenesis. By the late 1980s it had become clear that these complications were not common and that the recurrence rate after nonprosthetic herniorrhaphies was much higher than generally appreciated, especially outside specialized centers (population-based studies). Modern hernia specialists such as Lichtenstein in 1986 and Gilbert in 1987 reported their techniques of "tensionless and sutureless" repairs, which involved placing a synthetic polypropylene mesh either deep to or in front of the repaired transversalis fascia in addition to using a rolled-up strip of mesh to plug wide hernial defects. Surgeons at the Lichtenstein Institute initially applied their technique only for the repair of complicated groin hernias (large direct, pantaloon, and recurrent hernias). It was their observation of the low recurrence rate in this group that led them to apply the technique universally.

The preperitoneal space can also be used to repair an inguinal hernia. An open preperitoneal procedure was described by the ancient Hindus to relieve cases of strangulated hernia. Fruchard is credited with development of the concept that the root cause of all groin hernias is failure of the transversalis fascia to retain the peritoneum and its contents. The basis of preperitoneal repairs is to reinforce the space between the peritoneum and the transversalis fascia, thereby re-establishing the ability of the transversalis fascia to retain intra-abdominal viscera. In this model the difference between direct, indirect, and femoral hernias looses its significance because all hernias are treated the same by covering the entire myopectineal orifice. There are several different ways for the surgeon to enter the preperitoneal space for the purpose of performing the repair there. Read and Rives favor an anterior approach through a conventional groin incision. In contrast, Nyhus, Condon, and Wantz in the United States and Stoppa and others in France have been strong proponents of an extraperitoneal posterior approach, either a midline, high transverse or Pfannenstiel incision, especially for complicated or recurrent hernias. The introduction of therapeutic laparoscopy into general surgery in the early 1990s made a transabdominal approach to the same space more attractive.

EMBRYOLOGY

The processus vaginalis is a peritoneal diverticulum in the embryonic lower anterior abdominal wall that traverses the inguinal canal; in males it forms the tunica vaginalis testis. In the eighth week of fetal life, the processus vaginalis is open into the inguinal canal with an extraperitoneal gubernaculum, a mesenchymal column of tissue that connects the fetal testis to the developing scrotum and plays a role in testicular descent. The primitive testis and metanephros lie close together near the pelvic brim. As the trunk of the fetus elongates, the kidney migrates upward and the testis follows its anchoring gubernaculum downward. By the third trimester, it is located behind the processus vaginalis. At birth, 60% of infants still have an open processus. This figure drops by half after the first month. Although a persistent processus vaginalis is associated with an indirect inguinal hernia, it is important to realize that the processus vaginalis remains open in 25% of adult men, in most of whom an inguinal hernia never develops.[4] A persistent processus vaginalis in females is known as the canal of Nuck.

NATURAL HISTORY

It is impossible to obtain a completely accurate picture of the natural history of inguinal hernias because of the difficulty of finding a whole group of untreated patients. Most surgeons would repair a hernia at diagnosis, even if asymptomatic, to avoid potential complications. The commonly quoted 4% to 6% lifetime risk for strangulation of an inguinal hernia is probably more the result of speculation than fact. A probability of 0.037 hernia-related complications per patient per year was determined by studying a group of hernia patients from a Paris truss clinic in the 19th century at a time before inguinal herniorrhaphy was routinely performed. A similar figure was noted in a more recent Colombian government study. Using life table analysis and the probability calculated from these two studies, the lifetime risk for a hernia accident in an 18-year-old man is 20%, or 1 in 5 patients; for a 72-year-old, it is 4.0%, or 1 in 25 patients. Hair and colleagues provided some data concerning the likelihood of pain or incarceration by examining a prospectively maintained database of 699 patients.[5] Using Kaplan-Meier estimates, they were able to calculate that the probability of pain developing by 10 years was 90%, but this seemed to have minimal clinical significance because leisure activity was affected in only 29% and just 13% of the employed patients had to take time off of work because of hernia-related symptoms. Similarly, the cumulative probability of a hernia becoming irreducible rose from 6.5% at 12 months to 30% by 10 years, but only 10 patients in their series required an emergency operation and only 2 had to have strangulated contents resected. The U.S. Agency for Healthcare Related Quality of Life, in conjunction with the American College of Surgeons, sponsored a comprehensive clinical trial to compare a strategy of observation for asymptomatic patients with routine repair. The results of this study showed, on a 2-year observation period, that watchful waiting in minimally symptomatic patients is an acceptable option, and delaying repair until symptoms increase is safe because incarceration or strangulation occur rarely.[5a]

INCIDENCE

Seventy-five percent of all abdominal wall hernias occur in the groin. Approximately 750,000 inguinal herniorrhaphies are performed annually in the United States,

with indirect hernias outnumbering direct hernias by about 2:1. Reliable figures concerning the incidence and prevalence of hernias are not readily available, the major reason being a lack of objective criteria to consistently make an accurate diagnosis. The prevalence of an inguinal hernia in a male is clearly age dependent. In a recent study 32% of male children weighing less than 1500 g required a hernia operation by the age of 8 years. For an adult male, the incidence increases steadily with age and has been reported to approach 50% for men older than 75 years. Abramson and colleagues from Israel published a particularly helpful paper dealing with inguinal hernia epidemiology. They studied 455 men with inguinal hernias from a settlement community in the early 1950s. The patients were a mixture of native-born Israelis and immigrant Europeans, Americans, Asians, and Africans and were therefore thought to be representative of the population as a whole. From this group they were able to calculate a current prevalence rate (excluding repaired hernias) of 18% and a lifetime prevalence rate (including repaired hernias) of 24%.[6] However, it should be noted that there is considerable variance in reporting. A recent study by Akin et al.[7] in adult male military recruits revealed a 3.2% prevalence, much lower than that reported by Abramson et al.[6]

ETIOLOGY, BIOCHEMICAL BASIS, AND MECHANICAL STRESS

The cause of an inguinal hernia is undoubtedly multifactorial. In the evolution from a quadruped to a biped, the unprotected groin has become more vulnerable to changes in intra-abdominal pressure. Physical exertion is probably less important than commonly believed, as suggested by the fact that athletes and weightlifters do not seem to have an excessive incidence of inguinal hernias. Russel proposed the so-called saccular theory based on the presence of a patent processus vaginalis as the cause of an indirect inguinal hernia.[8] Opponents of this theory point out that autopsy studies have shown that patients can have a patent processus without clinical evidence of hernia and, conversely, that patients with an obliterated processus vaginalis have been noted to have an abdominal wall defect lateral to the epigastric vessels. Increased intra-abdominal pressure and relative weakness of the posterior inguinal wall are thought to be important in the development of direct inguinal hernias. Increased intra-abdominal pressure and the size and shape of the femoral ring contribute to the development of femoral hernias. Although the femoral vein laterally and Cooper's ligament inferiorly are fairly constant boundaries of the femoral ring, variations in attachment of the iliopubic tract anteriorly and medially account for the development of femoral hernias. The iliopubic tract normally inserts for a distance of 1 to 2 cm along the pectinate line between the pubic tubercle and the midportion of the superior pubic ramus. A femoral hernia can result if the insertion is less than 1 to 2 cm or if it is shifted medially. The myopectineal orifice is an area bounded superiorly by the internal oblique and transversus abdominis muscles, medially by the rectus muscle and sheath, laterally by the iliopsoas muscle, and inferiorly by Cooper's ligament. This funnel-shaped orifice is lined in its entirety by the fascia transversalis. As noted previously, Fruchaud's concept states that the fundamental cause of all groin hernias is failure of the transversalis fascia to retain the peritoneum. This led to the development of operations by some of his better-known students, such as Rives and Stoppa, in which a barrier (e.g., a mesh) was placed between the transversalis fascia and the peritoneum (i.e., the preperitoneal space) to address all types of groin hernias, thus rendering the distinction between direct indirect and femoral hernias less meaningful.

Familial predisposition and the role of connective tissue diseases in hernia development have received considerable attention in recent years. Various connective tissue disorders, such as osteogenesis imperfecta, Marfan's syndrome, Ehlers-Danlos syndrome, and congenital hip dislocation, are associated with hernias. Autosomal dominant polycystic kidney disease is characterized by abnormal production of extracellular matrix (ECM) and a 43% incidence of hernias. Individuals with hypermobile joints (e.g., circus contortionists) have been shown to have an abnormal increase in type III collagen and an increased risk for hernias. A similar phenomenon is observed in smokers.

Research at the molecular level has uncovered disturbances in collagen metabolism that are believed to contribute to hernia disease and high recurrence rates. Read performed biopsies of the rectus sheaths from adults with inguinal hernias. He found that equal-sized biopsy specimens were lighter in patients with hernias. He went on to show a striking decrease in hydroxyproline (a surrogate for collagen) in the hernia patients. Hydroxyproline makes up about 80% of the rectus sheath. Subsequently, he showed that fibroblasts cultured from the anterior rectus sheath of patients with inguinal hernias proliferated only half as well as those from individuals without herniation. The patients with direct herniation in this study had the longest generation time in the reproduction of fibroblasts. Furthermore, he demonstrated decreased incorporation of radioactive proline in the rectus sheath samples of individuals with hernias and a reduced hydroxyproline-to-proline ratio. Peacock and Madden suggested that the metabolic abnormality in patients with inguinal herniation might involve increased collagenolysis.[9] Cannon and Read coined the term "metastatic emphysema" based on their finding that elastase activity was increased in patients with direct hernias and elastase inhibitory activity measured by serum antitrypsin levels was decreased, with remarkably low levels seen in smokers.[10] Further evidence of the role of collagen abnormality is the increased incidence of inguinal herniation in patients with lathyrism and several congenital connective tissue diseases.

Recent studies dealing with the development of a hernia have focused on the ECM. The ECM is in a dynamic balance of synthesis and degradation by matrix metalloproteinases (MMPs). Within the transversalis fascia, an alteration in collagen composition leads to increased tissue elasticity. Whereas type I collagen confers predominantly tensile strength, type III collagen consists of thinner fibers and is regarded as a temporary matrix during tissue remodeling. A decreased ratio of type I to type III collagen can be detected in fascial and skin specimens from patients with incisional hernia disease at both the mRNA and protein levels. Further analysis of the collagen content of mesh samples that were removed at the time of repair of a recurrence demonstrated a significantly decreased collagen type I–to–type III ratio. The MMP family consists of zinc-dependent proteases secreted as latent proenzymes with substrate specificity.[11] Recent studies by Bellon et al. revealed MMP-2 overexpression in the fibroblasts of patients with direct inguinal hernias, whereas Klinge et al. detected MMP-13 overexpression in patients with recurrent inguinal hernias.[12,13]

Herniogenetics is rapidly developing as a science and has the goal of unraveling the secrets of genes that might contribute to the tendency for development of an inguinal hernia. Currently, hernia disease is believed to be a polygenetic trait, with penetrance of the hernia phenotype being dependent on complex interactions between environmental factors and multiple genes. The most likely candidate genes for genetic studies are those that are responsible for the production of fibrillar type I and type III collagen and MMPs. Polymorphisms occurring not only within the coding sequences but also within the regulatory and promoter sequences might be of importance in disease manifestation. Microarray analysis of ECM-related genes in patients with hernias and healthy subjects will help determine the susceptibility genes for hernia development.

Bendavid has recently proposed a "unified theory" of hernia formation that links anatomic, chemical, genetic, environmental, and metabolic etiologies of inguinal hernias. He makes the point that the final common denominator in all these proposed etiologies is the collagen matrix.[14]

ANATOMY

A surgeon who is attempting to repair a hernia with an open technique as opposed to one using a laparoscopic approach views the abdominal wall anatomy differently. Surgical anatomy is discussed from both perspectives in this chapter. The abdominal wall spans the space between the lower ribs and the pelvis. The diaphragm is the superior border of the abdominal cavity, whereas inferiorly the abdominal cavity is continuous with the pelvic cavity. The anterior abdominal wall is formed above by the lowest ribs and below by the rectus abdominis, external oblique, internal oblique, and transversus abdominis muscles and their aponeuroses. Posteriorly, the abdominal wall is made up in the midline of the lumbar vertebrae and their intervertebral disks; laterally, the gap between the 12th rib and the upper part of the pelvis is bridged by the psoas muscles, quadratus lumborum muscles, and the aponeurosis of the transversus abdominis muscles.

Anterior Abdominal Wall

Skin, Fascia, Vessels, and Nerves

The lines of cleavage in the skin run horizontally around the trunk, and this is clinically important when planning operative incisions. Camper's fascia is the superficial fatty layer that lies below the skin; it is continuous below with the outer layers of fascia covering the perineum and genitalia and also contains the dartos muscle fibers of the scrotum. The superficial circumflex iliac and superficial epigastric vessels, tributaries of the femoral vessels, are the major blood vessels of the superficial fascia. The lymphatic channels that traverse this fascia drain to the axillary nodes above the umbilicus and to the inguinal nodes below. The lymphatic channels cross the inguinal ligament and are potentially located in the surgical field for an inguinal herniorrhaphy. A second fascial layer in the superficial abdominal wall is the deep fascia of Scarpa, which is composed of compressed fibrous components of the superficial fascia. After forming the suspensory ligament of the penis (or clitoris), it fuses with the membranous layer of the superficial fascia, or Colles' fascia, in the perineum. Scarpa's fascia is thin and fades out above and laterally, where it becomes continuous with the superficial fascia of the thorax and back, respectively. Scarpa's fascia also fuses with the deep fascia investing the external oblique muscle. This fascia is bound inferiorly to the inguinal ligament and pubis before continuing onto the thigh, where it blends with the fascia lata to seal the space beneath and inferior to the inguinal ligament, which is the inferior portion of the myopectineal orifice. This portion of the inguinal region includes Hesselbach's triangle superiorly and is therefore the weakest aspect of the groin.

The cutaneous nerve supply to the anterior abdominal wall is derived from the anterior rami of the lower six thoracic and the first lumbar nerves in the familiar dermatomal pattern. Because of considerable overlap in dermatomal fields, disruption of one of these nerves is rarely clinically significant in postoperative patients. The cutaneous branches reach the subcutaneous layer by coursing between the flat lateral muscles and by piercing the sheath of the rectus abdominis.

Muscles, Ligaments, and Aponeurosis

The great lateral muscles of the anterior abdominal wall are composed of large aponeuroses and variable amounts of muscle. From exterior to interior they are the external oblique, internal oblique, and transversus abdominis. On either side of the midline anteriorly are the wide vertical muscles, the rectus abdominis muscles. The aponeuroses of the lateral muscles form the sheath of the rectus abdominis. The linea alba is the midline decussation of the three aponeuroses. In the lower part of the rectus sheath there may be a small muscle called the pyramidalis. The cremaster muscle is derived from the lower fibers of the internal oblique and passes inferiorly, covering the spermatic cord.

External Oblique Muscle and Associated Ligaments

The external oblique arises from the posterior aspect of the lower eight ribs (Fig. 45–2). The direction of the muscle fibers varies from nearly horizontal in its upper portion to oblique in the middle and lower portions. The fibers fan out and insert into the xiphoid process, linea alba, pubic crest, pubic tubercle, and anterior half of the iliac crest. The obliquely arranged anteroinferior fibers of insertion fold on themselves to form the inguinal ligament. The most posterior fibers passing down to the iliac crest form a posterior free border, which together with the anterior fibers of the latissimus dorsi and the iliac crest form the inferior lumbar triangle of Petit.

The more medial fibers of the external oblique aponeurosis divide into medial and lateral crura and form the superficial inguinal ring. The spermatic cord (or round ligament), the ilioinguinal nerve, and the genital branch of the genitofemoral nerve pass through this opening. The crural margins give origin to the external spermatic fascia.

The inguinal ligament is important because of its role as both a landmark and an integral component of many groin hernia repairs. It is the incurved free edge of the external oblique aponeurosis between its origin on the iliac crest and its insertion at the pubis. The ligament has a caudally directed convexity as a consequence of its connection to the fascia lata of the thigh. The ligament bridges the muscular and vascular structures that leave the pelvis inferiorly. This area deep to and above the inguinal ligament, including Hasselbach's triangle (see later), is called the *myopectineal orifice*. At its insertion to the pubic tubercle, the fibers of the inguinal ligament flare out in a fan-like fashion and fuse with the anterior rectus sheath and fibers from the opposite inguinal ligament along the upper border of the pubic bone to form the superior pubic ligament. The inguinal ligament continues downward to the superior pubic ramus to form the lacunar (Gimbernat's) ligament and courses laterally along the pectineal line as Cooper's ligament.

Internal Oblique and Transversus Muscles and Aponeurosis

The internal oblique is also a broad, thin, muscular sheet that lies deep to the external oblique. It arises from the lumbar fascia, the anterior two thirds of the iliac crest, and the lateral two thirds of the inguinal ligament. The muscle is inserted into the lower three ribs and their costal cartilages, the xiphoid process, the linea alba, and the symphysis pubis (Fig. 45–3). The transversus muscle runs horizontally deep to the internal oblique. It arises from the deep surface of the lower six costal cartilages, the lumbar fascia, the anterior two thirds of the iliac crest, and the lateral third of the inguinal ligament. The medial aponeurotic fibers of the transversus abdominis contribute to the rectus sheath and insert on the pecten pubis and the crest of the pubis to form the falx inguinalis. These fibers are infrequently joined by a

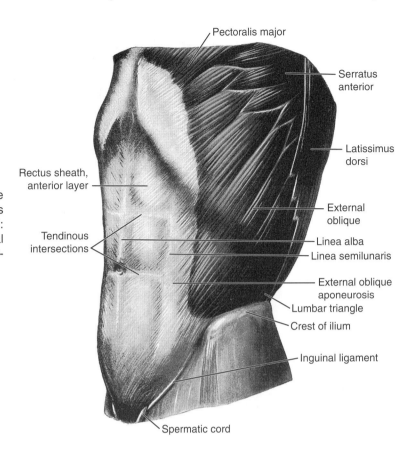

Figure 45–2. Left anterolateral view of the abdominal wall muscles showing the anterior rectus and external oblique muscles. (From Standring S: Gray's Anatomy: The Anatomical Basis of Clinical Practice, 39th ed. London, England, Churchill Livingstone, 2005. Fig 67.8, p 1108.)

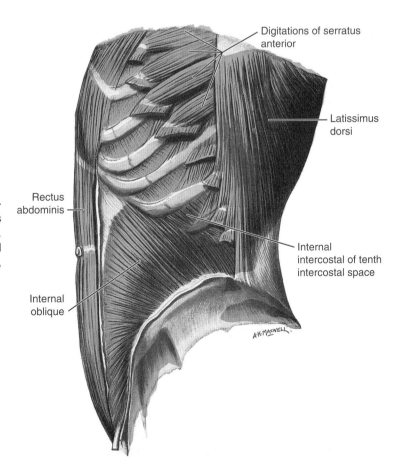

Figure 45–3. Left anterolateral view of the abdominal wall with the external oblique and anterior rectus muscles removed to show the internal oblique muscle. (From Standring S: Gray's Anatomy: The Anatomical Basis of Clinical Practice, 39th ed. London, England, Churchill Livingstone, 2005. Fig 67.9, p 1108.)

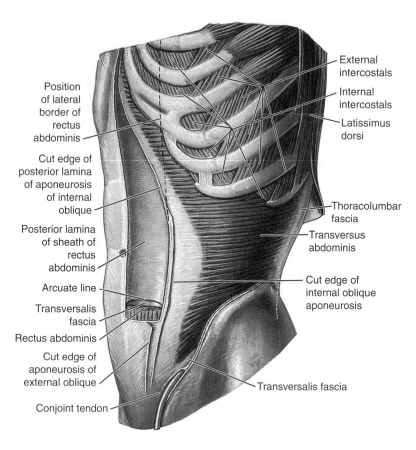

Position
of lateral
border of
rectus
abdominis

Cut edge of
posterior lamina
of aponeurosis
of internal
oblique

Posterior lamina
of sheath of
rectus
abdominis

Arcuate line

Transversalis
fascia

Rectus abdominis

Cut edge of
aponeurosis of
external oblique

Conjoint tendon

External
intercostals

Internal
intercostals

Latissimus
dorsi

Thoracolumbar
fascia

Transversus
abdominis

Cut edge of
internal oblique
aponeurosis

Transversalis fascia

Figure 45–4. Left anterolateral view of the abdominal wall muscles with the rectus and internal oblique muscles removed to show the posterior rectus sheet, transversus abdominis muscles, and conjoint tendon. (From Standring S: Gray's Anatomy: The Anatomical Basis of Clinical Practice, 39th ed. London, England, Churchill Livingstone, 2005. Fig 67.11, p 1109.)

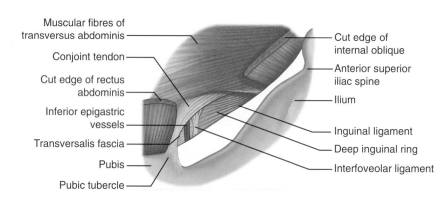

Muscular fibres of
transversus abdominis

Conjoint tendon

Cut edge of rectus
abdominis

Inferior epigastric
vessels

Transversalis fascia

Pubis

Pubic tubercle

Cut edge of
internal oblique

Anterior superior
iliac spine

Ilium

Inguinal ligament

Deep inguinal ring

Interfoveolar ligament

Figure 45–5. Anterior view of the muscles of the groin area (the internal oblique has been removed and the conjoint tendon is highlighted). (From Standring S: Gray's Anatomy: The Anatomical Basis of Clinical Practice, 39th ed. London, England, Churchill Livingstone, 2005. Fig 67.16, p 1111.)

portion of the internal oblique aponeurosis; only then is a true conjoint tendon formed (Fig. 45–4). What is commonly referred to as the conjoint tendon in many texts might better be termed the aponeurotic arch. Contraction of the transversus abdominis causes this structure to move down toward the inguinal ligament in a kind of shutter mechanism that reinforces the weakest area of the groin when intra-abdominal pressure is elevated (Fig. 45–5).[15]

Rectus Abdominis and Rectus Sheath

The rectus abdominis is a long muscle that arises from the symphysis pubis and pubic crest and is inserted into the fifth, sixth, and seventh costal cartilages and the xiphoid process (see Fig. 45–2). Three tendinous inter-

sections, one at the xiphoid, one at the umbilicus, and one halfway between the two, usually divide it segmentally. The rectus sheath is a long fibrous sheath that encloses the rectus abdominis and pyramidalis muscle (a small muscle found in front of the lower part of the rectus abdominis). Above the costal margin the anterior wall is formed by the external oblique aponeurosis, and the fifth, sixth, and seventh costal cartilages and their intercostal spaces form the posterior wall. Between the costal margin and the anterior superior iliac spine, the internal oblique aponeurosis splits to enclose the rectus muscle. The external oblique muscle is directed in front and the transversus aponeurosis is directed behind the muscle. Between the level of the anterior superior iliac spine and the pubis, the sheath does not have a posterior wall and the aponeurosis of all three muscles forms

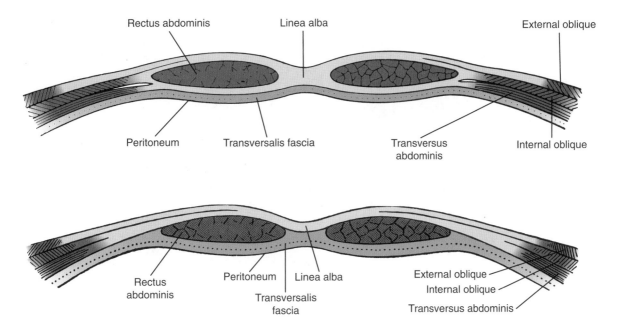

Rectus abdominis   Linea alba   External oblique

Peritoneum   Transversalis fascia   Transversus abdominis   Internal oblique

Rectus abdominis   Peritoneum   Linea alba   External oblique

Transversalis fascia   Internal oblique

Transversus abdominis

Figure 45–6. Transverse view of the abdominal wall above and below the arcuate line. (From Standring S: Gray's Anatomy: The Anatomical Basis of Clinical Practice, 39th ed. London, England, Churchill Livingstone, 2005, p 1105.)

the anterior wall. The curved free lower border of the posterior wall is called the arcuate line, and it allows passage of the deep inferior epigastric vessels into the sheath (Fig. 45–6).

Laparoscopic Anatomy of the Inguinal Region

Surgeon preparation for laparoscopic herniorrhaphy mandates relearning inguinal anatomy from the preperitoneal perspective.[16] Surgeons unaccustomed to the unique viewpoint encountered during laparoscopic procedures find the images to be quite disorienting. The anatomy of the groin area and anterior wall can easily be mastered if several relatively consistent anatomic landmarks are noted. Details of laparoscopic anatomy are discussed in Chapter 46, Laparoscopic Inguinal Hernia Repair, and only a brief overview follows here.

Deep Aspects of the Anterior Abdominal Wall, Peritoneal Folds, and Associated Structures

Distending the peritoneal cavity with gas allows identification of the umbilical peritoneal folds, which are prominent and easily identifiable landmarks in most individuals. The single median umbilical fold extends from the umbilicus to the urinary bladder and covers the fibrous remnant of the allantois, the urachus. The urachus may be partially or completely patent and may open onto the umbilical scar in newborns or form a cystic remnant along the course of the median umbilical ligament. The medial umbilical fold, on either side, is formed by the underlying obliterated portion of the fetal umbilical artery, a branch of the anterior division of the internal iliac artery. The patent proximal portion of this artery supplies the superior vesical artery to the bladder. The lateral umbilical fold covers the inferior epigastric

arteries as they course toward the posterior rectus sheath, which they enter approximately at the level of the arcuate line. The *supravesical fossa* is the depression found between the medial and median umbilical ligaments. This is also the site for hernias of the same name. The *medial fossa* is the space between the medial and lateral ligaments and is the site of direct inguinal hernias. The *lateral fossa* is less well delineated than the others. The lateral umbilical ligament and the rectus abdominis form the medial border of the fossa. This fossa does not have a lateral border; rather, the concavity slowly attenuates and is the site of congenital or indirect inguinal hernias.

Nerve injury during laparoscopic hernia repair may cause considerable and often persistent postoperative pain. The iliohypogastric, ilioinguinal, genitofemoral, lateral femoral cutaneous, and femoral nerves are all at risk. Two anatomic danger zones in regard to nerve and vessel injury are described and must be avoided. The first danger zone is the so-called *triangle of doom*, which is an area bounded laterally by the gonadal vessels and medially by the vas deferens with its apex orientated superiorly at the internal ring. The inferior border is arbitrary because it is the interface between dissected and nondissected peritoneum after preperitoneal dissection (Fig. 45–7). Within this triangle are the external iliac artery and vein, the deep circumflex iliac vein, the genital branch of the genitofemoral nerve, and the femoral nerve. The second anatomic danger zone is referred to as the *triangle of pain* or the *electrical hazard zone*. The medial border is constant and is formed by the internal spermatic vessels. It is questionably accurate to call this zone a triangle inasmuch as the lateral and inferior borders are nebulous because the entire space lateral to the internal spermatic vessels where critical nerves pass is included. The "triangle" contains the lateral femoral cutaneous nerve, the femoral branch of the

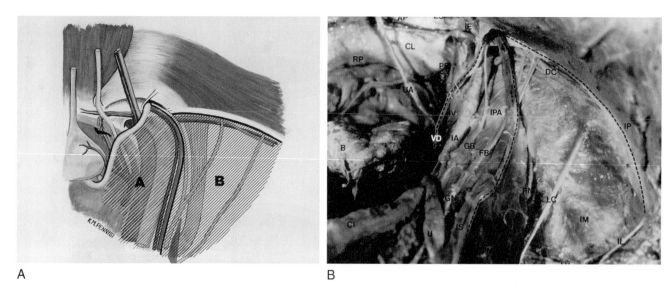

A   B

Figure 45–7. **A,** Preperitoneal view of the right side of the groin depicting the so-called triangle of doom (A) and the triangle of pain or the electrical hazard zone (B). **B,** Cadaveric preparation showing the structures included within these triangles that could be damaged during preperitoneal herniorrhaphy. AP, anterior pubic branch and iliopubic vein; B, bladder (reflected posteriorly); CI, common iliac artery; CL, Cooper's ligament; DC, deep circumflex iliac vessels; ES, external spermatic vessels; FB, femoral branch of the genitofemoral nerve; FN, femoral nerve; GB, genital branch of the genitofemoral nerve; GN, genitofemoral nerve; IA, external iliac artery; IE, inferior epigastric vessels; IL, ilioinguinal nerve; IM, musculus iliacus; IP, iliopubic tract; IPA, iliopectineal arch; IS, internal spermatic vessels; IV, external iliac vein; LC, lateral femoral cutaneous nerve; LV, iliolumbar vessels; PB, anastomotic pubic branch; PM, musculus psoas major; RP, retropubic vein; U, ureter; UA, umbilical artery; VD, vas deferens. (From Greene FL, Ponsky JL: Endoscopic Surgery. Philadelphia, WB Saunders, 1994, p 365.)

genitofemoral nerve, and the femoral nerve. Avoidance of electrosurgical energy, dissection, or the application of staples within these triangles is crucial to prevent nerve injury, entrapment, or vascular injury. The genitofemoral nerve is especially at risk during laparoscopic herniorrhaphy, as is the lateral femoral cutaneous nerve.

Transversalis Fascia and Its Derivatives

Harrison in 1922 was the first to stress the importance of the fascia transversalis in the pathology and repair of inguinal hernias. The transversalis fascia is a continuous sheet that extends throughout the extraperitoneal space. It is defined as the deep or endoabdominal fascia covering the internal surface of the transversus abdominis, the iliacus, the psoas muscles, the obturator internus, and portions of the periosteum. One variant of this convention is the use of terms specific to the muscle covered by the fascia (e.g., obturator fascia). Most hernia specialists believe that the transversalis fascia is bilaminar. There is a posterior fatty preperitoneal component (referred to as the preperitoneal fascia by some) and an anterior lamina that is adherent to the deep surface of the transversus and rectus abdominis muscles. The transversalis fascia is essentially a vascular envelope that encloses between these two laminae the arterial and venous plexuses that supply the muscles of this region (Fig. 45–8). The extraperitoneal space of Bogros lies behind the posterior lamina. It is important that in any preperitoneal approach the prosthesis be placed deep to the posterior lamina of the transversalis fascia, but superfi-

cial to the vas deferens and the parietalized spermatic vessels lying in the extraperitoneal fat.

At its attachments to the pubis and at points where it is penetrated by neurovascular or cord structures the transversalis fascia thickens to form important derivatives: the iliopectineal arch, the iliopubic tract, and the crura of the deep inguinal ring. The superior and inferior crura form a sling around the deep inguinal ring, a structure shaped like a "monk's hood." When the transversus abdominis contracts, the crura of the ring are pulled upward and laterally, which results in a valvular action that helps prevent the formation of an indirect hernia. With the increasing use of laparoscopy the iliopubic tract has become a more important surgical landmark. It is the thickened band of transversalis fascia formed at the zone of transition between the deep surfaces of the iliac and transversus abdominis muscles. It is not obviously visible in every patient from a laparoscopic perspective, but its location should be immediately known to the surgeon because of its constant relationship to other landmarks in the area. Anatomically, the tract courses parallel to the more superficially located inguinal ligament and is attached to the iliac crest laterally and the pubic tubercle medially. It forms a portion of the inferior crus of the deep ring and the anterior and medial walls of the femoral sheath. The tract fuses with the inguinal ligament to form a portion of the inferior wall of the inguinal canal. The pectineal ligament is reinforced by fibers of the iliopubic tract that are reflected downward off the pubic tubercle. The branches of the lumbar plexus run inferior to this tract. In fully 42% of

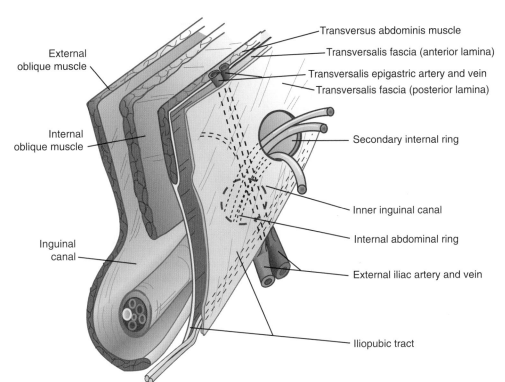

Figure 45–8. Parasagittal view of the right midinguinal area demonstrating the two laminae of the transversalis fascia. (From Read RC: The transversalis and peritoneal fasciae—a re-evaluation. In Nyhus LM, Condon RE [eds]: Hernia, 4th ed. Philadelphia, JB Lippincott, 1995, pp 57-63.)

Labels in figure:
External oblique muscle
Internal oblique muscle
Inguinal canal
Transversus abdominis muscle
Transversalis fascia (anterior lamina)
Transversalis epigastric artery and vein
Transversalis fascia (posterior lamina)
Secondary internal ring
Inner inguinal canal
Internal abdominal ring
External iliac artery and vein
Iliopubic tract

examined specimens in a recent study, the iliopubic tract was a substantial structure suitable for use in hernia repair. The iliopectineal arch, also a derivative of the fascia transversalis, separates the vascular compartment (lacuna vasorum) containing the femoral vessels from the neuromuscular compartment (lacuna musculorum) containing the iliopsoas muscle, femoral nerve, and lateral femoral cutaneous nerve. It joins the iliopubic tract in contributing to the femoral sheath. The femoral sheath itself is a downward protrusion into the thigh of the fascial envelope lining the abdominal walls, as previously alluded to. The sheath surrounds the femoral vessels and lymphatics for about 1 inch below the inguinal ligament. The vascular compartment is further divided by septa into compartments for the vessels and the femoral branch of the genitofemoral nerves. The medial border of the femoral sheath follows the transversus abdominis aponeurosis to its insertion just lateral to that of the lacunar ligament and extends inferiorly to eventually fuse with the medial septum and adventitia of the femoral vein. The resultant cone-shaped cul-de-sac is the femoral canal, which often contains a large lymph node referred to as Cloquet's node. The femoral ring is the extraperitoneal opening of the canal. Its boundaries are the lacunar ligament medially, the femoral vein and its connective tissue septum laterally, the inguinal ligament anteriorly, and Cooper's ligament posteriorly reinforced by fibers from the iliopubic tract. The roof of the femoral ring (i.e., the iliopubic tract) is not reinforced by the tough transversalis fascia, which is diverted to form the femoral sheath in this location, and this predisposes to hernia formation, especially in female subjects (see Fig. 45–8).

Hesselbach's Triangle and the Spermatic Cord

The inguinal (Hesselbach's) triangle is formed by the rectus abdominis medially, the inferior epigastric vessels superolaterally, and the inguinal ligament at the base. It is the site of direct inguinal herniation. Only the peritoneum and transversalis fascia cover the triangle in this area. The aponeurotic arch, which is formed from the transversus abdominis muscle, crosses the apex of this triangle and reinforces this area of weakness when one strains. A high arch may predispose to the formation of direct inguinal hernias by offering less reinforcement. The cord structures include the ductus deferens, the pampiniform venous plexus, the testicular artery, and the genital branch of the genitofemoral nerve, a branch of the lumbar plexus.

Innervation and Blood Supply of the Abdominal Wall

The lumbar plexus is formed in the psoas muscle from the anterior rami of the upper four lumbar nerves. The branches of the plexus emerge from the lateral and medial borders of the muscle and its anterior surface. The iliohypogastric, ilioinguinal, lateral cutaneous nerve of the thigh, and femoral nerves emerge from the lateral border of the psoas, in that order from above downward. The genitofemoral nerve is the most anterior of the nerves encountered. The genital branch travels with the spermatic cord and ultimately innervates the cremaster muscle and the lateral aspect of the scrotum. Most studies show that the branches of the lumbar plexus destined for the thigh run beneath the iliopubic tract, which

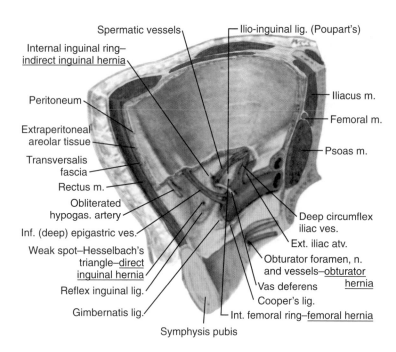

Spermatic vessels

Ilio-inguinal lig. (Poupart's)

Internal inguinal ring–
indirect inguinal hernia

Peritoneum

Iliacus m.

Femoral m.

Extraperitoneal
areolar tissue

Psoas m.

Transversalis
fascia

Rectus m.

Obliterated
hypogas. artery

Inf. (deep) epigastric ves.

Deep circumflex
iliac ves.

Ext. iliac atv.

Weak spot–Hesselbach's
triangle–direct
inguinal hernia

Obturator foramen, n.
and vessels–obturator
hernia

Reflex inguinal lig.

Vas deferens

Gimbernatis lig.

Cooper's lig.

Int. femoral ring–femoral hernia

Symphysis pubis

Figure 45–9.   Posterior and sagittal view of the right inguinal area demonstrating the inguinal, femoral, and obturator orifices and their relationships. (From Read RC: Basic features of abdominal wall herniation and its repair. In Zuidema GD, Yeo CJ [eds]: Shackelford's Surgery of the Alimentary Tract, vol 5, 5th ed. Philadelphia, WB Saunders, 2002, p 92.)

has important implications for a surgeon working in the preperitoneal space. This is not universally accepted, however, because anomalous routes for some of the nerves above the iliopubic tract have been described. The femoral branch of the genitofemoral nerve innervates the proximal midthigh skin. The iliohypogastric and ilioinguinal nerves (L1) enter the lateral and anterior abdominal walls. The iliohypogastric nerve crosses the iliac fossa just inferior to the kidney and pierces the transversus abdominis. The subsequent course of the nerve carries it between the transversus and the internal oblique until it pierces the aponeurosis of both obliques just above the external inguinal ring. The ilioinguinal nerve normally crosses the iliac fossa just inferior to the iliohypogastric nerve. The nerve pierces the transversus and internal oblique above the iliac crest and subsequently enters the inguinal canal. The iliohypogastric nerve supplies the skin of the lower part of the anterior abdominal wall, and the ilioinguinal nerve passes through the inguinal canal to supply the skin of the groin and the scrotum or labium majus. The lateral cutaneous nerve crosses the iliac fossa under the iliac fascia and pierces the inguinal ligament to enter the thigh. The femoral nerve lies immediately below the lateral aspect of the psoas muscle and is not routinely encountered in laparoscopic surgery, although there are some reports of injury to this nerve.

The primary blood supply to the deep anterior abdominal wall is from the inferior epigastric artery, a branch of the external iliac artery. Aberrant obturator vessels may arise from the inferior epigastric vessels, arch inferiorly over Cooper's ligament, and join the normal obturator circulation to form the corona mortis; copious bleeding can result during careless dissection of Cooper's ligament or when one attempts to release a tight femoral hernial neck by incising the lacunar ligament. It is questionable whether the finding of a corona

mortis should be considered anomalous because the variant is so common. Other veins in this area are larger than the accompanying arteries and are also prone to injury. The external iliac artery and vein are the vessels in the vascular compartment of the deep inguinal region. The deep circumflex iliac artery and vein pierce the transversalis fascia and run along the iliac fossa to anastomose with the deep lumbar system. As they course along the iliopubic tract, they can be inadvertently stapled or otherwise injured during laparoscopic herniorrhaphy (Fig. 45–9).

SYMPTOMS AND DIAGNOSIS

Patients with groin hernias have a wide range of clinical manifestations ranging from no symptoms at all to a life-threatening condition caused by strangulation of incarcerated intestinal contents. Asymptomatic patients are detected during routine physical examination or seek medical attention for a painless groin bulge. Indirect hernias are more likely to produce symptoms than direct ones are, with patients describing a heavy feeling or dragging sensation that tends to be worse as the day wears on. Radiation of pain into the testicle is not rare. Although some patients describe the pain as intermittent, others complain of a sharper pain that is either localized or diffuse. It is important to distinguish groin strain with a coexistent asymptomatic hernia from a truly symptomatic hernia. If the hernia is improperly determined to be a cause of the patient's pain, the stage is set for a post-herniorrhaphy pain syndrome.

Physical examination is the best way to determine the presence or absence of an inguinal hernia. The diagnosis may be obvious by simple inspection when a visible bulge is present. Nonvisible hernias require digital examination of the inguinal canal, which is best done in both the lying and standing positions. This invagination test helps distinguish a true hernia from a normal expansile bulge of muscle. Classic teaching is that an indirect hernia will push against the fingertip whereas a direct hernia will push against the pulp of the finger. Many authors, however, do not believe that direct and indirect inguinal hernias can be distinguished clinically.[17] The ring occlusion test is based on the premise that fingertip pressure over the midinguinal point will prevent an indirect hernia from protruding but will not be able to control a direct hernia. The differential diagnosis for groin hernias includes groin malignancies, ectopic and undescended testicles, psoas abscess, epididymitis, hydrocele, enlarged lymph nodes, saphenous varix, and femoral aneurysms.

Almost all groin hernias in women are either indirect or femoral. The stronger transversalis fascia in the floor of the inguinal canal, as a result of childbearing, makes direct herniation unusual. The indirect sac is the nonobliterated portion of the prenatal peritoneal evagination, known in females as the canal of Nuck, that runs along and partly covers the round ligament. In repair of these hernias most authors recommend ligation of both the sac and the round ligament at the level of the deep ring and anchoring of the round ligament stump to the internal oblique for support of the uterus. A femoral hernia appears as a swelling below the inguinal ligament and just lateral to the pubic tubercle. Femoral hernias need to be distinguished from a prominent femoral fat pad, the so-called femoral pseudohernia. Femoral hernias account for less than 10% of all groin hernias, but 40% are initially manifested as emergencies because of incarceration or strangulation. They are more common in older patients and in men who have previously undergone an inguinal hernia repair. Although the absolute number of femoral hernias in males and females is about the same, the incidence in females is four times that in males because of the lower overall frequency of groin hernia in women (male-to-female ratio of 7:1)

Sliding hernias constitute about 1.5% of all inguinal hernias. One wall of the sac, the posterior and lateral, is formed by a hollow viscus, usually the cecum on the right and the sigmoid colon on the left. The bladder may be present. The danger of these hernias is that the viscus may be mistaken for a sac and opened. They occur more commonly in the elderly, especially those with long-standing herniation. Characteristically, they can be only partially reduced during physical examination. A preperitoneal approach to the groin, whether open or laparoscopic, enables easier reduction and repair of these difficult hernias.

Irreducibility and incarceration may persist for years or decades without great inconvenience as a result of adhesions developing between the contents and the sac. Recent onset of incarceration is a potentially dangerous condition because it may result in strangulation and gangrene of the contents and is an indication for urgent repair. Bowel obstruction is more common in indirect, recurrent, and femoral hernias and is of the closed loop type. As a result of blockage at both the entry and exit of the intestine at the level of the internal ring, the pres-

sure in the intestinal lumen and accompanying vasculature and lymphatics cannot be dissipated, and perforation and gangrene of the bowel follow in neglected cases. Plain roentgenograms of the abdomen can be diagnostic. Taxis can be attempted in the absence of signs of strangulation. Taxis is performed with the patient sedated and in the Trendelenburg position. The hernia sac neck is grasped with one hand while the other applies pressure on the most distal part of the hernia. The goal is to elongate the neck of the hernia so that the contents of the hernial sac can be reduced with a rocking movement. Mere pressure on the most distal part of the hernia causes bulging of the hernia contents around the neck, which can occlude the neck and prevent reduction. Taxis should be performed only by a surgeon who is willing to observe the patient after successful reduction because of the slight possibility that gangrenous bowel might be reduced into the abdomen, viable hernia contents might be perforated, or the phenomenon known as en masse reduction might occur, which is defined as displacement of a hernia mass without relief of incarceration or strangulation secondary to a constricting fibrous ring. Strangulation is a life-threatening condition. The irreducible hernia is tense and tender, and the overlying skin may be discolored with a reddish or bluish tinge. The patient is often febrile, dehydrated, and toxic. Laboratory investigations often reveal metabolic acidosis and leukocytosis with a left shift.

Radiologic investigations are sometimes warranted to correctly diagnose the cause of groin pain. Herniography, though invasive, helps avoid unnecessary surgical exploration. Ultrasound is useful, especially in acute manifestations of groin swelling, to distinguish incarcerated bowel from acute lymphadenitis. It is, however, operator dependent.

Cross-sectional imaging techniques such as magnetic resonance imaging (MRI) and computed tomography (CT) are increasingly being used for the investigation of groin pain and swelling. Hernias are visualized as anteroposterior ballooning of the inguinal canal with simultaneous protrusion of fat or bowel. Van den Berg et al. looked at a group of patients scheduled to undergo elective laparoscopic herniorrhaphy for either unilateral or bilateral hernias detected on physical examination.[18] Blinded interpreters examined ultrasound and MRI scans and looked at not only the affected but also the opposite side; laparoscopy was considered the final arbitrator of the groin pathology on either side. The sensitivity and specificity were 74.5% and 96.3% for physical examination, 92.7% and 81.5% for ultrasound, and 94.5% and 96.3% for MRI. With the development of fast imaging scanners that allow dynamic imaging during straining, the addition of intraperitoneal contrast, and tweaking of the best weighting for images along with improved understanding of the technology, MRI is likely to become the imaging modality of choice in investigating groin pathology.

CLASSIFICATION

Surgeons have traditionally classified inguinal hernias as direct or indirect and groin hernias as inguinal or

| Table 45–1 | Inguinal Hernia Classification Systems | | | |

Modified	Traditional	Nyhus-Stoppa	Modified Gilbert	Schumpelick/Aachen
IA	Indirect small	I	1	L1
IB	Indirect medium	II	2	L2
IC	Indirect large	IIIB	3	L3
IIA	Direct small	IIIA	5	M1
IIB	Direct medium	IIIA	—	M2
IIC	Direct large	—	4	M3
III	Combined	IIIB	6	Mc
IV	Femoral	IIIC	7	F
0	Other	—	—	—
R	Recurrent	IV A, B, C, D	—	—

femoral, and that is the convention used in this chapter. However, this classification is not universally accepted, with many surgeons considering the terms groin hernia and inguinal hernia to be synonymous and inclusive of direct, indirect, and femoral hernias. Although it was Cooper who devised the concept of direct and indirect, it was Hesselbach who used the inferior epigastric vessels as the defining boundary between these two areas. With the advent of a new generation of herniorrhaphies in the 1950s there arose interest in devising a more scientific classification of groin hernias. Harkins developed a grading system to classify groin hernias. Grade I consists of indirect infant hernias, whereas grade 2 represents simple indirect hernias in older children and healthy young adults. Grade 3 hernias are "intermediate" types of hernia (larger indirect hernias, inguinal hernias in young adults or small hernias in older patients with strong tissue, or direct inguinal hernias in older patients with strong tissue or narrow necks). Grade 4 hernias include recurrent, femoral, direct, and indirect hernias not specifically falling within the earlier grades.

The primary purpose of a classification system for any disease is to stratify for severity so that reasonable comparisons can be made between various treatment strategies. However, with the multiplicity of operative techniques and approaches for repair of groin hernias, no single classification system has been accepted by all practitioners. The reason why it is so difficult to develop a classification system that all surgeons can agree on is that in the final analysis, physical examination represents an important component and no one has been able to eliminate its subjectivity. The more commonly applied classification systems are summarized in Table 45–1. The advantage of the modified traditional classification system, as proposed by Zollinger, is that it includes all the classes or grades within the other commonly used classification systems.[19] It separates the Nyhus IIIA and IIIB groups into distinct components, and it accounts for the direct (medium) hernias missing from Gilbert's system (Fig. 45–10). Finally, the modified traditional method allows for an "other" group rather than forcing the user to imprecisely classify an unusual hernia and separately classifies recurrent hernias, as does Nyhus. Kingsnorth

has developed a clinical classification system that groups patients according to grades of predicted technical difficulty. A score of 2 to 8 for prediction of the grade of difficulty of repair can be generated from the size of the hernia (H1 to H4) and the subscapular skin fold (F1 to F4) and enables preoperative stratification into groups of difficulty to match the competency level of the operator. The subscapular skin fold thickness correlates well with groin fat thickness, a marker of technical difficulty.[20] Future classification systems will probably include modifiers such as contents, associated abnormality, and reducibility of the hernia and will also be applicable from a laparoscopic perspective.

SURGERY

Indications and Alternatives

Strangulation and bowel obstruction are sometimes referred to as hernia accidents and are absolute indications for surgery. Unlike an adhesive bowel obstruction, obstruction caused by an inguinal hernia is almost never partial. Therefore, semiurgent surgery is indicated. Resuscitation includes bowel decompression, intravenous fluids to correct dehydration and electrolyte imbalance and ensure optimal urine output, followed by immediate surgery. All significantly symptomatic hernias should be repaired to improve quality of life.[21] Nonoperative treatment is applicable only for asymptomatic and minimally symptomatic hernias. Patients are counseled about the signs and symptoms of complications from their hernia so that they may promptly contact their physician in case of an adverse event. Nonoperative treatment remains controversial, and most standard surgical texts continue to recommend surgical repair of all inguinal hernias at diagnosis. However, a recent randomized controlled trial has provided strong evidence that supervised observation is safe.[5a] Women early in pregnancy should undergo surgery, whereas those who are about to deliver should have their hernia dealt with after delivery. Infants and young children should undergo prompt repair of groin herniation because their

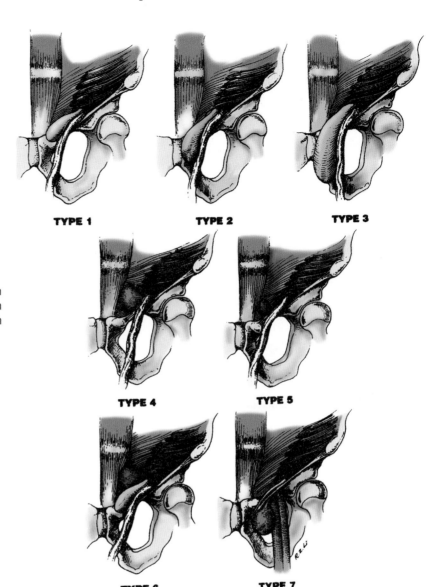

TYPE 1   **TYPE 2**   **TYPE 3**

TYPE 4   **TYPE 5**

TYPE 6   **TYPE 7**

Figure 45–10.   Gilbert's hernia classification (From Rutkow IM, Robbins AW: Classification systems and groin hernias. Surg Clin North Am 78:1122-1124, 1998.)

clinical course is unpredictable. Patients starting peritoneal dialysis commonly became more symptomatic, and therefore prophylactic herniorrhaphy is a good option. Predisposing pathologies of hernia accidents, such as liver disease with ascites and colon cancer, should be considered in the appropriate clinical setting.

A truss is a mechanical appliance consisting of a belt with a pad that is applied to the groin after spontaneous or manual reduction of a hernia and has been used for centuries (Fig. 45–11). It serves to maintain reduction and possibly prevents enlargement of the hernia. There are insufficient studies to determine how effective trusses actually are and whether they are as good as surgery for control of symptoms. Most patients find them cumbersome to use and difficult to keep clean. With prolonged use, atrophy of the spermatic cord has been reported, and eventual surgical repair is made more difficult because of fibrosis of the tissues. However, some patients do achieve symptomatic relief.

Preoperative Preparation

Most patients require no special preparation and can be safely treated as outpatients (day care surgery). Significant comorbid illness should be addressed, as with any surgical procedure. A single dose of preoperative intravenous antibiotics is preferred by many, especially if a prosthesis is to be used. However, there is no conclusive evidence that administration of antibiotics decreases the incidence of wound infection. With large groin hernias, one must be cognizant of the fact that replacement of hernia contents into the abdominal cavity during herniorrhaphy could be followed by respiratory embarrassment or abdominal compartment syndrome, or both. The term "loss of domain" refers to this clinical scenario and can be addressed by establishment of pneumoperitoneum in preparation for hernia surgery. A CT scan allows the surgeon to determine the extent of domain loss and make a final decision about the need for pneu-

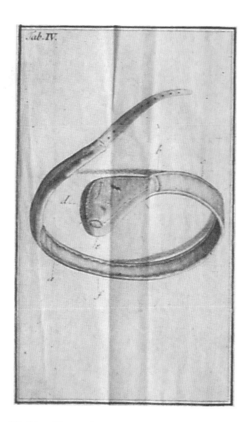

Figure 45–11. Illustration of an older style truss from the 18th century. (From Rutkow IM: A selective history of hernia surgery in the late eighteenth century: The treatises of Percivall Pott, Jean Louis Petit, D. August Gottlieb Richter, Don Antonio de Gimbernat, and Pieter Camper. Surg Clin North Am 83:1021-1044, 2003.)

Anesthesia

Although general anesthesia is almost always recommended for laparoscopic hernia repairs, the choice of anesthesia for open inguinal herniorrhaphy depends on the personal preference of the surgeon. Local anesthesia, when used in adequate doses and far enough in advance, proves very effective, especially in combination with short-acting amnesic and anxiolytic agents such as propofol. The local anesthetic should be injected before preparing and draping the patient for best results. One of the biggest advantages of local anesthesia is that the patient can be aroused from sedation at intervals to perform Valsalva maneuvers and test the repair. Regional anesthesia in the form of spinal or epidural anesthesia can also be used successfully in experienced hands. If general anesthesia is used, a local anesthetic should be administered at the end of the procedure as an adjunct to reduce postoperative pain.

Choice of Prosthetic Material

As far back as 1878, Billroth envisioned that prosthetic material would be the best solution for the problem of inguinal herniation. Numerous randomized comparative trials, as well as meta-analyses and comprehensive reviews, have unequivocally proved the superiority of prosthetic repairs over pure tissue repairs in terms of recurrence.[22] Tissue repairs are associated with an irreducible recurrence rate of 5% to 10%. The modern era of hernia repair has seen a progressive decrease in recurrence rates because of improvement in surgical technique and prosthetics. Most authorities agree that prosthetic herniorrhaphy will decrease the recurrence rate by approximately 50% when compared with tissue methods. The properties of the ideal prosthetic material are listed in Box 45–1.[23] Materials that have emerged as suitable for routine use in hernia surgery and fulfill Cumberland's classic ideal characteristics include polypropylene, either monofilament (Marlex, Prolene) or polyfilament (Surgipro), Dacron (Mersilene), and

moperitoneum. The objective of pneumoperitoneum, which is applied in successive sessions, is to increase the amount of room in the peritoneal cavity. Many techniques have been described, including daily needle puncture, placement of an indwelling catheter by a percutaneous system or minilaparotomy, or a completely implanted system involving a tunneled peritoneal catheter and a venous access reservoir. Room air is inflated into the abdominal cavity on a once- or twice-daily timetable to patient tolerance as determined by abdominal discomfort or shortness of breath. Usually, 1 to 2 L is insufflated at each session. Upright chest roentgenography is useful because the level of the diaphragm is a measurable objective monitor.

Potential complications include infection and visceral or vascular injury during placement of the catheter. Furthermore, pneumoperitoneum is not always successful because the insufflated air may preferentially enter the hernia sac and have minimal effect on the abdominal cavity. In addition, pneumoperitoneum has been shown to diminish lower extremity venous return, which could translate into a higher risk for thromboembolic complications. Deep venous thrombosis prophylaxis is prudent when one is considering this approach.

expanded polytetrafluoroethylene (ePTFE) (Gore-Tex). An absorbable prosthesis has no role in groin hernia surgery. The newer biologic prostheses made of human cadaver skin, porcine cross-linked dermal collagen, or porcine small intestinal submucosa are more expensive and have no proven advantage over synthetic prostheses in uncomplicated groin hernia surgery. However, they can be useful in infected groin hernia wounds.[24,25] Recently, the development of prostheses that modulate ECM expression by incorporating basic fibroblast growth factor has attracted the attention of investigators.[26]

Although foreign body reaction, infection, erosion into surrounding structures, rejection, increased incidence of postherniorrhaphy pain, and even carcinogenesis remained an early concern with the use of prostheses, after nearly 50 years of use it is obvious that these fears are without foundation. Metal prostheses have largely been abandoned in the United States because of many of the aforementioned complications. Cost of prostheses is still an issue in many parts of the world, but with the skyrocketing increases in overall operating room charges in the West, the cost of the mesh pales in significance. The incidence of postherniorrhaphy pain is lower with mesh repairs than with pure tissue repairs. When it occurs, however, it can occasionally be relieved by removal of the prosthesis. Sarcomatous transformation has been observed in animals after polypropylene implantation; however, no such transformation has been noted in humans, but one should remain vigilant. Another issue that has recently emerged is the possibility of injury to the vas deferens caused by a reaction to a prosthesis that resulted in infertility in a small subset of patients. This consideration demands careful follow-up. Ironically, one of the major arguments for the routine use of mesh in inguinal hernia surgery is to preserve fertility. The theory is that by decreasing the generally accepted recurrence rate in the general population from 10% to 15%, as seen with the Bassini repair and its variants, to less than 5% with the mesh tension-free approach, reoperative surgery with its heavy toll of testicular loss is avoided.

Approaches to Repair of Groin Hernias

Groin hernia repairs can be performed conventionally (anterior or preperitoneal) or laparoscopically. For conventional operations one can use a prosthesis or a pure tissue technique for repair. Whereas prosthetic approaches are by definition tension-free, avoidance of tension in nonprosthetic repairs is accomplished by relaxing incisions. Table 45–2 summarizes the more common herniorrhaphy procedures. Numerous modifications of inguinal hernia repairs, usually associated with a specific surgeon's name, have been described over time. Laparoscopic herniorrhaphy is dealt with in Chapter 46, Laparoscopic Inguinal Hernia Repair.

Conventional Anterior, Nonprosthetic

Many elements are common to all of the herniorrhaphy procedures, and they will be summarized initially in this section. Subsequently, the distinguishing features of prominent individual operations will be presented.

The initial skin incision is horizontal along the lines of Langer for cosmetic reasons. The incision is deepened through Camper's and Scarpa's fascia to the external oblique aponeurosis. This structure is incised medially to and through the external ring. The superior flap of the external oblique is bluntly swept off the internal oblique muscle laterally and superiorly. The ilioinguinal and iliohypogastric nerves are identified and preserved. The cord structures are then separated from the inferior flap of the external oblique aponeurosis by blunt dissection to expose the shelving edge of the inguinal ligament and the iliopubic tract. The cord structures are lifted en masse with the fingers at the pubic tubercle so that the index finger can be passed underneath to meet the index finger of the other hand. A Penrose drain is placed around the cord for retraction. Most surgeons would now avoid complete division of the cremasteric muscle and instead open it longitudinally to expose the inguinal floor. This avoids testicular descent in the postoperative period. High ligation of the sac performed by formal

---

| Table 45–2 | Commonly Recognized Conventional Inguinal Hernia Repairs |

	Anterior	**Preperitoneal**		**Combined**
Nonprosthetic	Marcy Bassini Moloney darn Shouldice McVay–Cooper's ligament repair Miscellaneous	Original Nyhus-Condon (historical interest only now)		
Prosthetic	Lichtenstein tension-free Hernioplasty Mesh plug and patch	Anterior approach Read-Rives	Posterior approach GPRVS Kugel Nyhus-Condon	Bilayer repair

GPRVS, great prosthesis for reinforcement of the visceral sac.

division and transfixion or simply inverting the sac into the preperitoneal space follows. The latter technique avoids injury to unrecognized incarcerated sac structures and decreases the risk for adhesive complications. It is questionable whether pain is lessened by the simple inversion technique, which avoids incision of the richly innervated peritoneum. A small indirect inguinal hernia sac is completely mobilized and excised or inverted into the preperitoneal space. For a larger indirect hernia or an inguinal-scrotal hernia, the sac should be divided in the inguinal canal. The proximal end can be inverted or excised, but the distal end should not be removed to avoid injury to the testicular blood supply. The anterior wall of this distal sac needs to be opened as far distally as convenient. Contrary to popular opinion in the urologic literature, this technique does not increase the incidence of hydrocele formation. Tanner described a relaxing incision in the anterior rectus sheath that extends from the pubic tubercle superiorly for a variable distance as determined by the tension. This incision works by allowing the various components of the abdominal wall to displace laterally and inferiorly. The rectus muscle itself is strong enough to prevent future herniation. The external oblique fascia is closed to reconstruct the superficial ring tight enough to avoid a so-called industrial hernia, but loose enough to avoid strangulation of the cord structures. The term industrial hernia refers to the presence of a dilated external ring that an inexperienced examiner confuses with a hernia.

The Bassini Repair The Bassini repair involves division of the cremaster muscle lengthwise, followed by resection of the indirect sac while simultaneously exposing the floor of the inguinal canal to assess for a direct hernia. The transversalis fascia in the floor of the inguinal canal is divided along its full length. This ensures adequate inspection for a femoral hernia and results in preparation of the deepest layer of Bassini's famous triple layer (the transversalis fascia, the transversus abdominis, and the internal oblique muscle). After high ligation of the sac, the posterior wall is reconstructed by suturing this triple layer medially to the inguinal ligament and possibly the iliopubic tract laterally. Classically, the first stitch in the repair includes the triple layer superiorly and the periosteum of the medial side of the pubic tubercle along with the rectus sheath. Most surgeons would now avoid the periosteum of the pubic tubercle to decrease the incidence of osteitis pubis. Laterally, the repair ends with closure of the internal ring. In the classic Bassini procedure the suture material used for the repair was silk placed in interrupted fashion. As described earlier, the Bassini operation could be considered a preperitoneal repair, but the American version does not involve opening the transversalis fascia (inguinal floor), hence its classification as a conventional anterior procedure. In lieu of opening the floor, forceps are used to blindly grasp tissue in the hope of including the transversalis fascia and the transversus abdominis muscle. The layer is then sutured along with the internal oblique muscle to the reflected part of the inguinal ligament. Because of anatomic variations among individuals, the structures grasped superiorly are not always consistent. Students of

Bassini believe that it is this variability that accounts for the inferior results achieved with this procedure in North America.[27,28] Perhaps the need to develop better herniorrhaphies would not have been so pressing if Bassini's operation had been practiced as he described it. The McVay Cooper's repair is similar to the Bassini repair except that Cooper's ligament is used instead of the inguinal ligament for the medial portion of the repair. Interrupted sutures beginning at the pubic tubercle and continuing laterally along Cooper's ligament progressively narrow the femoral ring, and this is the most common application (i.e., treatment of a femoral hernia). The last stitch into Cooper's ligament is known as a transition stitch and it includes the inguinal ligament. The stitch effectively narrows the femoral ring and allows a step-up to the inguinal ligament over the femoral vessels so that the repair can be continued laterally similar to the Bassini procedure. A Tanner slide (a relaxing incision on the anterior rectus sheath) is essential because there is considerable tension associated with this repair. It is indicated for the repair of femoral hernias or large direct inguinal hernias with extensive destruction of the inguinal floor when a mesh would be contraindicated, such as infection.

The Moloney Darn The Moloney darn and its variant the Abramson darn use nonabsorbable suture to form a meshwork over the inguinal floor. The interstices of this meshwork fill with fibrous connective tissue that buttresses the weakened area of the inguinal canal. The initial layer consists of a continuous nylon suture to appose the transversalis fascia and the transversus abdominis, rectus, and internal oblique muscles medially to the reflected portion of the inguinal ligament laterally, similar to a Bassini repair. A difference is that the first suture is continued into the muscle about the cord, woven in and out to form reinforcement around the cord, and finally tied to the inguinal ligament on the lateral side of the internal ring. The darn is a second layer with sutures applied in a crisscross fashion through muscular tissue medially to the inguinal ligament. Abramson stresses the importance of leaving the suture loose and not forcing the edges of the repair together during the darn, thereby allowing a "tension-free" repair and maintaining the meshwork structure.[29] The darn must be carried well over the medial edge of the inguinal canal onto the anterior rectus sheath.

The Shouldice Technique The Shouldice Clinic in Toronto serves as a model specialty clinic where hernia repairs are combined with weight reduction and exercise programs. The initial approach is similar to the Bassini repair, with particular importance placed on freeing the cord from its surrounding adhesions, resection of the cremaster muscle, high dissection of the hernia sac, and division of the fascia transversalis. Continuous monofilament steel wire is used to repair the floor to ensure even distribution of tension and avoid the defects that could potentially occur between interrupted sutures. The repair is started at the pubic tubercle by approximating the iliopubic tract laterally to the undersurface of the lateral edge of the rectus muscle. The suture is continued laterally to approximate the iliopubic tract to the medial flap, which is made up of the transversalis fascia, transversus abdominis, and internal oblique. The running suture is continued to the internal ring, where the lateral stump of the cremaster muscle is picked up to form a new internal ring. The direction of the suture line is then reversed toward the pubic tubercle to approximate the medial edge of the internal oblique and transversus abdominis muscles to Poupart's ligament, and the wire is tied to itself. The second wire suture is started near the internal ring and approximates the internal oblique and transversus muscles to a band of external oblique aponeurosis superficial and parallel to the inguinal ligament, in effect creating a second artificial inguinal ligament. The suture is then reversed and a fourth suture line is constructed in a similar manner, superficial to the third line. The cribriform fascia is always incised in the thigh, parallel to the inguinal ligament, to make the inner side of the lower flap of the external oblique aponeurosis available for these multiple layers. When performed by experienced surgeons at the Shouldice Clinic, the operation has a recurrence rate of less than 1% and was the gold standard against which other operations were compared. The major criticisms are that it is difficult to teach and it is hard for surgeons to understand what is really being sewn to what. This is further compounded by the fact that modifications outside the Shouldice Clinic have resulted in different versions.

Conventional Anterior, Prosthetic

Lichtenstein Technique The Lichtenstein Clinic is dedicated to hernia repairs. The herniorrhaphy is performed under local anesthesia with sedation. The initial steps are similar to those of the Bassini repair. After the external oblique aponeurosis has been opened from just lateral to the internal ring through the external ring, the upper leaf is freed from the underlying anterior rectus sheath and internal oblique aponeurosis in an avascular plane from a point at least 2 cm medial to the pubic tubercle to the anterior superior iliac spine laterally. The cord with its cremaster is swept off the pubic tubercle and separated from the inguinal floor. The ilioinguinal nerve, external spermatic vessels, and genital branch of the genitofemoral nerve all remain with the cord structures. The effect is to create a large space for eventual placement of the prosthesis and at the same time provide excellent visualization of the nerves.

High ligation is performed by dissecting the sac from the surrounding cord structures after incising the cremaster muscle longitudinally. Direct hernias are separated from the surrounding structures and reduced back into the preperitoneal space. Dividing the superficial layers of the neck of the sac circumferentially facilitates reduction and aids in maintaining the reduction while the prosthesis is being placed. A suture can also be placed to allow the repair to proceed unencumbered by the sac protruding into the operative field. A mesh prosthesis with a minimum size of 15 by 8 cm is positioned over the inguinal floor. The medial end is rounded to correspond to the patient's anatomy and secured to the

anterior rectus sheath a minimum of 2 cm medial to the pubic tubercle. The mesh is secured on either side of the pubic tubercle, and then the suture is continued along the shelving edge in a running locking fashion. The suture is tied at the internal ring.

Two tails, a wide one (two thirds) above and a narrower (one third) below, are created by making a slit at the lateral end of the mesh. The tails are positioned around the cord structures and placed beneath the external oblique laterally, with the upper tail placed on top of the lower. The lower edge of the superior tail is anchored to the lower edge of the inferior tail by a single suture to re-create the shutter valve at the internal ring. This step is considered crucial for preventing the indirect hernia recurrence that is seen when simple reapproximation of the tails is performed. This shutter valve suture should also pass through the shelving edge to allow the mesh to buckle medially over the direct space and avoid tension when the patient stands upright. A few interrupted sutures are then placed to secure the superior and medial aspects of the mesh to the underlying internal oblique and fascia (Fig. 45–12A and B). Care should be taken to avoid placing anchoring suture through the iliohypogastric nerve. Sufficient laxity should be maintained in the prosthesis to account for the difference in tension between the supine and prone positions and to compensate for mesh shrinkage. The only potential drawback of this procedure is that a femoral hernia could be missed because the inguinal floor is not opened. If one is detected, the posterior surface of the mesh is sutured to Cooper's ligament after the inferior edge has been attached to the inguinal ligament.

Plug and Patch (Rutkow) Technique The mesh plug technique was developed by Gilbert and then modified by Robbins and Rutkow.[30,31] The sac is dissected away from the surrounding structures and reduced into the preperitoneal space after a standard anterior approach. A plug made of rolled polypropylene mesh or prefabricated in the configuration of a flower is inserted into the defect and secured to its edges by interrupted suture. Millikan suggests that the internal petals be sewn to the preperitoneal side of the ring of the defect, which forces the outside of the prosthesis underneath the inner side of the defect and makes it act like a preperitoneal underlay. For an indirect hernia, the plug is held in place with three or four sutures around the defect (Fig. 45–13). For direct hernias, the transversalis fascia is opened to facilitate plug placement (Fig. 45–14). The patch portion is optional and involves placing a flat piece of polypropylene in the conventional inguinal space so that it widely overlaps the plug in a fashion similar to the Lichtenstein procedure (Fig. 45–15). The technique is not only fast but also easy to teach in both academic and private centers.

Conventional Preperitoneal Prosthetic

The key to preperitoneal prosthetic repairs is placement of a large prosthesis in the preperitoneal space between the transversalis fascia and the peritoneum, in effect replacing the transversalis fascia. This preperitoneal

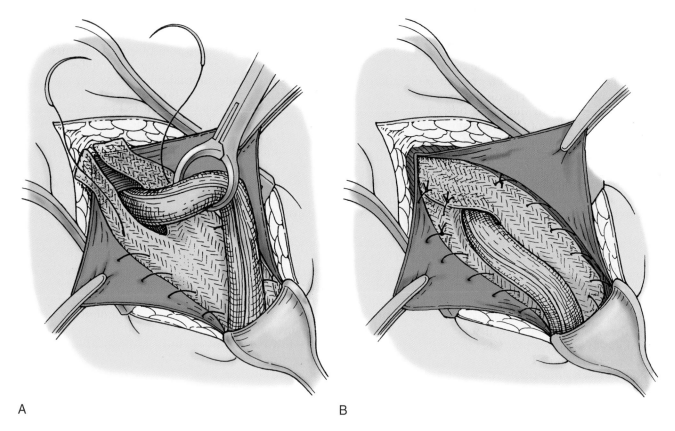

A   B

Figure 45–12.   Lichtenstein repair. **A,** One of the sutures demonstrates approximation of the inferior edge of the prosthesis to the inguinal ligament. The second suture will include the inferior surface of the superior tail and the inferior surface of the inferior tail just lateral to the internal ring, as well as the inguinal ligament, to create a shutter valve. (From Surg Clin North Am 83:1110-1111, 2003.) **B,** The "shutter" valve has been completed, and the superior and medial surfaces have been sutured to the underlying internal oblique muscle and anterior rectus sheath, respectively. This older illustration shows continuous suture on the superior medial border of the prosthesis, but interrupted sutures are now preferred by most surgeons to minimize the incidence of nerve entrapment. (From Kurzer M, Belsham PA, Kark AE: The Lichtenstein repair for groin hernias. Surg Clin North Am 83:1099-1117, 2003. Courtesy of Gillian Lee.)

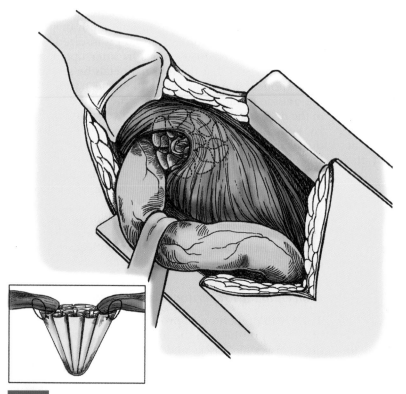

Figure 45–13.   Plug and patch technique: plug placement for an indirect inguinal hernia. The *inset* shows a sagittal view of the implanted plug. (From Rutkow IM: The PerFix plug repair for groin hernias. Surg Clin North Am 83:1079-1098, 2003.)

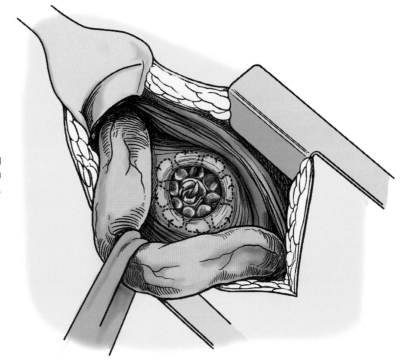

Figure 45–14. Plug and patch technique: plug placement for a direct inguinal hernia. (From Rutkow IM: The PerFix plug repair for groin hernias. Surg Clin North Am 83:1079-1098, 2003.)

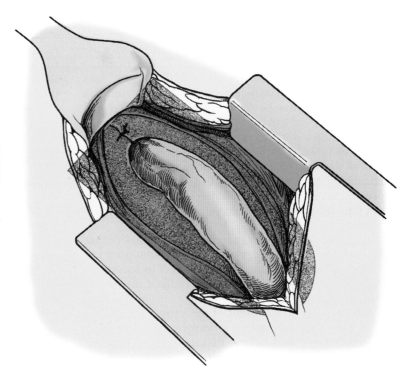

Figure 45–15. Tails of the mesh encircling the spermatic cord. One or two sutures are placed where the tails of the mesh cross lateral to the cord to ensure a snug fit. (From Kurzer M, Belsham PA, Kark AE: The Lichtenstein repair for groin hernias. Surg Clin North Am 83:1099-1117, 2003. Courtesy of Gillian Lee.)

space can be entered from either the anterior or the posterior aspect. In the anterior approach a groin incision is made and the space is entered directly through the inguinal floor. A midline, Pfannenstiel, or paramedian incision can be used to enter the space from the posterior aspect. The transabdominal approach as advocated by LaRoque has returned to popularity because of the ease of entering the space laparoscopically.

Anterior Approach (Read/Rives) This operation starts like a classic Bassini procedure, including opening the inguinal floor. The inferior epigastric vessels are identified and the preperitoneal space is completely dissected. The spermatic cord is parietalized by separating the ductus deferens from the spermatic vessels. A 12- by 16-cm mesh is positioned in the preperitoneal space deep to the inferior epigastric vessels and secured with three sutures: one each to the pubic tubercle, Cooper's ligament, and the psoas laterally. The transversalis fascia is closed over the prosthesis and the cord structures replaced before closure.

Posterior Approach

Great Prosthesis for Reinforcement of the Visceral Sac The procedures described by Wantz, Stoppa, and Rives are grouped together under the heading of great prosthesis for reinforcement of the visceral sac because they have only minor variations. These repairs are used for bilateral hernias, recurrent hernias, and diffuse abdominal wall weakness associated with collagen disorders. A lower midline, transverse or Pfannensteil incision can be used according to surgeon preference. If a transverse incision is chosen, it should extend from the midline 8 to 9 cm in each direction laterally and 2 to 3 cm below the level of the anterior superior iliac spine, but above the level of the internal ring. The anterior rectus sheath and the oblique muscles are incised for the length of the skin incision. The lower flap of these structures is retracted inferiorly toward the pubis. The preperitoneal space is entered by incising the fascia transversalis along the lateral edge of the rectus muscle or by incising the fascia overlying the space of Retzius. The preperitoneal space is completely dissected to a point lateral to the anterior superior iliac spine. The symphysis pubis, Cooper's ligament, and iliopubic tract are identified. The spermatic cord is "parietalized" (completely dissected) to provide adequate length to displace it laterally. Direct sacs are reduced in the course of this dissection. Indirect sacs are mobilized from the cord structures and reduced back into the peritoneal cavity. Large sacs may be difficult to mobilize and may be divided so that the distal part of the sac is left in situ and the proximal portion of the sac is dissected away from the cord structures. Care should be taken during the course of this dissection to avoid damage to the testicular vessels. It must be particularly emphasized that the dissection should proceed in the relatively avascular plane between the fascia transversalis and the peritoneum to avoid a bloody procedure.

Stoppa and Wantz recommend that the abdominal wall defect be left alone, but other surgeons prefer to plicate the fascia transversalis in the defect by suturing it to Cooper's ligament to prevent a bulge caused by a seroma in the undisturbed sac.

The next step is placement of the prosthesis. Dacron mesh is preferred over polypropylene by many European surgeons because they believe that it conforms better to the preperitoneal space. The size of the prosthesis for unilateral repairs is approximately the distance between the umbilicus and the anterior superior iliac spine minus 1 cm for the width, with the height being approximately 14 cm. Because of his extensive parietalization of the cord structures, Stoppa does not think that it is necessary to split the prosthesis laterally to accommodate the cord structures, and this avoids potential recurrence through the keyhole. Wantz recommends cutting the prosthesis eccentrically, with the lateral side longer than the medial, to achieve the best fit in the preperitoneal space. Rignault, on the other hand, prefers a keyhole defect in the

mesh to encircle the spermatic cord in the belief that this technique provides the prosthesis with enough security that fixation sutures or tacks can be avoided. Minimizing fixation in this area is important because of the numerous anatomic elements in the preperitoneal space that could be inadvertently damaged during suture or tack placement. For Wantz's technique, three absorbable sutures are used to attach the superior border of the prosthesis to the anterior abdominal wall well above the defect. The three sutures are placed near the linea alba, semilunar line, and anterior superior iliac spine in a medial-to-lateral direction. A Reverdin suture needle facilitates such placement. Subsequently, the mesh is positioned to cover the iliac fossa and the parietalized cord structures and iliopsoas muscle laterally; the pubic ramus, obturator fossa, and iliac vessels medially; and the space of Retzius in the middle. The size of the mesh for the Stoppa technique to repair bilateral hernias is the distance between the two anterior superior iliac spines minus 2 cm for the width, and the height is equal to the distance between the umbilicus and the pubis. The wound is closed in layers.[32]

Nyhus/Condon (Iliopubic Tract Repair) These two authorities performed extensive cadaver dissections and pointed out the importance of the iliopubic tract. A transverse lower abdominal incision is made two fingerbreadths above the pubic symphysis. The anterior rectus sheath is opened on its lateral side to allow the rectus muscle to be retracted medially, and the two oblique and the transversus abdominis muscles are incised to expose the fascia transversalis. A combination of sharp and blunt dissection inferiorly opens the preperitoneal space and exposes the posterior inguinal floor. Direct or indirect defects are repaired similarly after the peritoneal sac has been reduced or divided and closed proximally. The transverse aponeurotic arch is sutured to the iliopubic tract inferiorly, with Cooper's ligament occasionally included in the medial portion of the repair. The internal ring, if large, is also narrowed by placing a suture lateral to it. For femoral hernias the iliopubic tract is sutured to Cooper's ligament. Once the defect has been formally repaired, a tailored mesh prosthesis can be sutured to Cooper's ligament and the transversalis fascia for reinforcement.[33]

Kugel/Ugahary Repair These operations were devised to compete with laparoscopy by using a small 2- to 3-cm skin incision 2 to 3 cm above the internal ring. Kugel locates this point by making an oblique incision one third lateral and two thirds medial to a point halfway between the anterior superior iliac spine and the pubic tubercle. The incision is deepened through the external oblique aponeurosis, and the internal oblique fibers are bluntly spread. The transversalis fascia is opened vertically about 3 cm, but the internal ring is not violated. The inferior epigastric vessels are identified to ensure that the dissection is in the correct plane. The vessels are left adherent to the overlying transversalis fascia. The cord structures are thoroughly parietalized, and anatomic landmarks, including the iliac vessels, Cooper's ligament, pubic bone, and hernia defect, are identified by palpation. Most direct and small indirect sacs are reduced by such dissection; large indirect sacs are often divided with the distal end being left in situ while the proximal end is reduced. A specifically designed 8- by 12-cm prosthesis made of two pieces of polypropylene is deformed and fit through the small incision. It then springs open to regain its normal shape and provides wide overlap of the myopectineal orifice. Ugahary's operation is similar, but a special prosthesis is not needed.[34,35]

Combination Anterior and Preperitoneal Approaches (Bilayer Technique)

This repair depends on a dumbbell-shaped device consisting of two flat pieces of polypropylene mesh connected by a cylinder of the same material. The basis of this design is to take advantage of the benefits of both the anterior and posterior approaches, with prosthetic material being placed in both the preperitoneal space and the conventional inguinal canal. The preperitoneal space is entered through the hernia defect. The deep layer of the prosthesis is deployed in the preperitoneal space, whereas the superficial layer of the device occupies the conventional anterior space in a manner similar to the Lichtenstein repair. It is slit laterally to accommodate the cord structures and then sutured with three or four interrupted sutures to the area of the pubic tubercle, the middle of the inguinal ligament, and the internal oblique muscle.

COMPLICATIONS

Complications specific to laparoscopic herniorrhaphy are presented in Chapter 46, Laparoscopic Inguinal Hernia Repair. General complications such as urinary retention, paralytic ileus, and cardiorespiratory compromise can follow any operative procedure, and inguinal herniorrhaphy is no exception.[36,37] The most common is urinary retention, especially after general anesthesia. Complications specific to the herniorrhaphy itself are summarized in Box 45–2.

Chronic Postherniorrhaphy Pain Syndromes

Chronic postherniorrhaphy groin pain is defined as pain that lasts longer than 3 months after hernia repair. The overall incidence is about 25%, with 10% fitting the definition of moderate or severe pain that prevents the subject from returning to the preoperative level of functioning or is frankly incapacitating. Patients are difficult to categorize because of the heterogeneous description of their pain; nevertheless, an attempt should be made to assign them to one of two groups to help determine therapeutic options: (1) nociceptive pain caused by tissue injury, which is further subdivided into somatic and visceral, and (2) neuropathic pain secondary to nerve damage.

Somatic pain is usually caused by damage to ligaments, tendons, and muscles and includes osteitis pubis and

---

| Box 45–2 | Postherniorrhaphy Complications After Conventional Repair |

Recurrence
Chronic groin pain
 Nociceptive
 Neuropathic
Cord and testicular
 Hematoma
 Ischemic orchitis
 Testicular atrophy
 Injury to the vas deferens
 Hydrocele
 Testicular descent
Bowel and bladder injury
Osteitis pubis
Prosthetic complications
 Contraction
 Erosion
 Infection
 Rejection
 Fracture
Miscellaneous complications
 Seroma
 Hematoma
 Wound infection
General complications

---

adductor tenoperiostitis. Visceral pain refers to specific visceral dysfunction such as dysejaculation and urinary dysfunction. The principles of treating patients with nociceptive pain are similar to those for patients with groin pain but no obvious hernia.

Division, stretching, contusion, crushing, entrapment, or electrical injury to the nerve causes neuropathic groin pain. The nerves most commonly injured during conventional herniorrhaphy are the ilioinguinal and iliohypogastric. The classic manifestation is pain or paresthesia (or both) in the distribution of one of the major nerves. Precise diagnosis of nerve involvement is difficult because of dermatomal overlap. Physical activity aggravates the pain, and a recumbent position with hip flexion relieves it. Reassurance plus conservative treatment with anti-inflammatory medications and local nerve blocks is preferred initially. At least 1 year of conservative treatment should be tried before offering neuroma excision or neurectomy.

Recurrent Hernias

The hernia recurrence rate with the use of prosthetic material is less than 1%. This rate is probably an underestimation of the problem because patients frequently do not return to their original surgeon. It still translates to a hefty number because of the size of the denominator. A recurrent hernia is usually manifested as a bulge with a cough impulse. Occasionally, the initial symptom is pain. In this situation, a consistent definition of recurrent hernia does not exist because of difficulty differentiating a lipoma of the cord, a seroma, or an expansile bulge of the internal oblique muscle from true hernia recurrence. Imaging in the form of CT, MRI, or ultrasound should be obtained to unequivocally document recurrence. Causes of recurrence include (1) failure to perform high ligation or reduce the peritoneal sac with an indirect hernia, (2) inadequate closure of the internal ring, (3) missed hernias, (4) continuing failure of the floor of the canal, and (5) infection. The general principle for managing recurrent hernias depends on the original repair. The logical approach is to perform herniorrhaphy in the space that has not been dissected. If the patient has previously undergone a conventional repair, a preperitoneal repair is best chosen. On the other hand, if the index operation was a preperitoneal one, a repair that is performed in the conventional inguinal space is best.

Cord and Testicular Injury

Ischemic orchitis is defined as postoperative inflammation of the testicle that occurs within 1 to 5 days after surgery. It is thought to result from thrombosis of veins draining the testicle secondary to extensive dissection of the spermatic cord. It is much more common after repair of recurrent hernias. Initial symptoms include a low-grade fever with painful enlargement of the testicle. Management is supportive and consists of scrotal support and anti-inflammatory agents. Ischemic orchitis usually resolves without sequelae but may occasionally progress to testicular atrophy. It is generally accepted that dividing rather than excising large indirect inguinal-scrotal hernia sacs and leaving the distal part of the sac open in situ can decrease the incidence of testicular complications.

The dysejaculation syndrome is defined as a burning, searing, painful sensation occurring just before, during, or after ejaculation (or any combination). A stenotic lesion in the vas deferens probably causes it. The condition is usually self-limited, and thus the initial treatment is expectant. Injury to both vasa is a potentially devastating complication after bilateral hernia repair. If injury to the vas is recognized during herniorrhaphy, reanastomosis should be attempted if paternity is an issue. Even unilateral injury to the vas can result in infertility as a result of the development of sperm antibodies in response to extravasated sperm. Scrotal hematomas can occur after herniorrhaphy as a consequence of cremasteric or vascular hemostatic errors. Postherniorrhaphy hydroceles can develop, but the cause is not known. Although the urologic literature suggests that hydroceles develop as a result of the practice of leaving the distal sac in situ, most experienced hernia surgeons do not accept this theory. Treatment is the same as for any other hydrocele.

Prosthetic Complications

Shrinkage of prosthetic material because of scarification of the recipient's tissues should be anticipated during herniorrhaphy. Sufficient overlap in anticipation of 20% contracture is recommended. Mesh migration of polypropylene plugs into nearby organs such as the bladder has been reported but is rare. Intra-abdominal placement of a mesh prosthesis should be avoided in favor of an ePTFE or biologic prosthesis to avoid fistulation or bowel obstruction. Local erosion into cord structures has been reported. Rejection because of allergic reactions is extremely rare and is probably a manifestation of chronic infection. The ideal prosthetic material characteristics are enunciated in Box 45–1.

Bowel and Bladder Injury

Bladder and bowel injury is unusual with conventional anterior herniorrhaphy unless a sliding hernia goes unrecognized during repair. The bladder is at much greater risk during preperitoneal procedures, especially in the setting of previous surgery in the space of Retzius. Previous surgery in this space can be considered a relative contraindication to preperitoneal repair. Bladder injuries need to be repaired in two layers with absorbable suture, followed by extended Foley decompression until a cystogram confirms bladder integrity.

Wound Infection

The groin appears to be a protected area inasmuch as wound infection after inguinal herniorrhaphy occurs in less than 5% of patients. However, this figure may be an underestimation of the true incidence because of a delayed manifestation in many cases. In a recent study from the United Kingdom, the median interval between repair and infection was 4 months (range, 2 weeks to 39 months).[38] Most surgeons in North America would recommend prophylactic broad-spectrum antibiotics, although studies by the Cochrane group have shown no benefit.[39] Whereas infection after nonprosthetic repairs can be managed by open drainage and dressing changes, prosthetic removal is commonly required in addition to routine wound care after prosthetic procedures. In general, ePTFE prostheses always have to be removed, but true meshes can on occasion be salvaged with conservative wound care and antibiotic treatment. The late recurrence rate is much higher after a postoperative wound infection.

SUGGESTED READINGS

Annibali R, Quinn TH, Fitzgibbons RJ Jr: Anatomy of the inguinal region from the laparoscopic perspective: Critical areas for laparoscopic repair. In Bendavid R (ed): Prosthesis and Abdominal Wall Hernias. Austin, TX, RG Landes, 1994, pp 82-103.

Bendavid R: The unified theory of hernia formation. Hernia 8:171-176, 2004.

Condon RE, Nyhus LM: Complications of groin hernia. In Condon RE, Nyhus LM (eds): Hernia, 4th ed. Philadelphia, JB Lippincott, 1995, pp 269-282.

EU Hernia Trialists Collaboration: Repair of groin hernia with synthetic mesh: Meta analysis of randomized controlled trials. Ann Surg 235:322-332, 2002.

Jansen PL, Mertens PR, Klinge U, Schumpelick V: The biology of hernia formation. Surgery 136:1-4, 2004.

REFERENCES

1. Rutkow IM: A selective history of hernia surgery in the late eighteenth century: The treatises of Percivall Pott, Jean Louis Petit, D. August Gottlieb Richter, Don Antonio de Gimbernat, and Pieter Camper. Surg Clin North Am 83:1021-1044, 2003.
2. Bassini E: Nuovo metodo per la cura radicale dell'ernia inguinale. Atti Congr Assoc Med Ital 2:179, 1887.
3. Bassini E: Sopra 100 casi di cura radicale dell'ernia inguinale operata col metodo dell'autore. Arch Ed Atti Soc Ital Chir 5:315, 1885.
4. Kitchen WH, Doyle LW, Ford GW: Inguinal hernia in very low birth-weight children: A continuing risk to age 8 years. J Paediatr Child Health 27:300-301, 1991.
5. Hair A, Paterson C, Wright D, et al: What effect does the duration of an inguinal hernia have on patient symptoms? J Am Coll Surg 193:125-129, 2001.
5a. Fitzgibbons RJ Jr, Giobbie-Hurder A, Gibbs JO, et al: Watchful waiting vs repair of inguinal hernia in minimally symptomatic men: A randomized clinical trial. JAMA 295:285-292, 2006.
6. Abramson JH, Gofin J, Hopp C, et al: The epidemiology of inguinal hernia. A survey in western Jerusalem. J Epidemiol Community Health 32:59-67, 1978.
7. Akin ML, Karakaya M, Batkin A, Nogay A: Prevalence of inguinal hernia in otherwise healthy males of 20 to 22 years of age. J R Army Med Corps 143:101-102, 1997.
8. Russel RH: The saccular theory of hernia and the radical operation. Lancet 3:1197-1208, 1906.
9. Peacock EE Jr, Madden JW: Studies on the biology and treatment of recurrent inguinal hernia. II. Morphological changes. Ann Surg 179:567-571, 1974.
10. Canon DJ, Read RC: Metastatic emphysema: A mechanism for acquiring inguinal herniation. Ann Surg 194:270-278, 1981.
11. Jansen PL, Mertens PR, Klinge U, Schumpelick V: The biology of hernia formation. Surgery 136:1-4, 2004.
12. Bellon JM, Bajo A, Ga-Honduvilla N: Fibroblasts from the transversalis fascia of young patients with direct inguinal hernias show constitutive MMP-2 over expression. Ann Surg 233:287-291, 2001.
13. Klinge U, Zheng H, Si ZY, et al: Synthesis of type I and III collagen, expression of fibronectin and matrix metalloproteinases-1 and -13 in hernial sacs of patients with inguinal hernia. Int J Surg Invest 1:219-227, 1999.
14. Bendavid R: The unified theory of hernia formation. Hernia 8:171-176, 2004.
15. Condon RE: The anatomy of the inguinal region and its relation to the groin hernia. In Nyhus LM, Condon RE (eds): Hernia, 3rd ed. Philadelphia, JB Lippincott, 1989, pp 18-64.
16. Anniballi R, Quinn TH, Fitzgibbons RJ Jr: Anatomy of the inguinal region from the laparoscopic perspective: Critical areas for laparoscopic repair. In Bendavid R (ed): Prosthesis and Abdominal Wall Hernias. Austin, TX, RG Landes, 1994, pp 82-103.
17. Cameron AE: Accuracy of clinical diagnosis of direct and indirect inguinal hernia. Br J Surg 81:250, 1994.
18. Van den Berg JC, de Valois JC, Go PM, Rosenbusch G: Detection of groin hernia with physical examination, ultrasound, and MRI compared with laparoscopic findings. Invest Radiol 34:739-743, 1999.
19. Zollinger MZ: Classification systems for groin hernias. Surg Clin North Am 83:1053-1063, 2003.
20. Kingsnorth AN: A clinical classification for patients with inguinal hernia. Hernia 8:283-284, 2004.
21. Report of a working party convened by the Royal College of Surgeons of England: Clinical guidelines on the management of groin hernias in adults. London, Royal College of Surgeons of England, 1993.
22. EU Hernia Trialists Collaboration: Repair of groin hernia with synthetic mesh: Meta analysis of randomized controlled trials. Ann Surg 235:322-332, 2002.
23. Cumberland VH: A preliminary report on the use of a prefabricated nylon weave in the repair of ventral hernia. Med J Aust 1(5):143-144, 1952.
24. Read RC: Prosthesis in abdominal wall hernia surgery. In Bendavid R (ed): Prosthesis and Abdominal Wall Hernias. Austin, TX, RG Landes, 1994, pp 2-6.
25. Read RC: The milestones in the repair of hernia surgery: Prosthetic repair. Hernia 8:8-14, 2004.
26. Dunbay DA, Wang X, Kuhn MA, et al: The prevention of incisional hernia formation using a delayed-release polymer of basic fibroblast growth factor. Ann Surg 240:179-186, 2004.
27. Rutkow IM: A selective history of groin herniorrhaphy in the 20th century. Surg Clin North Am 73:395-411, 1993.
28. Castrini G, Pappalardo G, Trentino P et al: The original Bassini technique in the surgical treatment of inguinal hernia. Int Surg 71:141-143, 1986.
29. Lifschutz H: The inguinal darn. Arch Surg 121:717-718, 1986.
30. Gilbert AI: Sutureless repair of inguinal hernia. Am J Surg 163:331-335, 1992.
31. Robbins AW, Rutkow IM: Mesh plug repair and groin hernia surgery. Surg Clin North Am 78:1007-1023, vi-vii, 1998.
32. Wantz GE, Fischer E: Unilateral giant prosthetic reinforcement of the visceral sac. In Fitzgibbons RJ Jr, Grenburg AG (eds): Nyhus and Condon's Hernia, 5th ed. Philadelphia, Lippincott, Williams & Wilkins, 2002, pp 219-227.
33. Nyhus LM: Iliopubic tract repair of inguinal and femoral hernia. The posterior (preperitoneal) approach. Surg Clin North Am 73:487-499, 1993.
34. Kugel RD: Minimally invasive, nonlaparoscopic, preperitoneal, and sutureless, inguinal herniorraphy. Am J Surg 178:298-302, 1999.
35. Ugahary F: The gridiron hernioplasty. In Bendavid R, Abrahamson J, Flament JB, Phillips EH (eds): Hernias of the Abdominal Wall: Principles and Management. New York, Springer-Verlag, 2001 pp 407-411.
36. Bendavid R: Complications of groin hernia surgery. Surg Clin North Am 78:1089-1103, 1998.
37. Condon RE, Nyhus LM: Complications of groin hernia. In Condon RE, Nyhus LM (eds): Hernia, 4th ed. Philadelphia, JB Lippincott, 1995, pp 269-282.
38. Kumar S, Foo Wong P, Melling A, Leaper DJ: Surgical site repair after groin hernia repair. Br J Surg 91:105-111, 2004.
39. Sanchez-Manuel FJ, Seco-Gil JL: Antibiotic prophylaxis for hernia repair. Cochrane Database Syst Rev 2:CD003769, 2003.

46

Laparoscopic Inguinal Hernia Repair

Varun Puri · Alene J. Wright · Robert J. Fitzgibbons, Jr.

Laparoscopic techniques and procedures were introduced into mainstream general surgery in the 1980s with the development of laparoscopic cholecystectomy. Since then, the laparoscopic approach has been adapted for numerous conventional general surgical operations, and many ingenious surgeons have devised new operations using videoscopic principles. Inguinal hernia surgery is no exception. The two most commonly performed laparoscopic inguinal hernia repairs, the *transabdominal preperitoneal* (TAPP) repair and the *totally extraperitoneal* (TEP) repair, have been modeled after the conventional open preperitoneal inguinal hernia repairs. The *intraperitoneal onlay mesh* (IPOM) repair, however, is a novel laparoscopic approach and is the only truly minimally invasive laparoscopic herniorrhaphy because radical dissection of the preperitoneal space is avoided. The other advancement that has defined the development of modern-day hernia surgery, though not limited to laparoscopic techniques, is the development of newer and better prosthetics.

APPLIED ANATOMY OF THE REGION

A detailed understanding of the anatomy of the deep inguinal region and the posterior aspect of the anterior abdominal wall is necessary to perform a laparoscopic inguinal hernia repair. Mastery of this knowledge is especially important because the region contains a number of major blood vessels and nerves that may be exposed to injury. Anatomic background descriptions for traditional repairs have defined the anatomy from the superficial to the deep aspect because this is the perspective that the surgeon will use when performing a herniorrhaphy. Understanding the same from the opposite perspective was the first challenge that laparoscopists faced. What follows is a description of the anatomy from the peritoneal surface to the skin.

Peritoneal Folds and Fascia Transversalis

The umbilical folds in most patients are quite prominent and easily identified. They have been referred to as ligaments in some texts but do not possess the true structure of a ligament. The unpaired median umbilical fold covers the urachus, the fibrous remnant of the fetal allantois, and extends from the urinary bladder to the umbilicus. The urachus may be patent for a variable length along its course, usually close to the urinary bladder in adults and close to the umbilicus in children. The paired medial umbilical folds are created by the obliterated fetal umbilical arteries. The artery, like the urachus, may be patent in its proximal course and may contribute to the superior vesical artery. The paired lateral umbilical folds are created by the peritoneal coverings over the inferior epigastric vessels. The inferior epigastric artery arises from the external iliac artery and supplies the anterior abdominal wall. It enters the rectus sheath at about the level of the arcuate line. Injury to this vessel may occur during accessory trocar placement. The fossa lying between the median and medial umbilical folds is called the supravesical fossa. The fossa formed between the medial and lateral ligaments is the medial fossa and is the site of direct inguinal hernias. The lateral fossa extends lateral to the lateral umbilical fold and is the site of indirect inguinal hernias (Fig. 46–1).

The transversalis fascia is the deep or endoabdominal fascia covering the internal surface of the transversus abdominis, iliacus, psoas, and obturator internus muscles and portions of the periosteum of the pelvis. Some authors believe that this fascia consists of two layers or laminae. The importance of the transversalis fascia for laparoscopic hernia surgeons is due to its derivatives or analogues: the iliopectineal arch, iliopubic tract, and crura of the deep inguinal ring. The iliopectineal arch, a condensation of the transversalis fascia, is situated at the medial border of the iliacus muscle and is continuous with the fascia iliaca, or the endoabdominal fascia

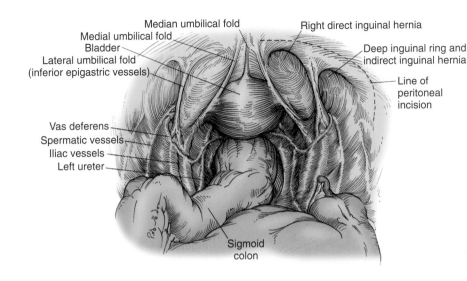

Median umbilical fold
Medial umbilical fold
Bladder
Lateral umbilical fold
(inferior epigastric vessels)

Right direct inguinal hernia

Deep inguinal ring and
indirect inguinal hernia

Line of
peritoneal
incision

Vas deferens
Spermatic vessels
Iliac vessels
Left ureter

Sigmoid
colon

Figure 46–1. Laparoscopic view of groin anatomy before incision of the peritoneum. (From Eubanks S: Hernias. In Sabiston DC Jr, Lyerly HK [eds]: Sabiston Textbook of Surgery: The Biological Basis of Modern Surgical Practice, 15th ed. Philadelphia, WB Saunders, 1997, p 1226.)

covering the iliacus. The iliopectineal arch divides the vascular compartment containing the iliac vessels from the neuromuscular compartment containing the iliopsoas muscle, femoral nerve, and lateral femoral cutaneous nerve. The iliopubic tract is a condensation of the transversalis fascia that is attached to the iliac crest laterally, crosses over the femoral vessels, and inserts on the pubic tubercle medially. It serves as an important landmark for laparoscopic surgeons, and its location should always be established during preperitoneal dissection. Branches of the lumbar plexus (T12, S1-S4) are located inferior to this tract. Mesh fixation or excessive dissection in this location can lead to nerve damage/entrapment and result in long-term morbidity. The superior and inferior crura of the deep inguinal ring are derived from the transversalis fascia and form a fascial sling. When the transversus abdominis contracts, the crura of the deep ring are pulled upward and laterally, thereby creating a valve-like action at the deep ring that prevents the formation of indirect hernias.

Important Nerves and Vessels

The lumbar plexus is formed by nerve roots from the 12th thoracic and 1st through 4th lumbar nerves. Five branches of this plexus, which have cutaneous innervation, can be seen to course across the iliacus muscle and are encountered during laparoscopic inguinal hernia repair (Fig. 46–2). The nerve branches, which may quite variable in course in different subjects, lie in the so-called triangle of pain bordered medially by the psoas muscle, anteriorly and inferiorly by the iliopubic tract, and laterally by the iliac crest.[1] This region lateral to the spermatic cord and posterior to the level of the iliopubic tract, where the cutaneous nerves reside, has also been referred to as the "electrical hazard zone."[2] The use of electrocautery is best avoided in this area.

The most anterior nerve seen is the genitofemoral nerve. The genital branch travels with the spermatic cord and innervates the cremaster muscle and the medial aspect of the scrotum, whereas the femoral branch innervates the skin of the proximal aspect of the midthigh. The femoral nerve lies deep to the lateral psoas muscle and is not routinely encountered during dissection. The lateral femoral cutaneous nerve crosses the iliac fossa deep to the iliacus fascia and the iliopubic tract and pierces the inguinal ligament to enter the thigh. The iliohypogastric nerve arises from the first lumbar trunk and courses across the iliac fossa to pierce the transversus abdominis. It then courses between the transversus and internal oblique muscles and becomes superficial by piercing the aponeuroses of both the internal and external oblique muscles just above the superficial inguinal ring. The ilioinguinal nerve, also arising from the first lumbar nerve root, runs parallel and just inferior to the iliohypogastric nerve in the iliac fossa. It usually pierces the transversus abdominis and internal oblique muscles to eventually enter the inguinal canal.

The inferior epigastric artery, a branch of the external iliac artery, supplies the deep anterior abdominal wall (Fig. 46–3). In some individuals, more frequently than previously thought, an artery called the "aberrant" obturator artery arises from the inferior epigastric artery, arches over Cooper's ligament, and joins the "normal" obturator artery to complete a vascular ring. It is referred to as the "corona mortis." Injury to this ring may be sustained while working in the region of Cooper's ligament and results in severe bleeding. The internal spermatic vessels and the ductus deferens approach the deep inguinal ring from different directions. As the two structures approach, they form the apex of the "triangle of doom,"[3] so called because deep to it, hidden under the peritoneum and transversalis fascia, are the external iliac vessels. Identification of the ductus deferens may not be easy in all subjects, thus rendering it and the adjacent iliac vessels at risk during mesh fixation. Another vessel of some importance in this region is the deep circumflex artery. Its origin may be variable, but it usually courses along the iliopubic tract, pierces the transversalis fascia, and runs across the iliac fossa. It may sustain injury during mesh fixation close to the iliopubic tract.

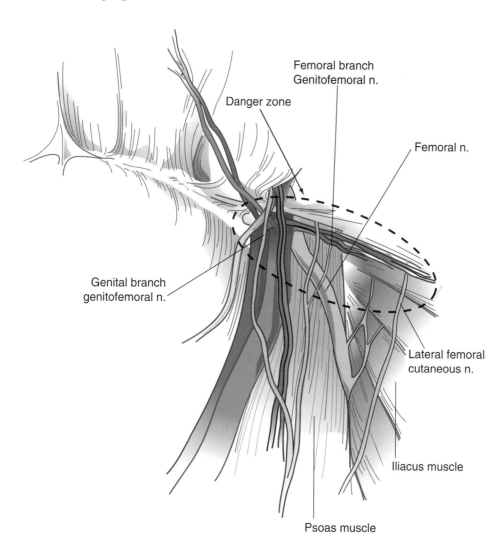

Femoral branch
Genitofemoral n.

Danger zone

Femoral n.

Genital branch
genitofemoral n.

Figure 46–2. Important nerves and their relationship to inguinal structures (the right side is illustrated).

Lateral femoral
cutaneous n.

Iliacus muscle

Psoas muscle

LAPAROSCOPIC OR CONVENTIONAL INGUINAL HERNIORRHAPHY

Over the past decade a number of randomized trials have been conducted to compare laparoscopic and conventional hernia repairs (Table 46–1). These trials, along with meta-analyses of pooled data, have indicated that patients undergoing laparoscopic hernia repair experience less pain in the early postoperative period, have lower analgesic and narcotic requirements and better cosmesis, and return to normal activities sooner.[26,27] These improvements are even more marked if we compare laparoscopic repairs with tissue-based/sutured conventional repairs (Table 46–2). Opinion about the laparoscopic approach leading to earlier return to work is divided. Social factors such as workers' compensation issues complicate objective evaluation.

The advantages attributed to the laparoscopic approach must be weighed against its potential disadvantages, which include complications related to laparoscopy such as major vascular injury or bowel injury, possible adhesion formation at trocar sites or where the prosthesis is placed, increased cost because of expensive equipment, increased operating room time, and the need for general anesthesia. Conversely, open/conventional inguinal herniorrhaphy can be performed under local anesthesia, with minimal risk for vascular or bowel injury. Many of the recent randomized trials show a recurrence rate with laparoscopic repair comparable to that of conventional tension-free repair. However, most have been conducted at single centers with a keen interest in laparoscopic surgery. A notable exception to these trials is a recently published multicenter trial conducted in the Veterans' Administration system in which laparoscopic preperitoneal hernia repair (mostly TEP) was compared with tension-free anterior (Lichtenstein) repair.[25] Recurrence was significantly more common after laparoscopic repair than after open repair of primary hernias (10.1% percent versus 4.0%), but rates of recurrence after repair of recurrent hernias were similar in the two groups. This particular study holds importance for surgeons practicing outside a specialty laparoscopic center and has caused many to suggest that the laparoscopic approach should be performed only at centers with a special interest. The early and delayed complication rates of the laparoscopic and conventional approaches are similar, but the seriousness of complications in the laparoscopic approach can be far greater.

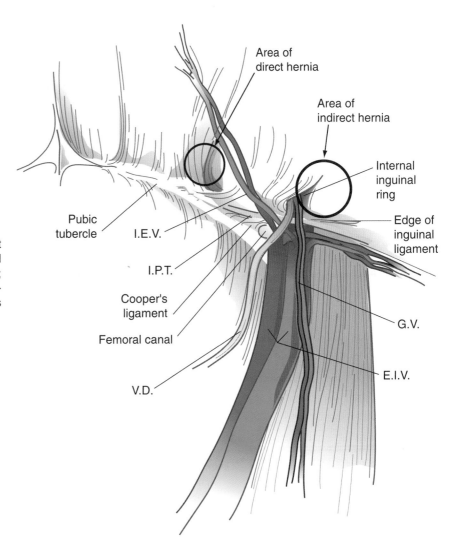

Area of
direct hernia

Area of
indirect hernia

Internal
inguinal
ring

Edge of
inguinal
ligament

Pubic
tubercle

I.E.V.

I.P.T.

Cooper's
ligament

Femoral canal

G.V.

E.I.V.

V.D.

Figure 46–3. Anatomy of the important preperitoneal structures in the right inguinal iliopubic tract. EIV, external iliac vessels; GV, gonadal vessels; IEV, inferior epigastric vein; IPT, iliopubic tract; VD, vas deferens.

The hospital cost of laparoscopic repair is significantly higher than that of conventional repair, but it may be somewhat compensated by the higher productivity attributable to earlier return to work.

Patient Selection

Laparoscopic inguinal herniorrhaphy is technically more challenging than a tension-free anterior repair and thus has a steep learning curve. Consequently, patient selection for the procedure is heavily dependent on the surgeon's experience and skills. If laparoscopic and conventional repairs have equivalent complication and recurrence rates in the hands of a particular surgeon, any patient with an inguinal hernia who can undergo a general anesthetic is a candidate for laparoscopic repair. The laparoscopic approach is particularly useful for bilateral or recurrent hernias. Absolute contraindications include intra-abdominal infection and uncorrectable coagulopathy. Previous surgery in the retropubic space, intra-abdominal adhesions, and the presence of ascites are relative contraindications. Adhesions and suprapubic operations make retroperitoneal dissection difficult and

can result in bladder injury or peritoneal tears leading to exposed mesh. An incarcerated inguinal-scrotal hernia is also a relative contraindication, especially when the colon is involved because of the risk for bowel injury during the dissection. Many laparoscopic herniorrhaphists find that sliding hernias, especially when reducible, are more effectively approached endoscopically than conventionally. However, in the absence of considerable experience, a conventional approach may be preferred.

Operative Strategies

The terminology used in the description of laparoscopic inguinal hernia repair can be confusing because terms such as *preperitoneal* have been used in conventional hernia repairs as well. For the purpose of this chapter, a laparoscopic hernia repair in which the peritoneal cavity is initially entered and the preperitoneal space is entered by another incision into the peritoneum from within the abdomen is called a *transabdominal preperitoneal,* or TAPP, repair. The next commonly used type of laparoscopic inguinal hernia repair is the *totally extraperitoneal,* or TEP,

Table 46–1 Comparative Trials of Laparoscopic and Open Inguinal Hernia Repair Using Mesh

Author	Hernias (n) LH vs. OH	Intervention	Recurrence Rate (%)	Salient Results
Horeyseck et al., 1996[4]	100 vs. 100	TAPP vs. Lichtenstein	8 vs. 0	Higher recurrence, higher cost
Zieren et al., 1996[5]	86 vs. 105	TAPP vs. PP	2.3 vs. 0	Higher recurrence, higher cost, similar complications
Sarli et al., 1997[6]	64 vs. 66	TAPP vs. Lichtenstein	0 vs. 0	Similar complications, missed contralateral hernias in OH group
Champault et al., 1997[7]	50 vs. 50	TAPP vs. Stoppa	6 vs. 2	Lower morbidity, higher patient comfort, higher recurrence rate
Khoury, 1998[8]	169 vs. 146	TAPP vs. MP	2.5 vs. 3	Similar recurrence rates, earlier return to normal activity, lower nerve complications
Paganini et al., 1998[9]	52 vs. 56	TAPP vs. Lichtenstein	2 vs. 0	Similar return to normal activity, higher cost
Aitola et al., 1998[10]	24 vs. 25	TAPP vs. Lichtenstein	13 vs. 8	Similar return to work, higher recurrence rates
Picchio et al., 1999[11]	53 vs. 52	TAPP vs. Lichtenstein	Not mentioned	Higher pain scores, similar recovery periods
Kumar et al., 1999[12]	25 vs. 25	TEP vs. Lichtenstein	4 vs. 8	*Nonrandomized,* lower pain score, fewer local complications
Johansson et al., 1999[13]	613 total	TAPP vs. preperitoneal mesh vs. conventional	2 vs. 5.5 vs. 2	Earlier resumption of normal activity and return to work, higher cost
MRC group, 1999[14]	468 vs. 460	TEP vs. mainly tension-free	1.9 vs. 0	Earlier resumption of normal activity, less long-term pain, higher recurrence rate
Beets et al., 1999[15]	56 vs. 52	TAPP vs. Stoppa	12.5 vs. 1.9	Less pain, fewer early complications
Sarli et al., 2001[16]	40 vs. 46	TAPP vs. Licttenstein	0 vs. 4.3	Less pain, earlier return to work
Wright et al., 2002[17]	145 vs. 151	TEP vs. mostly Lichtenstein	2 vs. 2	Similar recurrences, similar missed contralateral hernias
Pikoulis et al., 2002[18]	309 vs. 234	TAPP vs. MP	1.9 vs. 0.4	*Nonrandomized,* higher cost, higher recurrence rate
Mahon et al., 2003[19]	60 vs. 60 (all bilateral or recurrent)	TAPP vs. Lichtenstein	6.7 vs. 1.7	Shorter operative time, less pain, earlier return to work
Andersson et al., 2003[20]	81 vs. 87	TEP vs. Lichtenstein	2.5 vs. 0	Similar complications, earlier return to work, less pain, higher recurrence rate
Douek et al., 2003[21]	122 vs. 120	TAPP vs. Lichtenstein	1.6 vs. 2.5	Less groin pain, less frequent paresthesias
Bringman et al., 2003[22]	Total N = 298	TEP vs. MP vs. Lichtenstein	1.3 vs. 1.3	Shorter sick leave period, less time to full recovery
Lal et al., 2003[23]	25 vs. 25	TEP vs. Lichtenstein	0 vs. 0	Earlier return to work better cosmesis, similar recurrence rate
Heikkinen et al., 2004[24]	62 vs. 61	TAPP vs, Lichtenstein	8 vs. 3.2	Similar recurrence rate, less long-term groin pain
Neumayer et al., 2004[25]	862 vs. 834	TAPP/TEP vs. Lichtenstein	10.1 vs. 4	Less pain, higher recurrence rate for primary hernias

IPOM, intraperitoneal onlay mesh repair; LH, laparoscopic hernia repair; MP, mesh plug repair; OH, open hernia repair; PP, patch plug repair; TAPP, transabdominal preperitoneal hernia repair; TEP, totally extraperitoneal repair.

Table 46–2   Comparative Trials of Laparoscopic and Open Tissue-Based Inguinal Hernia Repair

Author	Hernias (n) LH vs. OH	Intervention	Recurrence Rate (%)	Salient Results
Lawrence et al., 1995[28]	58 vs. 57	TAPP vs. Maloney darn	Not mentioned	Less pain, higher cost, similar return to work
Vogt et al., 1995[29]	30 vs. 32	IPOM vs. Bassini/McVay	3 vs. 6	Lower analgesic requirement, earlier return to normal activity
Liem et al., 1997[30]	487 vs. 507	TEP vs. mostly tissue repairs	3 vs. 6	Rapid recovery, shorter time to return to work, fewer recurrences
Dirksen et al., 1998[31]	114 vs. 103	TAPP vs. Bassini	6 vs. 21	Less pain, earlier resumption of normal activity, fewer recurrences
Tanphiphat et al., 1998[32]	60 vs. 60	TAPP vs. modified Bassini	1.5 vs. 0	Higher cost, less pain, earlier return to full activity, similar work leave
Zieren et al., 1998[33]	80 vs. 80 vs. 80	TAPP vs. MP vs. Shouldice	0 vs. 0 vs. 0	Less pain, less restriction of activity
Juul et al., 1999[34]	138 vs. 130	TAPP vs. Shouldice	2.9 vs. 2.3	Lower analgesic requirement, early return to work, similar recurrence rates
Leibl et al., 2000[35]	48 vs. 43	TAPP vs. Shouldice	2 vs. 5	Greater patient satisfaction, similar recurrence rates
Tschudi et al., 2001[36]	51 vs. 49	TAPP vs. Shouldice	3.9 vs. 10.2	Less pain, earlier return to full activity, fewer recurrences
Wennstrom et al., 2004[37]	131 vs. 130	Tep vs. Shouldice	Similar	Similar pain, hospital stay, complications, and recurrence rates

IPOM, intraperitoneal onlay mesh repair; LH, laparoscopic hernia repair; MP, mesh plug repair; OH, open hernia repair; TAPP, transabdominal preperitoneal hernia repair; TEP, totally extraperitoneal repair.

repair. Strictly speaking, the peritoneal cavity is not entered in this approach, and thus true laparoscopy is not performed; however, because a laparoscope and related instruments are used, it is appropriate to discuss this operation here. An inguinal hernia repair that is performed by placing mesh intraperitoneally over the defect via a laparoscopic approach is labeled an *intraperitoneal onlay mesh,* or IPOM, repair.

Transabdominal Preperitoneal Repair

The TAPP procedure is begun with placement of a Hasson cannula at the umbilicus under direct vision. Thorough diagnostic laparoscopy is performed to rule out any unrelated pathology, and both myopectineal orifices are inspected. Two additional 5-mm laparoscopic ports are placed on either side of the umbilical cannula just lateral to the rectus sheath (Fig. 46–4). This assumes the availability of a 5-mm fastening device. If a 10-mm instrument is to be used for this purpose, one of the lateral cannulas will need to be 10 mm. If the hernia is unilateral, a transverse incision of the peritoneum is begun on the lateral side of the medial umbilical ligament. The lateral leaf of the ligament is opened and the peritoneum is incised to a point medial to the anterior superior iliac spine while staying approximately 2 cm above the internal inguinal ring and the hernia defect. The medial umbilical ligament can be divided if needed and the remnant of the obliterated fetal umbilical artery

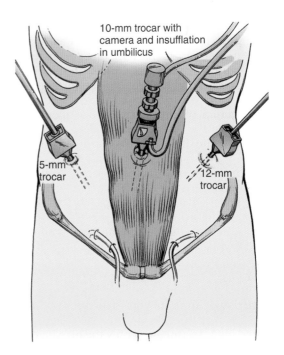

10-mm trocar with camera and insufflation in umbilicus

5-mm trocar

12-mm trocar

Figure 46–4. Trocar placement for a transabdominal preperitoneal laparoscopic hernia repair.

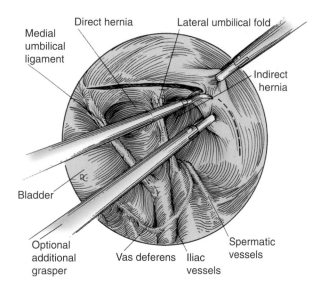

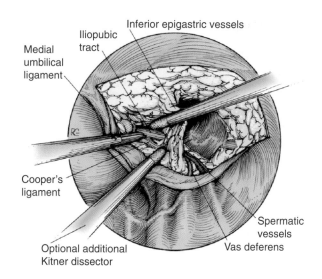

Figure 46–5. A transverse curvilinear peritoneal incision is made cephalad to the internal inguinal ring. The incision extends from the medial umbilical ligament to a point 2 to 3 cm lateral to the internal inguinal ring. The incision may be made in a medial-to-lateral or lateral-to-medial direction. Counteraction on the peritoneum inferior to the line facilitates dissection and reduces the risk of injury to underlying structures (e.g., inferior epigastric vessels). (From Eubanks S: Hernias. In Sabiston DC Jr, Lyerly HK [eds]: Sabiston Textbook of Surgery: The Biological Basis of Modern Surgical Practice, 15th ed. Philadelphia, WB Saunders, 1997, p 1226.)

Figure 46–6. Blunt dissection of the inguinal floor. (From Eubanks S: Hernias. In Sabiston DC Jr, Lyerly HK [eds]: Sabiston Textbook of Surgery: The Biological Basis of Modern Surgical Practice, 15th ed. Philadelphia, WB Saunders, 1997, p 1226.)

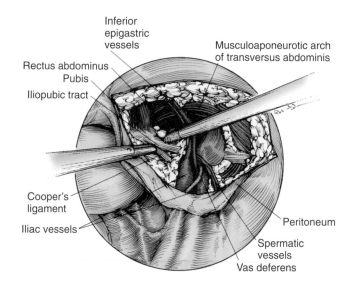

Figure 46–7. Completed dissection of the inguinal floor skeletonizes Cooper's ligament, the iliopubic tract, the lateral edge of the rectus abdominis, and the transversus abdominis aponeurotic arch. (From Eubanks S: Hernias. In Sabiston DC Jr, Lyerly HK [eds]: Sabiston Textbook of Surgery: The Biological Basis of Modern Surgical Practice, 15th ed. Philadelphia, WB Saunders, 1997, p 1226.)

controlled with electrocautery. Extensive, mostly blunt dissection is performed in the preperitoneal space. The use of electrocautery to prevent bleeding is especially helpful because bleeding interferes with adequate visualization by absorbing the light. It is important to dissect beyond the symphysis to the contralateral side to achieve sufficient overlap of all medial hernia openings. Both pubic tubercles, the inferior epigastric vessels, Cooper's ligament, and the iliopubic tract are identified (Figs. 46–5 to 46–8). The spermatic cord structures are mobilized and the peritoneal flap is dissected well proximal to the bifurcation of the vas deferens and the internal spermatic vessels. If the inferior peritoneal flap is not adequately mobilized, the mesh is prevented from laying flat or the inferior edge of the mesh will roll up when the peritoneum is closed. This has been identified as an important mechanism of recurrence with the TAPP procedure. A direct hernia sac is easily reduced during the preperitoneal dissection. A small indirect hernia sac can be dissected away from he cord structures and reduced. A larger sac needs to be divided at a suitable point distal to the deep inguinal ring, with only the proximal portion dissected away from the cord structures. No effort is made to disturb the distal part of the sac because it may lead to unnecessary vascular disruption, which can result in hematoma formation, ischemic orchitis, testicular atrophy, or any combination of these complications.

A large piece of prosthesis (at least 15 × 10 cm) is placed so that the entire myopectineal orifice is gener-

ously covered. At this point one must not forget about the femoral space. Slitting of the mesh laterally to create a new deep ring is optional. There is no conclusive evidence that such slitting confers any advantage over the technique of simply placing the unslit mesh over the internal ring. However, if the mesh is slit, it is important that it be adequately repaired around the cord structures because this step has been incriminated in recurrence.[38]

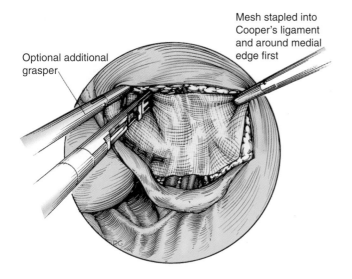

Optional additional grasper

Mesh stapled into Cooper's ligament and around medial edge first

Figure 46–8. The mesh is secured to the anatomic frame with a hernia stapler. (From Eubanks S: Hernias. In Sabiston DC Jr, Lyerly HK [eds]: Sabiston Textbook of Surgery: The Biological Basis of Modern Surgical Practice, 15th ed. Philadelphia, WB Saunders, 1997, p 1226.)

The need for mesh fixation is another controversial subject. Most surgeons believe that the possibility of mesh shrinkage or migration mandates the use of staples, tacks, anchors, or biologic glue. Others think that if a large enough piece of mesh is used, fixation become unnecessary, thereby avoiding complications associated with trauma related to the fixation device.[39] If fixation is chosen, it is begun at the contralateral pubic tubercle and extended medially onto the anterior abdominal wall at least 2 cm superior to the hernia defect, to the anterior superior iliac spine laterally, and to the tissue just above Cooper's ligament inferiorly. Staples, tacks, or anchors should never be placed below the iliopubic tract when lateral to the internal spermatic vessels because of the possibility of nerve damage and neuralgias. For the superior border of the mesh, staples are placed in horizontal fashion to prevent trauma to the ilioinguinal and iliohypogastric nerves, which also run horizontally. Lateral staples are oriented vertically because the femoral branch of the genitofemoral nerve and the lateral cutaneous nerve of the thigh run in this direction. Meticulous peritoneal coverage of the prosthesis is essential, and hence lowering the pressure of the pneumoperitoneum and further undermining of the inferior peritoneal flap may be necessary. The goal is isolation of the prosthesis from the viscera, and if it is not possible to reapproximate the superior and inferior peritoneal flaps, the inferior flap should be tacked to the transversalis fascia after ensuring complete mesh coverage. If all else fails, omentum can be used to cover the exposed mesh.

For bilateral inguinal hernias, both preperitoneal spaces are dissected. The median umbilical ligament is left undisturbed to avoid the theoretical complication of dividing a patent urachus. However, because both preperitoneal spaces communicate with each other

above the symphysis pubis, a single large piece of mesh (at least 30×10 cm) can be used to cover the entire lower portion of the pelvis. Some surgeons prefer two separate pieces of mesh for ease of handling, and there does not appear to be a significant increase in the recurrence rate.[40]

Totally Extraperitoneal Repair

A three-trocar approach for the TEP repair is also used. A 10-mm umbilical incision is deepened to either the ipsilateral or the contralateral anterior rectus sheath, depending on the preference of the surgeon. The rectus sheath is opened and the rectus muscle retracted laterally. The posterior sheath is visualized. Blunt dissection is now begun between the rectus muscle and the posterior rectus sheath with a blunt dissector or a finger while aiming toward the symphysis pubis. A blunt Hasson cannula with a laparoscope is introduced into the space between the rectus abdominis muscle and the posterior rectus sheath. It is aimed beyond the superior third of the distance between the umbilicus and the pubic symphysis. This allows the tip of the trocar to be placed inferior to the arcuate line. The cannula is now advanced at a 30-degree angle off the midline toward the side of the hernia. Gentle side-to-side movements of this assembly are used to dissect this preperitoneal space. Care must be taken to avoid aiming too far posteriorly because the bladder may be injured. Once adequate space has been created, two more ports are placed, one approximately 5 cm above the pubis symphysis and the other midway between the umbilicus and the pubis symphysis. Dissection of the preperitoneal space is now completed under direct vision. Popular technical variations include the use of a saline- or air-filled balloon to dissect the preperitoneal space and placement of the two accessory ports on either side of the midline as in the TAPP repair (Fig. 46–9). One of the advantages of the balloon device is that the preperitoneal space can be visualized through the transparent structure of the balloon. A disadvantage is a higher incidence of dissection in front of the inferior epigastric vessels, which causes them to be reduced with the peritoneal flap. This can complicate exposure. Once the preperitoneal space has been completely developed, treatment of the hernia sac and its contents, parietalization, and placement of the mesh proceed in an fashion identical to that for the TAPP repair.

Potential advantages of the TEP procedure are avoidance of complications associated with entering the peritoneal cavity, including visceral injury, intra-abdominal vascular injury, adhesion formation, and trocar site hernias. Perhaps most important, peritoneal closure does not have to be performed, which eliminates one of the more difficult aspects of the TAPP repair and greatly speeds up the operation. However, the operative space is limited and the anatomy is less easily understood than with the TAPP procedure, thus leading to a slower learning curve. Previous lower abdominal surgery can be a relative contraindication to the TEP repair. Studies comparing the TAPP and TEP repairs have not shown consistent superiority of one approach over the other. A comparison of recent studies of the various methods of

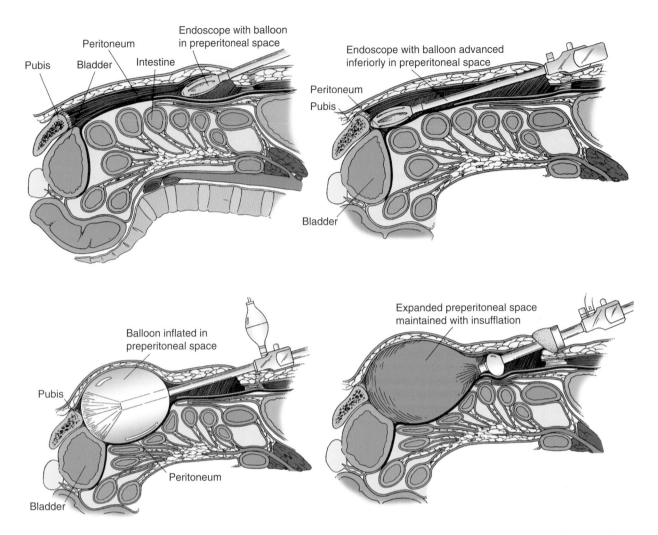

Figure 46–9.   The totally extraperitoneal approach for laparoscopic hernia repair is demonstrated. Access to the posterior rectus sheath is gained in the periumbilical region. **A,** A balloon dissector is placed on the anterior surface. **B,** The balloon dissector is advanced to the posterior surface of the pubis in the preperitoneal space. **C,** The balloon is inflated, thereby creating an optical cavity. **D,** The optical cavity is insufflated with carbon dioxide, and the posterior surface of the inguinal floor is dissected. (From Shadduck PP, Schwartz LB, Eubanks WS: Laparoscopic inguinal herniorrhaphy. In Pappas TN, Schwartz LB, Eubanks WS [eds]: Atlas of Laparoscopic Surgery. Philadelphia, Current Medicine, 1996. Copyright © 1996 by Current Medicine. Reproduced by permission of the publisher.)

laparoscopic hernia repair is presented in Table 46–3. Surgeon expertise with a particular procedure may be the key to consistent good results.

Intraperitoneal Onlay Mesh Repair

Only a thin layer of peritoneum separates the abdominal cavity from the preperitoneal space. The rationale for the IPOM repair is to place a prosthesis directly onto the peritoneum so that radical preperitoneal dissection can be avoided. Initial laparoscopy, port placement, and landmark identification are the same as for the TAPP repair. A large prosthesis is introduced into the peritoneal cavity and secured in place with tacks, staples, or sutures. Some surgeons open the peritoneum over

Cooper's ligament to ensure adequate fixation in this area.

This repair has been less popular than the TAPP and TEP approaches because of concern among surgeons about placing a prosthesis directly in contact with intraperitoneal structures. Many believe that it should be considered an experimental operation. In addition, the results in several series have not been as good as the results of other laparoscopic repairs, with a higher incidence of neuralgia and recurrence, but this may be more a reflection of experience than the operation itself.[45,49] The IPOM repair represents the only truly minimally invasive herniorrhaphy because radical dissection of the preperitoneal space is avoided. The development of a totally inert prosthesis might renew interest in the future.

Table 46–3 Comparative Trials of Different Types of Laparoscopic Inguinal Hernia Repair

Author	Hernias (n)	Intervention	Recurrence Rate (%)	Salient Results
Fitzgibbons et al., 1995[41]	Total 869	TAPP vs. IPOM vs. TEP	4.5 vs. 4.5 vs. 4.5	Similar complication and recurrence rates
Khoury, 1995[42]	60 vs. 60	TAPP vs. TEP		Longer hospital stay and higher analgesic requirement with TAPP
Ramshaw et al., 1996[43]	300 vs. 300	TAPP vs. TEP	2 vs. 0.3	Increased vascular injury and recurrence with TAPP
Kald et al., 1997[44]	393 vs. 98	TAPP vs. TEP	1.5 vs. 1	Higher major complications and recurrences with TAPP
Sarli et al., 1997[45]	59 vs. 56	TAPP vs. IPOM	0 vs. 11.1	Fewer neuralgias and recurrences with TAPP
Van Hee et al., 1998[46]	33 vs. 58	TAPP vs. TEP	2.7 vs. 2.8	Similar complication and recurrence rates
Cohen et al., 1998[47]	108 vs. 100	TAPP vs. TEP	1.9 vs. 0	Similar local complication and recurrence rates, TAPP technically easier
Lepere et al., 2000[48]	1290 vs. 682	TAPP vs. TEP	1 vs. 1	Similar local complication and recurrence rates

IPOM, intraperitoneal onlay mesh repair; TAPP, transabdominal preperitoneal hernia repair; TEP, totally extraperitoneal repair.

COMPLICATIONS OF LAPAROSCOPIC INGUINAL HERNIA REPAIR

The overall incidence of morbidity after laparoscopic inguinal hernia repair has been quite variable (Table 46–4). Complication rates vary from 3%[50] to 25%,[27] depending largely on the thresholds set for categorizing an event as a complication. Fortunately, serious complications are quite uncommon. One may classify these complications according to whether they are related to

Laparoscopy
Hernia repair
Prosthesis
Patient factors

It is also important to classify complications in relation to their timing: immediate (at the time of initial surgery), early (days to weeks), and delayed (months to years).

Complications Associated with the Laparoscopic Approach

Major Vascular Injury

The risk of major vascular injury requiring operative repair is 0.08%.[51] Many authors believe that this incidence is seriously underestimated because such injuries commonly go unreported. Access to the peritoneal cavity is the most crucial phase of laparoscopy, and over three quarters of major vascular injuries occur during insertion of the Veress needle or the trocars at the beginning of the procedure.[52] The vessels most frequently involved include the aorta, inferior vena cava, and the iliac artery and vein. Mesenteric and omental vessels, splenic vessels,

and renal vessels have been injured occasionally. Epigastric vessels running in the rectus sheath may be injured during the placement of secondary trocars. The use of disposable trocars with safety shields, optical trocars, and blunt-tipped cannulas has not eliminated this dramatic complication. It has even been described during the open approach with the Hasson cannula used for initial access.

Knowledge of the anatomic relationships between the anterior abdominal wall and the retroperitoneum, careful introduction of the Veress needle, and avoidance of the Trendelenburg position during initial access have been reported to decrease the incidence of this complication. Major vascular injury is manifested as either hemoperitoneum or retroperitoneal hematoma. Mortality has been estimated to be as high as 36%. Expeditious laparotomy with repair of the vessel is usually required. Lacerations of the epigastric vessels can be controlled by applying pressure applied with a cannula. Occasionally, suture ligation is required, which is now possible with the use of an "exit device" for transfascial suture placement.

Bowel Injury

The incidence of bowel injury and bowel perforation in laparoscopic operations is about 0.13%.[53] Up to half of these injuries occur during the access phase of laparoscopy. The small bowel is the most frequently injured segment (56%). About two thirds of these injuries are detected intraoperatively. The injury can be repaired laparoscopically if the operator is experienced in intracorporeal suturing or the injury is amenable to a stapled repair without compromising luminal diameter. Patients with missed bowel injury typically manifest

| Table 46–4 | Complications of Laparoscopic Hernia Repair |

Associated with Laparoscopy	Associated with the Patient	Associated with the Hernia Repair	Associated with the Prosthesis
Major vascular injury (I)	Ileus (E)	Recurrence (D)	Contraction (D)
Retroperitoneal	Urinary retention (E)	Trocar site problems	Erosion (D)
Intra-abdominal	DVT (E)	Hematoma (E)	Folding (E)
Abdominal wall	Cardiopulmonary	Infection (E)	Infection (E, D)
Bowel injury (I, E)	complications (I, E)	Hernia (D)	Rejection (D)
Bladder injury (I, E)		Keloid (D)	Pain (E, D)
Gas embolism (I)		Seroma (E)	
Bowel obstruction (E, D)		Hematoma (I, E)	
Shoulder pain (E)		Groin	
Subcutaneous/preperitoneal		Scrotal	
emphysema (I, E)		Retroperitoneal	
Diaphragmatic dysfunction (E)		Hydrocele (E, D)	
Arrhythmias (I)		Orchitis (E)	
		Infertility (D)	
		Neurologic (D)	
		Groin pain	
		Anesthesia	
		Paresthesias	
		Dysejaculation (D)	

D, delayed manifestation (weeks to years); DVT, deep venous thrombosis; E, early manifestation (hours to days); I, immediate/intraoperative manifestation.

peritoneal signs and sepsis 1 day to 1 week after the index operation. The overall mortality rate with this complication is about 4%.[53]

Bladder Injury

Injury to the bladder may occur from suprapubic trocar placement or from dissection during the course of the operation. Bladder injury may be obvious when blood and gas collect in the drainage bag if a Foley catheter is in place. When there is any doubt about bladder injury, methylene blue dye may be instilled into the bladder to look for leakage.[54] Bladder injury recognized during laparoscopy should be repaired laparoscopically if the experience of the surgeon is sufficient, followed by bladder drainage for 7 to 10 days. Bladder injury may be manifested in delayed fashion as hematuria and lower abdominal discomfort. A retrograde cystogram generally confirms the diagnosis. Small defects may be managed with urinary drainage, whereas larger defects necessitate repair.

Gas Embolism

Gas embolism is a very rare, but potentially life-threatening complication. Carbon dioxide can be introduced into a large vein, most likely the result of inadvertant cannulation by the Veress needle, and trapped in the right ventricle, where it causes outflow obstruction into the pulmonary artery and sudden circulatory collapse. Careful insertion of the Veress needle

and the usual confirmatory tests of its intraperitoneal position should keep the incidence of air embolism low.

Intestinal Obstruction

During the developmental years of laparoscopic inguinal hernia repair the importance of closing all fascial defects greater then 5 mm was not recognized. This resulted in the development of Richter's hernia with bowel obstruction in occasional patients.[55] Several devices that can be used to close fascial defects larger than 5 mm are now routinely available commercially. Inadequate peritoneal closure over the prosthesis after the TAPP repair may leave gaps that allow bowel to migrate into the preperitoneal space and thereby result in bowel obstruction. Operative strategies to minimize this complication have been described in the section on operative techniques. With the advent of the TEP repair it was hoped that bowel-related complications would be minimized or eliminated. However, frequently unrecognized peritoneal defects are common after the TEP repair, especially in patients with previous lower abdominal surgery, and intestinal obstruction has been reported.[56] Delayed adhesive small bowel obstruction is theoretically possible because of the intra-abdominal dissection. Fortunately, this complication is exceedingly rare.

Shoulder Pain

Shoulder pain is commonly seen after any laparoscopic procedure and can be quite troublesome to the patient.

It is commonly assumed that residual carbon dioxide in the peritoneal cavity is trapped under the diaphragm and causes diaphragmatic irritation and referred pain to the shoulder, but this has never been proved. Nevertheless, it is standard practice to completely deflate the pneumoperitoneum at the conclusion of laparoscopic inguinal herniorrhaphy with the patient still in the Trendelenburg position. A low-pressure pneumoperitoneum has also been recommended.[57]

Subcutaneous and Preperitoneal Emphysema

Subcutaneous emphysema is usually harmless and resolves spontaneously, aided by massaging the swollen anterior abdominal wall toward the nearest trocar site. Preperitoneal emphysema is due to a malpositioned Veress needle and can be frustrating to the surgeon. It can be avoided by using a Hasson cannula for primary access.

Diaphragmatic Dysfunction

Diaphragmatic dysfunction has been described after a variety of laparoscopic procedures. Its exact etiology is unclear, but the effects are transient and generally resolve spontaneously by 24 hours.

Cardiac Arrhythmia

Bradycardia may occasionally follow the creation of pneumoperitoneum. It is a reflex vagal response to peritoneal distention. It can usually be managed by stopping the inflow of carbon dioxide temporarily and administering an anticholinergic drug. Once the heart rate has recovered, pneumoperitoneum can be re-created gradually.

Complications Associated with the Patient

Ileus

Ileus is somewhat more common after a laparoscopic inguinal hernia repair than after a conventional repair. It is a self-limited problem but occasionally requires nasogastric decompression.

Urinary Retention

Older age, general anesthesia, aggressive hydration, narcotics for pain relief, and a history of prostatic symptoms predispose to urinary retention after hernia repair. Intermittent catheterization or temporary placement of an indwelling urinary catheter is usually adequate therapy. Prophylactic use of prazosin after herniorrhaphy may significantly reduce the incidence of urinary retention and catheterization.[58]

Deep Venous Thrombosis

The incidence of deep venous thrombosis after laparoscopic procedures is about 0.33%.[59] Thromboprophylaxis for laparoscopy should be the same as for conventional surgery, that is, tailored to individual risk and continued for a minimum of 7 to 10 days. Graduated compression stockings, sequential intermittent compression devices, maintenance of relatively low insufflation pressure, keeping use of the reverse Trendelenburg position to a minimum, and intermittent release of the pneumoperitoneum in longer procedures are other measures that can decrease the incidence of deep venous thrombosis.

Complications Associated with Hernia Repair

Recurrence

The often-quoted rate of recurrence after a laparoscopic repair is on the order of 3%.[27] Similar recurrence rates are also routinely seen after the open tension-free repair. Most of these data are from specialty centers, however, and the overall recurrence rate after laparoscopic herniorrhaphy may be closer to 10%.[25]

Hernia recurrences may be difficult to distinguish clinically from lipoma of the cord, a seroma, or a bulge in the internal oblique muscle and may require imaging with ultrasound, CT, or MRI. Definitive identification of recurrence is especially important to avoid unnecessary surgery in those with groin pain. It is logical to approach the recurrence through a previously undissected plane, and thus many surgeons prefer to perform an open anterior tension-free repair for a hernia previously repaired laparoscopically. Laparoscopic preperitoneal herniorrhaphy after a previous failed endoscopic herniorrhaphy is controversial. A strong argument can be made that this procedure should not be performed except in cases in which failure has occurred in both the conventional and the preperitoneal space. Nevertheless, surgeons are confronted with patients who request a laparoscopic repair regardless. This situation most commonly comes up when the patient has previously undergone conventional repair on the opposite side. In the hands of experienced laparoscopists, this would appear to be an acceptable approach. However, it is a technically demanding procedure with the potential for serious complications for the uninitiated, most notably bladder injury. Therefore, referral to a specialty center by the practicing surgeon should be considered in such cases. The TAPP procedure is the safest laparoscopic herniorrhaphy for these recurrent hernias inasmuch as a significant series using the TEP approach has not been reported.

Infertility

Injury to the vas deferens or the testes can cause infertility. The incidence of injury to the vas deferens during inguinal hernia repair is 0.3% in adults and up to 2% in children.[60] The vas deferens may be injured during dissection and mobilization or during fixation of the mesh. Traction injuries to muscular wall of the vas deferens sustained during mobilization may interfere with transfer of spermatozoa.[61] Unilateral injury to the cord can lead to exposure of spermatozoa to the immune system and the formation of antisperm antibodies, thus causing infertility.[62]

Ischemic Orchitis

Interruption of blood flow to the testis because of inguinal herniorrhaphy may result in ischemic orchitis and subsequent testicular atrophy. It is manifested 1 to 3 days after surgery as a painful, enlarged, firm testicle accompanied by low-grade fever. Its incidence in large series of TAPP repairs was 0.11%.[63] Complete excision of all indirect inguinal hernia sacs is thought to be an important cause secondary to trauma to the testicular blood supply, especially the delicate venous plexuses. Large indirect inguinal-scrotal hernia sacs should be divided just distal to the internal ring. The proximal portion of the sac is ligated and the distal part is opened on its anterior surface as far distally as convenient. Contrary to popular opinion in the urologic literature, this technique does not result in an excessive rate of postoperative hydrocele formation.[64] Treatment is largely supportive and consists of elevation and anti-inflammatory medication.

Groin Pain

Chronic groin pain is a major cause of morbidity after inguinal hernia surgery. Its incidence may be as high as 53% at 1 year of follow-up.[65] Evaluation of postherniorrhaphy groin pain involves ruling out a myriad of causes, including muscle injury, adductor strain, osteitis pubis, and lumbosacral disorders. The superior soft tissue resolution offered by MRI makes it the most useful diagnostic modality for evaluation of postherniorrhaphy groin pain. The etiology of this groin pain can be

Nociceptive—as a result of direct tissue damage
Somatic
Visceral
Neuropathic—as a result of nerve damage.

Nociceptive pain is further subdivided into (1) somatic, which is the most common and includes ongoing preoperative pathology that was the real cause of the patient's pain, usually related to ligament or muscle injury, new ligament or muscle injury caused by the operation, scar tissue, osteitis pubis, or a reaction to prosthetic material, and (2) visceral pain, which is pain related to a specific visceral function and includes urinary problems and the dysejaculation syndrome. Neuropathic pain is caused by damage to nerves or incorporation by staples or suture material during the repair. The nerves that may commonly be involved are the genital and femoral branches of the genitofemoral nerve and the lateral femoral cutaneous nerve. Treatment of all three types of pain is initially conservative and consists of reassurance, anti-inflammatory medications, cryotherapy, physical therapy, and local nerve blocks, except when sudden severe groin pain is present immediately after surgery, which suggests a stapled or sutured nerve. Such a patient can benefit from immediate re-exploration. Otherwise, groin exploration should be reserved as a last resort because the results are often less than satisfactory. Our approach when groin exploration is the only option is to perform a combined laparoscopic and conventional groin exploration with fluoroscopic capability to maximize the chance of removing as much mesh and as many fastening devices as possible. Neurectomy, neuroma excision, and adhesiolysis are performed if indicated. The hernia is then repaired in the conventional space.

Wound Infection

Wound infection rates of up to 3% have been described with the laparoscopic approach,[66] but this problem is fortunately quite rare. Although antibiotic prophylaxis is quite commonly used for inguinal herniorrhaphy, its role in preventing infection is not clear.[67]

Seromas

Seromas are common and are almost entirely due to the use of prosthetic materials. Treatment is aspiration for symptomatic benefit, and one must weigh the risk of possibly introducing infection in a otherwise sterile collection.

Other Complications

Testicular descent is a complication related to complete division of the cremasteric fibers. The problem is sometimes described by patients as a "testicle dropping into the toilet." Avoiding complete transection of the cremaster prevents this problem. A hydrocele may occasionally develop, possibly related to a remnant of the hernia sac left in the scrotum, but this relationship has not been conclusively proved. Regardless, treatment is similar to that for a hydrocele unrelated to hernia surgery.

Mesh contraction by up to 20% has been described and may account for some of the recurrences after hernia repair.[68] The entity of mesh rejection is of doubtful significance and is probably a manifestation of prosthetic infection. Prosthetic erosion into cord structures or intra-abdominal viscera has been seen rarely.

REFERENCES

1. Annibali R, Quinn TH, Fitzgibbons RJ Jr: Anatomy of the inguinal region from the laparoscopic perspective: Critical areas for laparoscopic hernia repair. In Bendavid R (ed): Prostheses and Abdominal Wall Hernias. Austin, TX, RG Landes, 1994, p 82.
2. Tarpley JL, Holzman MD: Groin hernia. In Cameron JL (ed): Current Surgical Therapy. Philadelphia, Elsevier, 2004, p 545.
3. Spaw AT, Ennis BW, Spaw LP: Laparoscopic hernia repair: The anatomic basis. J Laparoendosc Surg 1:269, 1993.
4. Horeyseck G, Roland F, Rolfes N: "Tension-free" repair of inguinal hernia: Laparoscopic (TAPP) versus open (Lichtenstein) repair. Chirurg 67:1036, 1996.
5. Zieren J, Zieren HU, Wenger FA, Muller JM: Laparoscopic or conventional repair of inguinal hernia with synthetic mesh? Langenbecks Arch Chir 381:289, 1996.
6. Sarli L, Pietra N, Choua O, et al: Prospective randomized comparative study of laparoscopic hernioplasty and Lichtenstein tension-free hernioplasty. Acta Biomed Ateneo Parmense 68:5, 1997.
7. Champault GG, Rizk N, Catheline JM, et al: Inguinal hernia repair: Totally preperitoneal laparoscopic approach versus Stoppa operation: Randomized trial of 100 cases. Surg Laparosc Endosc 7:445, 1997.

8. Khoury N: A randomized prospective controlled trial of laparoscopic extraperitoneal hernia repair and mesh-plug hernioplasty: A study of 315 cases. J Laparoendosc Adv Surg Tech A 8:367, 1998.

9. Paganini AM, Lezoche E, Carle F, et al: A randomized, controlled, clinical study of laparoscopic vs open tension-free inguinal hernia repair. Surg Endosc 12:979, 1998.

10. Aitola P, Airo I, Matikainen M: Laparoscopic versus open preperitoneal inguinal hernia repair: A prospective randomised trial. Ann Chir Gynaecol 87:22, 1998.

11. Picchio M, Lombardi A, Zolovkins A, et al: Tension-free laparoscopic and open hernia repair: Randomized controlled trial of early results. World J Surg 23:1004, 1999.

12. Kumar S, Nixon SJ, MacIntyre IM: Laparoscopic or Lichtenstein repair for recurrent inguinal hernia: One unit's experience. J R Coll Surg Edinb 44:301, 1999.

13. Johansson B, Hallerback B, Glise H, et al: Laparoscopic mesh versus open preperitoneal mesh versus conventional technique for inguinal hernia repair: A randomized multicenter trial (SCUR Hernia Repair Study). Ann Surg 230:225, 1999.

14. MRC group: Laparoscopic versus open repair of groin hernia: A randomised comparison. The MRC Laparoscopic Groin Hernia Trial Group. Lancet 354:185, 1999.

15. Beets GL, Dirksen CD, Go PM, et al: Open or laparoscopic preperitoneal mesh repair for recurrent inguinal hernia? A randomized controlled trial. Surg Endosc 13:323, 1999.

16. Sarli L, Iusco DR, Sansebastiano G, Costi R: Simultaneous repair of bilateral inguinal hernias: A prospective, randomized study of open, tension-free versus laparoscopic approach. Surg Laparosc Endosc Percutan Tech 11:262, 2001.

17. Wright D, Paterson C, Scott N, et al: Five-year follow-up of patients undergoing laparoscopic or open groin hernia repair: A randomized controlled trial. Ann Surg 235:333, 2002.

18. Pikoulis E, Tsigris C, Diamantis T, et al: Laparoscopic preperitoneal mesh repair or tension-free mesh plug technique? A prospective study of 471 patients with 543 inguinal hernias. Eur J Surg 168:587, 2002.

19. Mahon D, Decadt B, Rhodes M: Prospective randomized trial of laparoscopic (transabdominal preperitoneal) vs open (mesh) repair for bilateral and recurrent inguinal hernia. Surg Endosc 17:1386, 2003.

20. Andersson B, Hallen M, Leveau P, et al: Laparoscopic extraperitoneal inguinal hernia repair versus open mesh repair: A prospective randomized controlled trial. Surgery 133:464, 2003.

21. Douek M, Smith G, Oshowo A, et al: Prospective randomised controlled trial of laparoscopic versus open inguinal hernia mesh repair: Five year follow up. BMJ 326:1012, 2003.

22. Bringman S, Ramel S, Heikkinen TJ, et al: Tension-free inguinal hernia repair: TEP versus mesh-plug versus Lichtenstein: A prospective randomized controlled trial. Ann Surg 237:142, 2003.

23. Lal P, Kajla RK, Chander J, et al: Randomized controlled study of laparoscopic total extraperitoneal versus open Lichtenstein inguinal hernia repair. Surg Endosc 17:850, 2003.

24. Heikkinen T, Bringman S, Ohtonen P, et al: Five-year outcome of laparoscopic and Lichtenstein hernioplasties. Surg Endosc 18:518, 2004.

25. Neumayer L, Giobbie-Harder A, Jonasson O, et al: Open mesh versus laparoscopic mesh repair of inguinal hernia. N Engl J Med 350:1819, 2004.

26. Grant AM: EU Hernia Trialists Collaboration. Laparoscopic versus open groin hernia repair: Meta-analysis of randomised trials based on individual patient data. Hernia 6:2, 2002.

27. Memon MA, Cooper NJ, Memon B, et al: Meta-analysis of randomized clinical trials comparing open and laparoscopic inguinal hernia repair. Br J Surg 90:1479, 2003.

28. Lawrence K, McWhinnie D, Goodwin A, et al: Randomized controlled trial of laparoscopic versus open repair of inguinal hernia: Early results. BMJ 311:981, 1995.

29. Vogt DM, Curet MJ, Pitcher DE, et al: Preliminary results of a prospective randomized trial of laparoscopic onlay versus conventional inguinal herniorrhaphy. Am J Surg 169:84, 1995.

30. Liem MS, van der Graaf Y, van Steensel CJ, et al: Comparison of conventional anterior surgery and laparoscopic surgery for inguinal-hernia repair. N Engl J Med 336:1541, 1997.

31. Dirksen CD, Beets GL, Go PM, et al: Bassini repair compared with laparoscopic repair for primary inguinal hernia: A randomised controlled trial. Eur J Surg 164:439, 1998.

32. Tanphiphat C, Tanprayoon T, Sangsubhan C, Chatamra K: Laparoscopic vs open inguinal hernia repair. A randomized, controlled trial. Surg Endosc 12:846, 1998.

33. Zieren J, Zieren HU, Jacobi CA, et al: Prospective randomized study comparing laparoscopic and open tension-free inguinal hernia repair with Shouldice's operation. Am J Surg 175:330, 1998.

34. Juul P, Christensen K: Randomized clinical trial of laparoscopic versus open inguinal hernia repair. Br J Surg 86:316, 1999.

35. Leibl BJ, Daubler P, Schmedt CG, et al: Long-term results of a randomized clinical trial between laparoscopic hernioplasty and Shouldice repair. Br J Surg 87:780, 2000.

36. Tschudi JF, Wagner M, Klaiber C, et al: Randomized controlled trial of laparoscopic transabdominal preperitoneal hernioplasty vs Shouldice repair. Surg Endosc 15:1263, 2001.

37. Wennstrom I, Berggren P, Akerud L, Jarhult J: Equal results with laparoscopic and Shouldice repairs of primary inguinal hernia in men. Report from a prospective randomised study. Scand J Surg 93:34, 2004.

38. Lowham AS, Filipi CJ, Fitzgibbons RJ Jr, et al: Mechanisms of hernia recurrence after preperitoneal mesh repair. Traditional and laparoscopic. Ann Surg 225:422, 1997.

39. Smith AI, Royston CM, Sedman PC: Stapled and nonstapled laparoscopic transabdominal preperitoneal (TAPP) inguinal hernia repair. A prospective randomized trial. Surg Endosc 13:804, 1999.

40. Kald A, Domeij E, Landin S, et al: Laparoscopic hernia repair in patients with bilateral groin hernias. Eur J Surg 166:210, 2000.

41. Fitzgibbons RJ Jr, Camps J, Cornet DA, et al: Laparoscopic inguinal herniorrhaphy. Results of a multicenter trial. Ann Surg 221:3, 1995.

42. Khoury N: A comparative study of laparoscopic extraperitoneal and transabdominal preperitoneal herniorrhaphy. J Laparoendosc Surg 5:349, 1995.

43. Ramshaw BJ, Tucker JG, Conner T, et al: A comparison of the approaches to laparoscopic herniorrhaphy. Surg Endosc 10:29, 1996.

44. Kald A, Anderberg B, Smedh K, Karlsson M: Transperitoneal or totally extraperitoneal approach in laparoscopic hernia repair: Results of 491 consecutive herniorrhaphies. Surg Laparosc Endosc 7:86, 1997.

45. Sarli L, Pietra N, Choua O, et al: Laparoscopic hernia repair: A prospective comparison of TAPP and IPOM techniques. Surg Laparosc Endosc 7:472, 1997.

46. Van Hee R, Goverde P, Hendricx L, et al: Laparoscopic transperitoneal versus extraperitoneal inguinal hernia repair: A prospective clinical trial. Acta Chir Belg 98:132, 1998.

47. Cohen RV, Alvarez G, Roll S, et al: Transabdominal or totally extraperitoneal laparoscopic hernia repair? Surg Laparosc Endosc 8:264, 1998.

48. Lepere M, Benchetrit S, Debaert M, et al: A multicentric comparison of transabdominal versus totally extraperitoneal laparoscopic hernia repair using Parietex meshes. JSLS 4:147, 2000.

49. Kingsley D, Vogt DM, Nelson MT, et al: Laparoscopic intraperitoneal onlay inguinal herniorrhaphy. Am J Surg 176:548, 1998.

50. Bittner R, Schmedt CG, Schwarz J, et al: Laparoscopic transperitoneal procedure for routine repair of groin hernia. Br J Surg 89:1062, 2002.

51. Schafer M, Lauper M, Krahenbuhl L: A nation's experience of bleeding complications during laparoscopy. Am J Surg 180:73, 2000.

52. Roviaro GC, Varoli F, Saguatti L, et al: Major vascular injuries in laparoscopic surgery. Surg Endosc 16:1192, 2002.

53. van der Voort M, Heijnsdijk EA, Gouma DJ: Bowel injury as a complication of laparoscopy. Br J Surg 91:1253, 2004.

54. Raut V, Shrivastava A, Nandanwar S, Bhattacharya M: Urological injuries during obstetric and gynaecological surgical procedures. J Postgrad Med 37:21, 1991.

55. Boughey JC, Nottingham JM, Walls AC: Richter's hernia in the laparoscopic era: Four case reports and review of literature. Surg Laparosc Endosc Percutan Tech 13:55, 2003.

56. Rink J, Ali A: Intestinal obstruction after totally extraperitoneal laparoscopic inguinal hernia repair. JSLS 8:89, 2004.

57. Sarli L, Costi R, Sansebastiano G, et al: Prospective randomized trial of low-pressure pneumoperitoneum for reduction of shoulder-tip pain following laparoscopy. Br J Surg 87:1161, 2000.

58. Gonullu NN, Dulger M, Utkan NZ, et al: Prevention of postherniorrhaphy urinary retention with prazosin. Am Surg 65:55, 1999.

59. Catheline JM, Turner R, Gaillard JL, et al: Thromboembolism in laparoscopic surgery: Risk factors and preventive measures. Surg Laparosc Endosc Percutan Tech 9:135, 1999.

60. Sheynkin YR, Hendin BN, Schlegel PN, Goldstein M: Microsurgical repair of iatrogenic injury to vas deferens. J Urol 159:139, 1998.

61. Ceylan H, Karakok M, Guldur E, et al: Temporary stretch of the testicular pedicle may damage the vas deferens and the testis. J Pediatr Surg 38:1530, 2003.

62. Matsuda T, Muguruma K, Horii Y, et al: Serum antisperm antibodies in men with vas deferens obstruction caused by childhood inguinal herniorrhaphy. Fertil Steril 59:1095, 1993.

63. Leibl BJ, Schmedt CG, Schwarz J, et al: A single institution's experience with transperitoneal laparoscopic hernia repair. Am J Surg 175:446, 1998.

64. Fong Y, Wantz GE: Prevention of ischemic orchitis during inguinal hernioplasty. Surg Gynecol Obstet 174:399, 1992.

65. Poobalan AS, Bruce J, Smith WC, et al: A review of chronic pain after inguinal herniorrhaphy. Clin J Pain 19:48, 2003.

66. Wellwood J, Sculpher MJ, Stoker D, et al: Randomised controlled trial of laparoscopic versus open mesh repair for inguinal hernia: Outcome and cost. BMJ 317:103, 1998.

67. Sanchez-Manuel FJ, Seco-Gil JL: Antibiotic prophylaxis for hernia repair. Cochrane Database Syst Rev 2:CD003769, 2003.

68. Amid PK: How to avoid recurrence in Lichtenstein tension-free hernioplasty. Am J Surg 184:259, 2002.

Ventral Herniation in Adults

Andrew G. Harrell · Yuri W. Novitsky ·
Kent W. Kercher · B. Todd Heniford

*A surgeon can do more for the community by operating on
hernia cases and seeing that his recurrence rate is low than
he can by operating on cases of malignant disease.*

Sir Cecil Wakely
President, Royal College of Surgeons, 1948

Some of the first medical writings from thousands of
years ago describe the anatomy and morbidity of hernias.
Changes in their management have followed our understanding of their origins and, perhaps more importantly,
our failures in their repair. Sutured repair continues to
play a valuable role in herniorrhaphy, but suturing a
defect under tension or using tissues of questionable
strength results in a repair that is doomed to fail. Bridging a hernia with prosthetic mesh has established a valid
position not only in the repair of large or recurrent
hernias but also in small, primary repairs. The need for
a strong prosthetic that is well tolerated by the human
body is not a new thought or concept. In the mid-1800s,
Bilroth stated, "If we could artificially produce tissue of
the density and toughness of fascia and tendon, the
secret of the radical cure of the hernia repair would be
discovered." Nearly 150 years later we understand the
importance of that statement. Industry also recognizes
its worth, both in improving patient outcomes and in
providing materials to a million-cases-a-year market.
Research in the area of prosthetic mesh has soared over
the last decade, with materials engineered for placement
inside the abdomen and outside the abdomen, "nonstick" surfaces, mesh preformed for left- or right-sided
laparoscopic inguinal hernias (in small, medium, or
large sizes), umbrella-like "plugs," and other innovations.
Natural material, such as that developed from cadaveric
skin or porcine intestinal submucosa, has also seen a
growth in interest. A perfect biomaterial is not currently
available, but some very good and well-tolerated choices
exist. There is little question that they have helped
reduce rates of recurrence and morbidity in the most
common operations performed by general surgeons.

DEFINITIONS

The term *ventral hernia* is used to describe any protrusion
of abdominal viscera through the anterior abdominal
wall. There are two categories of ventral hernia: spontaneous or primary hernias and incisional hernias. Ventral
hernias can also be subdivided by location. Subxiphoid
refers to the area just inferior to the xiphoid process.
Epigastric hernias also overlap this area to some degree
but include spontaneous hernias through the linea alba
down to the umbilicus. Umbilical hernias are a special
class of spontaneous or congenital ventral hernia that are
located at the umbilicus. Hypogastric hernias are rare,
spontaneous hernias inferior to the umbilicus. Suprapubic and parailiac hernias occur along the pelvic brim
adjacent to their respective bony prominences. Spontaneous hernias along the semilunar line are termed
spigelian; Adriaan van der Spiegel was a Belgian
anatomist who first described the area. Traumatic hernias
can occur almost anywhere in the anterior abdominal
wall when fascial planes are disrupted after blunt or penetrating abdominal force.

Any hernia of the anterior abdominal wall that
occurs through a previous surgical incision is naturally
termed an incisional hernia. Two additional conditions
apply to an anterior abdominal wall that appears to
have a hernia but does not. Eventration of the anterior
abdominal wall is a bulging that occurs from either
paralysis of a portion of the abdominal musculature
or congenital absence. There is no definable hernia
sac or fascial defect; however, a bulge results from the
lack of muscle tone. Similarly, diastasis recti is manifested
as a midline bulge. The linea alba is broadened or
stretched, which causes the medial margins of the rectus
abdominis muscles to separate. Again, there is no hernia
sac or fascial defect, and most are completely asymptomatic. If a diastasis results in significant symptoms, the
abdominal wall can be reconstructed, but most often
it is not a simple procedure. Incarceration describes
the irreducible contents of a hernia sac. If not addressed,
this process can compromise blood flow to the incarcer-

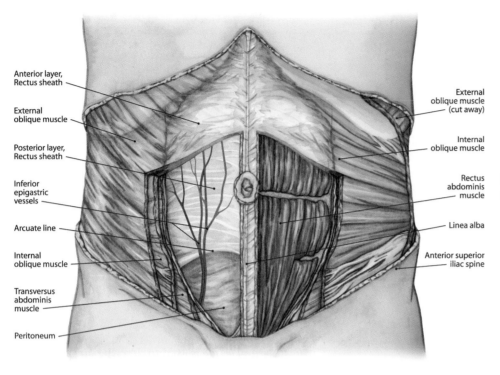

Anterior layer,
Rectus sheath

External
oblique muscle

Posterior layer,
Rectus sheath

Inferior
epigastric
vessels

Arcuate line

Internal
oblique muscle

Transversus
abdominis
muscle

Peritoneum

External
oblique muscle
(cut away)

Internal
oblique muscle

Rectus
abdominis
muscle

Linea alba

Anterior superior
iliac spine

Figure 47–1. Layers of the abdominal wall.

ated hernial contents and potentially lead to necrosis or strangulation.

ANATOMY

The anterior abdominal wall is a complex layering of muscles, aponeuroses, and fascia (Fig. 47–1). The most obvious feature is the umbilicus, which represents the cicatricial remnants of the former umbilical cord and vessels. Typically, it lies at the midpoint between the xiphoid process and the pubis, depending on the amount of subcutaneous adipose tissue. The midline is further defined by the linea alba, which extends from the xiphoid to the symphysis pubis. It can be seen as a linear furrow in the anterior abdominal wall of muscular patients and is situated between the medial borders of the rectus abdominis muscles. The linea alba is composed of dense, crisscross fibrous bands from the blending aponeuroses of the external oblique, internal oblique, and transversalis muscles.[1] The linea alba is quite broad at the xiphoid, measuring 1 to 2.5 cm, as the rectus sheath fibers diverge to insert on the fifth, sixth, and seventh costal cartilages. Below the level of the umbilicus, the linea alba narrows to a fine line between the rectus muscles as it inserts on the pubis. Several tendinous intersections extend from the linea alba medially to the convex lateral rectus sheath border, the linea semilunaris, and firmly adhere the rectus muscles to the anterior rectus sheath.

The rectus sheath houses the rectus muscles and is a complex weaving of aponeuroses from the flat abdominal muscle. The anterior sheath is formed from fusion of the external oblique aponeurosis and the anterior lamina of the internal oblique aponeurosis. The posterior internal oblique lamina fuses with the transversus abdominis aponeurosis to generate the posterior sheath. Medially, these layers interlace to form the linea alba. Midway between the umbilicus and the pubis, the three aponeurotic layers fuse into one anterior sheath. The arcuate line marks the crescentic end of the posterior sheath.[2]

The spigelian fascia is a true aponeurosis formed by fusion of the internal oblique and transversus abdominis aponeurosis. It extends from the cartilage of the eighth rib to the pubis, lateral to the edge of the rectus muscle, and medial to the semilunar line. Below the umbilicus, the fibers of this aponeurosis run in parallel fashion, thus making it vulnerable to separation. At the level of the semicircular line of Douglas, the spigelian fascia is the weakest. The inferior epigastric vessels contribute to the weakness of that area by traversing the posterior aspect of the rectus abdominis. A spigelian hernia is a partial defect of the abdominal wall, with the preperitoneal fat or peritoneal sac protruding through the internal oblique but remaining posterior to the external oblique aponeurosis. Although it can occur anywhere along the semilunar line, 90% of hernias occur in the so-called spigelian belt, a 6-cm area of the aponeurosis extending cranially from the line between anterior superior iliac spines. This broad and weak region of the spigelian fascia is bounded by the semilunar line laterally, the inferior epigastric vessels medially, and the arcuate line superiorly (Fig. 47–2).

The lateral abdominal wall is composed of three layered flat muscles. The external oblique, the most superficial, courses inferior from its lower costal origins to its insertion on the iliac crest and medially to fuse

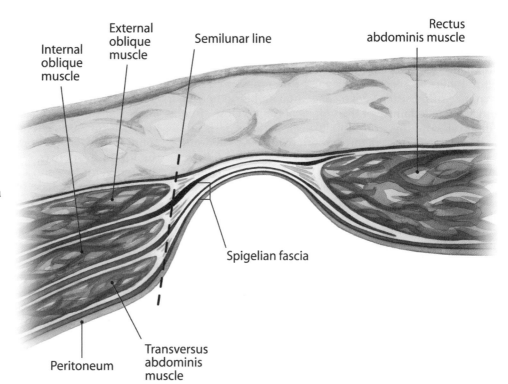

Figure 47–2. Spigelian fascia and location of hernias.

with the internal oblique. The intermediate abdominal muscle, the internal oblique, originates from the lateral half of the inguinal ligament and courses perpendicular to the external oblique superior and anteriorly. There is a significant contribution to the inguinal anatomy from this muscle layer. The innermost muscle layer, the transversus abdominis, courses horizontally and joins medially with the internal oblique aponeurosis. As with the internal oblique, many inferior fibers contribute to the inguinal region. The preperitoneal space separates the deep fascia layer from the peritoneum; this space often contains fat, which is more prominent in the lower part of the abdomen.

The blood supply to the anterior abdominal wall is derived from multiple sources. The upper part of the abdomen receives blood from the superior epigastric artery, the terminal branch of the internal thoracic artery, in combination with collateral branches of the lower intercostal arteries. The lower part of the abdomen is supplied by the inferior epigastric and deep circumflex iliac arteries, which are branches of the external iliac vessels. The superior and inferior epigastrics are continuous with each other deep to the rectus muscle. Nerves supply the anterior abdominal wall by running between the internal oblique and transversus abdominis muscles. The nerves then pierce superficially through the rectus sheath as anterior cutaneous nerves. Branches originate from the lower thoracic nerve roots (T7-T9) superior to the umbilicus, T10 innervates the periumbilical skin, and T11-L1 supplies the infraumbilical area. Several small blood vessels and nerves that penetrate the linea alba and umbilicus are occasional sites of spontaneous or acquired hernia.

ETIOLOGY

The formation of ventral hernias is a multifactorial and complex process. Three types of ventral hernias are recognized: spontaneous, congenital, and incisional hernias. Congenital hernias are just that, congenital, and are most often treated during the pediatric period of life. Spontaneous ventral hernias are most commonly found along the midline linea alba. Although they are typically supraumbilical in location, they can occur anywhere along this structure, and more than one hernia may be found. As previously described, the interlacing fibers of the aponeuroses in this portion of the linea alba are pierced by small blood vessels and nerves.[1] Through these openings, extraperitoneal areolar tissue may herniate and produce an epigastric (linea alba) hernia. The hernia opening is usually 1 cm in size or smaller. Extrusion of extraperitoneal fat may or may not be accompanied by a sac of the subjacent peritoneum. Though frequently referred to as lipomas, the fatty tissue is not a tumor; it is a mushroom-like mass of preperitoneal encapsulated fat with a feeding artery that usually comes through a tight, small defect. When a sac is present, it is generally small and barely protrudes through the opening in the fascia. This sac may not become apparent until the surrounding preperitoneal fat is removed. If the hernia contains only the preperitoneal fat of the falciform ligament, the hernia opening is almost always just to the right of midline. If the hernia does not contain fat from the falciform ligament, the opening is nearly always to the left, but occasionally in the midline. Small epigastric hernias increase in size slowly because the fascial ring through which they protrude is strong and unyielding. If a larger sac is present, it may contain omentum, intestine, and other viscera.

Umbilical hernias are relatively common in the adult population and are another example of a spontaneous ventral hernia. Occasionally they can represent reappearance or persistence of a congenital umbilical hernia and are due to failure of the umbilical ring to close after umbilical cord ligation. In 90% of patients it is an acquired defect that is a direct result of increased abdominal pressure.[3] Causes of this increase in abdominal pressure include multiparous status, obesity, and cirrhosis with ascites.[4] Umbilical hernias are more common in females and often develop in the forth to fifth decade of life. The fascial ring that constitutes the neck of the hernia can be dense and is formed by gradual yielding of the cicatricial tissue closing the umbilical ring.[5] These hernias tend to enlarge with time and will not resolve spontaneously.

Numerous patient-related factors may lead to the formation of ventral hernias and include obesity,[6] older age,[7] male gender,[7] sleep apnea,[6] emphysema and other chronic lung conditions, prostatism,[8] abdominal distention, steroids,[8] and jaundice,[9,10] although some of these causes are controversial. Some evidence suggests that certain biochemical processes, including the metalloproteinases, may lead to both aneurysmal disease and hernia formation. These collagen defects have also been implicated in a higher rate of incisional hernia formation after aortic surgery.[11] The concept of "metastatic emphysema," that is, the same processes that break down pulmonary tissue disturb normal fascia, was introduced by Dr. Raymond Read and appears to be well founded.[12]

Every year, 4 to 5 million laparotomies are performed, with a hernia developing in 2% to 36% of these incisions.[13-15] This gives rise to well in excess of 150,000 ventral hernia repairs each year. Surgery-related factors may lead to subsequent incisional hernia formation. Wound infection, closure technique, suture material, and incision type have all been described as possible factors.[7] Primary closure of midline abdominal incisions has been the subject of numerous clinical trials. The two main variables compared are absorbable versus nonabsorbable suture and continuous versus interrupted closure technique. Ideally, the suture material used should retain high tensile strength until substantial wound healing has occurred and be a monofilament to prevent bacterial attachment among the fibers. Some additional evidence exists that absorbable suture eliminates the suture material as a nidus of infection,[9] although we have seen this regardless of the suture's permanence. A recent meta-analysis sought to answer the question of suture permanence.[16] In this study, the principal investigators divided suture material into rapidly absorbable, slowly absorbable, and nonabsorbable types. They included only prospective randomized controlled trials with at least 100 patients and follow-up of at least 1 year in their analysis. They identified 6566 patients from 15 studies. Closure of the midline abdominal incision by continuous, rapidly absorbable suture resulted in a statistically higher rate of incisional hernias than did closure by either continuous, slowly absorbable suture ($P < .009$) or nonabsorbable suture ($P = .001$). Although

closure by continuous, slowly absorbable suture versus nonabsorbable suture was not statistically different ($P = .75$), patients with nonabsorbable suture had more suture sinuses ($P = .02$). No significant differences were noted when comparing continuous and interrupted closure techniques, except that continuous closure is more expeditious; again, there was no difference in hernia formation. These data led to a conclusion that a continuous, slowly absorbable fascial closure may lead to the lowest incidence of incisional hernia.[17] The ratio of suture length to wound length appears to be 4:1.[18] This allows a 2-cm purchase of fascia on each side of the incision followed by a 1-cm advance.

As laparoscopic techniques have become popular in nearly all aspects of abdominal surgery, it appears intuitive that the incidence of ventral hernias should decrease. Laparoscopic trocar site hernias are not rare and occur at a rate between 0.6% and 2.8%.[19] It appears that fascial defects larger than 5 mm should be closed in adults. However, there is debate, but little evidence, that dilating, noncutting trocar sites up to 10 mm do not need to be closed with suture. It is true that any size incision, given infection, poor tissue healing, increased abdominal pressure, and other factors, can give rise to a hernia. Additionally, closing only the anterior fascia can result in the rare Richter hernia or preperitoneal hernia, which can be difficult to diagnose without repeat laparoscopy or laparotomy.[20]

SYMPTOMS

Ventral hernias are often noted by the patient as an abdominal bulge. They can be exacerbated by any action that raises intra-abdominal pressure, such as coughing, performing a Valsalva maneuver, lifting weights, or elevating the head or legs. Rest or reduction of the incarcerated hernia may offer temporary relief. Smaller hernias are often asymptomatic or produce intermittent complaints. Discomfort or a ventral bulge is the most common initial symptom, but bowel obstruction can also be the first symptom that forces a patient to seek medical attention. Incarceration and strangulation are more common if the hernia neck defect is small.

INDICATIONS FOR SURGERY

Abdominal wall hernias in adults do not spontaneously heal or close, and nearly all enlarge with time. In most patients, if they are an appropriate surgical candidate, the presence of a hernia is an indication for repair, which allows the potentially dangerous sequelae of incarceration, obstruction, or strangulation to be avoided. As stated, hernias tend to enlarge over time; thus, delay can make repairing them more difficult.

PREPARATION

A standard patient evaluation consisting of a thorough history and physical examination should be undertaken. Pulmonary and cardiac comorbid conditions, diabetes, and other medical problems need to be identified and addressed. The physical examination may be straightforward in patients who have hernias with well-defined fascial borders; however, a computed tomography scan can also be helpful when the presence of a hernia is questionable, such as in an obese patient, if it is located in an unusual location, or if there have been several failed attempts at repair. A cleansing bowel preparation is not often required, but it should be considered for patients at greater risk of enterotomy; such patients might include those with multiple previous surgeries and patients with recurrent hernias and intra-abdominal mesh. Questions concerning the hernia should include any symptoms of incarceration, such as pain, nausea, vomiting, and constipation. As much information as possible about the original or previous operations should be obtained, including the type of surgery, any postoperative wound complications, and if the patient has a recurrent hernia, the previous hernia size and location and the type and location of any prosthetic mesh. Obese patients have a higher risk for recurrence and should be considered for weight loss techniques or counseling before or around the time of hernia repair. The majority, however, will not be able to lose weight.

At the time of surgery, most patients should receive a first-generation cephalosporin, which should be dose-adjusted according to patient weight and repeated if the operation lasts longer than 2 hours. Compression stockings or another form of deep venous thrombosis prophylaxis is warranted. Placement of a gastric or bladder catheter should be considered, depending on the operative location, length of surgery, and extent of intestinal manipulation.

PROSTHETICS

Prosthetic mesh products have radically changed the repair of ventral hernias. The ideal characteristics of a prosthetic were popularized by Cumberland[21] and Scales.[22] These properties include chemical inertness, resistance to mechanical stress, pliability, lack of physical modification by the body's tissues, capability of being sterilized, no carcinogenic potential, no or limited inflammatory or foreign body reaction, and hypoallergenic nature. To date, no prosthetic has been able to attain all these properties. Early metallic prosthetics included tantalum gauze and stainless steel mesh. Numerous difficulties arose from their use, including lack of flexibility, fatigue fractures with subsequent herniation through these fractures or migrating fragments resulting in fistulas, loss of structural integrity, and need for abdominal wall resection if these materials became infected. These meshes never gained wide acceptance. In 1958, Usher et al. reported on the newly developed polypropylene mesh Marlex (C. R. Bard, Cranston, NJ).[23] The introduction of Marlex was a major change in available prosthetics (Fig. 47–3). Apart from it now being knitted instead of woven, the mesh used today has largely remained unchanged over the past 45 years. Several brands of heavyweight polypropylene mesh such as this are available and have become the standard mesh used

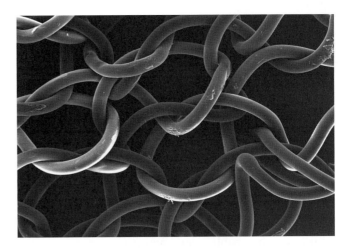

Figure 47–3. Scanning electron micrograph of Marlex mesh.

in the United States. The large pores (600 nm) allow for ingrowth of native fibroblasts, but it does evoke an inflammatory reaction that can cause scarring and limit incorporation into the surrounding fascia or other tissues. It is flexible, but various manufacturing techniques give it various forms of rigidity. Because of the potential intestinal adhesions, ingrowth, and scarring around this mesh, it is not for use in an intra-abdominal location unless omentum or other tissue can be interposed between the mesh and the bowel. When placed against the intestine, the development of enterocutaneous fistulas is well documented and may eventually occur in more than 2% of patients.[24,25]

One concern regarding the long-term implantation of a heavy polypropylene mesh is the concept of decreased abdominal wall compliance. This prosthetic, though chemically inert, does generate an intense inflammatory reaction. The result is a rigid scar plate produced by pronounced perifilamentous fibrosis and deposition of collagen fibers.[26] Two observations are noted: the abdominal wall becomes stiff or exhibits decreased compliance, and the mesh prosthetic shrinks as much as 30% to 46%.[27,28] This decrease in compliance can lead to a sensation of stiffness and discomfort in many patients. Additionally, areas of the abdominal wall that have previous incisions but lack mesh coverage may experience an increase in herniation as the abdominal pressure is no longer distributed evenly. Ultrasound examination and three-dimensional stereography have been used to compare the effects of different concentrations of polypropylene mesh. As the amount of polypropylene decreases and the pore size increases, compliance of the abdominal wall appears to improve.[29] The curvature of the abdominal wall increased over time with the lighter weight meshes but not with the heavyweight polypropylene mesh.

The force required to burst the abdominal cavity is difficult to measure directly. In cadaveric models the maximum abdominal wall force has been calculated to be 16 N/cm.[30] When standard (heavyweight) polypropylene is tested, the bursting force is 40 to 100 N/cm.[31] In this same study, vertical distention of the abdominal wall at the maximum of 16 N/cm is only 25% ± 7%. This measure of elasticity or compliance was severely reduced with the use of prosthetics; however, lightweight polypropylene biomaterials more closely resembled the natural distensibility of the abdominal wall at 21% to 31% relative distention.[32] This evidence suggests that the standard polypropylene mesh is "overengineered" and that a reduced-weight polypropylene material may offer several advantages without compromising the strength of the hernia repair. These findings have been confirmed in long-term animal studies.[27]

Lightweight polypropylene mesh products are now available. Reduced-mass polypropylene alone, however, can be so light and flexible that handling during surgery can be difficult. To correct this problem, the concept of adding an absorbable component to increase its initial stiffness has been adopted. Both Vicryl and Monocryl suture materials have been incorporated in this fashion. Vypro and Ultrapro (Ethicon, Somerville, NJ) are examples of this technology.

Polyester is a popular mesh choice in Europe, especially in France. This mesh is supple, has a grainy texture, and induces a rapid fibroblastic tissue response.[33] The supple handling properties of this mesh allow it to conform easily to curvatures in the abdominal wall. Infection rates with polyester mesh have been documented to be 12% or greater.[34] When placed in the intra-abdominal position, however, the fistula rate can exceed 15%.[24]

The first expanded polytetrafluoroethylene (ePTFE) hernia repair biomaterial was developed and introduced in 1983. This product now exists in several forms. There are perforated versions that are used for extraperitoneal and inguinal repairs and a solid version with two distinctly different sides that is intended for intra-abdominal use (DualMesh, W.L. Gore and Associates, Flagstaff, AZ) (Fig. 47–4). The mesh made for intra-abdominal use has a unique design; one side is smooth and microporous, resists tissue ingrowth, and as such, is ideal to face or touch the intestine. The opposite side is rough and has wide pores that allow intense tissue incorporation; this side is made for placement against the abdominal wall. This material conforms well to the abdominal wall and has minimal shrinkage and good long-term compliance. DualMesh Plus is the same ePTFE, but one side is impregnated with silver carbon-

ate and chlorhexidine diacetate. These two agents act synergistically to inhibit bacterial colonization of the device for up to 10 days after implantation.[35]

Composite or combination mesh types have also increased in popularity. These products layer more than one type of material to form one mesh. By doing so, manufacturers attempt to take advantage of the different biomaterials. Most often, composite meshes are developed for intra-abdominal use, with a protective non–tissue ingrowth side facing the intestine and a tissue-incorporating mesh against the abdominal wall. One such product (Composix E/X, Bard, Cranston, NJ) layers polypropylene and ePTFE on top of one another. The ePTFE surface is positioned toward the abdominal contents and serves as a protective interface against the bowel. The polypropylene side faces the abdominal wall to be incorporated into the native peritoneum and fascial tissue. Other examples of these composite products add an absorbable "nonstick" layer to a standard polypropylene or polyester mesh. Such products include Proceed (Ethicon, Somerville, NJ) and Parietex Composite (Sofradim, Villfranche-sur-Saône, France), which apply a collagen-based material to inhibit intestinal adhesions. At present, no clinical data on the use of these products are available.

There have been several advances in tissue engineering that have introduced several new products into the market for hernia repair. The premise in all these products is a decellularization and protein stabilization process of human or porcine tissue to preserve the structural architecture of the tissue of origin but remove any cells that could precipitate a foreign body reaction. These products, essentially a collagen implant, allow remodeling by the host via native fibroblast migration with subsequent collagen deposition. In vitro studies demonstrate that fibroblasts grow rapidly through these meshes.[36] Surgisis Gold (Cook Biotech, West Lafayette, IN) is manufactured from porcine small intestinal submucosa, Permacol (Tissue Science Laboratories, Covington, GA) is porcine dermal collagen, and AlloDerm (LifeCell, Branchburg, NJ) is an acellular dermal matrix from cadaveric skin. FortaGen (Organogenesis, Canton, MA) is a highly purified type I collagen. All these products are considered biologic mesh prosthetics. They are extremely expensive, and long-term studies demonstrating the effectiveness of these products in hernia repair are currently not available. However, they appear to have advantages in abdominal closure involving complex or infected wounds. Early, short follow-up case series involving the use of these "tissue meshes" in contaminated wounds are encouraging.

PRINCIPLES OF SURGICAL HERNIA REPAIR

The Mayo repair, "vest over pants," was once thought to represent a major advance in the repair of incisional hernias. It involves overlapping layers of normal fascia and securing with a double row of mattress sutures (Fig. 47–5).[37] The operation is performed by incising the skin and dissecting the hernia sac free of surrounding tissue.

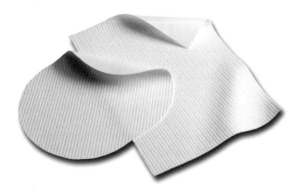

Figure 47–4. Photograph of DualMesh.

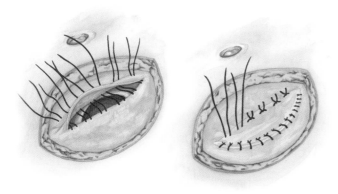

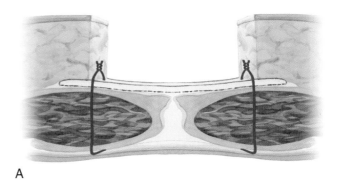

A

Figure 47–5. Mayo vest-over-pants technique.

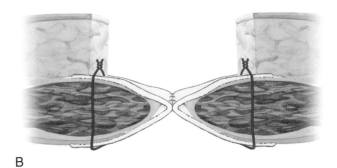

B

Figure 47–6. Mesh repair techniques. **A,** Onlay. **B,** Wrap-around.

The fascial edges are cleared of overlying tissue. Once free, the sac is opened carefully and the contents examined. Adhesions and scar to the sac are released if needed, and the hernia sac is resected. The classic description includes closing the peritoneum with absorbable suture. The fascia is then overlapped with a double row of nonabsorbable mattress sutures. Once completed, the skin is reapproximated. Relaxing incisions along the lateral rectus sheath reduce tension on the wound edges.[3] However, long-term studies have shown that this has not been an effective repair. Recurrence rates of up to 54% at 10 years have been reported and are similar to the rates of a standard, simple fascial reapproximation.[38] The inability to place strong fascia in apposition without tension in all hernias prevents this repair from attaining universal success. Other patient factors, as previously described, can significantly contribute to failure of hernia repair. Even relatively small defects repaired primarily had high recurrence rates in these series.

To determine the superior repair method, Luijendijk et al. performed a prospective randomized trial comparing suture repair with mesh repair for incisional hernias.[8] The 3-year cumulative rate of recurrence was 43% for suture repair and 24% for mesh repair ($P = .02$). One of the shortfalls in this study was that the mesh was essentially sewn to the edges of the fascia with little overlap, which possibly resulted in the higher than expected overall failure rate in the mesh group. A very important finding was discovered when smaller hernias were compared. When hernias less than 10 cm^2 were repaired with suture, their recurrence rate was greater than 40%; in contrast, the recurrence rate was only 6% when repaired with mesh. It is elementary that large hernias require mesh implantation for an adequate repair. However, it appears that the use of a prosthetic may be as important for small defects. The 10-year cumulative recurrence rate again confirms a 50% reduction in hernia recurrence if a prosthetic is used.[13]

The development of hernia prosthetics has led to a variety of techniques for placing the mesh. The onlay technique involves primary closure of the fascial defect and subsequent reinforcement by placing the mesh prosthetic on top of the fascial repair (Fig. 47–6A). Supporters of this technique promote the separation of

the mesh from intra-abdominal contents as a major advantage in avoiding complications. The mesh is secured to the anterior rectus sheath with sutures or fascial staples. The onlay technique has several disadvantages. Significant subcutaneous dissection is needed to place the mesh, which can lead to devitalized tissue with seroma formation or infection. The superficial location of the mesh also puts it in danger of becoming infected if there is a superficial wound infection. The primary repair is often under tension, which can contribute to recurrence. Ideally, the transfascial sutures are placed before primary closure of the fascial defect to avoid the potential bowel injury that can occur if the sutures are placed blindly. Long-term studies are not available to accurately describe the recurrence rate with this technique, but retrospective review suggests a rate of 28%.[39]

Another variation of mesh placement is the wrap-around, or cuff, technique (see Fig. 47–6B). The mesh is wrapped around the anterior and posterior rectus sheath and secured with penetrating sutures. Unfortunately, these sutures can lead to underlying muscle necrosis and can be very painful if placed very tightly.[40] The prosthetic-reinforced edges of the fascia are then closed in the midline. Unfortunately, closure may not be possible without tension. In addition, the mesh on the underside of the abdominal wall is exposed to the intestines; if it is a macroporous mesh such as polypropylene or polyester, intestinal adhesion or possibly a fistula may result.

The French surgeons Rives and Stoppa revolutionized hernia repair by popularizing a retrorectus

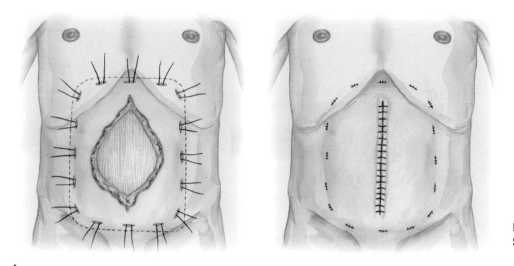

A

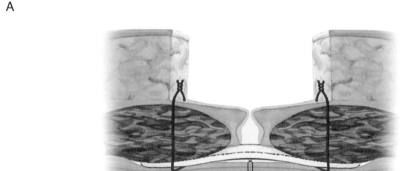

B

Figure 47–7. **A** and **B,** The Stoppa repair technique.

extraperitoneal repair with prosthetics.[34,41] This technique was additionally popularized in the United States by George Wantz.[33] The prosthetic is placed preperitoneally below the arcuate line or just superficial to the posterior rectus sheath above the umbilicus. The sutures ends are individually placed through the mesh and out through the abdominal wall with the knots buried in subcutaneous tissue.[33] In addition to a mesh repair the midline fascia is closed, which can restore the previously displaced abdominal muscle into a more anatomic and functional position (Fig. 47–7). Drains are placed above the prosthetic. This method has a documented recurrence rate of approximately 14%.[34] The advantages of a large mesh with significant overlap placed under the muscular abdominal wall can be explained by Pascal's principles of hydrostatics. The intra-abdominal cavity functions as a cylinder, and therefore the pressure is distributed uniformly to all aspects of the system. Consequently, the same forces that are attempting to push the mesh through hernia defects are also holding the mesh in place against the intact abdominal wall (Fig. 47–8). In this manner, the prosthetic is held firmly in place by intra-abdominal pressure. The mechanical strength of the prosthetic prevents protrusion of the peritoneal cavity through the hernia because the hernia sac is indistensible against the mesh. Over time, the prosthetic is incorporated into the fascia and unites the abdominal wall, now without an area of weakness. Lateral fixation

sutures are again necessary to keep the mesh in position until fibrous ingrowth has occurred.

Laparoscopic Operative Method

The principles of retrorectus prosthetic reinforcement have been adapted for laparoscopic ventral hernia repair. Instead of applying the mesh in a preperitoneal position, an intraperitoneal onlay with wide coverage of the hernia defect is performed. The mesh is fixed in position with transfascial sutures and metallic staples or tacks. This wide overlap and combination fixation technique has been developed so that it mimics the open retrorectus or preperitoneal repair previously described. This technique also takes advantage of Pascal's principle of hydrostatics to provide a secure hernia repair.

Laparoscopic ventral hernia repair is usually performed with a 30- or 45-degree angled laparoscope. A minimal number of laparoscopic bowel graspers, dissectors, scissors, and blunt graspers are also necessary. Currently, 5-mm fixation devices (spiral tacks or anchors) are commonly used. A suture-passing device (W. L. Gore and Associates, Flagstaff, AZ) is used for full-thickness transabdominal wall sutures. This repair requires an intraperitoneal prosthetic to be in contact with the viscera. At this time, ePTFE is the best studied and most commonly used mesh for laparoscopic repair.

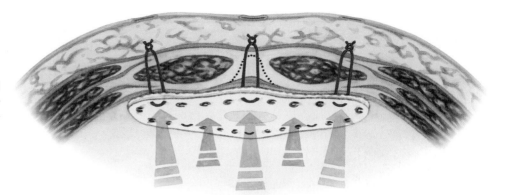

Figure 47–8. Intra-abdominal forces illustrating Pascal's principle of hydrostatics.

To establish pneumoperitoneum, an open abdominal access technique or Veress needle can be used safely. A window of access between the costal margin and the iliac crest on one side or the other is usually present, even in a multiply operated abdomen. After inserting the first trocar, the abdominal cavity is viewed, and under direct visualization, additional trocars are placed as far laterally as possible. Usually, three trocars are placed on the operative side for an in-line view and a two-handed technique for dissection, mesh deployment, and fixation. An additional trocar or two on the contralateral side is occasionally required.[42]

The most difficult and time-consuming portion of the procedure is adhesiolysis. Serious, albeit rare complications from this procedure are related to bowel injury; therefore, meticulous dissection technique must be used. Sharp dissection should be performed as much as possible to avoid thermal spread from electrothermal (cautery) and ultrasonic energy. The adhesions to the anterior abdominal wall surrounding the hernia and within the hernia sac are lysed, and the hernia contents are reduced. The peritoneal sac is left in situ.

To correctly size the mesh prosthesis, the hernia defect must be measured, which may be accomplished externally or internally. If the hernia margins are measured externally, the abdomen should be desufflated to more accurately delineate the actual size of the hernia; if not, a thick abdominal wall or large hernia can result in overestimation of the mesh needed to fix the hernia. Measuring the hernia internally is performed with a disposable plastic ruler that is brought through a trocar into the abdomen. The length and width of the hernia defect are determined inside the abdominal cavity. In this manner the size of the hernia can be very accurately measured. These measurements, whether obtained inside or outside the abdomen, are used to choose an appropriately sized prosthetic mesh that will overlap all margins of the defect by approximately 4 cm.

Four nonabsorbable, size 0 monofilament or ePTFE sutures (approximately 30 cm in length) are placed at the midpoint of each side (Fig. 47–9). Exit sites for the sutures are predetermined on the abdominal wall and marked 4 or more cm beyond the margin of the hernia. The mesh is rolled like a scroll from the superior and

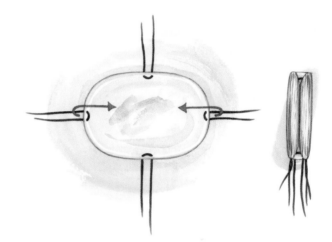

Figure 47–9. Orientation sutures for intra-abdominal mesh and rolling the mesh for insertion through the abdominal wall.

inferior ends and compressed and pulled or pushed into the peritoneal cavity through a 10-mm port site.[40]

The mesh is unfurled within the abdomen. The sutures are individually pulled through the abdominal wall with a suture passer at the previously marked positions. The individual strands of each suture are brought out through separate fascial punctures but through the same skin incisions so that full-thickness abdominal wall "bites" are taken to fix the mesh in position (Fig. 47–10). The initial marked sites may need to be modified further radially to allow for taut placement of the mesh; it is important that the mesh be taut when the abdomen is insufflated. The sutures are individually tied with the knots left buried in subcutaneous tissue. The perimeter of the mesh is then secured with spiral tacks or staples placed 1 cm apart or so. The tacks are positioned close to the mesh edge to prevent infolding of the mesh and exposure of the rough, woven side to bowel (see Fig. 47–10). Additional full-thickness, nonabsorbable sutures are placed in the mesh every 4 to 7 cm circumferentially with the suture passer. The tacks ensure that bowel will not herniate between the sutures. They do add some security

| Table 47–1 | Comparison Studies of Laparoscopic and Open Ventral Hernia Repairs |

Name	Year	No. of Patients		Morbidity (%)		Mesh Infection (%)		Infection (%)		Recurrence (%)	
		Lap	Open	Lap	Open	Lap	Open	Lap	Open	Lap	Open
McGreevy[48]	2003	65	71	8	21	3	0	0	10	—	—
Raftopoulos[49]	2003	50	22	28	45	2	0	2	5	2	18
Wright[50]	2002	90	90	17	34	1	1	1	9	1	6
Robbins[51]	2001	18	31	—	—	6	13	6	0	—	—
DeMaria[46]	2000	21	18	62	72	5	11	5	22	5	0
Carbajo[47]	1999	30	30	67	20	0	10	0	17	3	7
Ramshaw[52]	1999	79	174	19	26	1	3	8	1	3	21
Park[25]	1998	56	49	18	37	4	2	0	4	11	35
Holzman[53]	1997	21	16	24	31	0	6	5	0	10	13
Totals		430	501	23	30	2	4	3	6	4	16.5

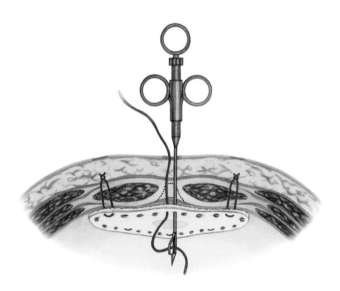

Figure 47–10. Full-thickness transfascial sutures placed with a suture passer device and tacks.

to the repair but do not provide enough strength to serve as the only points of fixation. Drains are not used.[43,44]

Minimally Invasive Versus Open Mesh Ventral Hernia Repair

The laparoscopic approach to ventral hernia repair has been the subject of numerous publications. The benefits of laparoscopy may include a reduction in postoperative pain, shorter length of stay, decreased morbidity and especially wound infections, and improvements in recurrence rates as compared with the open procedure.[42,45] Only two studies have been performed in a prospective, randomized fashion to compare laparoscopic and open ventral hernia repair. Carbajo et al. and DeMaria et al.

published their trials in 1999 and 2000, respectively.[46,47] Carbajo et al. randomly assigned 60 patients to receive either laparoscopic ventral hernia repair or the open procedure. The two groups were matched for incisional hernia type, size of defect, age, and sex distribution. Postoperative hospital stay and operative time were significantly shorter in the laparoscopic ventral hernia repair group.[47] They also reported that the laparoscopic ventral hernia repair group had fewer complications and a reduced hernia recurrence rate (3% versus 6.7%) during their 27-month follow-up period.[47] DeMaria and associates similarly compared laparoscopic and open ventral hernia repair prospectively at a tertiary care, university setting. Thirty-nine consecutive patients were enrolled in their study. Ninety percent of the laparoscopic group was treated on an outpatient basis as compared with only 7% in the open group. The incidence of complications and the recurrence rate were not different between the two groups.[46] The laparoscopic repair was also statistically less expensive than the open repair. Retrospective studies appear to apply additional evidence to support the use of laparoscopic techniques to repair abdominal hernias.

Based on the data from the comparative studies (Table 47–1), postoperative complications are less frequent (23.2% versus 30.2%), wound and mesh infections are lower, and recurrence rates are reduced (4.0% versus 16.5%) in laparoscopic versus open repairs. Long-term follow-up data from the larger laparoscopic series continue to demonstrate potential advantages.[42,45] A randomized prospective trial with sufficient power is needed to truly answer the question of whether an open or laparoscopic repair is the safest and most durable.

Perioperative Considerations

Repair of smaller hernias may be performed on an outpatient basis, but larger repairs require inpatient stay. Feeding is advanced as tolerated and is frequently accomplished on the first postoperative day. In both open and laparoscopic surgery, early ambulation is encouraged and emphasized for resolution of atelectasis, reduction of venous stasis, bowel motility, and general recovery. The use of a first-generation cephalosporin perioperatively is recommended. Frequently, it is continued for the first 24 hours after surgery, but the effectiveness of this practice has not been verified. Routine deep venous thrombosis prophylaxis is started before surgery with sequential compression devices and continued in the postoperative period. Low-molecular-weight heparin can be used as an additional adjunct in patients with greater than average risk.

Extensive lysis of adhesions is commonly required during incisional ventral herniorrhaphy. Small bowel injuries during adhesiolysis can be catastrophic, especially if they are missed.[54] Nearly a fifth of open adhesiolysis operations may result in inadvertent enterotomy.[55] Enterotomy has been reported in an average of 1% of patients in all large series of laparoscopic ventral hernia repair.[42,45,56,57] Prompt recognition of a bowel injury is needed to avoid serious morbidity. Management of a recognized intraoperative enterotomy varies according to the type and extent of the injured intestine and the type of mesh available. Small lacerations in the small intestine or bladder without significant contamination may not be an absolute contraindication to mesh placement, either laparoscopically or by open means. In the event of fecal spillage, the bowel should be repaired and the adhesiolysis completed, and a delayed hernia repair is generally warranted if a prosthetic is required. The patient is usually placed on a regimen of antibiotics and returned to the operating room in 3 or 4 days for definitive repair if there are no signs of infection, or the procedure may be aborted all together. Primary repair of the hernia defect, with the anticipated higher recurrence rate, is another option. This may be a place for biologic or natural tissue, although the long-term durability of these repairs has not been established. Placement of standard mesh in the presence of significant contamination is contraindicated.

A patient-controlled analgesia device is often quite useful until the patient can be transitioned to oral analgesics. Postoperative pain when an open retrorectus or laparoscopic repair has been performed is frequently noted at sites of full-thickness transfascial sutures. Persistent suture site discomfort, lasting 2 to 4 weeks postoperatively, may be effectively treated by subfascial injection of a local anesthetic.[58] Its efficacy is perhaps due to the anesthetic's ability to block the affected nerve's afferent signal temporarily and allow the hypersensitivity to subside.[58] Few patients complain of this problem in the long term, and rates after laparoscopic repair vary from 2% to 4%. It appears that with the recent advent of minimal access techniques and heightened patient expectations, surgeons have paid greater attention to even minor incisional discomfort and ways to prevent and treat it.

Seromas develop in many patients undergoing ventral herniorrhaphy. Regardless of whether a laparoscopic or open approach is used, most hernia surgery results in a potential space that is filled with serous fluid in the post-operative period. Most often drains are recommended with open repairs. Nonetheless, seromas are common but rarely require any intervention. Seromas are ubiquitous in the early postoperative period after laparoscopic ventral herniorrhaphy. Expectant management is our preferred approach to all asymptomatic seromas. We reserve aspiration of fluid for patients with significant or persistent symptoms or if there is a question regarding infection. Long-term problems associated with seromas are rare.

Large abdominal incisions, wide tissue dissection with the creation of large flaps, and placement of a prosthetic (foreign body) result in a 12% to 18% rate of wound complications after open prosthetic repair.[24,34] The laparoscopic approach to incisional hernias has dramatically reduced wound-related morbidity. The consequences of any mesh infection are severe regardless of how the prosthetic was originally placed. Traditional surgical teaching has advocated removal of contaminated or exposed prosthetics, although the morbidity associated with resection is high. In addition, mesh removal almost always results in recurrence, an open wound, and a larger hernia that will require reoperation. Fortunately, mesh removal is not mandatory. Infected polypropylene, polyester, and ePTFE mesh is often capable of being salvaged with a combination of intravenous antibiotics, local wound débridement, vacuum-assisted closure, and subsequent soft tissue coverage of the granulated mesh.[59]

Special Considerations

Umbilical Hernia

Repair of an umbilical hernia as described by William Mayo's vertical fascial overlap technique was discussed previously.[37] This operation or simple fascial closure is still performed frequently today by many surgeons. These repairs are effective and may be the preferred technique for small umbilical hernias with no tension after fascial approximation, but larger hernias have been shown to have a recurrence rate of up to 28%.[60]

The introduction of mesh prosthetics has appropriately had an impact on umbilical hernia repair. These tension-free repairs, which have been popularized for other ventral hernias, may have a role in umbilical hernia repair. In 2001, Arroyo et al. published a randomized controlled trial comparing primary suture repair and mesh repair in 200 patients with umbilical hernias.[4] The two patient groups were comparable with regard to age, sex, hernia defect size, and American Society of Anesthesiologists class. Operative times and complications were not statistically different. The mean follow-up was 64 months. The major difference was the recurrence rate of 11% in the suture repair group versus 1% in the mesh repair group ($P = .0015$). Other studies using mesh implantation as a sublay or plug have also shown low recurrence rates.[61]

Laparoscopic techniques have recently been proposed for umbilical hernias as well. The technical aspects are essentially the same as applied to other ventral hernia defects. The laparoscopic approach took longer to perform, tended to have fewer complications, and had no recurrences reported in a small retrospective group.[50] Criticism of the laparoscopic approach is the need for general anesthesia to establish pneumoperitoneum and the increased length of operating time. Conversely, placement of trocars around and not through the umbilicus has the potential to avoid the wound-related complications associated with an incision directly over the mesh.

There are many effective methods to repair umbilical hernias. Each patient must be evaluated individually, and one method of repair may not apply to all cases. Small primary umbilical defects in low-risk patients can probably be repaired with sutures alone and achieve good results. As the defect size increases, a mesh prosthetic should be considered. Whether the repair is better performed via an open or laparoscopic approach is controversial because prospective data are not available. Improvements in mesh prosthetics may continue to guide the ideal approach.

Spigelian Hernias

Adriaan van der Spiegel, a Belgian anatomist, was the first to describe the semilunar line as a concave region at the lateral border of the rectus muscle formed by the aponeurosis of the internal oblique. More than a hundred years later, in 1764, Klinkosh identified the "hernia of the Spigelian line" as a distinct entity.[62]

Although spigelian hernias are rare, accounting for 0.1% to 2% of all abdominal wall hernias, its diagnostic incidence has been rising because of improved imaging technology and incidental identification during laparoscopy. Spigelian hernias usually occur in the sixth and seventh decades and affect both sexes and sides equally. Most are acquired, and nearly 50% of patients with spigelian hernias have a history of previous laparotomy or laparoscopy.[63] Other factors that have been implicated in contributing to the development of these hernias are alterations in compliance of the abdominal wall as a result of morbid obesity, multiple pregnancies, prostatic enlargement, chronic pulmonary disease, and rapid weight loss in obese patients.[63]

A spigelian hernia is a challenge to diagnose and requires a high index of suspicion. Pain is the most common initial complaint. The fascial defect is masked by the intact overlying external oblique aponeurosis, thus complicating physical examination.[64] In addition, a palpable mass, when present, may mimic an abdominal wall lipoma or desmoid tumor. Although abdominal imaging may be helpful, the findings of unusual abdominal complaints in the proper anatomic location should alert one to the possibility of a spigelian hernia. Nevertheless, more than half of all spigelian hernias are diagnosed intraoperatively.[63]

Given the small neck of these hernias, 20% to 30% require emergency intervention.[63,64] Thus, even incidental spigelian hernias should be repaired electively to avoid incarceration. Surgical management of these hernias has typically been accomplished via a transverse incision and primary repair. Primary repairs have been associated with a low, but real recurrence rate of about 4%.[64] As expected, mesh repairs have been successfully applied to treat spigelian hernias. Few or no recurrences at long-term follow-up have been reported by several investigators.[62,64] More recently, laparoscopic repair of spigelian hernias has also been reported.[65,66] Evidence-based surgical recommendations are limited by the rarity of this condition, and a recommendation regarding suture- or mesh-based repair, either open or laparoscopic, is not clear at present for the treatment of spigelian hernias.

Components Separation

Large incisional hernias often occur in patients who have experienced traumatic injuries or intra-abdominal catastrophes and are at times left with an open abdomen. Damage control laparotomy and early recognition and treatment of abdominal compartment syndrome have improved survival, but at times patients are left with massive ventral hernias because the fascia is unable to be reapproximated. Subsequent skin closure alone or skin grafting directly to granulating abdominal viscera provides coverage. Over time, the musculature of the anterior abdominal wall, although anatomically present, retracts laterally and enlarges the hernia. The defects remaining after excision of the skin grafts are most often not amenable to primary closure, and prosthetic closure may be difficult as well. In addition, these cases have a high incidence of fistula formation and infection, which complicates the placement of prosthetics.

Native tissue transfer is a possibility for closure of these wounds. A vascularized and innervated muscle flap is ideal for maintaining support of the abdominal wall. Free flap tissue transfer has been used for this repair, but it may include the morbidity of a separate donor site in addition to potential vascular flow issues that can lead to flap necrosis. The flap is also denervated, and this leads to muscular atrophy and laxity in the new site, which are not ideal properties for abdominal hernia repair. Tissue expanders under the external oblique can be useful; however, they call for an additional surgical procedure, and the device requires a prolonged expansion phase and is associated with an inherent risk of infection, expander extrusion, and failure.[67] "Components separation techniques" have been developed to provide a tension-free and, most often, prosthetic-free repair of the abdominal wall.

The ideal timing of this procedure depends on the patient. The appropriate time is when complete healing of the abdomen has occurred and the overlying skin or graft is freely movable from the underlying viscera, which typically requires 6 to 12 months. Another benefit of delayed repair is to permit the most intense part of the inflammatory response to resolve and allow "softening" of the ubiquitous intra-abdominal adhesions. Aggressive nutritional support to achieve preinjury status is also essential.

The first goal in this technique is to acquire access to the abdominal cavity and lyse the necessary adhesions. Adhesions to the anterior abdominal wall skin or grafts should be cleared laterally to the anterior axillary line. Interloop adhesions need not be divided; however, any omentum that can be freed can be used later to protect the bowel from a prosthetic if one is required.[68] If an abdominal skin graft is present, it is excised. This initial phase of the operation can be lengthy, depending on the density of the adhesions.

Once the adhesiolysis is complete, mobilization of the muscle or fascial flaps (or both) is started. The subcutaneous tissue is mobilized free of the superficial fascia and the dissection carried laterally to the anterior axillary line if needed. This in and of itself releases the muscular fascia somewhat and may provide enough additional length to close the fascial defect without tension. The dissection is typically stopped at the point when the fascia is approximated tension-free. If this first maneuver does not add sufficient medial mobilization to the fascia, component separation is performed. In the technique described by Ramirez et al., the external oblique fascia is incised lateral to the semilunar line from the costal margin to the pubis.[67] The plane between the external oblique muscle and the internal oblique fascia can be developed laterally to the anterior axillary line. The blood supply to the external oblique muscle enters between the posterior and anterior axillary line, so dissection medial to this point does not endanger the neurovascular bundle. After this maneuver has been completed, the posterior rectus fascia is incised just lateral to the linea alba. The muscle can then be freed from the posterior fascia while taking care to preserve the blood supply, which enters posteriorly near the central portion of the muscle. These techniques applied to both sides of the abdominal wall can yield up to 20 cm of combined medial mobilization of the fascia. Many other modifications of this procedure have been proposed, with similar results (Fig. 47–11).

An important aspect to be emphasized again is the necessity for a tension-free repair. If this cannot be achieved, a prosthetic material can be inserted. Peak inspiratory pressure can also be monitored during fascial closure to limit the pressure to less than 40 cm H_2O.[68] Because this procedure results in significant areas of dissection, a closed suction drain is placed to limit seroma formation. Hernia recurrence after this operation has been reported to be as high as 32%.[67,69] Wound complication rates also range from 5.7% to 33%.[69,70] The components separation technique offers ventral hernia repair to patients who have complicated courses and in whom prosthetics are often contraindicated. Although the presence of infection and fistula add morbidity to this patient population, many patients can undergo successful hernia repair.

Suprapubic Hernias

The abdominal oblique aponeurosis, rectus abdominis musculature, and rectus sheath insert on the symphysis pubis. Suprapubic hernias result from disruption of these musculotendinous elements of the lower abdominal wall and usually occur after blunt abdominal trauma or pelvic surgery. The origin of traumatic suprapubic hernias is often through a ruptured rectus muscle at or near its insertion to the pubic bone. In contrast, incisional suprapubic hernias develop as a result of apical pubic osteotomy or iatrogenic detachment of the rectus muscle from its pubic insertion to improve visualization during pelvic surgery. Inadequate tissue purchase inferiorly during closure may result in hernia formation, although infection and other patient factors may also play a role.

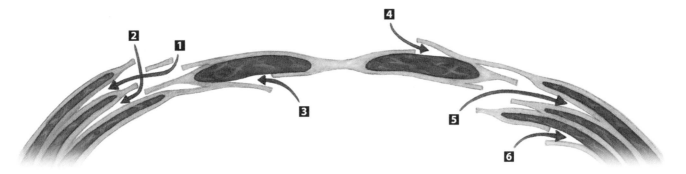

Technique	Author (Year)	Steps Involved
Components Separation Release	Ramirez (1990)	1 3
External Oblique Release	Shestak (2000)	1
External & Internal Oblique Release	Levine (2001)	1 2
"Sliding Door" Release	Kuzbari (1998)	1 3 4
External Oblique/Transversus Abdominis Release	Thomas (1993)	1 6
External Oblique/Anterior Rectus Release	Lucas (1998)	1 4
Anterior Rectus Fascia Release	Yeh (1996)	4
"Lateral" Release	Mathes (2000)	5
Modified Components Separation Release	Fabian (1994)	1 2 3

Figure 47–11. Components separation techniques.

Radical prostatectomy is the most common operative procedure that leads to the development of a suprapubic defect. Similar defects are also seen after operations involving the uterus, urinary bladder, and sigmoid colon.[71]

Suprapubic hernias may be manifested as vague lower abdominal discomfort, urinary symptoms such as frequency, or a palpable mass. The diagnosis of a suprapubic hernia may be missed because of the similarity of features with more common inguinal hernias. However, a thorough physical examination will demonstrate close proximity of the mass or defect, or both, to the pubis and not the external inguinal ring. Although suprapubic hernias may be a source of significant abdominal pain, bowel incarceration requiring emergency repair is extremely rare.

Primary repair of traumatic suprapubic hernias may be a viable alternative if the herniorrhaphy is undertaken without delay. With time, the rectus muscle retracts, which can lead to significant tension if primary repair is performed. Thus, a mesh repair is preferred for most traumatic and incisional suprapubic hernia repairs. Several approaches to mesh placement for suprapubic hernias have been described. An onlay repair involves placement of the mesh anterior to the defect and subsequent fixation to Cooper's ligament, the arcuate ligament, and the anterior abdominal wall fascia. Although this technique may require limited or no intra-abdominal dissection, it may impair visualization of the inferior aspect of the defect and lead to a high rate of hernia recurrence. On the other hand, the preperitoneal approach provides excellent delineation of the bladder and pubis and thus fixation of the inferior aspect of the mesh. The laparoscopic approach to suprapubic herniorrhaphy also allows for a definitive repair. This approach does require mobilization of the bladder, much like a transabdominal, preperitoneal inguinal hernia repair. In our series of 36 patients who underwent laparoscopic repair of a suprapubic hernia, the recurrence rate was 5.5% at nearly 2 years of follow-up; no major perioperative complications were documented, and there was one conversion to open surgery.[72] The dissection can be complex, whether open or laparoscopic, because of the close proximity of these hernias to bony, vascular, and nerve structures and the bladder (Fig. 47–12).

Ventral Hernia and Obesity

Obesity has long been considered a risk factor for the development of both primary and incisional ventral hernias. Medical comorbidity, increased intra-abdominal pressure, and technically difficult fascial closure are all likely contributors to the development of postoperative incisional hernias in overweight patients. The incidence of wound infections, perhaps the most important risk factor for the development of an incisional hernia, is also higher in the obese.[24,51,73-76] Sugerman et al. reported obesity to be the greatest risk factor for hernia recurrence.[6] Indeed, open ventral hernia repair in the obese has been marked by a recurrence rate of up to 50%.[15]

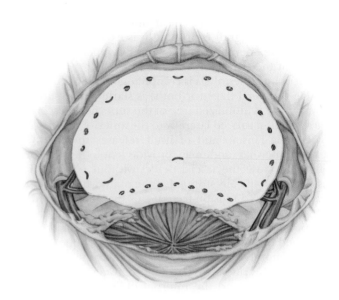

Figure 47–12.   Suprapubic repair technique.

Weight loss may reduce the risk of hernia recurrence in obese patients. As a result, several alternative approaches combining ventral herniorrhaphy with bariatric or plastic surgery procedures have been proposed. Although several investigators reported low rates of hernia recurrence, the evidence remains inconclusive. At present, larger series with longer follow-up are still necessary to establish the long-term durability of herniorrhaphy combined with bariatric procedures and abdominoplasty.

The use of a laparoscopic approach to ventral hernia repair in obese patients has been shown to possibly reduce perioperative complications and improve failure rates. In a series of 167 obese and morbidly obese patients who underwent a laparoscopic ventral hernia repair, we found a 12.3% rate of perioperative morbidity and a low 5.5% recurrence rate at long-term follow-up.[77] These results were confirmed in a larger, multi-institutional trial.[42] In this study, obese patients had a significantly higher rate of recurrence than did patients of normal weight, but they also had larger and more frequently recurrent hernias. The results indicate the safety of the laparoscopic approach in the obese patients with complex hernias. A success rate of up to 94.5% may suggest improved outcomes with the minimally invasive technique when compared with historical open controls.[42]

CONCLUSION

Ventral hernia repair continues to evolve as new technologies and new techniques are developed. The past decade illustrates this point with the introduction of new prosthetics and new open and laparoscopic repair methods. The search for the ideal repair technique with low long-term recurrence rates is ongoing. Until ventral hernias can be prevented, surgical repair of hernias will remain an important issue for the general surgeon.

SUGGESTED READINGS

Heniford BT (ed): Problems in General Surgery: Abdominal Hernias, vol 19, issue 4. Philadelphia, Lippincott Williams & Wilkins, 2002, pp 1-108.

Heniford BT, Park A, Ramshaw BJ, Voeller G: Laparoscopic repair of ventral hernias: Nine years' experience with 850 consecutive hernias. Ann Surg 238:391-399, discussion 399-400, 2003.

Luijendijk RW, Hop WC, van den Tol MP, et al: A comparison of suture repair with mesh repair for incisional hernia. N Engl J Med 343:392-398, 2000.

Stoppa RE: The treatment of complicated groin and incisional hernias. World J Surg 13:545-554, 1989.

Wantz GE: Incisional hernioplasty with Mersilene. Surg Gynecol Obstet 172:129-137, 1991.

REFERENCES

1. Kingsnorth AN, LeBlanc KA: Management of Abdominal Hernias, 3rd ed. London, Arnold, 2003.
2. Moore KL: Clinically Oriented Anatomy, 3rd ed. Baltimore, Williams & Wilkins, 1992.
3. Muschaweck U: Umbilical and epigastric hernia repair. Surg Clin North Am 83:1207-1221, 2003.
4. Arroyo A, Garcia P, Perez F, et al: Randomized clinical trial comparing suture and mesh repair of umbilical hernia in adults. Br J Surg 88:1321-1323, 2001.
5. Perrakis E, Velimezis G, Vezakis A, et al: A new tension-free technique for the repair of umbilical hernia, using the Prolene Hernia System—early results from 48 cases. Hernia 7:178-180, 2003.
6. Sugerman HJ, Kellum JM Jr, Reines HD, et al: Greater risk of incisional hernia with morbidly obese than steroid-dependent patients and low recurrence with prefascial polypropylene mesh. Am J Surg 171:80-84, 1996.
7. Bucknall TE, Cox PJ, Ellis H: Burst abdomen and incisional hernia: A prospective study of 1129 major laparotomies. Br Med J (Clin Res Ed) 284:931-933, 1982.
8. Luijendijk RW, Hop WC, van den Tol MP, et al: A comparison of suture repair with mesh repair for incisional hernia. N Engl J Med 343:392-398, 2000.
9. Santora TA, Roslyn JJ: Incisional hernia. Surg Clin North Am 73:557-570, 1993.
10. Lamont PM, Ellis H: Incisional hernia in re-opened abdominal incisions: An overlooked risk factor. Br J Surg 75:374-376, 1988.
11. Pleumeekers HJ, De Gruijl A, Hofman A, et al: Prevalence of aortic aneurysm in men with a history of inguinal hernia repair. Br J Surg 86:1155-1158, 1999.
12. Cannon DJ, Read RC: Metastatic emphysema: A mechanism for acquiring inguinal herniation. Ann Surg 194:270-278, 1981.
13. Burger JW, Luijendijk RW, Hop WC, et al: Long-term follow-up of a randomized controlled trial of suture versus mesh repair of incisional hernia. Ann Surg 240:578-583, discussion 583-585, 2004.
14. Mudge M, Hughes LE: Incisional hernia: A 10 year prospective study of incidence and attitudes. Br J Surg 72:70-71, 1985.
15. Hesselink VJ, Luijendijk RW, de Wilt JH, et al: An evaluation of risk factors in incisional hernia recurrence. Surg Gynecol Obstet 176:228-234, 1993.
16. van't Riet M, Steyerberg EW, Nellensteyn J, et al: Meta-analysis of techniques for closure of midline abdominal incisions. Br J Surg 89:1350-1356, 2002.
17. Rucinski J, Margolis M, Panagopoulos G, Wise L: Closure of the abdominal midline fascia: Meta-analysis delineates the optimal technique. Am Surg 67:421-426, 2001.
18. Jenkins TP: The burst abdominal wound: A mechanical approach. Br J Surg 63:873-876, 1976.
19. Tonouchi H, Ohmori Y, Kobayashi M, Kusunoki M: Trocar site hernia. Arch Surg 139:1248-1256, 2004.
20. Matthews BD, Heniford BT, Sing RF: Preperitoneal Richter hernia after a laparoscopic gastric bypass. Surg Laparosc Endosc Percutan Tech 11:47-49, 2001.
21. Cumberland VH: A preliminary report on the use of prefabricated nylon weave in the repair of ventral hernia. Med J Aust 1:143-144, 1952.
22. Scales JT: Tissue reactions to synthetic materials. Proc R Soc Med 46:647-652, 1953.
23. Usher FC, Ochsner J, Tuttle LL Jr: Use of Marlex mesh in the repair of incisional hernias. Am Surg 24:969-974, 1958.
24. Leber GE, Garb JL, Alexander AI, Reed WP: Long-term complications associated with prosthetic repair of incisional hernias. Arch Surg 133:378-382, 1998.
25. Park A, Birch DW, Lovrics P: Laparoscopic and open incisional hernia repair: A comparison study. Surgery 124:816-821, discussion 821-822, 1998.
26. Klinge U, Klosterhalfen B, Muller M, Schumpelick V: Foreign body reaction to meshes used for the repair of abdominal wall hernias. Eur J Surg 165:665-673, 1999.
27. Cobb WS, Burns JM, Peindl RD, et al: Textile analysis of heavyweight, midweight, and lightweight polypropylene mesh in a porcine ventral hernia model. Paper presented at the 38th Annual Meeting of the Association for Academic Surgery, 2004, Houston.
28. Klinge U, Klosterhalfen B, Muller M, et al: Shrinking of polypropylene mesh in vivo: An experimental study in dogs. Eur J Surg 164:965-969, 1998.
29. Welty G, Klinge U, Klosterhalfen B, et al: Functional impairment and complaints following incisional hernia repair with different polypropylene meshes. Hernia 5:142-147, 2001.
30. Klinge U, Klosterhalfen B, Conze J, et al: Modified mesh for hernia repair that is adapted to the physiology of the abdominal wall. Eur J Surg 164:951-960, 1998.
31. Klinge U, Conze J, Limberg W, et al: [Pathophysiology of the abdominal wall.] Chirurg 67:229-233, 1996.
32. Junge K, Klinge U, Prescher A, et al: Elasticity of the anterior abdominal wall and impact for reparation of incisional hernias using mesh implants. Hernia 5:113-118, 2001.
33. Wantz GE: Incisional hernioplasty with Mersilene. Surg Gynecol Obstet 172:129-137, 1991.
34. Stoppa RE: The treatment of complicated groin and incisional hernias. World J Surg 13:545-554, 1989.
35. Carbonell AM, Matthews BD, Dreau D, et al: The susceptibility of prosthetic biomaterials to infection. Surg Endosc 19:430-435, 2005.
36. Harold KL, Kercher KW, Heniford BT: In-vitro fibroblastic adherence to standard hernia meshes. Paper presented at the Annual Meeting of the American Hernia Society, Tucson, AZ, May 8-12, 2002.
37. Mayo WJ: Radical cure of umbilical hernia. JAMA 1842, 1907.
38. Luijendijk RW, Lemmen MH, Hop WC, Wereldsma JC: Incisional hernia recurrence following "vest-over-pants" or vertical Mayo repair of primary hernias of the midline. World J Surg 21:62-65, discussion 66, 1997.
39. de Vries Reilingh TS, van Geldere D, Langenhorst B, et al: Repair of large midline incisional hernias with polypropylene mesh: Comparison of three operative techniques. Hernia 8:56-59, 2004.
40. Millikan KW: Incisional hernia repair. Surg Clin North Am 83:1223-1234, 2003.
41. Rives J, Pire JC, Flament JB, et al: [Treatment of large eventrations. New therapeutic indications apropos of 322 cases.] Chirurgie 111:215-225, 1985.
42. Matthews BD, Bui HT, Harold KL, et al: Thoracoscopic sympathectomy for palmaris hyperhidrosis. South Med J 96:254-258, 2003.
43. Heniford BT, Park A, Voeller G: Laparoscopic ventral hernia repair. Surgical Prospectus 1-11, 1999.
44. LeBlanc KA: The critical technical aspects of laparoscopic repair of ventral and incisional hernias. Am Surg 67:809-812, 2001.

45. LeBlanc KA, Whitaker JM, Bellanger DE, Rhynes VK: Laparoscopic incisional and ventral hernioplasty: Lessons learned from 200 patients. Hernia 7:118-124, 2003.

46. DeMaria EJ, Moss JM, Sugerman HJ: Laparoscopic intraperitoneal polytetrafluoroethylene (PTFE) prosthetic patch repair of ventral hernia. Prospective comparison to open prefascial polypropylene mesh repair. Surg Endosc 14:326-329, 2000.

47. Carbajo MA, Martin del Olmo JC, Blanco JI, et al: Laparoscopic treatment vs open surgery in the solution of major incisional and abdominal wall hernias with mesh. Surg Endosc 13:250-252, 1999.

48. McGreevy JM, Goodney PP, Birkmeyer CM, et al: A prospective study comparing the complication rates between laparoscopic and open ventral hernia repairs. Surg Endosc 17:1778-1780, 2003.

49. Raftopoulos I, Vanuno D, Khorsand J, et al: Comparison of open and laparoscopic prosthetic repair of large ventral hernias. JSLS 7:227-232, 2003.

50. Wright BE, Niskanen BD, Peterson DJ, et al: Laparoscopic ventral hernia repair: Are there comparative advantages over traditional methods of repair? Am Surg 68:291-295, discussion 295-296, 2002.

51. Robbins SB, Pofahl WE, Gonzalez RP: Laparoscopic ventral hernia repair reduces wound complications. Am Surg 67:896-900, 2001.

52. Ramshaw BJ, Esartia P, Schwab J, et al: Comparison of laparoscopic and open ventral herniorrhaphy. Am Surg 65:827-831, discussion 831-832, 1999.

53. Holzman MD, Purut CM, Reintgen K, et al: Laparoscopic ventral and incisional hernioplasty. Surg Endosc 11:32-35, 1997.

54. Berger D, Bientzle M, Muller A: Postoperative complications after laparoscopic incisional hernia repair. Incidence and treatment. Surg Endosc 16:1720-1723, 2002.

55. Van Der Krabben AA, Dijkstra FR, Nieuwenhuijzen M, et al: Morbidity and mortality of inadvertent enterotomy during adhesiotomy. Br J Surg 87:467-471, 2000.

56. Ben-Haim M, Kuriansky J, Tal R, et al: Pitfalls and complications with laparoscopic intraperitoneal expanded polytetrafluoroethylene patch repair of postoperative ventral hernia. Surg Endosc 16:785-788, 2002.

57. Egea DA, Martinez JA, Cuenca GM, et al: Mortality following laparoscopic ventral hernia repair: Lessons from 90 consecutive cases and bibliographical analysis. Hernia 8:208-212, 2004.

58. Carbonell AM, Harold KL, Mahmutovic AJ, et al: Local injection for the treatment of suture site pain after laparoscopic ventral hernia repair. Am Surg 69:688-691, discussion 691-692, 2003.

59. Kercher KW, Sing RF, Matthews BD, Heniford BT: Successful salvage of infected PTFE mesh after ventral hernia repair. Ostomy Wound Manage 48:40-42, 44-45, 2002.

60. Celdran A, Bazire P, Garcia-Urena MA, Marijuan JL: H-hernioplasty: A tension-free repair for umbilical hernia. Br J Surg 82:371-372, 1995.

61. Kurzer M, Belsham PA, Kark AE: Tension-free mesh repair of umbilical hernia as a day case using local anaesthesia. Hernia 8:104-107, 2004.

62. Vos DI, Scheltinga MR: Incidence and outcome of surgical repair of spigelian hernia. Br J Surg 91:640-644, 2004.

63. Montes IS, Deysine M: Spigelian and other uncommon hernia repairs. Surg Clin North Am 83:1235-1253, viii, 2003.

64. Larson DW, Farley DR: Spigelian hernias: Repair and outcome for 81 patients. World J Surg 26:1277-1281, 2002.

65. Tarnoff M, Rosen M, Brody F: Planned totally extraperitoneal laparoscopic Spigelian hernia repair. Surg Endosc 16:359, 2002.

66. Moreno-Egea A, Carrasco L, Girela E, et al: Open vs laparoscopic repair of spigelian hernia: A prospective randomized trial. Arch Surg 137:1266-1268, 2002.

67. Ramirez OM, Ruas E, Dellon AL: "Components separation" method for closure of abdominal-wall defects: An anatomic and clinical study. Plast Reconstr Surg 86:519-526, 1990.

68. Jacobs DG, Pratt BL, Capizzi PJ: Reconstruction of the massive posttraumatic abdominal wall hernia. Probl Gen Surg 19:73-83, 2002.

69. de Vries Reilingh TS, van Goor H, Rosman C, et al: "Components separation technique" for the repair of large abdominal wall hernias. J Am Coll Surg 196:32-37, 2003.

70. DiBello JN Jr, Moore JH Jr: Sliding myofascial flap of the rectus abdominis muscles for the closure of recurrent ventral hernias. Plast Reconstr Surg 98:464-469, 1996.

71. Bendavid R: Incisional parapubic hernias. Surgery 108:898-901, 1990.

72. Carbonell AM, Kercher KW, Matthews BD, et al: The laparoscopic repair of suprapubic ventral hernias. Surg Endosc 19:174-177, 2005.

73. White TJ, Santos MC, Thompson JS: Factors affecting wound complications in repair of ventral hernias. Am Surg 64:276-280, 1998.

74. Houck JP, Rypins EB, Sarfeh IJ, et al: Repair of incisional hernia. Surg Gynecol Obstet 169:397-399, 1989.

75. Rios A, Rodriguez JM, Munitiz V, et al: Factors that affect recurrence after incisional herniorrhaphy with prosthetic material. Eur J Surg 167:855-859, 2001.

76. Rios A, Rodriguez JM, Munitiz V, et al: Antibiotic prophylaxis in incisional hernia repair using a prosthesis. Hernia 5:148-152, 2001.

77. Novitsky YW, Cobb WS, Kercher KW, et al: Laparoscopic ventral hernia repair in obese patients: A new standard of care. Arch Surg 141:57-61, 2006.

48

Lumbar and Pelvic Hernias

Nir Wasserberg · Howard S. Kaufman

Lumbar and pelvic floor hernias, including obturator and sciatic hernias, present difficulties in diagnosis and treatment because of the deep position of the sac and the surrounding layers of muscle, fascia, and bone. Lumbar hernias have been described in children as well as adults and originate in an area of weakness in the parietal wall of the torso, namely, the superior triangle of Grynfeltt-Lesshaft and the inferior triangle of Petit. Obturator hernias are uncommon and occur most frequently in thin elderly women. In contrast, other pelvic floor hernias, such as those associated with advanced pelvic floor relaxation, occur more commonly in multiparous women. Obesity is a risk factor for hernias associated with pelvic relaxation. These hernias may be accompanied by entrapment of the rectum and symptoms of obstructed defecation, pelvic bulging, heaviness, pain, or any combination of these symptoms. Though more common, they may also produce diagnostic and therapeutic challenges.

Advances in both static and dynamic imaging techniques with computed tomography (CT), magnetic resonance imaging (MRI), and fluoroscopic pelvic floor imaging with cystocolpoproctography (with or without enteral or peritoneal contrast) have enhanced the clinician's ability to diagnose both lumbar and pelvic hernias. Moreover, laparoscopy has become a useful diagnostic tool, and many hernias may be approached and repaired via minimally invasive techniques. Overall, the low incidence of lumbar and pelvic hernias limits the opportunity to study different techniques of repair prospectively, and individual surgeon experience in their treatment is usually limited.

In the last edition of this text, DeMeester and Magnuson performed a comprehensive rewrite of this chapter.[1] Many of the historical and anatomic sections have not changed, and therefore we are grateful to them for their permission to reuse many of these sections. However, many advances in imaging, laparoscopic surgery, and graft materials have occurred in the past 5 years, and these areas will be highlighted.

As a general rule, the principle of tension-free repair should apply for most lumbar and pelvic floor hernias.

However, discrete levator ani hernias may not be amenable to such an approach. A variety of synthetic and biologic materials are frequently used for hernia repairs, and a basic understanding of the biomechanical properties of synthetic and biologic grafts will aid the surgeon in choosing the best prosthesis for a given indication. Synthetic materials can be divided into absorbable and nonabsorbable, flat, single component, and combination. Types of mesh differ in pore size, weave variation, thickness, pliability, and weight. All are available in various sizes and can be cut and fashioned for a specific use. Biologic materials range from autologous tissues such as *tensor fascia lata* and allografts to xenografts. AlloDerm (LifeCell Corporation, Branchburg, NJ) is an acellular human dermal graft used for repair of a variety of soft tissue defects. Commonly used collagen/elastin xenograft materials include porcine submucosa (Surgisis, Cook Biotech Incorporated, West Lafayette, IN) and a variety of porcine dermal grafts (Pelvicol and PelviSoft, C.R. Bard, Inc, Covington, GA). Although most elective hernia repairs are clean cases, patients may have intestinal obstruction or compromised bowel and require concomitant intestinal resection. Though still debated, an increasing body of evidence supports the reasonably safe use of prosthetic materials in clean-contaminated and even contaminated cases.[2,3]

HISTORICAL BACKGROUND

The first description of a lumbar hernia is attributed to Barbette in 1672. Garangeot described the first incarcerated lumbar hernia, which was found at autopsy, and Ravanton was the first to perform surgical reduction of a lumbar hernia. Petit delineated the anatomic boundaries of the inferior lumbar triangle in 1783. Initially, all lumbar hernias were believed to arise from Petit's triangle. However, in 1866 Grynfeltt and Lesshaft independently described the anatomic landmarks of the superior lumbar triangle; therefore, a hernia at this region became known as a Grynfeltt-Lesshaft hernia.[4] The superior triangle was also described by Geiss and Saletta in

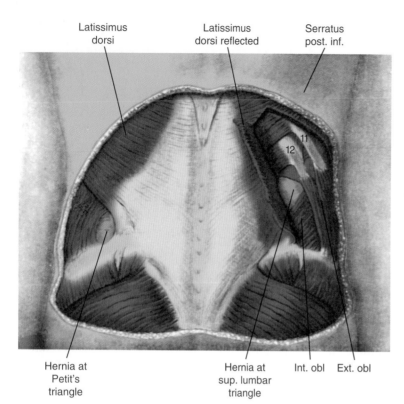

Latissimus dorsi Latissimus dorsi reflected Serratus post. inf.

11 12

Hernia at Petit's triangle Hernia at sup. lumbar triangle Int. obl Ext. obl

Figure 48–1. The anatomy of lumbar hernias, posterior view. On the *left* is Petit's triangle; on the *right* is the superior lumbar triangle of Grynfeltt-Lesshaft. (From Watson LF: Hernia, 3rd ed. St Louis, CV Mosby, 1948.)

1869, who referred to a defect in this area as a hernia. Despite this long history of anatomic descriptions, only 300 cases have been reported in the literature.

Obturator and perineal hernias were originally described by the French physicians Rene Jacques Croissant de Garengeot and Roland Arnaud de Ronsil in the 1700s.[5] For this reason, an obturator hernia was for some time referred to as "the French hernia." Watson, in his classic text on hernias, claimed a sciatic hernia to be the rarest of all hernias, with only 35 documented reports in the literature though 1948.[6] He credited the original description of a sciatic hernia to both Verdier (1753) and Papen (1750).

LUMBAR HERNIAS

Anatomic Considerations of the Lumbar Region

The borders of the lumbar region are defined by the 12th rib superiorly, the crest of the iliac bone inferiorly, the erector spinae muscles medially, and the external oblique muscle laterally (Fig. 48–1). Although many areas of weakness may occur within the lumbar region, the two most commonly described areas are the superior lumbar triangle of Grynfeltt-Lesshaft and the inferior lumbar triangle of Petit. The superior lumbar triangle of Grynfeltt-Lesshaft is an inverted triangle bounded by the free border of the internal oblique muscles laterally, the erector spinae muscle group medially, and the inferior margin of the 12th rib superiorly. This triangle is larger and more constant in shape than the inferior triangle.

The roof of this triangle is formed by the latissimus dorsi muscle, and the floor is formed by the transversalis fascia along with the aponeurosis of the transversus abdominis muscle. Collectively, these boundaries make up what is known as the lumbocostal abdominal space. The weakest aspect of this space is at its upper portion immediately below the 12th rib, where the 12th intercostal neurovascular bundle exists.

The inferior lumbar triangle described by Petit is upright in configuration and less constant in size and shape than the superior triangle is. Its base is formed by the crest of the iliac bone. The medial border is formed by the lateral border of the latissimus dorsi muscle, and the lateral border is the posterior free margin of the external oblique. The floor of the inferior triangle is formed by the lumbodorsal fascia, which is contiguous with the aponeurosis of the internal oblique and transversus abdominis muscles. Occasionally, the iliohypogastric or the ilioinguinal nerves pierce the lumbodorsal fascia and cause an additional weak area within the floor. In cadaveric studies, the inferior triangle ranges in size from nonexistent to up to 6 cm in width at the base and up to 8 cm in height.[7] Lesshaft, also studying cadavers, found the inferior triangle to be present in 77% of adults and 25% of children.[8]

Clinical Features and Diagnosis

Most lumbar hernias develop gradually, and there are no pathognomonic symptoms or signs. The patient often complains of a dragging sensation that disappears when supine. Occasionally, palpation of the hernia can result in referred pain along the distribution of the sciatic nerve and to the testes or thigh. With time, the hernia defect grows and becomes more symptomatic, as well as cosmetically noticeable and displeasing to the patient. The most common manifestation is a unilateral bulge in the flank region discovered by the patient, which may be visible to the examiner only with the patient standing. Because the roof of the superior triangle prevents the protrusion of a discrete hernia mass, a more subtle bulge in the latissimus dorsi muscle bed may be palpable and tender. Pain may also be referred to the anterior aspect of the abdomen if viscera become entrapped in the hernia defect. On standing, the bulge may become more tense and large, and coughing produces an impulse over the hernia. The hernia may recede entirely if the patient is placed in the supine position. In children, a lumbar hernia gives rise to a large, soft mass that increases in size as the child cries. The hernia is usually reducible by palpation. On percussion, the hernia may be tympanitic.

Incarceration and strangulation of lumbar hernias are not common because of the large size of the hernia defect and the broad neck of the sac. In a review of 186 cases of lumbar hernia, Watson noted that strangulation was present in only 8% of all hernias.[6] Alternatively, strangulation occurred in 18% of cases of spontaneously acquired lumbar hernias. Goodman and Speese noted a 24% incidence of incarceration within a spontaneous lumbar hernia.[7] The most common cause of strangulation in this series was either the occurrence of volvulus within the sac or constriction at the neck of the sac.

The differential diagnosis of a flank bulge, with or without pain, includes lipoma; soft tissue tumor, including fibroma, rhabdomyoma, and sarcoma; hematoma; abscess; renal tumors; muscular hernia; pannicular lumbosacroiliac hernia (herniation of fascia but no true sac); and panniculitis. Indeed, most masses within the lumbar region do not prove to be a lumbar hernia.

The diagnosis of a lumbar hernia is easily made by CT of the abdomen and associated lumbar region (Fig. 48–2). The use of oral contrast may aid in the diagnosis. Barium enema, nuclear medicine testing (with tracer accumulating within the herniated bowel), and ultrasonography have also been used to diagnose a posterior abdominal wall hernia. MRI may assist in determining the cause of referred sciatic nerve pain or unexplained back pain in patients with a lumbar hernia.

Classification

Lumbar hernias have been classified according to their contents, cause, and site of protrusion. In general, the most accepted classification system, as proposed by Swartz,[9] is based on cause of the defect. In this classification system, all lumbar hernias that occur in infants and children with obvious musculoskeletal defects in the lumbar region are defined as *congenital* lumbar hernias, and all lumbar hernias not defined as congenital are termed *acquired*. With these simple criteria, about 20% of lumbar hernias are congenital and 80% are acquired.

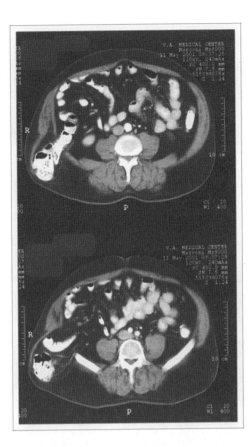

Figure 48–2. Intravenous and oral contrast-enhanced computed tomographic images of a right inferior lumbar hernia after iliac bone harvest. (From Patten LC, Awad SS, Berger DH, Fagan SP: A novel technique for the repair of lumbar hernias after iliac crest bone harvest. Am J Surg 188:85, 2004.)

Acquired defects are further subdivided into *primary* and *secondary* hernias. Primary acquired lumbar hernias occur spontaneously and represent about 55% of reported cases. Factors contributing to the development of a spontaneously acquired lumbar hernia include older age, excessive weight loss, and pulmonary disease. Primary hernias are found mostly on the left side, more often on the upper triangle, and two thirds of them have been documented in men. In contrast, secondary hernias are usually associated with trauma, infection, or previous surgical intervention in this region. Approximately 25% of all lumbar hernias are considered secondary. Iliac crest bone harvesting has been associated with a 5% to 9% postoperative incidence of lumbar hernia formation.[10] Blunt trauma to the torso is another cause; however, only 66 cases have been reported in the English literature.[11] Most of these (70%) occurred in the inferior lumbar triangle. When the hernia defect encompasses both the superior and inferior triangle, it is termed a *diffuse* lumbar hernia. Common operative interventions in the lumbar region resulting in a postoperative hernia defect include iliac

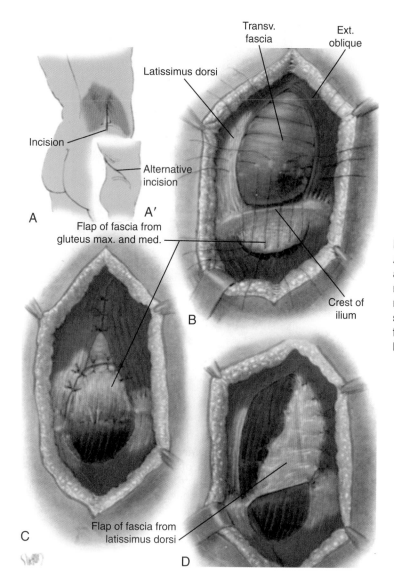

Figure 48–3. Dowd's operation for lumbar hernia. **A,** Line of incision. **B,** Turning up a flap of the fascia lata and aponeurosis of the gluteus maximus and medius muscles and suturing it to the lumbar fascia and external oblique and latissimus dorsi muscles. **C,** The flap sutured. **D,** Closing the remaining gap with a flap of fascia from the latissimus dorsi. (From Watson LF: Hernia, 3rd ed. St Louis, CV Mosby, 1948.)

crest bone harvest, open nephrectomy, adrenalectomy, and renal biopsy.

Treatment

The prognosis of lumbar hernias is generally good, with or without surgery. However, as they enlarge, they become more difficult to repair. It is therefore recommended that all lumbar hernias be repaired early. The exception is newborns with a lumbar hernia, in whom repair should be delayed until the child reaches at least 6 months of age so that anatomic landmarks are easier to identify. Any suggestion of strangulation, including erythema and increasing pain, should lead to consideration of emergency operative intervention.

The preoperative preparation of a patient undergoing repair of a lumbar hernia defect should include an imaging study to demonstrate the position of the urogenital and gastrointestinal tracts in relation to the hernia defect. Contrast-enhanced CT or MRI should provide this information. If bowel contents are found within the hernia and the hernia defect is large, preop-

erative mechanical bowel preparation should be performed. Obese patients may be counseled to lose weight before undergoing repair.

A variety of surgical approaches and techniques for repair have been described. The patient should be placed in the lateral position, which provides the best access to all structures necessary for repair. The upper part of the leg is extended over the flexed lower part of the leg, the operating room table is flexed, and the kidney rest is elevated. Adequate padding and stabilization are essential in this position. These maneuvers increase the distance from the 12th rib to the iliac crest and therefore increase exposure. The operation is divided into two steps: exploration and repair.

Exploration and reconstruction are best accomplished through an oblique incision beginning posteriorly at the 12th rib and directed anteriorly toward the iliac crest (Fig. 48–3). During exploration, the hernia mass is carefully separated from the surrounding fatty tissue. If mesocolon is inadvertently mistaken for preperitoneum, injury to the colonic blood supply could result.

Small or moderately sized hernias in the superior or inferior triangles can be repaired securely by approximation of the transversalis fascia to the fascia of the transversus abdominis muscle. Repair of a defect in the superior lumbar triangle should include approximation of the transversalis fascia to the lumbocostal ligament and the periosteum along the undersurface of the 12th rib. In moderate-sized to large hernias, additional support is necessary for adequate repair. In 1907, Dowd popularized the use of a generous aponeurotic flap from the gluteus maximus muscle.[12] Ravdin subsequently popularized the use of free fascia lata grafts for the repair of large traumatic superior lumbar triangle hernias.[13] Given the availability of synthetic and biologic grafts, most of these techniques of autologous tissue transfer have been abandoned. Common to most of these procedures is an extraperitoneal approach with fixation of the prosthesis beyond the borders of the aponeurotic defect. When a pelvic iliac bony defect exists, the closure must be modified. The iliopsoas muscle has been used as a pedicle graft to replace lost soft tissue mass. However, more recently, corkscrew bone anchors have been used successfully to anchor mesh to the remnant of the iliac crest after harvest of bone grafts.[10] If extensive mobilization of flaps has occurred, a closed suction drainage system should be used.

Burick and Parascandola were the first to describe a laparoscopic approach for the repair of a traumatic lumbar hernia in 1996.[14] Arca and colleagues reported seven cases of laparoscopic lumbar hernia repair with mesh.[15] Complications included only one failed repair secondary to infection of the mesh. More recently, Moreno-Egea et al. published a nonrandomized prospective study of 16 patients who underwent laparoscopic ($n = 9$) versus open ($n = 7$) repair of secondary lumbar hernias.[16] Patients chosen for the laparoscopic approach had smaller hernias, but they also had a lower mean operating time, postoperative morbidity, length of stay, analgesic use, and time to return to normal activities. Hernias recurred in three patients in the open group, whereas there were no recurrences in the laparoscopic group between 1 and 4 years after surgery.

OBTURATOR HERNIA

An obturator hernia is an uncommon entity that represents less than 0.1% of all hernias. Because of the unyielding structures of the obturator foramen, these hernias have a high incidence of strangulation and may cause up to 0.4% of cases of small intestinal obstruction. Though initially reported by Le Maire in 1718, it was Pierre Roland Arnaud de Ronsil who published the first case report in 1724. The first successful repair has been attributed to Obre in 1851.[17] Through 2005, approximately 700 cases of obturator hernia have been described in the literature. The hernia results from the protrusion of a sac (often containing small intestine) through the obturator foramen and canal along the pathway of the obturator nerve and vessels. The classic example is a thin, frail, multiparous elderly woman with small bowel obstruction of unclear etiology.

Anatomy

The obturator foramen is located within the anterolateral aspect of the pelvis. This is the largest foramen in the body, and it is usually larger in the female pelvis. The foramen is almost completely closed off by the obturator membrane, a fibrous covering that is an extension of the periosteum of the bony pelvis and tendinous attachments of the internal and external obturator muscles. Embryologically, the foramen and its membrane are an area of potential bone formation that has not been completed. The obturator canal is a 2- to 3-cm-long tunnel that begins in the pelvis, exits through the obturator foramen, and passes obliquely downward to end in the obturator region of the thigh (Figs. 48–4 and 48–5). The canal is bounded superiorly and laterally by the pubic bone and inferiorly by the obturator membrane and internal and external obturator muscles.

The obturator nerve, artery, and vein enter the canal through an opening in the anterosuperior aspect of the obturator membrane and pass through the canal, thereby creating a pathway for the protrusion of a hernia sac. The obturator nerve lies superior to the obturator artery within the canal and divides immediately on exiting the canal into anterior and posterior branches. The anterior branch of the obturator nerve emerges between the adductor longus and adductor brevis muscles and supplies sensory innervation to the medial aspect of the thigh, hip joint, and knee joint and motor innervation to the adductor longus, adductor brevis, gracilis, and pectineus muscles. The posterior division emerges between the adductor brevis and adductor magnus muscles to supply motor innervation to the obturator externus, adductor magnus, and occasionally the adductor brevis muscles.

Anatomically, there are three potential hernia pathways. The first and most common route is protrusion of the sac and contents through the external orifice of the obturator canal, accompanied by the anterior division of the obturator nerve. The sac lies in front of the obturator externus and underneath the pectineus. In the second type, the hernia emerges between the middle and superior fasciculi of the obturator externus along with the posterior division of the nerve. In this type the sac is posterior to the adductor brevis. In the third and most rare type, the sac emerges between the internal and external obturator muscles and membranes. Recognition of the three variants is important when repair is attempted through the thigh, but it has no bearing on emergency cases when the hernia is approached through the abdomen.

Clinical Features and Diagnosis

An obturator hernia is called "the skinny old lady hernia" because thin, elderly, multiparous and debilitated women are at greatest risk for the development of an obturator hernia. The female-to-male ratio for an obturator hernia is 6:1, and the female preponderance in this condition is thought to be secondary to the larger and more oblique incline of the obturator canal in the female pelvis. Though generally unilateral, bilateral obturator

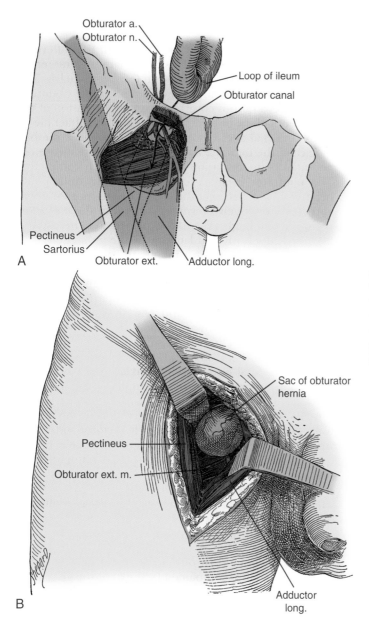

A

B

Figure 48–4. Anatomy of an obturator hernia. **A,** The structures passing through the obturator canal, in order of their superposition behind the hernial sac, are the obturator nerve, artery, and vein. **B,** Hernia in the obturator canal, the most common type of obturator hernia. The sac lies on the obturator externus muscle and is covered by the pectineus. The obturator nerve is seen directly behind the sac. (From Watson LF: Hernia, 3rd ed. St Louis, CV Mosby, 1948.)

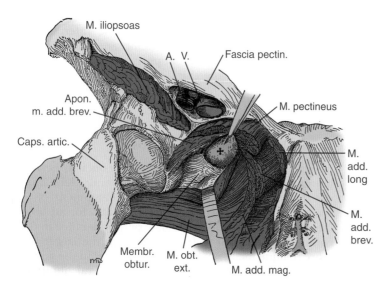

Figure 48–5. Obturator region: dissection carried to the level of the obturator membrane and obturator canal. The hernia sac can be seen protruding (marked by a *plus sign*). (From Watson LF: Hernia, 3rd ed. St Louis, CV Mosby, 1948.)

hernias have been described in 6% of cases. Obturator hernias occur more frequently on the right side, which is thought to be due to the physical presence of the sigmoid colon overlying the obturator foramen in the left side of the pelvis. Predisposing factors include constipation, chronic obstructive pulmonary disease, multiparity, and ascites, all of which lead to increased intra-abdominal pressure and defects in collagen metabolism. Rapid weight loss with a decrease in fatty tissue surrounding the obturator foramen also predisposes to obturator hernia formation.

Formation of an obturator hernia consists of three stages: a prehernia stage, which involves preperitoneal fat, or "pilot tags"; a second stage, with formation of a true sac; and a third stage in which the hernia becomes clinically significant.[18] Diagnosis during the first two stages is uncommon. However, in the third or symptomatic stage, intestinal obstruction results from involvement of the jejunum or ileum within the hernia sac. Up to 90% of cases are initially seen because of obstruction, either intermittent or acute and complete.[19] Approximately 50% of patients have an incomplete obstruction secondary to a Richter-type hernia.

Three clinical signs are specific to incarceration of an obturator hernia. Obturator neuralgia is manifested as cramping or as hypoesthesia or hyperesthesia extending from the inguinal crease to the anteromedial aspect of the thigh. The *Howship-Romberg* sign is characterized by pain radiating down the medial aspect of the thigh to the knee and less often to the hip. The pain is a result of compression of the obturator nerve (anterior division) by the hernia sac within the canal and is relieved by flexion and external rotation of the thigh and exacerbated by extension, adduction, and medial rotation of the leg. The Howship-Romberg sign is considered pathognomonic for an incarcerated obturator hernia and is present in 25% to 50% of patients. The *Hannington-Kiff* sign is absence of the obturator reflex in the thigh, which is caused by compression on the obturator nerve. This reflex can usually be elicited by placing an extended index finger across the adductor muscle approximately 5 cm above the knee and percussing over the finger. Muscle contraction should be seen or felt with an intact reflex. If the patellar reflex of the ipsilateral side is present in the absence of an obturator reflex, it is highly likely that the obturator nerve is compressed. Occasionally, a mass may be palpated in the groin region. The optimal position for palpation of a mass is with the patient supine and the thigh flexed, abducted, and externally rotated. Transrectal or transvaginal palpation of the obturator canal may demonstrate a tender mass, which is indicative of possible strangulation.

A variety of modalities can assist in diagnosing an obturator hernia, including ultrasonography, CT, MRI, herniography, and laparoscopy.[19-23] Both CT and ultrasound (transvaginal or inner thigh views) (Fig. 48-6) have been shown to be useful in the diagnosis of obturator hernia in patients coming to the emergency room with bowel obstruction and predisposing risk factors. Kammori and colleagues recently reported improved diagnosis, treatment, morbidity, and mortality in the era of CT scanning for the diagnosis and treatment of

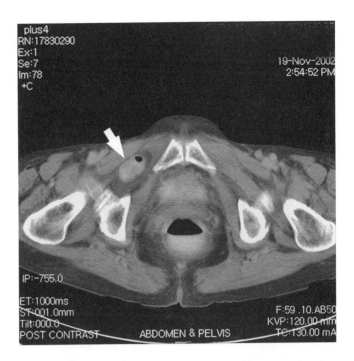

Figure 48–6. Pelvic computed tomographic scan showing bowel *(arrow)* protruding outside the right obturator foramen. (From Kim JJ, Jung H, Oh SJ, et al: Laparoscopic transabdominal preperitoneal hernioplasty of bilateral obturator hernia. Surg Laparosc Endosc Percutan Tech 15:106, 2005.)

obturator hernias.[24] MRI has been shown to be as good as but not superior to CT.[25] An abdominal radiograph obtained for the evaluation of a patient with suspected intestinal obstruction may show air in the obturator region (Fig. 48-7). Herniography, or the instillation of contrast material by infraumbilical injection into the peritoneal cavity, can be useful in the diagnosis of groin pain in adults with an inconclusive examination.[26] This method has no place in emergency diagnosis and is of questionable utility in the era of axial imaging. Laparoscopy may be used as a diagnostic tool, as well as a treatment modality.

Treatment

In more than half of suspected cases, an obturator hernia is found intraoperatively when the surgeon is performing a diagnostic laparoscopy or laparotomy. In patients with a preoperative diagnosis of obturator hernia, a variety of approaches for repair have been suggested, including abdominal, retropubic, obturator, inguinal, and laparoscopic. Historically, the preferred approach has been through a midline lower abdominal incision. With the patient in the Trendelenburg position, both obturator canals can easily be inspected, the diagnosis made quickly, and bowel resection performed if necessary. In the abdominal approach, both obturator foramina should be inspected and palpated to exclude bilateral herniation. If a dimple is found in the peritoneum of the obturator region and there is no defect palpable under

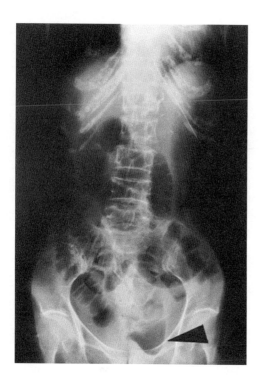

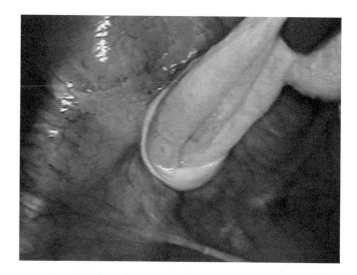

Figure 48–8. Laparoscopic view of a left obturator hernia with the sac reduced into the abdominopelvic cavity. (From Kim JJ, Jung H, Oh SJ, et al: Laparoscopic transabdominal preperitoneal hernioplasty of bilateral obturator hernia. Surg Laparosc Endosc Percutan Tech 15:106, 2005.)

Figure 48–7. Abdominal radiograph in a patient with small bowel obstruction caused by an incarcerated obturator hernia. There is a gas shadow in the obturator foramen *(arrow)*. (From Nishina M, Fujii C, Ogino R, et al: Preoperative diagnosis of obturator hernia by computed tomography in six patients. J Emerg Med 20:277, 2001.)

the ischiopubic area, a decision must be made regarding whether to dissect the obturator region for possible herniation of preperitoneal fat. When incarcerated or strangulated bowel is present, the obturator ring can be gently stretched with the surgeon's fingers or incised inferiorly. Care should be taken with the obturator vessels, which although variable, usually lie lateral to the hernia sac.

Bowel reduction must be done carefully because necrotic bowel may rupture. Bowel resection is indicated in nearly half of all cases. The sac may contain omentum, uterus and adnexal organs, bladder, and appendix. Traditionally, simple opposition plus direct repair of a small defect has a low recurrence rate. The repair can be further reinforced with an autogenous fascial flap or by patching an adjacent structure with round ligament or uterus. Optimal repair generally involves the use of prosthetic mesh, or Teflon, with a final covering provided by closure of the peritoneum. Stoppa and Warlaumont[27] have championed the use of large prosthetic sheets of mesh for bilateral and recurrent inguinal hernias; such mesh may also be used to treat obturator hernias as well. Both totally extraperitoneal (TEP) and transabdominal preperitoneal polypropylene (TAPP) laparoscopic approaches were reported to be feasible and highly effective in the treatment of obturator hernia.[28] During laparoscopy, the sac may be easily identified (Fig. 48–8) and the defect repaired with a synthetic or biologic mesh. In the presence of frank peritonitis, the contralateral side must be routinely explored for an asymptomatic hernia that may cause problems in the future.

The retropubic, obturator, and inguinal approaches avoid the peritoneal cavity. These alternative approaches may be appropriate in a nonemergency setting when there is no evidence of strangulation and a palpable mass is felt in the obturator region. When an obturator or inguinal approach is used, a mass is palpable in the obturator region, and an incision is made just above this mass. The first structure encountered is fascia lata. On division of fascia lata, two muscles, the adductor longus and pectineus, are exposed. Drawing back these muscles allows visualization of the hernia sac (see Fig. 48–5). To strengthen the repair, the pectineus muscle is usually sutured to the periosteum of the ischium.

PERINEAL HERNIA

Classification of Perineal Hernias

The pelvic floor is a sling of muscles and connective tissue that connect the pubic and ischial bones to the greater sacrosciatic ligaments and the tip of the coccyx posteriorly and to the ischial tuberosities laterally. These tissues converge centrally on the perineal body and support the sphincter mechanisms, which allows for continence of urine and stool, and the paravaginal tissues, which allows for parturition. A perineal hernia is the protrusion of intra-abdominal or pelvic viscera or fat through a defect in the pelvic floor musculature and fascia.

Perineal or levator hernias are classified as either primary or secondary. A primary perineal hernia results from a congenital or acquired defect between the muscles and fascia that form the pelvic floor. Acquired

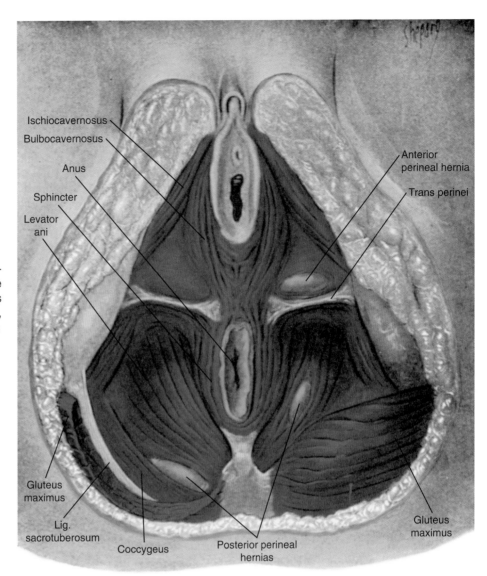

Figure 48–9. Anatomy of a perineal hernia in a woman with the points of exit of perineal hernias shown. (From Watson LF: Hernia, 3rd ed. St Louis, CV Mosby, 1948.)

defects are much more common and often result from vaginal childbirth, aging, obesity, and chronic constipation with straining. Secondary perineal hernias are true incisional hernias that occur as a result of extensive perineal procedures, including abdominoperineal resection of the rectum, pelvic exenteration, parasacral–trans-sphincteric rectal resection, vaginal hysterectomy, and perineal prostatectomy.[29,30] Hernias of the perineum are further divided into two types, anterior and posterior. This classification is based on the position of the hernia in relation to the superficial perineal muscles (Fig. 48–9). In an anterior perineal hernia, the defect passes through the urogenital diaphragm and is bounded by the bulbocavernosus muscles medially, the ischiocavernosus muscles laterally, and the superficial perineal muscles posteriorly.

If the hernia is associated with a labial mass arising between the ischiopubic bone and the vagina, it is called a *pudendal* hernia (Fig. 48–10). Anterior perineal hernias are not believed to occur in men. Posterior perineal hernias protrude through the levator ani muscles or between the levator ani and coccygeus muscles in a plane posterior to the superficial transverse perineal muscles. A congenital anatomic defect that may lead to the development of a posterior perineal hernia is known as the *hiatus of Schwalbe,* which is a result of failure of the levator ani muscle to anchor to the obturator fascia. At times, a central perineal hernia may exist. Central defects are usually associated with detachment of the perineal body from the distal rectovaginal fascia or more extensive disruption of the perineal body. Fat, rectum, sigmoid colon, or small intestine may fill this distally dissecting hernia sac. Clinically, patients with a central perineal defect have symptoms associated with the syndrome of the descending perineum, including bothersome bulging accompanied by fecal or urinary incontinence or obstruction.

Perineal hernias may be associated with pelvic organ prolapse, a primary defect acquired as a consequence of relaxation of the supporting structures of the pelvic floor. Risk factors include multiparity, older age, obesity, connective tissue disease, and previous pelvic surgery. It is

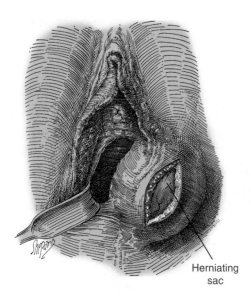

Herniating
sac

Figure 48–10. Anterior perineal hernia. When the hernia descends only into the posterior portion of the labium majus, it is known as a pudendal or vaginolabial hernia. (From Watson LF: Hernia, 3rd ed. St Louis, CV Mosby, 1948.)

estimated that 50% of parous women have some degree of pelvic organ prolapse. Population-based data from the Kaiser group in Oregon suggest that a woman's lifetime risk of requiring surgery for prolapse or incontinence approaches 11% by the age of 80, with a reoperation rate of nearly 30% after primary repair.[31] This condition may involve any of the pelvic or abdominal viscera, including the small bowel (enterocele), vagina, urethra, bladder (cystocele), and anorectum (rectocele and rectal prolapse).

Although the topic of distal rectocele will be discussed, a complete discussion of all types of rectocele repair, as well as hernias that include the bladder, vagina, uterus, and cervix, is beyond the scope of this chapter. Rectal prolapse is discussed elsewhere.

Anatomy

The pelvic support anatomy is complex and includes a network of muscles and fascia (Fig. 48–11). Because most disorders of pelvic support occur in women, specific reference will be made to the female pelvic anatomy, although the muscles are similar in men. Grossly, the front of the pelvis is bounded by the internal surface of the pubic symphysis, whereas the sides are formed by the obturator internus muscles. The sacrum occupies a central position of the posterior pelvis, with the piriformis muscles bounding the posterior pelvis more laterally. The levator ani muscles form a sling within these boundaries. These muscles contain both slow- and fast-twitch fibers and are innervated by sacral efferents from S2-S4 on the pelvic side and by branches of the pudendal nerves on the perineal side. The slow-twitch fibers maintain resting tone of the pelvic floor, whereas the fast-twitch fibers contract during increases in intra-abdominal pressure.[32,33]

The levator ani muscle complex is composed of three muscle groups, the iliococcygeus, pubococcygeus, and puborectalis. A condensation of the parietal fascia overlying the obturator internus serves as the lateral origin of the iliococcygeus, which then inserts into the lateral aspect of the coccyx. The pubococcygeus arises from the superior ramus of the pubic bone and inserts onto the coccyx and anococcygeal raphe. The pubococcygeus muscle surrounds the lower third of the vagina. Most centrally, the puborectalis muscle arises from the superior and inferior pubic rami and forms a sling around the rectum. This muscle draws the anorectal junction anteriorly when contracted, thereby helping maintain fecal continence. When relaxed, the puborectalis allows for the formation of a more obtuse anorectal angle to facilitate defecation. A condensation of the parietal fascia of the levator ani complex, the arcus tendineus fasciae pelvis, stretches from the pubic arch to the ischial spine on each side. This important "white line" forms the basis for the lateral attachments of the pubocervical fascia and rectovaginal fascia.

The most distal and superficial supporting structure of the pelvic floor is the centrally located perineal body, which is located between the posterior aspect of the vaginal introitus and the anus. The perineal body is flat underneath the skin and extends in a pyramidal shape up into the distal portion of the rectovaginal septum, to which it attaches. The perineal body (and therefore pelvic floor support) is further stabilized through its connections via the rectovaginal fascia to the uterosacral ligaments and the sacrum. Other structures that condense and attach to the perineal body include the bulbocavernosus muscles, the superficial transverse perineal muscles, the distal central portion of the levator ani complex, and the external anal sphincter muscle complex.

Clinical Features and Diagnosis

Primary hernias occur most commonly in women older than 40 years. The female preponderance of perineal hernias is again related to the broader female pelvis and weakening of pelvic floor muscles during pregnancy and childbirth. Moreover, the growing epidemic of obesity is also associated with symptoms related to constant pressure on the muscles involved in pelvic floor support. A primary perineal hernia initially comes to medical attention because of the physical presence of a bulge or because of associated bowel or genitourinary dysfunction. Symptoms commonly associated with perineal hernias include obvious bulging, pain, heaviness, urinary or fecal incontinence, obstructed urination or defecation, constipation, and sexual dysfunction. Obstructed defecation may result from anterior or lateral rectocele formation with entrapment of the rectum through the levator defect (Fig. 48–12).

Patients should be examined both in the left lateral decubitus position and in the lithotomy position. The pelvic floor should be systematically palpated with the patient at rest and then with the patient attempting to expel the examiner's finger. This maneuver allows for the

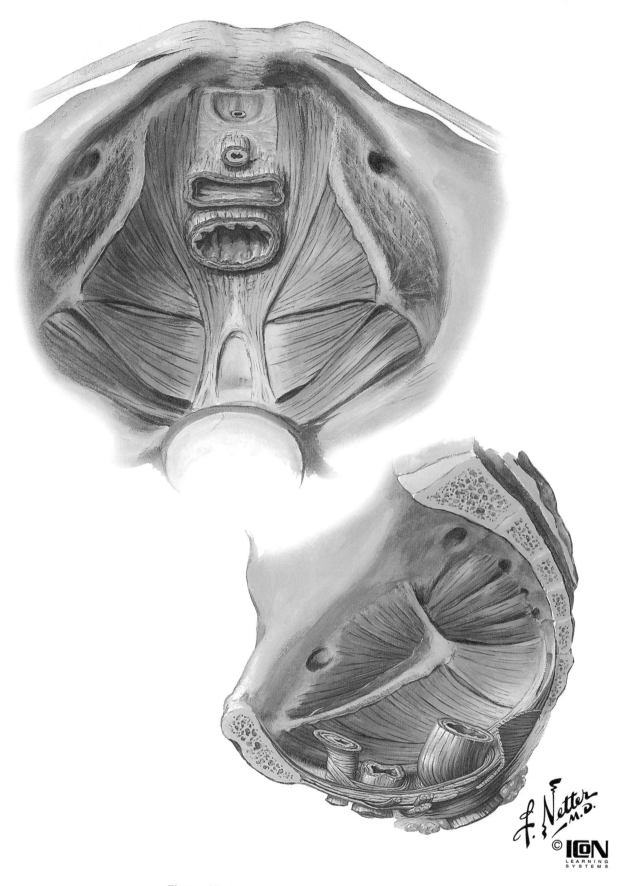

Figure 48–11. Muscles of the pelvis (female shown).

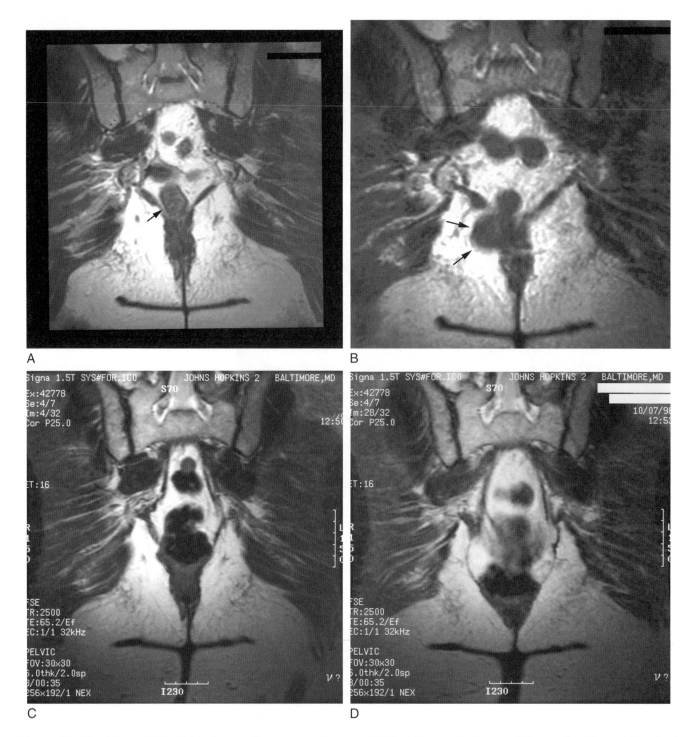

Figure 48–12.   Coronal T2-weighted magnetic resonance images. **A,** Rest image showing a midline rectum *(arrow)* in patient with obstructed defecation. **B,** Strain image demonstrating the rectum *(arrows)* herniating through a defect in the right levator ani complex. **C,** Postoperative rest image after a combined abdominoperineal approach to simple levator hernia repair with no absorbable sutures. **D,** The rectum remains midline after hernia repair, and the patient's symptoms of obstructed defecation were resolved. (From Kaufman HS, Buller JL, Thompson JR, et al: Dynamic pelvic MR imaging and cystocolpoproctography alter surgical management of pelvic floor disorders. Dis Colon Rectum 44:1575, discussion 1584, 2001.)

detection of posterolateral levator defects, which become apparent with this bellowing of the pelvic floor. Moreover, paradoxical contraction of the puborectalis can be appreciated during this maneuver because an improperly functioning puborectalis will deflect the examiner's finger anteriorly. While the patient is in the lithotomy position, associated pelvic organ prolapse should be noted in relation to an anatomic landmark, such as the hymenal ring, at rest and during straining. It may be helpful to examine a woman while she is standing to rule

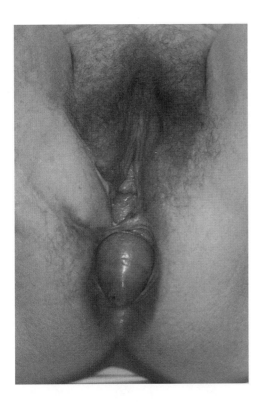

Figure 48–13. Perineal hernia after proctocolectomy for Crohn's disease. The patient has complete uterocervical procidentia. These skin bridges are seen attached to a previous harvest site of a gracilis flap.

out distal dissection of an enterocele, sigmoidocele, or rectocele high at the level of the cuff or more distally into the perineal body. Physical examination findings along with patient symptoms and complementary studies will help define the treatment modality.

Factors that may contribute to the formation of secondary perineal hernias include removal of the coccyx bone as part of an operative procedure, postoperative perineal infections, and complications of pelvic radiation therapy. A secondary perineal hernia is usually manifested as a palpable perineal mass that may cause the patient discomfort while sitting (Fig. 48–13). If the mesentery of the small bowel is long enough, the hernia defect may contain small bowel. Secondary perineal hernias most commonly develop within 1 year of an operation.[30]

Current imaging methods for evaluation of pelvic floor hernias include dynamic MRI, cystocolpoproctography, peritoneography, ultrasound, and CT. Additional anorectal physiologic and urodynamic testing may be required for associated symptoms of incontinence or obstruction (or both). Several investigations may be necessary to demonstrate pelvic floor abnormalities, especially in reoperative situations. Sentovich and colleagues described the use of dynamic proctography with peritoneography for pelvic floor disorders, and this imaging technique changed their operative plan in 85% of 13 women studied.[20] Dynamic MRI has been touted as a quick, noninvasive technique that demonstrates both pelvic visceral prolapse and the configuration of the

pelvic floor musculature.[34] Kaufman et al. demonstrated that dynamic MRI and cystocolpoproctography were concordant with physical examination findings in only 41% of 22 patients with advanced pelvic floor disorders who underwent both tests.[35] Moreover, the use of these imaging studies changed operative management in 9 of the 22 patients (41%). Gearhart and colleagues[36] identified a total of 16 levator hernias (8 unilateral, 4 bilateral) in 12 of 80 patients (15%) evaluated at a tertiary center for advanced pelvic floor disorders. Levator hernias were not more frequent in women who had undergone previous pelvic surgery, nor was they associated with any specific symptoms. However, the finding of perineal descent on physical examination was associated with the presence of a levator hernia by dynamic MRI.

Treatment

The natural history of a primary perineal hernia is not one of incarceration and strangulation but, rather, progressive enlargement and destruction of the pelvic floor. Compromise of the pelvic floor may lead to difficulty voiding and defecating, and formal evaluation of these functions should be considered. Breakdown of the perineum is rare but has also been an indication for surgery. Abdominal, perineal, and combined abdominoperineal approaches have been described for the repair of primary and secondary perineal hernias. The size of the defect, the contents of the sac, and the magnitude of the patient's symptoms usually dictate the approach for repair. Repair of secondary perineal hernias (see Fig. 48–13) often requires an abdominoperineal approach for reduction and support of herniated viscera and subsequent reinforcement of the pelvic floor.

If preoperative imaging does not suggest incarceration of a small levator hernia, an attempt may be made to repair it primarily through a perineal approach. Pudendal or vaginolabial hernias may also be approached in this manner. Similarly, most distal rectoceles that produce perineal bulging can be repaired via the discreet defect approach described by Richardson.[37] Debate continues in the urogynecologic and colorectal surgery literature about the preferred approach for rectocele repair.[38-40] Options include the aforementioned transvaginal discrete defect approach,[37,41,42] with or without an onlay graft (Fig. 48–14), the traditional transvaginal posterior colporrhaphy with midline levator plication,[38] and the transanal approach with rectal wall plication.[39] The presence of additional symptoms of pelvic relaxation should be investigated and ruled out before rectocele repair because more complex surgery to repair coexisting pelvic organ prolapse may be indicated. If the rectovaginal fascia is attenuated beyond repair, posterior fascial replacement with a biologic graft may be performed transvaginally (Fig. 48–15).[41] In addition, laparoscopic abdominal sacral colpoperineopexy has been used to attach a graft from the sacrum to the perineal body, which not only will fix the rectocele but will also primarily compensate for the central endopelvic fascial disruption associated with perineal descent (Fig. 48–16).[43]

The use of mesh or bioprostheses in pelvic floor surgery is frequently directed toward supporting pelvic viscera when the pelvic floor can no longer support these structures. Discrete hernias may not necessarily exist in the setting of global pelvic floor weakness (often with perineal descent). Sullivan et al. have described a total pelvic mesh repair with Marlex in these situations.[44] The procedure involves a strip of Marlex mesh secured between the perineal body and the sacrum; the strip may be partially wrapped around the rectum to treat rectal prolapse (Fig. 48–17). Two additional strips are tunneled laterally to support the vagina, bladder, and urethra. This procedure usually involves a multidisciplinary team of colorectal, urologic, and gynecologic surgeons. Sullivan and colleagues reported total mesh repair in 236 females with combined pelvic organ prolapse and a levator hernia. Satisfaction with correction of symptoms was achieved in 74% at greater than 6 years' follow-up. The main complication was mesh erosion to the vagina and bowel in 5% of patients.

SCIATIC HERNIA

Sciatic hernias are rare, with fewer than 100 cases reported in the literature. A sciatic hernia is defined as

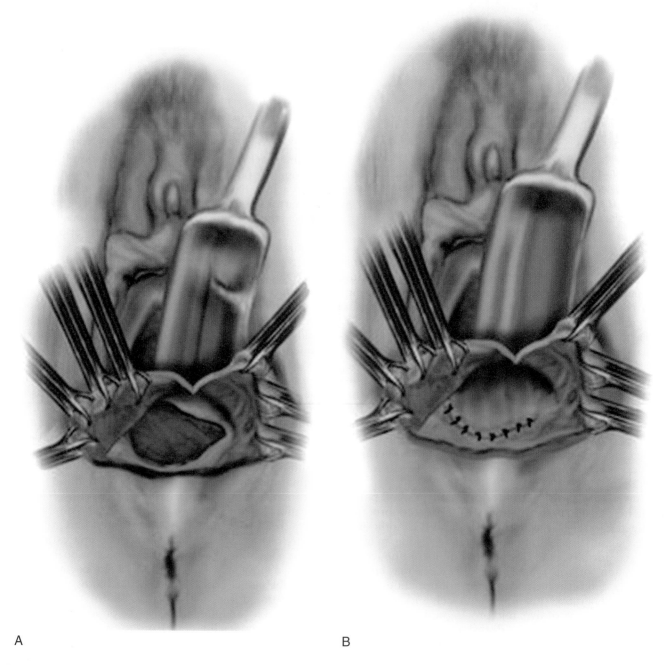

A   B

Figure 48–14. Site-specific rectocele repair of a distal defect with separation of the rectovaginal fascia from the perineal body. **A,** Dissection of a discrete defect. **B,** Repair of the defect to the perineal body.

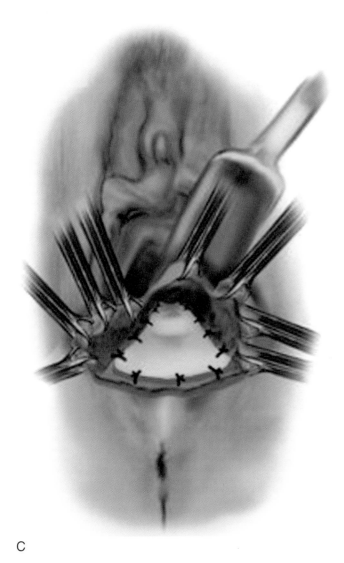

C

Figure 48–14, cont'd. C, Onlay dermal graft attached to the levators laterally, the rectovaginal fascia apically, and the perineal body distally. (From Kohli N, Miklos JR: Dermal graft–augmented rectocele repair. Int Urogynecol J 14:146, 2003.)

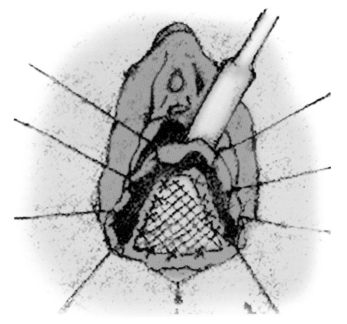

Figure 48–15. A meshed porcine dermal graft, PelviSoft (C.R. Bard, Inc, Covington, GA), replacing the posterior fascia for a large rectocele with inadequate host tissue for repair. (From Dell JR, O'Kelley KR: PelviSoft BioMesh augmentation of rectocele repair: The initial clinical experience in 35 patients. Int Urogynecol J 16:44, 2005.)

protrusion of a peritoneal sac and its contents through the greater or lesser sciatic foramen. They occur more frequently in women than in men, and the diagnosis should be considered in women with chronic pelvic pain. The development of a sciatic hernia is thought to be the direct result of piriform muscle atrophy, which allows the peritoneum to sag into the greater sciatic foramen. The sac may contain small bowel, ovary, fallopian tube, ureter, and occasionally bladder and colon. Classification of a sciatic hernia is based on anatomic relationships. Treatment consists of surgical repair.

Anatomy

Sciatic hernias have been classified according to the anatomic site of exit from the pelvis, either the greater or lesser sciatic foramen. The greater sciatic foramen is formed by a broad ligamentous band, the sacrotuberous ligament, which stretches across the greater sciatic notch on its way from the coccyx to the ischial tuberosity (Fig. 48–18). The lesser sciatic notch is converted to the lesser sciatic foramen by the bony attachments of the sacrospinous ligament. Greater sciatic hernias are further classified by their anatomic relationship to the piriformis muscle, either *suprapiriformis* or *infrapiriformis*. All vessels and nerves entering the gluteal region pass through the greater sciatic foramen. The course of the nerves and vessels entering the greater sciatic foramen is altered by the presence of the piriformis muscle. The superior gluteal artery, vein, and nerve can be found above the piriformis, whereas the inferior gluteal vessels and nerve and the internal pudendal vessels and nerve course below it. Importantly, the sciatic nerve also leaves the pelvis below the piriformis muscle near the ischial border of the greater sciatic notch.

Clinical Features and Diagnosis

Sciatic hernias are usually accompanied by varying degrees of pelvic, buttock, and posterior thigh pain. Because of the bulk of the gluteus muscles, there is rarely a palpable gluteal mass. The symptoms may be similar to those of classic sciatica with pain radiating down the back of the leg and aggravated by dorsiflexion, as well as the development of muscle weakness. A sciatic hernia may also cause pain as a result of incarceration or strangulation of bowel within the hernia sac. The patient

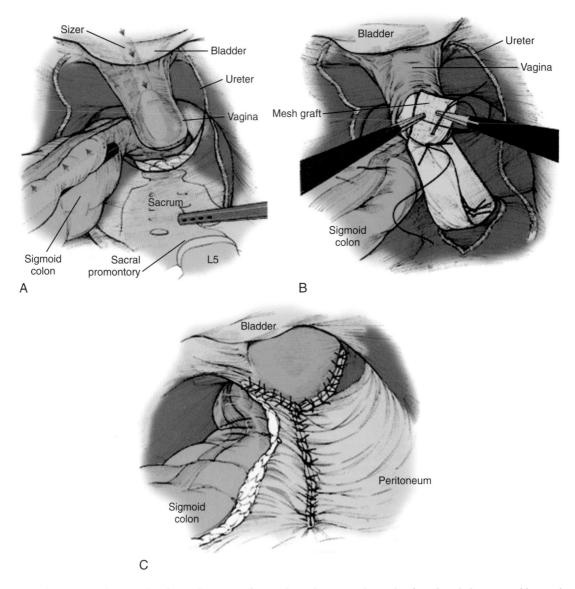

Figure 48–16. Laparoscopic sacral colpoperineopexy for vault prolapse and repair of perineal descent with mesh. **A,** Initial laparoscopic view with a sizer in the vagina showing the position of the vaginal apex and sacral promontory. **B,** Suturing graft material to the anterior aspect of the vagina. The posterior graft has been taken down to the perineal body. **C,** Completion with culdoplasty and exclusion of the graft from the peritoneal cavity. (From Link RE, Su LM, Bhayani SB, Wright EJ: Laparoscopic sacral colpoperineopexy for treatment of perineal body descent and vaginal vault prolapse. Urology 64:145, 2004.)

may have signs and symptoms of bowel or ureteral obstruction. On rare occasion, a gluteal mass may be palpable and appear more prominent with standing, straining, and coughing but diminished with lying down. If the gluteal mass is not reducible, however, one must entertain the diagnosis of a lipoma, cyst, abscess, aneurysm, or malignant tumor.

The presence of acute small bowel obstruction in the setting of a hernia warrants urgent or emergency surgery. The diagnosis may be made with ultrasound or CT (Fig. 48–19).[45] In more elective settings, especially in women with chronic pelvic pain, laparoscopy may allow both diagnosis and treatment. Miklos et al. have identified and repaired sciatic hernias laparoscopically in 20 of 1100 women with chronic pelvic pain over a 46-month period.[46]

Treatment

Definitive surgery should be performed soon after the diagnosis of a sciatic hernia has been made. There are two standard approaches: transabdominal and transgluteal. A transabdominal approach is mandatory in the presence of intestinal obstruction or evidence of strangulation. The transabdominal approach allows for easier identification of the important neurovascular structures that lie next to the hernia sac. When the diagnosis is certain and the hernia sac is reducible, a transgluteal approach may be used. Miklos et al. suggested that women with a history of chronic pelvic pain of more than 6 months' duration should be considered for diagnostic laparoscopy and, if a sciatic hernia is diagnosed, laparoscopic repair should be performed.[46] In 20 patients who

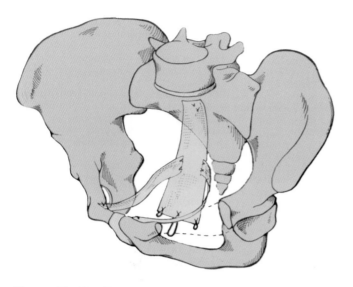

Figure 48–17. Total pelvic mesh repair as described by Sullivan et al. Mesh supports are used centrally from the upper part of the sacrum to the perineal body, and then two additional strips are tunneled laterally to support the vagina, bladder, and urethra. (From Sullivan ES, Longaker CJ, Lee PY: Total pelvic mesh repair: A ten-year experience. Dis Colon Rectum 44:857, 2001.)

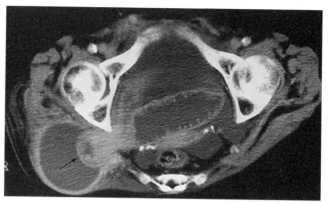

Figure 48–19. Computed tomographic scan showing incarcerated bowel *(arrow)* through the right sacral foramen and surrounding ascites in the right subgluteal region. (From Yu PC, Ko SF, Lee TY, et al: Small bowel obstruction due to incarcerated sciatic hernia: Ultrasound diagnosis. Br J Radiol 75:381, 2002.)

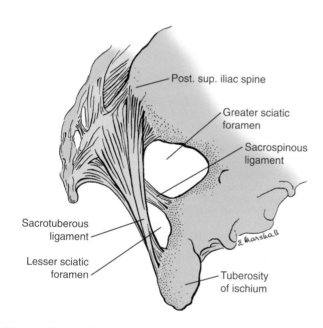

Figure 48–18. Posterolateral view of the pelvis showing the greater and lesser sciatic foramina and their ligamentous and osseous boundaries. (From Watson LF: Hernia, 3rd ed. St Louis, CV Mosby, 1948.)

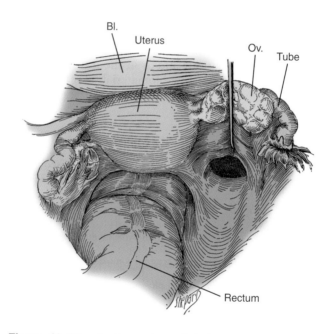

Figure 48–20. Anatomy of a sciatic hernia. In women, the sciatic opening is found behind the broad ligament. (From Watson LF: Hernia, 3rd ed. St Louis, CV Mosby, 1948.)

were found to have a sciatic hernia, the hernia was reduced laparoscopically, the peritoneum overlying the sciatic hernia was opened, and a polypropylene mesh plug was placed within the space created by the atrophic piriformis muscle. A second piece of mesh was secured as an onlay patch and the overlying peritoneum closed. All 20 women treated in this fashion were reported to

have total relief or improvement of chronic pelvic pain at a median follow-up of 13 months (range, 3 to 36 months).

In an open transabdominal sciatic hernia repair, the patient is placed in the Trendelenburg position, and a lower midline incision is made. The abdomen is explored and the viscera inspected for evidence of incarceration or strangulation. In women, the internal opening of a sciatic hernia is posterior to the broad ligament and above the uterosacral ligament (Fig. 48–20). In men, the location of the internal opening is similar to that in women, in the lateral aspect of the pelvis between the bladder and rectum. If a ring is constricting the hernia sac and thus precludes easy reduction, the ring can be manually dilated or sharply incised. With a suprapiriformis hernia, the most common type of sciatic hernia, the sac is usually lateral to the vessels. Therefore, the sac should be separated and excised in a posterior, lateral, and inferior direction. In the less common infrapiriformis sciatic hernia, the sac lies medial to the vessels and nerves and should therefore be separated and incised in a medial and superior direction.

For small hernia defects, repair may be performed by primary closure of the fascia of the piriformis muscle to the periosteum of the iliac bone. If the defect is larger or if the fascia of the piriformis muscle is weak, the hernia sac can be folded on itself and sutured to the piriformis muscle and the periosteum of the iliac bone. Greater durability can be achieved with the use of a synthetic mesh or biologic graft to close the defect.

In the transgluteal approach, the patient is placed in the prone position. This approach is best reserved for palpable masses and allows the surgeon to make an incision across the mass starting from the greater trochanter. The hernia sac is dissected free, opened, and inspected for any sign of strangulation. Once reduced, the hernia defect is closed by approximating the fascia of the piriformis muscle to the fascia of the gluteus maximus and medius. Alternatively and as in the transabdominal approach, synthetic mesh or biomaterials may be used to close the defect.

REFERENCES

1. DeMeester SL, Magnuson TH: Lumbar and pelvic hernias. In Zuidema GD, Yeo CJ (eds): Surgery of the Alimentary Tract, 5th ed. Philadelphia, 2002, p 165.
2. Campanelli G, Nicolosi FM, Pettinari D, Contessini Avesani F: Prosthetic repair, intestinal resection, and potentially contaminated areas: Safe and feasible? Hernia 8:190, 2004.
3. Stringer RA, Salmek JR: Mesh herniorrhaphy during elective colorectal surgery. Hernia 9:26, 2005.
4. Grynfeltt J: Quelques mots sur la hernie lombaire. Montpellier Med 16:323, 1866.
5. de Garengeot RJC: Mimoire sur plusieurs hernies singulieres. Mem Acad R Chir Paris 1:699, 1743.
6. Watson LF: Hernia, 3rd ed. St Louis, CV Mosby, 1948.
7. Goodman EH, Speese J: Lumbar hernia. Ann Surg 63:548, 1916.
8. Lesshaft P: Lumbalgegren in Anatomisch. Chirurgischer Himsicht Anat Physiol Wissensch Med 264, 1870.
9. Swartz WT: Lumbar hernia. In Nyhus LM, Condon RE (eds): Hernia. Philadelphia, JB Lippincott, 1978, p 409.
10. Patten LC, Awad SS, Berger DH, et al: A novel technique for the repair of lumbar hernias after iliac crest bone harvest. Am J Surg 188:85, 2004.
11. Burt BM, Afifi HY, Wantz GE, et al: Traumatic lumbar hernia: Report of cases and comprehensive review of the literature. J Trauma 57:1361, 2004.
12. Dowd CN: Congenital lumbar hernia at the triangle of Petit. Ann Surg 45:245, 1907.
13. Ravdin IS: Lumbar hernia through Grynfeltt and Lesshaft's triangle. Surg Clin North Am 3:267, 1923.
14. Burick AJ, Parascandola SA: Laparoscopic repair of a traumatic lumbar hernia: A case report. J Laparoendosc Surg 6:259, 1996.
15. Arca MJ, Heniford BT, Pokorny R, et al: Laparoscopic repair of lumbar hernias. J Am Coll Surg 187:147, 1998.
16. Moreno-Egea A, Torralba-Martinez JA, Morales G, et al: Open vs laparoscopic repair of secondary lumbar hernias: A prospective nonrandomized study. Surg Endosc 19:184, 2005.
17. Bjork KJ, Mucha P Jr, Cahill DR: Obturator hernia. Surg Obstet Gynecol 167:217, 1988.
18. Skandalakis LJ, Androulakis J, Colborn GL, et al: Obturator hernia. Embryology, anatomy, and surgical applications. Surg Clin North Am 80:71, 2000.
19. Chang SS, Shan YS, Lin YJ, et al: A review of obturator hernia and a proposed algorithm for its diagnosis and treatment. World J Surg 29:450, 2005.
20. Sentovich SM, Rivela LJ, Thorson AG, et al: Simultaneous dynamic proctography and peritoneography for pelvic floor disorders. Dis Colon Rectum 38:912, 1995.
21. Yokoyama T, Mulnakata Y, Ogiwara M, et al: Preoperative diagnosis of strangulated obturator hernia using ultrasonography. Am J Surg 174:76, 1997.
22. Yokoyama Y, Yamaguchi A, Isogai M, et al: Thirty-six cases of obturator hernia: Does CT contribute to the postoperative outcome? World J Surg 23:214, 1999.
23. Nishina M, Fujii C, Ogino R, et al: Preoperative diagnosis of obturator hernia by computed tomography in six patients. J Emerg Med 20:277, 2001.
24. Kammori M, Mafune K, Hirashima T, et al: Forty-three cases of obturator hernia. Am J Surg 187:549, 2004.
25. Schmidt PH, Bull WJ, Jeffery KM, et al: Typical versus atypical presentation of obturator hernia. Am Surg 67:191, 2001.
26. Jones RL, Wingate JP: Pictorial review: Herniography in the investigation of groin pain in adults. Clin Radiol 53:805, 1998.
27. Stoppa RE, Warlaumont CR: The preperitoneal approach to prosthetic repair of a groin hernia. In Nyhus LM, Condon RE (eds): Hernia, 3rd ed. Philadelphia, JB Lippincott, 1989, p 199.
28. Shapiro K, Patel S, Choy C, et al: Totally extraperitoneal repair of obturator hernia. Surg Endosc 18:954, 2004.
29. Beck D, Fazio VW, Jagelman DG, et al: Postoperative perineal hernia. Dis Colon Rectum 30:21, 1987.
30. Bok-yan SJ, Palmer MT, Shellito PC: Postoperative perineal hernia. Dis Colon Rectum 40:954, 1997.
31. Olsen AL, Smith VJ, Bergstrom JO, et al: Epidemiology of the surgical management of pelvic organ prolapse and urinary incontinence. Obstet Gynecol 89:501, 1997.
32. Wall LL: The muscles of the pelvic floor. Clin Obstet Gynecol 36:910, 1993.
33. DeLancey JOL: The anatomy of the pelvic floor. Curr Opin Obstet Gynecol 6:313, 1994.
34. Kelvin FM, Maglinte DD, Hale DS, et al: Female pelvic organ prolapse. A comparison of triphasic dynamic MR imaging and triphasic fluoroscopic cystocolpoproctography. AJR Am J Roentgenol 174:81, 2000.
35. Kaufman HS, Buller JL, Thompson JR, et al: Dynamic pelvic MR imaging and cystocolpoproctography alter surgical management of pelvic floor disorders. Dis Colon Rectum 44:1575, 2001.
36. Gearhart SL, Pannu HK, Cundiff GW, et al: Perineal descent and levator ani hernia: A dynamic magnetic resonance imaging study. Dis Colon Rectum 47:1298, 2004.
37. Richardson AC: The rectovaginal septum revisited: Its relationship to rectocele and its importance in rectocele repair. Clin Obstet Gynecol 36:976, 1993.
38. Kahn MA, Stanton SL: Posterior colporrhaphy: Its effects on bowel and sexual function. Br J Obstet Gynaecol 104:82, 1997.
39. Roman H, Michot F: Long-term outcomes of transanal rectocele repair. Dis Colon Rectum 48:510, 2005.
40. Maher C, Baessler K: Surgical management of posterior vaginal wall prolapse: An evidence-based literature review. Int Urogynecol J Pelvic Floor Dysfunct May 25, 2005 [Epub ahead of print].
41. Dell JR, O'Kelley KR: PelviSoft BioMesh augmentation of rectocele repair: The initial clinical experience in 35 patients. Int Urogynecol J 16:44, 2005.
42. Kohli N, Miklos JR: Dermal graft–augmented rectocele repair. Int Urogynecol J 14:146, 2003.
43. Link RE, Su LM, Bhayani SB, et al: Laparoscopic sacral colpoperineopexy for treatment of perineal body descent and vaginal vault prolapse. Urology 64:145, 2004.
44. Sullivan ES, Longaker CJ, Lee PY: Total pelvic mesh repair: A ten-year experience. Dis Colon Rectum 44:857, 2001.
45. Yu PC, Ko SF, Lee TY, et al: Small bowel obstruction due to incarcerated sciatic hernia: Ultrasound diagnosis. Br J Radiol 75:381, 2002.
46. Miklos JR, O'Reilly MJ, Saye WB: Sciatic hernia as a cause of chronic pelvic pain in women. Obstet Gynecol 91:998, 1998.

49

Hernias and Congenital Groin Problems in Infants and Children

Walter Pegoli, Jr.

Surgically significant problems involving the structures in the groin and scrotum are common in infants and children. The epicenter of this group of anomalies is geographically located in the area surrounding the ilioinguinal ligament. The problems most often encountered by general pediatric surgeons are inguinal hernia (direct and indirect), femoral hernia, and an undescended testis. An acute scrotum (most commonly the result of an incarcerated/strangulated inguinal hernia or testicular torsion), though rare, is a diagnostic challenge and requires real-time surgical decision making and intervention.

EMBRYOLOGY

The inguinal canal forms as the result of mesenchymal consolidation around the gubernaculum. The gubernaculum is then invaginated by an outpouching of peritoneum, the processus vaginalis.[1] At the start of the third trimester, the distal portion of the gubernaculum extends beyond the abdominal wall into the scrotum. The processus elongates proportionally within the gubernaculum to facilitate testicular descent.[2] Scrotal migration of the testicle begins during the seventh month of intrauterine life and is complete by 35 weeks' gestation. Persistent patency of the processus vaginalis is the principal factor required for the development of a hydrocele or indirect inguinal hernia. The difference between hernia and hydrocele is based on the size and content of the resultant sac. A hydrocele has a narrow sac neck and contains peritoneal fluid. Indirect inguinal hernias exhibit a wider neck and may contain intraperitoneal or retroperitoneal organs.

Normally, the processus vaginalis obliterates spontaneously from the internal ring to the testis. The distal end of the processus survives as the tunica vaginalis of the testis. Incomplete obliteration predisposes to the development of hydrocele or hernia. However, postnatal patency does not uniformly result in surgically significant disease. Postmortem studies in adults without clinical evidence of hernia have found patency of the processus vaginalis in 15% to 37% of groins examined.[3]

Any disruption in normal testicular descent can result in cryptorchidism. The location of the cryptorchid gonad is dependent on the timing of arrest along the natural path of testicular descent. Intra-abdominal testis are uncommon, being noted in only 5% to 10% of boys with undescended testes.[4] In most cases the testicle is located at the apex of the scrotum or slightly lateral to the external inguinal ring, within the superficial inguinal pouch. In such cases there is notable patency of the processus vaginalis 85% to 90% of the time.

A number of conditions have been identified as factors contributing to the development of indirect inguinal hernias. In infants with abdominal wall defects such as gastroschisis, omphalocele, and bladder exstrophy, congenital hernia or cryptorchidism, or both, may develop.[5] Patients with elevated peritoneal fluid volume as a consequence of ventriculoperitoneal shunting or peritoneal dialysis are at increased risk for the development of bilateral inguinal hernia.

INCIDENCE

The incidence of inguinal hernia in children ranges from 0.8% to 4.4% and is notably higher in infants.[6] It is highest during the first year of life, with a peak during the first months. The incidence is greatest in former premature infants, in whom it is reported to range from 16% to 25%.[7] Boys are affected six times more often than girls.[8] Right-sided hernias predominate. Rowe and Clatworthy reported that children manifest 60% of hernias on the right, 30% on the left, and 10% on both sides.[9]

The incidence of undescended testes in infants has been reported to be approximately 4%.[10] Spontaneous descent has been documented for the first 3 months after birth but rarely beyond that time. A British study reported an incidence of 1.58% at 1 year of age.[11] The frequency of undescended testes is significantly higher in premature infants. However, these testes have been noted to descend postnatally, and if monitored over time as a function of postconceptual age, the incidence decreases to nearly normal.[12]

CLINICAL FEATURES OF INGUINAL HERNIAS AND HYDROCELES

Most commonly, inguinal hernias are manifested as a bulge in the groin that may extend down into the scrotum with increased intra-abdominal pressure. Congenital inguinal hernias contain an abdominal or retroperitoneal organ, whereas hydroceles contain only fluid. In communicating hydroceles, the processus vaginalis is in continuity with the peritoneal cavity. Noncommunicating hydroceles are walled off from the peritoneal cavity and therefore do not change in size with crying or straining.

Examination of the groin should take place in the supine and, if possible, the erect position. Struggling infants naturally increase their intra-abdominal pressure, which may result in spontaneous protrusion of abdominal contents into the hernia sac. Older, more cooperative children can perform the Valsalva maneuver and produce the hernia.

Palpation of a thickened spermatic cord as it exits the external inguinal ring and crosses the pubic tubercle may be a useful clinical finding. Rolling of the spermatic cord beneath the examining finger may mimic the sensation of rubbing two pieces of silk together (silk glove sign). The silk glove sign is a useful diagnostic aid when a hernia is suspected but not clinically evident.[13]

Scrotal swelling that historically changes over time, is not associated with a mass in the groin, and slowly evacuates with compression is suggestive of a communicating hydrocele. Scrotal swelling that has been present since birth, is static, and does not evacuate with compression is most likely a noncommunicating hydrocele. A nontender scrotal mass that transilluminates brightly is probably a hydrocele. Noncommunicating hydroceles that are evident shortly after birth and bilateral have a high likelihood of spontaneous resolution.[14]

An incarcerated hernia contains viscera that cannot be returned to the abdominal cavity. When the contents of the sac cannot be reduced and are ischemic or gangrenous, the hernia is strangulated. Early on, the contents of an incarcerated hernia are compressed by the rigid confines of the internal ring. Initially, compression leads to impaired lymphatic and venous return. Over time, pressure within the sac increases and arterial inflow is interrupted. If the herniated material is intestine, progressive ischemia results in gangrene and perforation. Concomitant testicular ischemia can result from compression of the spermatic cord by the strangulated hernia.[15]

The reported incidence of incarceration ranges between 12% and 17% in patients younger than 10 years.[16,17] The greatest risk for incarceration is in infancy, with reports ranging from 24% to 31% in children younger than 6 months.[18,19] Rates of incarceration have been noted to be lower in premature infants. Krieger et al. reported a 17% rate of incarceration in 52 premature infants.[20] The authors speculate that the reduced incidence in premature infants is due to an internal ring that is proportionately larger than in their full-term counterparts.

Irritability and vomiting, which may be bilious in nature, are typical in infants with incarcerated hernias. On examination, a firm, well-defined mass is present in the groin, and it often extends into the scrotum. If the mass has been present for some time, there is often edema and erythema of the overlying skin. Tenderness to palpation progresses over time.

The mass may transilluminate, but not brightly. Radiographs of the abdomen may show air-filled bowel in the scrotum. In addition, radiographic findings consistent with partial or complete bowel obstruction may be apparent. In a nonacute scrotum, ultrasound evaluation of the mass may differentiate hernia from hydrocele.

The initial management of an incarcerated but not strangulated indirect inguinal hernia is nonoperative.[21] More than 80% of incarcerated hernias are reducible without surgery.[22] An attempt at manual reduction of an incarcerated hernia in a crying infant is not usually successful. In an agitated infant, sedation and analgesia are often required. Relaxation reduces intra-abdominal pressure and decreases the extrinsic compression of the neck of the sac by the internal inguinal ring. Placement of the infant in the Trendelenburg position plus observation in a warm, dark, quiet room often results in spontaneous reduction. In the absence of spontaneous reduction, manual reduction should be attempted. Simultaneous pressure at the base of the hernia sac and the external ring applied over a period of several minutes produces the best clinical result. Isolated compression of the base of the sac causes the contents of the sac to ride over the external ring and markedly reduces the likelihood of a successful reduction. After reduction, definitive surgical intervention should be delayed 24 to 48 hours to allow for resolution of edema in the structures surrounding the hernia sac. When the hernia cannot be reduced, immediate surgical intervention is indicated to prevent further ischemic damage.

OPERATIVE MANAGEMENT OF AN INDIRECT INGUINAL HERNIA

The principle objective of repair of an indirect inguinal hernia in infants and children is high ligation of the sac at the internal inguinal ring. In most cases, the procedure requires general anesthesia. In infants, endotracheal anesthesia is preferred to secure the airway. In older children, in whom the airway is less problematic, facial or laryngeal mask anesthesia is adequate.

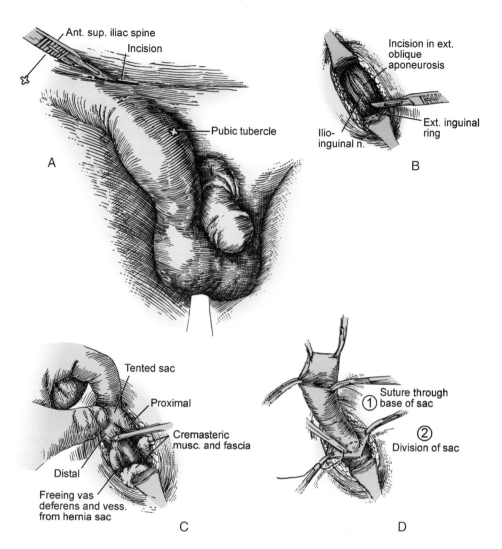

Figure 49–1. Indirect inguinal hernia repair. **A,** Skin incision in the groin crease. **B,** Incision in the external oblique aponeurosis. **C,** Dissection of the vas deferens and testicular vessels from the hernia sac. **D,** High ligation of the hernia sac. (From White JJ, Haller JA Jr: Groin hernia in infants and children. In Nyhus LM, Condon RE [eds]: Hernia, 2nd ed. Philadelphia, JB Lippincott, 1978, p 101.)

A transverse groin crease incision lateral to the pubic tubercle offers adequate exposure to the components of the inguinal canal (Fig. 49–1A). The length of the incision should be dictated by the size of the patient and the expected anatomic pathologic changes. In general, the incision should be long enough to provide adequate exposure to the spermatic cord and the totality of the inguinal canal. Scarpa's fascia is easily identified by gentile blunt separation of the subcutaneous fat. Visible vessels in the subcutaneum should be retracted aside, not transected, to prevent bleeding complications. Scarpa's fascia is then incised sharply to expose the external oblique aponeurosis. The external inguinal ring is identified just lateral to the pubic tubercle. The external oblique aponeurosis is then divided in the direction of its fibers to the external inguinal ring (see Fig. 49–1B). Care must be taken to not injure the underlying ilioinguinal nerve. In an infant, it may not be necessary to incise the external oblique aponeurosis to gain adequate access to the contents of the inguinal canal. In a newborn, the internal inguinal ring is almost directly subjacent to the external inguinal ring, thus allowing access to the cord structures at the level of the internal inguinal ring. With time, the inguinal canal elongates, and the inguinal rings become progressively farther apart.[23]

Dissection below the flaps of the incised external oblique aponeurosis exposes the spermatic cord. The spermatic cord is gently dissected free from the inguinal canal and elevated into the wound. The spermatic cord is stretched over fine forceps. Normally, the indirect inguinal hernia sac is found to lie anteromedial to the vas deferens and the testicular vessels.

Gentle separation of the cord structures from the hernia sac is accomplished by sweeping the vas deferens and testicular vessels laterally with nontoothed forceps (see Fig 49–1C).

The vas deferens should be carefully inspected. Failure to identify a vas deferens at surgery should prompt investigation for associated anomalies. The incidence of indirect inguinal hernia in patients with cystic fibrosis is reported to be 6% to 15%.[24] In cystic fibrosis, abnormalities range from atresia to complete absence of the vas deferens, and the anomalies are often bilateral. Absence of the vas deferens may be associated with ipsilateral renal agenesis and should prompt an investigation to rule out upper urinary tract abnormalities.

Once the distal sac is identified, it is elevated to expose the neck of the hernia sac. Traction on the sac aids in the dissection. With large sacs, hemisection aids in exposure. A short sac can be freed entirely to the internal ring.

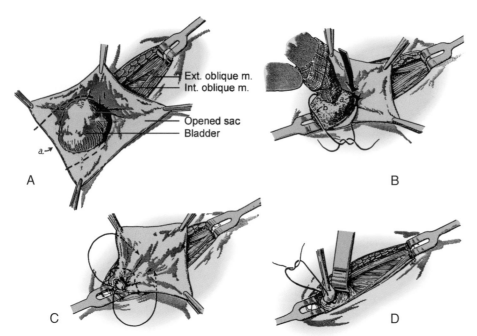

Figure 49–2. Sliding hernia repair. **A,** The bladder forms the medial wall of an open indirect inguinal hernia sac. **B,** Bladder turned down into the residual hernia sac. **C,** Purse-string suture of the sac at the internal ring. **D,** Invagination of the ligated residual sac. (From Golliday ES, White JJ: Hernias and congenital groin problems in infants and children. In Yeo CJ [ed]: Shackelford's Surgery of the Alimentary Tract, 5th ed. Philadelphia, Elsevier, 1996, p 196.)

The cord structures are dissected away to the level of the properitoneal fat. The sac is then inspected to confirm that it is empty. If the sac contains abdominal or retroperitoneal organs, reduction is accomplished by gentle compression of the base of the sac. When empty, the sac is twisted two to three times. This maneuver strengthens the sac to provide better purchase for transfixing sutures and narrows the internal inguinal ring. The sac is ligated high at the internal ring with one to two suture ligatures of absorbable material. Hernia sacs with large necks may require a purse-string suture technique to achieve satisfactory closure (see Fig. 49–1D).

Management of the distal segment of the hemisected hernia sac is controversial. Some pediatric surgeons cite the incidence of postsurgical scrotal hydrocele and recommend removal of the distal sac. Others are wary of increasing the risk of injury to the cord structures and the possibility of bleeding with the development of a scrotal hematoma. These surgeons recommend leaving the distal sac in situ.

After high ligation of the hernia sac the internal ring should be inspected. In infants with large indirect inguinal hernia sacs, the internal ring is often patulous and the floor of the inguinal canal attenuated. The internal ring may be plicated and the floor of the inguinal canal reconstructed by suturing the transversalis fascia to the shelving portion of the inguinal ligament. In infants, normal anatomy is best re-created by closing the floor over the spermatic cord. In children and adolescents, the floor is repaired under the spermatic cord.

The objective of surgical repair in girls is identical to that in boys: high ligation of the hernia sac. However, up to 20% of girls have a sliding component to the hernia sac.[25] On occasion, the fallopian tube, ovary, or uterus may make up a portion of the wall of the sac. The sac is routinely opened to evaluate for the presence of a sliding component. Empty sacs are ligated high. After high ligation, Bastionelli recommends securing the remaining sac to the undersurface of the conjoined tendon to maintain lateral uterine support.[26]

The surgical principles of sliding hernia repair are gender and organ neutral. Sliding hernias of the intestine, bladder, uterus, and fallopian tube are managed via similar surgical techniques (Fig. 49–2A). Redundant hernia sac is excised to the wall of the organ down to the level of the internal ring. The viscera and the remaining sac are invaginated through the internal ring (see Fig. 49–2B). At the level of the internal ring, the seromuscular segment of viscera and the inverted sac are secured with a purse-string suture (see Fig. 49–2C). The internal ring may be plicated to reinforce the repair (see Fig. 49–2D).[27]

At completion of the critical portion of the repair, gentle traction on the testis returns the testicle to the base of the scrotum and seats the spermatic cord within the inguinal canal. The external oblique aponeurosis and Scarpa's fascia are closed with several interrupted absorbable sutures. The skin is approximated with subcuticular absorbable suture and reinforced with adhesive strips or collodion.

Before closure of the superficial layers of the wound, administration of local anesthesia is highly recommended to aid in postoperative pain management. Local infiltration and ilioinguinal nerve blocks with 0.25% bupivacaine (maximum recommended dose of 1 ml/kg or 2 mg/kg) has been shown to significantly reduce postoperative pain after inguinal hernia repair.[28] Oral acetaminophen or nonsteroidal anti-inflammatory agents are excellent analgesics during the first few days of convalescence. Older children are encouraged to return to school after 2 or 3 days and may return to full, unrestricted activity in 3 to 4 weeks.

CONTRALATERAL INGUINAL EXPLORATION

The advantage of contralateral inguinal exploration is the diagnosis and repair of a patent processus vaginalis or indirect inguinal hernia that was not discernible at the time of physical examination. In the event of a patent processus vaginalis, it prevents the development of a future indirect inguinal hernia and the need for an additional general anesthetic for repair.

The major surgical risk involved in contralateral inguinal exploration is injury to the vas deferens or the testicular blood supply. The risk of proven injury to the vas deferens, based on finding a segment of the vas in the surgical specimen, has been reported to be 1.6%.[29] The risk of testicular atrophy after routine inguinal hernia repair, assumed to be the result of injury to the testicular vessels, is approximately 1%.[30] With an incarcerated inguinal hernia, the blood supply to the testis may be compromised by extrinsic compression at the internal inguinal ring. The incidence of testicular atrophy with incarceration ranges from 2.6% to 5%.[31,32]

In a review of published data, Rowe et al. concluded that in infants with a unilateral inguinal hernia, the processus vaginalis obliterates within the first 2 years of life in 40% of patients. Of note, a surgically significant contralateral indirect inguinal hernia eventually developed in half of these children. The remaining 20% were found to have a patent processus vaginalis that was clinically silent.[33] These data suggest that contralateral exploration will be negative in two of five infants and three of five children.

In a recent review of practicing pediatric surgeons, 40% limited contralateral exploration to infants younger than 1 year and 39% to children younger than 2 years.[34] Female gender was thought to increase the incidence of bilateral indirect inguinal hernias. However, the incidence of a positive contralateral exploration has been shown to be no different from that in boys.[35]

The risk of contralateral hernia developing after unilateral herniorrhaphy is low, and data suggest that the contralateral hernia rate is no higher than that of the general childhood population.[36] A growing number of practicing surgeons do not recommend routine contralateral exploration. However, there are exceptional circumstances that warrant contralateral exploration. Children who are at high anesthetic risk, such as those with cystic fibrosis, are candidates for contralateral exploration. In addition, children with conditions known to increase intra-abdominal pressure (ascites, ventriculoperitoneal shunts, peritoneal dialysis) should undergo contralateral exploration.

OPERATIVE MANAGEMENT OF UNDESCENDED TESTIS

Treatment of an undescended testis is based on the assumption that the best environment for testicular function is the base of the scrotum. Studies suggest that elevated temperature can result in testicular degeneration. The scrotal testis is 4° C cooler than core temperature, and this cooler temperature has been shown to be an essential requirement for normal testicular development.[37] Degeneration, which has been demonstrated at the electron microscopic level in the second year of life, has been shown to progress to gross atrophy in school-aged children.[38] As a result of the growing body of evidence that testicular degeneration begins in infancy, the recommended age for orchidopexy has decreased. Presently, the recommended age for orchiopexy ranges from 6 to 24 months.[39]

For an inguinal undescended testis, the initial steps in the operation mirror those of indirect inguinal hernia repair. An ipsilateral groin crease incision is made and carried down to the external oblique aponeurosis. The external ring is identified, and then the external oblique aponeurosis is divided to the level of the external ring to expose the inguinal canal and its contents.

A widely patent processus vaginalis, or an indirect inguinal hernia, has been reported in more than 70% of patients with canalicular undescended testes.[40] As described previously, the hernia sac most often lies anteromedial to the vas deferens and the testicular vessels (Fig. 49–3A). In a high undescended testis, the sac may contain the testicle, and the cord structures are intimately associated with the wall of the sac. The method of sac separation is similar to that used during indirect inguinal hernia repair. Separation of the critical cord structures from the sac proceeds to the level of the internal inguinal ring. At the internal inguinal ring the cord structures diverge from the vas deferens, with the cord structures coursing medially and the testicular vessels laterally. At this level, the sac is ligated and divided.

The most common impediment to reaching the scrotum is insufficient length of the testicular vessels. In most cases adequate length may be obtained by blunt dissection of the testicular vessels from the fibrous bands that fix the vessels within the retroperitoneum. If necessary, the dissection can be extended up the retroperitoneum to the inferior pole of the kidney. If an additional 1 to 2 cm of length is required, the cord can be translocated medially (see Fig. 49–3B). This maneuver requires ligation and division of the inferior epigastric vessels, along with incision of the transversalis fascia, which forms the posterior wall of the inguinal canal. The vas deferens is usually of sufficient length and reaches the scrotum without any special manipulation.

If after thorough dissection the testis cannot be made to reach the scrotum, a staged procedure should be performed. The testis is sutured to the pubis or the lowest portion of the scrotum that can be reached without undo tension. The second stage is performed 6 to 12 months later. Successful scrotal positioning via the two-stage procedure can be expected in 70% to 90% of children.[41]

When adequate length has been achieved, the testicle should be fixed in the scrotum. The most common technique anchors the testicle to the dartos fascia in a pouch located just below the scrotal skin.[42] A transverse skin incision is made at the base of the scrotum, and a subcutaneous pouch is developed between the skin and dartos fascia (see Fig. 49–3C). Once the pouch is large enough to accommodate the testicle, a small incision is made in the dartos fascia. A clamp is then passed

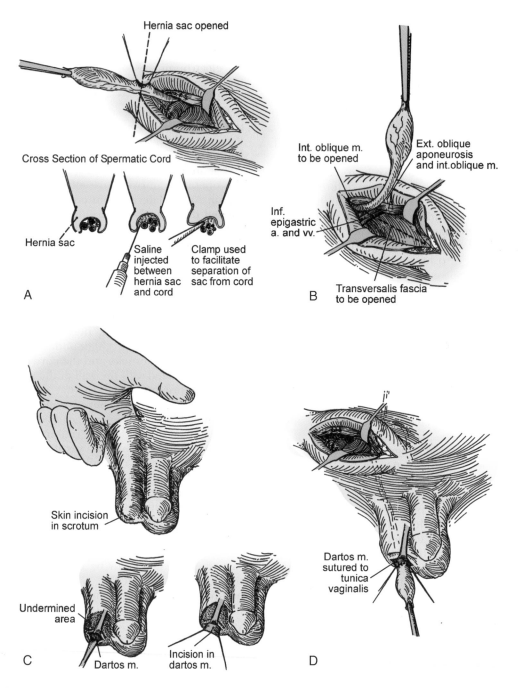

Figure 49–3. Dartos pouch orchidopexy. **A,** Hernia sac dissected free from the vas deferens and testicular vessels. **B,** Incision of the transversalis fascia to improve cord length. **C,** Tunnel to the scrotum created with the index finger and creation of the dartos pouch. **D,** Testicle brought through the defect created in the dartos fascia. The dartos fascia is sutured to the tunica to secure the testicle within the scrotum. (From Fonkalsrud EW: The undescended testis. In Ravitch MM, Benson CD, Mustard WT, et al [eds]: Current Problems in Surgery. Year Book, Chicago, 1978.)

retrograde from the scrotum into the inguinal canal, and the testicle is grasped and pulled into the scrotum. Care must be taken to avoid twisting the cord structures during this portion of the procedure. The testicle is secured in the scrotum by suturing the dartos fascia to the tunica albuginea with fine absorbable sutures (see Fig. 49–3D). The inguinal and scrotal incisions are closed in routine fashion.

Approximately 10% of undescended testes are not palpable.[43] An impalpable testicle may reside within the abdomen or may be absent. Intrauterine torsion of the spermatic cord can lead to testicular atrophy, or the "vanishing testis."[44] In such cases, the remaining testicle is grossly hypertrophic, which is a helpful physical sign and can be of use in determining the cause of the contralateral empty scrotum.[45]

Laparoscopy is a useful adjunct in the evaluation of an impalpable testis. The technique is highly effective in confirming the presence and location of the testicle. In addition, minimally invasive surgery can be used to remove or manipulate an abdominal or canalicular testis into the scrotum.

A laparoscope is inserted into the abdomen, and the anatomy on the side of the descended testicle is inspected to provide a reference. The testicular vessels and the vas deferens should converge at the internal ring. Normally, the internal ring should be closed and the peritoneum well coapted. On inspection of the involved side, if the testicular vessels and vas deferens end abruptly at the internal inguinal ring, the diagnosis of vanishing testis is made and the procedure terminated. In approximately 3% to 5% of children, a normal-appearing vas deferens and testicular vessels traverse the internal ring and a testis is probably present within the inguinal canal.[46] This finding mandates open inguinal exploration. In approximately half of these cases, the testicle is atrophic and should be removed because of the associated increase risk for malignancy. If the testicle is normal, orchidopexy should be performed.

An abdominal testicle visualized at laparoscopy may be approached via minimally invasive or open maneuvers. The Fowler-Stevens procedure offers the best opportunity to position a viable gonad in the scrotum.[47] The procedure requires the presence of a long, looping vas deferens to be successful. The testicular vessels are ligated and divided in the abdomen. The testicle is then brought down on the vas deferens supplied by collateral circulation derived from the inferior epigastric vessels and the gubernaculum.

The Fowler-Stevens operation is most often a two-stage procedure. In the first stage, the testicular vessels are ligated or clipped. Six months later, the testis is mobilized, with care taken to not disturb the collateral blood supply, through the inguinal canal into the scrotum. In long-term follow-up of the two-stage procedure, a 70% to 90% success rate has been reported.[48]

TORSION OF THE TESTIS

Twisting or torsion of the testis can produce occlusion of testicular blood flow and result in gonadal necrosis. The time frame for ischemic injury is variable. Loss of spermatogenesis occurs after 6 hours of torsion, loss of Leydig cells within 10 hours, and necrosis in as little as 2 hours, but mostly after 24 hours of ischemia.[49]

The most common form of torsion is intravaginal, and intravaginal torsion is predisposed by a high investment of the spermatic cord by the tunica vaginalis. The testis is pendulous and tends to lie horizontally within the scrotum. This position exposes the testicle to environmental conditions that can lead to twisting.

Extravaginal torsion is less common and confined to the newborn period. During testicular descent, the testis is loosely adherent to the surrounding structures. Inadequate fixation can allow the entire testis and spermatic cord to twist.

The incidence of testicular torsion is highest in infancy and adolescence. The peak incidence occurs in boys 13 to 16 years old. Patients complain of a sudden onset of pain in the scrotum, groin, or lower part of the abdomen. The pain may be associated with nausea or vomiting. On examination, the testis often lies horizontally within the scrotum and is extremely tender to palpation. The scrotum rapidly becomes edematous and erythematous. Over time the testis infarcts and the scrotum takes on a bluish discoloration.

Several clinical conditions can mimic the scrotal findings seen in testicular torsion. A child with torsion of the appendix testis has testicular pain that is of sudden onset. This condition occurs in younger adolescent boys, with a peak at age 11.[50] A blue dot may be seen at the upper pole of the testis. Palpation of this area results in severe pain, whereas the testicle itself is not tender.

Infectious conditions of the testis can produce significant inflammatory changes within the scrotum. Mumps virus has a predilection for the postpubertal testis. Epididymitis is usually the result of retrograde infection via the vas deferens in children with an *Escherichia coli* urinary tract infection. Children with underlying urinary tract anomalies or those who require intermittent catheterization are at increased risk.

Early diagnosis is the cornerstone of successful management of testicular torsion. Progressive ischemia mandates urgent clinical decision making. Doppler ultrasound and radioisotope scans have been used to determine whether there is blood flow to the testis in the acute scrotum.[51] In a small prepubescent testis, the volume of the gonad decreases accuracy and limits clinical utility. In older adolescents, a radioisotope scan can help differentiate between torsion and epididymo-orchitis. Blood flow is increased in infectious conditions, whereas it is markedly reduced in testicular torsion. Because of the time constraints imposed by progressive testicular ischemia, diagnostic delay and clinical indecision should not inhibit prompt surgical intervention.

Operative Management of Testicular Torsion

Treatment of testicular torsion is immediate scrotal exploration with a midline incision overlying the scrotal septum. The involved hemiscrotum is entered and the testicle is inspected. If the testis is twisted, it is untwisted and viability assessed. This maneuver usually results in the return of blood flow to the testis within several minutes. In some cases the testis appears congested or hemorrhagic, and it may be difficult to determine viability. A Doppler flow probe can prove helpful in determining the presence of testicular blood flow.

A viable testis should be fixed within the scrotum. The testis should be sutured to the septum with several nonabsorbable sutures. However, management of a testis of questionable viability remains a controversial issue. It has been shown that ischemia damages the blood-testis barrier and can expose the child to autoimmunization against his own sperm.[52] This risk is low in children younger than 10 years because there is no blood-testis barrier and spermatogenesis is dormant.[53] Thus, the current recommendation is to preserve a compromised testis in children younger than 10 years and proceed with orchiectomy in older children. The contralateral scrotum should be explored because the defect in fixation is usually bilateral. Regardless of the clinical findings, the contralateral testis is also fixed within the scrotum to prevent future torsion.

FEMORAL HERNIA

Femoral hernias are rare in children. They are often clinically misdiagnosed as direct inguinal hernias or as recurrent indirect inguinal hernias. In a large review of patients with groin hernias, femoral hernias were found in only 0.2% of the patient population, with a girl-to-boy ratio of approximately 2:1.[54] The symptoms and signs associated with femoral hernias are nonspecific and may mimic those of inguinal hernia. The initial surgical exposure is also the same. A low inguinal crease incision is made and carried down to the inguinal ligament. In femoral hernias, a mass is identified in the femoral canal. The mass is reduced and the canal obliterated. The Cooper ligament repair closes the canal by suturing the inguinal ligament to the pectineal ligament and pectineal fascia. An alternative repair involves the use of a plug of prosthetic material sutured to the surrounding fascia to obliterate the orifice of the femoral canal.

SUGGESTED READINGS

Benson CD, Lofti MW: The pouch technique in the surgical correction of cryptorchidism in infants and children. Surgery 62:967, 1967.

Grosfeld JL: Current concepts in inguinal hernia in infants and children. World J Surg 13:506, 1989.

Fonkalsrud EW, Mengal W: The Undescended Testis. Chicago, Year Book, 1981.

Fowler R, Stephens FD: The role of testicular vascular anatomy in the salvaged high undescended testis. Aust N Z J Surg 29:92, 1959.

Rowe MI, Clatworthy HW: Incarcerated and strangulated hernias in children. Arch Surg 101:136, 1970.

REFERENCES

1. Backhouse KM: Embryology of testicular descent and maldescent. Urol Clin North Am 9:315, 1982.
2. Heyns CF: The gubernaculum during testicular descent in the human fetus. J Anat 153:93, 1987.
3. Morgan EH, Anson BJ: Anatomy of region of inguinal hernia IV. The internal surface of the parietal layers. Q Bull Northwestern Univ Med School 16:20, 1942.
4. Bloom DA: Symposium: What is the best approach to the non-palpable testis? Contemp Urol 4:39, 1992.
5. Kaplan LM, Koyle MA, Kaplan GW, et al: Association between abdominal wall defects and cryptorchidism. J Urol 136:645, 1986.
6. Bronsther B, Abrams MW, Elbolm C: Inguinal hernias in children—a study of 1,000 cases and a review of the literature. J Am Med Womens Assoc 27:524, 1972.
7. Rajput A, Gawderer MWL, Hack M: Inguinal hernia in very low birth weight infants: Incidence and timing of repair. J Pediatr Surg 27:1322, 1992.
8. Peevy KJ, Speed FA, Hoff JC: Epidemiology of inguinal hernia in preterm neonates. Pediatrics 7:246, 1986.
9. Rowe MI, Clatworthy HW: The other side of the pediatric inguinal hernia. Surg Clin North Am 51:1371, 1971.
10. Scorer CG: The descent of the testis. Arch Dis Child 39:605, 1964.
11. John Radcliffe Hospital Cryptorchidism Study Group: Cryptorchidism: An apparent substantial increase since 1960. BMJ 293:1401, 1986.
12. Fonkalsrud EW, Mengel W: The Undescended Testis. Chicago, Year Book, 1981.
13. Gilbert M, Clatworthy HW: Bilateral operations for inguinal hernia and hydrocele in infancy and childhood. Am J Surg 97:255, 1959.
14. Rowe MI, Marchildon MB: Inguinal hernia and hydrocele in infants and children. Surg Clin North Am 61:2237, 1981.
15. Walc L, Bass J, Rubin S, Walton M: Testicular fate after incarcerated hernia repair and/or orchidopexy performed in patients under 6 months of age. J Pediatr Surg 30:1195, 1995.
16. Rowe MI, Clatworthy HW: Incarcerated and strangulated hernias in children. Arch Surg 101:136, 1970.
17. Stephens BJ, Rice WT, Koucky CJ, Gruenberg JC: Optimal timing of elective indirect inguinal hernia repair in healthy children: Clinical considerations for improved outcome. World J Surg 16:952, 1992.
18. Rescorla FJ, Grosfeld JL: Inguinal hernia repair in the perinatal period and early infancy: Clinical considerations. J Pediatr Surg 19:832, 1984.
19. Misra D, Hewitt G, Potts SR, et al: Inguinal herniotomy in young infants with emphasis on premature neonates. J Pediatr Surg 29:1496, 1994.
20. Krieger NR, Shochat SJ, McGowan V, Hartman GE: Early hernia repair in the premature infant: Long-term follow-up. J Pediatr Surg 29:978, 1994.
21. Grosfeld JL: Current concepts in inguinal hernia in infants and children. World J Surg 13:506, 1989.
22. Davies N, Najmaldin A, Burge DM: Irreducible inguinal hernia in children below two years of age. Br J Surg 77:1291, 1990.
23. Duckett JW: Treatment of congenital inguinal hernia. Ann Surg 135:879, 1952.
24. Holsclaw DS: Incarcerated incidence of inguinal hernia, hydrocele and undescended testis in males with cystic fibrosis. Pediatrics 48:442, 1971.
25. Goldstein IR, Potts WJ: Inguinal hernia in female infants and children. Ann Surg 148:819, 1958.
26. Wright JE: Direct inguinal hernia in infancy and childhood. Pediatr Surg Int 9:161, 1994.
27. Shaw A, Santulli TV: Management of sliding hernias of the urinary bladder in infants. Surg Gynecol Obstet 124:1314, 1967.
28. Broadman LM, Belman AB, Hannallah RS, et al: Comparison of caudal and ilioinguinal/iliohypogastric nerve blocks for control of post-orchiopexy pain in pediatric ambulatory surgery. Anesthesiology 66:832, 1987.
29. Sparkman RS: Bilateral exploration in inguinal hernia in juvenile patients. Surgery 51:393, 1962.
30. Fahlstrom C, Holmberg L, Johansson H: Atrophy of the testis following operations upon the inguinal region on infants and children. Acta Chir Scand 126:221, 1963.
31. Murdoch RWG: Testicular strangulation from incarcerated inguinal hernia in infants. J R Coll Surg Edinb 24:95, 1979.
32. Palmer BV: Incarcerated inguinal hernia in children. Ann R Coll Surg Engl 60:121, 1978.
33. Rowe MI, Copelson LW, Clatworthy HW: The patient processus vaginalis and the inguinal hernia. J Pediatr Surg 4:102, 1969.
34. Wiener ES, Touloukian RJ, Rogers BM, et al: AAP Section on Surgery Hernia Survey Proceedings of the 47th Annual Meeting of the American Academy of Pediatrics, October 1995, San Francisco.
35. Given JP, Rubin SZ: Occurrence of contralateral inguinal hernia following unilateral repair in a pediatric hospital. J Pediatr Surg 24:963, 1989.
36. Surana R, Puri P: Is contralateral exploration necessary in infants with unilateral inguinal hernia? J Pediatr Surg 28:1026, 1993.
37. Mieusset R, Fouda PJ, Vaysse P, et al: Increase in testicular temperature in case of cryptorchidism in boys. Fertil Steril 59:1319, 1993.
38. Kogan SJ: Testis and andrology. Curr Opin Urol 2:409, 1992.
39. Hutson JM: Orchiopexy. In Spitz L, Coran AG (eds): Pediatric Surgery, Rob & Smith's Operative Surgery, 5th ed. London, Chapman & Hall, 1995.

40. White JJ, Shaker IJ, Oh KS et al: Herniography: A diagnostic refinement in the management of cryptorchidism. Am Surg 39:624, 1973.

41. Hazebrook FWJ, Molenaar JC: The management of the impalpable testis by surgery alone. J Urol 148:629, 1992.

42. Benson CD, Lofti MW: The pouch technique in the surgical correction of cryptorchidism in infants and children. Surgery 62:967, 1967.

43. Canavese F, Lalla R, Linari A, et al: Surgical treatment of cryptorchidism. Eur J Pediatr 152(Suppl 2):S43, 1993.

44. Diamond DA, Caldamone AA, Elder JS: Prevalence of the vanishing testis in boys with a unilateral impalpable testis: Is the side of presentation significant? J Urol 152:502, 1994.

45. Huff DS, Snyder HM, Hadzilelimoovic F: An absent testis is associated with contralateral testicular hypertrophy. J Urol 148:627, 1992.

46. Bloom DA, Semm K: Advances in genitourinary laparoscopy. Adv Urol 4:167, 1991.

47. Fowler R, Stephens FD: The role of testicular vascular anatomy in the salvaged high undescended testes. Aust N Z J Surg 29:92, 1959.

48. Elder JS: Two-stage Fowler-Stephens orchiopexy in the management of intra-abdominal testes. J Urol 148:1239, 1992.

49. Kaplan GW, King CR: Acute scrotal swelling in children. J Urol 104:219, 1970.

50. Skuglund RW, McRoberts JN, Ragde H: Torsion of testicular appendages: Presentation of 43 new cases and a collective review. J Urol 104:598, 1970.

51. Morgagni GB: Torsion of the testis and its appendages during childhood. Arch Dis Child 37:214, 1982.

52. Puri P, Barton D, O'Donnell B: Prepubertal testicular torsion: Subsequent fertility. Pediatr Surg 20:598, 1985.

53. Urry RL, Carrell DT, Starr NT, et al: The incidence of antisperm antibodies in infertility patients with a history of cryptorchidism. J Urol 151:381, 1994.

54. Fonkalsrud EW, deLorimier A, Clatworthy HW Jr: Femoral and direct inguinal hernias in infants and children. JAMA 192:101, 1965.

Stomach and
Small Intestine

Daniel T. Dempsey

50

Anatomy and Physiology of the Stomach

David W. Mercer • James W. Suliburk

ANATOMY

Divisions

The stomach originates as a dilatation in the tubular embryonic foregut during the fifth week of gestation. By the seventh week, it assumes its normal anatomic shape and position by descent, rotation, and further dilatation, along with disproportionate elongation of the greater curvature. After birth, the stomach is easily recognizable as the pear-shaped, most proximal abdominal organ of the alimentary tract. The stomach is divided into four anatomic regions, and although these divisions are useful to the surgeon when describing anatomic resections, they do not necessarily denote histologic or physiologic division of the organ (Fig. 50–1). The region of the stomach that attaches to the esophagus is called the cardia. Proximal to the cardia is the physiologically competent lower esophageal sphincter. The pylorus connects the distal stomach (antrum) to the proximal duodenum. Although the stomach is fixed at the gastroesophageal junction (GEJ) and the pylorus, the large midportion is mobile. The superior-most part of the stomach is the floppy, distensible fundus. It is bounded superiorly by the diaphragm and laterally by the spleen. The largest portion of the stomach is the body (corpus). The body contains the bulk of the gastric parietal cells and is bounded on the right by the relatively straight lesser curvature and on the left by the longer greater curvature. At the angularis incisura, the lesser curvature abruptly angles to the right. This point marks the end of the body and the beginning of the antrum, which extends to the pylorus. Another important anatomic angle (angle of His) is the one that the fundus forms with the left margin of the esophagus.

Anatomic Relationships

Most of the stomach is in the left upper quadrant of the abdomen (Fig. 50–2). The GEJ is normally about 2 to 3 cm below the diaphragmatic esophageal hiatus in the horizontal plane of the seventh chondrosternal articulation, a plane only slightly cephalad to that containing the pylorus. The left lateral segment of the liver usually covers a large portion of the stomach anteriorly. The remainder is bounded by the diaphragm, chest, and abdominal wall.

The relationship of the stomach to other intra-abdominal organs has important implications in disease. Adjacent organs include the pancreas and liver, which lie dorsal and ventral, as well as the spleen, which lies immediately to the left of the greater curvature. Inflammation of the pancreas may interfere with gastric emptying, whereas enlargement by neoplasm may cause an increased sensation of satiety or even obstruction of the gastric outlet. The transverse colon lies caudal and may interfere with function as a result of neoplastic invasion. The stomach itself may affect adjacent organs via perforation from peptic ulceration. Additionally, another closely related structure is the biliary tree, which runs posterior to the first portion of the duodenum, within centimeters of the gastric outlet, and can be injured during gastrectomy.

The stomach is anchored within the abdominal cavity to adjacent organs via a variety of flexible attachments known as ligaments. The gastrocolic ligament connects the greater curvature of the stomach and the transverse colon and runs along with the greater omentum, which hangs freely in the peritoneal cavity from the transverse colon. The lesser omentum is a double layer of peritoneum extending from the porta hepatis of the liver to the lesser curvature of the stomach and the first portion of the duodenum. The lesser omentum forms the anterior wall of the lesser sac and makes up the hepatogastric and hepatoduodenal ligaments; it contains the left and right gastric vessels, and its right free margin contains the hepatic artery, bile duct, and portal vein. The hepatogastric ligament attaches the stomach to the liver along the lesser curvature. The gastrosplenic ligament extends from the left portion of the greater curvature of the stomach to the hilum of the spleen and contains the short gastric vessels and the left gastroepiploic vessels. Finally, the gastrophrenic ligament runs from the upper portion of the greater curvature to the diaphragm.

Blood Supply

The stomach derives the bulk of its blood supply (Fig. 50–3) from the celiac axis through four arteries: the left and right gastric arteries running along and supplying the lesser curvature and the left and right gastroepiploic arteries running along and supplying the greater curvature. A substantial quantity of blood may be supplied to the proximal part of the stomach by the inferior phrenic

arteries and by the vasa brevia (short gastric arteries) from the spleen. The left gastric artery is the largest artery to the stomach. It originates from the celiac axis, generally courses cephalad and left, runs toward the gastric cardia, and gives off esophageal and hepatic branches before turning to the right and coursing along the lesser curvature of the stomach and the lesser omentum. It is also not uncommon (15% to 20%) for an aberrant left hepatic artery to originate from the left gastric artery. Occasionally, this vessel represents the only arterial flow to the left hepatic lobe. Proximal ligation of the left gastric artery, under these circumstances, could therefore result in acute left-sided hepatic ischemia. The right gastric artery arises from the hepatic artery but may occasionally come from the gastroduodenal artery. The right gastroepiploic artery provides blood supply to the wall of the greater curvature of the stomach, as well as the greater omentum, and originates from the gastro-duodenal artery behind the pyloric channel. It usually runs along the greater curvature of the stomach and terminates in an anastomosis with the left gastroepiploic artery, which originates from the splenic artery. The anastomotic connection between these major vessels ensures that in most cases the stomach will survive if three of four arteries are ligated, provided that the arcades along the lesser and greater curvatures are not disturbed, an important surgical consideration in patients undergoing gastric resection. Generally, the veins of the stomach parallel the arteries. The left gastric (coronary) and right gastric veins usually drain to the portal vein. The right gastroepiploic vein drains into the superior mesenteric vein (a useful anatomic landmark), whereas the left gastroepiploic vein drains into the splenic vein.

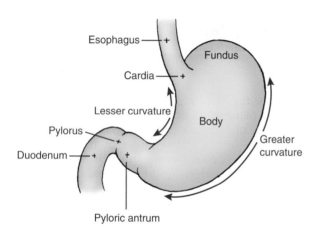

Figure 50–1.   Divisions of the stomach.

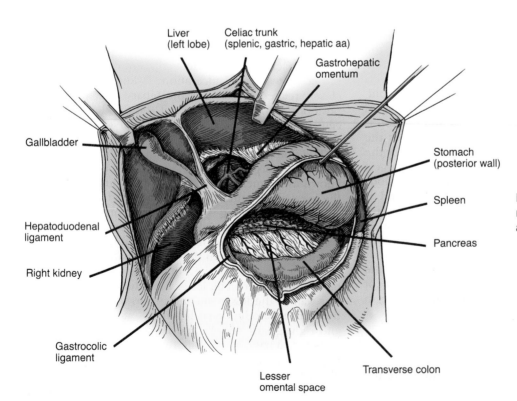

Figure 50–2.   The stomach in relation to some of the deeper, adjacent structures.

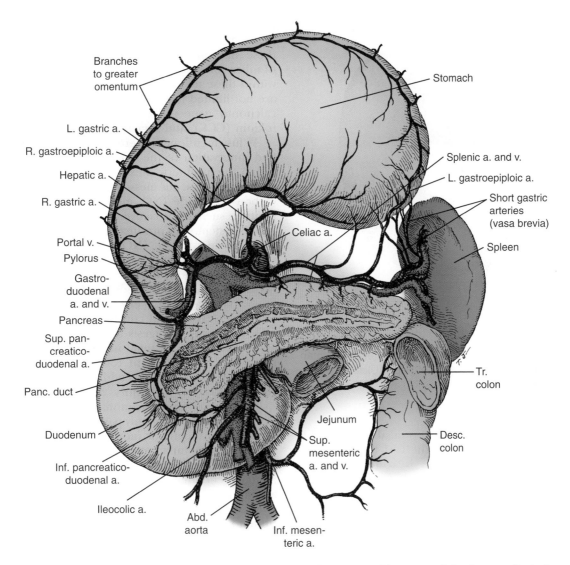

Figure 50–3. Blood supply of the stomach, duodenum, spleen, and pancreas. The stomach is shown reflected upward, and the pancreatic duct is exposed.

Lymphatic Drainage

The lymphatic drainage of the stomach usually parallels the vasculature. The cardia and medial half of the body drain to the left gastric nodes. The lesser curvature sides of the distal antrum and pylorus drain to the right gastric nodes. The greater curvature half of the distal 60% of the stomach drains into the right gastroepiploic nodal chain, whereas the proximal greater curvature drains into the left gastroepiploic chain. These four groups of nodes all drain to the celiac group, from which lymph drains into the thoracic duct. Although intraoperative and postmortem studies appear to corroborate this scheme of lymph drainage, it is widely recognized that a gastric cancer anywhere in the stomach may metastasize to any of the four nodal groups. The rich submucosal plexus of lymphatics accounts for the fact that there is often microscopic evidence of malignant cells several centimeters from the resection margin of gross disease. The anatomy of the lymph drainage of the stomach has received renewed interest as reports suggest that there may be improved survival with extended lymph node dissection in patients undergoing gastrectomy for primary gastric cancer, although this comes at a cost of increased morbidity with the more extensive procedure except when performed in high-volume centers.[1] Definitive randomized controlled trials are ongoing to determine the purported survival advantage.

Innervation

The extrinsic innervation of the stomach is both parasympathetic through the vagus and sympathetic through the celiac plexus (Fig. 50–4). From the vagal nucleus in the floor of the fourth ventricle, the vagus traverses the neck in the carotid sheath and enters the mediastinum, where it divides into several branches around the esophagus. These branches coalesce above the esophageal hiatus to form the left and right vagus nerves.

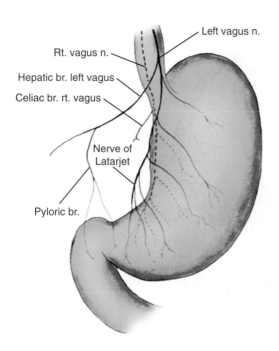

Left vagus n.

Rt. vagus n.

Hepatic br. left vagus

Celiac br. rt. vagus

Nerve of
Latarjet

Pyloric br.

Figure 50–4. Diagram of vagal innervation of the human stomach. (From Menguy R: Surgery of Peptic Ulcer. Philadelphia, WB Saunders, 1976.)

Commonly, there are more than two vagal trunks at the distal end of the esophagus. At the GEJ the *l*eft vagus is *a*nterior, and the *r*ight vagus is *p*osterior (LARP mnemonic). Near the cardia, the left (anterior) vagus gives off a branch to the liver and then continues along the lesser curvature as the anterior nerve of Latarjet. The antral and pyloric portions of this nerve (crow's foot) must be preserved during a highly selective vagotomy so that gastric emptying is not compromised. The "criminal" nerve of Grassi is the first branch of the posterior vagus nerve. This branch has been recognized as a cause of recurrent ulcers when left undivided. The right (posterior) nerve also gives a branch off to the celiac plexus and then continues posteriorly along the lesser curvature. The majority of vagal fibers are afferent and carry stimuli from the gut to the brain. The vagal efferent fibers originate in the dorsal nucleus of the medulla and synapse with neurons in the myenteric and submucosal plexuses. These neurons use acetylcholine as their neurotransmitter and influence gastric motor function and gastric secretion. In comparison, the sympathetic nerve supply comes from T5-T10 and travels in the splanchnic nerve to the celiac ganglion. Postganglionic fibers then travel with the arterial system to innervate the stomach.

The intrinsic or enteric nervous system of the stomach consists of neurons in Auerbach's (myenteric plexus located between the longitudinal and circular muscle layers) and Meissner's (submucosal plexus located between the muscularis mucosa and circular muscle) autonomic plexuses. Cholinergic, serotonergic, and peptidergic neurons are present in addition to a newly identified system of neurons that use a nonadrenergic noncholinergic (NANC) pathway. There are probably more neurons in the intrinsic gastric nervous system than there are gastric vagal efferent fibers.[2] The function of these neurons is still poorly understood, although a number of neuropeptides have been demonstrated within these neurons. These neuropeptides include but are not limited to acetylcholine, serotonin, substance P, calcitonin gene–related peptide, bombesin, cholecystokinin (CCK), and somatostatin.

As just mentioned, there is a third and newly identified innervation of the stomach via an NANC pathway within the myenteric plexus. Signals in this pathway are mediated by gaseous messengers such as nitric oxide and carbon monoxide (NO and CO), in addition to other peptides such as vasoactive intestinal polypeptide (VIP). In this system, NO production occurs via activity of the nitric oxide synthase (NOS) enzyme system, of which there are two constitutive calcium-dependent isoforms, neuronal (n) and endothelial (e), as well as an inducible (i) calcium-independent isoform. CO is derived from the heme-oxygenase (HO) enzyme system, which itself has inducible (HO-1) and constitutive isoforms (HO-2 and HO-3). Research suggests that NO and CO expression may be regulated by vagal nerve nicotinic synapses and that they have important roles in modulating smooth muscle contractility in addition to the stomach's response to stress and injury.[3,4,5]

Thus, it is an oversimplification to think of the stomach as containing only parasympathetic (cholinergic input) and sympathetic (adrenergic input) supply. Moreover, the parasympathetic system contains adrenergic as well as cholinergic neurons, and the sympathetic system contains cholinergic as well as adrenergic neurons. In addition to these complex interactions, the exact mechanisms by which the NANC pathways are mediated continue to be the focus of ongoing research.

Gastric Morphology

The stomach is covered by peritoneum except for the exact lesser and greater curvatures and a small posterior area at the proximal cardia and distal pyloric antrum. The peritoneal coat forms the outer serosa. Below this is the thicker muscularis propria, or muscularis externa, which consists of three layers of smooth muscle (Fig. 50–5). The middle layer of smooth muscle is circular and is the only complete muscle layer of the stomach wall. This middle circular muscle layer becomes progressively thicker toward the pylorus, where it becomes impressively thick as a true anatomic sphincter. The outer muscle layer is longitudinal and continuous with the outer layer of longitudinal esophageal smooth muscle. Within the layers of the muscularis externa is Auerbach's myenteric plexus. Between the muscularis externa and the mucosa lies the submucosa, a collagen-rich layer of connective tissue that is the strongest layer of the gastric wall. The rich anastomotic network of blood vessels and lymphatics mentioned earlier lies in this layer, and it also contains Meissner's plexus.

The mucosa consists of surface epithelium, lamina propria, and muscularis mucosae. The latter is on the luminal side of the submucosa and is probably responsi-

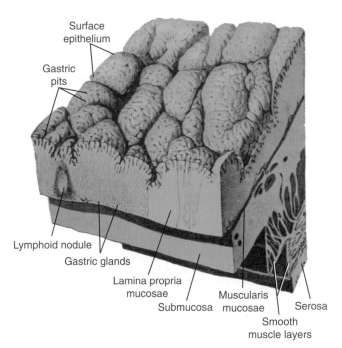

Surface
epithelium

Gastric
pits

Lymphoid nodule

Gastric glands

Lamina propria
mucosae

Submucosa

Muscularis
mucosae

Smooth
muscle layers

Serosa

Figure 50–5. Surface of the gastric mucosa of a man (drawing based on a binocular microscope view). The cut surfaces are slightly diagrammatic. At the *left* is the normal distribution of gastric glands; to the *right,* only a few are indicated. Glands, *orange*; gastric pits, *black* (×17). (From Fawcett DW: Bloom and Fawcett's Textbook of Histology, 11th ed. Philadelphia, WB Saunders, 1986.)

Cells	Location	Function
Parietal	Body	Secretion of acid, ghrelin, leptin, and intrinsic factor
Mucus	Body, antrum	Mucus
Chief	Body	Pepsin and leptin
Surface epithelial	Diffuse	Mucus, bicarbonate, and prostaglandins
ECL	Body	Histamine
G	Antrum	Gastrin
D	Body, antrum	Somatostatin
Gastric mucosal interneurons	Body, antrum	Gastrin-releasing peptide
Enteric neurons	Diffuse	CGRP, others

Table 50–1 Gastric Cell Types, Location, and Function

CGRP, calcitonin gene–related peptide; ECL, enterochromaffin-like.

ble for the rugae that greatly increase epithelial surface area. It also marks the microscopic boundary for invasive and noninvasive gastric carcinoma. The lamina propria is a small connective tissue layer that contains the capillaries, vessels, lymphatics, and nerves necessary to support the surface epithelium.

Gastric Glandular Organization

The gastric mucosa consists of columnar glandular epithelia. The functions of the glands and the types of cells lining them vary according to the region of the stomach in which they are found (Table 50–1). It should be noted that the endocrine cells, of which gastrin (G) cells and somatostatin (D) cells are best known, can be either open or closed. Open cells have microvilli on their apical membranes, which allows direct contact with the gastric contents. The microvilli probably possess chemical and pH sensors that signal the cell to secrete its prestored peptides. In contrast, closed cells do not have microvilli in contact with the gastric lumen. In the antrum, G cells and D cells are both of the open type, whereas in the fundus and body, the D cells are of the closed type and are in direct contact with the acid-secreting parietal cells. The glandular organization in the gastric mucosa differs, depending on the region of stomach examined. In the cardia, the mucosae are arranged in branched glands that secrete mostly mucus,

and the pits are short. In the fundus and body, the glands are more tubular, and the pits are long. The fundus has an elaborate network of glands that arise from the base of the mucosa in groups of four or five and join together at the bottom of the gastric pit, or foveola. In the antrum, the glands are again more branched. The luminal ends of the gastric glands and pits are lined with mucus-secreting surface epithelial cells that extend down into the necks of the glands for variable distances. The glands at the cardia are predominantly mucus secreting. In the body, the glands are lined from the neck to the base mostly with parietal and chief cells (Fig. 50–6). There are a few parietal cells in the fundus and proximal antrum, but none are present in the cardia or prepyloric antrum. Stomach biopsy specimens have shown that parietal cells account for 13% of the epithelial cells, chief cells for 44%, mucous cells for 40%, and endocrine cells for 3%.

PHYSIOLOGY

Gastric Peptides

Gastrin

Synthesis and Action Gastrin is produced by G cells located in the gastric antrum. It is synthesized as a pre-propeptide and undergoes post-translational processing to produce biologically active gastrin peptides. Several molecular forms of gastrin exist in the stomach. G-34 (big gastrin), G-17 (little gastrin), and G-14 (mini-gastrin) have all been identified. However, 90% of the antral gastrin produced is released as the 17–amino acid peptide, although G-34 predominates in the circulation because its metabolic half-life is longer than that of G-17.[6] The biologically active component of gastrin is the

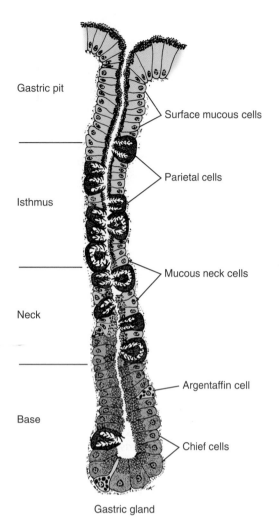

Figure 50–6. A gastric gland. (From Ito S, Winchester RJ: The fine structure of the gastric mucosa in the bat. J Cell Biol 16:541, 1963.)

The following labels appear in the figure:

- Gastric pit
- Surface mucous cells
- Isthmus
- Parietal cells
- Mucous neck cells
- Neck
- Argentaffin cell
- Base
- Chief cells
- Gastric gland

significantly blunted after the administration of H$_2$ receptor antagonists.[7] In addition to its acid secretory effects, gastrin has considerable trophic effects on parietal and gastric ECL cells. In fact, prolonged hypergastrinemia from any cause (e.g., gastrinoma, antisecretory drugs, atrophic gastritis) leads to mucosal hyperplasia, as well as an increase in the number of ECL cells; under some circumstances, it is associated with the development of gastric carcinoid tumors.[8] Finally, both exogenous gastrin and the release of endogenous gastrin have been shown to prevent the damaging effects of luminal irritants on gastric mucosa, thus suggesting that gastrin also plays a role in the intrinsic gastric mucosal defense system.[9]

Hypergastrinemia   The hypergastrinemia that results from the administration of antisecretory agents is an appropriate response caused by a loss of feedback inhibition of gastrin release by luminal acid. Lack of acid causes a reduction in somatostatin release, which in turn causes increased release of gastrin from antral G cells. Hypergastrinemia also develops as a result of gastric atrophy, such as occurs with pernicious anemia or uremia, as well as after surgical procedures such as vagotomy or retained gastric antrum after gastrectomy. In contrast, gastrin levels increase inappropriately in patients with gastrinoma (Zollinger-Ellison syndrome). These gastrin-secreting tumors are typically located in the head of the pancreas, duodenal wall, or regional lymph nodes and secrete gastrin autonomously.

Somatostatin

Synthesis and Action   Somatostatin is produced by D cells and exists endogenously as either a 14– or 28–amino acid peptide.[10] In the stomach, the predominant molecular form is somatostatin 14. Somatostatin is produced by diffuse neuroendocrine cells located in both the fundus and the antrum of the stomach. In these locations, their cytoplasmic extensions have direct contact with parietal cells and G cells, thus suggesting that somatostatin exerts its actions primarily through paracrine effects on acid secretion and gastrin release.[10] Somatostatin directly inhibits acid secretion by parietal cells but also inhibits gastrin release and down-regulates histamine release from ECL cells, which indirectly inhibits acid secretion. Antral acidification is the principal stimulus for somatostatin release, and acetylcholine from vagal fibers inhibits its release.

Effects of *Helicobacter pylori* on Somatostatin   Basal and stimulated gastrin concentrations are significantly increased in patients infected with *H. pylori*. It has been proposed that *H. pylori* causes a decrease in antral D cells. The resultant decrease in somatostatin levels causes disinhibition of antral G cells and hence leads to increased gastrin in the antrum and serum.[11] Eradication of *H. pylori* restores the antral D-cell population, with a consequent increase in antral somatostatin and a decrease in gastrin levels.[11] Thus, it is tempting to speculate that infection with *H. pylori* decreases antral D cells and somatostatin levels, thereby increasing gastrin release

pentapeptide sequence contained at its carboxyl terminus, which is identical to that found on another gut peptide, CCK. The two peptides differ in the location of tyrosine sulfation. A major stimulant for the release of gastrin is protein, as well as the digestion products of protein. Its release is inhibited by the presence of luminal acid. Somatostatin (see later) has paracrine actions on antral G cells and acts as a local inhibitor of gastrin release. In the antrum, somatostatin and gastrin release is functionally linked, and an inverse reciprocal relationship exists between these two peptides. Furthermore, somatostatin exerts a tonic inhibitory effect on gastrin release and probably mediates the inhibitory effects of luminal acid on gastrin release.

Gastrin is the major hormonal regulator of the gastric phase of acid secretion after a meal. Although parietal cells possess receptors to gastrin and exogenous gastrin elicits gastric acid secretion when given in physiologic doses, it is likely that histamine, released from enterochromaffin-like (ECL) cells, is the principal mediator of this action. Evidence supporting this concept is the finding that gastrin-stimulated gastric acid secretion is with a resultant increase in gastric acid secretion. However, although *H. pylori*–infected patients with duodenal ulcer disease usually have enhanced acid secretion, *H. pylori*–positive healthy volunteers with no peptic ulcer disease have either an increase of lesser magnitude or no increase at all when compared with *H. pylori*–negative volunteers. Nevertheless, cure of the infection in patients with duodenal ulcers has been demonstrated by some but not all investigators to diminish acid secretion.[11]

Gastrin-Releasing Peptide

Bombesin was isolated 20 years ago from an extract prepared from skin of the amphibian *Bombina bombina*. Its mammalian counterpart is gastrin-releasing peptide (GRP). GRP-staining immunoreactivity is particularly prominent in nerves ending in the acid-secreting and the gastrin-secreting portions of the stomach, as well as in the circular muscular layer.[12] In the antral mucosa, GRP stimulates gastrin and somatostatin release by binding to receptors located on G and D cells. GRP is rapidly cleared from the circulation by neutral endopeptidase and has a half-life of only 1.4 minutes.[12] Interestingly, exogenous GRP that is given peripherally stimulates gastric acid secretion, whereas central administration in the ventricles blunts gastric acid secretion induced by a variety of secretagogues.[12] The inhibitory pathway activated is not mediated by a humoral factor, is unaffected by vagotomy, and appears to involve the sympathetic nervous system. Research indicates that bombesin also possesses potent gastroprotective action mediated through an increase in gastric mucosal blood flow. This effect is most pronounced during times of stress and injury and acts to provide additional nutrients and remove toxins from the mucosa. This action is probably mediated via both NOS and COX (cyclooxygenase) enzyme systems.[12]

Histamine

Histamine plays a prominent role in parietal cell stimulation. H_2 receptor antagonists almost completely abolish gastrin-stimulated acid secretion and significantly blunt stimulated acid secretion induced by acetylcholine.[7] These findings suggest that histamine is a necessary intermediary of gastrin- and acetylcholine-stimulated acid secretion. Histamine is stored in the acidic granules of ECL cells, as well as in resident mast cells. ECL cells have been shown to possess receptors for gastrin, acetylcholine, and epinephrine, all of which stimulate histamine release. The ECL cell also has receptors for somatostatin, which inhibits gastrin-stimulated histamine release. Thus, the ECL cell plays a central role in parietal cell activation and possesses both stimulatory and feedback pathways that modulate the release of histamine and, consequently, acid secretion.

Ghrelin

Ghrelin is a recently discovered 28–amino acid acylated peptide secreted by oxyntic cells in the fundus of the stomach. Ghrelin is the first gut peptide found to have orexigenic (appetite stimulating) properties and appears to play a major role in energy homeostasis. Ghrelin levels have been shown to increase preprandially, coinciding with the development of feeling hungry, and then decrease postprandially after a satiating meal has been consumed.[13] Ghrelin appears to increase food intake through stimulation of ghrelin receptors located in the hypothalamic areas of the brain, such as the paraventricular nucleus and lateral hypothalamic area, as well as areas of the brainstem (all areas of major integration for the control of feeding behavior, energy expenditure, and gastrointestinal function) where neuropeptide Y (NPY)-expressing neurons and agouti-related protein (AgRP)-expressing neurons are localized.[14] This ghrelin-induced activation of NPY acts as a powerful orexigenic signal that results in increased food intake, decreased energy expenditure, and stimulation of peripheral glucocorticoid and insulin secretion, which favors the deposition of fat into adipose tissue.[15] Interestingly, gastrectomy and gastric bypass procedures significantly reduce plasma ghrelin levels, thus underscoring the importance of the stomach as an endocrine organ intimately involved in the maintenance of body weight and energy metabolism.[16] Additionally, it appears that the afferent vagus nerve fibers play an important role in transducing some of the effects of ghrelin inasmuch as vagotomy abolishes some of these effects.[17] Research further indicates that a complex signaling system involving the gut peptides leptin, CCK, pancreatic polypeptide, and peptide YY, along with ghrelin, works to control energy expenditure, although the exact interactions among these different peptides remain to be defined.[18]

Leptin

Leptin is a 14-kD protein discovered in 1994 that is also intimately involved in the regulation of metabolism and body weight.[19] Though mostly synthesized by adipocytes of white fat, another important source of leptin is the chief cells of the stomach because it is not found anywhere else in the gastrointestinal tract.[20] Like ghrelin, leptin exerts its influence on energy and appetite via stimulation of hypothalamic neurons expressing AgRP and NPY. When initially discovered, the elegant mechanism proposed indicated that levels of leptin rose in proportion to the amount of adipose tissue and signaled satiety to the hypothalamus with a resultant reduction in food intake. Thus, the actions of leptin seem to oppose those of ghrelin in that leptin acts as an antiobesity hormone that decreases appetite and increases metabolism by acting as a "satiety signal" as opposed to the "hunger signal" mediated by ghrelin. However, as the knowledge base has expanded, the effects of leptin have been found to be much more complex, and differential interactions among the pathways controlling both ghrelin and leptin probably play a major role in weight regulation. Additional data suggest that the vagus nerve may mediate gastric secretion of leptin and that short-term regulation of appetite may be due to differential alterations between systemic, plasma, and local gastric mucosal levels of leptin caused by the ingestion of enteral nutrients—again underscoring the important role of the stomach as an endocrine organ in the maintenance of body weight.[21,22]

Outside of its effects on appetite, leptin also has numerous other effects on the body. For example, leptin is a powerful gastroprotective agent against damage caused by luminal irritants and has effects on insulin sensitivity, inflammation and immune function, bone formation, and angiogenesis.[23-26] These additional actions of leptin outside its effects on energy balance are probably due to local rather than systemic effects and appear to be mediated via JAK-STAT phosphorylation protein kinases.[26]

Gastric Acid Secretion

In all vertebrates, gastric acid secretion by the parietal, or oxyntic, cell is regulated by three local stimuli: acetylcholine, gastrin, and histamine. These three stimuli account for basal and stimulated gastric acid secretion. Acetylcholine, released from the vagus and parasympathetic ganglion cells, is the principal neurotransmitter modulating acid secretion. In addition to innervating parietal cells, vagal fibers innervate G cells and ECL cells. Gastrin has hormonal (i.e., endocrine) effects on the parietal cell and causes release of histamine. Histamine, in turn, has paracrine-like effects on the parietal cell and is produced by ECL cells that receive additional endocrine (gastrin) and neural (acetylcholine) input. As shown in Figure 50–7, the ECL cell plays a central role in the regulation of acid secretion by the parietal cell. The model depicted also illustrates the inhibitory actions of somatostatin on gastric action secretion. The presence of intraluminal acid to a pH of 3 elicits the release of somatostatin from antral D cells, which inhibits gastrin release through paracrine effects and also modifies histamine release from ECL cells.[27] This negative feedback response is defective in some patients with peptic ulcer disease.[28] Thus, the precise state of acid secretion is dependent on the overall influence of these positive and negative stimuli.

Basal or Interprandial Acid Secretion

The secretory status of the parietal cell in the absence of food varies among species. Humans maintain a basal level of acid secretion that is roughly 10% of maximal acid output. Basal acid secretion also exhibits a circadian variation, with nighttime acid secretion being greater than daytime. Under basal conditions, 1 to 5 mmol of hydrochloric acid is secreted, and this amount is reduced by 75% to 90% after vagotomy or administration of atropine. These findings suggest that acetylcholine plays a significant role in basal secretion. However, H_2 receptor blockade also diminishes the magnitude of acid secretion by 90%, which suggests that histamine is also an important intermediary. Thus, it appears likely that basal acid secretion is the result of a combination of cholinergic and histaminergic input.

Stimulated Acid Secretion

The physiologic stimulus for acid secretion is ingestion of food. The acid secretory response that occurs after a meal has traditionally been described in three phases: cephalic, gastric, and intestinal. These three phases are interrelated and occur concurrently, not consecutively.

Cephalic Phase   The vagal, or cephalic, phase originates with the sight, smell, thought, or taste of food, which excites neural centers in the cortex and hypothalamus. Although the exact mechanisms by which senses stimulate acid secretion remain to be fully elucidated, it is hypothesized that several sites are stimulated in the brain. Sensitive sites include the dorsal vagal complex, nucleus tract solitarius, and dorsal motor nucleus, with secretion of thyrotropin-releasing hormone possibly involved in stimulation. Signals are transmitted from these higher centers to the stomach by the vagus nerves via release of acetylcholine, which in turn activates muscarinic receptors located on target cells. Acetylcholine directly increases acid secretion by parietal cells and can both inhibit and stimulate gastrin release, the net effect being a slight increase in gastrin levels.[29] Vagal stimulation in humans by sham feeding (chew and spit) results in an increase in acid secretion to about 50% of the maximal acid response to exogenous gastrin or histamine. Although the intensity of the acid secretory response in the cephalic phase surpasses that of the other phases, because the duration of the cephalic phase is brief, it accounts for only 20% to 30% of the total volume of gastric acid produced in response to a meal in humans.

Gastric Phase   The gastric phase of acid secretion begins when food enters the gastric lumen. Chemical components contained within the ingested food interact with the microvilli of antral G cells to stimulate gastrin release. Protein digests and amino acids are particularly effective at stimulating gastrin release, with the aromatic amino acids phenylalanine and tryptophan being the most potent. In addition, food stimulates acid secretion by causing mechanical distention of the stomach. Gastric distention activates stretch receptors in the stomach to elicit the long vagovagal reflex arc. It is abolished by proximal gastric vagotomy and is, at least in part, independent of changes in serum gastrin levels. However, antral distention does cause gastrin release in humans, and this reflex has been called the pyloro-oxyntic reflex.[30] It has been estimated from human studies that mechanical distention of the stomach results in about 30% to 40% of the maximal acid secretory response to a peptone meal, with the remainder being due to gastrin release. The entire gastric phase accounts for most (60% to 70%) of the meal-stimulated acid output because it lasts until the stomach is empty.

Intestinal Phase   The intestinal phase of gastric secretion is still poorly understood but is initiated by entry of chyme into the small intestine. It occurs after gastric emptying and lasts as long as partially digested food components remain within the proximal part of the small bowel. It accounts for roughly 10% of the acid secretory response to a meal and does not appear to be mediated by serum gastrin levels. It is thought to be mediated by a distinct acid stimulatory peptide hormone (enterooxyntin) that is released from small bowel mucosa.

Cellular Basis of Acid Secretion

Parietal Cell Receptors

Gastrin Receptors CCK and gastrin initiate their biologic actions by activation of surface membrane receptors. These receptors are members of the classic G protein–coupled seven transmembrane–spanning receptor family and have been classified as either type A or type B CCK receptors. Type A CCK receptors have high affinity for sulfated CCK analogues and low affinity for gastrin.[9] Type B CCK receptors, on the other hand, have high affinity for both gastrin and CCK. The gastrin or CCK-B receptor has been cloned from a parietal cell library, and binding of ligand with receptor was found to be coupled to elevated intracellular calcium levels.[31]

Muscarinic Receptors The actions of acetylcholine on the parietal cell are mediated via the M_3 subtype of the muscarinic receptor family. This receptor is also coupled to increased levels of intracellular calcium, which is mediated by phospholipase-induced production of inositol triphosphate (IP_3).[31]

Histamine Receptors Histamine belongs to the same family of G protein–coupled seven transmembrane–spanning receptors. The receptor on the parietal cell is the H_2 subtype. Coupling with histamine causes activation of adenylate cyclase, which leads to an increase in intracellular cyclic adenosine monophosphate (cAMP) levels.

Somatostatin Receptors At least five different types of somatostatin receptors have been cloned. These receptors are also members of the seven transmembrane–spanning receptors and are coupled to one or more inhibitory guanine nucleotide binding proteins. The different somatostatin receptors also appear to have divergent pharmacologic effects because one somatostatin receptor may associate with an inhibitory G protein whereas another may not.[10] In the stomach, parietal cell somatostatin receptors have been identified and appear to be a single subunit of glycoproteins with a molecular weight of 99 kD and equal affinity for somatostatin 14 and somatostatin 28.[10] Inhibition of parietal cell secretion by somatostatin occurs through both G protein–dependent and G protein–independent mechanisms. However, the ability of somatostatin to exert its inhibitory actions on cellular function is primarily thought to be mediated by inhibition of adenylate cyclase with a resultant reduction in cAMP levels.

Second Messengers Stimulation of acid secretion by parietal cells is primarily mediated by increased levels of intracellular cAMP and calcium. The production of these two second messengers in turn activates a variety of protein kinases. However, although these protein kinases become activated and result in the phosphorylation of parietal cell proteins within the cytosol, little is known about the precise phosphorylation pathways that result in activation of the proton pump, which is ultimately responsible for acid secretion. Nonetheless, the intracellular events following ligand binding to receptors on the

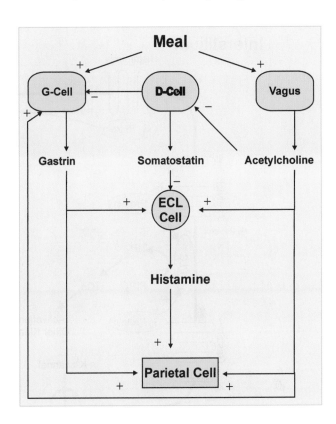

Figure 50–7. The central role of the enterochromaffin-like (ECL) cell in regulation of acid secretion by the parietal cell is depicted. As shown, after ingestion of a meal, vagal fibers are stimulated and release acetylcholine (cephalic phase). Acetylcholine binds to M_3 receptors located on the ECL cell, parietal cell, and G cell to cause the release of histamine, hydrochloric acid, and gastrin, respectively. Acetylcholine also interacts with M_3 receptors located on the D cell to inhibit somatostatin release. Food within the gastric lumen also stimulates the G cell to release gastrin, which in turn binds to type B cholecystokinin receptors located on the ECL cell and parietal cell and causes the release of histamine and hydrochloric acid, respectively (gastric phase). Somatostatin released from the D cell inhibits histamine release from the ECL cell and gastrin release from the G cell. Somatostatin also inhibits acid secretion by the parietal cell (not shown). The principal stimulus for activation of the D cell is antral luminal acidification (not shown).

parietal cell are demonstrated in Figure 50–8. As shown, histamine causes intracellular cAMP levels to increase, which activates protein kinases to initiate a cascade of phosphorylation events that culminate in the activation of H^+,K^+-adenosine triphosphatase (ATPase). In contrast, acetylcholine and gastrin stimulate phospholipase C, which converts membrane-bound phospholipids into IP_3 to mobilize calcium from intracellular stores. Increased intracellular calcium activates other protein kinases that ultimately activate H^+,K^+-ATPase to begin secretion of hydrochloric acid.

Activation and Secretion by the Parietal Cell The final common pathway for gastric acid secretion by the

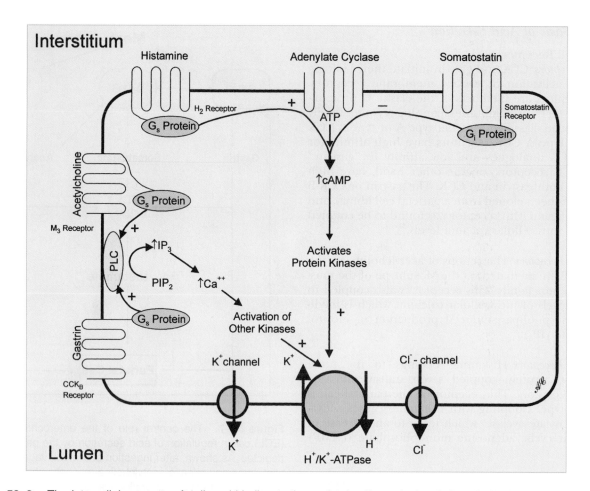

Figure 50–8. The intracellular events after ligand binding to the parietal cell are depicted. Gastrin binds to the type B cholecystokinin (CCK) receptor and acetylcholine binds to M_3 receptors to stimulate phospholipase C (PLC) through a G protein—linked mechanism. Activated phospholipase C converts membrane-bound phospholipids into inositol triphosphate (IP_3), which stimulates the release of intracellular calcium from intracellular calcium stores. The increase in intracellular calcium leads to the activation of protein kinases, which activate H^+,K^+-ATPase. Histamine binds to its H_2 receptor to stimulate adenylate cyclase, which also occurs through a G protein—linked mechanism. Activation of adenylate cyclase leads to an increase in intracellular cyclic adenosine monophosphate (cAMP) levels, which activates protein kinases. Activated protein kinases stimulate a phosphorylation cascade that results in increased levels of phosphoproteins, which activate the proton pump. Activation of the proton pump leads to extrusion of cytosolic hydrogen in exchange for extracytoplasmic potassium. In addition, chloride is secreted through a chloride channel located at the luminal side of the membrane. ATP, adenosine triphosphate; ATPase, adenosine triphosphatase; G_s, stimulatory guanine nucleotide protein; G_i, inhibitory guanine nucleotide protein; PIP_2, phosphatidylinositol 4,5-diphosphate.

parietal cell is H^+,K^+-ATPase. The enzyme is composed of a catalytic α (relative molecular weight [M_r], $\approx$100 kD) subunit and a glycoprotein β (M_r, $\approx$60 kD) subunit. During the resting or nonsecreting state, gastric parietal cells store H^+,K^+-ATPase within intracellular tubulovesicular elements. For acid secretion to increase in response to stimulatory factors, cellular relocation of the acid pump through cytoskeletal rearrangements must occur. Binding of secretagogues causes fusion of the tubulovesicles with the apical plasma membrane. This is an essential process, and research indicates that alkalinization of the gastric environment during critical illness may be due to failure of rearrangement of the cytoskeleton of the cell.[32] The subsequent insertion and heterodimer assembly of the H^+,K^+-ATPase subunits into the microvilli of the

secretory canaliculus cause an increase in gastric acid secretion.[31] In addition, a potassium chloride (KCl) efflux pathway must exist to supply potassium to the extracytoplasmic side of the pump. H^+,K^+-ATPase secretes cytosolic hydrogen in exchange for extracytoplasmic potassium (see Fig. 50–8), which is an electroneutral exchange and therefore does not contribute to the transmembrane potential difference across the parietal cell. Chloride is secreted through a chloride channel that moves chloride from the cytoplasm to the gastric lumen. The secretion/exchange of hydrogen for potassium, however, does require energy in the form of ATP because hydrogen is being secreted against a gradient of more than 1 million–fold. Because of this large energy requirement, the parietal cell also has the largest mitochondrial content of any mammalian cell, with the mitochondrial compartment representing 34% of its cell volume. In contrast to stimulated acid secretion, cessation of acid secretion requires endocytosis of H^+,K^+-ATPase with regeneration of cytoplasmic tubulovesicles containing the subunits, and this occurs through a tyrosine-based signal.[33] The tyrosine-containing sequence is located on the cytoplasmic tail of the β subunit and is highly homologous to the motif responsible for internalization of the transferrin receptor.

The normal human stomach contains more than 1 billion parietal cells that secrete about 20 mmol of hydrochloric acid per hour in response to a protein meal. Each individual parietal cell secretes 3.3 billion hydrogen ions per second, and there is a linear relationship between maximal acid output and parietal cell number. Gastric acid secretory rates are altered in patients with upper gastrointestinal diseases. For example, gastric acid is increased in patients with duodenal ulcer or gastrinoma, whereas it is decreased in patients with pernicious anemia, gastric atrophy, gastric ulcer, or gastric cancer. The lower secretory rates observed in patients with gastric ulcer are typically for proximal gastric ulcers, whereas distal, antral, or prepyloric ulcers are associated with acid secretory rates similar to those found in patients with duodenal ulcer.

Pharmacologic Regulation of Gastric Acid Secretion

Gastric acid secretion can be blunted by the administration of site-specific receptor antagonists for histamine or gastrin, as well as by muscarinic receptor antagonists. These receptor antagonists inhibit gastric acid secretion by competitive inhibition of the receptor. The best known of the site-specific antagonists is the group collectively known as the H_2 or histamine receptor antagonists. The most potent of the H_2 receptor antagonists is famotidine, followed by ranitidine, nizatidine, and cimetidine. The half-life of famotidine is 3 hours, with an approximately 1.5-hour half-life for the others. All undergo hepatic metabolism, are excreted by the kidney, and do not differ much in bioavailability. The substituted benzimidazoles are another class of antisecretory agents, of which omeprazole, esomeprazole, rabeprazole, and lansoprazole are examples. These agents are more complete inhibitors of acid secretion because they act at the final step of gastric acid secretion to irreversibly inhibit the proton pump. The proton pump inhibitors are weak acids with a pK_a of 4.0 and therefore become selectively localized in the secretory canaliculus of the parietal cell, which is the only structure in the body with a pH lower than 4. After oral administration, these agents are absorbed into the bloodstream as prodrugs and then selectively concentrate in the secretory canaliculus. At low pH, they become ionized and then activated by the formation of an active sulfur group. For this reason, patients consuming substituted benzimidazoles should not take additional antisecretory agents because they will raise gastric pH and prevent activation of the benzimidazoles. Because the proton pump is located on the luminal surface, the transmembrane pump proteins are also exposed to acid or low pH. The cysteine residues on the α subunit form a covalent disulfide bond with acti-

vated benzimidazoles that irreversibly inhibits H^+,K^+-ATPase. Because of the covalent nature of this bond, omeprazole and agents like it exhibit more prolonged inhibition of gastric acid secretion than H_2 blockers do. It is quite likely that recovery of acid secretion after administration of these compounds requires the synthesis of new enzyme. Furthermore, the covalent bond causes a longer duration of action than the plasma half-life, with intragastric pH being maintained above 3 for 18 hours or more.

One side effect of the proton pump inhibitors is an elevation in serum gastrin levels, which also occurs in response to the other antisecretory agents. However, 24-hour plasma gastrin levels are greater with proton pump inhibitors than with H_2 receptor antagonists, and this effect is accompanied by hyperplasia of G cells and ECL cells when these agents are administered chronically. The effect is reversed after discontinuation of these agents, provided that gastric acidity returns to normal levels. Under long-term administration of omeprazole, it was also noted that ECL cell hyperplasia could progress to carcinoid tumors in rats.[8] These tumors were more common in females than in males and occurred only when the rats were at the end of their natural life span. This sequence of events was not specific for omeprazole and was reproduced by other agents that caused prolonged inhibition of acid secretion and resultant hypergastrinemia.

Functions of Gastric Acid

Gastric acid plays a critical role in the digestion of a meal. It is required to convert pepsinogen (see later) into pepsin, which is necessary for the hydrolysis of proteins into polypeptides. Gastric acid also elicits the release of secretin from the duodenum, which results in pancreatic bicarbonate secretion. Furthermore, gastric acid functions to limit colonization of the upper gastrointestinal tract by bacteria. Colonization of the stomach and duodenum is known to occur in patients with achlorhydria and those receiving antisecretory agents. In addition, there is evidence of causation between gastric colonization and the subsequent development of nosocomial pneumonia in the intensive care unit (ICU).[34] Gastric luminal alkalinization attenuates the natural bactericidal effect of gastric acid and thus creates an environment conducive to bacterial overgrowth. Interestingly, the pathogens involved in nosocomial pneumonia, the principal infection of patients with multiple organ failure in the ICU, are frequently found in gastric aspirates and appear to temporally colonize the stomach before the development of clinical pneumonia.[35] However, some studies challenge the importance of increased gastric colonization with bacterial pathogens in the subsequent development of nosocomial pneumonia.[36]

Other Gastric Secretory Products

Gastric Juice

Gastric juice is the result of secretions by parietal cells, chief cells, and mucous cells, in addition to swallowed

Table 50–2	Gastric Electrolyte Composition in the Human Whole Stomach

Parietal						
[H]	[Na]	[K]	[All Cations]	[HCO₃]	[Cl]	[All Anions]
148.9	—	16.9	165.8	—	166.3	166.3

Nonparietal						
[H]	[Na]	[K]	[All Cations]	[HCO₃]	[Cl]	[All Anions]
—	136.7	6.4	143.1	25.0	117.8	142.8

saliva and duodenal refluxate. The electrolyte composition of parietal and nonparietal gastric secretions (Table 50–2) varies with the rate of gastric secretion. Parietal cells secrete an electrolytic solution that is isotonic with plasma and contains 160 mmol/L. The pH of this solution is 0.8. The lowest intraluminal pH commonly measured in the stomach is 2 because of secretions that also contain sodium, potassium, and bicarbonate.

Intrinsic Factor

Intrinsic factor is a 60,000-dalton mucoprotein secreted by the parietal cell that is essential for the absorption of vitamin B_{12} in the terminal ileum. Intrinsic factor is secreted in amounts that far exceed what is necessary for vitamin B_{12} absorption. However, the gastric mucosa is the critical site of production for intrinsic factor, and thus patients undergoing gastrectomy or proximal stomach resection may require a monthly injection of vitamin B_{12}. Its secretion parallels that of gastric acid secretion, yet the secretory response is not necessarily linked to acid secretion. For example, proton pump inhibitors do not block secretion of intrinsic factor in humans, nor do they alter the absorption of labeled vitamin B_{12}. Deficiency of intrinsic factor can develop in the setting of pernicious anemia, and these patients also require vitamin B_{12} supplementation.

Pepsinogen

Pepsinogens are proteolytic proenzymes with a molecular weight of 42,500 that are secreted by the glands of the gastroduodenal mucosa. In general, two types of pepsinogens are secreted. Group 1 pepsinogens are secreted by chief cells and by mucous neck cells located in the glands of the acid-secreting portion of the stomach. In contrast, group 2 pepsinogens are produced by surface epithelial cells throughout the acid-secreting portion of the stomach, as well as the antrum and proximal duodenum. As a result, group 1 pepsinogens are secreted by the same glands that secrete acid, whereas group 2 pepsinogens are secreted by acid-secreting and gastrin-secreting mucosa. In the presence of acid, both forms of pepsinogen are converted to pepsin by removal of a short amino-terminal peptide. Pepsins become inactivated at a pH higher than 5, although group 2 pepsinogens are active over a wider range of pH values than the group 1 pepsinogens are.[37] Consequently, group 2 pepsinogens may be involved in peptic digestion in the setting of increased gastric pH, which commonly occurs with stress or in patients with gastric ulcer.

Mucus and Bicarbonate

Mucus and bicarbonate combine to neutralize gastric acid at the gastric mucosal surface. Both are secreted by surface mucous cells and by mucous neck cells located in the acid-secreting portion of the stomach and the antrum. Mucus is a viscoelastic gel that contains approximately 85% water and 15% glycoproteins and provides a mechanical barrier to injury by contributing to the unstirred layer of water found at the luminal surface of the gastric mucosa. It provides some impediment to ion movement from the lumen to the apical cell membrane and is relatively impermeable to pepsins. It is also in a constant state of flux because it is secreted continuously by mucosal cells on the one hand and solubilized by luminal pepsin on the other. Research suggests that both prostaglandins derived from the constitutive cyclooxygenase-1 enzyme and nitric oxide from the eNOS and nNOS systems are critical to maintenance of the protective mucous layer and may act as important molecular mediators of the protective mucous layer.[38] Vagal stimulation, cholinergic agonists, prostaglandins, and some bacterial toxins stimulate mucus production, whereas anticholinergic drugs and nonsteroidal anti-inflammatory drugs (NSAIDs) inhibit its secretion. H. pylori, however, secretes various proteases and lipases that break down mucin, thereby impairing the protective function of the mucous layer.[39] Newer research techniques have shown that neither chief nor parietal cells have a significant amount of differential transcription expression in the presence of H. pylori whereas the mucous cell exhibits profound changes in its transcription patterns because of H. pylori. Furthermore, the genes that are differentially expressed upon infection are implicated in proinflammatory and mucosal defense responses, as well as modulation of angiogenesis, iron availability, and tumor suppression.[40]

In the acid-secreting portion of the stomach, bicarbonate secretion is an active process, whereas in the antrum, both active and passive secretion of bicarbonate occurs. It is noteworthy that the magnitude of bicarbonate secretion is considerably less than that of acid secretion, yet although the luminal pH is 2, the pH observed at the surface epithelial cell layer is usually 7. The pH gradient found at the epithelial surface is the result of the aforementioned unstirred layer of water contained within the mucous gel and the continuous secretion of bicarbonate by the surface epithelial cells. Gastric cell surface pH remains greater than 5 until the luminal pH is less than 1.4. However, luminal pH in patients with duodenal ulcer is frequently less than 1.4, so the cell surface is exposed to lower pH in these patients. This reduction in pH may reflect a decrease in gastric bicarbonate secretion, as well as decreased duodenal bicarbonate secretion, and may explain why some patients with duodenal ulcer have a higher relapse rate after treatment.[41]

Gastric Barrier Function and Peptic Ulcer Disease

Gastric barrier function depends on a number of physiologic and anatomic factors, including but not limited to cell membranes, tight junctions, cell renewal processes, mucus secretion, alkaline secretion, and gastric pH. Microvascular blood flow also plays a role in gastric mucosal defense by providing nutrients and delivering oxygen to ensure that the intracellular processes that underlie mucosal resistance to injury can proceed unabated. Decreased gastric mucosal blood flow has minimal effects on lesion production until it approaches 50% of normal. When blood flow is reduced by more than 75%, marked mucosal injury results and is exacerbated in the presence of luminal acid. Once damage occurs, injured surface epithelial cells are replaced rapidly by migration of surface mucous cells located along the basement membrane. This process is referred to as restitution or reconstitution.[42] It occurs within minutes and does not require cell division.

Exposure of the stomach to noxious agents causes a reduction in the potential difference across the gastric mucosa. In normal gastric mucosa, the potential difference across the mucosa is −30 to −50 mV and results from the active transport of chloride into the lumen and sodium into the blood whose gradients are maintained by the activity of Na^+/K^+-ATPase. Damage disrupts the tight junctions between mucosal cells and causes the epithelium to become leaky to ions (i.e., Na^+ and Cl^-), with a resultant loss of the high transepithelial electrical resistance normally found in gastric mucosa. In addition, damaging agents such as NSAIDs or aspirin possess carboxyl groups that are nonionized at low intragastric pH because they are weak acids. Consequently, they readily enter the cell membranes of gastric mucosal cells because they are now lipid soluble, whereas they will not penetrate the cell membranes at neutral pH because they are ionized. On entry into the neutral pH environment found within the cytosol, they become reionized, will not exit the cell membrane, and are toxic to the mucosal cells.

Duodenal ulcer disease is a disease of multiple causes. The only relatively absolute requirements are secretion of acid and pepsin in conjunction with *H. pylori* infection or ingestion of NSAIDs. Gastric acid secretory rates are usually increased in patients with duodenal ulcer disease. Both basal gastric acid output and peak pentagastrin-stimulated acid output are increased in duodenal ulcer patients when compared with controls, although there is extensive overlap between groups. Mean parietal cell numbers have also been shown to be increased in duodenal ulcer patients when compared with controls.[43] In contrast, the mean parietal cell number is not increased in patients with gastric ulcer disease, which is also not associated with excess gastric acid secretion. Pepsin secretion has likewise been found to be increased in duodenal ulcer patients and is associated with an increase in the peptic cell mass responsible for synthesizing pepsinogens. When compared with the level in control patients, serum pepsinogen 1, but not pepsinogen 2, was found to be increased in patients with duodenal ulcer.[44]

Gastric Motor Function

Gastric motility is regulated by extrinsic and intrinsic neural mechanisms, as well as by myogenic control. The extrinsic neural controls are mediated through parasympathetic (vagus) and sympathetic pathways, and the intrinsic controls involve the enteric nervous system already discussed in the "Anatomy" section. In contrast, myogenic control resides within the excitatory membranes of the gastric smooth muscle cells. When the cell membrane potential exceeds its threshold potential, an action potential is generated that results in muscle contraction. The resting potential changes in gradient from −48 mV in the gastric pacemaker interstitial cells of Cajal (ICCs), located in the proximal part of the stomach, to a resting gradient of −75 mV in the pylorus. This change in resting potential may be responsible in part for the reduced rate of contractions observed in the distal end of the stomach when compared with that in the proximal end. ICCs are critical for the generation of sequential contractions and probably receive input from a variety of mechanical as well as biochemical sources. Future research on ICCs will most likely yield important knowledge about the pathogenesis of gastric dysfunction.[45]

Fasting Gastric Motility

The electrical basis of gastric motility begins with depolarization of the pacemaker cells located in the midbody of the stomach along the greater curvature. Once initiated, slow waves travel at three cycles per minute in a circumferential and antegrade fashion toward the pylorus.[46] In addition to these slow waves, gastric smooth muscle cells are capable of producing action potentials, which are associated with larger changes in membrane potential than slow waves are. When compared with slow waves, which are not associated with gastric contractions, action potentials are associated with actual muscle contractions. During fasting, the stomach goes through a cyclic pattern of electrical activity that has been termed the myoelectric migrating complex (MMC). Each MMC cycle lasts 90 to 120 minutes and is made up of four phases. Phase I of the MMC is the quiescent phase, in which slow waves are present without action potentials; this phase results in an increase in gastric tone but no gastric contraction. In phase II of the MMC, the motor spikes are associated with slow waves and occasional gastric contractions. During phase III, motor spike activity is associated with each slow wave, and forceful gastric contractions are produced every 15 to 20 seconds. The net effect of phase III MMC activity is clearance of large undigestible food substances contained within the stomach. Phase IV activity is characterized as a brief period of recovery before the next MMC cycle. The net effects of the MMC are frequent clearance of gastric contents during periods of fasting. The exact regulatory mechanisms of MMC activities are unknown, but these activities remain intact after vagal denervation.

Postprandial Gastric Motility

Ingestion of a meal results in a decrease in the resting tone of the proximal stomach and fundus, referred to as receptive relaxation and gastric accommodation. Because these reflexes are mediated by the vagus nerves, interruption of vagal innervation to the proximal part of the stomach, such as by truncal vagotomy or proximal gastric vagotomy, can eliminate these reflexes with resultant early satiety and rapid emptying of ingested liquids.[47] In addition to its storage function, the stomach is responsible for the mixing and grinding of ingested solid food particles. This activity involves repetitive forceful contractions of the midportion and antral portion of the stomach, which causes food particles to be propelled against a closed pylorus with subsequent retropulsion of solids and liquids. The net effect is a thorough mixing of solids and liquids and a sequential shearing of solid food particles to a size less than 1 mm.

The emptying of gastric contents is under the influence of well-coordinated neural and hormonal mediators. Systemic factors such as anxiety, fear, depression, and exercise can affect the rate of gastric motility and emptying. Additionally, the chemical properties, mechanical properties, and temperature of the intraluminal contents can influence the rate of gastric emptying. In general, liquids empty more rapidly than solids, and carbohydrates empty more readily than fats. Increases in the concentration or acidity of liquid meals cause a delay in gastric emptying. In addition, hot and cold liquids tend to empty at a slower rate than ambient-temperature fluids do. These responses to luminal stimuli are regulated by the enteric nervous system. Osmoreceptors and pH-sensitive receptors in the proximal part of the small bowel have also been shown to be involved in the activation of feedback inhibition of gastric emptying. Inhibitory peptides proposed to be active in this setting include CCK, glucagon, VIP, and gastric inhibitory polypeptide.

Abnormal Gastric Motility

Symptoms of abnormal gastric motility are nausea, fullness, early satiety, and abdominal pain and discomfort. Although mechanical obstruction can and should be ruled out with upper endoscopy or radiographic contrast studies (or both), objective evaluation of a patient with a suspected motility disorder can be accomplished with gamma scintigraphy, real-time ultrasound, and magnetic resonance imaging. The gastric motility disorders that are most commonly encountered in clinical practice are gastric dysmotility after vagotomy, delayed gastric emptying associated with diabetes mellitus, and gastric motility dysfunction related to *H. pylori* infection. Vagotomy results in the loss of receptive relaxation and gastric accommodation in response to meal ingestion, with resultant early satiety, postprandial bloating, accelerated emptying of liquids, and a delay in emptying of solids. Clinical manifestations of diabetic gastropathy can occur in insulin-dependent or insulin-independent patients and closely resemble the clinical picture of postvagotomy gastroparesis. Furthermore, structural changes have been identified in the vagus nerves of patients with diabetes, thus suggesting that diabetic autonomic neuropathy may be responsible. However, the metabolic effects of diabetes have also been implicated. Specifically, hyperglycemia has been shown to cause a decrease in contractility of the gastric antrum, an increase in pyloric contractility, and suppression of phase III activity of the MMC. Suppression of phase III MMC activity is thought to be responsible for the accumulation of gastric bezoars seen in some diabetics. In contrast, hyperinsulinemia, which is often associated with non–insulin-dependent diabetics, may play a role in the gastroparesis seen in non–insulin-dependent diabetics because it also leads to suppression of phase III MMC activity.[48]

Critically ill patients are also predisposed to gastric dysfunction. These patients frequently have impaired gastric emptying because of profound changes in their systemic physiology. Acidosis, sepsis, electrolyte derangements, and shock combine to impair the normal mechanisms that control emptying of the stomach. This impairment in emptying, when combined with an increase in reflux from the duodenum to the pylorus, results in increased gastric residual volumes. Additionally, these patients are frequently maintained nutritionally by enteral nasogastric tube feedings. The increased volume of gastric fluid combined with alkalinization of the gastric environment because of dysfunction of H^+,K^+-ATPase predisposes to bacterial colonization of the normal environment. Furthermore, aspiration of this increased gastric fluid, now colonized with pathogenic bacteria, may easily occur and result in the development of nosocomial pneumonia as previously mentioned.[34,35]

H. pylori–infected patients with non–ulcer-associated dyspepsia have also been demonstrated to have impaired gastric emptying that is accompanied by a reduction in gastric compliance.[49] In rats, lipopolysaccharide derived from *H. pylori* causes a delay in gastric emptying of a liquid meal for up to 12 hours by an unknown mechanism. Regardless of the cause of gastroparesis, treatment consists of prokinetic agents such as metoclopramide and erythromycin. Both have been shown to have some benefit, although the evidence is more compelling in diabetics.[50]

SUGGESTED READINGS

Ahima RS, Flier JS: Leptin. Annu Rev Physiol 62:413-437, 2000.

Cummings DE, Weigle DS, Frayo RS, et al: Plasma ghrelin levels after diet-induced weight loss or gastric bypass surgery. N Engl J Med 346:1623-1630, 2002.

Dunn BE: Pathogenetic mechanisms of *Helicobacter pylori*. Gastroenterol Clin North Am 22:43-57, 1993.

Shah V, Lyford G, Gores G, Farrugia G: Nitric oxide in gastrointestinal health and disease. Gastroenterology 126:903-913, 2004.

Walsh JH, Dockray GJ (eds): Gut Peptides: Biochemistry and Physiology. New York, Raven Press, 1994.

REFERENCES

1. Sano T, Sasako M, Yamamoto S, et al: Gastric cancer surgery: Results of morbidity and mortality of a prospective randomized controlled trial (JCOG 9501) comparing D2 and extended para-aortic lymphadenectomy. J Clin Oncol 22:2767-2773, 2004.
2. Furness JB, Costa M: Types of nerves in the enteric nervous system. Neuroscience 5:1-20, 1980.
3. Nakamura K, Takahashi T, Taniuchi M, et al: Nicotinic receptor mediates nitric oxide synthase expression in the rat gastric myenteric plexus. J Clin Invest 101:1479-1489, 1998.
4. Shah V, Lyford G, Gores G, Farrugia G: Nitric oxide in gastrointestinal health and disease. Gastroenterology 126:903-913, 2004.
5. Xue L, Farrugia G, Miller SM, et al: Carbon monoxide and nitric oxide as coneurotransmitters in the enteric nervous system: Evidence from genomic deletion of biosynthetic enzymes. Proc Natl Acad Sci U S A 97:1851-1855, 2000.
6. Berson SA, Yalow RS: Nature of immunoreactive gastrin extracted from tissues of gastrointestinal tract. Gastroenterology 60:215-222, 1971.
7. Berglindh T: The mammalian gastric parietal cell in vitro. Annu Rev Physiol 46:377-392, 1984.
8. Carney JA, Go VLW, Fairbanks VF, et al: The syndrome of gastric argyrophil carcinoid tumors and nonantral gastric atrophy. Ann Intern Med 99:761-766, 1983.
9. Mercer DW, Cross JM, Smith GS, et al: Protective action of gastrin-17 against alcohol-induced gastric injury in the rat: Role in mucosal defense. Am J Physiol 273:G365-G373, 1997.
10. Chiba T, Yamada T: Gut somatostatin. In Walsh JH, Dockray GJ (eds): Gut Peptides: Biochemistry and Physiology. New York, Raven Press, 1994, pp 123-145.
11. Queiroz DMM, Mendes EN, Rocha GA, et al: Effect of *Helicobacter pylori* eradication on antral gastrin- and somatostatin-immunoreactive cell density and gastrin and somatostatin concentrations. Scand J Gastroenterol 28:858-864, 1993.
12. West SD, Mercer DW: Bombesin-induced gastroprotection. Ann Surg 241:227-231, 2005.
13. Kojima M, Hosoda H, Date Y, et al: Ghrelin is a growth-hormone–releasing acylated peptide from stomach. Nature 402:656-660, 1999.
14. Tschop M, Statnick MA, Suter TM, Heiman ML: GH-releasing peptide-2 increases fat mass in mice lacking NPY: Indication for a crucial mediating role of hypothalamic agouti-related protein. Endocrinology 143:558-568, 2002.
15. Jeanrenaud B, Rohner-Jeanrenaud F: Effects of neuropeptides and leptin on nutrient partitioning: Dysregulations in obesity. Annu Rev Med 52:339-351, 2001.
16. Cummings DE, Weigle DS, Frayo RS, et al: Plasma ghrelin levels after diet-induced weight loss or gastric bypass surgery. N Engl J Med 346:1623-1630, 2002.
17. Date Y, Murakami N, Toshinai K, et al: The role of the gastric afferent vagal nerve in ghrelin-induced feeding and growth hormone secretion in rats. Gastroenterology 123:1120-1128, 2002.
18. Inui A, Asakawa A: Leptin and gastric neuroendocrine system. Gastroenterology 123:1751, 2002.
19. Halaas JL, Gajiwala KS, Maffei S, et al: Weight-reducing effects of the plasma protein encoded by the obese gene. Science 269:543-546, 1995.
20. Sobhani I, Bado A, Vissuzaine C, et al: Leptin secretion and leptin receptor in the human stomach. Gut 47:178-183, 2000.
21. Sobhani I, Buyse M, Goiot H, et al: Vagal stimulation rapidly increases leptin secretion in human stomach. Gastroenterology 122:259-263, 2002.
22. Wang J, Liu R, Hawkins M, et al: A nutrient-sensing pathway regulates leptin gene expression in muscle and fat. Nature 393:684-688, 1998.
23. Lord GM, Matarese G, Howard JK, et al: Leptin modulates the T-cell immune response and reverses starvation-induced immuno-suppression. Nature 394:897-901, 1998.
24. Sierra-Honigmann MR, Nath AK, Murakami C, et al: Biological action of leptin as an angiogenic factor. Science 281:1683-1686, 1998.
25. Cohen B, Novick D, Rubinstein M: Modulation of insulin activities by leptin. Science 274:1185-1188, 1996.
26. Ahima RS, Flier JS: Leptin. Annu Rev Physiol 62:413-437, 2000.
27. Schubert ML, Edwards NF, Makhlouf GM: Regulation of gastric somatostatin secretion in the mouse by luminal acidity: A local feedback mechanism. Gastroenterology 94:317-322, 1988.
28. Walsh JH, Richardson CT, Fordtran JS: pH dependence of acid secretion and gastrin release in normal and ulcer subjects. J Clin Invest 55:462-468, 1975.
29. Lucey MR, Wass JAH, Fairclough PD, et al: Autonomic regulation of postprandial plasma somatostatin, gastrin and insulin. Gut 26:683-688, 1985.
30. Debas HT, Konturek SJ, Walsh JH, Grossman MI: Proof of a pyloro-oxyntic reflex for stimulation of acid secretion in the dog. Gastroenterology 66:526-523, 1974.
31. Sach G: The gastric H, K-ATPase: Regulation and structure/function of the acid pump of the stomach. In Johnson LR (ed): Physiology of the Gastrointestinal Tract, 3rd ed. New York, Raven Press, 1994, pp 1119-1138.
32. Helmer KS, West SD, Vilela R, et al: Lipopolysaccharide-induced changes in rat gastric H/K-ATPase expression. Ann Surg 239:501-509, 2004.
33. Courtois-Country N, Roush D, Rajendran V, et al: A tyrosine-based signal targets H/K-ATPase to a regulated compartment and is required for the cessation of gastric acid secretion. Cell 90:501-510, 1997.
34. Heyland D, Mandell LA: Gastric colonization by gram-negative bacilli and nosocomial pneumonia in the intensive care unit patient. Evidence for causation. Chest 101:187-193, 1992.
35. Driks MR, Craven DE, Celli BR, et al: Nosocomial pneumonia in intubated patients given sucralfate as compared with antacids or histamine type 2 blockers. The role of gastric colonization. N Engl J Med 317:1376-1382, 1987.
36. Tryba M, Zevounou F, Torok M, Zenz M: Prevention of acute stress bleeding with sucralfate, antacids, or cimetidine. A controlled study with pirenzepine as a basic medication. Am J Med 27(2C):55-61, 1985.
37. Samloff IM: Peptic ulcer: The many proteinases of aggression. Gastroenterology 96(2 Suppl):586-595, 1989.
38. Helmer KS, West SD, Shipley G, et al: Gastric nitric oxide synthase expression during endotoxemia: Implications in mucosal defense in rats. Gastroenterology 123:173-186, 2002.
39. Dunn BE: Pathogenic mechanisms of *Helicobacter pylori*. Gastroenterol Clin North Am 22:43-57, 1993.
40. Mueller A, Merrell DS, Grimm J, Falkow S: Profiling of microdissected gastric epithelial cells reveals a cell type–specific response to *Helicobacter pylori* infection. Gastroenterology 127:1446-1462, 2004.
41. Quigley EM, Turnberg LA: pH of the microclimate lining human gastric and duodenal mucosa in vivo. Studies in control subjects and in duodenal ulcer patients. Gastroenterology 92:1876-1884, 1987.

42. Silen W, Ito S: Mechanisms for rapid re-epithelialization of the gastric mucosal surface. Annu Rev Physiol 47:217-229, 1985.

43. Cox AJ: Stomach size and its relation to chronic peptic ulcer. Arch Pathol 54:407-422, 1952.

44. Rotter JI, Sones JQ, Samloff IM, et al: Duodenal-ulcer disease associated with elevated serum pepsinogen 1: An inherited autosomal dominant disorder. N Engl J Med 300:63-66, 1979.

45. Huizinga JD: Physiology and pathophysiology of the interstitial cell of Cajal: From bench to bedside: II. Gastric motility: Lessons from mutant mice on slow waves and innervation. Am J Physiol Gastrointest Liver Physiol 281:G1129-G1134, 2001.

46. Hinder RA, Kelly KA: Human gastric pacesetter potential: Site of origin, spread, and response to gastric transection and proximal gastric vagotomy. Am J Surg 139:29-33, 1977.

47. Azpiroz F, Malagelada JR: Gastric tone measured by an electronic barostat in health and postsurgical gastroparesis. Gastroenterology 92:934-943, 1987.

48. Abrahamsson H: Gastrointestinal motility disorders in patients with diabetes mellitus. J Intern Med 237:403-409, 1995.

49. Saslow SB, Thumshirn M, Camilleri M, et al: Influence of *H. pylori* infection on gastric motor and sensory function in asymptomatic volunteers. Dig Dis Sci 42:258-264, 1998.

50. Peeters TL: Erythromycin and other macrolides as prokinetic agents. Gastroenterology 105:1886-1899, 1993.

51

Diagnostic and Therapeutic Endoscopy of the Stomach and Small Bowel

Jeffrey M. Marks · Jeffrey L. Ponsky

Utilization of flexible endoscopic techniques for the diagnosis of gastrointestinal (GI) diseases of the stomach and small bowel has become the gold standard. Advances in instrumentation have also allowed for therapeutic interventions such that many problems previously requiring surgery are now managed in a less invasive fashion. In addition, newer technologies have facilitated further endoscopic diagnosis of small intestinal disease that had always been somewhat elusive to the flexible endoscope. Finally, further evolution of endoscopic procedures may eventually allow transvisceral access to the peritoneal cavity to perform appendectomy, organ removal, anastomoses, or treatment of gastroesophageal reflux disease, morbid obesity, and cancer.

DIAGNOSTIC ENDOSCOPY OF THE STOMACH

Indications

Common indications for diagnostic endoscopy include evaluation of pain that persists despite medical therapy, evaluation of symptoms in the postoperative stomach, assessment of hematemesis or GI bleeding from a suspected upper GI source, evaluation of an abnormal radiographic study, or follow-up for previously biopsied gastric ulcers. Other indications requiring upper endoscopy for evaluation of the esophagus include long-standing reflux disease, dysphagia, odynophagia, or work-up of identified cervical lymph node metastasis. Esophagoscopy is discussed in Chapter 6. Anatomic abnormalities of the stomach such as paraesophageal hernias, volvulus, or outlet obstruction can also be evaluated endoscopically. Finally, diagnostic esophagogastroduodenoscopy (EGD) may be used for sampling of gastric/jejunal tissue or fluid, surveillance of patients with familial adenomatous polyposis, or follow-up for symptoms of suspected organic disease and weight loss.

Indications for therapeutic endoscopy of the stomach include treatment of bleeding, dilation of gastric outlet obstruction, and resection of gastric tumors by either polypectomy or endoscopic mucosal resection. Laparoscopic-assisted therapeutic endoscopy has also been used for the management of GI stromal tumors. In addition, future technologies of transgastric intra-abdominal surgery are being developed for the management of appendicitis, cholecystitis, and alimentary tract obstruction.

EGD is not indicated in patients with chronic, non-progressive, and atypical symptoms without evidence of organic disease. It is also not indicated in patients with metastatic adenocarcinoma of an unknown primary when identification of the primary tumor will not result in alteration of management. EGD is contraindicated when the risk to the patient outweighs the most likely expected benefit of the procedure, when adequate patient cooperation cannot be achieved, or if a perforated viscus is already known or suspected.

Endoscopic Instrumentation and Patient Preparation

Flexible endoscopes initially contained fiberoptic bundles for transmission of light to the tip of the scope and return of a real image back to the endoscopist's eye. With advancement in video monitors and computer processors, flexible endoscopes now use fiberoptics only for transmission of light, and the image is transmitted via a CCD (charge-coupled device) computer chip at the tip of the endoscope. Similar to laparoscopy, multiple observers and assistants can observe a similar image, thereby permitting enhanced assistance when performing advanced therapeutic procedures. It also provides better opportunities for education.

Flexible endoscopes with smaller outer diameters and larger biopsy channels have resulted in better patient tolerance and comfort and the performance of complex interventions. Double-channel endoscopes allow "two-handed techniques" such as mucosal resection and tissue approximation in the absence of more effective endoscopic suturing devices. Early prototypes of robotic arms placed on the outside of the endoscope have been used in an animal model and are hoped to some day solve the limitations of present instrumentation in performing advanced transgastric intra-abdominal procedures.

Preparation for diagnostic and therapeutic endoscopy of the stomach requires merely 6 to 8 hours of fasting before the procedure.[1] Patients with gastric outlet obstruction or profound gastroparesis require a longer period of fasting, and tube decompression before the procedure may be prudent. Fasting before the procedure may not be feasible in emergency situations such as GI bleeding, caustic ingestion, or foreign body removal. In these situations, one may consider the use of general anesthesia and endotracheal intubation to protect the airway and prevent aspiration. Otherwise, in the majority of cases, conscious sedation with the combination of a narcotic and a benzodiazepine delivered intravenously and titrated slowly is used to achieve acceptable patient sedation and comfort.

Delivery of conscious sedation requires adequate monitoring with pulse oximetry, blood pressure recordings, and regular documentation of respiration. In patients with extensive upper GI bleeding, placement of a large-bore orogastric tube is necessary for saline lavage to clear clots and old blood. Whether cold or warm water should be used has been debated, without identification of actual clinical benefit from one or the other. It should be noted that lavage of ice water may lead to hypothermia in patients with massive GI hemorrhage, possibly accentuating a coagulopathic state.

After delivery of conscious sedation and placement of the patient in the left lateral decubitus position, the endoscope is passed under direct visualization into the esophagus. Inspection of the vocal cords is important to rule out polyps or upper airway obstruction (Figs. 51–1 and 51–2). The endoscope is advanced posterior to the arytenoid processes, and with careful pressure and instillation of air, the endoscope is passed beyond the upper esophageal sphincter into the cervical esophagus under direct visualization. Asking the patient to swallow, as well as placing the head in a flexed position, may assist in this portion of the procedure. The endoscope is then advanced with direct view of the lumen at all times. The esophagus can be somewhat tortuous in older patients, and the endoscopist must be aware that anatomic changes such as cervical ribs or an esophageal diverticulum may increase the risk for complications such as perforation.

The squamous mucosa of the esophagus is somewhat shiny and whitish in coloration. Endoscopic findings in the esophagus and their management are discussed in Chapter 6. After advancement of the endoscope into the stomach, air is insufflated to distend the stomach. As the

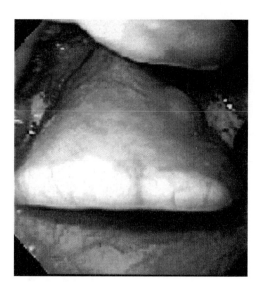

Figure 51–1.   Initial view of the epiglottis before passage of the endoscope into posterior part of the pharynx.

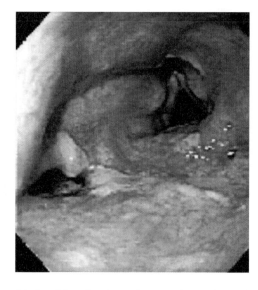

Figure 51–2.   Visualization of normal vocal cords during esophagogastroduodenoscopy (EGD) is a vital part of a complete EGD.

endoscope advances into the stomach, it assumes a "greater curve position," with the posterior wall at 3 o'clock, the greater curvature at 6 o'clock, the anterior wall at 9 o'clock, and the lesser curvature in the 12-o'clock position. When the scope is initially advanced into the stomach, rugal folds are identified in the fundus and body and are typically absent at the junction of the distal body and antrum (Figs. 51–3 and 51–4). As the scope is advanced further, the pylorus comes into view and appears round, but it may have different contours as a result of associated inflammatory diseases (Figs. 51–5 and 51–6). By continuing to look upward beyond the pylorus, a retroflex view will be obtained with visualization of the incisura and fundus of the stomach (Fig.

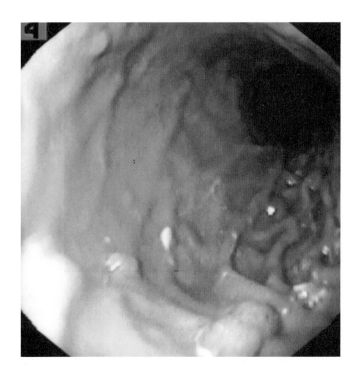

Figure 51–3. Appearance of the proximal part of the stomach with the presence of numerous rugal folds. Several small fundic gland polyps are also seen.

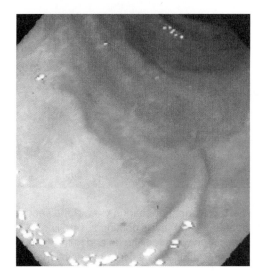

Figure 51–4. As the endoscope is advanced into the distal end of the stomach at the juncture of the body and antrum, the rugal folds become less pronounced.

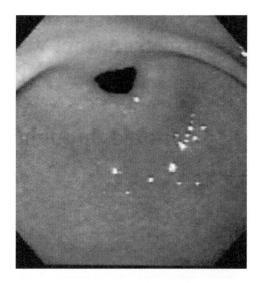

Figure 51–5. Normal-appearing distal antrum and pylorus.

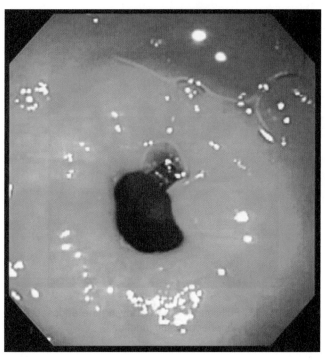

Figure 51–6. Notched pylorus secondary to a previous inflammatory process.

51–7). Withdrawing the endoscope at this time results in paradoxical movement and allows complete circumferential visualization of the fundus and cardia (Fig. 51–8). Full evaluation should be performed and the fundic pool should be aspirated to allow completion of this endoscopic evaluation. Evaluation of the angularis is important to rule out type I gastric ulcers.

The endoscope should then be advanced through the pylorus into the pyloric channel with assessment of all surfaces circumferentially to rule out duodenal ulcers (Fig. 51–9). Advancement of the scope into the second portion of the duodenum is possible by merely looking up and to the right and trolling back on the endoscope. This maneuver places the scope in what is called a "lesser curve" or "short" position and provides paradoxical advancement of the endoscope further down into the second and third portions of the duodenum (Fig. 51–10). With a forward-viewing scope, visualization of the ampullary complex may be somewhat difficult, but it may

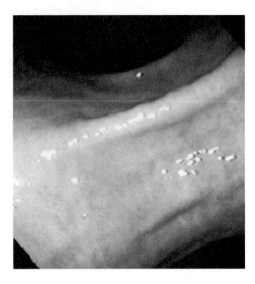

Figure 51–7. Retroflex view in the stomach showing the antrum and fundus simultaneously, separated by the angularis.

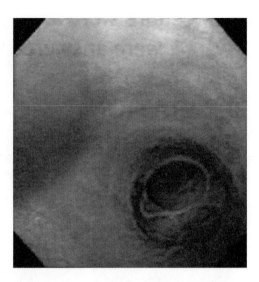

Figure 51–9. The smooth surfaces of the duodenal bulb are visualized after advancing through the pylorus. No valvulae conniventes (folds) are present in the bulb.

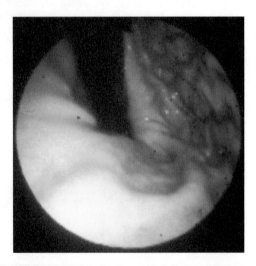

Figure 51–8. Full retroflex view showing the endoscope as it traverses the esophagogastric junction.

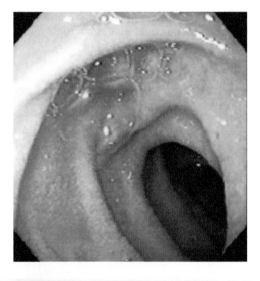

Figure 51–10. Normal-appearing view of the second portion of the duodenum. This view is obtained by trolling back (pulling out) the endoscope while looking up and to the right; the endoscope is left in a "short" or lesser curve position.

be seen at the 9-o'clock position. A side-viewing endoscope is necessary to obtain a full endoscopic view of this portion of the duodenum. The endoscope can then be withdrawn back into the stomach, and the luminal surfaces should again be reinspected for any abnormalities. The stomach is quite full at this juncture and should be evacuated of air before withdrawing the endoscope. If the vocal cords had not been inspected on intubation, they should be inspected during withdrawal of the endoscope. At completion of the procedure, patients are observed during resolution of the conscious sedation, and a clear liquid diet is started. Usually within 30 to 60 minutes patients should be stable for discharge from the endoscopy unit.

Gastric Pathology

The ability to differentiate normal from abnormal findings at the time of endoscopy is vital to ensure appropriate patient care. Normal variations, though possibly peculiar in appearance, may not require any intervention. Gastric lesions that can be identified at the time of endoscopy include inflammatory processes, benign and malignant neoplasia, vascular abnormalities, postoperative deformities, congenital lesions, and foreign bodies. Inflammatory changes of the gastric mucosa are the most common finding at the time of diagnostic endoscopy. Inflammatory changes in the stomach may be secondary

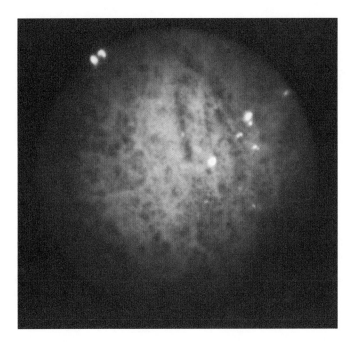

Figure 51–11. Diffuse gastritis in the body of the stomach. Testing for *Helicobacter pylori* must always be done in this situation.

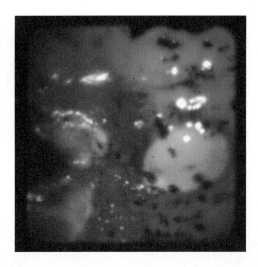

Figure 51–12. Coffee ground material secondary to bleeding seen in conjunction with multiple ulcerations in the distal part of the stomach.

to medications, infections, caustic agents, postoperative changes in the upper digestive tract, or severe physiologic stress secondary to sepsis, hypoxia, or hypoperfusion (Fig. 51–11). A thorough physical examination and history are required, including identification of comorbid diseases, exogenous stress, previous surgery, and a social history of drugs, alcohol, and tobacco use.

Initial endoscopic evaluation must include documentation of the location and extent of the inflammatory process, associated anatomic changes, and intraluminal contents such as excessive bile, coffee ground material, undigested food, or blood (Fig. 51–12). Bleeding may be commonly associated with these conditions and may vary from minor occult bleeding with associated iron deficiency anemia all the way to severe active bleeding with hemodynamic compromise. Identification of the presence of *Helicobacter pylori* infection is also important for providing appropriate and complete treatment. Numerous tests are available for identification of *H. pylori*, including histology, urease testing (CLO test), serologic antibody testing, and the carbon-labeled urea breath test.[2] Eradication of *H. pylori* with antibiotic therapy is important when treating inflammatory lesions of the stomach. Antibiotic therapy minimizes the risk for recurrence in patients with *H. pylori*–associated inflammatory diseases of the stomach.[3]

Gastric ulcers may be identified in the prepyloric, body, and fundic portions of the stomach (Fig. 51–13). In addition, peptic ulcers may also hide on the angularis, and thus endoscopic evaluation of the entire stomach, including retroflex views, is important to discern these processes. Gastric ulcers found at the time of endoscopy require aggressive biopsy of all margins at the junction of the edges of the base and surrounding gastric mucosa

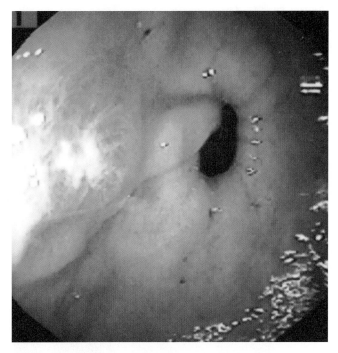

Figure 51–13. Prepyloric ulcer with surrounding induration of the gastric mucosa.

(Fig. 51–14). Suspicion of malignancy may be supported by the presence of heaped edges, deeper ulcerated bases, or diffuse infiltrative processes. Follow-up endoscopy within 8 to 12 weeks is necessary for ulcers that are benign by initial biopsy but have an atypical appearance, are larger than 2 cm, appear suspicious pathologically, or are leading to persistent symptoms. Absence of healing at the time of second endoscopy may be an indication for surgical excision (Fig. 51–15).

Congenital lesions of the stomach are also frequently identified at the time of endoscopy. Hiatal hernias are

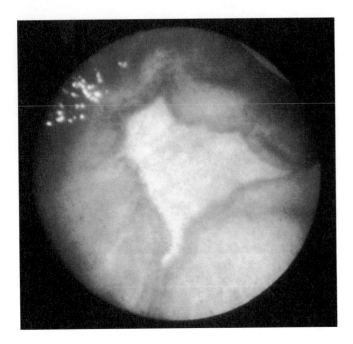

Figure 51–14. Large benign gastric ulcer seen on the greater curvature of the stomach.

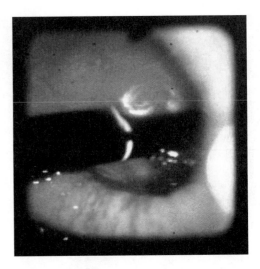

Figure 51–16. Type I sliding hiatal hernia seen on a retroflex view.

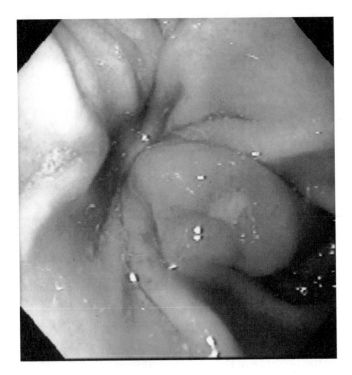

Figure 51–15. A chronic nonhealing gastric ulcer seen after 12 weeks of medical therapy. Multiple biopsy specimens of the periphery of the ulcer base are required again, and even with benign results on biopsy, surgical resection must be strongly considered.

the most frequently encountered deformity of the stomach and may be identified during passage of the endoscope from the esophagus into the stomach or on the retroflex view (Fig. 51–16). These hernias may play no clinical role in a patient's symptoms but are commonly associated with reflux disease or dysphagia. Careful measurements from the incisors to the gastroesophageal junction, Z-line (squamous columnar junction), and diaphragmatic incursion on the stomach are important markers with implications for surgical intervention in this process. In patients with large paraesophageal hernias, entry into the stomach may be inhibited by incarceration of the stomach in an intrathoracic position. Commonly, paradoxical movement of the endoscope occurs when one tries to advance the endoscope into a gastric lumen complicated by a paraesophageal hernia. The endoscope will most likely not be able to be advanced into the body of the stomach, and the pylorus will not be visualized. Rarely, advancement of the endoscope may allow reduction of the stomach back into an intra-abdominal position, and temporary fixation can be provided at that time via percutaneous endoscopic gastrostomy.

Other congenital lesions identified may include antral webs or pyloric stenosis. Antral webs mimic the appearance of the pylorus but occur in the more proximal part of the antrum, and one may visualize the associated antral ring. Pyloric stenosis is more commonly seen in children, although it can be identified in adults. The diagnosis is made when the endoscope cannot be advanced beyond the pyloric channel and there is no associated inflammatory changes (Fig. 51–17). One final congenital lesion occasionally discovered, a pancreatic rest, is typically found in the antrum or duodenum and appears as a 5- to 10-mm raised donut-shaped lesion with a central punctate center (Fig. 51–18). These processes are benign, and biopsy will prove these rests to be of pancreatic origin.

Upper GI bleeding is quite common, and endoscopic identification of vascular abnormalities such as gastric

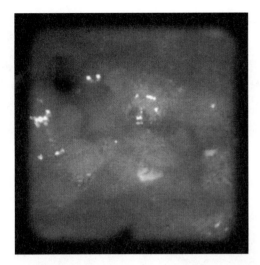

Figure 51–17. Pyloric stenosis.

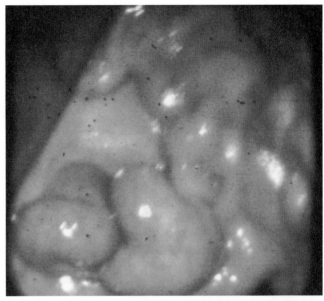

Figure 51–19. Gastric varices in the cardia of the stomach.

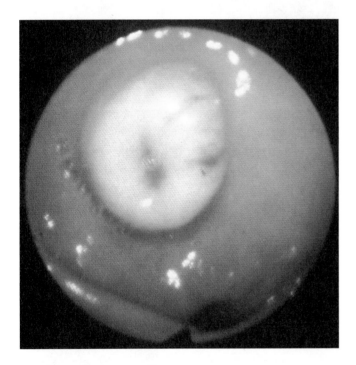

Figure 51–18. A pancreatic rest in the distal body of the stomach. No intervention is required for this benign congenital process.

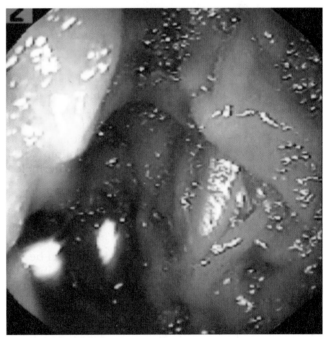

Figure 51–20. Arteriovenous malformation of the proximal part of the small bowel.

varices, angiodysplasia, and ulcerative lesions may require endoscopic therapy. Gastric varices are related to portal hypertension and are most commonly due to splenic vein thrombosis secondary to either pancreatitis or pancreatic neoplasms. Gastric varices may or may not be associated with esophageal varices and are most frequently found in the fundus (Fig. 51–19). Absence of esophageal varices is more pathognomonic of splenic vein than portal vein thrombosis. Gastric varices appear as serpentine folds crossing over the normally positioned gastric rugal folds. As opposed to rugal folds, varices are easily compressed when palpated with an endoscopic

instrument. In addition, endoscopic ultrasound may be useful in the diagnosis of varices. Prophylactic therapy in patients without bleeding is debatable and may not alter overall survival. Angiodysplasia and arteriovenous malformations appear as red discolorations with tortuous feeding vessels at their base (Fig. 51–20). They may or may not have active bleeding at the time of endoscopy, and they are usually multicentric. A subset of angiodysplasia termed gastric antral vascular ectasia (GAVE)

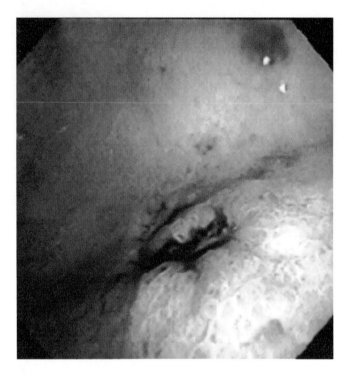

Figure 51–21. Dieulafoy's ulcer of the proximal part of the stomach.

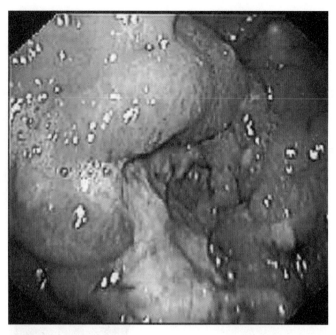

Figure 51–22. Diffuse gastric carcinoma of the distal end of the stomach.

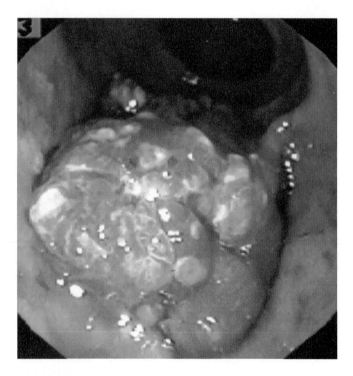

Figure 51–23. Inflammatory polyp with overlying mucosal irregularities.

refers to the presence of numerous vascular lesions throughout the antrum in a linear fashion and is also commonly referred to as watermelon stomach. GAVE was first identified by Jabbari et al. in 1984, and the term was used to describe the striped vascular lesions seen in watermelon stomach.[4] Argon plasma coagulation (APC) has been shown to be an effective therapy for watermelon stomach.[5-7]

Dieulafoy's lesions are superficial ulcerations with underlying exposed arterial structures that are commonly found in the upper portions of the stomach; they can be the source of massive upper GI bleeding (Fig. 51–21). If not actively bleeding, these lesions can be discriminated by endoscopic ultrasound or identified by visualizing bleeding stigmata of an exposed vessel in a small-caliber ulcer base. Gastric varices and GAVE syndrome are much less common than other sources of upper GI bleeding, such as gastritis and ulcers. It should be noted that most of these vascular lesions identified at the time of endoscopy can be managed with therapeutic maneuvers involving either thermal or nonthermal techniques.

Neoplasms of the stomach may be either benign or malignant. Cancer of the stomach has a wide variety of endoscopic appearances, including fungating, ulcerating, infiltrating, and exophytic (Fig. 51–22). Polypoid lesions may be inflammatory or adenomatous. Inflammatory polyps can be quite numerous, and although they may grow extremely large, they carry no malignant potential (Fig. 51–23). Fundic gland-type polyps are included in this category (Fig. 51–24). Adenomatous polyps of the stomach are also predominantly benign but should be removed because they have a small malignant potential similar to polyps in the colon. Other benign lesions include leiomyomas, lipomas, carcinoid, and pancreatic rests (Fig. 51–25). Leiomyomas, or gastrointestinal stromal tumors, are commonly found in the cardia of the stomach adjacent to the gastroesophageal junction (Fig. 51–26). They may lead to occult blood loss and have

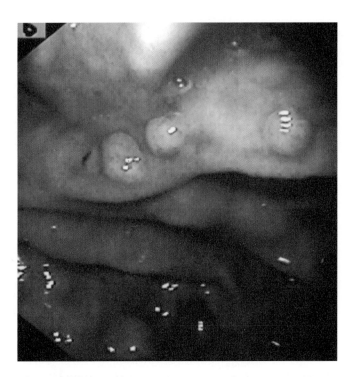

Figure 51–24. Multiple fundic gland polyps seen in the proximal part of the stomach. Random sampling is all that is required.

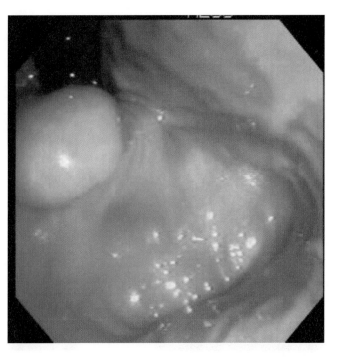

Figure 51–26. Gastrointestinal stromal tumor adjacent to the gastroesophageal junction.

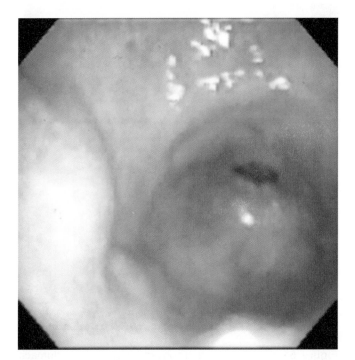

Figure 51–25. A submucosal mass identified in the distal end of the stomach eventually proved to be a gastrointestinal stromal tumor.

malignant potential based on size, mucosal invasion, and mitotic activity. Because of extension of leiomyomas through the entire gastric wall, endoscopic resection may result in full-thickness perforation or bleeding. A combined endoscopic and laparoscopic or intraluminal laparoscopic approach may be warranted. Benign submucosal lesions such as lipomas may require intervention before they lead to obstruction.

Standard endoscopic imaging can be enhanced with several techniques to improve visualization of obscure GI disease. Several staining solutions, including Lugol's solution, methylene blue, acetic acid, and indigo carmine, have been used to enhance discrimination of normal and abnormal tissue. Inflammatory tissue does not stain with Lugol's solution, and methylene blue is readily absorbed into absorptive epithelium such as intestinal metaplasia of the stomach or esophagus. Magnification endoscopy may also allow for more accurate identification of intestinal metaplasia and dysplasia, although it requires extended time for endoscopy and has quite variable sensitivity and specificity.[8]

Management of Bleeding

Endoscopic techniques for the management of bleeding can be divided into thermal and nonthermal modalities. Thermal modalities include bipolar and monopolar contact probes, APC, and laser therapy. Contact probes use direct tissue delivery of current and provide a deeper source of energy than APC does (Fig. 51–27). Hemostasis of an active bleeding site in the stomach may best be handled by initial injection sclerotherapy followed by delivery of thermal energy. Contact probes provide an

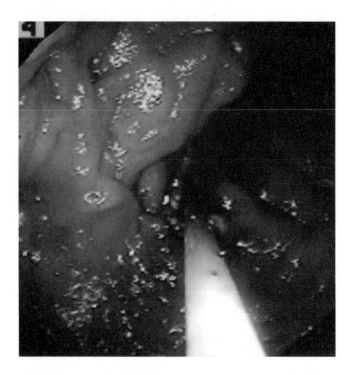

Figure 51–27. Cauterization of a small bowel arteriovenous malformation with an endoscopic contact probe.

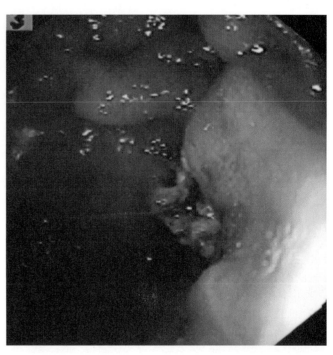

Figure 51–28. Appearance of mucosa after treatment of an arteriovenous malformation with contact probe therapy.

advantage in certain situations because of the ability to provide direct tamponade at the time of energy delivery (Fig. 51–28). APC provides a more superficial depth of penetration and may therefore be associated with a smaller risk of perforation than is the case with contact probes. In addition, APC can be applied over broader surface areas, similar to spray paint, as opposed to the single site of therapy provided by contact probes.[5-7]

Before any endoscopic management of gastric bleeding, adequate preparation of the stomach must be provided with gastric lavage via a large oral gastric tube (Fig. 51–29). Airway control with endotracheal intubation should be considered in patients with massive GI bleeding before initiating endoscopic treatment. Endoscopic management of gastric bleeding should be considered the first line of therapy, and reports have shown less morbidity and mortality than with initial surgical intervention when endoscopy has been used for both the initial episode of bleeding and the scenario of recurrent GI bleeding. Even if the patient requires surgical intervention, as long as endoscopy can be provided quickly and efficiently, the patient will benefit if the source of bleeding can be identified and slowed before an emergency surgical procedure. Flexible endoscopy will also guide the appropriate surgical therapy and is vital in differentiating the varied causes of gastric bleeding.

Nonthermal techniques for the management of gastric bleeding continue to be developed and improved. Injection sclerotherapy was probably the first nonthermal modality and is effective in achieving tissue hemostasis on the basis of several pathways. Injectable agents such as sodium morrhuate lead to vessel sclerosis, whereas vasoconstriction and local compression can be

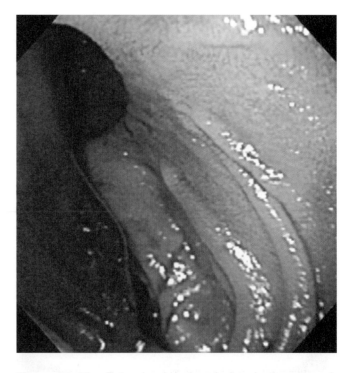

Figure 51–29. Extensive blood and clots in the stomach from a bleeding duodenal ulcer, which will limit the endoscopic examination and treatment if not adequately cleared with pre-endoscopic gastric lavage.

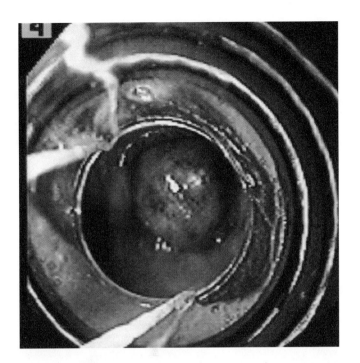

Figure 51–30. Image through the endoscopic band ligator after placement of a band.

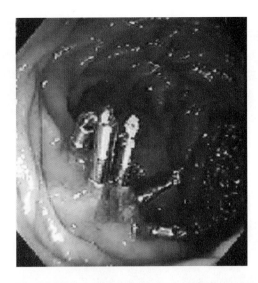

Figure 51–31. Endoscopic clips placed on a bleeding duodenal ulcer for hemostasis.

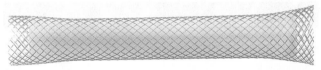

Figure 51–32. Self-expanding metal stent that can be used for palliation of an enteric stricture. These types of stents are considered unremovable and are predominantly used for malignant disease.

provided by other injected components such as saline, alcohol, or epinephrine. Injection therapy may be one of the best ways to provide initial hemostasis through the combination of these three factors, but one must be careful to avoid extensive tissue destruction because perforation may result. Perforation is more common in the thin-walled areas of the small bowel and colon, as opposed to the stomach. Combination contact probes and injection sclerotherapy needles are now available and provide efficient endoscopic management of GI bleeding without having to use numerous tools.

Other endoscopic nonthermal tools include clips, detachable loops, band ligators, and endoscopic suturing devices. A combination of thermal and nonthermal techniques may provide the best chance for resolution of GI bleeding. Detachable snares similar to laparoscopic Endoloops can be used to encircle structures and, after ligation, provide hemostasis. They are commonly used on stalks of pedunculated polyps that bleed after polypectomy. Endoscopic band ligation was first used for the management of esophageal varices, but it may also be used in the gastric lumen on gastric varices or Dieulafoy lesions (Fig. 51–30). Endoscopic clips provide mucosal approximation, as well as superficial vessel closure (Fig. 51–31). They usually fall off within 4 to 7 days. Novel endoscopic suturing devices are probably still too cumbersome to be used in patients with active GI bleeding, but they can be used to provide mucosal approximation over exposed submucosal surfaces after endoscopic resection. In the future, it is hoped that suturing technology will mimic that of open surgery.

Nonoperative management of alimentary tract obstruction has been performed since 1885 when Charter Simonds was able to relieve an esophageal

obstruction with a short hollow wooden tube. Since that time, advancements in stent materials have allowed the development of smaller-diameter delivery systems (Fig. 51–32). In addition, the higher expansile force of these stents has led to increased patency. Endoscopic balloon dilation for benign alimentary tract strictures such as congenital pyloric stenosis or peptic ulcer–induced stenosis is now available. Balloon dilation via hydrostatic force can provide resolution, although complex strictures may require multiple serial dilations to achieve success. The risk for perforation is lower with hydrostatic balloons than with the pneumatic balloon dilators used previously. In patients with gastric emptying abnormalities, pyloric dilation may also be beneficial. Another endoscopic technique that has been investigated in small series for the treatment of gastroparesis or chronic gas/bloating syndromes is botulinum toxin treatment of the pylorus.[9] In a study by Bromer et al., more than 40% of patients had a short-term response.

Palliation of intrinsic and extrinsic lesions secondary to gastric, duodenal, or pancreatic cancer can be provided by endoscopic techniques, including laser debulking, dilation, or endoscopic stent placement. Self-expanding metallic stents have been shown to provide decreased complication rates (Figs. 51–33 and 51–34). In a multicenter study of palliation of patients with malignant gastric outlet obstruction, deployment of

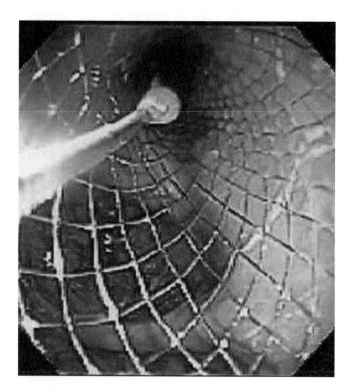

Figure 51–33. Endoscopic image after deployment of a self-expanding metal stent for malignant gastric outlet obstruction.

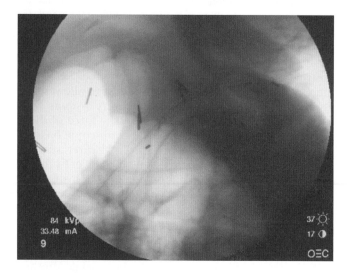

Figure 51–34. Fluoroscopic image of a self-expanding metal stent deployed across malignant gastric outlet obstruction.

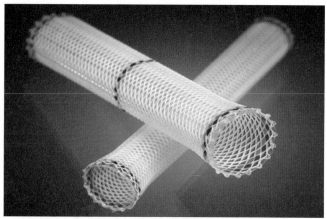

Figure 51–35. Covered self-expanding plastic stent that can be used for the treatment of strictures or fistulas. Unlike metal stents, these stents are to be removed after 2 to 3 months.

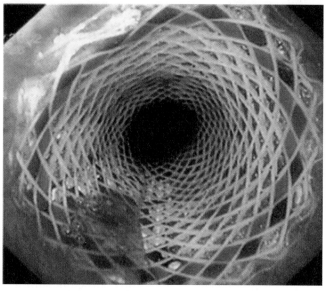

Figure 51–36. Endoluminal view after deployment of a self-expanding plastic stent.

self-expanding metallic stents was technically successful in 173 of 176 patients.[10] Eighty-four percent of patients resumed oral intake. It should be noted that expandable plastic stents that are removable have been used in small series for benign disease (Figs. 51–35 and 51–36). The longevity of relief of obstruction from stenting of benign gastric and duodenal strictures is not truly known, and dilation may be more beneficial. Overall, these patients may be better served by either resective therapy or operative gastroenteric bypass.

The role of endoscopy in the management of gastric neoplasia has advanced from a solely diagnostic use to a therapeutic technique over the past decade. Endoscopic mucosal resection techniques have allowed the removal of benign masses, as well as early gastric cancer. With the use of a double-lumen gastroscope, mucosal resection can be performed with a modified needle knife sphincterotome. Mucosal defects can then be reapproximated with endoscopic clips. Other techniques such as saline-lift or cap-assisted snare endoscopic mucosal resection also allow for larger segments of tissue to be removed safely. Submucosal masses such as GI stromal tumors and carcinoid tumors can likewise be removed with endoscopic resective techniques. A concern with this approach, however, is the resultant full-thickness injury. One of the great limitations to fully endoscopic resective techniques is the ability to suture because endoscopic suturing techniques are still very primitive.

The combination of endoscopic and laparoscopic approaches for deeper tumors or those higher up on the cardia of the stomach can be beneficial. Laparoscopic evaluation at the time of endoscopic resection can identify the presence of a full-thickness defect, as well as provide access for repair. An alternative to the combined endoscopic and laparoscopic approach is intragastric laparoscopic techniques with ports placed in the gastric lumen.

Transgastric Endoscopic Surgery

Natural orifice transvisceral endoscopic surgery procedures have been investigated in animal models and performed in several small human series. Cholecystectomy, cholecystogastric anastomosis, gastroenteric anastomosis, appendectomy, and tubal ligation have all been attempted with transgastric techniques.[11-14] There are numerous inherent limitations in the use of transgastric techniques, including gastrotomy creation, reliable gastrotomy closure, abdominal insufflation, tissue retraction/exposure, tissue approximation, and difficulties with imaging. Other transvisceral techniques, or natural orifice surgeries, via the colon or vagina could possibly allow for a more direct avenue into the upper part of the abdomen. All these technologies need to be further investigated for efficacy and risk. One concern is intraperitoneal infectious complications related to visceral violation. These technologies may eventually require a combination of transvisceral and transabdominal laparoscopic techniques with an endoscope advanced via natural access in combination with microlaparoscopy devices for tissue manipulation or retraction. As endoscopic tools are improved, transvisceral techniques may find a role in the management of numerous intra-abdominal disease processes.

DIAGNOSTIC ENDOSCOPY OF THE SMALL BOWEL

Endoscopic evaluation plus treatment of lesions of the small bowel has always been very challenging. Transoral and transanal routes have been used and provide the ability to see the most proximal and most distal aspects of the small bowel, respectively. Push enteroscopy can be a valuable tool to identify mucosal abnormalities, as well as sources of bleeding in patients with an unidentified cause (Figs. 51–37 and 51–38). Push enteroscopy allows for biopsy and in some cases actual therapeutic interventions for bleeding. The use of an overtube permits advancement of the endoscope without the normal buckling of the scope in the greater curve position of the stomach. The overall diagnostic yield of push enteroscopy is about 30% in most series.[15-17]

Recently developed endoscopic modifications, as well as novel imaging devices, have allowed improved visual-

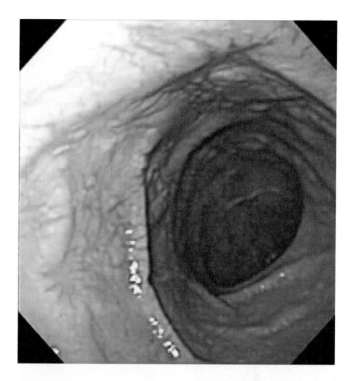

Figure 51–37. Small bowel sprue identified by push enteroscopy.

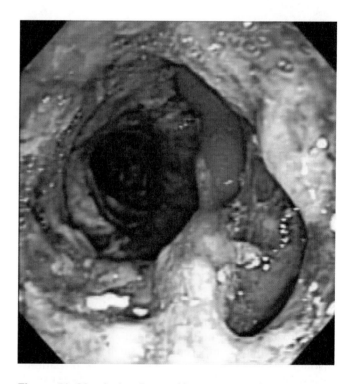

Figure 51–38. Ischemic enteritis seen on push enteroscopy.

ization of small bowel disease. Wireless capsule endoscopy has rapidly emerged as a safe and well-tolerated tool for assessment of small bowel lesions (Fig. 51–39). Capsule endoscopy can be used for the diagnosis of obscure GI bleeding, as well as inflammatory bowel

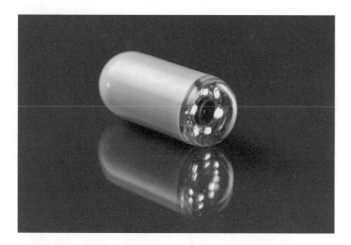

Figure 51–39. Capsule used for wireless endoscopy.

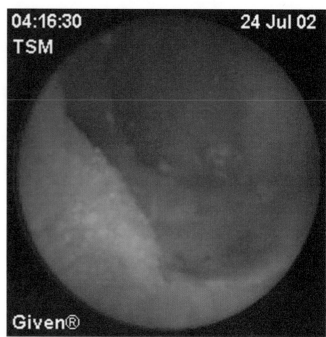

Figure 51–41. Arteriovenous malformation seen on capsule endoscopy.

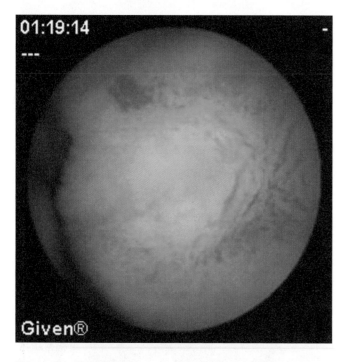

Figure 51–40. Wireless capsule endoscopic view of a small bowel arteriovenous malformation.

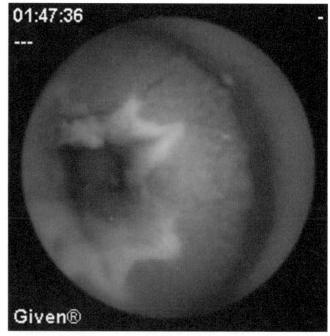

Figure 51–42. Wireless capsule endoscopic image revealing small bowel ulceration and stricture secondary to Crohn's disease.

disease (Figs. 51–40 to 51–42).[18-29] Small bowel tumors have also been identified with capsule endoscopy (Fig. 51–43).[30] When compared with small bowel follow-through, capsule endoscopy identified 29% of patients with small bowel polyps as compared with 12% via small bowel follow-through. In another series comparing capsule endoscopy with push enteroscopy and entero-clysis, capsule endoscopy detected more lesions than the other two modalities did, and this led to a change in management in 70% of these patients.[31] Capsule endoscopy, however, is only a diagnostic tool and must be carefully used in patients with suspected small bowel obstruction or strictures.

The ability of intraoperative enteroscopy via enterotomy to identify occult small bowel sources of bleeding ranges from 70% to 100%.[32-39] Intraoperative enteroscopy, however, can be associated with a higher rate of complications, including wound infection,

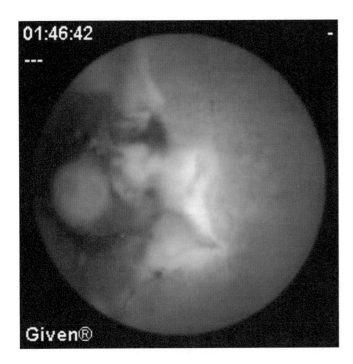

Figure 51–43. Polypoid mass in the small bowel seen on capsule endoscopy.

intestinal ischemia, mucosal laceration, and mesenteric hematoma. In one series comparing intraoperative enteroscopy as the gold standard with capsule endoscopy, capsule endoscopy had a sensitivity of 95% and a positive predictive value of 95%.[40]

Another novel technology being evaluated for the investigation of small bowel disease is double-balloon endoscopy. Peroral double-balloon enteroscopy has both diagnostic and therapeutic potential but is a time-consuming procedure requiring advanced endoscopic skills. In one case report, double-balloon endoscopy was used to identify a bleeding polyp in the distal end of the small bowel that was managed by a saline-lift polypectomy technique. At 8 months' follow-up, the patient had no evidence of recurrent bleeding.[41] Because these technologies are still in an evolutionary phase, therapeutic interventions for most small bowel lesions still commonly require a combination of endoscopic and surgical approaches with either intraoperative endoscopy and laparoscopy or endoscopic evaluation via enterotomy at the time of laparotomy.

CONCLUSION

Over the past several decades, flexible endoscopy has gained numerous therapeutic options that have now supplanted many surgical procedures for the management of GI disease. As these technologies continue to evolve in the future, it is imperative for GI surgeons to be skilled in these techniques, as well as maintain an understanding of the limitations, indications, and complications associated with these modalities.

REFERENCES

1. American Society of Gastrointestinal Endoscopists: Preparation of patients for gastrointestinal endoscopy [publication No. 1015]. Gastrointest Endosc 34:32s, 1988.
2. Cutler AF, Hvstad S, Ma C, et al: Accuracy of invasive and noninvasive tests to diagnose *Helicobacter pylori* infection. Gastroenterology 109:136, 1995.
3. Sung JJY, Chung SCS, Ling TKW, et al: Antibacterial treatment of gastric ulcers associated with *Helicobacter pylori*. N Engl J Med 332:139, 1995.
4. Jabbari M, Cherry R, Lough JO, et al: Gastric antral vascular ectasia: The watermelon stomach. Gastroenterology 87:1165, 1984.
5. Yusoff I, Brennan F, Ormonde D, et al: Argon plasma coagulation for treatment of watermelon stomach. Endoscopy 34:407, 2002.
6. Roman S, Saurin JC, Dumortier J, et al: Tolerance and efficacy of argon plasma coagulation for controlling bleeding in patients with typical and atypical manifestations of watermelon stomach. Endoscopy 35:1024, 2003.
7. Ginsberg GG, Barkun A, Bosco J, et al: The argon plasma coagulator. Gastrointest Endosc 55:807, 2002.
8. Sharma P: Magnification endoscopy. Gastrointest Endosc 61:435, 2005.
9. Bromer M, Friedenberg F, Miller L, et al: Endoscopic pyloric injection of botulinum toxin A for the treatment of refractory gastroparesis. Gastrointest Endosc 61:833, 2005.
10. Telford JJ, Carr-Locke DL, Baron TH, et al: Palliation of patients with malignant gastric outlet obstruction with the enteral Wallstent: Outcomes from a multicenter study. Gastrointest Endosc 60:916, 2004.
11. Jagannath S, Kantsevoy S, Vaughn C, et al: Peroral transgastric endoscopic ligation of fallopian tubes with long-term survival in a porcine model. Gastrointest Endosc 61:449, 2005.
12. Kalloo A, Singh V, Jagannath S, et al: Flexible transgastric peritoneoscopy: A novel approach to diagnostic and therapeutic interventions in the peritoneal cavity. Gastrointest Endosc 60:114, 2004.
13. Fritscher-Ravens A, Mosse C, Muckherjee D, et al: Transluminal endosurgery: Single lumen access anastomotic device for flexible endoscopy. Gastrointest Endosc 58:585, 2003.
14. Park P, Bergstrom M, Ikeda K, et al: Experimental studies of transgastric gallbladder surgery: Cholecystectomy and cholecystogastric anastomosis. Gastrointest Endosc 61:601, 2005.
15. Lepere C, Cuilerier E, Gossum A, et al: Predictive factors of positive findings in patients explored by push enteroscopy for unexplained GI bleeding. Gastrointest Endosc 61:709, 2005.
16. Bouhnik Y, Bitoun A, Coffin B, et al: Two way push videoenteroscopy in investigation of small bowel disease. Gut 43:280, 1998.
17. Landi B, Tkoub M, Gaudric M, et al: Diagnostic yield of push-type enteroscopy in relation to indication. Gut 42:421, 1998.
18. Iddan G, Meron G, Glukhovsky A, et al: Wireless capsule endoscopy. Nature 25:405, 2000.
19. Lewis B, Swain P: Capsule endoscopy in the evaluation of patients with suspected small intestinal bleeding: Results of a pilot study. Gastrointest Endosc 56:349, 2002.
20. Ell C, Remke S, May A, et al: The first prospective controlled trial comparing wireless capsule endoscopy with push enteroscopy in chronic gastrointestinal bleeding. Endoscopy 34:685, 2002.
21. Costamagna G, Shah A, Ricconi M, et al: A prospective trial comparing small bowel radiographs and video capsule endoscopy for suspected small bowel disease. Gastroenterology 123:999, 2002.
22. Scapa E, Jacob H, Lemkowicz S, et al: Initial experience of wireless capsule endoscopy for evaluating occult gastrointestinal bleeding and suspected small bowel pathology. Am J Gastroenterol 97:2776, 2002.
23. Hartmann D, Schilling D, Bolz G, et al: Capsule endoscopy versus push enteroscopy in patients with occult gastrointestinal bleeding. Z Gastroenterol 41:377, 2003.
24. Saurin J, Delvaux M, Gaudin J, et al: Diagnostic value of endoscopic capsule in patients with obscure bleeding: Blinded comparison with video push enteroscopy. Endoscopy 35:576, 2003.
25. Mylonaki M, Fritscher-Ravens A, Swain A: Wireless capsule endoscopy: A comparison with push enteroscopy in patients with gastroscopy and colonoscopy negative gastrointestinal bleeding. Gut 52:1122, 2003.

26. Mata A, Bordas J, Feu F, et al: Wireless capsule endoscopy in patients with obscure bleeding: A comparative study with push enteroscopy. Aliment Pharmacol Ther 20:189, 2004.

27. Fireman Z, Mahajna E, Broide E, et al: Diagnosing small bowel Crohn's disease with wireless capsule endoscopy. Gut 52:390, 2003.

28. Eliakim R, Fischer D, Suissa, A, et al: Wireless capsule video endoscopy is a superior diagnostic tool in comparison to barium follow through and computerized tomography in patients with suspected Crohn's disease. Eur J Gastroenterol Hepatol 15:363, 2003.

29. Liangpunsakuo S, Chadalawada V, Rex D, et al: Wireless capsule endoscopy detects small bowel ulcers in patients with normal results from state of the art enteroclysis. Am J Gastroenterol 98:1295, 2003.

30. de Mascarenhas-Saraiva M, da Silva Araujo Lopes L: Small bowel tumors diagnosed by wireless capsule endoscopy: Report of five cases. Endoscopy 35:865, 2003.

31. Chong AKH, Taylor A, Miller A, et al: Capsule endoscopy vs. push enteroscopy and enteroclysis in suspected small-bowel Crohn's disease. Gastrointest Endosc 61:255, 2005.

32. Douard R, Wind P, Panis Y, et al: Intraoperative endoscopy for diagnosis and management of unexplained gastrointestinal bleeding. Am J Surg 180:181, 2000.

33. Szold A, Katz L, Lewis B: Surgical approach to occult gastrointestinal bleeding. Am J Surg 163:90, 1992.

34. Lau W, Fan S, Wong S, et al: Preoperative and intraoperative localization of gastrointestinal bleeding of obscure origin. Gut 28:869, 1987.

35. Lewis B, Wenger J, Waye J: Small bowel enteroscopy and intraoperative enteroscopy for obscure gastrointestinal bleeding. Am J Gastroenterol 86:171, 1991.

36. Ress A, Benacci J, Sarr M: Efficacy of intraoperative enteroscopy in diagnosis and prevention of recurrent occult gastrointestinal bleeding. Am J Surg 163:94, 1992.

37. Desa L, Ohri S, Hutton K, et al: Role of intraoperative enteroscopy in obscure gastrointestinal bleeding of small bowel origin. Br J Surg 78:192, 1991.

38. Lopez M, Cooley J, Etros J, et al: Complete intraoperative small bowel endoscopy in the evaluation of occult gastrointestinal bleeding using the sonde enteroscope. Arch Surg 131:272, 1996.

39. Bowden T, Hooks V, Mansberger A: Intraoperative gastrointestinal endoscopy. Ann Surg 191:680, 1980.

40. Hartman D, Schmidt H, Bolz G, et al: A prospective two-center study comparing wireless capsule endoscopy with intraoperative enteroscopy in patients with obscure bleeding. Gastrointest Endosc 61:826, 2005.

41. Kita H, Yamamoto H, Nakamura T, et al: Bleeding polyp in the mid small intestine identified by capsule endoscopy and treated by double-balloon endoscopy. Gastrointest Endosc 61:628, 2005.

52

Intubation of the Stomach and Small Intestine

Sean P. Harbison

Intubation of the gastrointestinal (GI) tract occurs frequently in the course of patient care for a variety of reasons. Enteral access, whether gastric or intestinal, nasal or percutaneous, is procured in the vast majority of instances for either decompression or nutrition. To a lesser extent, indications for intestinal intubation are both diagnostic and therapeutic for various disorders, such as upper GI bleeding. Despite the large number of devices and techniques for enteral intubation and the ubiquity of their use in modern medical and surgical practice, intestinal tubes are not always innocuous. Serious, even potentially fatal complications may result from placement or management complications of enteral tubes. Proper determination of the feasibility, timing, and route of access of intestinal tubes is essential for successful placement and use.

The treating surgeon must weigh the potential benefits of tube placement against possible morbidity. The time-honored practice of postoperative gastric decompression is being re-evaluated by evidence-based analysis. The conventional practice of postoperative gastric decompression via a nasogastric tube for patients undergoing laparotomy may not be required. The benefit of gastric decompression carries a concomitant risk of aspiration and sinusitis. Numerous studies, including a meta-analysis of more than 3000 postoperative patients, suggest that a selective approach to postoperative nasogastric decompression is more advantageous. Significantly more pulmonary complications occurred in patients with nasogastric tubes placed routinely, although there was no difference in wound-related complications when compared with selective placement of tubes for vomiting and gastric distention.[1]

Occasionally, patients undergoing laparotomy may not be able to tolerate intragastric feeding in the early postoperative period. Similar to GI intubation for decompression, the benefit of accessing the GI tract for feeding must be weighed against the potential risk associated with placement of a nasogastric or intraoperative feeding tube. The feasibility of placement, potential length of use, and route of enteral access are equally important considerations in determining the optimal intestinal intubation for nutrition. Gastric access for feeding may be of little value or even detrimental, such as in patients with a high risk for aspiration, impaired gastric emptying, or pancreatitis. It is imperative that the underlying medical and comorbid conditions, the anticipated length of time that enteral access will be required, and the setting in which it will occur be taken into account. Thoughtful consideration of these factors is needed to determine selection of the optimal device, route of access, and method of tube placement. Certain conditions create difficulty or completely preclude enteral intubation for decompression or nutrition. Obstruction of the nasopharynx, esophagus, or proximal part of the stomach is an absolute contraindication to nasoenteric intubation or endoscopically or fluoroscopically placed tubes. Coagulopathy, ascites, obesity, previous abdominal surgery, and esophagogastric varices are all relative contraindications to enteral tube placement by any method (Table 52–1).

Careful consideration of these factors and clear understanding of the risks and benefits of GI intubation lead to proper choice of materials and methods for appropriate enteral access.

NASOGASTRIC AND NASOENTERIC INTUBATION

GI intubation is a well-established diagnostic and therapeutic modality that has been in common use for centuries. The earliest descriptions of nasogastric tubes and intestinal intubation date from the 17th century.[2] Modern tubes are known eponymously for the individuals who introduced them into clinical practice. In 1921 Levin described a single-lumen catheter fenestrated at the distal end for decompression (low intermittent

| Table 52-1 | Enteral Access: Common Indications and Contraindications |

Route	Indications	Contraindications
Nasogastric	Decompression, ileus, obstruction, upper gastrointestinal bleeding, toxic ingestion	Nasopharyngeal obstruction, varices, coagulopathy, thrombocytopenia, craniofacial injury
Nasoenteric	Short-term feeding, nutritional support, partial small bowel obstruction	Long term nutritional need >7-10 days, craniofacial injury
Gastric: percutaneous endoscopic gastrostomy	Malnutrition, head and neck cancer, cerebrovascular accident, trauma, prolonged intubation, respiratory failure	Gastroesophageal reflux disease, gastroparesis, gastric outlet obstruction, pancreatitis, recent foregut surgery
Gastric: open, Stamm	Inability to perform endoscopy, above indications	Above contraindications, recent foregut surgery
Intestinal: jejunal	Recent surgery, gastric outlet obstruction, gastroparesis, pancreatitis, fistula	Short-bowel syndrome, fistula, distal obstruction, inability to provide continuous infusion

suction or gravity drainage) or feeding.[3] A 1960s modification of the Levin tube is now widely used and known as a "Salem sump" tube (Fig. 52–1A). The Salem tube has a second lumen that allows air to be drawn into the stomach, or "sump," during suctioning, thereby avoiding adherence to the gastric mucosa. This tube is used most commonly today for GI decompression (e.g., ileus, partial small bowel obstruction) and is available in various sizes.

Long nasoenteric tubes designed for decompression are also available as single-lumen or multilumen tubes. Generally, long tubes have weighted or balloon-tipped ends and are intended to pass distally to provide intestinal rather than gastric decompression. Because of difficulty passing tubes through the pylorus, some authors espouse postpyloric endoscopic placement.[4] Others have shown little or no difference in the efficacy of long versus short decompressive tubes.[5] In 1934 Miller and Abbott first introduced a long, balloon-tipped intestinal tube designed to pass into the intestine via gentle advancement and peristalsis; subsequent modifications included percutaneous, weighted, multilumen, and silicone models (Baker, Cantor tubes) (see Fig. 52–1B and C).[6]

Nasoenteric tubes designed for feeding are similar to long tubes in that they are intended to pass distal to the pylorus, but in contradistinction to decompression tubes, they are generally of smaller caliber and made of softer plastic polymers than standard nasogastric or nasoenteric tubes are. These tubes often require a stiffening wire for passage and manipulation. The most familiar and widely used tube, introduced by Dobbie and Hoffmeister in the 1970s, is the now familiar Dobbhoff tube (see Fig. 52–1D).[7] The weighted, enlarged, radiopaque distal end purportedly facilitates spontaneous duodenal passage; however, evidence suggests that such is not usually the case.[8-10] Transpyloric passage may occur spontaneously in only limited instances. Silk and associates reported their experience with over 800 intubations and found that less than 4% spontaneously passed

beyond the stomach.[10] Proper placement distal to the pylorus can be difficult and vexing and may require manipulation or endoscopic or radiologic maneuvers.

Indications

The most common indication for nasogastric and nasoenteric intubation is decompression of the stomach or intestine. It is used less frequently for diagnostic and therapeutic modalities such as gastric lavage and evacuation of gastric contents in the initial management of upper GI bleeding or toxic ingestion. Diagnostic uses are numerous and include aspiration to determine the presence of drugs or toxins; measurement of gastric secretion, volume, or pH; and procurement of specimens for culture of *Mycobacterium* or *Helicobacter pylori*. Decompression is by far the most common indication for nasointestinal intubation and includes decompression of air or enteric contents (or both) in the setting of ileus, partial or complete intestinal obstruction, gastric dilatation, perioperative gastric drainage, and reduction of the risk for aspiration. Routine postoperative nasogastric drainage after abdominal surgery is a time-honored practice, but the current literature and evidence-based medicine do not support such use. Studies suggest that selective use in patients for indications such as gastric distention, nausea, and vomiting is associated with fewer pulmonary complications than routine postoperative nasogastric tube decompression is.[11] Nasogastric and nasoenteric decompression is integral to the therapeutic and diagnostic management of intestinal obstruction. In terms of decompressive treatment of intestinal obstruction, placement of a nasogastric tube is often sufficient to relieve the obstruction. In the case of partial intestinal obstruction, decompression usually effects relief of the obstruction within 48 hours. If the obstruction is persistent, further diagnostic investigation and exploration should be considered. In patients with suspected

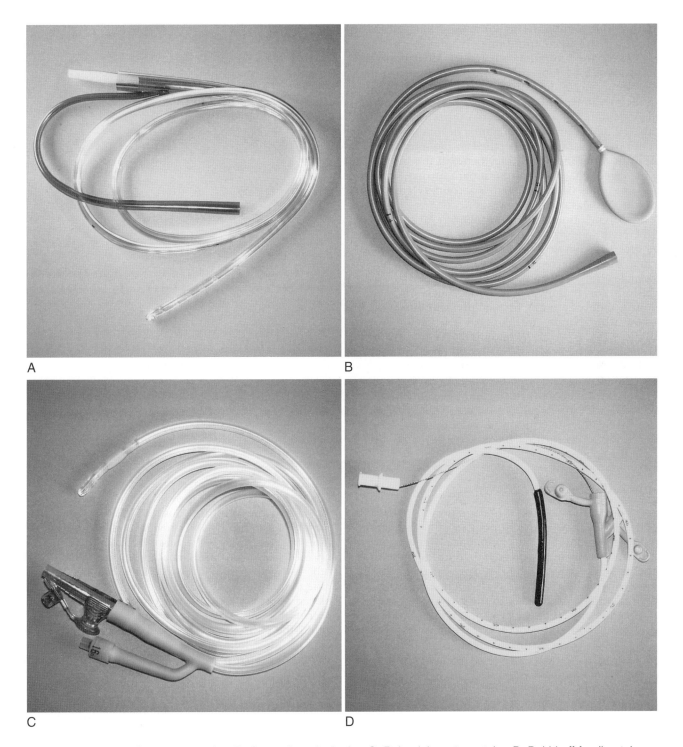

Figure 52–1.   A, Salem sump tube. **B,** Cantor intestinal tube. **C,** Baker jejunostomy tube. **D,** Dobbhoff feeding tube.

complete intestinal obstruction, nasogastric intubation is important in the preoperative resuscitative period to decompress the stomach and minimize aspiration.

Long intestinal tubes (Miller-Abbott, Cantor, Baker) are available in numerous designs and sizes and are placed nasoenterically or operatively. The theoretical advantage of these tubes is that they decompress the small intestine distally at the site of obstruction. Long tubes use either an air-filled or weighted balloon to achieve transpyloric passage and rely on peristalsis for

distal positioning. Long tubes are most effective and have been successful in the treatment of partial obstruction but have little, if any role in complete obstruction.[5] Limitations of long tubes and lack of clear superiority over nasogastric decompression have led to sparse use, mostly in specific clinical circumstances, such as in patients with significant operative comorbidity or malignant partial obstruction. Long tubes must be passed through the pylorus and then distally to the site of obstruction, both of which take time and may pose significant obstacles requiring intervention. In addition, most long tubes do not have a gastric decompression port and therefore may allow emesis and aspiration from gastric dilatation. The superiority of long tubes has not been proved prospectively. Numerous authors have reported successful non-operative treatment of partial small bowel obstruction with long tubes.[12] One randomized prospective study that compared nasogastric with long tube decompression for partial intestinal obstruction failed to demonstrate any significant difference in efficacy between the tubes.[5] In the management of partial intestinal obstruction, long tubes must still be considered a secondary treatment option to nasogastric decompression.

The aforementioned intestinal tubes are large bore (14 to 18 French) and designed to provide distal decompression; they are only occasionally used for gastric or jejunal feeding. Nasojejunal feeding tubes (e.g., Dobbhoff tubes) are smaller caliber (7 to 9 French) and softer and used exclusively for therapeutic purposes, such as feeding and drug administration in patients with functioning intestine who require nutrition but are unable to eat orally (see Fig. 52–1D). Distal enteral feeding through soft, small-bore tubes (Dobbhoff) positioned beyond the ligament of Treitz is thought to present a lower risk of aspiration than intragastric feeding does. Level 1 evidence does not exist to support this hypothesis. Some authors have shown that the risk for aspiration is not affected by the site of feeding. In critically ill patients maintained by either intragastric or jejunal feeding, there was no difference in the incidence of aspiration.[13-16]

Contraindications

Strong contraindications to nasoenteric intubation include nasopharyngeal or esophageal obstruction, recent foregut surgery, and craniofacial injuries. Orogastric intubation is the preferred route of intubation in the presence of facial injuries or trauma, and it also temporarily facilitates stomach decompression when a patient is under anesthesia or in the event of toxic ingestion. Coagulopathy is a relative contraindication to nasogastric intubation and should lead to consideration of the orogastric route to avoid epistaxis. Patients with esophagogastric varices who require nasoenteric or oroenteric intubation should have tubes placed with caution and only for short periods to minimize the risk for variceal injury or erosion (see Fig. 52–1).

Methods of Intubation

Nasoenteric intubation is easily accomplished at the bedside and has several basic requirements for success, ease, and safety. As with many bedside procedures, the process can be divided into several phases, in this case three, to achieve the objectives of patient comfort, ease of placement, and minimal complications.[2,17] The insertion technique is identical for nasogastric and nasoenteric tubes. The steps are preparing the patient, passing the tube, and confirming position of the tube. If the patient is awake, explanation of the procedure pays dividends by alleviating anxiety and facilitating placement because patient cooperation simplifies the procedure.

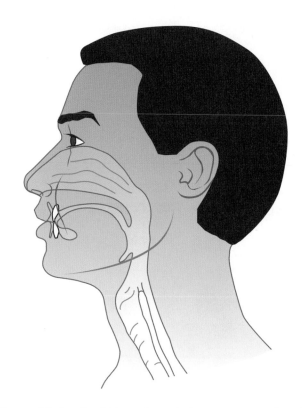

Figure 52–2. Sagittal section of the upper aerodigestive tract.

Nasogastric intubation is easiest with the patient in the Fowler or upright sitting position with the neck flexed forward in the "sniffing" position. This position places the trachea anteriorly and provides a gentle curve for the tube to pass through the nasopharynx, often the most uncomfortable and problematic site through which the tube must be passed. Before placement, the length of tube that must be passed is gauged. Generally, tubes are placed approximately 50 cm from the nares so that they lie comfortably within the stomach. In the majority of adults the gastroesophageal junction is 40 cm from the incisors. Most tubes are marked to provide an approximation of proper placement. The length of insertion for blank tubes can be estimated by measuring from the patient's nares to the earlobe and then to the xiphoid (Fig. 52–2).

After consideration of the general contraindications to nasoenteric intubation (discussed in the previous section), each naris should be checked for obstruction. Both the nostril and the distal tip of the tube should be lubricated with water-soluble lubricant or, better yet, 2% viscous lidocaine. Topical anesthetic spray may also be used to anesthetize the posterior nasopharynx for improved patient comfort. The tube is inserted into the nostril aimed directly posterior toward the angle of the jaw or earlobe. A common mistake is to direct the tube in a cephalad direction, which may cause curling of the tube or trauma resulting in epistaxis. Placing the tip of the tube in ice for several minutes stiffens and may decrease curling of the tube, thereby facilitating passage. This practice is usually unnecessary, however, and can easily cause discomfort or trauma. As the tube reaches the posterior nasopharynx and is redirected inferiorly, there is usually mild resistance. Gentle pressure is all that is required to turn the tube as it is redirected inferiorly and passes through the pharynx into the esophagus. Tubes should never be forced against resistance, which if encountered, is an indication to abandon the attempt and start anew. In awake and cooperative patients, a useful strategy is to enlist their involvement and have them sip water from a straw. Participation in the procedure helps alleviate anxiety, and sipping water closes the trachea and helps the patient swallow the tube. Placing the patient in the sniffing position helps direct the tube posteriorly and avoid tracheal intubation. Gagging, coughing, respiratory distress, or resistance should raise suspicion of tracheal intubation or misplacement and prompt immediate withdrawal of the tube.

Small-caliber (7 to 9 French) nasoenteric tubes used for feeding (Dobbhoff tubes) are softer and require a wire stylet for placement. Common wisdom holds that once removed, the stylet should never be replaced because it may result in perforation of the tube, mucosal damage, or both. Others, however, recommend routine reinsertion of the stylet as a means of transpyloric placement. With the tube successfully placed in the stomach, the stylet is removed and bent at a 30-degree angle several centimeters from its tip. The stylet is then reinserted and rotated; "corkscrewing" the tube while advancing it directs the tube toward and through the pylorus. Authors have reported this technique to be successful in more than 90% of insertions.[18-20]

Confirmation of proper tube placement should be accomplished before use for either aspiration or feeding. Placement is most often assessed by air insufflation into the tube during auscultation of the left upper quadrant. This routine method is certainly not foolproof; there are many reports of false-positive results.[2,21-23] Aspiration of enteric contents is helpful when large-bore, stiffer tubes are used, but again, this is not absolute proof of placement. Radiographic evidence of proper positioning of enteric tubes is most definitive. X-ray evidence of placement is prudent for all tubes placed with any degree of difficulty and should be considered necessary for all tubes before instituting feeding.

If the methods described fail, nasoenteric tubes can be successfully placed fluoroscopically or endoscopically into the duodenum in greater than 98% of cases.[24] Tubes should be anchored to the nose loosely after ascertaining placement to prevent inadvertent dislodgement and avoid undue pressure on the nasal ala.

Complications

Nasoenteric intubation is ubiquitous in the course of modern patient care but certainly is not always inconsequential. Complications associated with tubes and intubation have been reported in up to 15% of hospitalized patients undergoing nasoenteric intubation and range from minor to life-threatening.[17,21,25,26] The most serious complications occur in patients least able to compensate and protect themselves: those with impaired tracheo-

pharyngeal defense mechanisms, impaired sensorium, or advanced age. Frequent complications associated with nasoenteric tubes include emesis, gagging, epistaxis, sinusitis, alar pressure necrosis, odynophagia, nasopharyngitis, and otitis. The litany of complications is more than merely annoying; apparently minor complications may easily progress or contribute to more serious conditions. Complications can be avoided by assiduous attention to proper placement and maintenance of tubes. Aspiration pneumonia is the most common serious complication associated with nasoenteric intubation. Malfunctioning tubes and simply the presence of a stent through the gastroesophageal junction are contributing factors. Some authors suggest that the incidence of tube-related aspiration approaches 50%.[27] Placing the patient's bed in the 30-degree head-up position and attention to proper function of the tube help prevent this potentially devastating complication. Less common, but equally serious complications include esophageal stricture or perforation, laryngeal injury, pulmonary complications, and insertion of the tube into the cranium through the cribriform plate. Proper insertion technique, assessment of placement, and management of the tube minimize complications. A common complication of small tubes is occlusion by solidified feeding matter or crushed drugs. Flushing solutions such as soda, cranberry juice, or enzyme solutions have met with only limited success.[28] Assiduous care of tubes, frequent flushing, limited aspiration, and use of pumps for feeding when indicated minimize occlusion. Replacement of the tube obviates the problem of occlusion and may be necessary but subjects the patient to discomfort and the risk of another procedure.

ENTERIC FEEDING

Feeding via the GI tract is preferable to nutrition via the parenteral route in patients who require nutritional support. Patients with functioning GI tracts who are nutritionally depleted or unable to swallow or who have inadequate food intake for their ongoing metabolic requirements benefit from enteral feeding.[29] Enteral nutrition is less expensive, easier to administer, safer, and more physiologic for the patient.[30] Animal evidence confirms that subjects maintained with parenteral nutrition succumb more easily to septic challenges than do those fed enterally.[31] Human studies confirm that enteral nutrition preserves the histologic structure and physiologic viability of the gut better than parenteral supplements do.[32] In contradistinction to total parenteral nutrition, enteral feeding is additionally beneficial to the patient because it helps maintain the immune system and the nutritional-metabolic axis.[33]

Intubation of the GI tract for nutritional support is frequent but not always innocuous. There are several considerations for optimal implementation and effect. The feasibility of enteral support depends on general patient considerations, the timing of tube placement, and the route of access. Any patient who is malnourished or expected to have inadequate oral intake for 5 to 7 days should be considered for enteral access for nutritional

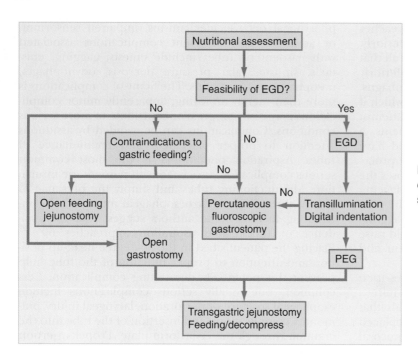

Figure 52–3. Algorithm for placement of tube enterostomies. EGD, esophagogastroduodenoscopy; PEG, percutaneous endoscopic gastrostomy.

support. Patients being considered for nutritional support within this very broad definition should subsequently undergo a clinical nutritional assessment, including a history, physical examination, and pertinent laboratory indices, to judge their nutritional status and anticipated needs. The route of nutritional support— enteral versus parenteral—should be part of the assessment. The GI tract should be used whenever possible. Patients with existing malnutrition, hypoalbuminemia (<3.3 g/dl), or recent significant weight loss (10% to 15% of pre-illness weight loss within 6 months) should be considered for immediate nutritional support. Nourished patients who have had insufficient intake for 5 to 7 days or are expected to have poor oral intake for 5 to 7 days subsequently should also be considered for nutritional support. Normally nourished or even mildly malnourished individuals requiring major operations do not usually require nutritional support if the procedure is prompt and the postoperative course is uncomplicated.[34] When a determination is made to provide nutritional support, initiation should be prompt. A small-bore nasoenteric (Dobbhoff) tube can easily and effectively provide short-term nutritional support and may temporize until a patient is capable of oral intake. If the GI tract is functional and longer-term nutritional support is required (>10 to 14 days), GI intubation via a gastrostomy (percutaneous or open) or jejunostomy should be considered. Moderately or severely malnourished patients undergoing open laparotomy should be considered for concomitant placement of gastrostomy or jejunostomy tubes at the time of surgery. Facilitated relatively easily during laparotomy, enteral access may pay dividends in the postoperative period if a patient is nutritionally depleted or requires ongoing support through postoperative recovery. Clinical judgment must be applied because placement of enteral access has its own risk-benefit balance. GI access should be prompt in

patients requiring longer-term nutritional support without imminent surgery. Temporization with a soft small-bore nasoenteric tube (Dobbhoff) is an effective alternative until more effective access can be obtained. Soft, small-bore tubes are associated with difficult placement, frequent extubation, and a higher incidence of tube-related complications, which serve to impair or delay nutritional support. Feeding via nasogastric or nasoenteric tubes may be necessary but predisposes to aspiration. Authors have reported documented aspiration of enteric contents in up to 44% of critically ill patients receiving tube feeding regardless of whether it is delivered by the gastric or jejunal route.[13] Any candidate for nutrition via enteral access through any route should be evaluated the same as those requiring intestinal intubation for other indications. The patient's underlying medical and comorbid conditions, contraindications, and nutritional and ancillary needs, including the expected length of time that access will be required, are used to determine the method, route of placement, and choice of tube (Fig. 52–3).

Gastric Access for Nutrition

Currently, the most desirable—and common—route for enteral support is via a percutaneously placed gastrostomy. Authors have shown intragastric feeding to be more physiologic than parenteral nutritional support for several reasons.[35] The stomach provides a reservoir that allows cyclic bolus feeding, dilution of hyperosmolar solutions, and acidification of nutrients, which is bactericidal and improves the absorption of some nutrients. Cyclic feedings cause variations in insulin levels, thereby promoting lipolysis and anabolism. Other beneficial effects of feeding into the stomach include decreased gastric atony and bile stasis.

Gastric intubation is easier to accomplish than jejunal intubation because percutaneous gastrostomy does not require operative intervention and can be performed in sedated patients at the bedside. Technical, pathologic, and clinical impediments to gastric access may exist, however. Pharyngoesophageal obstruction, recent foregut surgery, or ascites may preclude gastric intubation by any method. Clinical conditions precluding use of the stomach include an inability to accommodate feeding, delayed gastric emptying, gastroesophageal reflux, ongoing pancreatitis, ileus, and intrinsic disease of the GI tract, including inflammatory bowel disease and radiation enteritis. These conditions should lead to abandonment of gastric intubation and consideration of jejunal or parenteral nutrition. If dictated by the clinical situation, combined gastric and jejunal tubes are available and can provide the advantage of postpyloric feeding and simultaneous gastric decompression. The only caveat is that combination tubes usually require placement by the open method and thus a small laparotomy.

TUBE ENTEROSTOMIES

Gastrostomy

Intubation of the stomach (exclusive of the nasogastric route) results in a planned gastrocutaneous fistula. Most commonly, simply placing the gastrostomy tube as a communicating stent from the gastric lumen to the exterior creates a temporary fistula with serosal lining. The anterior gastric wall and parietal peritoneum are held in direct contact by sutures or the tube itself. The Stamm or standard open gastrostomy, laparoscopic gastrostomy, and percutaneous endoscopic gastrostomy (PEG) are common examples of serosal gastrostomies and have the advantages of a low leak rate, ease of placement, and spontaneous closure when removed. One disadvantage is that inadvertent tube removal may result in rapid and premature loss of enteral access. These three methods—especially the PEG method—have been shown to be efficient and safe and represent the vast majority of gastrostomies placed today.[24,36] In unusual circumstances, a permanent gastrocutaneous fistula may be created in which part of the stomach wall is used to fashion a mucosa-lined tube between the lumen and exterior (Janeway-type gastrostomy).

Open Gastrostomy: Stamm Method

The Stamm, or open, gastrostomy is considered the gold standard for transabdominal gastric access and presents minimal risk. It requires a small laparotomy that can be performed under local anesthesia if necessary. The stomach is accessed via a small upper midline incision. The omentum or transverse colon is identified and retracted inferiorly. The appearance and arrangement of vessels along the greater curvature can identify the stomach. A relatively avascular site is chosen along the anterior wall of the stomach well away from the antrum and pylorus. The site should reach the planned

abdominal wall exit site in the left upper quadrant to avoid undue tension on the tube and allow contact of the stomach serosa and parietal peritoneum of the abdominal wall.

The chosen tube, usually a large-bore (22 to 24 French) tube, often with a balloon or mushroom tip, is placed through the abdominal wall via a separate stab incision. One or two purse-string sutures are placed in the seromuscular layer of the anterior wall of the stomach at the prospective site. Creating a gastrotomy in the middle of the purse-string suture allows access for insertion of the tube several centimeters into the gastric lumen. If the tube is equipped with a distal balloon, it is inflated and the purse-string sutures tied securely. The anterior wall of the stomach is then affixed to the abdominal wall entry site with several sutures and the tube secured to the skin. The abdominal incision is closed in standard fashion (Fig. 52–4).

Laparoscopic Gastrostomy

Intragastric access is feasible with minimally invasive operative techniques. General anesthesia and pneumoperitoneum are required; open gastrostomy and PEG placement may actually be less invasive and therefore more attractive. Laparoscopic suturing may be used to replicate the open technique described in the previous section. Alternatively, approximation of the stomach to the abdominal wall is accomplished with T-fasteners placed percutaneously under laparoscopic visualization through the gastric wall into the lumen. Four T-fasteners placed around the prospective gastrostomy site are used to pull and maintain the anterior stomach wall in contact with the abdominal wall in the left upper quadrant. A gastrostomy tube is then placed percutaneously through the center of the T-fasteners into the gastric lumen. The stomach can be affixed to the abdominal wall via T-fasteners or sutures and further held in place with an intraluminal balloon. The need for general anesthesia and pneumoperitoneum and the technical requirements have rendered this method less often used than standard open (Stamm type) or percutaneous approaches.

Percutaneous Gastrostomy

Gastric access via a percutaneous endoscopic technique was developed and reported by Ponsky et al. in 1980.[37] The method allows safe, efficient transabdominal placement of a gastrostomy tube under local anesthesia at the bedside while avoiding laparotomy. Percutaneous gastrostomy has few absolute contraindications. Strong deterrents to PEG placement are recent upper abdominal surgery, especially on the foregut, and to a lesser extent any recent abdominal surgery. Two variations of this technique are used commonly and described in this section. Both techniques involve the use of esophagogastroduodenoscopy, air insufflation of the stomach, and transillumination of the anterior stomach wall through the abdominal wall. Transillumination and visualization of a probing finger indenting the stomach suggest that the transverse colon is displaced, the stomach is immediately adjacent to the abdominal wall,

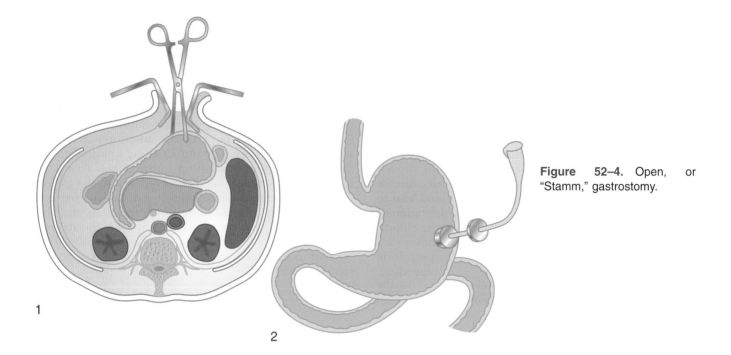

1

2

Figure 52–4. Open, or "Stamm," gastrostomy.

and percutaneous access is safe. A site should be chosen along the anterior aspect of the greater curvature within the stomach lumen well away from the pylorus. The skin site should be sufficiently distant from the costal margin in the left upper quadrant to minimize patient discomfort. The gastric lumen is accessed percutaneously with a small angiocatheter-type trocar under direct endoscopic vision. A guidewire is passed through the trocar into the gastric lumen and grasped with an endoscopic snare. The endoscope and wire are withdrawn through the esophagus, oropharynx, and mouth. Using the most common "pull" method originally described by Ponsky, the guidewire is pulled through the mouth and affixed to the gastrostomy tube. The abdominal end of the guidewire is then pulled to draw the gastrostomy tube through the mouth, pharynx, and esophagus so that it lies within the stomach. The preceding end of the tube is tapered to dilate the abdominal wall tract as the tube is passed. Tubes are equipped with a mushroom tip and gradations along the length. Initial placement can be estimated by determining the approximate thickness of the abdominal wall or the point where resistance is encountered. A second gastroscopy for ascertaining proper placement must be performed and can be facilitated by tightening the wire snare onto the "mushroom" end of the gastrostomy catheter.

The alternative "push" method, a variant of the Seldinger technique, is similar in all respects to the "pull method" except that the long tapered end of the gastrostomy tube is hollow and advanced over a guidewire while being pushed through the pharynx, esophagus, stomach, and abdominal wall. The tapered end of the tube effects dilatation of the abdominal wall tract. Direct visualization of the tube should be accomplished with either method to ascertain proper placement.

Procedure-related complications are divided into early (within 14 days) or late (after 14 days). Minor

complications are generally tube related and include dislodged tubes, leaks, wound infections requiring wound care, mucosal obstruction or "buried bumper syndrome," and fever. Aspiration, bleeding, infection requiring antibiotic therapy, and abdominal emergencies (acute abdomen, peritonitis, gastric or colonic perforation) are major complications.[24] Percutaneous gastrostomy is well established and safe and can be done at the bedside with a minimum of anesthesia and complications.[38] Large clinical studies suggest that the technical success rate is greater than 99% with procedure-related mortality approaching 0%.[39] Barring contraindications, PEG is currently the method of choice for gastric intubation for nutritional support (Fig. 52–5).[40]

Combination Tubes

Multilumen tubes designed to provide postpyloric feeding and concomitant gastric decompression are a useful adjunct to standard gastric or jejunal tubes. Endoscopic, fluoroscopic, or open techniques have been used to place transgastric jejunal tubes. Transgastric jejunostomy tubes are more difficult to place, however, because the distal tube must pass through the pylorus and is thus usually placed operatively without endoscopy or fluoroscopy. Even with an initial open procedure, multiple procedures (endoscopy or fluoroscopy) may be required to successfully place the jejunal lumen of the tube in a postpyloric position. Care must be taken to avoid duodenal or jejunal perforation. Occasionally, clinical circumstances require conversion of a gastrostomy to a jejunostomy for more distal enteral feeding, such as in patients with gastric outlet obstruction or atony. Several options are available to accomplish conversion. Depending on the needs of the patient and the resources available, a percutaneous jejunostomy may be placed with a

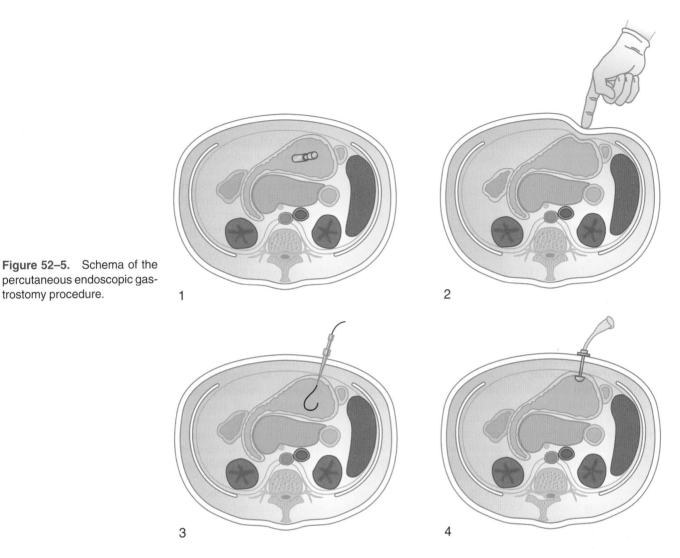

Figure 52–5. Schema of the percutaneous endoscopic gastrostomy procedure.

1

2

3

4

technique identical to the Ponsky PEG method after visualizing the proximal jejunum with an enteroscope. Other options include open or laparoscopic placement of a Witzel-type jejunostomy and endoscopic or fluoroscopic conversion of a gastrostomy to a transgastric jejunostomy tube.

Jejunostomy

Patients requiring enteral support in which gastric intubation or feeding is contraindicated for any reason may benefit from small intestinal access, or a jejunostomy. Enteral feeding distal to the ligament of Treitz is thought to decrease but does not eliminate the risk of aspiration.[14] Some authors hypothesize that distal feeding does not decrease aspiration and have shown similar documented aspiration rates in subsets of critically ill patients regardless of the route and site of feeding.[13] Witzel jejunostomy is the time-tested gold standard; the enteral access tube is incorporated in an oblique serosal or "Witzel" tunnel for several centimeters parallel to the small bowel lumen to prevent leakage of enteral con-

tents. Placement of a Witzel-type jejunostomy requires laparotomy accomplished via a small upper midline incision. The site chosen for the jejunostomy is 15 to 20 cm distal to the ligament of Treitz. A purse-string suture is placed on the antimesenteric aspect of the jejunum. The chosen tube—usually a 14-French Silastic tube—is passed through an adjacent stab incision in the left upper quadrant. An enterotomy is created through the purse-string suture, and the tube is passed distally into the jejunal lumen. The purse-string suture is tightened, and a serosal tunnel is created proximally for approximately 3 to 5 cm by placing Lembert sutures over the tube along the antimesenteric border of the bowel. Care should be taken to avoid narrowing the jejunal lumen while creating the Witzel tunnel. Several sutures are used to affix the jejunum to the parietal peritoneum of the anterior abdominal wall at its exit site (Fig. 52–6).

Needle catheter jejunostomy, an alternative technique, is a method of access in which a large-bore needle is placed in the bowel lumen instead of a tube. The needle catheter is inserted identically to standard jejunostomy tubes via the Witzel method. The method has been used extensively in the critical care and trauma

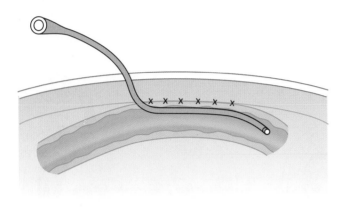

Figure 52–6.   "Witzel" jejunostomy.

patient population. The small-bore catheter is easily removed when no longer needed but occludes easily.

Minimally invasive techniques similar to laparoscopic gastrostomy placement may easily be applied to jejunostomy tube placement. Identical technique using T-fasteners placed into the antimesenteric small bowel lumen under direct laparoscopic visualization allows fixation of the jejunum. An introducer with a peel-away sheath is placed through the abdominal wall and thence into the jejunum. The T-fasteners are cut at skin level 10 to 14 days later. Similar to laparoscopic gastrostomy, this technique is less often used because of technical requirements and tube-related complications. Alternatively, laparoscopic suturing expertise may allow the surgeon to mimic the open technique described earlier.

Enteral tubes may be placed by the same endoscopic techniques as used for PEG tubes, although it is substantially more difficult. Most often a PEG is placed first or a preexisting PEG is converted to a transgastric jejunal tube. Transpyloric placement of a guidewire is accomplished under direct endoscopic visualization. The jejunal tube is then advanced over the wire through the duodenum into the small bowel. This technique is fraught with difficulty and potential serious complications, such as perforation as a result of placing a relatively stiff tube through the curved duodenum. An alternative method of distal tube placement is to use fluoroscopic imaging to guide the tube through the pylorus.

MANAGEMENT AND COMPLICATIONS OF INTESTINAL TUBES FOR NUTRITION

There is great variability in the literature regarding when nutritional support can be initiated after GI intubation. The literature has suggested that early feeding, even within 2 to 3 hours, is feasible and does not result in an increased incidence of complications when compared with initiation of feeding at 24 hours.[10] Typically, with either gastric or jejunal tubes, feeding can be started safely within 24 hours of placement regardless of the method if certain criteria are met. Reasonable criteria for initiating enteral feeding include tube output or residual volume measured at less than 200 ml/8 hr and no abdominal distention, abdominal wall tube site leakage,

or surrounding erythema. It is acceptable to begin full-strength feeding solutions at a low rate and progressively increase until the goal volume is reached.

Intestinal access tubes are placed and used almost without complications. In the relatively unusual circumstance that they occur, serious morbidity or even fatality may result, and thus they should be treated promptly. Postoperative and tube-related complications are similar for jejunal and gastric tubes. All tubes are subject to mechanical tube-related complications such as occlusion and tube displacement. Periodic flushing and proper use prevent catheter clogging. Assiduous attention to the tube itself minimizes dislodgement, although inadvertent extubation remains commonplace in the hospital setting.

Aspiration pneumonia has been documented in up to 44% of critically ill patients and is directly related to enteral feeding.[15] Measures to prevent aspiration should be instituted for all patients with intestinal intubation or those receiving enteral feeding regardless of the site. The literature has shown no difference in the rate of aspiration in critically ill patients fed into the stomach or small intestine.[13,23]

Dislodgement of gastrostomy or jejunostomy tubes is a common complication that is usually merely annoying but can be life-threatening. Tubes that are completely dislodged should be replaced with caution only if the transabdominal tract is well established (>14 days). A well-lubricated, small-bore tube or even a flexible guidewire may be used to access the intestinal lumen. A radiologic contrast study should be performed to confirm tube placement, especially before using a recently replaced tube.[41] In the absence of a well-established transabdominal tract, the more prudent course may be to leave the tube out and replace it formally at another setting because reinsertion risks inadvertent intraperitoneal placement.

Peritonitis from leakage of enteric contents or feeding formula, or both, may occur as a result of separation of the bowel from the abdominal wall with or without tube dislodgment. An acute abdomen or presumed peritonitis mandates prompt, urgent intervention. Bowel obstruction is a complication encountered both early and late after intestinal tube placement from various causes. Balloon-tipped catheters may cause obstruction by migration or simply lodge in a disadvantageous position. Jejunostomy catheters placed via the Witzel technique may become obstructed from a too tight Witzel tunnel or angulation of the jejunal loop as it apposes the abdominal wall. Additionally, tube or tube placement complications such as hematoma, contained leak, or abscess may cause either mechanical or functional obstruction. Volvulus or internal herniation of small intestine around a tube insertion site resulting in obstruction is a less frequent occurrence and may require operative repair. Regardless of the cause of obstruction, timely investigation and intervention are warranted.

SUMMARY

The two common broad indications for intestinal intubation—decompression and nutrition—are ubiquitous in the course of care of surgical patients. Many options exist for establishing intestinal access. The practitioner must use clinical judgment and knowledge to choose the safest, most suitable method for the individual patient.

REFERENCES

1. Cheatham ML, Chapman WC, Key SP, et al: A meta-analysis of selective v. routine nasogastric decompression after elective laparotomy. Ann Surg 221:469, 1995.
2. Boyes RJ, Kruse JA: Nasogastric and nasoenteric intubation. Crit Care Clin 8:865, 1992.
3. Levin AL: A new gastroduodenal catheter. JAMA 76:1007, 1921.
4. Gowen GF: Long tube decompression is successful in 90% of patients with adhesive small bowel obstruction. Am J Surg 185:512, 2003.
5. Fleshner PR, Siegman MG, Slater GI, et al: A prospective randomized trial of short v. long tubes in adhesive small-bowel obstruction. Am J Surg 170:366, 1995.
6. Matarese LE: Enteral alimentation: Equipment part III. Nutr Support Serv 2:48, 1982.
7. Dobbie RP, Hoffmeister JA: Continuous pump-tube enteric hyperalimentation. Surg Gynecol Obstet 143:273, 1976.
8. Levenson R, Turner WW Jr, Dyson A, et al: Do weighted nasoenteric feeding tubes facilitate duodenal intubations? JPEN J Parenter Enteral Nutr 12:135, 1988.
9. Rees RGP, Payne-James JJ, King C, Silk DB: Spontaneous transpyloric passage and performance of "fine-bore" polyurethane feeding tubes: A controlled clinical trial. JPEN J Parenter Enteral Nutr 12:469, 1988.
10. Silk DBA, Rees RG, Keohane PP, Attrill H: Clinical efficacy and design changes of "fine bore" nasogastric feeding tubes. A seven-year experience involving 809 intubations in 403 patients. JPEN J Parenter Enteral Nutr 11:378, 1987.
11. Wolff BG, Pemberton JH, van Heerden JA, et al: Elective colon & rectal surgery without nasogastric decompression. A prospective randomized trial. Ann Surg 209:670, 1989.
12. Wolfson PJ, Bauer JJ, Gelernt IM, et al: Use of the long tube in the management of patients with small-intestinal obstruction due to adhesion. Arch Surg 120:1001, 1985.
13. Strong RM, Condon SC, Solinger MR, et al: Equal aspiration rates from postpylorus and intragastric-placed small-bore nasoenteric feeding tubes: A randomized prospective study. JPEN J Parenter Enteral Nutr 16:59, 1992.
14. Gomes GF, Pisani JC, Marcedo ED, Campos AC: The nasogastric feeding tube as a risk factor for aspiration and aspiration pneumonia. Curr Opin Clin Nutr Metab Care 7:327, 2003.
15. Fox KA, Mularski RA, Sarfati MR, et al: Aspiration pneumonia following surgically placed feeding tubes. Am J Surg 170:564, discussion 566, 1995.
16. Mullan H, Roubenoff RA, Roubenoff R, et al: Risk of pulmonary aspiration among patients receiving enteral nutrition support. JPEN J Parenter Enteral Nutr 16:160, 1992.
17. Broughton WA, Green AE Jr: The technique of placing a nasoenteric tube. A revised protocol to avoid serious complication. J Crit Illness 5:1101, 1990.
18. Zaloga GP: Bedside method for placing small bowel feeding tubes in critically ill patients. A prospective study. Chest 100:1643, 1991.
19. Coulfield KA, Page OP: Technique for intraduodenal placement of transnasal enteral feeding catheters. Nutr Clin Pract 6:23, 1991.
20. Thurlow PM: Beside enteral feeding tube placement into duodenum and jejunum. JPEN J Parenter Enteral Nutr 10:104, 1986.
21. McClave SA, Chang WK: Complications of enteral access. Gastrointest Endosc 58:739, 2003.
22. Salasidis R, Fleiszer T, Johnston R: Air insufflation technique of enteral tube insertion. A randomized controlled trial. Crit Care Med 26:1036, 1998.
23. Broughton WA, Green AE, Hall MW, Bass JB: Nasoenteric tube placement: Users guide to possible complications. J Crit Illness 5:1085, 1990.
24. Cosenti EP, Sautner T, Gnant M, et al: Outcomes of surgical percutaneous endoscopic and percutaneous radiologic gastrostomies. Arch Surg 133:1076, 1998.
25. Bohnker BK, Artman LE, Hoskins WJ: Narrow bore nasogastric feeding tube complications. Nutr Clin Pract 2:203, 1987.
26. Davis RM: Complications of nasoenteric tubes. JAMA 254:54, 1985.
27. Hussain T, Roy U, Young PJ: Incidence and immediate respiratory consequence of pulmonary aspiration of enteral feed as detected using a modified glucose oxidase test. Anesth Intensive Care 31:272, 2003.
28. Marcuard SP, Stegall KL: Clearing obstructed feeding tubes. JPEN J Parenter Enteral Nutr 13:81, 1989.
29. Russell TR, Brotman M, Norris F: Percutaneous gastrostomy: A new simplified and cost-effective technique. Am J Surg 148:132, 1984.
30. Turosian MH, Rombeau JL: Feeding by tube enterostomy. Surg Gynecol Obstet 150:918, 1980.
31. Kudsk KA, Stone JM, Carpenter G, Sheldon GF: Enteral and parenteral feeding influences mortality after Hgb *E coli* peritonitis in normal rats. J Trauma 23:605, 1983.
32. Johnson LR, Copeland EM, Dudrick SJ, et al: Structural and hormonal alterations in the gastrointestinal tract of parenterally fed rats. Gastroenterology 68:1177, 1975.
33. Daly JM, Reynolds J, Sigal RK, et al: Effect of dietary protein and amino acids on immune function. Crit Care Med 18:586, 1990.
34. Henderson JM, Strodel WE: Limitations of percutaneous endoscopic jejunostomy. JPEN J Parenter Enteral Nutr 17:546, 1993.
35. Cass OW, Steinberg SE, Onstad G: A long-term follow-up of patients with percutaneous endoscopic gastrostomy or surgical (Stamm) gastrostomy. Gastrointest Endosc 32:144, 1986.
36. Grant JP: Percutaneous endoscopic gastrostomy initial placement by single endoscopic technique and long term follow up. Ann Surg 217:168, 1993.
37. Gauderer MWL, Ponsky JL, Izant RJ Jr: Gastrostomy without laparotomy: A percutaneous endoscopic technique. J Pediatr Surg 15:872, 1980.
38. Ponsky JL, Gauderere MWL: Percutaneous endoscopic gastrostomy. Arch Surg 118:913, 1983.
39. Loser C: Clinical aspects of long term enteral nutrition via percutaneous endoscopic gastrostomy (PEG). J Nutr Health Aging 4:47, 2000.
40. Moran BJ, Taylor MB, Johnson CD: Percutaneous endoscopic gastrostomy. Br J Surg 77:858, 1990.
41. Kohn CL, Keithley JK: Enteral nutrition: Potential complications and patient monitoring. Surg Clin North Am 24:339, 1989.

53

Injuries to the Stomach, Duodenum, and Small Bowel

Amy J. Goldberg · Mark Seamon · Abhijit S. Pathak

GASTRIC INJURIES

Historical

Throughout history, abdominal visceral wounds were generally considered fatal. It was not until the late 19th century, with improved surgical techniques and antisepsis, that intra-abdominal operations began to be performed on a widespread basis. By the early 20th century, laparotomy for abdominal penetration, including successful repair of gastric wounds, was being reported.[1] During World War I the role of surgery in penetrating abdominal trauma was further defined, and mandatory surgery for all penetrating abdominal wounds was an established principle by World War II.[2]

Anatomy and Physiology

The stomach is located in the superoanterior portion of the peritoneal cavity and is relatively well protected by its location and mobility. The inferior thoracic cage provides some protection laterally and anteriorly. Even though the stomach is tethered at the esophageal and duodenal junctions, it can descend into the lower part of the abdomen in an erect patient. The central location of the stomach in the upper part of the abdomen increases its risk for injury with thoracoabdominal penetration. Furthermore, if the esophagogastric junction and pylorus are constricted, the stomach, especially if distended or full, is at risk for rupture in blunt trauma.

Several upper abdominal viscera are in close relation to the stomach and can sustain an associated injury when blunt, penetrating, or corrosive injuries to the stomach occur. Both lobes of the liver overlap the stomach anteriorly, whereas posteriorly, the stomach is in close proximity to the pancreas, left kidney, and adrenal gland. Also in close proximity are the aorta, celiac trunk, and renal and splenic vessels. Most importantly, the stomach is in

very close relation to the spleen posterolaterally and attached to it by the short gastric arteries. Superiorly, the left lobe of the liver overlaps the gastric fundus and is closely related to the left hemidiaphragm. During normal ventilation, the diaphragm rises and falls. In deep expiration, the left hemidiaphragm can rise as high as the fifth costal cartilage, thereby placing the stomach at risk for injury from thoracic penetration. Because the posterior gastric wall lies within the lesser sac, injuries to this region may not produce the usual signs of peritoneal irritation.

The stomach has a rich blood supply with extensive collateralization. The major vessels supplying the stomach include the left gastric artery, a branch of the celiac trunk; the right gastric and gastroepiploic arteries, which are branches of the hepatic artery; and the short gastric and left gastroepiploic arteries, which are distal branches of the splenic artery. Because of this extensive vascular supply, ligation of two major vessels and many times three vessels in young patients is well tolerated. In addition, the submucosa is highly vascular, and injuries that extend through this layer have the potential to cause life-threatening hemorrhage (Fig. 53–1).

The stomach has two major functions: storage of foodstuff and digestion. These important physiologic roles are also responsible for both its vulnerability to injury and the postinjury consequences. The stomach stores foodstuff and regulates passage of chyme into the duodenum. A distended, postprandial stomach is susceptible to both penetrating and blunt trauma. A rapid elevation in intragastric pressure when the lower esophageal sphincter and pylorus are contracted can lead to either partial- or full-thickness injury of the organ.

The stomach secretes HCl and the zymogen pepsinogen, which is converted to the proteolytic enzyme pepsin in the presence of acid. Pulmonary aspiration of acid-peptic contents can induce a florid chemical pneumonitis, a principal danger in trauma. Peritoneal spillage of gastric contents from a full-thickness injury can induce

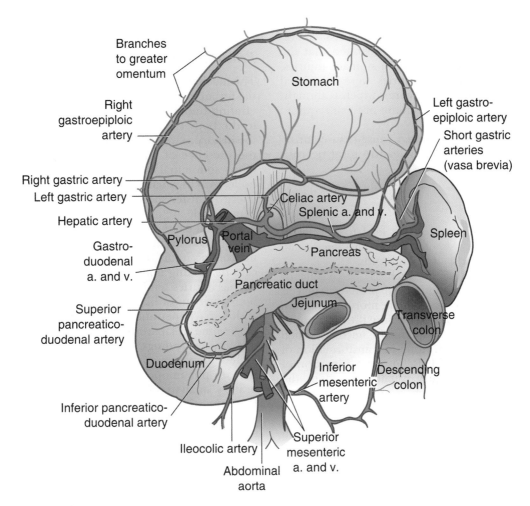

Figure 53–1. Anatomy of the stomach, duodenum, and pancreas. (From Zuidema G: Shackelford's Surgery of the Alimentary Tract, 4th ed. Philadelphia, WB Saunders, 1995.)

acute chemical peritonitis. If not immediately recognized, the subsequent inflammatory response leads to massive exudation of extracellular fluid into the peritoneal cavity. A delay in the diagnosis of gastric perforation will lead to intra-abdominal infection and sepsis. Even though the stomach has a low bacterial count, spillage of food particles enhances the virulence of these small numbers of bacteria.

Patterns of Injury

Penetrating Injuries

The incidence of gastric injury with penetrating abdominal trauma is anywhere from 5% to 20%.[3,4] As mentioned previously, its location and mobility, as well as its size, place the stomach at risk from penetrating injury. Missile injuries to the anterior abdominal, thoracoabdominal, or thoracic region can injure the stomach, depending on the trajectory. Stab wounds to the stomach are usually isolated injuries, whereas gunshot wounds generally have associated injuries. These associated

injuries are mainly responsible for and strongly influence mortality because isolated gastric wounds are rarely fatal.[5,6]

Blunt Injuries

Blunt gastric injuries are fairly uncommon and have been reported in less than 1% of cases of blunt abdominal injury.[5,7] The pathophysiology of gastric rupture is related to constriction of the esophagogastric junction and pylorus with an increase in intragastric pressure and subsequent rupture, especially with a distended or full stomach. According to Laplace's law, gastric rupture would be predicted to occur along the greater curvature; however, this is not the general rule.[8] Blunt injuries usually occur as single lesions, with the most common site being the anterior wall (40%), followed by the greater curvature (23%), the lesser curvature (15%), and the posterior wall (15%).[9] Most blunt gastric injuries occur after rapid-deceleration motor vehicle collisions and are associated with significant concomitant injuries. Splenic and thoracic injuries are the two most commonly associated with stomach injuries. Indeed, the multicenter hollow viscus injury study by the Eastern Association for Surgery in Trauma (EAST) demonstrated that the highest mortality rate was recorded for stomach injuries, 28.2%.[7] Furthermore, gastric injuries were associated with the highest injury severity scores, which is thought to be related to the significant amount of force required to cause gastric rupture.[7]

Besides rupture, blunt force may cause devascularization of the stomach and thereby lead to focal necrosis and delayed perforation.[10]

Caustic Injuries

Ingestion of caustic substances can lead to significant gastric injury. The most common corrosive agents fall into two major categories: alkali and acids.

Ingestion of alkaline agents such as lye (NaOH or KOH), which is found in household products such as drain cleaner, leads to injuries that are more severe than those caused by ingestion of acid because the mechanism of injury in alkali ingestion is liquefactive necrosis, which progresses over time and can result in transformation of the necrotic tissue to a liquid viscous mass. Ingestion of crystalline lye results in injury usually limited to the upper aerodigestive tract, such as the pharynx and esophagus. Ingestion of liquid lye can produce injury not only to the aforementioned structures but also to the esophagus and stomach. Severe gastric injury is unusual in the absence of significant esophageal injury. The duodenum and pancreas can be injured as well.

Gastric injury after acid ingestion is less common. Ingestion of acid leads to a coagulative necrosis that generally results in preservation of the general tissue architecture and is less severe than liquefactive necrosis. The stratified squamous epithelium of the pharynx and esophagus is relatively resistant to acid injury; however, the gastric columnar epithelium is not, and significant injury may occur. Transmural gastric necrosis is rare after acid ingestion, with the more common pattern of injury being mucosal ulceration and hemorrhage. Late sequelae of gastric acid injury may be manifested as gastric outlet obstruction from severe fibrosis.

Emetogenic Injuries

Emetogenic injuries of the stomach occur when there is a sudden increase in intragastric pressure that results in tearing of the mucosa or submucosa, usually near the esophagogastric junction. Also known as a Mallory-Weiss tear, these injuries can be a common cause of upper gastrointestinal (GI) bleeding.[11]

Iatrogenic Injuries

Iatrogenic gastric injuries can occur as a result of endoscopy or surgery or even after cardiopulmonary resuscitation or the Heimlich maneuver.[12-14] Delayed gastric necrosis has been reported after splenectomy and highly selective vagotomy, probably secondary to devascularization of the stomach.[15,16]

Diagnosis

Penetrating and Blunt Injuries

The mechanism of injury may help determine the potential for an intra-abdominal injury. In cases involving penetrating trauma, the external wound will draw attention to the body cavity most likely injured. In blunt trauma, the history as well as the mechanism of injury will suggest the presence of an intra-abdominal injury. Patterns of blunt abdominal trauma that may result in injury to a hollow viscus, such as the stomach, usually involve high energy transfer such as motor vehicle collisions and as a general rule are associated with other injuries as well.

Physical examination, especially in a multiply injured patient, can be unreliable, particularly in patients with neurologic injury, drug or alcohol ingestion, or significant distracting injury.[17] As mentioned previously, penetrating injuries tend to draw attention to the underlying body cavity most likely injured. Indeed, in patients with abdominal penetration, gastric injury is usually identified at the time of laparotomy.

Clinical findings that may suggest gastric injury include hematemesis, aspiration of blood from a gastric tube, or pneumoperitoneum on plain films. Routine laboratory analysis may be neither sensitive nor specific for diagnosing a gastric injury.[18] Other diagnostic studies available include computed tomography (CT), contrast-enhanced upper GI series, and diagnostic peritoneal lavage (DPL). Focused assessment of sonography in trauma (FAST) has gained wide acceptance as an adjunctive diagnostic modality in a blunt trauma victim. Its usefulness in blunt trauma is limited to identifying the presence or absence of free fluid within the peritoneal cavity, which in the majority of cases represents blood. It cannot distinguish between blood and other fluids and is therefore not specific in its ability to diagnose a hollow viscus injury.[19]

The role of CT scanning in trauma has emerged to the forefront in the past 15 to 20 years, especially for the evaluation of a hemodynamically stable blunt trauma patient and even for penetrating torso injuries.[20] CT scanning has proved to be useful in the diagnosis of blunt solid organ injury, thereby allowing subsequent nonoperative management of these injuries. The ability of CT to diagnose hollow viscus injuries is relatively limited. A delay in diagnosis of blunt hollow viscus injuries such as gastric injuries, though rare, can lead to increased morbidity and mortality.[7,21] The presence of free, low-density fluid without a solid organ injury should alert the surgeon that a hollow viscus injury may be present. Extravasation of oral contrast into the peritoneal cavity or pneumoperitoneum implies injury to a hollow viscus as well.

Water-soluble contrast studies of the upper GI tract can be used to detect gastric perforation, but their main use is for the diagnosis of gastric and duodenal hematoma. DPL is generally used for the evaluation of a hemodynamically unstable blunt trauma victim with equivocal or negative FAST results. Although it is a technique primarily for the diagnosis of intra-abdominal hemorrhage, DPL can provide evidence of hollow viscus injury with high sensitivity. In particular, a white blood cell (WBC) count of greater than 500 WBCs/mm³ in the lavage effluent or the presence of bile or food particles denotes a hollow viscus injury.

The role of laparoscopy in trauma has been mainly for evaluation of stable patients with penetrating torso wounds in whom absolute indications for exploration are not present and the work-up has not sufficiently eliminated peritoneal violation. Therefore, laparoscopy is frequently used to aid in the identification of diaphragmatic lacerations and peritoneal violation after penetrating wounds.[22] In particular, thoracoabdominal penetrating wounds and tangential gunshot wounds may be evaluated with this technique. Once identified, some injuries, such as diaphragm and gastric lacerations, have been repaired laparoscopically.[23] The drawback of laparoscopy for assessment of penetrating trauma has been its relatively low sensitivity for the identification of hollow viscus injuries and evaluation of the retroperitoneum.[22,24-26] Hence, its role as a therapeutic tool is still limited mainly to repair of anterior gastric and diaphragm injuries. It should be emphasized that caution should be exercised when using laparoscopy for identification and exclusion of hollow viscus injuries.

Caustic Ingestion

The most useful modality for the diagnosis of caustic injuries is endoscopy. After the ingestion of alkali, endoscopy is usually terminated at the point where deep, circumferential burns are identified because with second- or third-degree circumferential injury, further passage of the endoscope can produce additional injury.[27]

Treatment

Penetrating and Blunt Injuries

Initial care of a trauma patient centers on the standard advanced trauma life support (ATLS) principles. Once a gastric injury is suspected or confirmed, laparotomy is indicated. Patients should receive preoperative prophylactic antibiotics directed against GI flora. Preparation of the patient for surgery should include antisepsis and draping from the chin to the knees. A midline laparotomy incision from the xiphoid to the pubis is created and the abdominal cavity entered. After control of significant hemorrhage, contamination from the GI tract is addressed. Any hollow viscus perforations can initially be controlled with Babcock clamps.

Examination of the stomach must be thorough, and to do so, mobilization of the stomach is needed for visualization. A gastric tube should be placed for decompression and to facilitate exposure. It may be necessary to divide the left triangular ligament of the liver with medial retraction of the lateral segment of the left liver lobe to expose the gastroesophageal (GE) junction. The lesser sac and posterior surface of the stomach should be visualized by dividing the avascular portion of the gastrocolic omentum. A technique we find useful for

evaluation of the posterior aspect of the stomach is to place a Deaver retractor along the posterior gastric wall after division of the gastrocolic omentum and apply posterior and caudal retraction on the pancreas with a sponge stick. The gastric retractor is directed cranially and the Deaver retractor is carefully withdrawn to allow visualization from the posterior GE junction proximally to the antrum distally. Any hematoma of the stomach wall should be evacuated and thoroughly explored. The presence of a single anterior wound should prompt a search for a second wound (especially posteriorly). A useful intraoperative adjunct for the diagnosis of small perforations or injuries in areas difficult to visualize is the intragastric instillation of methylene blue dye, which will stain the surrounding tissues.

Because of the stomach's large size and generous blood supply, most wounds are amenable to primary repair by either hand-sewn or stapling techniques. Narrowing the lumen is rarely a concern. Intramural hematomas are repaired with an interrupted Lembert suture technique after evacuation of the hematoma. Small lacerations can be repaired in two layers after adequate débridement. The inner layer should be a full-thickness hemostatic absorbable suture and the outer layer, an interrupted seromuscular suture. Alternatively, a TA stapler can be used to resect the gastric laceration.

Repair of wounds near the GE junction or pylorus may result in stenosis. A pyloric wound might require conversion to a pyloroplasty. Some wounds may be extensive and necessitate either proximal or distal gastrectomy. The standard principles of gastric resection are safely applied in these circumstances. If a vagus nerve injury is encountered, a drainage procedure should be performed.

Caustic Injuries

Laparotomy may be indicated in patients with severe gastric injury and suspected full-thickness necrosis. The entire stomach should be inspected and all areas of gastric necrosis resected, which may require subtotal or total gastrectomy. Reconstruction is based on the degree of resection: Billroth I or II for antrectomy and Roux-en-Y for total gastrectomy. Usually, if significant gastric injury is present, there may be an associated severe esophageal injury, especially with lye ingestion. In theses cases, total esophagectomy and gastrectomy with creation of a feeding jejunostomy may be needed.

Emetogenic Injuries

Bleeding from most emetogenic injuries is self-limited. Endoscopy generally identifies these injuries, which are located near the GE junction. Furthermore, gastroscopy is not only diagnostic but can also be therapeutic. Endoscopic treatment includes the injection of sclerosing agents and epinephrine, as well as electrocautery. Arteriography with the infusion of vasopressin or embolization of the left gastric artery can effectively provide hemostasis.

If surgery is indicated for refractory bleeding, a vertical gastrotomy on the anterior body of the stomach will allow visualization of the injury. The injury is repaired and closed with running nonabsorbable suture.

Complications

As mentioned previously, isolated gastric injuries are rarely fatal. The associated injuries usually carry high morbidity and mortality. Specific complications relating to penetrating gastric wounds include postoperative bleeding, intra-abdominal abscess, sepsis, and gastric fistulas. A delay in the diagnosis of gastric wounds and extensive spillage of gastric contents at surgery increase the frequency of intra-abdominal infections and sepsis. Based on the current literature it seems reasonable that surgery should be performed within 8 hours of injury in patients with hollow viscus injuries to avoid the increase in morbidity.[21] Meticulous débridement of the gastric wound plus thorough cleansing of the peritoneal cavity of any spilled enteric contents is essential. When both diaphragm and gastric injuries are present, the incidence of empyema is increased. Therefore, if the pleural space has been contaminated by enteric contents, the pleural cavity should be irrigated through the diaphragmatic defect.[4] The presence of a gastric injury in addition to a colon injury has been shown to have a synergistic effect on the rate of postoperative infection.[28]

An intra-abdominal abscess may be manifested as postoperative fever, leukocytosis, ileus, and signs of sepsis. CT usually confirms the diagnosis, and most abscesses can be managed by percutaneous drainage and broad-spectrum antibiotics. Consideration of fungal elements such as *Candida* species should not be overlooked in patients who appear to be refractory to appropriate management. A leak from a repair or anastomosis, which is often the cause of the abscess, is usually of low output and can be managed with adequate drainage, antibiotics, and nutritional support.

Early postoperative bleeding after gastric repair is generally a technical error. Reoperation may be necessary if the bleeding continues despite adequate correction of any metabolic and coagulopathic abnormalities. Late (>7 days) bleeding is generally mild, self-limited, and caused by sloughing of the inner layer of the gastric repair.

DUODENAL INJURIES

History

Management of penetrating abdominal injuries was nonoperative until the late 19th century. Larrey probably provided the first description of a penetrating duodenal injury in 1811 when he reported a 17-year-old patient who was stabbed above the umbilicus.[29] He described eviscerated omentum, persistent hematemesis, and sepsis, but the patient was treated nonoperatively. Later, autopsy reports from the American Civil War described five soldiers with duodenal shot wounds.[30] All injuries were treated without surgery. It was not until 1896 that Herczel reported the first repair of a duodenal injury.[31] Sporadic reports and small series followed, but a nonoperative approach persisted until World War I, when surgeons began to use exploratory laparotomy to diagnose and treat penetrating abdominal injuries. Mortality remained substantial despite routine operative intervention for penetrating abdominal injuries in World War II. Cave et al. reported the first large military series (118 cases) of duodenal injuries after World War II and described a 55.9% mortality rate despite attempts at operative repair.[31] Since the mid-20th century, advances in operative technique, nutrition, antibiotics, and critical care have reduced the mortality associated with duodenal injuries.

Anatomy

The duodenum is the first portion of the small bowel and measures 25 to 30 cm in adults. The duodenum is divided into four portions. The first portion stretches from the pylorus to the gastroduodenal artery superiorly and the common bile duct inferiorly. The second, or descending, portion extends from the gastroduodenal artery and common bile duct to the ampulla of Vater. The third portion courses transversely and superiorly and extends from the ampulla to the superior mesenteric vessels. The final, or fourth, portion of the duodenum continues from the mesenteric vessels to the duodenojejunal flexure at the ligament of Treitz, located to the left of the second lumbar vertebra. Overall, the duodenum assumes a C shape and overlies the first three lumbar vertebrae (see Fig. 53–1). With the exception of the anterior half of the first portion, the duodenum is a retroperitoneal structure that lies in close proximity to numerous vital structures. In addition to the vertebral bodies, the posterior surface of the duodenum rests on the aorta, inferior vena cava, portal vein, right kidney, and psoas muscles. The common bile duct passes deep to the duodenum, between the first and second portions, and enters the posterior aspect of the pancreatic head in most patients. Anterior to the duodenum are the liver, gallbladder, hepatic flexure, transverse mesocolon, and stomach. The pancreas lies within the confines of the duodenal C loop. The mesenteric vessels protrude from the inferior aspect of the pancreas to lie atop the duodenum. Blood supply is shared between these two intimately associated organs. Arterial supply to the duodenum includes the gastroduodenal artery, superior and inferior pancreaticoduodenal arteries, supraduodenal artery, and retroduodenal artery. This close proximity to numerous organs and major vascular structures accounts for the high incidence of associated injuries, morbidity, and mortality common in patients with duodenal injuries.

Physiology

Each day, approximately 10 L of digestive fluids passes though the duodenum. It is here that the chyle, bile, and pancreatic secretions initially mix together. The duodenum is partially responsible for absorption of carbohydrates, protein, fats, water, ions, and vitamins. Although digestion of carbohydrates begins in the mouth, the majority of digestion occurs when chyle mixes with pancreatic amylase in the duodenum. Further digestion by brush border enzymes in the small bowel takes place before carbohydrates are ultimately absorbed as monosaccharides. Protein digestion begins in the stomach through the enzymatic action of pepsin, but once again, the majority of digestion occurs in the upper portion of the small intestine. Once the duodenal brush border enzyme enterokinase comes in contact with chyle, trypsin is formed from inactive trypsinogen, and the remainder of pancreatic proteases (chymotrypsin, elastase, carboxypeptidase, etc.) are secreted into the duodenal lumen and activated. Most proteins are absorbed in the proximal part of the small bowel. Fats are emulsified through the action of bile salt– and lecithin-containing bile once excreted from the ampulla. Pancreatic lipase further digests triglycerides, which are ultimately absorbed in the proximal part of the small intestine. Whereas water is absorbed by simple diffusion, calcium and iron are absorbed by active processes in the duodenum. Importantly, this large volume of chyle and enzymatically active digestive secretions further contributes to the morbidity associated with failure of a duodenal repair—namely, a duodenal fistula.

Mechanisms

Deep in the retroperitoneum, the duodenum is protected from superficial injuries. Both blunt trauma and penetrating duodenal trauma are uncommon and account for just 3% to 5% of all abdominal injuries. Blunt injuries constitute roughly 22% of all duodenal injuries and are usually caused by motor vehicle collisions, assaults, or falls.[32] Motor vehicle collisions are responsible for 77% of blunt duodenal injuries, whereas assaults and falls each account for 10%.[32] The remaining 3% of blunt injuries are caused by various injury mechanisms. Overall, 78% of duodenal injuries are penetrating.[32] Of these penetrating injuries, 75% are inflicted by gunshots, 19% by stab wounds, and 6% by shotgun wounds.[32] Injuries may be further classified by anatomic location. Whereas penetrating injuries may be distributed more equally among the four duodenal segments, blunt mechanisms predominantly injure the second and third portions of the duodenum. When both blunt and penetrating mechanisms are considered, the second portion of the duodenum is the most commonly injured (33%), followed by third and fourth portions (19% each), first portion (15%), and multiple sites (14%).[32]

Penetrating mechanisms are responsible for the majority of duodenal injuries. Knife wounds are usually simple duodenal lacerations, but gunshot wounds are created by missiles that impart their kinetic energy on tissues and thereby create a pathway of tissue destruction. Associated injuries are commonplace. Asensio et al., in a review of 11 series, analyzed 1153 patients with duodenal injuries and found 86.9% to have associated injuries.[32] The liver was the most common organ to sustain associated injury, but injury to the pancreas, small bowel, major vascular structures, and colon was also common.

Blunt duodenal injuries are caused by a complex series of forces that may crush, burst, or shear the duodenum. Crush injuries are due to a blow to the anterior abdominal wall, which then crushes the duodenum against the underlying vertebral column. This injury pattern is commonly caused by a steering wheel in a head-on–type of collision. Simultaneous closure of the pylorus and contraction of the ligament of Treitz during a powerful blow to the abdomen can result in a bursting-type injury to the fluid- and air-filled duodenum. A shearing-type injury may also occur. Although the duodenum is anatomically fixed by the common bile duct and ligament of Treitz, the remainder of the duodenum remains highly mobile. Sudden changes in acceleration (e.g., falls) may shear the mobile segments of the duodenum from the fixed portions. Occasionally, these complex crushing or shearing forces rupture the small vessels within the submucosal layers and cause an intramural duodenal hematoma.

Diagnosis

The diagnosis of blunt duodenal injuries remains challenging. Information obtained from emergency medical service personnel present at the injury scene is essential to elucidate the injury mechanism and pattern of forces involved. Data should include the direction of collision, the use of restraints, airbag deployment, condition of the steering wheel, and whether extrication was necessary. However, less violent injury mechanisms such as falls and assaults may also injure the duodenum, but such injury is less often suspected. Given its retroperitoneal location, physical examination is often unimpressive despite frank duodenal perforation. The injured patient may have only vague or mild complaints. Peritonitis becomes evident later, only after retroperitoneal contents leak into the peritoneal cavity. Signs and symptoms of duodenal hematomas are even less convincing. Copious bilious vomiting may be observed in cases of nearly complete obstruction, but such symptoms are often late in onset. For these reasons, the diagnosis and treatment of blunt duodenal injuries are frequently delayed despite knowledgeable practitioners.

Laboratory data are of little diagnostic benefit. Although serum amylase is elevated in a majority of patients with pancreatic injuries, the level may be normal or only mildly elevated in those with duodenal injuries. Several reports have questioned the prognostic significance of a single serum amylase level, but work by Lucas and Ledgerwood found that serial amylase levels may improve the diagnostic yield.[33] Indeed, the presence of a normal amylase value does not preclude duodenal injury.

Plain films of the abdomen are equally unhelpful. Often described but present in less than a third of patients, evidence of duodenal injury on plain film includes air visualized around the right kidney, right psoas, or cecum; obliteration of the right psoas shadow; and scoliosis of the spine to the left. Free air is seen in less than 10% of patients with duodenal rupture.[33,34] An upper GI study with diatrizoate meglumine given either orally or via nasogastric tube improves the diagnostic yield. *A coiled spring* or *stacked coin* sign may indicate a duodenal intramural hematoma, whereas extraluminal

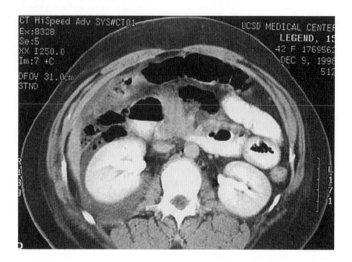

Figure 53–2. Computed tomography scan demonstrating retroperitoneal air and edema. (From Hoyt DB, Coimbra R, Potenza B: Management of acute trauma. In Townsend CM, Beauchamp RD, Evers BM, Mattox KL [eds]: Sabiston Textbook of Surgery, 17th ed. Philadelphia, WB Saunders, 2004, p 516.)

contrast or air indicates perforation. Both DPL and FAST are unreliable adjuncts for the diagnosis of duodenal injuries.

CT scanning with intravenous and intraluminal contrast is presently the diagnostic study of choice for hemodynamically stable patients with suspected retroperitoneal injury. CT has a unique ability to visualize the retroperitoneum, and findings consistent with blunt duodenal injury include bowel wall thickening or hematoma; extraluminal gas, fluid, or contrast medium; and retroperitoneal air or edema (Fig. 53–2). However, findings consistent with duodenal perforation (extravasation of contrast or the presence of retroperitoneal air) are infrequent, even in patients with documented full-thickness perforation. CT scans with subtle findings should be followed by an upper GI series. Patients with evidence of full-thickness duodenal perforations should undergo urgent operative exploration.

The diagnosis of penetrating duodenal injuries is usually made intraoperatively during laparotomy. All wound trajectories near the duodenum require full mobilization and visualization of the duodenum to ensure the absence of injury.

Management

Intramural hematomas are a rare subset of duodenal injuries with distinctly different management practices. Although operative intervention is the rule for most duodenal injuries, the majority of duodenal hematomas are managed nonoperatively. Hematomas generally resolve within a week with nasogastric decompression, bowel rest, and parenteral nutrition. Patients with prolonged complete obstruction or a deteriorating clinical condition may warrant laparotomy. A longitudinal seromuscu-

lar incision is made over the hematoma, and the contents are expressed. A careful search for occult perforations is then made, and complete hemostasis is achieved. The seromuscular wound is repaired with interrupted silk Lembert suture. However, most operations for duodenal injuries are performed to repair full-thickness perforations, not evacuate hematomas. Total exposure of the duodenum is essential before repair.

Exploratory laparotomy through a generous midline incision, from the xyphoid to the pubic symphysis, allows full inspection of the abdomen in cases of suspected duodenal injury. The abdomen is packed, and the zones of the retroperitoneum are quickly explored. Life-threatening hemorrhage and spillage of enteric contents are controlled. A methodical, organ-by-organ inspection then ensues. Evidence of paraduodenal injury such as hematoma, bilious staining, edema, or enteric contents mandates complete duodenal exposure. All duodenal hematomas must be thoroughly explored to exclude the possibility of an occult perforation.

Complete exposure of the duodenum is achieved with the aid of the Kocher and Cattell-Braasch maneuvers. The duodenum is kocherized by incising its lateral attachments while lifting the duodenum and pancreas medially until the superior mesenteric artery is approached. This procedure should completely expose the underside of the first, second, and third portions of the duodenum. The Cattell-Braasch maneuver consists of complete mobilization of the hepatic flexure, ascending colon, and small bowel from the right lower quadrant to the ligament of Treitz. With the bowel retracted cephalad, the entire third portion of the duodenum should now be visible (Fig. 53–3). Incision of the ligament of Treitz exposes the fourth portion of the duodenum (Fig. 53–4). All aspects of the duodenum must be fully inspected. Two options exist for patients with suspected injury but without evidence of obvious perforation. First, the abdomen may be filled with warm saline after a nasogastric tube is guided into the proximal part of the duodenum. Air is then instilled through the nasogastric tube as the surgeon watches for air bubbles arising from the duodenum. Methylene blue may also be instilled through the nasogastric tube after the duodenum is surrounded by clean lap sponges. Evidence of blue staining on the sponges indicates full-thickness perforation.

Before proceeding to duodenal repair, a careful assessment of the general condition of the patient should be made, with inspection for associated injuries to structures such as the pancreas, common bile duct, and ampulla. Diagnostic maneuvers such as cholangiography or pancreatography must be performed when a ductal injury is questioned. The presence of these high-grade injuries warrants more complex repairs and therefore may be more suitable for a subsequent operation in a hypothermic, coagulopathic, acidotic patient.

Still, the majority of duodenal wounds may be repaired by simple suture techniques.[32,35,36] Partial-thickness injuries may be either observed or buttressed with silk seromuscular Lembert sutures. Full-thickness wounds must be débrided back to healthy tissue. Adjacent wounds caused by a tangential trajectory are connected to create a single suture line. Wounds should be

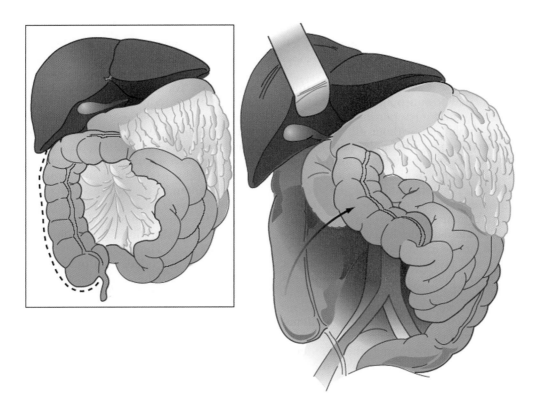

Figure 53–3. The Cattell-Braasch maneuver provides adequate exposure to the retroperitoneal structures. (From Hirshberg A, Mattox KL: Vascular trauma. In Townsend CM, Beauchamp RD, Evers BM, Mattox KL [eds]: Sabiston Textbook of Surgery, 17th ed. Philadelphia, WB Saunders, 2004, p 2041. Illustration by Jan Redden © Kenneth L. Mattox.)

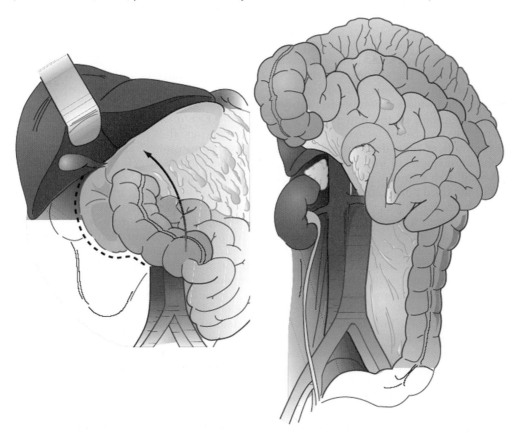

Figure 53–4. The Kocher maneuver provides adequate exposure and mobilization of the duodenum. (From Hirshberg A, Mattox KL: Vascular trauma. In Townsend CM, Beauchamp RD, Evers BM, Mattox KL [eds]: Sabiston Textbook of Surgery, 17th ed. Philadelphia, WB Saunders, 2004, p 2041. Illustration by Jan Redden © Kenneth L. Mattox.)

repaired transversely and may be one or two layered, interrupted or continuous, depending on surgeon preference. No study to date has conclusively shown the superiority of one technique over another.

Several repair options are available for larger wounds when simple repair may compromise the duodenal lumen. The first, third, and fourth portions of the duodenum are usually mobilized without difficulty. For destructive injuries to these portions, mobilization, resection, and primary end-to-end anastomosis may be performed. Because of tethering by the adjacent pancreas and several small vessels, mobilization of the second portion of the duodenum is more difficult, and as a result, resection with primary anastomosis is often impossible. In these cases, an end-to-side, Roux-en-Y duodenojejunostomy may be necessary. A jejunal Roux limb is brought up in retrocolic fashion if the patient's clinical condition permits, and a mucosa-to-mucosa anastomosis is performed. The duodenum requires only minimal mobilization, and the wound is repaired without tension. A serosal patch is another option for larger duodenal wounds. Originally described by Kobold and Thal, this method of repair involves overlaying the duodenal wound with a loop of jejunum.[37] The margins of the duodenal wound are sutured directly to the jejunal serosa to provide wound closure. All duodenal wound repairs should be externally drained. Closed-suction drains are placed adjacent to, but not touching repairs. In the unfortunate event of repair breakdown and duodenal fistula, adjacent closed-suction drains will better control the process and allow diagnostic imaging.

Duodenal fistulas are perhaps the most serious complication of duodenal injuries. Over the years, surgeons have developed several innovative procedures to prevent duodenal fistulas and convert them from a lateral to a more controllable end type of fistula. One adjunctive procedure to limit fistula formation is tube decompression. By preventing distention of the new repair, duodenostomy tubes may prevent fistula formation in severe injuries. Several methods of tube decompression have been described, the most simple of which is lateral tube duodenostomy. A small stab wound is made in the most dependent aspect of the third portion of the duodenum, through which a drainage catheter is placed. The catheter is then secured with a purse-string suture and brought out laterally along the retroperitoneum to exit the peritoneal cavity in the midaxillary line. This method, though efficient, unfortunately requires the addition of yet another wound to an already injured duodenum. Alternatively, a nasogastric tube may be fed under direct guidance to a postpyloric location, adjacent to the repair. Nasogastric tubes, however, are uncomfortable and are often removed by the patient before clinically indicated. Although tube decompression does not completely divert the digestive secretion stream, the suture line is protected and decompressed.

Perhaps the most protective form of tube decompression is the triple-tube ostomy described by Stone in 1966 and 1979.[34,34a] In their original work, the authors compared fistula rates in patients repaired without triple-tube drainage (44 patients) and those repaired with triple-tube drainage (237 patients). Eight duodenal fistulas were reported in the group repaired without triple-tube drainage, but only one duodenal fistula occurred in the tube decompression group. These encouraging results have never been duplicated, and reports since have been conflicting. Ivatury and Cogbill separately reported increases in both duodenal complications and mortality in patients treated by adjunctive triple-tube ostomy.[38,39]

The surgical technique of triple-tube drainage is straightforward. A standard gastrostomy tube is placed, after which two separate jejunal tubes are inserted. The proximal tube is threaded in retrograde fashion into the duodenum to decompress the suture line, whereas the distal tube is placed as for standard jejunal feeding access. This adjunctive procedure has several drawbacks. Three new perforations are required in the already injured GI tract. The decompressive tubes frequently do not drain as intended to protect the fresh duodenal repair. Finally, if the drainage tubes are inadvertently removed, the open perforation is a set up for a fistula— the very scenario that the surgeon had hoped to prevent. Although this method offers superior protection over single-tube decompression, procedures for complete diversion of the GI stream were soon developed.

Berne and Donovan first reported duodenal diverticulization in 1968.[40,41] As originally described, the procedure consists of vagotomy, antrectomy, oversewing of the duodenal stump, duodenostomy tube placement, T-tube biliary drainage, and gastrojejunostomy. Although the procedure completely diverts GI secretions away from the healing duodenal suture line, duodenal diverticulization is a fairly complex operation. In critically injured patients, this labor-intensive procedure is time-consuming. Diverticulization is seldom performed today and has largely been replaced by the pyloric exclusion technique. First described by Vaughan et al. in 1977, pyloric exclusion does not involve resection of normal, healthy tissue as is the case with duodenal diverticulization, but instead it consists of duodenal repair, oversewing the pylorus through a gastrotomy, and gastrojejunostomy.[42] The gastrotomy is made proximal to the pylorus, which is then grasped and closed with suture. Closure may be accomplished in a purse-string or running fashion, and use of a variety of suture materials has been described. The gastrotomy wound is then fashioned into a gastrojejunostomy (Fig. 53–5). Today, the pyloric exclusion technique is often performed by applying a noncutting stapler immediately distal to the pylorus. Stapled exclusion is quicker than the hand-sewn version and may be more permanent.

Despite its technical simplicity, pyloric exclusion with gastrojejunostomy permanently alters the GI tract in a predominantly young, healthy population. Although reports indicate that the pylorus reopens within 3 weeks in more than 90% of patients, pyloric exclusion remains an ulcerogenic operation.[42,43] Postoperative marginal ulceration rates range from 0% to 33%, with most studies indicating marginal ulcers in approximately 10% of patients who underwent surveillance.[43,44] Truncal vagotomy in addition to pyloric exclusion has been advocated by some but is not routinely performed in critically injured patients. With these problems in mind, several authors have attempted to define which

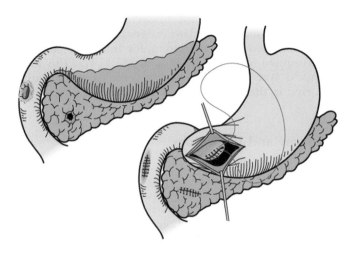

Figure 53–5. Pyloric exclusion. A gastrotomy is created and the pylorus is oversewn. The gastrotomy is then fashioned into a gastrojejunostomy. (From Steer ML: Exocrine pancreas. In Townsend CM, Beauchamp RD, Evers BM, Mattox KL [eds]: Sabiston Textbook of Surgery, 17th ed. Philadelphia, WB Saunders, 2004, p 1675.)

duodenal injuries may require these more sophisticated procedures.

Much time has been devoted to defining which duodenal injuries are in fact complex and which injuries may require the addition of these adjunctive procedures. Snyder and colleagues classified duodenal injuries as either mild or severe.[45] Severe injuries were characterized by one or more of the following criteria: missile injury, damage to greater than 75% of the duodenal wall circumference, involvement of the first or second portion of the duodenum, longer than 24 hours from injury to repair, and common bile duct injury. American Association for the Surgery of Trauma (AAST) grading may be used to classify duodenal injury severity, but it has not been a proven predictor of mortality.[46] Most authors consider grade III injuries (50% to 75% circumferential laceration) or greater to be severe, although there remains no clear consensus on the best operative treatment of these injuries. Timaran et al. showed that duodenal injury grade is not a risk factor predicting either duodenal fistula or mortality and that hypotension and shock are the most important predictors of outcome.[47] They concluded that even minor duodenal injuries compounded by hemorrhagic shock should be considered complex. Other authors consider a concomitant vascular or pancreatic injury an indication for a more sophisticated repair. Combined pancreaticoduodenal injuries deserve special mention.

Although injuries to the duodenum and body or tail of the pancreas may be managed separately, injuries to the duodenum and head of the pancreas require a unified approach. The first priority in these cases of combined pancreaticoduodenal injury is to fully examine the wound tract. Tracts in the vicinity of the common bile

duct, main pancreatic duct, or ampulla are scrutinized and merit further diagnostic evaluation. Intraoperative cholangiography is required to completely examine the common bile duct. A cholangiocatheter is introduced into the cystic duct and contrast is injected. Dye is visualized throughout the common bile duct, into the main pancreatic duct, and into the duodenum. Cholecystectomy is then performed. Although the cholangiocatheter may be introduced into the common bile duct or gallbladder, these options are less appealing. Whereas complete visualization of the bile ducts is frequently achieved with cholangiography, the pancreatic duct is poorly visualized.

Several methods of pancreatography have been described, none of which are ideal. Thorough examination of the ampullary complex is imperative in all injuries involving the second portion of the duodenum. This inspection is accomplished through the duodenal wound. In patients with wound tracts adjacent to the ampulla, the ampulla should be thoroughly palpated and probed to ensure integrity of the structure. If the ampulla is visualized through the duodenal wound, a catheter may be introduced under direct vision for pancreatography. However, if the wound is not adjacent to the ampulla, a new duodenotomy may be created for placement of the catheter. Once again, this method involves further injury to an already wounded duodenum. Alternatively, the tail of the pancreas may be transected and pancreatography performed in retrograde fashion. This controversial maneuver has been widely criticized. After the healthy tissues in the pancreatic tail are transected, the duct is often exceedingly small and difficult to cannulate at this location. Perhaps the best option for complete visualization of the bile and pancreatic ducts is intraoperative endoscopic retrograde cholangiopancreatography (ERCP). At many centers, ERCP is either impractical or unavailable during afterhours. In the end, sound surgical judgment and wisdom are the tools that the surgeon often relies on to decide whether the main pancreatic duct is injured.

Unreconstructable ductal injury in the pancreatic head is one of the few possible indications for pancreaticoduodenectomy. Today, the trauma Whipple procedure is rarely performed. At our own institution, pancreaticoduodenectomy was performed for 1 of 54 duodenal injuries over the past 10 years.[48] Other institutions echo the same hesitation to perform this complex, time-consuming operation in critically ill patients—and with good reason. The value of pancreaticoduodenectomy for severe bleeding in the pancreatic head is questionable. The patient is probably better served by a so-called damage control laparotomy followed by a definitive procedure once the patient is warmed and resuscitated. Asensio et al. reviewed 52 series in the literature involving 172 patients who underwent pancreaticoduodenectomy and noted a 33% mortality rate.[32] Some small single series have revealed better mortality rates, but these same series used more liberal indications for pancreaticoduodenectomy, thus making interpretation difficult.

Currently, the trauma Whipple procedure is reserved for destructive, devascularizing, unreconstructable wounds to the second portion of the duodenum and pancreatic head or for extensive injuries to the ampullary complex, distal common bile duct, and proximal main pancreatic duct that prevent reconstruction. As Walt once stated, "In the massively destructive lesions involving the pancreas, duodenum, and common bile duct, the decision to do a pancreaticoduodenectomy is unavoidable; and, in fact, much of the dissection may have been done by the wounding force" (p 641).[49]

Morbidity and Mortality

Complication rates remain significant for duodenal injuries despite improvements in perioperative care and operative technique. The morbidity and mortality related to duodenal injuries depend on the severity of injury, the presence of associated injuries, the general physiologic condition of the patient, the injury mechanism, and the elapsed interval between injury and repair. Several complications have been described, including duodenal fistula, abdominal abscess, pancreatitis, pancreatic fistula, duodenal or small bowel obstruction, and biliary fistula.

Perhaps the most serious and well described complication of duodenal repair is duodenal fistula. Asensio and colleagues reviewed 15 series involving 1408 patients and found an overall duodenal fistula rate of 6.6%.[32] The cornerstones of treatment of these fistulas remain drainage; nutritional support, ideally through a jejunostomy tube; skin protection; and antibiotics, if necessary. The somatostatin analogue octreotide may be used to decrease fistula output, but this agent has not yet been proved to promote spontaneous fistula closure. Unrelenting, high-output, lateral-type fistulas may require reoperation if spontaneous closure does not occur within a few weeks. At reoperation, the fistulous tract is resected, the duodenal repair is excluded from the GI stream, and feeding access is established. Nonoperative management of early postoperative duodenal and small bowel obstruction is the rule, but a gastrojejunostomy may be required for persistent duodenal obstruction.

In the extensive review by Asensio et al. involving 17 series in literature from 1968 to 1990, the overall mortality rate for duodenal injuries was 17%.[32] Roughly half of these deaths occurred early and were attributed to associated vascular injuries and exsanguination. When deaths caused by associated injuries are excluded, the mortality rate for duodenal injury remains an appreciable 6.5% to 12.5%.[32]

SMALL BOWEL INJURIES

History

Small bowel perforation from blunt abdominal trauma was first recognized by Aristotle.[50] Hippocrates was the first to report intestinal perforation from penetrating abdominal trauma. Before the late 19th century, the dismal results of surgical intervention for small bowel perforation led to the abandonment of laparotomy, even with obvious intestinal injury in war.[51] The routine use of exploratory laparotomy for suspected intestinal injury did not take place until late in World War I. Mortality rates associated with laparotomy for intestinal perforation dropped from 75% to 80% in World War I to 14% in World War II.[52] Further improvements in mortality occurred in the Korean and Vietnam wars.

Anatomy and Physiology

The small intestine includes the duodenum, jejunum, and ileum. This segment of the chapter focuses on the jejunum and ileum. The jejunum measures approximately 100 to 110 cm, whereas the ileum measures 150 to 160 cm. The major function of the small intestine is to serve as a surface for the absorption and digestion of proteins, carbohydrates, fat, water, and electrolytes. Proximal jejunal resections are better tolerated than distal ileal resections. A shorter length of small intestine is required for absorption if resection spares the ileocecal valve. Roughly 80 cm of small intestine is required to prevent short-bowel syndrome if the ileocecal valve is left in continuity. About 100 cm of small intestine is required to prevent short-bowel syndrome if the ileocecal valve has been resected.[53] The blood supply to the small intestine is the superior mesenteric artery and its branches. The superior mesenteric vein provides venous drainage into the portal system.

Mechanism

The small intestine is the most frequently injured organ after sustaining a penetrating injury. Stab wounds injure by direct contact, in contrast to gunshot wounds, which injure by both direct contact and transfer of energy from the bullet to the surrounding bowel.

After the spleen and liver, the small bowel is the third most common organ injured in blunt abdominal trauma. Approximately 5% to 20% of patients who require surgical exploration for blunt trauma have small bowel injuries.[54]

Blunt abdominal trauma can be due to motor vehicle crashes, falls, or assaults with blunt objects. Blunt injury to the small bowel can occur by one of three mechanisms. The small bowel can be crushed between the blunt object and the vertebral bodies. Sudden deceleration as a result of a fall from a height or a high-speed motor vehicle crash can lead to shearing of the small bowel at three fixed points: at the ligament of Treitz, at the ileocecal valve, and around the mesenteric artery. A bursting or blowout injury to the small bowel can occur secondary to an increase in intraluminal pressure in a functionally closed loop of bowel.

The presence of a seat belt sign on a patient who sustained a motor vehicle crash should lead the trauma surgeon to investigate for a Chance fracture of the lumbar vertebral body and subsequent small bowel injury.[55,56] In the EAST multi-institutional study, the seat belt sign was associated with a 4.7-fold increase in relative risk for small bowel perforation in patients after motor vehicle crashes.[57]

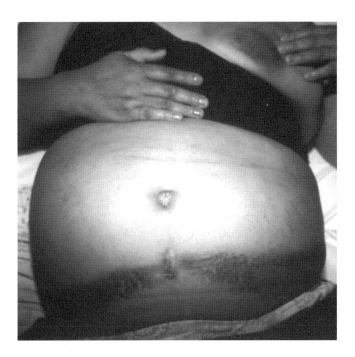

Figure 53–6. Abdominal wall ecchymoses secondary to seat belt deceleration.

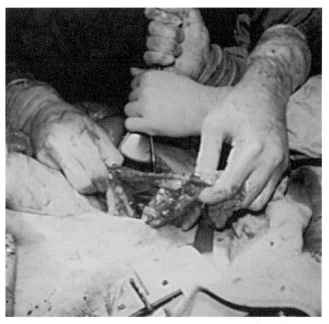

Figure 53–7. Small bowel and mesenteric injury from seat belt trauma.

Iatrogenic perforation of the small bowel by cauterization or direct injury during laparoscopic procedures should be treated by immediate laparotomy and repair.

Diagnosis

The key to successful management of small bowel injuries is prompt recognition and treatment, which can be challenging with the increasing use of nonoperative management of blunt solid organ injuries. Delay in diagnosis of perforated small bowel injuries is associated with significantly increased mortality.[7,21]

The ability to arrive at a successful diagnosis of small bowel injury caused by either blunt or penetrating trauma begins with a thorough focused history. If the patient is evaluated after having sustained penetrating trauma, a description of the wounding instrument is obtained, as well as the handedness of the assailant. The time that the injury occurred is also critical. Rapid transit from the scene may lead to the patient arriving before peritoneal inflammation has time to develop. If the patient has sustained blunt trauma, a thorough description of the scene can be invaluable when provided by the emergency medical services staff.

A thorough physical examination should be performed. Examination begins with measurement of the vital signs: heart rate, blood pressure, and respiratory rate. Inspection for gunshot wounds and stab wounds is critical, and total exposure of the patient is required. Seat belt marks and abrasions are also noted on patients who have sustained blunt trauma. The presence of a seat belt sign should raise suspicion for enteric and mesenteric injuries (Fig. 53–6). In fact, in a published study by Velmahos et al., 23% of patients with a seat belt sign had

intra-abdominal injuries.[58] Chandler et al. found that 21% of patients with abdominal seat belt signs had a small bowel perforation[59] (Fig. 53–7).

Loss of bowel sounds during auscultation could signify ileus secondary to injury to a hollow viscus. Tenderness to percussion and abdominal rigidity, guarding, and rebound suggest peritoneal irritation and warrant immediate exploration. Of special note, the abdominal examination may be compromised by alcohol or drug ingestion, as well as by head injury.

Radiographic work-up with an upright chest or abdominal radiograph may reveal free air; however, this sign can be rare.[60] Computed axial tomography (CAT) of the abdomen and pelvis with intravenous contrast only (oral contrast has recently been shown to offer no additional benefit, yet carries a risk for aspiration) can reveal findings suggestive of small bowel and mesenteric injury.[61,62] Such findings are free air, free fluid with no solid organ injury, small bowel wall thickening, mesenteric fat streaking, or mesenteric hematoma with extravasation of intravenous contrast.[63,64] (Fig. 53–8) Reports of the sensitivity and specificity of CAT scans in revealing small bowel injury have been quite varied. The experience of the Presley Regional Trauma Center with new-generation helical CAT scan evaluation for blunt bowel and mesenteric injuries indicates a sensitivity as high as 88.3%.[17] However, results from the EAST multi-institutional hollow viscus injury trial revealed that 13% of patients with a perforated small bowel found at the time of exploratory laparotomy had a normal preoperative abdominal CAT scan.[60]

The trauma surgeon must be cautious when the radiologist describes CAT scan findings in terms of general surgical diagnoses. The presence of mesenteric fat streaking and bowel wall thickening may be appropriate for a

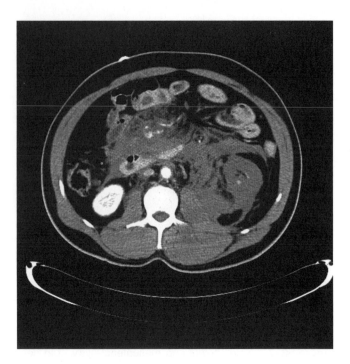

Figure 53–8. Computed axial tomographic scan of the abdomen and pelvis showing thickened loops of small bowel with extravasation of intravenous contrast into the mesentery.

patient with diverticulitis, but not for a patient who has sustained significant blunt abdominal trauma.

DPL has been replaced by FAST in the evaluation of unstable trauma patients. There is still a role for DPL in a blunt abdominal trauma patient who remains hypotensive after a repeat FAST examination fails to reveal free fluid. DPL would also be appropriate for a patient who sustains blunt abdominal trauma and is found to have free fluid on a CAT scan of the abdomen and pelvis with no solid organ injury. DPL revealing a WBC count of $500/mm^3$ or greater would mandate exploration to rule out small bowel injury. As an initial study, DPL may yield false-negative results when patients have been rapidly transported to the hospital and have had minimal time for leakage of enteric contents into the peritoneal cavity.

Diagnostic laparoscopy may be used as a diagnostic tool to determine peritoneal violation, as well as small bowel injury. However, the trauma surgeon must have the technical ability to evaluate the small bowel from the ligament of Treitz to the ileocecal valve. Once an injury is found, conversion to an open procedure would be recommended.

Operative Management

Exploration of the peritoneal cavity should be performed in a methodical, organized fashion. A midline incision is made, and all four quadrants of the peritoneal cavity should be packed. Control of hemorrhage is always the first priority. Once hemorrhage control is achieved, the next priority is to stop any ongoing enteric spillage.

The entire small bowel should be evaluated from the ligament of Treitz to the ileocecal valve. Attention should be particularly paid to both sides of the mesentery, as well as both sides of the bowel wall, mesenteric and anti-mesenteric. As injuries are discovered, control should be achieved with Babcock clamps. Hematomas of the bowel wall should be carefully unroofed and explored to assess for full-thickness injury. Hematomas of the mesentery should also be explored thoroughly as well. Any bleeding encountered should be controlled. Adequate evaluation of the small bowel to assess for viability should be performed, if necessary, with a Doppler probe. If there is any question about the viability of the small bowel, second-look laparotomy is always an option if the surgeon is not convinced of adequate blood supply or viability.

Grade I intramural hematomas may be repaired with inverted 3-0 silk seromuscular Lembert suture. Small wounds or wounds encompassing less than half the circumference of the small bowel can be managed by débridement if necessary and primary repair in two-layer fashion. Wounds involving more than half the circumference of the small bowel or multiple wounds of the small bowel should be managed by resection and primary anastomosis either in a two-layer hand-sewn manner or via stapled anastomosis.

In damage control situations, the bowel should be quickly repaired or resected. Definitive repair or primary anastomosis should not be performed until the patient returns to the operating room after all physiologic parameters have been corrected. Primary anastomosis can then be undertaken safely.

Adjacent through-and-through gunshot wounds or stab wounds to the small bowel may be joined, débrided, and closed primarily in the transverse direction. Use of the standard principles of a tension-free anastomosis with adequate blood supply will ensure proper healing.

Postoperative Management and Complications

The patient should receive 24 hours of antibiotics effective against gram-negative and anaerobic organisms. The first dose of antibiotics should be given as close to the time of injury as possible.

More commonly, complications are related to associated injuries and to delay in diagnosis and subsequent operative intervention of the small bowel injury. Postoperative complications can consist of wound infection, anastomotic leakage, intra-abdominal abscess formation, enteric fistula formation, and bowel obstruction. Anastomotic leakage requires return to the operating room if fever, tachycardia, an elevated WBC count, or peritonitis is found on physical examination. An intra-abdominal abscess can be treated by percutaneous drainage under CAT scan guidance.

If significant amounts of ileum have been resected, vitamin B_{12} deficiency may develop, as well as disruption of the enterohepatic recirculation of bile salts and subsequent fat malabsorption and hence fat-soluble vitamin deficiencies.

Short-bowel syndrome is usually seen after significant resections of the small bowel. Jejunal resections are better tolerated than ileal resections.

REFERENCES

1. Fenner ED: Report of six cases of penetrating wounds of the abdomen submitted to abdomen section. Ann Surg 35:15, 1902.
2. Wolf LH: Wounds of the stomach. In Surgery in World War II, vol 2, General Surgery. Washington, DC, Office of the Surgeon General, Department of the Army, 1955.
3. Blaisdell FW: General assessment, resuscitation and exploration of penetrating and blunt abdominal trauma. In Blaisdell FW, Trunkey OP (eds): Trauma Management: Abdominal Trauma, vol 1. New York, Thieme-Stratton, 1982, p 1.
4. Durham RM, Olson S, Weigelt JA: Penetrating injuries to the stomach. Surg Gynecol Obstet 172:298-302, 1991.
5. Courcey PA, Brotman S: Gastric rupture from blunt trauma. A plea for minimal diagnosis and early surgery. Am Surg 50:424-427, 1984.
6. Yajko RD, Seydel F, Trimble C: Rupture of the stomach from blunt abdominal trauma. J Trauma 15:177-183, 1975.
7. Watts, DD, Fakhry SM, East Multi-Institutional Hollow Viscus Injury Research Group: Incidence of hollow viscus injury in blunt trauma: An analysis from 257,557 trauma admissions from the EAST multi-institutional trial. J Trauma 54:289-294, 2003.
8. Brunsting LA, Morton JH: Gastric rupture from blunt abdominal trauma. J Trauma 27:887-891, 1987.
9. Nanji SA, Mock C: Gastric rupture resulting from blunt abdominal trauma and requiring gastric resection. J Trauma 47:410-412, 1999.
10. Garfinkle SE, Matolo WM: Gastric necrosis from blunt abdominal trauma. J Trauma 16:405-407, 1976.
11. Mallory GK, Weiss S: Hemorrhage from lacerations of cardiac orifice of stomach due to vomiting. Am J Med Sci 178:506, 1929.
12. Cowan M, Bardole J, Dlesk A: Perforated stomach following the Heimlich maneuver. Am J Emerg Med 5:121-122, 1987.
13. McDonnell PJ, Hutchins GM, Hruban RH, Brown CG: Hemorrhage from gastric mucosal tears complicating cardiopulmonary resuscitation. Am J Emerg Med 13:230-233, 1984.
14. Vinen JD, Gavdry PL: Pneumoperitoneum complicating cardiopulmonary resuscitation. Anaesth Intensive Care 14:193-196, 1986.
15. Harrison BJ, Glanges E, Sparkman RS: Gastric fistula following splenectomy: Its cause and prevention. Ann Surg 185:210-213, 1977.
16. Kennedy T, Magill P, Johnston GW, Parks TG: Proximal gastric vagotomy, fundoplication, and lesser curve necrosis. BMJ 1:1455-1456, 1979.
17. Malhotra AK, Fabian TC, Katsis SB, et al: Blunt bowel and mesenteric injuries: The role of screening computed tomography. J Trauma 48:991-998, discussion 998-1000, 2000.
18. Alyono D, Perry JF Jr: Value of quantitative cell count and amylase activity of peritoneal lavage fluid. J Trauma 21:345-348, 1981.
19. Rozycki GS, Ochsner MG, Jaffin JH, Champion HR: Prospective evaluation of surgeon's role of ultrasound in the evaluation of trauma patients. J Trauma 34:516-526, discussion 526-527, 1993.
20. Miller LA, Shanmuganathan K: Multidetector CT evaluation of abdominal trauma. Radiol Clin North Am 43:1079-1095, viii, 2005.
21. Fakhry SM, Brownstein M, Watts DD, et al: Relatively short diagnostic delays (<8 hrs) produce morbidity and mortality in blunt small bowel injury: An analysis of time to operative intervention in 198 patients from a multicenter experience. J Trauma 48:408-414, discussion 414-415, 2000.
22. Zantut LF, Ivatury RR, Smith RS, et al: Diagnostic and therapeutic laparoscopy for penetrating abdominal trauma: A multicenter experience. J Trauma 42:825-829, discussion 829-831, 1997.
23. Kawahara N, Zantut LF, Poggetti RS, et al: Laparoscopic treatment of gastric and diaphragmatic injury produced by thoracoabdominal stab wound. J Trauma 45:613-614, 1998.
24. Ivatury RR, Simon RJ, Stahl WM: A critical evaluation of laparoscopy in penetrating abdominal trauma. J Trauma 34:822-827, discussion 827-828, 1993.
25. Guth AA, Pachter HL: Laparoscopy for penetrating thoracoabdominal trauma: Pitfalls and promises. JSLS 2:123-127, 1998.
26. Elliott DC, Rodriguez A, Moncure M, et al: The accuracy of diagnostic laparoscopy in trauma patients: A prospective, controlled study. Int Surg 83:294-298, 1998.
27. Kirsh MM, Ritter F: Caustic ingestion and subsequent damage to the oropharyngeal and digestive passage. Ann Thorac Surg 21:74-82, 1976.
28. O'Neill PA, Kirton OC, Dresner LS, et al: Analysis of 162 colon injuries in patients with penetrating abdominal trauma: Concomitant stomach injury results in a higher rate of infection. J Trauma 56:304-312, discussion 312-313, 2004.
29. Larrey DJ: Memoirs of Military Surgery and Campaigns [translated from the French by RW Hall], vol 3. Baltimore, Joseph Cushing, 1814, pp 309-389.
30. Otis GA: Medical and Surgical History of the War of Rebellion, part 2, vol 2. Washington, DC, Government Printing Office, 1876, pp 158-161.
31. Cave WH: Duodenal injuries. Am J Surg 72:26-31, 1946.
32. Asensio JA, Feliciano DV, Britt LD, et al: Management of duodenal injuries. Curr Probl Surg 30:1023-1093, 1993.
33. Lucas CE, Ledgerwood AM: Factors influencing outcome after blunt duodenal injury. J Trauma 15:839-846, 1975.
34. Stone HH, Fabian TC: Management of duodenal wounds. J Trauma 19:334-339, 1979.
34a. Stone HH, Garoni WJ: Experiences in the management of duodenal wounds. South Med J 59:864, 1966.
35. Ivatury RR, Nassoura ZE, Simon RJ, et al: Complex duodenal injuries. Surg Clin North Am 76:797-812, 1996.
36. Carrillo EH, Richardson DJ, Miller FB: Evolution in the management of duodenal injuries. J Trauma 40:1037-1046, 1996.
37. Kobold EE, Thal AP: A simple method for the management of experimental wounds of the duodenum. Surg Gynecol Obstet 116:340-344, 1963.
38. Ivatury RR, Nallathambi M, Gaudino J, et al: Penetrating duodenal injuries: Analysis of 100 consecutive cases. Am J Surg 2:153-158, 1985.
39. Cogbill TH, Moore EE, Feliciano DV, et al: Conservative management of duodenal trauma: A multicenter perspective. J Trauma 30:1469-1475, 1990.
40. Berne CJ, Donovan AJ, Hagen WE: Combined duodenal pancreatic trauma: The role of end-to-side gastrojejunostomy. Arch Surg 96:712-722, 1968.
41. Berne CJ, Donovan AJ, White EJ, et al: Duodenal "diverticulization" for duodenal and pancreatic injury. Am J Surg 127:503-507, 1974.
42. Vaughan GD III, Frazier OH, Graham DY, et al: The use of pyloric exclusion in the management of severe duodenal injuries. Am J Surg 134:785-790, 1977.
43. Martin TD, Feliciano DV, Mattox KL, et al: Severe duodenal injuries: Treatment with pyloric exclusion and gastrojejunostomy. Arch Surg 118:631-635, 1983.
44. Buck JR, Sorensen VJ, Fath JJ, et al: Severe pancreatico-duodenal injuries: The effectiveness of pyloric exclusion with vagotomy. Am Surg 58:557-561, 1992.
45. Snyder WH III, Weigelt JA, Watkins WL, et al: The surgical management of duodenal trauma. Arch Surg 115:422-429, 1980.
46. Moore EE, Cogbill TH, Malangoni MA, et al: Organ injury scaling II: Pancreas, duodenum, small bowel, colon and rectum. J Trauma 30:1427-1429, 1990.
47. Timaran CH, Martinez O, Ospina JA: Prognostic factors and management of civilian penetrating duodenal trauma. J Trauma 47:330-335, 1999.
48. Seamon MJ, Pathak AS, Goldberg AJ, et al: Unpublished data, 2005.
49. Walt AJ: Penetrating injuries to the duodenum. In Ivatury RR, Cayten CG (eds): The Textbook of Penetrating Trauma. Baltimore, Williams & Wilkins, 1996, p 641.
50. Loria FL: Historical aspects of penetrating wounds of the abdomen. Int Abstr Surg 87:521, 1948.
51. Bailey H (ed): Surgery of Modern Warfare, vol 2, 3rd ed. Baltimore, Williams & Wilkins, 1944.
52. Surgery in World War II, vol 2, General Surgery. Washington, DC, Office of the Surgeon General, Department of the Army, 1955.
53. Sundaram A, Koutkia P, Apovian CM: Nutritional management of short bowel in adults. J Clin Gastroenterol 34:207-220, 2002.
54. Hoyt DB, Coimbra R, Potenza B: Management of acute trauma. In Townsend CM, Beauchamp RD, Evers BM, Mattox KL (eds): Sabis-

ton Textbook of Surgery, 17th ed. Philadelphia, Elsevier, 2004, pp 518-519.

55. Appleby JP, Nagy AG: Abdominal injuries associated with the use of seatbelts. Am J Surg 157:457-458, 1989.

56. Rutledge R, Thomason M, Oller D, et al: The spectrum of abdominal injuries associated with the use of seat belts. J Trauma 31:820-825, discussion 825-826, 1991.

57. Watts D, Fakhry S, Pasquale M, et al: Motor vehicle crash (MVC) and abdominal seatbelt mark as risk factors for perforating small bowel injury (SBI): Results from a large multi-institutional study [abstract]. J Trauma 51:1232, 2001.

58. Velmahos GC, Tatevossian R, Demetriades D: The "seat belt mark" sign: A call for increased vigilance among physicians treating victims of motor vehicle accidents. Am Surg 65:181-185, 1999.

59. Chandler CF, Lane JS, Waxman, KS: Seatbelt sign following blunt trauma is associated with increased incidence of abdominal injury. Am Surg 63:885-888, 1997.

60. Fakhry SM, Watts DD, Luchette FA, East Multi-Institutional Hollow Viscus Injury Research Group: Current diagnostic approaches lack sensitivity in the diagnosis of perforated blunt small bowel injury: Analysis from 275,557 trauma admissions from the EAST multi-institutional HVI trial. J Trauma 54:295-306, 2003.

61. Allen TL, Mueller MT, Bonk RT, et al: Computed tomographic scanning without oral contrast solution for blunt bowel and mesenteric injuries in abdominal trauma. J Trauma 56:314-322, 2004.

62. Holmes JF, Offerman SR, Chang CH, et al: Performance of helical computed tomography without oral contrast for the detection of gastrointestinal injuries. Ann Emerg Med 43:120-128, 2004.

63. Nghiem HV, Jeffrey RB Jr, Mindelzun RE: CT of blunt trauma to the bowel and mesentery. Semin Ultrasound CT MR 16:82-90, 1995.

64. Akiyoshi H, Tesuo Y, Michihiro S et al: Early diagnosis of small intestine rupture from blunt abdominal trauma using computed tomography: Significance of the streaky density within the mesentery. J Trauma 38:630, 1995.

54

Small Intestinal Diverticula

Michael C. Stoner ▪ Joanna C. Arcuni ▪ John M. Kellum

Small intestinal diverticula are protrusions of various layers of the intestinal wall through the serosa and onto the mesenteric or peritoneal aspects of the bowel. In contrast to congenital diverticula, such as Meckel's diverticulum, which include all layers of the normal intestinal wall, the more common acquired diverticula, the pseudodiverticula, lack the muscularis propria. Although small intestinal diverticula are frequently asymptomatic, they can cause life-threatening complications. This chapter includes a discussion of duodenal, jejunoileal, and Meckel's diverticula.

In order of frequency, diverticula of the gastrointestinal tract occur in the colon, ileum (Meckel's diverticulum), duodenum, pharynx and esophagus, stomach, jejunum, appendix, and ileum (other than Meckel's).[1] Thus, for pseudodiverticula, the duodenum, after the colon, is the most common site, whereas the jejunum and ileum, excluding Meckel's diverticulum, are rarely the location of small intestinal diverticula.

DUODENAL DIVERTICULA

Small intestinal diverticula are difficult to demonstrate either radiographically or anatomically because of their frequent location in the mesentery. Consequently, their incidence is underestimated. The reported incidence of duodenal diverticula ranges from 0.2% to 7.1% based on radiologic contrast studies,[2,3] 9% to 20% by upper gastrointestinal endoscopy,[2] and 3% to 22% according to autopsies.[2] The lesion is most common in the fifth decade of life, with a 2:1 female preponderance.[3-5] Extraluminal duodenal diverticula are much more common than the intraluminal type. Most of the former are pseudodiverticula located on the pancreatic aspect (Fig. 54–1). Four percent to 12% of diverticula occur in the first portion of the duodenum, 56% to 80% in the second portion, and 4% to 36% in the third and fourth portions[4,6-9] (Fig. 54–2). Two thirds to three fourths of duodenal diverticula occur within 2 cm of the ampulla of Vater. Most patients with immediately juxtavaterian diverticula have ampullae entering the duodenum at the superior margin rather than through the diverticulum itself[3] (Fig. 54–3).

Although most duodenal diverticula occur on the medial aspect, 4% to 16% are on the lateral or anterior wall. Most of these latter lesions are true diverticula. Diverticula on the medial aspect of the duodenum may be embedded within the substance of the pancreas.[10] An autopsy study by Suda and colleagues[11] demonstrated that 18 of 27 diverticula in the second portion of the duodenum penetrated the pancreas.

Intraluminal diverticula are congenital webs that arise near the ampulla of Vater. They are caused by incomplete recanalization of the duodenum. As a result of stretching and peristalsis, they are transformed into diverticula. On contrast radiography, they give a typical *windsock* effect (Fig. 54–4). Only slightly more than 100 have been described in the world literature. Most attach to less than half the circumference of the duodenal lumen, but a few attach to the entire circumference. They all have an opening, usually located near the apex. Without an opening, they are manifested in neonatal life as duodenal obstruction.[12]

Pathogenesis

Because duodenal diverticula are often associated with colonic and jejunal diverticula, it is postulated that pulsion forces lead to herniation of mucosal or submucosal outpouchings through the muscularis of a weakened intestinal wall. Because most of these pseudodiverticula form on the concave (pancreatic) side of the duodenum, the pulsion theory postulates that diverticula occur at points of penetration of the duodenal wall by blood vessels or by the ampulla of Vater. As Roses and associates[13] noted, the pulsion theory is supported by the increasing incidence of diverticula with age and by the usual absence of muscularis in the wall of the diverticulum.

Horton and Mueller[1] noted that the pancreas often penetrates the longitudinal wall of the concave aspect of the duodenum, with only the circular muscle separating

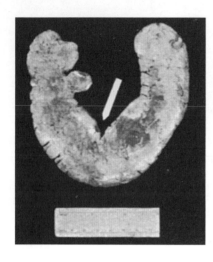
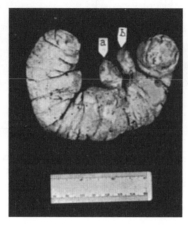

Figure 54–1. Plaster casts of diverticula in the second, third, and fourth portions of the duodenum. The *arrow* in the figure on the *left* marks the papilla of Vater. (From Ackerman W: Diverticula and variations of the duodenum. Ann Surg 117:403, 1943.)

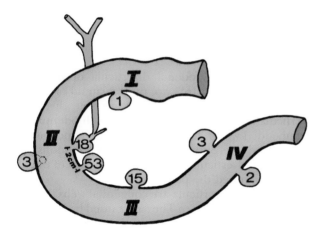

Figure 54–2. Distribution of duodenal diverticula within the four portions of the duodenum. (The *circled numbers* indicate how many cases were seen.) (From Townsend CM, Thompson JCT: Small intestine. In Schwartz SI [ed]: Principles of Surgery, vol 2, 6th ed. New York, McGraw-Hill, 1993, p 1178.)

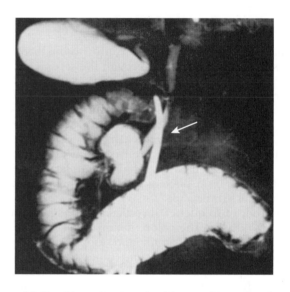

Figure 54–3. Air-contrast study of the small intestine demonstrating a diverticulum of the second part of the duodenum with the pancreatic duct and common bile duct entering directly into the diverticulum *(arrow)*. (From Wolfson NS, Miller FB: Anatomic relationship of insertion of the common bile duct into primary duodenal diverticula. Surg Gynecol Obstet [now J Am Coll Surg] 146:628, 1978. By permission of *Surgery, Gynecology and Obstetrics*.)

it from the mucosa. Less commonly, pancreatic tissue penetrates both muscular layers and produces an intrinsically weak segment of duodenal wall. They postulated that either situation favored the development of diverticula.

An increased incidence of duodenal and jejunoileal diverticula has been reported in diseases associated with disorders of smooth muscle or the myenteric plexus and in systemic immunologic diseases. They have been reported as having a higher incidence in scleroderma, rheumatoid arthritis, ulcerative colitis, and myxedema after thyroiditis.[14,15]

Associated Disease

Duodenal diverticula have been associated with colonic diverticulosis (26% to 30%), gallbladder disease (18% to 22%), hiatal hernia (16% to 18%), and pancreatic

disease (3%). Furthermore, duodenal diverticula frequently coexist with diverticula of the jejunum or ileum. It has been reported that jejunal and ileal diverticula are present in 6% to 13% of patients with duodenal diverticula whereas duodenal diverticula are noted in 22% to 44% of patients with jejunal diverticula.[16,17]

Uomo and colleagues[18] investigated the relationship of periampullary extraluminal duodenal diverticula and acute pancreatitis. They retrospectively reviewed 439 patients (58 with periampullary diverticula) who underwent successful endoscopic retrograde cholangiopancreatography (ERCP) over a 3-year period. When compared with the 375 control subjects (i.e., those without diverticula), the patients with periampullary diverticula were

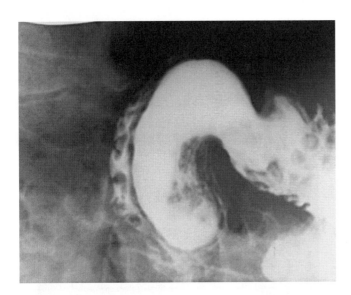

Figure 54–4. Demonstration of the windsock effect caused by an intraluminal duodenal diverticulum. (Courtesy of M. A. Turner, Medical College of Virginia.)

significantly older ($P < .0001$), had a significantly higher incidence of biliary lithiasis (65.5% versus 40.8%; $P < .0001$), and more frequently had a recent attack of acute pancreatitis as the indication for ERCP (62% versus 24.8%; $P < .0001$). On the other hand, they found that the prevalence of gallstone pancreatitis was not significantly different between the two groups. Noting a significantly ($P < .04$) higher incidence of idiopathic acute pancreatitis in the 58 patients, they postulated an autonomous etiologic role for periampullary duodenal diverticula in acute pancreatitis (see Fig. 54–3). We think it more likely that the periampullary diverticula, by disrupting the normal physiologic ampullary emptying mechanisms, contributed to both a higher incidence of biliary stasis and microlithiasis and, secondarily, a higher incidence of acute pancreatitis.

Another study in patients who had undergone cholecystectomy more than 2 years earlier noted a significantly increased incidence of recurrent biliary calculi in those with perivaterian diverticula as compared with those without. In our opinion, however, a causal relationship of duodenal diverticula to biliary tract stones has not been demonstrated.[3]

Miyazawa and associates[19] studied 115 patients with common duct stones. Most underwent simple choledochotomy with stone extraction and T-tube drainage. The 85 patients who still had their gallbladders also underwent cholecystectomy. Of the five in whom recurrent common duct stones developed, all had pigment stones and coexisting periampullary duodenal diverticula. We propose that end-to-side Roux-en-Y choledochojejunostomy be considered in patients with these two factors.

Symptoms

Neill and Thompson[20] reported that only 10% of people with small bowel diverticula have symptoms attributable to them. When symptoms do occur, they are usually secondary to obstruction of the diverticulum with subsequent stasis, bacterial overgrowth, pouch distention, and inflammation, or they result from compression of adjacent structures, such as the intestinal lumen or the pancreatic or bile duct. Jones and Merendino[17] and Chitambar[4] examined the frequency of symptoms in patients known to have duodenal diverticula. According to these authors, postprandial pain, usually epigastric or right upper quadrant in location, with radiation to the subscapular or costovertebral locations, occurred in half the patients referred to them. It will be obvious to the reader that these patients referred to clinicians were selected as having symptoms in the first place. The pain varied from mild abdominal distress to gnawing, crampy, sharp pain and generally occurred 2 to 4 hours after meals. In some cases, the pain was relieved by changing position and presumably draining the diverticulum. In addition, vague abdominal complaints such as bloating, belching, and flatulence have commonly been reported in this patient population. Nausea and vomiting, sometimes associated with weight loss, have been reported in 17% to 34% of patients. Christiansen and Thommesen[7] found a high incidence of gastroesophageal reflux and biliary calculi and recommended an evaluation for reflux and biliary disease in patients known to have duodenal diverticula with upper abdominal symptoms. Both diarrhea and constipation have been reported in these patients.

Duodenal diverticula can cause serious problems when complications such as ulceration with hemorrhage, obstruction of the neck, perforation into adjacent structures or the peritoneal cavity, or compression of adjacent structures occur. In these cases, the condition may mimic a perforated or bleeding duodenal ulcer or acute pancreatitis. Handelsman and co-workers[16] noted hematemesis, melena, or both in 32% of patients undergoing laparotomy for duodenal diverticula. Duodenocolic fistula secondary to rupture of a diverticulum into the transverse colon may cause malabsorption and diarrhea.[21,22]

Intraluminal, or congenital, duodenal diverticula are most often detected between the ages of 20 and 40 years. Twenty percent of these patients have had some upper abdominal discomfort since childhood. Two thirds have symptoms of duodenal obstruction, including postprandial epigastric or periumbilical crampy pain with or without bilious vomiting. Other manifestations include hemorrhage and pancreatitis. The latter, which is the initial symptom in as many as 20% of patients, is thought to arise from obstruction of the ampulla by the diverticulum. Many are discovered when the opening in the diverticulum is obstructed by food, gallstones, clots, ingested medications, or foreign bodies.[12,23-25]

Diagnosis

Duodenal diverticula are usually diagnosed by contrast-enhanced upper gastrointestinal radiographs or at laparotomy. They are occasionally difficult to demonstrate radiographically. Case[26] emphasized the importance

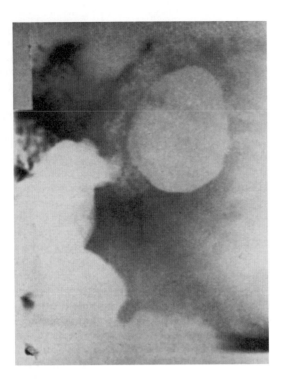

Figure 54–5. Large diverticulum arising from the second portion of the duodenum. (From Chitambar IA: Duodenal diverticula. Surgery 33:768, 1954.)

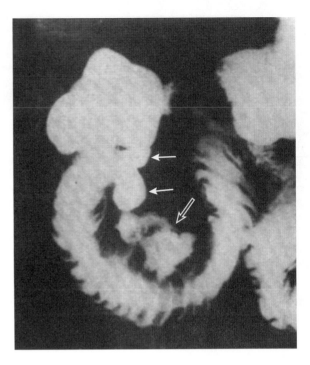

Figure 54–6. Upper gastrointestinal examination showing a lobulated periampullary diverticulum *(arrows)* and a large irregular collection of contrast material within an inflamed diverticulum *(open arrow)*. It has a deformed lumen with ulcerated mucosa, and the adjacent duodenal folds are thickened because of peridiverticular inflammation. (From Gore RM, Ghahremani GG, Kirsch MD: Diverticulitis of the duodenum: Clinical and radiological manifestations of seven cases. Am J Gastroenterol 86:982, 1991.)

of manual palpation of the abdomen with pressure exerted over the pylorus and duodenojejunal junction to facilitate filling of the diverticula under fluoroscopy. Fluoroscopy is important because when the ostium is relatively large, duodenal diverticula often empty rapidly. When the ostium is narrow, the diverticulum fills poorly and can be missed as a result of rapid transit through the duodenal lumen. Hypotonic duodenography with the use of drugs that retard duodenal motility has also been advocated for the demonstration of diverticula not amenable to conventional techniques.[27]

During upper gastrointestinal contrast radiologic examination, duodenal diverticula appear as one or more collections of barium continuous with the duodenal lumen (Figs. 54–5 and 54–6). Residual barium after emptying may outline round, oval, or multiloculated radiolucencies corresponding to diverticula. Because emptying is often slow, delayed films are frequently recommended after 24 hours. Case[26] noted that retention extended 48 hours with some periampullary diverticula. Radiologic findings in patients with intraluminal duodenal diverticula include a collection of barium within the duodenal lumen surrounded by a narrow band of barium with a thin rim of radiolucency in between, the so-called windsock appearance[28] (see Fig. 53–4).

Stone and associates[29] examined computed tomography (CT) of the abdomen for evaluation of small intestinal diverticula. They noted that the presence of air with or without contrast was the most consistent finding. In cases of duodenal diverticula, the air-, contrast-, or fluid-filled mass was often in the region of the pancreas, mimicking a pseudocyst or abscess (Fig. 54–7).

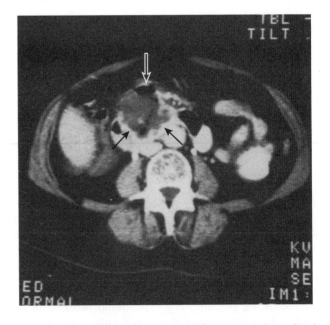

Figure 54–7. Computed tomography scan through the center of duodenal diverticulitis showing its markedly distorted margins *(arrows)* and a mixture of secretions, debris, and gas within its lumen *(open arrow)*. (From Gore RM, Ghahremani GG, Kirsch MD: Diverticulitis of the duodenum: Clinical and radiological manifestations of seven cases. Am J Gastroenterol 86:982, 1991.)

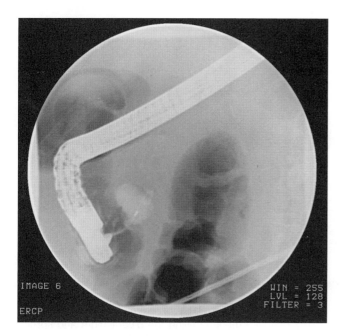

Figure 54–8. Endoscopic retrograde cholangiopancreatography demonstrating filling of a periampullary diverticulum with contrast. (Courtesy of M. A. Turner, Medical College of Virginia.)

Upper gastrointestinal endoscopy has become popular as a means of diagnosing and classifying duodenal diverticula. In many instances, intraluminal diverticula can be treated endoscopically by excision or by incision and widening of the ostium.[28] Endoscopy can also differentiate duodenal abnormalities noted on contrast radiography. After the diagnosis of a periampullary duodenal diverticulum, ERCP can be performed to delineate the relationship of the diverticulum to the pancreatic and common bile ducts in cases of pancreatitis or biliary sepsis[28,30] (Fig. 54–8).

Angiography may be indicated in cases of hemorrhage associated with diverticula. Tisnado and colleagues[31] reported the first angiographic demonstration of a bleeding jejunal diverticulum (Fig. 54–9). The same principles apply to duodenal diverticula, although they bleed less frequently than jejunal or ileal diverticula do. The characteristic feature is pooling of the material in a smooth-walled collection during the arterial and capillary phases, followed by spread of the contrast material into the lumen during the venous phase.

Complications

Serious complications occur in about 5% to 10% of patients with duodenal diverticula. Bleeding, perforation, and diverticulitis are all rare, but the morbidity and mortality are high because of delay in diagnosis as a result of lack of suspicion of the underlying condition. The diagnosis is seldom made preoperatively.[3]

A progressive inflammatory reaction within duodenal diverticula may lead to ulceration with associated duodenitis and pancreatitis. Perforation of an inflamed diverticulum may result in peritonitis, retroperitoneal abscess, or fistulization into the colon, adjacent segment of duodenum, or even the aorta. Stasis within a diverticulum may predispose to enterolith formation with subsequent obstruction of the diverticular neck and inflammation; stasis may also result in a blind-loop syndrome with resultant malabsorption. In addition, stasis can cause passive distention of diverticula with resultant obstruction of the intestinal lumen, common bile duct, or pancreatic duct.

Perforation

Perforation of duodenal diverticula is rare, with only slightly more than 100 cases reported in the world literature.[21] Perforation of a duodenal diverticulum is suggested when the surgeon observes retroperitoneal edema lateral to the duodenum, bile-stained phlegmon in the paraduodenal area, retroperitoneal crepitus or pus, or a right subhepatic abscess with no obvious primary source of infection. Only 13 of 101 cases of perforated duodenal diverticula were correctly diagnosed preoperatively.[21] The differential diagnosis includes perforated peptic ulcer, cholecystitis, pancreatitis, appendicitis, intestinal obstruction, and myocardial infarction. CT scanning has led to an increased frequency of correct preoperative diagnosis.[32]

Gross peritonitis is not characteristic of perforated duodenal diverticula. Because duodenal diverticula emanating from the concave aspect of the duodenum are partially supported by the pancreas, those arising from the lateral (convex) aspect are more likely to perforate, most commonly into the retroperitoneal space. Zeifer and Goersch[33] reported 23 cases of perforated duodenal diverticula. The mean patient age was 61 years, and men were affected twice as often as women. The second portion of the duodenum was the site of perforation in 19 of the patients. In 6 of the patients, the diagnosis was not made at surgery. The overall mortality rate was 48%. In a review of the world literature, Duarte and colleagues[21] defined the most common causes of duodenal diverticular perforation as being diverticulitis (57%), enterolithiasis (12%), ulceration (9%), and other rarer causes, including foreign bodies and trauma. Five cases of duodenocolic fistula have been reported as complications of perforated duodenal diverticula.[21,22]

Obstruction

Duodenal obstruction occurs primarily as a result of intraluminal duodenal diverticula, when the ostium of the diverticulum becomes obstructed by substances such as food and medication. The clinical picture is that of a high small intestinal obstruction with bilious vomiting; plain abdominal radiographs demonstrate dilation of the stomach and proximal duodenum but not the remaining small intestine. Upper endoscopy can usually confirm the diagnosis in such cases.

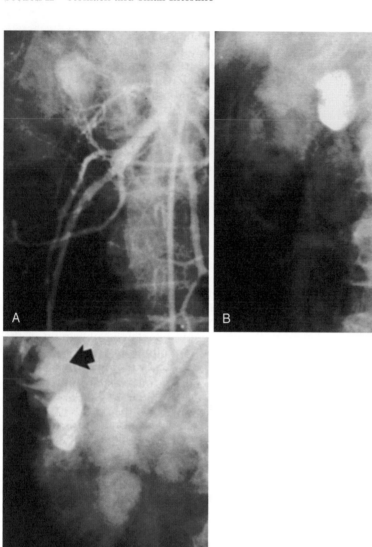

Figure 54–9. Angiographic study demonstrating a bleeding jejunal diverticulum. **A,** Arterial injection phase (2 seconds). **B,** Capillary phase showing a distinct smooth-walled lake of extravasation. **C,** Contrast medium filling the diverticulum and spreading into the lumen of the intestine *(arrow).* (From Tisnado J, Konerding KF, Beachley MC, et al: Angiographic diagnosis of a bleeding jejunal diverticulum. Gastrointest Radiol 4:291, 1979.)

Hemorrhage

When hemorrhage is a complication of duodenal diverticula, it may be manifested as hematemesis, melena, or both. Preoperative diagnosis can be made by upper endoscopy or arteriography (see Fig. 54–9). Bleeding has been described with ulceration,[34] cavernous hemangioma,[35] or angiodysplasia[36] within the diverticulum.

Biliary-Pancreatic Complications

Periampullary diverticula have been implicated in the pathogenesis of calculus formation and obstructive biliary tract disease. Stasis and inflammation within these periampullary diverticula may cause edema of the papilla of Vater and consequent insufficiency of the sphincter of Oddi with reflux of duodenal contents and bacterial colonization. Using endoscopic pull-through techniques

with biliary manometry, Lotveit and co-workers[30] and Kubota and associates[37] showed that patients with juxtapapillary diverticula have dysfunction and insufficiency of the choledochal sphincter. Periampullary duodenal diverticula filled with debris and stones have been associated with biliary pancreatitis and obstructive jaundice.[38]

The incidence of biliary disease varies between 13% and 22% in patients with duodenal diverticula,[4,16,17,39] but it may rise as high as 50% if only juxtavaterian diverticula are considered.[5,40] These diverticula are over twice as likely to be associated with gallstones as diverticula more distal in the duodenum.[39] Furthermore, lending credence to the bacterial overgrowth theory, patients with juxtapapillary diverticula are more likely to have pigment stones, whereas those without diverticula are more apt to have cholesterol gallstones.[19,41] Recurrent stone disease or postcholecystectomy syndrome is more likely to develop after cholecystectomy. In addition, Lotveit and co-workers[5,30] found diverticula in 17 of 75 patients with acute pancreatitis as compared with an incidence of 4.2% in a comparable control group.

Management

Nonoperative Treatment

Several approaches have been used for the nonoperative management of symptomatic duodenal diverticula. Cattell and Mudge[6] suggested that patients with presumed symptomatic duodenal diverticula be treated with trials of antacids, antispasmodics, a low-fat diet, and barbiturates. According to these authors, such a trial should last as long as 1 year. Most authors agree that medical treatment should be reserved for patients without complications of diverticula and those in whom other causes of the symptoms have been excluded by a thorough diagnostic evaluation.

Several nonsurgical approaches have been advocated for periampullary diverticula causing symptoms of biliary obstruction. Willcox and Costopoulous[42] reported on three patients treated endoscopically with common duct dilators. Urakami and colleagues[43] treated common duct stones associated with periampullary diverticula in 33 patients by endoscopic papillotomy. Endoscopic visualization and control of bleeding from duodenal diverticula have also been described.[44]

Operative Therapy

It is widely agreed that surgical treatment is indicated only for patients with serious complications of duodenal diverticula. These diverticula are difficult to treat surgically because of their frequent intimate association with the bile and pancreatic ducts. The mortality rate associated with surgical resection of uncomplicated diverticula has been reported to be 8% to 10%.[6,9,16] On the other hand, symptomatic improvement after surgical therapy has been disappointing, with 47% of the patients in Cattell and Mudge's series[6] having either fair or poor results.

Many intraluminal duodenal diverticula can be treated endoscopically by incision, excision, or dilation of the aperture. When ERCP cannot clearly delineate the biliary and pancreatic ducts, however, open duodenotomy with surgical excision remains the gold standard and offers better protection against ductal injury or iatrogenic pancreatitis.[45]

In cases of bleeding, duodenotomy with inversion and mucosal excision has been successful, but Slater reported a 28% mortality rate from this complication.[46] Excision is best reserved for patients in whom the diverticulum arises from the lateral aspect of the duodenum and the margins of the neck are clearly delineated. *In cases in which the diverticulum arises in the periampullary region, it is imperative that the ductal structures be protected whether excision or oversewing of a bleeding site is being performed.* In many cases, transduodenal sphincteroplasty should be performed, with fine suturing of the duodenal mucosa to the bile duct mucosa accomplished under direct vision (Figs. 54–10 and 54–11). The authors advocate a

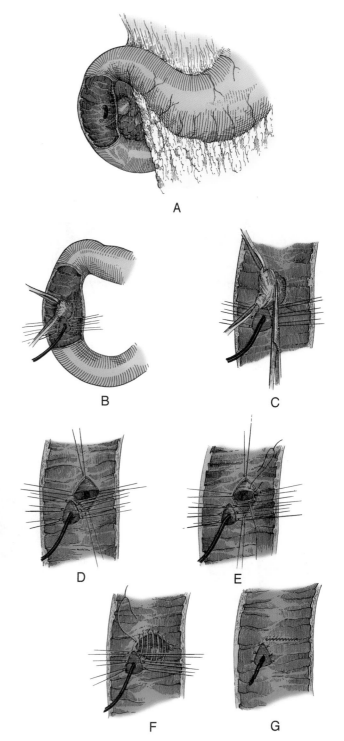

Figure 54–10. Technique for excising juxta-ampullary duodenal diverticula. **A,** Identification of a diverticulum through a duodenotomy. **B,** Eversion of the fundus of a diverticulum with Babcock forceps. **C,** Resection of the mucosa of the diverticulum. **D,** Stay sutures in the edges of the mucosa. **E,** Suture of the muscle layers. **F,** Transverse suture of the mucosa. **G,** Placing an intrapancreatic drain through the papilla. Observe the suture of the mucosal layer after diverticulectomy. (From Pinotti HW, Tacla M, Pontes JF, et al: Surgical procedures upon juxta-ampullar duodenal diverticula. Surg Gynecol Obstet [now J Am Coll Surg] 135:11, 1972. By permission of *Surgery, Gynecology and Obstetrics.*)

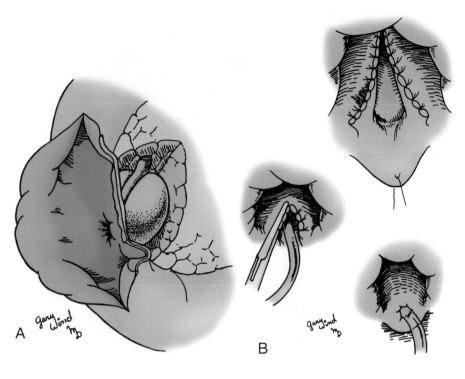

Figure 54–11. A, Anatomy of a juxtapapillary diverticulum. The relationship of the diverticulum to the pancreas makes transduodenal excision hazardous. **B,** When the wall between the diverticulum and the bile duct is divided, flow is established, thereby relieving stasis in both the duct and the diverticulum. (From Kaminsky HH, Thompson WR, Davis B: Extended sphincteroplasty for juxtapapillary duodenal diverticulum. Surg Gynecol Obstet [now J Am Coll Surg] 162:281, 1986. By permission of *Surgery, Gynecology and Obstetrics.*)

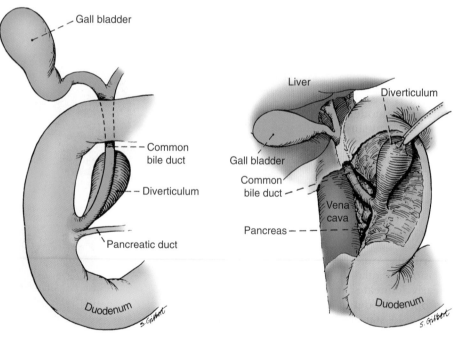

Figure 54–12. Usefulness of the Kocher maneuver in demonstrating duodenal diverticula. (From Jones TW, Merendino KA: The perplexing duodenal diverticulum. Surgery 48:1068, 1960.)

generous Kocher maneuver to adequately visualize the relationship of the diverticulum to ductal structures (Fig. 54–12).

Handelsman and co-workers[16] emphasized the high morbidity and mortality associated with excision of juxtavaterian diverticula. This morbidity was primarily the result of the frequent occurrence of bile duct injury, duodenal fistula, or fulminant postoperative pancreatitis. These authors strongly advocated bypass procedures to avoid such potentially lethal complications.

Critchlow and colleagues[47] proposed Roux-en-Y duodenojejunostomy as treatment of pancreaticobiliary disease associated with perivaterian duodenal diverticula (Fig. 54–13). They note that this procedure has the advantage of removing the diverticulum from the food stream, thereby relieving stasis and stasis-induced problems such as cholangitis and pancreatitis. If the problem is that of recurrent choledochal stones after cholecystectomy or multiple choledochal pigment stones, even before cholecystectomy, end-to-side Roux-en-Y choledo-

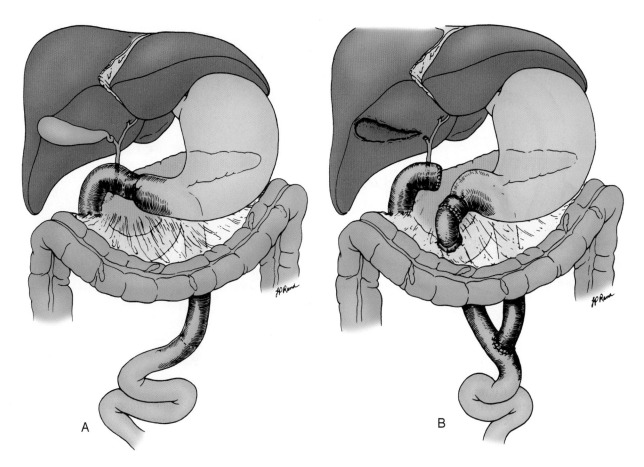

Figure 54–13.   A, Anatomy before reconstruction. *Dashed lines* indicate proposed sites of division of the intestine. **B,** Anatomy after reconstruction. The gallbladder has been removed. The Roux limb has been brought through the mesocolon, the duodenojejunostomy has been completed, and the mesentery has been closed. (From Critchlow JF, Shapiro ME, Silen W: Duodenojejunostomy for the pancreaticobiliary complications of duodenal diverticulum. Ann Surg 202:56, 1985.)

chojejunostomy, as advocated by Miyazawa and colleagues,[19] is probably the preferred option because it more directly relieves biliary stasis (Fig. 54–14).

The authors of this chapter strongly concur that these bypass procedures are preferable to excision in patients with pancreaticobiliary complications of juxtavaterian duodenal diverticula. In addition, if excision, partial excision, or oversewing is necessary for such problems as ulceration, bleeding, or perforation, when possible, patients should be referred to experienced pancreaticobiliary surgeons.

JEJUNOILEAL DIVERTICULA

Incidence

By small bowel contrast-enhanced radiographic series, the incidence of jejunoileal diverticula in the general adult population ranges from 0.02% to 1.3%.[48] At autopsy, the incidence of jejunal diverticulosis has been cited to be as high as 7.1%.[49] Small bowel diverticula are difficult to demonstrate radiographically or anatomically, and therefore the incidence is probably much higher.

Associated Diseases

Jejunoileal diverticula are most commonly identified in the sixth and seventh decades of life and are more common in men than women. We previously alluded to the association of jejunoileal diverticulosis with other gastrointestinal diverticula. Concurrent diverticulosis of the colon and duodenum is particularly common.[50] Less commonly, urinary bladder and esophageal diverticula have been described as synchronous lesions.[51] Theories of this association with systemic disorders that affect muscle tone imply that diverticula can be a secondary manifestation of dysmotility.[15]

Pathogenesis

Jejunoileal diverticula, occasionally referred to as nonmeckelian diverticula, are generally considered to be acquired diverticula, although familial cases have been reported.[52] The familial distribution of diverticula may be related to a motility disorder or congenital weakness of the intestinal muscularis.[4] They are pseudodiverticula and lack a muscular wall. These lesions are pulsion-type

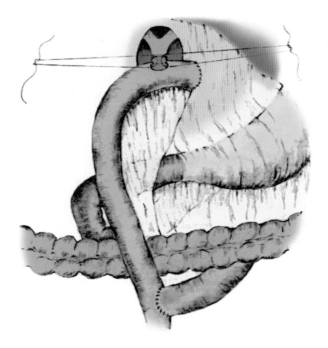

Figure 54–14. Roux-en-Y choledochojejunostomy to remove a diverticulum from the food stream and relieve biliary stasis. (From Schwartz SI: Current modalities in surgery. In Surgery: Excision of Extrapancreatic Bile Ducts and Hepaticojejunostomy. Marlton, NJ, Innovative Publishing, 1985, p 2.)

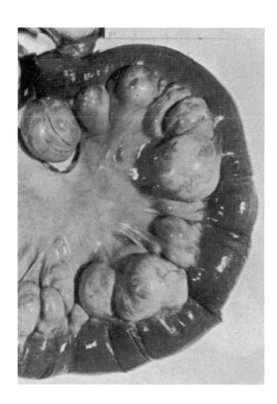

Figure 54–15. Formol-saline–preserved specimen demonstrating multiple jejunal diverticula. (From Badenoch J, Bedford P, Evans JR: Massive diverticulosis of the small intestine with steatorrhea and megaloblastic anemia. Q J Med 24:321, 1955.)

diverticula and are thought to result from a weakened intestinal wall.[13] An attenuated muscularis is associated with aging and with hereditary neuromuscular disorders. In addition, it has been postulated that local weakness exists at the points where the vasa recta penetrate the intestinal wall. This theory is supported by observations that small intestinal diverticula occur more commonly along the mesentery, with an increased frequency in the proximal jejunum and distal ileum, where the caliber of the blood vessels is greatest (Fig. 54–15).

Symptoms

Previously, it was thought that most cases remain asymptomatic throughout the patient's life. More recent studies have suggested that upward of 90% of patients with jejunoileal diverticula may manifest nonspecific symptoms.[53] This fact must be remembered when jejunoileal diverticula are incidentally found on diagnostic studies or at surgery. Because of the associated dysmotility, the most common symptoms of jejunoileal diverticulosis are nonspecific and include chronic abdominal pain, bloating, and early satiety. Diverticulitis is manifested as acute abdominal pain and may cause symptoms of a febrile illness, but this is rare. Obstructive symptoms, bleeding, and peritonitis occur at an incidence of 10% and are an indication that operative management is required.[54]

Diagnosis

Classically, the diagnosis of small bowel diverticula is made radiographically by small bowel contrast series or by an enteroclysis study (Fig. 54–16). A variety of techniques have been described to facilitate the diagnosis, but current consensus is that enteroclysis is the most accurate.[27,55] Preoperative diagnosis is unusual, however, because the symptoms overlap those of more common causes of acute abdominal pain. CT demonstrating extraluminal air within the small bowel mesentery should raise suspicion of a perforated diverticula.

Complications

Even though most patients with jejunoileal diverticula do not have symptoms and will never experience complications of their disease, there are potentially serious outcomes related to these lesions. The overall complication rate may be higher than the previously estimated 10% to 30%.[56]

Hemorrhage

Massive hemorrhage may be a sequela and can sometimes be fatal.[57,58] Hemorrhage is less common with jejunoileal diverticula than with other small bowel diverticula; it occurred in only 12% of patients according to a

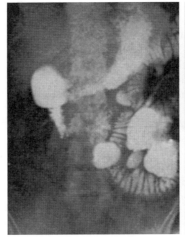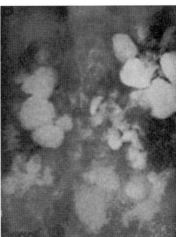

Figure 54–16. Multiple jejunal diverticula demonstrated on small intestine contrast examination. (From Altemeier WA, Bryant LR, Wulsin JH: The surgical significance of jejunal diverticulosis. Arch Surg 86:732, 1963. Copyright © 1963, American Medical Association.)

1996 series.[56] As a cause of gastrointestinal hemorrhage, a bleeding jejunoileal diverticulum is rare.[53] A radioscintigraphic bleeding scan or angiography may be useful in identifying the bleeding diverticulum in these patients. When angiography is performed, vital dyes can be introduced intraoperatively through angiographic catheters placed selectively in branches of the superior mesenteric artery that feed the involved segment and be used to guide the surgeon to the exact location of the bleeding lesion.[31]

Perforation

Perforation is a serious condition with a mortality rate that approaches 50% in some historical series. With modern perioperative care and intraoperative monitoring, this mortality rate should be much lower.[56] Perforation is the most common complication of jejunoileal diverticular disease and is a sequela of diverticulitis.[59] A perforated diverticulum can be difficult to identify at laparotomy because the peritonitis may be confined to the leaves of the mesentery. Astute intraoperative observation, often combined with a preoperative CT scan, is required if this potentially fatal complication is to be diagnosed correctly.[4] Signs of mesenteric inflammation with either retroperitoneal air or air within the mesentery should raise suspicion for this complication. Abscess formation is an obvious outcome of perforation in patients who do not succumb to sepsis.

Obstruction

Small bowel obstruction secondary to jejunoileal diverticula is well described and is identified at laparotomy.[54,60] Obstruction is typically cited as a less common complication, with an estimated incidence of 5% and only 27 cases described in the modern literature. This low incidence is a result of the liquid nature of the small bowel contents and the relatively large ostia of most intestinal diverticula. When obstruction does occur, it is usually due to enterolith formation. Nonmechanical obstruc-

tion, or pseudo-obstruction, may occur and is related to the dyskinesia associated with this condition.[61]

Malabsorption

Malabsorption is primarily reported to occur with jejunoileal diverticular disease.[53] Diverticular disease eventually leads to the physiologic equivalent of a blind-loop syndrome with ensuing bacterial overgrowth. Bacterial overgrowth within the diverticulum may then lead to symptoms associated with malabsorption and may contribute to cases of diverticulitis or perforation.

Management

Nonoperative Treatment

The role of antibiotics is agreed on for patients with bacterial overgrowth and is controversial for patients with evidence of perforation.[21] Metronidazole, tetracyclines, and ciprofloxacin are among the antibiotics recommended for bacterial overgrowth.[62] Isolated reports in the literature suggest that perforated diverticula can be managed with supportive measures. The combination of parenteral antibiotics, intravenous fluids, and close observation is acceptable treatment of isolated small bowel diverticulitis, although as stated previously, this diagnosis is difficult to make.

Nonoperative management of asymptomatic disease is based on increasing dietary fiber to decrease the intraluminal forces associated with peristalsis.[12] With the onset of symptoms, recommendations include small, frequent meals and rest in a supine position for 1 hour after each meal. Close observation is required to identify patients who may require surgical treatment.

Operative Therapy

Conservative management is the rule in the operative treatment of jejunoileal diverticular disease. Incidental, asymptomatic diverticula should be left alone. In patients with hemorrhage or perforation, segmental resection of the affected bowel is indicated. Because of the mesenteric location of the diverticulum, simple diverticulectomy may impair blood flow and therefore lead to anastomotic breakdown or fistula formation.[63] In addition, local excision may be difficult because of inflammation.[64] Obstruction is best managed by resection as well, but in cases of enterolith impaction, simple enterotomy with stone extraction has been advocated in some reports.[54,65] Controversy persists regarding whether surgery should be performed for symptomatic, but uncomplicated lesions. Given the generally benign natural history of these acquired lesions, surgery should probably be reserved for complicated cases.

MECKEL'S DIVERTICULUM

Incidence

Meckel's diverticulum is the most commonly encountered congenital anomaly of the small intestine, with autopsy studies estimating the incidence to be 2%,[66,67] and it found with equal frequency in men and women.

Pathogenesis

Meckel's diverticulum is a true diverticulum; that is, it contains all layers of the bowel wall because it is derived from an intact embryologic vitelline duct (omphalomesenteric duct) that does not undergo normal obliteration during the fifth to ninth weeks of gestation.[68,69] Persistence of this duct results in (1) a fibrous cord between the umbilicus and the ileum, which represents an obliterated duct and its vessels; (2) an umbilical sinus when the umbilical side of the duct does not fully obliterate; (3) Meckel's diverticulum secondary to failure of the intestinal end to close; (4) a fistula between the umbilicus and the ileum when the entire duct remains patent; or (5) any combination of these abnormalities.[70,71]

Meckel's diverticulum usually arises from the antimesenteric border of the ileum, within 100 cm of the ileocecal valve, and derives its blood supply from persistent vitelline vessels that are present within a distinct mesentery.[72] The length and diameter vary from 1 to 12 cm. The embryologic cells lining the vitelline duct retain their pluripotential capability, and thus it is not uncommon to find heterotopic tissue within the diverticulum. Gastric mucosa is present in 30% to 50%,[73] and although Meckel's diverticula are usually benign incidental findings at laparotomy, 75% of patients with symptoms have gastric mucosa within their diverticula. The incidence of pancreatic tissue approximates 5%, and even though colonic mucosa, lipoma, leiomyoma, neurofibroma, angioma, and their malignant counterparts have been reported, these findings are uncommon.[74] Consideration must be given to these tumors, however, not only for their oncologic significance but also as lead points for intussusception.

Symptoms

About 4% of patients with Meckel's diverticulum have symptoms within their lifetime, and in more than half of these patients the symptoms occur before 2 years of age.[67] The average mortality rate in patients in whom symptoms develop is 6%,[67] and it is disproportionately high in elderly patients. Symptomatic manifestations are secondary to hemorrhage (23%), small bowel obstruction (31%), diverticulitis (14%), intussusception (14%), perforation (10%), and miscellaneous umbilical abnormalities and tumors (8%).[75]

Diagnosis

In patients who have ectopic gastric mucosa in Meckel's diverticulum, technetium scanning is a useful diagnostic aid. ^{99m}Tc-pertechnetate is taken up by gastric mucosa, and the uptake can be detected scintigraphically (Fig. 54–17). Pentagastrin given subcutaneously 20 minutes before the study has been shown to enhance uptake within the gastric mucosa.[73] Cimetidine, a histamine H_2 receptor blocker, has a similar effect and may enhance the intraluminal release of pertechnetate.[73] The sensitivity of this scan for detecting Meckel's diverticulum with ectopic gastric mucosa has been found to be 85%, with a specificity of 95% and an accuracy of 90% in surgically proven diagnoses.[73] A negative test excludes a diverticu-

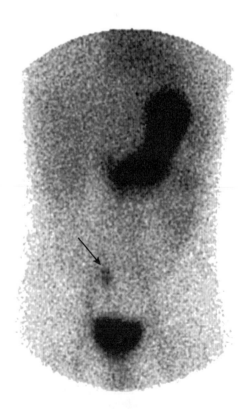

Figure 54–17. ^{99m}Tc-pertechnetate scintigraphy demonstrates ectopic gastric mucosa, indicative of Meckel's diverticulum *(arrow)*. (Courtesy of P. R. Jolles, Medical College of Virginia.)

lum in more than 90% of patients who have none.[76,77] Meckel's diverticulum can also sometimes be detected by enteroclysis, in which a large volume of contrast medium is introduced through a fluoroscopically directed nasointestinal tube directly into the jejunum to induce distention, which makes morphologic abnormalities easier to visualize.[55] When the diverticulum itself is not visualized, a mass effect is sometimes noted and can lead to a correct diagnosis.[55] In some cases, the demonstration of intussusception is associated with an inverted Meckel's diverticulum as the lead point.

Complications

Hemorrhage

Hemorrhage is the most common symptom in children 2 years or younger with Meckel's diverticulum[73,78]; it is usually manifested as painless bright red blood from the rectum, with intermittent episodes persisting without treatment. The usual source of the bleeding is an ileal ulcer located adjacent to a Meckel diverticulum containing gastric mucosa. Diagnosis of a diverticulum containing gastric mucosa can be made via ^{99m}Tc-pertechnetate radioisotope scanning. The use of pentagastrin stimulation before the scan decreases false-negative results by enhancing uptake of the isotope by the gastric mucosa.[73] Although the diagnostic accuracy of this test approaches 90% because of a high index of suspicion in young children with painless rectal bleeding,[73] the scan is not as useful in adults, in whom enteroclysis has a high incidence of accurate diagnosis.[55]

Obstruction

Obstructive symptoms are common with Meckel's diverticulum and may be due to volvulus, intussusception, or incarceration of the diverticulum in an inguinal hernia (Littre's hernia). The most common of these causes is acute volvulus, in which the small bowel kinks around a fibrous band running from the tip of the diverticulum to the umbilicus.[70] Strangulation of the involved bowel may ensue if not suspected. Intussusception results from a broad-based diverticulum invaginating and being carried forward by peristalsis. The intussusception may be ileoileal or ileocolic[70] and is manifested as acute obstruction with early vomiting, an urge to defecate, and occasionally the classic currant-jelly stools. Reduction can be achieved with a barium enema; however, reduction is not as successful as in non-Meckel's intussusception (Fig. 54–18). Resection is indicated regardless of success with hydrostatic reduction.[74]

Diverticulitis

Diverticulitis accounts for 10% to 20% of symptomatic cases[70] and is more common in older patients (Fig. 54–19). It is the third most frequent complication in adults after obstruction and bleeding. Clinically indistinguishable from appendicitis, if not considered it may lead to perforation or peritonitis. If during exploration for appendicitis the appendix is found to be normal, inspection of the distal 100 cm of ileum for Meckel's diverticulum is crucial. The indications for resection in this clinical setting parallel those of appendectomy. Inflamed diverticula and diverticula found incidentally when other causes of the acute abdomen are not obvious should undergo resection.[72]

Umbilical Anomalies

Eight percent to 10% of patients with Meckel's diverticulum have umbilical abnormalities, including fistulas, cysts, sinuses, and fibrous bands.[75] Identification of such abnormalities is not usually difficult and may be signaled by the presence of intestinal mucosa at the skin level or a persistently draining fistula. Cannulation and injection of the enterocutaneous fistula draining at the umbilicus can delineate the fistula, after which elective surgical exploration and resection can be performed.[75] If a fibrous band is found at laparotomy, it is generally recommended that the diverticulum be resected because of the risk for internal herniation and volvulus.[67] Should a situation arise in which resection is not safe, simple division of the band is sufficient.

Management

Operative Therapy

Management of Meckel's diverticulum discovered incidentally at laparotomy for another condition is controversial. Supporters of incidental diverticulectomy state that minimal postoperative complications occur with removal.[66,79] It is generally agreed that diverticula that appear to have heterotopic mucosa on physical examination should be resected, given their higher risk for subsequent complications.[72,80] Age younger than 40 years, diverticula longer than 2 cm,[72] and fibrous bands to the umbilicus or mesentery are risk factors for complications and relative indications for resection. Resection of asymptomatic diverticula in children at laparotomy is also generally recommended.

In 1976, Soltero and Bill[67] estimated a 4.2% lifetime risk for complications from Meckel's diverticulum with the use of population-based life-table analysis. They used previously published mortality rates after resection of symptomatic and asymptomatic diverticula and estimated that 800 asymptomatic diverticula would need to be resected to save the life of one patient with an asymptomatic Meckel's diverticulum. Assuming Von Hendenberg's morbidity rate of 9% after incidental removal,[81] these authors opposed prophylactic diverticulectomy. Cullen and colleagues,[66] however, reported an epidemiologic, population-based study of 145 patients undergoing resection of Meckel's diverticulum in which 87 were incidentally found; they calculated a 6.4% lifetime risk for complications of Meckel's diverticulum. These authors reported an operative morbidity rate of 2% after resection of diverticula found incidentally and, in contrast to Soltero and Bill[67] and others[80] who demonstrated a greater complication rate occurring in patients of

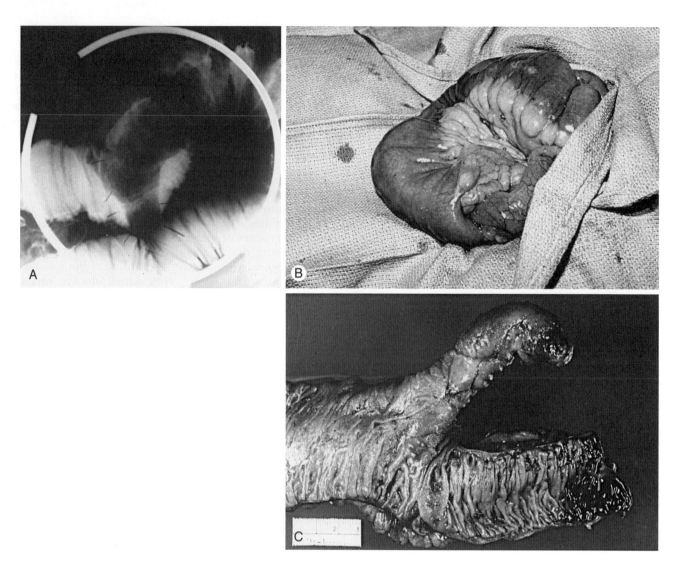

Figure 54–18.   A case of small bowel obstruction secondary to intussusception of Meckel's diverticulum. A preoperative barium study **(A)** demonstrates a diverticulum. An intraoperative view **(B)** and specimen **(C)** show the relationship of the diverticulum to the small bowel. (Courtesy of J. M. Kellum, Medical College of Virginia.)

younger age, showed no trend consistent with age. The risk for long-term complications included a 2% risk for adhesive small bowel disease as compared with a 7% risk in patients undergoing resection of complicated diverticular disease. The authors of this study concluded that incidentally discovered diverticula should be resected in the absence of peritonitis or other conditions precluding the safe performance of this operation.[66] In summary, the standard of care in recent decades has been selective resection of incidentally discovered diverticula based on estimated risks for future complications. Studies conducted since the advent of laparoscopy demonstrate that performance of prophylactic diverticulectomy under appropriate operative conditions is safe and may be beneficial.

Patients experiencing a complication of Meckel's diverticulum should be treated by diverticulectomy.

Resection in this setting is associated with a 5% to 10% mortality rate. A simple diverticulectomy can be performed in which the diverticulum is divided at its junction with the small intestine and the defect in the small intestine is closed with sutures or staples; alternatively, wedge excision of a portion of the ileal wall with the diverticulum can be performed. Finally, some patients require excision of the segment of ileum containing the diverticulum with an enteroenteric anastomosis.

The choice of operation depends, in part, on the condition of the diverticulum and the adjacent ileum. In general, the worse the condition, the more extensive the resection. In patients with hemorrhage from adjacent ileal ulcers, simple diverticulectomy does not remove the ulcer, and postoperative bleeding may recur. Segmental resection is also advocated in small children who have broad-based diverticula, in whom postoperative ileal

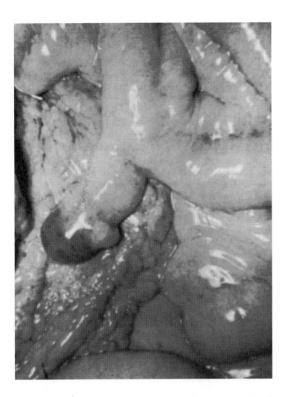

Figure 54–19. Meckel's diverticulitis. The tip of the diverticulum is reddened because of peptic ulceration secondary to a rest of gastric epithelium. (From Robbins SL, Cotran RS, Kumar V: Pathologic Basis of Disease, 3rd ed. Philadelphia, WB Saunders, 1984.)

stenosis is a risk. Recent reports demonstrate the feasibility of laparoscopic removal[78,82,83]; however, long-term results of these techniques are not available. With increasing use of diagnostic laparoscopy, further controversy regarding the management of asymptomatic diverticula is inevitable.

REFERENCES

1. Horton BT, Mueller SC: Duodenal diverticula. Proc Staff Meet Mayo Clin 7:185, 1932.
2. Afridi SA, Fichtenbaum CJ, Taubin H: Review of duodenal diverticula. Am J Gastroenterol 86:935, 1991.
3. Townsend CM, Thompson JCT: Small intestine. In Schwartz SI (ed): Principles of Surgery. New York, McGraw-Hill, 1993, p 1178.
4. Chitambar I: Duodenal diverticula. Surgery 33:768, 1953.
5. Lotveit T, Osnes M: Duodenal diverticula. Scand J Gastroenterol 19:579, 1994.
6. Cattell R, Mudge T: The surgical significance of duodenal diverticula. N Engl J Med 246:317, 1952.
7. Christiansen T, Thommesen P: Duodenal diverticula demonstrated by barium examination. Acta Radiol Diagn 27:419, 1986.
8. Eggert A, Teichmann W, Wittmann DH: The pathologic implication of duodenal diverticula. Surg Gynecol Obstet 154:62, 1982.
9. Waugh JM, Johnston EV: Primary diverticula of the duodenum. Ann Surg 141:193, 1955.
10. Ackermann W: Diverticula and variations of the duodenum. Ann Surg 117:403, 1943.
11. Suda K, Mizuguchi K, Matsumoto M: A histopathological study of the etiology of duodenal diverticulum related to the fusion of the pancreatic anlage. Am J Gastroenterol 78:335, 1983.
12. Karoll MP, Ghahremani GG, Port RB: Diagnosis and management of intraluminal duodenal diverticulum. Dig Dis Sci 28:411, 1983.
13. Roses D, Gourge T, Scher K: Perforated diverticula of the jejunum and ileum. Am J Surg 132:649, 1976.
14. Krishnamurthy S, Kelly MM, Rohrmann CA: Jejunal diverticulosis: A heterogeneous disorder caused by a variety of abnormalities of smooth muscle and myenteric plexus. Gastroenterology 85:538, 1983.
15. Milanes-Gonzalez A, Herrera-Esparza R, Arguelles R: Multiple duodenal-jejunal diverticula in a case of scleroderma [letter]. Clin Exp Rheumatol 4:289, 1986.
16. Handelsman JC, Murphy G, Fishbein R: Duodenal diverticulum: Clinical significance and surgical treatment. Am Surg 26:272, 1960.
17. Jones TW, Merendino KA: The perplexing duodenal diverticulum. Surgery 48:1068, 1960.
18. Uomo G, Manes G, Ragozzino A, et al: Periampullary extraluminal duodenal diverticula and acute pancreatitis: An underestimated etiological association. Am J Gastroenterol 91:1186, 1996.
19. Miyazawa Y, Okinaga K, Nishida K, Okano T: Recurrent common bile duct stones associated with periampullary duodenal diverticula and calcium bilirubinate stones. Int Surg 80:120, 1995.
20. Neill SA, Thompson NW: The complications of duodenal diverticula and their management. Surg Gynecol Obstet 120:1251, 1965.
21. Duarte B, Nagy K, Cintron J: Perforated duodenal diverticulum. Br J Surg 79:877, 1992.
22. Kellum JM, Boucher JC, Ballinger WF: Serosal patch repair for duodenocolic fistula. Am J Surg 13:607, 1976.
23. Abdel-Hafiz AA, Birkett DH, Ahmed MS: Congenital duodenal diverticula: A report of three cases and a review of the literature. Surgery 104:74, 1988.
24. Adams DB: Endoscopic removal of entrapped coins from an intraluminal duodenal diverticulum 20 years after ingestion. Gastrointest Endosc 2:415, 1986.
25. Soreide JA, Seime S, Soreide O: Intraluminal diverticulum: Case report and update of the literature 1975-1986. Am J Gastroenterol 83:988, 1988.
26. Case JT: Diverticula of small intestine other than Meckel's diverticulum. JAMA 75:1463, 1920.
27. Nagi B, Khandelwal N, Gupta R: Role of enteroclysis in acquired small bowel diverticula. Indian J Gastroenterol 10:31, 1991.
28. Ravi J, Joson PM, Ashok PS: Endoscopic incision of intraluminal duodenal diverticulum. Dig Dis Sci 38:762, 1993.
29. Stone EE, Brant WE, Smith GB: Computed tomography of duodenal diverticula. J Comput Assist Tomogr 13:61, 1989.
30. Lotveit T, Skar V, Osnes M: Juxtapapillary duodenal diverticula. Endoscopy 20:175, 1988.
31. Tisnado J, Konerding K, Beachley M: Angiographic diagnosis of a bleeding jejunal diverticulum. Gastrointest Radiol 4:291, 1979.
32. Gore RM, Ghahremani GG, Kirsch MD: Diverticulitis of the duodenum: Clinical and radiological manifestations of seven cases. Am J Gastroenterol 86:981, 1991.
33. Zeifer HD, Goersch H: Duodenal diverticulitis with perforation. Arch Surg 82:746, 1961.
34. Herrington JL Jr: Perforation of acquired diverticula of the jejunum and ileum: Analysis of reported cases. Surgery 51:426, 1962.
35. Eid A, Gur H, Fish A: Recurrent upper gastrointestinal bleeding from a cavernous hemangioma in a duodenal diverticulum [letter]. J Clin Gastroenterol 8:698, 1985.
36. Balkissoon J, Balkissoon B, Leffall LD: Massive upper gastrointestinal bleeding in a patient with a duodenal diverticulum: A case report and review of the literature. J Natl Med Assoc 84:365, 1992.
37. Kubota K, Itoh T, Shibayama K: Papillary function of patients with juxtapapillary duodenal diverticulum. Scand J Gastroenterol 24:140, 1989.
38. Caos A: Biliary pancreatitis and jaundice associated with obstructed periampullary duodenal diverticulum [letter]. Am J Gastroenterol 84:982, 1989.
39. Landor JH, Fulkerson CC: Duodenal diverticula: Relationship to biliary tract disease. Arch Surg 93:182, 1966.
40. Kennedy RH, Thompson MH: Are duodenal diverticula associated with choledocholithiasis? Gut 29:1003, 1988.
41. Viceconte G, Viceconte GW, Bogliolo G: Endoscopic manometry of the sphincter of Oddi in patients with and without juxtapapillary duodenal diverticula. Scand J Gastroenterol 19:329, 1984.

42. Willcox GI, Costopoulos LB: Entry of common bile and pancreatic ducts into a duodenal diverticulum. Arch Surg 98:447, 1969.

43. Urakami Y, Kishi S, Seifert E: Endoscopic papillotomy (EPT) in patients with juxtapapillary diverticula. Gastrointest Endosc 25:10, 1979.

44. Sim EKW, Goh PMY, Isaac JR: Endoscopic management of a bleeding duodenal diverticulum. Gastrointest Endosc 37:634, 1991.

45. Adams DB: Management of the intraluminal duodenal diverticulum: Endoscopy or duodenotomy? Am J Surg 151:524, 1986.

46. Slater RB: Duodenal diverticulum treated by excision of mucosal pouch only. Br J Surg 58:198, 1971.

47. Critchlow JF, Shapiro ME, Silen W: Duodenojejunostomy for the pancreaticobiliary complications of duodenal diverticulum. Ann Surg 202:56, 1985.

48. Scully R, Mark E: Case records of the Massachusetts General Hospital. N Engl J Med 322:1796, 1990.

49. Palder S, Frey C: Jejunal diverticulosis. Arch Surg 123:889, 1988.

50. Wilcox R, Shatney C: Surgical implications of jejunal diverticula. South Med J 81:1386, 1988.

51. Benson R, Dixon C, Waugh J.: Non-meckelian diverticula of the jejunum and ileum. Ann Surg 118:337, 1943.

52. Anderson L, Schjoldager B, Halver B: Jejunal diverticulosis in a family. J Gastroenterol 23:672, 1988.

53. Chow D, Babaian M, Taubin H: Jejunoileal diverticula. Gastroenterologist 5:78, 1997.

54. Harris L, Volpe C, Doerr R: Small bowel obstruction secondary to enterolith impaction complicating jejunal diverticulitis. Am J Gastroenterol 92:1538, 1997.

55. Nolan DJ: The true yield of the small-intestinal barium study. Endoscopy 29:447, 1997.

56. Akhrass R, Yaffe M, Fischer C, et al: Small-bowel diverticulosis: Perceptions and reality. J Am Coll Surg 184:383, 1996.

57. Bokhari M, Fitzgerald S, Vernava A, Longo W: Hemorrhagic efferent limb diverticulosis: An unusual cause for postgastrectomy bleeding. J Clin Gastroenterol 18:174, 1994.

58. Schackelford R, Marcus W: Jejunal diverticula: A cause for gastrointestinal hemorrhage. Ann Surg 151:930, 1960.

59. Leon C, Iniguez S: Jejunal diverticulitis: An unusual cause of acute abdomen. Am J Gastroenterol 91:393, 1995.

60. Mughal S, Hasan N: Retroperitoneal jejunal diverticulum: Cause of intestinal obstruction. J Pediatr Surg 27:1587, 1992.

61. Brown J, Woolverton W, Pearce C: Jejunal dyskinesia: Case report and review of the literature. South Med J 62:1102, 1969.

62. Husebye E: Gastrointestinal motility disorders and bacterial overgrowth. J Intern Med 237:419, 1995.

63. Longo W, Vernava A: Clinical implications of jejunoileal diverticular disease. Dis Colon Rectum 35:381, 1992.

64. Nobles E. Jejunal diverticula. Arch Surg 102:172, 1971.

65. Phelan M, Kaufman H, Becker H: Small bowel obstruction by jejunal enterolith. Surgery 121:119, 1997.

66. Cullen JJ, Kelly KA, Moir CR, et al: Surgical management of Meckel's diverticulum: An epidemiologic, population-based study. Ann Surg 220:564, discussion, 568, 1994.

67. Soltero MJ, Bill AH: The natural history of Meckel's diverticulum and its relation to incidental removal: A study of 202 cases of diseased Meckel's diverticulum found in King County, Washington, over a fifteen year period. Am J Surg 132:168, 1976.

68. DiGiacomo JC, Cottone FJ: Surgical treatment of Meckel's diverticulum. South Med J 86:671, 1993.

69. Moore K: The Developing Human: Clinically Oriented Embryology. Philadelphia, WB Saunders, 1988, p 235.

70. Cullen JJ, Kelly KA: Current management of Meckel's diverticulum. Adv Surg 29:207, 1996.

71. Moore TC: Omphalomesenteric duct malformations. Semin Pediatr Surg 5:116, 1996.

72. Mackey WC, Dineen P: A fifty year experience with Meckel's diverticulum. Surg Gynecol Obstet 156:56, 1983.

73. Heyman S: Meckel's diverticulum: Possible detection by combining pentagastrin with histamine H_2 receptor blocker. J Nucl Med 35:1656, 1994.

74. Clary BM, Lyerly HK: Meckel's dverticulum. In Sabiston DC (ed): Sabiston Textbook of Surgery. Philadelphia, WB Saunders, 1997, p 946.

75. Freeman NV, Burge DM, Griffiths DM, Malone PSJ: Surgery of the Newborn. Edinburgh, Churchill Livingstone, 1994.

76. Cooney D, Duszynski D, Camboa E, et al: The abdominal technetium scan (a decade of experience). J Pediatr Surg 17:611, 1982.

77. Wine C, Nahrwold D, Waldhausen J: Role of the technetium scan in the diagnosis of Meckel's diverticulum. J Pediatr Surg 8:885, 1974.

78. Huang CS, Lin LH: Laparoscopic Meckel's diverticulectomy in infants: Report of three cases. J Pediatr Surg 28:1486, 1993.

79. Michas C, Cohen S, Wolfman E: Meckel's diverticulum: Should it be excised incidentally at operation? Am J Surg 129:682, 1975.

80. Bemelman WA, Bosma A, Wiersma PH, et al: Role of *Helicobacter pylori* in the pathogenesis of complications of Meckel's diverticula. Eur J Surg 159:171, 1993.

81. Von Hendenberg C: Surgical indications in Meckel's diverticulectomy. Acta Chir Scand 135:530, 1969.

82. Fansler RF: Laparoscopy in the management of Meckel's diverticulum. Surg Laparosc Endosc 6:231, 1996.

83. Teitelbaum DH, Polley TZ Jr, Obeid F: Laparoscopic diagnosis and excision of Meckel's diverticulum. J Pediatr Surg 29:495, 1994.

55

Operations for Peptic Ulcer

Ali Tavakkolizadeh • Stanley W. Ashley

Gastroduodenal peptic ulcer disease (PUD) is a common problem, with an estimated 2% of the U.S. population having a symptomatic ulcer at any given time. A recent review of Medicare records estimates nearly 900,000 peptic ulcer–related hospital admissions per year, with an annual cost of $4.8 billion and an overall ulcer-related mortality rate of 4.5%.[1] With the identification of *Helicobacter pylori (H. pylori)* and recognition of nonsteroidal anti-inflammatory drugs (NSAIDs) as etiologic factors, our understanding of the disease has improved significantly, which has lead to the introduction of more potent and successful therapeutic regimens. Before the introduction of histamine H_2 receptor antagonists and proton-pump inhibitors (PPIs), operations for chronic intractable PUD were common. With the advent of successful medical therapy, the role of elective surgery in this field has diminished. Based on a population study from Finland, the number of elective peptic ulcer procedures fell from 11.9 to 1.3 per 100,000 population between 1987 and 1999, an 89% reduction.[2] This reduction has also been confirmed by large epidemiologic studies from Iceland and the United Kingdom.[3,4]

Complications of ulcer disease will develop in 10% to 20% of people during the course of their disease, and operative intervention is often required when such complications occur. Although the new drug regimens have reduced the number of elective operations for PUD, the number of admissions and surgical interventions for complications of this disease has remained unchanged.[5] In fact, epidemiologic data from the United Kingdom suggest that the incidence of duodenal ulcer bleeding and perforation has increased in older age groups. Interestingly, this increase has been documented during a period when there has been a 50-fold increase in the prescription of PPIs and a lower prevalence of *H. pylori* infection in the cohort.[3] This finding has led to the conclusion that the increased prevalence of PUD complications is due to the wider use of ulcerogenic drugs such as NSAIDs, low-dose aspirin, and selective serotonin reuptake inhibitors. The mortality rate for those undergoing surgery has also remained unchanged, which in part reflects the population that is undergoing surgery: the sickest and eldest individuals, in whom such problems eventually develop.

Current indications for surgical intervention are

1. Bleeding—most common complication of PUD, with an incidence of approximately 100 per 100,000 population
2. Perforation—with an annual incidence of 11 operations per 100,000 population
3. Obstruction—occurs as a result of scarring of prepyloric and duodenal ulcers
4. Failed medical therapy—in the era of PPIs, an uncommon indication for surgery
5. Risk for malignancy—of particular importance with regard to large gastric ulcers

The goals of surgical procedures are to

1. Permit ulcer healing
2. Prevent or treat ulcer complications
3. Address the underlying ulcer etiology
4. Minimize postoperative digestive consequences

No single procedure satisfies all these objectives. To choose the best operation, the surgeon must consider the characteristics of the ulcer (location, chronicity, type of complication), the probable cause (acid hypersecretion, drug induced, possible role of *H. pylori*), the patient (age, nutrition, comorbid illness, condition at initial evaluation), and the operation (mortality rate, side effects). In some respects, all ulcer operations represent a compromise: the morbidity of ulcer disease is replaced by the morbidity of the operation. Finally, surgeon experience must play a role in the choice of operation; today, most surgical residents complete their training with significantly less experience in more complex procedures, which undoubtedly influences their choices for both elective and emergency operations.

In this chapter we first discuss elective surgery for intractable peptic ulcers before discussing emergency procedures to deal with complications of ulcer disease.

ELECTIVE SURGERY FOR PEPTIC ULCER DISEASE

Elective Surgery for Intractable Duodenal Ulcer Disease

With the identification of *H. pylori*, the recognition that greater than 95% of duodenal ulcers are associated with this organism, and the fact that eradication of the pathogen results in cure rates in excess of 95% without the need for chronic acid suppression, medical therapy for duodenal ulcer has shifted away from an antisecretory/antacid approach to an antimicrobial strategy. This change has resulted in a dramatic reduction in the number of elective procedures performed for intractable, noncomplicated disease. However, when operative intervention is being considered, the strategy continues to be based on reduction of acid secretion. Acid secretion by the parietal cells is normally stimulated by acetylcholine from the vagus nerve and release of gastrin from the antrum. Surgeons attempt to reduce this acid secretion by sectioning the vagus (vagotomy) and eliminating hormonal stimulation from the antrum (antrectomy). Each of these maneuvers has effects on acid secretion and consequences in terms of the normal physiology of the upper gastrointestinal tract that tend to be amplified when procedures are combined (e.g., vagotomy and antrectomy). In the past, the choice of operation involved weighing rates of recurrent ulceration with the risk for postoperative complications and long-term sequelae (postgastrectomy syndromes). This decision dilemma prompted a large number of trials comparing the procedures in the surgical literature. Recently, improvements in medical therapy, particularly treatment of *H. pylori*, have markedly reduced the risk for ulcer recurrence, thus rendering much of these data obsolete. Consequently, surgical decision making has become confusing, with few quality data available from the post–*H. pylori* era. The choices of surgical intervention for intractable duodenal ulcer disease, however, have remained unchanged:

1. A form of vagotomy
2. ± A drainage procedure
3. ± Gastric resection/anterectomy

Here we discuss the choices available within each category.

Vagotomy

Technically speaking, the term *vagotomy* implies transection of the vagus nerve and thus interruption of sensory, secretory, and motor impulses to the stomach and other gastrointestinal organs. In common practice, a 1- to 2-cm section of each nerve is actually resected and sent to the pathologist, who confirms that it is nerve tissue. Although the proper term for the resection should be *vagectomy, vagotomy* is the much more commonly used term. The rationale for vagotomy is the elimination of direct cholinergic stimulation of acid secretion. In the stomach, vagal fibers innervate the mucosa and play a major role in the cephalic phase of gastric acid secretion

by releasing acetylcholine; once released, acetylcholine stimulates acid secretion via a specific receptor on the parietal cell. The distal portions of the anterior and posterior trunks send branches to the antrum and pylorus that serve primarily a motor function. The celiac branch of the posterior vagus stimulates small intestinal motility. Gastric motility is affected not just by the antral and pyloric branches of the vagus, which stimulate peristaltic activity of the antrum and relaxation of the pylorus; the vagus also stimulates receptive relaxation of the fundus, which results in accommodating intake without a corresponding increase in pressure.

Vagotomy results in a variety of physiologic alterations in the stomach. Acid secretion is drastically reduced because of diminished cholinergic stimulation of parietal cells, and the cephalic phase of gastric secretion is essentially eliminated. There is a 75% decrease in basal acid secretion and a 50% decrease in maximum acid output. After vagotomy, the parietal cells are less responsive to histamine and gastrin, with a resultant increase in serum gastrin levels and gastrin cell hyperplasia. Because of loss of reflex relaxation of the gastric fundus, increased gastric volume after eating is accompanied by an increase in pressure, which results in rapid emptying of liquids. Similarly, vagotomy adversely affects distal stomach motility and thereby results in difficulty emptying solids. As a result of the latter alterations, gastric atony develops in approximately 20% of patients and leads to stasis, chronic abdominal pain, and distention. For that reason, it is recommended that after truncal vagotomy patients undergo a drainage procedure to counteract the nonrelaxing pylorus, which acts as an obstruction. The various drainage procedures available are discussed later. Four types of vagotomy have been described in the surgical literature: *truncal, selective, highly selective,* and *supradiaphragmatic.* Truncal and highly selective vagotomy are commonly used to treat PUD, whereas selective and supradiaphragmatic vagotomies are used infrequently.

Truncal Vagotomy Truncal vagotomy involves division of the anterior and posterior vagal trunks after they emerge below the diaphragm (Fig. 55–1). As part of truncal vagotomy, all branches of the two trunks that lie on the esophagus, between the diaphragm and gastroesophageal junction, should be sought and transected as well. This procedure not only completely denervates the stomach but also eliminates vagal innervation to the pancreas, small intestine, proximal part of the colon, and hepatobiliary tree. Although truncal vagotomy significantly reduces acid secretion, it also markedly alters gastric motility by impairing both receptive relaxation of the stomach and the process of antral grinding and pyloric sphincter coordination, which permits gastric emptying. As discussed earlier, some form of gastric-emptying procedure should be performed. This procedure is often combined with antrectomy, but in the event of an emergency, pyloroplasty or gastroenterostomy is performed.

Selective Vagotomy Selective vagotomy was developed in an attempt to decrease the incidence of postvagotomy diarrhea and ameliorate the increased incidence of gallbladder stasis, which leads to increased gallstone forma-

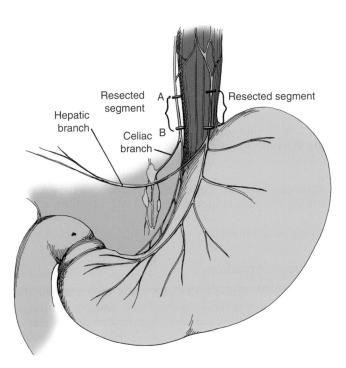

Figure 55–1. Truncal vagotomy involves resecting a 2- to 3-cm section of the anterior and posterior nerve trunks between the gastroesophageal junction and diaphragm. (From Zollinger RM: Atlas of Surgical Operations. New York, Macmillan, 1975.)

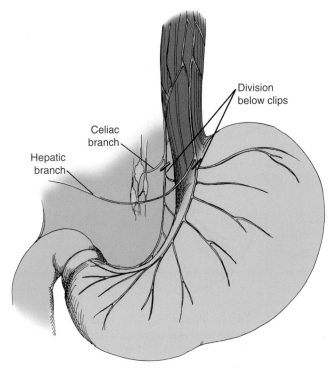

Figure 55–2. Selective vagotomy involves a bilateral vagotomy distal to the takeoff of the hepatic and celiac vagal brunches. (From Zollinger RM: Atlas of Surgical Operations. New York, Macmillan, 1975.)

tion and cholecystitis. The vagal fibers are divided distal to the takeoff of the hepatic branches (from the anterior vagus) and the celiac branches (from the posterior vagus) (Fig. 55–2). This procedure is technically more demanding than truncal vagotomy and requires more careful and meticulous dissection. The effectiveness of this procedure, when performed carefully, is borne out by reported ulcer recurrence rates as low as 2%. This low recurrence rate is in part due to the meticulous periesophageal dissection that is performed. This technique spares vagal innervation to the gallbladder and intestine while completely denervating the stomach. Because vagal pyloric innervation is also eliminated, a drainage procedure is still required. The drainage procedure could take the form of a pyloroplasty, or the procedure may be combined with antrectomy. Unlike truncal vagotomy, after which antrectomy is recommended, trials have shown that selective vagotomy, when performed in conjunction with pyloroplasty or antrectomy, results in similar recurrence rates. The main reason for the evolution of this technique, however, was its presumed lower side effect profile. Nonetheless, a prospective randomized study failed to show substantial benefit for selective vagotomy over truncal vagotomy. Although the incidence of diarrhea after selective vagotomy appeared to be lower, it did not reach statistical significance.

The introduction of highly selective vagotomy (HSV) with a lower side effect profile and the need for a drainage procedure with selective vagotomy resulted in limited use of selective vagotomy as a therapeutic option.

Highly Selective Vagotomy HSV is also known as *parietal cell vagotomy* and *proximal gastric vagotomy*. The rationale for HSV is to eliminate vagal stimulation to the acid-secreting portion of the stomach without interrupting motor innervation to the antrum and pylorus. The operation involves severing all branches of the vagus nerve along the lesser curvature that innervate the corpus and fundus of the stomach while preserving the hepatic and celiac branches, as well as the distal vagal branches extending to the antrum and pylorus (Fig. 55–3). The end result of this technically demanding and somewhat tedious procedure is the same reduction in acid secretion that occurs after truncal vagotomy (basal and stimulated acid secretion is reduced by more than 75% and 50%, respectively), but without the troublesome stasis and gastric atony. Because the distal motor nerves are preserved, emptying of solids is normal; however, the nerves affecting receptive relaxation are divided, and thus some rapid emptying of liquids may occur. The alteration in liquid emptying is usually minimal. This procedure is associated with the lowest morbidity rate of all vagotomy procedures and became the operation of choice in many centers despite an ulcer recurrence rate of 5% to 20%. A meta-analysis of 12 trials has confirmed that HSV has a higher recurrence rate than truncal vagotomy with pyloroplasty, but fewer long-term side effects.[6] HSV has also been compared with truncal vagotomy in a randomized trial, in which it was shown to have a lower incidence of dumping syndrome and weight loss. Although ulcer recurrence rates were higher with HSV,

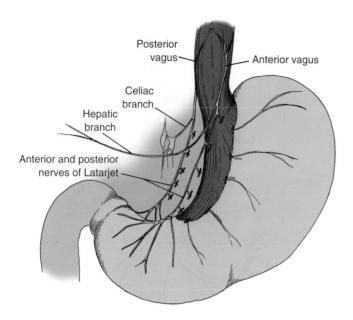

Figure 55–3. Highly selective vagotomy involves dividing the vagal branches to the fundus and corpus of the stomach while preserving the motor branches to the antrum and pylorus. (From Zollinger RM: Atlas of Surgical Operations. New York, Macmillan, 1975.)

this was not significant when prepyloric ulcers (for which HSV is now known to be an inadequate operation) were excluded.[7]

Both truncal vagotomy with antrectomy and selective vagotomy with antrectomy are more effective than HSV in curing PUD and would have been regarded as the gold standard were it not for their higher incidence of side effects.

It was assumed that when duodenal scarring is present and pyloroplasty or gastroenterostomy is needed, HSV is unlikely to offer any benefit and the procedure was abandoned in favor of the simpler truncal vagotomy. Several studies have, however, shown that this simplified thinking is incorrect and that HSV offers symptomatic advantages over vagotomy even when performed with a drainage procedure. Preservation of antral innervation is thought to preserve antral motility and prevent bile accumulation in the stomach, as well as minimize early dumping in patients.[8]

HSV is a complex and lengthy procedure, and to help simplify the procedure, several variations have been described. They usually consist of a posterior truncal vagotomy and a more selective ablation of the anterior vagal fibers to the gastric fundus and body. Hill and Baker performed posterior truncal vagotomy with anterior HSV (Hill-Baker procedure). Taylor combined posterior truncal vagotomy with anterior lesser curve seromyotomy (Taylor procedure). Randomized studies have confirmed superiority of the Taylor procedure over truncal vagotomy[9] and have documented outcomes equal to those of HSV with a shorter operative time.[10] With the decreased incidence of elective ulcer surgery, these operations are not commonly performed.

However, such approaches have proved popular for laparoscopic treatment of ulcer disease (see Laparoscopic Surgery, later).

Supradiaphragmatic Vagotomy This type of vagotomy is performed primarily in patients for whom attempts at complete vagotomy via an abdominal approach have failed; it is thought that further attempts to find the missed trunks in a reoperated abdomen may be difficult and thus a thoracic approach is advised. This operation involves performing a thoracotomy or thoracoscopy, identifying the two large nerve trunks, and then performing truncal vagotomy.

The surgical technique for various vagotomies is covered in Chapter 56.

Drainage Procedures

In Dragstedt's initial series of truncal vagotomy for the treatment of duodenal ulcer disease without drainage, nearly a third of his patients experienced postoperative nausea, vomiting, and distention. Further investigations revealed that truncal vagotomy denervated the antrum and pylorus, which resulted in loss of the antral pump mechanism and failure of the pylorus to reflexively relax and allow emptying into the duodenum. The end result was a functional gastric outlet obstruction. It became apparent that a drainage procedure was necessary to avoid the symptoms of gastric stasis. Accordingly, any patient being treated by truncal, selective, or supradiaphragmatic vagotomy should undergo a drainage procedure to facilitate gastric emptying. Drainage procedures fall into two categories—pyloroplasty and gastrojejunostomy. Pyloroplasty is the preferred approach because it perpetuates the original anatomy, is a simple procedure, and is associated with less bile reflux than gastrojejunostomy. More than 90% of all drainage procedures performed today are variations of pyloroplasty.

Pyloroplasty In children with pyloric hyperplasia, a pyloromyotomy is performed to divide the pylorus muscle and relax the pyloric sphincter while leaving the mucosa intact. Such an approach in adults is often unsuccessful because the duodenal mucosa is adherent to the muscle layer and the intestinal lumen is often entered during the myotomy. Thus, a pyloroplasty is performed. Three different types of pyloroplasty have been described (Fig. 55–4).

Heineke-Mikulicz This procedure was described independently by two surgeons, Heineke and Mikulicz, in 1888, years before it found routine application as the most commonly performed drainage procedure. The technique is popular because it is simple, applicable to many clinical ulcer scenarios, and associated with few complications. The procedure may be performed with single- or double-layer closure, with the latter being more commonly used. The Heineke-Mikulicz pyloroplasty entails making a longitudinal incision through the pylorus (thus interrupting the circular muscle) and reconstructing the duodenotomy in a transverse fashion. It is the most

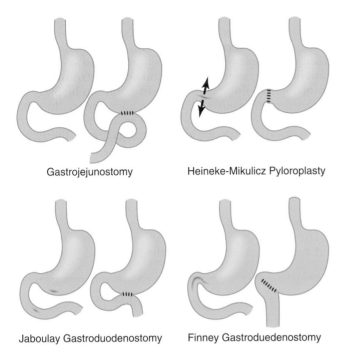

Gastrojejunostomy　　Heineke-Mikulicz Pyloroplasty

Jaboulay Gastroduodenostomy　　Finney Gastroduedenostomy

Figure 55–4. Drainage procedures used with truncal or selective vagotomy. (From Matthews JB, Silen W: Operations for peptic ulcer disease and early operative complications. In Sleisenger MH, Fordtran JS [eds]: Gastrointestinal Disease. Philadelphia, WB Saunders, 1993.)

commonly performed drainage procedure, and when conducted carefully and in a technically sound fashion, obstruction is rare. Candidates for this procedure include patients who have a mobile, uninvolved anterior pylorus and those who have no evidence of a severely distorted or edematous pylorus. A variety of postgastrectomy complications may occur after pyloroplasty, including dumping, diarrhea, alkaline reflux gastritis, anemia, and marginal ulceration. Such complications may be seen on a temporary basis in up to 50% of patients after surgery, but they resolve within 6 to 8 months in most, and only 5% to 7% of patients have a persistent, symptomatic postoperative complication such as dumping.

Finney This uncommonly used pyloroplasty is indicated primarily for patients with a J-shaped stomach or extensive scarring and narrowing of a significant portion of the duodenal bulb, thus making Heineke-Mikulicz pyloroplasty untenable. Use of this drainage procedure makes a larger lumen possible and involves a fairly long incision from the stomach, through the pylorus, and well into the duodenal bulb, with closure of the inferior duodenum to the inferior stomach and the superior duodenum to the superior stomach (see Fig. 55–4). It is a much more complicated procedure than the Heineke-Mikulicz technique, involves a great deal more suturing, and has more potential for complications.

Jaboulay Gastroduodenostomy This drainage procedure is the only one of the three described here that does not

transect the pyloric muscle. As the name implies, the procedure involves anastomosis of the distal part of the stomach to the first and second portions of the duodenum, thus bypassing the pylorus (see Fig. 55–4). The procedure is rarely used and is indicated primarily for a severely scarred or deformed pylorus or duodenal bulb that would be too treacherous to operate on. Use of the Jaboulay procedure may also be associated with increased bile reflux because the anastomosis is close to the ampulla of Vater.

Gastrojejunostomy This procedure was first performed alone in 1881 and was plagued by two problems: ulcers (because no vagotomy was performed) and vomiting, which was thought to be due to kinking with excessive length of the afferent limb of jejunum. The two problems have been overcome with the addition of vagotomy and construction of a shorter afferent jejunal segment (see Fig. 55–4). Gastrojejunostomy is most commonly indicated as a drainage procedure when there is duodenal obstruction and the duodenal bulb is so scarred, inflamed, and edematous that pyloroplasty would not be safe or would be technically demanding. A vagotomy should always be performed when using gastrojejunostomy as a drainage procedure for the treatment of PUD. Older patients with achlorhydria and atrophic gastritis secrete little acid, and thus a vagotomy may not be necessary, especially in the setting of malignant obstruction. A decision that has to be made when creating a gastrojejunostomy is whether the anastomosis will be antecolic or retrocolic. In most circumstances, it is desirable to perform the anastomosis in a retrocolic manner because there is likely to be less tension and less interference with gastric emptying when the colon becomes distended. The antecolic approach is generally used when there are no well-defined mesenteric windows and the blood supply to the colon might be compromised by attempts to create a window. In addition, many prefer this approach when bypassing a malignant obstruction, which might invade a more posterior retrocolic limb.

The surgical technique for various drainage procedures is detailed in Chapter 56.

Gastric Resection Procedures

Although subtotal gastrectomy was used for the treatment of duodenal ulcer disease in the past, today it is most commonly performed for gastric ulcer and distal gastric malignancies. A more common gastric resection performed for intractable duodenal ulcer is antrectomy (35% distal gastrectomy), combined with truncal or selective vagotomy. The simultaneous effects of vagotomy and antrectomy remove both the cholinergic and the gastrin stimulus to acid secretion. Basal acid secretion is virtually abolished, and stimulated secretion is reduced by nearly 80%. After antrectomy, gastrointestinal continuity must be restored by some form of reconstruction. The remnant is anastomosed either to the duodenum (Billroth I) or, after closing the duodenal stump, to the jejunum distal to the ligament of Treitz (Billroth II)

(Fig. 55–5). Billroth I reconstruction has several theoretical advantages:

1. Restores normal gastrointestinal continuity
2. Leaves specialized duodenal mucosa next to the gastric mucosa
3. Avoids problems with an afferent and efferent limb
4. Allows easier performance of endoscopic retrograde cholangiopancreatography and endoscopic examination of the bowel
5. Is associated with a reduced incidence of gastric cancer in the remnant stomach[11]

Despite the theoretical physiologic advantages, no important functional differences have ever been demonstrated between these reconstructions. Although studies have shown larger fecal fat loss after a Billroth II procedure, this is unlikely to be of any significance. The difference in cancer risk is real, but significant only after a long follow-up period (>15 years). Typically, the choice is based on the degree of scarring of the duodenum and the ease with which the duodenum and gastric remnant can be brought together. Several variations of the Billroth I and Billroth II operations have been described and are summarized in Figures 55–6 and 55–7.

The Billroth reconstructions can lead to bile reflux, which can result in disabling symptoms. To avoid such complications, some favor a Roux-en-Y reconstruction. Unfortunately, Roux-en-Y reconstruction can be plagued by Roux stasis syndrome. Studies have shown that the Braun variation of Billroth II (see Fig. 55–7) is associated with a lower incidence of bile reflux[12] and therefore has been recommended as the standard reconstruction technique by some authors. Others, however, promote the uncut Roux-en-Y reconstruction (Fig. 55–8), but this technique has not gained widespread use because of reports of staple line dehiscence leading to severe alkaline reflux.

The surgical techniques for the various gastrectomies and reconstructions are described in detail in Chapter 57.

Choice of Operation for Intractable Duodenal Ulcer

As can be seen from the foregoing descriptions, a variety of surgical operations are available for patients with intractable duodenal ulcers. Reliable data on the results of the various procedures for duodenal ulcer were generated by a series of trials during the latter half of the 20th century. Published series in general used different criteria for patient selection and for estimating the incidence of side effects. Table 55–1 summarizes the data on the three most commonly performed procedures: vagotomy and antrectomy, vagotomy and drainage, and HSV. Mortality and early morbidity were highest for the resection procedures and lowest for HSV, which avoids opening the gastrointestinal tract. Recurrence rates were significantly lower for vagotomy with antrectomy. Truncal vagotomy plus pyloroplasty is virtually never indicated as an elective procedure because it has the disadvantages of both a high incidence of postgastrectomy complications and a high ulcer recurrence rate (10% to 15%).

Historically, an important factor when considering the choice of surgery would have been the ulcer recurrence rate. However, with identification of *H. pylori*, it is believed that recurrences are for the most part

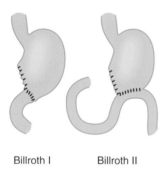

Billroth I   Billroth II

Figure 55–5. Reconstruction techniques after partial gastrectomy: Billroth I gastroduodenostomy and Billroth II gastrojejunostomy. (From Matthews JB, Silen W: Operations for peptic ulcer disease and early operative complications. In Sleisenger MH, Fordtran JS [eds]: Gastrointestinal Disease. Philadelphia, WB Saunders, 1993.)

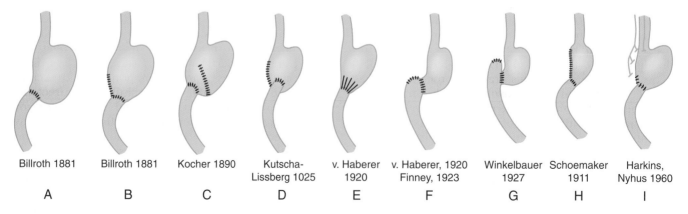

| Billroth 1881 | Billroth 1881 | Kocher 1890 | Kutscha-Lissberg 1025 | v. Haberer 1920 | v. Haberer, 1920 Finney, 1923 | Winkelbauer 1927 | Schoemaker 1911 | Harkins, Nyhus 1960 |
| A | B | C | D | E | F | G | H | I |

Figure 55–6. Variations of Billroth I reconstructions. (From Siewert JR, Bumm R: Billroth I gastrectomy. In Baker RJ, Fischer JE [eds]: Mastery of Surgery. Philadelphia, Lippincott, Williams & Wilkins, 2001.)

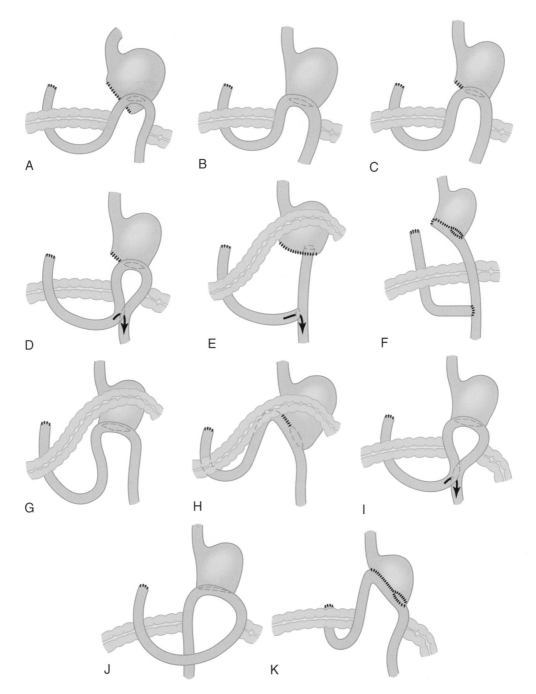

Figure 55–7. Variations of Billroth II reconstruction. (From Wastell C, Davis PA: Billroth II gastrectomy. In Baker RJ, Fischer JE [eds]: Mastery of Surgery. Philadelphia, Lippincott, Williams & Wilkins, 2001.)

eliminated, although no data in this setting have yet been generated. Consequently, HSV, which is associated with fewer postoperative sequelae, is the preferred acid-reducing procedure in patients with intractable ulcer symptoms. One trial randomized 248 patients with stable PUD to truncal vagotomy and drainage, selective vagotomy and drainage, or HSV. At 11 to 15 years after surgery, HSV was associated with a reduction in the incidence of severe postvagotomy symptoms such as dumping, diarrhea, and dyspepsia. Interestingly, this study did not show

a significant difference in ulcer recurrence rates between the three groups.[13] Although this would more strongly favor HSV, today's experience with this more complex procedure is limited. In a review of the experience of surgical chief residents in the United States, the average number of vagotomies performed by each resident has decreased dramatically during the 1990s.[14] In addition, most patients undergoing operation now are elderly and debilitated, conditions favoring the most expeditious procedure, usually truncal vagotomy and antrectomy.

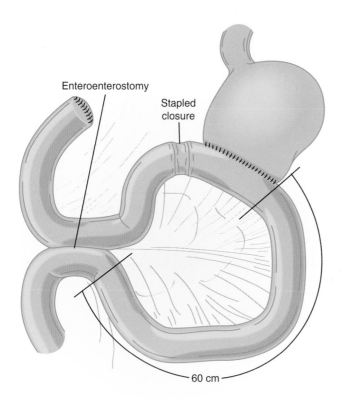

Enteroenterostomy

Stapled closure

60 cm

Figure 55–8. "Uncut" Roux-en-Y reconstruction after partial gastrectomy. A jejunoduodenostomy with a 60-cm efferent limb is constructed. The afferent limb is occluded with a staple line. (From van Stiegmann G, Goff, JS: An alternative to Roux-en-Y for treatment of bile reflux gastritis. Surg Gynecol Obstet [now J Am Coll Surg] 166:69, 1988.)

Table 55–1 Ulcer Recurrence Rates for the Three Common Acid-Reducing Procedures

Surgical Procedure	Ulcer Recurrence Rate	Risk for Side Effects
Truncal vagotomy and drainage	15%	Highest
Truncal vagotomy and antrectomy	2%	High
Highly selective vagotomy	15%	Low

Figure 55–9 summarizes the recommended surgical approach to a patient with a chronic duodenal ulcer.

Recurrent Peptic Ulcer Disease

Supradiaphragmatic vagotomy is used almost exclusively for the treatment of ulcer recurrence after previous acid-reducing surgery that included vagotomy. The

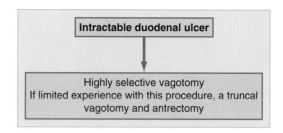

Intractable duodenal ulcer

Highly selective vagotomy
If limited experience with this procedure, a truncal vagotomy and antrectomy

Figure 55–9. Treatment algorithm for intractable duodenal ulcer.

most common cause of ulcer recurrence after an acid-reducing procedure is a missed vagus. If attempts to find the missed nerve are unsuccessful through the densely scarred upper abdomen, thoracic truncal vagotomy may be used successfully. The procedure can now be performed with minimally invasive techniques that include the use of a thoracoscope.

Laparoscopic Surgery

An increasing number of reports indicate the feasibility of laparoscopic approaches to operations for duodenal ulcer disease. Although most open procedures have been attempted laparoscopically, including the more difficult HSV, the Taylor procedure (anterior seromyotomy with posterior truncal vagotomy) seems to be the simplest option. The Taylor procedure was reported in 1982 as an open procedure. Although the open approach is not widely performed, the technique is very suitable for a laparoscopic approach. This procedure begins with a posterior truncal vagotomy followed by a seromyotomy that should start approximately 6 cm from the pylorus. The circular muscle is incised 1.5 cm from the lesser curve and the muscle fibers divided with a hook coagulator. The dissection is continued caudally as far as the gastroesophageal junction. All the circular muscle fibers along the length of the myotomy are divided, but it is not necessary to divide the deeper thin layer of the oblique muscle. Air is injected through a nasogastric tube to ensure that no leaks are present. The seromyotomy is then closed with overlapping running suture. The serosal myotomy can be performed as a stapled anterior linear gastrotomy, which helps expedite the procedure[15] (Fig. 55–10). Other groups have used the Hill-Baker procedure with good results.[16]

Elective Surgery for Intractable Gastric Ulcer Disease

Although both gastric and duodenal ulcers are peptic lesions, fundamental differences between these entities affect surgical strategy. The most important is that a gastric ulcer may harbor malignancy and must therefore be excised or generous biopsy specimens taken. Acid hypersecretion, which is important in pathogenesis of duodenal ulcers, does not have a role in the pathogenesis of many gastric ulcers. A classification system

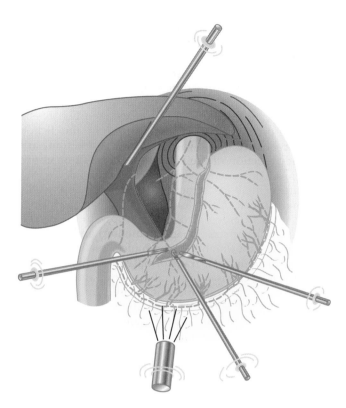

Figure 55–10. Laparoscopic anterior seromyotomy as part of the Taylor procedure. (From Dubois F: New surgical strategy for gastroduodenal ulcer: Laparoscopic approach. World J Surg 24:270, 2000.)

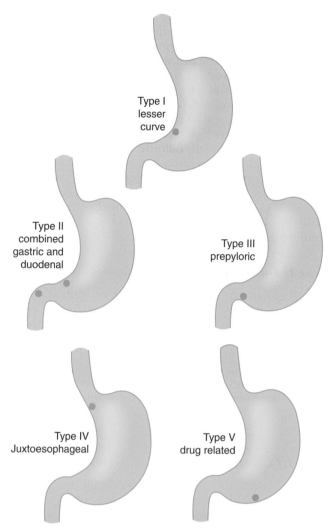

Figure 55–11. Classification of gastric ulcer based on anatomic location. (From Matthews JB, Silen W: Operations for peptic ulcer disease and early operative complications. In Sleisenger MH, Fordtran JS [eds]: Gastrointestinal Disease. Philadelphia, WB Saunders, 1993.)

Table 55–2 Modified Johnson Classification of Gastric Ulcers

Type	Location	Acid Secretion
I	Lesser curvature	Low
II	Body of the stomach and duodenum	High
III	Prepyloric (within 2-3 cm of the pylorus)	High
IV	High on the lesser curve, near the gastroesophageal junction	Low
V	Anywhere, induced by medication	Low

developed by Johnson that is based on anatomic location and acid secretory potential provides a useful basis for considering operative treatment of gastric ulcer (Table 55–2) (Fig. 55–11).

Type I Gastric Ulcer

Type I ulcers are the most common form. They occur along the lesser curvature at the junction of fundic and antral mucosa and develop in the setting of acid hyposecretion. Distal gastrectomy with Billroth I or II reconstruction is recommended for most patients because this approach removes the ulcer and the diseased antrum. Partial gastrectomy also eliminates the risk of missing a malignancy, which can occur with biopsy, and reduces the acid secretory potential. Earlier recommendations of performing a biopsy of the ulcer combined with vagotomy and drainage have now become outdated because of high ulcer recurrence rates.[17] Low recurrence rates (5%) and excellent symptomatic relief are usually achieved with a distal gastrectomy alone. Experience from the Cleveland Clinic has shown that the addition of truncal vagotomy to gastric resection offers no additional benefit to the patient.[18] Reported mortality rates for elective surgery have generally been less than 5%; however, because formal gastric resection can add to the morbidity and mortality of the operation, some have tried less disruptive surgical procedures for type I gastric ulcers, including ulcer excision combined with HSV. The value of HSV in treating gastric ulcer may derive from its ability to decrease acid secretion while maintaining adequate gastric emptying and minimizing postoperative duodenogastric reflux. The procedure is performed with the addition of a gastrotomy to excise or biopsy the ulcer bed. In one series of 48 patients, HSV combined with mucosal ulcerectomy produced an excellent clinical outcome in most patients with a recurrence rate of 6.5% and few side effects.[19] A Swedish randomized study in which gastrectomy with Billroth I reconstruction was compared with ulcer excision and HSV has shown equal outcomes in terms of complications and ulcer recurrence.[20] Ulcer size and location may make this operative approach untenable for some patients in whom ulcer-induced inflammation, edema, or scarring may obscure accurate dissection.

Type II Gastric Ulcer

Type II gastric ulcers occur synchronously with scarring or ulceration in the duodenum or pyloric channel. They tend to be large, deep ulcers with poorly defined margins. They frequently occur in younger men and are associated with increased acid secretion. Preoperative endoscopic examination of such ulcers must include biopsy of the lesion to rule out an underlying malignancy. Treatment is similar to that for duodenal ulcer, with vagotomy plus antrectomy or HSV being the preferred approach.

Type III Gastric Ulcer

Type III ulcers are prepyloric, although no precise anatomic definition exists. They occur in the setting of increased acid secretion and are approached in a manner similar to that for duodenal ulcer and type II gastric ulcer. Curiously, HSV (as well as medical therapy with H_2 receptor antagonists) has been associated with poor results in type III gastric ulcer, with recurrence rates ranging from 16% to 44% in various series.[6] This finding plus the observation that these lesions may harbor gastric malignancy makes vagotomy and antrectomy the most prudent approach. Early consideration of surgical referral is advisable for resistant ulcers or those causing obstructive symptoms.

Type IV Gastric Ulcer

Type IV gastric ulcer is distinguished by its anatomic location high along the lesser curvature, close to the gastroesophageal junction. Antral mucosa may extend to within 1 to 2 cm of the gastroesophageal junction; thus, type IV ulcers may simply represent a subset of type I gastric ulcer. Type IV ulcers are associated with gastric hyposecretion and come to attention early as a result of dysphagia and reflux. Large ulcer size, the degree of surrounding inflammation, and proximity to the gastroesophageal junction render operative management difficult and potentially dangerous. If the integrity of the distal end of the esophagus can be ensured, subtotal gastric resection (including the ulcer bed) is considered optimal. Lesions close to the cardia, however, pose a particular challenge, and to help avoid total gastrectomy and an esophageal anastomosis, other surgical approaches have been described. Such alternatives include the Schoemaker procedure (a modification of Billroth I resection with tube-shaped resection of high gastric ulcers and anastomosis of the duodenum to the greater curvature side of the stomach; see Fig. 55–6), Pauchet's procedure[21] (a modification of the Schoemaker procedure that involves a lower gastrectomy and freehand resection of the ulcer with scissors), or nonresective procedures in which the ulcer itself is not excised. The latter includes procedures such as the Kelly-Madlener procedure (a distal gastrectomy is performed but the ulcer is left in place, after biopsy, to avoid compromise of the gastroesophageal junction) and vagotomy plus pyloroplasty, which has a high ulcer recurrence rate. The risk for malignant transformation or missed malignancy (despite biopsies) is small but real, and thus nonresective procedures should not be used routinely.

Although there is no consensus in the literature, some have suggested that for ulcers 5 cm below the cardia, Pauchet's procedure should be used, whereas for lesions within 2 cm of the cardia, the Kelly-Madlener procedure (nonresective) or the Csendes procedure should be attempted[22] (Fig. 55–12). The Csendes procedure involves a near-total gastrectomy and an esophagogastrojejunostomy for reconstruction. The principle of this operation is to remove the high gastric ulcer such that the circumference of the esophageal mucosa remains intact. The reconstruction involves a Roux-en-Y loop 30 cm distal to the ligament of Treitz. The end of the loop is closed and a terminolateral esophagogastrojejunostomy is created. The reconstruction is completed by forming a jejunojejunostomy 40 cm distal to the gastric anastomosis.

Type V Gastric Ulcer

These lesions can occur anywhere in the stomach and are induced by the use of medications such as NSAIDs. A definitive antisecretary operation is recommended for these ulcers, especially if treatment with the offending medications cannot be stopped.

Figure 55–13 summarizes the recommended approach to chronic intractable gastric ulcers. The surgical technique for various gastrectomies and reconstructions is described in detail in Chapter 57.

EMERGENCY SURGERY FOR COMPLICATED PEPTIC ULCER DISEASE

Such operations are most often performed in the elderly and the sick. Patients may have bleeding, perforation, or obstruction. The objectives of surgery in these cases follow:

1. Deal with the complication that necessitated surgical intervention.
2. Reduce the risk for future ulcer recurrence.
3. Perform a safe, quick, and effective operation.

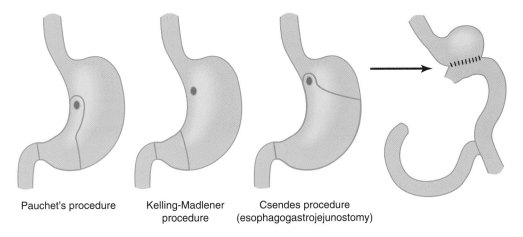

Pauchet's procedure

Kelling-Madlener
procedure

Csendes procedure
(esophagogastrojejunostomy)

Figure 55–12. Operations for a type IV gastric ulcer. (Modified from Seymour NE: Operations for peptic ulcer and their complications. In Feldman M, Scharschmidt BF, Sleisenger MH [eds]: Gastrointestinal Disease. Philadelphia, WB Saunders, 1998.)

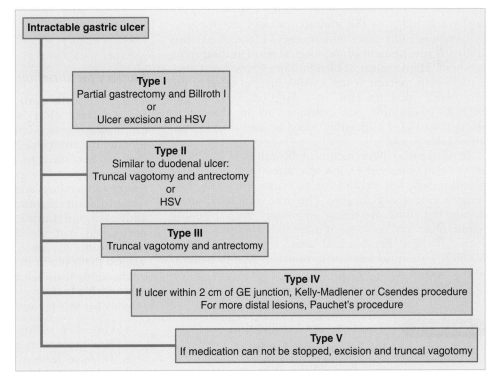

Figure 55–13. Algorithm for the surgical treatment of intractable gastric ulcers. GE, gastroesophageal; HSV, highly selective vagotomy.

4. Minimize long-term effects on the gastrointestinal tract
5. Establish the *H. pylori* status of the patient

Usually, the biggest intraoperative dilemma is whether to proceed with a definitive antiulcer operation (to reduce the risk for recurrence), in addition to addressing the specific ulcer complication. This issue has received considerable attention over the past several decades but remains unsettled. Shifting ulcer epidemiology, recognition of the role of *H. pylori,* and improvements in medical therapy have confused this issue considerably, and the decision must be individualized.

Omission of an acid-reducing ulcer procedure carries a risk for recurrent ulcer symptoms and complications; this risk is variable in the literature, but not negligible. Recent evidence would suggest that this risk may be considerably reduced by treatment of *H. pylori* postoperatively, but obviously only if the patient is *H. pylori* positive. Unfortunately, there is no reliable, rapid test for *H. pylori* status at the time of surgery to help guide this decision making. A definitive procedure is always more appropriate in the setting of NSAIDs, especially if the patient is unlikely to be able to stop the treatment because of an underlying medical condition. On the other hand, inclusion of an acid-reducing ulcer procedure may result in serious gastrointestinal sequelae in patients who may not have required the intervention. Definitive surgery is generally avoided during emergency procedures in patients with major underlying medical illness or intraoperative hemodynamic instability.

Bleeding

Most patients with a bleeding upper gastrointestinal lesion undergo an endoscopic examination of the stomach and the first and second portions of the duodenum. This procedure enables identification of the site of bleeding and allows therapeutic attempts at stopping the bleeding. An estimated 10% to 20% of patients admitted with bleeding peptic ulcers, however, fail medical therapy and require emergency surgical intervention. Despite endoscopic advances, the mortality rate has remained stable at 5% to 10%. In fact, recent epidemiologic data suggest that the incidence and mortality rate of bleeding duodenal ulcers may be increasing in older women.[3] The ability to predict the risk for rebleeding is important to the endoscopist and the surgeon because it permits closer monitoring of high-risk patients and early involvement of the surgical team in their management. High recurrent bleeding rates have been associated with a spurting vessel, a visible arterial vessel in the ulcer bed, adherent clot, or a large ulcer bed. The Forrest classification was developed in an attempt to assess the risk for rebleeding based on endoscopic findings (Table 55–3).

In those who have recurrent bleeding, it has been shown that a second endoscopic attempt at control of bleeding will fail in 25% of patients, who will then require emergency surgery. This has stimulated some debate regarding the timing of surgery for a bleeding peptic ulcer and the role of a second attempt at endoscopic therapy. Randomized prospective studies have, however, shown no increase in mortality rate in patients who undergo a second therapeutic endoscopic procedure versus surgery after the first failed endoscopy. Therefore, most clinicians would encourage a second attempt at endoscopic control.[23]

Current indications for surgery for peptic ulcer hemorrhage include the following:

1. Hemodynamic instability despite vigorous resuscitation (transfusion of >3 units)
2. Failure of endoscopic techniques to arrest hemorrhage
3. Recurrent hemorrhage after initial stabilization (with up to two attempts at obtaining endoscopic hemostasis)
4. Shock associated with recurrent hemorrhage
5. Continued slow bleeding with a transfusion requirement exceeding 3 U/day

Secondary or relative indications include a rare blood type or difficult crossmatch, refusal of transfusion, shock on initial evaluation, advanced age, severe comorbid disease, and a bleeding chronic gastric ulcer. These criteria also apply to elderly patients, in whom prolonged resuscitation, large-volume transfusion, and periods of hypotension are poorly tolerated.

Surgery for Bleeding Duodenal Ulcer

The first priority during emergency surgery for a bleeding duodenal ulcer is control of the bleeding site. If esophagogastroduodenoscopy has failed to precisely identify the source of hemorrhage, pyloroduodenotomy may be necessary to inspect the duodenal bulb and gastric antrum. The gastroduodenal artery is the usual source of bleeding, and it should be controlled by placement of suture ligatures. Once the bleeding has been addressed, a definitive acid-reducing operation may be performed. With the identification of *H. pylori*, the utility of vagotomy has been questioned. The data, however, suggest that even in the era of *H. pylori* and our ability to eradicate it, truncal vagotomy should be performed in those with a bleeding duodenal ulcer. There are several reasons for this recommendation:

1. Only 40% to 70% of patients with a bleeding duodenal ulcers are positive for *H. pylori*.
2. *H. pylori* testing in the setting of acute bleeding is less reliable, with the CLO (*Campylobacter*-like organism) test having a false-negative rate of 18% versus 1% in those not actively bleeding.[24]
3. If an acid-reducing procedure is not performed, up to 50% of patients are at risk for recurrent bleeding.

Our inability to determine the *H. pylori* status in the case of acute bleeding and a lower prevalence of *H. pylori* infection for patients with bleeding reinforce the need to perform an acid-reducing operation at the time of initial surgery. In contrast to other situations, the argument for performing a less aggressive operation in the face of massive bleeding exposes the patient to a high rebleeding risk after surgery.

Because it is simple to open the pylorus in longitudinal fashion, truncal vagotomy with pyloroplasty is the

| Table 55–3 | The Forrest Classification for Endoscopic Findings and Rebleeding Risk |

Classification	Description	Rebleeding Risk
Grade Ia	Active, pulsatile bleeding	High
Grade Ib	Oozing, nonpulsatile bleeding	Low/Intermediate
Grade IIa	Nonbleeding visible vessel	High
Grade IIb	Adherent clot	Low/Intermediate
Grade IIc	Black dot	Low
Grade III	No signs of recent bleeding	Low

most frequently used operation for a bleeding duodenal ulcer.

The procedure starts with a midline laparotomy to enter the peritoneal cavity. A Kocher maneuver is then performed to mobilize the duodenum. This will give better exposure and relieves any tension on the subsequent suture line. Careful palpation reveals the firm, rubbery pylorus at the junction between the stomach and duodenum. The pyloric vein of Mayo is virtually always present on the anterior surface of the inferior pylorus. Two 3-0 silk traction sutures are placed astride the anterior pylorus and parallel to each other. While lifting up on the traction sutures, a longitudinal incision is made through the pyloric muscles and extended 2 to 3 cm proximally into stomach and distally into duodenum. The duodenal mucosa is inspected for any evidence of active bleeding, ulceration, or induration. If active bleeding is encountered, it is controlled by digital pressure, which in addition to controlling the bleeding, gives time for fluid resuscitation of the patient. The bleeding vessel is then ligated. This vessel is often the gastroduodenal artery, which at the level of the posterior duodenal wall has a three-vessel junction. It is important to suture-ligate the gastroduodenal artery superiorly and inferiorly, followed by ligation of the medial transverse pancreatic branches with a U-stitch (Fig. 55–14). Care should be taken to avoid injury to the common bile duct during suture placement. If no bleeding is encountered on opening the lumen, the mucosa should be carefully inspected for an ulcer. If identified, the ulcer base should be cleaned to help identify a visible vessel, which if seen should be ligated. In situations in which no active bleeding is seen, it is important to carry out a careful inspection of the mucosa to look for other potential bleeding ulcers, even if a nonbleeding ulcer is identified. This inspection can be done by manual palpation of the lumen with a finger. In cases in which preoperative endoscopy has failed to identify a specific location, it is reasonable to start with a duodenotomy, which can be extended proximally or distally to allow further exploration. On occasion, a second gastrostomy near the esophageal junction is needed to inspect the proximal part of the stomach.

After gaining control of the bleeding, a pyloroplasty is performed, most often a Heineke-Mikulicz pyloroplasty. The traction sutures initially placed are used as superior and inferior edges of the closure, with the longitudinal opening converted to a horizontal one. If the duodenum is soft, pliable, and minimally deformed, running closure of the inside layer is performed with absorbable suture in an inverting fashion. Either a baseball stitch or whip stitch (inside-out, outside-in) works well. It is imperative that tension be kept on the suture while closing this layer and that adequate purchase of the duodenal side be obtained. An outside Lembert layer of 4-0 silk suture in interrupted fashion completes the procedure. Care is needed to not turn in too much serosa in the Lembert layer because an obstruction could result; however, such obstruction rarely occurs. Some prefer single-layer closure because of the potential risk for obstruction associated with a two-layer closure. The single-layer closure (Weinberg variation) could be done as a single layer of

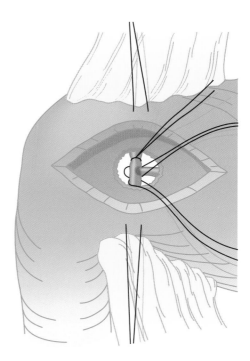

Figure 55–14. Technique of suture control of a bleeding duodenal ulcer. After making a longitudinal pyloric incision and identifying the bleeding vessel, figure-of-eight sutures are placed at the cephalic and caudal aspects of the ulcer deep enough to occlude the gastroduodenal artery. An additional U-stitch is placed to control small transverse pancreatic branches from the main vessel. (From Debas HT, Mulvihill SJ: Complications of peptic ulcer. In Zinner MJ, Schwartz SJ, Ellis H [eds]: Maingot's Abdominal Operations. Stamford, CT, Appleton & Lang, 1997.)

inverting 3-0 silk suture (Gambee stitch) (Fig. 55–15). The procedure is then completed by performing truncal vagotomy as described in Chapter 56.

In experienced hands, HSV may be the best therapy for a bleeding duodenal ulcer. Several reports have shown that even in the setting of acute bleeding, HSV can be performed safely with good long-term results.[25,26] However, because endoscopic hemostatic techniques have reduced the total number of surgical referrals and because many patients who do require surgery are bleeding so massively that they are unstable or have refractory hemorrhage after multiple attempts at endoscopic control, undertaking a procedure that takes longer to perform is not recommended unless the surgeon has significant experience with the operation. As a result, more traditional expedient operations with proven efficacy, such as truncal vagotomy with pyloroplasty, are recommended over HSV. A recent survey of surgeons in the United Kingdom, however, has shown that although they were more likely to perform a vagotomy for a bleeding ulcer than for a perforated duodenal ulcer, 40% of those surveyed would refrain from performing a vagotomy in the acute setting.[27] This highlights the issue of shrinking clinical experience with vagotomy and the reluctance of

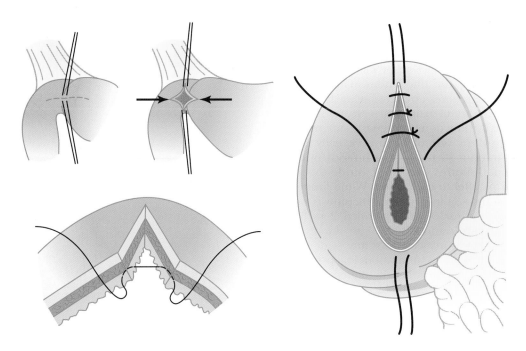

Figure 55–15.   Heineke-Mikulicz closure with a single-layer technique using the Gambee stitch. (From Schirmer BD, Kouretas PC: Bleeding duodenal ulcer. In Baker RJ, Fischer JE [eds]: Mastery of Surgery. Philadelphia, Lippincott, Williams & Wilkins, 2001.)

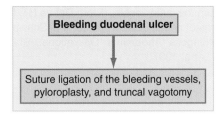

Figure 55–16. Recommended surgical procedures for bleeding duodenal ulcer.

many to perform it in an acute setting. Figure 55–16 summarizes the recommended surgical therapy for a bleeding duodenal ulcer.

Bleeding Gastric Ulcer

For bleeding gastric ulcers, distal gastrectomy with Billroth I or II reconstruction is preferred. This approach permits excision and histologic evaluation of the ulcer to rule out malignancy. In high-risk patients or those with ulcers that are high, excision of the ulcer and vagotomy plus pyloroplasty may be considered.

Perforation

Smoking and NSAIDs are important etiologic factors for ulcer perforation, and recent epidemiologic studies have documented an increasing rate of perforation, particularly in older women. The outcome of patients with a perforated ulcer depends on the following:

1. Delay from initial evaluation to treatment: recent data suggest increasing delay until surgical treatment, in part because of more extensive diagnostic work-up.
2. Site of perforation: gastric perforations are associated with a poorer prognosis.
3. Patient's age: elderly patients, who often have associated comorbid conditions, have a worse outcome.
4. Presence of hypotension at initial evaluation (systolic blood pressure <100 mm Hg).

Recent studies have shown that in carefully selected groups of patients, perforation can be treated conservatively with nasogastric decompression and antibiotics. Such treatment should, however, be used only if a water-soluble contrast study has confirmed that the ulcer is sealed with no extravasation of contrast into the peritoneal cavity. These patients should be monitored closely with regular physical examination and, if their abdominal examination or laboratory findings indicate progressive sepsis, undergo surgery. This approach is generally used for individuals who have had a perforated ulcer for 24 hours or longer, and are stable. It should be noted that although this approach is often used for elderly patients with comorbid conditions, studies have shown that the risk for failure of conservative treatment is highest in the elderly, and thus close observation of such patients is recommended. Because perforated gastric ulcers have a higher rate of reperforation and complications, conservative therapy in situations in which the source of the perforation is known to be gastric is not recommended.

Perforated Duodenal Ulcer

An acute perforation is estimated to occur in 2% to 10% of patients with a duodenal ulcer. Surgeons have traditionally performed either simple patch closure or truncal vagotomy with pyloroplasty (incorporating the perforation). The natural history of those treated by simple repair has been documented in a paper that followed the course of 122 such patients over a 25-year period. In total, 48% of the original study population required additional ulcer treatment in the form of prolonged medical therapy or further surgery.[28] Therefore, truncal vagotomy with pyloroplasty had been recommended as the minimal therapy required. A recent study reported the outcomes of 159 patients who were monitored more than 10 years after vagotomy and pyloroplasty for perforated duodenal ulcer.[29] Perioperative mortality was 5.5%, ulcers recurred in 8.8%, and postoperative digestive sequelae, notably diarrhea and dumping, developed in 16%. Nevertheless, the overall results were good to excellent in almost 90% of cases. HSV with patch closure does at least as well. Boey et al., in a prospective study of 101 patients randomized to simple closure, truncal vagotomy and pyloroplasty, or HSV, reported 39-month recurrence rates of 63.3%, 11.8%, and 3.8%, respectively. Operative time was significantly longer for HSV, but no deaths occurred in any of the groups. The study, however, excluded the elderly (>70 years) and patients with preoperative shock, which may account for the low mortality rates.[30] Another randomized study by the same group in which HSV was compared with simple closure documented recurrence rates of 10.6% and 36.6% (half requiring surgical intervention) at 3 years. Again, there was a sample bias in the group because unstable and elderly patients were excluded.[31] Another report of 107 patients with perforated pyloroduodenal ulcers documented minimal morbidity, low mortality, and excellent patient satisfaction for omental patching and HSV, with a recurrence rate of 3.7% for duodenal ulcer; the recurrence rate for pyloric and prepyloric ulcer was substantially higher at 16%.[32] Chronic pyloroduodenal scarring is considered a relative contraindication to the use of HSV in this setting because it may be associated with delayed gastric emptying after surgery.

With the identification of *H. pylori,* the ideal surgical approach has once again been questioned. A recent study has shown that 81% of patients with a perforated duodenal ulcer are *H. pylori* positive. In this study all patients underwent simple closure of the perforation. The *H. pylori*–positive patients were then randomized postoperatively to a 4-week course of PPIs alone versus *H. pylori* eradication therapy. The ulcer recurrence rate at 1 year was 5% in the *H. pylori*–eradicated group versus 38% in the PPI-treated group, as determined by repeat endoscopy. Notably, the 5% recurrence rate is equivalent to the recurrence rate in those who undergo a definitive antiulcer procedure.[33] These data have provided good evidence for the practice of simple closure of perforated duodenal ulcers in the acute setting. However, at the time of surgery, the *H. pylori* status of the patient is often unknown, and in the absence of a reliable intraoperative test, the merits of a definitive antisecretory procedure

have to be considered. This may be particularly important in patients with a previous history of peptic ulcer surgery, *H. pylori* eradication, or chronic ulcer symptoms despite the use of PPIs or in those taking NSAIDs in whom this therapy cannot be discontinued. In general, simple patch closure is appropriate for patients with the following:

1. Acute NSAID-related perforation (provided that use of the drugs can be discontinued postoperatively) and for patients who have never been treated for PUD and can be treated with PPIs and *H. pylori* eradication
2. Perforation in the setting of ongoing shock, delayed evaluation, considerable comorbid disease, or marked peritoneal contamination

Figure 55–17 summarizes the recommended approach to a perforated duodenal ulcer.

To perform the patch procedure, a midline laparotomy is carried out and the intra-abdominal organs inspected. The presence of bilious fluid in the peritoneal cavity suggests an upper gastrointestinal perforation. Once a duodenal perforation has been confirmed, pads are placed around the perforation to contain any further spillage, and 3-0 silk or PDS sutures are placed across the perforation. Usually, three to four sutures are needed. It is important to take bites of appropriate width (0.5 to 1 cm) to prevent the sutures from cutting through the inflamed duodenal tissue. To ensure bites that are full thickness, it is recommended that one pass the needle through the wall of the duodenum on one side of the ulcer, retrieve the needle through the perforation, and then pass it through the wall on the other side of the perforation (Fig. 55–18). These sutures should not be tied to approximate the ulcer; rather, the adjacent omentum should be mobilized on an intact vascular pedicle and brought up. Sutures are tied over this omental pedicle to secure the omentum in place. These sutures should not be tied too tightly to avoid strangulation of the omental patch (Fig. 55–19). Sewing the ulcer closed before placing the omental pedicle over the perforation is discouraged because it reduces surface contact of the omentum with the duodenal mucosa (Fig. 55–20).

After closure of the ulcer, irrigation of the peritoneal cavity with warm saline solution should be carried out. There is no evidence to suggest that the use of antibiotic or iodine solutions helps in any way. The abdomen is then closed in standard fashion. Drains are not needed and their use is discouraged.

There is a growing body of literature on laparoscopic suture patch repair, as well as laparoscopic sutureless techniques with fibrin glue to repair a perforated ulcer. These studies have demonstrated the feasibility of minimally invasive approaches. The first randomized study on this issue showed that laparoscopic suture and sutureless repair of perforated ulcers is equal to open repair of perforated ulcers in terms of hospital stay and time to resume normal diet, with less postoperative analgesia being required.[34] A subsequent randomized trial has documented a shorter operative time, shorter hospital stay, and fewer pulmonary complications with the laparoscopic approach.[35] Conversion rates for such laparoscopic procedures have been between 15% and 20%.

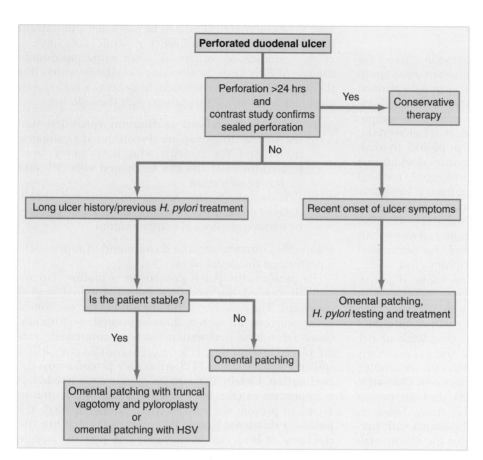

Figure 55–17. Treatment algorithm for surgical treatment of perforated duodenal ulcers. HSV, highly selective vagotomy.

Perforated Gastric Ulcer

A perforated gastric ulcer is associated with greater overall mortality that may range from 10% to 40% and increases significantly with age (>65 years).[36] There has been debate in cases of perforated type I and IV gastric ulcers over whether to perform partial gastrectomy or proceed with simple patching of the perforation. Partial gastrectomy is the preferred approach unless the patient is at unacceptably high risk because of advanced age, comorbid disease, intraoperative instability, or severe peritoneal soilage.[37] Even in this high-risk group who may initially be in shock, there is increasing evidence that definitive surgery can be tolerated as well as the simpler and quicker patching technique.[38,39] It is therefore recommended that a patient with a perforated type I gastric ulcer undergoes partial gastrectomy unless the patient is unstable with significant comorbid conditions. Biopsy and patch closure may be an appropriate approach for the treatment of a high type IV ulcer, where more extensive resection may lead to total gastrectomy in a critically ill patient. If closure techniques are to be used, patch closure is favored over simple suturing and closure of the ulcer, which has a reported mortality of greater than 60%.[40] Because the pathophysiology of such ulcers does not involve acid hypersecretion, an antacid procedure is not required. It is important to perform an adequate four-quadrant biopsy of ulcers that are not excised.

For type II ulcers the treatment algorithm should be similar to that for perforated duodenal ulcers because the pathophysiology of the disease is very similar. This means that the ulcers should be patched, the *H. pylori* status of the patient determined by intraoperative biopsy, and the patient treated appropriately. For such ulcers, it is important to obtain an intraoperative biopsy to rule out malignancy, which can be associated with these gastric ulcers. Similar to a perforated duodenal ulcer, an acid-reducing procedure is not required unless the patient has a history of recurrent ulcer disease and has been previously treated for *H. pylori*. In circumstances in which a definitive antiulcer procedure is deemed appropriate because of the chronicity of symptoms and lack of response to PPIs, HSV or truncal vagotomy and antrectomy should be considered.

Type III ulcers are thought to have a pathogenesis similar to that of duodenal ulcers; however, their treatment in the event of acute perforation deserves particular attention. Patch repair of such prepyloric ulcers is associated with a high incidence of gastric outlet obstruction,[40] and HSV has been shown to be associated with a high recurrence rate for these ulcers. Therefore, antrectomy and vagotomy may be the best surgical approach.

Figure 55–21 summarizes the proposed surgical approaches to a perforated gastric ulcer.

Gastric Outlet Obstruction

This problem accounts for 5% to 8% of ulcer-related complications and results in an estimated 2000

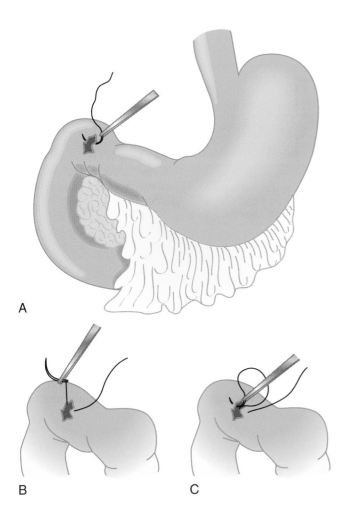

A

B   C

Figure 55–18. **A** to **C,** Perforated duodenal ulcers. Repair is begun by placing sutures through the full thickness of the bowel wall in two steps. This allows the use of smaller tapered needles and reduces the risk for inadvertent penetration of the posterior duodenal wall. (From Baker RJ: Perforated duodenal ulcer. In Baker RJ, Fischer JE [eds]: Mastery of Surgery. Philadelphia, Lippincott, Williams & Wilkins, 2001.)

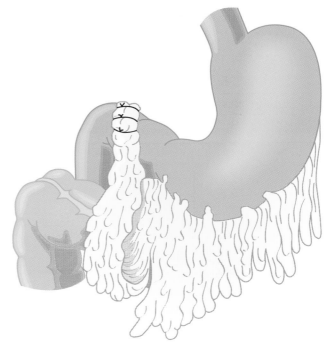

Figure 55–19. The omentum, which has been mobilized on a vascular pedicle, is secured in place with sutures tied loosely enough to prevent tissue strangulation. This technique allows effective closure of the perforation without narrowing the duodenal lumen. (From Baker RJ: Perforated duodenal ulcer. In Baker RJ, Fischer JE [eds]: Mastery of Surgery. Philadelphia, Lippincott, Williams & Wilkins, 2001.)

operations per year in the United States.[41] Patients with gastric outlet (pyloric) obstruction as a result of a duodenal ulcer typically have symptoms of gastric retention, including early satiety, bloating, indigestion, anorexia, nausea, vomiting, epigastric pain, and weight loss. They are frequently malnourished and dehydrated and have a metabolic alkalosis, factors that increase operative risk. Nevertheless, surgery is generally indicated if the obstruction fails to resolve despite 48 to 72 hours of adequate intravenous fluid replenishment, antisecretory therapy, and nasogastric tube decompression. In less acute settings, where the obstruction is not complete, balloon dilatation of the scarred pylorus has been attempted, with an unacceptably high recurrence rate over the short term and a morbidity rate of 0% to 6%. The most serious complication is perforation. If balloon dilatation is being attempted, it is important to rule out

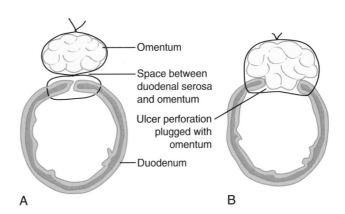

A   B

Figure 55–20. When the sutures are initially tied to approximate the edges of the ulcer and the omentum is placed above these knots **(A),** there is less intimate apposition of the duodenal serosa to the omentum. By performing the procedure as described, the omentum plugs the hole **(B)** and is closely applied to the serosa, thereby ensuring a watertight closure. (From Baker RJ: Perforated duodenal ulcer. In Baker RJ, Fischer JE [eds]: Mastery of Surgery. Philadelphia, Lippincott, Williams & Wilkins, 2001.)

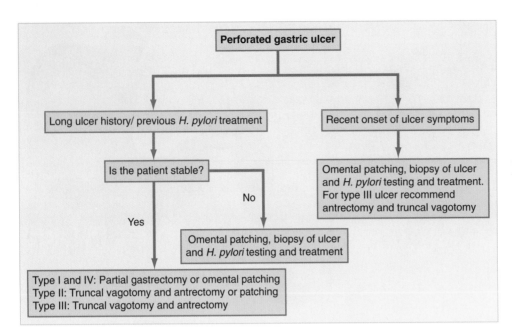

Figure 55–21. Recommended treatment algorithm for the surgical management of perforated gastric ulcers.

an underlying malignancy because cancer has been identified in more than 50% of patients who have gastric outlet obstruction.[24]

Truncal vagotomy and antrectomy is the ideal procedure for this condition. Placement of a feeding jejunostomy tube at the time of surgery is usually recommended, both because of preoperative malnutrition and because the chronic gastric outlet obstruction predisposes to delayed postoperative gastric emptying. The inflammation and scarring at the duodenal bulb may at times prevent safe performance of an antrectomy. In this setting, truncal vagotomy with drainage is the preferred approach. Again, in such a procedure in which the ulcer is not being excised, biopsy of the lesion to rule out an underlying malignancy is important.

Debate persists regarding the optimal drainage procedure. The Jaboulay side-to-side duodenoplasty has gained popularity as a result of its technical simplicity and because the anastomosis is performed in healthy tissue, distinct from the ulcer bed. In one report of 19 patients treated with this procedure combined with HSV, there was a high degree of patient satisfaction (100% modified Visick grade I or II), universal weight gain, and no operative mortality or ulcer recurrence at mean follow-up of 31 months.[42] However, these benefits have not been noted in all reports. One trial randomized 90 consecutive patients with gastric outlet obstruction secondary to duodenal ulcer to HSV with gastrojejunostomy, HSV with Jabouley duodenoplasty, or selective vagotomy with antrectomy. There were no differences in the postoperative course or reduction in gastric acid secretion; however, both HSV with gastrojejunostomy and selective vagotomy with antrectomy produced clinical results superior to those of HSV with Jaboulay pyloroplasty.[43]

As already mentioned, HSV with drainage has been used in the setting of obstructing ulcer. Although the need for pyloric reconstruction or bypass would theoretically negate several advantages of HSV over other options, maintenance of antropyloric innervation may preserve controlled gastric emptying and minimize bile reflux.[8]

With the identification of *H. pylori*, its role in the pathogenesis of gastric outlet obstruction has been evaluated. Studies have shown that the incidence of *H. pylori* infection in this population is low (33% to 57%).[41] In those infected with the organism, however, eradication therapy and balloon dilatation may result in long-term symptomatic relief and alleviate the need for surgery. In general, surgery should be the standard of therapy in this group (in particular, *H. pylori*–negative patients) until further studies define the role of conservative therapy in *H. pylori*–positive patients.

COMPLICATIONS OF ULCER OPERATIONS

Postgastrectomy Syndromes

After operations on the stomach, a variety of chronic undesirable sequelae may develop. Although some of these conditions are related more to vagotomy than to resection, they have been referred to collectively as postgastrectomy syndromes. Virtually all patients note a change in their digestive habits postoperatively, and about 20% are significantly affected. Most are able to adapt with time; lifelong symptoms develop in only 5%, and 1% are significantly debilitated by these syndromes. The following is a summary of the main issues with regard to postgastrectomy syndromes, and a more detailed discussion is provided in Chapter 59.

Early Satiety Early satiety may develop as a result of postsurgical atony, gastric stasis secondary to denervation, or the small gastric remnant related to resection. Symptoms consist of epigastric fullness with meals, often followed by emesis. Atony can be identified with a solid food–emptying test and may respond to prokinetic agents such as metoclopramide and erythromycin. If these measures fail, although there is some anecdotal evidence that gastric pacing may prove useful, completion gastrectomy is the procedure of choice for atony. The small gastric remnant syndrome will usually improve with small frequent feedings and time.

Postvagotomy Diarrhea After truncal vagotomy, postvagotomy diarrhea develops in approximately 30% of patients. Its pathogenesis is unclear, but it may be related to the rapid passage of unconjugated bile salts from the denervated biliary tree into the colon, where they stimulate secretion. Most cases are self-limited; oral cholestyramine, which binds bile salts, can be effective in persistent cases.

Dumping Syndrome Dumping syndrome is a constellation of postprandial symptoms that occurs in about 20% of patients after gastrectomy or vagotomy and drainage. Although the exact mechanism has eluded definition, it appears to be related to rapid emptying of hyperosmolar chyme, particularly carbohydrate, into the intestine. The symptoms may occur within 30 minutes of eating, referred to as *early dumping*, or 2 to 3 hours after the meal, referred to as *late dumping*. The symptoms vary in intensity, and the syndrome varies from a mild nuisance to disabling.

Early Dumping Rapid introduction of hyperosmolar chyme into the bowel lumen draws fluid into the intestine and probably releases one or more vasoactive hormones such as serotonin and vasoactive intestinal polypeptide. This is associated with epigastric distention, cramps, nausea, vomiting, dizziness, flushing, and palpitations. In most patients, the symptoms tend to resolve as they learn to avoid foods that aggravate the problem. Frequent small meals low in carbohydrate may eliminate the problem. In the most refractory cases, octreotide may be of benefit.

Late Dumping This condition is a reactive hypoglycemia that occurs 2 to 3 hours after the meal in response to excess insulin release. Symptoms of late dumping are relieved by the administration of sugar.

Alkaline Reflux Gastritis After operations that eliminate the pyloric sphincter, reflux of bile into the stomach is common. Alkaline reflux gastritis, a syndrome of persistent burning epigastric pain and chronic nausea that is aggravated by meals, develops in about 2% of patients. The diagnosis is one of exclusion, although endoscopy may reveal gastritis and a technetium biliary scan can demonstrate increased reflux of bile into the stomach. A variety of medical therapies have been reported, but none has proved particularly effective, although there is enthusiasm for the use of ursodeoxycholic acid (Actigall). In debilitating cases, conversion of the original drainage procedure to a Roux-en-Y anastomosis, in which bile is diverted 45 to 60 cm from the gastric remnant, has proved effective in selected patients.

Afferent and Efferent Loop Syndromes These syndromes develop after Billroth II reconstruction or gastroenterostomy. They are related to mechanical obstruction of the limbs by kinking, anastomotic narrowing, or adhesions. Afferent loop syndrome is typically associated with postprandial epigastric pain and nonbilious vomiting, which is then relieved by projectile bilious vomiting. Detection of a distended afferent loop on computed tomography is diagnostic. Conversion to a Roux-en-Y anastomosis is necessary to treat this problem. Several different surgical reconstructions have been proposed to help reduce the incidence of afferent loop syndrome after a Billroth II reconstruction, including the Braun variation of Billroth II and the uncut Roux-en-Y reconstruction.

Efferent loop syndrome is associated with epigastric pain, distention, and bilious vomiting; surgery to relieve the obstruction is the treatment of choice.

Roux Stasis Syndrome Roux stasis syndrome occurs after a Roux-en-Y reconstruction. It consists of chronic abdominal pain, nausea, and intermittent vomiting. The etiology of this syndrome is unknown, and treatment is often difficult. The uncut Roux-en-Y reconstruction previously mentioned has been shown to reduce the incidence of Roux stasis syndrome and may be a better reconstruction technique.[44]

Gastric Cancer In patients who have undergone gastric resection for gastric but not duodenal ulcers, an increased risk for gastric cancer has been documented. This risk is twofold at 15 years and increases with time after partial gastrectomy.[45] The risk for development of gastric cancer is higher after a Billroth II than after a Billroth I reconstruction.[11]

SUGGESTED READINGS

Ashley SW, Soper NJ: Gastric surgery. Probl Gen Surg 14:1, 1997.

Millat B, Fingerhut A, Borie F: Surgical treatment of complicated duodenal ulcers: Controlled trials. World J Surg 24:299, 2000.

Ohmann C, Imhof M, Roher HD: Trends in peptic ulcer bleeding and surgical treatment. World J Surg 24:284, 2000.

Sawyers JL, Richards WO: Selective vagotomy and pyloroplasty. In Baker RJ, Fischer JE (eds): Mastery of Surgery. Philadelphia, Lippincott, Williams & Wilkins, 2001.

Svanes C: Trends in perforated peptic ulcer: Incidence, etiology, treatment, and prognosis. World J Surg 24:277, 2000.

REFERENCES

1. Xu W, Hood HM, Burgess PA: The description of outcomes in Medicare patients hospitalized with peptic ulcer disease. Am J Gastroenterol 95:264, 2000.

2. Paimela H, Paimela L, Myllykangas-Luosujarvi R, et al: Current features of peptic ulcer disease in Finland: Incidence of surgery, hospital admissions and mortality for the disease during the past twenty-five years. Scand J Gastroenterol 37:399, 2002.

3. Higham J, Kang JY, Majeed A: Recent trends in admissions and mortality due to peptic ulcer in England: Increasing frequency of haemorrhage among older subjects. Gut 50:460, 2002.

4. Thors H, Svanes C, Thjodleifsson B: Trends in peptic ulcer morbidity and mortality in Iceland. J Clin Epidemiol 55:681, 2002.

5. Bardhan KD, Williamson M, Royston C, et al: Admission rates for peptic ulcer in the Trent region, UK, 1972-2000. Changing pattern, a changing disease? Dig Liver Dis 36:577, 2004.

6. Chan VM, Reznick RK, O'Rourke K, et al: Meta-analysis of highly selective vagotomy versus truncal vagotomy and pyloroplasty in the surgical treatment of uncomplicated duodenal ulcer. Can J Surg 37:457, 1994.

7. Jordan PH, Thornby J: Twenty years after parietal cell vagotomy or selective vagotomy antrectomy for treatment of duodenal ulcer. Final report. Ann Surg 220:283, 1994.

8. Donahue PE, Griffith C, Richter HM: A 50-year perspective upon selective gastric vagotomy. Am J Surg 172:9, 1996.

9. Taylor TV, Lythgoe JP, McFarland JB, et al: Anterior lesser curve seromyotomy and posterior truncal vagotomy versus truncal vagotomy and pyloroplasty in the treatment of chronic duodenal ulcer. Br J Surg 77:1007, 1990.

10. Oostvogel HJM, van Vroonhoven TJMV: Anterior lesser curve seromyotomy with posterior truncal vagotomy versus proximal gastric vagotomy. Br J Surg 75:121, 1988.

11. Tersmette AC, Offerhaus GJ, Tersmette KW, et al: Meta-analysis of the risk of gastric stump cancer: Detection of high risk patient subsets for stomach cancer after remote partial gastrectomy for benign conditions. Cancer Res 50:6486, 1990.

12. Vogel SB, Drane WE, Woodward ER: Clinical and radionuclide evaluation of bile diversion by Braun enteroenterostomy: Prevention and treatment of alkaline reflux gastritis. An alternative to Roux-en-Y diversion. Ann Surg 219:458, 1994.

13. Hoffmann J, Jensen HE, Christiansen J, et al: Prospective controlled vagotomy trial for duodenal ulcer. Results after 11-15 years. Ann Surg 209:40, 1989.

14. Espat NJ, Ong ES, Helton WS, et al: 1990-2001 US general surgery chief resident gastric surgery operative experience: Analysis of paradigm shift. J Gastrointest Surg 8:471, 2004.

15. Dubois F: New surgical strategy for gastroduodenal ulcer: Laparoscopic approach. World J Surg 24:270, 2000.

16. Croce E, Olmi S, Russo R, et al: Laparoscopic treatment of peptic ulcers. A review after 6 years experience with Hill-Barker's procedure. Hepatogastroenterology 46:924, 1999.

17. Duthie HL, Moore TH, Bardsley D, et al: Surgical treatment of gastric ulcers. Controlled comparison of Billroth-I gastrectomy and vagotomy and pyloroplasty. Br J Surg 57:784, 1970.

18. McDonald MP, Broughan TA, Hermann RE, et al: Operations for gastric ulcer: A long-term study. Am Surg 62:673, 1996.

19. Jordan PH: Type I gastric ulcer treated by parietal cell vagotomy and mucosal ulcerectomy. J Am Coll Surg 182:388, 1996.

20. Emas S, Grupcev G, Eriksson B: Ten-year follow-up of a prospective, randomized trial of selective proximal vagotomy with ulcer excision and partial gastrectomy with gastroduodenostomy for treating corporeal gastric ulcer. Am J Surg 167:596, 1994.

21. Lewis A, Qvist G: Operative treatment of high gastric ulcer with special reference to Pauchet's method. Br J Surg 59:1, 1972.

22. Csendes A, Braghetto I, Calvo F, et al: Surgical treatment of high gastric ulcer. Am J Surg 149:765, 1985.

23. Lau JY, Sung JJY, Lam Y, et al: Endoscopic retreatment compared with surgery in patients with recurrent bleeding after initial endoscopic control of bleeding ulcers. N Engl J Med 340:751, 1999.

24. Behrman SW: Management of complicated peptic ulcer disease. Arch Surg 140:201, 2005.

25. Miedema BW, Torres PR, Farnell MB, et al: Proximal gastric vagotomy in the emergency treatment of bleeding duodenal ulcers. Am J Surg 161:64, 1991.

26. Hoffmann J, Devantier A, Koelle T, et al: Parietal cell vagotomy as an emergency procedure for bleeding peptic ulcer. Ann Surg 206:583, 1987.

27. Gilliam AD, Speake WJ, Lobo DN, et al: Current practice of emergency vagotomy and *Helicobacter pylori* eradication for complicated peptic ulcer in the United Kingdom. Br J Surg 90:88, 2003.

28. Griffin GE, Organ CH: The natural history of the perforated duodenal ulcer treated by suture plication. Ann Surg 183:382, 1976.

29. Robles R, Parrilla P, Lujan JA, et al: Long-term follow-up of bilateral truncal vagotomy and pyloroplasty for perforated duodenal ulcer. Br J Surg 82:665, 1995.

30. Boey J, Lee NW, Koo J, et al: Immediate definitive surgery for perforated duodenal ulcers: A prospective controlled trial. Ann Surg 196:338, 1982.

31. Boey J, Branicki FJ, Alagaratnam TT, et al: Proximal gastric vagotomy. The preferred operation for perforations in acute duodenal ulcer. Ann Surg 208:169, 1988.

32. Jordan PH, Thornby J: Perforated pyloroduodenal ulcers. Long-term results with omental patch closure and parietal cell vagotomy. Ann Surg 221:479, 1995.

33. Ng EK, Lam YH, Sung JJ, et al: Eradication of *Helicobacter pylori* prevents recurrence of ulcer after simple closure of duodenal ulcer perforation: Randomized controlled trial. Ann Surg 231:153, 2000.

34. Lau WY, Leung KL, Kwong KH, et al: A randomized study comparing laparoscopic versus open repair of perforated peptic ulcer using suture or sutureless technique. Ann Surg 224:131, 1996.

35. Siu WT, Chau CH, Law BK, et al: Routine use of laparoscopic repair for perforated peptic ulcer. Br J Surg 91:481, 2004.

36. Hewitt PM, Krige J, Bornman PC: Perforated gastric ulcers: Resection compared with simple closure. Am Surg 59:669, 1993.

37. McGee GS, Sawyers JL: Perforated gastric ulcers. A plea for management by primary gastric resection. Arch Surg 122:555, 1987.

38. Hodnett RM, Gonzalez F, Lee WC, et al: The need for definitive therapy in the management of perforated gastric ulcers. Review of 202 cases. Ann Surg 209:36, 1989.

39. Di Quinzio C, Phang PT: Surgical management of perforated benign gastric ulcer in high-risk patients. Can J Surg 35:94, 1992.

40. Turner WW, Thompson WM, Thal ER: Perforated gastric ulcers. A plea for management by simple closures. Arch Surg 123:960, 1988.

41. Gibson JB, Behrman SW, Fabian TC, et al: Gastric outlet obstruction resulting from peptic ulcer disease requiring surgical intervention is infrequently associated with *Helicobacter pylori* infection. J Am Coll Surg 191:32, 2000.

42. Dittrich K, Blauensteiner W, Schrutka-Kolbl C, et al: Highly selective vagotomy plus Jaboulay: A possible alternative in patients with benign stenosis secondary to duodenal ulceration. J Am Coll Surg 180:654, 1995.

43. Csendes A, Maluenda F, Braghetto I, et al: Prospective randomized study comparing three surgical techniques for the treatment of gastric outlet obstruction secondary to duodenal ulcer. Am J Surg 166:45, 1993.

44. Noh SM: Improvement of the Roux limb function using a new type of "uncut Roux" limb. Am J Surg 180:37, 2000.

45. Hansson LE: Risk of stomach cancer in patients with peptic ulcer disease. World J Surg 24:315, 2000.

56

Vagotomy and Drainage

Timothy J. Broderick · Jeffrey B. Matthews

VAGOTOMY AND DRAINAGE IN THE MODERN ERA

Recognition of the roles that *Helicobacter pylori* and nonsteroidal anti-inflammatory drugs (NSAIDs) play in peptic ulcer disease has revolutionized the care of patients who suffer from gastroduodenal ulcer. Research over the last decade confirmed that *H. pylori* infection and NSAID use are highly associated with peptic ulcer disease.[1-4] Recent data suggest that less than 1% of all duodenal ulcers and 4% of all gastric ulcers are *not* associated with either *H. pylori* infection or NSAID use.[5] Medical therapy has become significantly more effective with targeted treatment of *H. pylori,* improved antisecretory medications (histamine H_2 receptor antagonists and, subsequently, proton pump inhibitors), and the introduction of NSAIDs that have less effect on mucosal integrity. Endoscopic diagnosis and therapy have also improved in the past decade.

Classically, complications of peptic ulcer disease requiring surgery included intractability, obstruction, perforation, and hemorrhage. With more effective medical therapy, intractable peptic ulcer and peptic gastric outlet obstruction have become an uncommon indication for elective surgery,[6-9] but perforated or bleeding peptic ulcers have remained a relatively common indication for urgent surgery.[6-8] Recent data confirm that surgical treatment of peptic ulcer disease has evolved from elective surgery for medically refractory ulcer disease to urgent surgery for the treatment of perforation or hemorrhage.[6-8,10]

Although *H. pylori* eradication has significantly decreased the need for elective surgery, it has also changed the selection of which procedures are commonly performed in the treatment of ulcer complications. Local procedures such as suture duodenorrhaphy and gastrorrhaphy were used in 25% of operations for peptic ulcer disease in 1987 and in 90% of such operations in 1999 in Finland.[7,8] Additional studies from the United Kingdom demonstrated that most surgeons in the United Kingdom no longer perform vagotomy for peptic ulcer complications.[11,12] A recent study from the United States suggests that surgical treatment of peptic ulcer disease has similarly evolved.[13] The indication for and selection of operations for peptic ulcer disease have evolved, and the majority of surgeons now choose the simplest and quickest operation that will address the ulcer complication while minimizing postoperative gastrointestinal side effects. The decrease in ulcer recurrence provided by definitive acid reduction surgery has been replaced by *H. pylori* eradication, tailored NSAID therapy, and proton pump inhibitor therapy.[8,11,12,14]

Traditional operations such as vagotomy and drainage remain effective in addressing complications of peptic ulcer disease. However, modern medical therapy that effectively treats the underlying ulcer diathesis and the occasional patient who is crippled by the unpleasant digestive side effects of vagotomy and drainage argue for limited use of this procedure in modern treatment of peptic ulcer. The historical, anatomic, and physiologic basis for the recommendation of limited application of vagotomy and drainage in the treatment of select patients suffering from complications of peptic ulcer is discussed in the remainder of this chapter. Additional investigation is needed to determine the optimal combination of medical, endoscopic, and surgical therapy in the treatment of peptic ulcer disease in the modern era.

PATHOGENESIS OF PEPTIC ULCER DISEASE

Surgical treatment of peptic ulcer has been based on the assumed central role of acid and pepsin in its pathogenesis. The notion of autodigestion of the stomach as the cause of ulceration dates back at least as far as John Hunter in 1772.[15] The epidemiologic evidence supporting a role for acid and pepsin in the pathogenesis of duodenal ulcer is abundant. Elevated basal, nocturnal, induced, and maximal levels of gastric acid output have been demonstrated in duodenal ulcer patients in comparison to the normal population,[16,17] and this increased capacity to secrete HCl has been correlated with increased parietal cell mass.[18] The oxyntic cells of duodenal ulcer patients appear to be more sensitive to stimulation because the dose of pentagastrin necessary to induce a maximal secretory response is reduced in ulcer patients as compared with controls.[19]

Consequently, the development of surgical procedures for the treatment of duodenal ulcer had its foundation in the reduction of acid-peptic aggression. The works of Pavlov, Brodie, Jabouley, and Bircher in identifying the vagus as the anatomic effector of the cephalic phase of acid secretion provided the foundation for surgical vagotomy in the treatment of ulcer disease. Dragstedt and Edkins established that the gastric phase of acid secretion is derived from the gastrin-producing antrum, and this concept supported the use of distal gastrectomy to achieve a greater reduction in secretory capacity. The importance of acid and pepsin in mucosal injury is illustrated convincingly by the therapeutic efficacy of antacids, H_2 receptor antagonists, and proton pump inhibitors and supports the use of vagotomy and other forms of acid reduction surgery in surgical therapy.

Impaired mucosal defense mechanisms may also contribute to ulcerogenesis. Normal mucosal defense systems against acid-peptic aggression are dynamic, multifactorial, and multilayered. Pre-epithelial factors include the intrinsic surface hydrophobicity of mucosal surfaces and the physiochemical ability of mucus to retard acid diffusion. The epithelial cell itself confers a degree of resistance against the harmful effects of luminal acid by secreting mucus and bicarbonate ions and precisely regulating its intracellular pH. Moreover, the apical membrane and intracellular junctions have limited permeability to protons. Subepithelial defenses include bicarbonate production, which balances parietal cell proton secretion and provides a rich source of neutralizing base to the surface epithelium. Furthermore, rapid epithelial restitution allows repair of the superficial damage incurred from daily chemical and physical surface trauma.

The pathogenesis of chronic gastric ulceration is even less well understood than duodenal ulcer disease, but "impaired mucosal defenses" are often cited as an etiologic factor,[20-22] although this notion is rather vague and hence unhelpful. Gastric ulcer affects older patients without a sex predilection and occurs in the setting of atrophic gastritis. It is associated with normal or decreased acid secretory capacity and pepsin levels, and this epidemiologic factor has led some to suggest that gastric ulcer represents a fundamentally different disease process. Despite this concept, surgical procedures for the treatment of gastric ulcer to a large degree resemble procedures used for duodenal ulcer to reduce acid-peptic aggression. Yet in the absence of a coherent theory of gastric ulcerogenesis, it is difficult to account for their efficacy. It has been reasoned that the gastric mucosa of patients in whom ulcers develop in the setting of normal or decreased secretion must have inherently increased sensitivity to autodigestion. This concept has provided justification for distal gastrectomy with the removal of susceptible mucosa in the surgical treatment of gastric ulceration.

The paradigm for modern medical therapy has tended to shift away from combating acid-peptic aggression toward enhancing mucosal defenses. Maintenance of adequate gastroduodenal blood flows appears to be important in preventing mucosal damage in experimental injury,[23] and new data suggest a possible therapeutic role for growth factors and angiogenesis factors in accelerating the reparative processes crucial for ulcer healing. Medical efforts to bolster defenses by using so-called cytoprotective agents have met with mixed results. For example, synthetic prostaglandin analogues, which enhance mucosal self-protective mechanisms at a number of levels (e.g., production of mucus, bicarbonate secretion, and mucosal blood flow[24]), have been shown to prevent or reverse mucosal injury associated with NSAID use but have been effective in duodenal ulcer disease only when given at antisecretory doses. Altered gastrointestinal motility has been implicated in ulcer genesis in that rapid emptying of acidic gastric contents has been hypothesized to overwhelm duodenal neutralization capacity[25] and duodenogastric reflux of bile salts is thought to promote mucosal injury.[26]

No discovery has so profoundly altered the fundamental concepts of ulcerogenesis and dramatically altered approaches to therapy as the isolation of *H. pylori* by Warren and Marshall in 1983.[27] A causal relationship between *H. pylori* infection and chronic gastritis is well established,[28] but the mechanistic basis for the association of *H. pylori* infection with duodenal ulcer disease has proved more difficult to elucidate. In some cohorts, greater than 95% of patients with duodenal ulcer and 75% with gastric ulcer harbor *H. pylori*.[29,30] Duodenal ulcers develop far more frequently in the setting of established infection than they do de novo,[31,32] and eradication of the pathogen markedly reduces the ulcer recurrence rate, in some series from 60% to less than 15%.[33-35] Furthermore, a modest acceleration in ulcer healing has been observed when *H. pylori* treatment is combined with standard antisecretory therapy.[28] Although much of the evidence suggesting a pathogenic role for *H. pylori* is circumstantial, it is also quite compelling. A recent National Institutes of Health consensus conference concluded that ulcer patients with demonstrated infection should be treated with antisecretory drugs and adjuvant antimicrobial agents, even in the setting of NSAID-induced ulceration.[28] It must be noted that only a small proportion of patients transition from antral gastritis to the development of gastric or duodenal ulceration and that infection or colonization is frequently asymptomatic.[36] Furthermore, primary healing of ulcers in the setting of active *H. pylori* infection is achieved in a majority of patients with drug regimens that do not include antimicrobials.

VAGAL ANATOMY

The vagus nerve originates in the medulla oblongata, and most of its fibers are involved in forming the parasympathetic division of the autonomic nervous system. The vagus nerve is the longest of the cranial nerves, and it has an extended distribution with branches

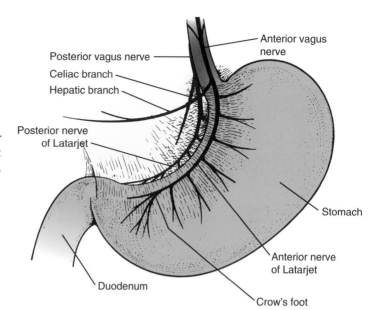

Figure 56–1. Anatomy of the vagus nerve on the lower part of the esophagus and stomach. (From Lawrence PF: Essentials of General Surgery. Philadelphia, Lippincott, Williams, & Wilkins, 2000.)

to the cervical, thoracic, and abdominal regions. Multiple branches extend to both thoracic (esophagus, heart, lungs, and bronchi) and abdominal (stomach, gallbladder, small intestine, colon, and other viscera) structures. After leaving the plexus surrounding the hilum of the lung, the vagal fibers reunite in two large lateral bundles on the left and right sides of the esophagus.

A clockwise rotation of the nerves as they course inferiorly results in the left vagus nerve appearing anteriorly and the right appearing posteriorly as the trunks enter the abdominal cavity. Gastric branches run from both the anterior and posterior trunks as they course parallel and superior to the lesser curvature of the stomach and finally extend to the pylorus (Fig. 56–1). Additional branches given off in the abdomen include hepatic branches from the anterior vagus and celiac branches from the posterior vagus. There may be substantial variation in vagus nerve distribution around the esophagus as the trunks pass beyond the diaphragm into the abdomen (Fig. 56–2). Although the great majority of individuals (80%) have a single large anterior and posterior trunk, other variations include multiple branches, fusing of branches, tangential branches, and plexiform branches. Awareness of these variations should result in a careful circumferential search of the mobilized esophagus for any additional branches after presumed complete truncal vagotomy.

VAGAL PHYSIOLOGY

The pioneering work of Pavlov, Brodie, and Latarjet elucidated the role of the vagus nerve in gastric acid secretion. The vagus nerves provide somatic and visceral afferent fibers that innervate the mucosa of the stomach and play a major role in the cephalic phase of gastric acid secretion by releasing acetylcholine. Release of acetylcholine stimulates acid secretion via a specific receptor on the parietal cell. Vagotomy diminishes direct cholin-

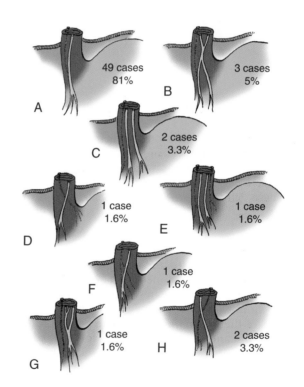

Figure 56–2. Illustrations of the high degree of variability in vagus nerve distribution along the lower part of the esophagus. (From Dragstedt LR, Fournier HJ, Woodward ER, et al: Transabdominal gastric vagotomy. A study of the anatomy of the vagus nerves at the lower portion of the esophagus. Surg Gynecol Obstet [now J Am Coll Surg] 85:461, 1947.)

ergic stimulation of the parietal cell and eliminates vagally mediated release of gastrin.[37] The parietal cell becomes generally less responsive to gastrin stimulation.[19,38,39] As a result, basal acid secretion is reduced by up to 85% and stimulated secretion by 50%.[40] Vagotomy also reduces pepsin secretion by the chief cell.[41]

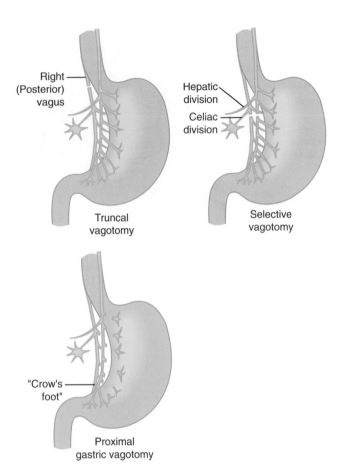

Figure 56–3. Schematic representation of the three standard forms of vagotomy. (From Sleisenger MH, Fordtran JS: Operations for peptic ulcer disease and early postoperative complications. In Sleisenger MH, Fordtran JS: Gastrointestinal Disease, 5th ed. Philadelphia, WB Saunders, 1993.)

The distal portions of the anterior and posterior trunks send branches to the antrum and pylorus that serve primarily a motor function. The celiac branch of the posterior vagus stimulates small intestinal motility. Gastric motility is affected by the antral and pyloric branches of the vagus, which stimulate peristaltic activity of the antrum and relaxation of the pylorus; in addition, the vagus stimulates receptive relaxation of the fundus, which results in accommodating liquid intake without a corresponding increase in pressure. The impaired gastric emptying seen after truncal vagotomy reflects not only impaired relaxation of the pyloric sphincter[42] but also disturbances in antral grinding and propulsive function,[43] as well as loss of fundic receptive relaxation.[44]

VAGOTOMY

Vagotomy is defined as transection of the vagus nerve or its branches, thus interrupting sensory, secretory, and motor impulses to the stomach and other gastrointestinal organs. The most commonly used vagotomies have been truncal, selective, and proximal gastric vagotomy. The various types of vagotomies are illustrated in Figure 56–3.

Dragstedt and Owens introduced transthoracic truncal vagotomy as treatment of duodenal ulcer in 1943.[45] Although two main vagal trunks in the chest make transthoracic vagotomy easy to perform, the postoperative gastric retention and ulceration that occurred in approximately a third of patients necessitated a transabdominal approach to add a concomitant procedure for improvement of gastric drainage.[46] In modern practice, transthoracic vagotomy may be performed thoracoscopically, but this approach is generally reserved for rare refractory cases of recurrent ulceration in which incomplete previous vagotomy has been demonstrated.

Transabdominal truncal vagotomy requires division of the two main vagal trunks, as well as division of the multiple small vagal branches that are often present at the distal esophageal level. The procedure is begun with a high midline incision and division of the triangular ligament of the left lateral hepatic segment. The hiatus is exposed and the nasogastric tube is palpated within the abdominal esophagus. The peritoneum overlying the distal esophagus is incised, and the index finger is used to begin gentle blunt dissection around the esophagus until it meets the thumb on the other side. A Penrose drain is then placed around the distal esophagus for anterior and inferior retraction. The distal end of the esophagus is dissected free from surrounding connective tissue to delineate the anterior (left) and posterior (right) vagi. Sharp dissection is used to free the vagal trunks, and a 3-cm segment of the nerves is excised. Some surgeons recommend placement of metal clips to mark the superior and inferior vagal remnants, as well as confirmation of nerve division via pathologic evaluation. The posterior (right) vagus is more difficult to find, and the surgeon must be particularly attentive in this dissection. A careful search of the distal esophagus excludes any additional branches, which must be resected if encountered. It must be emphasized that multiple small branches of both the anterior and posterior trunks are generally found at this level; if only the main anterior and posterior trunks are severed, the vagotomy will almost certainly be incomplete. In cases of recurrent ulcer after vagotomy, histologic review of the number of vagal nerve specimens from the original procedure is advisable.

Truncal vagotomy sacrifices the vagal innervation of not only the entire stomach but also the hepatobiliary system, pancreas, small intestine, and proximal part of the colon. A number of the adverse sequelae of ulcer operations have been blamed on vagotomy, particularly diarrhea and cholelithiasis.[47] Truncal vagotomy cures the majority of patients of their duodenal ulcer diathesis but does not entirely eliminate the problem of recurrent ulceration. Moreover, to obviate the problem of postoperative gastric retention, the pyloric sphincter must be bypassed (gastroduodenostomy or gastrojejunostomy), destroyed (pyloroplasty), or resected (antrectomy). The evolution, description, and indications for the use of "drainage" procedures are discussed in detail in a subsequent section.

In an effort to decrease the incidence of these postoperative side effects, selective vagotomy (with preservation of the hepatic and celiac divisions of the anterior and posterior vagus nerves) was introduced in 1948.[48,49] In selective gastric vagotomy, the anterior and posterior nerves of Latarjet are divided distal to the branching of the hepatic and celiac divisions. This procedure denervates the antropyloric region of the stomach, and gastric reservoir function and gastric emptying are impaired to the same extent as with truncal vagotomy. In a comparison of truncal and selective vagotomy, controlled studies have demonstrated a similar incidence of postoperative diarrhea,[50,51] postoperative dumping symptoms,[52] and recurrent ulceration with the use of selective or truncal vagotomy. Because selective gastric vagotomy offers little advantage over truncal vagotomy and is technically more difficult to perform, there remain few advocates of this procedure. Selective vagotomy will not be discussed further in this chapter.

Proximal gastric vagotomy has been called by a variety of names: highly selective vagotomy, superselective vagotomy, and parietal cell vagotomy. We prefer proximal gastric vagotomy and will use that term throughout the remainder of this chapter. Based on the anatomic studies of Griffith and Harkins,[53] proximal gastric vagotomy was introduced in the late 1960s by groups from Great Britain, Germany, and Scandinavia[54-56] as a method of vagotomy that limits the field of denervation to the fundus of the stomach and preserves vagal innervation of the antrum and pylorus. By preserving the antropyloric motor apparatus, proximal gastric vagotomy avoids the need for concomitant drainage or resection. For the most part, the details of the technique of proximal gastric vagotomy are well established. The nerves of Latarjet course along the lesser curvature of the stomach within the anterior and posterior leaves of the gastrohepatic (lesser) omentum. Starting from the incisura angularis, these fibers are divided systematically at their attachment to the stomach wall. The dissection is carried proximally to the gastroesophageal junction, and the distal 4 to 7 cm of esophagus is meticulously cleared of all vagal fibers. Small branches of the vagus nerve extend to the gastric cardia in this region and are easily overlooked.[57] The distal antral branches of the nerves of Latarjet (the "crow's foot"), as well as the hepatic and celiac divisions of the main vagal trunks, are preserved, and as a result, antropyloroduodenal innervation remains intact and gastric stasis and biliary reflux are minimized. To minimize the risk for the unusual, but life-threatening complication of lesser curvature necrosis, the lesser curvature should be imbricated.

Anterior lesser curve seromyotomy along with posterior truncal vagotomy was introduced by Taylor et al.[58] as a means of decreasing the technical difficulty of proximal gastric vagotomy. In this procedure, a seromyotomy along the anterior aspect of the lesser curve divides the branches of the anterior nerve of Latarjet that course through the superficial seromuscular layer of the stomach before penetrating the gastric wall to innervate the parietal cell mass. Posterior truncal vagotomy is performed to denervate the entire posterior gastric wall. Despite such denervation, normal antral motility seems to be preserved[59] because neural impulses appear to be adequately transmitted from the distal antral branches of the anterior branch of the nerve of Latarjet to the pos-

terior wall via intramural arcs.[60] There does not appear to be an increased incidence of postoperative diarrhea and dumping symptoms after this procedure despite the loss of vagal innervation to the pancreas and proximal portion of the small bowel,[61,62] again attesting to the central role that emptying procedures appear to play in the development of diarrhea.

Minimally invasive versions of vagotomy have been reported in recent years and include truncal vagotomy and pyloric stretch, truncal vagotomy and pyloromyotomy, posterior truncal vagotomy and anterior seromyotomy, and posterior truncal vagotomy with anterior highly selective vagotomy. Enthusiasm for these approaches should continue to be tempered with skepticism. Laparoscopic proximal gastric vagotomy has met with some promising results, although is unlikely to find wide application because of its technical demands.[63] The minimally invasive version of the Taylor procedure may prove to be a better alternative. Anecdotal results with this approach have been reported,[63] but until long-term follow-up becomes available, the role of minimally invasive vagotomy in the treatment of duodenal ulcer disease remains to be established. As previously mentioned, thoracoscopic truncal vagotomy has been reported[65] and may be useful in the setting of recurrent ulceration secondary to incomplete truncal vagotomy.

DRAINAGE PROCEDURES

In Dragstedt's initial series of truncal vagotomy for the treatment of duodenal ulcer disease, nearly a third of his patients experienced postoperative nausea, vomiting, and distention. As described earlier, further investigations revealed that truncal vagotomy denervated the antrum and pylorus and thereby resulted in a functional gastric outlet obstruction. Gastrojejunostomy was the drainage procedure originally explored but was later supplanted by pyloroplasty[66] and then by antrectomy.[67]

Gastrojejunostomy remains a useful and effective option for providing gastric drainage in the setting of an extensive scarred or acutely inflamed pylorus, particularly in patients with obstruction. First performed in 1881, gastrojejunostomy was originally plagued by two problems: marginal ulcers and vomiting. The two problems were subsequently overcome with the addition of vagotomy and construction of a shorter afferent jejunal limb. Gastrojejunostomy is currently most commonly performed for the treatment of benign and malignant duodenal obstruction. In peptic ulcer disease, gastrojejunostomy is performed for duodenal obstruction when the duodenal bulb is so scarred, inflamed, and edematous that pyloroplasty would not be safe or would be excessively technically demanding. A vagotomy should be performed when using gastrojejunostomy as a drainage procedure for the treatment of peptic ulcer disease. Obstruction as a result of pancreatic cancer is another common indication for palliative gastrojejunostomy. In many cases, the pancreatic cancer patient is elderly, secretes little hydrochloric acid, and does not require a vagotomy to accompany the bypass.

Gastrojejunostomy begins with taking down the greater omentum of the transverse colon to open the lesser sac and access the posterior aspect of the stomach. A site in the distal part of the stomach that is posterior and close to the greater curve is selected for the anastomosis to ensure dependent drainage of the stomach. A decision is then made with regard to whether the anastomosis will be antecolic or retrocolic. In the setting of peptic obstruction, many surgeons perform the anastomosis in a retrocolic manner. The antecolic approach is preferred when bypassing a malignant obstruction to avoid possible invasion of the more posterior retrocolic limb. A site approximately 15 to 20 cm from the ligament of Treitz is selected on the jejunum, a generous window is made in the mesocolon, and the stomach is pushed through the window until it lies next to the selected jejunal site (Fig. 56–4A).

The afferent limb of the proximal jejunum at the site should be attached to the lesser curve of the distal stomach. A posterior row of interrupted silk sutures is then placed to attach the serosa of the jejunum to the serosa of the stomach. A gastrotomy and enterotomy of equal size (4 to 5 cm) are then made 5 to 6 cm lateral to the Lembert layer. Running absorbable suture is used to close the inside layer while making certain that full-thickness tissue bites are procured. A final layer of interrupted Lembert silk sutures completes the anterior outside layer (see Fig. 56–4B). So that no torsion occurs, it is usually wise to fix the jejunal limb in one additional place to either the stomach or the liver capsule with a single suture. The defect in the mesocolon is then closed with absorbable suture to obviate internal hernia. A stapled anastomosis may also be performed, but it is unwise to use the stapler in extremely edematous or scarred tissue.

Pyloroplasty is used for approximately 90% of all drainage procedures. Pyloroplasty is the most popular drainage procedure for peptic ulcer disease because it is simple to perform and is associated with less bile reflux than gastrojejunostomy is. A number of methods for performing pyloroplasty have been described, the sheer variety attesting to a general unspoken dissatisfaction with the procedure.[68] The Heineke-Mikulicz pyloroplasty is the most widely practiced,[69] although no firm data support its superiority over other methods.

Heineke-Mikulicz Pyloroplasty

This procedure was described independently by two surgeons, Heineke and Mikulicz, in 1888, years before it found routine application as the most commonly performed drainage procedure. The technique is popular because it is technically straightforward, applicable to many clinical ulcer scenarios, and associated with few complications if performed correctly. The procedure may be performed with a single- or a double-layer closure, with the latter being performed more commonly. Careful palpation reveals the firm, rubbery pylorus at the junction between the stomach and duodenum. The pyloric vein of Mayo is virtually always present on the anterior surface of the inferior pylorus. If helpful, a Kocher maneuver to mobilize the duodenum

may be performed, but it is usually not necessary. Two silk traction sutures are placed astride the anterior pylorus and parallel to each other. While lifting up on the traction sutures, a longitudinal incision is made through the pyloric muscles and extended 2 to 3 cm proximally into the stomach and distally into the duodenum (Fig. 56–5, part 1). With the incision open, careful palpation with the index finger in the lumen of the stomach and duodenum rules out obstruction, tumor, active bleeding, or additional ulcers.

After careful inspection, the inside layer of the closure is initiated by selecting the midpoint of the longitudinal incision and pulling it laterally to convert the longitudinal opening into a horizontal one (thus opening up the pyloric muscle). If the duodenum is soft, pliable, and minimally deformed, a running closure of the inside layer is begun with absorbable suture in an inverting fashion (see Fig. 56–5, part 2). An outside layer of Lembert silk sutures in an interrupted fashion completes the procedure (see Fig. 56–5, part 3). Caution must be exercised to not turn in too much serosa while placing the Lembert layer to avoid the rare complication of obstruction. With scarring, edema, or deformation of the pylorus and duodenal bulb, the running technique on the inside layer described earlier may not be possible. When these conditions are present, an interrupted, simple layer of absorbable suture may be placed while making certain that adequate purchase of both the stomach and duodenum is obtained. A final, interrupted Lembert layer can then be completed if the tissue is sufficiently pliable. Many surgeons prefer a single layer of interrupted suture to close the pyloroplasty, and this technique is likely to be sufficient in the vast majority of cases. To make certain that the outlet is of adequate size, the initial longitudinal incision should be approximately 5 to 7 cm in length. Some surgeons recommend extension of the gastric portion of the incision approximately 1 cm longer than the duodenal portion.

Finney Pyloroplasty

This uncommonly used pyloroplasty is primarily performed in patients with a J-shaped stomach or extensive scarring and narrowing of a significant portion of the duodenal bulb, thus making a Heineke-Mikulicz pyloroplasty untenable. Use of this drainage procedure makes a larger lumen possible and involves a fairly long incision from the stomach, through the pylorus, and well into the duodenal bulb with closure of the inferior duodenum to the inferior stomach and superior duodenum to the superior stomach. It is a more complicated undertaking than the Heineke-Mikulicz procedure and has more potential for complications.

The procedure is begun by identifying the pylorus and performing a duodenum-mobilizing Kocher maneuver. After placement of silk traction sutures through the pylorus on the anterior duodenum, an incision is made through the pylorus and extended 5 to 7 cm onto the stomach and 5 to 7 cm onto the duodenum. After the careful exploration previously described, closure is initiated by using absorbable suture to begin a running

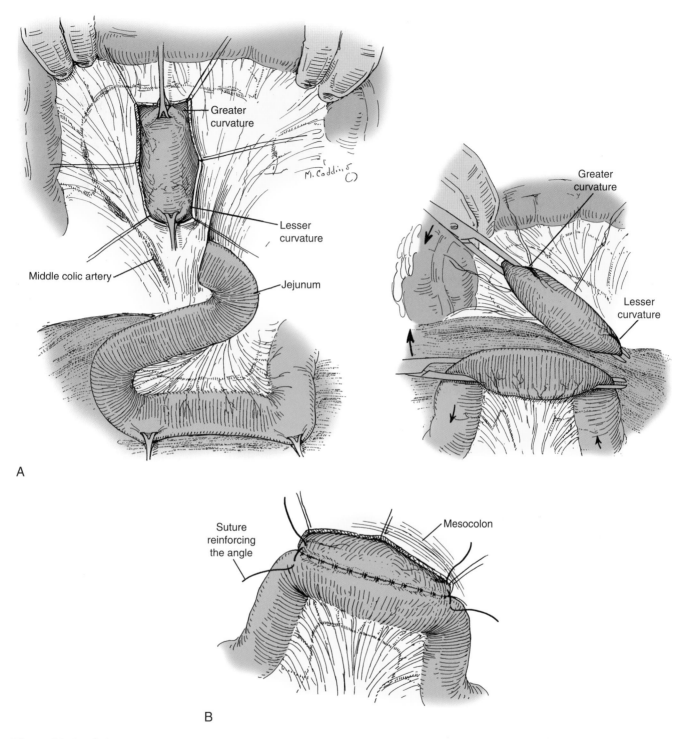

A

B

Figure 56–4.   Schematic representation of a gastrojejunostomy. A site approximately 15 to 20 cm from the ligament of Treitz is selected on the jejunum, a generous window is made in the mesocolon, and the selected jejunal site is pushed through the window until it lies next to the selected gastric site **(A).** A final layer of interrupted Lembert silk sutures completes the anterior outside layer **(B).** (From Zollinger RM: Atlas of Surgical Operations. New York, Macmillan, 1975.)

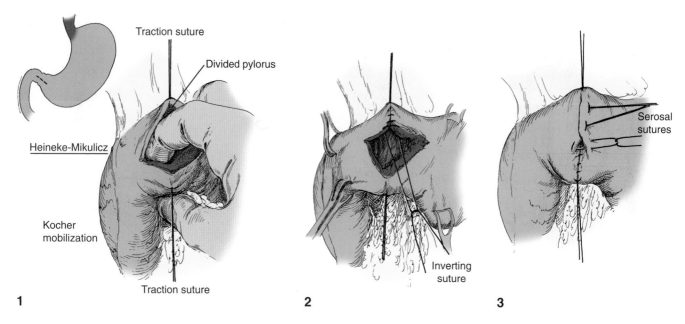

Figure 56–5.   Schematic representation of Heineke-Mikulicz pyloroplasty. While lifting up on the traction sutures, a longitudinal incision is made through the pyloric muscles and extended 2 to 3 cm proximally into the stomach and distally into the duodenum *(part 1)*. If the duodenum is soft, pliable, and minimally deformed, a running closure of the inside layer is begun with absorbable suture in an inverting fashion *(part 2)*. An outside layer of Lembert silk sutures in an interrupted fashion completes the procedure *(part 3)* (From Zollinger RM: Atlas of Surgical Operations. New York, Macmillan, 1975.)

closure (Fig. 56–6, part 4). The repair begins at the pylorus with suture being used to sew the inferior duodenum to the inferior stomach and, as the closure moves superiorly, the superior duodenum to the superior stomach. A final, interrupted row of silk sutures is then placed in Lembert fashion to complete the pyloroplasty (see Fig. 56–6, Part 5).

Jaboulay Gastroduodenostomy

The Jaboulay gastroduodenostomy is infrequently used in modern practice. This drainage procedure does not transect the pyloric muscle but instead involves an anastomosis of the distal end of the stomach to the first and second portions of the duodenum. The procedure is rarely performed, but when used, it is indicated primarily for a severely scarred or deformed pylorus or duodenal bulb. The procedure begins with adequate duodenal mobilization through a Kocher maneuver. The first and second portions of the duodenum are then folded back on the distal end of the stomach, and a posterior row of interrupted Lembert silk sutures is used to attach the duodenum to the distal stomach. Equal-size incisions approximately 4 to 5 cm in length are then made in the distal stomach and proximal duodenum (Fig. 56–7, part 6). An inside posterior running absorbable suture is placed to approximate the inferior duodenum to the inferior stomach. As the closure moves inferiorly, the superior duodenum is sewn to the superior stomach. A final anterior, outside layer of interrupted Lembert silk sutures is then placed to complete the gastroduodenostomy (see Fig. 56–7, part 7).

A variety of gastrointestinal complications may occur after gastric drainage, including dumping, diarrhea, bezoar formation, alkaline reflux gastritis, anemia, and marginal ulcers. These complications may develop in up to 50% of patients after surgery, but they resolve within 6 to 8 months in most patients. Five percent to 7% of patients have a persistent, symptomatic postoperative complication such as dumping. Should ulcers recur and a distal gastrectomy become necessary, the Finney and Jaboulay drainage procedures make reoperation more difficult. The choice of operation for the treatment of recurrent postoperative peptic ulcer is described in detail later in this chapter. Use of the Jaboulay procedure may also be associated with increased bile reflux because the anastomosis is close to the ampulla of Vater.

SURGICAL TREATMENT OF PEPTIC ULCER DISEASE

The fundamental goals of surgical treatment of peptic ulcer are to treat ulcer complications, address the ulcer diathesis, and minimize physiologic disturbances. No single procedure satisfies all the stated goals or is universally applicable to all surgical candidates. In choosing the most appropriate procedures, the surgeon must consider the characteristics of the ulcer (location, chronicity, presence of complications), the characteristics of the patient (age, nutritional status, comorbid illness, condition at initial evaluation), and the characteristics of the procedure itself (mortality rates and potential postoperative sequelae). This choice is heavily influenced by the surgeon's training, personal experience, and biases.

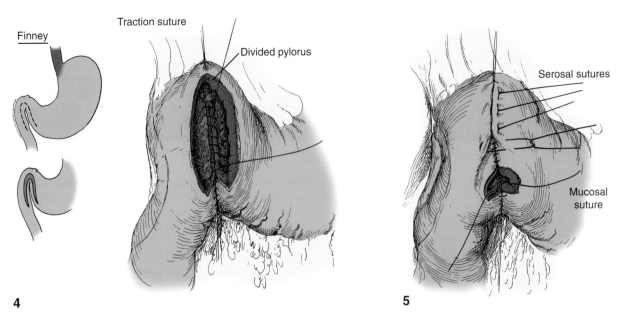

Figure 56–6. Schematic representation of the Finney pyloroplasty. After the careful exploration previously described in Figure 55–5, closure is initiated by using absorbable suture to begin a running closure *(part 4)*. A final, interrupted row of silk sutures is then placed in Lembert fashion to complete the pyloroplasty *(part 5)*. (From Zollinger RM: Atlas of Surgical Operations. New York, Macmillan, 1975.)

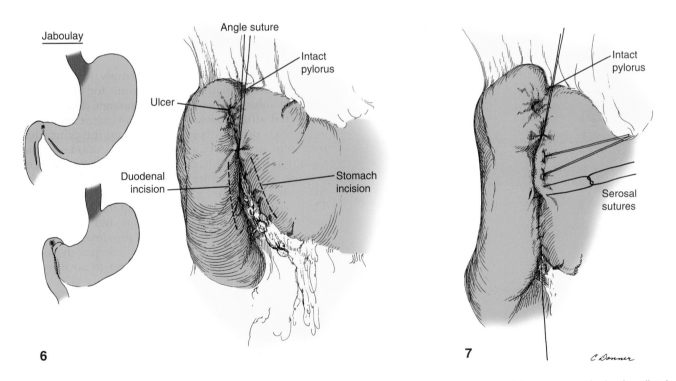

Figure 56–7. Schematic representation of the Jaboulay gastroduodenostomy. Equal-size incisions are made in the distal stomach and proximal duodenum approximately 4 to 5 cm in length *(part 6)*. A final anterior, outside layer of interrupted Lembert silk sutures is then placed to complete the gastroduodenostomy *(part 7)*. (From Zollinger RM: Atlas of Surgical Operations. New York, Macmillan, 1975.)

Gastric Ulcer

It is useful to consider a classification system modified after Johnson,[70] one based on anatomic location and acid secretory potential, when discussing operative therapy for gastric ulcer. This classification system is illustrated in Figure 56–8. Of importance, it may be impossible to distinguish between benign and malignant gastric ulcers purely on clinical or radiographic grounds, and 5% of ostensibly benign ulcers are found to harbor foci of malignancy.[71] A type I gastric ulcer is typically located along the lesser curvature of the stomach, usually at the antral-fundic junction, and is associated with acid hyposecretion. A type II ulcer is also found on the lesser curvature, but it occurs in younger patients in conjunction with active or healed duodenal ulcer disease. A type III gastric ulcer occurs in the prepyloric region. Both type II and type III ulcers are associated with high acid secretory capacity. A type IV ulcer encroaches on the gastro-

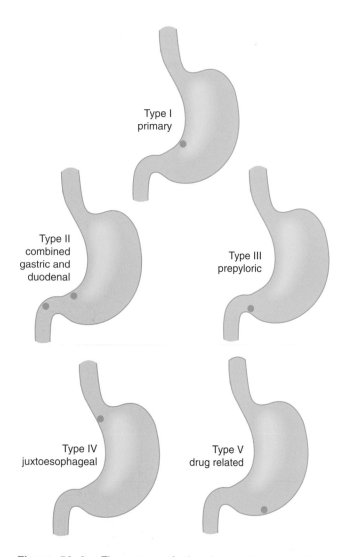

Figure 56–8. Five types of chronic gastric ulcer. (From Sleisenger MH, Fordtran JS: Operations for peptic ulcer disease and early postoperative complications. In Sleisenger MH, Fordtran JS: Gastrointestinal Disease, 5th ed. Philadelphia, WB Saunders, 1993.)

esophageal junction along the lesser curvature. A type V gastric ulcer is the result of chronic aspirin or NSAID use and may occur anywhere in the stomach.

Type I ulcers account for up to 60% of all gastric ulcers and occur in the setting of acid hyposecretion. Primary gastric ulceration occurs at the junction of the fundic and antral mucosa, often at or near the incisura, and almost always on the lesser curvature. The standard approach to these ulcers is a distal gastrectomy that encompasses the ulcer itself, followed by Billroth I or II reconstruction. Recurrence rates are very low,[72-74] and excellent symptomatic relief is usually achieved.[73,75] In general, closure of the duodenal stump is almost never a problem in the setting of a type I ulcer because the duodenal bulb is usually normal. Distal gastrectomy removes not only the ulcer itself but also much of the remaining susceptible mucosa, excises the diseased antrum, reduces acid secretory potential, and speeds gastric drainage. Distal gastrectomy also removes a major mucosal colonization site for *H. pylori*.

Because acid hypersecretion is not a major pathogenetic factor in gastric ulcer disease, it is unnecessary to add vagotomy to distal gastrectomy for a type I ulcer, which serves to only increase postoperative sequelae. Truncal vagotomy with drainage, when compared with distal gastrectomy in prospective series, carries greater morbidity, as well as higher recurrence and reoperation rates for gastric ulcer.[76-78] Furthermore, because the ulcer is left in situ, extensive biopsy is necessary to exclude malignancy. Consequently, vagotomy with pyloroplasty has a limited role in the treatment of this disease and should be reserved for high-risk patients requiring an expedient operation.[76]

Type II ulcers occur synchronously with duodenal ulcer disease or diathesis and account for up to 25% of all gastric ulcers. They exhibit pathologic derangements associated with duodenal rather than gastric ulcers, such as acid and pepsin hypersecretion, and the principles of treatment are analogous to those for duodenal ulcer. Vagotomy plus antrectomy is frequently preferred because it reliably addresses the duodenal ulcer, removes the gastric ulcer, and excises susceptible antral mucosa. There are advocates for truncal vagotomy and drainage in conjunction with ulcer excision, but no consensus exists in the literature. The use of proximal gastric vagotomy for type II ulcers has not been adequately assessed, but the data of Jordan[70] would appear to advise against its use in this setting.

A type III gastric ulcer refers to lesions situated in the prepyloric region of the stomach, although no precise anatomic definition exists. Accounting for 20% of all gastric ulcers, they also occur in the setting of increased acid and pepsin secretion and should be approached in a manner similar to duodenal ulcer. Truncal vagotomy plus antrectomy is probably superior to truncal vagotomy, drainage, and ulcer excision for these lesions. Proximal gastric vagotomy in this setting has been associated with excessively high recurrence rates approaching 35% and is therefore not recommended.[79-81]

Type IV ulcers are high-lying ulcers located within 1 to 2 cm of the gastroesophageal junction. Pathophysiologically, type IV ulcers are associated with gastric hyposecretion and represent a subset of primary gastric ulcers that occur in antral mucosa and extend high along the lesser curvature. The technical difficulty involved in their surgical treatment accounts for their separate categorization. If distal esophageal integrity can be ensured, subtotal gastric resection, including the ulcer bed, is considered optimal.[69] A variety of techniques have been proposed to address ulcers whose proximity to the gastroesophageal junction makes standard resection problematic. A Roux-en-Y jejunal segment (Csende procedure) may be useful for reconstruction. Other alternatives include the Pauchet procedure (a distal gastrectomy that is extended along the lesser curve to include the ulcer) and the Kelling-Madlener procedure (in which a distal gastrectomy is performed with the ulcer left in situ after biopsy). Safe management of type IV ulcers requires mature surgical judgment.

Drug-associated type V gastric ulcer lesions are best treated by withdrawal of the offending agent and only in rare circumstances come to surgery in the absence of severe complications.

As previously mentioned, chronic postoperative morbidity inevitably affects a significant minority of patients. The most common adverse digestive side effects of ulcer operations are epigastric fullness and episodic diarrhea, each occurring in about 20% to 35% of patients after classic ulcer operations. Many patients also experience nausea, heartburn, and intermittent vomiting of bile or food. "Dumping" symptoms (postprandial faintness, sweating, and other vasomotor symptoms) occur in approximately 10%. The incidence and severity of these postoperative sequelae must be considered when comparing various surgical options and should be discussed in detail with patients during the planning stages of elective surgery.

Historically, the functional outcome after antiulcer surgery has been assessed by a four-grade system introduced by Visick in 1948[82] and subsequently modified by Goligher et al.[83] Patients are categorized as "excellent" (grade 1, asymptomatic), "good" (grade 2, mild symptoms but no disability), "satisfactory" (grade 3, moderate symptoms not easily controlled and producing some disability), or "unsatisfactory" (grade 4, severe postoperative symptoms with considerable disability). The Visick system has a number of obvious shortcomings, most notably the fact that it relies heavily on subjective evaluation by both the patient and surgeon. Moreover, all cases of recurrent ulceration are classified as grade 4 regardless of whether the ulcer is symptomatic or easily treated by medication. Rates of postoperative ulcer recurrence vary widely and depend on not only the surgical technique but also the vigilance with which recurrence is sought. Many series report only symptomatic recurrences despite the fact that endoscopic surveillance indicates that as many as half of recurrences are asymptomatic.[84] Most would agree that trials of ulcer surgery performed in the pre-endoscopy era greatly underestimate the true incidence of recurrence.

Since the introduction of truncal vagotomy with antrectomy as an alternative to gastrojejunostomy or pyloroplasty by Smithwick in 1945,[67] surgeons have repeatedly argued about the indications for use of vagotomy and drainage. Although proponents of truncal vagotomy with pyloroplasty have maintained that the incidence of postoperative sequelae is greater with resection than with drainage, this has not been demonstrated. In fact, a number of trials were performed in the 1960s that compared the results of subtotal gastrectomy, truncal vagotomy with drainage, and truncal vagotomy with resection. The several series reported from the Leeds-York group,[66,83,85] as well as prospective studies by Price et al.[86] and by Jordan and Condon,[87] uniformly demonstrate that the resectional procedures yielded the lowest recurrence rates (1% to 2% versus up to 10% with drainage procedures) without a clear difference among these procedures in the incidence of postoperative functional disturbances. Operative mortality was generally somewhat higher with resection than with drainage procedures, and even ardent supporters of antrectomy tend to avoid gastric resection in high-risk or elderly patients.[88] Because of concern of leakage from the duodenal suture line, antrectomy is also avoided in the presence of extensive duodenal inflammation.

When compared with truncal vagotomy and drainage, proximal gastric vagotomy preserves the antropyloric motor apparatus, avoids the need for concomitant drainage or resection, and minimizes the complications of dumping, diarrhea, malnutrition, anemia, bile gastritis, and weight loss.[84,88-96] Because the stomach is not entered during the course of the procedure and no suture lines are created, infectious complications are few and problems of afferent or efferent loop obstruction (by definition) do not occur. Mortality from proximal gastric vagotomy has been estimated to be less than 0.3%.[97]

Proximal gastric vagotomy was initially slow to gain popularity in the United States, largely because of fears that preservation of an innervated antrum would result in hypergastrinemia and continued nonvagal stimulation of the parietal cell mass. Additionally, concern was raised over the adequacy of gastric emptying after the procedure. That these additional procedures are unnecessary was established in a prospective study reported by Holle.[56] In practice, these concerns have not been realized. Postoperative gastrin levels are comparable to those measured after total vagotomy,[98] and meal-stimulated acid secretion approximates that of selective vagotomy.[99] Gastric emptying approaches normal. In fact, the degree of postoperative digestive disturbances with this procedure is quite minimal. The percentage of patients who are categorized as Visick grade I after this procedure is nearly indistinguishable from normal control populations after exclusion of patients with ulcer recurrence.[100,101] The symptoms of postoperative diarrhea and dumping are vanishingly small. The fact that these sequelae are commonly seen after selective gastric vagotomy but not after proximal gastric vagotomy strongly suggests that it is the emptying procedure and not the vagotomy that is responsible for the postvagotomy diarrhea and dumping.

The greatest concern with proximal gastric vagotomy is the high rate of recurrent ulceration. Long-term follow-up data from prospective studies have reported recurrence rates approaching 40% with this procedure.[51] Part of this may be due to the close scrutiny that this procedure has received and the vigilance with which recurrences (many of them minimally symptomatic or silent) have been sought, particularly since the beginning of the modern endoscopic era. Technical familiarity and expertise with this procedure are clearly important,[57,102] the major problem being inadequate denervation of the acid-secreting regions. Some investigators, notably Jordan,[103] also attribute the high rate of recurrence to the inclusion of patients with pyloric channel or prepyloric ulcers. Although these patients, as a population, are acid hypersecretors and should benefit from vagotomy, the incidence of recurrent ulceration is particularly high in this subset. This high rate of recurrence may be due to a degree of gastric outlet obstruction associated with the presence of a local inflammatory reaction in the region of the pylorus. Based on these data, proximal gastric vagotomy is probably best avoided in patients with prepyloric or channel ulcers.

Laparoscopic proximal gastric vagotomy has met with some promising results, although it is unlikely to find wide application because of its technical demands.[63] The minimally invasive version of the Taylor procedure may prove to be a better alternative. Anecdotal results with the use of this approach have been reported.[64] Most surgeons agree that the trade-off between ulcer recurrence and postoperative digestive sequelae tends to weigh in favor of proximal gastric vagotomy for the few patients who require elective ulcer surgery. Recurrences after proximal gastric vagotomy are frequently mild and generally easily managed medically, particularly when antisecretory agents can be combined with antimicrobials in the setting of *H. pylori* infection. Numerous clinical series, including several prospective randomized trials, have demonstrated its superiority to other acid-reducing operations in terms of postoperative morbidity.[79,91,94,96,100,102,104-106]

The results of Taylor's anterior lesser curve seromyotomy and posterior truncal vagotomy are comparable to those of proximal gastric vagotomy with regard to reduction in acid secretion and ulcer recurrence. The great advantage of this procedure is its relative technical simplicity in comparison to proximal gastric vagotomy. Siriwardena and Gunn[107] reported an experience involving 241 patients in which they observed a 14% recurrence rate in 5 years. Eighty-one percent of their patients were classified as Visick grade I or II, and only 10% experienced significant postoperative symptoms (heartburn, distention, or flatulence). There were no instances of dumping or significant diarrhea. Taylor and colleagues performed a prospective randomized trial comparing this procedure with truncal vagotomy plus pyloroplasty.[108] Both procedures produced similar reductions in the acid secretory response to provocative insulin challenge (Hollander test). As with proximal gastric vagotomy, anterior lesser curve seromyotomy with posterior truncal vagotomy was associated with more recurrences but substantially fewer undesired postoperative effects. Ulcer recurrence rates appear to be equivalent to the results of proximal gastric vagotomy. A small subset of patients have experienced delayed gastric emptying that has required reoperation for a drainage procedure.[63]

CURRENT INDICATIONS FOR VAGOTOMY AND DRAINAGE

Although truncal vagotomy plus pyloroplasty is infrequently performed in the elective treatment of intractable peptic ulcer, it is useful in select patients suffering from perforated and especially bleeding duodenal and type II and III gastric ulcers. Vagotomy with drainage (pyloroplasty and gastrojejunostomy) also remains useful in the treatment of select patients with peptic gastric outlet obstruction. These recommendations are explained in detail in the following section.

Peptic Ulcer Intractability

Few patients have peptic ulcers that are absolutely refractory to optimal medical management. The duration and severity of symptoms, a history of patient noncompliance, or the frequency of recurrences may render elective surgery an excellent therapeutic alternative in some patients. Most patients who require surgery for duodenal ulcer are seen in the context of ulcer complications (hemorrhage, perforation, or obstruction), either as surgical emergencies or semi-electively after nonoperative management of a severe complication. Occasionally, patients who have suffered frequent recurrences, have chronic blood loss, or are at high risk for ulcer complications (e.g., renal transplant patients) will become appropriate candidates for elective surgical treatment. Elective surgery is indicated for many patients with giant gastric ulcers, which are more difficult to heal with medical therapy and carry a greater risk for complications and malignancy. Finally, patients who cannot tolerate the side effects of antiulcer drug regimens, particularly those used for the treatment of *H. pylori* infection, should be considered for elective ulcer surgery.

In the absence of concomitant complications, vagotomy plus drainage is not recommended for the treatment of intractable peptic ulcer. We recommend proximal gastric vagotomy as the procedure of choice in the elective treatment of intractable duodenal and type II and III gastric ulcers. Intractable type I and IV gastric ulcers are best treated by resection without concomitant vagotomy. The results of a prospective randomized controlled trial conducted by Gear[109] are interesting in the context of patient selection for elective surgery. Patients with endoscopically proven severe duodenal ulcers were treated by either proximal gastric vagotomy or H$_2$ receptor antagonists and underwent yearly endoscopic evaluation. After 1 to 4 years (which included maintenance H$_2$ receptor antagonist therapy for patients on the medical arm), 90% of the surgically treated patients versus 46% of the medically treated patients were found to be Visick grade I or II. The ulcer recurrence rate for vagotomy was 10% as compared with 54% for maintenance medical therapy. Based on this experience, it is reasonable to suggest that for severely symptomatic ulcer patients, surgery offers efficient and arguably more effective primary therapy.

Although the effect of long-term H$_2$ blockade on the incidence of ulcer complications remains undetermined because studies of maintenance medical therapy have had limited follow-up or insufficient sample size,[110] it has been demonstrated that within the first 6 weeks of medical therapy for a newly diagnosed ulcer, complications of hemorrhage, perforation, or obstruction develop in 3% to 6% of patients.[111] Indeed, since the introduction of H_2 receptor antagonists there has been a somewhat paradoxical increase in the complications and mortality attributable to peptic ulcer disease.[112] In contrast, in a 14- to 18-year follow-up of patients treated by proximal gastric vagotomy,[91] despite a troubling 30% ulcer recurrence rate, there were no instances of bleeding or perforation, even though 30% of the patients initially had hemorrhage as the indication for surgery. In a study of 779 patients with surgically treated peptic ulcer disease and a minimum follow-up of 15 years, none of the 360 deaths were related to ulcer disease.[113] These findings suggest that surgical therapy offers excellent protection against life-threatening complications of ulcer disease.

A similar line of reasoning has led Taylor[112] to suggest that surgical therapy should have a more prominent role early in the management of patients who exhibit the strongest ulcer diathesis and are at the greatest risk for morbid complications. He has defined candidate patients as those who frequently relapse on maintenance therapy with H_2 receptor antagonists, those who relapse early after two or more 2-month courses of medical therapy, or those who have relapsed after three or more courses of treatment at or about the age of 50.

Peptic Ulcer Perforation

In general, the incidence rates of emergency surgery, hospital admissions, and mortality for perforated peptic ulcer have remained stable throughout the last 2 decades. In older patients, admission rates for duodenal ulcer perforation increased and gastric ulcer perforation decreased in the last decade. Duodenal perforation currently accounts for approximately 75% of peptic perforations. Of note, the mortality rate for perforated ulcer is higher in the elderly and higher after gastric than after duodenal perforation. A recent study reported a 19% postoperative mortality rate in patients with perforated peptic ulcer but 41% in the elderly.[114] Factors such as concomitant diseases, shock on admission, delayed surgery (greater than 24 hours), resectional surgery, and postoperative abdominal and wound infections have been associated with increased morbidity and mortality in patients with perforated ulcer.[115-118] For decades, delay in operative treatment has remained a primary determinant of morbidity, mortality, and cost.

The mean prevalence of H. pylori infection in patients with perforated peptic ulcer is approximately 60%, as opposed to the 90% to 100% figure reported for uncomplicated ulcer disease. However, if NSAID use is excluded, the prevalence of infection is similar to that found in patients with nonperforating ulcer disease—approximately 90%.[119] In addition to H. pylori infection and NSAID use, smoking and alcohol consumption are also associated with perforated peptic ulcer.

In patients who do not have generalized peritonitis, hemodynamic instability, or free peritoneal perforation on a diatrizoate meglumine (Gastrografin) upper gastrointestinal study, nonoperative management can be considered. Retrospective and prospective randomized studies suggest that conservative management is effective in properly selected patients.[120-124]

Over the last decade, much has been published regarding the minimally invasive approach to peptic ulcer disease. Although essentially all of the procedures used to treat peptic ulcer disease have been performed laparoscopically, the more complicated procedures are challenging laparoscopic procedures even in the elective setting. Fortunately, open management of peptic ulcer disease has evolved such that most surgeons currently perform simple closure for perforated duodenal ulcer and do not routinely add complex acid reduction procedures. Simple closure translates well from the open to the laparoscopic approach for surgeons with advanced laparoscopic skills.

In the H. pylori era, a perforated duodenal ulcer is routinely closed with interrupted suture. The point of perforation is usually easily recognized in the proximal anterior aspect of the duodenum. If not apparent, exploration of the remainder of the duodenum, the anterior and posterior gastric walls, and the jejunum is undertaken. Omentum is laid over the closure and secured with the ends of the previously placed sutures. Additional sutures can be placed as necessary to plicate the omentum about the closure. When combined with postoperative H. pylori eradication, morbidity, mortality, and ulcer recurrence after closure and omental onlay have been shown to be acceptably low.[125-127]

Most surgeons agree that a laparoscopic diagnosis of perforated ulcer is readily apparent in the majority of cases. Laparoscopic surgery has not been as widely used as expected for perforated ulcer because of concern regarding the technical challenge of two-handed manipulation and intracorporeal suturing of indurated and friable tissue. Recent studies have confirmed the appropriateness of the laparoscopic approach for treating perforated peptic ulcer in appropriately selected patients.[128-135] Laparoscopic duodenal ulcer closure with an omental patch combined with postoperative H. pylori eradication and proton pump inhibitor therapy has been shown to be technically feasible and associated with low morbidity and mortality and appropriately low ulcer recurrence.

Laparoscopic closure of perforated duodenal ulcer has also been shown to be a simple and safe procedure. Although initial reports of laparoscopic closure of perforated duodenal ulcer demonstrated little difference in comparison to open duodenal ulcer closure, recent data demonstrate that the laparoscopic approach is safe and maintains the benefits of the minimally invasive approach.[128,130-135] Specifically, laparoscopic closure of perforated duodenal ulcer has been associated with shorter operating time, less postoperative pain, a shorter postoperative hospital stay, and earlier return to normal daily activities than the conventional open repair has. Patients in shock, with delayed evaluation, or with a high Acute Physiology and Chronic Health Evaluation

(APACHE) II score are better served by expeditious open closure of the ulcer.[129]

Postoperatively, patients should be treated with anti-secretory medications and antibiotics to eradicate *H. pylori*. A number of regimens are effective in eradicating *H. pylori*.[136,137] Treatment should be started during the immediate postoperative period, and eradication should be confirmed at the conclusion of therapy. Eradication of *H. pylori* after ulcer closure has been shown to significantly decrease ulcer recurrence in patients with *H. pylori*–associated perforated ulcers.[125] Current practice contrasts with the previous recommendation to add a concomitant acid reduction procedure to ulcer closure. Because there is no significant alteration in gastrointestinal anatomy with ulcer closure, patients suffer no postvagotomy or postgastrectomy side effects after this procedure.

Ulcer closure without a concomitant acid reduction procedure is especially indicated in patients with generalized peritonitis, shock, perforation for longer than 24 hours, or no significant symptoms for 3 months before perforation. However, in patients with perforated duodenal ulcers, truncal vagotomy and drainage could be of value in the unusual situation in which an unclear diagnosis mandates gastroduodenotomy for intraluminal exploration, a concomitant complication such as obstruction mandates drainage, or the patient has a chronic ulcer refractory to medical therapy. It should be reiterated that the benefit of definitive acid reduction surgery over closure and antibiotic therapy has not been demonstrated, and vagotomy plus drainage is not routinely used in treatment of perforated duodenal ulcer.

In patients with gastric ulcer perforation, the clinical condition and comorbid disease dictate which surgical procedure should be chosen. Truncal vagotomy with drainage is not routinely used in the treatment of perforated gastric ulcer. Commonly used procedures include simple closure with biopsy, excision and closure, and resection. Most perforated gastric ulcers are prepyloric. Prepyloric and pyloric ulcers are best treated with distal gastric resection because this technique avoids the 15% incidence of postoperative gastric obstruction seen with simple closure and also allows histologic assessment.[138] If a gastric ulcer is difficult to include in a resection, generous biopsy samples should be taken to exclude malignancy, and the ulcer is primarily closed or patched with omentum.

Peptic Ulcer Bleeding

Bleeding ulcers not associated with *H. pylori* or NSAIDs are uncommon. Recent data demonstrate that a negative biopsy urease test is unreliable for exclusion of *H. pylori* infection during the acute phase of ulcer bleeding and that bleeding peptic ulcers are not associated with *H. pylori* or NSAIDs in approximately 4% of patients.[139] Approximately half of patients with peptic ulcer bleeding use NSAIDs.

The incidence of peptic ulcer hemorrhage has decreased over the past decade. For example, in the Netherlands the incidence was 62 per 100,000 persons in 1993 and 48 per 100,000 in 2000.[140] Interestingly, despite changing treatment patterns during the 1990s, mortality rates from gastrointestinal bleeding have been relatively stable.[140,141] The incidence remained stable for both duodenal and gastric ulcer bleeding, but it was higher in patients of more advanced age. Bleeding from peptic ulcer disease most often occurs in the sixth decade of life. Epidemiologic data suggest that the incidence of emergency surgery has not changed over the last decade despite major improvements in endoscopic treatment.[142] Similarly, rebleeding (15% to 22%) and mortality (14% to 15%) in the modern endoscopic era remain unchanged.[140]

Ulcer bleeding is still a frequent cause of upper gastrointestinal bleeding and has been estimated at approximately 40% to 46%.[140] However, a recent study from the United States suggests that the percentage of patients with peptic ulcer as the source of upper gastrointestinal bleeding is decreasing.[143] A review of endoscopic data from 7822 patients with upper gastrointestinal bleeding from December 1999 until April 2001 in the national Clinical Outcome Research Initiative database demonstrated that peptic ulcer was the source of upper gastrointestinal bleeding in 20% of patients and a nonbleeding visible vessel was present in only 7% of the ulcers.

Increasing age, the presence of shock on initial evaluation, severe comorbidity, and rebleeding are associated with higher mortality in patients with bleeding ulcers.[140] The cause of death is usually multiple-system organ failure and not exsanguinating hemorrhage. Elderly patients with a hemorrhagic gastric ulcer have a high incidence of severe ulcer disease and concomitant medical problems.[144,145] Although initial endoscopic diagnosis and therapy for hemorrhagic peptic ulcer disease in the elderly are agreed on, debate exists regarding the advisability of early surgical intervention in elderly patients who have stopped bleeding.[142,146-150]

The optimal surgical management of patients with a bleeding peptic ulcer is debated. Most surgeons agree that patients with a profusely bleeding peptic ulcer associated with hemodynamic instability require aggressive resuscitation, endotracheal intubation to protect their airway, and emergency exploration to control the hemorrhage. However, the necessity and timing of surgical intervention to prevent or treat recurrent bleeding are less clear.[142,148] Some surgeons offer elderly patients with comorbid disease and an ulcer with stigmata worrisome for recurrent bleeding a semi-elective surgical procedure as soon as the initial bleeding spontaneously stops or is endoscopically controlled.[147,149,150] The role of angiographic embolization in the control of recurrent or intractable hemorrhage remains unclear. Further investigation is required to delineate the optimal medical, endoscopic, and surgical treatment of acute peptic ulcer bleeding.

A bleeding duodenal ulcer is approached through an upper midline incision. A longitudinal duodenotomy is performed to locate the ulcer, which is usually situated in the posterior duodenal bulb. As necessary, the duodenotomy is extended proximally across the pylorus or

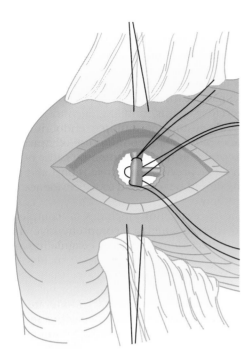

Figure 56–9. Technique of suture control of a bleeding duodenal ulcer. Through a longitudinal pyloric incision, figure-of-eight sutures are placed at the cephalad and caudad aspect of the ulcer deep enough to occlude the gastroduodenal artery. An additional U stitch is placed to control small transverse pancreatic branches of the gastroduodenal artery. (From Zinner M: Maingot's Abdominal Operations, 10th ed. New York, McGraw-Hill, 1997.)

distally beyond the first portion of the duodenum to find the ulcer. The bleeding is controlled with digital pressure and suture ligation. Figure-of-eight sutures are applied at the cephalad and caudad margins of the ulcer to ligate the gastroduodenal artery. A U stitch is placed in the ulcer base to occlude pancreatic branches of the gastroduodenal artery. The technique suggested for suture control of ulcer bleeding is illustrated in Figure 56–9. After hemostasis is obtained, the duodenal bulb and prepyloric stomach are examined for additional ulcers. As necessary, the duodenotomy is extended to control bleeding from additional ulcers. A small duodenotomy is closed primarily and longer duodenotomies are closed via a Heineke-Mikulicz or a Finney pyloroplasty.[151]

In the past, the addition of a truncal vagotomy has been recommended to decrease recurrent bleeding. As described earlier, surgeons are less likely to add vagotomy to pyloroplasty in the *H. pylori* era. Although a vagotomy is not recommended, further study of bleeding duodenal ulcer is required to validate this recommendation. In the past, many surgeons favored the aggressive addition of a truncal vagotomy and antrectomy to duodenal ulcer oversewing in the hope of further decreasing the incidence of recurrent bleeding and ulceration. Studies of vagotomy and antrectomy without *H. pylori* treatment suggest that the morbidity and mortality of antrectomy for a bleeding duodenal ulcer are equal to that of pyloroplasty and that antrectomy decreases the incidence of

recurrent bleeding.[152] Regardless of which procedure is performed, patients with a bleeding duodenal ulcer will probably have a lower rebleeding rate if *H. pylori* is eradicated than if they are treated by surgery alone. NSAID use should also be limited.

Surgical treatment of a bleeding gastric ulcer is determined by the clinical status of the patient, as well as the gastric ulcer type. In general, the recommended surgical treatment of a bleeding gastric ulcer mirrors the surgical treatment previously described for intractable gastric ulcers. In type I ulcers, the pathogenesis is not clearly understood and surgical recommendations include excision of the ulcer. At this point on the lesser curve, wedge excision is difficult and a partial gastrectomy is recommended unless the patient is unstable. If the patient is unstable, the ulcer should be excised and closed. In extreme instability, the ulcer is biopsied and oversewn and the gastrotomy is closed. Vagotomy plus pyloroplasty has previously been recommended in high-risk patients requiring urgent operations for bleeding type I gastric ulcers. However, the functional outcome of vagotomy and pyloroplasty is worse than that of vagotomy and distal gastrectomy. In addition, the lesser curve ulcer should be excised, and this makes vagotomy and pyloroplasty less attractive. Because the duodenal dissection is usually easy in patients who do not have duodenal ulceration, distal gastrectomy is recommended over vagotomy and pyloroplasty.

There is no consensus regarding surgical treatment of type II and type III bleeding ulcers. Because of concern for malignancy in gastric ulcers, excision of these gastric ulcers is recommended. The anatomy, inflammation, and patient condition at surgery dictate selection of the procedure. Excision with primary closure is acceptable when technically feasible. When simple closure would narrow the gastric outlet or multiple ulcers are present, distal gastrectomy is recommended. If significant duodenal inflammation would make distal gastrectomy technically challenging, gastric ulcer excision with vagotomy and pyloroplasty is performed. When combined with gastric ulcer excision, proximal gastric vagotomy is less appealing and has been associated with a high recurrence rate. Postoperatively, patients should have *H. pylori* infection eradicated and avoid the use of NSAIDs.

Peptic Ulcer Obstruction

In peptic ulcer disease, gastric outlet obstruction is less common than perforation or bleeding. Obstruction from a duodenal ulcer is the most common cause of peptic outlet obstruction and occurs in approximately 2% of patients with chronic duodenal ulcer. Although prepyloric, pyloric, and duodenal ulcers previously caused up to 80% of gastric outlet obstructions, it is likely that the percentage of outlet obstructions caused by ulcer disease has significantly decreased. This putative decrease has not been confirmed, however. Malignancy and chronic pancreatitis continue to cause gastric outlet obstruction and must be considered in all patients with a clinical picture suggestive of gastric outlet obstruction.

Risk factors for the development of peptic gastric outlet obstruction are similar to those for other complications of peptic ulcer disease and include NSAID use and *H. pylori* infection. Therefore, in patients with peptic gastric outlet obstruction, *H. pylori* should be eradicated and NSAID use should be limited as much as possible. Fortunately, experience has shown that many cases of gastric outlet obstruction will resolve with such treatment. Although recurrent gastric outlet obstruction has been a significant problem in the past, anecdotal clinical experience suggests that improved medical treatment of peptic ulcer disease has decreased recurrent peptic gastric outlet obstruction. However, in a number of cases, obstruction is associated with significant irreversible cicatrix formation, and nonoperative management will not provide lasting resolution of obstruction.

The recommended operation is vagotomy and antrectomy with insertion of a feeding jejunostomy tube to provide postoperative enteral nutritional support. In cases of severe inflammation that precludes safe resection of the duodenum, vagotomy plus gastrojejunostomy is recommended. A prolonged preoperative period of obstruction suggests that a gastrostomy tube could help decompress the stomach and avoid the need for prolonged use of a nasogastric tube in the postoperative period. Recent data suggest that the morbidity and mortality of elective surgical treatment of intractable gastric outlet obstruction have decreased. Interestingly, in one small series, *H. pylori* infection was present in a minority of patients with peptic gastric outlet obstruction who required surgical intervention. Endoscopic balloon dilation was used in a number of these patients without success. Operative morbidity was low and mortality was zero. Importantly, patient satisfaction was positive by the Visick scale.[153] Further investigation is required to determine the optimal combination and timing of medical, endoscopic, and surgical treatment in patients with peptic gastric outlet obstruction.

RECURRENT POSTOPERATIVE PEPTIC ULCER AFTER VAGOTOMY AND DRAINAGE

Recurrent postoperative ulceration after peptic ulcer surgery has become an increasingly uncommon problem in the last decade. Primary treatment of peptic ulcer disease with *H. pylori* eradication, NSAIDs with fewer gastrointestinal side effects, and proton pump inhibitors have decreased the incidence of peptic surgery, as well as the use of acid reduction procedures such as vagotomy and drainage. Despite less aggressive surgical procedures, postoperative recurrence rates are low because of improved medical treatment in the postoperative period. The contribution of incomplete vagotomy and gastrinoma to the development of recurrent ulcer disease requires further study in the *H. pylori* era. Because the incidence of acid reduction surgery has decreased and the incidence of gastrinoma has remained stable, it is likely that the percentage of postoperative patients with gastrinoma will increase from the 2% previously described.

Evaluation of recurrent ulceration after vagotomy and drainage begins with a thorough history and physical examination. The patient should be asked and the medical record should be reviewed regarding the initial operative indication and the procedure performed. Furthermore, past treatment of *H. pylori,* use of NSAIDs, use of antisecretory agents, smoking, alcohol consumption, and a family history of multiple endocrine neoplasia should be explored. Surreptitious use of aspirin or other NSAIDs is probably the most common cause of recurrent ulceration. The previous operative report and pathology specimens should be reviewed to seek evidence of incomplete vagotomy.

Laboratory evaluation includes a complete blood count to detect anemia, comprehensive metabolic profile to detect dehydration, a coagulation profile to detect coagulopathy in the presence of bleeding, and a gastrin level. Gastrin levels greater than 1000 pg/ml are diagnostic of a gastrinoma, and normal levels below 100 pg/ml exclude gastrinoma.[154] Moderate hypergastrinemia should be further evaluated with a secretin stimulation test. An increase in gastrin secretion greater than 100 pg/ml with secretin administration suggests gastrinoma. Previous vagotomy and G-cell hyperplasia are not associated with a significant increase in gastrin levels with secretin administration. Protein meal–stimulated gastrin levels greater than 300 pg/ml suggest G-cell hyperplasia or retained gastric antrum in patients who have previously undergone gastrectomy. Measurement of postoperative acid secretory function and sham feeding to evaluate the completeness of vagotomy are infrequently necessary and have little clinical relevance in the modern era.

Upper gastrointestinal barium study and upper endoscopy are useful in the evaluation of recurrent postoperative ulcer. Upper endoscopy can help make the diagnosis of recurrent ulcer disease, as well as localize the ulcer. Biopsy specimens are taken to assess for the presence of *H. pylori* and malignancy. Malignant ulceration is more common in gastric ulcers and is surprisingly uncommon in duodenal or jejunal ulcers. Barium studies help delineate the postoperative anatomy and functional abnormalities. However, barium studies are less sensitive and specific for recurrent ulcer disease than endoscopy is.[155,156]

Management of patients with recurrent ulcer disease after vagotomy and drainage consists of antibiotics directed at *H. pylori* if present, limitation of NSAID use, treatment with an antisecretory medication, smoking cessation, and limitation of alcohol intake. Ulcer disease refractory to such treatment is unusual. If the ulcer persists for longer than 3 months despite eradication of *H. pylori,* or maintenance antisecretory therapy for the ulcer is associated with perforation, bleeding, or obstruction, surgery is indicated. Although few data exist regarding therapeutic endoscopy for the treatment of a complicated postoperative recurrent ulcer, endoscopic control of bleeding and dilatation of the obstruction are routinely applied in a manner similar to the preoperative setting.

The choice of surgery for a recurrent ulcer after vagotomy and drainage depends on the indication for the initial operation, the original operation performed, the cause of the recurrence, and patient comorbidity.[157] Because these ulcers have recurred despite previous peptic ulcer disease surgery and maximal medical therapy, surgery should be appropriately aggressive. Persistent ulcers are worrisome for malignant disease and should be resected. After previous vagotomy and drainage, reoperation should include repeat vagotomy and antrectomy. Of note, the functional results after reoperative peptic surgery are not as good as those after primary surgery, with good to excellent results achieved in only 60% to 70% of patients.[158-160] Fortunately, even in the pre–*H. pylori* era, second recurrences were unusual and developed in less than 10% of patients managed by gastric resection.[160]

SUMMARY

The fundamental goals of surgical treatment of peptic ulcer are to treat ulcer complications, address the ulcer diathesis, and minimize physiologic disturbances. No single procedure satisfies all the stated goals or is universally applicable to all surgical candidates. In choosing the most appropriate procedures, the surgeon must consider the characteristics of the ulcer, the patient, and the procedure, as well as previous surgical training. Vagotomy plus drainage is infrequently performed in the modern era, but it remains a valuable procedure in the surgical armamentarium. Although vagotomy plus pyloroplasty is not routinely performed for the treatment of intractable peptic ulcer, it is useful in select patients suffering from perforated and especially bleeding duodenal and type II and III gastric ulcers. Vagotomy with drainage (pyloroplasty and gastrojejunostomy) also remains useful in the treatment of select patients with peptic gastric outlet obstruction.

REFERENCES

1. NIH Consensus Development Panel: *Helicobacter pylori* in peptic ulcer disease. JAMA 272:65-69, 1994.
2. Huang JQ, Sridhar S, Hunt RH: Role of *Helicobacter pylori* infection and non-steroidal anti-inflammatory drugs in peptic-ulcer disease: A meta-analysis. Lancet 359:14-22, 2202.
3. Hawkey CJ, Naesdal J, Wilson I, et al: Relative contribution of mucosal injury and *Helicobacter pylori* in the development of gastroduodenal lesions in patients taking non-steroidal anti-inflammatory drugs. Gut 51:336-343, 2002.
4. Garcia Rodriguez LA, Hernandez-Diaz S: Risk of uncomplicated peptic ulcer among users of aspirin and nonaspirin nonsteroidal anti-inflammatory drugs. Am J Epidemiol 159:23-31, 2004.
5. Arroyo MT, Forne M, de Argila CM, et al: The prevalence of peptic ulcer not related to *Helicobacter pylori* or non-steroidal anti-inflammatory drug use is negligible in southern Europe. Helicobacter 9:249-254, 2004.
6. Schwesinger WH, Page CP, Sirinek KR, et al: Operations for peptic ulcer disease: Paradigm lost. J Gastrointest Surg 5:438-443, 2001.
7. Paimela H, Paimela L, Myllykangas-Luosujarvi R, et al: Current features of peptic ulcer disease in Finland: Incidence of surgery, hospital admissions and mortality for the disease during the past twenty-five years. Scand J Gastroenterol 37:399-403, 2002.
8. Paimela H, Oksala NK, Kivilaakso E: Surgery for peptic ulcer today. A study on the incidence, methods and mortality in surgery for peptic ulcer in Finland between 1987 and 1999. Dig Surg 21:185-191, 2004.
9. Gibson JB, Behrman SW, Fabian TC, et al: Gastric outlet obstruction resulting from peptic ulcer disease requiring surgical intervention is infrequently associated with *Helicobacter pylori* infection. J Am Coll Surg 191:32-37, 2000.
10. Kleeff J, Friess H, Buchler MW: How *Helicobacter pylori* changed the life of surgeons. Dig Surg 20:93-102, 2003.
11. Johnson AG: Proximal gastric vagotomy: Does it have a place in the future management of peptic ulcer? World J Surg 24:259-263, 2000.
12. Gilliam AD, Speake WJ, Lobo DN, et al: Current practice of emergency vagotomy and *Helicobacter pylori* eradication for complicated peptic ulcer in the United Kingdom. Br J Surg 90:88-90, 2003.
13. Towfigh S, Chandler C, Hines OJ, et al: Outcomes from peptic ulcer surgery have not benefited from advances in medical therapy. Am Surg 68:385-389, 2002.
14. Millat B, Fingerhut A, Borie F: Surgical treatment of complicated duodenal ulcers: Controlled trials. World J Surg 24:299-306, 2000.
15. Hunter J: On the digestion of the stomach after death. Philos Trans R Soc Lond 62:447-454, 1772.
16. Feldman M, Richardson CT: Total 24-hour gastric acid secretion in patients with duodenal ulcer. Gastroenterology 90:540-544, 1986.
17. Kirkpatrick JR, Lawrie JH, Forrest AP, et al: The short pentagastrin test in the investigation of gastric disease. Gut 10:760-762, 1969.
18. Cox AJ: Stomach size and its relation to chronic peptic ulcer. Arch Pathol 54:407-422, 1952.
19. Roland M, Berstad A, Liavag I: Acid and pepsin secretion in duodenal ulcer patients in response to greater doses of pentagastrin or pentagastrin and carbocholine before and after proximal gastric vagotomy. Scand J Gastroenterol 9:511-518, 1974.
20. Mertz HR, Walsh JH: Peptic ulcer pathophysiology. Med Clin North Am 75:799-814, 1991.
21. Davenport HW: Is the apparent hyposecretion of acid of patients with gastric ulcer a consequence of a broken barrier to the diffusion of hydrogen ions into the gastric mucosa? Gut 6:513, 1965.
22. Debas HT, Orloff SL: Surgery for peptic ulcer disease and postgastrectomy syndromes. In Yamada T (ed): Textbook of Gastroenterology. Philadelphia, JB Lippincott, 1995, pp 1523-1543.
23. Schwartz K: Uber penetrierende magen- und jejunal Geschwure. Beitr Klin Chir 76:96-128, 1910.
24. Leung FW, Itoh M, Hirabayashi K, et al: Role of blood flow in gastric and duodenal mucosal injury in the rat. Gastroenterology 88:281-289, 1985.
25. Malagelada JR, Longstreth GF, Deering TB, et al: Gastric secretion and emptying after ordinary meals in duodenal ulcer. Gastroenterology 73:989-994, 1977.
26. Niemela S, Heikkila J, Lehtola J: Duodenogastric bile reflux in patients with gastric ulcer. Scand J Gastroenterol 19:896-898, 1984.
27. Warren JR, Marshall B: Unidentified curved bacilli on gastric epithelium in active chronic gastritis. Lancet 1:1273-1275, 1983.
28. *H pylori* in peptic ulcer disease—NIH consensus conference. JAMA 272:265-268, 1994.
29. Blaser MJ: Gastric *Campylobacter*-like organisms, gastritis, and peptic ulcer disease. Gastroenterology 93:371-383, 1987.
30. Soll AH: Pathogenesis of peptic ulcer and implications for therapy. N Engl J Med 322:909-916, 1990.
31. Sipponen P, Seppala K, Aarynen M, et al: Chronic gastritis and gastroduodenal ulcer: A case control study on risk of co-existing duodenal or gastric ulcer in patients with gastritis. Gut 30:922-929, 1989.
32. Cullen DJE, Collins BJ, Christiansen KJ, et al: Long term risk of peptic ulcer disease in people with *H pylori* infection—community based study. Gastroenterology 60(Suppl A):104, 1991.
33. Marshall BJ, Goodwin CS, Warren JR, et al: Prospective double-blind trial of ulcer relapse after eradication of *Campylobacter pylori*. Lancet 2:1437-1442, 1988.
34. Hentschel E, Brandstatter G, Dragosics B, et al: Effect on ranitidine and amoxicillin plus metronidazole on the eradication of *Helicobacter pylori* and the recurrence of duodenal ulcer. N Engl J Med 328:308-312, 1993.
35. Rauws EAJ, Tytgat GNJ: Cure of duodenal ulcer associated with eradication of *Helicobacter pylori*. Lancet 335:1233-1235, 1990.

36. Clearfield HR: *Helicobacter pylori:* Aggressor or innocent bystander? Med Clin North Am 75:815-829, 1991.

37. Lee SK, Thirlby RC, Thompson W, et al: Acute effect of experimental truncal vagotomy on serum gastrin concentrations. Ann Surg 211:136-140, 1990.

38. Csendes A, Ornsholt J, Venturelli A, et al: Dose response studies of acid secretion after administration of tetragastrin. Am J Surg 139:832-837, 1980.

39. Blair AJ, Richardson CT, Walsh JH, et al: Effect of parietal cell vagotomy on acid secretory responsiveness to circulating gastrin in humans. Gastroenterology 90:1001-1007, 1986.

40. Debas HT: Peripheral regulation of gastric acid secretion. In Johnson LR (ed): Physiology of the GI Tract, 2nd ed. New York, Raven Press, 1987, p 931.

41. Grossman MI: Secretion of acid and pepsin in response to distension of vagally innervated fundic gland area in dogs. Gastroenterology 42:718-721, 1962.

42. Papsova M: Sphincteric function. In Schultz SG, Wood JD, Rauner BB (eds): Handbook of Physiology, vol I, pt 2. Baltimore, Waverly Press, 1989, p 987.

43. Sheiner HJ, Quinlan MF, Thompson IJ: Gastric motility and emptying in normal and post-vagotomy subjects. Gut 21:753-759, 1980.

44. Hartley MN, Mackie CR: Gastric adaptive relaxation and symptoms after vagotomy. Br J Surg 78:24-27, 1991.

45. Dragstedt LR, Owens FM: Supradiaphragmatic section of the vagus nerve in the treatment of duodenal ulcer. Proc Soc Exp Biol Med 53:152-154, 1943.

46. Dragstedt LR, Harper PV, Tovee EB, et al: Section of the vagus nerve to the stomach in the treatment of peptic ulcer: Complications and end results after 4 years. Ann Surg 126:687-708, 1947.

47. Griffith CA: Long-term results of selective vagotomy and pyloroplasty: 12 to 17 year follow-up. Am J Surg 139:608-615, 1980.

48. Jackson RG: Anatomic study of the vagus nerves, with a technique of transabdominal selective gastric vagus section. Arch Surg 57:333-352, 1948.

49. Franksson C: Selective abdominal vagotomy. Acta Chir Scand 96:409, 1948.

50. Kennedy T, Connell AM: Selective or truncal vagotomy? A double-blind randomized controlled trial. Lancet 1:899-901, 1969.

51. Hoffman J, Jensen H, Christiansen J, et al: Prospective controlled vagotomy trial for duodenal ulcer: Results after 11-15 years. Ann Surg 209:40-45, 1989.

52. Humphrey CS, Johnston D, Walker BE, et al: Incidence of dumping after truncal and selective vagotomy with pyloroplasty and highly selective vagotomy without drainage procedure. BMJ 3:785-788, 1972.

53. Griffith CA, Harkins HN: Partial gastric vagotomy: An experimental study. Gastroenterology 32:96-102, 1957.

54. Johnston D, Wilkinson A: Selective vagotomy with innervated antrum without drainage for duodenal ulcer. Br J Surg 56:626, 1969.

55. Amdrup E, Jensen H: Selective vagotomy of the parietal cell mass preserving innervation of the undrained antrum. Gastroenterology 59:522-527, 1970.

56. Holle F: New method for surgical treatment of gastroduodenal ulceration. In Harkins HM, Nyhus LM (eds): Surgery of the Stomach and Duodenum, 2nd ed. Boston, Little, Brown, 1969, pp 629-634.

57. Hallenbeck GA, Gleysteen JJ, Aldrete JS, et al: Proximal gastric vagotomy: Effects of two operative techniques on clinical and gastric secretory results. Ann Surg 184:435-442, 1976.

58. Taylor TV, Gunn AA, Macleod DAD: Anterior lesser curve seromyotomy and posterior truncal vagotomy in the treatment of chronic duodenal ulcer. Lancet 2:846-848, 1982.

59. Taylor TV, Holt S, Heading RC: Gastric emptying after anterior lesser curve seromyotomy and posterior truncal vagotomy. Br J Surg 72:620-622, 1985.

60. Daniel EE, Sarna SK: Distribution of excitatory vagal fibers in canine gastric wall to central motility. Gastroenterology 71:608-613, 1976.

61. Taylor TV, Gunn AA, Macleod DAD, et al: Mortality and morbidity after anterior lesser curve seromyotomy and posterior truncal vagotomy for duodenal ulcer. Br J Surg 72:950-951, 1985.

62. Oostvogel JHM, van Vroonhoven TJMV: Anterior lesser curve seromyotomy with posterior truncal vagotomy versus parietal gastric vagotomy. Br J Surg 75:121-124, 1988.

63. Cuschieri A: Laparoscopic vagotomy: Gimmick or reality? Surg Clin North Am 72:357-367, 1992.

64. Katkhouda N, Mouiel J: A new technique of surgical treatment of chronic duodenal ulcer without laparotomy by videocelioscopy. Am J Surg 161:361-364, 1991.

65. Wittmoser R: Thoracoscopic sympathectomy and vagotomy. In Cuschieri A, Buess G, Perissat J (eds): Manual of Operative Endoscopic Surgery. Berlin, Springer-Verlag, 1992, pp 110-133.

66. Goligher JC, Pulvertaft CN, Irvin TT, et al: Five- to eight-year results of truncal vagotomy and pyloroplasty for duodenal ulcer. BMJ 1:7-13, 1972.

67. Farmer DA, Smithwick RH: Hemigastrectomy combined with resection of the vagus nerve. N Engl J Med 247:1017-1022, 1952.

68. Matthews JB, Silen W: Operations for peptic ulcer disease and early postoperative complications. In Sleisenger MH, Fordtran JS (eds): Gastrointestinal Disease. Philadelphia, WB Saunders, 1993, pp 713-730.

69. Weinberg JA, Stempien SJ, Movius HJ, et al: Vagotomy and pyloroplasty in the treatment of duodenal ulcer. Am J Surg 92:202-207, 1956.

70. Johnson HD: Gastric ulcer: Classification, blood group characteristics, secretion, pathogenesis. Ann Surg 162:996-1004, 1965.

71. Podolsky I, Storm PR, Richardson CT, et al: Gastric adenocarcinoma masquerading endoscopically as benign gastric ulcer: A five-year experience. Dig Dis Sci 33:1057-1063, 1988.

72. Walters W, Lynn TE: The Billroth I and Billroth II operations. Arch Surg 74:680-685, 1957.

73. Thomas WEG, Thompson MH, Williamson RCN: The long-term outcome of Billroth I partial gastrectomy for benign gastric ulcer. Ann Surg 195:189-195, 1982.

74. Sapala JA, Ponka JL: Operative treatment of benign gastric ulcer. Am J Surg 125:19-28, 1973.

75. Duthie HL, Kwong NK: Vagotomy and gastrectomy for gastric ulcer. BMJ 4:79-81, 1973.

76. Kraft RO: Long term results of vagotomy and pyloroplasty in the treatment of gastric ulcer. Surgery 95460-466, 1984.

77. Madsen P, Schousen P: Long-term results of truncal vagotomy and pyloroplasty for gastric ulcer. Br J Surg 69:651-654, 1982.

78. Duthie HL, Moore KTH, Bardsley D, et al: Surgical treatment of gastric ulcers: Controlled comparison of Billroth I gastrectomy and vagotomy and pyloroplasty. Br J Surg 57:784-787, 1970.

79. Sawyers JL, Herrington JL: Vagotomy and antrectomy. In Nyhus LM, Wastell C (eds): Surgery of the Stomach and Duodenum, 3rd ed. Boston, Little, Brown, 1977, pp 343-369.

80. Poppen B, Delin A: Proximal gastric vagotomy for duodenal and pyloric ulcers. I. Clinical factors leading to failure of the operation. Am J Surg 141:323-329, 1981.

81. Hollingshead JW, Smith RC, Gillett DJ: Proximal gastric vagotomy: Experience with 114 patients with prepyloric or duodenal ulcer. World J Surg 6:596-602, 1982.

82. Visick AH: A study of the failures after gastrectomy. Ann R Coll Surg Engl 3:266-284, 1948.

83. Goligher JC, Pulvertaft CN, deDombal FT, et al: 5 to 8 year results of Leeds/York controlled trial of elective surgery for duodenal ulcer. BMJ 2:781-787, 1968.

84. von Holstein CG, Graffner H, Oscarson J: 100 patients 10 years after parietal cell vagotomy. Br J Surg 74:101-103, 1987.

85. Goligher JC, Pulvertaft CN, deDombal FT, et al: Clinical comparison of vagotomy and pyloroplasty with other forms of elective surgery for duodenal ulcer. BMJ 2:787-789, 1968.

86. Price WE, Grizzle JE, Postlethwait RW, et al: Results of operation for duodenal ulcer. Surg Gynecol Obstet 131:233-244, 1970.

87. Jordon PH, Condon RE: A prospective evaluation of vagotomy-pyloroplasty and vagotomy-antrectomy for treatment of duodenal ulcer. Ann Surg 172:547-563, 1970.

88. Herrington JL: A possible solution to the vagotomy-antrectomy and vagotomy-pyloroplasty controversy. Am J Surg 121:215-216, 1971.

89. Macintyre IMC, Millar A, Smith AN, et al: Highly selective vagotomy 5-15 years on. Br J Surg 77:65-69, 1990.

90. Herrington JL, Davidson J, Shumway SJ: Proximal gastric vagotomy: Follow-up of 109 patients for 6-13 years. Ann Surg 204:108-113, 1986.

91. Hoffman J, Oleson A, Jensen HE: Prospective 14- to 18-year follow-up study after parietal cell vagotomy. Br J Surg 74:1056-1059, 1987.

92. Sawyers JL, Herrington JL, Burney DP: Proximal gastric vagotomy compared with vagotomy and antrectomy and selective gastric vagotomy and pyloroplasty. Ann Surg 186:510-517, 1978.

93. Byrne DJ, Brock BM, Morgan G, et al: Highly selective vagotomy: A 14-year experience. Br J Surg 75:869-867, 1988.

94. Goligher JC, Hill GL, Kenny TE, et al: Proximal gastric vagotomy without drainage for duodenal ulcer: Results after 5-8 years. Br J Surg 65:145-151, 1978.

95. Gonzalez EM, Arnau BN, Dupont TC, et al: Proximal gastric vagotomy: A prospective study of 829 patients with four-year follow-up. Acta Chir Scand 149:69-76, 1983.

96. Gorey TF, Lennon F, Heffernan SJ: Highly selective vagotomy in duodenal ulceration and its complications: A 12-year review. Ann Surg 200:181-184, 1984.

97. Johnston D: Operative mortality and postoperative morbidity of highly selective vagotomy. Br J Surg 4:545-547, 1975.

98. Thompson JC, Fender HR, Watson LC, et al: The effects on gastrin and gastric secretion of five current operations for duodenal ulcer. Ann Surg 183:599-608, 1976.

99. Johnston D, Humphrey CS, Smith RB, et al: Should the gastric antrum be vagally denervated if it is well drained and in the acid stream? Br J Surg 58:725-731, 1971.

100. Kennedy T, Johnston GW, Macrae KD, et al: Proximal gastric vagotomy: Interim results of a randomized controlled trial. BMJ 2:301-303, 1975.

101. Johnston GW, Spenser EFA, Wilkinson AJ, et al: Proximal gastric vagotomy: Follow-up at 10-20 years. Br J Surg 78:20-23, 1991.

102. Blackett RL, Johnston D: Recurrent ulceration after highly selective vagotomy for duodenal ulcer. Br J Surg 68:705-710, 1981.

103. Jordan PH: Indications for parietal cell vagotomy without drainage in gastrointestinal surgery. Ann Surg 210:29-41, 1989.

104. Jensen HE, Amdrup E: Follow-up of 100 patients five to eight years after parietal cell vagotomy. World J Surg 2:525-532, 1978.

105. de Miguel J: Late results of proximal gastric vagotomy without drainage for duodenal ulcer: 5-9 year follow-up. Br J Surg 69:7-10, 1982.

106. Jordan PH, Thornby J: Should it be parietal cell vagotomy or selective vagotomy-antrectomy for treatment of duodenal ulcer? Ann Surg 205:572-590, 1987.

107. Siriwardena AK, Gunn AA: Anterior lesser curve seromyotomy and posterior truncal vagotomy for chronic duodenal ulcer: The results at five years. Br J Surg 75:866-868, 1988.

108. Taylor TV, Lythgoe JP, McFarland JB, et al: Anterior lesser curve seromyotomy and posterior truncal vagotomy versus truncal vagotomy and pyloroplasty in treatment of chronic duodenal ulcer. Br J Surg 77:1007-1009, 1990.

109. Gear MLW: Proximal gastric vagotomy versus long term maintenance therapy with cimetidine for chronic duodenal ulcer: A prospective randomised trial. Br Med J (Clin Res Ed) 286:98-99, 1983.

110. Isenberg JI, McQuaid KR, Laine L, et al: Acid peptic diseases. In Yamada T (ed): Textbook of Gastroenterology. Philadelphia, JB Lippincott, 1995, p 1408.

111. Katkhouda N: Peptic ulcer surgery in 1994. Endosc Surg 2:87-90, 1994.

112. Taylor TV: Current indications for elective peptic ulcer surgery. Br J Surg 76:427-428, 1989.

113. McLean Ross AH, Smith MA, Anderson JR, et al: Late mortality after surgery for peptic ulcer. N Engl J Med 307:519-522, 1982.

114. Uccheddu A, Floris G, Altana ML, et al: Surgery for perforated peptic ulcer in the elderly. Evaluation of factors influencing prognosis. Hepatogastroenterology 50:1956-1958, 2003.

115. Noguiera C, Silva AS, Santos JN, et al: Perforated peptic ulcer: Main factors of morbidity and mortality. World J Surg 27:782-787, 2003.

116. Hermansson M, Stael von Holstein C, Zilling T: Surgical approach and prognostic factors after peptic ulcer perforation. Eur J Surg 165:566-572, 1999.

117. Testini M, Portincasa P, Piccinni G, et al: Significant factors associated with fatal outcome in emergency open surgery for perforated peptic ulcer. World J Gastroenterol 9:2338-2340, 2003.

118. Svanes C: Trends in perforated peptic ulcer: Incidence, etiology, treatment, and prognosis. World J Surg 24:277-283, 2000.

119. Gisbert JP, Legido J, Garcia-Sanz I, Pajares JM: *Helicobacter pylori* and perforated peptic ulcer prevalence of the infection and role of non-steroidal and anti-inflammatory drugs. Dig Liver Dis 36:116-120, 2004.

120. Crofts TJ, Park KG, Steele RJ, et al: A randomized trial of non-operative treatment for perforated peptic ulcer. N Engl J Med 320:970-973, 1989.

121. Berne TV, Donovan AJ: Nonoperative treatment of perforated duodenal ulcer. Arch Surg 124:830-832, 1989.

122. Keane TE, Dillon B, Afdhal HH, et al: Conservative management of perforated duodenal ulcer. Br J Surg 75:583-584, 1988.

123. Donovan AJ, Berne TV, Donovan JA: Perforated duodenal ulcer: An alternative therapeutic plan. Arch Surg 133:1166-1171, 1998.

124. Marshall C, Ramaswamy P, Bergin FG, et al: Evaluation of a protocol for the non-operative management of perforated peptic ulcer. Br J Surg 86:131-134, 1999.

125. Ng EK, Lam YH, Sung JJ, et al: Eradication of *Helicobacter pylori* prevents recurrence of ulcer after simple closure of duodenal ulcer perforation: Randomized controlled trial. Ann Surg 231:153-158, 2000.

126. Gisbert JP, Pajares JM: *Helicobacter pylori* infection and perforated peptic ulcer prevalence of the infection and role of antimicrobial treatment. Helicobacter 8:159-167, 2003.

127. Kate V, Ananthakrishnan N, Badrinath S: Effect of *Helicobacter pylori* eradication on the ulcer recurrence rate after simple closure of perforated duodenal ulcer: Retrospective and prospective randomized controlled studies. Br J Surg 88:1054-1058, 2001.

128. Katkhouda N, Mavor E, Mason RJ, et al: Laparoscopic repair of perforated duodenal ulcers: Outcome and efficacy in 30 consecutive patients. Arch Surg 134:845-848, 1999.

129. Lee FY, Leung KL, Lai PB, et al: Selection of patients for laparoscopic repair of perforated peptic ulcer. Br J Surg 88:133-136, 2001.

130. Bergamaschi R, Marvik R, Johnsen G, et al: Open vs laparoscopic repair of perforated peptic ulcer. Surg Endosc 13:679-682, 1999.

131. Khoursheed M, Fuad M, Safar H, et al: Laparoscopic closure of perforated duodenal ulcer. Surg Endosc 14:56-58, 2000.

132. Arnaud JP, Tuech JJ, Bergamaschi R, et al: Laparoscopic suture closure of perforated duodenal peptic ulcer. Surg Laparosc Endosc Percutan Tech 12:145-147, 2002.

133. Siu WT, Leong HT, Law BK, et al: Laparoscopic repair for perforated peptic ulcer: A randomized controlled trial. Ann Surg 235:313-319, 2002.

134. Siu WT, Chau CH, Law BK, et al: Routine use of laparoscopic repair for perforated peptic ulcer. Br J Surg 91:481-484, 2004.

135. Malkov IS, Zaynutdinov AM, Veliyev NA, et al: Laparoscopic and endoscopic management of perforated duodenal ulcers. J Am Coll Surg 198:352-355, 2004.

136. McMahon BJ, Hennessy TW, Bensler JM, et al: The relationship among previous antimicrobial use, antimicrobial resistance, and treatment outcomes for *Helicobacter pylori* infections. Ann Intern Med 139:463-469, 2003.

137. Duck WM, Sobel J, Pruckler JM, et al: Antimicrobial resistance incidence and risk factors among *Helicobacter pylori*–infected persons, United States. Emerg Infect Dis 10:1088-1094, 2004.

138. McGee GS, Sawyers JL: Perforated gastric ulcers: A plea for management by primary gastric resection. Arch Surg 122:555-561, 1987.

139. Chan HL, Wu JC, Chan FK, et al: Is non–*Helicobacter pylori*, non-NSAID peptic ulcer a common cause of upper GI bleeding? A prospective study of 977 patients. Gastrointest Endosc 53:438-442, 2001.

140. van Leerdam ME, Vreeburg EM, Rauws EA, et al: Acute upper GI bleeding: Did anything change? Time trend analysis of incidence and outcome of acute upper GI bleeding between 1993/1994 and 2000. Am J Gastroenterol 98:1494-499, 2003.

141. Lewis JD, Bilker WB, Brensinger C, et al: Hospitalization and mortality rates from peptic ulcer disease and GI bleeding in the 1990s: Relationship to sales of nonsteroidal anti-inflammatory

drugs and acid suppression medications. Am J Gastroenterol 97:2540-2549, 2002.

142. Ohmann C, Imhof M, Roher HD: Trends in peptic ulcer bleeding and surgical treatment. World J Surg 24:284-293, 2000.

143. Boonpongmanee S, Fleischer DE, Pezzullo JC, et al: The frequency of peptic ulcer as a cause of upper-GI bleeding is exaggerated. Gastrointest Endosc 59:788-794, 2004.

144. Yamaguchi Y, Yamato T, Katsumi N, et al: Endoscopic treatment of hemorrhagic gastric ulcer in patients aged 80 years or more. Hepatogastroenterology 48:1195-1198, 2001.

145. Fowler SF, Khoubian JF, Mathiasen RA, et al: Peptic ulcers in the elderly is a surgical disease. Am J Surg 182:733-737, 2001.

146. Imhof M, Ohmann C, Roher HD, et al: Endoscopic versus operative treatment in high-risk ulcer bleeding patients—results of a randomised study. Langenbecks Arch Surg 387:327-336, 2003.

147. Schoenberg MH: Surgical therapy for peptic ulcer and nonvariceal bleeding. Langenbecks Arch Surg 386:98-103, 2001.

148. Barkun A, Bardou M, Marshall JK, et al: Consensus recommendations for managing patients with nonvariceal upper gastrointestinal bleeding. Ann Intern Med 139:843-857, 2003.

149. Monig SP, Lubke T, Baldus SE, et al: Early elective surgery for bleeding ulcer in the posterior duodenal bulb. Own results and review of the literature. Hepatogastroenterology 49:416-418, 2002.

150. Imhof M, Schroders C, Ohmann C, et al: Impact of early operation on the mortality from bleeding peptic ulcer—ten years' experience. Dig Surg 15:308-314, 1998.

151. Knight CD Jr, van Heerden JA, Kelly KA: Proximal gastric vagotomy: Update. Ann Surg 197:22-26, 1983.

152. Millat B, Hay JM, Valleur P, et al: Emergency surgical treatment for bleeding duodenal ulcer: Oversewing plus vagotomy versus gastric resection, a controlled randomized trial. French Associations for Surgical Research. World J Surg 17:568-573, 1993.

153. Gibson JB, Behrman SW, Fabian TC, et al: Gastric outlet obstruction resulting from peptic ulcer disease requiring surgical intervention is infrequently associated with *Helicobacter pylori* infection. J Am Coll Surg 191:32-37, 2000.

154. McGuigan JE, Wolfe MM: Secretin injection test in the diagnosis of gastrinoma. Gastroenterology 79:1324-1331, 1980.

155. Mosiman F, Donovan IA, Alexander-Wiliams J: Pitfalls in the diagnosis of recurrent ulceration after surgery for peptic ulcer disease. J Clin Gastroenterol 7:133-136, 1985.

156. Turnage RH, Sarosi G, Cryer B, et al: Evaluation and management of patients with recurrent peptic ulcer disease after acid-reducing operations: A systematic review. J Gastrointest Surg 7:606-626, 2003.

157. Schirmer BD, Meyers WC, Hanks JB, et al: Marginal ulcer: A difficult surgical problem. Ann Surg 195:653-661, 1982.

158. Stabile BE, Passaro E Jr: Recurrent peptic ulcer. Gastroenterology 70:124-135, 1976.

159. Koo J, Lam SK, Ong GB: Cimetidine versus surgery for recurrent ulcer after gastric surgery. Ann Surg 195:406-412, 1982.

160. Hoffman J, Shokouh-Amiri MH, Klarskov P, et al: Gastrectomy for recurrent ulcer after vagotomy: Five to nineteen-year follow-up. Surgery 99:517-522, 1986.

57

Gastric Resection and Reconstruction

Douglas J. Turner • Michael W. Mulholland

PREOPERATIVE PREPARATION

A first- or second-generation cephalosporin is adequate coverage for the majority of gastric operations, with a broader-spectrum antibiotic used in patients with achlorhydria or gastric outlet obstruction. The intravenous delivery is completed before skin incision. Pneumatic compression boots are worn for prophylaxis of deep vein thrombosis.

A bowel preparation is useful only in complicated cases and will both aid exposure through decompression and lessen the bacterial load if an intestinal bypass is required. In this instance, oral erythromycin and neomycin are administered in 1-g preparations at 1 PM, 2 PM, and 11 PM for a morning surgery planned for the next day. Polyethylene glycol solutions are administered to mechanically cleanse the bowel.

After a general anesthetic agent is administered, the patient is placed in the supine position, with the operating surgeon on the right side of the patient. Some degree of reverse Trendelenburg positioning will also facilitate exposure. A midline incision from the xiphoid to the umbilicus is adequate for most gastric operations and can easily be extended bidirectionally in obese patients and those for whom better exposure is mandated.

On entering the abdomen, the surgeon should perform a routine exploration of the abdominal cavity. A nasogastric tube for decompression of the stomach should be placed by the anesthetist, if not already in place, to allow orientation within the abdomen. Although it is often maintained postoperatively, routine nasogastric decompression has not been shown to affect outcomes in postgastrectomy patients in several reports.

PROCEDURES

Truncal Vagotomy

The steps involved in truncal vagotomy include the following sequence: exposure of the esophagogastric junction (Figs. 57–1 to 57–4), exposure of the anterior vagus nerve (Fig. 57–5), ligation of the nerve trunk (Fig. 57–6), exposure and isolation of the posterior vagus nerve (Fig. 57–7), and ligation of the nerve trunk (Fig. 57–8).

Proximal Gastric Vagotomy

The steps involved in proximal gastric vagotomy include the following sequence: interior anterior dissection (Figs. 57–9 and 57–10), neurovascular ligation (Fig. 57–11), periesophageal and posterior dissection (Figs. 57–11 and 57–12), and esophageal skeletonization (Figs. 57–13 and 57–14).

Highly Selective Vagotomy

The steps involved in highly selective vagotomy include the following sequence: port placement (Fig. 57–15), exposure of the gastroesophageal junction (Fig. 57–16), division of the gastrohepatic omentum (Fig. 57–17), isolation of the posterior trunk (Fig. 57–18), division of the posterior trunk (Fig. 57–19), identification of the anterior trunk (Fig. 57–20), and division of the vagal branches (Fig. 57–21).

Pyloroplasty

The steps involved in pyloroplasty include the following sequence: (1) incision (Figs. 57–22 and 57–23) and closure (Figs. 57–24 and 57–25) for the Heineke-Mikulicz pyloroplasty; (2) incision (Fig. 57–26), posterior closure (Fig. 57–27), and anterior closure for the Finney pyloroplasty (Figs. 57–28 and 57–29); and (3) incision (Figs. 57–30 and 57–31) and closure (Fig. 57–32) for the Jaboulay pyloroplasty.

Text continued on p. 845

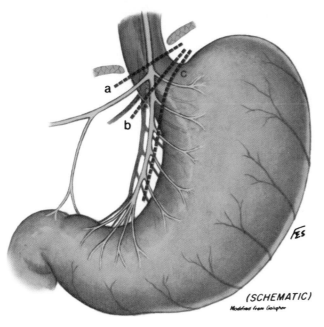

(SCHEMATIC)

Modified from Gallagher

Figure 57–1. Depiction of normal vagal anatomy and the traditional incision sites for standard vagotomies. Truncal vagotomy, shown as the incision at level *a*, involves transection of the nerves as they traverse the diaphragmatic hiatus. Selective vagotomy *(b)* severs the vagal trunks after the takeoff of the hepatic and celiac branches. Proximal gastric vagotomy (also highly selective vagotomy and parietal cell vagotomy) *(c)* incises the esophagogastric vagal branches at the level of the stomach while preserving the hepatic and celiac branches, as well as innervation to the antrum and pylorus (the "crow's foot" of the nerves of Latarjet). (From Braasch JW: Truncal vagotomy and Heineke-Mikulicz pyloroplasty including selective vagotomy. In Braasch JW, Sedgewick CE, Veidenheimer MC, Ellis FH Jr [eds]: Atlas of Abdominal Surgery. Philadelphia, WB Saunders, 1991, p 48.)

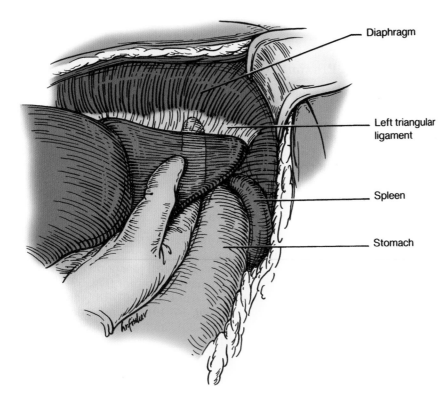

Diaphragm

Left triangular ligament

Spleen

Stomach

Figure 57–2. The left lateral segment of the liver should be mobilized to allow full exposure of the gastroesophageal junction. The surgeon's right hand retracts the left lateral segment inferiorly to expose the left triangular ligament, which is thin and translucent. This ligament can be divided by electrocautery; mobilization need proceed only to the midline for adequate exposure. Care should be taken to avoid the inferior phrenic vein as the midline is approached. (From Mulholland MW: Atlas of gastric surgery. In Bell RH Jr, Rikkers LF, Mulholland MW [eds]: Digestive Tract Surgery. Philadelphia, Lippincott-Raven, 1996, p 306.)

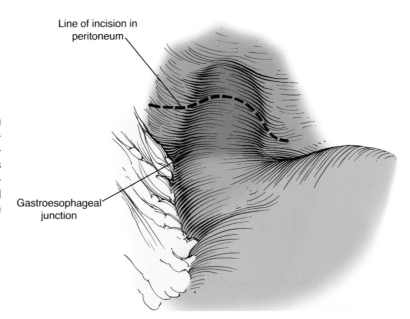

Figure 57–3. Line for incision of the peritoneum to expose the distal esophagus and gastroesophageal junction. Palpation of the preoperatively placed nasogastric tube ensures that this location is correct. (From Pappas TN: Truncal vagotomy. In Sabiston DC Jr [ed]: Atlas of General Surgery. Philadelphia WB Saunders, 1994, p 330.)

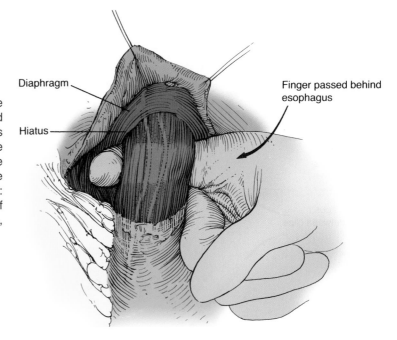

Figure 57–4. Blunt, gentle encirclement of the esophageal hiatus after exposure should be attempted as cephalad as possible to capture the posterior vagus in the encirclement. Palpation of the nasogastric tube before this maneuver will help avoid errors. A Penrose drain or umbilical tape is then placed around the esophagus to aid in retraction. (From Pappas TN: Truncal vagotomy. In Sabiston DC Jr [ed]: Atlas of General Surgery. Philadelphia, WB Saunders, 1994, p 330.)

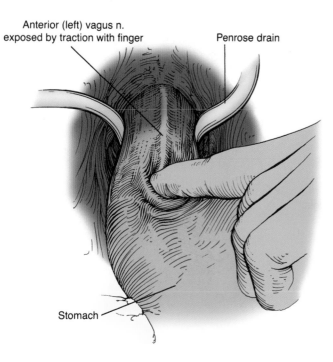

Anterior (left) vagus n.
exposed by traction with finger

Penrose drain

Stomach

Figure 57–5. Exposure of the anterior vagus nerve. This structure is often likened to a bowstring and is palpated by passing a finger across the distal end of the esophagus. If the anterior vagus is not palpable, it usually becomes more prominent, as shown here, with gentle downward traction on the stomach. If the nerve cannot be found with these maneuvers, gentle downward traction can be placed on the hepatic branch of the anterior vagus nerve, which will expose the anterior trunk. The hepatic branch is usually visible within the gastrohepatic ligament. (From Pappas TN: Truncal vagotomy. In Sabiston DC Jr [ed]: Atlas of General Surgery. Philadelphia, WB Saunders, 1994, p 331.)

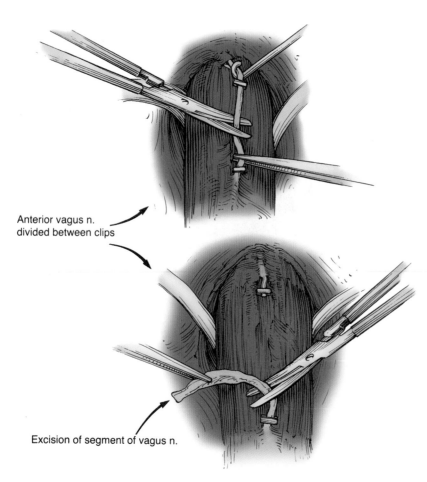

Anterior vagus n.
divided between clips

Excision of segment of vagus n.

Figure 57–6. Ligation and excision of the anterior vagus nerve. A 2-cm length of nerve is excised and sent to the pathology laboratory for histologic confirmation. (From Pappas TN: Truncal vagotomy. In Sabiston DC Jr [ed]: Atlas of General Surgery. Philadelphia, WB Saunders, 1994, p 331.)

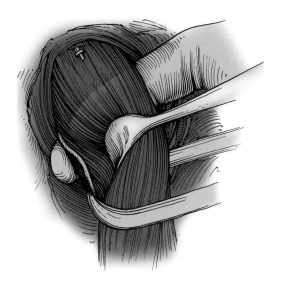

Figure 57–7.   Exposure of the posterior vagus nerve, which usually lies between the esophagus and the right crus of the diaphragm. The esophagus is retracted to the left and anteriorly to expose the right crus. The Penrose drain should contain the posterior vagus nerve if the blunt encirclement was performed at or above the level of the diaphragm. With slight rotation of the esophagus, the nerve is identified by the surgeon's finger and delivered into view. If the vagus cannot be found, palpation of the esophagus should be performed to locate the nerve before separating it from the esophagus. Alternatively, one could retract the celiac division of the posterior vagus if it is easily seen. (From Pappas TN: Truncal vagotomy. In Sabiston DC Jr [ed]: Atlas of General Surgery. Philadelphia, WB Saunders, 1994, p 332.)

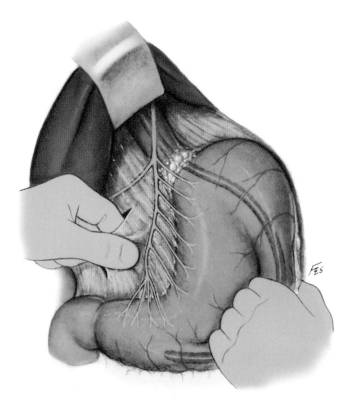

Figure 57–9.   Initial exposure for proximal gastric vagotomy. The gastrohepatic ligament is opened after confirmation of the absence of a replaced left hepatic artery. The anterior nerve of Latarjet is tented to expose its gastric branches. The hepatic branch is identified and preserved. The first assistant stabilizes the stomach to prevent avulsion of the short gastric vessels and consequent splenic injury. (From Rossi RL: Parietal cell vagotomy [highly selective vagotomy]. In Braasch JW, Sedgewick CE, Veidenheimer MC, Ellis FH Jr [eds]: Atlas of Abdominal Surgery. Philadelphia, WB Saunders, 1991, p 56.)

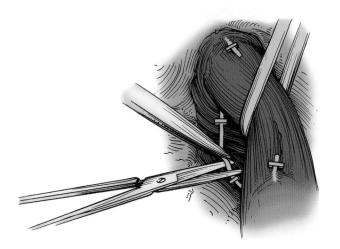

Figure 57–8.   Ligation of the posterior vagus, with excision of a 2-cm portion that is sent to the pathology laboratory. (From Pappas TN: Truncal vagotomy. In Sabiston DC Jr [ed]: Atlas of General Surgery. Philadelphia, WB Saunders, 1994, p 332.)

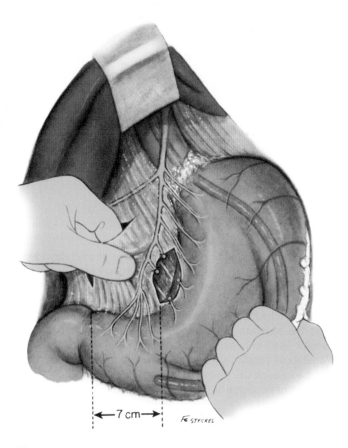

Figure 57–10. Dissection is initiated 7 cm proximal to the pylorus, which will allow preservation of the anterior nerve of Latarjet and maintain antral and pyloric innervation. (From Rossi RL: Parietal cell vagotomy [highly selective vagotomy]. In Braasch JW, Sedgewick CE, Veidenheimer MC, Ellis FH Jr [eds]: Atlas of Abdominal Surgery. Philadelphia, WB Saunders, 1991, p 57.)

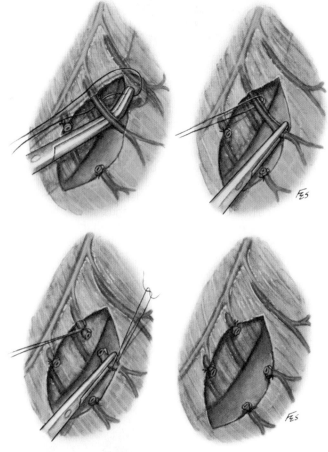

Figure 57–11. Ligation of the neurovascular bundles, which proceeds cephalad toward the gastroesophageal junction and continues completely over the esophagus toward the angle of His to completely skeletonize the stomach body and fundus. (From Rossi RL: Parietal cell vagotomy [highly selective vagotomy]. In Braasch JW, Sedgewick CE, Veidenheimer MC, Ellis FH Jr [eds]: Atlas of Abdominal Surgery. Philadelphia, WB Saunders, 1991, p 56.)

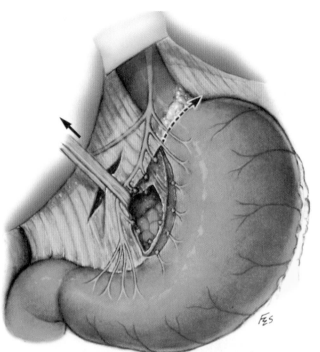

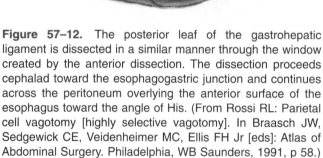

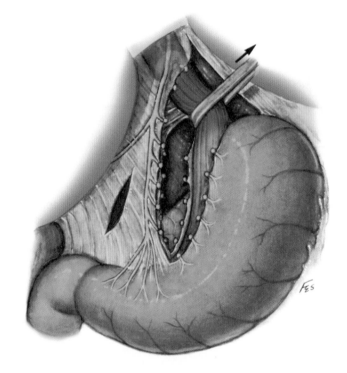

Figure 57–12. The posterior leaf of the gastrohepatic ligament is dissected in a similar manner through the window created by the anterior dissection. The dissection proceeds cephalad toward the esophagogastric junction and continues across the peritoneum overlying the anterior surface of the esophagus toward the angle of His. (From Rossi RL: Parietal cell vagotomy [highly selective vagotomy]. In Braasch JW, Sedgewick CE, Veidenheimer MC, Ellis FH Jr [eds]: Atlas of Abdominal Surgery. Philadelphia, WB Saunders, 1991, p 58.)

Figure 57–13. Fibers from the anterior vagus are gently swept off the anterior surface of the esophagus and divided. The distal end of the esophagus is skeletonized for 6 to 8 cm to completely divide the vagal efferents, some of which travel intramurally to innervate the proximal part of the stomach. Special attention should be directed toward division of the "criminal" nerves of Grassi, which loop off the posterior vagus and travel posteriorly to innervate the superior fundus. (From Rossi RL: Parietal cell vagotomy [highly selective vagotomy]. In Braasch JW, Sedgewick CE, Veidenheimer MC, Ellis FH Jr [eds]: Atlas of Abdominal Surgery. Philadelphia, WB Saunders, 1991, p 59.)

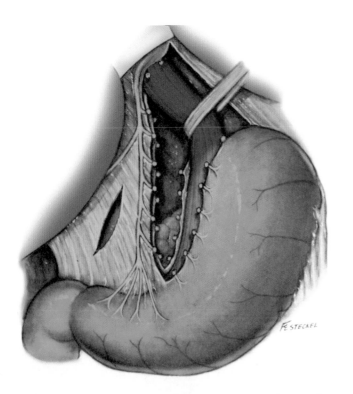

Figure 57–14. Completed dissection demonstrating sparing of the anterior and posterior trunks, as well as innervation to the antrum. (From Rossi RL: Parietal cell vagotomy [highly selective vagotomy]. In Braasch JW, Sedgewick CE, Veidenheimer MC, Ellis FH Jr [eds]: Atlas of Abdominal Surgery. Philadelphia, WB Saunders, 1991, p 59.)

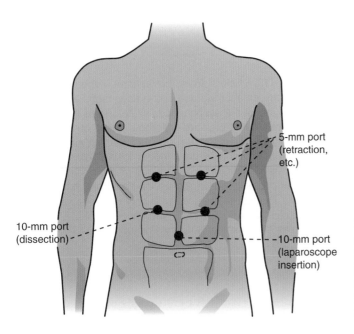

Figure 57–15. Sites of port placement for laparoscopic highly selective vagotomy. Pneumoperitoneum is established in standard fashion. The camera is introduced through the umbilical port, retractors for the liver and the stomach are placed through the two superior ports, and the remaining ports are used for the dissection. Reverse Trendelenburg positioning is used to aid in exposure.

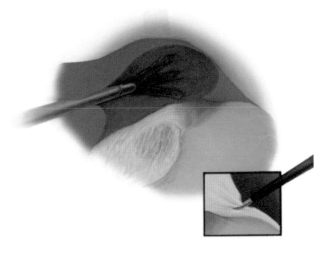

Figure 57–16. A fan-type retractor is used to retract the left lateral segment of the liver away from the gastroesophageal junction. Partial division of the left triangular ligament *(inset)* allows for optimal retraction. (From Bailey RW, Zucker KA, Flowers JL: Vagotomy. In Ballantyne GA, Leahy PF, Modlin IM [eds]: Laparoscopic Surgery. Philadelphia, WB Saunders, 1994, p 409.)

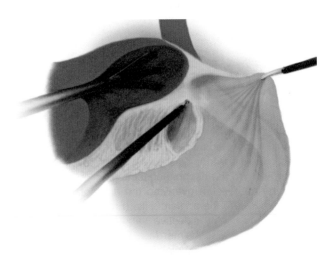

Figure 57–17. A window is created in the avascular portion of the gastrohepatic ligament along the lesser curvature to approach the posterior aspect of the gastroesophageal junction. The stomach is retracted toward the left to aid in this dissection. (From Bailey RW, Zucker KA, Flowers JL: Vagotomy. In Ballantyne GA, Leahy PF, Modlin IM [eds]: Laparoscopic Surgery. Philadelphia, WB Saunders, 1994, p 409.)

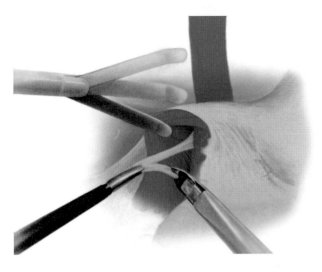

Figure 57–18. The right crus of the diaphragm is retracted to the patient's right to allow identification of the posterior vagal trunk behind the esophagus. The nerve is isolated and exposed for ligation. (From Bailey RW, Zucker KA, Flowers JL: Vagotomy. In Ballantyne GA, Leahy PF, Modlin IM [eds]: Laparoscopic Surgery. Philadelphia, WB Saunders, 1994, p 411.)

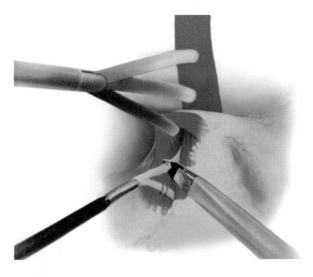

Figure 57–19. The main trunk of the posterior vagus is clipped and ligated; the proximal extent of ligation should be as close as possible to the esophageal hiatus. (From Bailey RW, Zucker KA, Flowers JL: Vagotomy. In Ballantyne GA, Leahy PF, Modlin IM [eds]: Laparoscopic Surgery. Philadelphia, WB Saunders, 1994, p 411.)

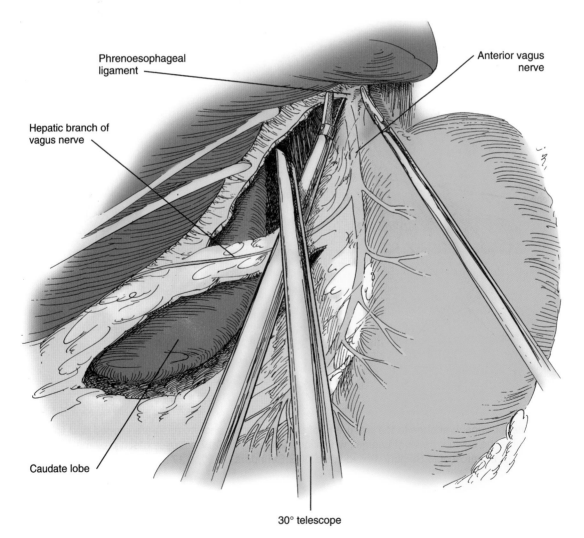

Figure 57–20. The anterior vagal trunk is located in the peritoneum on the anterior surface of the esophagus and then gently elevated to provide optimal exposure. (From Ballantyne GH: Atlas of Laparoscopic Surgery. Philadelphia, WB Saunders, 2000, p 167.)

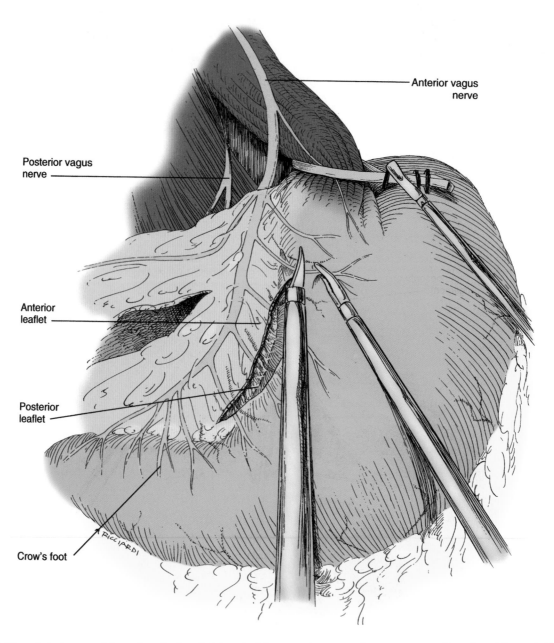

Figure 57–21. Anterior vagal branches to the distal end of the esophagus and stomach are clipped and ligated. This continues caudally but spares the anterior nerve of Latarjet, which innervates the distal 7 cm of stomach proximal to the pylorus. (From Ballantyne GH: Atlas of Laparoscopic Surgery. Philadelphia, WB Saunders, 2000, p 171.)

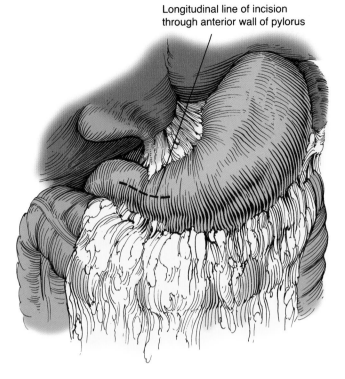

Longitudinal line of incision through anterior wall of pylorus

Figure 57–22. The Heineke-Mikulicz procedure is the most widely used pyloroplasty. In a strict sense, a Heineke-Mikulicz pyloroplasty is a two-layer closure, whereas most surgeons actually perform the one-layer modification: the Weinberg pyloroplasty. This procedure is acceptable if there is minimal scarring at the pylorus and no foreshortening of the proximal end of the duodenum. After kocherization of the duodenum, a longitudinal incision is centered over the anterior pylorus and extends 2 to 3 cm proximally and distally. (From Meyers WC: Heineke-Mikulicz pyloroplasty. In Sabiston DC Jr [ed]: Atlas of General Surgery. Philadelphia, WB Saunders, 1994, p 251.)

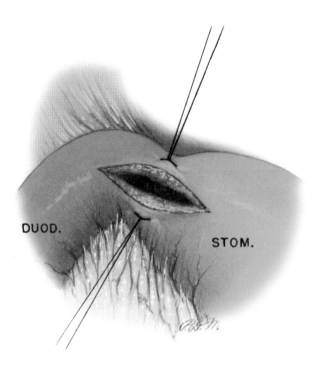

DUOD.   STOM.

Figure 57–23. After the incision, silk sutures are placed superiorly and inferiorly at the pylorus for traction and orientation. (From Braasch JW: Truncal vagotomy and Heineke-Mikulicz pyloroplasty including selective vagotomy. In Braasch JW, Sedgewick CE, Veidenheimer MC, Ellis FH Jr [eds]: Atlas of Abdominal Surgery. Philadelphia, WB Saunders, 1991, p 51.)

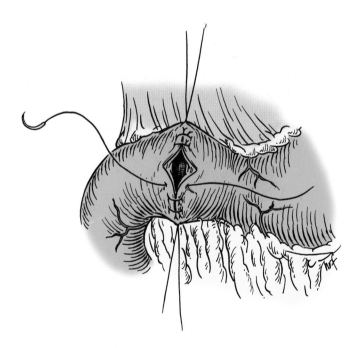

Figure 57–24. The longitudinal incision is closed transversely, which widens the pyloric channel. The closure is usually performed with a single layer of interrupted nonabsorbable sutures, each placed as shown. (From Mulholland MW: Atlas of gastric surgery. In Bell RH Jr, Rikkers LF, Mulholland MW [eds]: Digestive Tract Surgery. Philadelphia, Lippincott-Raven, 1996, p 316.)

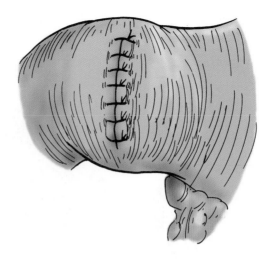

Figure 57–25. Completed Heineke-Mikulicz pyloroplasty. (From Soybel DI, Zinner MJ: Stomach and duodenum: Operative procedures. In Zinner MJ, Schwartz SI, Ellis H [eds]: Maingot's Abdominal Operations. Stamford, CT, Appleton & Lange, 1997, p 1095.)

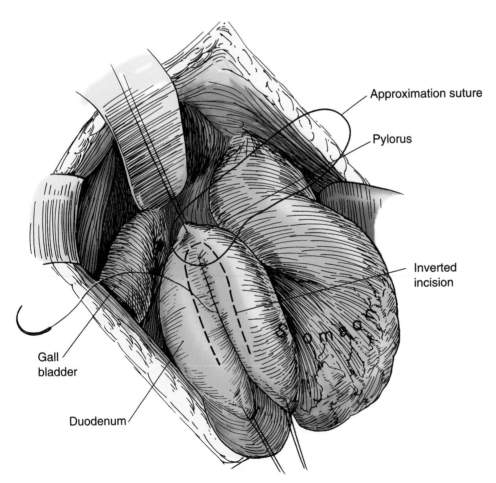

Figure 57–26. Orientation for a Finney pyloroplasty. After kocherization of the duodenum, a single stay stitch is placed superiorly for traction. A posterior row of sutures is used to appose the duodenum to the distal antrum with 3-0 silk sutures. An inverted U-shaped incision is made between the aligned duodenum and stomach. (From Soybel DI, Zinner MJ: Stomach and duodenum: Operative procedures. In Zinner MJ, Schwartz SI, Ellis H [eds]: Maingot's Abdominal Operations. Stamford, CT, Appleton & Lange, 1997, p 1096.)

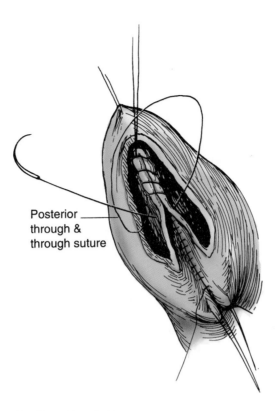

Figure 57–27. Absorbable suture is used to anastomose the mucosa of the stomach to that of the duodenum. This suture line starts posteriorly and continues anteriorly. (From Soybel DI, Zinner MJ: Stomach and duodenum: Operative procedures. In Zinner MJ, Schwartz SI, Ellis H [eds]: Maingot's Abdominal Operations. Stamford, CT, Appleton & Lange, 1997, p 1096.)

Figure 57–28. The mucosal stitch is continued anteriorly to complete the anastomosis. (From Mulholland MW: Atlas of gastric surgery. In Bell RH Jr, Rikkers LF, Mulholland MW [eds]: Digestive Tract Surgery. Philadelphia, Lippincott-Raven, 1996, p 318.)

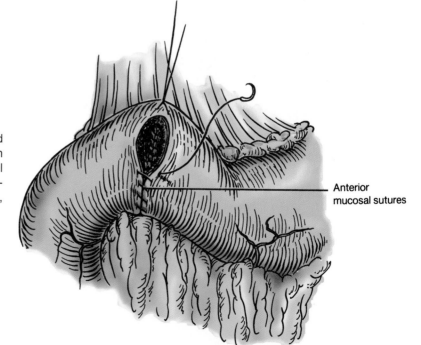

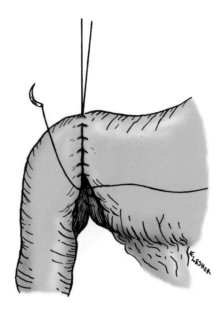

Figure 57–29. Nonabsorbable sutures are placed in Lembert fashion over the closure to complete the anastomosis. (From Sawyers JL: Selective vagotomy and pyloroplasty. In Nyhus LM, Baker RJ, Fischer JE [eds]: Mastery of Surgery. Boston, Little, Brown, 1997, p 888.)

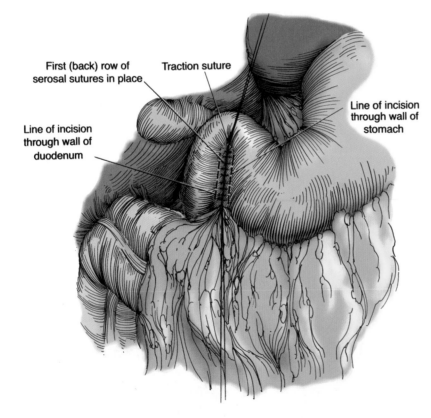

First (back) row of serosal sutures in place

Traction suture

Line of incision through wall of stomach

Line of incision through wall of duodenum

Figure 57–30. A Jaboulay pyloroplasty is used when pylorus is too scarred to attempt to manipulate it. In actuality, a Jaboulay pyloroplasty is a gastroduodenostomy that does not traverse the pylorus. After a Kocher maneuver to mobilize the duodenum, traction sutures are placed to allow the normal duodenum distal to the scarring to be apposed to the distal antrum. Interrupted silk sutures are placed posteriorly before matching incisions are made. (From Meyers WC: Jaboulay pyloroplasty. In Sabiston DC Jr [ed]: Atlas of General Surgery. Philadelphia, WB Saunders, 1994, p 259.)

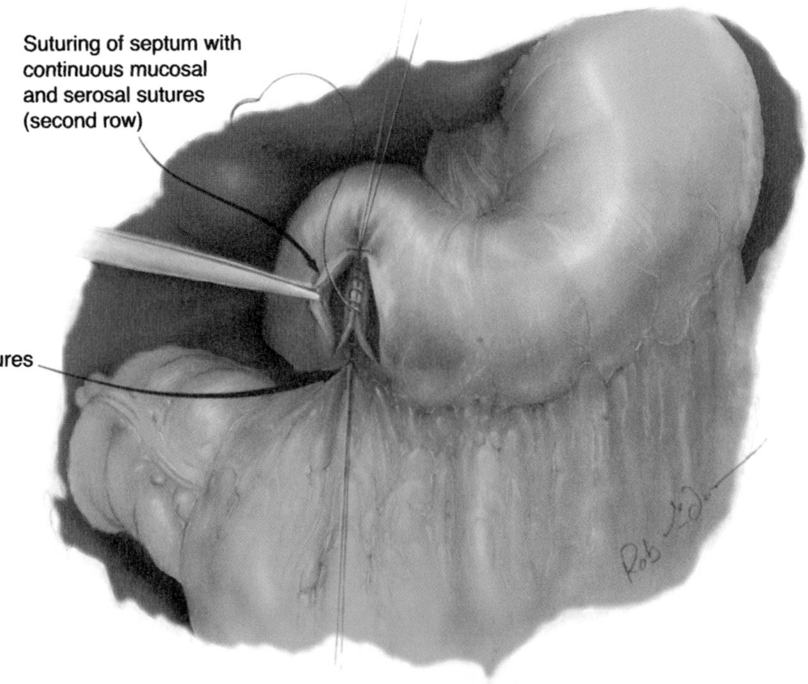

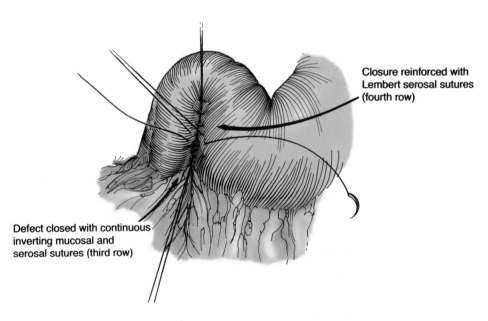

Figure 57–31. Parallel incisions are made in the duodenum and stomach and closed in two layers with mucosal absorbable suture and outer nonabsorbable suture. The pylorus is not incised or dilated. (From Meyers WC: Jaboulay pyloroplasty. In Sabiston DC Jr [ed]: Atlas of General Surgery. Philadelphia, WB Saunders, 1994, p 260.)

Suturing of septum with continuous mucosal and serosal sutures (second row)

First row of serosal sutures

Closure reinforced with Lembert serosal sutures (fourth row)

Figure 57–32. Lembert serosal sutures complete the anastomosis. (From Meyers WC: Jaboulay pyloroplasty. In Sabiston DC Jr [ed]: Atlas of General Surgery. Philadelphia, WB Saunders, 1994, p 260.)

Defect closed with continuous inverting mucosal and serosal sutures (third row)

Gastrojejunostomy

The steps involved in gastrojejunostomy include the following sequence: creation of a transverse mesenteric window (Fig. 57–33), selection of the site for anastomosis (Figs. 57–34 and 57–35), completion of a two-layer anastomosis (Figs. 57–35 to 57–39), and closure of the mesenteric defect.

Distal Gastrectomy

The steps involved in distal gastrectomy include the following sequence: division of the gastrocolic omentum

(Fig. 57–40); division of the gastroepiploic vessels (Fig. 57–41); ligation of the right gastric vessels and dissection of the lesser curvature (Fig. 57–42); division of the duodenum (Fig. 57–43); division of the proximal end of the stomach (Fig. 57–44); reconstruction by gastrojejunostomy, sutured technique (Figs. 57–45 to 57–48) and stapled technique (Figs. 57–49 and 57–50); and reconstruction via gastroduodenoscopy, sutured technique (Figs. 57–51 to 57–54) and stapled technique (Figs. 57–55 to 57–57).

Text continued on p. 857

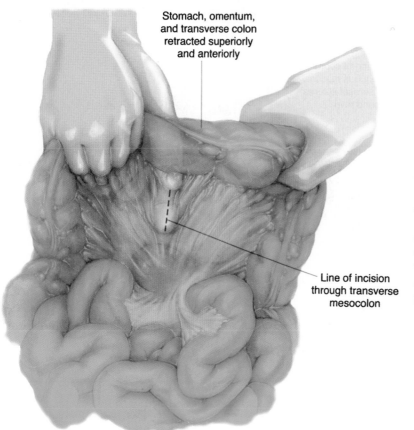

Figure 57–33. Selection of the site in the transverse mesentery to create a window for the gastrojejunostomy. The transverse colon is retracted upward to allow inspection for identification of an avascular area to the left of the middle colic vessels. A vertical incision is created to allow delivery of the distal end of the stomach. (From Peete WPJ: Gastrojejunostomy. In Sabiston DC Jr [ed]: Atlas of General Surgery. Philadelphia, WB Saunders, 1994, p 348.)

Stomach, omentum, and transverse colon retracted superiorly and anteriorly

Line of incision through transverse mesocolon

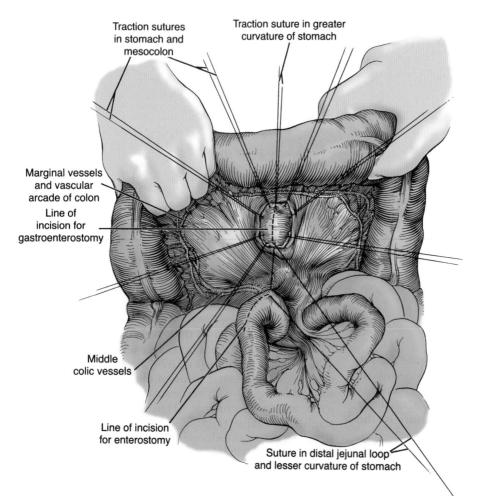

Figure 57–34. The gastric site that is chosen for anastomosis should be in the distal antrum for optimal drainage, be of normal tissue, and be free of large vessels. The stomach is delivered through the mesenteric defect and secured in place with interrupted sutures between the transverse mesocolon and the antrum. These sutures also close the mesenteric defect. The most proximal portion of jejunum that reaches the antrum without tension is placed in apposition to the stomach. (From Peete WPJ: Gastrojejunostomy. In Sabiston DC Jr [ed]: Atlas of General Surgery. Philadelphia, WB Saunders, 1994, p 349.)

Traction sutures in stomach and mesocolon

Traction suture in greater curvature of stomach

Marginal vessels and vascular arcade of colon

Line of incision for gastroenterostomy

Middle colic vessels

Line of incision for enterostomy

Suture in distal jejunal loop and lesser curvature of stomach

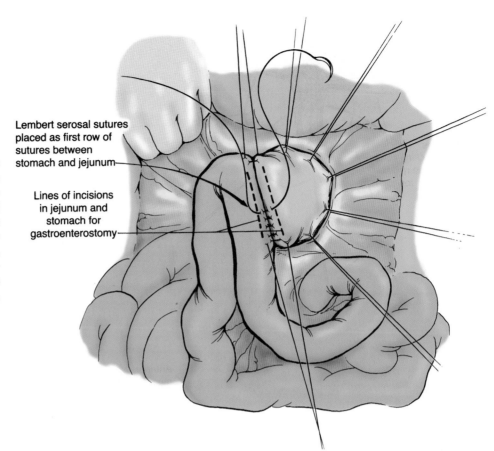

Figure 57–35. The jejunum is fixed in position with traction sutures. Interrupted nonabsorbable sutures are then placed in seromuscular fashion from the inferior gastric wall to the antimesenteric border of the jejunum. (From Peete WPJ: Gastrojejunostomy. In Sabiston DC Jr [ed]: Atlas of General Surgery. Philadelphia, WB Saunders, 1994, p 350.)

Lembert serosal sutures placed as first row of sutures between stomach and jejunum

Lines of incisions in jejunum and stomach for gastroenterostomy

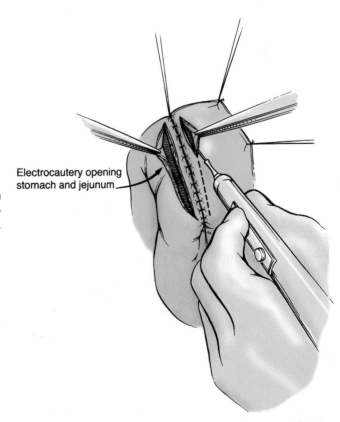

Electrocautery opening stomach and jejunum

Figure 57–36. Matching incisions in the stomach and jejunum are created with electrocautery. (From Peete WPJ: Gastrojejunostomy. In Sabiston DC Jr [ed]: Atlas of General Surgery. Philadelphia, WB Saunders, 1994, p 351.)

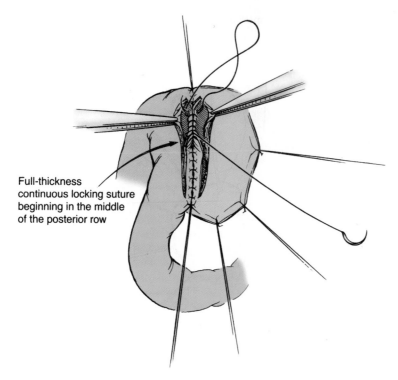

Full-thickness
continuous locking suture
beginning in the middle
of the posterior row

Figure 57–37. A continuous mucosal suture with 3-0 absorbable material is placed. The suture starts posteriorly and is performed most easily with a double-armed stitch. (From Peete WPJ: Gastrojejunostomy. In Sabiston DC Jr [ed]: Atlas of General Surgery. Philadelphia, WB Saunders, 1994, p 351.)

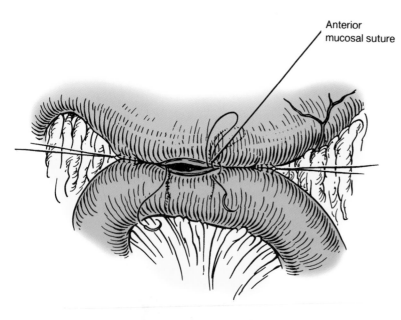

Anterior
mucosal suture

Figure 57–38. The anastomosis continues anteriorly. (From Mulholland MW: Atlas of gastric surgery. In Bell RH Jr, Rikkers LF, Mulholland MW [eds]: Digestive Tract Surgery. Philadelphia, Lippincott-Raven, 1996, p 325.)

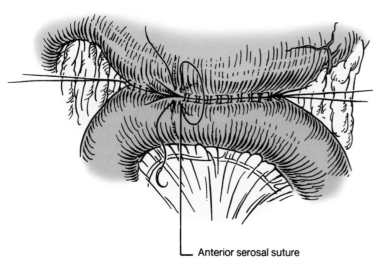

Figure 57–39. The double-layer anastomosis is completed with an anterior seromuscular layer of interrupted silk 3-0 sutures. (From Mulholland MW: Atlas of gastric surgery. In Bell RH Jr, Rikkers LF, Mulholland MW [eds]: Digestive Tract Surgery. Philadelphia, Lippincott-Raven, 1996, p 326.)

Anterior serosal suture

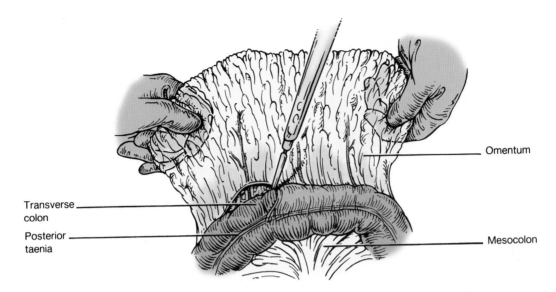

Figure 57–40.   Partial gastrectomy is initiated with a full Kocher maneuver that mobilizes the duodenum. The next goal is entry into the lesser sac to allow early evaluation of the posterior surface of the stomach and to aid in division of the greater omentum. With cephalad retraction of the greater omentum, an avascular plane above the transverse colon can be entered. The maneuver is performed left of midline to avoid encroachment on the middle colic vessels. (From Mulholland MW: Atlas of gastric surgery. In Bell RH Jr, Rikkers LF, Mulholland MW [eds]: Digestive Tract Surgery. Philadelphia, Lippincott-Raven, 1996, p 342.)

Figure 57–41. The gastrocolic omentum is then dissected from the stomach. The dissection begins at the pylorus with ligation of the right gastroepiploic artery and proceeds cephalad along the greater curvature. The gastroepiploic vessels may be preserved with benign disease. For a 50% gastric resection, the dissection ends halfway between the pylorus and the esophagogastric junction and spares the left gastroepiploic vessels and the short gastric vessels. For subtotal gastrectomy, the left gastroepiploic vessels are divided, as well as a portion of the short gastric vessels. The posterior antrum is then separated from the anterior pancreas and base of the transverse mesocolon by division of fine connective tissue attachments. (From Jones RS: Gastric resection: Billroth I anastomosis. In Sabiston DC Jr [ed]: Atlas of General Surgery. Philadelphia, WB Saunders, 1994, p 263.)

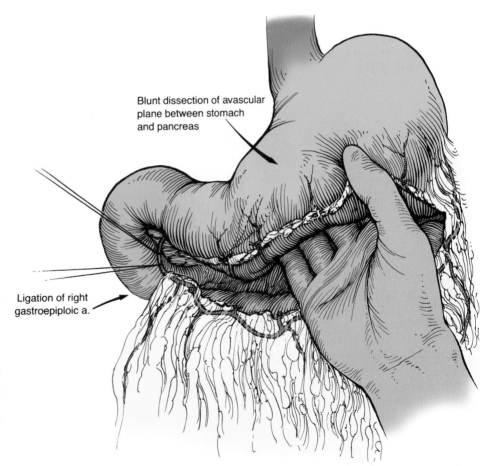

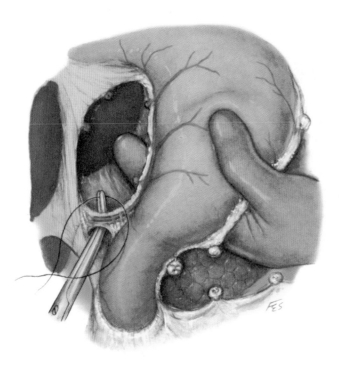

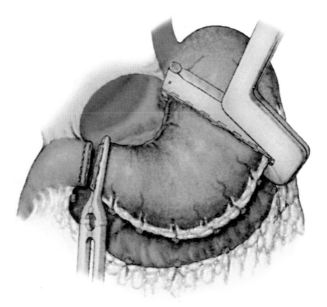

Figure 57–42. The gastrohepatic ligament is incised, and the lesser curvature is dissected. The right gastric vessels are ligated close to the stomach. In patients with pyloric inflammation, care must be taken to avoid injury to both the hepatic artery and the common bile duct. (From Sedgewick C: Gastrectomy. In Braasch JW, Sedgewick CE, Veidenheimer MC, Ellis FH Jr [eds]: Atlas of Abdominal Surgery. Philadelphia, WB Saunders, 1991, p 37.)

Figure 57–44. The proximal end of the stomach is divided with a TA-90 stapling device. Gastric resection can also be accomplished with two applications of a GIA stapling device. (From Stapling Techniques in General Surgery. Norwalk, CT, United States Surgical Corporation, 1988, p 59. Trademark of United States Surgical. Copyright © 1974, 1980, 1988, 2001 United States Surgical. Reprinted with permission of United States Surgical, a Division of Healthcare Group LP.)

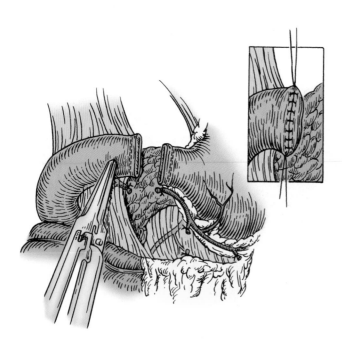

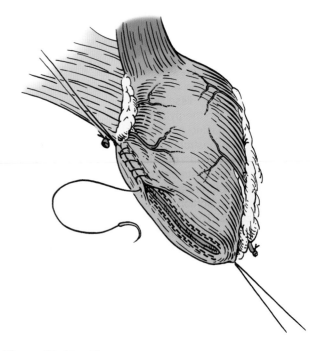

Figure 57–43. The proximal duodenum is divided with care to avoid injury to the common bile duct. The closure is reinforced with interrupted 3-0 silk sutures at the discretion of the surgeon. (From Mulholland MW: Atlas of gastric surgery. In Bell RH Jr, Rikkers LF, Mulholland MW [eds]: Digestive Tract Surgery. Philadelphia, Lippincott-Raven, 1996, p 348.)

Figure 57–45. The gastric staple line is oversewn superiorly with either continuous or running suture. Traction sutures are useful to steady the remnant within the operative field. (From Mulholland MW: Atlas of gastric surgery. In Bell RH Jr, Rikkers LF, Mulholland MW [eds]: Digestive Tract Surgery. Philadelphia, Lippincott-Raven, 1996, p 350.)

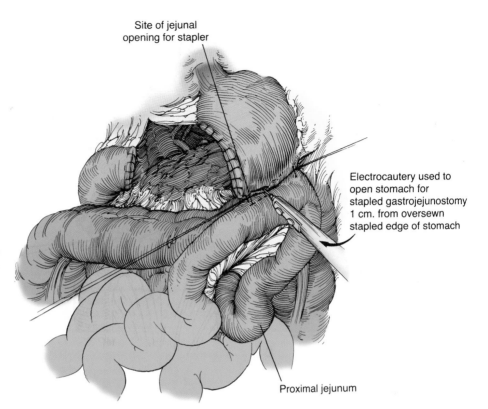

Figure 57–46. A proximal loop of jejunum is apposed to the stomach. The jejunum can be delivered through an incision in the transverse mesocolon or anterior to the transverse colon. Interrupted sutures are placed in seromuscular fashion between the posterior gastric wall and the antimesenteric border of the jejunum. (From Jones RS: Gastric resection: Billroth II. In Sabiston DC Jr [ed]: Atlas of General Surgery. Philadelphia, WB Saunders, 1994, p 284.)

Site of jejunal opening for stapler

Electrocautery used to open stomach for stapled gastrojejunostomy 1 cm. from oversewn stapled edge of stomach

Proximal jejunum

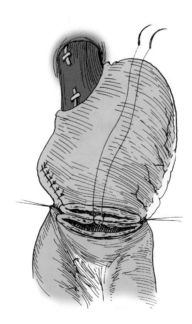

Figure 57–47. Matching incisions are made with electrocautery in the jejunum and stomach, with the latter involving partial excision of the stapled gastric closure. The posterior mucosal closure is initiated with a continuous suture of absorbable material on a double arm. Corner stitches include the anterior gastric wall, the posterior gastric wall, and the jejunum. (From Soybel DI, Zinner MJ: Stomach and duodenum: Operative procedures. In Zinner MJ, Schwartz SI, Ellis H [eds]: Maingot's Abdominal Operations. Stamford, CT, Appleton & Lange, 1997, p 1112.)

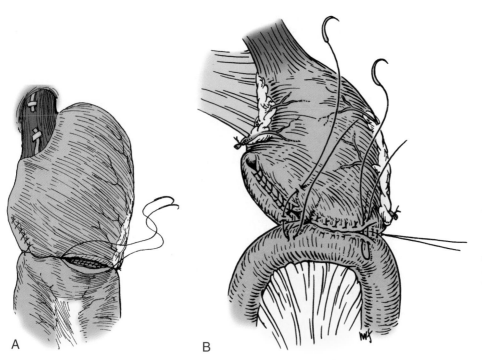

A   B

Figure 57–48. **A,** The mucosal suture is continued along the length of the anterior aspect of the anastomosis. **B,** An anterior layer of interrupted silk sutures completes the anastomosis. (**A** from Soybel DI, Zinner MJ: Stomach and duodenum: Operative procedures. In Zinner MJ, Schwartz SI, Ellis H [eds]: Maingot's Abdominal Operations. Stamford, CT, Appleton & Lange, 1997, p 1112; **B** from Mulholland MW: Atlas of gastric surgery. In Bell RH Jr, Rikkers LF, Mulholland MW [eds]: Digestive Tract Surgery. Philadelphia, Lippincott-Raven, 1996, p 352.)

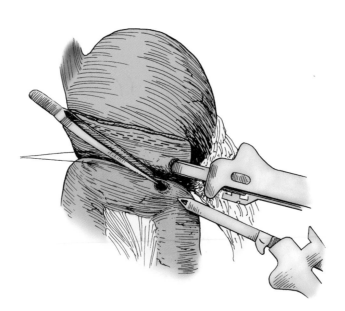

Figure 57–49. A stapled gastrojejunostomy can be created with a GIA stapling device. The posterior gastric wall is apposed to the antimesenteric surface of the jejunum with traction sutures. The site on the posterior gastric wall is usually 2 to 3 cm proximal from the stapled closure. Matching gastrotomy/enterotomy incisions are made with electrocautery to allow insertion of the GIA limbs. After the stapler is fired, the device is withdrawn and the staple line inspected for hemostasis. (From Soybel DI, Zinner MJ: Stomach and duodenum: Operative procedures. In Zinner MJ, Schwartz SI, Ellis H [eds]: Maingot's Abdominal Operations. Stamford, CT, Appleton & Lange, 1997, p 1131.)

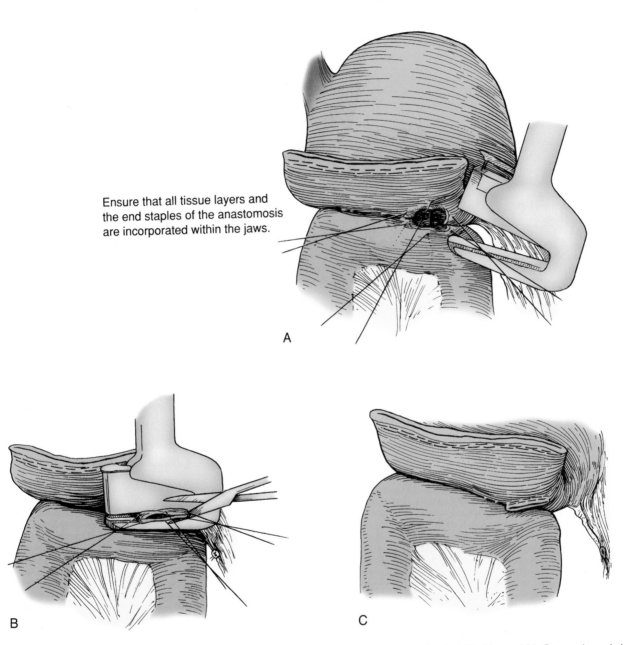

Ensure that all tissue layers and the end staples of the anastomosis are incorporated within the jaws.

A

B

C

Figure 57–50. The GIA defect is closed with the application of a TA stapler. (From Soybel DI, Zinner MJ: Stomach and duodenum: Operative procedures. In Zinner MJ, Schwartz SI, Ellis H [eds]: Maingot's Abdominal Operations. Stamford, CT, Appleton & Lange, 1997, p 1114.)

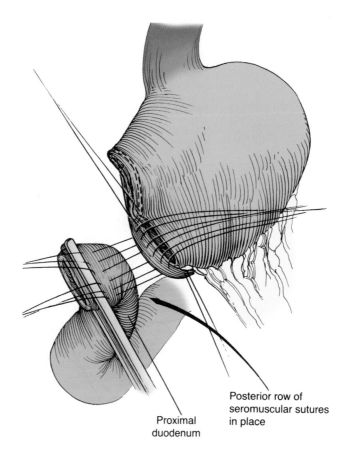

Posterior row of
seromuscular sutures
in place

Proximal
duodenum

Figure 57–51. For gastroduodenostomy reconstruction, the duodenum and the inferior gastric staple line are apposed through the placement of a posterior serosal layer of interrupted silk sutures. (From Jones RS: Gastric resection: Billroth I. In Sabiston DC Jr [ed]: Atlas of General Surgery. Philadelphia, WB Saunders, 1994, p 267.)

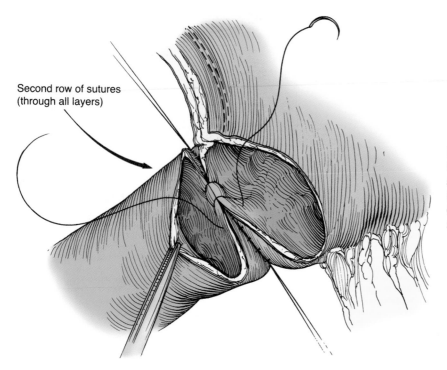

Second row of sutures
(through all layers)

Figure 57–52. An inner mucosal closure is initiated with a continuous absorbable suture. (From Jones RS: Gastric resection: Billroth I. In Sabiston DC Jr [ed]: Atlas of General Surgery. Philadelphia, WB Saunders, 1994, p 268.)

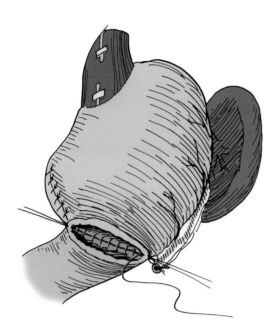

Figure 57–53. The mucosal suture continues anteriorly. (From Soybel DI, Zinner MJ: Stomach and duodenum: Operative procedures. In Zinner MJ, Schwartz SI, Ellis H [eds]: Maingot's Abdominal Operations. Stamford, CT, Appleton & Lange, 1997, p 1105.)

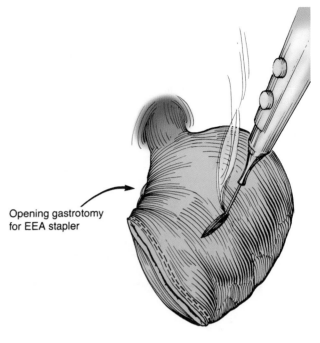

Opening gastrotomy for EEA stapler

Figure 57–55. For a stapled gastroduodenostomy, a gastrotomy is created with electrocautery on the anterior surface of the stomach at least 3 cm proximal to the staple closure. (From Siegler HF: Gastric resection: Billroth I anastomosis [stapler]. In Sabiston DC Jr [ed]: Atlas of General Surgery. Philadelphia, WB Saunders, 1994, p 274.)

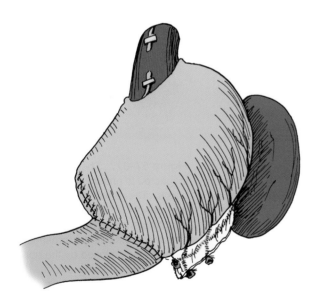

Figure 57–54. An anterior serosal layer is placed with interrupted silk seromuscular sutures. (From Soybel DI, Zinner MJ: Stomach and duodenum: Operative procedures. In Zinner MJ, Schwartz SI, Ellis H [eds]: Maingot's Abdominal Operations. Stamford, CT, Appleton & Lange, 1997, p 1105.)

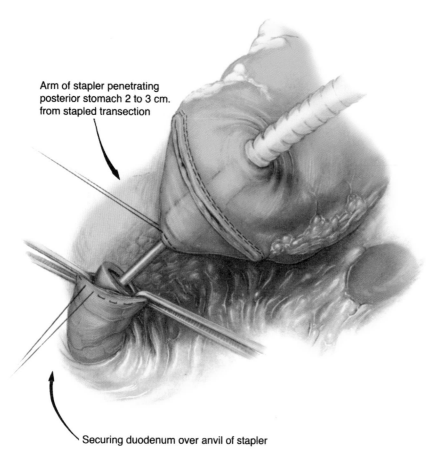

Arm of stapler penetrating
posterior stomach 2 to 3 cm.
from stapled transection

Securing duodenum over anvil of stapler

Figure 57–56. The end-to-end stapling device, without the anvil, is passed into the anterior gastrotomy with the rod advancing through the posterior gastric wall, again 3 cm proximal to the stapled edge. The anvil is introduced into the duodenum after placement of a purse-string suture with an automatic device. The EEA is closed, fired, and withdrawn. (From Siegler HF: Gastric resection: Billroth I anastomosis [stapler]. In Sabiston DC Jr [ed]: Atlas of General Surgery. Philadelphia, WB Saunders, 1994, p 275.)

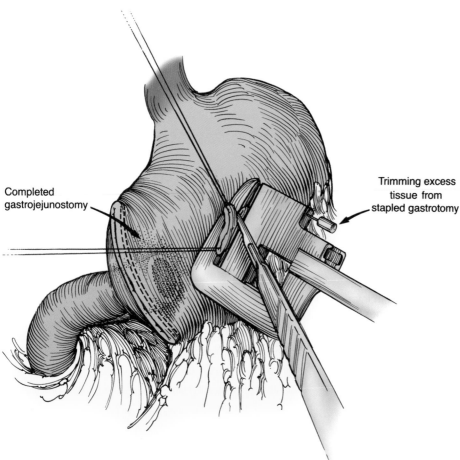

Completed
gastrojejunostomy

Trimming excess
tissue from
stapled gastrotomy

Figure 57–57. The anastomosis is inspected to ensure adequate hemostasis. The anvil is then removed and checked to ensure that tissue doughnuts from both the duodenum and the stomach are present. The gastrotomy is closed by the application of a TA stapling device. (From Siegler HF: Gastric resection: Billroth I anastomosis [stapler]. In Sabiston DC Jr [ed]: Atlas of General Surgery. Philadelphia, WB Saunders, 1994, p 276.)

Total Gastrectomy

The steps involved in total gastrectomy include the following sequence: division of the short and left gastric vessels (Figs. 57–58 to 57–60), purse-string suture and division of the esophagus (Fig. 57–61), creation of a Roux-en-Y limb (Fig. 57–62), use of the EEA stapling device (Figs. 57–63 and 57–64), completion of the anastomosis (Fig. 57–65), and enteroenterostomy.

Stamm Gastrostomy

The steps involved in the Stamm gastrostomy include the following sequence: placement of purse-string sutures (Fig. 57–66), insertion of a Foley catheter (Fig. 57–67), and placement of anchoring sutures (Fig. 57–68).

POSTOPERATIVE MANAGEMENT

Postoperative patients will often experience ileus and should undergo nasogastric decompression until bowel function returns. At this time, a diet can be initiated as well.

The incision will be closed unless a contamination event has occurred intraoperatively. Perioperative antibiotics should continue for 24 hours unless there are indications to lengthen this period.

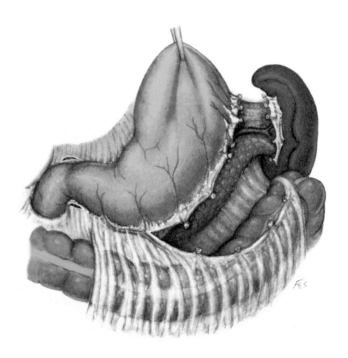

Figure 57–58. The initial steps in total gastrectomy are similar to those of distal gastrectomy. Total gastrectomy mandates a complete omentectomy. In total gastrectomy, the dissection continues cephalad to include division of the left gastroepiploic artery, as well as the short gastric vessels. (From Sedgewick C: Gastrectomy. In Braasch JW, Sedgewick CE, Veidenheimer MC, Ellis FH Jr [eds]: Atlas of Abdominal Surgery. Philadelphia, WB Saunders, 1991, p 36.)

Figure 57–59. The gastrohepatic ligament is entered as in a distal gastrectomy, with ligation of the right gastric artery. The inferior phrenic vein is ligated if encountered within the gastrohepatic ligament. (From Mulholland MW: Atlas of gastric surgery. In Bell RH Jr, Rikkers LF, Mulholland MW [eds]: Digestive Tract Surgery. Philadelphia, Lippincott-Raven, 1996, p 360.)

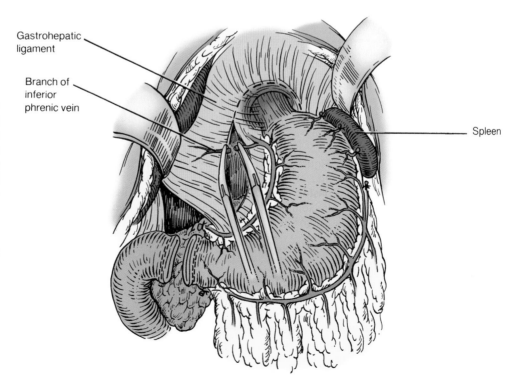

Gastrohepatic ligament

Branch of inferior phrenic vein

Spleen

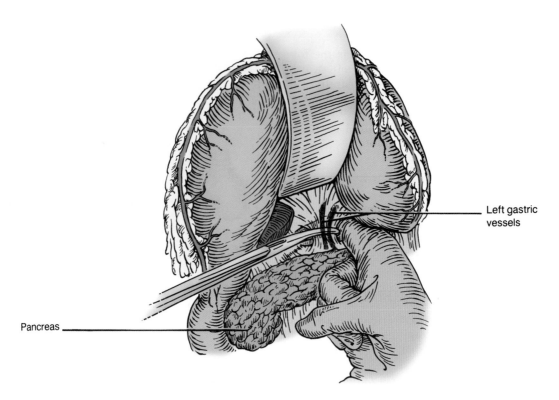

Figure 57–60.   Identification and ligation of the left gastric artery is best accomplished with cephalad retraction of the stomach. (From Mulholland MW: Atlas of gastric surgery. In Bell RH Jr, Rikkers LF, Mulholland MW [eds]: Digestive Tract Surgery. Philadelphia, Lippincott-Raven, 1996, p 361.)

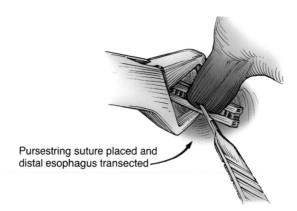

Figure 57–61.   A purse-string device is placed on the distal end of the esophagus. The esophagus is divided, and the gastric specimen is removed. (From Siegler HF: Total gastrectomy [stapler]. In Sabiston DC Jr [ed]: Atlas of General Surgery. Philadelphia WB Saunders, 1994, p 309.)

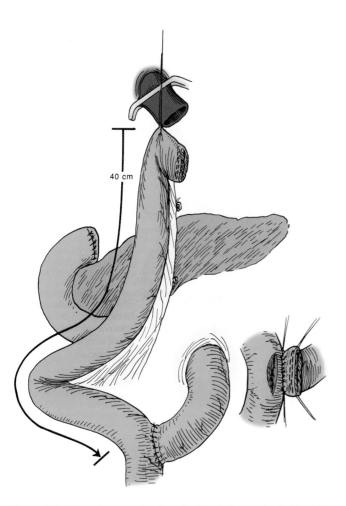

Figure 57–62. The proximal end of the jejunum is divided 10 to 20 cm distal to the ligament of Treitz. A Roux limb is delivered to the distal end of the esophagus and is 40 cm long. An end-to-side enteroenterostomy (*inset*) is performed to complete the Roux-en-Y. (From Soybel DI, Zinner MJ: Stomach and duodenum: Operative procedures. In Zinner MJ, Schwartz SI, Ellis H [eds]: Maingot's Abdominal Operations. Stamford, CT, Appleton & Lange, 1997, p 1121.)

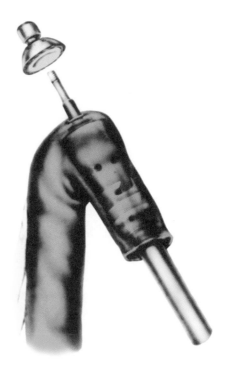

Figure 57–63. An EEA stapling device is introduced through the open end of the Roux-en-Y limb, and the rod exits 3 cm proximally along the antimesenteric border of the jejunum. The EEA device can be properly sized before the gastric resection by introducing the sizing instruments through a proximal gastrotomy just before removing the specimen. (From Ravitch MM, Steichen FM: Principles and Practice of Surgical Stapling. Chicago, Year Book, 1987, p 229.)

Figure 57–64. After EEA device placement, the anvil is positioned through the purse string and into the distal end of the esophagus. After the purse string is secured, the EEA is fired to create an end-to-side esophagojejunostomy. The EEA is carefully removed and inspected for tissue doughnuts from the esophagus and the jejunum. The anastomosis is inspected to ensure adequate hemostasis, and the open end of the jejunum is closed with a TA stapler. The nasoenteric tube is gently guided through the anastomosis. Anastomotic integrity is tested by insufflating air via the nasogastric tube after the operative field is filled with saline. The absence of bubbling from the anastomosis suggests an intact anastomosis. (From Ravitch MM, Steichen FM: Principles and Practice of Surgical Stapling. Chicago, Year Book, 1987, p 230.)

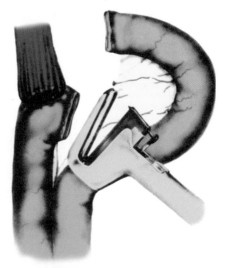

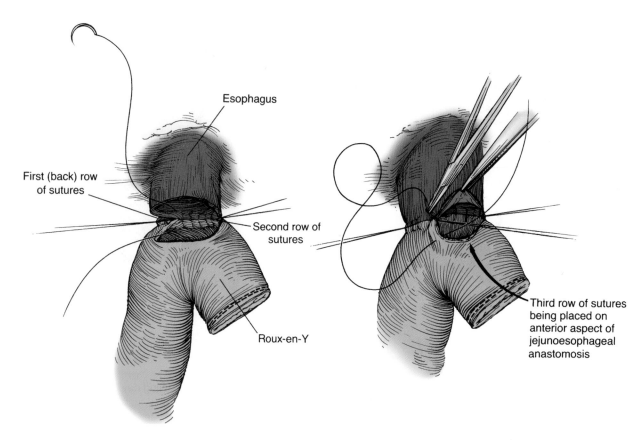

Figure 57–65. Alternatively, hand-sewn esophagojejunostomy can be performed. This is typically performed with two layers of 3-0 silk in interrupted fashion. (From Meyers WC: Total gastrectomy. In Sabiston DC Jr [ed]: Atlas of General Surgery. Philadelphia, WB Saunders, 1994, p 304.)

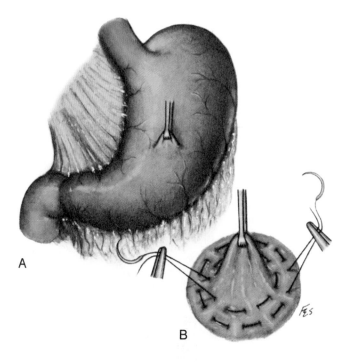

Figure 57–66. Open gastrostomy is performed either primarily or as an adjunct to a separate abdominal procedure **(A)**. The selected site on the anterior gastric wall is grasped with an Allis clamp, and two concentric purse-string sutures are placed with nonabsorbable material **(B)**. Electrocautery is used to create the gastrotomy within the purse strings. (From Sedgewick C: Gastrectomy. In Braasch JW, Sedgewick CE, Veidenheimer MC, Ellis FH Jr [eds]: Atlas of Abdominal Surgery. Philadelphia, WB Saunders, 1991, p 26.)

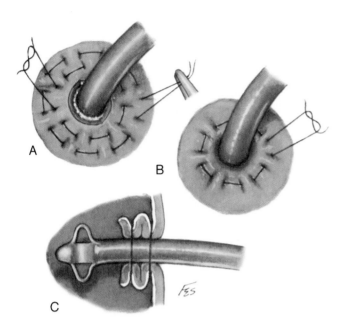

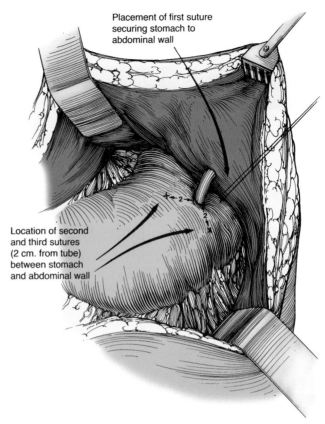

Placement of first suture securing stomach to abdominal wall

Location of second and third sutures (2 cm. from tube) between stomach and abdominal wall

Figure 57–67.   A large mushroom-tipped or Foley catheter is placed, and the purse strings are tied. (From Sedgewick C: Gastrectomy. In Braasch JW, Sedgewick CE, Veidenheimer MC, Ellis FH Jr [eds]: Atlas of Abdominal Surgery. Philadelphia, WB Saunders, 1991, p 27.)

Figure 57–68.   The tube is brought out through the abdominal wall at a site where the stomach will reach without tension. Three or four tacking sutures are placed through the abdominal wall and the seromuscular surface of the stomach. The sutures are tied to secure the stomach to the abdominal wall around the tube. (From Grant JP: Stamm gastrostomy. In Sabiston DC Jr [ed]: Atlas of General Surgery. Philadelphia, WB Saunders, 1994, p 232.)

SUGGESTED READINGS

Adachi Y, Shirasishi N, Shiromizu A, et al: Laparoscopy-assisted Billroth I gastrectomy compared with conventional open gastrectomy. Arch Surg 135:806-810, 2000.

Callahan MA, Christos PJ, Gold HT, et al: Influence of surgical subspecialty training on in-hospital mortality for gastrectomy and colectomy patients. Ann Surg 238:629-636, 2003.

Doglietto GB, Papa V, Tortorelli AP, et al: Nasojejunal tube placement after total gastrectomy: A multicenter prospective randomized trial. Arch Surg 139:1309-1313, 2004.

Donahue PE, Griffith C, Richter HM: A 50-year perspective upon selective gastric vagotomy. Am J Surg 172:9-12, 1996.

Lehnert T, Buhl K: Techniques of reconstruction after total gastrectomy for cancer. Br J Surg 91:528-539, 2004.

Nichols RL: Surgical antibiotic prophylaxis. Med Clin North Am 79:509-522, 1995.

Roberts JP, Debas HT: A simplified technique for rapid truncal vagotomy. Surg Gynecol Obstet 168:539-541, 1989.

So JB, Yam A, Cheah WK, et al: Risk factors related to operative mortality and morbidity in patients undergoing emergency gastrectomy. Br J Surg 87:1702-1707, 2000.

Thomas WEG, Thompson MH, Williamson RCN: The long-term outcome of Billroth I partial gastrectomy for benign gastric ulcers. Ann Surg 195:189-195, 1982.

Urschel JD, Blewett CJ, Bennett WF, et al: Handsewn or stapled esophagogastric anastomoses after esophagectomy for cancer: Meta-analysis of randomized controlled trials. Dis Esophagus 14:212-217, 2001.

Yoo CH, Son BH, Han WK, Pae WK: Nasogastric decompression is not necessary in operations for gastric cancer: Prospective randomized trial. Eur J Surg 168:379-383, 2002.

Zucker KA, Bailey RW: Laparoscopic truncal and selective vagotomy for intractable ulcer disease. Semin Gastrointest Dis 5:128-139, 1994.

Zollinger-Ellison Syndrome

James P. Dolan • Jeffrey A. Norton

In 1955, Zollinger and Ellison[1] first reported the occurrence of unusual, severe jejunal peptic ulcer disease associated with gastric acid hypersecretion and islet cell tumors of the pancreas. After vagotomy, antrectomy, and hemigastrectomy, recurrent peptic ulceration still developed and required total gastrectomy for control of symptoms. In consideration of the patients' complex clinical course, they postulated that the pancreatic tumor was the cause of the peptic ulcer diathesis. Subsequently, in 1972 Oberhelman and others noted that the syndrome did not require a pancreatic neuroendocrine tumor and described duodenal gastrinoma as a cause of Zollinger-Ellison syndrome (ZES).[2] We now know that ZES is caused by both pancreatic and duodenal tumors, but the most common causative tumor is a duodenal neuroendocrine tumor that elaborates excessive and unregulated amounts of the hormone gastrin.

ZES is one of many functional duodenal or pancreatic neuroendocrine syndromes. It occurs in both sporadic (80% of cases) and familial or inherited (20% of cases) forms. The familial form is associated with multiple endocrine neoplasia type I (MEN-I) syndrome, which consists of primary hyperparathyroidism and pituitary tumors in association with duodenal or pancreatic neuroendocrine tumors, of which most functional tumors are gastrinomas.[3] Although the precise incidence is unknown, it is estimated that gastrinomas develop in 1 to 3 persons per 1 million each year.[4] Furthermore, gastrinomas are the underlying cause of peptic ulcer disease in approximately 0.1% to 1% of patients.[5]

Although slow growing, more than 60% of gastrinomas are malignant, with patients having lymph node, liver, or distant metastatic disease at laparotomy.[6] In 25% of cases the tumor pursues an aggressive course.[7,8] As screening of patients with peptic ulcer disease for hypergastrinemia has become more common, a larger proportion of localized, nonmetastatic tumors are being discovered and treated.

SYMPTOMS AND SIGNS

The mean age at diagnosis of ZES is 50 years, although children as young as 7 years and adults as old as 90 years have been identified. There is a male preponderance, with a male-to-female ratio of approximately 2:1. In patients with MEN-I syndrome, ZES is usually diagnosed at the age of 20 to 30 years, whereas in the sporadic form it occurs at approximately 50 years of age.[3,6,8] The clinical manifestations are related to excessive secretion of gastric acid; the most common symptoms are epigastric pain, diarrhea, heartburn, and dysphagia (Table 58–1). The majority of patients with ZES (80% to 90%) are found to have peptic ulceration, and the proximal duodenum is the most common site of ulcer. Moreover, some patients still have multiple peptic ulcers or ulcers in unusual locations, such as the distal duodenum (14%) and jejunum (11%), or even recurrent ulceration after surgery.[9] In 7% to 10% of patients, a perforated peptic ulcer is the initial sign of ZES.[9] Gastric acid hypersecretion also leads to secretory diarrhea, which occurs in up to 40% of patients with ZES and may be the sole initial complaint in 20% of individuals.[9] In patients with diarrhea, malabsorption may be manifested as weight loss and malnutrition. Approximately 10% of patients with ZES have signs and symptoms of gastroesophageal reflux disease (GERD). Endoscopy shows evidence of lower esophageal inflammation, ulceration, and even stricture if the reflux symptoms are long-standing. As a large primary tumor burden develops or metastases occur, symptoms such as bleeding or obstruction may be related to the tumor itself.

DIAGNOSIS

Evidence suggests that in most cases there is a delay in diagnosis of ZES, with a mean period of 6 years from initial symptoms to diagnosis.[4] This delay occurs for a

Table 58–1	Usual Symptoms and Signs of Zollinger-Ellison Syndrome

Symptom or Sign	Patients (%)
Dyspepsia	80
Gastroesophageal reflux disease	60
Dysphagia	30
Diarrhea	40
Duodenal ulceration	80-90

Box 58–1 Differential Diagnosis of Hypergastrinemia

With excessive gastric acid formation (ulcerogenic)
  Zollinger-Ellison syndrome
  Gastric outlet obstruction
  Retained gastric antrum (after Billroth II reconstruction)
  G-cell hyperplasia
Without excessive gastric acid formation (nonulcerogenic)
  Pernicious anemia
  Atrophic gastritis
  Renal failure
  Postvagotomy status
  Short-gut syndrome (after significant intestinal resection)

Box 58–2 Situations in Which the Diagnosis of Zollinger-Ellison Syndrome Should Be Considered

When standard antiulcer and *Helicobacter pylori* treatments fail and surgery is being considered
Secretory diarrhea
Peptic ulcer disease in conjunction with diarrhea
Recurrent peptic ulceration after acid reduction surgery
Ulcers in unusual locations
Gastric rugal hypertrophy
Multiple ulcers
Peptic ulceration and reflux esophagitis
Reflux esophagitis with stricture
Peptic ulceration at a young age
Perforation or bleeding from peptic ulceration
Family history of peptic ulceration or endocrine tumors
Ulcers and primary hyperparathyroidism

number of reasons. First, although excessive gastrin secretion is the hallmark of the ZES, hypergastrinemia may also occur as a consequence of other diseases or conditions, most of which do not lead to excessive gastric acid secretion and ulcer formation (Box 58–1). Second, because ZES is uncommon, there may be resistance or failure to consider the diagnosis of ZES in the face of clinical, endoscopic, radiologic, and biochemical findings suggestive of it. In this regard, ZES should be considered in all patients with one or more symptoms referable to the upper gastrointestinal tract or in those with primary hyperparathyroidism and nephrolithiasis or a family history suspicious for MEN (Box 58–2).

In general, ZES can be accurately diagnosed in all patients by measurement of an elevated fasting serum level of gastrin in association with an increase in basal acid output (BAO). The diagnosis can be confirmed by the addition of a secretin stimulation test. Measurement of the fasting serum level of gastrin is the initial study to diagnose ZES. Of patients with ZES, virtually 100% will have a fasting serum gastrin level greater than 100 pg/ml. Patients should not be taking antisecretory medications for 3 to 7 days before the determination because medications that reduce gastric acid secretion (e.g., H_2

blockers or omeprazole) cause an elevation in serum gastrin levels. It should be noted that fasting serum gastrin levels in individuals with renal failure, pernicious anemia, or atrophic gastritis may exceed 300 pg/ml, and therefore concomitant measurement of BAO is necessary to confirm the diagnosis of ZES. In this case, a BAO greater than 15 mEq/hr in most patients and greater than 5 mEq/hr in patients with previous surgery to decrease gastric acid secretion unequivocally confirms the diagnosis. Alternatively, a gastric pH less than 2 is also consistent with ZES. With a working diagnosis of ZES, confirmatory provocative testing with secretin should be undertaken. The *secretin stimulation test* is the test of choice because it has a sensitivity of 85% or greater.[10] With this test, a 2-U/kg bolus of secretin is administered intravenously, and fasting serum levels of gastrin are measured before and 2, 5, 10, and 15 minutes after administration. An increase of 200 pg/ml in the gastrin level after secretin administration is consistent with a diagnosis of ZES (Fig. 58–1). However, in our experience the secretin test is positive in only 80% of ZES patients, so it is not absolutely required for diagnosis.[11]

TUMOR CHARACTERISTICS

Because of the small size of the tumor, even the most sensitive preoperative localization study for gastrinoma may prove falsely negative. Gastrinomas may be single, multiple, or metastatic and range in size from less than 1 cm to more than 3 cm. When associated with MEN-I, gastrinomas are usually multiple and commonly found within the duodenum.[12,13] Although it has been suggested that

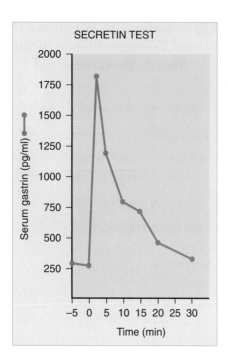

Figure 58–1. Secretin test for the diagnosis of Zollinger-Ellison syndrome (ZES). The patient had an elevated basal fasting serum level of gastrin, 260 pg/ml (normal, <100 pg/ml). After he received 2 U/kg intravenous secretin at time 0, serum gastrin levels increased to 1800 pg/ml at 5 minutes. This increment in serum gastrin level with secretin administration (>200 pg/ml) is diagnostic of ZES. However, these clearly abnormal results occur only in approximately 80% of patients with ZES.

the tumors found in patients with MEN-I have a lower potential for metastasis, they appear to metastasize with a frequency similar to that of regional lymph nodes, thus necessitating careful dissection of periduodenal and pancreatic lymph nodes. Furthermore, some tumors in patients with MEN-I may still act aggressively and be malignant.[8]

Approximately 80% of gastrinomas are found within the *gastrinoma triangle,* an area that includes the first, second, and third portions of the duodenum and the head of the pancreas.[14] In addition to the duodenum and pancreas, primary gastrinomas have been found in the jejunum, stomach, liver, spleen, mesentery, ovary, and heart.[15,16] A particularly confusing tumor is one that is found to be both extrapancreatic and extraintestinal within a lymph node. Though uncommon, it is now clear that some patients have been biochemically cured of ZES after excision of solitary gastrinomas that appear to have arisen within a lymph node. Patients have remained disease-free for more than 10 years. This strongly supports the possibility that there is a *lymph node primary gastrinoma.*[17] Gastrinomas of the duodenum and pancreas appear to have a similar incidence of metastases; however, pancreatic gastrinomas have a higher incidence of liver metastases than duodenal tumors do, and duodenal tumors have a higher incidence of lymph node metastases than pancreatic tumors do. Liver metastases

are the rate-limiting step in long-term survival in that patients in whom liver metastases develop generally die of tumor whereas lymph node metastases do not adversely affect survival. This leads to decreased long-term survival in patients with primary pancreatic gastrinomas.[7]

LOCALIZATION PROCEDURES

Preoperative localization of tumor in patients with ZES continues to be imprecise. No solitary imaging or localization study can clearly identify the total extent of tumor. In general, preoperative imaging includes multiphasic computed tomography (CT), magnetic resonance imaging (MRI), somatostatin receptor scintigraphy (Octreoscan), and endoscopic ultrasound (EUS). More invasive localization studies, including portal venous sampling for gastrin levels or intra-arterial injection of secretin with hepatic venous sampling for gastrin levels, provide functional localization to a region of the pancreas. However, because most occult gastrinomas are in the gastrinoma triangle,[14] these invasive regional localization studies are seldom indicated.

The accuracy of *CT scanning* is dependent on the size of the gastrinoma. Tumors smaller than 1 cm are seldom visualized. With current advanced helical multiphasic CT sequences, most tumors between 2 and 3 cm are seen. CT can detect primary and metastatic tumors larger than 3 cm. Overall, CT imaging can identify approximately 80% of pancreatic and 35% of extrahepatic gastrinomas.[18] *MRI* may be useful in identifying small lesions and, in particular, liver metastases. It is also useful in distinguishing metastatic liver neuroendocrine tumors from benign hemangiomas. However, MRI images only about 25% of primary gastrinomas.[19]

Somatostatin receptor scintigraphy (Fig. 58–2) with ^{111}In-labeled diethylenetriamine pentaacetic acid (DPTA)-D-Phe[1]-octreotide was first evaluated in 1993.[20] It is the imaging test of choice for localizing both primary and metastatic gastrinomas, although it may not image small duodenal gastrinomas. The radiolabeled somatostatin analogue has high affinity for the type 2 somatostatin receptor, which is expressed in more than 90% of gastrinomas. Ninety percent of tumors can be imaged with this modality, with a specificity approaching 100%.[21,22] In the setting of ZES, when clinical suspicion of gastrinoma is high, it has a positive predictive value of 100% and can have a sensitivity exceeding that of all other imaging studies combined.[20] However, it may still miss some small duodenal tumors (<1 cm).

EUS is an observer-dependent method of localizing neuroendocrine tumors, including gastrinomas. It is invasive because an endoscope is positioned in the duodenum or stomach to image tumors with a high-frequency ultrasonic transducer. EUS has achieved its best results in imaging small intrapancreatic islet cell tumors such as insulinomas.[23] Tumors appear sonolucent, as opposed to the more echo-dense pancreas. The procedure has had difficulty in reliably identifying small duodenal tumors, possibly because of the mixed echogenicity of the duodenum, which contains both

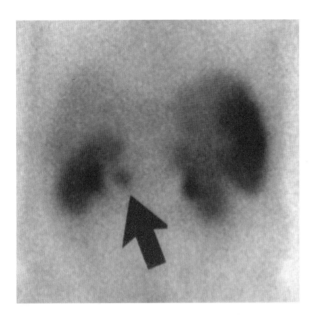

Figure 58–2. Somatostatin receptor scintigraphy showing a lesion that is consistent with a gastrinoma *(arrow)* within the area of the gastrinoma triangle. On exploration, the lesion was found in the medial wall of the duodenum.

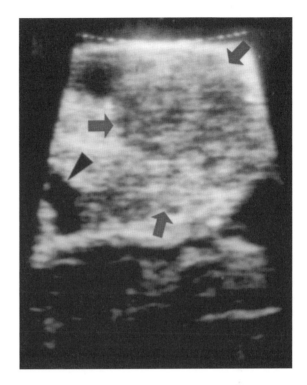

Figure 58–3. Intraoperative ultrasound showing the echogenic characteristics of a gastrinoma within the head of the pancreas *(arrows)*. The mass itself is about 2 cm in diameter. The pancreatic duct is seen in the lower left of the screen *(arrowhead)*.

liquid and gas within a thin solid wall. In addition, EUS may have difficulty differentiating normal lymph nodes from those containing tumor because the sonographic appearance is similar. One study found the sensitivity of EUS to be 50% to 75% for duodenal, 75% for pancreatic, and 63% for lymph node gastrinomas.[24]

Because noninvasive studies may fail to image the gastrinoma, regional localization studies have also been used. The *selective infusion of secretin was combined with angiography* in an attempt to identify the region of the pancreas that contained the gastrinoma. This approach became popular because it obviated the need for transhepatic portal venous sampling. In this study, secretin is selectively and sequentially injected into arteries that supply specific regions of the pancreas and liver. Gastrin levels are then measured in the hepatic vein. A substantial increase in hepatic vein gastrin levels localizes the gastrinoma to the area supplied by the injected artery.[25] However, this study seldom identifies tumors outside the gastrinoma triangle and appears to add little new information.[14] One advantage is that it can be used to identify patients who would probably be cured by Whipple pancreaticoduodenectomy.[26]

Intraoperative methods have been used to localize tumors not imaged preoperatively and to confirm preoperative findings. In this regard, *intraoperative ultrasound (IOUS)* has proved to be most useful for pancreatic neuroendocrine tumors.[27] It images gastrinomas within the pancreas as sonolucent masses (Fig. 58–3) and facilitates the removal of these tumors by showing the relationship of the tumor to the pancreatic duct and other structures. IOUS has not been effective in imaging duodenal gastrinomas, so *opening the duodenum (duodenotomy)* was developed (Fig. 58–4).[28] With duodenotomy, duode-

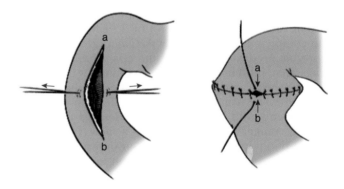

Figure 58–4. Duodenotomy for intraoperative localization of duodenal gastrinomas. The duodenum is opened longitudinally *(left panel),* and the wall is palpated and the mucosa examined. Gastrinomas feel like firm nodules within the wall, and they dimple the mucosa. The duodenum is closed transversely *(right panel)* so that the lumen is not narrowed.

nal wall tumors appear as firm nodules within the wall of the duodenum that dimple the mucosa. Opening the duodenum has been able to identify more duodenal gastrinomas than any other method. It has resulted in an increased cure rate and prolonged survival.[29] The tumor is removed with a small rim of normal duodenum to allow complete resection.

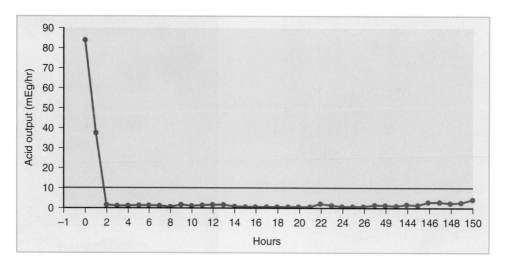

Figure 58–5. Intravenous pantoprazole to control gastric acid hypersecretion in a patient with Zollinger-Ellison syndrome (ZES). Gastric acid output needs to be kept below 10 mEq/hr at all times *(solid purple line)*. The patient's basal acid output is 85 mEq/hr, which is markedly elevated (normal, <15 mEq/hr), consistent with ZES. After being administered 80 mg of pantoprazole intravenously, his acid output drops to 2 mEq/hr within 2 hours and remains less than 10 mEq/hr for more than 24 hours. Therefore, to control the gastric acid hypersecretion of this patient with ZES, he needs 80 mg of pantoprazole intravenously every 24 hours. The oral dose is equally effective.

MEDICAL MANAGEMENT

Gastric acid hypersecretion can be effectively controlled with medications in all patients with ZES. Originally, total gastrectomy was the procedure of choice for the control of gastric acid hypersecretion, but it is no longer indicated. With the advent of proton pump inhibitors, all patients can experience control of acid hypersecretion and complete relief of symptoms. Omeprazole and pantoprazole are two members of the class of antisecretory drugs that inhibit gastric acid secretion by inhibiting parietal cell apical H^+,K^+-adenosine triphosphatase (ATPase). The usual dosage is 20 to 40 mg twice a day, and patients with ZES may require dosages in the 80-mg/day range.[30] Pantoprazole is a new intravenous proton pump inhibitor that has been shown to be effective in control of gastric acid secretion in ZES patients. It is especially useful during surgery or acute hospitalization. The usual dose is 40 to 80 mg intravenously every 12 hours (Fig. 58–5).[30]

Measurement of BAO is necessary to adjust the dose of proton pump inhibitor for effective medical treatment of individual cases. Furthermore, relief of symptoms is not a reliable indicator of overall medical control of ZES. To allow healing of ulceration and to prevent recurrences, gastric acid secretion should be maintained below 10 mEq/hr before the next dose of medication and should be kept below 5 mEq/hr if previous ulcer surgery has been performed or in patients with GERD and esophageal stricture. Even with long-term medical control of ZES, there are the associated risks of sustained achlorhydria. In particular, diffuse malignant gastric carcinoid tumors have developed in some patients with MEN-I after prolonged treatment with omeprazole.[31] It is therefore necessary to perform periodic gastric sur-

veillance endoscopy on patients with MEN-I who are treated with proton pump inhibitors for long periods.

SURGICAL MANAGEMENT

Medical control of symptoms allows time for localization and nonemergency surgical treatment of gastrinoma. It also obviates the need for total gastrectomy. With the results of a number of long-term studies, it is evident that the malignant potential of the tumor itself becomes the main determinant of survival (Fig. 58–6).[32] Therefore, all patients with sporadic (nonfamilial) gastrinoma should be considered candidates for tumor localization and exploratory laparotomy for cure of ZES.[11] Management of patients with MEN-I and ZES is controversial and more complex. In patients with MEN-I and primary hyperparathyroidism, the usual parathyroid pathology is multigland disease or hyperplasia. It has been shown that successful neck exploration for resection of parathyroid hyperplasia can significantly ameliorate the end-organ effects of hypergastrinemia (Fig. 58–7). In patients with MEN-I, ZES, and primary hyperparathyroidism, neck exploration should be performed before resection of gastrinoma.[33] Removal of pancreatic and duodenal tumors seldom cures MEN-I patients of ZES.[11,34] It has been shown that resection of primary gastrinomas in all patients decreases the likelihood of liver metastases[35]; however, surgical resection of localized gastrinoma has not been demonstrated to prolong survival of patients with ZES.[35] The goals of surgical management, therefore, are resection of the primary tumor for potential cure and prevention of malignant progression. This latter goal is desired whether the patient has a sporadic gastrinoma or one in the setting of MEN-I syndrome. Operative

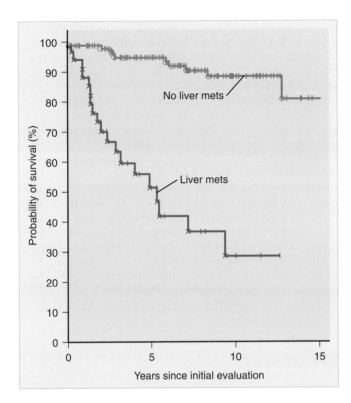

Figure 58–6. Kaplan-Meier survival curve for patients with gastrinoma in the presence or absence of liver metastasis (mets). Data are derived from follow-up of a cohort of patients who were evaluated and treated at the National Institutes of Health.

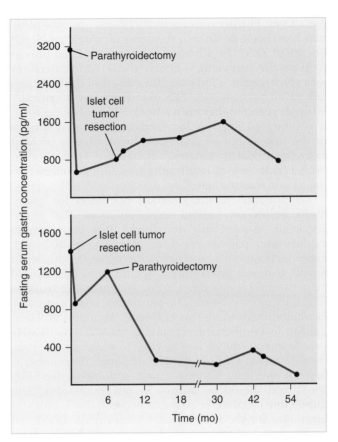

Figure 58–7. Effect of parathyroidectomy on the fasting serum levels of gastrin in two patients with multiple endocrine neoplasia type I. In each case, resection of parathyroid disease significantly reduced serum gastrin levels regardless of the timing of islet cell tumor resection.

management of patients with MEN-I and gastrinoma is complicated by the fact that within this setting the tumors tend to be multiple and small (4 to 6 mm), usually involve the duodenum,[13] and spread early to lymph nodes. In these patients the controversy centers on the fact that surgery is seldom curative,[11,34] yet it may be effective in treating the potential malignant disease and preventing liver metastases.[36]

Recommendations for management of MEN-I ZES patients have ranged from medical management to aggressive surgery, without a clear consensus for a single ideal therapy.[3,36] We have operated on patients with MEN-I when the primary tumor is imaged at 3 cm or larger.[34] This decision is based on the fact that the presence of liver metastases correlates with primary tumor size: liver metastases develop in 4% of patients with primary gastrinomas smaller than 1 cm as compared with 28% of patients with tumors between 1 and 3 cm and 61% with tumors larger than 3 cm.[7] After a review of current data, it seems more prudent to operate on patients with MEN-I who have smaller, but clearly identifiable pancreatic and duodenal gastrinomas (2 cm in size) because this should decrease the probability of hepatic metastases considerably.[36]

Approximately 95% of patients with sporadic ZES will have gastrinomas found at surgery, and 60% to 68% will be cured.[11,29] Importantly, duodenotomy has increased the tumor detection and cure rate (see Fig. 58–4).[29]

Surgery is also effective treatment of localized metastatic liver gastrinoma because it appears to prolong survival and cure some patients.[37,38] In patients with MEN-I and gastrinoma, identification of all tumor foci is problematic, and surgery results in a much lower cure rate.[11,34] Paradoxically, although patients with gastrinoma associated with MEN-I may be identified at a younger age, have multiple small duodenal tumors, and undergo abdominal exploration without surgical cure, liver metastases develop at a lower rate than in their sporadic counterparts, and they have excellent survival.[3] However, recent studies have shown that in some (25%) the activity of pancreatic neuroendocrine tumors is significant and survival is dependent on the aggressive behavior of the pancreatic tumor.[8]

In general, in MEN-I patients with ZES, if 2-cm tumors are clearly imaged on preoperative studies, surgery is indicated to remove these tumors, which may be malignant.[36] In patients with sporadic ZES who have no clear imageable tumor[11] or localized primary or metastatic[37,38] tumor, laparotomy is also indicated because duodenotomy will find duodenal tumors and imageable tumors (even when metastatic) can usually be completely resected. Surgery for gastrinoma requires careful dissection of the regional lymph nodes that may contain metastases. Furthermore, primary lymph node gastrinomas have been described, resection of which can result in cure of ZES.[17] Enucleation of pancreatic head tumors is generally sufficient, whereas distal pancreatectomy with splenectomy is indicated for tumors of the body and tail. In all patients with ZES, duodenotomy is critical.[29] Whipple resection has been advocated by some; however, it is indicated only for localized large (>3 cm) tumors in the duodenum or pancreatic head, with or without extensive nodal metastases.[39] It has also been used in MEN-I patients with locally advanced tumor confined to the gastrinoma triangle.[40]

Performance of the standard operation for gastrinoma relies on careful exploration of the entire abdomen, as previously described.[11] It is important to explore and palpate the liver, stomach, small bowel, mesentery, pancreas, and pelvis, including the ovaries in female patients. An extended Kocher maneuver should be performed to mobilize the duodenum and gain access to the pancreatic head. The pancreatic body and tail is examined by dividing the gastrocolic ligament. IOUS is used to image the pancreas and liver. A 7.5- to 10-mHz near-field transducer is necessary to examine the pancreas, whereas a 2.5- to 5-mHz wide-angle transducer is best for the liver. Tumors appear sonolucent (see Fig. 58–3) and should be imaged in two dimensions. The duodenum can then be palpated between the thumb and forefinger for the presence of a tumor mass. Duodenal gastrinomas feel like sharply defined, small firm nodules within the wall. A longitudinal duodenotomy is indicated in all cases (see Fig. 58–4) because it permits visualization, as well as more careful palpation of the entire duodenal wall, particularly its medial portion. Suspicious nodules on the medial wall should not be excised until after clear identification of the nodule and its relationship to the ampulla of Vater and pancreatic duct. The duodenum is preferably closed transversely in two layers to minimize the risk for leakage or obstruction (see Fig. 58–4). If a long duodenotomy is necessary, longitudinal closure may be necessary. The peripancreatic, porta hepatis, and celiac lymph nodes are also sampled and excised for pathologic review. Reoperation for recurrent localized gastrinoma is indicated if the tumor can be clearly imaged, and it results in complete resection of all tumor in nearly every patient and complete remission in 30%.[41]

METASTATIC DISEASE

With successful control of gastric acid hypersecretion and the indolent growth pattern of the gastrinoma, distant metastatic disease is the most important determinant of survival (see Fig. 58–6).[7] A histologic diagnosis of cancer is impossible to make pathologically, and malignancy is diagnosed by identifying lymph node and distant visceral metastases. Previously, about 60% of patients had metastatic disease at diagnosis. However, with more widespread availability of biochemical testing and earlier diagnosis, that percentage has decreased to 25%.[6] The long-term survival rate for patients with distant metastatic disease is approximately 20%, and chemotherapy has

not been helpful.[7,42] In patients with completely resected localized liver metastases, the 5-year survival rate is 80%.[38] In contrast, patients with unresectable hepatic disease have a 5-year survival rate of 20% to 38%.[32] Most recently, lesser surgical procedures than open resection have been used to effectively deal with liver metastases from neuroendocrine tumors. Laparoscopic radiofrequency ablation (RFA) of liver metastases from pancreatic neuroendocrine tumors is associated with a liver tumor control rate of 90%.[43] Because of the indolent nature of these tumors and the lack of other effective treatments, surgical resection has been the main treatment of recurrent or metastatic gastrinoma (or both), and the results have been encouraging. Furthermore, growth of tumor can be suppressed by somatostatin analogues.[44] If a tumor is imaged by Octreoscan and expresses somatostatin receptors, we combine surgical resection or RFA with long-term high-dose somatostatin analogues (Sandostatin LAR, 30 mg intramuscularly every 3 weeks). This regimen has provided excellent results in terms of symptom-free survival.

REFERENCES

1. Zollinger RM, Ellison EH: Primary peptic ulceration of the jejunum associated with islet cell tumors of the pancreas Ann Surg 142:709, 1955.
2. Oberhelman HA Jr: Excisional therapy for ulcerogenic tumors of the duodenum: Long-term results. Arch Surg 104:447, 1972.
3. Veldhuis JD, Norton JA, Wells SA Jr, et al: Surgical versus medical management of multiple endocrine neoplasia (MEN) type I. J Clin Endocrinol Metab 82:357, 1997.
4. Meko JB, Norton JA: Management of patients with Zollinger-Ellison syndrome. Annu Rev Med 46:395, 1995.
5. Isenberg JI, Walsh JH, Grossman MI: Zollinger-Ellison syndrome. Gastroenterology 65:140, 1973.
6. Norton JA: Gastrinoma: Advances in localization and treatment. Surg Oncol Clin North Am 7:845, 1998.
7. Weber HC, Vernon DJ, Lin JT, et al: Determinants of metastatic rate and survival in patients with Zollinger-Ellison syndrome: A prospective long-term study. Gastroenterology 108:1637, 1995.
8. Gibril F, Venzon DJ, Ojeauburu JV, et al: Prospective study of the natural history of gastrinoma in patients with MEN1: Definition of an aggressive and nonaggressive form. J Clin Endocrinol Metab 86:5282, 2001.
9. Norton JA: Advances in the management of Zollinger-Ellison syndrome. Adv Surg 27:129, 1994.
10. Slaff JI, Howard JM, Maton PN, et al: Prospective assessment of provocative gastrin tests in 81 consecutive patients with Zollinger-Ellison syndrome. Gastroenterology 90:1637, 1986.
11. Norton JA, Fraker DL, Alexander HR, et al: Surgery to cure the Zollinger-Ellison syndrome. N Engl J Med 341:635, 1999.
12. Thompson NW: Surgical treatment of the endocrine pancreas and Zollinger-Ellison syndrome in the MEN 1 syndrome. Henry Ford Hosp Med J 40:195, 1992.
13. Pipeleers-Marichal M, Somers G, Willems G, et al: Gastrinomas in the duodenum of patients with multiple endocrine neoplasia type 1 and Zollinger-Ellison syndrome. N Engl J Med 322:723, 1990.
14. Stabile BE, Morrow DJ, Passaro E Jr: The gastrinoma triangle: Operative implications. Am J Surg 147:25, 1984.
15. Gibril F, Curtis LT, Termanini B, et al: Primary cardiac gastrinoma causing Zollinger-Ellison syndrome. Gastroenterology 112:567, 1997.
16. Maton PN, Mackem SM, Norton JA, et al: Ovarian carcinoma as a cause of Zollinger-Ellison syndrome: Natural history, secretory products, and response to provocative tests. Gastroenterology 97:468, 1989.
17. Norton JA, Alexander HR, Fraker DL, et al: Possible lymph node primary gastrinomas: Occurrence, natural history, and predictive

factors: A prospective study. Ann Surg 237:650, discussion 657, 2003.

18. Wank SA, Doppman JL, Miller DL, et al: Prospective study of the ability of computed axial tomography to localize gastrinomas in patients with Zollinger-Ellison syndrome. Gastroenterology 92:905, 1987.

19. Pisegna JR, Doppman JL, Norton JA, et al: Prospective comparative study of ability of MR imaging and other imaging modalities to localize tumors in patients with Zollinger-Ellison syndrome. Dig Dis Sci 38:1318, 1993.

20. Krenning EP, Kwekkeboom DJ, Bakker WH, et al: Somatostatin receptor scintigraphy with [^{111}In-DTPA-D-Phe^1]- and [^{123}I-Tyr^3]-octreotide: The Rotterdam experience with more than 1000 patients. Eur J Nucl Med 20:716, 1993.

21. Gibril F, Reynolds JC, Doppman JL, et al: Somatostatin receptor scintigraphy: Its sensitivity compared with that of other imaging methods in detecting primary and metastatic gastrinomas: A prospective study. Ann Intern Med 125:26, 1996.

22. Gibril F, Doppman JL, Jensen RT: Comparative analysis of tumor localization techniques for neuroendocrine tumors. Yale J Biol Med 70:481, 1997.

23. Thompson NW, Czako PF, Fritts LL, et al: Role of endoscopic ultrasonography in the localization of insulinomas and gastrinomas. Surgery 116:131, 1994.

24. Ruszniewski P, Amouyal P, Amouyal G, et al: Localization of gastrinomas by endoscopic ultrasonography in patients with Zollinger-Ellison syndrome. Surgery 117:629, 1995.

25. Thom AK, Norton JA, Doppman JL, et al: Prospective study of the use of intra-arterial secretin injection and portal venous sampling to localize duodenal gastrinomas. Surgery 112:1002, 1992.

26. Kato M, Immamura M, Hosotani R, et al: Curative resection of microgastrinomas based on the intraoperative secretin test. World J Surg 24:1425, 2000.

27. Sugg SL, Norton JA, Fraker DL, et al: A prospective study of intraoperative methods to diagnose and resect duodenal gastrinomas. Ann Surg 218:138, 1993.

28. Thompson NW, Vinik AI, Eckhauser FE: Microgastrinomas of the duodenum: A cause of failed operations for the Zollinger-Ellison syndrome. Ann Surg 209:396, 1989.

29. Norton JA, Alexander HR, Fraker D, et al: Does the use of routine duodenotomy (DUODX) affect rate of cure, development of liver metastases or survival in patients with Zollinger-Ellison Syndrome (ZES)? Ann Surg 239:617, 2004.

30. Metz DC, Forsmark C, Lew EA, et al: Replacement of oral proton pump inhibitors with intravenous pantoprazole to effectively control gastric acid secretion in patients with Zollinger-Ellison syndrome. Am J Gastroenterol 96:3274, 2001.

31. Norton JA, Melcher ML, Gibril F, Jensen RT: Gastric carcinoid tumors in multiple endocrine neoplasia-1 patients with Zollinger-Ellison syndrome can be symptomatic, demonstrate aggressive growth, and require surgery. Surgery 136:1267, 2003.

32. Sutliff VE, Doppman JL, Gibril F, et al: Growth of newly diagnosed, untreated metastatic gastrinomas and predictors of growth patterns. J Clin Oncol 15:2420, 1997.

33. Norton JA, Cornelius MJ, Doppman JL, et al: Effect of parathyroidectomy in patients with hyperparathyroidism, Zollinger-Ellison syndrome, and multiple endocrine neoplasia type I: A prospective study. Surgery 102:958, 1987.

34. Norton JA, Alexander HR, Fraker DL, et al: Comparison of surgical results in patients with advanced and limited disease with multiple endocrine neoplasia type 1 and Zollinger-Ellison syndrome. Ann Surg 234:495, 2001.

35. Fraker DL, Norton JA, Alexander HR, et al: Surgery in Zollinger-Ellison syndrome alters the natural history of gastrinoma. Ann Surg 220:320, 1994.

36. Norton JA, Jensen RT: Resolved and unresolved controversies in the surgical management of patients with Zollinger-Ellison syndrome. Ann Surg 240:757, 2004.

37. Norton JA, Doherty GM, Fraker DL, et al: Surgical treatment of localized gastrinoma within the liver: A prospective study. Surgery 124:1145, 1998.

38. Norton JA, Warren RS, Kelly MG, et al: Aggressive surgery for metastatic liver neuroendocrine tumors. Surgery 134:1057, 2003.

39. Delcore R, Friesen SR: Role of pancreaticoduodenectomy in the management of primary duodenal wall gastrinomas in patients with the Zollinger-Ellison syndrome. Surgery 112:1016, 1992.

40. Lairmore TC, Chen VY, DeBenedetti MK, et al: Duodenopancreatic resections in patients with multiple endocrine neoplasia type 1. Ann Surg 231:909, 2000.

41. Jaskowiak NT, Fraker DL, Alexander HR, et al: Is reoperation for gastrinoma excision indicated in Zollinger-Ellison syndrome? Surgery 120:1055, discussion 1062, 1996.

42. von Schrenck T, Howard JM, Doppman JL, et al: Prospective study of chemotherapy in patients with metastatic gastrinoma. Gastroenterology 94:1326, 1988.

43. Berber E, Flesher N, Siperstein AE: Laparoscopic radiofrequency ablation of neuroendocrine liver metastases. World J Surg 26:985, 2002.

44. Arnold R, Trautmann MF, Creutzfeldt W, et al: Somatostatin analogue octreotide and inhibition of tumor growth in metastatic endocrine gastroenteropancreatic tumors. Gut 38:430, 1996.

59

Postgastrectomy Syndromes

Thomas A. Miller · Jeannie F. Savas

Before the late 1970s, surgical management of acid-peptic diseases of the stomach and duodenum was relatively commonplace. Depending on the site of the ulcer, its chronicity, and what role acid hypersecretion was thought to play in its pathogenesis, surgical options varied from vagotomy and gastric drainage with some form of pyloroplasty to more radical procedures in which substantial portions of the distal part of the stomach were removed. The derangements in gastric function induced by these various operations were not infrequently associated with a variety of postoperative sequelae that have collectively been called the "postgastrectomy syndromes."

With the commercial introduction of cimetidine (Tagamet) in 1977, management of peptic ulcer disease radically changed. For the first time, effective treatment of the ulcer diathesis was now possible with a pharmacologic agent. Shortly after the introduction of this H_2 receptor blocker, several other similar blockers appeared on the market. In addition, by the late 1980s, proton pump inhibitors were also released and made inhibition of acid secretion even more effective than had previously been observed with the H_2 receptor blockers. Such pharmacologic manipulation resulted in most forms of acid-peptic disease being effectively managed nonoperatively. Concomitant with these developments was the further observation that a bacterium known as *Helicobacter pylori* was probably responsible for most forms of duodenal ulcer disease and a significant proportion of gastric ulceration. Surprisingly, it now became possible to actually eradicate peptic ulceration with antibiotic therapy in a large majority of patients. Thus, as we entered the 21st century, peptic ulcer disease has become a predominantly medical disease that can be effectively managed in most patients with nonsurgical interventions. Only when complications occur that are resistant to medical therapy, such as perforation, uncontrolled hemorrhage, and gastric outlet obstruction, is the surgeon called on to offer expertise in the management of peptic ulceration.

Along with these advances in peptic ulcer therapy has been a steady decline in the incidence of gastric cancer in the United States and most areas of Western Europe. Thus, the radical surgical procedures that were previously used to manage this malignancy have likewise become less radical. In fact, with early surveillance by upper endoscopy, gastric cancer is now being diagnosed in many patients at much earlier stages of development, and less radical procedures are required for cure.

All these advances have resulted in a major decrease in patients with postgastrectomy problems, and many surgeons have actually had minimal experience managing them. Because a sufficient number of patients with refractory ulcer disease and more advanced gastric cancer still require ablative procedures for effective management, the small, but consistent number of patients who will still be subject to postgastrectomy problems require that the surgeon of the early 21st century be cognizant of their management until other treatment modalities evolve that make gastric operations a relative thing of the past. This chapter highlights the major postgastrectomy syndromes that still occur and demand thoughtful management by the treating surgeon. Three types of causes have been identified: gastric reservoir dysfunction, vagal denervation, and aberrations in surgical reconstruction. Discussion of their pathogenesis and management forms the basis of this chapter.

GASTRIC RESERVOIR DYSFUNCTION

Dumping Syndrome

The human stomach possesses a remarkable capability of adapting to large volumes of orally administered liquids and solids through a process known as receptive relaxation.[1] These intragastric contents are then acted on by secreted acid and pepsin along with muscular churning to prepare an isosmotic gastric chyme that is then slowly discharged into the upper part of the gut for subsequent processing so that effective digestion and absorption can occur throughout the small bowel. If a portion of the stomach has been previously removed or the normal pyloric sphincter mechanism has been deranged, the ingested meal is not as effectively processed by the stomach and is prematurely discharged into the upper intestine. Depending on the speed of this discharge and the osmolarity of the contents being discharged, a variety of symptoms may result that have been referred to as the *dumping syndrome*. Both an early and late form of this disorder have been identified.

The early form of dumping syndrome is by far the more common and usually occurs within 10 to 30 minutes after the ingestion of a meal. A constellation of postprandial symptoms have been described that range in severity from annoying to disabling. The classic gastrointestinal (GI) symptoms include nausea and vomiting, epigastric fullness, eructations, abdominal cramping, and occasionally, explosive diarrhea. Cardiovascular symptoms are often associated with these GI complaints and include tachycardia, palpitations, diaphoresis, and a feeling of lightheadedness and flushing that may be accompanied by blurred vision. This symptom complex may occur while the patient is still seated at the table eating; more commonly, however, it occurs shortly after completing the meal. The precise mechanism or mechanisms responsible for early dumping are still being debated, but most investigators are in general agreement that rapid passage of food of high osmolarity from the stomach into the small intestine is the basic cause.[2,3] Thus, the previous gastric resection or interrupted pyloric sphincter mechanism no longer enables the intact stomach to prepare its contents and deliver them into the proximal part of the bowel in the form of small particles in isosmotic solution. The rapid discharge of this hyperosmotic chyme then induces a rapid shift of extracellular fluid into the intestinal lumen so that the newly received gastric chyme is brought to a state of isotonicity. Accordingly, the gut distention and autonomic responses induced by the changes in plasma volume are thought to be responsible for the underlying symptomatology.

A variety of clinical conditions may give rise to early dumping. As many as 5% to 10% of patients experience dumping symptoms after operations involving the pyloric sphincter, such as pyloroplasty or pyloromyotomy, or after varying degrees of distal gastric resection.[4,5] The type of GI reconstruction after distal gastrectomy also appears to play a role because dumping after partial gastrectomy with a Billroth II reconstruction is especially common, as opposed to a Billroth I gastrectomy, in which this condition is less frequently observed.[6] The role that various neuroendocrine responses may play in its pathogenesis remains to be defined. A variety of hormonal abnormalities have been observed in early dumping, including aberrations in serotonin, vasoactive intestinal peptide, cholecystokinin, neurotensin, peptide YY, enteroglucagon, renin-angiotensin-aldosterone, and atrial natriuretic peptide.[7-12]

In contrast to early dumping, which usually occurs within 30 minutes of eating, late dumping is delayed until 2 to 3 hours after the ingestion of a meal. It is also much less common than its early counterpart. The basic pathophysiology appears to be the same, namely, rapid discharge of hypertonic chyme from the stomach into the upper part of the gut. This form of dumping, however, seems to be specifically related to carbohydrates such as monosaccharides and disaccharides. After rapid delivery of these sugars into the small intestine, hyperglycemia results from their relatively quick absorption. The pancreas is subsequently triggered to release insulin to control the elevated blood sugar and, in the process of doing so, actually "overshoots" so that marked hypoglycemia is induced. This insulin shock condition then activates the adrenal gland to release catecholamines, which cause a constellation of symptoms, among which are tachycardia, tachypnea, diaphoresis, and lightheadedness. Why late dumping develops in some patients whereas the majority have an early expression of this syndrome remains unknown.

In most patients in whom dumping develops after gastric surgery, medical management is usually successful. The simple dictum of limiting the amount of liquids ingested during a meal has greatly improved symptoms in many patients. Certainly, hyperosmolar substances such as ice cream or liquids such as milkshakes should be cautiously avoided because these substances may prove to be particularly troublesome. Sometimes, measures as simple as avoiding certain foods, eating small meals more frequently, separating liquids from solids, or lying down when symptoms start to occur may be all that is necessary to control or significantly alleviate the symptomatology. In some instances, carbohydrate gelling agents such as pectin, when taken with a meal, have proved to be successful.[13] The α-glucosidase inhibitor acarbose has proved to be particularly helpful in ameliorating the symptoms of late dumping.[14,15] If dumping continues after instituting these various measures, octreotide has proved useful in many patients.[16,17] Administered subcutaneously in a 100-μg dose twice daily, this somatostatin inhibitor has been shown to ameliorate many of the hormonal abnormalities seen in patients with dumping syndrome, as well as restore a fasting motility pattern in the small intestine known as the migratory motor complex. If this low dose is not successful, it can be increased to as high as 500 μg twice daily.

Fortunately, the majority of patients with dumping symptoms will respond to these conservative measures. In only 1% or less of patients will operative intervention be required. Great care should be taken in selecting patients who might benefit from surgery. Every effort should be made to define the severity of the patient's symptoms, whether disciplined nonoperative measures have been used to alleviate the symptoms, and whether some associated stressful situation (such as divorce or financial problems) is contributing to the symptomatology and would very likely not be altered by operative intervention. If surgery has been judged to be the best alternative for management, the type of procedure previously performed and the amount of gastric reservoir that still exists will influence the operative approach. If no stomach has been previously resected and the dumping has resulted primarily from pyloric dysfunction, pyloric reconstruction can often be performed in these patients. The advantage of this technique is that it is quite safe and does not require irreversible maneuvers such as gastric resection or vagotomy. Cheadle and associates[18] performed pyloric reconstruction in a

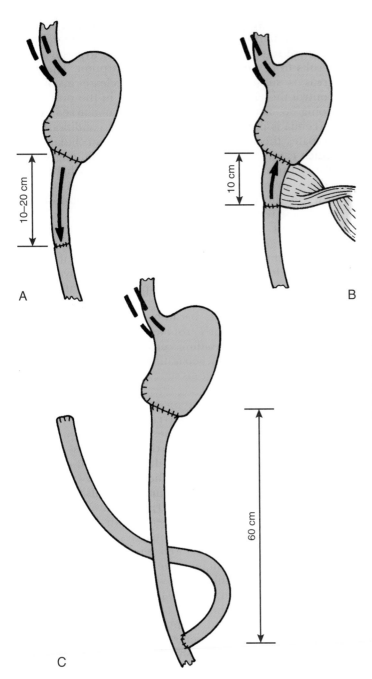

Figure 59–1. Surgical approaches to treat dumping syndrome. **A,** A 10- to 20-cm loop of jejunum is interposed between the stomach and small intestine in an isoperistaltic fashion. **B,** A 10-cm loop of jejunum is twisted on its mesentery so that its distal end is anastomosed to the stomach and its proximal end to the small intestine in an antiperistaltic fashion. **C,** Long-limb Roux-en-Y anastomosis in which the jejunojejunostomy is fashioned approximately 60 cm from the gastrojejunostomy. (From Miller TA, Mercer DW: Derangements in gastric function secondary to previous surgery. In Miller TA [ed]: Modern Surgical Care: Physiologic Foundations and Clinical Applications, 2nd ed. St Louis, Quality Medical, 1998, p 400.)

number of patients with severe dumping after vagotomy and pyloroplasty (Visick 4 score) and were able to demonstrate considerable symptomatic improvement so that their new scores were reduced to 2 or 3. Although Frederiksen and associates had similar results in a small series with disabling diarrhea or dumping after vagotomy and pyloroplasty,[19] other experienced gastric surgeons have not been as successful.[20] If a previous gastric resection and Billroth II reconstruction gave rise to the dumping, simple takedown of this anastomosis and converting it to a Billroth I reconstruction may be all that is needed.[21]

Two other options have also been used to surgically treat dumping syndrome (Fig. 59–1). The first has involved the use of isoperistaltic or antiperistaltic jejunal segments interposed between the stomach and small intestine. The rationale behind these procedures is that the 10- or 20-cm loop of jejunum used for interposition slows down gastric emptying. Although early results with both procedures suggested considerable benefit, amelioration of severe dumping has not been consistently demonstrated in the long term.[20] Furthermore, such interposition operations have often led to obstruction, thereby necessitating a reoperation.[20]

The most durable procedure has been the Roux-en-Y-gastrojejunostomy (see Fig. 59–1). This procedure delays gastric emptying, probably on the basis of disordered motility in the Roux limb as shown by Cullen and Kelly[22] in a study in which electrical and mechanical activity in the Roux limb was found to advance toward the stomach rather than in an aboral direction. In a series of 22 patients treated over a period of 13 years, Vogel and colleagues showed that this operative approach successfully managed the dumping syndrome, with complete resolution of symptoms in 19 of these individuals.[20]

Metabolic Aberrations

Three metabolic disturbances may occur after gastric surgery, including anemia, bone disease, and weight loss. Although any type of gastric procedure can induce such problems, gastric resection is more commonly associated with them than vagotomy is, and the incidence after gastrectomy with a Billroth II reconstruction is greater than that encountered with a Billroth I approach.[23]

Of the causes of anemia, a deficiency in iron is clearly the most commonly encountered. As many as 30% to 50% of patients experience this type of anemia after gastrectomy. Although iron absorption takes place primarily in the proximal portion of the gut, it requires an acidic environment for this action to maximally occur. Thus, any gastric procedure that alters acidity can contribute to this problem. Vagotomy is known to decrease both fasting and stimulated acid production, and antrectomy removes an important source of the hormone gastrin, which physiologically contributes to gastric acid production. If a larger portion of stomach is resected than the antrum, not only is the gastrin source removed, but some of the parietal cell mass is also absent. If iron deficiency develops, the problem is easily corrected by the addition of iron supplements to the patient's diet.

The other common anemia is related to a deficiency of vitamin B_{12}. Because intrinsic factor, which is made by the parietal cells of the stomach, is essential for the enteric absorption of vitamin B_{12}, any gastric procedure that alters parietal cell mass can contribute to this problem.[23] Furthermore, vitamin B_{12} bioavailability is also facilitated by an acidic environment. Thus, any patient who has undergone vagotomy or gastrectomy (even if only partial) should be periodically monitored by hematocrit, red cell indices, iron, transferrin, and vitamin B_{12} to be sure that an incipient anemia is not developing. Although folate deficiency can also occur after gastric resection, it is quite uncommon in comparison to the other types described. It is usually related to inadequate oral intake rather than a defect in absorption, as occurs with iron and vitamin B_{12} deficiencies. Finally, it needs to be emphasized that in all patients who have undergone total gastrectomy, vitamin B_{12} deficiency will invariably develop, and thus they must be given an intramuscular injection of cyanocobalamin every 3 to 4 months for the rest of their lives because oral administration is not a reliable route for absorption.

Calcium and vitamin D metabolism may also be perturbed by previous gastric surgery. Fat malabsorption is not uncommon after gastric resection with a Billroth II reconstruction as a result of the inefficient mixing of food, bile, and pancreatic enzymes. Because vitamin D is a fat-soluble vitamin, this circumstance can significantly affect its absorption.[24] Of equal importance, calcium absorption, which predominantly occurs in the duodenum, can also be adversely affected by gastrectomy and Billroth II reconstruction.[23,24] The metabolic bone disease that can occur in patients under these circumstances is usually insidious and may require many years to manifest itself. Unexplained aches and pains in the back or bones may be the initial symptomatology. Occasionally, a spontaneous fracture indicates the presence of bone disease. Patients suspected of having this problem should undergo a bone density study. Skeletal monitoring of patients at risk (i.e., elderly men and women, postmenopausal women) may prove useful in identifying skeletal deterioration, which may be arrested with appropriate treatment. In selected patients, dietary supplementation of calcium and vitamin D appears to be useful in preventing these complications.

Weight loss is a frequent finding after surgical procedures on the stomach. Often, it is temporary, and once the patient adjusts to the dietary aberrations evoked by the operation, sufficient protein/calorie nutrition commonly results so that no clinically significant problem develops. In patients who have had either all or substantial portions of their stomach removed, considerable malnutrition may occur, particularly in thin women. Thus, great care should be taken to avoid a gastric procedure for benign disease in a woman who is marginally normal in terms of weight. In a patient who has lost weight after gastric surgery, it is important to determine whether it is related to an alteration in dietary intake or is a consequence of malabsorption. If a stool stain for fecal fat is negative, decreased caloric intake is the probable cause. Usually, an improvement in nutritional balance can be accomplished by changing one's diet to multiple small feedings if dumping-like symptomatology occurs with regular feeding. If intractable problems with weight loss become chronic, a surgical procedure to delay gastric emptying or enhance the gastric reservoir effect, as discussed under "Dumping Syndrome," may become the most prudent means of management.

VAGAL DENERVATION

Diarrhea

At least 30% of patients who undergo gastric surgery will complain of diarrhea postoperatively if carefully questioned.[5] As already indicated in the section on dumping syndrome, diarrhea is frequently a component of this entity. Regardless of cause, for most patients the diarrhea is not severe and often abates within several months of the operation. Even in patients with dumping syndrome, the diarrhea usually improves as patients adjust their diet to modify intake of food that may trigger this response. Distinct from other causes of diarrhea, vagotomy by itself may induce changes in postoperative bowel function that may range from a simple increase in stool frequency to frank, explosive bowel movements that could result in soiling of clothing if the patient does not find a toilet in time. Fortunately, clinically significant postvagotomy diarrhea occurs in only 5% to 10% of patients, and over time this problem also corrects itself in the majority of individuals.

Despite scores of studies by multiple investigators, the precise mechanisms responsible for postvagotomy diarrhea have not been elucidated. It was originally thought that this problem occurred only in patients with truncal vagotomy and that maintaining vagal innervation of the small bowel with more selective vagotomy approaches would obviate this problem. Long-term follow-up of this latter group of patients has not borne out this contention, so intestinal dysmotility and accelerated transit secondary to vagal denervation are only partially responsible for the diarrhea, if at all.[25,26] Other proposed mechanisms include bile acid malabsorption, rapid gastric emptying, and bacterial overgrowth.[26-29] The latter problem is known to be facilitated by the decreased gastric acid secretion after vagotomy; furthermore, bacterial overgrowth can be confirmed in many postvagotomy diarrhea patients, and anecdotal reports indicate that the diarrhea has abated or markedly decreased after antibiotic therapy. Whether this proves a cause-and-effect relationship can be debated. Interestingly, a subset of patients with postvagotomy diarrhea have been shown to respond to cholestyramine.[30] This anionic exchange resin absorbs bile salts and renders them inactive. Moreover, it has been shown experimentally that the total bile acid content in the stools of patients with postvagotomy diarrhea, though not significantly greater than in those without this problem, has more than twice the amount of chenodeoxycholic acid.[29] Such findings lend support to the hypothesis that bile acid malabsorption may contribute to postvagotomy diarrhea in some patients.

Fortunately, no more than 1% of all patients undergoing vagotomy will experience a sustained problem with diarrhea. Over time, the problem seems to abate. In patients not responsive to cholestyramine, codeine or loperamide may prove useful. In patients who have incapacitating diarrhea for at least a year after the initial operation that is unresponsive to medical management, remedial surgery is an appropriate treatment option. The operation of choice is to interpose a 10-cm segment of reversed jejunum placed in continuity 70 to 100 cm from the ligament of Treitz (Fig. 59–2). In patients requiring operative intervention, this approach has been associated with sustained relief from the diarrheal problem.[21]

Gastric Stasis

It is not unusual for some degree of delayed gastric emptying to occur after vagotomy, particularly if the major vagal trunks were transected (i.e., both truncal and selective vagotomy). This circumstance is not surprising because the nerves of Latarjet are denervated in both these procedures, thus disrupting the normal function of the vagus nerve in adjusting gastric tone to changes in gastric volume so that normal peristalsis and emptying are coordinated properly.[22] The atonic stomach that results from these procedures is not a problem with parietal cell vagotomy because this approach to vagal transection does not disrupt antral innervation and

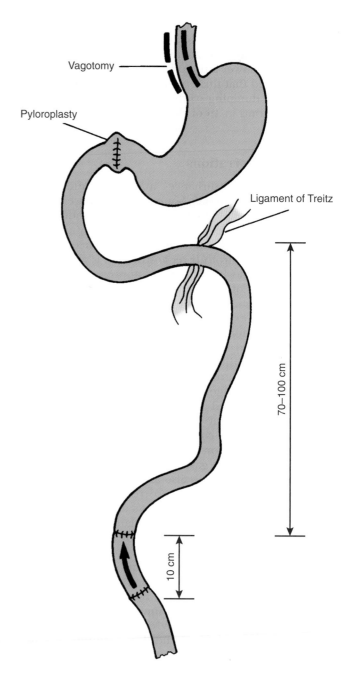

Figure 59–2. Surgical management of postvagotomy diarrhea. (From Miller TA, Mercer DW: Derangements in gastric function secondary to previous surgery. In Miller TA [ed]: Modern Surgical Care: Physiologic Foundations and Clinical Applications, 2nd ed. St Louis, Quality Medical, 1998, p 407.)

accordingly allows propulsive activity of the distal part of the stomach to be maintained.

In patients subjected to truncal or selective vagotomy and in whom gastric stasis occurs, treatment is determined by the degree of symptomatology. Often, the only significant symptom is a feeling of fullness in the epigastric region, which at worst is simply a nuisance. Fortunately, this problem usually abates within several weeks after vagotomy as the patient resumes more normal alimentation. In other individuals, marked abdominal pain may occur, and in rare individuals a functional gastric outlet obstruction may develop.

In evaluating a patient with presumed postvagotomy gastroparesis, other causes of delayed gastric emptying must be excluded. Medical causes include diabetes mellitus, electrolyte imbalance, toxicity to drugs, and neuromuscular diseases. Mechanical causes include postoperative adhesions, anastomotic stricture, afferent or efferent loop obstruction, and internal adhesions if a gastroenterostomy or a concomitant gastric resection and Billroth II reconstruction were done in conjunction with the vagotomy. At the very least, evaluation should include esophagogastroduodenoscopy and some type of gastric emptying study with either barium or a scintigraphic agent.[31] In most individuals, gastric emptying is best quantified clinically with scintigraphic techniques that give half-lives for liquid and solid emptying. If the underlying problem responsible for gastric stasis is thought to be a disorder of intrinsic motor function, additional techniques such as electrogastrography and GI manometry may prove helpful.[32]

Assuming that mechanical obstruction has been excluded, short-term treatment with various pharmacologic agents has proved successful in most cases of motor dysfunction. Such treatment includes a combination of dietary modification and various pharmacotherapeutic agents that enhance promotility. One of several gastrokinetic agents, such as metoclopramide, domperidone, and erythromycin, will generally prove efficacious in a given patient. Metoclopramide is a dopamine antagonist that works on the stomach by facilitating acetylcholine release from enteric cholinergic neurons.[33] Domperidone works on both the stomach and the intestine by facilitating acetylcholine release from the mesenteric plexus of the gut.[34] Erythromycin is a motilin agonist that works on both the stomach and intestine by binding to motilin receptors on GI smooth muscle.[35] One of the agents mentioned is usually sufficient to enhance gastric tone so that improved gastric emptying results. Unfortunately, cisapride, a very effective prokinetic agent that works similar to domperidone, was taken off the market by the Food and Drug Administration because of associated cardiac problems in a small subset of patients with underlying heart disease.

In the rare patient recovering from gastric surgery, persistent nausea and vomiting prevent removal of the nasogastric tube. If one is patient, even such individuals can usually be nursed through this turbulent experience. If the nasogastric tube cannot be removed within a period of 7 to 10 days after surgery, a gastrostomy may be placed either laparoscopically or endoscopically. Alimentation can then be given via a J-tube extension placed during one of these techniques. If the gastric remnant is not of sufficient size to accommodate these approaches, a decompressing gastric tube can often be passed retrograde through the efferent limb and exited through the skin via a Witzel technique. Distal to this placement, another tube may be placed antegrade as a Witzel feeding jejunostomy. In patients in whom these enteral approaches to alimentation are not possible, total parenteral nutrition is still an alternative. In any event,

reoperative surgery should generally be delayed for at least 3 months because the majority of patients will regain satisfactory GI function. Only after this period should re-exploration be considered.

Gallstones

The role of vagal denervation in causing gallstone formation has been debated for more than 30 years. The argument in favor of this contention is that division of the hepatic branches of the anterior vagal trunk (as occurs during truncal vagotomy and is frequently done during antireflux and bariatric operations) increases gallstone formation by the creation of gallbladder dysmotility.[36] Both experimental and clinical evidence can be provided that support and challenge this hypothesis. For most forms of gastric surgery in which concomitant vagotomy is anticipated, prophylactic cholecystectomy is not justified. It should be seriously considered only if the gallbladder appears abnormal and if subsequent cholecystectomy is likely to be difficult, as would occur in a patient undergoing gastric bypass for morbid obesity. Obviously, if preoperative evaluation reveals sludge or gallstones in a patient scheduled for gastric surgery and no other complicating problems are anticipated, concomitant cholecystectomy should probably be performed.

ABERRATIONS IN RECONSTRUCTION

A variety of disorders may occur after gastric resection that are greatly influenced by the type of reconstruction performed to re-establish GI continuity. By far, the majority of problems develop in patients who have previously undergone a Billroth II gastrectomy.

Bile Reflux Gastritis

Bile reflux commonly occurs after gastric surgery regardless of the procedure performed. Bile in the stomach on endoscopic examination is often seen when the pyloric sphincter has been ablated or resected; it is even more commonly encountered if a portion of the distal part of the stomach has been resected, regardless of whether a Billroth I or Billroth II reconstruction has been fashioned. Because most patients have no symptoms that can be definitely linked to bile reflux, the attribution of symptomatology to this event has been challenged by many clinicians. Nonetheless, it is generally accepted that in a small subset of patients such reflux is associated with marked, unrelenting epigastric pain, nausea, bilious vomiting, and quantitative evidence of excessive enterogastric reflux.[37,38] For reasons that are not clear, these symptoms may be delayed for months or years after the initial operation. Interestingly, the bilious vomiting may occur anytime during the day or night and not infrequently awakens a patient who is sleeping comfortably. In patients in whom this condition develops, endoscopic examination of the stomach demonstrates a beefy red and friable mucosa with diffuse, superficial erosions that may involve the entire stomach with extension into the distal end of the esophagus. The parietal and gastrin cell mass may be greatly decreased, and hemorrhage, atrophy, and intestinalization of the epithelial surface are often demonstrable microscopically. In some patients achlorhydria may be present, which is indicative of a profound effect on parietal cell mass. Depending on the chronicity of this problem, weight loss is often a part of the initial symptomatology, as is iron deficiency anemia.

Although bile reflux (also called alkaline reflux) gastritis has been reported in patients after undergoing a Billroth I gastrectomy or gastroenterostomy as a drainage procedure following vagotomy, the large majority of patients have previously undergone gastric resection with restoration of GI continuity via a Billroth II approach.[37,38] For reasons that are unclear, asymptomatic patients may demonstrate the same histologic and endoscopic changes in the gastric epithelium as those with bile reflux gastritis. Furthermore, a clear correlation between the volume of bile reflux, the type of bile acid components in this reflux, and which of these components is more likely to induce alkaline gastritis remains to be delineated. Thus, great care must be exercised in attributing symptomatology to reflux when other problems may be at fault, such as afferent or efferent loop obstruction, gastric stasis, or small bowel obstruction from adhesion formation. If radiologic or endoscopic evaluation excludes these other possibilities, a diagnosis of bile reflux as the cause of the symptomatology is on much firmer ground.

Quantification of bile reflux by gastric analysis or scintigraphy (bile reflux scan) is essential for diagnosis.[39] Marked abnormalities in either or both of these studies strengthen the diagnosis. Medical treatment, including acid secretory inhibitors, anticholinergic drugs, and cholestyramine, has been used in an attempt to attenuate the symptoms but unfortunately has not consistently demonstrated any substantial benefit.[37,38] Accordingly, patients with unrelenting or intractable symptoms are best managed with surgery. The physiologic principle underlying surgical intervention should be to divert the bile and pancreatic secretions away from the stomach. Several procedures have been recommended, each with its proponents.[37,40-43] These procedures include Roux-en-Y gastrojejunostomy (Fig. 59–3), interposition of a 40-cm

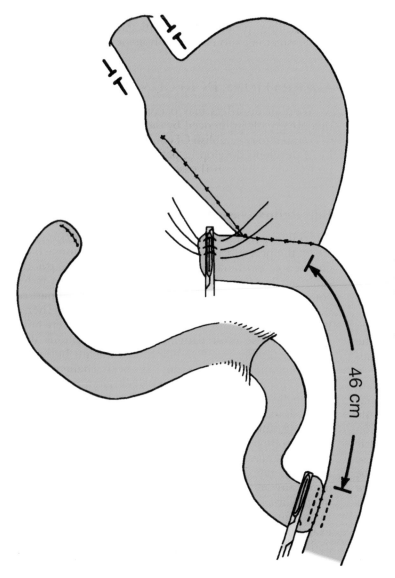

Figure 59–3. Roux-en-Y gastrojejunostomy for the treatment of alkaline reflux gastritis. Note the generous distal gastrectomy and truncal vagotomy. Adequate Roux length minimizes bile reflux. (From Fromm D: Ulceration of the stomach and duodenum. In Fromm D, ed: Gastrointestinal Surgery. New York, Churchill Livingstone, 1985.)

46 cm

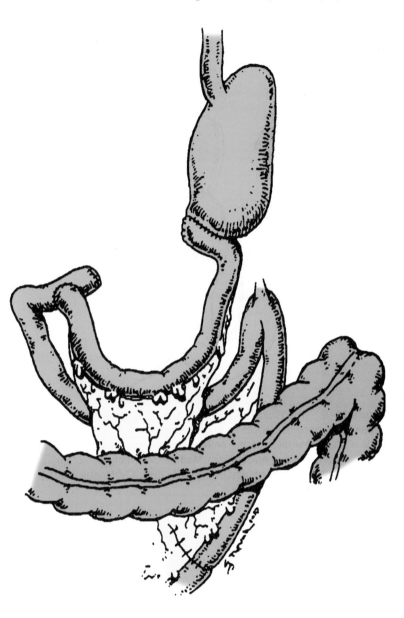

Figure 59–4.   Interposition of a 40-cm isoperistaltic jejunal segment between the stomach and duodenum to treat alkaline reflux gastritis. (From Aronow JS, Matthews JB, Garcia-Aquilar J, et al: Isoperistaltic jejunal interposition for intractable postgastrectomy alkaline reflux gastritis. J Am Coll Surg 180:648, 1995.)

isoperistaltic jejunal loop between the gastric remnant and the duodenum (Henley loop) (Fig. 59–4), and revision of a Billroth II gastrojejunostomy, if previously performed, with a Braun enteroenterostomy (anastomosis between the afferent and efferent limbs) (Fig. 59–5). All of these procedures have proved successful to varying degrees. It is our belief that a Roux-en-Y gastrojejunostomy in which the Roux limb is at least 45 cm in length is the most consistent in relieving symptoms, promoting weight gain, and reversing the findings associated with bile gastritis.

Afferent and Efferent Loop Obstruction

Afferent loop obstruction, known as the *afferent loop syndrome,* is a mechanical problem resulting from the inability of this loop to empty its contents. A variety of causes can give rise to this syndrome, all resulting in partial obstruction of the afferent limb, as shown in Figure 59–6. The afferent limb is nearly always greater than 30 to 40 cm in length for such obstruction to occur; the longer the afferent limb, the more likely obstruction will occur.

Although both acute and chronic forms of afferent loop syndrome have been described, chronic, intermittent obstruction is by far the more common clinical manifestation.[44,45] Typically, increasingly severe epigastric pain develops secondary to the presence of food in the gastric remnant and efferent loop; this food elicits various neurohumoral mechanisms that induce bile secretion and pancreatic enzyme secretion involved in the normal digestive process. As these secretions become more and more pronounced, the obstructed duodenum and proximal jejunum become more distended, and approximately 30 to 60 minutes after eating, copious, often projectile bilious vomiting occurs and provides dramatic relief of pain as the intraluminal pressure in the afferent limb overcomes the obstruction and shoots bile into the gastric remnant. The reason that the vomitus is

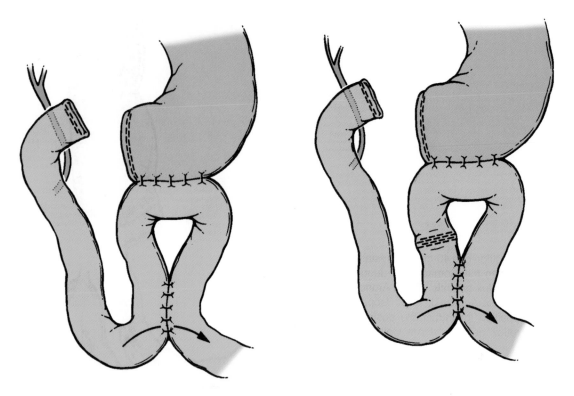

Figure 59–5. The Braun procedure is one of the oldest attempts at bile diversion. The figure on the *left* shows the original procedure with gastrojejunostomy and "downstream" enteroenterostomy to divert bile distally. A recent modification (on the *right*) adds a staple line distal to the enteroenterostomy in an effort to further divert the duodenal contents distally. It has been designated the uncut Roux-en-Y. (From Madura JA: Postgastrectomy problems: Remedial operations and therapy. In Cameron JL [ed]: Current Surgical Therapy, 7th ed. St Louis, CV Mosby, 2001.)

bilious in nature is because the food has already passed into the efferent limb. If the obstruction is severe enough, the distended afferent loop may not be able to sufficiently discharge its contents, and a clinical picture of "closed loop obstruction" manifested as an acute abdomen will result. If this condition is not recognized in its early stages, the afferent loop may actually perforate and result in peritonitis. Obviously, urgent surgery is necessary to correct this problem.

Occasionally, diarrhea may be part of the symptomatology associated with an obstructed afferent limb. It occurs because of bacterial overgrowth, which ultimately binds with vitamin B_{12} and deconjugates the bile acids. The net result of this process is a systemic deficiency of vitamin B_{12}, development of megaloblastic anemia, inefficient micelle formation necessary for fat digestion, and ultimately, steatorrhea if not corrected. This situation can be an especially complex problem if a long afferent loop was created in a more distal segment of the small intestine. Gastroileostomy is the extreme example of this problem. Not only are the aforementioned abnormalities present, but any acid produced by the gastric remnant is also less buffered when it enters distally in the small bowel, thereby leading to a potentially high incidence of marginal ulceration with the long afferent loop.

In contrast to the relatively stereotypical manifestation of afferent loop obstruction, efferent loop obstruction generally mimics proximal small bowel obstruction. It can be caused by intra-abdominal adhesions, like most small bowel obstruction, or can result from herniation of the limb behind the gastrojejunostomy anastomosis, usually in a right-to-left direction. Such herniation occurs because a space generally exists posterior to the anastomosis regardless of whether the initial procedure was antecolic or retrocolic.[46] Because the gastrojejunostomy is usually positioned to the left of the main mass of the small intestine, it is mechanically easier for herniation to occur in a right-to-left direction.

In diagnosing afferent or efferent loop obstruction, it is of utmost importance to remember that obstruction can occur in any patient who previously underwent a Billroth II gastrectomy, no matter how experienced the operating surgeon might have been. In any patient with bilious vomiting, especially if projectile and associated with eating, the possibility of an afferent loop syndrome must be considered. Helpful diagnostic tests include esophagogastroduodenoscopy, computed tomography (CT), upper GI series, and a hepato-iminodiacetic acid (HIDA) scan (not necessarily in that order). Furthermore, if it is known that the afferent loop is long and the Billroth II anastomosis was performed in an anticolic

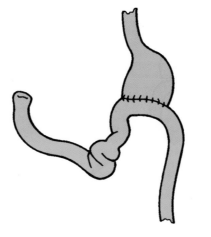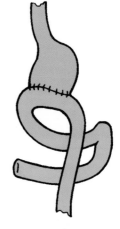

Kinking and
angulation

Internal
herniation behind
efferent limb

Figure 59–6.   Causes of afferent loop syndrome. (From Miller TA, Mercer DW: Derangements in gastric function secondary to previous surgery. In Miller TA [ed]: Modern Surgical Care: Physiologic Foundations and Clinical Applications, 2nd ed. St Louis, Quality Medical, 1998, p 402.)

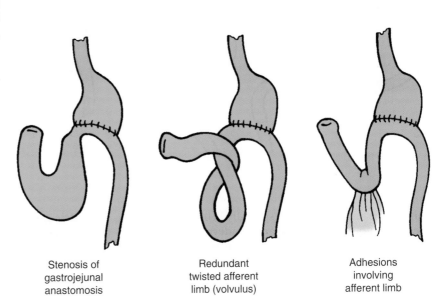

Stenosis of
gastrojejunal
anastomosis

Redundant
twisted afferent
limb (volvulus)

Adhesions
involving
afferent limb

fashion, the diagnostic possibility of an obstructed afferent loop is strengthened, especially if the clinical picture supports this diagnosis. Because there is no medical means of managing this problem, a reoperation will always be needed. The underlying reason for the obstruction will dictate the surgical procedure performed. Possible approaches to management are illustrated in Figure 59–7. If an efferent limb obstruction is the cause of the patient's problem, simple lysis of adhesions may be all that is necessary. If herniation of the limb behind the gastrojejunostomy is responsible for the obstruction, suture closure of the retroanastomotic space may be effective therapy. An alternative approach is to anastomose the two limbs (i.e., afferent and efferent) together to create an enteroenterostomy so that a retroanastomotic hernia would be less likely to occur from a mechanical standpoint. Finally, the Billroth II anastomosis may be converted to a Billroth I.

Jejunogastric Intussusception

Jejunogastric intussusception is a rare complication of gastrojejunostomy. It may occur after a Billroth II gastrectomy but has most commonly been seen after simple gastroenterostomy. In the majority of cases, the efferent limb becomes intussuscepted into the stomach. The clinical manifestation is acute upper abdominal pain and vomiting. Not infrequently, fresh or old blood is identified in the vomitus. The patient is often acutely ill, and a palpable mass may be present in the upper part of the abdomen. Even though both acute and chronic forms of this condition have been described, the possibility that the intussusceptum may incarcerate and eventually strangulate makes it a true surgical emergency more commonly than not. Although the diagnosis is often difficult to make, it should be considered in any patient with a gastrojejunal anastomosis who has severe abdominal

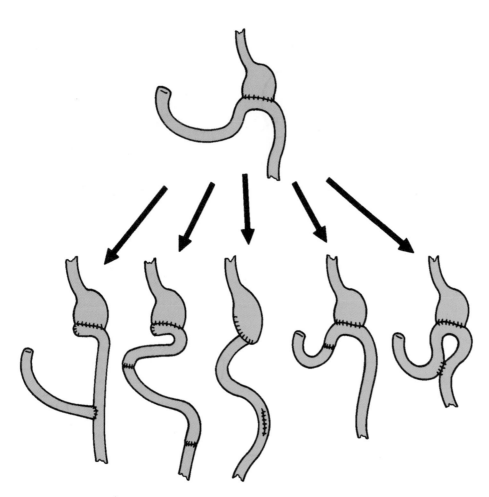

Figure 59–7. Surgical management of afferent loop syndrome. (From Miller TA, Mercer DW: Derangements in gastric function secondary to previous surgery. In Miller TA [ed]: Modern Surgical Care: Physiologic Foundations and Clinical Applications, 2nd ed. St Louis, Quality Medical, 1998, p 404.)

pain, persistent vomiting (especially if bloody), a palpable upper abdominal mass, and tenderness over the epigastrium.[47] The operation of choice is resection of the intussuscepting small bowel if there is any question regarding strangulation. If the intussuscepted intestine is viable, the afferent and efferent limbs of jejunum may be fixed to adjacent tissue such as the mesocolon, colon, or stomach to prevent recurrence. An alternative operative approach is to convert the Billroth II anastomosis to a Billroth I.

The Roux Syndrome

Occasionally, a patient who has undergone distal gastrectomy with a Roux-en-Y reconstruction will have difficulty with gastric emptying along with symptoms such as gastric vomiting, epigastric pain, and weight loss. Endoscopically, the gastric remnant may be dilated as well as the Roux limb, but no evidence of mechanical obstruction can be identified on CT or upper GI series. The only significant finding with this latter study is a delay in gastric emptying. This constellation of clinical findings has been called the *Roux syndrome.*[48]

The cause of this syndrome appears to be an abnormality in motility.[22,49] Key findings include abnormal propulsive activity in the Roux limb that proceeds toward the stomach rather than away from it; in some patients

gastric motility is also perturbed. This disordered motility appears to occur in all patients after this procedure, but why the Roux syndrome develops in only a small subset remains unknown. Furthermore, it seems to be more common in patients with a large gastric remnant and in those who have previously undergone truncal vagotomy.

Some patients benefit with promotility agents. Many, however, require surgical intervention. If gastric motility appears to be a major contributing factor, the gastric remnant should be pared down; in some patients 95% gastrectomy has been performed.[50] If the Roux limb is unusually dilated or flaccid, it too should be resected. Various approaches to re-establishing GI continuity include another Roux limb, a Billroth II anastomosis with an enteroenterostomy between the afferent and efferent limbs, or an isoperistaltic jejunal interposition between the stomach and the duodenum.[42] Because this syndrome is relatively rare, data supporting one surgical approach in preference to another are limited, and selection of the approach has often been dictated by surgeon preference.

REFERENCES

1. Abrahamsson H, Jansson G: Vago-vagal gastro-gastric relaxation in the cat. Acta Physiol Scand 88:289, 1973.

2. Linehan IP, Weinman J, Hobsley M: The 15 min dumping provocation test. Br J Surg 73:810, 1986.

3. Snook JA, Wells AD, Prytherch DR, et al: Studies on the pathogenesis of the early dumping syndrome by intraduodenal instillation of hypertonic glucose. Gut 30:1716, 1989.

4. Carvajal SH, Mulvihill SJ: Postgastrectomy syndromes: Dumping and diarrhea. Gastrointest Clin North Am 23:261, 1994.

5. Goligher JC, Feather DB, Hall R, et al: Several standard elective operations for duodenal ulcer: Ten to 16 year clinical results. Ann Surg 189:18, 1979.

6. Miller TA, Mercer DW: Derangements in gastric function secondary to previous surgery. In Miller TA (ed): Modern Surgical Care: Physiologic Foundations and Clinical Applications. St Louis, Quality Medical, 1998, p 398.

7. Lawaetz O, Blackburn AM, Bloom SR, et al: Gut hormone profile and gastric emptying in the dumping syndrome: A hypothesis concerning the pathogenesis. Scand J Gastroenterol 18:73, 1983.

8. Miholic J, Reilmann L, Meyer HJ, et al: Extracellular space, blood volume, and the early dumping syndrome after total gastrectomy. Gastroenterology 99:923, 1990.

9. Tulassy Z, Tulassay T, Gupta R, Rascher W: Decreased activity of atrial natriuretic peptide in dumping syndrome after gastric surgery. Dig Dis Sci 36:1177, 1991.

10. Yamashita Y, Toge T, Adrian TE: Gastrointestinal hormones in dumping syndrome and reflux esophagitis after gastric surgery. J Smooth Muscle Res 33:37, 1997.

11. Reichle FA, Brigham MP, Reichle RM, Rosemond GP: The effect of gastrectomy on serotonin metabolism in the human portal vein. Ann Surg 172:585, 1970.

12. Sagor GR, Bryant MG, Ghatei MA, et al: Release of VIP in the dumping syndrome. BMJ 282:507, 1981.

13. Jenkins DJA, Bloom SR, Albuquerque RH, et al: Pectin and complications after gastric surgery. Gut 21:574, 1980.

14. Speth PAJ, Jansen JBMJ, Lammers CBHW: Effect of acarbose, pectin, or a combination of acarbose with pectin, and placebo on post-prandial reactive hypoglycemia after gastric surgery. Gut 24:798, 1983.

15. Hasegawa T, Yoneda M, Nakamura K, et al: Long-term effect of alpha-glucosidase inhibitor on late dumping syndrome. J Gastroenterol Hepatol 13:1201, 1998.

16. Richards WO, Geer R, O'Dorisio TM, et al: Octreotide acetate induces fasting small bowel motility in patients with dumping syndrome. J Surg Res 49:483, 1990.

17. Geer RJ, Richards WO, O'Dorisio TM, et al: Efficacy of octreotide acetate in treatment of severe postgastrectomy dumping syndrome. Ann Surg 212:678, 1990.

18. Cheadle WG, Baker PR, Cuschieri A: Pyloric reconstruction for severe vasomotor dumping after vagotomy and pyloroplasty. Ann Surg 202:568, 1985.

19. Frederiksen HJ, Johansen TS, Christiansen PM: Postvagotomy diarrhea and dumping treated with reconstruction of the pylorus. Scand J Gastroenterol 15:245, 1980.

20. Vogel SB, Hocking MP, Woodward ER: Clinical and radionuclide evaluation of Roux-Y diversion for postgastrectomy dumping. Am J Surg 155:57, 1988.

21. Steffes C, Fromm D: Postgastrectomy syndromes. In Ritchie WD (ed): Shackelford's Surgery of the Alimentary Tract, 4th ed. Philadelphia, WB Saunders, 1996.

22. Cullen JJ, Kelly KA: Gastric motor physiology and pathophysiology. Surg Clin North Am 73:1145, 1993.

23. Alexander-Williams J, Donovan IA: Postgastrectomy and postvagotomy syndromes and their management. In Glass GBJ, Sherlock P (eds): Progress in Gastroenterology, vol 4. New York, Grune & Stratton, 1983.

24. Tovey FI, Hall ML, Ell PJ, Hobsley M: A review of postgastrectomy bone disease. J Gastroenterol Hepatol 7:639, 1992.

25. Kennedy T: The vagus and the consequences of vagotomy. Med Clin North Am 58:1231, 1974.

26. Ladas SD, Isaccs PE, Quereshi Y, Sladen G: Role of the small intestine in post-vagotomy diarrhea. Gastroenterology 85:1088, 1983.

27. Cuschieri A: Post-vagotomy diarrhea: Is there a place for surgical management? Gut 31:245, 1990.

28. Browning GC, Buchanan KA, Mackay C: Clinical and laboratory study of post-vagotomy diarrhea. Gut 15:644, 1974.

29. Allan JC, Gerskovitch VP, Russell RI: The role of bile acids in the pathogenesis of post-vagotomy diarrhea. Br J Surg 61:516, 1974.

30. Duncombe YM, Bolin TD, Davis AE: Double blind trial of cholestyramine in post-vagotomy diarrhea. Gut 18:531, 1977.

31. Behrns KE, Sarr MG: Diagnosis and management of gastric emptying disorders. Adv Surg 27:233, 1994.

32. Hocking MP, Vogel SB, Sninsky CA: Human gastric myoelectric activity and gastric emptying for gastric surgery and with pacing. Gastroenterology 103:1811, 1992.

33. McClelland RN, Horton JW: Relief of acute, persistent post-vagotomy atony by metoclopramide. Ann Surg 188:439, 1978.

34. Davis RH, Clench MH, Mathias JR: Effects of domperidone in patients with chronic unexplained upper gastrointestinal symptoms. Dig Dis Sci 33:1505, 1988.

35. Tack J, Janssens J, Vantrappen G, et al: Effect of erythromycin on gastric motility in controls and in diabetic gastroparesis. Gastroenterology 103:72, 1992.

36. Pankin GJ, Smith RB, Johnston D: Gallbladder volume and contractibility after truncal, selective and highly selective vagotomy in man. Ann Surg 178:581, 1973.

37. Ritchie WP Jr: Alkaline reflux gastritis: An objective assessment of its diagnosis and treatment. Ann Surg 192:288, 1980.

38. Ritchie WP Jr: Alkaline reflux gastritis: A diagnosis in search of a disease. J Clin Surg 1:414, 1982.

39. Xynos E, Vassilakis JS, Fountos A, et al: Enterogastric reflux after various types of antiulcer gastric surgery: Quantitation by 99m TC-HIDA scintigraphy. Gastroenterology 101:991, 1991.

40. Miedema BW, Kelly KA: The Roux operation for postgastrectomy syndromes. Am J Surg 161:256, 1991.

41. Van Stiegmann G, Goff JS: An alerative to Roux-en-Y for treatment of bile gastritis. Surg Gynecol Obstet 166:69, 1988.

42. Vogel SB, Drane WE, Woodward ER: Clinical and radionuclide evaluation of bile diversion by Braun enteroenterostomy: Prevention and treatment of alkaline reflux gastritis: An alternative to Roux-en-Y diversion. Ann Surg 219:458, 1994.

43. Aronow JS, Mathews JB, Garcia-Aquilar J, et al: Isoperistaltic jejunal interposition for intractable postgastrectomy alkaline reflux gastritis. J Am Coll Surg 180:648 1995.

44. Jordon GL Jr: The afferent loop syndrome. Surgery 38:1027, 1955.

45. Mitty WE Jr, Grossi C, Nealon TF Jr: Chronic afferent loop syndrome. Ann Surg 172:996, 1970.

46. Rutledge RH: Retroanastomotic hernias after gastrojejunal anastomoses. Ann Surg 177:547, 1973.

47. Foster DG: Retrograde jejunogastric intussusception—rare cause of hematemesis. Arch Surg 73:1009, 1956.

48. Hollands MJ, Filipe I, Edwards S, et al: Clinical and histological sequelae of Roux-en-Y diversion. Br J Surg 76:481, 1989.

49. Van der Milje HCJ, Kleibeuker JH, Limber AJ, et al: Manometric and scintigraphic studies of the relation between motility disturbances in the Roux limb and the Roux-en-Y syndrome. Am J Surg 166:11, 1993.

50. Eckhauser F, Knol JA, Roper SA, Guice KS: Completion gastrectomy for post-surgical gastroparesis syndrome. Ann Surg 208:345, 1988.

60

Miscellaneous Benign Lesions and Conditions of the Stomach, Duodenum, and Small Intestine

Emil L. Popa[†] · Daniel T. Dempsey

STOMACH

The gastrointestinal tract accounts for more neoplastic disease than any other organ system in the human body. A variety of pathologic lesions can occur in the stomach (Table 60–1), many of them polyps, but like in other segments of the digestive tract, adenoma is the only lesion that is truly neoplastic and carries a threat for the development of cancer. The risk is related most closely to the histologic type, size, and number of polyps. Variations in these three factors account for the wide range in reported risk associated with gastric polyps. Other benign lesions found in the stomach are also discussed.

Benign Mucosal (Epithelial) Hypertrophy and Hyperplasia

Benign Focal Mucosal Hypertrophy and Hyperplasia

The principal causes of focal or multifocal thickening of the gastric mucosa are polyps, the presence of heterotopic tissue, and the localized effects of inflammation and repair (Table 60–2).

Benign Polyps The term *polyp* (from the Greek πολυπους, or "morbid excrescence") refers to a macroscopic nodular lesion that protrudes above the mucosal surface of a hollow organ into its lumen. Benign gastric polyps may be neoplastic or non-neoplastic, and their nature can be determined only by histologic examination. The first report of a gastric polyp is believed to have probably been made in 1557. In 1761, Morgagni described a pedunculated polyp near the pylorus, and in 1835, Cruveilhier mentioned the possibility of a polyp causing obstruction or becoming malignant.[1] In 1888, Ménétrier described and illustrated in detail the formation process and malignant transformation of gastric polyps and classified them for the first time.

One of today's classifications is based on the location of the bulk of the lesion in relation to the wall of the stomach: intraluminal or intramural. Such a distinction is clinically relevant. Intraluminal polyps are usually mucosal lesions, which may bleed if their surface is eroded or obstruct if their location is near the orifices of the stomach and their size is large. Intramural polyps are generally submucosal and asymptomatic if small, but if large, the covering mucosa may become ulcerated and bleed as well; a large intramural mass may also become obstructive, depending on its location.

Gastric polyps are not common, with an incidence varying between 0.4% in autopsy series[2] and 3% to 5% in endoscopy series.[3-5] Polyps account for 3.1% of all gastric tumors,[6] and their frequency increases to almost 90% of benign tumors in patients who have undergone upper endoscopy with biopsy, thus making them at present the most common benign tumor of the stomach.

Non-neoplastic Benign Polyps Non-neoplastic benign polyps represent localized expansions of the mucosa and are usually composed of hyperplastic epithelial elements, mainly surface-foveolar mucous cells and pyloric glands,

†Deceased.

Table 60–1   Incidence of Benign Lesions of the Stomach

Type of Lesion	%	Tissue of Origin
Epithelial polyps	41	Epithelium
Leiomyomas (GIST)	37	Smooth muscle
Inflammatory polyps	<5	Inflammatory
Heterotopic tissues	<5	Pancreas
Lipomas	<4	Fat tissue
Neurogenic tumors (GIST)	3	Neural elements
Vascular tumors	2	Vascular tissue
Eosinophilic granulomas	2	Lymphoid tissue
Fibromas	1.5	Connective tissue
Miscellaneous lesions	1	Other

GIST, gastrointestinal stromal tumor.
Modified from Ming SC, Goldman H: Pathology of the Gastrointestinal Tract, 2nd ed. Philadelphia, Lippincott Williams & Wilkins, 1998.

together with varying amounts of edema, inflammatory cells, and proliferating stromal cells of the lamina propria.[7,8]

Hyperplastic or Regenerative Polyps   The most common gastric polyps are hyperplastic or regenerative polyps, which occur in 0.5% to 1% of the general population and account for 70% to 80% of all gastric polyps in most series. Regenerative polyps frequently occur in the setting of gastritis and have low (<1%), if any malignant potential. Hyperplastic polyps contain an overgrowth of histologically normal-appearing gastric epithelium. Atypia is rare. Size of the polyp does not appear to be an important factor. Because *Helicobacter pylori* is a major cause of gastritis, its relationship with hyperplastic polyps has been studied: in a report by Varis et al., *H. pylori* was present in 81% of stomachs with inflammatory polyps and in 45% to 48% of stomachs with hyperplastic polyps or foveolar hyperplasia, respectively.[9] A well-developed hyperplastic polyp is a distinct oval lesion. The polyps are usually single but can be multiple and exceptionally confluent in their appearance. The incidence of hyperplastic polyps is particularly high in the gastric remnant after partial gastrectomy. Enterogastric reflux is common in

Table 60–2   Benign Focal Mucosal Hypertrophy of the Stomach

Type of Benign Hypertrophy	%	Tissue of origin
Non-neoplastic benign polyps		Epithelium
Hyperplastic/regenerative	70-90	Foveolae and pyloric-type glands
Focal polypoid hyperplasia		
Hyperplastic regenerative polyp		
Hyperplastic adenomatous polyp		
Inflammatory	20-33	Inflammatory, pauciepithelial
Inflammatory pseudopolyp		
Inflammatory/retention polyp		
Inflammatory fibroid polyp	3	
Eosinophilic granulomas	2	Lymphoid tissue
Hamartomatous		Epithelium and mesenchyme
Peutz-Jeghers polyp		
Juvenile polyp		
Gardner's polyp		
Familial adenomatous polyposis coli		
Fundic gland polyp	1	Epithelial cells, lymphoid tissue
Heterotopic/ectopic polyp	2-4	
Ectopic pancreatic (±biliary) tissue		Acinary pancreas ± bile ducts
Brunner's gland hyperplasia	1	Duodenal exocrine glands
Adenomyoma		Ductal cells and smooth muscle
Nodular mucosal remnants		
Neoplastic benign polyps = adenomatous	10-15	Adenomatous epithelium
Flat/tubular adenomas		
Papillary/villous adenomas		
Benign inflammatory lesions		Inflammatory
Edema		
Regeneration		

Modified from Ming SC, Goldman H: Pathology of the Gastrointestinal Tract, 2nd ed. Philadelphia, Lippincott Williams & Wilkins, 1998.

these patients, but its role in polyp formation is not certain. Polyps were present in 20% to 66% of gastric stumps 20 years after gastrectomy.[10,11] Finally, hyperplastic polyps may enlarge, shrink, or disappear, but in most cases they remain stationary.

Most people with hyperplastic polyps are asymptomatic. Dyspepsia and vague epigastric discomfort are the most common complaints, although coexistent gastroduodenal disease is also frequently identified. Complications are unusual and gastric hemorrhage occurs in less than 20%.

Inflammatory Polyps   Inflammatory polyps are heterogeneous and encompass several entities. They account for a fifth to a third of gastric polyps.[4] A polyp made of inflammatory tissue can be properly called an *inflammatory pseudopolyp* because glandular tissue is either lost or absent. A special form of inflammatory polyp known as *inflammatory fibroid polyp* occurs most commonly in the stomach, mainly the distal region and the pylorus, and constitutes 3% of gastric polyps. It is the name given collectively to group expansile, mainly submucosal lesions that contain a mixture of spindle cells, small vessels, and inflammatory cells.[12]

An inflammatory polyp with prominent cystic glands may be called a *retention polyp* because of the dilated glands that are filled with retained mucus; such polyps are rare in the stomach. Polyps associated with Cronkhite-Canada syndrome (CCS) are of retention type. This syndrome is characterized by diffuse gastrointestinal polyposis associated with ectodermal changes. Polyps are common in the stomach of patients with CCS; they are 0.5 to 1.5 cm in diameter and either are long and finger-like or resemble a hydatid mole.[13,14] In CCS, the lesions first appear late in adult life, with 80% of patients being in their sixth decade. The male-to-female ratio is close to 1:1.

Hamartomatous Polyps   Hamartomatous polyps are tumor-like nodules composed of tissue present in the location, but in a disorganized arrangement. Because the stomach consists of many different types of cells, the composition of hamartomatous polyps is not uniform. They are encountered most commonly in association with hereditary gastrointestinal polyposis syndromes, including generalized juvenile polyposis (15% of patients), Peutz-Jeghers syndrome (25% to 50% of patients), familial adenomatous polyposis coli (FAP), and the related Gardner syndrome.[15-18] In these syndromes the polyps are located more commonly in the intestine than in the stomach, so they will be discussed more extensively in that segment. It is noteworthy that gastric and intestinal polyps in the same disease may be of different types. For instance, whereas intestinal polyps in Gardener's syndrome and FAP are mostly adenomas, the most common form of gastric polyp in these syndromes is hamartomatous, and it involves mainly the fundic mucosa. Although the polyps in both Peutz-Jeghers syndrome and juvenile polyposis are hamartomatous, they have different histologic characteristics. Finally, hamartomatous polyps may be seen in patients without other characteristics of these syndromes.

Fundic Gland Polyps   Also known as fundic gland hyperplasia or glandular cysts, the less common fundic gland polyps occur in the oxyntic mucosa of the stomach.[19,20] These lesions are composed of fundic pits, or glands lined with increasing numbers of normal-appearing parietal and chief cells with prominent cystically dilated, tortuous changes, and benign lymphoid polyps, or localized areas of marked lymphoid hyperplasia.[21] Fundic gland polyps have been found in patients with Gardner's syndrome, as well as in FAP patients.[22,23] Histologically, the constituent cells of the polyp appear normal and the polyp may regress and disappear, thus suggesting that these lesions may not be hamartomatous.

Heterotopic Pancreatic Polyps   More commonly, heterotopic polyps are made of tissue from the neighboring pancreas and duodenum. Ectopic foci of mature pancreatic tissue may be observed in the stomach, more often in the distal, prepyloric portion.[24-27] The gastric implants consist of pancreatic elements alone—exocrine glands and ducts—or occur in combination with varying amounts of biliary elements (bile ducts epithelia, smooth muscle). The lesions are usually small and primarily confined to the gastric submucosa, but they may enlarge and extend into the mucosal region.

Endoscopic examination reveals slightly raised, umbilicated, or nipple-like nodules. The umbilication represents the outlet of the exocrine duct. Biopsy samples are generally too superficial to detect the heterotopic glandular tissue. The lesions are asymptomatic, with no malignant potential, but if they are large, ulceration and bleeding are common manifestations. In children, pancreatic heterotopia can be manifested as peptic ulcer or intermittent pyloric obstruction.

Brunner's Gland Polyps   Brunner's gland hyperplasia has been called *adenoma* because of the tightly packed glands, whereas in reality, only hyperplasia is present and the glands are normal. Some categorize it as a hamartoma because of its stationary appearance. The lesion accounts for only about 1% of gastric polyps,[28] and it always occurs in the prepyloric region.[29,30] Brunner's glands, normally found in the duodenal submucosa, secrete an alkaline, bicarbonate-rich fluid and mucus that serves to neutralize acidified luminal contents arriving from the stomach.

Because of its presence in the prepyloric region, obstruction is the common manifestation.

Adenomyomas   A rare benign gastric lesion related to heterotopic tissue is adenomyoma or adenomyosis, which is composed of a mixture of ducts lined by columnar cells and bundles of smooth muscle in a haphazard arrangement. Pancreatic tissue or Brunner's glands, or both, may also be present. Most of the lesions are smaller than 2 cm, but some are as large as 5 cm in diameter.[31]

Inflammatory, hamartomatous, and heterotopic polyps have negligible malignant potential.

Adenomatous or Neoplastic Polyps   Neoplastic or adenomatous polyps constitute about 10% to 15% of gastric polyps and are composed of immature and dysplastic cells. On the basis of their architectural pattern and the cytologic appearance of cells, adenomas are subdivided into a flat (tubular) type and a papillary (villous and tubulovillous) type. Rarely, dysplastic or adenomatous lesions are present in hyperplastic polyps. Among patients with FAP, gastric polyps are common in 33% to 60%, whereas gastric adenoma occurs in 15%.[32,33] Affected individuals are usually in the seventh decade of life. The incidence of gastric adenoma increases with age, from only 0.1% in the third decade to 3.7% in the ninth decade. Men are affected more often then women (2:1 to 3:1). The adenomas are generally solitary lesions. They may arise anywhere in the stomach, with about 50% at the lesser curvature and only 5% in the upper third of the stomach; the preferred location is the distal portion of the stomach, particularly the antrum.[34] In gastric adenomas, mucosal atypia is frequent and mitotic figures are more common than in hyperplastic polyps. Gastric adenomas may undergo malignant transformation, similar to adenomas in the other segments of the gastrointestinal tract. The frequency of malignant transformation ranges from 5% to 75% in different series,[35,36] with an average of 10% to 20%, and is greatest for polyps larger than 2 cm in diameter. Multiple adenomatous polyps increase the risk for cancer. The presence of an adenomatous polyp is also a marker indicating an increased threat for the development of cancer in the remainder of the gastric mucosa. Gastric flat adenomas have a lower incidence of malignant changes; the incidence increases with the grade of dysplasia, the papillary pattern, and the size of the lesion.[34]

Flat Adenomas Flat adenomas are the most common form of adenoma in the stomach, especially in Japan.[37] Their gross appearance resembles that of early gastric carcinoma. Most flat adenomas are slightly elevated lesions with an irregular, but flat surface, or they show varying degrees of nodularity. Some adenomas, however, have a smooth surface that is even with the surface of the surrounding mucosa. The histologic features of gastric flat adenomas are unique; whereas the atypical cells in other adenomas extend through the entire thickness of the mucosa, in gastric adenomas they occupy only the upper third to half of the gastric mucosa and maintain a two-layer structure. Depressed adenomas, however, usually occupy the entire thickness of the mucosa. The two-layer architecture and relative indolence of the immature epithelial cells are hallmarks distinguishing flat adenomas from papillary adenomas. The possibility that flat adenomas are earlier forms of papillary adenoma has not been confirmed; most flat adenomas appear stationary. Despite the lack of growth, flat adenomas are clearly neoplastic, as evidenced by cellular atypism and a relatively high incidence (10%) of malignant change within the lesion. As a neoplasm, a flat adenoma is a sharply delimited lesion that spreads horizontally within the confines of the epithelium, thereby resulting in a demarcation between the lesion and the neighboring non-neoplastic epithelium.

Symptoms are similar to those for non-neoplastic polyps.

Papillary Adenomas Papillary adenomas of the stomach are sessile or broad-based nodular lesions with a lobulated contour and deep crevices. The average size of papillary adenomas is 4 cm, although lesions as large as 15 cm have been reported.[38] Gastric papillary adenomas are located mostly in the antrum. Fixation to deep tissue indicates carcinomatous changes with invasion. In contrast to the relative uniformity of cells in gastric flat adenomas, pleomorphism and mitosis are common in papillary adenomas. The neoplastic cells end abruptly at the junction with the neighboring epithelium. Adenomas with malignant change are positive for carcinoembryonic antigen.[39]

On endoscopy, the lesions are soft and freely mobile and have a velvety appearance. On radiologic examination, barium trapped in the crevices gives a pathognomonic finding of a "soap bubble" or "paint brush" appearance because of rounded radiolucent areas intermixed with a meshwork of radiopaque material. Esophagogastroduodenoscopy (EGD) with biopsy is appropriate after a positive result on a radiologic study.

All types of the aforementioned polyps that are symptomatic, larger than 2 cm, or adenomatous should be resected, usually by endoscopic snare polypectomy. Consideration should also be given to removing hyperplastic polyps for histologic examination, especially if large, and such treatment should be sufficient. Endoscopic resection is adequate for the pedunculated adenomatous type if the polyp is completely removed and shows no evidence of invasive cancer on histologic examination. Larger or sessile lesions should be removed by laparoscopic wedge resection when present on the anterior gastric wall or by a laparoscopic intragastric approach for lesions present in other areas (posterior wall, lesser curvature, gastroesophageal junction). Polyps with biopsy-proven invasive carcinoma, if not amenable to laparoscopic resection, may need open surgical removal. Repeat EGD for surveillance of the gastric mucosa should be done after removal of adenomatous polyps and perhaps after removal of hyperplastic polyps as well.

Benign Inflammatory Lesions These lesions are most often observed adjacent to ulcers and appear as uniform elevations of the mucosa or as deformed folds. Mucosal biopsy is frequently performed to confirm the inflammatory nature of such areas and to exclude other more significant lesions such as neoplasms.

Benign Diffuse Mucosal Hypertrophy and Hyperplasia

Rugae are limited to the gastric fundus and corpus region and are composed of both mucosal and submucosal tissue. Enlargement of rugae can be readily appreciated by radiographic and gross endoscopic examination, and the diagnosis of a normal variation depends on noting that the rugae are simply enlarged, not deformed in any way, and excluding any associated inflammation or hypersecretory state. More significant causes of diffuse mucosal hypertrophy in the stomach include Zollinger-Ellison syndrome (hyperplasia of the parietal cells), Ménétrier's disease (hyperplasia of the surface-foveolar mucous cells), or some sort of combination. The disorders must be distinguished from a variety of inflammatory (tuberculosis, syphilis, sarcoidosis, allergic gastroenteritis, etc.) and neoplastic (lymphoma) conditions that can also infiltrate and expand the mucosal region.

Ménétrier's Disease (Hypertrophic Gastropathy)

Ménétrier's disease, originally described in 1888, is a rare clinical syndrome characterized by diffuse epithelial hyperplasia leading to giant cerebriform enlargement of the rugal folds in the proximal part of the stomach, usually with sparing of the antrum. The etiology and pathogenesis are unclear, although a frequent association with previous respiratory infections has been noted in cases in children.[40] The disorder is characteristically associated with protein-losing gastropathy resulting in hypoalbuminemia and with hypochlorhydria. Mucosal biopsy shows diffuse hyperplasia of the surface mucus-secreting cells with accompanying glandular atrophy. The reduction in gastric acid may be related to dilution by mucous secretions or to loss of parietal cells secondary to expansion of foveolar cells—this issue has not been decided yet. There is also a hyperplastic hypersecretory variant of Ménétrier's disease characterized by normal or increased acid secretion and no protein loss. There may be an increased risk for gastric cancer, although the present literature suggests that the risk for cancer in patients with Ménétrier's disease may have been exaggerated in the past because of confusion with other cases of chronic gastritis. The tendency has been to consider all cases with giant folds in the proximal part of the stomach, with the exception of Zollinger-Ellison syndrome, as potential examples of Ménétrier's disease, without further consideration of their histologic and functional features.

Symptoms and Diagnosis   Most patients with Ménétrier's disease are men (M/F = 3:1) 30 to 60 years of age with complaints of epigastric discomfort or pain, weight loss, diarrhea, and hypoalbuminemia/hypoproteinemia with possible peripheral edema. Familial cases have been recorded rarely.[41] Bleeding related to superficial rugal erosions can also be an initial sign. In some cases the disease regresses spontaneously.[42,43]

Definitive diagnosis of Ménétrier's disease requires documentation of foveolar hyperplasia without significant inflammation, lack of increased acid production, and the presence of protein loss from the mucosa.

Treatment   Medical treatment is limited mainly to albumin replacement and maintenance of adequate nutrition. Gastric resection may be indicated for bleeding, severe hypoproteinemia, or cancer in some patients with this rare problem.

Childhood Cases of Ménétrier's Disease

Although many children have an antecedent history of a respiratory infection and peripheral blood eosinophilia, the exact etiology and pathogenesis have not been established. When compared with the clinical course in adults, Ménétrier's disease in children is self-limited and

regresses spontaneously after several weeks. This disease neither recurs nor is associated with carcinoma.

Symptoms and Diagnosis   The major differential diagnosis is allergic gastroenteritis, manifestations of which include enlarged gastric folds and protein loss.[44] In the allergic condition, however, the lesions are typically located in the gastric antrum, blood loss and anemia are often evident, and an increased number of eosinophils is noted in biopsy tissue.

Treatment   Because the condition is self-limited and regresses spontaneously after several weeks, surgical excision is not required.

Benign Mesenchymal (Nonepithelial) Lesions

Vascular Lesions

"Watermelon Stomach" (Gastric Antral Vascular Ectasia)

Gastric antral vascular ectasia is a rare entity characterized by the presence of both inflammatory and vascular components in the mucosa. Gross endoscopic examination reveals prominent longitudinal folds with parallel striking red stripes atop the mucosal folds of the distal part of the stomach, much like the rind of a watermelon. Histologically, the disorder is distinguished by dilated mucosal blood vessels in the lamina propria, often containing thrombi, with no evidence of vascular malformation on angiographic and morphologic examination. Mucosal fibromuscular hyperplasia and hyalinization are often present. The histologic appearance can resemble portal gastropathy, but "watermelon stomach" predominantly affects the distal portion of the stomach, whereas the former usually affects the proximal portion. Patients with gastric antral vascular ectasia are generally elderly women with chronic bleeding. Most have an associated autoimmune connective tissue disorder, and at least 25% have chronic liver disease.

Symptoms and Diagnosis   Patients typically have iron deficiency anemia and chronic gastrointestinal blood loss requiring transfusions. The diagnosis of gastric antral vascular ectasia is based on the typical endoscopic and biopsy appearance of the mucosa, together with angiographic findings and a compatible clinical history.

Treatment   The lesions are treated by endoscopic cautery. Antrectomy is not ordinarily necessary but may be required to control blood loss. In patients with portal hypertension, a transvenous intrahepatic portosystemic shunt (TIPS) should be considered first.

Dieulafoy's Disease (Gastric Congenital Arteriovenous Malformation)

Dieulafoy's disease is a rare condition characterized by an unusually large (1 to 3 mm in diameter) tortuous artery that courses through the submucosa of the proximal part of the stomach for a variable distance.[45] Erosion of the gastric mucosa overlying the vessel results in necrosis of the arterial wall and brisk hemorrhage. The mucosal defect is usually small (2 to 5 mm) and without evidence of chronic inflammation. This condition typically occurs in middle-aged (sixth decade of life) and elderly men, although younger men and women can be affected.[46] The lesion occurs twice as frequently in men as in women. No significant association has been found with alcohol abuse or antecedent symptoms.[46]

Symptoms and Diagnosis Recurrent painless hematemesis and melena are the typical symptoms at initial evaluation. Recurrent bleeding with spontaneous cessation is likewise common.[46] Massive gastric hemorrhage can also occur.[47]

The diagnosis is most frequently made endoscopically by demonstrating arterial bleeding from a pinpoint mucosal defect. Occasionally, a small arterial vessel may be seen protruding from the gastric mucosa. Characteristically, the lesions are located within 6 cm of the gastroesophageal junction along the lesser curvature, although they may occur at other sites. When a relatively small ulcer is noted together with a single large bleeding artery during endoscopy for upper gastrointestinal hemorrhage, the possibility of a Dieulafoy vascular malformation of the stomach should be considered.

Treatment Most patients can be managed by endoscopic electrocoagulation of the bleeding vessel.[48] If operative excision is required, a combined endoscopic and surgical approach may be useful.[49]

Angiodysplasia Angiodysplastic lesions may occur throughout the gastrointestinal tract, but they are found most commonly in the stomach and duodenum. The lesions are frequently multiple rather than single. They appear as minute flat or slightly raised red lesions with round or stellate shapes. The margins are characteristically sharp with a pale mucosal halo surrounding the lesion. They are all arteriovenous malformations, microscopically visible as dilated, distorted, thin-walled vessels (small arteries, capillaries, and veins). The etiology of angiodysplasia is unknown, but the lesions are considered degenerative lesions.[50]

Symptoms and Diagnosis These lesions may be diagnosed by endoscopy, although their minute size and sessile nature complicate detection. Because the lesions are mostly submucosal, endoscopic mucosal biopsy is often not diagnostic. The lesions may be mistaken for submucosal hemorrhage associated with acute gastritis or trauma artifacts from a nasogastric tube or endoscope. The mainstay of diagnosis of angiodysplastic lesions is selective arteriography, which often features an early filling vein, a densely opacified and slowly emptying, dilated, tortuous vein, and a vascular tuft.[49]

Treatment Endoscopic injection of sclerosants, electrocoagulation, and laser photocoagulation have all been used to treat gastroduodenal angiodysplasia with good results. The multiplicity of lesions often necessitates several courses of therapy to eliminate recurring hemorrhage. Surgical resection of the gastric wall containing the lesion and oversewing of the bleeding lesion have been reported to control hemorrhage successfully.

Telangiectasia Telangiectasia is a localized dilation of arterioles, capillaries, and venules. Multiple congenital lesions may occur in the gastrointestinal tract in Osler-Weber-Rendu syndrome and Turner's syndrome. As acquired lesions, they occur in the CRST syndrome (calcinosis cutis, Raynaud's phenomenon, sclerodactyly, telangiectasia).

Congenital Telangiectasia Osler-Weber-Rendu syndrome (hereditary hemorrhagic telangiectasia) is inherited as an autosomal dominant disorder. Telangiectases arise from simple dilation of normal vascular structures because of congenital thinning of the muscular layer and elastic fibers in the arteriolar wall. Telangiectases occur in many places, including the skin, mucous membranes, and internal organs, and result in recurrent hemorrhage. Gastrointestinal bleeding is present in about 15% of patients. The vascular lesions may be stellate or nodular; they are punctate, red to purple noncompressible lesions that vary in diameter from 1 to 4 mm. The mucocutaneous lesions usually become clinically apparent in the second and third decades of life and are later manifested as chronic bleeding, usually in the fourth decade. It should be noted that vascular anomalies also occur in other organs: the meninges, spinal cord, eyes, liver, and genitourinary tract.

Turner's syndrome (ovarian dysgenesis) is associated with hemorrhage from telangiectases present mostly lower in the gastrointestinal tract and is discussed later.

Acquired Telangiectasia Telangiectases are also present in patients with systemic sclerosis, especially the CRST syndrome. Gastrointestinal hemorrhage may result from lesions in the stomach, as well as lesions in the rectum and colon.[51] Most frequently, the lesions are found on the hands, lips, face, and tongue.

Treatment Frequently, endoscopy with electrocoagulation, a heater probe, or neodymium:yttrium-aluminum-garnet (Nd:YAG) laser can adequately treat these lesions.

Hemangiomas Whether gastrointestinal hemangiomas are true neoplasms or represent hamartomas continues to be a subject of controversy and debate. Gastric hemangiomas are very infrequent and not hereditary, whereas hemangiomas in the small intestine account for about 10% of all benign small bowel tumors. Because of these aspects, the subject is discussed more extensively under the duodenum and small intestinal segment.

Diffuse gastrointestinal hemangiomatosis is an entity in which as many as 100 lesions involving the stomach, small bowel, and colon are encountered. Bleeding or anemia in childhood usually leads to diagnosis of this condition.

Lymphangiomas Lymphangiomas of the gastrointestinal tract are extremely rare. They have been reported beside the stomach and in the small intestine (mostly jejunum) and esophagus, as well as in the colon.[52] They are usually soft, submucosal polypoid lesions with a broad base, and cystically dilated lymph vessels are seen on microscopic examination.

Glomus Tumors   These benign neoplasms are composed of uniform round cells that ultrastructurally are mature smooth muscle cells. In the gastrointestinal tract, glomus tumors occur almost exclusively within the stomach, especially the antral region, where they appear grossly as intramural circumscribed masses.[12] A few have been described in the esophagus and even fewer in the small intestine. Most tumors are about 2 to 2.5 cm in size, but they may grow to 4 cm in diameter. The bigger lesions are likely to ulcerate. Microscopically, glomus tumors lie mostly within the muscularis propria; the mucosa is never infiltrated. The monotonous cells are arranged in sheets, cords, or clusters, usually intimately applied to the walls of capillaries.

The major differential diagnosis for such a small intramural round cell tumor is an epithelioid cell stromal tumor.

Leiomyomas

In recent years, what used to be called leiomyoma is now termed gastrointestinal stromal tumor (GIST) because it has been recognized that these tumors may arise not just from smooth muscle but from other components of the wall as well.[53] GIST may arise from pluripotential mesenchymal cells within the muscular wall of the gastrointestinal tract, most commonly those supposed to become smooth muscle or neural cells. Gastric leiomyomas are well-differentiated benign GISTs arising from the smooth muscle in the stomach wall. The typical leiomyoma is submucosal and firm.

Symptoms and Diagnosis   Lesions smaller than 2 cm are usually asymptomatic and benign. Larger lesions have greater malignant potential and a greater likelihood of causing symptoms such as bleeding, obstruction, or pain. If ulcerated, they have an umbilicated appearance and may bleed.

Treatment   Asymptomatic lesions smaller than 2 cm may be observed. Larger lesions and symptomatic lesions should be removed by wedge resection—often possible laparoscopically or by a laparoscopic intragastric approach. When these lesions are observed rather than resected, the patient should be made aware of their presence and the small possibility for malignancy.

Neurogenic Benign Tumors

Neurogenic tumors are too rare in the stomach to be of concern, and they account for less than 3% of all gastric neoplasms. Patients with von Recklinghausen's multiple neurofibromatosis commonly have gastric and intestinal involvement, sometimes taking the form of neurofibromas with a plexiform pattern. Less commonly, diffuse neurofibromas extend from the submucosa across the muscularis mucosae into the mucosa, where they expand and distort the crypts and produce a picture resembling the mucosa of patients with incipient juvenile polyps. The occurrence of a typical neurofibroma of the stomach in the absence of von Recklinghausen's disease is too rare to discuss. It is important to remember that GISTs of the typical or usual type may also occur in patients with von Recklinghausen's multiple neurofibromatosis.[54]

Neurilemomas originating from nerve sheaths and ganglioneuromas arising from components of the sympathetic nervous system are other tumors originating from neural tissue. These tumors can also be associated with von Recklinghausen's disease. When these proliferations are confined to the mucosa, they result in the formation of polyps or plaques. The Schwann cells also present distort them, and such distortions again resemble those encountered in juvenile polyps.

Symptoms and Diagnosis   Pain, intestinal bleeding, and obstruction occur as the initial complaint with equal frequency.

Treatment   Symptomatic lesions are treated by local excision.

Lipomas

These circumscribed intramural yellow masses attenuate the overlying mucosa. In the case of larger lesions, the mucosa can become ulcerated with secondary fibrotic and hemorrhagic changes at the ulcer base. The bigger the tumors, the more likely they are to produce bleeding, pain, or obstruction. Microscopically, these submucosal masses of rather uniform adipose cells compress the muscularis mucosae and often cause thinning of the overlying mucosa.

Symptoms and Diagnosis   Descriptions of gastrointestinal lipomas are especially prevalent in the radiologic literature because of a set of fairly characteristic features, including pliability, which allows for changing shape of the tumor, and their low density, as noted on computed tomography (CT).

Treatment   Many gastric lipomas are discovered as incidental findings during endoscopic procedures and can be amputated completely at that time if they are large or pedunculated. Otherwise, small tumors less than 2 cm can be safely observed. Excision is necessary in symptomatic patients with bleeding or obstruction, and treatment is by local excision. Resection can be accomplished by either open or laparoscopic techniques. Larger or growing lesions should be resected to rule out malignant liposarcoma.

Fibromas

Fibromas are large, well-circumscribed tumors consistent with dense collagen bundles and a variable number of mature fibroblasts. They occur in the submucosa, muscularis, or serosa of the stomach. Fibromas are difficult to distinguish from scar tissue. They usually occur in adults 50 to 60 years of age.

Symptoms and Diagnosis   Most tumors are asymptomatic and discovered at exploratory laparotomy performed for other reasons or at autopsy.

Treatment Small tumors can be safely observed. Local excision provides satisfactory treatment of symptomatic lesions.

Congenital Lesions

Duplication Cysts Gastric duplication cysts are tubular or cystic lesions surrounded by smooth muscle that is continuous with the muscle of the stomach.[55,56] The underlying mechanism of formation that has been suggested is adherence or fusion (or both) of proliferating gastric longitudinal folds during fetal development.[57] The lining of duplication cysts most frequently represents a mixture of gastric epithelia, with possible pancreatic heterotopia. Sometimes the lining can be destroyed by inflammation. These lesions occur most often along the greater curvature in children, typically infants, and can be detected incidentally. Most of the cystic lesions range in size from 3 cm to less than 12 cm, whereas the tubular forms communicate with the stomach. True congenital gastric diverticula with full muscular walls that are manifested in childhood may be considered gastric duplication cysts that have incompletely separated. Associated malformations include other foregut complete duplications or malformations, vertebral anomalies, but most frequently, esophageal duplication.

Symptoms and Diagnosis These lesions can be detected incidentally or be manifested as bleeding with extrinsic compression and obstruction of the stomach and vomiting. They can also cause symptoms as a result of perforation or fistulization into other adjacent organs.

Treatment Although isolated duplication cysts can be removed surgically, even when extensive, complex malformations are harder to manage and can be fatal.

DUODENUM AND SMALL INTESTINE

Even though the small intestine constitutes 70% to 80% of the total length of the gastrointestinal tract and more than 90% of its inner mucosal surface area, it is the site of only 5% to 7% of neoplasms that arise. This discrepancy is thought to be due to the rarity of non-neuroendocrine epithelial tumors in the small bowel.[58] Moreover, little consensus has been reached regarding the relative incidence rates of small bowel tumors in the United States or worldwide. Noticeably, geographic variations are found around the world. Given the rarity of small intestinal tumors and the wide variety of histologic types, the actual reported numbers are small even in the largest series, so reliable comparisons are difficult and incidence rates are impossible to confirm. Primary small bowel tumors are 40 to 60 times less common than colonic neoplasms, and they are found in 0.2% to 0.3% of autopsies, which is 15 times higher than the operative incidence. The frequency of benign small bowel tumors generally increases from the duodenum to the ileum. However, per unit area, the proximal 20 cm of intestine has the greatest number. Therefore, the duodenum, which constitutes less than 10% of the small intestine, contributes a disproportionately higher percentage of tumors.

Benign neoplasms of the small bowel can occur at any age, but the average age at diagnosis is 62 years. The incidence of small intestinal neoplasms is about equal in men and women.

Benign neoplasms can arise from all constituent tissues of the small intestine. The most frequently encountered benign tumors of the small intestine are leiomyomas (25% to 50% in different series) and adenomas (11% to 35% in different series), followed by lipomas (15% to 25%), lymphangiomas (2% to 12%), hemangiomas (<10%), fibromas (<6%), and others that occur less commonly (Table 60–3).[59-61] Hamartomas usually occur as part of Peutz-Jeghers syndrome, whereas schwannomas of the small intestine occur most frequently in the clinical setting of von Recklinghausen's disease. Hemangiomas and telangiectasia are often associated with Osler-Weber-Rendu syndrome and, to a lesser extent, Turner's syndrome.

Symptoms and Diagnosis

Tumors of the small intestine, besides being uncommon, are also insidious in manifestation and frequently represent a diagnostic challenge.[62] Benign tumors generally cause vague, nonspecific symptoms, but about half are asymptomatic (Table 60–4). They are often encountered as incidental findings at laparotomy or autopsy. Therefore, the relative distribution of benign tumors of the small intestine is affected by whether the reported series is based on clinical or autopsy findings. Thus, in clinical series, two thirds of small bowel tumors reported are malignant. The converse is true in autopsy series, in which benign tumors account for more than three fourths of all tumors.

When symptomatic, benign tumors of the small intestine are usually associated with either abdominal pain or symptoms of iron deficiency anemia secondary to occult gastrointestinal hemorrhage. Indeed, small bowel tumors are the second most common cause of obscure gastrointestinal bleeding and account for 5% to 10% of all cases of chronic blood loss; in patients younger than 50 years, small bowel tumors are the single most common lesion with occult digestive bleeding.[58] The abdominal pain is usually due to episodes of intermittent obstruction secondary to transient intussusception of the small bowel, with the tumor serving as the lead point.[63] Finally, benign periampullary duodenal neoplasms may initially be manifested as obstructive jaundice.

The diagnosis of small bowel tumors requires a high index of suspicion. Bowel obstruction in a patient without previous abdominal surgery should raise suspicion for a neoplasm. An accurate preoperative diagnosis is made in only about a third of patients. The history and physical examination, though essential, are usually nonspecific and unrevealing. In a minority of patients laboratory data may reveal iron deficiency anemia that is due to intestinal bleeding.

Evaluation of patients with gastrointestinal bleeding thought to be secondary to a small bowel neoplasm can be particularly difficult. Diagnostic methods for small bowel tumors include enteroclysis, visceral arteriography, CT scanning, magnetic resonance imaging, and enteroscopy.

Table 60–3   Incidence of Benign Tumors of the Small Intestine

Type of Lesion	%	Tissue of Origin
Leiomyomas (GIST)	25-50	Smooth muscle
Adenomas	11-35	Epithelium
Tubular		
Villous	<1	
Lipomas	15-25	Fat tissue
Hemangiomas	7-10	Vascular tissue
Neurogenic tumors (GIST)	<5-10	Neural elements
Schwannomas		Peripheral neural elements
Neurilemomas		Nerve sheath
Ganglioneuromas		Sympathetic nervous system
Fibromas	0-6	Connective tissue
Hamartomas	0-6	Various elements
Lymphangiomas	2-3	Lymphoid tissue
Ectopic tissue	Rare	
Pancreatic tissue		Pancreas
Endometriosis		Endometrium
Dermoid cysts	Rare	
Eosinophilic "granulomas"	Rare	Nonspecific inflammation with eosinophils
Angiodysplasia	Rare	Vascular
Hyperplastic polyps	Rare	Mucosal crypts

GIST, gastrointestinal stromal tumor.
Modified from Greenfield LJ, Mulholland MW, Oldham KT, et al: Surgery, Scientific Principles and Practice, 3rd ed. Philadelphia, Lippincott Williams & Wilkins, 2001.

Table 60–4   Clinical Findings in Patients with Benign Tumors of the Small Intestine

Symptom	%
Asymptomatic	47-60
Abdominal pain	24-50
Acute gastrointestinal bleeding	29-44
Anemia	28-58
Intermittent obstruction	12-28
Jaundice	<2
Nausea and/or vomiting	Rare
Abdominal mass	Rare
Perforation	—
Weight loss	—

Modified from Greenfield LJ, Mulholland MW, Oldham KT, et al: Surgery, Scientific Principles and Practice, 3rd ed. Philadelphia, Lippincott Williams & Wilkins, 2001.

Radiologic studies are the cornerstone of diagnosis for small bowel neoplasms. Plain abdominal radiographs indicating obstruction are not specific in terms of the cause. CT scanning of the abdomen with oral administration of contrast is a valuable technique for both demonstrating the primary lesion and defining any extraluminal extension. In patients with partial obstruction or those undergoing elective evaluation, barium contrast examination of the small bowel is the diagnostic procedure of choice. Enteroclysis study or small bowel enema with direct instillation of contrast material into the small bowel is preferred over standard upper gastrointestinal series with small bowel follow-through.[64] In the enteroclysis study, air-contrast techniques and fluoroscopic observation of the flow of contrast through the bowel improve the sensitivity for detection of subtle mucosal lesions. However, this technique can sometimes produce false-positive results.

Standard contrast-enhanced radiologic studies are useful in detecting tumors only if they are of substantial size. Tagged red blood cell radionuclide scans may localize the bleeding site to the small intestine but generally lack sensitivity. Visceral angiography can be useful in diagnosing and localizing the site of bleeding, but only in situations in which the hemorrhage is rapid (>0.5 ml/min).

Upper endoscopic examination or *total colonoscopy with ileal intubation* is useful in patients with duodenal or terminal ileal neoplasms. Direct visualization of tumors and endoscopic biopsy can often be obtained. *Endoscopic ultrasound examination* may be useful in the staging of periampullary duodenal tumors. *Push enteroscopy* can identify tumors in the jejunum with high effectiveness and efficiency. Nevertheless, the fact that exploration is restricted to the jejunum is a limitation of the method. In some patients, laparotomy with intraoperative push endoscopy may be required. Experience using enteroscopy and push endoscopy to visualize the entire small bowel is limited. *Sonde enteroscopy* can potentially identify tumors throughout the small intestine. Although encouraging results have been reported in small series, these techniques are not widely available.[65,66]

Benign Mucosal (Epithelial) Lesions

Non-neoplastic Benign Polyps

Non-neoplastic benign polyps of the small intestine include Peutz-Jeghers polyps, juvenile polyps, lymphoid polyps, and inflammatory fibroid polyps. Peutz-Jeghers polyps are discussed later, under the section on polyposis and small intestinal hamartomas, juvenile polyps under juvenile polyposis of the small bowel segment, and lymphoid polyps under intestinal lymphoid polyposis.

Inflammatory Fibroid Polyps

Inflammatory fibroid polyps are benign tumor masses that occur in the stomach and the small and large intestine. These uncommon lesions occur at all ages and have a worldwide distribution.[67] Their cause is unknown and they are not associated with any known syndromes; however, they have been reported in ileal pouches or the terminal ileum in patients with ulcerative colitis[68] and Crohn's disease.[69] They are also named eosinophilic granulomas, submucosal fibromas, hemangiopericytomas, inflammatory pseudotumors, and fibromas. Inflammatory fibroid polyps can occur at any age from 3 to 80 years. They range in size from 1.5 to 13 cm. These lesions must be distinguished from malignant mesenchymal tumors. Inflammatory fibroid polyps may penetrate the bowel wall with a pattern of dissection between the muscle fibers that causes splitting of the muscle layer; in contrast, mesenchymal neoplasms infiltrate and push the muscle layers aside.[67]

Symptoms and Diagnosis   In decreasing order of incidence, symptoms include episodic abdominal pain, vomiting, melena or hematochezia, diarrhea, constipation, abdominal distention, and weight loss. Inflammatory fibroid polyps can also cause intussusception. The vast majority of these lesions are found in the small intestine, mainly in the ileum, but they can occur less commonly in the colon.

Treatment   Inflammatory fibroid polyps are benign, and surgical resection is curative.

Adenomas or Neoplastic Polyps

Adenomas are the most common benign tumors of the small bowel with malignant potential and account for up to 35% of all benign small intestinal tumors. The most frequent location is the duodenum, and they typically occur in the periampullary region; however, each type has a characteristic pattern of occurrence. They vary in size from a few millimeters to several centimeters in diameter and can be sessile or pedunculated. The villous or tubulovillous architecture is prevalent in the small bowel, perhaps in relation to the normal villous anatomy of the mucosa in this segment. The premalignant potential of small intestinal adenomas is reliably attested, and histologic evidence indicates malignant transformation of adenomatous tissue.[70]

Even though all adenocarcinomas of the intestinal tract arise in adenomatous polyps, not all polyps evolve into carcinoma. The malignant potential of adenomas is related to polyp size and histologic characteristics. From the point of view of histologic characteristics, the malignant potential of an adenomatous polyp correlates with its degree of villous architecture. These features are interdependent, however, because large polyps tend to be villous and dysplastic. Diminutive polyps that measure 5 mm or less in diameter are most often tubular adenomas and are not likely (<0.5%) to contain high-grade dysplasia or invasive carcinoma. Only 1% to 2% of adenomatous polyps smaller than 1 cm contain carcinoma. Adenomas larger than 2 cm should be considered worrisome for malignancy; autopsy studies suggest that 40% of adenomas larger than 2 cm contain cancer.

Adenomas may occur in association with polyposis syndromes (FAP, Gardner's syndrome) or sporadically. In FAP, duodenal adenomas are extremely common. It is still uncertain whether patients with duodenal adenomas without FAP are at greater risk for colorectal neoplasia than the general population is.

Tubular Adenomas   Tubular adenomas can occur anywhere in the small intestine but are found most frequently in the ileum, followed by the duodenum and jejunum. They may be solitary or multiple and are usually pedunculated. There is an increased incidence of adenomatous polyps in the small intestine in patients with familial polyposis syndromes. Tubular adenomas are characterized by a complex network of branching adenomatous glands.

Symptoms and Diagnosis   Although most tubular adenomas are asymptomatic, they may be the source of gastrointestinal bleeding. The blood loss tends to be chronic and results in iron deficiency anemia rather than major acute hemorrhage. If the polyps become particularly large, episodes of intestinal obstruction can occur, generally with the polyp serving as the lead point for intussusception.

Treatment   Duodenal adenomas can often be removed by endoscopic snare polypectomy. Side-viewing endoscopic examination may be necessary for the diagnosis of ampullary adenomas. Most adenomas of the duodenal papillae without intraductal extension can also be fully resected by snare papillectomy. Today, endoscopic therapy appears to be a reasonable alternative to surgery for the management of these papillary tumors because it is relatively safe and easily performed. However, adenomas recur in about a third of patients (32% to 42%) by 3 years after index polypectomy, so longer follow-up is needed. The 3-year recurrence rate in patients with a known history of adenomas was higher (42%). In the case of adenomas with intraductal expansion, however, the traditional approach with surgical excision should be considered.[70]

Tumors present in the jejunum or ileum require laparotomy or laparoscopy with either enterotomy and local excision or limited segmental sleeve resection. Endoscopic resection and submucosal excision via operative enterotomy may be appropriate, depending on the size and location of the lesion. Intraoperative examination of the small bowel with careful palpation and the use of enteroscopy to evaluate suspected abnormalities is essential to rule out synchronous lesions. If intussusception is found at laparotomy for intestinal obstruction, the involved segment should be reduced to determine its viability. If compromised, this segment should be resected.

Villous Adenomas   Villous adenomas occur predominantly in the periampullary duodenum and account for less than 1% of all small intestinal tumors. They are almost always sessile and may attain quite large size before becoming symptomatic. Malignant degeneration is common and occurs in roughly 25% to almost half of these tumors. Villous adenomas contain glands that extend straight down from the surface to the base of the polyp. Frequently, both histologic types, adenomatous and villous, coexist in a mixed tubulovillous adenoma. The malignant potential of an adenomatous polyp correlates with its degree of villous architecture.

Symptoms and Diagnosis   Most villous adenomas cause chronic gastrointestinal bleeding, but tumors in the periampullary area may also be associated with obstructive jaundice secondary to biliary obstruction. The diagnosis of duodenal villous adenomas can be suggested by upper gastrointestinal series and confirmed by upper gastrointestinal endoscopy with biopsy. On radiologic examination, as in the case of gastric lesions, the "soap bubble" or "paint brush" appearance is pathognomonic. CT may be helpful to differentiate adenoma from carcinoma because an adenoma is not associated with thickening of the bowel wall. EGD with biopsy is appropriate after a positive result on a radiologic study. The accuracy of endoscopic biopsy is limited by sampling error, and a malignant neoplasm may be missed in up to 60% of cases.[71] Endoscopic ultrasound examination has recently proved to be particularly useful in determining the level of invasion, the presence of lymphadenopathy, and prediction of malignant versus benign tumors.

Treatment   Regardless of the preoperative diagnosis, complete excision of the entire lesion and thorough histologic evaluation are necessary. Endoscopic polypectomy with transduodenal excision of sessile lesions is adequate treatment if complete resection can be accomplished.[72] The entire lesion should be submitted for careful histologic examination for invasive carcinoma, which may be present in up to 50% of larger tumors.[73,74] If invasive carcinoma is found, major resection is indicated. A recent retrospective review demonstrated local recurrence rates of 40% at 10 years, with 25% of the recurrences being malignant. Based on these data, periampullary lesions usually require pancreaticoduodenectomy (Whipple procedure), whereas a pancreas-sparing duodenal resection can be performed for more distal lesions.[75] Patients who undergo local excision require annual surveillance with endoscopy.[76]

Brunner's Gland Adenomas   Brunner's gland adenomas are rare tumors that represent hyperplasia of the exocrine glands of the first portion of the duodenum. Brunner's glands, normally found in the duodenal submucosa, secrete alkaline mucus that aids in the neutralization of acidified luminal contents arriving from the stomach. These adenomas are usually solitary, always benign, and proximal to the ampulla. They have minimal, if any, malignant potential.

Symptoms and Diagnosis   Brunner's gland adenomas are generally asymptomatic and detected incidentally at endoscopic examination. The tumors may rarely bleed, and tumors of large size can cause duodenal obstruction.

Treatment   Endoscopic resection is adequate treatment of most Brunner's gland adenomas. Surgical management is indicated for larger tumors with local excision of a portion of the duodenal wall. If the lesion is so large that local resection is not technically possible, gastroenterostomy after histologic confirmation is appropriate treatment of the duodenal obstruction.

Ectopic Tissue Polyps   Ectopic gastric, pancreatic, and endometrial tissue usually involves the duodenum, but it can be seen in the subserosa of the small intestine in cases of trisomy, in intestinal duplication cysts, and in Meckel's diverticulum. In the small bowel, ectopic tissue can be manifested as a neoplasm.

Ectopic pancreatic tissue is generally found in the duodenum and jejunum and is asymptomatic, with no malignant potential.

Gastric heterotopia is a relatively common condition characterized by the presence of mature gastric fundic-corpus–type mucosa in ectopic locations throughout the gastrointestinal tract.[77] The proximal duodenum is the second most common place, after the esophagus and before the rectum. Nodules have also been noted in the jejunum, in Meckel's diverticulum, and in enteric and colonic duplication cysts, whereas they are rarely seen in the normal distal ileum and proximal part of the colon. The lesions are thought to arise from congenital rests. Such heterotopia in the intestine must be distinguished from the more common process of gastric metaplasia, which typically consists of the appearance of gastric pyloric glands or the surface-foveolar type of mucous cells and develops as a consequence of chronic inflammatory disorders such as peptic duodenitis, celiac disease, and Crohn's disease. Gastric heterotopia of the small intestine may be seen in either gender and occurs in all age groups.

Symptoms and Diagnosis   Most cases are asymptomatic and detected as incidental findings during endoscopic examination of the duodenum or as part of a pathologic study of excised diverticula or cysts, or both. Symptomatic cases appear to be more common in children. The specialized glandular cells are functional and secrete acid and proteolytic enzymes, but the occurrence of peptic injury is mainly related to the location of the lesions. Thus, ulceration of the adjacent unprotected mucosa is often observed when the gastric heterotopia involves relatively stagnant areas such as congenital diverticula and duplication cysts. Peptic injury is rarely seen

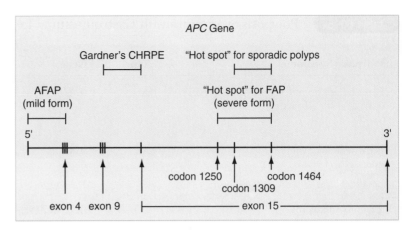

Figure 60–1. Schematic representation of the *APC* gene and its most important genotypic points of mutation with the corresponding phenotype expressions. AFAP, attenuated familial adenomatous polyposis; FAP, familial adenomatous polyposis; CHRPE, congenital hypertrophy of the retinal pigment epithelium. (Modified from Greenfield LJ, Mulholland MW, Oldham KT, et al: Surgery, Scientific Principles and Practice, 3rd ed. Philadelphia, Lippincott Williams & Wilkins, 2001.)

in cases affecting the duodenum, possibly because of prompt dilution of the acid by biliary secretions in this area. The gastric tissue in Meckel's diverticulum may show changes of reflux gastritis because of action of the adjacent intestinal secretions, similar to what is noted in the stomach after reflux of duodenal contents.

Treatment   Segmental intestinal excision is usually the best surgical treatment of perforation or recurrent bleeding. Meckel's diverticulectomy is indicated for incidental findings, with segmental resection if a peptic ulcer is found.

Endometriosis   Endometriosis can also occur on the surface of the small intestine and can cause either partial or complete bowel obstruction. Gastrointestinal involvement is noted in about 33% of cases of endometriosis. There are two major theories regarding the development of endometriosis. One suggests that endometrial tissue may extrude through the fallopian tubes at the time of normal menstruation, which would explain the concentration of lesions in pelvic tissues and on the peritoneal surfaces. Alternatively, it is known that the coelomic epithelium is capable of pluripotential differentiation and is the probable source of endometriosis in all regions, including those that are remote from the uterus. In either situation, the ectopic endometrial tissue can respond to the cyclic hormonal stimulation.

Symptoms and Diagnosis   In endometriosis, obstruction may be secondary to kinking, stenosis, fibrosis, volvulus, or intussusception. The diagnosis may be suggested by either barium enema or small bowel contrast study and is strongly suggested in a patient with known pelvic endometriosis.

Treatment   Segmental excision is usually the best surgical treatment, but hormonal therapy may also be helpful.

Intestinal Polyposis Syndromes

Familial Adenomatous Polyposis

FAP (Table 60–5) is a hereditary autosomal dominant disorder in which the large intestine and rectum are carpeted with multiple adenomas ranging from hundreds to thousands. No true case of FAP has fewer than 100 adenomas, and if less than 100, we are talking about attenuated FAP (see later).

The genetic defect is due to the chromosome allele loss 5q21, called the adenomatous polyposis coli *(APC)* gene (Fig. 60–1). The *APC* gene encodes 2844 codons, 1 for each amino acid, and is broken into 15 translated exons. *APC* is a tumor suppressor gene that encodes a large protein (311 kD) that binds to β-catenin and causes its degradation. The structure of the *APC* gene is unique in that the 15th exon makes up about 75% of the coding sequences of the gene. Because of its unusual length, the open reading frame is an easy target for the types of mutations that result in premature stop codons.[78] The portion of the *APC* gene that binds to β-catenin is represented in this 15th exon. The most common defects in *APC* are point mutations and microdeletions leading to truncated protein. Normal APC protein is localized in the cytoplasm and modulates extracellular signals that are transmitted to the nucleus through the cytoskeletal protein β-catenin, whereas mutant or truncated protein could disrupt this normal process. Mutations in a "hot spot" immediately downstream from the β-catenin binding site (see Fig. 60–1) result in a more virulent, profuse form of FAP. Abnormalities in the *APC* gene may also lead to disruption of normal cell-to-cell adhesions through interactions with the cellular adhesion molecule E-cadherin.

The lesions in FAP are adenomas and are histologically similar to those seen in patients without FAP, with flat/depressed adenomas representing 30% of the lesions. Originally described in association with FAP, *APC* gene mutations are found in more than 60% of sporadic adenomas.[79] Besides having colonic polyps, most patients with FAP also have upper gastrointestinal polyps: adenomatous changes in the duodenum in 60% to 90% of cases and fundic gland polyps or adenomas in the stomach. They are relatively rare in the bulb, whereas they are more frequent in the second and third portions of the duodenum,[80] where numerous sessile polyps are found, generally small in size but sometimes a few centimeters in diameter. There is a tendency for adenomas to involve the periampullary region, with 50% to 85% of patients having adenomatous alterations of the papilla of

Table 60–5 Polyposis Syndromes with Gastrointestinal Lesions

Polyposis Syndrome	Type	Gene	Locus	Polyp Type
Familial adenomatous polyposis (FAP)	AD	*APC*	5q21	Adenomas Lymphoid polyps Fundic gland polyps Hamartomas
Gardner's syndrome	AD	*APC*	5q21	Adenomas Lymphoid polyps Fundic gland polyps Hamartomas
Turcot's syndrome	AD	*APC, hPMS2, hMLH1*	5q21, 7p22, 3p21-23	Adenomas
Attenuated familial adenomatous polyposis (AFAP)	AD	*APC*	5q21	Hamartomas Adenomas
Hereditary flat adenoma syndrome (HFAS)			5q21-22	Flat adenomas Fundic gland polyps
Muir-Torre syndrome	AD	?	?	Adenomas
Juvenile polyposis syndrome	AD	*SMAD4, PTEN*	10q22-24, 18q21	Villous/papillary polyps Hyperplastic polyps Fundic gland polyps
Bannayan-Zonana (Bannayan-Ruvalcaba-Riley) syndrome	AD	*PTEN*		Hamartomas
Cowden's disease	AD	*PTEN/MMAC1*	10q22-23	Hamartomas Inflammatory polyps Ganglioneuromas Lipomas
Peutz-Jeghers syndrome	AD	*STK11/LKB1*	19p13	Hamartomas
Cronkhite-Canada syndrome (CCS)	NH			Juvenile polyps–like inflammatory polyps
Intestinal ganglioneuromatosis syndrome				Ganglioneuromas
Lymphoid polyposis syndrome				Lymphoid polyps
Hereditary mixed polyposis syndromes	AD	?	6q	Tubular adenomas Villous adenomas Flat adenomas Hyperplastic polyps Atypical juvenile polyp

AD, autosomal dominant; NH, nonhereditary.

Modified from Ming SC, Goldman H: Pathology of the Gastrointestinal Tract, 2nd ed. Philadelphia, Lippincott Williams & Wilkins, 1998; and Greenfield LJ, Mulholland MW, Oldham KT, et al: Surgery, Scientific Principles and Practice, 3rd ed. Philadelphia, Lippincott Williams & Wilkins, 2001.

Vater.[81,82] Staging of duodenal polyposis uses the Spigelman classification, with severity based on architectural parameters—villous status, grade of dysplasia, and number and size of polyps. Stage I indicates minimal duodenal disease, whereas stage IV represents advanced disease. The severity of duodenal polyposis increases with age, but progression may be especially rapid in patients at advanced stages of disease.[83] About 11% of patients have stage IV lesions; thus, it is not surprising that the risk for duodenal cancer in patients with FAP is about 100 times higher than in the general population.[84,85] Based on data from the John Hopkins Polyposis Registry,[85] it appears that the relative risk for adenocarcinoma of the duodenum developing in a patient with FAP is 331, whereas the relative risk for the development of

periampullary adenocarcinoma is 124. These neoplasms are thus the most important cause of mortality in patients already subjected to prophylactic colectomy, and they involve about 5% of cases.[86]

Finally, one should be aware of reports that patients with FAP may have benign lymphoid polyps of the terminal ileum.[87] Otherwise, little is known concerning the true prevalence of either polyps or cancer in the post-duodenal small intestine in FAP patients. Reports on the prevalence of polyps in the jejunum-ileum derive from the use of intraoperative enteroscopy.

Symptoms and Diagnosis The incidence of FAP has been estimated to be 1 in 8000 births, 20% of which are a new mutation in a family. The average age at detection in patients with symptoms is 36.5 years. In contrast, in patients who are examined because of a family history of FAP, the average age at detection is only 23.8 years. Adenomas do not usually appear before the age of 10. Adenocarcinoma will develop in all patients who are left untreated. The average age at diagnosis of adenocarcinoma in the FAP group is 39 years, which is at least 25 years younger than the average age at diagnosis of adenocarcinoma in the general population.

A clinical diagnosis of FAP is not generally difficult. When FAP is known to run in a family, relatives at risk should undergo surveillance sigmoidoscopy on an annual basis beginning in their mid-teenage years. Sigmoidoscopy is sufficient to detect carriers of the abnormal gene because the entire colon is at risk. If a single adenoma appears in a teenager at risk, the disease is strongly suspected. The lesion must be biopsied to confirm that it is an adenoma. In a family with FAP, each first-degree relative of an affected patient has a 50% likelihood of inheriting the mutated gene. With each passing year, negative sigmoidoscopy further reduces the probability that a patient carries the gene.

Endoscopic ultrasound and ultrasound miniprobe technology may increase the accuracy of duodenal staging, thus adding a further parameter to the decision-making process in advanced cases when surgery is not clearly indicated.

Treatment Because untreated FAP inevitably leads to colorectal adenocarcinoma, prophylactic colectomy is indicated. The clinical decision involves selection and timing of the operation because a delay of 20 years or more from appearance of the first adenoma to the development of cancer is typical. The safest surgical procedure is total proctocolectomy with ileoanal anastomosis. Any residual rectal mucosa that is left behind is at risk for the development of neoplasia and rectal carcinoma. Intraoperative enteroscopy in FAP patients should be carried out during surgical colectomy. Endoscopic screening of the upper gastrointestinal tract in FAP patients aims to identify high-risk individuals and to diagnose cancer at an early stage. The St. Mark's Hospital group[85] recommends beginning checkups at age 20. Subsequently, endoscopy should be repeated every 2 to 3 years for polyposis at Spigelman stages 0 to II. For stages III and IV, checkups should be performed every 12 months, mostly after the age of 30. Even if most duodenal adenomas appear to not change for considerable periods, it is prudent to remove most polyps and, above all, large ones or those showing rapid growth via routine upper endoscopy.

For periampullary surveillance, a side-viewing duodenoscope must be used. Biopsy samples must also be taken from the papilla of Vater, even if it has normal morphology. Various alternative therapies have been used for periampullary adenomas. Transduodenal submucosal excision with sphincteroplasty is beneficial only in the short term because of the high recurrence rate. On the other hand, snare ampullectomy and the Nd:YAG laser involve a risk for perforation. Highly selective thermal ablation via bipolar coagulation after sphincterotomy can be safer and may be preferable.[88,89] For patients at Spigelman stage IV, endoscopic laser photodynamic therapy appears to be promising,[90] but large case studies are not yet available.

If endoscopic snare polypectomy is appropriate for small or pedunculated lesions, as previously mentioned, pancreaticoduodenectomy may be required for adequate treatment of larger villous adenomas in the periampullary region.

Medical therapy with a nonsteroidal drug (sulindac) has been described.[91,92] Although colorectal adenomas have been found to regress in patients with FAP in response to sulindac, similar effectiveness was not found in the management of upper gastrointestinal tract neoplasia.

Gardner's Syndrome Polyposis

Gardener's syndrome (see Table 60–5) is presently thought to be a variant of FAP characterized by the triad of intestinal polyps, soft tissue abnormalities, and abnormalities of bones.[93] Also noted is congenital hypertrophy of the retinal pigment epithelium (CHRPE), which consists of single or multiple pigmented ovoid lesions occurring unilaterally or bilaterally. The retinal lesions occur when the mutations are between exons 9 and 15 on the APC gene (see Fig. 60–1). Traditionally, patients with signs and symptoms of FAP together with extraintestinal manifestations were historically considered to have Gardner's syndrome. It is now appreciated that no distinction can be made between families with Gardner's syndrome and those with FAP because extraintestinal manifestations have also been found in families with FAP. The genetic defect is identical to that for FAP. Similar to FAP, patients with Gardener's syndrome have upper gastrointestinal polyps,[93] and also as in FAP, the intestinal polyps are adenomas. This syndrome represents the variable expression of germline mutations in the APC gene. Benign lymphoid polyposis of the ileum has been associated with this syndrome.[94] At times, the soft tissue abnormalities, including epidermal cysts, fibromas, lipomas, and desmoid tumors, may precede the intestinal manifestations by years. The bony lesions are osteomas and cortical thickening of the long bones and ribs. In addition, dental abnormalities such as impacted teeth, supernumerary teeth, and dental cysts have been reported. There is an increased incidence of adenocarcinomas of the pancreaticoduodenal region, the thyroid gland, the adrenal gland, and the brain (particularly medulloblastomas). Malignant tumors of the colon are considered to be nearly inevitable.

Symptoms and Diagnosis CHRPE lesions may be seen in the general population but are small and usually single. Multiple, bilateral, and large CHRPE lesions are essentially diagnostic of FAP. The intestinal manifestations, number of adenomas, incidence of intestinal cancer, and methods of diagnosis have been described earlier under FAP syndrome.

Turcot's Syndrome Polyposis

Turcot's syndrome (see Table 60–5) is presently thought to also be a rare variant of FAP. The syndrome was originally described in 1959 in two siblings with polyposis coli in whom malignant brain tumors developed.[95] Traditionally, the occurrence of a malignant brain tumor in conjunction with intestinal polyposis was referred as Turcot's syndrome. Interestingly, one of the index families initially reported by Turcot did not have FAP but rather had hereditary nonpolyposis colorectal cancer (HNPCC), which is characterized by an excess of astrocytomas (glioblastoma multiforme). To date, evidence suggests that all of the aforementioned can result from two distinctive types of germline defects: the association with the *APC* gene mutation is a variant of FAP, whereas the association with mutation of a mismatch repair gene (*hPMS2*, *hMLH1*) is a variant of HNPCC. The lesions are adenomas and the malignant potential may be the same as for FAP. However, the true frequency of Turcot's syndrome may be difficult to assess because central nervous system tumors are associated with high mortality and may precede the detection of intestinal polyps or the onset of intestinal carcinoma. Like Gardner's syndrome, this syndrome represents variable expression of germline mutations in the *APC* gene.

Attenuated Familial Adenomatous Polyposis

Attenuated FAP (see Table 60–5) is a less severe form of polyposis with a lower number of adenomatous polyps, usually less than 100, but patients still have a high risk for intestinal cancer. The cancers usually develop 15 years later than in classic FAP patients, but 10 years earlier than in the sporadic cancer group.[79] Linkage to the *APC* gene has been found; the genetic defect is similar to that of FAP, linked to 5q21.[96,97] Four distinct mutations have been identified and described in a few families with attenuated FAP. These mutations predict truncated proteins; however, they differ from the situation in patients with classic *APC* base substitutions or small deletions in that the four mutated sites are very close to each other and to the 5′ end of the *APC* gene.

Hereditary Flat Adenoma Syndrome Polyposis

Hereditary flat adenoma syndrome (see Table 60–5) is presently thought to also be a variant of FAP with the genetic defect linked to 5q21-22. In contrast to FAP, the majority of adenomas are of the flat type. Signs of hereditary flat adenoma syndrome in patients consist of the following:

1. Multiple colorectal adenomas are present, but usually fewer than 100.
2. The adenomatous polyps tend to occur at a later age than in classic FAP.
3. The adenomatous polyps tend to show a more proximal location, so patients have adenomas and cancers of the stomach and duodenum.
4. Fundic gland polyps of the stomach are also noted, and in some patients they may be present in the absence of colorectal adenomas.[98,99]
5. The onset of intestinal cancer is later than with HNPCC and FAP.

Muir-Torre Syndrome Polyposis

Muir-Torre syndrome (see Table 60–5) is a rare autosomal dominant disorder with fewer than 100 adenomas that is typically present in the proximal part of the colon. Originally, Muir-Torre syndrome was subclassified as a form of FAP, but today it is believed that the syndrome is an HNPCC in which the intestinal adenomas are associated with skin lesions such as basal cell carcinoma, sebaceous carcinoma, and squamous cell carcinoma.

Juvenile Polyposis Syndrome

Juvenile polyposis syndrome (see Table 60–5) is a heterogeneous and complex group of disorders, with some patients expressing polyps limited to the colon, whereas others have polyps that also involve the stomach and small intestine; some cases are familial, whereas others are not; and some patients have coexisting separate adenomas, whereas others have juvenile polyps with adenomatous changes. Three different syndromic manifestations have been reported, but it is not known whether these are truly distinctive syndromes. They may consist of familial juvenile polyposis limited to the colon, familial juvenile polyposis limited to the stomach, and familial juvenile polyposis distributed throughout the gastrointestinal tract. To date, a unifying definition of juvenile polyposis syndrome considers juvenile polyps throughout the entire gastrointestinal tract, any number of juvenile polyps in a patient with a family history, or any patient with 3 or more, 5 or more, or 10 or more juvenile polyps. In general, 20% to 50% of patients have a familial or genetic history that indicates autosomal dominant inheritance. The genetic basis of this syndrome is not understood, but germline mutations in the *SMAD4* gene located on chromosome 18q21, which encodes an intracellular mediator in the transforming growth factor-β signaling pathway, have been identified in some affected patients. The *PTEN* gene located on chromosome 10q22-24 has also been linked to some cases. In juvenile polyposis the number of polyps ranges from dozens to hundreds; however, they are not as numerous as in FAP. Frequently, the polyps appear as pedunculated, cherry-red, edematous growths with a smooth surface and contour. From the literature, the reported distribution of juvenile polyps throughout the gastrointestinal tract shows 98% in the colorectum, 13.6% in the stomach, 2.3% in the duodenum, and 6.5% through the jejunum and ileum.[100] Extraintestinal congenital anomalies have been reported in 11% to 20% of both familial and nonfamilial cases.[100] Juvenile polyposis syndrome is diagnosed in infancy in most cases (75% occur in children younger than 10 years), with only 15% being detected initially in adults. Although juvenile polyps individually are not in themselves neoplastic, there is an increased risk for intestinal cancer ranging from 15% to 21% in patients with juvenile polyposis. The various anomalies associated with the syndrome and reported in the literature are gut malrotation, mesenteric lymphangioma, hypertelorism, amyotonia congenita, hydrocephalus, tetralogy of Fallot, coarctation of the aorta, thyroglossal duct cyst, and idiopathic hypertrophic subaortic stenosis.

There is a rare form of juvenile polyposis syndrome of infancy that consists of diarrhea, bleeding, protein-losing enteropathy, alopecia, and clubbing of the fingers and toes; it is often fatal and clinically mimics adult CCS.

Histologically, the lesions in juvenile polyposis syndrome are typical and atypical polyps. The typical ones are grossly round and smooth and are similar to solitary juvenile polyps. The atypical polyps often adopt a villous or papillary configuration. Separate hyperplastic polyps can also be seen.

Symptoms and Diagnosis Gastrointestinal bleeding, because these lesions are highly vascular, intussusception, and obstruction are typical manifestations of the disease. The passage of autoamputated lesions has been mentioned. Total colonoscopy, EGD, and small bowel enteroclysis are indicated for surveillance of these patients.

Treatment When surgery is necessary, careful examination of the entire small bowel with intraoperative enteroscopy should be performed, and larger polyps should be removed either endoscopically or surgically to prevent future intussusception, obstruction, or bleeding. It is important that the pathologist examine the lesions carefully for the presence of adenomatous tissue in the polyps because it indicates which lesions are premalignant. When mixed lesions are found, patients in these families should be subjected to colonoscopic surveillance, perhaps as often as every 2 years. In children with life-threatening protein-losing enteropathy, surgical resection of the affected segment of intestine is required.

Bannayan-Zonana (Bannayan-Ruvalcaba-Riley) Syndrome Polyposis

Bannayan-Zonana (Bannayan-Ruvalcaba-Riley) syndrome (see Table 60–5) is an inherited autosomal dominant disorder characterized by ileal and colonic hamartomatous polyps and lingual lesions. Other characteristics include ocular abnormalities, delayed motor development, lipid storage myopathy, and Hashimoto's disease. This disease is also linked to germline mutations in the *PTEN* gene and appears to be a variant of familial juvenile polyposis.

Cowden's Disease Polyposis

Cowden's disease (see Table 60–5) is an uncommon autosomal dominant disorder. This disease is discussed under the small bowel polyposis syndromes because of the presence of numerous colonic and small intestinal polyps. The disease is associated with facial trichilemmomas, acral keratosis, and oral mucosal papillomas, as well as with breast and thyroid cancer. Glycogenic acanthosis of the esophagus may also occur. Based on different authors, the lesions have been described as hamartomatous[101] or inflammatory or as lipomas or ganglioneuromas.[102] There is no increased risk for gastrointestinal cancer in this disorder. It is of interest that a germline

mutation in the *PTEN* gene on chromosome 10q22-23 has been identified in most families with Cowden's syndrome, the same locus affecting some families with juvenile polyposis.

Symptoms and Diagnosis The diagnosis of Cowden's syndrome should be considered in patients with multiple trichilemmomas. Gastrointestinal polyps are usually asymptomatic.

Treatment No specific therapy need be directed toward the gastrointestinal tract.

Peutz-Jeghers Syndrome Polyposis

Peutz-Jeghers syndrome (see Table 60–5) is a rare autosomal dominant inherited disorder associated with mutation in the *STK11/LKB1* gene and deregulation of mTOR. The gene responsible for the disease was mapped to chromosome 19p13 and encodes a serine/threonine kinase. Peutz first reported the syndrome in 1921, and Jeghers and colleagues described it anew in 1949. Multiple gastrointestinal polyps scattered throughout the entire gastrointestinal tract, but occurring primarily in the jejunum and ileum, and mucocutaneous melanotic pigmentation on the lips, oral mucosa, face, genitalia, and palmar surfaces characterize the disease. The number of polyps is usually counted in the dozens rather than in the hundreds as in FAP. In most patients the disorder is diagnosed in the twenties, and the male-to-female ratio is 1:1. On histologic examination these polyps are hamartomas and range from only few millimeters to several centimeters in diameter, but most often these lesions are less than 1 cm in diameter and are rarely large enough to cause symptoms. They are histologically distinct from juvenile polyps and show no inflammatory cell infiltrate. They may be found in the stomach, in the large bowel, and more frequently in the small intestine. Although the hamartomas are not premalignant, carriers of the *STK11* gene are at significant risk for the early onset of other malignant neoplasms, mainly pancreas, breast, lung, ovary, uterus, and sex cord tumors. In a series reported by Spigelman and associates,[103] another neoplasm developed in 23% of patients, 56% of which were gastrointestinal in origin. It is thought that neoplasia may arise from foci of adenomatous epithelium found in some Peutz-Jeghers polyps.

Symptoms and Diagnosis Peutz-Jeghers syndrome is manifested early and the diagnosis is made in the first 3 decades of life, with the clinical symptoms varying according to the location of the polyps. The larger hamartomas can cause obstruction as a result of intussusception and, less frequently, intestinal hemorrhage; obstruction and abdominal pain are also associated with small intestinal polyps because of its narrower diameter. Whereas surveillance of the upper and lower gastrointestinal tract is easily achieved through EGD and total colonoscopy with terminal ileoscopy, the small intestine is still an important and challenging problem. Enteroclysis can identify polyps and define the map of their distribution.

Treatment   The aim of management of these patients is to identify and remove the polyps endoscopically or surgically before they can cause complications. With EGD and total colonoscopy, the stomach, most of duodenum, and the entire large intestine can be kept free of polyps. Push enteroscopy allows only limited exploration of the jejunum but does permit operative procedures to be carried out further in the small bowel. Because the lesions are extensive in distribution, resection should be limited to the segment responsible for the symptoms. Since they have no malignant potential, no internal organ is at sufficient risk for cancer that a specific screening regimen is indicated, and prophylactic surgery or extensive resection of hamartomas is not justified. However, when surgery is necessary, careful examination of the entire small bowel with intraoperative enteroscopy should be performed and larger polyps removed either endoscopically or surgically to prevent future obstruction or intussusception. Most patients require several surgical intestinal resections during their lifetime and sometimes emergency operations at brief intervals, which may cause short-bowel syndrome. That is why some authors consider it necessary to schedule periodic radiologic and endoscopic checkups at intervals of 3 to 5 years or decide on a case-by-case basis. The clinician should be also aware of the extradigestive malignancy risk and should be particularly alert for the development of gonadal tumors.

Cronkhite-Canada Syndrome Polyposis

CCS (see Table 60–5) is an acquired, nonhereditary, nonfamilial gastrointestinal polyposis disorder associated with skin pigmentary changes, hair loss, and nail atrophy (onychodystrophy).[104,105] CCS is found worldwide and is characterized by the initial appearance of intestinal lesions in late adult life, with approximately 80% of patients being 50 years or older at onset. The male-to-female ratio is close to 1:1. The polyps in CCS are found in the stomach, small intestine, colon, and rectum and may be sessile or pedunculated. Histologically, the polyps are identical to juvenile polyps. There have been reports of adenomatous changes in these polyps.[106]

Symptoms and Diagnosis   The clinical symptoms (in decreasing order of frequency) are diarrhea, weight loss, abdominal pain, anorexia, weakness, and hematochezia. The physical findings, as already mentioned, are onycholysis, alopecia, and hyperpigmentation. The hair loss has been noted in all parts of the body, and hair regrowth has been mentioned during spontaneous remission and after therapy. Approximately 50% of cases are fatal, usually secondary to cachexia and anemia.

Treatment   Supportive therapy for CCS may provide long-term remission; it has been reported that polyps may decrease in size or number.[105] Primary attention should be drawn to treatment of the diarrhea and maintenance of nutritional status. In a number of cases, treatment of the bacterial overgrowth with antibiotics and maintenance of nutritional status have resulted in complete resolution of the cutaneous features. At present, surgery is recommended only for complications such as

prolapse, bowel obstruction, or malignancy. Present data on CCS indicate that the potential risk for development of intestinal cancer is not great enough to indicate colectomy, although there have been reported cases of colorectal malignancy in correlation with CCS.[106]

Intestinal Ganglioneuromatosis Syndrome Polyposis

The intestinal ganglioneuromatosis syndrome (see Table 60–5) is a familial disorder that has been associated with multiple endocrine neoplasia type IIB and with von Recklinghausen's disease.[107] There may be a diffuse proliferation of ganglioneuromatous elements that at times may be polypoid. In some instances, the syndrome has been found in association with juvenile polyposis.[107] See also the later discussion under "Neurogenic Benign Tumors."

Lymphoid Polyposis Syndrome

Benign lymphoid polyposis syndrome (see Table 60–5) occurs most often in children. The lesions are entirely benign and in some cases have been reported to disappear spontaneously. Histologically similar to solitary lymphoid polyps, lymphoid polyposis consists of prominent active lymphoid nodules in the mucosa and submucosa. In patients with a family history of polyps, it is essential to determine the exact histologic nature of the lesions so that unnecessary surgery is not performed.

As previously mentioned, benign lymphoid polyposis of the terminal ileum has been reported in patients with FAP and Gardner's syndrome.[94]

Hereditary Mixed Polyposis Syndrome

Hereditary mixed polyposis syndrome (see Table 60–5) is an autosomal dominant disorder that has been mapped to chromosome 6q. Five types of polyps have been described in the literature in individuals with this disorder: tubular adenomas, villous adenomas, flat adenomas, hyperplastic polyps, and atypical juvenile polyps. This disorder might be a variant of juvenile polyposis; however, in juvenile polyposis, only 2% of the polyps are adenomas, whereas in hereditary mixed polyposis, the majority of polyps are adenomas. In addition, in hereditary mixed polyposis the number of polyps is lower than seen in the juvenile syndrome, and hereditary mixed polyposis usually occurs 1 decade later than juvenile polyposis does.

Benign Mesenchymal (Nonepithelial) Lesions

Vascular Lesions

Angiodysplasia   The general aspects, symptoms and diagnosis, and treatment of angiodysplasia were described in detail earlier in the section on gastric angiodysplasia.

Telangiectasia   Telangiectases arise from simple dilation of normal vascular structures as a result of congenital thinning of the muscular layer and elastic fibers in the arteriolar wall. Multiple congenital lesions may occur in the gastrointestinal tract in Osler-Weber-Rendu syndrome and Turner's syndrome. Turner's syndrome (XO) is associated with gastrointestinal hemorrhage from telangiectases that may be found throughout the small and large bowel and mesentery, but it occurs most frequently in the small intestine.

Symptoms and Diagnosis Gastrointestinal bleeding is present in less than 15% of patients.

Treatment In Turner's syndrome, these vascular lesions tend to regress spontaneously; therefore, a conservative approach is generally warranted.[51] When necessary, intraoperative push enteroscopy with electrocoagulation or a heater probe can adequately treat these lesions.

Hemangiomas Hemangiomas are rare congenital lesions of the small intestine and account for about 7% to 10% of all benign small bowel tumors; they affect predominantly the jejunum and ileum. Arising from the submucosal vascular plexuses, hemangiomas are classified as capillary, cavernous, or mixed, depending on the size of the vessels primarily affected. Intestinal hemangiomas are usually solitary or, more rarely, multiple, and malignant degeneration is exceedingly rare. The appearance of the lesions may be quite varied, from bluish-colored areas to swollen bluish-colored polypoid lesions with a nodular surface and soft, elastic consistency.

Hemangiomas of the small bowel may also be associated with cutaneous lesions such as cavernous skin hemangiomas in the blue rubber bleb nevus syndrome or with capillary skin hemangiomas (port-wine stain) and soft tissue and bony hypertrophy in the Klippel-Trénaunay-Weber syndrome. In Peutz-Jeghers syndrome, intestinal hemangiomas without the presence of intestinal polyps has been reported. These cases are thought to represent incomplete penetrance of the gene responsible for the syndrome.[108]

Symptoms and Diagnosis Intestinal hemangiomas grow slowly, typically coming to medical attention in the third decade of life because of acute or chronic blood loss. Preoperative diagnosis may be achieved through angiography, but is usually difficult. Push enteroscopy and intraoperative enteroscopy have been used to diagnose hemangiomas of the small bowel.[58,109]

Treatment Depending on their size, hemangiomas may be locally excised or resected via limited small bowel resection. Efforts to manage intestinal hemangiomas with endoscopic or operative sclerotherapy or coagulation and operative or angiographic interruption of their arterial supply have been minimally successful.

Diffuse Gastrointestinal Hemangiomatosis As many as 100 lesions involving the stomach, small bowel, and colon can be encountered in patients with diffuse gastrointestinal hemangiomatosis. Bleeding or anemia in childhood usually leads to the diagnosis of this condition.

Symptoms and Diagnosis Patients often have hemangiomas of the skin and soft tissue of the head and neck. The gastrointestinal hemangiomas may be large enough to cause intussusception. In diffuse neonatal hemangiomatosis, angiography is probably the most reliable means of detecting the lesions.

Lymphangiomas Lymphangiomas are rare and account for less than 2% to 3% of benign small bowel neoplastic tumors. They are developmental lymphatic malformations and on microscopic examination consist of dilated submucosal lymphatic vessels. They are usually solitary, lobulated, and intramural and appear as circumscribed polypoid masses of soft consistency with an irregular surface and micronodules.

Symptoms and Diagnosis Almost all lymphangiomas are asymptomatic and discovered either incidentally or at autopsy. When symptomatic, they cause abdominal pain, obstruction, and more rarely, occult gastrointestinal bleeding. Cases of small bowel lymphangiomas responsible for bleeding have been reported, and their diagnosis was made with push enteroscopy[110] or sonde enteroscopy.[111]

Treatment Symptomatic lesions should be treated by segmental resection.

Leiomyomas

Leiomyoma is either the first or the second most common benign tumor of the small intestine, with some authors considering adenoma to be the most common.[40,112] It is the most frequent tumor of the postduodenal small intestine and occurs equally in the jejunum and in the ileum. Leiomyomas are the second most common small bowel neoplasms manifested by occult bleeding. As already mentioned under gastric leiomyomas, intestinal leiomyomas are well-differentiated benign GISTs that arise from smooth muscle in the small bowel wall. The GIST label is more appropriate in that the previous terminology—leiomyoma versus leiomyosarcoma—implied a clear definition between benign and malignant tumors. The distinction is often not clear at the time of original diagnosis and histologic examination. The incidence is equal in males and females. The peak incidence in both men and women is between the ages of 50 and 59 years. A relatively recent large review of the world's literature identified 2763 GISTs of the small bowel.[113] In this review approximately 40% were classified as benign and 60% as malignant, with the jejunum being the most frequent site of origin. Interestingly, a disproportionately high number of GISTs are located in Meckel's diverticulum.

The most frequent growth pattern is extraluminal (65%), whereas the form with intraluminal or intramural development is less frequent.[114] In gross appearance, leiomyomas are wide-based submucosal formations that are firm, gray, lobulated, and nonmobile on the underlying plane. Although well circumscribed, they are not encapsulated and frequently demonstrate cystic degeneration. Their biologic behavior is best correlated with the degree of mitotic activity and tumor size.[115-117]

Symptoms and Diagnosis As with gastric leiomyomas, most are asymptomatic, but many are associated with either bleeding or obstruction. Occasionally, the onset may consist of massive bleeding. Larger leiomyomas may outgrow their blood supply, thereby leading to central necrosis, ulceration, and intraluminal bleeding. Small bowel obstruction can occur either from luminal compression or more commonly from intussusception. Finally, patients may have an asymptomatic, yet palpable abdominal mass. The diagnosis can be made by contrast radiology, which shows a space-occupying lesion creating a smooth eccentric filling defect with intact small bowel mucosa. CT scanning is currently the most specific diagnostic study and often distinguishes a GIST with central necrosis from a lipoma, which would be of consistent fat density.

Treatment Because it is virtually impossible to differentiate benign from malignant lesions at laparotomy, even by frozen section, treatment of a small intestinal GIST should include segmental intestinal resection. Extensive lymph node dissection is not necessary because lymph node metastases are rare. Even if a tumor is asymptomatic, it should be resected because malignant behavior cannot be accurately predicted.

Neurogenic Benign Tumors

Neurogenic tumors are rare and account for less than 5% to 10% of all small intestinal neoplasms. They are GISTs with neural differentiation rather than being derived from smooth muscle like leiomyomas, leiomyosarcomas, or leiomyoblastomas. **Schwannomas** arise from peripheral neural elements, can be either solitary or multiple, and can occur at any age. Von Recklinghausen's disease is present in 15% of patients with schwannoma and is usually associated with multiple tumors.[118] Solitary tumors generally occur in the ileum. They appear as nodules of hard, elastic consistency, are mobile on the underlying plane, and are covered with smooth mucosa. Some nodules may demonstrate ulceration, which is responsible for the bleeding. **Neurilemomas** originating from nerve sheaths and **ganglioneuromas** arising from components of the sympathetic nervous system are other tumors originating from neural tissue. These tumors can also be associated with von Recklinghausen's disease.

Symptoms and Diagnosis Of patients with intestinal neurogenic tumors, symptoms will develop in approximately 70%.[119] Pain, intestinal bleeding, and obstruction occur as the initial complaint with equal frequency.

Endoscopic biopsy is not justified because it is not diagnostic. The diagnosis should be suspected in patients with von Recklinghausen's disease.

Treatment Symptomatic lesions are treated by local excision or segmental resection.

Lipomas

Lipomas, the third most common benign neoplasm of the small intestine, are submucosal fatty tumors and represent 15% to 25% of small intestinal benign tumors. Lipomas occur primarily in the distal portion of the small intestine: 60% are located in the ileum, with 20% present in the duodenum and 20% in the jejunum. They are most commonly found in older patients and in men. Occasional lipomas are pedunculated, and because they are also compressible, they may cause intussusception and obstruction. Lipomas may be multiple and are occasionally present diffusely throughout the small intestine. These rare cases of extremely numerous lesions have been termed *lipomatosis*. Microscopically, these submucosal masses of rather uniform adipose cells compress the muscularis mucosae and often cause thinning of the overlying mucosa. The bigger the tumors, the more likely they are to produce bleeding, pain, or obstruction.

Symptoms and Diagnosis Small intestinal lipomas are typically asymptomatic. In almost two thirds of patients, clinical symptoms are caused by intestinal obstruction; the most common point of obstruction is the ileocecal valve. Lipomas, which are usually asymptomatic, can be found incidentally on upper gastrointestinal series or EGD. The diagnosis can occasionally be made by barium enema with reflux into the terminal ileum or by a small intestinal contrast study. Contrast studies reveal a smooth, well-circumscribed, eccentric filling defect and intact mucosa. CT is particularly useful in the diagnosis of small intestinal lipomas because of the low density of the tumor as noted on studies. Endoscopically, they have a characteristic appearance, and there is also a distinctive appearance on endoscopic ultrasound.

Treatment Small tumors under 2 cm can be safely observed. Excision is unnecessary unless the patient is symptomatic. For lesions associated with bleeding or obstruction, treatment is by local excision, but segmental resection is usually necessary for larger tumors. Resection can be accomplished by either open or laparoscopic techniques. Larger or growing lesions should be resected to rule out malignant liposarcoma.

Lipohyperplasia (Lipomatous Hypertrophy) of the Ileocecal Valve In this condition, both sides of the ileocecal valve submucosa (ileal mucosal side and colonic mucosal side) contain adipose tissue in excess and produce a large, protruding valve that grossly resembles a uterine cervix.[120,121] The patients are more commonly middle-aged women; obesity does not provide an explanation.

Symptoms and Diagnosis Because the big valve protrudes in the cecal lumen, it can produce a dramatic radiographic filling defect resembling a neoplasm—cecal carcinoma. The condition is easily identified at colonoscopy and demonstrates adipose tissue covered by normal mucosa. Patients may have nonspecific clinical problems, such as constipation or abdominal pain, presumably the reasons for performing the radiographic or colonoscopic studies. In most cases the hypertrophic valves are found incidentally. Intestinal obstruction and bleeding from an ulcerated valve have been reported, but these cases are truly unusual.

Fibromas

Fibromas are large, well-circumscribed tumors consisting of dense collagen bundles and a variable number of mature fibroblasts. They occur in the submucosa, muscularis, or serosa. Fibromas are difficult to distinguish from scar tissue. They typically occur in adults 50 to 60 years of age and represent about 0% to 6% of all benign small intestinal tumors.

Symptoms and Diagnosis   Most tumors are asymptomatic and are discovered at exploratory laparotomy performed for other reasons or at autopsy.

Treatment   Local excision provides satisfactory treatment of symptomatic lesions.

Congenital Lesions

Duplication Cysts   Intestinal duplication cysts may be closed ovoid or spherical cystic structures that range in size from a few millimeters to 10 to 15 cm in diameter. As in the case of gastric duplication cysts, intestinal cysts may also appear as communicating tubular, elongated structures. Duplications are lined by functioning intestinal mucosa with a wall composed of smooth muscle. They are always dorsal to the intestine, usually within the mesentery between the spinal cords and the small bowel and sometimes intramural. Almost 50% of cases affect the terminal ileum and are generally single; however, they may be associated with multiple abdominal and thoracic duplications. Pathogenetically, they are thought to originate secondary to abnormal recanalization of the intestinal lumen obliterated by epithelial proliferation. Another likelihood is persistence of the outpouchings of the intestine that have been observed during embryogenesis and intrauterine intestinal ischemia. Their frequent association with vertebral clefts and rib anomalies suggests another possible explanation, such as failure of complete separation of the foregut and notochord. They occasionally communicate with the lumen of the bowel. Tubular duplication cysts generally lie parallel to the small bowel and share the muscular layer; they often communicate with the lumen of the intestine in their distal portion. Cases of extension along the entire small bowel have been reported.[122] Most duplications are manifested in the newborn period or early childhood, much less frequently in adult life. Gastrointestinal hemorrhage may be cause by peptic ulceration or by intestinal ischemia secondary to an altered blood supply by a mass effect or intussusception. The wall of a duplication cyst is thick and muscular and contains from one to three layers of smooth muscle with identifiable Auerbach's plexuses. The mucosal lining of the duplication may be gastric, intestinal, or pseudostratified ciliated columnar mucosa with occasional heterotopic pancreatic tissue. Peptic ulcers may occur within the duplication, usually at

the gastrointestinal mucosal junction or at its communication with normal bowel. Small intestine duplication cysts occur at a 22:10 female-to-male ratio.

Duplication cysts of the duodenum are rare. They are usually submucosal, generally noncommunicating, and separated by only a thin muscularis layer. They bulge into the lumen of the adjoining duodenum.

Symptoms and Diagnosis   When distended by mucous accumulations, cystic or tubular duplications may cause extrinsic compression of normal adjacent bowel and secondary intestinal obstruction or provoke intussusception (mostly seen with small intramural cysts) or volvulus. Small intestine duplication cysts may be palpable, and because they may be partially calcified, they are radiographically detectable as curvilinear densities on abdominal radiographs of children with associated intermittent pain, melena, or intussusception.

Treatment   Although isolated duplication cysts can be removed surgically, even when extensive, complex malformations are harder to manage and can be fatal.

REFERENCES

1. Spriggs EI: Polyps of the stomach and polypoid gastritis. Q J Med 12:1-60, 1943.
2. Ming SC: The classification and significance of gastric polyps. In Yardley JH, Morson BM (eds): The Gastrointestinal Tract. Baltimore, Williams & Wilkins, 1977, pp 149-175.
3. Ghazi A, Ferstenberg H, Shinya H: Endoscopic gastroduodenal polypectomy. Ann Surg 200:175-180, 1984.
4. Rosch W: Epidemiology, pathogenesis, diagnosis, treatment of benign gastric tumors. Front Gastrointest Res 6:167-184, 1980.
5. Laxen F, Sipponen P, Ihamaki T, et al: Gastric polyps; their morphological and endoscopical characteristics and relation to gastric carcinoma. Acta Pathol Microbiol Scand 90:221-228, 1982.
6. Ming SC: Tumors of the esophagus and stomach. In Atlas of Tumor Pathology, 2nd series, fascicle 7. Washington, DC, Armed Forces Institute of Pathology, 1973, pp 99-101.
7. Tomasulo J: Gastric polyps: Histologic types and their relationship to gastric carcinoma. Cancer 27:1346-1355, 1971.
8. Ming SC, Goldman H: Gastric polyps: A histogenetic classification and its relation to carcinoma. Cancer 18:721-726, 1965.
9. Varies O, Laxen F, Valle J: *Helicobacter pylori* infection and fasting serum gastrin levels in a series of endoscopically diagnosed gastric polyps. APMIS 102:759-764, 1994.
10. Koga S, Watanabe H, Enjoji M: Stomal polypoid hypertrophic gastritis: A polypoid gastric lesion at gastroenterostomy site. Cancer 43:647-657, 1979.
11. Stemmermann GN, Hayashi T: Hyperplastic polyps of the gastric mucosa adjacent to gastroenterostomy stomas. Am J Clin Pathol 71:341-345, 1979.
12. Lewin KJ, Appelman HD: Mesenchymal tumors and tumor-like proliferations of the esophagus, tumors of the esophagus and stomach. In Atlas of Tumor Pathology, 3rd series, vol 18. Washington, DC, Armed Forces Institute of Pathology, 1996.
13. Manousos O, Webster CU: Diffuse gastrointestinal polyposis with ectodermal changes. Gut 7:375-379, 1966.
14. Jarnum S, Jenson H: Diffuse gastrointestinal polyposis with ectodermal changes. A case with severe malabsorption and enteric loss of plasma proteins and electrolytes. Gastroenterology 50:107-118, 1966.
15. Sachatello CR, Pickren JW, Grace JT Jr: Generalized juvenile gastrointestinal polyposis. A hereditary syndrome. Gastroenterology 58:669-708, 1970.
16. Williams GT, Bussey HJR, Morson BC: Hamartomatous polyps in Peutz-Jeghers syndrome. N Engl J Med 299:101-102, 1978.

17. Watanabe H, Enjoji M, Yao T, Ohsato K: Gastric lesions in familial adenomatous polyposis coli: Their incidence and histological analysis. Hum Pathol 9:269-283, 1978.

18. Burke AP, Sobin LH: The pathology of Cronkhite-Canada polyps. A comparison to juvenile polyposis. Am J Surg Pathol 13:940-946, 1989.

19. Marcial MA, Villafana M, Hernandez-Denton J, et al: Fundic gland polyps: Prevalence and clinicopathologic features. Am J Gastroenterol 88:1711-1713, 1993.

20. Lee RG, Burt RW: The histopathology of fundic gland polyps of the stomach. Am J Clin Pathol 86:498-503, 1986.

21. Ranchod M, Lewin KJ, Dorfman RF: Lymphoid hyperplasia of the gastro-intestinal tract: A study of 26 cases and review of the literature. Am J Surg Pathol 2:383-400, 1978.

22. Snover DC: Benign epithelial polyps of the stomach. Pathol Annu 20:303-329, 1985.

23. Koch HK, Lesch R, Cremer M, et al: Polyp and polypoid foveolar hyperplasia in gastric biopsy specimens and their precancerous prevalence. Front Gastrointest Res 4:183-191, 1979.

24. Barbosa J de C, Dockerty MB, Waugh JM: Pancreatic heterotopia: Review of literature and report of 41 authenticated surgical cases, of which 25 were clinically significant. Surg Gynecol Obstet 85:527-542, 1946.

25. Taylor AL: The epithelial heterotopias of the alimentary tract. J Pathol 30:375-380, 1944.

26. Kaneda M, Yano T, Yamamoto T, et al: Ectopic pancreas on the stomach presenting as an inflammatory abdominal mass. Am J Gastroenterol 84:663-666, 1989.

27. Branch CD, Gross RE: Aberrant pancreatic tissue in GI tract. Surg Gynecol Obstet 82:527, 1946.

28. Stolte M, Sticht T, Eidt S, et al: Frequency, location, and age and sex distribution of various types of gastric polyp. Endoscopy 26:659-665, 1994.

29. Johnson CD, Bynum TE: Brunner gland heterotopia presenting as gastric and antral polyps. Gastrointest Endosc 22:210-211, 1976.

30. Williams AW, Michie W: Adenomatosis of the stomach of Brunner gland type. Br J Surg 45:259-263, 1957.

31. Stewart TW Jr, Mille LR: Adenomyoma of the stomach. South Med J 77:1337-1338, 1984.

32. Goedde TA, Rodriguez-Bigas MA, Herrera L, et al: Gastroduodenal polyps in familial adenomatous polyposis. Surg Oncol 1:357-361, 1992.

33. Marcello PW, Asbun HJ, Veidenhamer MC, et al: Gastroduodenal polyps in familial adenomatous polyposis. Surg Endosc 10:418-421, 1996.

34. Hirota T, Okada T, Itabashi M, et al: Histogenesis of human gastric cancer—with special reference to the significance of adenoma as a precancerous lesion. In Ming SC (ed): Precursors of Gastric Cancer. Philadelphia, Praeger, 1984, pp 233-252.

35. Nagayo T: Histogenesis and Precursors of Human Gastric Cancer. New York, Springer, 1986, pp 103-111.

36. Nakamura K, Sagakuchi H, Enjoji M: Depressed adenoma of the stomach. Cancer 62:2197-2202, 1988.

37. Nakamura T: Nakamura type III gastric polyp: History of the study. Proc 1st International Gastric Cancer Congress. Bologna, Italy, Monduzzi Editore, 1995, pp 209-212.

38. Meltzer AD, Ostrum BJ, Isard HJ: Villous tumors of the stomach and duodenum. Radiology 87:511-513, 1966.

39. Inaba S, Tanaka T, Okanoue T, et al: Villous tumors of the stomach associated with adenocarcinomas—a histochemical study of mucosubstances. Jpn J Clin Oncol 14:691-698, 1984.

40. Ming SC, Goldman H: Pathology of the Gastrointestinal Tract, 2nd ed. Philadelphia, Lippincott Williams & Wilkins, 1998, pp 579-584.

41. Larsen B, Tarp V, Kristensen E: Familial giant hypertrophic gastritis (Ménétrier's disease). Gut 28:1517-1521, 1987.

42. Walker FB IV: Spontaneous remission in hypertrophic gastropathy (Ménétrier's disease). South Med J 74:1273-1276, 1981.

43. Lesser PB, Falchuk KR, Singer M, et al: Ménétrier's disease: Report of a case with transient and reversible findings. Gastroenterology 68:1598-1601, 1975.

44. Teele RL, Katz AJ, Goldman H, et al: The radiographic features of eosinophilic gastroenteritis (allergic gastroenteropathy) of childhood. AJR Am J Roentgenol 132:575-580, 1979.

45. Katz PO, Salas L: Less frequent causes of upper gastrointestinal bleeding. Gastrointest Clin North Am 22:875-889, 1993.

46. Veldhuyzen van Zanten SJ, Bartelsman JF, Schipper ME, Tygat GN: Recurrent massive haematemesis from Dieulafoy vascular malformations—a review of 101 cases. Gut 27:213-222, 1986.

47. Mower GA, Whitehead R: Gastric hemorrhage due to ruptured arteriovenous malformation (Dieulafoy's disease). Pathology 18:54-57, 1986.

48. Baettig B, Haecki W, Lammer F, et al: Dieulafoy's disease: Endoscopic treatment and follow-up. Gut 34:1418-1421, 1993.

49. Grisendi A, Lonardo A, Della CG, et al: Combined endoscopic and surgical management of Dieulafoy vascular malformation. J Am Coll Surg 179:182-186, 1994.

50. Boley SJ, Sammartano R, Adams A, et al: On the nature and etiology of vascular ectasias of the colon: Degenerative lesions of aging. Gastroenterology 72:650-660, 1977.

51. Camilleri M, Chadwick VS, Hodgson HJF: Vascular anomalies of the gastrointestinal tract. Hepatogastroenterology 31:149-153, 1984.

52. Colizza S, Tiso B, Bracci F, et al: Cystic lymphangioma of stomach and jejunum: Report of one case. J Surg Oncol 17:169-176, 1981.

53. Erlandson RA, Klimstra DS, Woodruff JM: Subclassification of gastrointestinal stromal tumors based on evaluation by electron microscopy and immunohistochemistry. Ultrastruct Pathol 20:373-393, 1996.

54. Schaldenbrand JD, Appelman HD: Solitary solid stromal gastrointestinal tumors in von Recklinghausen's disease with minimal smooth muscle differentiation. Hum Pathol 15:229-232, 1984.

55. Wieczorek RL, Seidman I, Ranson JHC, et al: Congenital duplication of the stomach: Case report and review of the English literature. Am J Gastroenterol 79:597-602, 1984.

56. Abrami G, Dennison WM: Duplication of the stomach. Surgery 49:794-801, 1961.

57. Bremer JL: Diverticula and duplications of the intestinal tract. Arch Pathol Lab Med 38:132-140, 1944.

58. Rossini FP, Risio M, Pennazio M: Small bowel tumors and polyposis syndromes. Gastrointest Endosc Clin N Am 9:93-114, 1999.

59. Coit DG: Cancer of the small intestine. In DeVita VT Jr, Rosenberg SA, Hellman S (eds): Cancer: Principles and Practice of Oncology, vol 1, 4th ed. Philadelphia, JB Lippincott 1993, p 915.

60. Wilson JM, Melvin DB, Gray GF, Thorbjarnson B: Primary malignancies of the small bowel: A report of 96 cases and review of the literature. Ann Surg 180:175-179, 1974.

61. Ashley SW, Wells SA Jr: Tumors of the small intestine. Semin Oncol 15:116-128, 1988.

62. Wilson JM, Melvin DB, Gray GF, Thorbjarnson B: Benign small bowel tumors. Ann Surg 181:247-250, 1975.

63. Eisen LK, Cunningham JD, Aufses AH Jr: Intussusception in adults: An institutional review. J Am Coll Surg 188:390-395, 1999.

64. Bessette JR, Maglinte DDT, Kelvin FM, Chernish SM: Primary malignant tumors in the small bowel: A comparison of the small-bowel enema and conventional follow-through examination. AJR Am J Roentgenol 153:741-744, 1989.

65. Nakamura S, Iida M, Nakao Y, et al: Diagnostic value of push-type jejunal endoscopy in primary jejunal carcinoma. Surg Endosc 7:188-190, 1993.

66. Lewis BS, Kornbluth A, Waye JD: Small bowel tumors: Yield of enteroscopy. Gut 32:763-765, 1991.

67. Shimer GR, Helwig EB: Inflammatory fibroid polyps of the intestine. Am J Clin Pathol 81:708-714, 1984.

68. Tysk C, Schnurer LB, Wickbom G: Obstructing inflammatory fibroid polyp in pelvic ileal reservoir after restorative proctocolectomy in ulcerative colitis. Report of a case. Dis Colon Rectum 37:1034-1037, 1994.

69. Williams GR, Jaffe S, Scott CA: Inflammatory fibroid polyps of the terminal ileum presenting in a patient with active Crohn's disease. Histopatology 20:545-547, 1992.

70. Cheng CL, Sherman S, Fogel EL, et al: Endoscopic snare papillectomy for tumors of the duodenal papillae. Gastrointest Endosc 60:757-764, 2004.

71. Ryan DP, Schapiro RH, Warshaw AL: Villous tumors of the duodenum. Ann Surg 203:301-306, 1986.

72. Bjork KJ, Davis CJ, Nagorney DM, Mucha P Jr: Duodenal villous tumors. Arch Surg 125:961-965, 1990.

73. Rattner DW, Fernandez-del Castillo C, Brugge WR, Warshaw AL: Defining the criteria for local resection of ampullary neoplasms. Arch Surg 131:366-371, 1996.

74. Galandiu S, Hermann RE, Jagelman DG, et al: Villous tumors of the duodenum. Ann Surg 207:234-239, 1988.

75. Maher MM, Yeo CJ, Lillemoe KD, et al: Pancreas-sparing duodenectomy for infra-ampullary duodenal pathology. Am J Surg 171:62-67, 1996.

76. Farnell MB, Sakorafas GH, Sarr MG, et al: Villous tumors of the duodenum: Reappraisal of local vs. extended resection. J Gastrointest Surg 4:13-21, 2000.

77. Yokoyama I, Kozuka S, Ito K, et al: Gastric gland metaplasia in the small and large intestine. Gut 18:214-218, 1977.

78. Powell SM, Petersen GM, Krush AJ, et al: Molecular diagnosis of familial adenomatous polyposis. N Engl J Med 329:1982-1987, 1993.

79. Spirio L, Olschwang S, Groden J, et al: Alleles of the APC gene: An attenuated form of familial polyposis. Cell 755:951-957, 1993.

80. Jarvinen H, Nyberg M, Peltokallio P: Upper gastrointestinal tract polyps in familial adenomatosis coli. Gut 24:333-339, 1983.

81. Arrigoni A, Pennazio M, Rossini FP: Enteroscopy in small bowel neoplastic pathology. Acta Endosc 26:255-261, 1996.

82. Bertoni G, Sassatelli R, Pennazio M, et al: High prevalence of adenomas and microadenomas of the duodenal papilla and peri-ampullary region in patients with familial adenomatous polyposis. Eur J Gastroenterol 8:1201-1206, 1996.

83. Kashiwagi H, Spigelman AD, Debinski HS, et al: Surveillance of ampullary adenomas in familial adenomatous polyposis. Lancet 344:1582, 1994.

84. Iwama T, Mishima Y, Utsonomiya J: The impact of familial adenomatous polyposis on the tumorigenesis and mortality at the several organs: Its rational treatment. Ann Surg 217:101-108, 1993.

85. Offerhaus GJA, Giardiello FM, Krush AJ, et al: The risk of upper gastrointestinal cancer in familial adenomatous polyposis. Gastroenterology 102:1980-1982, 1992.

86. Nugent KP, Spigelman AD, Williams CB, et al: Surveillance of duodenal polyps in familial adenomatous polyposis: Progress report. J R Soc Med 87:704-706, 1994.

87. Dorazio RA, Whelan TJ Jr: Lymphoid hyperplasia of the terminal ileum associated with familial polyposis coli. Ann Surg 171:300-302, 1970.

88. Portwood GL, Morris AJ, Cotton PB: Obscure gastrointestinal bleeding: Role of small bowel enteroscopy. J S C Med Assoc 93:51-56, 1997.

89. Norton ID, Sorbi D, Geller A, et al: Endoscopic management of proximal small bowel adenomas in familial adenomatous polyposis [abstract]. Gastrointest Endosc 47:88, 1998.

90. Saurin JC, Ponchon T, Descos F, et al: Photodynamic therapy (PDT) targeted to the proximal duodenum in familial adenomatous polyposis (FAP) [abstract]. Gastrointest Endosc 47:38, 1998.

91. Nugent KP, Farmer KC, Spigelman AD, et al: Randomized controlled trial of the effect of sulindac on duodenal and rectal polyposis and cell proliferation in patients with familial adenomatous polyposis. Br J Surg 80:1618-1619, 1993.

92. Richard CS, Berk T, Bapat BV, et al: Sulindac for periampullary polyps in FAP patients. Int J Colorectal Dis 12:14-18, 1997.

93. Rustgi A: Hereditary gastrointestinal polyposis and nonpolyposis syndrome. N Engl J Med 331:1694-1702, 1994.

94. Thomford NR, Greenberger NJ: Lymphoid polyps of the ileum associated with Gardner's syndrome. Arch Surg 96:289-291, 1968.

95. Wennstrom J, Pierce ER, McKusik VA: Hereditary benign and malignant lesions of the large bowel. Cancer 34:850-857, 1974.

96. Spirio L, Otterud B, Stauffer D, et al: Linkage of a variant or attenuated form of adenomatous polyposis coli to the adenomatous polyposis coli (APC) locus. Am J Hum Genet 51:92-100, 1992.

97. Leppert M, Burt R, Hughes JP, et al: Genetic analysis of an inherited predisposition to colonic cancer in a family with a variable number of adenomatous polyps. N Engl J Med 322:904-908, 1990.

98. Lynch HT, Smyrk TC, Watson P, et al: Hereditary flat adenoma syndrome: A variant of familial adenomatous polyposis. Dis Colon Rectum 35:411-421, 1992.

99. Lynch HT, Smyrk TC, Lanspa SJ, et al: Upper gastrointestinal manifestations in families with hereditary flat adenoma syndrome. Cancer 71:2709-2714, 1993.

100. Desai DC, Neal KF, Talbot IC, et al: Juvenile polyposis. Br J Surg 82:14-17, 1995.

101. Carlson GJ, Nivatvongs S, Snover DC: Colorectal polyps in Cowden's disease. Am J Surg Pathol 8:763-770, 1984.

102. Weary PE, Gorlin RJ, Gentry WC Jr, et al: Multiple hamartoma syndrome: Cowden's disease. Arch Dermatol 106:682-690, 1972.

103. Spigelman AD, Murday V, Phillips RKS: Cancer and the Peutz-Jeghers syndrome. Gut 30:1588-1590, 1989.

104. Cronkhite LW, Canada WJ: Generalized gastrointestinal polyposis: An unusual syndrome of polyposis, pigmentation, alopecia, and onychodystrophy. N Engl J Med 252:1011-1015, 1955.

105. Daniel ES, Ludwig SL, Lew KJ, et al: The Cronkhite-Canada syndrome: An analysis of clinical and pathological features and therapy in 55 patients. Medicine (Baltimore) 61:293-309, 1982.

106. Katayama Y, Kimura M, Konn M: Cronkhite-Canada syndrome associated with rectal cancer and adenomatous changes in colonic polyps. Am J Surg Pathol 9:65-71, 1985.

107. Weidner N, Flanders DJ, Mitros FA: Mucosal ganglioneuromatosis associated with multiple colonic polyps. Am J Surg Pathol 8:779-786, 1984.

108. Camilleri M, Chadwick VS, Hodgson HJF: Vascular anomalies of the gastrointestinal tract. Hepatogastroenterology 31:149-153, 1984.

109. O'Mahony S, Morris AJ, Straiton M, et al: Push enteroscopy in the investigation of small intestinal disease. Q J Med 89:885-890, 1996.

110. Messer J, Romeu J, Waye J, et al: The value of proximal jejunoscopy in unexplained gastrointestinal bleeding [abstract]. Gastrointest Endosc 30:151, 1984.

111. Barquist ES, Apple SJ, Jensen DM, et al: Jejunal lymphangioma: An unusual cause of chronic gastrointestinal bleeding. Dig Dis Sci 42:1179-1183, 1997.

112. Spira R, Lewis B, Katz LB: Small bowel tumors presenting as occult GI bleeding [abstract]. Am J Gastroenterol 91:1961, 1995.

113. Blanchard DK, Budde JM, Hatch JF 3rd, et al: Tumors of the small intestine. World J Surg 24:421-429, 2000.

114. Starr GF, Dockerty MB: Leiomyomas and leiomyosarcomas of the small intestine. Cancer 8:101-111, 1995.

115. Ng EH, Pollock RE, Munsell MF, et al: Prognostic factors influencing survival in gastrointestinal leiomyosarcomas. Implications for surgical management and staging. Ann Surg 215:68-77, 1992.

116. Sanders L, Silverman M, Rossi R, et al: Gastric smooth muscle tumors: Diagnostic dilemmas and factors affecting outcome. World J Surg 20:992-995, 1996.

117. Ludwig DI, Traverso LW: Gut stromal tumors and their clinical behavior. Am J Surg 173:390-394, 1997.

118. Shaw RC: Von Recklinghausen's disease of the small intestine associated with skin lesions. Am J Surg 80:360-363, 1950.

119. Hochberg FH, Dasilva AB, Galdabini J, Richardson EP Jr: Gastrointestinal involvement in von Recklinghausen's neurofibromatosis. Neurology 24:1144-1151, 1974.

120. Skaane P, Eide TJ, Westgaard T, et al: Lipomatosis and true lipomas of the ileocecal valve. Rofo Fortschr Geb Rongenstr Neuen Bildgeb Verfahr 135:663-668, 1981.

121. Boquist L, Bargdahl L, Anderson A: Lipomatosis of the ileocecal valve. Cancer 29:136-140, 1972.

122. Gdanietz K, Wit J, Heller K: Complete duplication of the small intestine in childhood. Z Kinderchir 38:414-416, 1983.

61

Adenocarcinoma of the Stomach, Duodenum, and Small Intestine

Alexander A. Parikh · John M. Daly

GASTRIC ADENOCARCINOMA

Approximately 90% of all tumors of the stomach are malignant, the vast majority of which are gastric adenocarcinoma. Gastric cancer has been one of the leading causes of cancer-related mortality in the world for the past century and is currently the second most common cancer worldwide after lung cancer. Though still common in many parts of the world, particularly in the Eastern Hemisphere, the incidence has shown a dramatic decline in many parts of the Western world, including the United States. The incidence of proximal gastric cancers, however, is increasing. Surgical resection remains the only curative option, but the majority of patients in the United States are initially found to have unresectable disease. Advances in adjuvant therapies, including chemotherapy and radiotherapy, have improved survival rates in patients with resectable disease but remain palliative in patients who are not candidates for resection.

Epidemiology

In 2005 there will be an estimated 21,800 new cases of gastric cancer in the United States and approximately 13,000 deaths, which makes it the 14th most common malignancy and cause of cancer death in the United States.[1] Worldwide, gastric cancer remains the second or third most common malignancy (nearly 900,000 new cases annually) and the second most common cause of death (approximately 650,000 deaths).[2] The incidence of gastric cancer has significant geographic variation, with the highest incidence (75 to 100 per 100,000 men) occurring in Japan, Korea, and parts of South America and Eastern Europe and the lowest incidence (as low as 5 per 100,000 men) occurring in the United States and

Western Europe.[3,4] In the United States, gastric cancer is more prevalent in men than women (2:1) and is also more common in African Americans, Hispanics, and Native Americans.[3,4] The incidence also increases with age starting in the fourth decade of life and generally peaks in the seventh decade.[5]

The incidence of gastric cancer in the United States has dropped approximately 75% since the 1930s, when it was the leading cause of cancer-related death in men.[4] The mortality rate has also decreased significantly from approximately 31 per 100,000 in the 1930s to 7.8 per 100,000 by the mid-1980s.[3] Part of this decrease in mortality is due to an increase in the overall incidence, however. The decrease in incidence of gastric cancer from 1930 to 1976 was largely due to a decrease in distal gastric cancers. Interestingly, however, since 1976, the incidence of proximal (i.e., cardia and gastroesophageal [GE] junction) adenocarcinomas in the United States and Europe has increased at a rate exceeding that of any other malignancy, and it currently accounts for nearly half of all gastric cancers.[6-8] This trend is particularly concerning because proximal gastric cancers and distal esophageal cancers are generally more difficult to treat and are also associated with higher overall mortality than distal gastric cancers are. The reasons for this shift from distal to proximal cancers are unclear, but it has been suggested that factors such as increased body mass index, increased caloric intake, and GE reflux may play a role.[6-8]

The overall 5-year survival rate for all stages of gastric cancer in the United States from 1995 to 2000 was approximately 23%, with a range of 58% in patients with localized disease to below 5% in patients with distant metastases, thus making it one of the more lethal cancers.[9] In the United States, nearly two thirds of patients are initially seen at an advanced stage, and more than 80% have lymph node metastases. The overall

5-year survival rate has improved significantly, however, from only 15% in 1976 to 23% by 2000,[10] probably because of earlier and more accurate diagnosis and staging, improvements in surgical resectional technique, and significant improvements in adjuvant therapy regimens. In contrast, however, the overall 5-year gastric cancer survival rate in Japan and the Far East is about 50%, where earlier-stage disease is diagnosed in a far greater percentage of patients.[3,4]

Pathology

Adenocarcinomas constitute 95% of all gastric cancers in the United States, with gastric lymphoma, carcinoid, gastrointestinal (GI) stromal tumors, and squamous cell carcinomas making up the remaining 5%.[4] Several pathologic classifications have been devised to describe gastric adenocarcinoma. The Borrmann classification scheme categorizes gastric cancer into five types by its macroscopic appearance.[2,11] Type I consists of polypoid or fungating cancers, type II includes tumors that are fungating and ulcerated and surrounded by elevated borders, type III includes ulcerated lesions infiltrating the gastric wall, type IV cancers infiltrate diffusely, and type V consists of those that are unable to be classified.[12]

The Lauren classification is the most commonly used classification scheme and divides gastric cancers into two distinct types—intestinal and diffuse[3,13] (Box 61–1). The intestinal variant arises from the gastric mucosa and is glandular in origin. Intestinal-type tumors often arise

from precancerous lesions similar to other cancers of the GI tract. They are more common in men, in older patients, and in the distal part of the stomach. The intestinal variant is associated with *Helicobacter pylori* infection, chronic atrophic gastritis, intestinal metaplasia, and dietary factors (discussed in the next section).[5,11] In contrast, the diffuse-type pathology appears to arise from the lamina propria, is associated with an invasive growth pattern, and is less related to environmental factors.[5,11] Diffuse-type tumors are more common in younger patients and in the proximal part of the stomach. These tumors are characterized by noncohesive malignant cells diffusely infiltrating the stomach with minimal to no gland formation. They tend to spread rapidly in the submucosa, as well as by transmural extension and lymphatic invasion. Peritoneal metastases are also more common with diffuse-type gastric cancers. These cancers have increased in incidence and are associated with a worse prognosis than the intestinal variants are.[5,11]

The World Health Organization has further characterized gastric adenocarcinoma into five categories, depending on the degree of intestinal metaplasia. The classification includes adenocarcinoma (intestinal and diffuse), signet cell, mucinous, tubular, and papillary.[2,11]

Traditionally, most gastric cancers were found in the antrum; however, in the 1980s and 1990s, antral cancers declined and the proportion of proximal tumors and those of the cardia have increased.[4,14] In general, cancer of the lesser curve is more common than cancer of the greater curve. In almost 10% of cancers, the tumor can involve the entire stomach with malignant cells infiltrating beyond the apparent mass, a condition termed *linitis plastica*. This entity portends an especially poor prognosis, with 5-year survival being very unusual.[4,14]

Early gastric cancer is an entity characterized by tumor confined to the gastric mucosa or submucosa. In Japan, where extensive screening programs exist, early gastric cancer accounts for nearly 50% of all gastric cancers, whereas in the United States it is much less common (<10%).[4,15]

Risk Factors

Because there is such a pronounced difference in the incidence of gastric cancer in different areas of the world, many consider ethnic origin as a potential risk factor for the development of gastric cancer. In fact, the National Cancer Institute has categorized ethnic groups in three risk categories. Japanese, Koreans, Vietnamese, Native Americans, and Hawaiians are at the highest risk; Latino, Chinese, and blacks are at intermediate risk; and Filipinos and whites are at the lowest risk.[2] In addition, immigrants from high-risk to low-risk countries remain at high risk, but subsequent generations have a risk that is native to their new environment, thus suggesting that environmental factors may play a more important role.[5]

Several dietary factors have been found to be associated with an increased risk for gastric cancer (Box 61–2), including diets high in salt, cured and smoked foods, nitrates, and nitrites.[5,16] In contrast, diets high in fruits, vegetables, and antioxidants, as well as vitamins A and C

Box 61–1   Risk Factors and Protective Factors Involved in the Pathogenesis of Gastric Cancer

Intestinal Variant

Arises from precancerous areas (gastric atrophy, metaplasia)

5:1 Male-to-female ratio

Older population

Dominant histology in areas where stomach cancer is epidemic (environmental cause)

Declining in incidence

Diffuse Variant

Does not typically arise from a precancerous area

Women >> men

Younger patients

Higher association in familial occurrence (genetic cause)

Major histologic type in endemic areas

Worse overall prognosis

Box 61–2 **Characteristics of Intestinal and Diffuse Variants of Gastric Adenocarcinoma**

Acquired Factors

High-salt diet

High-nitrate diet

Smoked/cured food

Low vitamin A and C

Well water

Cigarette smoking

Helicobacter pylori

Epstein-Barr virus

Radiation exposure

Previous gastric surgery

Coal workers

Rubber workers

Genetic Factors

Type A blood

Pernicious anemia

Family history

Hereditary nonpolyposis colorectal cancer

Li-Fraumeni syndrome

Precursors

Adenoma

Atrophic gastritis

Dysplasia

Intestinal metaplasia

Ménétrier's disease

Protective Factors

Raw vegetables

Citrus fruits

Antioxidants—vitamins A and C

Selenium, zinc, iron

Green tea

Infection with *H. pylori* has also been associated with an increased risk for the development of gastric cancer. In a study by Parsonnet and colleagues, infection with *H. pylori* increased the risk for gastric cancer 3.6-fold as compared with noninfected patients. This increase in risk was present for the development of both intestinal- and diffuse-type cancers, but interestingly, there was no associated increase in risk for the development of GE junction tumors.[19] Similarly, a recent prospective cohort study from Japan showed a statistically significant increase in risk for gastric cancer in those infected with *H. pylori* as compared with controls. This risk was even higher in patients with severe atrophic gastritis, corpus-predominant gastritis, or intestinal metaplasia.[20] Epstein-Barr virus and medical conditions such as pernicious anemia, chronic atrophic gastritis, intestinal metaplasia, gastric villous adenoma, and obesity are also associated with an increased risk for gastric cancer.[3,4] Patients who have undergone partial gastrectomy for benign gastric ulcer disease are likewise at increased risk for gastric cancer in the stomach remnant. This risk for cancer also has a long latency period of about 15 years.[21,22]

Although most gastric cancers occur sporadically, approximately 10% have an inherited component.[23] Patients with hereditary nonpolyposis colon cancer syndrome and polyposis syndromes such as Peutz-Jeghers and familial adenomatous polyposis have an increased risk for the development of gastric cancer.[2] Gastric cancer can also develop in patients with germline mutations in p53 and *BRCA2*.[2] Finally, mutations in the cell adhesion protein E-cadherin lead to an increased risk for hereditary diffuse gastric cancer, and it has been recommended by some that prophylactic gastrectomy be considered in affected kindreds.[24]

Clinical Features

Early gastric cancer seldom produces symptoms, and when it does, they are usually nonspecific. Consequently, nearly 80% to 90% of patients are initially seen with locally advanced or metastatic disease. When early evaluation does take place, most patients complain of weight loss, anorexia, and abdominal pain. Anemia secondary to chronic blood loss is also common, but overt GI bleeding is not unless the tumors are large and ulcerated.[2,4] Dysphagia occurs predominantly in patients with proximal cancers, whereas nausea, vomiting, and symptoms of gastric outlet obstruction are more common with distal tumors that obstruct the lumen. Early satiety is especially prominent in patients with *linitis plastica* because of the nondistensibility of the stomach.[2,4,5]

Patients with early gastric cancer seldom have significant physical findings. Patients with more advanced disease may have a palpable abdominal mass, as well as ascites and cachexia.[2,4,5] Patients with metastatic disease may exhibit Blumer's shelf nodules or Krukenberg tumors (on rectal or pelvic examination), periumbilical lymphadenopathy or peritoneal metastases (Sister Mary Joseph's node), and palpable supraclavicular adenopathy (Virchow's node).[2,4,5]

and calcium, have been associated with a decreased risk for gastric cancer.[5,17] Smoking also appears to be a risk factor, but the role of alcohol is less clear.[17,18] In the United States, male gender, African American race, and low socioeconomic status, as well as occupational hazards in the metal-working, mining, and rubber-working industries, are all associated with a higher risk for gastric cancer.[3,4]

Diagnosis

Although mass screening, usually by upper endoscopy or double-contrast barium studies, for the detection of gastric cancer is recommended in endemic areas such as Japan, routine screening in Western countries such as the United States is not practical because of the low incidence. Once diagnosed, the National Comprehensive Cancer Network has developed consensus guidelines for the evaluation and staging of patients with suspected gastric cancer.[25] Patients with newly diagnosed gastric cancer should undergo a complete history and physical examination; laboratory studies, including a complete blood count, platelets, and chemistry profile; chest radiography; computed tomography (CT) of the abdomen (and the chest with proximal tumors); CT/ultrasonography of the pelvis in females; and upper endoscopy and biopsy with the goal of a tissue diagnosis and anatomic localization of the tumor.[25] Although double-contrast barium esophagography can still be very helpful in the detection and localization of gastric cancers,[26] it has largely been supplanted by esophagogastroduodenoscopy (EGD) and CT as a *routine* diagnostic modality.[3,27] Serum tumor markers, including carcinoembryonic antigen (CEA), CA 19-9, CA-125, CA 72-4, and β-human chorionic gonadotropin (β-HCG), can be elevated in patients with gastric cancer, although the individual sensitivities are generally low—in the 40% to 50% range.[28-30] The sensitivity of these tumor markers is significantly improved, however, when several are elevated.[31] Furthermore, in patients with known gastric cancer, markedly elevated tumor markers may also signify aggressive disease or tumor burden.

This work-up will usually allow one to classify patients into one of two groups—those with locoregional disease (stage I to III or M0) and those with systemic metastases (stage IV or M1). Patients with locoregional disease are further stratified according to resectability, functional status, and comorbid conditions, with further evaluation often including laparoscopy and endoscopic ultrasound (EUS). Patients with metastatic disease are considered for palliative therapy, depending on their symptoms and functional status.[25]

Upper GI endoscopy (EGD) with biopsy remains the modality of choice for the diagnosis of gastric cancer.[4] Tumor location and the size and extent of mucosal involvement are readily ascertained, provided that the gastric lumen is not obstructed by the tumor. In more than 95% of patients, four to six tissue biopsy specimens and brushings are sufficient to establish the diagnosis, although this can often be difficult in patients with linitis plastica.[27,32] In advanced disease, EGD can be a means to provide palliative therapy, including laser ablation, dilatation, and stenting, although the precise role of these modalities is still evolving.[3,4]

EUS has also become a valuable staging tool for patients with locoregional disease. In experienced hands, EUS can often accurately determine the depth of invasion and nodal status in patients with gastric cancer. The overall accuracy of EUS in staging is about 75% to 80%, but it is significantly operator and institution dependent. Staging of T1 (80%) and T3 (90%) lesions is quite accu-

rate, but EUS is limited in accurately staging T2 lesions (35% to 40%).[32,33] Nodal staging is also less accurate with EUS, but newer techniques have increased its accuracy 50% to 85%.[32,33] EUS-guided fine-needle aspiration for additional tissue diagnosis has also been performed, but experience with this technique is limited and usually confined to large referral centers.

CT of the abdomen and pelvis is also very useful and commonly used in the preoperative work-up of patients with gastric cancer. Contrast-enhanced CT can detect metastases to the liver and peritoneum, local invasion into adjacent structures, and regional and distal lymphadenopathy, as well as ascites suggesting peritoneal disease. The overall accuracy in assessing tumor stage is 66% to 77%, but its accuracy in correctly staging nodal disease is much more variable, from 25% to 86%. CT is also limited in detecting early gastric tumors or small (<5 mm) peritoneal or hepatic metastases.[34,35]

Magnetic resonance imaging (MRI) has also been shown to be as accurate as CT in the staging and detection of gastric cancer. Though expensive and associated with motion artifact, several studies have reported MRI as being slightly superior to CT in the T staging of tumors, with overall T staging accuracy between 73% and 88%.[36] Although MRI may also be superior to CT in N staging (73% versus 65%), both techniques suffer from under-staging. MRI has also been shown to be superior to CT in the detection of liver, bone, and peritoneal metastases.[37,38] Nevertheless, the continued improvement in CT scanning equipment and technique, combined with the expense and relative less availability of routine MRI, continues to result in CT being the preferred staging modality for gastric cancer at most institutions.

Positron emission tomography (PET) with [^{18}F]-fluorodeoxyglucose (FDG) is increasingly being used in the preoperative staging of GI cancers. Though fairly well established in the work-up of colorectal cancer and more recently esophageal cancer, experience with PET scanning in patients with gastric cancer is limited. Preliminary data suggest that PET may be very useful in identifying the primary gastric cancer (90% to 95% sensitivity) and perhaps in monitoring treatment response. Its usefulness in determining N stage is more variable, however (35% to 60% sensitivity), and in general, PET is more accurate in detecting N2- and N3-level nodes because they are further away from the primary tumor.[39,40] Nevertheless, additional studies are needed before PET scanning can be recommended as a *routine* diagnostic and staging tool for gastric cancer.

Diagnostic laparoscopy remains a popular diagnostic modality for the staging of gastric cancer and is especially helpful in detecting small-volume peritoneal and liver metastases. It has been demonstrated in several studies that the sensitivity of laparoscopy in detecting liver metastases is as high as 85% to 96%, though somewhat lower in detecting peritoneal disease. In general, between 23% and 37% of patients with gastric cancer are up-staged by the use of staging laparoscopy and therefore potentially spared a laparotomy.[41-45]

Laparoscopic ultrasound (LUS) has also been used in hope of further improving the capability of laparoscopic exploration.[46] The specific benefit of LUS over high-quality CT scanning and laparoscopy is unclear, however, and the use of LUS in the staging of gastric cancer remains limited.

Cytologic analysis of peritoneal washings may identify patients with occult carcinomatosis, and many institutions have adopted cytologic analysis of peritoneal washings obtained at laparoscopic staging or even during laparotomy as part of the diagnostic algorithm. Patients with positive findings on peritoneal cytology have a prognosis similar to those with occult visceral metastatic disease.[47,48] Cytologic analysis may result in false-positive results, however, and because some reports fail to confirm the prognostic significance of positive cytologic findings, it has not been universally adapted. At our institution, we use peritoneal cytology as an indication for systemic therapy, but not as an absolute contraindication to resection.

Staging

The most widely used staging system is the American Joint Commission for Cancer TNM system (Box 61–3), which involves standard evaluation of the tumor (T), regional lymph nodes (N), and the presence of metastatic disease (M). The T stage is divided into four levels, depending on the depth of invasion, with recent subdivision of the T2 level into T2a (invasion of the muscularis propria) and T2b (invasion of the subserosa). The N status reflects the number of lymph nodes involved, with the requirement that at least 15 lymph nodes be removed for the patient to be properly staged. Of note, N3 cancers (>15 metastatic lymph nodes) are considered stage IV. Studies from both the United States and Japan have validated the prognostic value of the number of lymph nodes involved in the TNM staging system. The Japanese staging system defines nodal stage by anatomic location and proximity to the tumor. This system is based on 16 nodal stations and is complicated and difficult to use, particularly in institutions where gastrectomies are rarely performed. However, because the TNM staging system has shown prognostic value and is simpler to use, it has largely supplanted the Japanese staging system for gastric cancer in the United States.[4]

Surgical Treatment

In the absence of metastatic spread, surgical resection remains the gold standard for the treatment of gastric cancer and the only chance for cure. The types of resection options vary according to the location, stage, and pattern of spread of the tumor, but in general they involve a wide enough resection to achieve negative microscopic margins (R0 resection), as well as en bloc resection of surrounding lymph nodes and any adherent organ or organs if required. In a study by Papachristou and associates, it was found that patients with a 2-cm gross margin had a 30% positive microscopic margin, those with a 4- to 6-cm gross margin had a 10% positive microscopic margin, and no patients with a 6-cm or larger gross margin had a positive microscopic margin.[49] Typically, a gross margin of 5 to 6 cm for intestinal and

---

Box 61–3 **AJCC Staging of Gastric Cancer**

Tumor

T1 Tumor invades the lamina propria or submucosa

T2 Tumor invades the muscularis propria (a) or submucosa (b)

T3 Tumor invades through the serosa without invading adjacent structures

T4 Tumor directly invades adjacent structures

Lymph Nodes

N0 0 lymph nodes
N1 1 to 6 positive lymph nodes
N2 7 to 15 positive lymph nodes
N3 >15 positive lymph nodes

Distant Metastases

M0 No distant metastases
M1 Distant metastases

TNM Grouping

Stage IA	T1, N0, M0
Stage IB	T1, N1, M0
	T2a, N0, M0
	T2b, N0, M0
Stage II	T1, N2, M0
	T2a, N1, M0
	T2b, N1, M0
	T3, N0, M0
Stage IIIA	T2a, N2, M0
	T2b, N2, M0
	T3, N1, M0
	T4, N0, M0
Stage IIIB	T3, N2, M0
Stage IV	Any T4 + any N1
	Any N3 or M1

Adapted from American Joint Commission for Cancer Staging Manual, 6th ed. New York, Springer, 2002, pp 114-115.

---

up to 8 to 10 cm for diffuse-type cancers is recommended, if possible, to ensure adequate negative margins by final histologic analysis.[50,51] Both positive microscopic (R1) and gross (R2) margins are associated with an increased recurrence rate and subsequent decrease in overall survival.[4]

Proximal Tumors

Proximal tumors and tumors of the GE junction represent 35% to 50% of all gastric cancers and require different considerations for resection and reconstruction. In general, these tumors are more advanced at initial evaluation, and therefore curative resection is often more difficult. The three types of GE junction tumors according to the Siewert classification include type I, or cancer associated with Barrett's esophagus or true esophageal carcinoma growing down to the GE junction; type II, or tumor at the true junction (within 2 cm of the squamocolumnar junction); and type III, or tumors of the subcardial region.[14,52] Patients with type I tumors are best considered for either a gastric pull-up to the neck or an Ivor-Lewis esophagogastrectomy.[4,14,52] Type II or III tumors can be resected by either total gastrectomy or proximal subtotal gastrectomy.[4,14,52] Total gastrectomy has been the traditional procedure of choice and may offer an advantage in that patients are unlikely to have reflux esophagitis after total gastrectomy and Roux-en-Y reconstruction.[53-55] In addition, the lymph nodes along the lesser curve, which is a common site of disease spread, may be more difficult to completely remove by proximal subtotal resection than by total gastrectomy.

An advantage of proximal subtotal gastrectomy is the presence of a gastric reservoir, and it has been reported to have similar mortality rates, hospital stay, and recurrence and survival rates as total gastrectomy in a retrospective study of nearly 100 patients with proximal gastric cancers from Memorial Sloan Kettering Cancer Center.[56] Nevertheless, other series have reported an increase in postoperative morbidity and mortality, as well as a poorer functional outcome and quality of life, in patients undergoing proximal versus total gastrectomy.[53-55] Although it is difficult to make definitive conclusions in the absence of a prospective randomized trial, it does appear that total gastrectomy is associated with a better functional outcome and fewer complications.

Midbody Tumors

Midstomach tumors account for 15% to 30% of all gastric cancers. Unless the tumor is very small, it is very difficult to achieve negative margins and leave enough residual stomach for adequate function. Total gastrectomy is therefore usually required.

Distal Tumors

For tumors of the distal part of the stomach, which represent about 35% of gastric cancers, there remains some controversy regarding the preferred approach, particularly for diffuse-type cancers, but in general, subtotal gastrectomy is performed when possible. A few prospective randomized studies have compared total versus subtotal gastrectomy for distal gastric cancers. A study from France involving 169 patients with antral cancer revealed a higher mortality rate (3.2% versus 1.3%) in patients undergoing total gastrectomy, but similar overall complication rates (34% versus 32%). There was no difference in overall 5-year survival between the two groups.[57] A prospective randomized trial by the Italian Gastrointestinal Tumor Study Group reported similar results. In a study of more than 600 patients with middle and distal cancers randomized to subtotal or total gastrectomy, 5-year survival rates were 65% and 62%, respectively. Patients who underwent subtotal gastrectomy had fewer complications, better nutritional status and overall

quality of life, and a shorter hospital stay.[58] Finally, a trial from Hong Kong in which subtotal gastrectomy with D1 lymphadenectomy (see later) was compared with total gastrectomy and D3 resection found no difference in overall survival.[59]

Numerous other studies have also reported higher mortality and morbidity rates for total gastrectomy, along with poorer functional results and quality of life.[60-62] Therefore, for distal and some midbody cancers, distal subtotal gastrectomy with at least a 5- to 6-cm gross margin and adequate remnant stomach should be performed whenever feasible.

Endoscopic Mucosal Resection

If diagnosed at an early stage, it may be possible to obtain a margin-negative resection (R0) without gastrectomy. Analogous to endoscopic polypectomy for colon adenomas, endoscopic mucosal resection (EMR) has been used, particularly in Japan, where nearly 50% of patients have early gastric cancer as a result of extensive screening programs.[3,4,14] Because nodal resection is not performed, this technique is appropriate for cancers with a low likelihood of nodal involvement, including well-differentiated tumors confined entirely to the mucosa, ultrasound T1 and Borrmann's type I (polypoid or fungating cancers), and type IIa and IIb (ulcerated lesions surrounded by elevated borders, but not infiltrating the gastric wall).[63,64] If EMR is performed, the specimen must be carefully examined with serial sectioning to evaluate for invasion of the submucosa. If the submucosa is involved, the chance of nodal involvement is higher and therefore gastric resection should be performed. Though used in Japan, experience in the United States is limited, but in experienced hands, EMR is certainly a suitable alternative for the small subset of patients with very early gastric cancer.

Extent of Lymphadenectomy

The extent of lymph node dissection in surgical resection of gastric cancer remains a very controversial issue despite the existence of several randomized clinical trials. The Japanese Research Society for Gastric Cancer, as well as other Asian counterparts, has advocated radical lymph node dissection, the so-called D2 lymphadenectomy, for the treatment of gastric cancer. Retrospective studies involving thousands of patients from Japan suggest that extended lymphadenectomy can improve survival, particularly in patients with stage II or III disease, with overall reported 5-year survival rates of greater than 60% as compared with 20% in most Western series.[65-68] The prevailing feeling among some Western surgeons, however, is that the presence of lymph node metastases represents a marker for systemic metastases and that radical lymphadenectomy will rarely improve the overall outcome but may instead be associated with a significant increase in morbidity and mortality. Lymphadenectomy is therefore viewed as a staging procedure rather than as part of a curative resection.

The incidence of lymph node involvement varies with the stage of the primary tumor. For tumors limited to the mucosa, the chance of lymph node involvement is less than 5%; for those involving the submucosa, it is up to 25%; and for stage III and IV, lymph nodes are involved in nearly 90%.[5,65-68] The extent of lymph node dissection is designated by "D." D1 dissection includes only the perigastric lymph nodes, usually within 3 cm of the stomach. D2 dissection also includes nodes along the hepatic, left gastric, celiac, and splenic arteries, as well as those in the splenic hilum, in addition to perigastric nodes farther than 3 cm from the primary tumor, along with omentectomy. D3 lymphadenectomy also includes nodes along the porta hepatis and hepatoduodenal ligament, retropancreatic nodes, and nodes along the base of the mesentery and periaortic regions (Fig. 61–1). For an absolute curative resection, it is often recommended that the level of lymph node resection be one level greater than the highest level of involved lymph nodes.[4,14] For grossly uninvolved nodes, Japanese surgeons typically advocate a standard D2 resection for most gastric cancers and have reported mortality rates of less than 2%, as well as improved stage-for-stage overall survival when retrospectively compared with lesser resections.[65-68]

Four prospective randomized trials have been conducted in an attempt to clarify the extent of lymphadenectomy most appropriate for gastric cancer (Table 61–1). In a small study from South Africa, only 43 of 400 evaluated patients were eligible for randomization. There was no benefit in overall survival, whereas operative time, blood loss, and hospital stay were all increased in the D2 group.[69] In a large trial started in 1989 by the Medical Research Council (MRC) in the United Kingdom, 400 patients (out of 737 who registered) were randomized to D1 versus D2 resection at the time of laparotomy. Perioperative mortality (13% versus 6.5%, $P < .04$) and morbidity (46% versus 28%, $P < .001$) were both significantly higher in the D2 group, whereas overall 5-year survival rates were similar (33% versus 35%).[70] Much of the increase in mortality and morbidity in this trial was associated with the routine use of distal pancreatectomy and splenectomy in the D2 group, and it is unclear how a D2 resection without distal pancreatectomy/splenectomy would compare with a D1 resection. Furthermore, the average number of nodes resected was 13 in the D1 group and 17 in the D2 group,

although the Japanese advocate the removal of at least 26 nodes for an adequate D2 resection.

Similarly, in the Dutch Gastric Cancer Group Study, approximately 1000 patients were randomized to D1 versus D2 resection.[71] In an attempt to monitor the quality of surgery, Professor Sasako from the National Cancer Center in Tokyo trained a group of Dutch surgeons, who subsequently supervised the resection techniques at the 80 participating centers. An R0 resection was achieved in 711 patients (380 in D1; 331 in D2), who

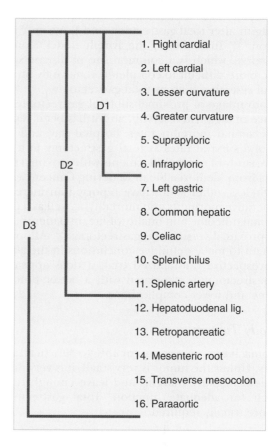

1. Right cardial
2. Left cardial
3. Lesser curvature
4. Greater curvature
5. Suprapyloric
6. Infrapyloric
7. Left gastric
8. Common hepatic
9. Celiac
10. Splenic hilus
11. Splenic artery
12. Hepatoduodenal lig.
13. Retropancreatic
14. Mesenteric root
15. Transverse mesocolon
16. Paraaortic

Figure 61–1. Lymph nodes removed in D1 versus D2 versus D3 lymphadenectomy during resection of gastric cancer.

| Table 61–1 | Prospective Randomized Trials of D1 Versus D2 Gastric Resection |

	D1				D2			
Study	*N*	**Morbidity**	**Mortality**	**5-yr Survival**	*N*	**Morbidity**	**Mortality**	**5-yr Survival**
Dent, 1988[69]	22	22%	0%	69%	21	43%	0%	67%
Robertson, 1994[59]	25	0%	0%	1511 days	30	59%*	3%	922 days
Cuschieri, 1999 (MRC)[70]	200	28%	6.5%	35%	200	46%*	13%*	33%
Bonenkamp, 1999 (Dutch)[71]	380	25%	4%	42%	331	43%*	10%*	47%

*$P < .05$ versus the D1 group.
MRC, Medical Research Council.

were therefore eligible for analysis in this trial. Similar to the British trial, perioperative morbidity and mortality were significantly higher in the D2 group (43% and 10% versus 25% and 4%, respectively, P = .004 for mortality, P < .001 for morbidity).[71,72] Moreover, there was no difference in overall 5-year survival (47% for D2, 42% for D1).[71] Several subsequent analyses and comments have been published regarding this trial. Perhaps most significant, despite having supervision, noncompliance (failure to remove the required number of lymph nodes) occurred in 51% of patients in the D2 group and 36% of patients in the D1 group. Similarly, contamination (removing additional unnecessary lymph nodes) occurred in 6% of the D1 group and 7% of the D2 group.[14,73] Because over half the patients in the D2 resection group did not undergo an adequate D2 resection, it is very difficult to make definite conclusions from this trial. Nevertheless, subsequent subset analysis of this trial revealed that patients with stage II and IIIA did appear to have a significant survival advantage. In addition, there was a significant decrease in local recurrence (41% versus 29%, P = 0.02) in the D2 group.[71]

In a report from Hong Kong, 55 patients were randomized to a D1 resection with subtotal gastrectomy or a D3 resection with total gastrectomy, distal pancreatectomy, and splenectomy. Operative time and hospital stay were longer in the D3 group, whereas median survival was significantly less. There was one death, which occurred in the D3 group.[59] The Japanese Cooperative Oncology Group, however, recently reported preliminary results of the JCOG 9501 trial in which D2 versus D3 resection was compared. More than 500 patients were randomized, and there was no difference in major complications between the groups. Overall mortality was less than 1% (two patients in each group).[74] Although recurrence and survival data are forthcoming, this study suggested that radical gastric resection, including extended lymphadenectomy, can be performed safely in experienced hands.

Several nonrandomized prospective trials in the United States and Europe from specialized centers have suggested an increase in survival with a D2 resection that approximates the results in Japan, particularly for stage II and III disease.[75-79] When the pancreas and spleen are preserved, the overall morbidity and mortality approach that of a more limited dissection.[75-79] One of the main problems with many of these studies is the continued noncompliance with D2 resection guidelines. Analysis of the INT-0116 adjuvant chemotherapy trial[80] (see later) in which a D2 resection was recommended but not required showed that only 10% of the patients actually underwent a true D2 resection, 36% underwent a D1 resection, and 54% underwent a D0 resection, as defined by Japanese staging criteria.[80] Although this may be the fault of surgical technique, the quality of pathologic evaluation of the specimen and lymph nodes is another potential concern.

In summary, although randomized prospective data on the extent of lymphadenectomy exist, controversy persists. Based on the available data, gastrectomy with a D2 resection, but without routine splenectomy/pancreatectomy, should be performed whenever possi-

ble, particularly for patients with stage II or III disease. Furthermore, in view of the morbidity and mortality data, these resections should also be performed at specialized centers whenever possible.

Reconstruction After Gastrectomy

After distal subtotal gastrectomy, several options exist for reconstruction, including Billroth I gastroduodenostomy, Billroth II gastrojejunostomy (either antecolic or retrocolic), and Roux-en-Y gastrojejunostomy (also either antecolic or retrocolic). All three methods have their advantages and disadvantages, and there is support in the literature for all of them.[54,81-89] A Billroth I reconstruction is often difficult to perform without creating undue tension on the anastomosis. A Billroth II reconstruction, with or without a Braun enteroenterostomy, is another option, particularly when a large remnant of stomach remains. In general, however, Roux-en-Y gastrojejunostomy is simpler and useful with a small stomach remnant and probably better in controlling dumping and bile reflux gastritis. In the absence of definite prospective randomized data, surgeon preference often dictates the reconstruction.

After total gastrectomy, options for reconstruction include a standard Roux-en-Y esophagojejunostomy, construction of a pouch, and jejunal interposition. Again, although there is no clear consensus on the preferred method of reconstruction,[54,81-89] Roux-en-Y esophagojejunostomy has the advantage of being simpler to construct and is usually associated with the least morbidity while providing generally equivalent functional outcome. The anastomosis is typically performed in an end of esophagus–to–side of jejunum manner. It can be done in a stapled fashion (usually circular, although linear has also been described) or hand sewn in one or two layers. Although leak rates are generally equivalent, there may be a higher rate of strictures and more difficulty in dilating strictures with a circular stapled technique.[4,14]

When constructing an esophagojejunostomy, one may use a jejunal pouch to provide for a neostomach reservoir. The pouch is constructed similar to an ileal J-pouch, with a linear stapler used to fashion the pouch. In addition, many surgeons prefer to leave a lip of undivided intestine at the end of the linear staple line to optimize blood supply to the esophageal anastomosis. The esophagojejunostomy is performed at the antimesenteric bend of the pouch with either the staple or hand-sewn technique. When constructing the pouch it is important that it not be longer than 15 cm to prevent stasis and ineffective clearing.[4,14]

Prognostic Factors and Patterns of Failure

The ability to achieve resection with a negative margin (R0) is the most important prognostic factor and determinant of survival, as has been shown in multiple studies throughout the world.[10,12,79,90,91] The pathologic stage also has valuable prognostic implications inasmuch as a higher T stage or N stage is associated with a higher chance of relapse and poorer overall survival.[12,79,92] As discussed earlier, location of the tumor is also related to prognosis, with proximal gastric cancers more likely to recur than distal cancers.

In patients who undergo curative resection, between 25% and 80% of cancers will recur locoregionally.[65,92,93] This large disagreement in the literature suggests that there are many factors governing recurrence, such as the adequacy of surgical and lymph node resection and tumor characteristics, including location, stage, and aggressiveness.

Adjuvant Therapy

Survival rates after resection for localized, node-negative gastric cancer approach 75% to 80% with surgery alone.[10,92,94] Unfortunately, however, most patients in the United States have node-positive disease, and survival rates drop to 10% to 30% with high local and distant recurrence rates.[10,92,94] This has generated great interest in developing effective adjuvant strategies to help decrease recurrence rates and provide long-term survival. Though initially somewhat disappointing and conflicting, recent studies using combined-modality therapy have shown significant improvement in survival rates in patients with gastric cancer. A continued problem with many studies is the inconsistent population groups and stages of gastric cancer, as well as the different surgical techniques, particularly the extent of lymph node dissection, as discussed earlier.

Adjuvant Chemotherapy

Numerous systemic chemotherapy trials have been published over the past few decades, with overall disappointing results and conclusions. Most of these trials were underpowered or poorly designed and have resulted in nonreproducible findings. Large meta-analyses of adjuvant chemotherapy trials have suggested only minimal benefit and in particular just in subgroups of node-positive or Asian patients.[95,96] Most single agents have response rates in the 15% to 20% range, and although some small trials have shown a survival benefit, it has not been reproducible.[14,92] Combination chemotherapy with agents such as 5-fluorouracil (5-FU), epirubicin, mitomycin, and methyl-CCNU have been associated with somewhat better response rates; however, in larger prospective trials, a clear benefit of combination chemotherapy has not been reproduced.[14,92] Several meta-analyses of the randomized clinical trials of adjuvant chemotherapy have also been published, and even though some have suggested a small survival benefit,[95,97,98] several others, as well as the majority of individual studies, failed to show a significant survival advantage.[2,14,92] In light of these nonconclusive results, routine adjuvant chemotherapy should be used only as part of a clinical trial.

Adjuvant Chemoradiotherapy

The combination of chemotherapy and radiotherapy has been extensively studied in the treatment of many GI cancers, including gastric cancer. Although early trials primarily using 5-FU and radiotherapy showed a small benefit,[99-101] it was very difficult to draw definitive conclusions because of their small patient numbers, lack of standardization of surgical technique, and heterogeneous populations. The largest gastric cancer adjuvant trial ever conducted in North America was recently published and updated. The Gastrointestinal Cancer Intergroup Trial (INT-0116)[80] randomized 556 eligible patients with stage IB to IV (M0) gastric cancer, who underwent margin-negative (R0) resection, to surgery alone or to surgery followed by bolus 5-FU/leucovorin (LV), followed by 45 Gy radiotherapy, followed by additional 5-FU/LV. Overall, 85% of patients were node positive and two thirds had T3 or T4 lesions. With more than 6 years of median follow-up, median disease-free survival was significantly improved in the adjuvant chemoradiotherapy group (30 versus 19 months, $P < .001$).[102] Overall median survival was also significantly improved in the adjuvant chemoradiotherapy group (35 versus 28 months, $P = .01$).[102] Given these results, postoperative chemoradiotherapy with this regimen has essentially become the standard of care for patients who have undergone curative resection for gastric cancer in the United States. Nevertheless, critics of the Intergroup trial point out that although a D2 resection was recommended, only 10% of patients underwent a D2 resection whereas 36% underwent a D1 resection and an alarming 54% underwent a *D0* resection.[80,92] Therefore, some believe that adjuvant therapy may have made up only for poor and inadequate surgical resection. For example, a randomized trial from Japan of 252 patients who underwent D2 or greater resection versus resection plus adjuvant mitomycin, 5-FU, and cytarabine failed to show any significant survival advantage for chemotherapy.[103] In this study it was noted that 98% of the patients underwent D2 or greater resection.[103]

In addition, the chemotherapy used in the Intergroup trial was bolus 5-FU, which was standard in the late 1980s when the trial was designed. Bolus 5-FU as a single agent has low response rates in gastric cancer, however, and newer agents and combinations, including the epirubicin, cisplatin, and 5-FU (ECF) regimen as discussed later,[104] have shown higher response rates and will need to be further studied in the adjuvant setting.

Adjuvant Intraperitoneal Therapy

Because a significant proportion of postoperative recurrences in patients who undergo resection for gastric cancer occur in the peritoneal cavity, intraperitoneal (IP) therapy has been an attractive option. An initial randomized trial from Japan comparing IP mitomycin C with no postoperative therapy showed a significant survival advantage of IP treatment.[14] Subsequent studies, both retrospective and randomized, failed to show a survival benefit of IP mitomycin C, however, and actually suggested a significant increase in postoperative complications and mortality.[105] A study from Korea randomized 248 patients to IP mitomycin and 5-FU versus observation. Morbidity and mortality were higher in the IP group, and although overall survival was not different, subset analysis did show a benefit for stage II and III disease.[106] Another randomized trial used IP cisplatin in both the adjuvant setting and patients with peritoneal carcinomatosis but failed to show a survival advantage.[3,14]

Similarly, continuous hyperthermic peritoneal perfusion (CHPP) has been used in patients with gastric cancer in both the adjuvant and palliative setting. This method relies on the synergistic effect of cytotoxic chemotherapy and hyperthermia. Several studies have reported on CHPP with mitomycin C after resection of gastric cancer. Although many of these trials are small, some of them have shown a survival advantage of CHPP versus surgery alone.[3,14]

Nearly all of these studies have compared IP or CHPP therapy with surgery alone rather than standard adjuvant therapy as discussed earlier. Future studies and newer agents will need to be compared against these systemic regimens before definitive conclusions can be made.

Neoadjuvant Therapy

Neoadjuvant or preoperative therapy has several theoretical advantages and has increasingly been used for the treatment of a variety of GI cancers. These advantages include improved patient tolerance, more effective delivery (increased oxygenation in the tumor bed), removal of treated tissue, early initiation of systemic therapy (in the case of preoperative chemotherapy), potential downsizing of the primary tumor, ability to achieve better margins at resection, and evaluation of response to therapy, thereby adding to prognostic information and assisting in the planning of future therapy.

Neoadjuvant Radiotherapy

Though seldom used without systemic chemotherapy, preoperative radiotherapy has shown promise in a few reports. A large randomized trial from China reported on 360 patients who underwent preoperative radiotherapy versus surgical resection alone. The radiotherapy group had a higher overall resection rate (89% versus 79%, $P < .01$) and 10-year survival rate (20% versus 13%, $P = .009$).[107] Tumor down-sizing and nodal down-staging were also noted, and there was no increase in operative mortality with the use of preoperative radiotherapy.[107] A smaller trial randomized 78 patients to preoperative radiotherapy, surgery and intraoperative radiotherapy, or surgery alone.[108] Patients with node-positive disease and T4 lesions had a significant survival advantage with the radiotherapy regimen, and again there was no increase in perioperative mortality or morbidity.[108]

Neoadjuvant Chemotherapy

Several phase II studies investigating systemic chemotherapy in the neoadjuvant setting have been reported and in general have suggested that preoperative chemotherapy can be given with acceptable toxicity and no increase in operative complications or mortality.[3,14,92] Furthermore, overall survival in these trials was generally improved when compared with historical controls. In addition, it has been suggested in several trials that the response to chemotherapy was a significant predictor of survival.[3,14,92]

The preliminary results of a small randomized trial of 107 patients randomized to receive neoadjuvant etoposide, cisplatin, and 5-FU or surgery alone were reported in 1996.[109] No significant differences in resectability rate or overall survival were noted.[109] More recently, preliminary results of the MAGIC trial from the United Kingdom were reported.[104] In this randomized controlled trial, 503 patients with adenocarcinoma of the stomach or lower esophagus were randomized to preoperative ECF, followed by surgery and postoperative ECF, versus surgery alone. No recommendation was given regarding the extent of lymphadenectomy because the results of the MRC and Dutch trials were unavailable at the start of this trial. The primary outcome was overall survival, and secondary outcomes were progression-free survival, surgical resectability, and quality of life. Patients in both groups were well matched in age, gender, performance status, site, and pretreatment size of tumor. Operative complications, mortality, and length of hospital stay were similar in both groups. A higher proportion of patients in the chemotherapy group underwent curative resection (79% versus 69%, $P = .018$) and were noted to have significantly smaller tumors at surgery, as well as significantly lower T and N stages.[104] Progression-free survival at 2 years was significantly improved in the ECF group (45% versus 30%, $P = .002$), but the improvement in overall survival did not quite reach statistical significance (48% versus 40%, $P = .063$; hazard ratio, 0.80; 95% confidence interval, 0.63 to 1.01).[104] Although these results are preliminary and a longer follow-up period is needed, they strongly suggest a benefit of perioperative chemotherapy with the ECF regimen in patients with operable gastric cancer.

Neoadjuvant Chemoradiotherapy

On the basis of the results of neoadjuvant chemoradiotherapy in the treatment of other cancers, including esophageal and rectal carcinoma, multimodality regimens involving preoperative chemotherapy and radiotherapy are currently under study. In a pilot phase II study at the M.D. Anderson Cancer Center, 24 patients were treated with 45 Gy of external beam radiotherapy with concurrent infusions of 5-FU.[110] Surgery was carried out 4 to 6 weeks later in 19 (79%) of the patients and consisted of D2 lymphadenectomy and intraoperative radiotherapy (10 Gy). Two (11%) patients had a complete pathologic response and 12 (63%) were noted to have a major treatment effect.[110] Another trial from M.D. Anderson involved 34 patients who were treated with 5-FU, folinic acid, and cisplatin, followed by 5-FU–potentiated radiotherapy (45 Gy).[111] Surgical resection after this preoperative regimen was safe, with a complete pathologic response in 30% and a partial pathologic response in 24%.[111] A phase II trial by the Radiation Therapy Oncology Group (RTOG 9904) investigated induction chemotherapy with cisplatin, 5-FU, and folinic acid, followed by radiotherapy with concomitant 5-FU in the preoperative setting and then surgical resection.[92] The trial is now closed, but the results are pending at this time. Because many of these trials are small and non-randomized in nature, however, it is difficult to make definitive recommendations until larger prospective randomized trials are performed, and thus patients with resectable disease should receive preoperative chemoradiation only as part of a clinical trial. Nevertheless, in view of these promising preliminary results, patients with locally advanced gastric cancer should also be considered for preoperative chemoradiotherapy in an attempt to down-size the tumor—although this remains unproved.

Management of Advanced Disease

More than 50% of patients with gastric cancer have unresectable or metastatic disease at initial evaluation, and therefore appropriate use of palliative techniques is important. Surgical palliation may include resection alone or in combination with endoscopic, percutaneous, or radiotherapeutic interventions. Other options for palliation include chemotherapy and radiotherapy. In the absence of prospective trials, the optimal choice for palliation is largely patient dependent.

Surgery for Palliation

Because survival in patients with advanced gastric cancer is so short, any attempt at palliative resection should not only provide symptomatic relief but also be associated with minimal morbidity and mortality. Although no randomized trials have been performed, several retrospective studies have been published. A study by Ekbom and Gleysteen compared palliative resection with intestinal bypass in 75 patients with advanced gastric cancer.[112] Operative mortality was similar, and 80% of patients had relief of their symptoms for a mean of 6 months in the bypass group, whereas 88% of patients experienced relief of symptoms for a mean of 14.6 months in the resection group.[112] Although patients with palliative resection appeared to have a longer duration of relief, this was not a randomized trial and selection bias may have accounted for the differences. In a similar report of 51 patients with advanced gastric cancer, palliative resection resulted in a higher percentage of patients having relief of symptoms and for a longer duration than with palliative bypass.[113] In a large review of nearly 250 patients from Italy who underwent exploratory laparotomy alone, GI bypass, or palliative resection, resection was associated with longer survival in patients with both local (8 versus 4.4 months) and distant (8 versus 3 months) spread of disease.[114]

Although these data are retrospective, they do suggest that for select patients with symptomatic advanced gastric cancer, palliative resection may offer relief of symptoms for a majority of patients with acceptable morbidity and mortality. The treatment options may also largely depend on the extent of resection required for adequate palliation; for example, total gastrectomy with possible resection of adjacent organs is not usually indicated for palliation of unresectable disease.

Endoscopic Palliation

In patients who are not good candidates for palliative resection but have symptoms of obstruction, endoscopic palliative techniques may be useful, including placement of metal expandable stents and laser recanalization. Although very limited prospective randomized data comparing endoscopic techniques and surgical bypass or resection are available, several studies suggest that both techniques are safe and can lead to some relief in many patients.[115,116] Endoscopic stenting may result in similar short-term relief of obstruction as surgical bypass and is certainly a less invasive option.[115] Long-term data, however, are unavailable. Laser therapy can also be used as a complement to stenting and has been shown to provide short-term relief of obstruction in some patients.[116,117] Although none of these techniques would be expected to improve survival, they are good alternatives in patients who are not candidates for palliative surgery but are suffering from signs of obstruction. After relief of obstruction, many of these patients can later receive palliative chemotherapy. Generally speaking, patients with peritoneal disease, hepatic or nodal metastases, or other poor prognostic factors will probably benefit most from endoscopic palliation, including laser recanalization, dilatation, and stent placement. For patients with a better prognosis and excellent performance status, consideration can be given to surgical resection if it can be accomplished with minimal morbidity.

Palliative Chemotherapy

Similar to the results of adjuvant therapy for resected gastric cancer, systemic chemotherapy for advanced gastric cancer has been demonstrated to be beneficial. Several randomized trials, albeit small, have shown that patients receiving systemic chemotherapy have a longer median survival (9 to 11 months versus 3 to 5 months) and better 1- and 2-year survival rates (35% to 40% versus 10% and 6% to 10% versus 0%, respectively) than with best supportive care alone.[3,14] More recently, combination chemotherapy with agents such as cisplatin, paclitaxel, and irinotecan have shown similar response rates and median survival times in several phase II studies.[118-121] Certainly, multiagent chemotherapy should be offered to all patients with advanced disease who have reasonable performance status.

Palliative Radiotherapy

Experience with radiotherapy in patients with advanced gastric cancer is much more limited. Although its use seems to be fairly effective in controlling symptoms such as bleeding and pain, most patients have diffuse metastatic disease, and the use of radiotherapy alone would not be expected to provide much increase in overall survival.[3,14] Nevertheless, in patients with advanced local disease precluding resection but with no distant metastases, radiotherapy in combination with chemotherapy could be considered, preferably as part of a clinical trial.

Summary

Although gastric cancer is decreasing overall worldwide, patterns have shifted toward more aggressive variants of the disease, including cancers of the proximal part of the stomach and GE junction. Aggressive surgical resection, including adjacent organs and extended lymphadenectomy, can lead to prolonged survival and is safe in experienced hands. Most patients in the United States, however, have advanced disease at initial evaluation. The use of adjuvant and neoadjuvant chemotherapy and chemoradiotherapy regimens has resulted in significant prolongation of survival in resected patients and has essentially become the standard of care in the United States, although continued prospective trials are needed in light of newer promising agents. For patients with advanced disease, control of symptoms is paramount, and options include surgical and endoscopic therapy, as well as a host of palliative chemotherapy and chemoradiotherapy regimens, again often as part of a clinical trial.

ADENOCARCINOMA OF THE DUODENUM AND SMALL INTESTINE

Small intestinal tumors are rare, and although the small bowel accounts for 80% of intestinal length, they make up only about 10% of GI tumors.[122,123] It is estimated that approximately 5000 cases of small bowel carcinoma are diagnosed per year in the United States.[124] Approximately two thirds of small bowel tumors are malignant (less than 5% of all GI malignancies), and nearly half of these are adenocarcinomas, the rest being carcinoid and GI stromal tumors and lymphomas.[123,125,126] Of the adenocarcinomas, approximately 40% occur in the duodenum, including the periampullary region, and the rest are distributed throughout the rest of the small intestine.[123,127-129] There is a slight male preponderance, and even though the incidence is low, there is a steady increase after the age of 30 years.[129]

Pathogenesis and Risk Factors

In general, small bowel malignancies are about 40 to 60 times less common than malignancies of the large intestine despite the increased length and absorptive capacity.[123,124] Several theories and hypotheses have been proposed to explain why such may be the case. The bacterial flora and count in the small bowel are significantly less active than in the colon,[130] transit time is faster, and the volume of enteric contents is much greater.[123] In addition, the small bowel contains many digestive enzymes, particularly in the proximal portion, which may help degrade potential carcinogens.[131,132] The presence of lymphatic tissue, especially Peyer's patches in the distal ileum, may also help provide immune surveillance against potential tumorigenesis.[123,125]

Because of overall duodenal length, adenocarcinoma of the duodenum, particularly the periampullary region, is much more common than that of the remaining small intestine. This may be due to increased susceptibility of the duodenal or ampullary mucosa to malignant transformation or be secondary to increased exposure to biliary and pancreatic secretions or ingested carcinogens and toxins, similar to pancreatic cancer.[125,133,134]

A few studies have reported some potential risk factors for the development of small bowel adenocarcinoma. One study reported on 430 patients with small bowel cancer and more than 900 patients who had died of other causes and found that increased consumption of red meat and salt-cured smoked foods was associated with an increased incidence, similar to other GI cancers.[135] Interestingly, however, smoking and alcohol use were not. Similarly, increased consumption of fat has also been reported as a risk factor, similar to colon cancer.[136] Small bowel cancers are also more likely (seven to nine times more likely) in patients with a history of colon cancer, and the converse is also true—patients with a history of small bowel carcinoma are at a higher risk for colon cancer.[137]

Small bowel adenocarcinomas are also thought to follow the adenoma-carcinoma sequence as in other GI organs. Studies have shown that adenomatous epithelium exists in many specimens of small bowel cancer. In addition, patients with Crohn's disease, celiac sprue, familial adenomatous polyposis, and cystic fibrosis are also at increased risk for the development of small bowel adenocarcinoma.[126,137,138]

Duodenal Adenocarcinoma

Approximately 50% of all small bowel adenocarcinomas occur in the duodenum, with 15% in the proximal, 40% in the middle, and 45% in the distal duodenum.[125,139,140] The most common initial symptoms include abdominal pain, nausea, and vomiting related to duodenal obstruction[125,140]; anemia from bleeding tumors; and biliary obstruction with ampullary lesions.[125,139,141] The diagnosis is usually made by upper endoscopy with biopsy or an upper GI study.[123,125]

Treatment of duodenal carcinoma is surgical resection, the details of which depend on the site of the tumor. In general, however, resectability rates for duodenal carcinoma are significantly higher than those for other upper GI cancers such as pancreatic, biliary, gastric, and esophageal cancer.[125,126] The overall 5-year survival rate is generally in the 25% to 60% range, also much better than that of other upper GI cancers.[125,126] For patients with cancer of the first or second portion of the duodenum, pancreaticoduodenectomy or a Whipple procedure is usually necessary to completely resect the cancer. For patients with tumors in the third or fourth portions of the duodenum, segmental duodenal resection with primary anastomosis is often possible, provided that negative proximal margins can be obtained. In either case, regional lymphadenectomy is recommended because up to 70% of patients may have nodal involvement and many of these patients survive 5 years.[125,139-141]

Adjuvant therapy after resection for duodenal cancer has not been well studied, although many patients are treated with 5-FU–based therapy, which is the standard for most GI cancers. Nevertheless, there is no clear evidence that chemotherapy prolongs survival,[126] and investigational therapies and participation in clinical trials using novel agents are often recommended. For patients with unresectable disease, palliative chemotherapy does appear to provide some survival advantage over best supportive care, and radiation therapy may help decrease ongoing blood loss.[125,126] Many patients with advanced cancer of the duodenum will become obstructed and therefore require palliative GI bypass or endoscopically placed stents.

Jejunal and Ileal Carcinoma

Jejunal and ileal carcinomas usually cause symptoms of obstruction or occult GI bleeding.[126,142,143] Because these lesions are located beyond the reach of a standard upper endoscopy scope, CT scanning and a small bowel series are usually the modes of diagnosis, but neither examination is very specific.[123,126] Many are found on exploration for obstruction or other GI symptoms. A majority (70% to 100%) of distal small bowel cancers are resectable,[126,143,144] although regional lymph nodes are usually involved.[126,145] The resection strategy is similar to that for colon cancer, specifically, obtaining negative proximal and distal margins and resection of the involved mesentery and corresponding lymph nodes.

Survival after resection largely depends on the histologic grade and stage of the disease, particularly lymph node status. Patients with a margin-negative resection and no nodal involvement have 5-year survival rates as high as 50% to 70%, whereas patients with nodal involvement have 5-year survival rates in the 10% to 15% range.[142,144] Most patients unfortunately have advanced disease at initial evaluation, and survival rates are generally in the 20% to 30% range.[126,142] Experience with adjuvant therapy is even more limited for jejunal and ileal cancers than for duodenal cancers, although 5-FU–based regimens are generally used. Radiation therapy, however, is not usually feasible because of the mobile nature of the small bowel.

For patients with metastatic disease, surgical resection or bypass is often required to relieve symptoms of obstruction and to provide enteral feeding if possible.

Summary

Cancers of the small bowel are rare, though more common in the duodenum. Although the diagnosis of duodenal cancer is usually made by EGD, diagnosis of more distal small bowel cancer is often more difficult. Surgical resection with negative margins plus resection of adjacent lymph nodes remains the only curative option and may also provide relief from symptoms, including bleeding and obstruction. Experience with adjuvant chemotherapy and chemoradiotherapy is very limited, although they are usually administered to appropriate patients.

REFERENCES

1. American Cancer Society: Cancer Facts and Figures 2005. Atlanta, American Cancer Society, 2005.
2. Dicken BJ, Bigham DL, Cass C, et al: Gastric adenocarcinoma: Review and considerations for future directions. Ann Surg 241:27-39, 2005.
3. Karpeh MS, Kelsen DP, Tepper JE: Cancer of the stomach. In DeVita VT, Hellman S, Rosenberg SA (eds): Cancer: Principles and Practice of Oncology. Philadelphia, Lippincott, Williams & Wilkins, 2001, pp 1092-1125.
4. Parikh AA, Mansfield P: Gastric adenocarcinoma. In Cameron JL (ed): Current Surgical Therapy, 8th ed. St. Louis, Mosby-Yearbook, 2004:95-100.
5. Gore RM: Gastric cancer. Clinical and pathologic features. Radiol Clin North Am 35:295-310, 1997.
6. Blot WJ, Devesa SS, Kneller RW, Fraumeni JF Jr: Rising incidence of adenocarcinoma of the esophagus and gastric cardia. JAMA 265:1287-1289, 1991.
7. Meyers WC, Damiano RJ Jr, Rotolo FS, Postlethwait RW: Adenocarcinoma of the stomach. Changing patterns over the last 4 decades. Ann Surg 205:1-8, 1987.
8. Salvon-Harman JC, Cady B, Nikulasson S, et al: Shifting proportions of gastric adenocarcinomas. Arch Surg 129:381-388, discussion 388-389, 1994.
9. Surveillance, Epidemiology and End Results Program, 1975-2001. Do.CCa.P Sciencesn (ed): National Cancer Institute, 2004. http://seer.cancer.gov/csr/1975_2001/results_merged/topic_seermap.pdf#search='surveillance%20epidemiology%20end%20results%20program%20197520%20national%20cancer%20institute'. Accessed June 7, 2006.
10. Hundahl SA, Phillips JL, Menck HR: The National Cancer Data Base Report on poor survival of US gastric carcinoma patients treated with gastrectomy: Fifth Edition American Joint Committee on Cancer staging, proximal disease, and the "different disease" hypothesis. Cancer 88:921-932, 2000.
11. Werner M, Becker KF, Keller G, Hofler H: Gastric adenocarcinoma: Pathomorphology and molecular pathology. J Cancer Res Clin Oncol 127:207-216, 2001.
12. Kim JP, Lee JH, Kim SJ, et al: Clinicopathologic characteristics and prognostic factors in 10 783 patients with gastric cancer. Gastric Cancer 1:125-133, 1998.
13. Lauren P: The two histological main types of gastric carcinoma: Diffuse and so-called intestinal-type carcinoma. An attempt at a histo-clinical classification. Acta Pathol Microbiol Scand 64:31-49, 1965.
14. Mansfield PF, Yao JC, Crane CH: Gastric cancer. In Holland J, Frie E (eds): Cancer Medicine 6. Hamilton, Ontario, BC Decker, 2003.
15. Kaneko E, Nakamura T, Umeda N, et al: Outcome of gastric carcinoma detected by gastric mass survey in Japan. Gut 18:626-630, 1977.
16. Ramon JM, Serra L, Cerdo C, Oromi J: Dietary factors and gastric cancer risk. A case-control study in Spain. Cancer 71:1731-1735, 1993.
17. Huang XE, Tajima K, Hamajima N, et al: Effects of dietary, drinking, and smoking habits on the prognosis of gastric cancer. Nutr Cancer 38:30-36, 2000.
18. Devesa SS, Blot WJ, Fraumeni JF Jr: Changing patterns in the incidence of esophageal and gastric carcinoma in the United States. Cancer 83:2049-2053, 1998.
19. Parsonnet J, Friedman GD, Vandersteen DP, et al: *Helicobacter pylori* infection and the risk of gastric carcinoma. N Engl J Med 325:1127-1131, 1991.
20. Uemura N, Okamoto S, Yamamoto S, et al: *Helicobacter pylori* infection and the development of gastric cancer. N Engl J Med 345:784-789, 2001.
21. Stalnikowicz R, Benbassat J: Risk of gastric cancer after gastric surgery for benign disorders. Arch Intern Med 150:2022-2026, 1990.
22. Tersmette AC, Offerhaus GJ, Tersmette KW, et al: Meta-analysis of the risk of gastric stump cancer: Detection of high risk patient subsets for stomach cancer after remote partial gastrectomy for benign conditions. Cancer Res 50:6486-6489, 1990.
23. La Vecchia C, Negri E, Franceschi S, Gentile A: Family history and the risk of stomach and colorectal cancer. Cancer 70:50-55, 1992.

24. Huntsman DG, Carneiro F, Lewis RF, et al: Early gastric cancer in young, asymptomatic carriers of germ-line E-cadherin mutations. N Engl J Med 344:1904-1909, 2001.
25. Gastric cancer. In Clinical Practice Guidelines in Oncology. National Comprehensive Cancer Network, 2006. http://www.nccn.org/professionals/physician_gls/PDF/gastric.pdf. Accessed June 7, 2006.
26. Halvorsen RA Jr, Yee J, McCormick VD: Diagnosis and staging of gastric cancer. Semin Oncol 23:325-335, 1996.
27. Sadowski DC, Rabeneck L: Gastric ulcers at endoscopy: Brush, biopsy, or both? Am J Gastroenterol 92:608-613, 1997.
28. Kodera Y, Yamamura Y, Torii A, et al: The prognostic value of pre-operative serum levels of CEA and CA19-9 in patients with gastric cancer. Am J Gastroenterol 91:49-53, 1996.
29. Nakane Y, Okamura S, Akehira K, et al: Correlation of preoperative carcinoembryonic antigen levels and prognosis of gastric cancer patients. Cancer 73:2703-2708, 1994.
30. Pectasides D, Mylonakis A, Kostopoulou M, et al: CEA, CA 19-9, and CA-50 in monitoring gastric carcinoma. Am J Clin Oncol 20:348-353, 1997.
31. Marrelli D, Pinto E, De Stefano A, et al: Clinical utility of CEA, CA 19-9, and CA 72-4 in the follow-up of patients with resectable gastric cancer. Am J Surg 181:16-19, 2001.
32. Karpeh MS Jr, Brennan MF: Gastric carcinoma. Ann Surg Oncol 5:650-656, 1998.
33. Willis S, Truong S, Gribnitz S, et al: Endoscopic ultrasonography in the preoperative staging of gastric cancer: Accuracy and impact on surgical therapy. Surg Endosc 14:951-954, 2000.
34. Kuntz C, Herfarth C: Imaging diagnosis for staging of gastric cancer. Semin Surg Oncol 17:96-102, 1999.
35. Ziegler K, Sanft C, Zimmer T, et al: Comparison of computed tomography, endosonography, and intraoperative assessment in TN staging of gastric carcinoma. Gut 34:604-610, 1993.
36. Motohara T, Semelka RC: MRI in staging of gastric cancer. Abdom Imaging 27:376-383, 2002.
37. Kim AY, Han JK, Seong CK, et al: MRI in staging advanced gastric cancer: Is it useful compared with spiral CT? J Comput Assist Tomogr 24:389-394, 2000.
38. Sohn KM, Lee JM, Lee SY, et al: Comparing MR imaging and CT in the staging of gastric carcinoma. AJR Am J Roentgenol 174:1551-1557, 2000.
39. Chen J, Cheong JH, Yun MJ, et al: Improvement in preoperative staging of gastric adenocarcinoma with positron emission tomography. Cancer 103:2383-2390, 2005.
40. Kole AC, Plukker JT, Nieweg OE, Vaalburg W: Positron emission tomography for staging of oesophageal and gastroesophageal malignancy. Br J Cancer 78:521-527, 1998.
41. Burke EC, Karpeh MS, Conlon KC, Brennan MF: Laparoscopy in the management of gastric adenocarcinoma. Ann Surg 225:262-267, 1997.
42. Romijn MG, van Overhagen H, Spillenaar Bilgen EJ, et al: Laparoscopy and laparoscopic ultrasonography in staging of oesophageal and cardial carcinoma. Br J Surg 85:1010-1012, 1998.
43. Stell DA, Carter CR, Stewart I, Anderson JR: Prospective compar-ison of laparoscopy, ultrasonography and computed tomography in the staging of gastric cancer. Br J Surg 83:1260-1262, 1996.
44. Lowy AM, Mansfield PF, Leach SD, Ajani J: Laparoscopic staging for gastric cancer. Surgery 119:611-614, 1996.
45. D'Ugo DM, Pende V, Persiani R, et al: Laparoscopic staging of gastric cancer: An overview. J Am Coll Surg 196:965-974, 2003.
46. Bartlett DL, Conlon KC, Gerdes H, Karpeh MS Jr: Laparoscopic ultrasonography: The best pretreatment staging modality in gastric adenocarcinoma? Case report. Surgery 118:562-566, 1995.
47. Burke EC, Karpeh MS Jr, Conlon KC, Brennan MF: Peritoneal lavage cytology in gastric cancer: An independent predictor of outcome. Ann Surg Oncol 5:411-415, 1998.
48. Ribeiro U Jr, Gama-Rodrigues JJ, Safatle-Ribeiro AV, et al: Prog-nostic significance of intraperitoneal free cancer cells obtained by laparoscopic peritoneal lavage in patients with gastric cancer. J Gastrointest Surg 2:244-249, 1998.
49. Papachristou DN, Agnanti N, D'Agostino H, Fortner JG: Histo-logically positive esophageal margin in the surgical treatment of gastric cancer. Am J Surg 139:711-713, 1980.
50. Bozzetti F: Principles of surgical radicality in the treatment of gastric cancer. Surg Oncol Clin N Am 10:833-854, ix, 2001.
51. Bozzetti F, Bonfanti G, Bufalino R, et al: Adequacy of margins of resection in gastrectomy for cancer. Ann Surg 196:685-690, 1982.
52. Siewert JR, Feith M, Stein HJ: Biologic and clinical variations of adenocarcinoma at the esophago-gastric junction: Relevance of a topographic-anatomic subclassification. J Surg Oncol 90:139-146, discussion 146, 2005.
53. Braga M, Molinari M, Zuliani W, et al: Surgical treatment of gastric adenocarcinoma: Impact on survival and quality of life. A prospec-tive ten year study. Hepatogastroenterology 43:187-193, 1996.
54. Buhl K, Schlag P, Herfarth C: Quality of life and functional results following different types of resection for gastric carcinoma. Eur J Surg Oncol 16:404-409, 1990.
55. Diaz De Liano A, Oteiza Martinez F, Ciga MA, et al: Impact of sur-gical procedure for gastric cancer on quality of life. Br J Surg 90:91-94, 2003.
56. Harrison LE, Karpeh MS, Brennan MF: Total gastrectomy is not necessary for proximal gastric cancer. Surgery 123:127-130, 1998.
57. Gouzi JL, Huguier M, Fagniez PL, et al: Total versus subtotal gas-trectomy for adenocarcinoma of the gastric antrum. A French prospective controlled study. Ann Surg 209:162-166, 1989.
58. Bozzetti F, Marabini E, Bonfanti G, et al: Subtotal versus total gas-trectomy for gastric cancer: Five-year survival rates in a multicen-ter randomized Italian trial. Italian Gastrointestinal Tumor Study Group. Ann Surg 230:170-178, 1999.
59. Robertson CS, Chung SC, Woods SD, et al: A prospective ran-domized trial comparing R1 subtotal gastrectomy with R3 total gastrectomy for antral cancer. Ann Surg 220:176-182, 1994.
60. Butler JA, Dubrow TJ, Trezona T, et al: Total gastrectomy in the treatment of advanced gastric cancer. Am J Surg 158:602-604, dis-cussion 604-605, 1989.
61. Paolini A, Tosato F, Cassese M, et al: Total gastrectomy in the treat-ment of adenocarcinoma of the cardia. Review of the results in 73 resected patients. Am J Surg 151:238-243, 1986.
62. Santoro E, Garofalo A, Carlini M, et al: Early and late results of 100 consecutive total gastrectomies for cancer. Hepatogastroen-terology 41:489-496, 1994.
63. Takekoshi T, Baba Y, Ota H, et al: Endoscopic resection of early gastric carcinoma: Results of a retrospective analysis of 308 cases. Endoscopy 26:352-358, 1994.
64. Yamao T, Shirao K, Ono H, et al: Risk factors for lymph node metastasis from intramucosal gastric carcinoma. Cancer 77:602-606, 1996.
65. Maruyama K, Okabayashi K, Kinoshita T: Progress in gastric cancer surgery in Japan and its limits of radicality. World J Surg 11:418-425, 1987.
66. Nakamura K, Ueyama T, Yao T, et al: Pathology and prognosis of gastric carcinoma. Findings in 10,000 patients who underwent primary gastrectomy. Cancer 70:1030-1037, 1992.
67. Otsuji E, Fujiyama J, Takagi T, et al: Results of total gastrectomy with extended lymphadenectomy for gastric cancer in elderly patients. J Surg Oncol 91:232-236, 2005.
68. Shimada S, Yagi Y, Honmyo U, et al: Involvement of three or more lymph nodes predicts poor prognosis in submucosal gastric car-cinoma. Gastric Cancer 4:54-59, 2001.
69. Dent DM, Madden MV, Price SK: Randomized comparison of R1 and R2 gastrectomy for gastric carcinoma. Br J Surg 75:110-112, 1988.
70. Cuschieri A, Weeden S, Fielding J, et al: Patient survival after D1 and D2 resections for gastric cancer: Long-term results of the MRC randomized surgical trial. Surgical Co-operative Group. Br J Cancer 79:1522-1530, 1999.
71. Bonenkamp JJ, Hermans J, Sasako M, et al: Extended lymph-node dissection for gastric cancer. N Engl J Med 340:908-914, 1999.
72. Bonenkamp JJ, Songun I, Hermans J, et al: Randomised compar-ison of morbidity after D1 and D2 dissection for gastric cancer in 996 Dutch patients. Lancet 345:745-748, 1995.
73. Bonenkamp JJ, Hermans J, Sasako M, van De Veldt CJ: Quality control of lymph node dissection in the Dutch randomized trial of D1 and D2 lymph node dissection for gastric cancer. Gastric Cancer 1:152-159, 1998.
74. Sano T, Sasako M, Yamamoto S, et al: Gastric cancer surgery: Morbidity and mortality results from a prospective randomized controlled trial comparing D2 and extended para-aortic lym-phadenectomy—Japan Clinical Oncology Group Study 9501. J Clin Oncol 22:2767-2773, 2004.

75. Baba H, Maehara Y, Takeuchi H, et al: Effect of lymph node dissection on the prognosis in patients with node-negative early gastric cancer. Surgery 117:165-169, 1995.

76. Marubini E, Bozzetti F, Miceli R, et al: Lymphadenectomy in gastric cancer: Prognostic role and therapeutic implications. Eur J Surg Oncol 28:406-412, 2002.

77. Otsuji E, Toma A, Kobayashi S, et al: Long-term benefit of extended lymphadenectomy with gastrectomy in distally located early gastric carcinoma. Am J Surg 180:127-132, 2000.

78. Roukos DH: Extended (D2) lymph node dissection for gastric cancer: Do patients benefit? Ann Surg Oncol 7:253-255, 2000.

79. Siewert JR, Bottcher K, Stein HJ, Roder JD: Relevant prognostic factors in gastric cancer: Ten-year results of the German Gastric Cancer Study. Ann Surg 228:449-461, 1998.

80. Macdonald JS, Smalley SR, Benedetti J, et al: Chemoradiotherapy after surgery compared with surgery alone for adenocarcinoma of the stomach or gastroesophageal junction. N Engl J Med 345:725-730, 2001.

81. Bozzetti F, Bonfanti G, Castellani R, et al: Comparing reconstruction with Roux-en-Y to a pouch following total gastrectomy. J Am Coll Surg 183:243-248, 1996.

82. Fuchs KH, Thiede A, Engemann R, et al: Reconstruction of the food passage after total gastrectomy: Randomized trial. World J Surg 19:698-705, discussion 705-706, 1995.

83. Horvath OP, Kalmar K, Cseke L: Aboral pouch with preserved duodenal passage—new reconstruction method after total gastrectomy. Dig Surg 19:261-264, discussion 264-266, 2002.

84. Kalmar K, Cseke L, Zambo K, Horvath OP: Comparison of quality of life and nutritional parameters after total gastrectomy and a new type of pouch construction with simple Roux-en-Y reconstruction: Preliminary results of a prospective, randomized, controlled study. Dig Dis Sci 46:1791-1796, 2001.

85. Liedman B: Symptoms after total gastrectomy on food intake, body composition, bone metabolism, and quality of life in gastric cancer patients—is reconstruction with a reservoir worthwhile? Nutrition 15:677-682, 1999.

86. Meyer HJ, Opitz GJ: [Stomach carcinoma. Optimizing therapy by stomach replacement or subtotal resection?] Zentralbl Chir 124:381-386, 1999.

87. Mochiki E, Kamimura H, Haga N, et al: The technique of laparoscopically assisted total gastrectomy with jejunal interposition for early gastric cancer. Surg Endosc 16:540-544, 2002.

88. Nakane Y, Michiura T, Inoue K, et al: A randomized clinical trial of pouch reconstruction after total gastrectomy for cancer: Which is the better technique, Roux-en-Y or interposition? Hepatogastroenterology 48:903-907, 2001.

89. Svedlund J, Sullivan M, Liedman B, et al: Quality of life after gastrectomy for gastric carcinoma: Controlled study of reconstructive procedures. World J Surg 21:422-433, 1997.

90. Hayashi H, Ochiai T, Suzuki T, et al: Superiority of a new UICC-TNM staging system for gastric carcinoma. Surgery 127:129-135, 2000.

91. Wanebo HJ, Kennedy BJ, Chmiel J, et al: Cancer of the stomach. A patient care study by the American College of Surgeons. Ann Surg 218:583-592, 1993.

92. Lim L, Michael M, Mann GB, Leong T: Adjuvant therapy in gastric cancer. J Clin Oncol 23:6220-6232, 2005.

93. Msika S, Benhamiche AM, Jouve JL, et al: Prognostic factors after curative resection for gastric cancer. A population-based study. Eur J Cancer 36:390-396, 2000.

94. Middleton G, Cunningham D: Current options in the management of gastrointestinal cancer. Ann Oncol 6(Suppl 1):17-25, discussion 25-26, 1995.

95. Earle CC, Maroun JA: Adjuvant chemotherapy after curative resection for gastric cancer in non-Asian patients: Revisiting a meta-analysis of randomised trials. Eur J Cancer 35:1059-1064, 1999.

96. Janunger KG, Hafstrom L, Nygren P, et al: A systematic overview of chemotherapy effects in gastric cancer. Acta Oncol 40:309-326, 2001.

97. Hu JK, Chen ZX, Zhou ZG, et al: Intravenous chemotherapy for resected gastric cancer: Meta-analysis of randomized controlled trials. World J Gastroenterol 8:1023-1028, 2002.

98. Mari E, Floriani I, Tinazzi A, et al: Efficacy of adjuvant chemotherapy after curative resection for gastric cancer: A meta-analysis of published randomised trials. A study of the GISCAD (Gruppo Italiano per lo Studio dei Carcinomi dell'Apparato Digerente). Ann Oncol 11:837-843, 2000.

99. Bleiberg H, Goffin JC, Dalesio O, et al: Adjuvant radiotherapy and chemotherapy in resectable gastric cancer. A randomized trial of the gastro-intestinal tract cancer cooperative group of the EORTC. Eur J Surg Oncol 15:535-543, 1989.

100. Dent DM, Werner ID, Novis B, et al: Prospective randomized trial of combined oncological therapy for gastric carcinoma. Cancer 44:385-391, 1979.

101. Moertel CG, Childs DS, O'Fallon JR, et al: Combined 5-fluorouracil and radiation therapy as a surgical adjuvant for poor prognosis gastric carcinoma. J Clin Oncol 2:1249-1254, 1984.

102. Macdonald JS, Smalley S, Benedetti J, et al: Postoperative combined radiation and chemotherapy improves disease-free survival and overall survival in resected adenocarcinoma of the stomach and gastroesophageal junction: Update of the results of Intergroup INT-0116 (SWOG 9008). Paper presented at the American Society of Clinical Oncology Gastrointestinal Cancers Symposium, 2004, San Francisco.

103. Nashimoto A, Nakajima T, Furukawa H, et al: Randomized trial of adjuvant chemotherapy with mitomycin, fluorouracil, and cytosine arabinoside followed by oral fluorouracil in serosa-negative gastric cancer: Japan Clinical Oncology Group 9206-1. J Clin Oncol 21:2282-2287, 2003.

104. Allum W, Cunningham D, Weeden S: Perioperative chemotherapy in operable gastric and lower oesophageal cancer: A randomized control trial (the MAGIC trial, ISRCTN 93793971) [abstract 998]. Paper presented at 22nd Annual Meeting of the American Society of Clinical Oncology, Chicago, Illinois, 2003, p 249.

105. Rosen HR, Jatzko G, Repse S, et al: Adjuvant intraperitoneal chemotherapy with carbon-adsorbed mitomycin in patients with gastric cancer: Results of a randomized multicenter trial of the Austrian Working Group for Surgical Oncology. J Clin Oncol 16:2733-2738, 1998.

106. Yu W, Whang I, Suh I, et al: Prospective randomized trial of early postoperative intraperitoneal chemotherapy as an adjuvant to resectable gastric cancer. Ann Surg 228:347-354, 1998.

107. Zhang ZX, Gu XZ, Yin WB, et al: Randomized clinical trial on the combination of preoperative irradiation and surgery in the treatment of adenocarcinoma of gastric cardia (AGC)—report on 370 patients. Int J Radiat Oncol Biol Phys 42:929-934, 1998.

108. Skoropad VY, Berdov BA, Mardynski YS, Titova LN: A prospective, randomized trial of pre-operative and intraoperative radiotherapy versus surgery alone in resectable gastric cancer. Eur J Surg Oncol 26:773-779, 2000.

109. Kang YK, Choi DW, Im YH: A phase III randomized comparison of neoadjuvant chemotherapy followed by surgery versus surgery for locally advanced stomach cancer. Paper presented at the 15th Annual Meeting of the American Society of Clinical Oncology, Philadelphia, 1996, p 215.

110. Lowy AM, Feig BW, Janjan N, et al: A pilot study of preoperative chemoradiotherapy for resectable gastric cancer. Ann Surg Oncol 8:519-524, 2001.

111. Ajani JA, Mansfield PF, Janjan N, et al: Multi-institutional trial of preoperative chemoradiotherapy in patients with potentially resectable gastric carcinoma. J Clin Oncol 22:2774-2780, 2004.

112. Ekbom GA, Gleysteen JJ: Gastric malignancy: Resection for palliation. Surgery 88:476-481, 1980.

113. Meijer S, De Bakker OJ, Hoitsma HF: Palliative resection in gastric cancer. J Surg Oncol 23:77-80, 1983.

114. Bozzetti F, Bonfanti G, Audisio RA, et al: Prognosis of patients after palliative surgical procedures for carcinoma of the stomach. Surg Gynecol Obstet 164:151-154, 1987.

115. Fiori E, Lamazza A, Volpino P, et al: Palliative management of malignant antro-pyloric strictures. Gastroenterostomy vs. endoscopic stenting. A randomized prospective trial. Anticancer Res 24:269-271, 2004.

116. Thompson AM, Rapson T, Gilbert FJ, Park KG: Endoscopic palliative treatment for esophageal and gastric cancer: Techniques, complications, and survival in a population-based cohort of 948 patients. Surg Endosc 18:1257-1262, 2004.

117. Spencer GM, Thorpe SM, Blackman GM, et al: Laser augmented by brachytherapy versus laser alone in the palliation of adenocarcinoma of the oesophagus and cardia: A randomised study. Gut 50:224-227, 2002.

118. Ajani JA, Fodor MB, Tjulandin SA, et al: Phase II multi-institutional randomized trial of docetaxel plus cisplatin with or without fluorouracil in patients with untreated, advanced gastric, or gastroesophageal adenocarcinoma. J Clin Oncol 23:5660-5667, 2005.

119. Moehler M, Eimermacher A, Siebler J, et al: Randomised phase II evaluation of irinotecan plus high-dose 5-fluorouracil and leucovorin (ILF) vs 5-fluorouracil, leucovorin, and etoposide (ELF) in untreated metastatic gastric cancer. Br J Cancer 92:2122-2128, 2005.

120. Shin SJ, Chun SH, Kim KO, et al: The efficacy of paclitaxel and cisplatin combination chemotherapy for the treatment of metastatic or recurrent gastric cancer: A multicenter phase II study. Korean J Intern Med 20:135-140, 2005.

121. Pozzo C, Barone C, Szanto J, et al: Irinotecan in combination with 5-fluorouracil and folinic acid or with cisplatin in patients with advanced gastric or esophageal-gastric junction adenocarcinoma: Results of a randomized phase II study. Ann Oncol 15:1773-1781, 2004.

122. Ellis H: Tumours of the small intestine. Semin Surg Oncol 3:12-21, 1987.

123. Torres M, Matta E, Chinea B, et al: Malignant tumors of the small intestine. J Clin Gastroenterol 37:372-380, 2003.

124. Ito H, Perez A, Brooks DC, et al: Surgical treatment of small bowel cancer: A 20-year single institution experience. J Gastrointest Surg 7:925-930, 2003.

125. Coit DG: Cancer of the Small Intestine. In DeVita VT, Hellman S, Rosenberg SA (eds): Cancer: Principles and Practice of Oncology. Philadelphia, Lippincott, Williams & Wilkins, 2001, pp 1204-1216.

126. Dabaja BS, Siki D, Pro B, et al: Adenocarcinoma of the small bowel: Presentation, prognostic factors, and outcome of 217 patients. Cancer 101:518-526, 2004.

127. Howe JR, Karnell LG, Menck HR, Scott-Conner C: The American College of Surgeons Commission on Cancer and the American Cancer Society. Adenocarcinoma of the small bowel: Review of the National Cancer Data Base, 1985-1995. Cancer 86:2693-2706, 1999.

128. Ojha A, Zacherl J, Scheuba C, et al: Primary small bowel malignancies: Single-center results of three decades. J Clin Gastroenterol 30:289-293, 2000.

129. Weiss NS, Yang CP: Incidence of histologic types of cancer of the small intestine. J Natl Cancer Inst 78:653-656, 1987.

130. Lowenfels AB: Why are small-bowel tumours so rare? Lancet 1:24-26, 1973.

131. Wattenberg LW: Studies of polycyclic hydrocarbon hydroxylases of the intestine possibly related to cancer. Effect of diet on benzpyrene hydroxylase activity. Cancer 28:99-102, 1971.

132. Wilson JM, Melvin DB, Gray GF, Thorbjarnarson B: Primary malignancies of the small bowel: A report of 96 cases and review of the literature. Ann Surg 180:175-179, 1974.

133. Ross RK, Hartnett NM, Bernstein L, Henderson BE: Epidemiology of adenocarcinomas of the small intestine: Is bile a small bowel carcinogen? Br J Cancer 63:143-145, 1991.

134. Lowenfels AB: Does bile promote extra-colonic cancer? Lancet 2:239-241, 1978.

135. Chow WH, Linet MS, McLaughlin JK, et al: Risk factors for small intestine cancer. Cancer Causes Control 4:163-169, 1993.

136. Lowenfels AB, Sonni A: Distribution of small bowel tumors. Cancer Lett 3:83-86, 1977.

137. Neugut AI, Jacobson JS, Suh S, et al: The epidemiology of cancer of the small bowel. Cancer Epidemiol Biomarkers Prev 7:243-251, 1998.

138. Stell D, Mayer D, Mirza D, Buckels J: Delayed diagnosis and lower resection rate of adenocarcinoma of the distal duodenum. Dig Surg 21:434-438, discussion 438-439, 2004.

139. Kerremans RP, Lerut J, Penninckx FM: Primary malignant duodenal tumors. Ann Surg 190:179-182, 1979.

140. Lai EC, Doty JE, Irving C, Tompkins RK: Primary adenocarcinoma of the duodenum: Analysis of survival. World J Surg 12:695-699, 1988.

141. Joesting DR, Beart RW Jr, van Heerden JA, Weiland LH: Improving survival in adenocarcinoma of the duodenum. Am J Surg 141:228-231, 1981.

142. Adler SN, Lyon DT, Sullivan PD: Adenocarcinoma of the small bowel. Clinical features, similarity to regional enteritis, and analysis of 338 documented cases. Am J Gastroenterol 77:326-330, 1982.

143. Williamson RC, Welch CE, Malt RA: Adenocarcinoma and lymphoma of the small intestine. Distribution and etiologic associations. Ann Surg 197:172-178, 1983.

144. Ouriel K, Adams JT: Adenocarcinoma of the small intestine. Am J Surg 147:66-71, 1984.

145. Lioe TF, Biggart JD: Primary adenocarcinoma of the jejunum and ileum: Clinicopathological review of 25 cases. J Clin Pathol 43:533-536, 1990.

62

Motility Disorders of the Stomach and Small Intestine

John E. Meilahn

GASTRIC MOTILITY

Normal gastric emptying reflects a coordinated function of the gastric fundus, corpus, antrum, pylorus, and duodenum. Proper gastric emptying thus involves a sequence of events involving all of these structures. Eating a meal causes receptive relaxation of the fundus for gastric storage. Subsequent fundic contraction is important for emptying liquids from the stomach. The gastric pacemaker is located in the body along the greater curvature and stimulates filling and mixing of food in the corpus and antrum. Food is sequentially mixed to and fro in the antrum against pyloric resistance in the process of trituration until food particles are ground down. Subsequent antral peristalsis, at the rate of three per minute, with associated pyloric relaxation allows small particles and liquids to pass to the duodenum. Therefore, the stomach may be thought of as three regions of motility that must act in a coordinated fashion to produce acceptable emptying of the stomach: the fundus, with relaxation and subsequent contraction; the body, with filling and mixing; and the antropyloroduodenal complex, with trituration and emptying into the duodenum as the pyloric sphincter opens.

Symptoms of abnormal gastric motility are nonspecific and generally include nausea, vomiting, epigastric fullness, postprandial bloating, and heartburn. The list of differential diagnoses includes gastroparesis, rapid gastric emptying as in dumping syndrome, functional dyspepsia with impaired fundic distention, ulcer, cancer, gastroesophageal reflux disease, rumination syndrome, cyclic vomiting syndrome, bulimia, and superior mesenteric artery (SMA) syndrome. Organic causes may be diagnosed with a combination of upper endoscopy, enteroscopy and enteroclysis, upper gastrointestinal (GI) series, or upper GI series with small bowel follow-through. If these studies are inconclusive, further testing along with gastroenterologic consultation is necessary to differentiate between nonorganic causes.

Gastroparesis

Gastroparesis is delayed gastric emptying in the absence of specific organic causes, such as stricture, ulcer, tumor, SMA syndrome, or mechanical obstruction, or of nonorganic causes, such as functional dyspepsia, rumination syndrome, cyclic vomiting syndrome, or bulimia/anorexia nervosa. Abnormal peristaltic contractile activity and abnormal electrical slow waves are usually present. Females are most often affected (about 80% female, 20% male), with the average age at onset of symptoms being about 34 years. Causes are evenly divided between diabetes and idiopathic (about 28% each), with other causes including postviral, postsurgical (especially with intended or inadvertent vagotomy), Parkinson's disease, scleroderma, and pseudo-obstruction. The predominant symptoms are nausea and vomiting with abdominal bloating and early satiety. Epigastric abdominal pain may be present in about half the patients, and some of them have become dependent on narcotics. Abdominal pain, in general, is not well treated by gastric electrical stimulation or by prokinetic drugs.[1]

The diagnosis of gastroparesis is usually made by the gastroenterologist after extensive testing to rule out other causes. Evaluation of gastric emptying by scintigraphy may be diagnostic of gastroparesis, with more than 50% of a solid meal being retained 2 hours after ingestion or more than 10% of a solid meal being retained at 4 hours. Liquid emptying, although quantifiable, is less accurate in the diagnosis of gastroparesis because liquids may empty normally even with an abnormal solid emptying scan. Either a ^{99m}Tc–sulfur colloid–labeled egg sandwich or an Eggbeaters meal is used as a test meal for the solid emptying scan. Though not commonly used in clinical settings, breath testing for gastroparesis can be performed with ^{13}C-labeled octanoate in a solid meal, which is absorbed in the small bowel after gastric emptying, metabolized there to $^{13}CO_2$, and then removed by respiration.[1]

General principles for the treatment of gastroparesis are to correct fluid and electrolyte abnormalities, as well as nutritional deficiencies, identify and treat any underlying causes, and suppress or eliminate symptoms such as nausea or vomiting. Diets may be changed toward softer solid foods and more toward liquid supplements, with smaller, more frequent meals. Total parenteral nutrition (TPN) may be necessary to provide the daily caloric intake for maintenance of body weight. In a diabetic patient, tight glucose control should be achieved because hyperglycemia may worsen gastroparetic symptoms. Hyperglycemia can impair both antral contractions and antropyloric coordination. The mainstay of medical treatment is the use of both antiemetic and prokinetic medications.[1]

Antiemetic agents useful in treating gastroparesis include prokinetic agents with antiemetic properties, such as metoclopramide (Reglan) or domperidone (Motilium). Phenothiazine derivatives, which antagonize dopamine receptors in the area postrema, include prochlorperazine (Compazine) and trimethobenzamide (Tigan). Antihistamines with H_1–receptor antagonist properties include diphenhydramine (Benadryl), promethazine, and meclizine (Antivert). Antiserotoninergics, which antagonize 5-hydroxytryptamine (5-HT$_3$) receptors, include ondansetron (Zofran), granisetron (Kytril), and dolasetron (Anzemet). Other agents include scopolamine, an anticholinergic, and aprepitant (Emend), a substance P/neurokinin-1 receptor antagonist.[1]

Not many effective prokinetic agents are currently available. Metoclopramide (Reglan) is the only Food and Drug Administration (FDA)-approved agent for gastroparesis, but it produces central nervous system side effects in 10% to 20% of patients. Cisapride (Propulsid) was approved only for the treatment of heartburn and was taken off the market in 2000 because of prolongation of the QT interval. Although domperidone (Motilium) has both prokinetic and antiemetic properties, it has not been approved by the FDA and is available only outside the United States. Erythromycin is useful as a motilin agonist, but it may have GI side effects of nausea, vomiting, and abdominal pain and is known to have decreasing effect as a result of tachyphylaxis.

Botulinum Toxin Injection

Because pyloric sphincter opening is the final step in gastric emptying, pyloric relaxation via injection of botulinum toxin A (Botox) into the pyloric sphincter may improve symptoms in those with idiopathic or diabetic gastroparesis. Botulinum toxin inhibits cholinergic neuromuscular transmission and has been used in multiple areas of the GI tract, including the lower esophageal sphincter to treat achalasia[2] and the anal sphincter to treat anal fissures. Multiple injections of botulinum toxin are placed circumferentially at endoscopy into the prepyloric area (within 2 cm of the pyloric channel). If there is a beneficial effect from injection, the process may be repeated at several-month intervals.

In a retrospective study at Temple University Hospital, 63 patients (53 females and 10 males with a mean age of 42 years) with gastroparesis were injected with botulinum toxin A.[3] Major symptoms were vomiting, nausea, and abdominal pain. Less than 10% had early satiety, decreased appetite, bloating, or weight loss as their major symptoms. None had a previous injection, and all had at least a 4-week follow-up after treatment (mean length of 9.3 months with a range of 1 to 37 months). Treatment consisted of five circumferential injections into the prepyloric area with a total of 100 to 200 U of botulinum toxin. There were no complications from endoscopy or the injection of toxin. Antiemetic and prokinetic agents were generally continued after injection, but gastric emptying studies were not usually performed. A positive symptomatic response was observed in 27 (42.9%) of the 63 patients, with a mean duration of response of 4.0 ± 2.7 months. Nine of the 27 responders had improvement for more than 6 months, all of whom were female. Fourteen of the 27 responders experienced complete resolution of all of their symptoms, with a duration of response of 5.1 ± 2.8 months. Females and patients older than 50 years had a better response rate than males and younger patients did.

Gastric Electrical Stimulation

Several different approaches have been used in gastric electrical stimulation in an effort to improve either gastric emptying or symptoms of gastroparesis. Because the intrinsic gastric pacemaker located along the greater curvature produces antral stimulation at 3 cycles per minute (cpm), low-frequency stimulation was used in an attempt to entrain and pace the gastric slow waves at 3.3 cpm to accelerate gastric emptying through possible activation of motor efferent nerves. Although the concept seems promising and has been reported in a small series of nine patients,[4] with improvement in both gastric emptying and symptoms of gastroparesis, this approach is not currently being used. *Sequential circumferential muscle stimulation* involves the use of bursts of suprahigh-frequency electrical stimulation to produce propagated antral contractions and to accelerate gastric emptying; however, this technology has not made the transition to actual clinical practice. In contrast, high-frequency stimulation is now being used in clinical practice for the treatment of both idiopathic and diabetic gastroparesis. With electrical stimulation at 12 cpm, symptoms improve in up to 60% of patients. It is thought that such stimulation activates sensory afferent nerves rather than increasing antral contractions. In addition, gastric emptying studies after stimulation may show little change in actual gastric emptying even though the gastroparetic symptoms may have improved.[5]

Medtronic (Enterra) Gastric Electric Stimulation Using high-frequency, low-energy, short-pulse electrical stimulation at 12 cpm, the Enterra stimulator with two electrical leads has been approved by the FDA for the treatment of patients with chronic, intractable (drug refractory) nausea and vomiting secondary to gastroparesis of diabetic or idiopathic origin. Ideally placed in patients who have previously undergone gastric surgery, the stimulator has also been used in those with an existing

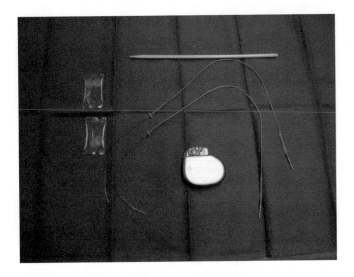

Figure 62–1. Enterra gastric electric stimulator system, with two Enterra leads, an introducer rod, plastic disks, and Enterra stimulator.

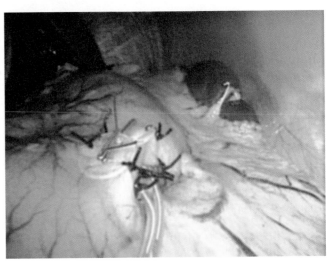

Figure 62–2. The Enterra leads are placed in the gastric wall 10 and 11 cm proximal to the pylorus and secured with plastic disks.

venting gastrostomy and feeding jejunostomy tubes. The beneficial effect of the stimulator may not be clinically apparent for several months, although some patients do report early improvement in well-being.

The stimulator package consists of a Medtronic Enterra stimulator (sized much like a cardiac pacemaker) and two insulated wire electrodes with an uninsulated metal tip connected to a monofilament suture with a straightened needle (Fig. 62–1). The two electrodes are positioned along the anterior greater curvature of the stomach, separated by about 1 cm. The most distal electrode is located about 10 cm proximal to the pylorus.[5] Both electrodes are placed parallel to each other, with partial-thickness penetration into the muscularis. The attached plastic flange of each electrode is sutured to the serosa to prevent dislodgement. Electrode placement may be done laparoscopically,[6] although needle and electrode passage in partial-thickness fashion is more difficult laparoscopically than with an open procedure, which can be performed through a small upper midline incision. In either case, upper endoscopy is recommended at the time of electrode placement to exclude full-thickness gastric wall penetration. If noted, the electrode can be repositioned and sutured (Fig. 62–2).

The stimulator itself is placed in a subcutaneous pocket on the abdominal wall in a location consistent with the patient's wishes, previous surgical procedures, and the potential need for future feeding tubes. The right side of the abdomen is preferred over the left for at least two reasons. First, space may need to be preserved for placement of a future venting gastrostomy tube or a feeding jejunostomy tube in the event that the stimulator does not reduce nausea, vomiting, or malnutrition. Second, if there are current venting/feeding tubes on the left, positioning the stimulator also on the left may increase the risk for contiguous spread of infection to the

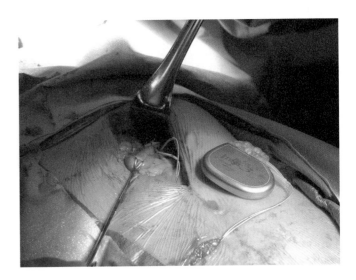

Figure 62–3. Open placement of the Enterra stimulator in a right lower quadrant pocket. Leads may be placed laparoscopically as well.

stimulator pocket if an infection or cellulitis develops at the tube site. A right upper quadrant location is easily facilitated unless the patient is short and thin, in which case the device may impinge on the costal margin when sitting. If a lower abdominal location is chosen, the stimulator should not be placed so low that it is forced upward when the patient sits. Both electrodes are brought through the abdominal wall with a trocar or provided tunneler and then connected to the stimulator (Fig. 62–3).

Next, the electrical resistance of the circuit through the gastric wall is determined before closure of the incisions. Transcutaneous interrogation of the stimulator is performed with a sterile plastic drape–wrapped transducer connected to the Enterra computer. A typical impedance value of less than 800 ohms is satisfactory. If the impedance is greater, the electrodes could be too far apart and may need to be positioned more closely together. After closure of the incisions, the stimulator may be left in the *off* position for the first day. Nausea and vomiting are common after surgery and anesthesia, and because the stimulator is unlikely to diminish these early symptoms, it may be psychologically better to delay activation for a day until the immediate postoperative symptoms subside.

Risks associated with the gastric electrical stimulator include full-thickness penetration of the gastric wall at the time of placement or erosion into the gastric lumen with subsequent infection or abscess. Dislodgement of the leads from the stomach is possible in the early postoperative period if the plastic flanges have been inadequately sutured. Moderate fibrosis subsequently covers the lead implant sites on the stomach, thus making dislodgement a remote possibility. The presence of two looping wire electrodes within the abdomen can lead to small bowel obstruction. This possibility is quite small with the omentum in its normal configuration because the electrodes are positioned in the upper part of the abdomen and on top of the omentum. However, previous major abdominal surgery such as colectomy or partial small bowel resection may predispose to small bowel obstruction unless the electrodes are sutured loosely to the upper abdominal wall at the time of placement. It is unusual for the electrodes to become adherent to the abdominal viscera, but if it does occur, subsequent dissection of the electrodes from surrounding attachments does risk cutting the insulating layer and negating the effect of the stimulator. Hematoma may develop in the subcutaneous pocket for the stimulator in the postoperative period, either from vessels within the pocket or from the abdominal wall as a result of passage of an electrode through it. Subsequent infection or abscess at the stimulator site mandates removal of it. Erosion of the stimulator through the skin, even without cellulitis, is also treated by removal. Placement of the stimulator in the lower portion of the abdomen is sometimes complicated by local pain when sitting, either from displacement of the stimulator upward in the sitting position or from pressure on local nerves. This problem is treated by relocation of the stimulator to a more cephalad position, with care taken to not position it under a skin fold of the abdomen. Magnetic resonance imaging (MRI) is not possible after stimulator placement. If there has been no therapeutic effect from placement of the stimulator and MRI is needed to evaluate another body area, the electrodes and stimulator are removed. Laparoscopy allows evaluation and dissection of the electrodes up to the gastric wall; traction alone usually allows removal of the leads with mechanical cutting of the wires at the stomach if necessary.

At Temple University Hospital, 28 patients with a mean age of 40 years underwent Enterra implantation over an 18-month study period, with an average follow-up of 148 days.[7] Of these 28 patients, 14 felt improved, 8 remained the same, and 6 worsened according to the validated Gastroparesis Cardinal Symptom Index (GCSI) questionnaire scoring. The overall GCSI score significantly decreased by 12% ± 7%, with improvement in nausea and vomiting but no improvement in bloating or abdominal pain. The decrease in GCSI score was greater for the 12 diabetic patients (18% ± 11%; $P < .05$) than for the 16 idiopathic patients (7% ± 9%; $P =$ NS). The subgroup of 22 patients with a chief complaint of nausea/vomiting had greater improvement (16% ± 9%; $P < .05$) than did the 6 patients with a chief complaint of abdominal pain (3% ± 11%; $P =$ NS). The 13 patients taking narcotic analgesics at the time of Enterra implantation had a poorer GSCI response (increasing by 9% ± 10%; $P =$ NS) than did the 15 who were not. As a result, three clinical parameters associated with a favorable clinical response to implantation were identified: diabetic rather than idiopathic gastroparesis, nausea/vomiting rather than abdominal pain as the primary symptom, and independence from narcotic analgesics before stimulator implantation.

Gastric Electrical Stimulation for Postsurgical Gastroparesis Gastric electrical stimulation is most commonly used on an intact stomach, without previous resection or surgery, except for prior gastrostomy tube placement. Postsurgical gastroparesis may develop in up to 10% of patients who have undergone vagotomy, in the absence of mechanical obstruction, and in up to 50% of those with chronic gastric outlet obstruction before surgery. Gastroparesis has been associated with partial gastrectomy, fundoplication, esophagectomy with colon interposition, and pylorus-preserving Whipple procedures. Gastric electrical stimulation is not usually thought to be suitable in these cases. However, McCallum et al. reported the application of electrical stimulation for postsurgical gastroparesis, including gastroparesis after Nissen fundoplication, vagotomy and pyloroplasty, Billroth I and vagotomy, Billroth II and vagotomy, spinal surgery, esophagectomy with colonic interposition, and cholecystectomy.[8] Sixteen patients (15 female, 1 male) with a diagnosis of gastroparesis for more than 1 year and refractoriness to antiemetics and prokinetics underwent implantation of the Enterra stimulator. In cases of antrectomy, the two electrodes were positioned within the muscularis propria 2 and 3 cm proximal to the gastric anastomosis. In those with an intact stomach, the electrodes were positioned in the usual manner at 10 and 11 cm proximal to the pylorus. Gastrostomy tubes were removed; however, feeding jejunostomy tubes were placed in 7 patients because of existing malnutrition. All patients were then monitored for at least 12 months. At 6 months after implantation, the severity and frequency of upper GI symptoms (vomiting, nausea, early satiety, bloating, postprandial fullness, and epigastric pain) were significantly reduced, and the improvement over the initial baseline state was sustained at 12 months ($P < .05$). Hospitalization for gastroparesis symptoms, which averaged 31 ± 13 days for the year preceding stimulator implantation, was reduced to 6 ± 2 days ($P < .05$) during the first year after implantation.

Gastric electrical stimulation in an intact stomach is not thought to generally improve symptoms by improvement in gastric emptying, verifiable by scintigraphy. However, some patients may demonstrate improvement or normalization of gastric emptying rates by scintigraphy.[6] Retrograde stimulation of the vagal nerves has been thought to be a possible mode of symptom improvement, and therefore it may be questioned whether improvement should be expected after placement of a stimulator in those in whom vagotomy or inadvertent vagal injury has already occurred. Although vagal nerve damage or disruption was thought to be part of the underlying pathophysiology of these 16 postsurgical patients, electrical stimulation was still effective in improving symptoms. Moreover, our experience at Temple is that in an intact stomach (with no divided vagus nerves), diabetic patients improve more than idiopathic gastroparetic patients. Some neuropathy is characteristic of diabetes, which implies that vagal dysfunction was present before stimulator implantation; it also implies that gastric electrical stimulation can be effective without normal vagal function.

Surgical Procedures

When prokinetic and antiemetic medications alone are not sufficient to maintain body weight, venting and feeding tubes are used. A percutaneous gastrostomy tube alone may reduce the incidence of vomiting through intermittent venting or by setting the tube at continuous external drainage. Previous upper abdominal surgical procedures may indicate the need for laparoscopic or open gastrostomy tube placement instead of the endoscopic approach. A combination transgastric gastrojejunal tube can vent the stomach and also provide proximal jejunal tube feeding. Although the concept is attractive, it is more difficult to place the tube properly and maintain correct placement in the proximal jejunum. In addition, this combination tube design is subject to proximal displacement of the jejunal tube, with repeated bouts of emesis. The jejunal end of the tube may be forced back into the duodenum or even back into the stomach with repeated vomiting.

Placement of a feeding jejunostomy tube allows the provision of both adequate nutrition and fluids and can help reduce the need for hospitalization for intravenous repletion of fluids. Placement of both a gastrostomy tube for gastric venting and a jejunostomy tube for fluids and nutrition allows many patients with gastroparesis to manage their symptoms and improve their quality of life. Enteral feeding is preferred over parenteral nutrition because of lower overall cost and avoidance of more severe complications from central intravenous access. Enteral feeding via the jejunostomy tube may be maintained for months or years. Potential complications of a feeding jejunostomy include tube dislodgement with closure of the opening, infection and cellulitis at the site, and leakage from the site if the tract enlarges, which would require the insertion of a larger-diameter feeding tube. If small bowel dysmotility accompanies the gastroparesis, tube feed rates may need to be limited because of the nausea, pain, or bloating that may occur with normal rates of feeding. If ongoing weight loss then

occurs, TPN is mandated via a PICC (percutaneous indwelling central venous catheter) line or tunneled central venous catheter. More aggressive surgical procedures have not been found to reliably reduce gastroparetic symptoms. Such procedures include pyloroplasty, gastrojejunostomy, and partial gastric resection. If gastric resection is chosen, a near-total gastrectomy with creation of a small proximal gastric pouch via a vertical staple line, as performed for a gastric bypass procedure, should be considered if blood supply is adequate. Additionally, a Roux gastrojejunostomy with at least a 15-mm opening, a short Roux limb, and a feeding jejunostomy should be performed.

Postsurgical Gastroparesis

After previous gastric procedures, complete evaluation of the gastric remnant and any anastomosis should be performed. An upper GI series will evaluate the overall morphology and may help assess for possible partial obstruction. Gastric emptying studies may be performed to evaluate the existing stomach if obstruction is not noted on the upper GI study. Endoscopic examination should be performed to examine the stomach for gastritis, the presence of *Helicobacter pylori*, ulcers, and the diameter and state of the anastomosis, as well as the possible presence of a marginal ulcer. If ulceration or friability is noted, medical treatment with proton pump inhibitors and sucralfate suspension and avoidance of nonsteroidal anti-inflammatory drugs may permit healing. A stricture may be balloon-dilated endoscopically if it is not overly fibrotic and if active inflammation is not present.[9] A perforation may occur if the dilation is overly aggressive, so limited dilation at one setting is advised. The dilation may be repeated one or more times for sequential enlargement of the anastomosis, up to 15 to 20 mm in diameter with current balloons. A wire-guided balloon catheter is safer for an initial dilation if the gastroscope cannot be passed through the anastomosis because the wire guide helps prevent perforation of the nonvisualized bowel distal to the stricture when the balloon is inflated. A gastroscope with a large working channel will be necessary if a wire-guided balloon is used.

If persistent marginal ulceration remains at the anastomosis after medical therapy (including treatment of *H. pylori* if present) or if an anastomotic stricture cannot be suitably dilated, surgical revision of the anastomosis should be considered. Revision should include completion vagotomy if there is a persistent ulcer, along with additional gastric resection. Before performing a larger operation, thoracoscopic truncal vagotomy should always be considered. If vagotomy and antrectomy have previously been performed, consider a subtotal (75%) gastrectomy. If subtotal gastrectomy has previously been performed, consider a near-total gastrectomy. If a recurrent ulcer is present after previous Roux gastroenterostomy, consider re-resection to a 95% gastrectomy with Roux gastrojejunostomy.[9,10]

In those with chronic postvagotomy, postgastrectomy gastric stasis, even aggressive resection with Roux reconstruction may not produce satisfactory outcomes. The results of near-total completion gastrectomy for severe postvagotomy gastric stasis in 62 patients (51 female, 11 male) at the Mayo Clinic were followed for more than 5 years.[11] In these patients the gastric remnant was largely resected, with a 1- to 2-cm remnant of gastric cardia left for the gastrojejunostomy. Despite a median of four previous gastric operations and symptoms of nausea, vomiting, postprandial pain, chronic abdominal pain, and chronic narcotic use, all or most symptoms were relieved in 43% of those operated on (Visick grade I or II). However, the rest remained in Visick grade III or IV. Although nausea, vomiting, and postprandial pain were improved, chronic pain, diarrhea, and dumping syndrome were not significantly improved.

Roux Stasis Syndrome

Roux stasis syndrome is a term that has been applied to symptoms of early satiety, vomiting, and postprandial pain occurring after distal gastrectomy with Roux gastrojejunostomy; it affects up to 30% to 50% of such patients.[9] It was postulated that ectopic pacemakers occur in the Roux limb and cause orally directed Roux limb contractions, as well as aboral contractions, thereby resulting in functional obstruction to gastric emptying. Most of these patients underwent vagotomy as part of their initial surgical procedure. Although Roux limb motility may be affected by division of its mesentery, it is also likely that gastric stasis plays a significant role in producing symptoms. Endoscopy may show gastric bezoar formation or dilation of the gastric remnant, as well as possible dilation of the Roux limb. Improvement after near-total gastrectomy in patients with previous vagotomy suggests that the gastric stasis component was more significant than the effect in the Roux limb itself.[9] Moreover, current experience with Roux gastric bypass procedures for morbid obesity tends to support this concept. In most gastric bypasses, vagotomy is not performed and a small gastric pouch not based on the fundus is retained. Postprandial pain and vomiting do not usually occur in these patients. Early satiety seems to be a function of the small pouch and the controlled size of the gastrojejunostomy. In patients with a dilated gastrojejunostomy in which food more rapidly enters the Roux limb from the pouch, early satiety and vomiting do not generally occur. Instead, more food can be ingested, and feelings of hunger usually return more quickly as a result. The Roux syndrome is therefore more likely to primarily be postoperative gastric atony.

INTESTINAL MOTILITY

In the fasting state, small intestinal motility is controlled by the migrating motor complex (MMC), which exhibits three phases. Phase I is a quiescent period and represents 20% to 30% of the total cycle length. Phase II accounts for 40% to 60% of the total cycle length and is characterized by intermittent and irregular contractions. In phase III, intense, rhythmic contractions develop and propagate from the proximal to the distal portion of the intestine over a 5- to 10-minute period. The MMC cycle occurs about every 90 minutes during the interdigestive period. However, after a meal, this fasting pattern of intestinal motility is changed to a postprandial pattern, with intermittent phasic contractions of irregular amplitude that are similar to the phase II contractions of the MMC.[12] Peristalsis occurs when a segment of circular muscle contracts as a result of excitatory motor neurons while the intestinal segment aboral to the contracted segment is simultaneously relaxed by inhibitory neurons.[13]

The interstitial cells of Cajal (ICCs) are known to be essential regulators of GI motility and seem to serve as pacemaker cells in the GI tract and mediators of neural regulation in GI motility. They lie in close proximity to smooth muscle cells and elements of the enteric nervous system. The generation of slow waves occurs within Auerbach's plexus and is an intrinsic property of ICCs; both circumferential intestinal contractions and longitudinal contractions are produced.[13] ICC abnormalities are increasingly being recognized in a number of GI tract disorders, such as chronic intestinal pseudo-obstruction, with findings of decreased ICCs or an abnormal ICC network.[14,15] Surgical procedures involving the small intestine produce disruption of ICC networks at the level of the myenteric and deep muscular plexuses, with resultant loss of slow waves and phasic contractions. This loss of intestinal motility, however, partially recovers within 24 hours after surgery.[16]

Because intestinal motility is controlled by interactions between smooth muscle, enteric nerves, extrinsic nerves, and humoral factors, abnormalities in each of these areas may result in intestinal dysmotility. Small intestinal dysmotility symptoms include abdominal bloating, distention, pain, nausea, and vomiting. Primary disorders of small intestinal dysmotility include inherited familial visceral myopathies, characterized by smooth muscle degeneration, and familial visceral neuropathies, characterized by the degeneration of enteric nerves. Secondary causes of small intestinal dysmotility include myopathic processes (scleroderma, muscular dystrophies, amyloidosis), neurologic diseases (Parkinson's disease, neurofibromatosis, Chagas' disease), endocrine disorders (diabetes mellitus, hyperthyroidism, hypothyroidism, hypoparathyroidism), celiac disease, and pharmacologic agents (anti-Parkinson medications, phenothiazines, tricyclic antidepressants, narcotics).[17]

Smooth muscle disease such as scleroderma frequently affects the GI tract, and small intestinal dysmotility develops in about 40% of such patients. Proximal involvement leads to megaduodenum or widemouth diverticula of the small bowel, with delayed transit, bacterial overgrowth, and malabsorption. Octreotide has been useful in treating stasis and the resultant bacterial overgrowth. Muscular dystrophies affect motility of the entire gut; although barium studies may be normal, small intestinal manometry may reveal a myopathic pattern. Amyloidosis produces infiltration of both smooth muscle and the autonomic nerves and affects the motility of the entire GI tract.[17]

Neurologic disease is most commonly seen with Parkinson's disease, with degeneration of the enteric nervous system and inhibition of intestinal motility by anti-Parkinson medications. Neurofibromatosis may produce dysmotility as a result of mechanical obstruction with GI tract tumor formation, but it is also associated with neuronal dysplasia of the enteric nervous system. Chagas' disease (infection with *Trypanosoma cruzi*) results in neuronal injury and is manifested as megaduodenum, megajejunum, or pseudo-obstruction.[17] Hirschsprung's disease or its allied disorders hypoganglionosis and intestinal neuronal dysplasia may produce small intestinal dysmotility.[18]

Endocrine disorders may give rise to intestinal dysmotility that may be treated. Hypothyroidism produces delayed transit, constipation, and pseudo-obstruction, which is reversible with thyroid hormone replacement. Hypoparathyroidism may be associated with small intestinal dysmotility and pseudo-obstruction, which improve with calcium repletion. Small intestinal complications of diabetes with autonomic neuropathy include delayed transit with bacterial overgrowth and diarrhea. Celiac sprue produces abdominal pain, distention, and malabsorption, with delayed intestinal transit, bacterial overgrowth, and pseudo-obstruction.[19] Both villous damage and small intestinal dysmotility improve with a gluten-free diet.[17]

GI motility is enhanced by the stimulation of distinct serotonin (5-HT) receptors on intestinal sensory nerves. 5-HT is released from mucosal enterochromaffin cells in response to mechanical and chemical stimuli within the intestine. 5-HT activates 5-HT$_4$ receptors on nerves synapsing in the myenteric plexus, which then results in motor responses and increased peristalsis and intestinal transit.[16] Tegaserod, a selective 5-HT$_4$ partial agonist, has been shown to significantly accelerate small bowel transit time, as well as gastric emptying.[20]

Diagnosis of Intestinal Dysmotility

After the history, physical examination, and conventional radiographic studies suggest the possibility of intestinal dysmotility, an upper GI study with small bowel follow-through should be performed. This study should suggest the possibility of obstructing lesions such as tumor, stricture, diverticula, or adhesions and, in their absence, may identify general small bowel dysmotility. Evaluation of small intestinal transit may be then done by small bowel scintigraphy, with imaging up to 6 hours after ingestion of a radiolabeled meal. Scintigraphy has a specificity of up to 75% for the diagnosis of dysmotility, but it does not differentiate between myopathic and neuropathic causes.

Small bowel manometry is then performed if abnormal small bowel transit is found to be present. In the interdigestive period the MMC is monitored to examine the cycle duration (interval between phase III events), the duration of each phase, including the amplitude and propagation velocity of phase III, and the rate of contraction of phase III. A motility disorder is present with abnormal bursts of phasic activity, low-amplitude con-

tractions, poorly coordinated activity, or absent, incomplete, or retrograde phase III activity. With eating, a change to typical postprandial activity is expected, with irregular, phasic contractions of variable amplitude as the intestinal contents are mixed and propelled distally. This postprandial period lasts for about 4 hours, and then a return to the interdigestive pattern should be noted. Whereas short-duration (2-hour) manometry studies may diagnose abnormalities while a patient is in the fed or postprandial state, longer study periods facilitate study in the interdigestive period as well. This concept has been extended to ambulatory study systems in an attempt to improve diagnostic accuracy. Manometry may also help distinguish myopathic causes of dysmotility from neuropathic causes.

Pharmacologic Treatment

Octreotide has been used to treat the chronic pseudo-obstruction and bacterial overgrowth seen with dysmotility from connective tissue diseases such as scleroderma. It induces phase III–like activity in the small intestine; however, it also decreases antral activity.[17] The addition of erythromycin, a motilin agonist, stimulates gastric emptying and also intestinal contractions at low doses. Tegaserod, a 5-HT$_4$ partial agonist, has been shown to accelerate small bowel transit time, as well as increase both gastric emptying and colonic transit.[17,20]

Surgical Treatment

Surgical options for the treatment of nonmechanical small intestinal dysmotility are limited. Mechanical causes of slow bowel transit, abdominal pain, or small intestinal dilation should first be investigated. The differential diagnosis includes luminal webs, polyps, carcinoid, duplication, internal hernias, intussusception, adhesions, malrotation, SMA syndrome, chronic gut ischemia, inflammatory bowel disease, radiation enteritis, and neoplasm. Radiographic modalities available for evaluation include upper GI series with small bowel follow-through and computed tomography with both oral and intravenous contrast. Transit studies with radiopaque markers may assess small intestinal motility. Upper endoscopy with enteroscopy allows evaluation of the proximal jejunum and also permits mucosal biopsy. Small intestinal manometry allows assessment of the MMC.

If radiologic and gastroenterologic studies have not enabled a diagnosis to be made, the surgeon may be requested to perform diagnostic laparoscopy. In a patient without extensive previous surgery, laparoscopy affords an adequate examination of the small intestine from the ligament of Treitz to the terminal ileum. Conversion to exploratory laparotomy may be indicated with previous surgery or with questionable findings at laparoscopy. If requested, a feeding jejunostomy tube may be placed and a full-thickness jejunal biopsy performed to evaluate for visceral myopathy or neurogenic causes of small bowel dysmotility and chronic intestinal pseudo-obstruction.[21]

Small bowel resection is uncommonly performed, although localized findings may justify segmental resection. Isolated megaduodenum (type I familial visceral myopathy) has been treated by either drainage or subtotal duodenal resection, with the posterior biliopancreatic duodenal wall left intact and the proximal jejunum used as an onlay patch.[17,22] Primary amyloidosis confined to the small intestine has been reported in the setting of persistent pseudo-obstruction and has been treated by partial jejunectomy.[23]

Chronic intestinal pseudo-obstruction in the pediatric population may occur as a result of short-gut syndrome after resection for intestinal aganglionosis or as a result of neuropathic or myopathic causes. When intestinal failure leads to permanent dependence on parenteral nutrition, patients are at risk for liver failure, eventual loss of central venous access, and catheter sepsis.[24] Small bowel transplantation with immunosuppressive treatment may be indicated for a subset of these patients and has resulted in improved outcomes. Early referral for transplantation should be considered once permanent TPN has become necessary. Multivisceral transplantation in children has also been reported, with 88.9% and 77.8% survival rates at 1 and 2 years, respectively, and all long-term survivors tolerating enteral feeding and off parenteral nutrition.[25] Intestinal and multivisceral (stomach, duodenum, pancreas, and intestine, with or without liver) transplantation has been extended to the adult population as well for short-bowel syndrome caused by intestinal infarction and for intestinal failure caused by chronic intestinal pseudo-obstruction.[26] With a mean age of 34.8 years and a mean TPN duration of 5.8 years, the 1-year graft survival rate was 88.4% for an isolated small bowel transplant and 42.8% for multivisceral transplants; the overall mortality rate was 18.5%.

REFERENCES

1. Parkman HP, Hasler WL, Fisher RS: American Gastroenterological Association technical review on the diagnosis and treatment of gastroparesis. Gastroenterology 127:1592-1622, 2004.
2. Miller LS, Szych GA, Kantor SB, et al: Treatment of idiopathic gastroparesis with injection of botulinum toxin into the pyloric sphincter muscle. Am J Gastroenterol 97:1653-1660, 2002.
3. Bromer MQ, Friedenberg F, Miller LS, et al: Endoscopic pyloric injection of botulinum toxin A for treatment of refractory gastroparesis. Gastrointest Endosc 61:833-839, 2005.
4. McCallum RW, Chen JD, Lin Z, et al: Gastric pacing improves emptying and symptoms in patients with gastroparesis. Gastroenterology 114:3456-3461, 1998.
5. Abell T, McCallum R, Hocking M, et al: Gastric electrical stimulation for medically refractory gastroparesis. Gastroenterology 125:421-428, 2003.
6. Mason RJ, Lipham J, Eckerling G, et al: Gastric electrical stimulation: An alternative surgical therapy for patients with gastroparesis. Arch Surg 140:841-848, 2005.
7. Maranki JL, Lytes V, Meilahn JE, et al: Predictive factors for clinical improvement with Enterra gastric electric stimulation treatment for refractory gastroparesis. Gastroenterology 130:A43, 2006.
8. McCallum R, Zhiyue L, Wetzel P, et al: Clinical response to gastric electrical stimulation in patients with postsurgical gastroparesis. Clin Gastroenterol Hepatol 3:49-54, 2005.
9. Schirmer BD: Mechanical and motility disorders of the stomach and duodenum. In Zuidema GD, Yeo CJ (eds): Shackelford's Surgery of the Alimentary Tract, 5th ed. Philadelphia, WB Saunders, 2002.
10. Meilahn JE, Dempsey DT: Postgastrectomy problems: Remedial operations and therapy. In Cameron JL (ed): Current Surgical Therapy, 8th ed, Philadelphia, Elsevier, 2004.
11. Forstner-Barthell AW, Murr MM, Nitecki S, et al: Near-total completion gastrectomy for severe postvagotomy gastric stasis: Analysis of early and long-term results in 62 patients. J Gastrointest Surg 3:115-121, 1999.
12. Xing J, Chen JDZ: Alterations of gastrointestinal motility in obesity. Obes Res 12:1723-1732, 2004.
13. Thomson ABR, Drozdowski L, Iordache C, et al: Small bowel review: Normal physiology, Part 2. Dig Dis Sci 48:1565-1581, 2003.
14. Kubota M, Kanda E, Ida K, et al: Severe gastrointestinal dysmotility in a patient with congenital myopathy: Causal relationship to decrease of interstitial cells of Cajal. Brain Dev 27:447-450, 2005.
15. Feldstein AE, Miller SM, El-Youssef M, et al: Chronic intestinal pseudoobstruction associated with altered interstitial cells of Cajal networks. J Pediatr Gastroenterol Nutr 36:492-497, 2003.
16. Yanagida H, Yanase H, Sanders KM, et al: Intestinal surgical resection disrupts electrical rhythmicity, neural responses, and interstitial cell networks. Gastroenterology 127:1748-1759, 2004.
17. Kuemmerle J: Motility disorders of the small intestine: New insights into old problems. J Clin Gastroenterol 31:276-281, 2000.
18. Tomita R, Ikeda T, Fujisaki S, et al: Upper gut motility of Hirschsprung's disease and its allied disorders in adults. Hepatogastroenterology 50:1959-1962, 2003.
19. Tursi A: Gastrointestinal motility disturbances in celiac disease. J Clin Gastroenterol 38:642-645, 2004.
20. Degen L, Petrig C, Studer D, et al: Effect of tegaserod on gut transit in male and female subjects. Neurogastroenterol Motil 17:821-826, 2005.
21. Arslan M, Bayraktar Y, Oksuzoglu G, et al: Four cases with chronic intestinal pseudo-obstruction due to hollow visceral myopathy. Hepatogastroenterology 46:349-352, 1999.
22. Endo M, Ukiyama E, Yokoyama J, et al: Subtotal duodenectomy with jejunal patch for megaduodenum secondary to congenital duodenal malformation. J Pediatr Surg 33:1636-1640, 1998.
23. Deguchi M, Shiraki K, Okano H, et al: Primary localized amyloidosis of the small intestine presenting as an intestinal pseudo-obstruction: Report of a case. Surg Today 31:1091-1093, 2001.
24. Bond GJ, Reyes JD: Intestinal transplantation for total/near-total aganglionosis and intestinal pseudo-obstruction. Semin Pediatr Surg 13:286-292, 2004.
25. Loinaz C, Mittal N, Kato T, et al: Multivisceral transplantation for pediatric intestinal pseudo-obstruction: Single center's experience of 16 cases. Transplant Proc 36:312-313, 2004.
26. Lauro A, Di Benedetto F, Masetti M, et al: Twenty-seven consecutive intestinal and multivisceral transplants in adult patients: A 4-year clinical experience. Transplant Proc 37:2679-2681, 2005.

Operations for Morbid Obesity

Robert E. Brolin · Christopher Kowalski

THE OBESITY EPIDEMIC

Prevalence

The term *epidemic* has frequently been used to describe the dramatic increase in the prevalence of both overweight and obesity in the United States. It was recently estimated that approximately two thirds of adults in the United States are overweight, with a body mass index (BMI) greater than 25kg/m^2, and that nearly half are obese, with a BMI greater than 30kg/m^2.[1] Other reports suggest that the most rapid increases in prevalence are seen in the most severely obese subgroups.[2] It is estimated that nearly 24 million Americans are severely obese, with a BMI greater than 35kg/m^2, and that more than 8 million are morbidly obese, with a BMI greater than 40kg/m^2.[3] The rate of obesity is increasing even more rapidly in children. It was recently estimated that more than 25% of children 17 years or younger are obese.[4] This percentage had more than doubled during the past decade. The prevalence of morbid obesity, a BMI greater than 40kg/m^2, may be increasing at a more rapid rate. There are a number of recent reports of severe obesity-related comorbid conditions in children, including type 2 diabetes, hypertension, hyperlipidemia, and sleep apnea syndrome.

Health Risk, Mortality

Entering the new millennium, it was estimated that obesity is the second leading cause of preventable deaths in the United States and that it accounts for approximately 300,000 deaths annually.[5] Moreover, it was projected that because of rapidly increasing prevalence, obesity would soon overtake cigarette smoking as the foremost cause of preventable deaths. The prevalence of complications related to severe obesity increases sharply

at a level corresponding to approximately 60% above desirable weight. At that level there is a twofold increase in morbidity and mortality. However, the slope of the "risk curve" rises almost exponentially above the 60% overweight level such that the complication rate corresponding to 100% above ideal weight is in the range of 13 to 14 times normal. Unfortunately, there is a paucity of actuarial statistics for adults who are more than 45 kg overweight. These data are particularly lacking in women, who are the most frequent subjects of obesity operations.

The mortality rate associated with *morbid* obesity, or a BMI greater than 40kg/mg^2, has not been accurately estimated. Until recently, only one study was focused on mortality differences between morbidly obese subjects and normal-weight individuals of similar age and gender. In 1980, Drenick et al. reported a markedly increased mortality rate in morbidly obese males versus age-matched normal-weight men (Fig. 63–1).[6] The most common causes of death in the overweight men in this study were myocardial infarction and stroke. More recently, there have been three published reports in which mortality was compared in surgically treated, morbidly obese patients and a similar age/gender group who did not have surgery. In 1997, MacDonald et al. reported a greater than sixfold increase in mortality among morbidly obese diabetics who for a variety of reasons did not undergo gastric bypass surgery after preoperative evaluation versus a similar age/gender mix of patients who underwent Roux-en-Y gastric bypass (RYGB).[7] In 2004, Flum and Dellinger reported a 1.5 times higher mortality rate over a 15-year period in 62,781 subjects who did not have surgery versus 3328 who had surgical treatment in Washington State.[8] The 1.9% operative mortality rate in the Washington report is at least twice as high as in most published series of bariatric surgical patients.[7,9,10] During the same year, Christou et al. reported 0.68% mortality in surgical patients versus

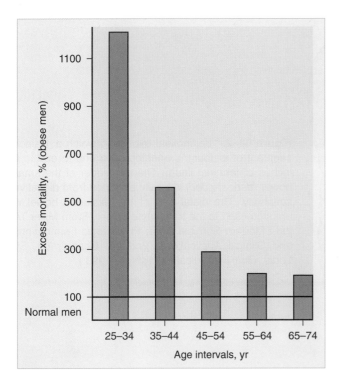

Figure 63–1. Comparison of excess mortality in men with morbid obesity *(red bars)* versus normal-weight men *(blue bars)* by age interval. (From Drenick EJ, Bale GS, Seltzer F, Johnson DG: Excessive mortality and causes of death in morbidly obese men. JAMA 243:443-335, 1980.)

| Table 63–1 | Diseases Associated with Severe Obesity |

Comorbidity	Incidence (%)
Hypertension	20-55
Obesity-hypoventilation/sleep apnea syndrome	20-50
Cholelithiasis	25-45
Degenerative osteoarthritis	20-50
Psychological depression	15-35
Hyperlipidemia	15-25
Diabetes mellitus	10-25
Asthmatic bronchitis	10-15
Coronary artery disease	5-15
Heart failure (right sided and/or left sided)	5-15
Stasis ulcers/venous insufficiency	5-15
Gastroesophageal reflux	5-15
Stress overflow urinary incontinence	5-15
Pseudomotor cerebri	1-2
Sexual hormone imbalance/infertility	—*
Malignancy (uterine, colon, gallbladder)	—*
Pulmonary embolism/thrombophlebitis	—*
Necrotizing subcutaneous infections	—*

Comorbid conditions are listed in the approximate order of reported frequency.
*Lack of specific numerical data in diseases known to be more common in obese patients.

a 6.17% death rate in a similar mix of nonoperative subjects monitored over a 16.5-year period, which represents a greater than 80% reduction in mortality risk in the surgical group.[11]

The health risk associated with severe obesity is intimately related to obesity-related illnesses. Table 63–1 shows a list of diseases associated with severe obesity. Although cardiovascular disease is reported as the leading cause of death in obese patients, the prevalence of cardiovascular symptoms in bariatric surgical cohorts is relatively low. Many obesity-related comorbid condition, such as degenerative arthritis, sleep apnea, and venous stasis, have a profoundly negative impact on *quality of life.*

Obesity-Related Cost

In 2000, the combined estimated direct and indirect costs associated with treatment of obesity and related comorbid conditions approached $117 billion.[1] At the same time, the annual expenditure in weight loss–related endeavors in the United States was conservatively estimated at $30 billion. Medicare is currently re-evaluating its policy on reimbursement for treatment of obesity because of the rapidly rising cost of obesity-related disability and medications used for the treatment of various comorbid diseases.

INDICATIONS FOR SURGERY

The primary premise as well as justification for surgical treatment of morbid obesity has been the compelling evidence that severe obesity is associated with a shortened life span and a variety of other serious medical problems. Severe obesity has been notoriously refractory to virtually every method of nonoperative treatment. The 2-year failure rate of diet and behavior modification in the morbidly obese approaches 100%. Many morbidly obese patients gain substantial weight after unsuccessful attempts at dieting. This so-called yo-yo syndrome is characterized by transient weight loss, followed by greater weight gain, and probably contributes to the refractoriness of nonsurgical treatment of severe obesity. A prospective randomized trial that compared a low-calorie diet with a now discarded method of stapled gastroplasty showed significantly better weight maintenance in the surgically treated group 2 years after intervention.[12] These results suggest that involuntary gastric restriction of oral intake is necessary for long-term weight control in morbidly obese patients.

In 1992 the National Institutes of Health Consensus Development Panel on gastrointestinal surgery for severe obesity recommended criteria for consideration of surgical treatment.[13] The panel recommended that surgical treatment be considered for any patient with a BMI of 40 kg/m² or higher who had failed serious attempts at nonsurgical treatment. The panel also recommended

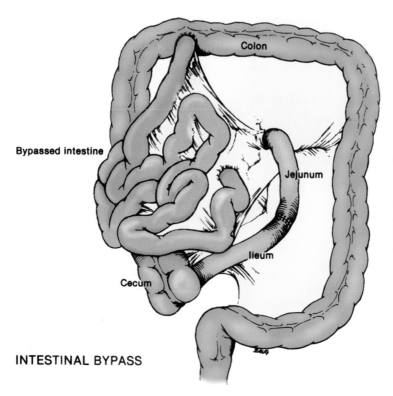

INTESTINAL BYPASS

Figure 63–2.   Jejunoileal bypass in which a 12-inch segment of jejunum is anastomosed end to end to 6 inches of terminal ileum. The remainder of the small bowel *(dark shaded)* is totally excluded from digestive continuity. The distal end of the excluded bowel is anastomosed to the transverse colon. (From Miller TA [ed]: Modern Surgical Care: Physiologic Foundations and Clinical Applications, 2nd ed. Chapter 68. St. Louis, Quality Medical Publishing, 1998.)

that surgery be considered for patients with a BMI of 35 kg/m² or greater who have serious coexisting medical problems such as diabetes, hypertension, hyperlipidemia, or sleep apnea.

Psychological stability should be assessed in some reliable manner before the operation, although standardized psychological tests and interviews with psychologists or psychiatrists have not reliably predicted postoperative outcome after obesity operations. However, many insurance carriers now require a formal psychological evaluation of prospective patients. Patients should also be carefully queried regarding the abuse of addictive drugs and alcohol before having surgery. All patients who undergo surgical treatment of obesity should be admonished that sustained long-term weight loss is not guaranteed merely by having an operation. This understanding is particularly important for patients who undergo gastric restrictive operations, which can be defeated by consuming large quantities of high-calorie liquids and soft junk food.

EARLY BARIATRIC OPERATIONS

Jejunoileal Bypass

The concept of surgery for morbid obesity was introduced by Kremen et al. in 1954 in the form of malabsorption-induced weight loss.[14] After experimenting with various lengths of jejunum and ileum, satisfactory weight loss was reported in patients in whom 30 to 35 cm of jejunum was anastomosed to 10 to 15 cm of terminal ileum (Fig. 63–2). During the 1960s and 1970s, thousands of intestinal bypasses were performed for the treatment of morbid obesity. However, by the mid-1970s, reports of serious late complications appeared in the

literature, including hepatic failure, urinary calculi, arthritis, and major nutritional deficiencies. Bacterial overgrowth of the distal bypassed bowel was suspected as the cause of the bypass enteritis syndrome, which was characterized by intermittent episodes of abdominal pain, bloating, arthralgia, rash, and diarrhea. The first public repudiation of jejunoileal bypass was delivered in 1979. Within less than 2 years jejunoileal bypass fell into a status of disrepute. Jejunoileal bypass is no longer recommended for the treatment of morbid obesity.[15]

Gastric Restrictive Operations

The concept of gastric restriction as treatment of morbid obesity was introduced by Mason and Ito in 1967.[16] All the current gastric operations are designed to restrict intake of solid food. Conversely, intake of liquids is not limited by these operations. In 1977, Mason et al. defined the anatomic parameters of restriction that were considered necessary for adequate weight loss with the gastric bypass operation, including a calibrated 1.2-cm-diameter gastrojejunostomy stoma and a small 50-ml-capacity upper gastric pouch.[17] Complication rates with gastric bypass decreased after introduction of the concept of stapling the stomach in continuity rather than dividing it. Use of the Roux-en-Y technique eliminated the problems with bile reflux esophagitis that were common after loop gastric bypass.

Stapled gastric partitioning was introduced in 1979. However, an unacceptably high incidence of early staple line failure led to a proliferation of modifications of gastric stapling in the hope of finding a more reliable technique. Gastroplasty techniques have evolved in favor of stapling in a vertical direction along the lesser curvature of the stomach. Stapling along the lesser curvature has also facilitated reinforcement of the outlet with prosthetic

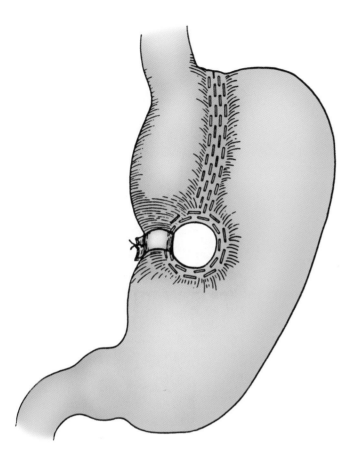

Vertical Banded Gastroplasty

Figure 63–3. Vertical banded gastroplasty in which an upper gastric pouch with a capacity of 15 to 20 ml empties into the remainder of the stomach through a calibrated stoma 5.0 cm in circumference. The stoma is reinforced with a strip of polypropylene (Marlex) mesh. The mesh is placed around the stoma through a "window" created by firing a circular stapling instrument alongside a 32-French bougie. (From Miller TA [ed]: Modern Surgical Care: Physiologic Foundations and Clinical Applications, 2nd ed. Chapter 68. St. Louis, Quality Medical Publishing, 1998.)

materials to prevent progressive stomal dilatation. Horizontal gastroplasty techniques have now been abandoned because of an unacceptably high incidence of staple line disruption, stomal dilation, and pouch dilation.

In 1982 Mason introduced vertical banded gastroplasty (VBG), as shown in Figure 63–3.[18] In VBG the stoma is reinforced with a strip of polypropylene (Marlex) mesh measuring 5.0 cm in circumference to create a stoma with an internal diameter of 1.0 to 1.2 cm. The mesh is placed around the stoma through a hole or window created by firing a circular stapling instrument alongside a 32-gauge-diameter bougie. The mesh is sutured to itself rather than the stomach, a modification that has greatly reduced the incidence of outlet stricture and leaks.

Morbidity and mortality rates with VBG have been low. An overall morbidity rate of less than 10% and a mortality rate of 0.25% were reported in a series of more than 1200 VBGs.[19] Early weight loss results have generally been

acceptable. MacLean et al. reported a mean 60% excess weight loss in 57 patients monitored for 5 years after VBG.[10] However, a substantial number of patients in this series required surgical revision for either complications or inadequate weight loss during the study period. There are remarkably few reports of long-term weight loss results after VBG. Weight loss maintenance after VBG has been somewhat problematic in that many patients regain at least 20% of their lost weight between 3 and 5 years postoperatively, perhaps in part because of increased intake of liquid or soft high-calorie foods that easily pass through the banded stoma.

CURRENT OPERATIONS

Roux-en-Y Gastric Bypass

RYGB is illustrated in Figure 63–4. Gastric bypass combines gastric restriction with a small amount of malabsorption. Many surgeons consider RYGB to be the "gold standard" bariatric operation because it has produced durable weight loss for most patients with an acceptable incidence of postoperative complications. Weight loss is in the range of 70% to 80% of the excess weight at 2 years with maintenance in the range of 50% to 60% after 5 years.[7,10] The East Carolina group showed maintenance of approximately 50% of the excess weight loss 14 years after RYGB.[7] No difference in weight loss has been found between the open and laparoscopic approach. There have been several large prospective randomized comparisons of RYGB with different gastric restrictive operations, each of which showed significantly better weight loss after gastric bypass and similar early morbidity rates.[9,20,21]

Currently, laparoscopic RYGB is the most commonly performed bariatric operation in the United States. RYGB was first performed via laparoscopy by Wittgrove and Clark in 1994.[22] Although the physiology and weight loss outcome of open and laparoscopic RYGB are essentially the same, there are considerable differences between the open and laparoscopic approach with respect to the required instrumentation and surgical skill set. Laparoscopic RYGB is a technically demanding procedure with a considerably longer learning curve than for the open approach.

Five distinct technical components are involved in performing laparoscopic RYGB: (1) abdominal access/trocar placement, (2) creation of the gastric pouch, (3) mobilization and positioning of the Roux limb, and (4) performance of the gastrojejunostomy and (5) jejunojejunostomy.

Most surgeons place five or six access ports in the upper part of the abdomen. The location of individual ports is influenced by the type of staplers to be used. Access is achieved with either a Veress needle or a 12-mm visualization port placed just below the left costal margin in the midclavicular line. After the abdomen is entered, CO_2 is insufflated at a pressure of 15 mm Hg. A 30-degree laparoscope is then inserted. The remaining ports are placed sequentially under direct visualization.

Creation of the upper gastric pouch begins by dividing the phrenoesophageal ligament at the angle of His with ultrasonic shears. The angle of His defines the end

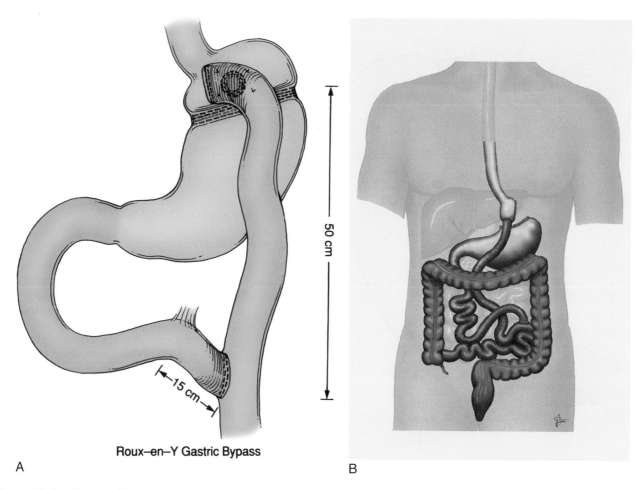

A   B

Figure 63–4.   Roux-en-Y gastric bypass (RYGB). **A,** The upper part of the stomach is stapled closed in continuity, which was typical of procedures performed in the 1980s and 1990s. An upper pouch with a capacity of 30 ml is created with exclusion of more than 95% of the stomach, all of the duodenum, and approximately 15 cm of proximal jejunum from digestive continuity. The Roux limb between the upper gastric pouch and jejunojejunostomy measures 50 cm in length. (From Brolin RE, Kenler HA, Gorman RC, Cody RP: The dilemma of outcome assessment after operations for morbid obesity. Surgery 105:337-346, 1989.) **B,** Transected retrocolic, antegastric RYGB typical of current laparoscopic techniques. (Courtesy of Inamed Health, Santa Barbara, CA.)

point of the gastric transection. Sliding-type hiatal hernias should be reduced before transection to prevent the creation of a large pouch. The lesser sac is then entered by dividing the vasa brevia along the lesser curvature of the stomach, starting 3 to 4 cm below the gastroesophageal junction. The stomach is then stapled horizontally with a 45-mm linear stapler. Subsequent stapling is directed vertically toward the angle of His until the stomach is completely transected. Usually, four or five firings of the 45-mm stapler are required to create a gastric pouch with a capacity of 15 to 30 ml.

The gastrojejunostomy can be performed with either a linear or a circular stapling device. In the circular approach, the anvil of the 21 mm or 25 mm EEA stapler is introduced into the gastric pouch either transorally attached to a percutaneous endoscopic gastrostomy (PEG)-type tube or with an endoscope or directly through a laparoscopic port site. In the transabdominal approach, a gastrotomy is required to place the EEA anvil into the gastric pouch before the stomach is completely transected. The gastrotomy site is then stapled shut after

the anvil is properly positioned within the pouch. Integrity of the gastrojejunostomy can be evaluated by several methods. Some surgeons pass an orogastric tube into the gastric pouch and instill 10 to 30 ml of a methylene blue dye/saline mixture. Others perform intraoperative upper endoscopy and air insufflation with the pouch submerged in normal saline. Anastomotic defects should be repaired immediately, after which a second test for integrity is performed.

The intestinal portion of the procedure begins with identification of the ligament of Treitz at the base of the transverse mesocolon. The jejunum is measured for a distance of 20 to 50 cm and divided with a 45-mm linear stapler. The Roux limb is then positioned in either an antecolic or retrocolic location before anastomosis to the gastric pouch. At this point the surgeon must avoid twisting the mesentery of the Roux limb. Division of the greater omentum is usually required when the antecolic route is chosen so that tension on the Roux limb is minimized. The circular stapler is placed in the abdomen via the left upper quadrant port site and inserted into the

Table 63–2	Complications After Open and Laparoscopic Gastric Bypass

	No. (%) of Patients		
Complication	**Open GBP**	**Laparoscopic GBP**	**_P_ Value**
Intraoperative			
Iatrogenic splenectomy	5/1218 (0.41)	Not reported	
Perioperative			
Anastomotic leak	42/2497 (1.68)	71/3464 (2.05)	.31
Bowel obstruction	Not reported	10/577 (1.73)	
Gastrointestinal tract hemorrhage	8/1334 (0.60)	11/570 (1.93)	.008
Pulmonary embolus	20/2577 (0.78)	11/2651 (0.41)	.09
Wound infection	34/513 (6.63)	97/3258 (2.98)	<.001
Pneumonia	5/1504 (0.33)	3/2075 (0.14)	.24
Death	24/2771 (0.87)	8/3464 (0.23)	.001
Late			
Bowel obstruction	53/2507 (2.11)	91/2887 (3.15)	.02
Incisional hernia	128/1492 (8.58)	14/2958 (0.47)	<.001
Stomal stenosis	12/2233 (0.67)	164/3464 (4.73)	<.001

Comparison of postoperative complications between open and laparoscopic gastric bypass (GPB).
Data from Podnos YD, Jimenez JC, Wilson SF, et al: Complications after laparoscopic gastric bypass. A review of 3464 cases. Arch Surg 138:957-961, 2003.

proximal end of the Roux limb. The spike of the circular stapler is advanced through the antimesenteric border of the Roux limb and engaged with the anvil protruding from the pouch. The stapler is fired and removed. The redundant open end of the Roux limb is then resected flush with the gastrojejunostomy with a linear stapler to avoid a long afferent limb, which can increase reservoir capacity.

Creation of the jejunojejunostomy begins by measuring the Roux limb distally for a distance of 75 to 150 cm from the gastrojejunostomy. Most surgeons perform a side-to-side, stapled anastomosis with a linear stapler. Several techniques can be used to close the enterotomies that remain after side-to-side stapling, including stapling in a perpendicular orientation to the previous stapling and laparoscopic suture closure. Alignment after stapled closure of the enterotomy defects must be precise to avoid kinking and obstruction. Several so-called antiobstruction stitches should be placed between the distal Roux limb and the biliopancreatic limb to prevent kinking at the anastomosis. Many surgeons are fastidious in closing mesenteric defects at the jejunojejunostomy site, including mesocolic defects (in the retrocolic technique) and Petersen's space. Closure of mesenteric defects should be performed with a nonabsorbable suture.

Postoperative morbidity and mortality rates observed with current techniques of RYGB are in the range of 10% and 1%, respectively. Table 63–2 shows a comparison of postoperative complications during open and laparoscopic RYGB.[23] The incidence of incisional hernia and wound infection is significantly lower with laparoscopic RYGB than with the open approach. Conversely, the incidence of bowel obstruction from internal hernia is significantly higher after the laparoscopic approach and ranges from 2% to 8%.[23] The majority of internal hernias occur in mesenteric defects at the jejunojejunostomy or at Petersen's space. Internal herniation can be manifested as mild intermittent distention with crampy abdominal pain or as complete bowel obstruction with or without bowel infarction. Symptoms may be intermittent. The single most useful radiologic test in evaluating the possibility of internal hernia, small bowel obstruction, or both in patients after RYGB is probably computed tomography (CT) with oral contrast. Prompt passage of oral contrast into the colon and absence of distention in the bypassed stomach and duodenum are reassuring signs that an internal hernia with obstruction is unlikely. Although radiographic imaging aids in diagnosis, persistent symptoms in the face of equivocal radiographs should prompt exploration.

Typical mortality statistics of large published series of bariatric surgical patients were challenged in an article by Flum et al., which showed 30-day and 1-year death rates of 2.0% and 4.6%, respectively, in a series of 16,155 Medicare patients who underwent bariatric operations between 1996 and 2002.[24] The 30-day and 1-year mortality rates in the age 65 and over Medicare patients were an astounding 4.8% and 11.1%, respectively. Mortality rates were significantly less for high-volume surgeons versus low-volume (≤35 procedures annually) surgeons. Two findings in this important study warrant emphasis:

1. The mortality rate of bariatric operations (and likely other complex surgical procedures) is lowest in the hands of the most experienced surgeons.
2. The mortality rate of bariatric operations published in peer-reviewed journals is considerably better than that of the community at large.

Gastric bypass is occasionally associated with symptoms of "dumping syndrome," including nausea, bloating, diarrhea, and colic. These symptoms are thought to be due to rapid emptying of the small gastric pouch directly into the small bowel. Vasomotor symptoms of dumping are associated with hypoglycemia and include lightheadedness, palpitations, and sweating. These symptoms occur in a smaller percentage of patients. The severity of dumping after gastric bypass is variable, with some patients reporting no symptoms, others having symptoms associated with eating specific foods such as milk products or sweets, and a few patients reporting troublesome symptoms after almost every meal.

Several metabolic complications are inherent in gastric bypass surgery, including iron, folate, and vitamin B_{12} deficiencies, each of which may result in anemia. Because of the relatively high incidence of these micronutrient deficiencies, prophylactic multivitamin/mineral supplements are routinely given to all patients who undergo gastric bypass. However, the efficacy of multivitamin supplements in prevention of both iron and calcium deficiency is problematic. In our experience, a daily multivitamin supplement does not consistently prevent the development of iron deficiency and anemia in women who have undergone gastric bypass. Additional supplements of specific vitamins or minerals in addition to multivitamins are frequently necessary to correct these deficiencies. Fortunately, the vast majority of vitamin and mineral deficiencies after gastric bypass are subclinical and easily corrected with oral supplements of the deficient micronutrients. Injection therapy is rarely required in patients who are willing to take oral supplements. Hospitalization for treatment of these vitamin and mineral deficiencies is rare.

Malabsorption of protein, carbohydrate, and fat has not been documented after conventional gastric bypass.

Gastric Banding

Gastric banding is the most commonly performed bariatric operation in Europe and Australia. Early techniques of gastric banding incorporated a premeasured strip of prosthetic material to restrict oral intake. However, these techniques lacked precision in measuring the volume of stomach above the band. The circumference of the band was generally in the range of 5.0 cm, similar to the measurements used for VBG. The band is sutured to both itself and the stomach to prevent "slipping." Complication rates with nonadjustable techniques of gastric banding were relatively high, with morbidity and mortality rates in the range of 30% and 3%, respectively.[25] Band erosion occurred in 10% to 15% of cases. Erosion occasionally resulted in leaks and obstruction that frequently required reoperation. The concept of an inflatable silicone band was introduced by Kuzmak in 1988.[26] The diameter of the inflatable band is adjusted by infusion of saline through a subcutaneous reservoir. The reported weight loss results and the complication rate with inflatable bands are better than those observed after nonadjustable banding techniques in which strips of polypropylene or Teflon were used.

Kuzmak's concept of adjustability was incorporated into laparoscopic approaches. Currently, there are two major brands of laparoscopic adjustable gastric bands: the Lap-Band (Inamed Health, Santa Barbara, California) and the Swedish adjustable gastric band (Obtech Medical, Baar, Switzerland). The Food and Drug Administration approved the Lap-Band device for use in the United States in June 2001. This device is illustrated in Figure 63–5. Adjustable gastric bands are placed laparoscopically via five or six access ports. The original technique used to position the adjustable gastric band involved perigastric dissection high along the lesser curvature of the stomach and entering the omenta bursalis. The band is passed around the upper part of the stomach through this space. Because the perigastric approach was associated with an excessive rate of pouch enlargement and prolapse, the pars flaccida technique was introduced.[27] Dissection with this technique begins at the angle of His, where the phrenoesophageal ligament is opened. The pars flaccida along the lesser curvature of the stomach is then incised to expose the anterior border of the right diaphragmatic crus. A grasper is advanced behind the upper part of the stomach toward the angle of His.

The adjustable band is then inserted into the abdomen. One end of the band is grasped at the angle of His, pulled behind the stomach, and locked anteriorly to create a small proximal gastric pouch. Several nonabsorbable stitches are then placed in the stomach to secure the band as shown in Figure 63–5. The tubing is pulled from the band through the subcutaneous tissue and connected to the access port. The port is secured to the abdominal wall fascia with four nonabsorbable sutures placed through the eyelets on the port. The presence of a hiatal hernia makes band placement more difficult because the normal anatomic landmarks are distorted. Some surgeons consider hiatal hernia an absolute contraindication to banding. Others recommend repair of the crus concomitant with band placement. The gastric band gradually forms a fibrous membrane that fixes its position around the stomach.

Adjustments begin approximately 6 to 8 weeks after placement and fixation of the band. These adjustments are essential for weight loss and regulate the amount of solid food that can be consumed at one sitting. Usually, four to six adjustments are required during the first year after placement.

Perioperative complications are rare after adjustable gastric banding, with the most common being infection at the access port, which occurs in about 1% of cases and usually requires removal of the port.[27,28] Occasionally, the tubing and band can be spared from port site infection by capping the tubing and reducing it intraperitoneally while the wound heals. After the infection has cleared, the tubing can be reconnected to a new port.

Late complications after adjustable laparoscopic banding are more common and include difficulty with accessing the subcutaneous port, tubing problems, gastric prolapse or "slip," band erosion, esophageal obstruction/dilatation, and dilatation of the gastric pouch. Tubing breaks and problems with access to the

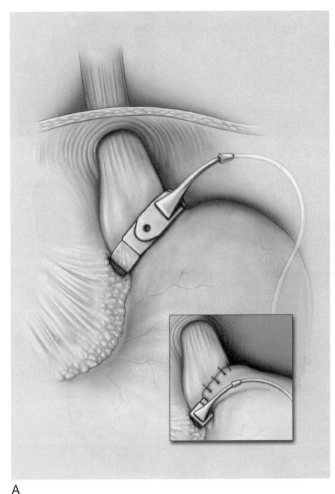

A

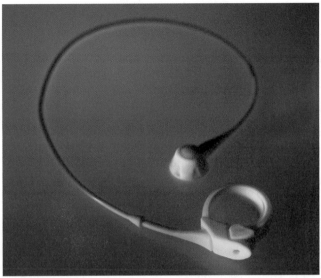

B

Figure 63–5. A, Lap-Band (Inamed, Santa Barbara, California) in situ just below the gastroesophageal junction. The *inset* shows imbricating sutures that fix the band to the stomach. **B,** Entire Lap-Band device, including tubing and access port. (Courtesy of Inamed Health, Santa Barbara, California.)

subcutaneous port for adjustments occur in 1% to 5% of patients.[28,29] The fixation sutures may occasionally become separated from the fascia and result in angling of the port away from the skin. Although fluoroscopy can facilitate access in these cases, some malrotated ports require repositioning or replacement.

"Slippage" of the band encompasses a spectrum of problems, including gastric pouch dilatation because of placement of the band too low on the stomach and prolapse of the distal part of the stomach beneath the band. Herniation of the distal fundus through the band with resulting necrosis is a rare life-threatening complication. Prolapse may occur on either the anterior or posterior aspect of the stomach. Causes of band prolapse include excessive perigastric dissection, the presence of a sliding hiatal hernia, and protracted, forcible vomiting. Another cause of gastric pouch dilatation is overinflation of the band. It is important to distinguish prolapse from gastric pouch dilatation because prolapse requires operative treatment. Conversely, deflation of the band frequently resolves simple dilatation. Widespread adoption of the pars flaccida technique has reduced the incidence of pouch enlargement and prolapse to approximately 1% and 3% of cases, respectively.[28-30]

Erosion or intragastric migration of adjustable gastric bands occurs in 1% to 3% of patients.[28,30] Possible causes include gradual pressure necrosis and subclinical injury to the stomach adjacent to the band. Band erosion requires operative removal of the band and repair of the residual defect. These procedures may be difficult because of intense inflammatory scarring.

Esophageal dilatation may occur either in the perioperative period or, more commonly, months to years after surgery. Acute esophageal obstruction is rare, whereas late dilatation of the esophagus may be relatively common.[31] The clinical significance of this problem is disputed because most cases are easily remedied by deflation of the band. Conversely, cases associated with dysphagia and complete esophageal obstruction have been reported. Band erosion should be ruled out as the cause of obstruction in these cases.

Weight loss with most techniques of gastric banding has been less consistent than weight loss reported after banded gastroplasty and RYGB. Weight loss after gastric banding is slower (3- to 5-lb weight loss per month) than after other bariatric procedures, but it tends to be protracted over a longer time frame (3 to 4 years).[28,30] Weight loss with the laparoscopic adjustable gastric band is better at international centers than in the United States. International series report mean percent excess weight loss ranging from 40% to 70% with a follow-up of 3 to 8 years.[28-30,32] Results in the United States have been mixed and range between 32% and 58% excess weight loss with a follow-up of 4 years.[31,32]

Biliopancreatic Diversion

Biliopancreatic diversion combines a modest amount of gastric restriction with substantial malabsorption. The concept of biliopancreatic diversion was introduced by Scopinaro during the late 1970s.[33] The technique includes performance of subtotal gastrectomy, with an approximately 400-ml-capacity gastric remnant anastomosed to the proximal ileum. All of the jejunum is excluded from digestive continuity and is anastomosed end to side to a "common channel" of ileum 50 cm proximal to the ileocecal junction. Because this degree of malabsorption predisposes to cholelithiasis, cholecystectomy is also routinely performed. In 1987 DeMeester introduced the duodenal switch procedure for treatment of refractory bile reflux gastritis.[34] Hess, Marceau, and colleagues independently modified this technique of biliopancreatic diversion for bariatric patients.[35,36] A conventional modification of the duodenal switch is illustrated in Figure 63–6. This procedure preserves enough parietal cells that vitamin B_{12} deficiency and marginal ulcers are unusual late complications.

Early postoperative complications are reported in 30% of patients who undergo biliopancreatic diversion, with a 1.3% mortality rate. However, the incidence of metabolic complications within the first postoperative year has been high, including a 30% incidence of anemia, an 8% to 10% incidence of marginal ulcers, and a 20% incidence of hospitalization for treatment of protein-calorie malnutrition.[33] Deaths from hepatic failure have been reported in patients who underwent biliopancreatic diversion. Weight loss results with biliopancreatic bypass have been almost uniformly good. A mean loss of 70% of preoperative weight was reported in a series of 57 patients monitored for more than 18 years, with excellent weight maintenance after stabilization.[37] Other surgeons have reported an average weight gain of only 5% from the point of maximum weight loss at 5 years after biliopancreatic diversion.[35]

REVISION OPERATIONS

Occasionally, bariatric operations require revision for either inadequate weight loss or late complications. The incidence of major postoperative complications after revision of bariatric procedures is high, with reports ranging from 15% to 60% and a mortality rate ranging from 0% to 15%. The reoperating surgeon must be aware of a persistent gastrogastric fistula and ischemic or undrained gastric remnants (or both). Patients who undergo revision operations for complications frequently have lost a sufficient amount of weight after their initial procedure. These patients should generally be offered a gastric restrictive rather than a malabsorptive procedure. Patients who require takedown of an intestinal bypass for metabolic complications and are no longer overweight are best managed by conversion to a banded gastroplasty for weight maintenance. Conversely, intestinal or biliopancreatic bypass patients who remain substantially overweight are best converted to RYGB in the hope of providing further weight loss through the added gastric restriction. Gastroplasty patients with stomal

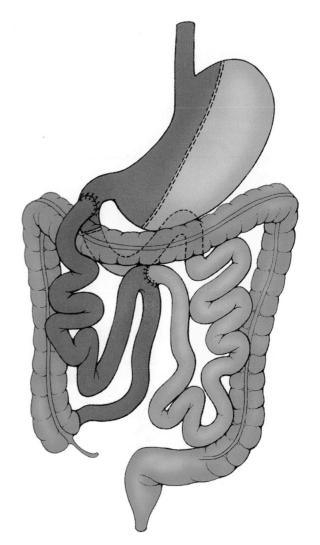

Duodenal Switch

Figure 63–6. Biliopancreatic diversion with duodenal switch. Two thirds of the stomach is excised along the greater curvature with linear staplers. The duodenum is dissected from the head of the pancreas for a distance of 5 cm beyond the pylorus and transected. The ileum is then transected at a point 250 cm proximal to the ileocecal junction. The distal end of the transected ileum *(shaded)* is anastomosed to the proximal duodenum. The remainder of the small bowel *(unshaded portion)* is diverted from the digestive stream. The distal end of the bypassed segment is reanastomosed to the ileum 100 to 150 cm proximal to the ileocecal junction to create the common channel. (From Miller TA [ed]: Modern Surgical Care: Physiologic Foundations and Clinical Applications, 2nd ed. Chapter 68. St. Louis, Quality Medical Publishing, 1998.)

stenosis and an intact staple line may undergo stomal dilatation by upper endoscopy. Endoscopic dilatation is usually performed with balloon-tip dilators. Unfortunately, less than 50% of patients with stomal stenosis obtain permanent relief with dilatation. Patients who do not respond to dilatation require operative revision, which is best accomplished by conversion to RYGB.

Reversal of bariatric operations without conversion to another weight reduction procedure is invariably associated with prompt regaining of previously lost weight. Gastroplasty patients with unsatisfactory weight loss are best converted to RYGB or, in some cases, biliopancreatic diversion. Gastroplasty or RYGB patients with staple line disruption require transection of the stomach between staple lines. There is a high incidence of subsequent staple line disruption in patients who undergo restapling in continuity. Gastric bypass patients with anatomically intact operations and unsatisfactory weight loss have almost certainly "outeaten" the operation. These patients may be converted to a biliopancreatic diversion procedure with anticipation of further weight loss. A small number of morbidly obese patients will "outeat" any bariatric operation or die trying. Whenever a patient has failed a second technically sound and intact operation, surgeons should approach the prospect of further revision with considerable caution and skepticism. Rejection of such patients for another operation is frequently a prudent decision.

PERIOPERATIVE CARE

All candidates for obesity operations should be interviewed in an outpatient setting before being considered for surgery. During the screening interview, the surgeon should provide prospective patients with a clear understanding of the risks and goals of the operation and explain the mechanism by which the proposed procedure produces weight loss. At the same time, the surgeon should obtain a complete medical history and make a preliminary assessment of the patient's operative risk. Psychological stability should also be evaluated, particularly in terms of the patient's willingness to adjust to the permanent postoperative side effects of gastric restriction and malabsorption. At the conclusion of the interview, the patient should have obtained sufficient information to give informed consent.

Routine preadmission tests include a complete blood count, Chem-21 screen, urinalysis, chest radiograph, electrocardiogram, testing for *Helicobacter pylori* antigen, and ultrasound of the gallbladder. *H. pylori* testing is performed to rule out a treatable cause of postoperative peptic ulcer disease. Patients with a positive test are treated with a combination of antibiotic and proton pump inhibitor therapy. Patients who have symptoms of gastroesophageal reflux disease or peptic ulcer disease should undergo upper endoscopy. An active peptic ulcer is a contraindication to bariatric surgery. The reported incidence of biliary tract disease in the morbidly obese ranges from 25% to 45%, which is three to four times higher than that in the normal-weight population. Hence, preoperative or intraoperative screening for gallstones is recommended in all bariatric surgical patients who have not undergone cholecystectomy. Ultrasonography is the most popular method of evaluation. The reported incidence of symptomatic cholelithiasis after obesity operations ranges from 3% to more than 50%, depending on the type of operation performed. Because symptomatic gallstones developed in more than 50% of patients after Scopinaro's biliopancreatic bypass, it has

been recommended that routine cholecystectomy be included as an integral part of that operation. The incidence of gallbladder disease after gastric restrictive operations varies from 3% to greater than 30%. Most surgeons do not perform prophylactic cholecystectomy during gastric restrictive operations, even though the risk of adding cholecystectomy to these procedures is negligible. Ultrasound of the gallbladder is performed to rule out unsuspected gallstones. Patients scheduled to have gastric or biliopancreatic bypass operations should also undergo testing for serum iron, iron-binding capacity, and vitamin B_{12}. Levels of fat-soluble vitamins should be obtained in patients before biliopancreatic diversion. All patients scheduled to undergo revision of a failed bariatric procedure should have blood cross-matched for possible transfusion because blood transfusion is often necessary in patients who undergo revision of failed gastric restrictive operations. All patients should be given intravenous (IV) prophylactic antibiotics during the perioperative period.

Although bariatric surgical patients do not require admission to the intensive care unit (ICU) postoperatively, all patients with sleep apnea, congestive heart failure, or severe asthmatic bronchitis should be considered for admission to the ICU for close monitoring of their cardiopulmonary status. Occasionally, patients who undergo open operations require overnight intubation. Conversely, virtually all patients who undergo laparoscopic operations are extubated within the first several hours postoperatively.

Because obesity is considered a risk factor for postoperative pulmonary embolism, a variety of methods of prophylaxis have been used in an attempt to prevent this feared complication, including subcutaneous low-dose heparin or enoxaparin (Lovenox), pneumatic compression stockings, IV low-molecular-weight dextran, and use of the Trendelenburg position intraoperatively. However, none of these methods have been proved to decrease the incidence of postoperative venous thromboembolism in bariatric surgical patients. Early postoperative ambulation is strongly encouraged and almost certainly contributes to the low incidence of postoperative venous thromboembolism reported in laparoscopic patients. All patients should get out of bed on the night of their operation and walk on the first postoperative day. Prophylactic superior vena cava filters should be considered in patients with a history of deep venous thrombosis or pulmonary embolism.

We routinely use IV patient-controlled analgesia (PCA) in postoperative bariatric patients. PCA provides more consistent pain relief than do intermittent intramuscular injections of narcotic analgesics. Oral narcotics are usually begun on the second or third postoperative day after administration of IV fluids has been stopped. All pills and tablets are crushed and administered as a slurry with a liquid beverage. Patients are instructed to not swallow whole pills during the first 4 weeks postoperatively.

A limited upper gastrointestinal contrast study is routinely performed on the first or second day to examine the integrity of the staple line and outlet stoma, although some experts have questioned the utility of this approach. If the contrast study is unremarkable, a clear liquid diet is begun. IV fluids are discontinued after clear liquids are tolerated without difficulty. A maximum 1000-calorie full-liquid diet is started on the next day, followed by a pureed diet shortly thereafter. Patients are usually discharged on the second or third postoperative day. Hospitalization for more than 4 days is unusual in the absence of major complications.

Severe distention of the bypassed stomach is an unusual, but serious complication that can be managed by percutaneous decompression or Stamm gastrostomy.

FOLLOW-UP AND DIETARY MANAGEMENT

Postoperative follow-up is extremely important in bariatric surgical patients. During the first year postoperatively, visits are scheduled at 1 week, at 4 weeks, and then at 3-month intervals thereafter. Two follow-up visits are scheduled at 6-month intervals during the second year, with subsequent annual visits. All patients should have easy access to both the operating surgeon and a clinical nutritionist.

Postoperative dietary counseling is essential to the long-term success of bariatric operations. Patients are instructed to follow a full liquid pureed diet for 4 weeks after discharge. A liquid or chewable multivitamin supplement is taken during this phase of the diet. The purpose of the pureed liquid diet is to (1) allow time for patients to adjust to their tremendously restricted stomach capacity by consuming foods that are relatively easy to chew and swallow and (2) minimize the likelihood of vomiting during the early postoperative period. Repeated episodes of vomiting during the early postoperative period have been associated with staple line disruption and leaks. Patients are started on a soft solid diet at the 4-week visit and then gradually progress to a normal diet. Patients can resume swallowing whole pills and tablets after solid food is well tolerated.

Patients who undergo gastric bypass or biliopancreatic diversion require periodic blood tests to check for possible nutritional deficiencies. These patients should take a multivitamin supplement with minerals daily for the rest of their lives. Menstruating women who have undergone gastric or biliopancreatic bypass should also take additional prophylactic iron supplements. Oral calcium supplementation of at least 1 g daily should be taken by all bypass patients. After biliopancreatic diversion, many patients require additional protein and other nutritional supplements, particularly fat-soluble vitamins.

AMELIORATION OF OBESITY-RELATED DISEASES

Amelioration of obesity-related medical problems is a primary goal of all bariatric operations. The incidence of type 2 diabetes mellitus in the morbidly obese ranges from 10% to 20%. Improvement or resolution of morbid obesity–associated diabetes, including a significant decrease in insulin resistance after weight reduction

surgery, has been reported by many investigators. Postoperative changes in glucose metabolism in morbidly obese diabetic patients have been studied extensively. Pories, Schauer, and colleagues independently reported that nearly 85% of patients with either overt diabetes or impaired glucose tolerance become euglycemic after open and laparoscopic RYGB.[38,39] Fasting insulin and glycosylated hemoglobin concentrations were also reduced to normal levels, whereas insulin release, insulin resistance, and utilization of glucose were substantially improved.

There is relatively little information about the effects of weight reduction surgery on obesity-related cardiovascular dysfunction. Echocardiography was used to measure a number of parameters of ventricular function in 63 morbidly obese patients. Surgically induced weight loss was associated with significant improvement in left ventricular ejection fraction and smaller, but measurable improvements in mean blood pressure, cardiac chamber size, and ventricular wall thickness.[40] Two groups have independently reported the response of blood pressure to weight loss in hypertensive patients after RYGB. Although each group noted improvement or resolution of high blood pressure in approximately 70% of patients after weight stabilization, there were conflicting results relative to the magnitude of the weight loss. One group found a significant correlation between improved blood pressure and proximity to ideal weight.[41] The other reported a correlation between improved blood pressure and the absolute quantity of weight lost.[42]

The ameliorative effects of weight reduction surgery on obesity-related hyperlipidemia have been documented by a number of investigators. Independent reports have demonstrated significant decreases in both total cholesterol and triglyceride levels after both gastroplasty and gastric bypass. Several investigators reported high-density lipoprotein/low-density lipoprotein ratios after gastric bypass and suggested that the risk for atherosclerosis may be decreased by surgically induced weight loss.[43] Our group and others have shown that these lipid reductions persist for as long as weight loss is satisfactorily maintained.[44] Occasionally, patients who regain a substantial portion of their lost weight are able to maintain the salutary changes in lipid profile.

Obesity-hypoventilation syndrome probably poses the greatest immediate risk to life of any of the obesity-related comorbid conditions. There have been a number of independent reports of complete resolution of sleep apnea symptoms and significant improvement in both arterial blood gas parameters and lung volumes after gastric restrictive operations. Significant reductions in mean pulmonary artery pressure have also been reported in patients with obesity-hypoventilation syndrome after RYGB.[45] Many patients in these reports were incapacitated by their condition preoperatively but, after losing weight, were able to lead normal lives.

Morbidly obese women of childbearing age are known to have a high incidence of infertility, as well as other menstrual and hormonal problems. Perioperative abnormalities have been reported in sex hormone–binding globulin (SHBG) in infertile morbidly obese women who were attempting pregnancy. However, after gastroplasty-induced weight loss, there were significant improvements in SHBG levels and a significantly decreased incidence of irregular menses.[46] A number of previously infertile women became pregnant and delivered normal babies after surgically induced weight loss. Similar results were reported by another group after gastric bypass. Despite restricted intake, both the mother and the developing fetus maintained adequate nutritional status. Pregnancy is not recommended during the period of active postoperative weight loss (the first 18 months postoperatively).

Although the proliferation in numbers of bariatric surgical procedures has slowed during the past 2 years, it appears that a need for surgical treatment will continue to exist in the absence of an effective alternative treatment. The current gastric restrictive operations appear to be safe and effective enough to justify their continued use. At present, surgery offers the only realistic hope for successful weight loss in the morbidly obese.

REFERENCES

1. Field AE, Barnoya J, Colditz GA: Epidemiology and health economic consequences of obesity. In Wadden TA, Stunkard AJ (eds): Handbook of Obesity Treatment. New York, Guilford, 2002, pp 3-18.
2. Storm R: Increases in clinically severe obesity in the United States, 1986-2000. Arch Intern Med 163:2146-2148, 2003.
3. Buchwald H, Avidor Y, Braunwald E, et al: Bariatric surgery: A systematic review and meta-analysis. JAMA 292:1724-1737, 2004.
4. Deckelbaum RJ, Williams CL: Childhood obesity: The health issue. Obes Res 9(Suppl):239-243, 2001.
5. Wolf AM, Colditz GA: Current estimates of the economic cost of obesity in the United States. Obes Res 6:97-106, 1998.
6. Drenick EJ, Bale GS, Seltzer F, Johnson DG: Excessive mortality and causes of death in morbidly obese men. JAMA 243:443-445, 1980.
7. MacDonald KG, Long SD, Swanson MS, et al: The gastric bypass operation reduces the progression and mortality of non–insulin dependent diabetes mellitus. J Gastrointest Surg 1:213-220, 1997.
8. Flum DR, Dellinger EP: Impact of gastric bypass operation on survival: A population-based analysis. J Am Coll Surg 199:543-551, 2004.
9. Sugerman HJ, Starkey JV, Birkenhauer R: A randomized prospective trial of gastric bypass versus vertical banded gastroplasty for morbid obesity and their effects on sweets versus non-sweets eaters. Ann Surg 205:613-624, 1987.
10. MacLean LD, Rhode BM, Sampalis J, Forse RA: Results of the surgical treatment of obesity. Am J Surg 165:155-160, 1993.
11. Christou NV, Sampalis JS, Lieberman M, et al: Surgery decreases mortality, morbidity, and health care use in morbidly obese patients. Ann Surg 240:416-424, 2004.
12. Andersen T, Larssen U: Dietary outcome in patients treated with a gastroplasty program. Am J Clin Nutr 50:1328-1340, 1989.
13. National Institutes of Health Consensus Development Panel: Gastrointestinal surgery for severe obesity. Am J Clin Nutr 55(Suppl):615-619, 1992.
14. Kremen AJ, Linner JH, Nelson CH: An experimental evaluation of the nutritional importance of proximal and distal small intestine. Ann Surg 140:439-448, 1954.
15. Griffen WO Jr, Bivins RA, Bell RM: The decline and fall of jejunoileal bypass. Surg Gynecol Obstet 157:301-308, 1983.
16. Mason EE, Ito C: Gastric bypass and obesity. Surg Clin North Am 47:1345-1352, 1967.
17. Mason EE, Printen KJ, Hartford CE, Boyd WE: Optimizing results of gastric bypass. Arch Surg 112:799-804, 1977.
18. Mason EE: Vertical banded gastroplasty for morbid obesity. Arch Surg 117:701-706, 1982.
19. Mason EE, Doherty C, Maher JW, et al: Super obesity and gastric reduction procedures. Gastroenterol Clin North Am 16:495-502, 1987.
20. Lechner GW, Callender K: Subtotal gastric exclusion and gastric partitioning: A randomized prospective comparison of one hundred patients. Surgery 90:637-644, 1981.
21. Hall JC, Watts JM, O'Brien PE, et al: Gastric surgery for morbid obesity. The Adelaide Study. Ann Surg 211:419-427, 1990.
22. Wittgrove AC, Clark GW, Tremblay LJ: Laparoscopic gastric bypass, Roux-en-Y: Preliminary report of five cases. Obes Surg 4:353-357, 1994.
23. Podnos YD, Jimenez JC, Wilson SF, et al: Complications after laparoscopic gastric bypass. A review of 3464 cases. Arch Surg 138:957-961, 2003.
24. Flum DR, Salem L, Broeckel Elrod JA, et al: Early mortality among Medicare beneficiaries undergoing bariatric surgical procedures. JAMA 294:1903-1908, 2005.
25. Granstrom L: Gastric banding: Study of one method for surgical treatment of massive obesity. Acta Chir Scand Suppl 1987;536:1-48.
26. Kuzmak LI: Gastric banding. In Dietel M (ed): Surgery for the Morbidly Obese Patient. Philadelphia, Lea & Febiger, 1989, p 225.
27. Fielding GA, Allan JW: A step-by-step guide to the placement of the Lap Band adjustable gastric banding system. Am J Surg 184:S26-S30, 2002.
28. Chapman AE, Kiroff G, Game P, et al: Laparoscopic adjustable gastric banding in the treatment of obesity: A systematic literature review. Surgery 135:326-351, 2004.
29. Fielding GA, Rhodes M, Nathanson LK: Laparoscopic gastric banding for morbid obesity. Surgical outcomes in 335 cases. Surg Endosc 13:550-554, 1999.
30. Weiner R, Blanco-Engert R, Weiner S, Matkowitz R, et al: Outcome after laparoscopic adjustable gastric banding—8 years experience. Obes Surg 13:427-434, 2003.
31. DeMaria EJ, Sugerman HJ: A critical look at laparoscopic adjustable gastric banding for surgical treatment of morbid obesity: Does it measure up? Surg Endosc 14:697-699, 2000.
32. Biertho L, Steffen R, Ricklin T, et al: Laparoscopic gastric bypass versus adjustable gastric banding: A comparative study of 1,200 cases. J Am Coll Surg 197:536-547, 2003.
33. Scopinaro N, Gianetta E, Friedman D, et al: Biliopancreatic diversion for obesity. Probl Gen Surg 9:362-379, 1992.
34. DeMeester TR, Fuchs KH, Ball CS, et al: Experimental and clinical results with proximal end-to-end duodenojejunostomy for pathologic duodenogastric reflux. Ann Surg 205:414-426, 1987.
35. Lagace M, Marceau P, Marceau S, et al: Biliopancreatic diversion with a new type of gastrectomy: Some previous conclusions revisited. Obes Surg 5:411-416, 1995.
36. Hess DS, Hess DW: Biliopancreatic diversion with duodenal switch. Obes Surg 8:267-282, 1998.
37. Scopinaro N, Gianetta E, Adami GF, et al: Biliopancreatic diversion for obesity at eighteen years. Surgery 119:261-268, 1996.
38. Pories WJ, Caro JF, Flickinger EG, et al: The control of diabetes mellitus (NIDDM) in the morbidly obese with the Greenville gastric bypass. Ann Surg 206:316-323, 1987.
39. Schauer PR, Barguera B, Ikramuddin S, et al: Effect of laparoscopic Roux-en-Y gastric bypass on type 2 diabetes mellitus. Ann Surg 238:467-484, 2003.
40. Alpert MA, Terry BE, Kelly DL: Effect of weight loss on cardiac chamber size, wall thickness and left ventricular function in morbid obesity. Am J Cardiol 56:783-786, 1985.
41. Carson JL, Ruddy ME, Duff AE, et al: The effect of gastric bypass surgery on hypertension in morbidly obese patients. Arch Intern Med 154:193-200, 1994.
42. Foley EF, Benotti PN, Borlace BC, et al: Impact of gastric restrictive surgery on hypertension in the morbidly obese. Am J Surg 167:392-399, 1992.
43. Gleysteen JJ, Barboriak JJ, Sasse EA: Sustained coronary-risk factor reduction after gastric bypass for morbid obesity. Am J Clin Nutr 51:774-778, 1990.
44. Brolin RE, Bradley LJ, Wilson AC, Cody RP: Lipid risk profile and weight stability after gastric restrictive operations. J Gastrointest Surg 4:464-469, 2000.
45. Sugerman HJ, Baron PL, Fairman RP, et al: Hemodynamic dysfunction in obesity-hypoventilation syndrome and the effects of treatment with surgically induced weight loss. Ann Surg 207:604-613, 1988.
46. Deitel M, Stone E, Kassam HA, et al: Gynecologic-obstetric changes after loss of massive weight following bariatric surgery. J Am Coll Nutr 7:147-153, 1988.

64

Foreign Bodies and Bezoars of the Stomach and Small Intestine

Karen A. Chojnacki

FOREIGN BODIES

Foreign bodies in the stomach and duodenum are relatively common, and nearly 80% of cases of foreign body ingestion occur in the pediatric population.[1] Such ingestion is usually inadvertent and a result of the natural oral curiosity of an infant or child. In several series, coins are the most commonly ingested objects by infants and children.[2-7] Other foreign bodies frequently found in this population are listed in Table 64–1. The foreign bodies most commonly ingested by adults are listed in Table 64–2. Several adult populations are at risk for foreign bodies in the gastrointestinal (GI) tract. The elderly, demented, and intoxicated have an increased risk for accidental foreign body ingestion. Denture wearers have decreased tactile sensation of the palate and are also at risk for accidental foreign body ingestion.[8,9] Psychiatric patients and prisoners are more apt to intentionally swallow foreign bodies for secondary gain. This population often swallows multiple objects on multiple occasions.[10]

Eighty percent to 90% of ingested foreign bodies pass through the GI tract spontaneously without injury,[11] 10% to 20% require endoscopic removal, and 1% require surgery.[11,12] Perforation, obstruction, and failure of an object to progress though the GI tract are all complications of foreign bodies that require surgical or endoscopic intervention. Obstruction and perforation can occur at any point along the GI tract. Obstruction is most likely to take place at the pylorus, the duodenal sweep, the ligament of Treitz, and the ileocecal valve. Objects greater than 5 cm in length or 2 cm in diameter are unlikely to pass through the pylorus.[13] Patients with a history of pyloric stenosis, previous pyloric surgery, or ulcer disease are at increased risk for obstruction.[14]

One percent of foreign body ingestions result in perforation of the GI tract. Perforation by a foreign body is often secondary to accidental ingestion of a sharp or pointed object such as a fish or chicken bone or a toothpick. The duodenal sweep is at increased risk for perforation from long or pointed objects (or both) because of its C shape.[4] In cases of perforation, the diagnosis of foreign body ingestion is often made intraoperatively because the patient is rarely aware of the ingestion.

Interestingly, once foreign bodies travel beyond the ligament of Treitz, complications are rare. In the small bowel lumen, objects are subject to axial flow and reflex relaxation of the muscle wall. This tends to orient objects with the blunt end leading and the sharp end trailing, thus decreasing the risk for bowel injury.[15] Within the colon, objects become centered in stool, which further protects the bowel wall and allows the objects to safely exit the GI tract.[16]

Diagnosis

The diagnosis of foreign bodies within the stomach and small intestine is established by patient history, radiology studies, or endoscopy (or any combination). Most communicative adults will be able to provide an accurate history of how, what, and when an object was ingested. Symptoms most commonly occur when the ingested object is in the esophagus and include dysphonia, dysphagia, and odynophagia. Retrosternal pain, pharyngeal discomfort, and respiratory compromise are also symptoms of a foreign body lodged in the esophagus. Patients will be able to localize an object when lodged at the cricopharyngeal muscle, but localization becomes less accurate as the object moves distally. Patients are able to accurately localize ingested foreign bodies in the esophagus in 30% to 40% of cases but are rarely able to localize objects when in the stomach.[17] Sudden resolution of symptoms often indicates that the object has passed to

Table 64–1	Foreign Bodies Found in Children Aged 3 Months to 10 Years	
Coins		33
Bones		4
Pins		4
Jacks/jackstones		2
Battery		1
Toy bell		1
Button		1
Marble		1
Meat		1
Metal clip		1
Tack		1
Total		50

From Pfau PR, Ginsberg GG: Foreign bodies and bezoars. In Feldman M, Friedman LS, Sleisenger MH, et al (eds): Gastrointestinal and Liver Disease. Philadelphia, WB Saunders, 2002: 386-398.

Table 64–2	Foreign Bodies Found in Older Children and Adults Aged 11 to 91 Years	
Meat		115
Bones		35
Fiber		13
Pills		6
Coins		5
Dental hardware		3
Batteries		2
Brush bristle		2
Brazil nut		1
Guitar pick		1
Herb		1
Miller-Abbott tube		1
Pencil		1
Popcorn husk		1
Potato		1
Razor blade		1
Splinter		1
Spoon		1
Wrapper		1
Total		192

From Pfau PR, Ginsberg GG: Foreign bodies and bezoars. In Feldman M, Friedman LS, Sleisenger MH, et al (eds): Gastrointestinal and Liver Disease. Philadelphia, WB Saunders, 2002: 386-398.

the stomach. Once a foreign body has reached the stomach, patients are usually asymptomatic unless perforation or obstruction develops.

The history and symptoms are less reliable with children and psychiatric patients. Most often the ingestion is a witnessed event or suspected by a caregiver. Recurrent foreign body ingestion is reported in 3.3% to 10% of psychiatric patients and prisoners.[4,18] Symptoms of foreign body ingestion in these patient populations include choking, vomiting, blood-stained saliva, respiratory distress, and stridor. Children may also fail to thrive or refuse to eat.[19] Thirty-three percent of children and infants may be asymptomatic after foreign body ingestion, but the true percentage may even be higher.[20]

All patients with suspected foreign body ingestion should have anteroposterior and lateral radiographs of the chest and abdomen taken to aid in determining the presence, type, and location of the foreign body. Plain films may also identify signs of perforation such as pneumoperitoneum, pleural effusion, or subcutaneous air.[4,21] Lateral films help distinguish between objects in the tracheobronchial tree versus the esophagus. Some objects, such as glass, bone, aluminum, plastic, and wood, are radiolucent and can be difficult to detect on plain radiography. If ingestion of one of these objects is suspected, flexible endoscopy is recommended to confirm and treat the ingestion.[4] In patients with a contraindication to endoscopy, a thin barium contrast study can be used to evaluate the upper GI system.[11] Barium esophagograms should not be performed if there is concern of perforation or obstruction.

Patients who remain symptomatic with normal imaging studies should undergo flexible endoscopy because it provides safe and effective management of foreign bodies in the upper GI tract. Multiple series report success rates for endoscopic management of foreign bodies in excess of 95%.[4,5,22,23]

Management

Once a foreign body has reached the stomach, the risk for complications diminishes greatly. Nearly 90% of objects in the stomach will progress through the GI tract without complication. Most patients can be managed conservatively. Patients who have ingested small or blunt objects, such as coins, can be observed with daily or weekly radiographs to document progression of the foreign body. Endoscopic removal of certain objects is recommended before passage from the stomach, as discussed in the next section. Surgery is indicated if signs or symptoms of perforation, hemorrhage, fistula formation, or obstruction of the small or large bowel develop. Failure of a sharp or pointed object in the small intestine to progress after 3 days is also an indication for surgery.[10] Several authors have reported success with laparoscopic removal of ingested foreign bodies.[24-26]

Certain foreign bodies deserve special consideration.

Sharp/Pointed or Long Foreign Bodies

Toothpicks, nails, needles, bones, razor blades, safety pins, and dental prostheses are the most commonly ingested sharp foreign bodies. Surgical intervention is most often required for bones and toothpicks.[21,27] The terminal ileum is the most frequent site of perforation by a sharp foreign body. Because 15% to 35% of these sharp foreign bodies will cause perforation, they should

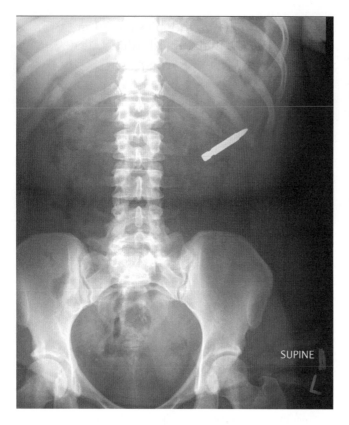

Figure 64–1.   A 36-year-old woman ingested a drill bit while working on home repairs. By the time that she arrived at the emergency department and this radiograph was taken, the bit had passed through the stomach into the small bowel.

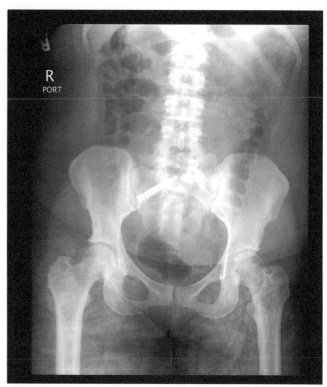

Figure 64–2.   After 24 hours, the drill bit had progressed to the terminal ileum. Here it lies in the right lower quadrant with the blunt end leading.

be removed by flexible endoscopy while still in the stomach. Objects longer than 5 cm are unlikely to pass through the duodenum and should also be removed.[13] Sharp or pointed objects that do pass through the duodenum into the small intestine can be treated conservatively unless symptoms of perforation or obstruction develop (Figs. 64–1 and 64–2). If the foreign body fails to reach the colon within 3 days, it should be surgically removed. When removing a sharp object with the endoscope, the foreign body should be positioned so that the sharp end trails distal to the endoscope.[10] This follows Jackson's axiom: "Advancing points puncture, trailing points do not" (Fig. 64–3).[28]

Button Batteries

Several common devices, such as hearing aids, calculators, cameras, computers, watches, and electronic games, are powered by small, often coin-like "button batteries." Ingestion of these batteries is widely reported.[29-33] Ten percent of ingested button batteries will become symptomatic. Batteries larger than 21 mm are more likely to cause problems. The most common battery systems contain an alkaline electrolyte solution that is a 26% to 45% solution of potassium or sodium hydroxide. This

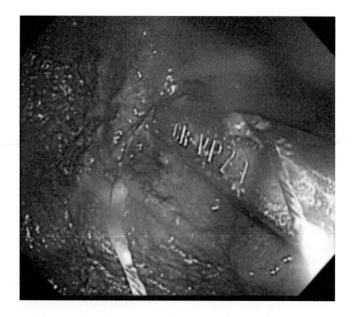

Figure 64–3.   The drill bit failed to progress into the colon over the next 3 days. It was removed by colonoscopy from the terminal ileum with a snare.

alkaline electrolyte can cause rapid liquefaction necrosis of tissues if it leaks into the GI tract. Batteries can also cause tissue damage by low-voltage burns and pressure necrosis.[31,34]

Button batteries lodged within the esophagus should be removed by endoscopy as soon as the diagnosis is established to prevent burn, perforation, or stricture of the esophagus. Once a battery has reached the stomach, it will usually pass without difficulty. Daily radiographs should be obtained. If the battery has not progressed beyond the pylorus by 36 to 48 hours, it should be retrieved by endoscopy. Emesis should not be induced to avoid aspiration of the battery into the trachea.[29,32,35] If symptoms of epigastric pain, fever, or peritonitis develop, the patient should be considered for surgical exploration.

Once in the small intestine, complications from an ingested button battery are quite rare. Only one complication has been reported in nearly 100 cases involving the intestine. In this case, the battery lodged in Meckel's diverticulum and caused perforation.[36] Most batteries will pass through the entire GI tract in 72 hours, with a range of 12 hours to 14 days.[29] After the battery has passed the pylorus, radiographs are obtained every 3 to 4 days. Surgery is warranted if the battery fails to progress or symptoms of perforation or obstruction develop.

Double AA and triple AAA alkaline batteries will usually pass from the stomach to the anus without complications.[4]

Illicit Drugs

Because of the ongoing popularity and profitability of heroin and cocaine, these drugs continue to be smuggled into the United States by "body packers" or "mules." Body packers ingest multiple small packages containing heroin or cocaine. The packets are usually condoms stuffed with 3 to 5 g of an illicit drug.[37] The packets are then swallowed so that they are concealed in the GI tract. Body packers often take high doses of anticholinergic drugs to postpone passage of the packets through the GI tract. Cocaine is lethal at a dose of 1 to 3 g; therefore, rupture of only one packet can be fatal.[38]

Body packers can have a variety of symptoms; however, they are often asymptomatic and are brought to medical attention by drug enforcement officials. These patients may also have signs and symptoms of bowel obstruction.[39] Plain radiographs will demonstrate the drug packets in 70% to 90% of cases (Fig. 64–4).[40] Patients may also have symptoms of toxicity from the carried drug, indicative of packet rupture. Patients with toxicity or obstruction, or both, should be stabilized and undergo urgent surgical evaluation. Gastrostomy, multiple enterotomies, or colotomies (or any combination) may be required to remove all drug packets.[41] Endoscopic retrieval is contraindicated because of the risk for perforation of the packet.[37] If a patient comes to medical attention within 24 hours of packet ingestion and is stable, conservative management can be attempted. These patients require close observation, whole-gut lavage, and serial radiographs to document evacuation of all packets.[42]

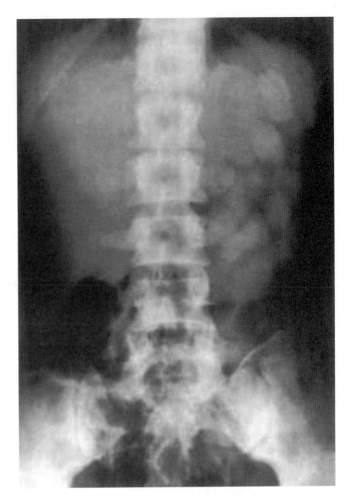

Figure 64–4. Plain abdominal radiograph showing multiple drug-containing packets within the bowel lumen. This patient is a "body packer" or "mule" attempting to smuggle drugs. (From Miller JS, Hendren SK, Liscum KR: Giant gastric ulcer in a body packer. J Trauma 45:617, 1998.)

BEZOARS

Bezoars are retained collections of indigestible foreign material that accumulate in the GI tract. Most bezoars are located in the stomach, but they may be encountered in the esophagus, small intestine, and rectum.[43] Altered gastric physiology with impaired gastric emptying and decreased acid production is often the cause of bezoar formation. These changes are usually consequences of previous gastric surgery, which is present in 70% to 94% of patients with bezoar formation.[44] Vagotomy with pyloroplasty or antrectomy is a predisposing factor for bezoar formation.[45] Patients with gastroparesis, diabetes, end-stage renal disease, and prolonged mechanical ventilation are at increased risk for bezoars.[46] In some patients, ingestion of large amounts of indigestible material is the only risk factor for bezoar formation.

There are four types of bezoars: phytobezoars, trichobezoars, pharmacobezoars, and lactobezoars. Phytobezoars are the most frequent type of bezoar and occur most commonly with the foods listed in Table 64–3.

Table 64–3	Contents of Various Bezoars	
Phytobezoar	**Trichobezoar**	**Pharmacobezoar**
Celery	Hair	Nifedipine
Pumpkin	Carpet fibers	Procainamide
Grape skins	String	Verapamil
Prunes	Clothing	Theophylline
Raisins		Cholestyramine
Leeks		Meprobamate
Beets		Sucralfate
Persimmons		Kayexalate resin
		Guar gum
		Enteral feeding formulas
		Vitamin C tablets
		Vitamin B_{12}
		Lecithin
		Ferrous sulfate

From Pfau PR, Ginsberg GG: Foreign bodies and bezoars. In Feldman M, Friedman LS, Sleisenger MH, et al (eds): Gastrointestinal and Liver Disease. Philadelphia, WB Saunders, 2002:386-398.

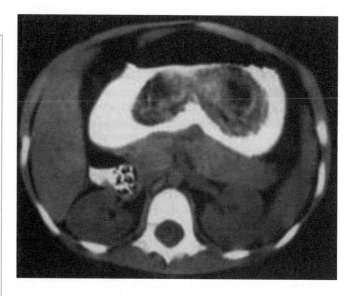

Figure 64–5. Computed tomography scan revealing a dilated stomach with an intraluminal mass consistent with a trichobezoar. (From Phillips MR, Zaheer S, Drugas GT: Mayo Clin Proc 73:653-656, 1998.)

These foods are composed of large amounts of nondigestible fiber such as cellulose, lignin, and fruit tannin.[47] A high concentration of tannins, exposed to gastric acid, can form a coagulum leading to bezoar formation.[48] Phytobezoars are typically dark brown, black, or green when visualized by endoscopy.

Trichobezoars are composed of hair or hair-like fibers (see Table 64–3). They are observed most commonly in children and women younger than 30 years.[49] Frequently, these patients have underlying mental retardation or psychiatric disorders. Trichotillomania is an impulse control disorder characterized by the repeated urge to pull out scalp and body hair. Trichophagia is the compulsion to eat or chew on hair. These behavioral disorders are associated with trichobezoar formation. Hair and fibers in the stomach become trapped in gastric folds. Trichobezoars are typically black regardless of the color of the hair ingested because of enzymatic oxidation of gastric acid on the hair fibers. Some gastric trichobezoars have a long extension of hair that trails into the duodenum, a condition known as the Rapunzel syndrome.[50] It has been reported to cause jaundice and pancreatitis as a result of obstruction of the ampulla of Vater by hair.[51,52]

Pharmacobezoars are composed of medications or vitamins (see Table 64–3). Resin-coated, extended-release products or other products designed to resist digestion are most often the nidus for this type of bezoar formation.[46] Pharmacobezoars can result in reduced medication efficacy because the active agent is trapped in the bezoar and cannot be absorbed. Alternatively, toxicity can result when the previously bound active agent is released in excessive amounts. Fatality secondary to pharmacobezoars has been reported. At autopsy the patient was found to have a serum theophylline concentration of 190.1 mg/ml (normal, 10 to 20 mg/ml). A 318-g pharmacobezoar containing 29 g of theophylline in sustained-release tablets was found within the stomach.[53]

Lactobezoars are a compact mass of undigested milk concretions located within the GI tract of infants and toddlers. These rare bezoars have been linked to nearly every commercially available infant formula and breast and cow milk.[54]

Symptoms and Signs of Bezoars

The most common symptom present in 80% of patients with bezoars is vague epigastric discomfort. Other symptoms include nausea, vomiting, anorexia, early satiety, and weight loss. If a bezoar reaches a large size and is present for a prolonged period, it may cause pressure necrosis and ulcers. Ulceration can lead to bleeding or obstruction. Once in the small bowel, bezoars most commonly result in obstruction.[55]

Physical examination is often unrevealing. Occasionally, a palpable mass may be present. Patients with trichotillomania and trichobezoars may have patchy baldness.[56]

Diagnosis

Bezoars can be demonstrated on plain films and computed tomography scans (Fig. 64–5). Barium studies will reveal a gastric filling defect (Fig. 64–6).[47] Up to 75% of bezoars may be missed on radiography. Endoscopy is the gold standard for the diagnosis of bezoars. The endoscopic appearance of phytobezoars consists of an amorphous mass of brown, green, or black material (Fig. 64–7). Trichobezoars are black, hard, and concrete-like. Pharmacobezoars contain whole pills or pill frag-

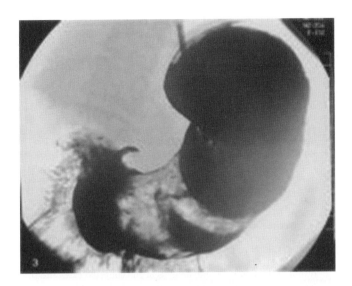

Figure 64–6. Barium study outlining a large gastric mass consistent with a bezoar. (From Zamir D, Goldblum C, Linova L, et al: J Clin Gastroenterol 38:873-876, 2004.)

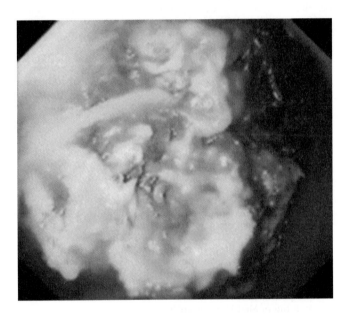

Figure 64–7. Endoscopic appearance of a phytobezoar. (From Sechopoulos P, Robotis JF, Rokkas T: Gastric bezoar treated endoscopically with a carbonated beverage: case report. Gastrointest Endosc 60:662-664, 2004.)

ments.[47,56] Lactobezoars are most commonly identified on contrast-enhanced upper GI series or ultrasound.[54]

Treatment

Treatment of bezoars involves removal of the mass and prevention of recurrence. Some small bezoars can be managed medically. Once a diagnosis is established by endoscopy, institution of a clear liquid diet and a prokinetic agent may clear the bezoar. Nasogastric lavage may be useful for these small bezoars.[57]

Most bezoars require endoscopic therapy. Using biopsy forceps or polypectomy snares, a bezoar can be fragmented and the pieces removed with multiple passes of the endoscope. The reported success rate of this technique is 85% to 90%. In addition to endoscopic fragmentation, success has been reported with the use of electrohydraulic lithotripsy, pulsed water jets, Nd:YAG laser, and needle-knife bezotome.[58-60] Enzymatic dissolution of bezoars has also been described with cellulose, papain (meat tenderizer), N-acetylcysteine, and Coca-Cola.[61-63]

Surgical intervention is required if endoscopic therapy fails or complications of bleeding, obstruction, or perforation occur. Trichobezoars are the most likely to require surgical management and can be removed by open or laparoscopic gastrostomy.[57,64] During surgery, the small bowel should be examined for a concomitant bezoar, which should be removed by enterostomy or milked into the cecum for passage through the large bowel.

In addition to removal of the bezoar, attempts must be made to prevent recurrence. Avoidance of foods causing a phytobezoar is necessary. Prophylactic treatment with cellulose can be considered. Patients with a motility disorder may benefit from prokinetic agents such as metoclopramide.[57] Patients with an underlying psychiatric disorder require specific therapy, which may include selective serotonin uptake inhibitors, hypnosis, or play therapy (children) to avoid recurrence.[65]

Lactobezoars are treated by withholding oral feedings and instituting intravenous hydration.[66] Gentle gastric lavage may decrease treatment time.[67] Although some recommend switching these infants to elemental formula, this may be unnecessary because recurrence has never been reported.[54]

REFERENCES

1. Webb WA: Management of foreign bodies of the upper gastrointestinal tract. Gastroenterology 94:204-216, 1988.
2. Shaffer HA, Delange EE: Gastrointestinal foreign bodies and strictures: Radiologic interventions. Curr Probl Diagn Radiol 23:205-249, 1994.
3. Kim JK, Kim SS, Kim JI, et al: Management of foreign bodies in the gastrointestinal tract: An analysis of 104 cases in children. Endoscopy 31:302-304, 1999.
4. Webb WA: Management of foreign bodies of the upper gastrointestinal tract. Gastrointest Endosc 41:39-51, 1995.
5. Vizcarrondo FJ, Brady PG, Nord HJ, et al: Foreign bodies of the upper gastrointestinal tract. Gastrointest Endosc 29:208-210, 1983.
6. Rosch W, Classen M: Fibroendoscopic foreign body removal from the upper gastrointestinal tract. Endoscopy 4:193-197, 1972.
7. Arana A, Houser B, Hachimi-Idrissi S, Vandenplas Y: Management of ingested foreign bodies in childhood and review of the literature. Eur J Pediatr 160:468-472, 2001.
8. Gunn A: Intestinal perforation due to swallowed fish or meat bone. Lancet 1:125-128, 1966.
9. Bunker PG: The role of dentistry in problems of foreign body in the air and food passage. J Am Dent Assoc 64:782-787, 1962.
10. Pfau PR, Ginsberg GG: Foreign bodies and bezoars. In Feldman M, Friedman LS, Sleisenger MH, et al (eds): Gastrointestinal and Liver Disease. Philadelphia, WB Saunders, 2002:386-398.
11. Schwartz GF, Polsky HS: Ingested foreign bodies of the upper gastrointestinal tract. Am Surg 42:236-238, 1976.

12. Bendig DW, Mackie GC: Management of smooth-blunt gastric foreign bodies in asymptomatic patients. Clin Pediatr (Phila) 29:642-645, 1990.
13. Koch H: Operative endoscopy. Gastrointest Endosc 24:65-68, 1977.
14. Caravati EM, Bennett DL, McElwee NE: Pediatric coin ingestion. A prospective study on the utility of routine roentgenograms. Am J Dis Child 143:549-551, 1989.
15. Davidoff E, Towne JB: Ingested foreign bodies. N Y State Med J 75:1003-1007, 1975.
16. Macmanus JE: Perforation of the intestine by ingested foreign body. Am J Surg 54:393-400, 1941.
17. Connolly AA, Birchall M, Walsh-Waring GI, Moore-Gillon V: Ingested foreign bodies: Patient-guided localization is a useful clinical tool. Clin Otolaryngol Allied Sci 17:520-524, 1992.
18. Rosenow EC: Foreign bodies of the esophagus. In Payne WS, Olsen AM (eds): The Esophagus. Philadelphia, Lea & Febiger, 1974, pp 158-170.
19. Chowdhurg CR, Bricknell MC, MacIver D: Oesophageal foreign body: An unusual cause of respiratory symptoms in a three-week baby. J Laryngol Otol 106:556-557, 1992.
20. Classen M, Farthmann EF, Seifert E, Wurbs D: Operative and therapeutic techniques in endoscopy. Clin Gastroenterol 7:741-763, 1978.
21. Maleke M, Evan WE: Foreign body perforation of the intestinal tract. Arch Surg 101:475-477, 1970.
22. Herranz-Gonzalez J, Martinez-Vidal J, Garcia-Sarandeses A, Vazquez-Barro C: Esophageal foreign bodies in adults. Otolaryngol Head Neck Surg 105:649-654, 1991.
23. Chaikhouni A, Kratz JM, Crawford FA: Foreign bodies of the esophagus. Am Surg 51:173-179, 1985.
24. Wishner JD, Roger AM: Laparoscopic removal of a swallowed toothbrush. Surg Endosc 11:472-473, 1997.
25. Furihata M, Tagaya N, Furihata T, Kubota K: Laparoscopic removal of an intragastric foreign body with endoscopic assistance. Surg Laparosc Endosc Percutan Tech 14:234-237, 2004.
26. Wichmann MW, Huttl TP, Billing A, Jauch KW: Laparoscopic management of a small bowel perforation caused by a toothpick. Surg Endosc 18:717-718, 2004.
27. Budnick LD: Toothpick-related injuries in the United States 1979 through 1982. JAMA 252:796-797, 1984.
28. Webb WA, McDaniel L, Jones L: Foreign bodies of the upper gastrointestinal tract: Current management. South Med J 77:1083-1086, 1984.
29. Litovitz TL: Battery ingestions: Product accessibility and clinical course. Pediatrics 75:468-476, 1985.
30. Votteler TP, Nash JC, Rutledge JC: The hazard of ingested alkaline disk batteries in children. JAMA 249:2504-2506, 1983.
31. Temple DM, McNeese MC: Hazards of battery ingestion. Pediatrics 71:100-103, 1983.
32. Maves MD, Carithers JS, Birck HG: Esophageal burns secondary to disc battery ingestion. Ann Otol Rhinol Laryngol 93:364-369, 1984.
33. Maves MD, Lloyd TV, Carithers JS: Radiographic identification of ingested disc batteries. Pediatr Radiol 16:154-156, 1986.
34. Litovitz TL: Button battery ingestions. JAMA 249:2495-2500, 1983.
35. Mofenson JC, Greensher J, Caraccio TR, Danoff R: Ingestion of small flat disc batteries. Ann Emerg Med 12:88-90, 1983.
36. Willis GA, Ho WC: Perforation of Meckel's diverticulum by an alkaline hearing aid battery. Can Med Assoc J 126:497-498, 1982.
37. Suarez CA, Arango A, Lester JL 3rd: Cocaine-condom ingestion: Surgical treatment. JAMA 238:1391-1392, 1977.
38. Price KR: Fatal cocaine poisoning. J Forensic Sci Soc 14:329-333, 1974.
39. Stack LB, Munter DW: Foreign bodies in the gastrointestinal tract. Emerg Med Clin North Am 14:493-521, 1996.
40. Caruana DS, Weinbach B, Goerg D, Gardner LB: Cocaine-packet ingestion. Diagnosis, management, and natural history. Ann Intern Med 100:73-74, 1984.
41. Aldrighetti L, Graci C, Paganelli M, et al: Intestinal occlusion in cocaine-packet ingestion. Minerva Chir 48:1233-1237, 1993.
42. Pollack CV Jr, Biggers DW, Carlton FB Jr, et al: Two crack cocaine body stuffers. Ann Emerg Med 21:1370-1380, 1992.
43. Byrme WJ: Foreign bodies, bezoars, and caustic ingestion. Gastointest Endosc Clin North Am 4:99-104, 1994.
44. Escamilla C, Robles-Campos R, Parrilla-Paricio P, et al: Intestinal obstruction and bezoars. J Am Coll Surg 179:285-288, 1994.
45. Robles R, Parrilla P, Escamilla C, et al: Gastrointestinal bezoars. Br J Surg 81:1000-1001, 1994.
46. Taylor JR, Streetman DS, Castle SS: Medication bezoars: A literature review and a report of a case. Ann Pharmacother 32:940-946, 1998.
47. Andru CH, Ponskky JL: Bezoars: Classification, pathophysiology, and treatment. Am J Gastroenterol 83:476-478, 1988.
48. Lee J: Bezoars and foreign bodies of the stomach. Gastrointest Endosc Clin N Am 6:605-619, 1996.
49. Debakey M, Oschner A: Bezoars and concretions: Comprehensive review of the literature with analysis of 303 collected cases and presentations of 8 additional cases. Surgery 5:132-160, 1939.
50. Vaughan ED Jr, Sawyers JL, Scott HW Jr: The rapunzel syndrome: An unusual complication of intestinal bezoar. Surgery 63:339-343, 1968.
51. Schreiber H, Filston HC: Obstructive jaundice due to gastric trichobezoar. J Pediatr Surg 11:103-104, 1976.
52. Shawis RN, Doig CM: Gastric trichobezoar associated with transient pancreatitis. Arch Dis Child 59:994-995, 1984.
53. Berstein G, Jehle D, Bernaski E, Braen GR: Failure of gastric emptying and charcoal administration in fatal sustained-release theophylline overdose: Pharmacobezoar formation. Ann Emerg Med 21:1388-1390, 1992.
54. DuBose TM 5th, Southgate WM, Hill GJ: Lactobezoars: A patient series and literature review. Clin Pediatr (Phila) 40:603-606, 2001.
55. Deitrich NA, Gau FC: Postgastrectomy phytobezoars: Endoscopic diagnosis and treatment. Arch Surg 120:432-435, 1985.
56. McGehee FT, Buchanan GR: Trichophagia and trichobezoar: Etiologic role of iron deficiency. J Pediatr 97:946-948, 1980.
57. Phillips MR, Zaheer S, Drugas GT: Gastric trichobezoar: Case report and literature review. Mayo Clin Proc 73:653-656, 1998.
58. Wang YG, Seitz U, Li ZL, et al: Endoscopic management of huge bezoars. Endoscopy 30:371-374, 1998.
59. Kuo JY, Mo LR, Tsai CC, et al: Nonoperative treatment of gastric bezoars using electrohydraulic lithotripsy. Endoscopy 331:386-388, 1999.
60. Klamer TW, Max MH: Recurrent gastric bezoars: A new approach to treatment and prevention. Am J Surg 145:417-419, 1983.
61. Walker-Renard P: Update on the medical management of phytobezoars. Am J Gastroenterol 88:1663-1666, 1993.
62. Zarling EJ, Moeller DD: Bezoar therapy: Complications using Adolph's meat tenderizer and alternatives from literature review. Arch Intern Med 141:1669-1670, 1981.
63. Sechopoulos P, Robotis JF, Rokkas T: Gastric bezoar treated endoscopically with a carbonated beverage: Case report. Gastrointest Endosc 60:662-664, 2004.
64. Siriwardana HPP, Ammori BJ: Laparoscopic removal of a large gastric bezoar in a mentally retarded patient with pica. Surg Endosc 17:834, 2003.
65. Christenson GA, Crow SJ: The characterization and treatment of trichotillomania. J Clin Psychiatry 57:42-49, 1996.
66. Wolf RS, Davis LA: Lactobezoar, a foreign body formed by the use of undiluted powdered milk substance. JAMA 184:782, 1963.
67. Singer JI: Lactobezoar causing an abdominal triad of colicky pain, emesis, and a mass. Pediatr Emerg Care 4:194-196, 1988.

Surgical Diseases of the Stomach and Duodenum in Infants and Children

Harsh Grewal · William H. Weintraub

Surgical diseases of the stomach and duodenum in infants and children are often the result of developmental anomalies. This chapter reviews congenital and acquired diseases of the stomach and duodenum in infants and children that a surgeon may encounter.

EMBRYOLOGIC DEVELOPMENT

At the beginning of the fourth week of development, the primordial gut forms from lateral and craniocaudal folding of the embryo. The distal part of the foregut dilates to form the stomach around the fourth to fifth week of development. During the 6th to 10th week, as the stomach enlarges, it also rotates 90 degrees in a clockwise direction. These differential rates of growth and subsequent rotation result in the stomach assuming its final position: the cranial part (gastric fundus) on the left and the caudal part (pylorus) on the right of the midline, the lesser curvature facing cranially and to the right, and the greater curvature located caudally.

The transition from foregut to midgut occurs at the second portion of the duodenum, just distal to the entry of the bile duct. The celiac arterial trunk supplies this part of the stomach and duodenum, whereas the superior mesenteric artery supplies the midgut (the bowel distal to the entry of the bile duct). The proximal duodenum moves superiorly and to the right as the distal duodenum rotates down and to the left, thereby resulting in the "C-loop" configuration of the duodenum around the 6th to 10th week of development. Elongation of the midgut around the fifth to sixth week causes herniation of the midgut into the umbilical cord (physiologic umbilical herniation). The midgut then rotates nearly 270 degrees counterclockwise around an axis formed by the superior mesenteric artery, which results

in fixation of the fourth portion of the duodenum to the left of the aorta. At the 10th to 12th week, the extraembryologic coelomic gut returns to the abdominal cavity. Subsequent shortening of the duodenal mesenteric base plus fusion with the parietal peritoneum fixes the duodenum in its retroperitoneal location at the ligament of Treitz to the left of the midline. The ampulla of Vater, in the second part of the duodenum, is medial and is the site where the common bile duct and often the pancreatic ducts enter into the duodenum.[1]

During this period of development, the proximal duodenum undergoes epithelial proliferation, and a transitional solid cord is created that obliterates the lumen. Around the eighth week, this transitional solid phase undergoes vacuolization with resultant recanalization. Vascular accidents or aborted recanalization can result in congenital duodenal obstruction. The pancreas develops from the rotation and fusion of paired buds arising from the dorsal and ventral duodenal entodermal epithelium, so abnormalities in development can result in an annular pancreas and in heterotopic pancreatic rests in the proximal duodenum or pylorus.[1]

INTESTINAL OBSTRUCTION IN THE NEWBORN

Because congenital and acquired diseases of the stomach and duodenum in the newborn may cause proximal intestinal obstruction, a brief review of the signs and symptoms and a diagnostic approach are presented in this section. Neonatal intestinal obstruction is often accompanied by bilious vomiting and alterations in the passage of meconium. Bilious vomiting in a newborn or infant should be presumed to be secondary to malrotation with midgut volvulus, and this condition should always be ruled out with an upper gastrointestinal (GI) study because untreated midgut volvulus can rapidly lead to intestinal ischemia and gangrene with loss of intestine and possibly death. The differential diagnosis of neonatal intestinal obstruction, especially with bilious vomiting, covers both proximal and distal obstructive lesions, including congenital gastric or duodenal obstruction, proximal and distal small intestinal atresia, meconium ileus secondary to cystic fibrosis, GI duplications, Hirschsprung's disease, colonic atresia, meconium plug syndrome, small neonatal left colon syndrome, and imperforate anus. Spontaneous gastric perforation and necrotizing enterocolitis may also be manifested as feeding intolerance and bilious vomiting. Clinically, neonatal sepsis with ileus may suggest intestinal obstruction.

Clinical Features and Diagnosis Proximal intestinal obstruction is usually accompanied by vomiting and a nondistended abdomen, whereas abdominal distention characterizes a distal intestinal obstruction; however, localized upper abdominal distention can suggest duodenal atresia or gastric outlet obstruction. Abdominal wall discoloration plus peritonitis may be associated with intestinal necrosis or perforation and indicates the need for immediate laparotomy. Plain abdominal radiography, followed by an upper GI series, is the usual sequence of studies in the evaluation of proximal intestinal obstruction. A plain film revealing pneumatosis suggests necrotizing enterocolitis. The "double bubble" from a distended stomach and duodenal bulb, with a gasless lower abdomen on a plain radiograph in a neonate, is suggestive of duodenal atresia. The presence of distal gas with a "double bubble" suggests malrotation with midgut volvulus. Distention of the small and large intestine is difficult to distinguish on plain radiographs in a newborn; therefore, differentiation of distal from proximal obstruction relies on the number of distended air-filled loops because with proximal obstruction there will be fewer air-filled loops. A prone cross-table lateral radiograph to determine the presence of gas in the distal end of the rectum may also help identify the level of obstruction.

Suspicion of a proximal obstruction will then suggest the need for an upper GI study, and distal obstruction, a lower GI study. In the absence of an acute abdomen on examination, an infant or newborn with bilious vomiting should have an upper GI study performed urgently to rule out malrotation with possible volvulus (Fig. 65–1A and B). The study should demonstrate the ligament of Treitz in its normal location to the left of the spine and at or above the level of the duodenal bulb to exclude malrotation. An upper GI study may also demonstrate malrotation without volvulus (see Fig. 65–1C), atresia, or stenosis, although in the absence of suspicion for midgut volvulus, it may not be necessary to perform this study urgently.

The following discussion of surgical diseases of the stomach and duodenum in infants and children is separated into congenital and acquired conditions.

CONGENITAL CONDITIONS

Gastric Duplications

Incidence and Etiology Duplications in the stomach and duodenum are uncommon and constitute less than 15% of all GI duplications. There are a number of theories on the embryogenesis of duplications, including the "split notochord" and "partial twinning" theory; additionally, duplications may be related to disordered recanalization of the solid-cord transitional embryonic phase. Duplications are usually found along the mesenteric border and share the blood supply of the adjacent functional stomach or intestine.[2,3]

Clinical Features In neonates or infants, gastric and duodenal duplications may be associated with signs and symptoms of gastric outlet obstruction. Less acute manifestations include a palpable mass or a mass detected on imaging (including fetal ultrasound), failure to thrive, abdominal discomfort, or GI bleeding. Duplications occasionally first come to attention as an emergency because of either a perforation or bleeding secondary to peptic ulceration. Gastric duplications are typically cystic, usually appear along the greater curve, and rarely communicate with the gastric lumen. Tubular duplications, which communicate with the gastric lumen and are also found along the greater curve, are less common. Communications between gastric duplications and intrathoracic esophageal duplications have been reported, and these patients may have respiratory symptoms such as effusions and occasionally vertebral anomalies.[2,4,5] Communications between a gastric duplication and the pancreatic ductal system have been reported and are associated with pancreatitis.[6] Duodenal duplications occur along the posterior aspect of the first or second part of the duodenum. Besides proximal intestinal obstruction and bleeding, duplications can obstruct the biliary and pancreatic ductal system and result in jaundice or pancreatitis. Malignant degeneration of the cyst lining to an adenocarcinoma or carcinoid tumor has been rarely reported in adults.[7,8]

Diagnosis Ultrasound, computed tomography (CT), or an upper GI study can define the duplication, which is usually cystic (Fig. 65–2A). Antenatal ultrasound may detect gastric duplication in a fetus. Technetium 99m imaging will identify duplications that contain ectopic gastric mucosa, which is more prone to bleeding; all histologic types of GI epithelia can be present ectopically in GI duplications.[2,3]

Management Resection of the cyst may be preferable (see Fig. 65–2B), but stripping of the mucosal lining and internal drainage into the duodenal lumen may be a safer alternative to avoid damage to the biliary and pancreatic ductal systems. Duodenal duplications may be drained into a Roux-en-Y jejunal limb. Recently, laparoscopic resection has been described for managing duplications in newborns and infants.[9]

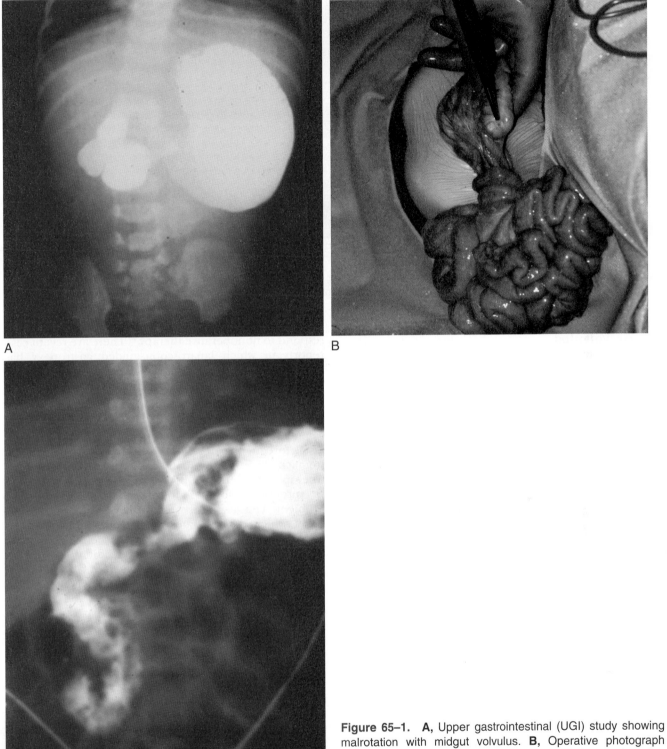

Figure 65-1. A, Upper gastrointestinal (UGI) study showing malrotation with midgut volvulus. **B,** Operative photograph showing midgut volvulus secondary to malrotation; the intestine is viable in this child. **C,** UGI study showing malrotation, with the ligament of Treitz to the right of the midline and no evidence of volvulus.

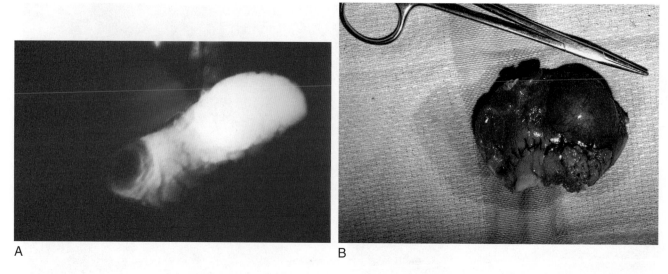

Figure 65–2. **A,** Upper gastrointestinal (UGI) study showing a gastric duplication in the antral region of the stomach. **B,** Resected specimen of a gastric duplication from the antral region of the stomach as seen on the UGI study.

Gastric Volvulus

Incidence and Etiology Gastric volvulus is a rare condition in childhood. It occurs more commonly as a chronic condition, but acute gastric volvulus can be a surgical emergency.[10-12] Anomalies in rotation and fixation of the stomach are responsible for most cases of childhood gastric volvulus; the presence of a wandering spleen or asplenia may be a predisposing factor.[12,13] The multiple ligamentous attachments of the stomach probably account for its rarity. The peritoneal attachments and the gastrophrenic, gastrosplenic, and gastrohepatic ligaments along with the retroperitoneal position of the duodenum stabilize its position in both the longitudinal and transverse axes. In organo-axial volvulus, the stomach remains fixed at the gastroesophageal junction and the duodenum, which allows it to twist along its longitudinal axis. Mesenterico-axial volvulus is a more common cause of acute gastric volvulus in children, with rotation around the transverse axis of the stomach through the greater and lesser curvatures.[11]

Clinical Features and Diagnosis Typical symptoms range from an acute proximal intestinal obstruction and gastric necrosis to a chronic picture of postprandial pain with intermittent volvulus. Plain radiographs and an upper GI study are used to make the diagnosis of gastric volvulus.

Management In acute gastric volvulus, hydration, correction of electrolyte abnormalities, and gastric decompression with nasogastric suction are essential; if not possible, emergency surgery is indicated. Derotation and anterior gastropexy along with crural repair may be sufficient if the stomach has no evidence of necrosis. If possible, gastric perforations are typically closed around a tube gastrostomy to fix the stomach to the anterior abdominal wall and create an anterior gastropexy. Management of chronic gastric volvulus is controversial, and some patients with intermittent primary volvulus may respond to nonoperative therapy.[10] There are recent case reports in which laparoscopic-guided gastropexy has been used for the management of gastric volvulus.[14,15]

Microgastria

Congenital microgastria is another rare condition of the distal foregut that results in a disproportionately small stomach. The infant initially has failure to thrive or gastroesophageal reflux (GER), or microgastria is observed at surgery performed for another intra-abdominal problem. The diagnosis is confirmed with an upper GI study, which demonstrates a dilated esophagus and a transverse lie of a small tubular stomach. Initial management includes multiple small feedings through a feeding tube and medical management of GER. If unsuccessful, surgery is indicated to provide adequate nutrition, but the size of the stomach limits the ability to perform an antireflux procedure and gastrostomy at the initial surgery. A feeding jejunostomy followed by creation of a jejunal reservoir (Hunt-Lawrence pouch) may be required.[16,17] Most of these children have multiple anomalies, including malrotation, situs inversus, megaesophagus, and asplenia, as well as cardiovascular, renal, and skeletal abnormalities.[18,19]

Gastric Outlet Obstruction

Incidence and Etiology Congenital gastric outlet obstruction, which may be caused by antral and pyloric webs, diaphragms, and atresia, is another uncommon cause of newborn obstruction. The embryologic cause of antral and pyloric atresia is not well understood.

Clinical Features Antral webs or partial diaphragms cause prepyloric obstruction and have varied clinical manifestations, depending on the severity or completeness of the obstruction. Pyloric atresia is usually ac-

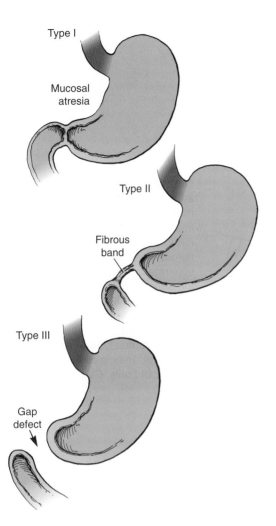

Type I

Mucosal
atresia

Type II

Fibrous
band

Type III

Gap
defect

Figure 65–3. Illustration showing the different types of congenital pyloric atresia. (From O'Neil JA Jr [ed]: Principles of Pediatric Surgery, 2nd ed. St Louis, CV Mosby, 2003, p 486.)

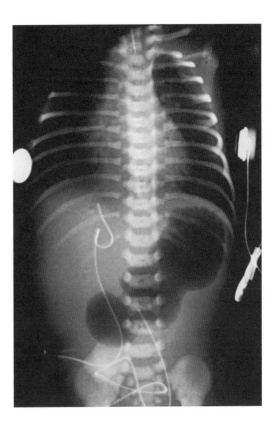

Figure 65–4. Classic plain film radiograph showing gastric outlet obstruction.

companied by nonbilious vomiting and gastric distention consistent with complete obstruction. If the diagnosis is delayed, a complete gastric outlet obstruction can become a surgical emergency with gastric perforation occurring within the first few days of life.[20] An incomplete web or diaphragm causes partial gastric outlet obstruction and may be associated with insidious findings of epigastric pain, failure to thrive, halitosis, and postprandial nonbilious vomiting; the diagnosis of an incomplete web may be delayed into adulthood.[21] The association of other anomalies, including epidermolysis bullosa with pyloric atresia, should be evaluated before surgery.[22,23]

Types Congenital pyloric anomalies are more frequent than antral anomalies. Pyloric webs are more common than atresia. The following three varieties of pyloric atresia have been described: type I, the most common type, is an intraluminal pyloric membrane or web; in type II, the pyloric channel is a solid cord; and in type III, there is a gap between the stomach and duodenum (Fig. 65–3).

Diagnosis The diagnosis may be indicated prenatally on ultrasound examination by the presence of polyhydramnios, a dilated stomach, and a narrowed gastric outlet. Postnatally, plain radiographs may show a large gastric bubble (Fig. 65–4); gastric outlet obstruction or the presence of a web may be seen on an upper GI study. Endoscopy is useful in the diagnosis of an incomplete web, especially if the results of radiographic studies are equivocal.

Management Nasogastric decompression and preoperative fluid and electrolyte resuscitation are indicated to correct the electrolyte abnormalities associated with gastric outlet obstruction. The type of congenital obstruction will dictate the surgical procedure.[20] Type I pyloric atresia requires a longitudinal gastrotomy to identify the web, followed by extension into the pylorus, excision of the web, and transverse closure of the pylorus as a pyloroplasty. Before closure, a catheter should be passed distally to ensure that no additional atresias are present. If there is difficulty in performing a transverse closure, a serosal or omental patch may be considered. Type II or III atresia is repaired by performing a gastroduodenal anastomosis or a pyloric reconstruction. Postoperatively, the stomach should be decompressed with a nasogastric tube; in patients with associated anomalies, a gastrostomy with a transanastomotic gastrojejunal feeding tube may be needed. Prepyloric membranes can become redundant and act as a "windsock" that produces an obstruction distal to the actual origin of the web; in

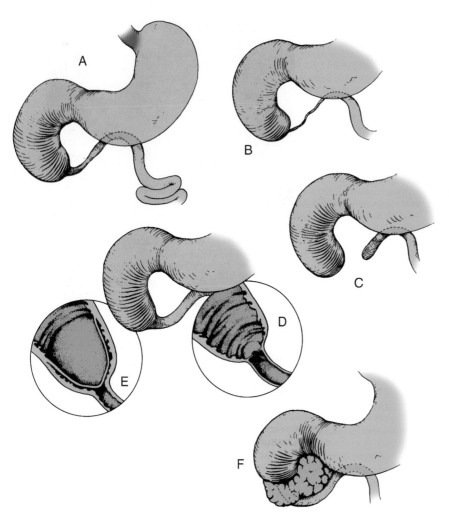

Figure 65–5.   Classification of anomalies causing duodenal obstruction. **A,** Type I atresia with intact membrane producing marked discrepancy in size between proximal and distal segments. **B,** Blind ends (type II) of duodenum connected by a fibrous cord. **C,** Blind ends (type III) are separated, and the mesentery is absent at the separation. **D,** Intraluminal membrane with a perforation. **E,** Windsock anomaly. An incision in the distal portion of the dilated segment is still beyond the obstruction. **F,** Annular pancreas. (From O'Neil JA Jr [ed]: Principles of Pediatric Surgery, 2nd ed. St Louis, CV Mosby, 2003, p 472.)

such instances the surgeon can mistakenly think that the obstruction is more distal. Longitudinal enterotomy, partial web excision, and transverse closure are sufficient. Incidentally noted ectopic pancreatic tissue or hamartomas in the pylorus should be excised.

The survival of infants and children with isolated congenital gastric outlet obstruction is excellent. In neonates with multiple anomalies, however, survival is lower. The presence of epidermolysis bullosa is associated with higher mortality and morbidity.[23]

Duodenal Obstruction

Incidence and Epidemiology   The overall incidence of congenital duodenal obstruction is approximately 1 in 5000 to 10,000 live births; it appears to be more common in males. The most common causes of congenital duodenal obstruction are atresia and stenosis. Duodenal atresia is associated with trisomy 21 in up to 30% of cases.[24-27] A rare familial duodenal atresia has been described as part of the "Feingold syndrome," which has associated microcephaly, limb anomalies, and tracheoesophageal anomalies; it appears to be autosomal dominant.

Embryology and Etiology   The embryonic duodenum is formed by the terminal part of the foregut and the cephalic portion of the midgut. Simultaneously, epithelial proliferation and recanalization occur in the duodenum. Vacuolization of the solid cord of proliferating epithelium results in recanalization. Abnormalities in recanalization or vascular accidents result in congenital duodenal anomalies, which may be associated with coexistent pancreatic and biliary anomalies. Around the third to fourth week the paired dorsal and ventral pancreatic buds originate from the duodenal entodermal epithelium and migrate to form the pancreas. The dorsal bud forms the body and tail; the ventral bud rotates 180 degrees and joins the dorsal gland to form the uncinate process. Abnormalities in rotation and fusion of the paired ventral buds around the pancreas result in an "annular" pancreas, which can cause extrinsic obstruction and may coexist with duodenal atresia.

Types   Duodenal obstruction can result from an intrinsic obstruction secondary to congenital atresia, stenosis, or a web, or it can result from an extrinsic obstruction secondary to GI duplications, compression by Ladd's bands, or an annular pancreas. The three morphologic types of intrinsic congenital duodenal obstruction are the following: type I, in which the duodenal wall is intact but there is an intraluminal membrane or web (Fig. 65–5A); type II, in which the atretic proximal and distal ends are connected by a fibrous cord (see Fig. 65–5B); and type

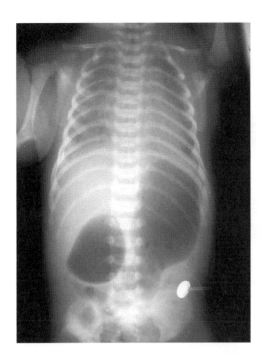

Figure 65–6. Classic plain film radiograph showing the "double bubble" in a patient with duodenal atresia. (Courtesy of Dr. Polly Kochan.)

III, in which there is a gap between the atretic ends, as well as a mesenteric defect (see Fig. 65–5C).

Clinical Features and Diagnosis Upper abdominal fullness with a flat or scaphoid lower abdomen is usual; feeding intolerance and bilious vomiting are classic signs. Congenital duodenal obstruction is associated with other congenital anomalies and trisomy 21, with more than 50% of patients having anomalies of the cardiac, renal, tracheoesophageal, anal, skeletal, and central nervous systems.[25-27] In addition, up to a third of these neonates may have an associated annular pancreas (see Fig. 65–5F) or malrotation. The diagnosis may be made prenatally by maternal ultrasound, which may also demonstrate polyhydramnios. Most often the diagnosis is made by the classic plain film radiographic image of a "double bubble" secondary to a distended stomach and duodenum (Fig. 65–6). Complete duodenal obstruction is associated with a gasless distal bowel. The presence of distal luminal air may indicate an incomplete membrane, a partially obstructing lesion, and most worrisome, a possible midgut volvulus causing the duodenal obstruction. In a neonate with a "double bubble" and distal air or one in whom it is uncertain whether the obstruction is related to a midgut volvulus, an urgent upper GI study needs to be performed because volvulus requires an immediate operation.

In the absence of any suspicion of volvulus, surgery can be performed less urgently. Patients with type I atresia can have a redundant intraluminal web that extends for a distance, thereby resulting in a windsock morphology (similar to antral or pyloric webs) (see Fig. 65–5E). Stenosis is usually secondary to an incomplete

diaphragm (Fig. 65–7A and B) or mucosal web with a central opening (see Fig. 65–5D). If the web has a larger opening, clinical detection may be delayed. Atresias usually cause postampullary obstruction, although up to 10% of cases can be preampullary.[24]

Management The stomach should be decompressed with an orogastric tube and all fluid and electrolyte abnormalities corrected. Associated anomalies should be investigated expeditiously before surgical repair. Chromosomal analysis for possible trisomy and a preoperative cardiology evaluation should be performed. A supraumbilical, right upper quadrant transverse incision is the usual surgical approach. Intestinal rotation is first inspected, and if malrotation is present, a "Ladd" procedure is performed before repair; if normal rotation is present, an extended "Kocher" maneuver is performed to expose the duodenum, pancreas, and root of the mesentery. The duodenum and distal bowel should be inspected to evaluate for additional coexisting distal atresia, which can occur in up to 5% of patients.

Type I atresias with a web and possible "windsock" should have the origin of the web confirmed by passage of an orogastric tube (Fig. 65–8A) or a balloon catheter into the duodenum or through a gastrotomy and withdrawal with the balloon inflated. A longitudinal duodenotomy is performed over the origin of the web (see Fig. 65–7B), and the location of the ampulla of Vater is identified; the web is then excised while taking care to avoid injury to the ampulla. The duodenotomy is closed transversely with interrupted sutures. The presence of distal atresia is excluded by passage of a balloon catheter distally through the duodenotomy.

Type II and III atresias may be repaired by a number of techniques, including side-to-side duodenoduodenostomy (see Fig. 65–8, C1), an end-to-side "diamond-shaped" duodenoduodenostomy (see Fig. 65–8, C2) and duodenojejunostomy (see Fig. 65–8B). The diamond-shaped duodenoduodenostomy appears to be the technique of choice and requires a transverse incision in the proximal duodenum with a longitudinal incision in the distal duodenum and an end-to-side duodenoduodenostomy (Fig. 65–8, C2). This technique results in a wider anastomosis that functions earlier and has reduced stasis from a blind loop or stenosis.[28] The side-to-side duodenoduodenostomy is often associated with delayed anastomotic transit times and megaduodenum.[29]

An annular pancreas causes duodenal obstruction in infancy and early childhood, although it is less frequent than intrinsic duodenal obstruction (see Fig. 65–5F).[26,30] A recent review of six case series since 1954 revealed a total of 66 reported cases of annular pancreas.[30] Such children are more likely to initially be seen in the neonatal period with nonbilious vomiting; they often have trisomy 21 and tracheoesophageal anomalies. Management is similar to that for type II and III duodenal atresia, with the diamond-shaped duodenoduodenostomy being the technique of choice to bypass the obstruction.[26,30] In the absence of significant comorbidity, the outcome is excellent.

Although we prefer using parenteral nutrition, enteral feeding after repair may be achieved early via a transanas-

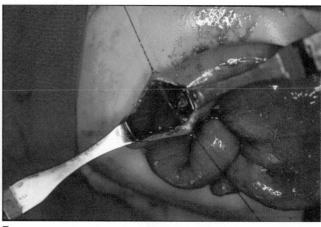

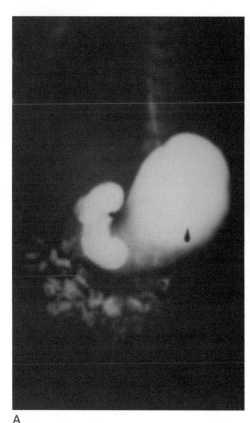

A

Figure 65–7.   A, Upper gastrointestinal study demonstrating a congenital type I duodenal web with incomplete obstruction of the duodenum. **B,** Operative photograph demonstrating a congenital type I duodenal web with incomplete obstruction of the duodenum visualized through the duodenotomy.

tomotic feeding tube because duodenal emptying is often delayed. Normal peristalsis is slow because of the dilated proximal duodenum, and in selected cases in which the proximal duodenum is markedly dilated, a tapering duodenoplasty is useful. A feeding gastrostomy is sometimes helpful in a complicated duodenal repair. The outcome depends on the associated comorbid conditions, such as congenital cardiac defects and chromosomal abnormalities.[25] Long-term follow-up studies have shown delayed morbidity in 12% and delayed mortality in 6% of patients undergoing repair of congenital duodenal anomalies.[29] GER disease and megaduodenum with upper GI motility disorders were the most common delayed morbidities identified in these studies. It appears that the dilated proximal duodenum is associated with disturbed transit.[31] Plication or a tapering duodenoplasty is recommended for the management of these delayed complications.[29,31]

ACQUIRED CONDITIONS

Hypertrophic Pyloric Stenosis

Incidence and Epidemiology Hypertrophic pyloric stenosis (HPS) is one of the most common disorders of the stomach and duodenum in infants that requires surgical correction. The reported incidence is 1 to 2 per 1000 live births.[32-34] It is more common in males at a 4 : 1 to 5 : 1 ratio and more common in white and Hispanic infants than in Asian and black infants. First-degree

relatives have an almost fivefold increase in risk for HPS.[35]

Etiology and Pathogenesis Hypertrophy of the pyloric muscle obstructs the passage of gastric contents through the pyloric canal. The pathogenesis has not been fully understood despite the frequency of its occurrence. A lack of nitric oxide synthase in pyloric muscle causes pylorospasm, and the loss of nitric oxide–mediated relaxation of smooth muscle may result in the hypertrophied and contracted pyloric muscle.[36] Abnormalities in peptide-containing nerve fibers, including a loss of peptide immunoreactivity in nerve fibers in the circular muscle, have also been described in the hypertrophied muscle.[37] Possible changes in hormonal control of pyloric sphincter function have been implicated, including abnormalities in gastrin and prostaglandins. Defects of the intestinal pacemaker (interstitial cells of Cajal), as well as abnormalities in extracellular matrix proteins and growth factors, are being reported as possible etiologic factors in the development of HPS.[38,39]

Clinical Features Typically, infants are 3 to 6 weeks old when they are initially evaluated for vomiting. They may start vomiting, however, as early as 2 weeks, or it may be delayed up to 12 weeks. The vomiting is usually nonbilious, postprandial, projectile, and progressive. HPS is most commonly seen in otherwise normal infants, but it occurs more frequently, at a 1% to 10% incidence, in patients who have undergone correction of esophageal

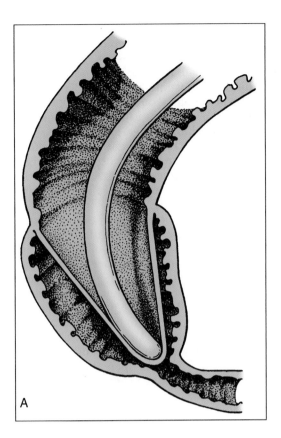

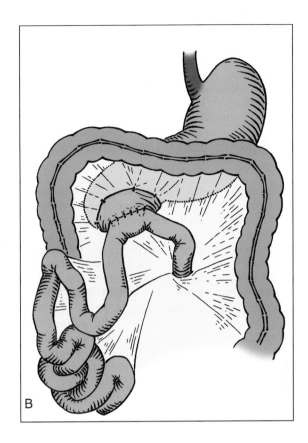

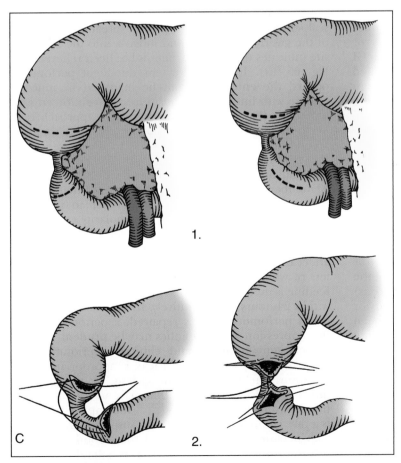

Figure 65–8. A, Pressure on the tube at the bottom of the web produces an indentation in the duodenal wall, indicating the point apex of the web. The incision should be placed at that point. **B,** Duodenojejunostomy. A loop of proximal jejunum is brought through an opening in the transverse mesocolon and anastomosed to the most dependent portion of the obstructed duodenum. This approach now is used only when direct duodenal anastomosis is not feasible. **C,** Duodenoduodenostomy. 1, Standard side-to-side anastomosis. 2, Diamond-shaped duodenoduodenostomy. (From O'Neil JA Jr [ed]: Principles of Pediatric Surgery, 2nd ed. St Louis, CV Mosby, 2003, p 474.)

atresia.[32,40] Intestinal malrotation and obstruction of the urinary tract also occur more frequently in association with this disorder.[32] A transient self-limited unconjugated hyperbilirubinemia secondary to a glucuronyl transferase deficiency similar to Gilbert's syndrome is seen in 1% to 2% of infants.[41] The differential diagnosis of non-bilious vomiting should include GER and overfeeding, gastroparesis, pylorospasm, other congenital gastric outlet obstruction (as discussed earlier in the chapter), and peptic ulcer disease.

Diagnosis An infant with a typical history and a palpable hypertrophic pylorus does not need additional diagnostic testing. The ability to successfully palpate a hypertrophic pylorus is variable, and this clinical ability appears to be decreasing with the increased reliance on imaging studies.[42] In a study of infants with HPS, for example, the pyloric mass was palpated in 87% during 1974 to 1977, as compared with 49% during 1988 to 1991.[43] In a more recent report (2000 to 2002), only 32% had a palpable "olive."[44] To successfully palpate the pyloric "olive," the infant needs to be quiet with a relaxed abdominal wall. One technique is to allow the infant to suck a pacifier, and while standing on the infant's left side and holding the legs flexed at the hips in the left hand, the fingertips of the right hand are gently swept from the liver edge toward the umbilicus. Increased serum bicarbonate and decreased serum chloride levels favor a diagnosis of HPS.[45]

In the absence of a palpable "olive," either an upper GI study or an ultrasonogram may be performed. An upper GI study is approximately 95% sensitive, although error rates of up to 11% have been reported.[46] On an upper GI study, a "string" sign indicating a narrowed elongated pyloric canal that does not relax is seen; a "shoulder" sign caused by the hypertrophied muscle indenting the antrum and a "double-track" sign caused by the redundant mucosa may be observed.[46,47] Real-time ultrasonography, however, appears to be the most reliable diagnostic test; it is almost 100% accurate in the hands of an experienced operator, it does not involve radiation exposure, and the examiner does not have to wait for the stomach to empty.[46,47] Sonographic measurements that are reported to be diagnostic include a pyloric wall thickness of at least 4 mm and a channel length of at least 17 mm.[48] The actual measurements may not be as important as evaluation of the overall morphology of the antrum and pylorus and evaluation of gastric emptying.[46] Measurement of the volume of gastric aspirate in a vomiting (nonbilious) infant can help determine whether an upper GI study or ultrasonography should be performed, and this has been suggested as a more cost-effective approach in deciding the appropriate imaging study.[49]

Management In an infant with normal fluid and electrolyte status, surgical correction with general anesthesia as soon as logistically feasible is appropriate. Some infants will need correction of their fluids and electrolytes, and about 10% to 15% will be significantly dehydrated and have a hyponatremic, hypochloremic, hypokalemic metabolic alkalosis.[42] In a severely dehydrated infant, initial resuscitation is begun with a 10- to 20-ml/kg bolus of normal saline. Correction of both electrolyte losses and intravascular depletion is essential before surgery because pyloric stenosis is not a surgical emergency. Once adequate hydration and normal urine output are achieved, potassium is added to the intravenous fluids. The metabolic alkalosis is chloride responsive; further fluids (5% dextrose with 0.45% saline and 20 mEq of potassium chloride per liter) are given at 150% of the maintenance requirement. A serum bicarbonate level of 28 mEq/L or lesser is usually the target for correction before surgical repair. Keeping the stomach empty before the repair by using a gastric tube may help limit further vomiting.

The procedure of choice is a Ramstedt-Fredet extramucosal pyloromyotomy performed with the infant under general anesthesia. A number of incisions to perform the pyloromyotomy have been described, including a transverse right upper quadrant incision, vertical midline incision, and circumumbilical incision (Fig. 65–9A-D),[50,51] as well as three-port laparoscopic approaches. There does not seem to be a significant difference in outcome between the laparoscopic and open approaches, although more complications may occur in the laparoscopic group.[52-54] In the open approach, after the peritoneum is opened and the hypertrophied pylorus is delivered to the surface, a seromuscular incision is made into the pyloric muscle. The pyloromyotomy incision extends from just proximal to the duodenum (pyloric vein) onto the antrum of the stomach. The initial myotomy is deepened bluntly with the back of a scalpel handle or a Benson pyloric spreader. Protrusion of the gastric submucosa and mucosa into the myotomy site indicates that the obstruction has been relieved (see Fig. 65–9D). If an inadvertent duodenal perforation occurs, the enterotomy can be managed by mucosal closure with fine absorbable suture and reinforced with omentum (Fig. 65–10A). An alternative approach is to perform a two-layer closure of the pylorus, followed by a second myotomy at a site rotated 90 to 180 degrees from the repair (see Fig. 65–10B). In an uncomplicated pyloromyotomy, feeding is resumed within 4 to 6 hours. A number of different feeding protocols that include incremental advances from sugar water to increased amounts of formula volume and osmolarity every 2 to 3 hours have been used. The type of feeding protocol may influence postoperative vomiting but does not appear to affect the time to full feeding or discharge.[55,56] Regardless of whether a feeding schedule or early ad libitum feeding is used, most infants will reach their feeding goal within 24 hours postoperatively. In an infant with a duodenal perforation that is repaired, a period of gastric decompression and antibiotics may be prudent. If there is persistent vomiting and clinical deterioration, an upper GI study to rule out a leak is appropriate. Complications include persistent emesis in up to 10%, mucosal perforation in less than 5%, and wound infection in up to 10% of infants.[42,56,57] Incomplete myotomy is a rare complication that may be suspected in an infant with persistent vomiting beyond the second week after pyloromyotomy. An upper GI study is helpful in showing the vomiting to be secondary to GER, which is a more likely diagnosis in this situation.

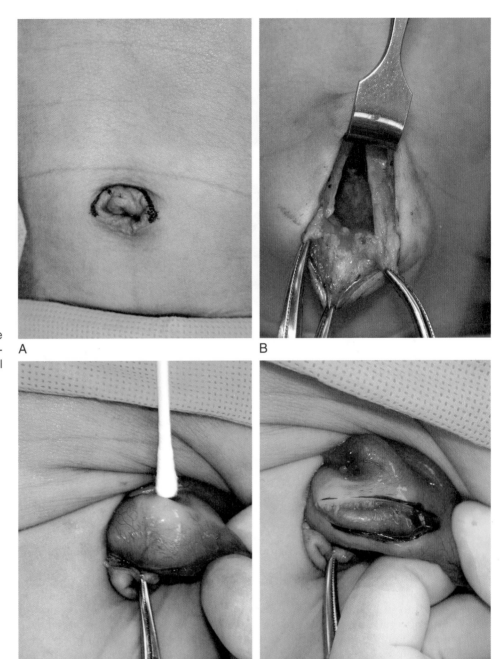

Figure 65–9. **A** to **D,** Operative photographs showing pyloromyotomy through a circumumbilical incision.

Neonatal Gastric Perforation

Incidence Gastric perforations are uncommon in neonates, but they may be seen in both term and preterm newborns and usually occur in the first week of life.[58-61] Perforations often occur in newborns who have undergone neonatal resuscitation.

Etiology There is no consensus regarding the cause of neonatal gastric perforation, and even whether these perforations are "spontaneous" or secondary to other factors is controversial.[58,59] "Mechanical" causes secondary to gastric dilatation from resuscitation and mechanical

ventilation, as well as "low-flow" or "ischemic" causes from hypoxia and prematurity, have been postulated.[59,61] The cause is probably multifactorial; possibly, the cause of perforation in a preterm newborn may be a low-flow state, whereas in a term newborn it may be a mechanical cause.[59-61]

Clinical Features and Diagnosis Gastric perforation may be manifested as feeding intolerance, abdominal distention, upper GI bleeding, respiratory distress, or a picture of "sepsis." The diagnosis of perforation is almost always evident on plain film radiographs with massive pneumoperitoneum. A cross-table lateral or decubitus film

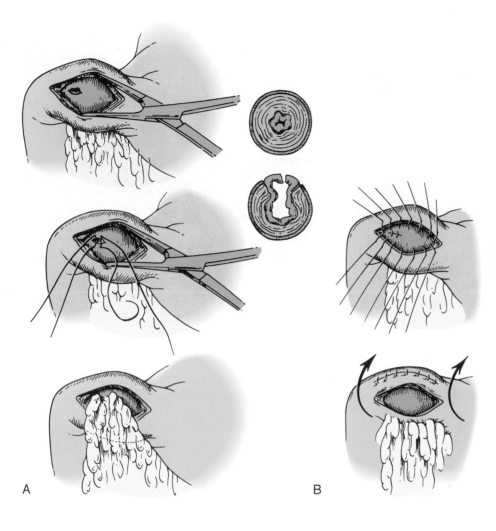

Figure 65–10.   A and **B,** Alternative techniques for closure of an inadvertent enterotomy.

may clarify the presence of pneumoperitoneum. In neonates with rapid deterioration and ventilation difficulty because of significant abdominal distention, decompressive peritoneocentesis may relieve the acute respiratory distress. There is usually a single perforation on the anterolateral aspect of the greater curvature near the fundus, although the perforation may be seen along the lesser curvature and rarely posteriorly near the gastroesophageal junction.[58-61] The differential diagnosis includes perforation from necrotizing enterocolitis, pyloric atresia, colonic atresia, and Hirschsprung's disease.

Management   Early surgical exploration is lifesaving, and the usual surgical approach is a transverse right supraumbilical incision. The posterior aspect of the stomach and the gastroesophageal junction should always be inspected by opening the lesser sac. Most isolated gastric perforations can be repaired primarily in one or two layers without major resection of the stomach. The addition of a gastrostomy or drain depends on individual preference. Cases of significant gastric necrosis from necrotizing gastritis may require subtotal gastrectomy. In up to 20% of infants with possible neonatal gastric perforation based on the clinical picture and radiographs, a perforation may not be identified at surgery and pre-

sumably a small perforation has sealed itself by the time that surgery is performed.[61] In preterm newborns maintained on ventilator support, air leaks can track from the lungs into the peritoneal cavity.[62] These newborns will usually have an obvious pneumomediastinum and pulmonary interstitial emphysema and do not show signs of sepsis from intestinal perforation. Despite the presence of perforation and peritonitis, most of these neonates have a good surgical outcome.

Gastric Tumors

Incidence   Gastric tumors are rare in infants and children.[63] A 10-year review of 1403 reports of gastric disease at a single institution revealed only three pediatric gastric tumors.[64] Another review of 39 children with gastrointestinal tumors over a 20-year period revealed one leiomyosarcoma of the stomach.[65]

Clinical Features and Diagnosis   Although rare, the most common gastric tumors are teratomas. They usually occur in males and are marked by a mass, abdominal distention, vomiting, and rarely, upper GI bleeding or perforation.[63,66] The diagnosis can be made with a combination of imaging modalities; usually, ultrasonog-

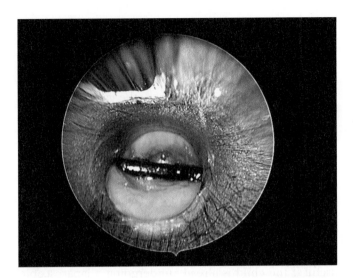

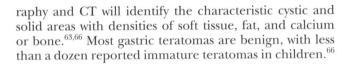

Figure 65–11. Endoscopic view of an impacted foreign body in the esophagus before removal. (Courtesy of Dr. Glenn Isaacson.)

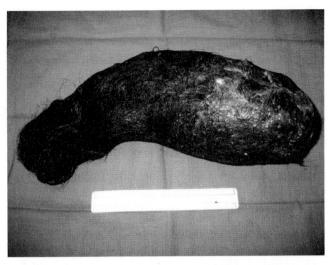

Figure 65–12. A large trichobezoar that caused gastric obstruction removed surgically.

raphy and CT will identify the characteristic cystic and solid areas with densities of soft tissue, fat, and calcium or bone.[63,66] Most gastric teratomas are benign, with less than a dozen reported immature teratomas in children.[66]

Management Treatment of gastric teratoma is complete surgical excision with reconstruction of the remaining stomach. In an immature gastric teratoma, a strategy of monitoring the α-fetoprotein level after resection seems prudent rather than giving these children chemotherapy.[66] After complete excision the prognosis for these benign tumors is excellent.

Foreign Bodies

Incidence Children swallow foreign bodies as a result of their exploration of the environment. The peak incidence is between 6 months and 3 years of age. Coins are the most commonly ingested objects. Most foreign bodies in the GI tract are asymptomatic and probably pass spontaneously in stool.

Clinical Features and Diagnosis Swallowed foreign bodies are diagnosed when plain radiographs are obtained for symptoms related to the airway or the esophagus. Transient coughing or choking, pain in the pharynx or retrosternal region, and excessive salivation, drooling, or retching are the common symptoms in a child with a foreign body in the esophagus. A plain radiograph, including a lateral view, can differentiate an esophageal from a tracheal foreign body; the lateral view demonstrates the foreign body's posterior relationship to the tracheal air column.

Management All esophageal foreign bodies confirmed by plain radiography should be removed by flexible or rigid esophagoscopy (Fig. 65–11).[67] If the foreign body passes into the stomach, extraction can usually be

avoided because most of these foreign bodies will pass spontaneously. Expectant management is appropriate for smaller rounded objects, with occasional serial radiographs taken after several weeks; exceptions include sharp objects and button batteries. If symptoms occur that are suggestive of obstruction or perforation or if the object remains lodged in the stomach for more than 4 weeks, endoscopic retrieval is recommended. Sharp objects, such as needles and safety pins, should be extracted if they are localized in the stomach because of the risk for perforation.[68] Button batteries are a special case, especially if they are larger than 15 mm, because of the risk of corrosive damage if lodged in the esophagus or the stomach.[69] Removal of an esophageal button battery as soon it is detected is recommended. Although most foreign bodies usually pass through the GI tract once they enter the stomach, button batteries should be extracted to avoid gastric perforation.[67]

Bezoars

Definition and Types Bezoars are foreign bodies in the lumen of the stomach or rarely the intestine that increase in size over time because of continued deposition of ingested food or fibers. There are principally three types: trichobezoars, composed of hair, are the most common; phytobezoars are composed of vegetable matter; and lactobezoars are derived from milk precipitates.

Clinical Features and Diagnosis Bezoars are an uncommon cause of gastric outlet obstruction and are associated with early satiety, abdominal pain, vomiting, and abdominal distention. They can usually be diagnosed by CT, upper GI study, or endoscopy.[70]

Management Although endoscopic and laparoscopic removal has been described, surgical removal is generally required because of their large size (Fig. 65–12).[71,72] Trichobezoars are often associated with trichotillomania, a psychiatric disorder associated with pulling and ingestion of hair, and psychiatric management is recommended to avoid recurrence. Phytobezoars can be digested with enzymes such as papain or fragmented endoscopically. Lactobezoars are often seen in newborns receiving formula feedings and usually respond to nasogastric lavage and decompression.

Gastrostomy

Short-term enteral access can be obtained in infants and children with a nasogastric tube; however, they occlude easily and can contribute to airway obstruction in an infant, who is an obligate nasal breather.

Indications The primary indication for a gastrostomy tube is the need for long-term enteral access for fluids and nutrition. Other indications include the need for gastric decompression in a neurologically impaired infant with a fundoplication, after repair of atresia, or the need for urgent gastric decompression in a newborn with a congenital tracheoesophageal fistula and ventilatory difficulty. A rare indication is for the management of gastric volvulus. A gastrostomy may be contraindicated in those with uncontrolled ascites and coagulopathy, and a relative contraindication is a terminal condition in an infant or child.

Types of Gastrostomy

Open Gastrostomy The Stamm gastrostomy, the most commonly used surgical gastrostomy, has the advantage of not requiring a surgical procedure for closure if the need for the gastrostomy is temporary. An upper midline or left paramedian muscle-splitting incision is used. A site on the anterior wall of the stomach at the junction of the body and antrum is chosen, not too close to the pylorus because the tube could act as an obstruction. Two concentric purse-string sutures are placed to invert the seromuscular layer of the anterior gastric wall around the tube, thus creating a tunnel. The exit site on the abdominal wall should be chosen so that it avoids tension between the stomach and abdominal wall; a separate stab incision is made for the exit site, or it may exit from the incision, and four-quadrant sutures secure stomach to the abdominal wall (see Chapter 52 for a detailed description). Usually, feeding can be started within 24 hours of gastrostomy placement. Any child who may need an esophageal replacement, such as those with long-gap esophageal atresia or a corrosive esophageal injury, should have the gastrostomy placed closer to the lesser curvature of the stomach to avoid injury to the gastroepiploic vessels because these vessels would be the blood supply for a potential gastric tube.

The Witzel gastrostomy is a modification of the Stamm gastrostomy that consists of imbrication of an additional anterior seromuscular layer of stomach over the tube to make a longer tunnel (see Chapter 52 for a detailed description).

The Janeway gastrostomy, the least common type of gastrostomy, is a permanent gastrostomy fashioned from a gastric flap that is tubularized (see Chapter 52 for a detailed description).

Percutaneous Endoscopic Gastrostomy A percutaneous, endoscopically assisted gastrostomy (PEG) was introduced by Gauderer et al. to allow placement of a feeding gastrostomy without laparotomy (see Chapter 52 for details).[73]

Once gastric access is obtained, the gastrostomy tube can be replaced by a gastrostomy button after 6 weeks (to ensure a mature gastrocutaneous tract). The gastrostomy button is a low-profile skin-level device with a valve that can also be placed primarily at the initial surgery.

Laparoscopic-Assisted Gastrostomy This technique involves percutaneously accessing the stomach for placement of a gastrostomy under visual control with the laparoscope. Sutures passed through the abdominal wall or "T-fasteners" are used to stabilize the anterior wall of the stomach while the tube is inserted. This technique is useful if the child is already undergoing a laparoscopic procedure; it may also be a safer alternative to PEG if there is concern regarding the anatomy of the colon.[74]

Percutaneous Image-Guided Gastrostomy There are a number of image-guided gastrostomy placement techniques. The retrograde percutaneous fluoroscopic technique is commonly used and involves fluoroscopic visualization of a needle puncture of the stomach followed by the creation of a tract over a guidewire.[75] A "pull" technique similar to PEG can also be used for image-guided gastrostomy.

Complications Gastrostomies have a number of reported complications. Major complications include dislodgement of the tube with peritonitis, inadvertent enteric perforation, gastrocolic fistula, GI bleeding, and peritonitis. Leakage around the gastrostomy occurs if the stomach separates from the abdominal wall. Placement close to the pylorus or inadvertent advancement of the tube toward the pylorus can cause gastric outlet obstruction. Local erythema, cellulitis, and tissue necrosis can occur if there is excess tension at the exit site. Surrounding tissue necrosis can result in an enlarging gastrostomy stoma with peristomal leakage. Granulation tissue often develops around the stoma and needs to be cauterized with silver nitrate. A review of PEG in children reported an overall 27% complication rate, including infection, abscess, vomiting, malposition of the gastrostomy, and one death.[76] A review of 208 children with image-guided gastrostomy or gastrojejunostomy tubes revealed a major complication rate of 5% and a minor complication rate of 73% after the insertion of gastrostomy and gastrojejunal tubes by the image-guided retrograde percutaneous route. Major complications included peritonitis, septicemia, abscess, GI bleeding, and death. Minor complications included tube dislodgement, leakage, skin infection, tube migration, and obstruction.[77]

There are reports of worsening GER after gastrostomy, which can be prevented by placing the gastrostomy closer to the lesser curve.[78] In neurologically impaired patients, an upper GI study and pH probe monitoring should be done, and in the absence of significant GER, a gastrostomy without a protective antireflux procedure is adequate. If GER is significant, some recommend that a fundoplication be performed along with the gastrostomy.[79]

The gastrocutaneous tract matures during a 3- to 6-week period. Removal of a Stamm-type gastrostomy can result in closure of the tract within 24 hours; therefore, immobilization of the tube at the exit site is important to avoid dislodgement. Inadvertent removal of the tube before a mature tract has formed warrants placement of a small catheter through the tract and confirmation of tube position by fluoroscopy and a water-soluble contrast study. If the tract cannot be safely accessed in the office, the tube should be replaced under fluoroscopic guidance.

Peptic Ulcer Disease

Definition and Types Clinically significant peptic ulcer disease is an uncommon condition in infancy and childhood, and with improved diagnosis and medical management, there are few indications for surgical therapy. The pediatric surgeon is usually consulted for complications of peptic ulcer disease, such as persistent life-threatening upper GI bleeding, acquired gastric outlet obstruction from chronic ulceration and scarring, and perforation.[80,81]

Peptic ulcers in infants and children are usually classified as primary or secondary ulcers. A primary ulcer occurs in the absence of any predisposing illnesses or factors and is often associated with gastric acid hypersecretion. A secondary ulcer is generally associated with increased stress from illness, trauma, burns, or medications such as steroids and nonsteroidal anti-inflammatory drugs (NSAIDs).

Etiology Primary ulcers may have a genetic basis and occur more frequently in association with blood group O. They are located in the duodenum and pyloric channel and are rarely seen in the stomach. Although increased or excessive acid secretion is important in the pathophysiology of primary peptic ulcer disease, no direct relationship has been established between consistently elevated levels of acidity in children with primary ulcer disease. There appears to be increasing evidence that the chronic relapsing ulcer disease characteristic of a primary peptic ulcer is linked to coexisting, chronic, active antral gastritis secondary to *Helicobacter pylori* infection.[82,83]

H. pylori is a gram-negative spiral-shaped organism that has been associated with the presence of chronic gastritis. *H. pylori* infection appears to be very common in developing countries, but it may also be seen in about 10% of children in the United States by the time that they are 10 years old.[82-84] It appears that up to 10% of cases of *H. pylori* gastritis will result in duodenal ulcers, especially in children older than 10 years.[83,84] In addition, it is a significant risk factor for the development of gastric cancer in adults. Eradication of *H. pylori* reduces the recurrence of ulcers to less than 5%.[86] Children with *H. pylori* infection and peptic ulcer disease should be treated with a 10- to 14-day triple-therapy regimen.[82,85,86]

Zollinger-Ellison syndrome, which results from a functional gastrinoma, G-cell hyperplasia, or G-cell hyper-

function, is a rare condition associated with acid hypersecretion. The increased gastrin levels lead to increased gastric acid output, which in turn results in diarrhea and multiple or recurrent peptic ulcers. These ulcers may also involve the proximal jejunum (see Chapter 58 for a discussion on Zollinger-Ellison syndrome).

Secondary peptic ulcers are more common in infants and children than primary ulcers are. They are also called "stress" ulcers because they occur with stresses that increase acid secretion or reduce mucosal defense mechanisms, or both. Drugs such as aspirin and NSAIDs decrease mucosal blood flow by inhibiting prostaglandin synthesis and stimulating inflammatory mediators. In addition, protective mucosal secretions can be inhibited by pharmacologic agents. Ulcers associated with head trauma are characterized by increased gastric acid secretion ("Cushing ulcer"); however, ulcers associated with thermal injury have normal gastric acid secretion (Curling's ulcer). Other stresses, such as sepsis, cardiac insufficiency, surgical trauma, and hypoxia, may result in ulcer disease. Secondary ulcers are usually located in the stomach, although they can occur in the duodenum as well. Secondary ulcers do not usually recur if they are treated and the associated factors are controlled.

Clinical Features Primary peptic ulcer disease in an older child is usually manifested as abdominal pain and vomiting and rarely as significant GI bleeding. In addition, iron deficiency anemia from occult blood loss may be an initial sign. Gastric outlet obstruction and perforation from peptic ulcer disease are rare in children. Stress ulcers are seen in critically ill infants and children, most often with GI bleeding from diffuse erosive mucosal lesions of the stomach. Perforation from stress ulceration is an unusual event, although more common than a perforated primary peptic ulcer in a child.

Diagnosis The diagnosis of peptic ulcer disease is based on endoscopic examination of the gastric and duodenal mucosa. Although an upper GI contrast study can be helpful in defining gastric outlet obstruction, it is inadequate for the diagnosis of mucosal ulceration. Antral and duodenal biopsy with the rapid urease test plus histopathologic examination is the current diagnostic standard for *H. pylori*.

Management The initial treatment of peptic ulcer disease is medical therapy. The goal is to heal the ulcer, prevent recurrence, and avoid the complications of bleeding, perforation, and obstruction. Secondary ulcers are treated by eliminating the stressful event; those related to NSAIDs are treated by discontinuing their use. Additionally, treatment involves the use of acid suppression and mucosal protection with antacids, H_2 blockers, proton pump inhibitors, or mucosal coating agents, alone or in combination. Secondary ulcers can be prevented by H_2 blockers or mucosal coating agents. In children with a diagnosis of *H. pylori* and documented peptic ulcer, it is essential to initiate a 7- to 14-day triple-therapy regimen. The traditional indications for surgical treatment include perforation, uncontrolled bleeding, gastric outlet obstruction, and intractable pain. Children with peptic ulcer disease may have complications requiring surgery in adulthood. Although the incidence of surgery has declined over time, the incidence of obstruction as an indication for surgery appears to be unchanged.[81] In a child with a refractory primary ulcer or multiple recurrences, or both, Zollinger-Ellison syndrome should be ruled out by evaluation of gastrin levels both at baseline and after secretin challenge. If a benign gastrinoma is suspected, localization and excision will result in cure.

Initial treatment of a bleeding peptic ulcer is medical and includes resuscitation, pharmacologic therapy, and diagnostic endoscopy. Endoscopic sclerotherapy or treatment with a heater probe is initiated by the gastroenterologist. Persistent bleeding after failed medical and endoscopic therapy, as indicated by the loss of half a blood volume in 8 hours or one blood volume in 24 hours, is an indication for surgery. The surgical approach is dictated by the location and the hemodynamic status and age of the patient. In a younger child with bleeding gastric ulcers, oversewing the ulcer along with intensive pharmacologic medical therapy is usually adequate. In an older child with a bleeding duodenal ulcer, management is similar to that for an adult: oversewing the bleeding ulcer and vagotomy with pyloroplasty or selective vagotomy. Perforations are treated by plication and an omental patch followed by intensive medical therapy; an acid reduction procedure is not usually needed in a child. Children with gastric outlet obstruction generally require vagotomy with a drainage procedure or vagotomy and antrectomy. Because of the lack of large series of children who have undergone these procedures, adult surgical recommendations are often extrapolated to these patients. A detailed description of the management of ulcer disease and vagotomy and drainage procedures may be found in Chapters 55 and 56.

REFERENCES

1. Moore KL, Persaud TVN: The digestive system. In Moore KL, Persaud TVN (eds): Before We Are Born. Essentials of Embryology and Birth Defects, 6th ed. Philadelphia, Elsevier, 2003, pp 201-227.
2. Holcomb GW 3rd, Gheissari A, O'Neill JA Jr, et al: Surgical management of alimentary tract duplications. Ann Surg 209:167-174, 1989.
3. Stringer MD, Spitz L, Abel R, et al: Management of alimentary tract duplication in children. Br J Surg 82:74-78, 1995.
4. Schochat SJ, Strand RD, Fellows KE: Perforated gastric duplication with pulmonary communication: A case report. Surgery 70:370-374, 1971.
5. Menon P, Rao KL, Saxena AK: Duplication cyst of the stomach presenting as hemoptysis. Eur J Pediatr Surg 14:429-431, 2004.
6. Moss RL, Ryan JA, Kozarek RA, et al: Pancreatitis caused by a gastric duplication communicating with an aberrant pancreatic lobe. J Pediatr Surg 31:733-736, 1996.
7. Kuraoka K, Nakayama H, Kagawa T, et al: Adenocarcinoma arising from a gastric duplication cyst with invasion to the stomach: A case report with literature review. J Clin Pathol 57:428-431, 2004.
8. Horie H, Iwasaki I, Takamashi M: Carcinoid in a gastrointestinal duplication. J Pediatr Surg 21:902-904, 1986.
9. Ford WD, Guelfand M, López PJ, Furness ME: Laparoscopic excision of a gastric duplication cyst detected on antenatal ultrasound scan. J Pediatr Surg 39(10):e8-e10, 2004.
10. Elhalaby EA, Mashaly EM: Infants with radiologic diagnosis of gastric volvulus: Are they over-treated? Pediatr Surg Int 17:596-600, 2001.
11. Miller DL, Pasquale MD, Seneca RP, Hodin E: Gastric volvulus in the pediatric population. Arch Surg 126:1146-1149, 1991.
12. Honna T, Kamii Y, Tsuchida Y: Idiopathic gastric volvulus in infancy and childhood. J Pediatr Surg 25:707-710, 1990.
13. Aoyama K, Tateishi K: Gastric volvulus in three children with asplenic syndrome. J Pediatr Surg 21:307-310, 1986.
14. Shah A, Shah AV: Laparoscopic gastropexy in a neonate for acute gastric volvulus. Pediatr Surg Int 19:217-219, 2003.
15. Cameron BH, Blair GH: Laparoscopic-guided gastropexy for intermittent gastric volvulus. J Pediatr Surg 28:1628-1629, 1993.
16. Velasco AL, Holcomb GW III, Templeton JM Jr, Ziegler MM: Management of congenital microgastria. J Pediatr Surg 25:192-197, 1990.
17. Neifeld JP, Berman WF, Lawrence W Jr, et al: Management of congenital microgastria with a jejunal reservoir pouch. J Pediatr Surg 15:882-885, 1980.
18. Kroes EJ, Festen C: Congenital microgastria: A case report and review of literature. Pediatr Surg Int 13:416-418, 1998.
19. Anderson KD, Guzzetta PC: Treatment of congenital microgastria and dumping syndrome. J Pediatr Surg 18:747-750, 1983.
20. Ilce Z, Erdogan E, Kara C, et al: Pyloric atresia. 15-year review from a single institution. J Pediatr Surg 38:1581-1584, 2003.
21. Blazek F, Boeckman CR: Prepyloric antral diaphragm: Delays in treatment. J Pediatr Surg 22:948-949, 1987.
22. Okoye BO, Parikh DH, Buick RG, et al: Pyloric atresia: Five new cases, a new association, and a review of the literature with guidelines. J Pediatr Surg 35:1242-1245, 2000.
23. Samad L, Siddiqui EF, Arain MA, et al: Pyloric atresia associated with epidermolysis bullosa—three cases presenting in three months. J Pediatr Surg 39:1267-1269, 2004.
24. Fonkalsrud EW, de Lorimier AA, Hays DM: Congenital atresia and stenosis of the duodenum. A review compiled from the members of the Surgical Section of the American Academy of Pediatrics. Pediatrics 43:79-83, 1969.
25. Grosfeld JL, Rescorla FJ: Duodenal atresia and stenosis: Reassessment of treatment and outcome based on antenatal diagnosis, pathologic variance, and long-term follow-up. World J Surg 17:301-309, 1993.
26. Stauffer UG, Schwoebel M: Duodenal atresia and stenosis-annular pancreas. In O'Neill JA Jr, Rowe MI, Grosfeld JL, et al (eds): Pediatric Surgery, 5th ed. St Louis, Mosby–Year Book, 1998, pp 1133-1143.
27. Dal la Vecchia LK, Grosfeld JL, West KW, et al: Intestinal atresia and stenosis: A 25-year experience with 277 cases. Arch Surg 133:490-497, 1998.
28. Kimura K, Mukohara N, Nashijima E, et al: Diamond-shaped anastomosis for duodenal atresia: An experience with 44 patients over 15 years. J Pediatr Surg 25:977-979, 1990.
29. Escobar MA, Ladd AP, Grosfeld JL, et al: Duodenal atresia and stenosis: Long-term follow-up over 30 years. J Pediatr Surg 39:867-871, 2004.
30. Jimenez JC, Emil S, Podnos Y, Nguyen N: Annular pancreas in children: A recent decade's experience. J Pediatr Surg 39:1654-1657, 2004.
31. Takahashi A, Tomomasa T, Suzuki N, et al: The relationship between disturbed transit and dilated bowel, and manometric findings of dilated bowel in patients with duodenal atresia and stenosis. J Pediatr Surg 32:1157-1160, 1997.
32. Applegate MS, Druschel CM: The epidemiology of infantile hypertrophic pyloric stenosis in New York State, 1983 to 1990. Arch Pediatr Adolesc Med 149:1123-1129, 1995.
33. Schechter R, Torfs CP, Bateson TF: The epidemiology of infantile hypertrophic pyloric stenosis. Paediatr Perinat Epidemiol 11:407-427, 1997.
34. Hedback G, Abrahamsson K, Husberg B, et al: The epidemiology of infantile hypertrophic pyloric stenosis in Sweden 1987-96. Arch Dis Child 85:379-381, 2001.
35. Mitchell LE, Risch N: The genetics of infantile hypertrophic pyloric stenosis: A reanalysis. Am J Dis Child 147:1203-1211, 1993.
36. Vanderwinden J, Mailleux P, Shiffmann S, et al: Nitric oxide synthase activity in infantile hypertrophic pyloric stenosis. N Engl J Med 327:511-515, 1992.

37. Wattchow DA, Cass DT, Furness JB, et al: Abnormalities of peptide-containing nerve fibers in infantile hypertrophic pyloric stenosis. Gastroenterology 92:443-448, 1987.
38. Ohishiro K, Puri P: Pathogenesis of infantile hypertrophic pyloric stenosis: Recent progress. Pediatr Surg Int 13:243-252, 1998.
39. Piotrowska AP, Solari V, Puri P: Distribution of heme oxygenase-2 in nerves and interstitial cells of Cajal in the normal pylorus and in infantile hypertrophic pyloric stenosis. Arch Pathol Lab Med 127:1182-1186, 2003.
40. Louhimo I, Lindahl H: Esophageal atresia: Primary results of 500 consecutively treated patients. J Pediatr Surg 18:217-229, 1983.
41. Schwartz MZ: Hypertropic pyloric stenosis. In O'Neill JA Jr, Rowe MI, Grosfeld JL, et al (eds): Pediatric Surgery, 5th ed. St Louis, Mosby–Year Book, 1998, pp 1111-1117.
42. Poon TS, Zhang AL, Cartmill T, Cass DT: Changing patterns of diagnosis and treatment of infantile hypertrophic pyloric stenosis: A clinical audit of 303 patients. J Pediatr Surg 31:1611-1615, 1996.
43. Macdessi J, Oates R: Clinical diagnosis of pyloric stenosis: A declining art. BMJ 306:553-555, 1993.
44. Helton KJ, Strife JL, Warner BW, et al: The impact of a clinical guideline on imaging children with hypertrophic pyloric stenosis. Pediatr Radiol 34:733-736, 2004.
45. Smith GA, Mihalov L, Shields BJ: Diagnostic aids in the differentiation of pyloric stenosis from severe gastroesophageal reflux during early infancy: The utility of serum bicarbonate and serum chloride. Am J Emerg Med 17:28-31, 1999.
46. Hernanz-Schulman M: Infantile hypertrophic pyloric stenosis. Radiology 227:319-331, 2003.
47. Cohen HL, Babcock DS, Kushner DC, et al: Vomiting in infants up to 3 months of age. American College of Radiology. ACR Appropriateness Criteria. Radiology 215(Suppl):779-786, 2000.
48. Teele RL, Smith EH: Ultrasound in the diagnosis of idiopathic hypertrophic pyloric stenosis. N Engl J Med 296:1149-1150, 1977.
49. Mandell GA, Wolfson PJ, Adkins ES, et al: Cost-effective imaging approach to the nonbilious vomiting infant. Pediatrics 103:1198-1202, 1999.
50. Tan KC, Bianchi A: Circumumbilical incision for pyloromyotomy. Br J Surg 73:399, 1999.
51. Misra D, Mushtag I: Surface umbilical pyloromyotomy. Eur J Pediatr Surg 8:81-82, 1998.
52. Sitsen E, Bax NMA, Van der Zee DC: Is laparoscopic pyloromyotomy superior to open surgery? Surg Endosc 12:813-815, 1998.
53. Campbell BT, McLean K, Barnhart DC, et al: A comparison of laparoscopic and open pyloromyotomy at a teaching hospital. J Pediatr Surg 37:1068-1071, 2002.
54. van der Bilt JD, Kramer WL, van der Zee DC, Bax NM: Laparoscopic pyloromyotomy for hypertrophic pyloric stenosis: Impact of experience on the results in 182 cases. Surg Endosc 18:907-909, 2004.
55. Gollin G, Doslouglu H, Flummerfeldt P, et al: Rapid advancement of feedings after pyloromyotomy for pyloric stenosis. Clin Pediatr (Phila) 39:187-190, 2000.
56. Michalsky MP, Pratt D, Caniano DA, et al: Streamlining the care of patients with hypertrophic pyloric stenosis: Application of a clinical pathway. J Pediatr Surg 37:1072-1075, 2002.
57. Hulka F, Harrison MW, Campbell TJ, et al: Complications of pyloromyotomy for infantile hypertrophic pyloric stenosis. Am J Surg 173:450-452, 1997.
58. Rosser SB, Clark CH, Elechi EN: Spontaneous neonatal gastric perforation. J Pediatr Surg 17:390-394, 1982.
59. Leone RJ Jr, Krasna IH: 'Spontaneous' neonatal gastric perforation: Is it really spontaneous? J Pediatr Surg 35:1066-1069, 2000.
60. Jawad AJ, Al-Rabie A, Hadi A, et al: Spontaneous neonatal gastric perforation. Pediatr Surg Int 18:396-399, 2002.
61. Kara CS, Ilce Z, Celayir S, et al: Neonatal gastric perforation: Review of 23 years' experience. Surgery Today 34:243-245, 2002.
62. Briassoulis GC, Venkataraman ST, Vasilopoulos AG, et al: Air leaks from the respiratory tract in mechanically ventilated children with severe respiratory disease. Pediatr Pulmonol 29:127-134, 2000.
63. Ford EG: Gastrointestinal tumors. In Andrassy RJ (ed): Pediatric Surgical Oncology. Philadelphia, WB Saunders, 1998, pp 289-304.
64. Murphy S, Shaw K, Blanchard H: Report of three gastric tumors in children. J Pediatr Surg 29:1202-1204, 1994.
65. Skinner MA, Plumley DA, Grosfeld JL, et al: Gastrointestinal tumors in children: An analysis of 39 cases. Ann Surg Oncol 1:283-289, 1994.
66. Corapcioglu F, Ekingen G, Sarper N, et al: Immature gastric teratoma of childhood: A case report and review of the literature. J Pediatr Gastroenterol Nutr 39:292-294, 2004.
67. Arana A, Hauser B, Hachimi-Idrissi S, et al: Management of ingested foreign bodies in childhood and review of the literature. Eur J Pediatr 160:468-472, 2001.
68. Stricker T, Kellenberger CJ, Neuhaus TJ, et al: Ingested pins causing perforation. Arch Dis Child 84:165-166, 2001.
69. Yardeni D, Yardeni H, Coran AG, et al: Severe esophageal damage due to button battery ingestion: Can it be prevented? Pediatr Surg Int 20:496-501, 2004.
70. Lynch KA, Feola PG, Guenther E: Gastric trichobezoar: An important cause of abdominal pain presenting to the pediatric emergency department. Pediatr Emerg Care 19:343-347, 2003.
71. Kanetaka K, Azuma T, Ito S, et al: Two-channel method for retrieval of gastric trichobezoar: Report of a case. J Pediatr Surg 38(2):e7, 2003.
72. Nirasawa Y, Mori T, Ito Y, et al: Laparoscopic removal of a large gastric trichobezoar. J Pediatr Surg 33:663-665, 1998.
73. Gauderer ML, Ponsky JL, Izant RJ Jr: Gastrostomy without laparotomy: A percutaneous endoscopic technique. J Pediatr Surg 15:872-875, 1980.
74. Rothenberg SS, Bealer JF, Chang JH: Primary laparoscopic placement of gastrostomy buttons for feeding tubes. A safer and simpler technique. Surg Endosc 13:995-997, 1999.
75. Chait PG, Weinberg J, Connolly BL, et al: Retrograde percutaneous gastrostomy and gastrojejunostomy in 505 children: A 4 1/2-year experience. Radiology 201:691-696, 1996.
76. Hament JM, Bax NM, van der Zee DC, et al: Complications of percutaneous endoscopic gastrostomy with or without concomitant antireflux surgery in 96 children. J Pediatr Surg 36:1412-1415, 2001.
77. Friedman JN, Ahmed S, Connolly B, et al: Complications associated with image-guided gastrostomy and gastrojejunostomy tubes in children. Pediatrics 114:458-461, 2004.
78. Wheatley MJ, Wesley JR, Tkach DM, Coran AG: Long term follow-up of brain-damaged children requiring feeding gastrostomy: Should an antireflux procedure always be performed? J Pediatr Surg 26:301-304, discussion 304-305, 1991.
79. Burd RS, Price MR, Whalen TV: The role of protective antireflux procedures in neurologically impaired children: A decision analysis. J Pediatr Surg 37:500-506, 2002.
80. Bickler SW, Harrison MW, Campbell JR: Perforated peptic ulcer disease in children: Association of corticosteroid therapy. J Pediatr Surg 28:785-787, 1993.
81. Azarow K, Kim P, Shandling B: A 45-year experience with surgical treatment of peptic ulcer disease in children. J Pediatr Surg 31:750-753, 1996.
82. Sherman PM: North American Society for Pediatric Gastroenterology and Nutrition. *Helicobacter pylori* infection in children: Recommendations for diagnosis and treatment. J Pediatr Gastroenterol Nutr 31:490-497, 2000.
83. Drumm B, Day AS, Gold B, et al: European Society for Paediatric Gastroenterology, Hepatology and Nutrition. J Pediatr Gastroenterol Nutr 39(Suppl 2):S626-S631, 2004.
84. Kato S, Nishino Y, Ozawa K, et al: The prevalence of *Helicobacter pylori* in Japanese children with gastritis or peptic ulcer disease. J Gastroenterol 39:734-738, 2004.
85. Chan KL, Zhou H, Ng DK, et al: A prospective study of a one-week nonbismuth quadruple therapy for childhood *Helicobacter pylori* infection. J Pediatr Surg 36:1008-1011, 2001.
86. Chan KL, Tam PK, Saing H: Long-term follow-up of childhood duodenal ulcers. J Pediatr Surg 32:1609-1611, 1997.

66

Anatomy and Physiology of the Duodenum

John M. Kellum · Roberto C. Iglesias · Jarrod Day

GROSS ANATOMY

The duodenum is so named because its length is approximately 12 fingerbreadths, or 20 to 30 cm. This first portion of the intestine begins at the end of the gastric pylorus, at the right of the spine, in the plane of the first lumbar vertebra. The duodenum then extends in a C-shaped curve around the head of the pancreas and connects with the jejunum to the left of the second lumbar vertebra. It is the most proximal portion of the intestine and the widest, shortest, and least mobile segment. The duodenum is divided into four parts: the first (or superior) portion, also known as the duodenal bulb or cap; the second, or the vertical or descending portion; the third, or the horizontal or transverse portion; and the fourth, or the oblique or ascending portion (Fig. 66–1).

The duodenal cap is freely mobile in the peritoneal cavity, and it is the area where 90% of duodenal ulcers occur. It has longitudinal mucosal folds, whereas the remainder of the duodenum displays prominent transverse folds. The anterior and posterior layers of the peritoneum join over the duodenal cap's upper aspect to form the hepatoduodenal ligament, which contains the portal triad (common bile duct, hepatic artery, and portal vein). The anterior border of the foramen of Winslow is formed by the free margin of this ligament (Fig. 66–2). Immediately above the duodenal cap are the gallbladder and the quadrate lobe of the liver. Below and behind the cap is the head of the pancreas. Also behind the bulb lies the gastroduodenal artery; thus, by eroding into this vessel, peptic ulcers can cause bleeding.

The mobility and circumferential serosal coating of the duodenal bulb facilitate operations on the pylorus and duodenum. Pyloroplasties and gastroduodenal resections are performed with greater ease when the pylorus and the adjoining second portion of the duodenum are mobilized forward into the abdominal cavity by Kocher's maneuver (Fig. 66–3). The proximity of the superior duodenum to the gallbladder explains the sometimes spontaneous passage of gallstones into the duodenum via a cholecystoduodenal fistula. The peritoneum covers the distal 2.5 cm of the first portion of the duodenum only ventrally. Its range of movement depends on the peritoneal coat. The posterior wall of the first portion of the duodenum is often intimately opposed to the structures of the hepatoduodenal ligament.

The second portion of the duodenum is retroperitoneal and fixed in position through fusion of its lateral visceral peritoneum to the parietal peritoneum of the lateral abdominal wall. By dividing the peritoneum at the right lateral edge of the segment (Kocher's maneuver), one mobilizes the descending duodenum to render the retroduodenal and intrapancreatic bile ducts surgically accessible. The right kidney and its hilar structures, the adrenal gland, and the vena cava lie posterior to the second portion of the duodenum (Fig. 66–4). Horizontally across the descending midpoint of the duodenum, folds of peritoneum come together from above and below to form the mesocolon. At the superior duodenal flexure, the descending second portion of the duodenum forms an acute angle with the first portion and descends about 7 to 8 cm to the inferior duodenal flexure. The transverse colon crosses it anteriorly and may or may not possess a mesocolon at this point. One must reflect the hepatic flexure of the colon anteromedially to fully mobilize the duodenum. About halfway down the posteromedial wall of the second portion of the duodenum is the papilla of Vater (see Fig. 66–1), which contains the opening of the common bile duct and the main pancreatic duct of Wirsung. The opening of the accessory pancreatic duct (of Santorini) is more proximal and may inadvertently be injured during gastrectomy for ulcer or distal gastric cancer. The superior pancreaticoduodenal branch of the gastroduodenal

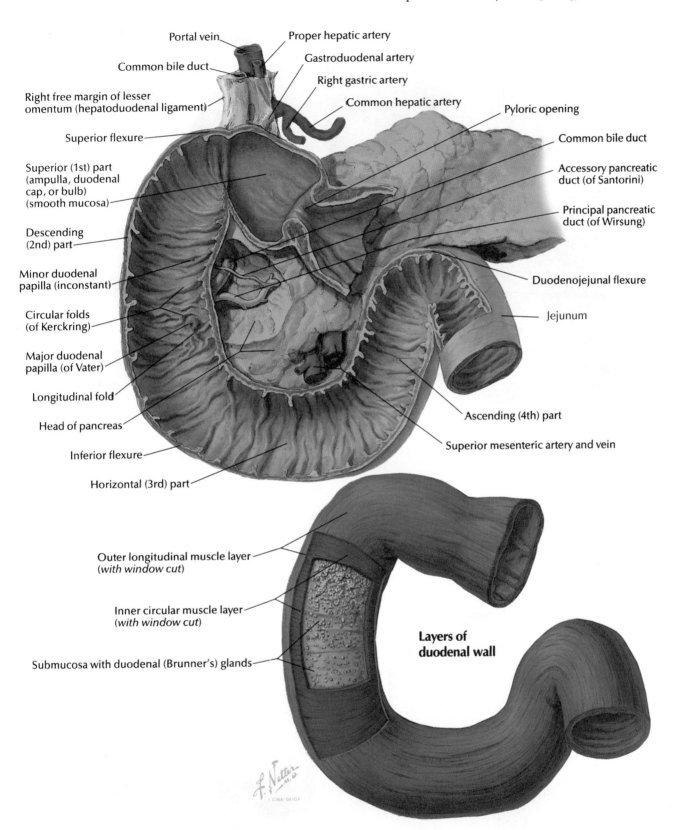

Figure 66–1.   The duodenum, the four portions, and their relationship to the bile duct and pancreas identified. (From Netter FH: Atlas of Human Anatomy. East Hanover, NJ, Ciba-Geigy, 1989, plate 262. Copyright, 1999. Icon Learning Systems, LLC, a subsidiary of Havas MediMedia USA Inc. Reprinted with permission from ICON Learning Systems, LLC, illustrated by Frank H Netter, MD. All rights reserved.)

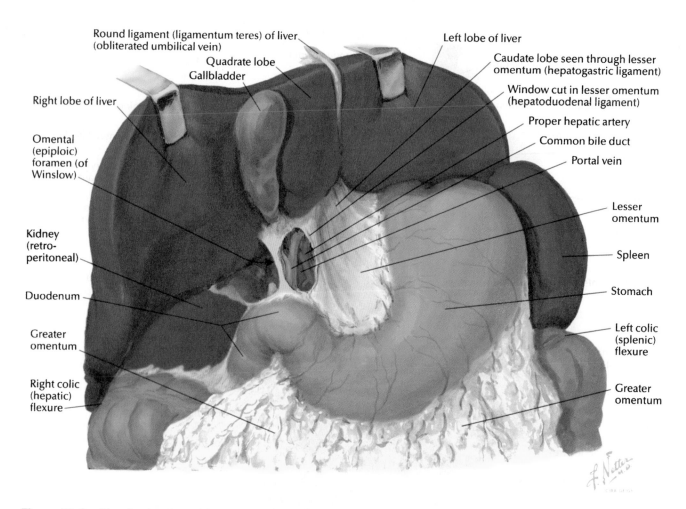

Round ligament (ligamentum teres) of liver
(obliterated umbilical vein)

Quadrate lobe
Gallbladder

Right lobe of liver

Omental
(epiploic)
foramen (of
Winslow)

Kidney
(retro-
peritoneal)

Duodenum

Greater
omentum

Right colic
(hepatic)
flexure

Left lobe of liver

Caudate lobe seen through lesser
omentum (hepatogastric ligament)

Window cut in lesser omentum
(hepatoduodenal ligament)

Proper hepatic artery

Common bile duct

Portal vein

Lesser
omentum

Spleen

Stomach

Left colic
(splenic)
flexure

Greater
omentum

Figure 66–2. The duodenum and its relationship to the foramen of Winslow and the hepatoduodenal ligament containing the portal triad. (From Netter FH: Atlas of Human Anatomy. East Hanover, NJ, Ciba-Geigy, 1989, plate 271. Copyright, 1999. Icon Learning Systems, LLC, a subsidiary of Havas MediMedia USA Inc. Reprinted with permission from ICON Learning Systems, LLC, illustrated by Frank H Netter, MD. All rights reserved.)

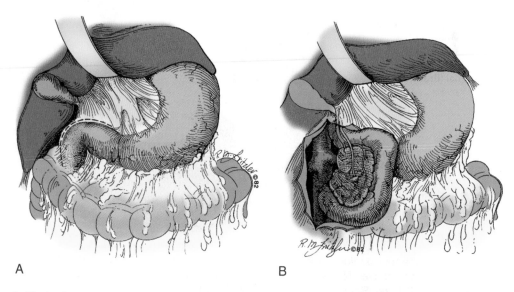

A   B

Figure 66–3. **A,** Kocher's maneuver begins by incising the peritoneum lateral to the first and second portions of the duodenum. **B,** By mobilizing the duodenum and head of pancreas medially, the posterior aspect of the head can be inspected. (From Nyhus LM, Baker RJ: Reparative procedures for the injured pancreas. In Mastery of Surgery, vol 2, 2nd ed. Boston, Little, Brown, 1992.)

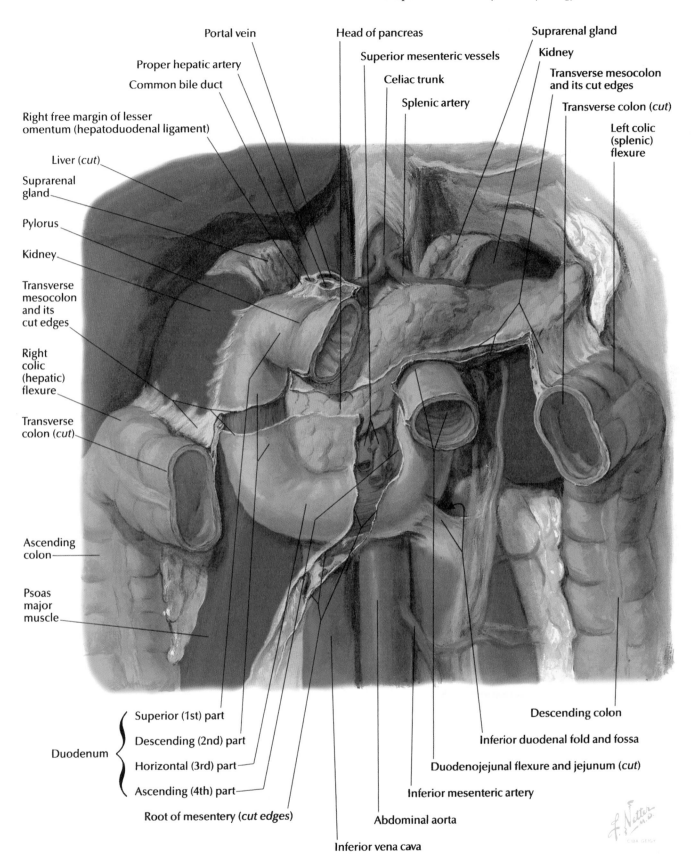

Figure 66–4. The abdominal contents as seen after removal of the stomach, jejunum, and ileum. The branches of the superior and inferior mesenteric arteries are shown. (From Netter FH: Atlas of Human Anatomy. East Hanover, NJ, Ciba-Geigy, 1989, plate 261. Copyright, 1999. Icon Learning Systems, LLC, a subsidiary of Havas MediMedia USA Inc. Reprinted with permission from ICON Learning Systems, LLC, illustrated by Frank H Netter, MD. All rights reserved.)

artery runs in the groove between the head of the pancreas and the descending duodenum; this intimate association of the duodenum with the pancreatic head generally mandates excision of the pancreatic head with attempted duodenum resection.

The third portion of the duodenum is about 12 to 13 cm in length; runs horizontally to the left in front of the aorta, inferior vena cava, lumbar column, and ureter; and ends at the left of the third lumbar vertebra. The root of the jejunoileum mesentery crosses it near its termination. The superior mesenteric artery runs downward over the anterior surface of the transverse duodenum to enter the root of the mesentery (Fig. 66–5). The inferior pancreaticoduodenal artery separates the pancreas from the upper border of this segment.

The fourth part of the duodenum runs upward and slightly to the left for 2 to 3 cm along the left side of the spine to the duodenojejunal angle at the root of the transverse mesocolon. At the left of the second lumbar vertebra, the terminal portion of the duodenum bends sharply downward, forward, and leftward to form the duodenojejunal flexure. At this point the suspensory ligament of the duodenum (ligament of Treitz) attaches (Fig. 66–6). This ligament is a small, triangular band of muscular and fibrous tissue that extends retroperitoneally, behind the pancreas and splenic vein, in front of the left renal vein, from the left or right crus of the diaphragm, to attach retroperitoneally to the upper margin of the terminal duodenum and sometimes to the adjacent jejunum. The ligament of Treitz is usually tenuous and is not invariably present. The duodenojejunal flexure is a readily recognized landmark that can be used to guide the search for obstruction in the small bowel and to locate a loop of upper jejunum for gastrojejunostomy. At laparotomy, it is found by passing the hand backward to the posterior abdominal wall below the transverse mesocolon and palpating upward along the left of the spine until the flexure is identified by its fixation. The bend is in contact with the inferior margin of the pancreas through the root of the transverse mesocolon.

Fusion of the pancreaticoduodenal visceral peritoneum with the primitive posterior parietal peritoneum anchors the entire duodenum, except part of the first portion. Variation in fusion of the duodenum to the posterior abdominal wall accounts for variation in mobility. The right colic flexure, the fixed portion of the transverse mesocolon, and vascular and ampullary connections anchor the duodenum still more firmly. In its deep position, the duodenum appears to be well protected from injury, yet it is sometimes crushed and even torn against the spine with severe blunt abdominal trauma, in part because of its comparatively unyielding peritoneal fixation.

Arterial Supply

The arterial supply of the duodenum is derived from the anterior and posterior pancreaticoduodenal arcades, which form a major arterial anastomosis between the celiac and superior mesenteric arterial circulations. The duodenum shares its blood supply with the proximal portion of the pancreas, thus making resection of either the duodenum or the pancreas alone usually impossible and always hazardous. The superior pancreaticoduodenal artery is a branch of the gastroduodenal artery, and the inferior pancreaticoduodenal is a branch of the superior mesenteric artery. These two arteries split and run in posterior and anterior grooves between the descending and transverse portions of the duodenum and the head of the pancreas, where they anastomose to form continuous anterior and posterior arcades (Fig. 66–7; see also Fig. 66–5). This rich periduodenal anastomotic network of arteries often frustrates attempts to control bleeding secondary to posterior duodenal ulcers.

Venous Supply

The veins that parallel the pancreaticoduodenal arteries are arranged in anterior and posterior pancreaticoduodenal arcades that accompany the arteries (Fig. 66–8). The posterior arcade ends in the portal vein above and the superior mesenteric vein (SMV) below. The posterosuperior pancreaticoduodenal vein may follow its companion artery anterior to the bile duct, or it may run behind the duct. The vein terminates inferiorly on the left border of the SMV. Here, it may be joined by a jejunal vein or by the anterior inferior pancreaticoduodenal vein. The gastrocolic trunk (Henle's trunk) drains most of the anterior arcade.[1] Several small branches drain the duodenal bulb and empty into the pancreaticoduodenal, right gastroepiploic, or portal vein; a key landmark for the pylorus is the prepyloric vein.

During pancreaticoduodenectomy, the SMV may be located by following the middle colic vein to its junction with the SMV just inferior to the neck of the pancreas. Sometimes, incision of the avascular peritoneum along the lower border of the gland to the left of the SMV facilitates identification. Superior to the pancreas, division of the common bile duct and gastroduodenal artery readily exposes the portal vein. Occasionally, a tortuous hepatic artery may be mistaken for the gastroduodenal artery; therefore, before ligation of the gastroduodenal artery, it should be transiently occluded with a vascular clamp or the surgeon's fingers while the hepatic artery pulse is palpated in the hilum of the liver.

Lymphatic Drainage

The lymphatic drainage of the duodenum generally parallels the vasculature. Lymph passes through several levels of lymph nodes that are located adjacent to the bowel wall, adjacent to the mesenteric arcades, and along the superior mesenteric and celiac arteries. Primary duodenal carcinomas may invade the pancreas via direct extension or lymphatic infiltration, but they usually first spread to the periduodenal lymph nodes and liver. Nodes at the superior duodenal flexure and retroduodenal nodes are commonly involved in metastatic pancreatic carcinoma.

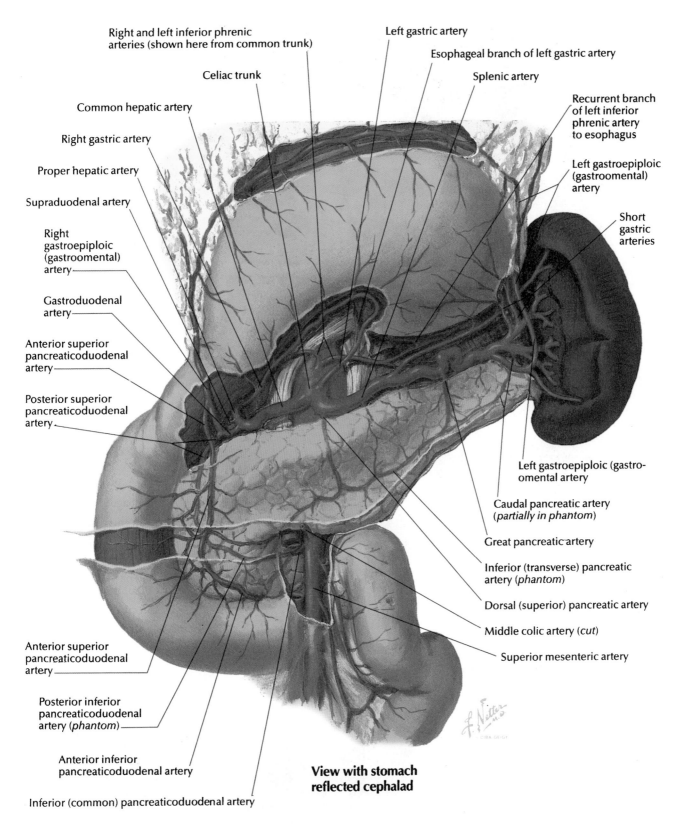

Right and left inferior phrenic arteries (shown here from common trunk)

Left gastric artery

Esophageal branch of left gastric artery

Celiac trunk

Splenic artery

Common hepatic artery

Recurrent branch of left inferior phrenic artery to esophagus

Right gastric artery

Left gastroepiploic (gastroomental) artery

Proper hepatic artery

Supraduodenal artery

Short gastric arteries

Right gastroepiploic (gastroomental) artery

Gastroduodenal artery

Anterior superior pancreaticoduodenal artery

Posterior superior pancreaticoduodenal artery

Left gastroepiploic (gastro-omental artery

Caudal pancreatic artery (*partially in phantom*)

Great pancreatic artery

Inferior (transverse) pancreatic artery (*phantom*)

Dorsal (superior) pancreatic artery

Anterior superior pancreaticoduodenal artery

Middle colic artery (*cut*)

Superior mesenteric artery

Posterior inferior pancreaticoduodenal artery (*phantom*)

Anterior inferior pancreaticoduodenal artery

View with stomach reflected cephalad

Inferior (common) pancreaticoduodenal artery

Figure 66–5. View of the arteries of the duodenum and pancreas, with the stomach reflected cephalad. (From Netter FH: Atlas of Human Anatomy. East Hanover, NJ, Ciba-Geigy, 1989, plate 283. Copyright, 1999. Icon Learning Systems, LLC, a subsidiary of Havas MediMedia USA Inc. Reprinted with permission from ICON Learning Systems, LLC, illustrated by Frank H Netter, MD. All rights reserved.)

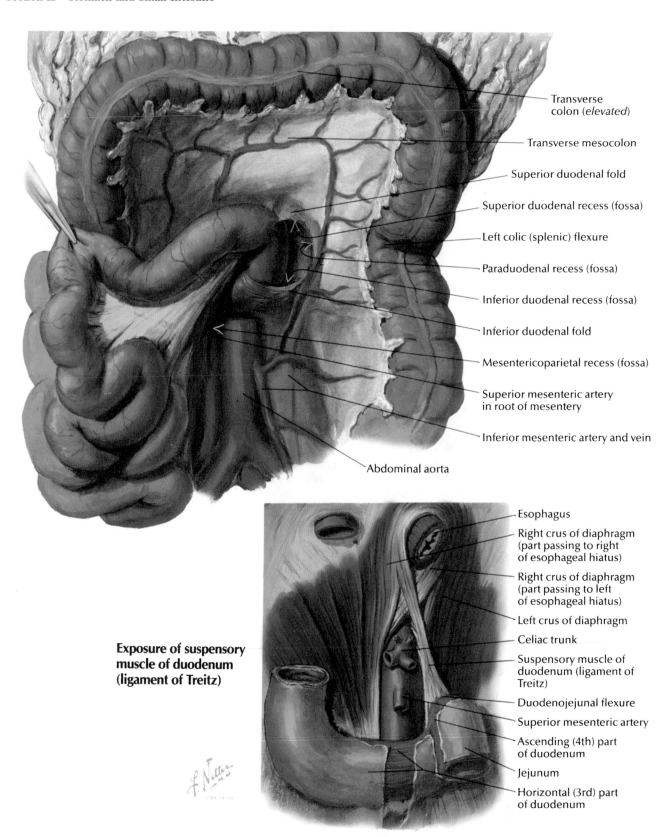

Exposure of suspensory muscle of duodenum (ligament of Treitz)

Labels (top figure):
- Transverse colon (*elevated*)
- Transverse mesocolon
- Superior duodenal fold
- Superior duodenal recess (fossa)
- Left colic (splenic) flexure
- Paraduodenal recess (fossa)
- Inferior duodenal recess (fossa)
- Inferior duodenal fold
- Mesentericoparietal recess (fossa)
- Superior mesenteric artery in root of mesentery
- Inferior mesenteric artery and vein
- Abdominal aorta

Labels (bottom figure):
- Esophagus
- Right crus of diaphragm (part passing to right of esophageal hiatus)
- Right crus of diaphragm (part passing to left of esophageal hiatus)
- Left crus of diaphragm
- Celiac trunk
- Suspensory muscle of duodenum (ligament of Treitz)
- Duodenojejunal flexure
- Superior mesenteric artery
- Ascending (4th) part of duodenum
- Jejunum
- Horizontal (3rd) part of duodenum

Figure 66–6. The duodenojejunal junction showing exposure of the suspensory ligament of Treitz. (From Netter FH: Atlas of Human Anatomy. East Hanover, NJ, Ciba-Geigy, 1989, plate 53. Copyright, 1999. Icon Learning Systems, LLC, a subsidiary of Havas MediMedia USA Inc. Reprinted with permission from ICON Learning Systems, LLC, illustrated by Frank H Netter, MD. All rights reserved.)

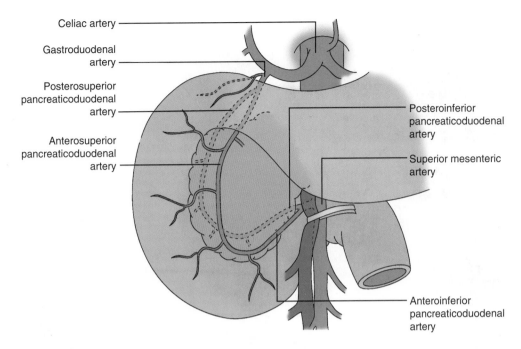

Figure 66–7. Arterial supply to the duodenum. (From Anatomy and physiology of the small intestine. In Greenfield LJ, Mulholland WM, Oldham KT, et al [eds]: Surgery: Scientific Principles and Practice, 3rd ed. Philadelphia, Lippincott Williams & Wilkins, 2001, p 788.)

Histology of the Duodenum

The wall of the duodenum is made up of four layers: an outer peritoneal coat, the serosa; a muscular coat made up of longitudinal and circular fibers, the muscularis; the submucosa; and the mucosa, which forms its inner lining (Fig. 66–9). Portions of the posterior and lateral walls of the duodenum are retroperitoneal and therefore lack the peritoneal or serosal coat. The serosa is an extension of the peritoneum. It consists of a single layer of flattened mesothelial cells overlying loose connective tissue.

Two layers of smooth muscle make up the muscularis, an outer or longitudinal layer and an inner or circular layer. The myenteric plexus of Auerbach lies between these two layers. Meissner's plexus is found in the submucosa along with a network of loose connective tissue rich in lymphatics and small blood vessels. Here, in the submucosa, are found the characteristic histologic features of the mammalian duodenum: the glands of Brunner, which empty into the crypts of Lieberkühn through small secretory ducts (Fig. 66–10). Brunner's gland secretion is viscous, alkaline (pH 8.2 to 9.3), and clear. These mucoid, viscous, alkaline secretions probably contribute to protection of the duodenal mucosa against the corrosive action of gastric juice.

The intestinal mucosa is thrown into numerous fingerlike projections, or villi, that greatly increase the mucosal surface area. The columnar cell–lined epithelium contains both mucus and HCO_3-secreting surface cells and absorptive cells. The mucosa can be divided into three layers: the deepest is the muscularis mucosae, the middle layer is the lamina propria, and the inner layer consists of a continuous sheet of a single layer of columnar epithelial cells lining both the crypts and the villi.

The main known functions of the crypt epithelium include (1) cell renewal; (2) exocrine, endocrine, water, and ion secretion; and (3) absorption of salt, water, and specific nutrients. The crypt epithelium is composed of at least four distinct cell types: Paneth, goblet, undifferentiated, and endocrine cells.

Innervation of the Duodenum

The gastrointestinal (GI) tract is innervated by the autonomic nervous system, which may be divided into extrinsic and intrinsic or enteric nervous systems. The extrinsic innervation of the duodenum is parasympathetic from the vagus nerves (anterior and celiac branches) and sympathetic from the splanchnic nerves of the celiac ganglion. Intrinsic innervation is from Auerbach's myenteric plexus and Meissner's submucosal plexus. Processes from these neurons innervate target cells such as smooth muscle, secretory, and absorptive cells, but they also connect to sensory receptors and interdigitate with processes from other neurons located both inside and outside the plexus. Thus, pathways within the enteric nervous system can be multisynaptic, and integration of activities can take place entirely within the enteric nervous system (Fig. 66–11).

Adult Anatomic Abnormalities That May Require Surgery

The main anatomic abnormalities of the duodenum that the surgeon may be asked to treat in adult patients are duodenal diverticula, vascular anomalies, and

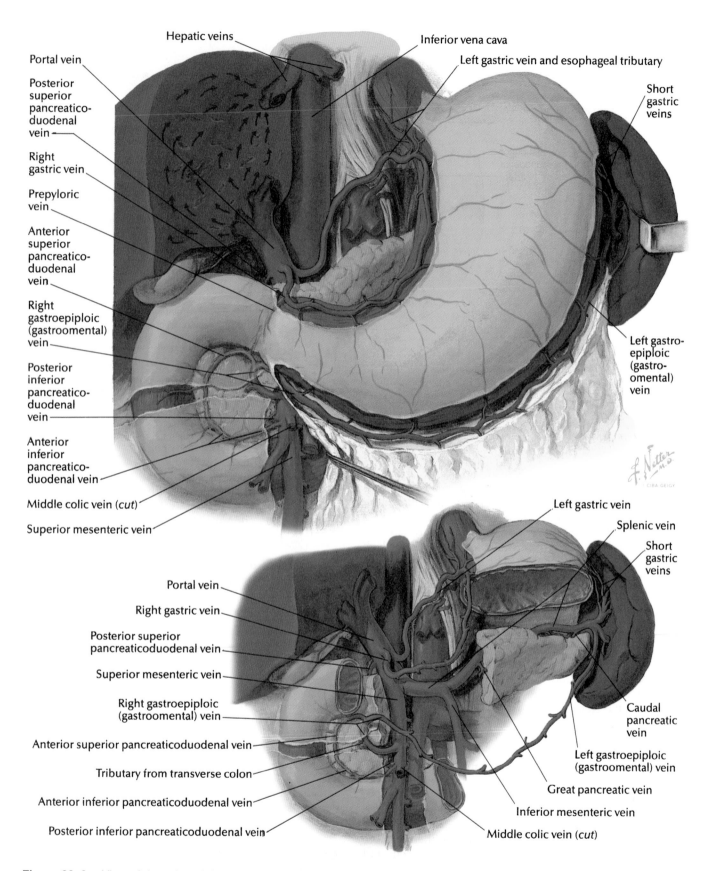

Figure 66–8. View of the veins of the duodenum and pancreas, with the stomach removed. (From Netter FH: Atlas of Human Anatomy. East Hanover, NJ, Ciba-Geigy, 1989, plate 294. Copyright, 1999. Icon Learning Systems, LLC, a subsidiary of Havas MediMedia USA Inc. Reprinted with permission from ICON Learning Systems, LLC, illustrated by Frank H Netter, MD. All rights reserved.)

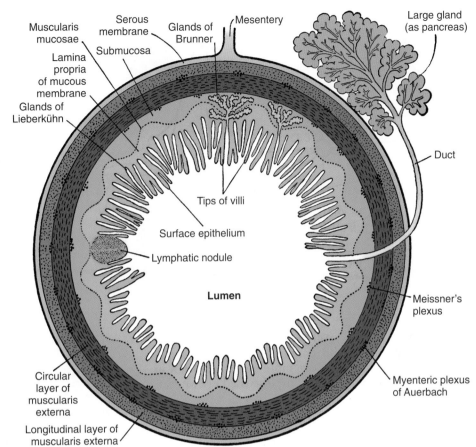

Figure 66–9. Schematic diagram of a cross section of the intestinal tract. (From Bloom WN, Fawcett DW: A Textbook of Histology. Philadelphia, WB Saunders, 1968.)

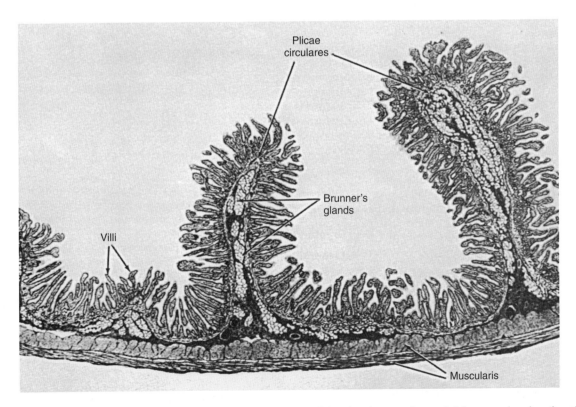

Figure 66–10. Drawing of a longitudinal section through the wall of the duodenum of an adult human showing the plicae circularis (valves of Kerckring), the villi, and the submucosal glands of Brunner. (From Bargmann W: Histologie und Mikroskopische Anatomie des Menschen, 6th ed. Stuttgart, Germany, Georg-Thieme Verlag, 1962.)

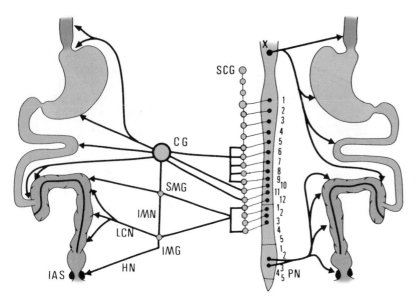

Figure 66–11. Schema of the extrinsic efferent innervation of the gut showing the sympathetic innervation *(left)* and the parasympathetic innervation *(right)*. This representation is a synthesis of various data and may present variations according to different species. CG, celiac ganglion; HN, hypogastric nerves; IAS, internal anal sphincter; IMG, inferior mesenteric ganglion; IMN, intermesenteric nerve; LCN, lumbar colonic nerves; PN, pelvic nerves; SCG, superior cervical ganglion; SMG, superior mesenteric ganglion; X, vagus dorsal motor nucleus and vagus nerve. (From Roman C, Gonella J: Extrinsic control of digestive tract motility. In Johnson LR [ed]: Physiology of the Gastrointestinal Tract, 2nd ed. New York, Raven Press, 1987, p 507.)

paraduodenal hernias. Although duodenal atresia or stenosis, malrotation, and annular pancreas are sometimes found in adults, they are more commonly seen in pediatric surgical patients and are discussed elsewhere.

Preduodenal Portal Vein

A rare, but important venous anomaly of which the duodenal surgeon should be aware is the preduodenal portal vein. In this congenital anomaly the portal vein passes anterior to the duodenum rather than lying in its normal posterior position. The anomaly is due to abnormal development of the vitelline veins, as described by Bower and Ternberg (Fig. 66–12).[2] The majority of cases reported in the literature involve infants or children, and there is a very high association with additional congenital anomalies such as (in decreasing order) malrotation, situs inversus, and cardiac lesions.[3] Most patients have acute or chronic high intestinal obstruction or symptoms of gastric outlet obstruction. The diagnosis is rarely made preoperatively.

At surgery, when the duodenum is found to be obstructed and a preduodenal portal vein is present, it is important to accurately determine whether the obstruction is caused by the anomalous vein, by associated anomalies, or by both. If the preduodenal portal vein is not causing obstruction, it is left undisturbed, and associated abnormalities are treated. If the anomalous vein is causing obstruction, relief can be obtained via one of two surgical procedures: (1) transection of the proximal duodenum with end-to-end duodenoduodenostomy anterior to the portal vein[2] or (2) duodenojejunostomy or gastrojejunostomy.[3] Both procedures have been used successfully.

Superior Mesenteric Artery Syndrome

Rokitansky first described compression and obstruction of the third portion of the duodenum by the superior mesenteric artery more than 100 years ago. Synonyms

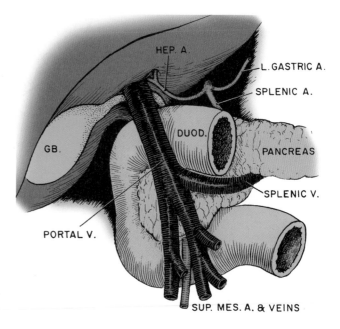

Figure 66–12. Anomalous preduodenal portal vein. GB, gallbladder. (From Edwards EA, Malone PD, MacArthur JD: Operative Anatomy of Abdomen and Pelvis. Philadelphia, Lea & Febiger, 1975.)

include Wilkie's syndrome, cast syndrome, and arteriomesenteric duodenal ileus or compression.[4] Despite intermittent waves of enthusiasm for this diagnosis, surgeons are generally reluctant to ascribe upper GI symptoms to this relatively rare abnormality (0.2% of 6000 upper GI examinations).[5] It is generally thought that for vascular compression to cause duodenal obstruction, some combination of three mechanical factors must be present: (1) an abnormally narrow aortomesenteric angle, (2) an abnormally highly fixed transverse duodenum, and (3) an abnormal course of the mesenteric

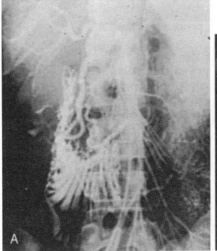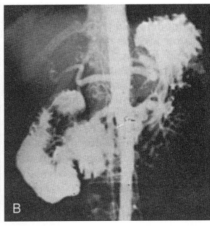

Figure 66–13. Combined gastrointestinal barium and aortography study revealing the point of compression and the abnormal course of the superior mesenteric artery. **A,** Narrow superior mesenteric-aortic angle. **B,** Aberrant course of the superior mesenteric artery. (From Mansberger AR: Vascular compression of the duodenum. In Sabiston DC [ed]: Textbook of Surgery, 13th ed. Philadelphia, WB Saunders, 1986, p 877.)

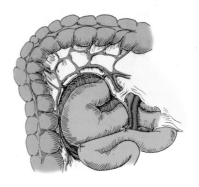

Figure 66–14. Duodenojejunostomy for vascular compression of the duodenum. (From Mansberger AR: Vascular compression of the duodenum. In Sabiston DC [ed]: Textbook of Surgery, 13th ed. Philadelphia, WB Saunders, 1986, p 877.)

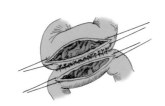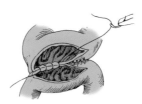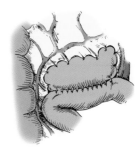

artery continuing inferiorly, anterior to the unyielding vertebral column (Fig. 66–13). Hyperextension of the spine (as may occur after the application of a body cast or skeletal traction) and weight loss (associated with depletion of retroperitoneal fat) further narrow the aortomesenteric angle and are associated with progressive symptoms of distal duodenal obstruction in patients with this diagnosis. This syndrome has also been described in patients with severe scoliosis after so-called spine-straightening surgery.

The preferred method of surgical treatment is duodenojejunostomy, which can be performed in side-to-side fashion between the dilated proximal jejunum after the mesocolon of the hepatic flexure has been opened (Fig. 66–14). Gastrojejunostomy is a poor second choice because it relies on retrograde decompression of the duodenum through the pylorus. A third option is extensive mobilization of the ligament of Treitz after mobilization of the hepatic flexure of the colon. After this maneuver, the distal duodenum and small bowel are passed under the mesenteric vessels, and the C loop of the duodenum is straightened out (Fig. 66–15). Although this third option does not involve opening the GI tract, it does require division of some small vessels to the distal duodenum. Segmental ischemia apparently has not been a problem.

Paraduodenal Hernia

Paraduodenal (or mesocolic) hernias and hernias of the foramen of Winslow are the two most frequent types of congenital internal hernia.[6] They most commonly cause symptoms of acute small bowel obstruction, and frequently plain radiographs of the abdomen are suggestive of the diagnosis. Some patients have symptoms of chronic intermittent obstruction for years before a definitive diagnosis is made. Bowel strangulation is commonly found at surgery for these disorders.

The most common paraduodenal hernia is the so-called left paraduodenal hernia (Fig. 66–16).[7] In this condition, variable amounts of small intestine herniate through the so-called vascular arch of Treitz formed by the inferior mesenteric vein and the left colic artery. The herniated small bowel is therefore posterior to the mesocolon. The cecum and terminal ileum are in their

normal anatomic configuration. Operative treatment of a left paraduodenal hernia involves opening the retroperitoneum just to the right of the inferior mesenteric vein and artery. The bowel can be reduced to its normal anatomic position, and the root of the mesentery of the left colon can be joined to the peritoneum anterior to the aorta to obliterate the arch of Treitz.

The more unusual right paraduodenal hernia is due to an abnormality in embryonic intestinal rotation.[8] The cecum is usually in the right upper quadrant, and Ladd's bands are apparent. In this hernia, the small bowel is trapped in a hernia sac, the anterior wall of which is formed by the mesentery of the small bowel. It is as though the herniated bowel has rotated under the superior mesenteric artery and is trapped in the right upper quadrant. The hernia is best approached by incising the attachments of the right colon rather than attempting to open the hernia sac from the medial side because this might involve the division of critical mesenteric arteries.

The least common paraduodenal hernia is a hernia of the foramen of Winslow.[9] It is almost always associated with an unusually patulous foramen of Winslow, which allows the bowel or right colon to herniate through the foramen into the lesser peritoneal sac (Fig. 66–17). The radiographic diagnosis is usually made in retrospect. Operative treatment involves gentle traction on the herniated bowel in an attempt at reduction. If reduction cannot be achieved, the lesser sac should be opened by incising the gastrocolic omentum, and the hernia can be reduced by both pulsion and traction. Rarely, strangulated bowel within the lesser peritoneal sac must be resected before reduction of the remaining contents. Once reduction has been completed, the patulous foramen of Winslow should be closed with interrupted sutures.

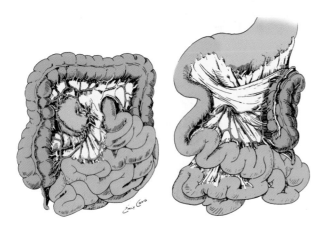

Figure 66–15. Operation to straighten the duodenum and return it to its prerotation position. (From Sabiston DC [ed]: Textbook of Surgery, 13th ed. Philadelphia, WB Saunders, 1986, p 877.)

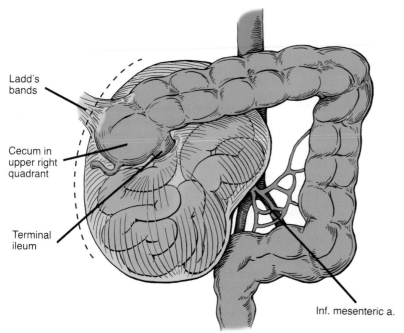

Ladd's bands

Cecum in upper right quadrant

Terminal ileum

Inf. mesenteric a.

Figure 66–16. Right mesocolic hernia. The prearterial segment *did not* rotate during the second stage. The postarterial segment *did* rotate and has trapped most of the small bowel behind the ascending mesocolon containing the ileocolic, right colic, and middle colic vessels. The *dashed line* shows the incision for release of the hernia. (From Nyhus LM, Harkins HN (eds): Hernia. Philadelphia, JB Lippincott, 1978, p 493.)

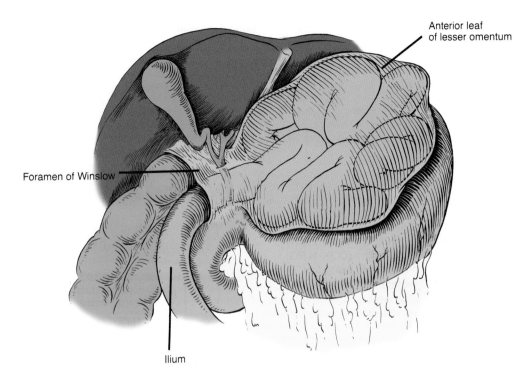

Figure 66–17. Diagrammatic illustration of a hernia into the lesser sac through the foramen of Winslow. (From Nyhus LM, Harkins HN [eds]: Hernia. Philadelphia, JB Lippincott, 1964, p 598.)

Duodenal Diverticula

Most duodenal diverticula are asymptomatic and come to the attention of the clinician during routine barium examination. They may be acquired or congenital, and up to 15% of the adult population is affected. Duodenal diverticula are probably true diverticula because the few resected specimens appear to have a complete, though attenuated, muscularis propria. The vast majority of patients with GI symptoms and duodenal diverticula have other causes for these symptoms, which is why excision should be undertaken with a great deal of circumspection. Another reason for caution is that most duodenal diverticula are located along the posteromedial surface of the second portion of the duodenum, where they are intimately related to the pancreatic head and occasionally contain the ampulla of Vater. About 20% occur in the third portion and 10% occur in the fourth portion of the duodenum.

Although usually asymptomatic, duodenal diverticula occasionally require emergency surgery because of perforation or association with massive hemorrhage.[10] Peri-Vaterian diverticula have been implicated in the pathogenesis of primary choledocholithiasis and pancreatitis. Elective surgery is occasionally undertaken because of chronic abdominal pain or symptoms of bacterial overgrowth. Bleeding is treated by excision and duodenal closure, although duodenal diverticularization, or duodenostomy, should be considered and peritoneal drainage of the paraduodenal space should always be performed.

DUODENAL PHYSIOLOGY

The duodenum is a complex organ with a unique set of structural and physiologic properties that differentiate it from the stomach and the remainder of the small intestine. It is here that the process of digestion and absorption truly begins, where meal contents are alkalinized and mixed with digestive enzymes and bile. The main functions of the duodenum are to (1) alkalinize acidic chyme from the stomach, (2) serve as a reservoir for pancreaticobiliary secretions, (3) be the main site of calcium and iron absorption, (4) further the breakdown of food products, and (5) exert neuroendocrine control of upper GI motility. Thus, duodenectomy can disrupt the relationship between cycles of both interdigestive GI motility and insulin secretion and can lead to anemia, secondary hyperparathyroidism, and other diseases caused by malabsorption.[11,12]

Exocrine Physiology

The duodenum is unique in that there are no tight junctions that provide inherent protection as in the stomach. Instead, it has a leaky epithelium between duodenocytes, and as a result, it must use alternative defense mechanisms against concentrated gastric acid and other irritants discharged by the stomach. Many compounds have been implicated in stimulating bicarbonate secretion after duodenocyte exposure to acid, including vagally produced acetylcholine; prostaglandins (especially

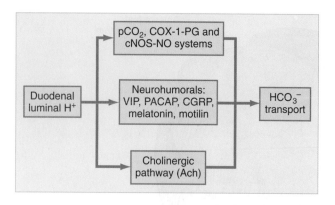

Figure 66–18. The mechanism of duodenal HCO_3^- secretion in response to gastric H^+ involves a variety of neurotransmitters, P_{CO_2}, cyclooxygenase-1–prostaglandin (COX-1–PG), and the constitutive nitric oxide synthase–nitric oxide (cNOS-NO) system. (From Konturek PC, Konturek SJ, Hahn EG: Duodenal alkaline secretion: Its mechanisms and role in mucosal protection against gastric acid. Dig Liver Dis 36:505-512, 2004.)

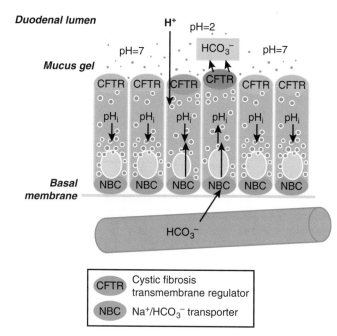

Figure 66–19. In the duodenocyte membrane transport system, HCO_3^- is exchanged for Cl^- at the apical cell membrane. This bicarbonate then neutralizes gastric acid entering the proximal duodenum. (From Konturek PC, Konturek SJ, Hahn EG: Duodenal alkaline secretion: Its mechanisms and role in mucosal protection against gastric acid. Dig Liver Dis 36:505-512, 2004.)

$PGE)^{13}$; vasoactive intestinal polypeptide (VIP) and its analogue PACAP (pituitary adenylate cyclase activating polypeptide); melatonin[14,15]; motilin; and P_{CO_2}, prostaglandin, and nitric oxide (NO) (Fig. 66–18).[16]

One defensive barrier lies in the bicarbonate secreted by the pancreas and liver in response to duodenal acidification and release of duodenal secretin; however, the majority of protection is inherent within the duodenal bulb, which coordinates a complex array of titrating mediators that ultimately produce neutralizing bicarbonate.

The duodenocyte membrane transport system is believed to be coordinated with phase II/III of the migrating motor complex (MMC) and functions as follows (Fig. 66–19)[16]:

1. Luminal H^+ diffuses into duodenocytes through their apical membrane and reduces their intracellular pH.
2. The acidification of duodenocytes promotes movement of extracellular bicarbonate into the cell through basolateral Na^+/HCO_3^- transporter (NBC) channels.
3. This base loading causes apical cystic fibrosis transmembrane conductance regulator (CFTR)-related HCO_3^-/Cl^- exchangers to transport bicarbonate into the duodenal lumen and thus further buffer the acid load.

Another alkaline-secreting mechanism relies on H^+ activation of capsaicin-sensitive afferent nerves within the axon-reflex pathway that stimulate the release of sensory neuropeptides such as enteroglucagon and calcitonin gene–related peptide (CGRP), which in turn activate the release of NO and cyclooxygenase-prostaglandin (COX-PG).[16] In addition, this system is self-perpetuating; as HCO_3^- is hydrolyzed to increase the partial pressure of

CO_2 (P_{CO_2}), duodenocytes further increase HCO_3^- secretion. The cumulative sum of these factors leads to the following (Fig. 66–20):

1. Stimulation of goblet cells and Brunner's glands to increase the thickness of the mucus gel layer
2. Stabilization of the pH gradient and prevention of acid from entering epithelial cells
3. NO-mediated mucosal vasodilation leading to hyperemia and increased blood flow

In support of this capsaicin–CGRP mechanism, COX inhibitors abolish this response and patients with duodenal ulcers have been shown to have decreased bicarbonate secretion as a result of *Helicobacter pylori* production of the NO inhibitor, asymmetric dimethylarginine (ADMA).[17] Finally, the last mechanism for maintaining cell integrity is repair from injury.

Absorption and Digestion

The duodenum receives largely undigested food particles from the stomach; it is the function of a duodenocyte's brush border to begin the process of nutrient absorption via a variety of complex transport systems. This process is aided by pancreaticobiliary secretion and a host of hormones that make the food content more manageable. The main nutrients absorbed are discussed.

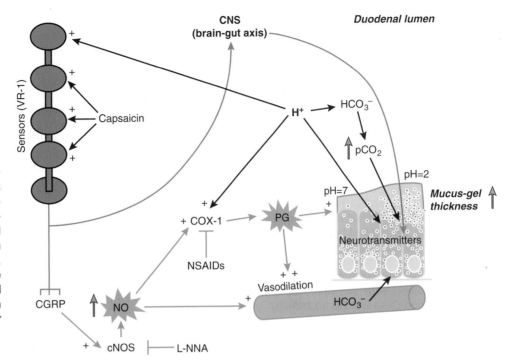

Figure 66–20. Involvement of capsaicin-sensitive nerves, calcitonin gene–related peptide (CGRP), nitric oxide (NO), prostaglandin (PG), and an increase in PCO_2 in the stimulation of mucus HCO_3^- secretion by duodenal mucosa in response to acidification. cNOS, constitutive nitric oxide synthase; CNS, central nervous system; COX-1, cyclooxygenase-1; L-NNA, $N(\omega)$-nitro-L-arginine; NSAIDs, nonsteroidal anti-inflammatory drugs. (From Konturek PC, Konturek SJ, Hahn EG: Duodenal alkaline secretion: Its mechanisms and role in mucosal protection against gastric acid. Dig Liver Dis 36:505-512, 2004.)

Calcium

The duodenum plays a major role in calcium absorption, especially when oral dietary calcium is low, at which time as much as 80% to 100% is absorbed through an active transport–dependent transcellular system that up-regulates and thus increases calcium absorption through three steps[18,19]: entry through the brush border, diffusion into the cytosol via the calcium binding protein calbindin D9k, and extrusion into blood through basal membrane Ca^{2+}-ATPase and Na^+/Ca^{2+} exchangers. This mechanism is confined to the duodenum and proximal jejunum and is dependent on vitamin D, which is essential for the biosynthesis of calbindin and possibly for increasing the number of extrusion pumps.[19]

Although calcium can also be absorbed through paracellular regulation throughout the small intestine, this mechanism is not as efficient because it absorbs only 20% to 60% and is time and concentration gradient dependent and thus most effective with high levels of dietary calcium intake or slow transient time.[18] The existence of this paracellular system ensures calcium absorption in the absence of vitamin D, as may be the case with northern winters, malabsorption, or inadequate oral intake.

The importance of this transcellular regulation mechanism is highlighted in patients in whom metabolic bone diseases develop after Roux-en-Y gastric bypass (RYGBP). Through bypassing the duodenum, this weight loss operation forces the body to become strictly dependent on paracellular regulation, which when not appropriately supported with a high-calcium diet, can result in calcium deficiency. In addition, the procedure can cause poor mixing of bile salts with fats and thus lead to malabsorption of fat-soluble vitamin D and, as a result, secondary hyperparathyroidism, osteoporosis, and osteomalacia.[20] Although the incidence of secondary hyperparathyroidism after RYGBP is unknown, Rhode and MacLean[21] reported elevated parathyroid hormone (PTH) in 14% and Amaral and colleagues[22] observed an increase in alkaline phosphatase in 34% of patients. Johnson et al.[23] found that elevated PTH was common after RYGBP and correlated with low vitamin D levels. The deficiency was progressive over time.

Iron

Another important function of duodenocytes is to serve as the main check point for iron homeostasis. Iron is an essential constituent of many important metabolic processes, including oxygen transport as a component of hemoglobin; however, too much iron can lead to free radical formation and thus toxic states such as hemochromatosis.

The mechanism by which duodenocytes regulate iron is a subject of debate. Whereas older theories support the programming of immature crypt cells to absorb more or less iron, depending on body stores,[24] more recent studies support the action of a number of molecules responsible for iron transport by mature enterocytes.[25]

The components of the current intestinal iron absorption pathway stem from direct action of the iron circulating inhibitor hepcidin on mature villus enterocytes; the process involves the following steps[25] (Fig. 66–21):
1. Dietary iron in the gut lumen is mainly in the Fe^{3+} form.
2. In the lumen, Fe^{3+} is reduced to Fe^{2+} by the ferrireductase Dcytb.
3. Fe^{2+} is transported intracellularly across the brush border membrane (BBM) by the divalent metal transporter DMT1.
4. Fe^{2+} is then transferred to the basolateral membrane (BLM) by the ferroxidase hephaestin.
5. Finally, Fe^{2+} is transferred across the BLM into the body by Ireg1.

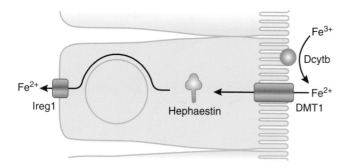

Figure 66–21. Components of the intestinal iron absorption pathway. (1) Luminal Fe^{3+} is reduced to Fe^{2+} by Dcytb. (2) Fe^{2+} is transported intracellularly across the brush border membrane (BBM) by the divalent metal transporter DMT1. (3) Fe^{2+} is transferred to the basolateral membrane (BLM) by hephaestin. (4) Fe^{2+} is transferred across the BLM into the body by Ireg1. (From Frazer DM, Anderson GJ: The orchestration of body iron intake: How and where do enterocytes receive their cues? Blood Cells Mol Dis 30:288-297, 2003.)

The complexity of this system is beyond the scope of this chapter; however, it is a negative feedback system dependent on continuous monitoring of transferrin levels by the liver, and it ultimately produces the so-called humoral factor hepcidin, which regulates Ireg1 expression. When iron stores are high, the liver increases hepcidin production and thus decreases Ireg1 expression, which in turn leads to decreased iron absorption.

The importance of the duodenum in iron absorption is highlighted in patients whose duodenum is bypassed during RYGBP, and the incidence of iron deficiency in such patients is at least 14% to 16% and up to 49% to 52%.[26,27] This deficiency is usually corrected by oral supplementation with multivitamins, but additional iron supplementation is frequently required, especially in menstruating females.

Macronutrients

Luminal macronutrients are absorbed via the BBM by a variety of transport systems.

Carbohydrates The duodenum plays a crucial role in the process of starch hydrolysis because pancreatic amylase is required, so by the time that the carbohydrate load reaches the proximal jejunum, this process is almost complete. After hydrolysis into simpler compounds, the monosaccharide fructose is passively absorbed through a GLUT5 transporter, whereas glucose and galactose are actively absorbed via the BBM sodium-glucose cotransporter SGLT-1.[28] Absorption occurs mostly in the early and midportion of the small intestine by mature enterocytes on the upper third of the villi.[29]

Protein Although protein digestion begins in the stomach by the action of pepsin, most proteolysis occurs in the proximal part of the small intestine. The duodenocyte brush border enzyme enteropeptidase (enterokinase) plays a key role in initiating proteolytic digestion

by converting trypsinogen into trypsin, which in turn activates all other pancreatic zymogens.[30] Furthermore, the majority of protein digestion occurs through dipeptide and tripeptide proton-coupled cotransporters, or PepT1, which are found mostly in the duodenum and jejunum.[31] As much as 50% of the protein ingested is digested and absorbed in the duodenum.

Lipids Most dietary fat is absorbed in the duodenum and upper jejunum. Entry of fat into the duodenum stimulates secretion of cholecystokinin (CCK) from the duodenal mucosa, which in turn promotes the release of pancreatic lipase. Duodenal hydrolysis of dietary lipids and biliary phospholipids and cholesterol is carried out by pancreatic lipase, colipase, phospholipase A_2, and cholesterol esterase. Bile acid solubilization starts in the duodenum and results in mixed micelles and liposomes, which are delivered to the brush border for passive diffusion of their lipid contents via fatty acid transport proteins.

Endocrine Physiology

The duodenum produces a diverse group of hormones that are crucial for initiating and coordinating digestion and absorption throughout the small intestine. Ingested nutrients stimulate the secretion of GI hormones that are necessary for the coordinated processes of digestion and absorption of food. The most clinically relevant are reviewed (Table 66–1).

Secretin

Bayliss and Starling[32] discovered secretin in 1902. Secretin is a helical peptide that shares structural similarities with pancreatic glucagons and VIP. It is released from S cells in the duodenal mucosa in response to fat, protein, and bile acids, but the most important is intraluminal acid, especially with a pH less than 3.0.[33] Release is neurally mediated by secretin-releasing peptide (SRP).[34,35]

Secretin is known as nature's antacid because it stimulates large volumes of alkaline pancreatic secretions. Other functions include (1) synergy with CCK in stimulating the exocrine pancreas; (2) stimulation of biliary bicarbonate, chloride, and water secretion; (3) decreasing the bile salt concentration; (4) stimulation of pepsin release; (5) antagonism of gastrin and thus acid production; (6) inhibition of gastric emptying, lower esophageal sphincter tone, and colonic contraction; and (7) increasing mucus production by gut mucosa.

Clinically, secretin paradoxically elevates gastrin levels in patients with Zollinger-Ellison syndrome and is thus often used as a diagnostic tool; it is also used to dilate the pancreatic duct for improved ductal evaluation during endoscopic retrograde cholangiopancreatography.

Cholecystokinin

CCK was discovered and named by Ivy and Oldberg,[36] who found that lipid infusion into the proximal part of

Table 66–1 Physiologic Functions of Gastrointestinal Hormones

CCK	Stimulates gallbladder contraction	Gastrin	Stimulates gastric acid secretion
	Stimulates exocrine pancreas secretion		Gastric trophic factor
	Growth of the pancreas	Ghrelin	Growth hormone secretagogue
	Satiety		Stimulates appetite
	Sphincter of Oddi relaxation	GRP	Stimulates gastrin release
	Inhibits gastric emptying	Melatonin	Stimulates bicarbonate secretion
GIP	Glucose-dependent insulin release		Antioxidant
	Inhibits gastric secretion	Neurotensin	Stimulates pancreas secretion
Motilin	Initiation of the migrating motor complex		Inhibits gastrointestinal motility
	Stimulates gastric emptying	NPY	Inhibits intestinal motility
	Stimulates pepsin secretion		Inhibits intestinal fluid/electrolyte absorption
NO	Smooth muscle relaxation		Vasoconstrictor
	Stimulates intestinal secretion	Opioids	Inhibit gastrointestinal motility
Secretin	Stimulates exocrine pancreaticobiliary function		Stimulate bicarbonate production
	Growth of the pancreas	PP	Stimulates GI and pancreaticobiliary secretion
	Stimulates gastric pepsin secretion		Causes satiety
	Stimulates colonic mucin		Stimulates UGI motility
	Inhibits gastric acid secretion	PYY	Causes satiety
	Inhibits gastrointestinal motility		Inhibits gastrointestinal motility
Serotonin	Gastric relaxation	Substance P	Stimulates GI motility
	Stimulates intestinal secretion		Smooth muscle contractility
	Stimulates intestinal motility		Immune activity
Somatostatin	Inhibits gastric acid and biliary secretions		Simulates GI secretion
	Inhibits pancreatic secretions		Stimulates CCK release
	Inhibits gastrointestinal secretion/motility		Gastric protection
	Inhibits gallbladder contraction	VIP	Stimulates water and electrolyte secretion
	Inhibits cell growth		Smooth muscle relaxation
			Inhibits intestinal absorption
			Immunomodulator

CCK, cholecystokinin; GI, gastrointestinal; GIP, gastric inhibitory polypeptide; GRP, gastrin-releasing peptide; NO, nitric oxide; NPY, neuropeptide Y; PP, pancreatic polypeptide; UGI, upper gastrointestinal; VIP, vasoactive intestinal polypeptide.

the small intestine resulted in gallbladder contraction. In 1943, Harper and Raper[37] found that the same physiologic stimulus resulted in pancreatic enzyme release and named it *pancreozymin*. It was not until 25 years later that Jorpes[38] sequenced these peptides and found that they were the same.

In a highly coordinated manner CCK regulates the ingestion, digestion, and absorption of nutrients. This hormone is a dipeptide produced by I cells and is present throughout the small intestine but concentrated in the duodenum and secreted into blood after the ingestion of proteins and fats. There are reports that acidification of the intestine can also release CCK. The physiologic actions of CCK include (1) stimulation of pancreatic enzyme secretion, (2) acetylcholine-mediated gallbladder contraction, (3) VIP/NO-mediated sphincter of Oddi relaxation, (4) potentiation of the pancreatic exocrine stimulatory effects of secretin, and (5) induction of satiety.[39]

Other less well known functions have been attributed to CCK, including relaxation of the lower esophageal

sphincter, VIP-mediated regulation of gastric emptying, and slowing of intestinal transit, which have been attributed to CCK-mediated interruption of the MMC. CCK may also function to decrease gastric acid release, stimulate insulin release, and stimulate pancreatic growth, and it has been found to be a central nervous system neurotransmitter responsible for panic and anxiety conditions.

Clinically, CCK has limited uses, but it has been suggested to reduce the incidence of acalculous cholecystitis and is being investigated as an anxiolytic. It can also be used during biliary imaging to stimulate gallbladder contraction.

Gastric Inhibitory Polypeptide (Glucose-Dependent Insulinotropic Peptide)

Gastric inhibitory polypeptide (GIP) was first purified and sequenced by Brown and Dryburgh in 1971,[40] who found it to have remarkable homology to secretin. GIP, along with glucagon-like peptide-1 (GLP-1), an enteroglucagon, is an incretin hormone, or a hormone responsible for endocrine enhancement of insulin secretion. Incretins, secreted from endocrine cells located in the intestinal mucosa, act to enhance meal-induced insulin secretion by the endocrine pancreas and are believed to inhibit meal-stimulated gastric secretion. They are stimulated by the presence of glucose and fat in the intestinal lumen. Direct contact of glucose and fat with these open-type K cells (GIP) and L cells (GLP-1) releases these hormones, although GIP release is postulated to be more dependent on the rate of absorption. K cells are found primarily in the duodenum but can be found throughout the small intestine; in contrast, L cells are found throughout the small intestine but predominately in the distal ileum.

Though not fully delineated, suggested mechanisms for neural modulation of incretin release include muscarinic, β-adrenergic, hormonal, and peptidergic (gastrin-releasing peptide [GRP]) fibers, and secretion is restrained by α-adrenergic stimulation, glucagon, insulin, peptide YY (PYY), and somatostatin.[41]

The importance of incretin hormones lies in their possible contribution to the early pathogenesis of type 2 diabetes in that it is believed that the incretin effect is greatly impaired in such patients. Thus, these hormones are being evaluated as potential treatment targets.[42]

Somatostatin

Somatostatin has been identified in nerves and cell bodies in the central and peripheral nervous system, including the intramural enteric nervous system and endocrine-like D cells of the stomach and small intestine.[43,44] It is a hormone present throughout the mammalian organism and has paracrine, endocrine, and neurocrine activity. Over two thirds of the circulating concentration of somatostatin is derived from the GI system, especially the distal part of the stomach, duodenum, jejunum, and pancreas. Although the mechanism of somatostatin secretion remains poorly understood, it has been shown that a significant increase occurs in response to the ingestion of a meal, more specifically, the presence of fat, protein, and to a lesser extent, carbohydrate in the distal portion of the stomach and duodenum. CGRP and catecholamines are also stimulants for somatostatin release. Release of acetylcholine from cholinergic neurons inhibits somatostatin release. Plasma somatostatin fluctuations are found during the interdigestive period and are controlled by a complex interplay between cholinergic and adrenergic neural input, prostaglandins, and circadian rhythms. Additional hormones affect circulating concentrations, including the stimulants gastrin, CCK, secretin, GIP, and bombesin.

A wide spectrum of GI actions has been attributed to somatostatin. In the stomach, somatostatin inhibits gastric acid and pepsin secretion by reducing the response to gastrin in addition to attenuating gastrin release. This effect is believed to be due to a paracrine effect of the hormone. Furthermore, it inhibits the absorption of amino acids in the duodenum and attenuates glucagon-induced jejunal water and electrolyte secretion. In the pancreas, somatostatin inhibits

enzymatic, but not bicarbonate secretion and blocks the response to CCK and secretin. Somatostatin reduces the frequency of the MMC of the stomach and small intestine, which may be due to direct inhibition of acetylcholine release from peripheral neurons. Because of its role as a universal inhibitor of GI activity, much research has been invested in the production of somatostatin analogues for the treatment of many GI diseases.

Motilin

Motilin is a regulatory polypeptide of 22 amino acid residues that originates in nonargentaffin endocrine cells, which are scattered in the absorptive epithelial cells covering the villi of the duodenum and upper jejunum.[45] It is released into the general circulation at about 100-minute intervals during the interdigestive state and is an important factor in initiation of phase III contractions in the stomach, also known as the MMC. Additionally, motilin has a stimulatory effect on gastric pepsin secretion and pancreatic exocrine secretion[46-48] while causing gallbladder contraction, including the sphincter of Oddi.[49,50] Previously, it was believed that changes in duodenal pH were stimulatory for motilin release (i.e., duodenal acidification). However, more recent data have refuted this theory.[51] Nevertheless, it is clear that the presence of nutrients in the duodenum, especially fat, is strongly inhibitory for motilin release.[52] Although the mechanism of action of motilin remains a mystery, it has generally been accepted that it exerts its effect on gastric smooth muscle by a vagal-dependent and vagal-independent pathway. Motilin has been shown to increase serum concentrations of insulin and pancreatic polypeptide (PP). Clinical application of motilin as a prokinetic agent has become possible since erythromycin and its derivatives were proved to be nonpeptide motilin receptor agonists.

Serotonin

Serotonin (5-hydroxytryptamine [5-HT]) is a nonpeptide hormone important in intestinal secretion and motility. Although it is now recognized to be localized throughout the enteric neuronal system, over 90% of total-body serotonin is contained in the enterochromaffin (EC) cells lining the mucosa of the intestine, including the duodenum.[53] It is widely accepted that in the GI tract serotonin acts as both a neurotransmitter and a mucosal signaling molecule. As a neurotransmitter, serotonin is involved in gastric relaxation through vagally induced activation of an inhibitory neural circuit containing serotoninergic neurons.[54] 5-HT also has a role in induction of the slow excitatory postsynaptic potentials in enteric neurons. As a mucosal signaling agent, the EC cell is purported to be a signal transducer such that mucosal distention or the presence of intraluminal nutrients (e.g., glucose, fat), or both, stimulates these cells to release 5-HT into the bowel wall, which initiates a cascade of physiologic events.[55-57] Included in these events are increased intestinal secretions via enhanced electrolyte transport and increased intestinal motility. The multitude of responses initiated by serotonin is attributed to the various serotonin receptor subtypes identified throughout the enteric smooth muscle, mucosal, and neuronal milieu. In fact, pharmacologic manipulation has become an area of intense investigation in the treatment of both constipation-prone and diarrhea-prone irritable bowel syndrome (IBD) inasmuch as serotonin is thought to be intricately involved in such pathologic phenomena. Serotonin is also a product of carcinoid tumors and is implicated in most of the symptoms seen in carcinoid syndrome.

Nitric Oxide

The inhibitory mechanism of nonadrenergic, noncholinergic (NANC) neurotransmission in the GI tract was discovered to be primarily mediated by NO.[58-60] First known as endothelium-derived relaxing factor, NO is an inorganic gas important in the neural and hormonal regulation of intestinal physiology. It is produced from the conversion of L-arginine to L-citrulline by nitric oxide synthase (NOS), an enzyme that exists as inducible and constitutive isoforms, the latter being present in neurons and the endothelium.[61] NO was first shown to be an inhibitory NANC neurotransmitter in isolated superperfused segments of canine intestine, in which it caused smooth muscle relaxation that was inhibited by NOS inhibitors. In the stomach, NO release is important in vagally mediated receptive relaxation and gastric distention–induced pyloric relaxation. NO is also an inhibitory neurotransmitter in duodenal and jejunal smooth muscle in the neuronal regulation of intestinal transit. In addition, it causes relaxation of the sphincter of Oddi, the pyloric sphincter, and the gallbladder smooth muscle. Moreover, NO has a role in intestinal secretion. It has been shown that the addition of NO donors to isolated rat gastric cells in suspension causes secretion.[62] Furthermore, in rat distal colon, NO has been suggested to be a secretomotor neurotransmitter responsible for increasing electrolyte transport initiated by serotonin.[63] Not only may NO be important in gastric acid secretion but also it has been implicated in pancreatic exocrine and endocrine function. In addition, it may serve to protect gastric mucosal integrity against various noxious intraluminal contents through inhibition of endothelial smooth muscle, thus increasing gastrin blood flow in times of stress.

Other Hormones

Other hormones are secreted by the duodenum but are not necessarily predominant in that region; such hormones include the following: VIP, neurotensin (NT), substance P (SP), GRP, ghrelin, enkephalins and endorphins, peptide tyrosine tyrosine (PYY), PP, neuropeptide Y (NPY), melatonin, and gastrin. Their relationships to the duodenal control of gastric and intestinal function remains poorly understood.

Vasoactive Intestinal Peptide VIP is a gut neuropeptide with similar structure to secretin and glucagon. It is released by intraduodenal hydrochloric acid, ethanol, fat, and vagal stimulation. VIP is a smooth muscle relaxant of blood vessels and sphincters, although it is best known for increasing intestinal secretion of water and electrolytes via stimulation of adenylate cyclase. Excess secretion of VIP into the blood by secretory tumors, which are most commonly localized in the pancreas, leads to the watery diarrhea hypokalemia achlorhydria (WDHA) syndrome, also known as a VIPoma or the Vernor-Morrison or *pancreatic cholera* syndrome. In addition, VIP is also known to inhibit intestinal absorption, increase bile flow, induce gallbladder relaxation, and inhibit acid and pepsin secretion, and it has a small glycogenolytic effect in the liver.[64] Recently, VIP has been recognized as an immunomodulator and possibly as a cytokine-like molecule[65]; a decrease in this function in the lamina propria and submucosa has been implicated in the pathophysiology of IBD.[66]

Neurotensin NT is most abundant in the ileum, with a lesser amount in the jejunum and duodenum; this tridecapeptide is also found in the brain to a lesser degree, where it has been linked to clinical disorders hypothesized to involve dopamine circuits, such as schizophrenia, Parkinson's disease, and drug abuse.[67] NT is present in the endocrine cells labeled N cells,[68] which are of the open type. NT is also present in nerves of the myenteric plexus, in the muscular layer, and in the submucosa of the stomach and duodenum. Release of NT is stimulated by intraluminal fat, and it functions to stimulate pancreatic secretion and inhibition of gastric and small bowel motility.

NT has been implicated in facilitating fatty acid translocation and stimulating the growth of various GI tissues, including cancer cells. It also stimulates colonic contraction and defecation; its release is accelerated in patients with dumping syndrome. The NT gene is developmentally regulated in the gut of both rats and humans in a distinctive temporally and spatially specific pattern[69]; therefore, this gene is an excellent model for defining differentiation pathways leading to gut development, maturation, and neoplasia. Some of the effects of NT are inhibited by COX inhibitors, thus suggesting prostaglandin-mediated release.

Substance P The first brain-gut peptide discovered, SP belongs to a group of neuropeptides called tachykinins, and it plays an important role as a neurotransmitter in the central and peripheral nervous system. In response to intraluminal food, SP leads to excitatory action on GI motor activity, which is seen virtually at all levels and in all layers of the mammalian gut, with the highest concentrations in the duodenum and jejunum. SP regulates smooth muscle contractility, epithelial ion transport, vascular permeability, and immune function in the GI tract.[70] It appears to increase the contraction of intestinal and gallbladder smooth muscle, reduce bile flow, and increase pancreatic juice outflow. This neurotransmitter has been suggested to play a role in the pathophysiology of inflammatory diseases such as arthritis, colitis, and intestinal inflammation. Elevated levels of SP have been reported in the rectum and colon of patients with IBD and correlate with disease activity. Preventing the proinflammatory effects of SP with tachykinin receptor antagonists may have therapeutic potential in inflammatory diseases such as asthma, sarcoidosis, chronic bronchitis, IBD, and rheumatoid arthritis. In gut-associated lymphoid tissue (GALT), the high concentrations of SP in intestinal nerve endings and expression of a specific SP receptor on T and B cells in murine Peyer's patches suggest that SP may act as a trophic factor, a homing factor, or a differentiation factor for IgA-secreting plasma cells.[71]

Gastrin-Releasing Peptide Bombesin was discovered in 1970 in extracts taken from the skin of amphibians.[72] It was later noted to have a mammalian counterpart that was named GRP, which has been detected throughout the digestive tract but is particularly prominent in both the acid- and gastrin-secreting portions of the stomach. It is known to modulate acid and gut peptide secretion, and it stimulates CCK release from the GI tract. Secretion of GRP causes the release of endogenous gastrin, which activates sensory neurons, and it is modified by somatostatin. Studies have shown that activation of sensory neurons causes increased production of NO through activation of constitutive NOS, thereby leading to increased gastric mucosal blood flow and thus protection from damage by irritants.[73] In addition to activation of capsaicin-sensitive sensory neurons, GRP requires endogenous prostaglandins to fully exert its gastroprotective actions.[74] This process is reminiscent of that described in protecting the duodenal mucosa. Clinically, GRP has been shown to improve maintenance of gut mucosal integrity after severe burns by decreasing burn-induced gut mucosal atrophy and epithelial cell apoptosis.[75]

Ghrelin *Ghrelin* is a recently identified peptide important in the peripheral regulation of energy balance. Endocrine cells of the gastric oxyntic mucosa are the primary site of production; they are responsible for over 70% of the circulating ghrelin concentration.[76] Through ultrastructural analysis these ghrelin cells are distinct from the histamine-producing enterochromaffin-like (ECL) cell, the somatostatin-producing D cell, and the serotonin-producing EC cell. Ghrelin cells have also been discovered in the small intestine and pancreas.[77] Ghrelin dose-dependently stimulates release of growth hormone from pituitary cells and is in fact the most potent growth hormone secretogogue discovered. Although the exact mechanism of action is not clearly defined, its orexigenic effect is well documented, and it increases appetite in a circadian fashion.[78] These findings suggest a role for ghrelin as a humoral signal from the stomach for meal initiation. This increase in appetite is associated with an increase in body weight via increased adipogenesis and reduced lipid metabolism.[79] It has been postulated that ghrelin may be a signal to the central nervous system regarding acute and chronic changes in food intake, metabolism, or body fat mass, thereby initiating efferent responses that regulate energy homeostasis.[80] Circulating levels of ghrelin are inversely related to body mass index, adipose tissue mass, and insulin plasma levels such that dysregulation of ghrelin gene expression may explain the impaired regulation of body weight in obesity.[81] Moreover, ghrelin has a motilin-like effect on gastric motility and stimulates the release of somatostatin and PP by increasing glucose and decreasing insulin levels.[80]

Endorphins and Enkephalins Endorphins and enkephalins are opioid peptides found in a variety of tissues. Though present in lower concentration in the gut than in the central nervous system, the proximal portion of the intestine has a particularly high concentration of enkephalins. Both are present in enteric nerves, especially in the myenteric plexus. Enkephalins are found in the intrinsic nerves of the stomach and innervate the pyloric sphincter; in contrast, endorphins have been found in pyloric antral G cells and in the submucosal plexus of the duodenum and ileum.[82]

Although their specific effects on the GI system are unknown, opioid peptides have been associated with several functions, including motility, acid secretion, and intestinal electrolyte and fluid transport. They have also been implicated in stimulating duodenocyte HCO_3^- production in response to duodenal acid. The antimotility effects of opioid drugs arise from changes in both motility and secretion caused by activation of opioid receptors located in the gut wall,[83] which leads to interruption of the enteric nerve pathways governing acetylcholine and other excitatory transmitters that stimulate muscle contraction. Allescher et al.,[84] in a naloxone-sensitive system, demonstrated that opioid-active drugs modify the peristaltic reflex by reducing the efficacy of the reflex response and modulating the timing of the ascending excitatory and descending inhibitory reflex pathway. Clinically, exogenous opioids, including morphine, have been well known to cause constipation, and other medications that interact with opioid receptors have been used for antidiarrheal therapy.

Peptide YY and Pancreatic Polypeptide PYY and PP belong to the NPY family, which contain several tyrosine residues within their homologous sequences. These peptides activate G protein–coupled Y receptors.

PP is restricted to endocrine cells mainly in the duodenal portion of the pancreas, but it is also found throughout the GI tract. It is released into blood in response to a meal rich in protein and especially fats. PP is known to stimulate gastric, pancreaticobiliary, and intestinal secretion, and it stimulates motility of the upper GI system. PP, along with PYY, has been implicated as an anorexigenic peptide promoting satiety.[85]

NPY is a neuropeptide widely distributed in the central and peripheral nervous system; its nerve fibers are widely located through the intestinal tract, with the largest numbers in the duodenum and upper part of the small intestine. Functionally, NPY is known to regulate large and small intestinal motility, vasoconstriction of surrounding vessels, and inhibition of small intestinal fluid and electrolyte secretion.

PYY is secreted in response to intraluminal carbohydrates and lipids, and it is expressed in both endocrine cells and enteric neurons throughout the gut. L cells that secrete GLP-1 also secrete PYY.[86] These cells predominate in the ileum, colon, and especially the rectum; however, enteric nerve fibers that innervate myenteric plexus smooth muscle are found in highest number in the stomach and duodenum.[87] The dual localization of PYY in endocrine cells and intestinal nerves suggests that it is important in several gut functions similar to NPY, including motility and secretion. Furthermore, its presence during early fetal development suggests that it may play a role in promoting development and maturation of the digestive tract.

Melatonin A product of intestinal EC cells and the pineal gland, melatonin is a potent stimulant of duodenal mucosal HCO_3^- secretion in the rat. Melatonin receptors are distributed throughout the GI tract. The effects of melatonin are mediated by specific high-affinity membrane-associated melatonin receptors that belong to the superfamily of G protein–coupled receptors. On the basis of pharmacologic evidence, three subtypes are reported. The total amount of melatonin in the alimentary tract is much higher (400-fold) than that in the central nervous system, but the role of melatonin in GI function has been largely unknown.[88] Melatonin may also exert a potent anti-inflammatory effect that may be useful in the treatment of IBD. These effects are attributed partly to its antioxidant property, which stems from eliminating NO in the inflamed colon.[89]

Gastrin A peptide hormone produced by G cells in the gastric antrum and duodenum, gastrin is induced by the presence of protein or calcium in the gastric lumen or by antral/duodenal distention. Gastrin stimulates gastric acid secretion by parietal cells in the stomach. Zollinger-Ellison syndrome is caused by a gastrinoma, or a gastrin-secretin tumor, which is usually localized in the pancreas or duodenum. Gastrin has also been documented to have trophic action and may contribute to the growth of gastric and colorectal carcinoma.[90] *H. pylori*–associated antrum gastritis produces hypergastrinemia by disinhibition of gastrin release and thereby contributes to hypersecretion of acid in *H. pylori*–associated gastritis and duodenal ulcer disease.[91] Pentagastrin, a gastrin analogue, is used clinically to measure maximal gastric secretion.

DUODENAL MOTILITY

Intrinsic Control

The intrinsic rhythm of small intestinal contractions probably originates from the MMC of the distal part of the stomach. It has been demonstrated that slow-wave and spike activities take place in preparations of neuron-free intestinal smooth muscle. The low-resistance junctions that exist between adjacent smooth muscle cells allow rapid propagation of electrical activity.[92] This intrinsic activity is modified by neural input and by hormones working in an endocrine, paracrine, or neurocrine pattern. Baseline duodenal peristalsis generally occurs at higher frequency (10 to 12/min) than in the jejunum or ileum. The electrical activity of duodenal smooth muscle is such that longitudinal waves of contraction continue for some distance down the small

bowel, possibly resulting in a strong propulsive forward movement of duodenal contents.

Extrinsic Control

Extrinsic control of duodenal motility is primarily regulated by the autonomic nervous system.[93] Afferent and efferent vagal fibers innervate the entire small intestine, including the duodenum. The sympathetic innervation consists of preganglionic neuronal processes originating from T9 and T10. These run in the splanchnic nerves and synapse with the celiac ganglia. Thus, the duodenum derives its sympathetic innervation from both celiac (proximal duodenum) and superior mesenteric (distal duodenum) ganglia. These fibers consist of both cholinergic and noradrenergic neurons; however, the sympathetic innervation of the stomach and duodenum is largely inhibitory.

The preganglionic vagal efferent neurons have cholinergic excitatory and inhibitory interneuronal connections before intestinal innervation. Therefore, the vagus nerve can elicit several responses in the stomach and duodenum, and there is a delicate interplay between stimulatory and inhibitory effects in the net response to vagal activity. In the stomach, vagal stimulation causes gastric acid secretion, and it has been shown that truncal vagotomy causes incoordination of antral contractions and loss of receptive relaxation and gastric emptying. In the duodenum, vagal stimulation has been linked to inhibition of duodenal motility. In addition, a large number of receptors have been identified on smooth muscle cells that are important in the initiation of contraction,[94] including receptors for CCK, gastrin, SP, bombesin, and acetylcholine. Other agents have been identified as smooth muscle relaxants, such as VIP and adenosine triphosphate. This is a testament to the complex interplay of local and extrinsic hormonal and neural input in the regulation of intestinal motility.

ACKNOWLEDGMENT

We would like to acknowledge the excellent work of the previous writers of this chapter, Vicky B. Tola and David I. Soybel; much of the material in the anatomy section has been retained.

REFERENCES

1. Edwards EA, Malone PD, MacArthur JD: Operative Anatomy of Abdomen and Pelvis. Philadelphia, Lea & Febiger, 1975.
2. Bower RJ, Ternberg JL: Preduodenal portal vein. J Pediatr Surg 7:579-584, 1972.
3. Braun P, Collin PP, Ducharme JC: Preduodenal portal vein: A significant entity? Report of two cases and review of the literature. Can J Surg 17:316-319, 322, 1974.
4. Schirmer BD: Vascular compression of the duodenum. In Sabiston DC (ed): Textbook of Surgery, 2nd ed. Philadelphia, WB Saunders, 1997, p 887.
5. Anderson JR, Earnshaw PM, Fraser GM: Extrinsic compression of the third part of the duodenum. Clin Radiol 33:75-81, 1982.
6. Jones TW: Paraduodenal hernia and hernias of the foramen of Winslow. In Nyhus LM, Harkins HN (eds): Hernia. Philadelphia, JB Lippincott, 1964, p 577.

7. Zollinger RM: Congenital mesocolic or paraduodenal hernias: An embryologic basis for classification and operative repair. In Nyhus LM, Harkins NH, Condon RE (eds): Hernia, 2nd ed. Philadelphia, JB Lippincott, 1978, p 491.

8. Willwerth BM, Zollinger RM Jr, Izant RJ Jr: Congenital mesocolic (paraduodenal) hernia. Embryologic basis of repair. Am J Surg 128:358-361, 1974.

9. Schneider WR, Hauck AE, Stone AH: Hernia through the foramen of Winslow. In Nyhus LM, Condon RE (eds): Hernia. Philadelphia, JB Lippincott, 1978, p 488.

10. Eggert A, Teichmann W, Wittmann DH: The pathological implication of duodenal diverticula. Surg Gynecol Obstet 154:62-64, 1982.

11. Suzuki H: Effects of duodenectomy on gastric motility and gastric hormones in dogs. Ann Surg 233:353-359, 2001.

12. Tanaka M, Sarr MG: Role of the duodenum in the control of canine gastrointestinal motility. Gastroenterology 94:622-629, 1988.

13. Pausawasdi N, Ramamoorthy S, Crofford LJ, et al: Regulation and function of COX-2 gene expression in isolated gastric parietal cells. Am J Physiol Gastrointest Liver Physiol 282:G1069-G1078, 2002.

14. Sjoblom M, Femstrom G: Melatonin in the duodenal lumen is a potent stimulant of mucosal bicarbonate secretion. J Pineal Res 34:288-293, 2003.

15. Bubenik GA: Localization, physiological significance and possible clinical implication of gastrointestinal melatonin. Biol Signals Receptors 10:350-366, 2001.

16. Konturek PC, Konturek SJ, Hahn EG: Duodenal alkaline secretion: Its mechanisms and role in mucosal protection against acid. Dig Liver Dis 36:505-512, 2004.

17. Bukhave K, Rask-Madsen J, Hogan DL, et al: Proximal duodenal prostaglandin E_2 release and mucosal bicarbonate secretion are altered in patients with duodenal ulcers. Gastroenterology 99:951-965, 1990.

18. Heller HJ: Calcium hemostasis. In Griffin JE, Ojeda SR (eds): Textbook of Endocrine Physiology, 5th ed. New York, Oxford University Press, 2004, p 362.

19. Bronner F: Mechanism and functional aspects of intestinal calcium absorption. J Exp Zool 300(A):47-52, 2003.

20. De Prisco C, Levine SN: Metabolic bone disease after gastric bypass surgery for obesity. Am J Med Sci 329:57-61, 2005.

21. Rhode B, MacLean D: Vitamin and mineral supplementation after gastric bypass. In Deitel M, Cowan GSM (eds): Update: Surgery for the Morbidly Obese Patient. Toronto, FD Communications, 2000, pp 161-170.

22. Amaral JF, Thompson WR, Caldwell MD, et al: Prospective metabolic evaluation of 150 consecutive patients who underwent gastric exclusion. Am J Surg 147:468-476, 1984.

23. Johnson JM, DeMaria EJ, Downs RJ, et al: The long-term effects of gastric bypass on vitamin D metabolism. Ann Surg 243:701-704, 2006.

24. Roy CN, Enns CA: Iron hemostasis: New tales from the crypt. Blood 96:4020-4027, 2000.

25. Frazer DM, Anderson GJ: The orchestration of body iron intake: How and where do enterocytes receive their cues? Blood Cells Mol Dis 30:288-297, 2003.

26. Brolin RE, Leung M: Survey of vitamin and mineral supplementation after gastric bypass and biliopancreatic diversion for morbid obesity. Obes Surg 9:150-154, 1999.

27. Brolin RE, LaMarca LB, Kenler HA, Cody RP: Malabsorptive gastric bypass in patients with superobesity. J Gastrointest Surg 6:195-203, 2002.

28. Takata K: Glucose transporters in the transepithelial transport of glucose. J Electron Microsc 45:275-284, 1996.

29. Wright EM, Martin MG, Turk E: Intestinal absorption in health and disease—sugars. Best Pract Res Clin Gastroenterol 17:943-956, 2003.

30. Jeno P, Green JR, Lentze MJ: Specificity studies on enteropeptidase substrates related to the N-terminus of trypsinogen. Biochem J 241:721-727, 1987.

31. Ogihara H, Saito H, Shin BC, et al: Immuno-localization of H^+/peptide cotransporter in rat digestive tract. Biochem Biophys Res Commun 220:848-852, 1996.

32. Bayliss WM, Starling EH: The mechanisms of pancreatic secretion. J Physiol 28:325, 1902.

33. Flemstrom G, Isenberg JI: Gastroduodenal mucosal alkaline secretion and mucosal protection. News Physiol Sci 16:23-28, 2001.

34. Li P, Lee KY, Chang TM, Chey WY: Mechanism of acid-induced release of secretin in rats: Presence of a secretin releasing factor. J Clin Invest 86:1474-1479, 1990.

35. Chey WY, Chang TM: Neural control of the release and action of secretin. J Physiol Pharmacol 54(Suppl 4):105-112, 2003.

36. Ivy AC, Oldberg E: A hormone mechanism for gallbladder contraction and evacuation. Am J Physiol 86:599, 1928.

37. Harper AA, Raper HS: Pancreozymin: A stimulant of the secretion of pancreatic enzymes in extracts of small intestine. J Physiol 102:115, 1943.

38. Jorpes JE: The isolation and chemistry of secretin and cholecystokinin. Gastroenterology 55:157-164, 1968.

39. Rehfeld J: Clinical endocrinology and metabolism. Cholecystokinin. Best Pract Res Clin Endocrinol Metabol 18:569-586, 2004.

40. Brown JC, Dryburgh JR: A gastric inhibitory polypeptide. II. The complete amino acid sequence. Can J Biochem 49:867-872, 1971.

41. Deacon CF: What do we know about the secretion and degradation of incretin hormones? Regul Pept 128:117-124, 2005.

42. Nauck MA, Baller B, Meier JJ: gastric inhibitory polypeptide and glucagon-like peptide-1 in the pathogenesis of type 2 diabetes. Diabetes 53(Suppl 3):S190-S196, 2004.

43. Walsh JH: Gastrointestinal hormones. In Jackson MJ (ed): Physiology of the Gastrointestinal Tract. Raven Press, Houston, 1987, pp 213-229.

44. Guillemin R, Gerich J: Somatostatin: Physiological and clinical significance. Annu Rev Med 27:379-388, 1976.

45. Brown JC: Presence of a gastric motor-stimulating property in duodenal extracts. Gastroenterology 52:225-229, 1967.

46. Nakaya M, Suzuki T, Arai H: Does motilin control interdigestive pepsin secretion in the dog? Peptides 4:439-444, 1983.

47. Keane F, DiMagno E, Dozois R: Relationships among canine interdigestive exocrine pancreatic and biliary flow, duodenal motor activity, plasma pancreatic polypeptide, and motilin. Gastroenterology 78:310-316, 1980.

48. Konturek SJ, Dembinski A, Krol R, Wunsch E: Effects of motilin on gastric and pancreatic secretion in dogs. Scand J Gastroenterol 39:57-61, 1976.

49. Itoh Z, Takahashi I: Periodic contractions of the canine gallbladder during the interdigestive state. Am J Physiol 240:G183-G189, 1981.

50. Muller E, Grace P, Conter R: Influence of motilin and cholecystokinin on sphincter of Oddi and duodenal mobility. Am J Physiol 253:G679-G683, 1987.

51. Kusano M, Sekiguchi T, Nishioka T: Gastric acid inhibits antral phase III activity in duodenal ulcer patients. Dig Dis Sci 28:824-831, 1993.

52. Mori K, Seino Y, Yanaihara N: Role of the duodenum in motilin release. Regul Pept 1:271-277, 1981.

53. Erspamer V: Occurrence of indolealkylamines in nature. In Erspamer V (ed): Handbook of Experimental Pharmacology: 5-Hydroxytryptamine and Related Indolealkylamines. New York, Springer-Verlag, 1966, pp 132-181.

54. Bulbring E, Gershon M: 5-Hydroxytryptamine participation in the vagal inhibitory innervation of the stomach. J Physiol (Lond) 192:23-46, 1967.

55. Bulbring E, Creena A: The release of 5-hydroxytryptamine in relation to pressure exerted on the intestinal mucosa. J Physiol (Lond) 146:18-28, 1959.

56. Kim M, Cooke H, Javed N: D-Glucose releases 5-hydroxytryptamine from human BON cells as a model of enterochromaffin cells. Gastroenterology 121:1400-1406, 2001.

57. Ponti FD: Pharmacology of serotonin: What a clinician should know. Gut 53:1520-1535, 2004.

58. Ignarro L, Buga G, Wood K: Endothelium-derived relaxing factor produced and released from artery and vein is nitric oxide. Proc Natl Acad Sci U S A 84:9265-9269, 1987.

59. Palmer R, Ferrige A, Moncada S: Nitric oxide release accounts for the biological activity of endothelium-derived relaxing factor. Nature 327:524-526, 1987.

60. Ignarro L, Byrns R, Wood K: Biochemical and pharmacological properties of endothelium-derived relaxing factor and its similarity to nitric oxide radical. In Vanhoutte P (ed): Vasodilation. New York, Raven Press, 1988, pp 427-435.

61. Bredt D, Snyder S: Isolation of nitric oxide synthetase, a calmodulin-requiring enzyme. Proc Natl Acad Sci U S A 87:682-685, 1990.

62. Brown J, Keates A, Hanson P: Nitric oxide generators and cGMP stimulate mucus secretion by rat gastric mucosal cells. Am J Physiol 265:G418-G422, 1993.

63. King B, Stoner M, Kellum J: Nitrergic secretomotor neurotransmitter in the chloride secretory response to serotonin. Dig Dis Sci 49:196-201, 2004.

64. Laburthe M, Couvineau A, Voisin T: Receptors for peptides of the VIP/PACAP and PYY/NPY/PP families. In Greeley GH (ed): Gastrointestinal Endocrinology. Totowa, NJ, Humana Press, 1999, pp 126-127.

65. Delgado M, Pozo D, Ganea D: The significance of vasoactive intestinal peptide in immunomodulation. Pharmacol Rev 56:249-290, 2004.

66. Kubota Y, Petras RE, Ottaway CA, et al: Colonic vasoactive intestinal peptide nerves in inflammatory bowel disease. Gastroenterology 102:1242-1251, 1992.

67. Kinkead B, Nemeroff CB: Neurotensin, schizophrenia, and antipsychotic drug action. Int Rev Neurobiol 59:327-349, 2004.

68. Reinecke M: Neurotensin. Immunohistochemical localization in central and peripheral nervous system and in endocrine cells and its functional role as a neurotransmitter and endocrine hormone. Prog Histochem Cytochem 16:1-172, 1985.

69. Evers BM: Expression of the neurotensin/neuromedin N gene in the gut: A potential model for gut differentiation. In Greeley GH (ed): Gastrointestinal Endocrinology. Totowa, NJ, Humana Press, 1999, p 425.

70. O'Connor TM, O'Connell J, O'Brien DI, et al: The role of substance P in inflammatory disease. J Cell Physiol 201:167-180, 2004.

71. Stanisz AM, Scicchitano R, Dazin P, et al: Distribution of substance P receptors on murine spleen and Peyer's patch T and B cells. J Immunol 139:749-754, 1987.

72. Erspamer V, Erspamer GF, Inselvini M: Some pharmacological actions of alytesin and bombesin. J Pharm Pharmacol 22:875-876, 1970.

73. West SD, Mercer DW: Bombesin-induced gastroprotection. Ann Surg 241:227-231, 2005.

74. Peskar B: Neural aspects of prostaglandin involvement in gastric mucosal defense. J Physiol Pharmacol 52:555-568, 2001.

75. Wu X, Spies M, Chappell VL, et al: Effect of bombesin on gut mucosal impairment after severe burn. Shock 18:518-522, 2002.

76. Jeon T, Lee S, Kim H: Changes in plasma ghrelin concentration immediately after gastrectomy in patients with early gastric cancer. J Clin Endocrinol Metab 89:5392-5396, 2004.

77. Kojima M, Hosoda H, Date Y: Ghrelin is a growth-hormone–releasing acylated peptide from stomach. Nature 402:656-660, 1999.

78. Cummings D, Purnell J, Frayo R: A preprandial rise in plasma ghrelin levels suggests a role in meal initiation in humans. Diabetes 50:1714-1719, 2001.

79. Inui A: Ghrelin: An orexigenic and somatotrophic signal from the stomach. Nat Rev Neurosci 2:551-560, 2001.

80. Otto B, Spranger J, Benoit S: The many faces of ghrelin: New perspectives for nutrition research? Br J Nutr 93:765-771, 2005.

81. Rindi G, Torsello A, Locatelli V: Ghrelin expression and actions: A novel peptide for an old cell type of the diffuse endocrine system. Exp Biol Med 229:1007-1016, 2004.

82. Beinfeld MC: Biosynthesis and processing of gastrointestinal peptide hormones. In Greeley GH (ed): Gastrointestinal Endocrinology. Totowa, NJ, Humana Press, 1999, pp 44-45.

83. Bianchi G, Ferretti P, Recchia M, et al: Morphine tissue levels and reduction of gastrointestinal transit in rats. Correlation supports primary action site in the gut. Gastroenterology 85:852-858, 1983.

84. Allescher HD, Storr M, Piller C, et al: Effect of opioid active therapeutics on the ascending reflex pathway in the rat ileum. Neuropeptides 34:181-186, 2000.

85. Stanley S, Wynne K, Bloom S: Gastrointestinal satiety signals III. Glucagon-like peptide 1, oxyntomodulin, peptide YY, and pancreatic polypeptide. Am J Physiol Gastrointest Liver Physiol 286:693-697, 2004.

86. Strader AD, Woods SD: Gastrointestinal hormones and food intake. Gastroenterology 128:175-191, 2005.

87. Ekblad E, Sundler F: Distribution of pancreatic polypeptide and peptide YY. Peptides 23:251-261, 2002.

88. Sjoblom M, Safsten B, Flemstrom G: Melatonin-induced calcium signaling in clusters of human and rat duodenal enterocytes. Am J Physiol Gastrointest Liver Physiol 284:G1034-G1040, 2003.

89. Mei Q, Xu JM, Xiang L, et al: Change of nitric oxide in experimental colitis and its inhibition by melatonin in vivo and in vitro. Postgrad Med J 81:667-672, 2005.

90. Walsh J: Gastrin. In Walsh JH, Dockray GJ (eds): Gut Peptides: Biochemistry and Physiology. New York, Raven Press, 1994, pp 75-121.

91. El-Omar E, Penman ID, Ardill JE, et al: *Helicobacter pylori* infection and abnormalities of acid secretion in patients with duodenal ulcer disease. Gastroenterology 109:681-691, 1995.

92. Nagai T, Prosser CL: Patterns of conduction in smooth muscle. Am J Physiol 204:910-914, 1963.

93. Roman C, Gonella J: Extrinsic control of digestive tract motility. In Johnson L (ed): Physiology of the Gastrointestinal Tract. New York, Raven Press, 1987, p 507.

94. Makhlouf GM: Isolated smooth muscle cells of the gut. In Johnson LR, Christensen J (eds): Physiology of the Gastrointestinal Tract, 2nd ed. New York, Raven Press, 1987, p 555.

67

Small Intestine

Mary F. Otterson ▪ David Binion ▪ Seth J. Karp ▪
David I. Soybel ▪ Edward C. Mun ▪ Jeffrey B. Matthews

ANATOMY

The duodenum, jejunum, and ileum make up the small intestine. The duodenum is anatomically distinct, but the jejunum (proximal two fifths) and ileum (distal three fifths) have no true anatomic border between them.

The duodenum is divided into four parts: the first portion or the bulb, the second or descending portion, the third or transverse portion, and the fourth or ascending portion. The first portion begins at the pylorus and sweeps to the right; it is anchored by the hepatoduodenal ligament and is referred to as the bulb of the duodenum. Just beyond the bulb, Kerckring's folds begin. These circular folds of mucosa and submucosa extend for the length of the small bowel. Radiographically, Kerckring's folds are referred to as the *valvulae conniventes*. Posterior to the bulb of the duodenum are the gastroduodenal artery and the pancreas. Blood supply is from the supraduodenal and gastroduodenal arteries; both arise from the hepatic artery. The second portion of the duodenum travels posteriorly and caudad to the level of the first lumbar vertebra, where it is retroperitoneal and attached to the head of the pancreas. Posterior is Gerota's fascia and the kidney, anterior is the hepatic flexure of the colon, and medial lies the inferior vena cava. The arterial supply is from the celiac axis through the gastroduodenal artery to the anterosuperior and posterosuperior pancreaticoduodenal arteries and from the superior mesenteric artery (SMA) through the anteroinferior and posteroinferior pancreaticoduodenal arteries. The common bile duct and the main pancreatic duct enter in the middle of the second portion of the duodenum, about 10 cm distal to the pylorus at the ampulla of Vater. The sphincter of Oddi surrounds and controls the ampulla of Vater. When an accessory pancreatic duct is present (6% of normal patients), it usually enters about 2 cm proximal to the ampulla.[1] The third portion begins as the duodenum sweeps to the left at the level of the third lumbar vertebra and ends at the aorta.

It is associated with the uncinate process of the pancreas and is dorsal to the superior mesenteric artery. Subtle anatomic anomalies can result from a high ligament of Treitz, prolonged immobilization, spinal surgery, rapid height gain, or scoliosis and can cause compression of the duodenum by the SMA and result in obstruction (variously called *SMA syndrome, cast syndrome, Wilkie's syndrome, duodenal ileus,* or *duodenal compression syndrome*).[2] The fourth portion of the duodenum begins at the aorta, extends to the left, and passes ventral to the left psoas. It emerges into the peritoneum at the duodenojejunal flexure, which is fixed to the posterior abdominal wall at the ligament of Treitz, striated fibromuscular tissue that arises from the right crus of the diaphragm. Defects in the mesentery of the flexure may give rise to internal hernias. Venous drainage from the duodenum is through the splenic, superior mesenteric, and portal veins.

The jejunum and ileum are suspended from the posterior aspect of the peritoneal cavity by mesentery that travels obliquely from the left upper quadrant to the right lower quadrant of the abdomen (Fig. 67–1). The mesentery begins at the ligament of Treitz, where a double fold of peritoneum is pulled up as the bowel exits the retroperitoneum. From a base of about 15 cm, this mesentery fans out to connect to the entire 2.5 m of small intestine. The intestinal blood supply, as well as fat and lymphatic tissue, resides within the mesentery. The blood supply of the jejunum and ileum derives from the SMA, which has an extensive anastomotic network (the vasa recta) near the mesenteric border of the bowel called the *marginal artery*. This artery runs along the length of the small bowel. At the ileal branch of the ileocolic artery, the marginal artery breaks up as the anastomotic network of the vasa recta increases in complexity. Venous drainage follows the course of the arteries.

Although there is no true anatomic distinction between the jejunum and ileum, a number of anatomic features progress in an orderly fashion over the course of the intestine and help distinguish the two portions of

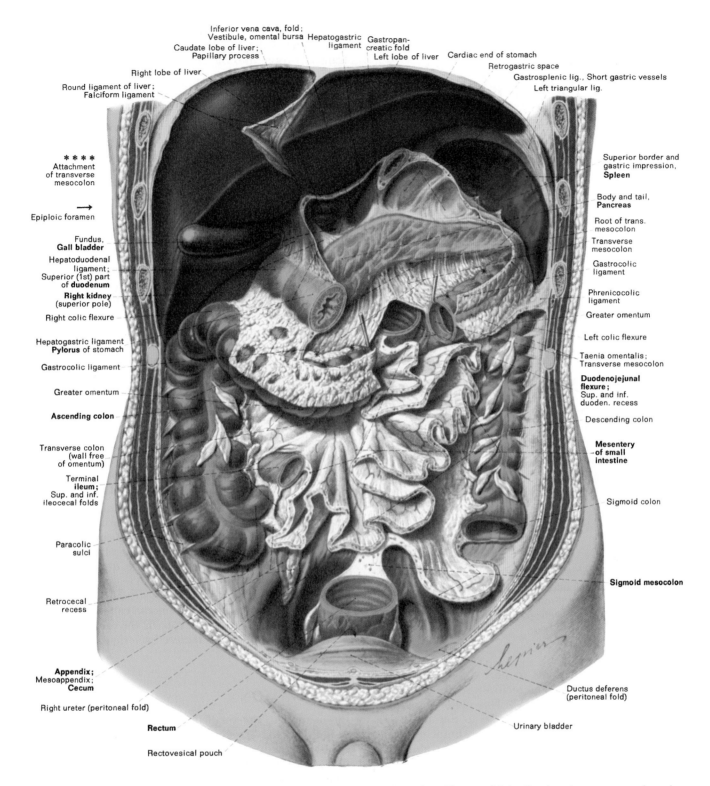

Figure 67–1. View of the mesentery and attachments of the small intestine. The small intestine has been removed, as has the sigmoid colon. (From Clemente CD: Anatomy: A Regional Atlas of the Human Body. Philadelphia, Lea & Febiger, 1975, plate 305.)

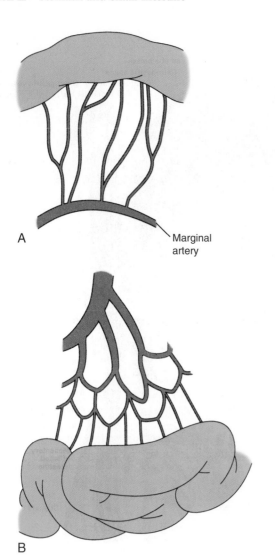

Figure 67–2. Schematic of the arterial network to different regions of the small intestine. **A,** Typical jejunal pattern. **B,** Typical ileal pattern. (From Greenfield LT, Mulholland MW [eds]: Surgery: Scientific Principles and Practice. Philadelphia, Lippincott-Raven, 1997, p 2036.)

bowel. The jejunum tends to have a single marginal artery from which arise long, relatively straight branches of the vasa recta (Fig. 67–2A). This pattern gradually blends into arcades that travel close to the mesenteric edge of the bowel and give rise to short branches in the ileum (see Fig. 67–2B). The amount of fat along the mesenteric border tends to increase distally, at times encroaching on the bowel in the distal aspects. The intestine tends to become thinner and paler distally, along with a decrease in diameter. Lymphatic tissues unique to the small intestine and called *Peyer's patches* are most numerous in the distal ileum, whereas plicae circulares are more prominent in the proximal jejunum. Small intestinal lymphatic drainage courses through a hierarchy of mesenteric nodes following the vascular arcades: through the wall of the small intestine into the mesenteric arcade and then to a lymphatic trunk around the SMA. The lymph ultimately drains into the *cisterna chyli.*

In addition to its usual reticuloendothelial function, the small intestinal lymphatic drainage serves as a major transport route into the circulation for absorbed lipid.

HISTOLOGY

The intestine has four distinct functional layers. The innermost is the mucosa, followed by the submucosa, muscularis, and serosa (Fig. 67–3). The mucosa is subdivided into three layers. Innermost is an epithelial layer, the middle layer is a lamina propria, and the outer layer is the muscularis mucosae. The epithelial layer consists of a single thickness of columnar cells supported by a basement membrane. The lamina propria consists of connective tissue, and the muscularis mucosae is a true muscular layer. Morphologically, the mucosa is arranged into finger-like projections called *villi* that serve to increase the surface area for absorption. Villi are covered with columnar cells and goblet cells. The former are responsible for absorption, and the latter secrete mucus. At the base of the villi, mucosal invaginations form crypts that contain secretory Paneth cells. The submucosa is the next layer radially outward and contains blood vessels, lymphatics, and nerves, including the parasympathetic ganglion, which make up Meissner's plexus. Continuing outward, the muscularis consists of an inner layer of circular muscle and an outer layer of longitudinal muscle. Between these muscular layers is the myenteric or Auerbach plexus. Finally, the serosa is an extension of the peritoneum and consists of a single layer of mesothelial cells and loose connective tissue.

The duodenum is distinguished histologically by the presence of Brunner's glands. These glands are spiral tubes that form an interconnected network beginning in the submucosa—below the lamina propria—and opening into the crypts between the villi. They secrete a thin, alkaline mucus that protects the duodenum and aids in acid neutralization. Additional features that mark the duodenum as a small intestinal structure include circular folds of mucosa and submucosa called *plicae circulares* or *Kerckring's valves.* Crypts in the small intestine termed *Lieberkühn's crypts* secrete bactericidal and digestive enzymes.

INNERVATION

Innervation to the small intestine is through the autonomic nervous system and includes sympathetic, parasympathetic, and enteric divisions. Sympathetic fibers arising from thoracic segments of the spinal cord synapse in the celiac ganglion before sending axons to the intestine. Parasympathetic fibers arise from the vagus nerve and synapse in the submucosal (Meissner's) and myenteric (Auerbach's) plexus. The myenteric plexus is responsible for basal electrical activity of the gut. Stimulation of the parasympathetic neurons in general prepares the intestine for activity by increasing blood flow, contractility, and secretion. These functions are antagonized by the sympathetic system.

The enteric nervous system is an integrative system distinct from the central nervous system (CNS) that

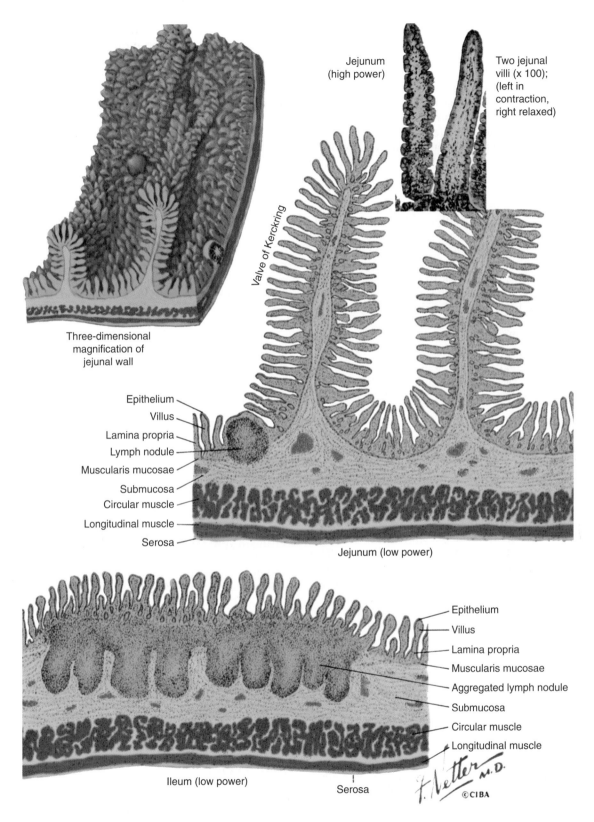

Figure 67–3. Schematic views of the histology of the jejunum and ileum. (Copyright, 1997. Icon Learning Systems, LLC, a subsidiary of Havas MultiMedia USA Inc. Reprinted with permission from ICON Learning Systems, LLC, illustrated by Frank H. Netter, MD. All rights reserved.)

ramifies throughout the submucosal and myenteric plexus of the gut. It senses the composition and characteristics of the luminal contents and integrates digestive functions that require motor or epithelial cell response. In particular, it regulates gut function by integrating smooth muscle tone and endocrine and exocrine secretion via input from afferent neurons sensitive to mechanical, chemical, osmotic, and thermal stimuli. Neurons of this system synthesize and secrete peptides that can act as neurotransmitters, paracrine factors, or endocrine factors.[3]

Pain from the small intestine is divided into visceral and somatic components. The clinical manifestations of each type of pain can be attributed to the type of innervation. Visceral pain occurs as a result of irritation of the visceral peritoneum, contraction of a tube against resistance, or distention of a tube and is carried by the autonomic nerves. Representation for these fibers is bilateral, and the pain tends to occur in the midline at the corresponding sensory level, which for the small bowel is in the epigastrium or periumbilical region. In general, this pain tends to be dull and deep in character. In contrast, parietal pain occurs as a result of irritation of the peritoneum lining the abdominal wall and is carried by somatic (spinal) nerves. This pain tends to be well localized, severe, and sharp.

LYMPHOID FUNCTIONS AND ARCHITECTURE

The intestine is protected from its tremendous bacterial load by mucosal defense mechanisms and a network of lymphatic tissue. At the mucosal level, three populations of lymphoid tissue form the first barrier to infection. Peyer's patches lie in the mucosa and submucosa and sample antigens to begin specific host responses. The lamina propria contains a separate collection of lymphoid cells consisting of T cells, B cells, and plasma cells. Intraepithelial lymphocytes form the final level of mucosal host defense. Three sets of nodes drain the small intestine. The first set lies in proximity to the mesenteric border, the second set is at the level of the arcades, and the third set is along the SMA.

MICROVASCULATURE

The vascular supply to the small intestine arises from the left side of the SMA.[4] The arterial branches derived from the SMA pass through the two layers of the mesentery into the gut at the mesenteric margin of the small bowel. Within the mesentery, the SMA branches into arcades that enter the gut wall via the vasa recta. In the jejunum, the arcades are comprised of long vasa recta (3 to 5 cm), whereas in the distal ileum the arcades are elongated and the vasa recta are relatively short. Venous drainage from the intestine parallels the arterial supply, with the superior mesenteric vein being the major venous collecting system; it also lies within the mesentery to the right of the SMA.

The vasa recta entering the bowel wall reach intramural distributive vessels located within the submucosa.

These vessels in the submucosa extend to the antimesenteric border of the intestine and form plexuses that are interconnected throughout the length and circumference of the small intestine. Blood supply to the outer muscle layers of the intestine is largely derived from this submucosal plexus, as is the venous drainage, although smaller direct branches from the vasa recta can also be demonstrated. Despite housing the submucosal vascular plexus, the submucosa itself is sparsely vascularized. This is in marked contrast to the mucosa, which contains a rich microvascular network. The extensive vascularization of the mucosa is arranged in microvascular capillary and venular arcades that form a subepithelial network within the small bowel villi.

The mucosal microvasculature in the small bowel differs from other vascular beds in the body by its high rate of blood flow, oxygen utilization, and transcapillary exchange of fluid and solutes. This distinct mucosal vascular physiology is thought to result from the high metabolic demand required by the epithelial layers, which receive up to 80% of intestinal blood flow during resting conditions.[5] The highly vascularized mucosal anatomy also accommodates the physiologic need demonstrated during nutritive function, when significant portions of cardiac output are shunted into the gut. Intestinal perfusion via the SMA ranges from a low of 29 to 70 ml/min/100 g intestinal tissue, whereas in the fed state, splanchnic hyperemia increases perfusion 28% to 132%. Resistance arterioles located in the submucosa beneath the muscularis mucosae play a major role in the regulation of intestinal perfusion. The molecular physiology underlying human intestinal microvascular function was assessed directly by Hatoum et al., who characterized vasodilator responses in isolated gut resistance arterioles 50 to 150 μm in diameter by measuring in vitro vasodilatory capacity in response to acetylcholine.[6] Normal intestinal microvessels vasodilate in response to acetylcholine via predominantly nitric oxide– and cyclooxygenase-dependent mechanisms. Interestingly, microvessels from patients with chronically inflamed inflammatory bowel disease (Crohn's disease, ulcerative colitis) and radiation enteritis demonstrated a significantly diminished vasodilator capacity in comparison to control microvessels.[6,7] These findings suggest that impaired vasodilator capacity is linked to an ischemic contribution found in both classic chronic inflammation (i.e., inflammatory bowel disease) and stricture formation (i.e., long-term complication of radiation enteritis).

EMBRYOLOGY

Gastrulation

Shortly after gastrulation specifies the three embryonic germ layers, the endoderm undergoes rapid elongation. At the rostral end of the embryo, invagination of the head fold results in formation of the foregut tube. In similar fashion, the hindgut is formed by invagination of the caudal aspect of the embryo. The midportion of the tube remains in broad communication with the yolk sac and is called the *midgut* (Fig. 67–4).[8] At 18 days'

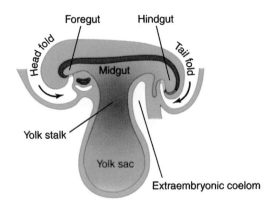

Figure 67–4. Schematic view of a 16-day-old human embryo showing the derivation of the foregut, midgut, and hindgut regions from endoderm. (From Moore KL, Persaud TVN: The Developing Human, 6th ed. Philadelphia, WB Saunders, 1998, p 84.)

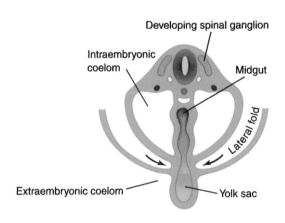

Figure 67–5. Schematic view of an 18-day-old embryo showing the derivation of the mesentery. (From Moore KL, Persaud TVN: The Developing Human, 6th ed. Philadelphia, WB Saunders, 1998, p 84.)

gestation, bilateral body folds ingress below the embryo and begin to separate it from the yolk sac. This causes splanchnic mesoderm to envelop the gut and defines the dorsal and ventral mesentery (Fig. 67–5).[8] The resulting increased distance between the neural tube and the gut may be important in preventing congenital gut duplications or diverticula, which occur at this time.[9] This separation may be necessary to remove the gut from the influence of secreted signaling molecules produced in the notochord. Consistent with this hypothesis, partial gut duplications can be induced in transgenic mice that overexpress one of these notochord-derived factors in the pancreatic region.[9]

At 28 days' gestation, continued elongation of the endoderm converts the open midgut into a tube with its midportion still connected to the yolk sac through the yolk stalk. The liver forms within the ventral mesentery, whereas the leaves of mesentery become the falciform

ligament; the dorsal mesentery gives rise to the adult mesentery and within it the blood supply to the gut.

At 35 days' gestation, the foregut, midgut, and hindgut all have a distinct blood supply, which serves to distinguish them throughout adult life. The foregut is supplied by the precursor of the celiac trunk and consists of the alimentary canal proximal to the ampulla of Vater. The midgut is supplied by the precursor of the SMA and consists of the small bowel distal to the ampulla and the proximal two thirds of the transverse colon. The hindgut consists of the distal third of the transverse, descending, and sigmoid colon and is supplied by the precursor of the inferior mesenteric artery. At this time, the yolk stalk separates from the intestine and the vitelline duct is obliterated. Failure of this process can result in diverticula (Meckel's diverticulum), cysts, cords, or combinations of these abnormalities.

At 42 days' gestation, the differentiated smooth muscle envelops the gut. This process is probably regulated by members of the "hedgehog" family of proteins secreted by the endoderm, which act as inductive signals on the mesoderm.[10] Mesodermal factors important in this process include members of the transforming growth factor-β family. There is evidence that these molecules initiate preprogrammed expression of *Hox* genes, which serve to establish the regional identity of the foregut, midgut, and hindgut.[10] At this point, elongation of the midgut is so rapid that the midgut can no longer be contained in the abdominal wall previously defined by the body folds and thus herniates out. The cecum is visible as a dilation of the midgut distal to the axis of the SMA. This location of the cecum distal to the SMA is important for understanding subsequent rotation. At about this time, innervation of the gut is under way, a process that is increasingly being appreciated as essential for normal gut development.

At 60 days' gestation, the herniated gut rotates counterclockwise 180 degrees around the axis of the SMA (Fig. 67–6). This rotation causes the cecal swelling to lie superior to the more proximal small bowel. If such rotation does not occur, the small bowel will lie on the right, with the cecum in the middle and the colon on the left.

At 10 weeks' gestation, the intestines return to the abdomen in a proximal-to-distal progression, with the proximal bowel being located in the dorsal aspect of the abdominal cavity and the cecum passing ventral to the small bowel. Failure of this return causes omphalocele. At this point a final additional 90 degrees of counterclockwise rotation sets the cecum in its final location in the right lower quadrant, with the transverse colon being ventral to the small bowel (see Fig. 67–6). Failure of this final rotation leads to a variety of anatomic anomalies.

At 12 weeks' gestation, the intestines become fixed in permanent position. The mesocolon of the ascending colon fuses with the parietal peritoneum to fix the ascending colon in a retroperitoneal position. In similar fashion, the left side of the mesocolon of the descending colon fuses with the parietal peritoneum of the dorsal body wall to fix the descending colon in a retroperitoneal location. Failure of this process can lead to spaces into which herniations can occur.

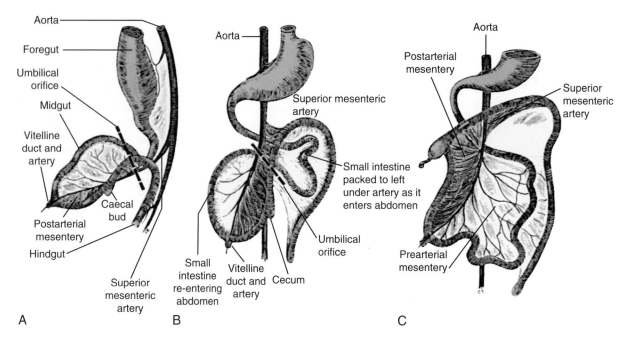

Figure 67–6.   Rotation of the midgut. **A,** First stage: the loop has rotated 90 degrees counterclockwise. **B,** Second stage: the physiologic umbilical hernia is reducing; the small gut is reentering the abdomen on the right side of the superior mesenteric vessels and passing to the left side of the abdomen behind the vessels. The cecum still lies outside the umbilicus. **C,** Completion of the second stage: the cecum is in contact with the posterior abdominal wall in the right pelvis; the midgut loop has rotated 270 degrees counterclockwise. (From Louw JH: Embryology and developmental abnormalities of the small and large intestines. In Bockus HL [ed]: Gastroenterology, vol 2. Philadelphia, WB Saunders, 1978, p 8.)

CLINICAL ASPECTS OF DEVELOPMENTAL ANOMALIES

Duplications

Duplications occur early during development as described previously. The duplication may communicate with the normal gut lumen and share its blood supply. Management of duodenal duplications can be particularly difficult because of the involvement of surrounding structures, including the biliary tree, pancreatic duct, and pancreas.[9] Small bowel duplications may serve as a lead point for intussusception or create a fixed axis for the development of volvulus. Enlargement of the duplication may cause compression of adjacent structures. These abnormalities frequently contain ectopic gastric mucosa whose acid secretion can cause bleeding, pain, or perforation.

Vitelline Duct Abnormalities (Meckel's Diverticulum and Others)

The vitelline duct connects the midgut to the yolk sac during development. Any portion of this duct can remain as either a tube or a fibrous cord (Fig. 67–7). Persistence of the entire duct results in an enterocutaneous fistula. If the intestinal portion does not obliterate, Meckel's diverticulum results, the most common gut malformation. It occurs on the antimesenteric border of the intestine and is present in about 2% of the population.

The diverticulum can be attached (25%) or unattached (75%) to the anterior abdominal wall by a remnant of the vitelline duct.[2] This abnormality generally occurs within 2 ft of the ileocecal valve and is always on the antimesenteric border of the intestine. Meckel's diverticulum is most commonly manifested as bleeding, usually resulting from acid-secreting ectopic gastric mucosa that causes ulceration of the nearby intestine. This abnormality also increases the risk for intussusception, with the diverticulum serving as the lead point. If the yolk sac side of the vitelline duct does not obliterate, an umbilical sinus results. Occasionally, a fibrous band with or without a cystic component (omphalomesenteric cyst) remains and can serve as an attachment point around which the bowel can rotate and lead to volvulus.

Omphalocele and Ventral Hernias

Failure of the intestine to return to the abdominal cavity can result in abdominal wall defects and omphalocele or gastroschisis. Omphalocele occurs when the intestines herniate through the anterior abdominal wall with only a peritoneal covering (Fig. 67–8). Most cases occur in association with other abnormalities, including those of the cardiac, neurologic, skeletal, or genitourinary system.[11] Gastroschisis occurs when an entire portion of the anterior abdominal wall is absent and abdominal viscera herniate without a peritoneal covering. Associated defects are much less common than with

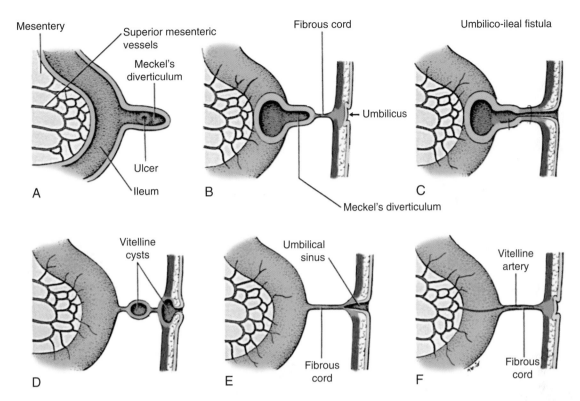

Figure 67–7. Meckel's diverticulum and other remnants of the yolk stalk. **A,** Section of the ileum and Meckel's diverticulum with an ulcer. **B,** Meckel's diverticulum connected to the umbilicus by a fibrous cord. **C,** Umbilicoileal fistula resulting from persistence of the entire intra-abdominal portion of the yolk stalk. **D,** Vitelline cysts at the umbilicus and in a fibrous remnant of the yolk stalk. **E,** Umbilical sinus resulting from persistence of the yolk stalk near the umbilicus. The sinus is not always connected to the ileum by a fibrous cord as illustrated. **F,** The yolk stalk has persisted as a fibrous cord connecting the ileum with the umbilicus. A persistent vitelline artery extends along the fibrous cord to the umbilicus. (From Moore K: The Developing Human: Clinically Oriented Embryology. Philadelphia, WB Saunders, 1982, p 245.)

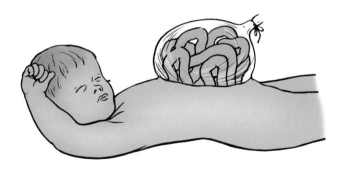

Figure 67–8. Exomphalos (omphalocele). The intestines fail to return to the abdomen in the first stage of intestinal rotation and fixation. (From Gray SW, Skandalakis JE: Embryology for Surgeons: Embryological Basis for Treatment of Congenital Defects. Philadelphia, WB Saunders, 1972, p 136.)

omphalocele and include intestinal abnormalities such as stenosis and atresia.[11]

Rotational Abnormalities

Midgut malrotation may occur in as many as 0.2% of live births.[12] These abnormalities are associated with a variety of other anomalies, including abdominal wall or diaphragmatic hernias, intestinal atresia, imperforate anus, and cardiac defects.[2] Down's syndrome is not as common with malrotation as with other anomalies, such as duodenal atresia.[2]

Rotational abnormalities of the small bowel can be divided into mixed rotation, nonrotation, and reversed rotation (Fig. 67–9).[2] In mixed rotation, partial failure of rotation may result in an abnormally high cecum or a duodenum that does not pass dorsal to the SMA. Such cases are often associated with adhesive bands (Ladd's bands) that course from the ligament of Treitz to the ileocecal junction. These bands may traverse the duodenum and can result in duodenal obstruction. This problem is associated with duodenal, pancreatic, and biliary abnormalities.

Nonrotation occurs when failure of rotation results in return of the bowel in a distal-to-proximal fashion; the small intestine is located on the right side of the abdomen with the cecum in the middle and the colon on the left. The mesentery is usually short, and fibrous bands are common. These bands may result in obstruction or volvulus.

Reversed rotation occurs when the initial counterclockwise rotation is only 90 degrees and subsequent rotation is 180 degrees clockwise. This results in a

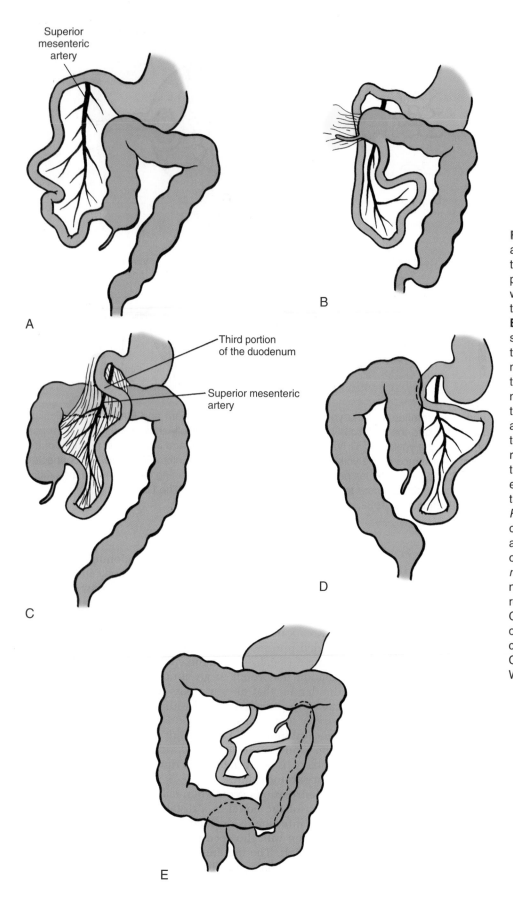

Superior mesenteric artery

A

B

Third portion of the duodenum

Superior mesenteric artery

C

D

E

Figure 67–9.   Different rotational abnormalities of the small intestine. **A,** *Nonrotation.* Return of the postarterial segment leaves the whole colon on the left and the small intestine on the right. **B,** *Mixed rotation.* The prearterial segment has failed to rotate, so the cecum is fixed to the abdominal wall and now lies anterior to the second portion of the duodenum. **C,** *Reversed rotation.* The third portion of the duodenum is anterior to the superior mesenteric artery, which in turn is anterior to the transverse mesocolon; the postarterial segment has entered the abdomen ahead of the prearterial segment. **D,** *Reversed rotation.* The colon occupies the right half of the abdomen, and the small intestine occupies the left half. **E,** *Hyperrotation.* The colon is longer than normal and the cecum has reached the splenic flexure. (From Gray SW, Skandalakis JE: Embryology for Surgeons: Embryological Basis for Treatment of Congenital Defects. Philadelphia, WB Saunders, 1972, p 178.)

transverse colon that passes dorsal to the duodenum and the SMA. Obstruction may result from various fibrous bands that may fix the colon.

Atresia and Stenosis

Atresias are divided into four types (Fig. 67–10).[2] Type I occurs when a membrane of mucosa and submucosa obstructs the bowel lumen. Type II is characterized by a fibrous band that replaces a portion of the intestine. In type III, the bowel is discontinuous, with proximal and distal blind ends. Type IV occurs when multiple areas of the intestine become fibrous bands. Duodenal atresia is probably due to failure of recanalization, whereas jejunal and ileal atresia is thought to occur as a result of intestinal ischemia. Patients with duodenal atresia have Down's syndrome in 30% of cases.[13] This abnormality is also associated with esophageal atresia, midgut malrotation, annular pancreas, imperforate anus, congenital anomalies of the heart, and intrauterine growth retardation.[13]

Internal Hernias

A variety of congenital hernias may result from abnormal rotation or fixation of the bowel on the abdominal wall. By far the most common type is a paraduodenal hernia, which results from abnormal fixation of the ascending or descending colon.

PHYSIOLOGY

The small intestine absorbs water, electrolytes, and nutrients. The process of digestion involves mechanical grinding of food, as well as chemical enzymatic digestion. For adequate absorption to occur, regulated fluid secretion and proper peristalsis must take place in concert to facilitate luminal surface hydration and mixing of food. The small intestine performs a number of other functions in addition to digestion. It is an important endocrine organ from which a host of gut-associated hormones are released. The epithelial barrier function of the small intestine protects the internal milieu against noxious luminal substances, such as bacteria and ingested toxins. The small intestine is also a major lymphoid organ where foreign antigens initially encounter the body's immune cells. The importance of the mucosal immune system is increasingly being appreciated as its involvement in the pathogenesis of intestinal disorders is elucidated.

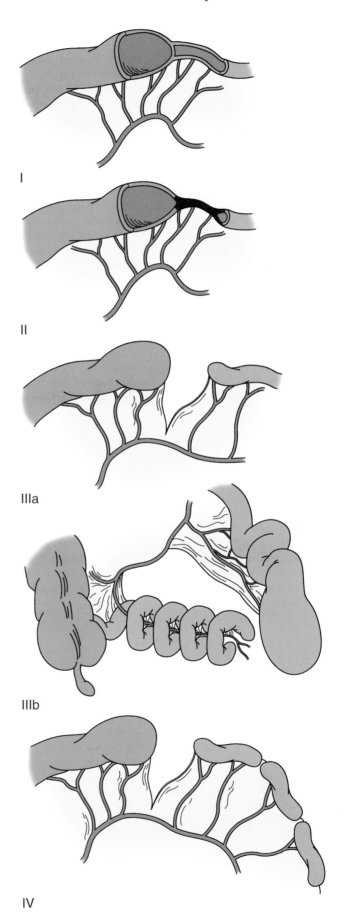

Figure 67–10. Different types of intestinal atresia. **Type I,** Continuity of mesentery and bowel with an incomplete web. **Type II,** The mesentery is intact, but the bowel has reduced to a fibrous cord. **Type IIIa,** The bowel and mesentery are focally disconnected. **Type IIIb,** The mesentery and bowel are completely separated, a so-called apple peel or Christmas tree deformity. **Type IV,** Multiple atresias (can be seen in combinations of type IIIa and IIIb). (From Welch KJ, Randolph JG, Ravitch MM, et al [eds]: Pediatric Surgery, 4th ed. Chicago, Year Book Medical Publishers, 1986.)

Layers of the Bowel Wall

The small bowel wall consists of the innermost *mucosa*, followed by the *submucosa, muscularis propria,* and the outermost *serosa.* The serosa is contiguous with the peritoneal lining and is absent in the posterior aspect of the duodenum because of its retroperitoneal location. The smooth muscle cells of the muscularis provide the motor activity necessary for intestinal peristalsis, and this smooth muscle consists of a thick inner circular layer and a thinner outer longitudinal layer. Gap junctions found on the plasma membrane of intestinal smooth muscle cells permit efficient propagation of peristaltic signal by allowing electrical coupling between adjacent cells. Ganglion cells and neural fibers form an extensive plexus throughout the layers of small intestine. The myenteric (Auerbach's) plexus is located between the circular and longitudinal layers of the muscularis.

The submucosa is a strong connective tissue layer that contains rich networks of vessels, nerves, and lymphoid tissue. The mucosa of the small intestine is structurally characterized by finger-like projections called *villi* and consists of three microscopic layers: the epithelium, the lamina propria, and the muscularis mucosae. The innermost epithelium is lined by a single layer of columnar epithelial cells of various types. The apical surface of these cells is covered by brush-border microvilli that project into the lumen of the intestine. The architectural arrangements of the villi and microvilli further contribute to the vast surface area of the small intestine. The lamina propria is located between the intestinal epithelium and the muscularis mucosae and consists of various connective tissue cell types and a rich microvascular network between artery and vein that enables efficient secretion and absorption of water, electrolytes, and nutrients. In addition, a central lymphatic vessel called a *lacteal* facilitates transport of fats and immunologic substances. The muscularis mucosae consists of a thin layer of smooth muscle cells between the mucosa and submucosa.

INTESTINAL EPITHELIUM AND ITS FUNCTIONS

Intestinal epithelial cells form a layer that separates the internal milieu from an external environment full of potentially harmful entities, such as luminal bacteria, toxins, digestive enzymes, xenobiotics, and ingested chemicals. The intestinal epithelium plays a central role in digestion and absorption of nutrients, as well as transport of water and electrolytes. Additionally, the epithelium is a major participant in intestinal immune function. These complexly regulated and multiple functions of the epithelium are accomplished by heterogeneous populations of specialized epithelial cells.

Architecture

The mucosal surface of the intestine is characterized by two structural features: villi and the crypts of Lieberkühn (Fig. 67–11). A single layer of simple columnar epithelial cells rests on a thin basement membrane overlying the lamina propria (Fig. 67–12). The lamina propria of the villus core contains numerous connective tissue cells, including fibroblasts, lymphocytes, plasma cells, eosinophils, smooth muscle cells, and nerve fibers. The function of the overlying epithelial cells is closely influenced by humoral factors released by cells in the lamina propria and by the matrix components of the basement membrane.

The intestinal epithelium is renewed continually, with an enterocyte life span of 3 to 7 days. Pluripotent stem cells located near the base of the crypt migrate along the so-called crypt-villus axis while differentiating into one of the four major cell types: absorptive enterocytes, enteroendocrine cells, goblet cells, and Paneth cells. Frequent mitoses are observed in the crypt zone as these cells differentiate into mature absorptive cells during their migration toward the villus tips. Villus enterocytes then undergo apoptosis and are subsequently shed from the epithelium. The spontaneous rate of apoptosis is lower in colonic epithelium than in the small intestine. The difference may reflect altered expression of the anti-apoptotic survival gene *bcl*-2 and may be one of many factors that contribute to the lower incidence of cancer in the small intestine.[14]

Several distinct cell types are found in the crypts. Enterochromaffin cells, also known as *enteroendocrine cells,* do not maintain direct contact with the intestinal lumen. The contents of their secretory granules are released into blood in response to regulatory stimuli. Paneth cells reside at the base of the crypts and are the only cell type to undergo downward migration from the proliferative zone. They resemble pancreatic or parotid acinar cells morphologically and may contribute to mucosal immunity by secreting antimicrobial peptides, including α-defensins.[15] Goblet cells are seen in both the villi and crypts and secrete a protective mucous layer onto the mucosal surface. Villus columnar epithelial cells are primarily responsible for the absorption of fluid and electrolytes, whereas secretion occurs mostly in the crypts, although recent observations suggest that villi and crypts can both absorb and secrete to some extent.[16,17] Microscopically, the luminal border of the villus cells has a fuzzy appearance (brush border) because of the presence of microvilli in the apical plasma membrane. In addition to increasing absorptive surface area, microvilli directly enhance digestion through the presence of high concentrations of membrane-associated digestive enzymes.

Barrier Function

One of the most distinctive functions of epithelial cells is the ability to establish a barrier or a seal at the interface between the external and internal environments of the tissue. In the intestine, the barrier function of the epithelium protects the internal milieu from the permeation of potentially harmful luminal substances. This function is attributed to several morphologically distinct components of the intercellular junctional complex, a structure that circumferentially seals adjacent epithelial cells.[18,19]

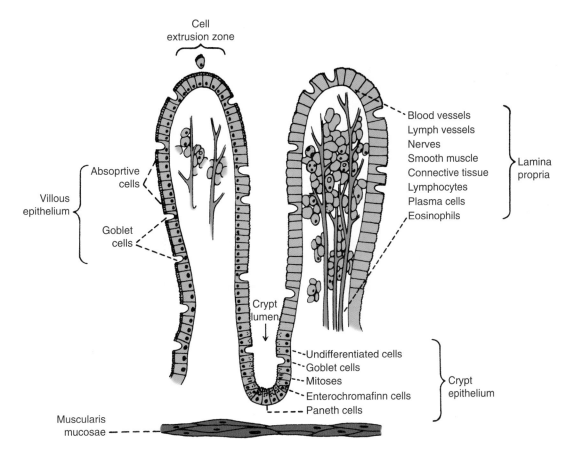

Figure 67–11. Schematic diagram of two sectioned villi and a crypt of the small intestinal mucosa. (From Trier JS, Winter HS: Anatomy, embryology, and developmental abnormalities of the small intestine and colon. In Sleisenger MH, Fordtran JS [eds]: Gastrointestinal Disease: Pathophysiology, Diagnosis, Management, 5th ed. Philadelphia, WB Saunders, 1993, p 796.)

The tight junction, or zonula occludens, forms a continuous contact at the apical-most aspect of the lateral membrane border between enterocytes (Fig. 67–13). The intercellular barrier is formed in part by the homotypic interactions of occludin between adjacent cells. *Occludin* is a transmembrane protein whose cytoplasmic tail is bound to a complex of cytoplasmic plaque proteins, including ZO-1 and ZO-2. A novel family of tight junction–associated transmembrane proteins known as *claudins* may account for the permselectivity characteristics of the intercellular junctional complex.[20] Adjacent and deep to the tight junction is the intermediate or adherens junction (zonula adherens), which also forms continuous contact by similar homotypic interaction of the transmembrane protein E-cadherin between adjacent cells. Intracellularly, E-cadherin associates directly with the cytoplasmic proteins α-, β- and γ-catenin and thereby with a contractile ring of actin and myosin that may regulate junctional permeability. Thick bands of perijunctional actin connect the adherens junction to the cytoplasmic plaque proteins of the tight junction. The tight junctions and adherens junctions are closely arranged spatially and behave as an integrated functional unit. Regulatory proteins of various tyrosine and serine-threonine kinase–based signaling pathways are localized in the vicinity of this apical junctional complex, thus reflecting the potential for regulatory control of junctional permeability by multiple cellular signaling mechanisms. Beneath the zonula occludens and zonula adherens are the desmosomes and gap junctions, which form focal contacts between neighboring cells.

The epithelial intercellular junctional complex does not present a static barrier. Solute permeability characteristics vary widely across different epithelia. The small intestine is classified as a "leaky" epithelium in comparison to the colon or urinary bladder. The influence of various humoral factors and other mediators on paracellular permeability is tissue and cell specific.[21,22] Tight junctions in absorptive cells become dilated by luminal glucose.[23-25] Physiologic regulation of junctional integrity can also occur in response to activation of Na$^+$-coupled transporters in the apical plasma membrane.[26] Intestinal barrier function is altered in many pathologic conditions. Bacterial toxins such as those elaborated by *Clostridium difficile* directly perturb intestinal barrier function by disrupting the interaction between junctions and the actin cytoskeleton.[27] ZO toxin from *Vibrio cholerae* has also been shown to disrupt actin and junctional integrity in a protein kinase C–dependent manner.[28] Translocation of bacteria and bacterial products as a result of increased intestinal paracellular permeability (associated with junctional disruption) in critically ill patients has

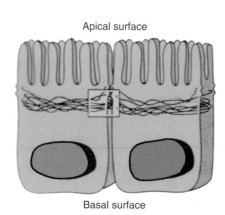

Lumen:

Dietary compounds
Alimentary secretions

Epithelium:

Local hormones
? Cell-cell interactions
? Lymphoid cell products

Basal lamina:

? Effects on epithelial polarity
and/or differentiation

Lamina propria:

Vessels – Regulation of
osmotic environment.
Distant horomones and
regulatory compounds
Nerves – Neurotransmitters
Non-epithelial cells –
Library of biologically
active products

Figure 67–12. Schematic illustration of some factors in the microenvironment of intestinal epithelial cells that may influence their function. With the exception of extravascular polymorphonuclear leukocytes, all elements are normally present at this site. (From Madara JL: Functional morphology of epithelium of the small intestine. In Handbook of Physiology: The Gastrointestinal System. Bethesda, MD, American Physiological Society, 1991, p 85.)

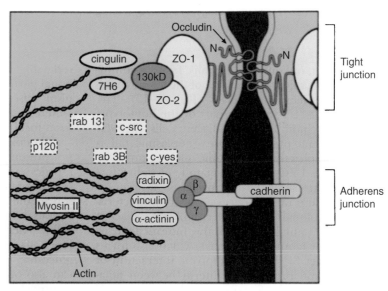

Figure 67–13. **Left,** Tight junctions are positioned as continuous contacts at the apical-lateral membrane borders between enterocytes. The *boxed region* is enlarged at the right. **Right,** Hypothetical model of protein interactions at the tight junction and adherens junction of two simple columnar epithelial cells. The intercellular barrier at the tight junction is formed by homotypic contacts of the transmembrane protein occludin, which is bound on the cytoplasmic surface directly to ZO-1. The ZO-1/ZO-2 heterodimer binds an uncharacterized 130-kD protein. Binding interactions of cingulin and the transmembrane protein cadherin are shown; they associate directly with the cytoplasmic proteins α-, β-, and γ-catenin. A thick band of perijunctional actin is positioned under the adherens junction with connections to tight junction plaques. (From Anderson JM, Van Itallie CM: Tight junctions and the molecular basis for regulation of paracellular permeability. Am J Physiol 269:G468, 1995.)

| Table 67–1 | Water and Electrolytes |

Nutrient	Receptor	Comment	References
Water	Aquaporins (AQP) Transcellular route for water transport	First described in the kidney AQP3: colon, small intestine AQP4: colon AQP5: salivary glands AQP7: small intestine AQP8: small intestine	33-40
Na^+/K^+	Na^+,K^+-ATPase	Absorption of Na^+ coupled to organic solutes (glucose, amino acids) Na^+ entry into the cell is dependent on the concentration gradient Cl^- entry is passive Co-entry of Na^+Cl^- through the Na^+/H^+ Cl^-/HCO_3^- exchanger operates in parallel. This accounts for Na^+ absorption between meals and is disrupted during diarrheal diseases	41
Na^+/K^+	Apical Na^+/H^+ exchangers (NHE)	NHE2: small intestine NHE3: small intestine (major functional brush-border isoform) NHE1: basolateral (important in intracellular pH homeostasis)	42-44

been postulated to underlie the development of a sepsis-like state in multiorgan failure. However, direct evidence in support of this hypothesis has been difficult to establish. Various cytokines have been shown to alter junctional permeability, including interferon-γ and tumor necrosis factor-α.[29,30]

Digestion and Absorption

The vast total surface area of the small intestine enables it to absorb large quantities of water, electrolytes, and nutrients. The small intestine receives 8 to 10 L of fluid daily, including 1 to 1.5 L of ingested fluid. The remainder consists of salivary, gastric, pancreaticobiliary, and small intestinal secretions. Most of this fluid load is absorbed by the small intestine before reaching the ileocecal valve. Absorption of specific luminal components is accomplished by complex mechanisms that consist, to varying degrees, of intraluminal processing, epithelial uptake, and transport into the portal or lymphatic circulation. These processes display distinct patterns of expression along the longitudinal axis of the gut.

Water

The absorptive capability of the small intestine is estimated to be 12 L/day. Water movement across the epithelial layer is driven by the active transport of Na^+ and Cl^- and by the absorption of small molecules such as glucose and amino acids. The principal energy for many of these transport processes derives from the Na^+ gradient generated by the action of a basolateral Na^+,K^+-

ATPase pump. The low intracellular Na^+ concentration maintained by this pump allows uptake of Na^+ and other solutes through coupled ion exchangers (Na^+/H^+ and Cl^-/HCO_3^-) and Na^+-coupled nutrient transporters. The precise route of water movement across an epithelium (transcellular, paracellular, or both) is controversial. The paracellular route (across the intercellular junctional complex) was previously thought to be the dominant pathway. However, this concept has been questioned on the basis of a number of recent observations, including attempts to directly measure water flow through junctions.[31] It is now recognized that water movement across plasma membranes can be greatly facilitated by members of a specialized family of proteins known as aquaporins (Table 67–1), which function as water channels.[32]

Another possible mechanism of bulk water transport has been proposed on the basis of observations that water may move in substantial quantities through the solute pocket of Na^+-coupled transporters. For example, water movement through the Na^+-glucose cotransporter SGLT1 appears to occur with a fixed stoichiometry of 2 Na^+, 1 glucose, and 210 H_2O in human SGLT1.[45] The physiologic relevance and relative contributions of these nonclassic routes of water transport in the intestine are not yet clear (see Table 67–1).

Sodium

Sodium absorption is driven by active transcellular uptake. Passive transport through the paracellular pathway also contributes to overall Na^+ absorption to a varying degree along the length of the gastrointestinal tract. A sizable, if not the major fraction of Na^+ and water

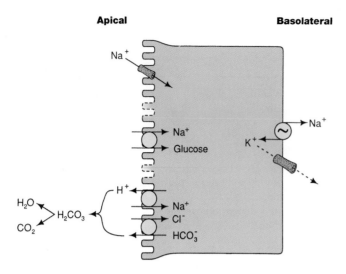

Figure 67–14. Apical sodium transporters. Luminal sodium enters the absorptive epithelial cell down an electrochemical gradient. Mechanisms for this transport include an ion-specific channel sensitive to amiloride, a carrier that couples the movement of sodium and nutrients (i.e., glucose), or a carrier that allows electroneutral entry of sodium in exchange for intracellular hydrogen (antiport). The common exit pathway across the basolateral membrane is the sodium pump. (From Sellin JH: Intestinal electrolyte absorption and secretion. In Sleisenger MH, Fordtran JS [eds]: Gastrointestinal Disease: Pathophysiology, Diagnosis, Management, 5th ed. Philadelphia, WB Saunders, 1993, p 960.)

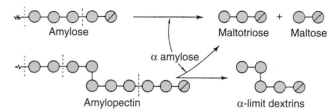

Figure 67–15. Action of α-amylase on amylose and amylopectin molecules. Because the a 1-6 link in the latter is resistant to amylase, the products include α-limit dextrin. (From Gray GM: Carbohydrate absorption and malabsorption. In Johnson LR [ed]: Physiology of the Gastrointestinal Tract. New York, Raven Press, 1981, p 1064.)

absorption in the proximal part of the small intestine occurs paracellularly across the relatively leaky and nonselective intercellular junctions. The junctions become "tighter" and more cation selective distally in the ileum and colon, which enables active transport mechanisms to absorb Na⁺ against a large osmotic gradient.

The engine driving active transcellular Na⁺ absorption is the Na⁺,K⁺-ATPase pump, which generates electric and chemical gradients by extruding Na⁺ in exchange for K⁺ in a 3:2 stoichiometry across the basolateral cell membrane (Fig. 67–14). This energy-dependent pump action establishes a transmembrane potential difference with the cell interior of about −35 mV and maintains a low intracellular Na⁺ concentration and a high intracellular K⁺ concentration. Na⁺ and Cl⁻ absorption across the apical membrane from the intestinal lumen involves three different mechanisms.

The apical Na⁺/H⁺ exchangers (NHEs) are members of the mammalian Na⁺/H⁺ exchanger gene family.[42,43] Among these exchangers, NHE2 and NHE3 are present in the apical membrane of human small intestinal epithelia, more specifically, the ileum.[44] NHE3 appears to be the major functional brush-border isoform in mammalian intestine, whereas the role of NHE2 is less clear (see Table 67–1).

Carbohydrates

Carbohydrates provide a major portion of adult dietary energy requirements. Human intestine is incapable of digesting and processing certain complex carbohydrates, such as cellulose-containing β-linked glucose molecules. Unlike the α bond found in starch, the β bond 1-4 is resistant to the digestive activity of amylase, although cellulose can be converted to absorbable fatty acids to some extent by colonic bacteria. Dietary fiber from "unavailable carbohydrates" also comes from pectins, gums, alginates, and lignins and helps reduce constipation by retaining water and increasing fecal bulk. Major dietary digestible carbohydrates include, in order of abundance, starch, sucrose, and lactose. Starch consists of amylose and the more abundant amylopectin. Sucrose is a disaccharide of glucose and fructose and is commonly found in fruit and sugar cane. The major source of lactose, a disaccharide consisting of glucose and galactose, is milk products.

Digestion of carbohydrates begins in the mouth, where salivary amylase is active. Ingested starch is broken down into smaller oligosaccharides by the action of amylase. The resulting digestive products therefore include maltose, maltotriose, short oligosaccharides, and α-dextrins, as well as short-branched oligosaccharides from amylopectin (Fig. 67–15). Because salivary amylase is promptly inactivated at low gastric pH, pancreatic amylase in the duodenum is thought to be the major enzyme for starch digestion. The resultant short-chain oligosaccharides from amylase digestion, along with ingested sucrose and lactose, are further digested into basic monosaccharides in the small intestine before absorption into enterocytes. The brush-border membrane of villus enterocytes contains three hydrolase activities: lactase, sucrase, and isomaltase. The final products of carbohydrate digestion consist primarily of three major diet-derived hexoses: glucose, galactose, and fructose.

Absorption of these major monosaccharides into enterocytes can occur by several different transport mechanisms. Glucose transporters are categorized into two broad categories: Na⁺ dependent (SGLT) and Na⁺ independent (GLUT, Table 67–2) (Fig. 67–16).[71]

Proteins

Although ingested dietary proteins constitute the main source of amino acids, a significant amount of the

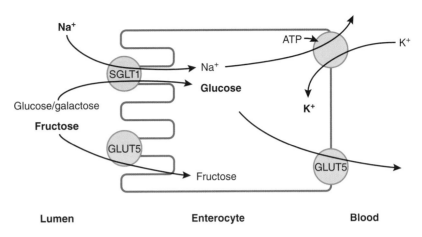

Figure 67–16. Schematic diagram for sugar transport across the enterocyte showing the brush-border SGLT1 and GLUT5 transporters and the basolateral Na^+-K^+ pumps and sugar transporter GLUT2. ATP, adenosine triphosphate. (From Wright EM: Genetic disorders of membrane transport. I. Glucose galactose malabsorption. Am J Physiol 275:G880, 1998.)

| Lumen | Enterocyte | Blood |

Table 67–2 Carbohydrates, Proteins, and Lipids

Nutrient	Receptor	Comment	References
Carbohydrates			
		The α bond (found in starch) is disrupted by amylase	
		The β bond (found in cellulose) is resistant to human digestive activity and contributes to dietary fiber	
Glucose	SGLT (Na+ dependent)	SGLT1 actively absorbs glucose and galactose against a concentration gradient	
	GLUT (Na+ independent)	GLUT2 is the major transporter for intestinal absorption (moves in the direction of the glucose concentration)	46-48
		GLUT5 absorbs fructose (fructose is also absorbed paracellularly through glucose-activated solution drag)	
Proteins			
Single amino acids (neutral, acidic and basic)	Na+-dependent active transport		49
Oligopeptides	Pep T-1	Transports dipeptides and tripeptides through H+-coupled active transport (very sensitive to luminal and intracellular pH; absorbed peptides are hydrolyzed by cytoplasmic peptidases)	50-62
Lipids			
Short- and medium-chain fatty acids		Diffusion into the cell	63, 64
Long-chain fatty acids	Fatty acid transport proteins (FATPs)	FATP4: apical membrane of mature enterocytes	65-67
	Fatty acid binding proteins (FABPs)	Promote the intracellular transport of fatty acids by decreasing the amount of fatty acids that my otherwise bind to immobile membranes	68-70

protein content in the intestinal lumen is derived from endogenous sources such as salivary, gastric, and pancreaticobiliary secretions, as well as desquamated epithelial cells. Digestion of proteins starts in the stomach by the action of pepsins, which are specialized proteolytic enzymes. Their precursor pepsinogens, released from chief cells, are converted into active enzyme pepsins with the truncation of a small peptide by low gastric pH.[72]

When in the duodenum, pepsins are irreversibly inactivated by the alkaline pH. Further digestion of luminal proteins is facilitated by the action of pancreatic proteases in the small intestine. Unlike amylase and lipase, which are secreted in their active forms, all pancreatic proteases are released as proenzymes that require proteolytic digestion for activation. Initiation of the activation cascade requires conversion of trypsinogen to trypsin by

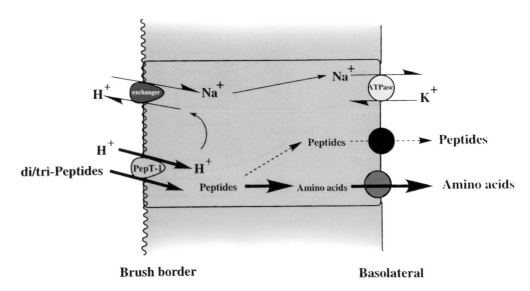

Figure 67–17.   Cellular processes that are involved for optimal function of the intestinal oligopeptide transporter (Pep T-1). (From Adibi SA: The oligopeptide transporter [PepT-1] in human intestine: Biology and function. Gastroenterology 113:336, 1997.)

brush-border enterokinase (enteropeptidase), which involves removal of a six–amino acid peptide from the proenzyme. Trypsin in turn activates other proteolytic enzyme precursors. Activated proteases are classified into two groups according to their relative site of action: endopeptidases and exopeptidases. Endopeptidases such as trypsin, chymotrypsin, and elastases display digestive activity against peptide bonds adjacent to specific amino acids within a polypeptide chain. Exopeptidases include carboxypeptidase A and B and release a single amino acid from the carboxyl terminal end. The digestive activities of these proteases in the small intestine result in the release of luminal amino nitrogen in the form of 30% single amino acids and 70% oligopeptides.[73]

Transport of luminal amino nitrogen involves the uptake of both single amino acids and oligopeptides. Multiple transport mechanisms exist for the 20 single amino acids, including carrier-mediated active transport, facilitated diffusion, and simple diffusion.[74] Separate Na^+-dependent active transport processes have been characterized for neutral, acidic, and basic amino acids. Since cloning of the first γ-aminobutyric acid and cationic amino acid transporters, the cDNA of more than 20 mammalian amino acid transporters has been isolated.[49] Facilitated diffusion may play a role, though a minor one, in the absorption of charged amino acids. Exit of absorbed intracellular amino acids through the basolateral membrane involves similar transport mechanisms.

The significance of the transport of oligopeptides in protein absorption has been demonstrated in several kinetic studies when it was shown to be more efficient than the absorption of single amino acids.[50-53] This oligopeptide transporter (Pep T-1) has recently been cloned as a 708–amino acid membrane protein[54] that transports only dipeptides and tripeptides through H^+-coupled active transport and thus is very sensitive to luminal and intracellular pH (Fig. 67–17, see Table 67–2).[55] In patients requiring enteral nutrition, Pep T-1

provides enhanced absorption of total protein in the form of dipeptides and tripeptides (1) through superior oligopeptide absorption over that of single amino acids, (2) by facilitating an alternative route of delivery of unstable glutamine and poorly soluble tyrosine, and (3) by decreasing the hypertonicity of elemental diets.[56] The clinical importance of Pep T-1 is further displayed by its ability to transport orally administered β-lactam antibiotics, whose structure resembles that of tripeptides.[57,58] Enterocytes consume about 10% of absorbed amino acids when glutamine appears to be a major source of energy.

Lipids and Cholesterol

Dietary fat, made up primarily of triglycerides, is an efficient source of energy that is derived from both animal and vegetable fat. A triglyceride consists of a glycerol backbone with three attached fatty acid chains of various length. Most dietary triglycerides consist of both saturated and unsaturated fatty acids of 16 and 18 carbons and include palmitic (C16:0), oleic (C18:1), stearic (C18:0), and linoleic (C18:2) fatty acids. About 10% of triglycerides consist of medium-chain (6 to 12 carbons) and short-chain (4 carbons) fatty acids. Phospholipids such as lecithin exist in smaller amounts.

Digestion of dietary fat begins in the stomach by acid hydrolysis and gastric lipase. Because of the insoluble nature of fat in water, however, digestion and absorption of lipids predominantly occur in the small intestine by emulsification. Optimal emulsion requires bile salts and phospholipids (either ingested or lecithin) and results in stable small emulsion droplets with a large surface area (Fig. 67–18). Triglycerides in this stable emulsion are then exposed to pancreatic lipase for hydrolysis in the duodenum. Binding of lipase to triglyceride, a prerequisite for hydrolysis, is inhibited by luminal bile salts. Colipase, secreted by the pancreas as an inactive proenzyme,

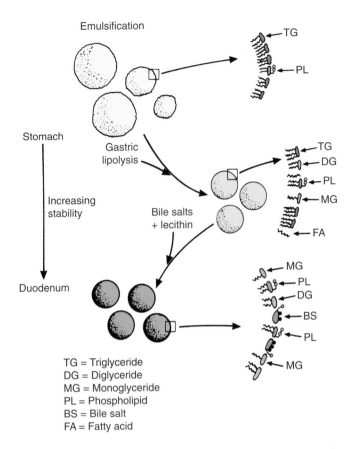

Emulsification

Stomach

Gastric
lipolysis

Increasing
stability

Bile salts
+ lecithin

Duodenum

TG
PL

TG
DG
PL
MG
FA

MG
PL
DG
BS
PL
MG

TG = Triglyceride
DG = Diglyceride
MG = Monoglyceride
PL = Phospholipid
BS = Bile salt
FA = Fatty acid

Figure 67–18. Diagram of steps leading to an increasingly stable emulsion. Gastric lipolysis yields fatty acids and diglyceride, which enhance emulsification, and this is further enhanced in the duodenum by bile salts and phospholipid. (From Tumberg LA, Riley SA: Digestion and absorption of nutrients and vitamins. In Sleisenger MH, Fordtran JS [eds]: Gastrointestinal Disease: Pathophysiology, Diagnosis, Management, 5th ed. Philadelphia, WB Saunders, 1993, p 984.)

is activated by luminal trypsin and facilitates exposure of the lipolytic site after binding to lipase in the presence of bile.[75] Sequential hydrolysis of the two outer ester bonds of the triglyceride molecule by the lipase-colipase complex yields two molecules of free fatty acid and a 2-monoglyceride molecule. Lipase helps present the products of hydrolysis to the mucosal absorptive surface by binding to the brush-border membrane. A specific lipase inhibitor, orlistat (tetrahydrolipstatin), is currently used clinically as a treatment of obesity. Ingested phospholipids are digested by pancreatic phospholipase A_2. Cholesterol is liberated from its esterified form by pancreatic cholesterol esterase.

For the products of lipolysis to be absorbed optimally, they must form micelles with bile salts because of their poor solubility in water. The amphipathic nature of bile salts allows solubilization of free fatty acids, monoglycerides, and cholesterol (but not triglyceride) within the lipophilic area of the micelles.[76] Micelles, shaped like disks, are much smaller (50 to 80 nm in diameter) than emulsion droplets and can form only when the bile salts

are above a critical concentration. Alternatively, droplets containing the products of lipolysis may form smaller spherical lipid droplets from their surface in the absence of an adequate bile salt concentration.[77,78] This nonmicellar lipid transport to the mucosal surface, though a minor mechanism, may account for significant triglyceride absorption when bile salts are absent.

At the brush border the lipid contents of the micelle pass into the enterocytes, whereas bile salts remain within the intestinal lumen. Liberation of fatty acids and glycerides at the surface of the brush border may in part be explained by the presence of an "unstirred water layer."[63] This layer is thin (about 40 μm[64]) and is thought to maintain an acidic microenvironment by the action of surface NHE. A low luminal pH in this layer decreases the solubility of the fatty acids in micelles and thus may enhance their liberation. Additionally, fatty acids are uncharged when protonated at an acidic pH and may thereby diffuse across lipid membrane more easily. Once inside cytoplasm, the near-neutral pH may trap them in their ionized form. Uptake of short-chain and medium-chain fatty acids across the brush-border membrane occurs predominantly by simple diffusion. Long-chain fatty acids (LCFAs), however, are transported into enterocytes by a saturable and specific uptake mechanism. Recently, a family of homologous fatty acid transport proteins (FATPs, see Table 67–2) has been identified and cloned, and these proteins were demonstrated to transport LCFAs across the plasma membrane.[65,66] Overexpression of FATP4 in nonenterocytes can facilitate uptake of LCFAs with the same specificity as enterocytes, whereas reduction of FATP4 expression in primary enterocytes inhibits fatty acid uptake significantly,[67] thus making such reduction a potential target for novel antiobesity therapy.

Once within the cell, fatty acids are transferred to the endoplasmic reticulum for re-esterification back to triglyceride. Intracellular movement of free fatty acids is facilitated through codiffusion with fatty acid binding proteins (FABPs, see Table 67–2), a group of low-molecular-weight cytosolic proteins capable of binding hydrophobic molecules.[68] In the endoplasmic reticulum, resynthesis of triglyceride can occur by two processes. The more predominant monoglyceride pathway involves sequential esterification to diglyceride and triglyceride by acetylcoenzyme A derived from activated fatty acids. The minor pathway involves acylation of α-glycerophosphate by glycerol and fatty acids and may become important during fasting.

After they are synthesized, triglycerides, along with cholesterol and phospholipids, coalesce with apoprotein to form a large lipoprotein complex called a *chylomicron*. During fasting, instead of chylomicrons, very-low-density lipoproteins with different apoproteins and fatty acids are mainly formed. Packaged vesicles containing chylomicrons from the Golgi apparatus then migrate to the basolateral membrane to be released by exocytosis (Fig. 67–19). Chylomicrons subsequently enter the lacteals and pass through the lymphatics into the system's venous circulation. Medium-chain fatty acids and polyunsaturated fatty acids are capable of passing directly into the portal circulation.

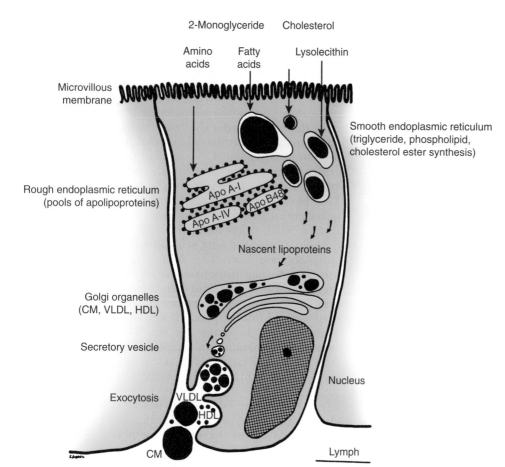

Figure 67–19. Enterocyte lipoprotein assembly. Lipid and amino acid products of digestion are absorbed from the intestinal lumen across the microvillous membrane, where they serve as substrates for the resynthesis of protein and lipid in the rough and smooth endoplasmic reticulum. Apolipoproteins are mobilized from the intracellular pool of protein to form nascent lipoproteins. Lipoproteins are progressively modified within Golgi organelles and secretory vesicles and then secreted into the intracellular space. Apo A-I, A-IV, and B$_{48}$, apolipoproteins A-I, A-IV, and B$_{48}$, respectively; CM, chylomicron; HDL, high-density lipoprotein; VLDL, very-low-density lipoprotein. (From Davidson NO, Magun AM, Glickman RM: Enterocyte lipid absorption and secretion. In Handbook of Physiology: The Gastrointestinal System. Bethesda, MD, American Physiological Society, 1991, p 516.)

Intestinal cholesterol absorption is dependent on luminal bile salts and follows steps similar to those for triglyceride absorption. Free cholesterol, derived from the hydrolysis of esterified cholesterol by pancreatic cholesterol esterase, is transported to the brush-border surface in micelles. After entering the cells by simple diffusion, cholesterol is re-esterified, mainly with oleic acid, and then incorporated into chylomicrons for subsequent lymphatic release. De novo cholesterol synthesis, particularly in the liver, increases when intestinal cholesterol absorption is reduced. Although cholesterol absorption is not significantly enhanced by increased intake of dietary cholesterol, certain dietary fats, such as saturated fats and short-chain fatty acids, may increase cholesterol absorption in the intestine.

Vitamins

Water-soluble vitamins were previously thought to be absorbed by simple passive diffusion; however, it is now clear that specific carrier-mediated mechanisms are involved. Additionally, some of these vitamins undergo hydrolysis before absorption because of attached conjugates or coenzymes.

Primates are incapable of synthesizing ascorbic acid (vitamin C) and thus require dietary supplementation.[75] In the small intestine, an active Na$^+$-dependent process transports vitamin C in the form of sodium ascorbate (Table 67–3).[80]

Folic (pteroylglutamic) acid is present in the diet in the form of polyglutamates and requires hydrolysis by a brush-border hydrolase (carboxypeptidase, see Table 67–3).[81] Ethanol inhibits the hydrolysis (but not uptake) of polyglutamates and may account for the folate deficiency seen in alcoholics.[82,83]

Vitamin B$_{12}$ (cobalamin; see Table 67–3) is derived almost entirely from animal sources and has a multistep process for absorption. Vitamin B$_{12}$ deficiency can therefore arise from multiple sources: loss of intrinsic factor (gastric resection), defective pancreatic proteolysis of cobalamin from R protein (pancreatic insufficiency or biliary obstruction), or loss of ileal receptors (distal ileal disease or resection).

Other water-soluble vitamins, such as thiamine, riboflavin, biotin, and pantothenic acid, also use specific Na$^+$-dependent active transport processes for their absorption.[74] After absorption into an enterocyte, thiamine exits through the basolateral membrane into the portal circulation. Ethanol decreases thiamine absorption by inhibiting this exit step, an effect that may account for thiamine deficiency in alcoholics.

Fat-soluble vitamins include vitamins A, D, E, and K, and they are primarily absorbed from the small intestine through passive diffusion, with absorption being dependent on their structure and hydrophobicity.[87] After they are absorbed, these vitamins enter the intestinal lymphatic system in chylomicrons and join the systemic venous circulation through the thoracic duct. Vitamin A

Table 67–3   Vitamins and Minerals

Nutrient	Receptor	Comment	References
Vitamins			
Ascorbic acid (vitamin C)		Na^+-dependent active absorption	79, 80
Folic acid (pteroylglutamic acid)		Hydrolysis by carboxypeptidase at the brush border (inhibited by ethanol)	81-83
		Hydrolysis is also inhibited in celiac sprue; subsequent uptake is carrier mediated and Na^+ dependent	
Cyanocobalamin (vitamin B_{12})	R protein Intrinsic factor	Bound to salivary binding protein (R protein) in the stomach until freed by hydrolysis in the duodenum	83a, 83b
		Binds to intrinsic factor (secreted by the parietal cells of the stomach) to protect B_{12} from proteolytic digestion	
		In the terminal ileum, specific brush-border receptors bind the cobalamin–intrinsic factor complex	
Thiamine	Na^+-dependent active transport	Exits through the basolateral membrane into the portal circulation (inhibited by ethanol)	74
Riboflavin	Na^+-dependent active transport		74
Biotin	Na^+-dependent active transport		74
Pantothenic acid	Na^+-dependent active transport		74
Vitamin A	Passive diffusion		87
Vitamin D	Passive diffusion		
Vitamin E	Passive diffusion		
Vitamin K	Passive diffusion		
Minerals			
Calcium	Passive paracellular process (throughout the small intestine)	Enhanced by vitamin D and luminal-associated increases in junctional permeability	
	Active, transcellular process (duodenum)	Occurs down its electrochemical gradient	84, 85
		Binds to calbindin and transported out of the cell across the basolateral membrane by calcium-dependent ATPase	
		Calbindin is up-regulated in villus enterocytes by vitamin D	
Magnesium	Passive diffusion, carrier-mediated process	Occurs primarily in the ileum	86
Iron	Non–transferrin receptor–mediated process	Modulated by the degree of transferrin receptor saturation	88, 89
Iron	Divalent cation transporter (DCT-1)		
Bile salts	Apical Na^+-dependent carrier transporter (ASBT)	Located on the luminal surface of ileal epithelial cells (ileal specific)	90, 91
	Liver Na taurocholate cotransporting polypeptide (NTCP)	Expressed on the basolateral membrane of hepatocytes	92

(retinol) is derived from dietary carotenoids, of which β-carotene is a principal form. β-Carotene undergoes hydrolysis by a brush-border oxygenase into two retinol molecules. Absorbed vitamin A is then released into the lymphatics in the form of retinyl palmitate. Two physiologically significant vitamin D sterols, vitamin D_2 (ergocalciferol) and vitamin D_3 (cholecalciferol), are converted from their precursor sterols by ultraviolet irradiation in skin. Vitamin E consists of several related tocopherols, of which the α-isomer is the most potent species. Dietary vitamin D and vitamin E are absorbed in the small intestine by simple diffusion and pass into the lymphatics largely unchanged. Vitamin K consists of two forms: plant-derived K_1 (phytomenadione) and colonic bacteria-produced K_2 (prenyl menaquinones). Absorption of vitamin K_1 occurs through a carrier-mediated process in the small intestine and is facilitated by luminal bile salts[93]; vitamin K_2 is passively absorbed in the ileum and colon.[94]

Minerals

Several essential divalent cations, such as calcium, magnesium, phosphorus, and iron, must be absorbed by the intestine; only trace amounts of other minerals are needed, such as zinc, copper, and selenium.

Intestinal absorption of calcium is mediated by two processes: an active, transcellular transport process occurring predominantly in the duodenum and passive, paracellular diffusion throughout the small intestine (see Table 67–3).[95] Magnesium, unlike calcium, is absorbed predominantly in the ileum, and its absorption involves both passive diffusion and a carrier-mediated process.[96]

Iron is an essential constituent of myoglobin and hemoglobin because of its flexible redox potential. Because excessive amounts of iron are toxic, sophisticated mechanisms exist for transport regulation and detoxification. Circulating iron in serum is tightly bound by transferrin, an 80-kD glycoprotein that can bind two molecules of ferric iron.[88] Because of the abundance of serum transferrin, full saturation of transferrin is seen only in pathologic conditions such as hereditary hemochromatosis and transfusion-related iron overload. Diferric transferrins bind to the transferrin receptor, a specific cell membrane protein ubiquitously present on cellular membranes. The receptor-ligand complex, along with bound iron, is then internalized by receptor-mediated endocytosis, a process regulated by posttranscriptional modulation of transferrin receptor mRNA expression.[89] The bulk of iron absorption from the intestine, however, appears to involve a non–transferrin receptor–mediated mechanism, although it is modulated through an unknown mechanism by the degree of transferrin receptor saturation.

Although mammalian divalent cation export systems have previously been characterized for zinc and copper,[97,98] only recently has a mammalian uptake system been identified. Divalent cation transporter 1 (DCT-1), an H^+-coupled divalent cation and metal ion transporter, has recently been characterized as the major iron transport protein in the intestine.[99-101] DCT-1 is a 561–amino acid transmembrane protein expressed highly in the proximal part of the duodenum and has a broad substrate specificity for many divalent metal ions, including Fe^{2+}, Zn^{2+}, Mn^{2+}, Co^{2+}, Cd^{2+}, Cu^{2+}, Ni^{2+}, and Pb^{2+}. In the intestine, dietary ferric (Fe^{3+}) iron is reduced to ferrous (Fe^{2+}) iron by ferrireductase or ascorbic acid and transported by DCT-1 into enterocytes of the villus tip.[102] Similar to regulation of transferrin receptor expression, iron levels appear to modulate the expression of DCT-1 mRNA.

The hemochromatosis (HFE) gene, which encodes a novel major histocompatibility complex class I–like protein, has also been cloned recently.[103] HFE protein interacts with transferrin receptor with high affinity at the plasma membrane and modulates the binding of diferric transferrin to the transferrin receptor.[103] HFE is prominently expressed in the crypt cells of the duodenum, where most iron absorption occurs. HFE protein in the duodenal crypts is thought to modulate the uptake of transferrin-bound iron, where these cells may act as sensors of the level of body iron stores (Fig. 67–20). In patients with a defect in the HFE gene, transferrin receptor–mediated iron uptake into crypt cells appears to be inappropriately modulated by HFE such that a false signal is sent that serum iron stores are low. Consequently, expression of DCT-1 and intestinal iron absorption are subsequently up-regulated, thereby leading to iron overload in these patients.

Bile Salts

Bile is synthesized from cholesterol in the liver as two primary bile salts: cholate and chenodeoxycholate. They are secreted into the small intestine conjugated with taurine or glycine. Bile salts in the intestinal lumen mix with ingested lipids and form micelles, thus facilitating their digestion. Reabsorption of bile acids from the lumen involves both passive and active reuptake, with active reabsorption in the ileum accounting for most of the total enterohepatic circulation. Absorbed bile salts return to the liver through the portal circulation and are resecreted into bile, thus completing the cycle of enterohepatic circulation. Active uptake of bile acids is mediated by an Na^+-dependent carrier transporter (apical Na^+-dependent bile acid transporter [ASBT]) located on the luminal surface of ileal epithelial cells.[90,91] A related, but distinct bile salt transporter (liver Na^+-taurocholate cotransporting polypeptide [NTCP]) is expressed on the basolateral membrane of hepatocytes.[92] Substrate (bile salt) specificity for ASBT is much narrower than that for NTCP, which suggests that in the lumen of the ileum, efficient recovery of bile acids accompanies elimination of non–bile acid metabolites and xenobiotics, whereas the multispecific transporter in the liver facilitates hepatic clearance of organic anion metabolites.[90] ASBT expression is ileal specific; this transporter is not induced in more proximal gut segments after resection.

Secretion

Intestinal fluid secretion is thought to derive primarily from cells lining the crypts and is dependent on the secondary active transcellular transport of Cl^-. This process facilitates the mixing of luminal nutrients for enhanced absorption and may be important in mucosal defense by diluting or "flushing" harmful toxins and organisms away from the epithelial surface. The driving force for epithelial secretion comes from Na^+,K^+-ATPase, which establishes a low intracellular Na^+ concentration (Fig. 67–21). Na^+ then enters the cell along this gradient coupled to the movement of K^+ and Cl^- through a basolateral Na^+-K^+-$2Cl^-$ cotransporter (NKCC1). Intracellular Cl^- is then extruded across the apical membrane through Cl^- channels, including the cystic fibrosis conductance regulator (CFTR). Na^+ and possibly water

Figure 67–20. Hypothesis of the regulation of iron absorption by the hemochromatosis gene *(HFE)*. An intestinal villus is shown with *insert* enlargements of an enterocyte on the villus tip (where iron is absorbed from the intestine) and a deep crypt cell (where the body iron stores are sensed by means of transferrin-mediated and HFE-modulated iron transport). Ferric iron is reduced in the intestine to ferrous iron and absorbed through the divalent metal transporter (DMT-1, also known as DCT-1) into the enterocyte on the villus tip. In the enterocyte, iron is oxidized to ferric iron and transported through an unidentified basolateral iron transporter into the circulation. In the deep crypt, HFE bound to the transferrin receptor (TfR) modulates the uptake of diferric transferrin. The level of cytoplasmic iron then acts through the binding of iron regulatory proteins (IRPs) to iron response elements (IREs) on the production of DMT-1 transporter mRNA. Mutations in *HFE* cause lack of cell surface expression of HFE, dysregulation of TfR-mediated iron uptake, and consequent alterations in DMT-1 production. (From Bacon BR, Powell LW, Adams PC, et al: Molecular medicine and hemochromatosis: At the crossroads. Gastroenterology 116:197, 1999.)

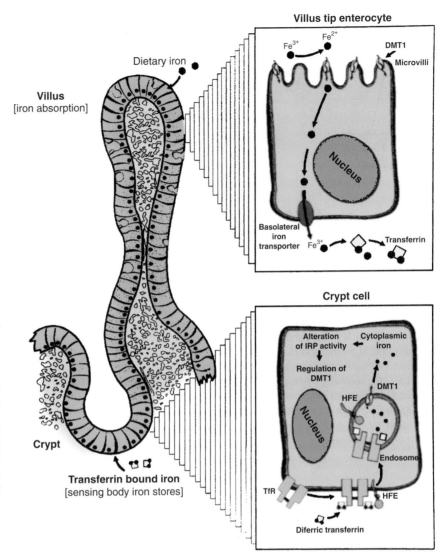

(see earlier) follow passively through the paracellular space into the lumen.

At least three major signal transduction pathways activate Cl⁻ secretion, including cyclic nucleotides (cyclic adenosine monophosphate [cAMP] and cyclic guanosine monophosphate [cGMP]), as well as intracellular calcium.[104] Vasoactive intestinal peptide (VIP), adenosine, prostaglandins, and certain bacterial enterotoxins elevate intracellular cyclic nucleotides, which leads to protein kinase A–dependent CFTR phosphorylation and subsequently to an increase in apical membrane permeability to Cl⁻. Secretory responses depend on the extent of the increase in cAMP and the duration of the stimulus. Calcium-dependent agonists such as histamine and acetylcholine, on the other hand, activate Cl⁻ secretion primarily through the opening of Ca^{2+}-activated K^+ channels in the basolateral membrane. Ca^{2+}-mediated secretory responses, in contrast to that activated by cyclic nucleotides, are transient in duration despite the continued presence of agonist and sustained elevation of intracellular Ca^{2+}.[104-106] Cyclic nucleotides and Ca^{2+} regu-

latory pathways are synergistic for secretion.[107,108] Overall secretory capacity may be largely determined by the activity of basolateral NKCC1, which may be affected at the level of gene transcription by multiple proinflammatory and anti-inflammatory factors.[109]

INTESTINAL IMMUNE SYSTEM

The human intestinal tract is the single largest organ of the immune system. The immune apparatus in the intestine has a dual role of modulating both local and systemic immune responses. Locally, the lymphoid tissue in the intestine plays an important role in defense against various toxic and pathogenic agents from the intestinal lumen. Both the epithelial cells per se and the various lymphoid cells in the lamina propria participate in the delicate balancing of mucosal defense with potential overstimulation of the immune system by the considerable foreign antigen load presented to the intestine daily.

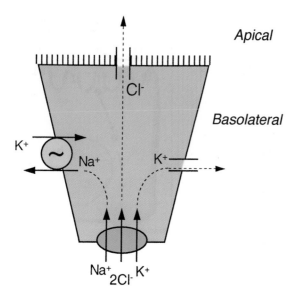

Apical

Basolateral

Figure 67–21. Chloride secretion. Na$^+$,K$^+$-ATPase generates the driving force for epithelial Cl$^-$ secretion by establishing a low intracellular Na$^+$ concentration. The Cl$^-$ entry step through the basolateral membrane Na$^+$-K$^+$-2Cl$^-$ (NKCC1) cotransporter involves the movement of sodium, potassium, and chloride in a 1:1:2 stoichiometry. Accumulated Cl$^-$ above its electrochemical equilibrium exits the cell across the apical membrane through a Cl$^-$ channel. Recycling of intracellular Na$^+$ and K$^+$ is facilitated by the sodium pump and a basolateral potassium channel, respectively.

Secretory Immunoglobulin A and Epithelial Immune Function

Immunoglobulins are synthesized and secreted by B lymphocytes. In the gut, immunoglobulin A (IgA) and IgM play a protective role of neutralizing luminal antigens. IgG antibodies in intestinal secretions are derived mainly from the serum, fix complement, and play an important role in inflammatory reactions and tissue injury. IgE appears to mediate the inflammatory response to antigens that penetrate the intestinal mucosa, as seen in bacterial invasion of the intestinal tract. The most abundant immunoglobulin secreted in the intestine is IgA, with IgM being secreted to a lesser extent. Their secretion into the lumen involves binding to the polymeric immunoglobulin receptor present on the basolateral membrane of the epithelial cells (Fig. 67–22). IgA interaction with microbial antigens prevents them from penetrating the epithelial layer. Although not lymphoid cells per se, intestinal epithelial cells (IECs) clearly participate to some degree in the immune function of the gut. These cells express major histocompatibility class I and II molecules on their surface, possess antigen-presenting activity for T cells,[110] produce cytokines to regulate the proliferation of mononuclear cells in the lamina propria,[111] and express functional receptors for several T-cell–derived cytokines and chemokines.[112] Thus, the epithelial cell layer may transmit important immune regulatory information to the underlying lymphocytes.

M Cells and Gut-Associated Lymphoid Tissue

The major route of passage of luminal antigens to resident lymphoid follicles occurs by means of specialized cells overlying Peyer's patches called *M cells*.[113] These cells rapidly internalize foreign antigens by the endosomal pathway through specialized apical membrane invaginations (Fig. 67–23). Lymphocytes and macrophages in these compartments then process the antigens from the delivered luminal substance. Antigen can also be taken up directly across the enterocytes by either transcellular or paracellular pathways. When the information from these antigen-processing cells reaches the underlying follicle, antigen-specific B-cell proliferation and subsequent IgA production occur. Antigen-specific B cells migrate from Peyer's patches to regional lymph nodes into the systemic circulation, from which they migrate back to the intestine to populate the mucosa diffusely within the lamina propria (Fig. 67–24). In Peyer's patches, B cells are segregated in the germinal centers from the T cells occupying the interfollicular area. Intraepithelial lymphocytes (IELs), however, are predominantly T lymphocytes. They are specialized T cells found in the paracellular space between absorptive enterocytes and are thought to mediate crosstalk between epithelial cells and the underlying immune cells of the lamina propria. Lamina propria lymphoid tissue contains numerous immune cell types, including plasma cells, mast cells, lymphocytes, and macrophages. These cells produce cytokines, chemokines, and immunoglobulins. In addition to these local actions, IgA-producing lymphocytes of Peyer's patches migrate to regional lymph nodes and into the systemic circulation.

Regulation of Gut Immune Activity

A remarkable feature of the mucosal immune system is its overall "hypoactive" or immunosuppressed tone. Despite the enormous antigenic load that passes through the gastrointestinal tract each day, spontaneous inflammatory responses are rare except in pathologic conditions such as inflammatory bowel diseases. This is partly explained by the production of secretory IgA, which unlike other immunoglobulins, does not participate in the proinflammatory response, fix complement, or serve as opsonizing antibody. Additionally, IELs appear to contribute to the overall tone of immunosuppression. Most IELs express the $\gamma\delta$-receptor instead of the $\alpha\beta$-receptor expressed in the more abundant T cells found in most peripheral lymphoid sites. Activation of the immune system by IECs that are capable of presenting antigen and triggering the immune response is also attenuated. The level of uptake and processing of antigens by IECs is quite low[114] because of the absence or minimal expression of appropriate processing enzymes (cathepsins) in the endosomal compartments. Even when the enzymes are present within normal epithelial cells, they are there in reduced amounts.[115] Thus, these cells may have only a limited ability to process intact protein antigens and elicit potent immune responses.

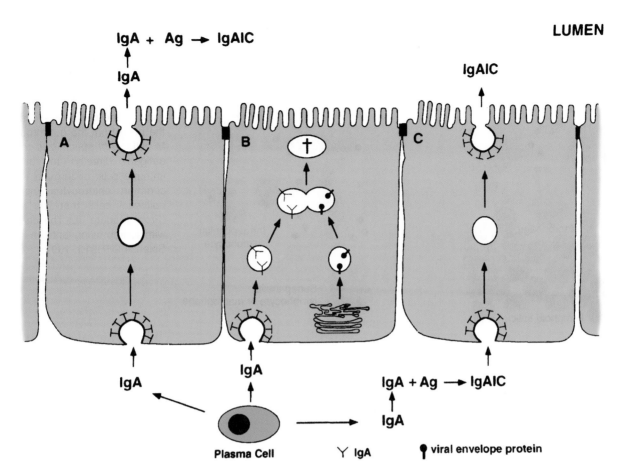

Figure 67–22. Compartments where immunoglobulin A (IgA) can potentially function in relation to mucosal epithelium. The lumen is above the layer of epithelial cells, which are interconnected by apical tight junctions. The lamina propria is below. Plasma cells (not drawn to scale) in the lamina propria secrete polymeric IgA. *Cell A* shows that polymeric IgA can be endocytosed at the basolateral surface (by pIgR), transcytosed, and secreted into the lumen, where it can combine with antigen (Ag) to form immune complexes (IgAIC). In *cell B,* which has been infected by a virus, it is suggested that a transcytotic vesicle containing IgA antibody to viral envelope protein can fuse with a post-Golgi vesicle containing newly synthesized envelope protein, which provides an opportunity for the antibody to disrupt the production of new virus. In the lamina propria below *cell C,* IgA antibody combines with antigen. The immune complex is endocytosed (by pIgR) and transported intact across the cell and into the lumen. (From Lamm ME: Current concepts in mucosal immunity. IV. How epithelial transport of IgA antibodies relates to host defense. Am J Physiol 274:G615, 1998.)

Immune Regulation of Gut Function

Intestinal epithelial function is also influenced by the gut immune system. Evidence for immune regulation of gastrointestinal water and electrolyte transport has recently accumulated. Mast cells play an important role in gut immune effector function and are distributed throughout the intestine but are most abundant in the small intestine. Mast cells secrete various mediators and cytokines upon degranulation after stimulation (e.g., IgE-mediated type I hypersensitivity reaction). Some of these mediators are preformed and stored in vesicles (e.g., histamine); others are newly synthesized as needed (e.g., prostaglandins, leukotrienes, interleukins). In the intestine, these mediators can affect smooth muscle function, vascular permeability, and the epithelial transport of electrolytes, water, acid, and mucin. Histamine acti-

vates H_1 receptors on the intestinal epithelial cell surface and stimulates chloride secretion. Histamine also synergistically enhances secretory responses to cAMP-dependent secretagogues such as adenosine, also a mast cell product. Important roles of mast cells in gut function are demonstrated by experimental manipulations of knockout animals. In genetically mast cell–deficient (W/W^v) mice, the intestinal secretory response associated with anaphylaxis is diminished.[116] They also exhibit reduced colonic mucin secretion from goblet cells and prostaglandin E_2 release in response to stress.[117] In addition, histamine-mediated intestinal epithelial chloride secretion plays an important role in parasitic nematode infections, in which mast cell hyperplasia is a predominant feature.

Immune regulation of intestinal epithelial water and electrolyte transport is manifested by the increased

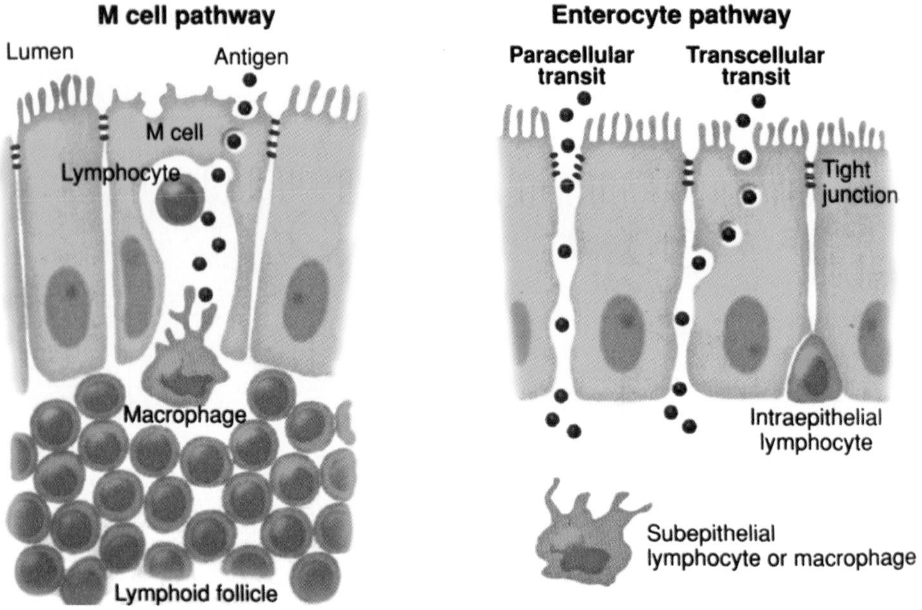

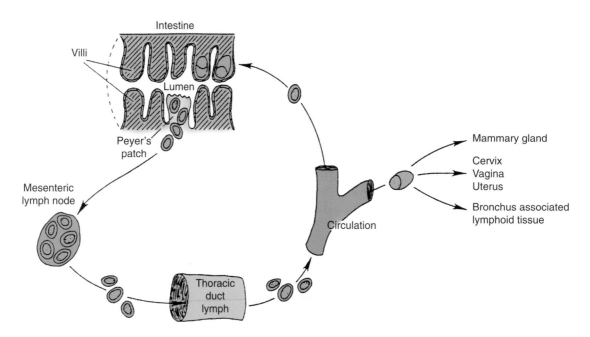

M cell pathway

Lumen
Antigen
M cell
Lymphocyte
Macrophage
Lymphoid follicle

Enterocyte pathway

Paracellular transit
Transcellular transit
Tight junction
Intraepithelial lymphocyte
Subepithelial lymphocyte or macrophage

Figure 67–23. Paths across the lining of the gut. Antigen can enter the body from the gut through rare M cells *(left)* specialized to deliver antigen directly to underlying immune cells or through the more common enterocytes *(right)*, the epithelial cells that line the gut. (From Madara JL: The chameleon within: Improving antigen delivery. Science 277:910, 1997.)

Intestine
Villi
Lumen
Peyer's patch
Mesenteric lymph node
Thoracic duct lymph
Circulation
Mammary gland
Cervix
Vagina
Uterus
Bronchus associated lymphoid tissue

Figure 67–24.   Migration of lymphoid cells from Peyer's patches. Lymphocytes travel from the mesenteric lymph nodes through the thoracic duct to the systemic circulation. These cells can disseminate to the lamina propria of the intestine or to extraintestinal sites, such as the mammary gland, female genital tract, and bronchus-associated lymphoid tissue. (From Kagnoff MF: Immunology of the digestive system. In Johnson LR [ed]: Physiology of the Gastrointestinal Tract. New York, Raven Press, 1981, p 1344.)

gastrointestinal fluid secretion and diarrhea seen in patients with food allergies, inflammatory bowel diseases, and various enteric infections.

MOTILITY OF SMALL INTESTINE

The primary goal of the small intestine, digestion, is facilitated by the contractile movements of the smooth muscle layers, which provide antegrade propulsion of the luminal contents combined with mixing action through segmentation. Organized periodic motor activity is present in the absence of luminal nutrients. Regulation of these motor activities in the intestine is complex and involves an autonomous intrinsic neural network that not only senses and responds to local mechanical and chemical signals but also communicates with central neurons in the spinal cord and brain.

Intestinal Smooth Muscle Cells

Smooth muscle cells form the outer longitudinal and inner circular muscle layers of the intestinal wall and the muscularis mucosae layer. Smooth muscle cells of the intestine derive their contractile force from the interaction between actin and myosin filaments. The actin content relative to myosin is much higher in smooth muscle cells than in skeletal muscle. Additionally, smooth muscle can maintain contractile tension at a lower rate of ATP hydrolysis. Smooth muscle cells of the small intestine display spontaneous electrical depolarizations and are able to propagate this signal to neighboring smooth muscle cells through gap junctions, thus resulting in a coordinated muscle contraction as a syncytium. The dominant intestinal pacemaker that initiates cyclic electrical impulses and contractions is localized in the proximal portion of the duodenum. Recently, the interstitial cell of Cajal (ICC) has been identified as the cell type responsible for the generation of pacemaker currents.[118,119] ICCs and smooth muscle cells originate from common mesenchymal precursor cells.[120-122] ICCs are found within the circular muscle layer of the intestinal wall and are interconnected by long processes containing gap junctions (Fig. 67–25).

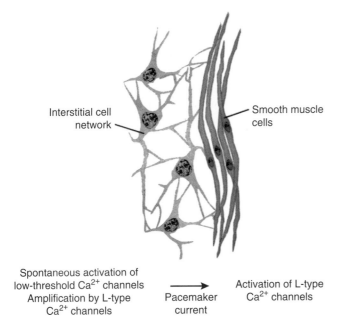

Figure 67–25. Model for initiation of pacemaker activity. Pacemaker activity appears to originate in the interstitial cell of Cajal. Spontaneous activation of low-threshold Ca^{2+} channels occurs near the resting potentials of these cells. As depolarization proceeds, L-type Ca^{2+} channels are also activated and amplify the current. The pacemaker current spreads to smooth muscle cells that are coupled through occasional gap junctions. In smooth muscle cells, L-type Ca^{2+} channels are activated, thus coupling the electrical activity to contraction. (From Sanders KM: A case for interstitial cells of Cajal as pacemakers and mediators of neurotransmission in the gastrointestinal tract. Gastroenterology 111:503, 1996.)

Patterns of Contractions

The small bowel accomplishes the absorption of ingested nutrients by using specific spatial and temporal patterns of contractile activity or motility. The contractions mix and propel ingested food at a rate that facilitates digestion; keep the intestinal tract clear of debris, secretions, and bacteria between meals; and in special situations, propel the intestinal contents rapidly over great distances. The contractile activity of the small intestine is under a variety of control mechanisms, including myogenic, neural, and chemical control.

Myogenic Control

Myogenic control refers to the electrical activity generated by the smooth muscle of the gut. Electrical control activity (ECA; slow waves, basic electrical rhythm, pacesetter potential)[123-126] is the omnipresent rhythmic depolarization of the cell membranes of the smooth muscle of the small intestine. This electrical activity may be recorded with either intracellular or extracellular electrodes. In humans, periodic depolarizations in membrane potential occur 11 to 13 times per minute in the proximal part of the small intestine and decrease to 8 to 10 times per minute in the ileum. With neural or chemical stimulation, membrane depolarization exceeds an excitation threshold and a contraction results. The electrical correlate of a contraction is called *electrical response activity* (ERA; spike burst, action potentials).[123-126] These ERA bursts have a 1:1 relationship with contractions. Because ERA occurs only during the depolarization phase of the ECA cycle, the frequency of contractions is limited to and determined by the frequency of ECA. Neural and chemical stimulation may not be present during each depolarization of ECA, and thus contractions then do not occur at the maximum possible frequency.

The spatial coordination of contractions along the small intestine is coordinated by ECA. Adjoining cells interact, and when electrical coupling is greater, ECA is phase locked such that oscillation of ECA between cells will occur with a fixed time lag. Cells with higher intrinsic frequency drive those with lower intrinsic frequency.

ECA frequency decreases as one progresses from the duodenum to the terminal ileum. There appears to be a *pacemaker region* in the proximal duodenum, similar to the pacemaker region of the stomach, that has an intrinsic ECA frequency that drives or paces the distal part of the small intestine.[127] In the duodenum and proximal jejunum, the electrical coupling is so strong that all the cells oscillate at the same frequency.[124,128] In the more distal portion of the small intestine, the electrical coupling between cells is not strong enough to entrain surrounding cells, and these cells have greater intrinsic frequency variation than do cells of the duodenum. Because individual contractions of the distal variable-frequency region[124,128] are not as coordinated and do not propagate over great distances in the proximal part of the gut, the transit time in the distal portion of the small intestine is longer than that of the proximal portion.[129]

Although both spatial and temporal patterns of contractile activity are ultimately under myogenic control, whether a contraction will occur at any given site depends on local neurochemical stimulation.

Neural Control

Small intestinal smooth muscle contractile activity is influenced by both extrinsic autonomic (parasympathetic and sympathetic) neural activity from the CNS and the intrinsic neurons of the enteric nervous system.

Extrinsic Neural Control The small intestine derives its parasympathetic innervation through the vagus nerve. The vagus nerve contains both afferent and efferent fibers. Efferent motor fibers arise from the dorsal motor nucleus in the region of the fourth ventricle. Relative to the intrinsic enteric neurons, the efferent potion of the vagus is really quite small; however, each vagal efferent fiber may influence about 2000 enteric neurons.[130,131]

In contrast, the sensory component of the vagus nerve is much greater. Sensory fibers account for 80% of all vagal fibers[132] and have their cell bodies primarily in the nodose ganglia. Vagal afferents detect both mechanical and chemical stimulation of the small intestine and relay this information centrally for processing.

Sympathetic innervation of the small intestine arises from the thoracic and lumbar spinal nerves (generally T5 through L3). These nerves pass through the paravertebral ganglia and form the splanchnic nerves, which go to the prevertebral ganglia—the celiac, superior mesenteric, and inferior mesenteric. Within these ganglia, cell bodies receive synaptic input from interganglionic mesenteric neurons. These ganglia intercommunicate and relay sensory information from the gut to the CNS, thereby allowing interactions between different areas of the gut. Stimulation of vagus fibers produces contractile activity within the upper part of the small intestine.[130,131] Electrical stimulation of the mesenteric sympathetic nerves releases norepinephrine and other neuroregulatory substances that inhibit small intestinal contractions.[133]

The enteric nervous system, or the "little brain" of the gut,[134] consists of an intricately coordinated network composed of all neurons having their cell bodies within the bowel wall. Though less well studied than the CNS, the enteric nervous system is quite complicated in that it contains nearly as many neurons as the CNS does.[135]

The enteric nervous system is made up of interconnected neural plexuses and ganglia, which contain the nerve cell bodies. The subserous plexus lies between the serosal and the external muscle of the small intestine. The longitudinal muscle plexus is made of fine nerve bundles that run parallel to the muscle cells and provide innervation to the longitudinal muscle. The myenteric (Auerbach's) plexus is located between the longitudinal and circular muscle layers. The myenteric plexus integrates sensory, extrinsic, and enteric neural information. As in the longitudinal muscle layer, the circular muscle layer has a plexus running parallel to the muscle fibers. This layer communicates with both the myenteric and the deep muscular plexus.[135,136] The deep muscular plexus is located in the inner aspect of the circular muscle layer and separates a thin layer of muscle cells from the bulk of the circular muscle. The fibers of this plexus originate with the myenteric ganglia. The submucosal (Meissner's) plexus also contains ganglia. The muscularis mucosae is a fine layer of smooth muscle just deep to the mucosa that contains a plexus of delicate nerve fibers. Finally, the mucosal plexus intertwines amid the lamina propria of the intestinal crypts and villi.

The majority of neurons controlling contractile activity in the small intestine have their cell bodies in the myenteric plexus.[137,138] Two classes of postsynaptic neurons innervate small intestinal smooth muscles: cholinergic excitatory and nonadrenergic noncholinergic (NANC) inhibitory neurons. Acetylcholine is the excitatory neurotransmitter, but NANC inhibitory neurotransmission is accomplished by nitric oxide,[139-144] ATP, and VIP.[145-148]

The enteric nervous system interfaces directly with the intestinal smooth muscle and provides moment-to-moment control of contractile activity. Neural isolation from the CNS has only a minor effect on the orderly propulsion of chyme within the small intestine.[149] Intrinsic neural pathways may extend 100 to 150 cm proximal and distal to any given point in the small intestine.[1501]

The *peristaltic* or *myenteric reflex* is a classic enteroenteric reflex. Bayliss and Starling[151] described excitation orad and relaxation aborad to the site of mechanical stimulation or chemostimulation. This reflex implies that chyme is propelled in an aborad direction. Although the precise significance of this reflex in normal postprandial contractile activity is uncertain, it reflects the coordinated neurocircuitry within the enteric nervous system.[152] Descending inhibition and ascending excitation are not seen with individual phasic contractions. However, in special situation such as giant migrating contractions (GMCs), both ascending and descending inhibition can be demonstrated.[153] It may be that the greater strength and duration of this special-situation contraction are needed to elicit the peristaltic reflex.

Chemical Control

Chemical control involves the stimulation or inhibition of smooth muscle contractile activity by humoral substances[124] that may act through either a neurocrine, paracrine, or endocrine mode. Examples of these regulatory substances include serotonin, histamine, opioids, cholecystokinin (CCK), motilin, somatostatin, VIP, and substance P. These and many other putative neuroregulatory substances administered exogenously can modulate contractile activity within the small intestine.

There is an intimate relationship between the immune system of the gut and the enteric nervous system that may extend to the motor activity of the small intestine. The best-recognized immune modulator is histamine, which is found within the mast cells of the gut. When mast cells degranulate in response to antigenic stimulation, the enteric nervous system is activated and specific patterns of contractile activity may be initiated.[154-157] Although the precise mechanism by which inflammatory cells and inflammatory mediators affect

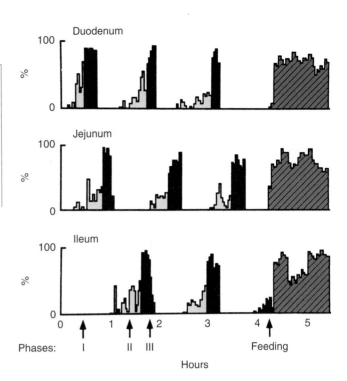

Box 67–1 Types of Contractions in the Small Intestine

Individual phasic contractions

Organized groups of contractions
   Migrating motor complexes
   Migrating clustered contractions

Special propulsive contractions
   Retrograde giant contractions
   Giant migrating contractions

Figure 67–26. The migrating motor complex. *Bars* are used to show the level of intensity in phases II *(open bars)* and III *(solid bars).* The periodicity of activity in fasting *(left)* is interrupted by feeding, when activity rises to a more constant level *(hatched bars).* (From Christensen J: Motility of the intestine. In Sleisenger MH, Fordtran JS [eds]: Gastrointestinal Disease: Pathophysiology, Diagnosis, Management, 5th ed. Philadelphia, WB Saunders, 1993, p 829.)

small intestinal motility is unknown, it is clear that an interaction exists.

Organization of Contractile Activity

Contractions of the small intestine may be divided into individual phasic contractions, organized groups of contractions, and special propulsive contractions (Box 67–1). The specific characteristics of these contractions or groups of contractions and how they relate to the previously described control mechanisms are explored in the following sections.

Individual Phasic Contractions

Individual phasic contractions are the basic contractile activity of the small intestine. They occur in both the fasted and the fed state. In the proximal portion of the small intestine, contractions occur more regularly and propagate caudally over a variable distance that tends to be greater than what occurs in the distal portion of the small intestine. Contractions in the distal part of the small intestine are much less coordinated, and consequently, the rate of propulsion in the distal part of the small bowel is less than that in the proximal part.

Oscillations of ECA directly determine the maximum frequency and duration of individual phasic contractions. When neurochemical stimulation is superimposed, a contraction occurs. Phasic contractile activity does occur without recordable ECA from extracellular electrodes. In this unique situation after drug administration and during some enteric infections, ECA gradually decreases in amplitude and becomes progressively unstable in the distal portion of the small intestine.[155,158] Rapidly migrating contractions may then occur without the tethering influence of ECA. These contractions are similar in amplitude and duration to individual phasic contractions, but they migrate at a velocity as great as 30 cm/sec over distances of up to 200 cm within the proximal part of the small intestine; these rapidly migrating contractions do not occur in the distal portion. Under these conditions, the absence of ECA has been called *amyogenesis.* This electrical and contractile pattern can be disrupted by an event such as feeding, and a special-situation contraction called a *GMC* frequently occurs.

Organized Groups of Contractions

Migrating Motor Complex The migrating motor complex (MMC) is a cyclic pattern of phasic contractile activity that occurs in the interdigestive state. The MMC originates in the proximal portion of the small intestine and migrates to the distal ileum, with cycling every 90 to 120 minutes (Fig. 67–26).[125,159] The MMC cycle is divided into four distinct phases. Phase I is an interval of contractile quiescence; phase II consists of intermittent contractions that eventuate into phase III, which consists of regular phasic contractions of large amplitude that occur at maximum frequency for approximately 6 to 8 minutes. Phase IV of the MMC consists of a short transition of intermittent contractions. In humans, the MMC occurs only during the fasted state (Fig. 67–27). Its purported function is to cleanse the small intestine of residual food, desquamated cells, and enteric secretions and keep bacterial growth to a minimum.[161] Many people refer to phase III of the MMC as "the MMC."

These patterns of small intestinal motor activity develop as the fetus matures.[161,162] Early in gestation, motor activity is irregular and disorganized, but as the fetus develops, the MMC pattern appears.[162] This maturation may occur postnatally in preterm infants.[161] MMCs are preserved in the small intestine throughout the process of aging.[163]

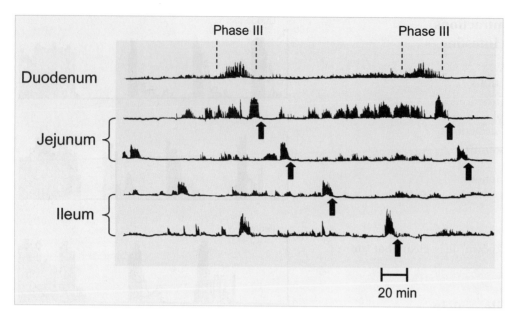

Figure 67–27. Migrating motor complex (MMC). The MMC migrates along the length of the small intestine from the duodenum to the terminal ileum. During the most intense period of contractile activity (phase III), contractions are occurring at their maximum frequency.

The MMC is not under direct CNS control. Truncal vagotomy,[126,164,165] superior and inferior mesenteric ganglionectomy,[166] sympathectomy,[135,167] and even total extrinsic denervation[149] do not abolish MMC cycling. It is likely, however, that the CNS modulates the MMC cycle, particularly during periods of stress.[168,169] Cyclic alterations of circulating regulatory peptides, in particular, motilin, appear to have an influence on the MMC.[170-172] When exogenous motilin is administered, a premature MMC cycle is initiated.[173] During spontaneous cycling of the MMC, plasma motilin concentrations are in their nadir during phase I, increase during phase II, and peak a few minutes after phase II in the duodenum.[174,175] Phase I of the MMC may be produced by ascending inhibition caused by the distally migrating phase III activity. This ascending inhibition may compete with other factors that stimulate contractile activity.

Overall control of the MMC appears to reside in periodic activation of the enteric nervous system, which initiates the cyclic contractile activity we recognized as the MMC. If a segment of the small intestine is isolated as in a loop of small intestine, MMCs cycle above and below as well as within the loop independent of one another.[176,177] Simple transection of the small intestine will disrupt normal migration of the MMC along its flanks.

Migrating Clustered Contractions Migrating or discrete clustered contractions last 1 to 3 minutes, and aboral migration over distances of 10 to 30 cm have been documented to occur.[178-181] Because they do not occur as regularly and predictably as MMCs, the mechanisms of initiation of propagation of the contractions have been less well studied. These migrating clustered contractions are highly effective at propulsion.[182] They usually occur during phase II of the MMC.

Special Propulsive Contractions

The small intestine usually propels chyme slowly in the aboral direction. In special situations, it is advantageous to the organism to expel ingested material rapidly. The small intestine is capable of generating special propulsive contractions to achieve rapid movement of chyme. If aboral propulsion is necessary, retrograde giant contractions (RGCs) occur. These small intestinal contractions immediately precede vomiting. When rapid aboral evacuation of the small bowel is necessary, GMCs rapidly propel chyme into the colon.

Retrograde Giant Contractions An RGC is a large-amplitude, long-duration contraction that originates in the midportion of the small bowel and rapidly propels the intestinal contents in the stomach for subsequent expulsion. It is one of the gastrointestinal motor correlates of vomiting. An RGC travels at a rapid velocity of 8 to 10 cm/sec.[183] By contrast, the MMC migrates at 2 to 8 cm/min.[125,159] RGCs have been extensively studied in the canine model.[183] RGCs also occur in primates but have not yet been documented in the human gastrointestinal tract. The powerful and rapid nature of this contraction may preclude recording with the manometric or solid-state methods currently used in human studies.

RGCs precede spontaneous or drug-induced emetic episodes but may also occur without subsequent vomiting.[183] This appears to be a dose-dependent response. For example, with low doses of an emetic agent, an RGC is initiated; higher doses generate an RGC followed by vomitus expulsion.

An RCG is associated with a series of unique electrical and contractile changes in the small intestine. The first to occur is the obliteration or disorganization of ECA.[183] This change inhibits normal phasic contractions of the

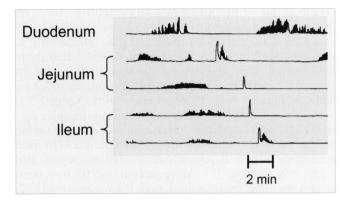

Figure 67–28. Giant migrating contraction. This giant migrating contraction begins in the proximal part of the small intestine and rapidly propels intestinal contents into the colon. In healthy humans, these contractions occur very infrequently and are limited to the distal end of the small intestine. In disease states, they may originate more proximally and are associated with the sensation of abdominal cramping.

small intestine, thus enhancing the propulsive efficiency of the subsequent RGC. An RGC then occurs and may or may not be followed by the somatomotor response of vomitus expulsion. The myoelectric correlate of an RCG is a large potential change, sometimes with a superimposed brief ERA burst.[183] RCGs are followed by a group of phasic contractions throughout the small intestine that last longer distally than proximally.[183] These contractions may propel distal intestinal contents into the colon just as the RGC propels proximal enteric contents into the stomach. Although an RGC itself is not controlled by ECA, the post-RGC phasic contractions are under myogenic control.

Spontaneous RGCs or those initiated by apomorphine or mucosal irritants are abolished by vagotomy.[183] Postvagotomy studies suggest that an RGC requires vagal involvement, but the actual mechanism for the initiation or propagation of an RGC exists within the intestinal wall, and they may be activated by high doses of the hormone CCK-8.[184] Atropine blocks the occurrence of RGCs, which suggests that the final neurotransmitter involved in the contraction is acetylcholine. Interestingly, atropine does not disrupt the ECA slowing and post-RGC phasic contractions, thus suggesting that other neurochemical transmitters may be involved.

Giant Migrating Contractions GMCs, also called *prolonged propagated contractions* (Fig. 67–28), are large-amplitude, long-duration contractions that propagate rapidly in an aboral direction. Their amplitude is approximately 1.5 times that of the phasic contractions of the MMC.[180,185] Once initiated, these contractions usually propagate uninterruptedly to the ileocolonic junction. GMCs are even more propulsive than the MMC.[182] In the normal, healthy state, these contractions occur intermittently in the distal part of the small intestine and are never seen postprandially. In pathologic states or after the administration of certain drugs, GMCs

are more frequent and originate more proximally in the small intestine.[153,155,157,185-187] In patients with irritable bowel syndrome, GMCs are associated with the sensation of abdominal cramping.[188] These powerful contractions may generate abdominal pain because they stimulate nociceptive receptors within the bowel wall above their threshold level and hence produce discomfort. Another theory is that effective propulsion of intestinal chyme by GMCs distends the distal intestinal wall and thereby produces pain.

A function of small intestinal GMCs may be to return fecal contents refluxed from the ileum into the colon.[186] In pathologic states, frequent GMCs may contribute to diarrhea by propelling bile and intestinal secretions rapidly through the gastrointestinal tract without allowing sufficient time for reabsorption.[155,187] Postprandial GMCs that propel undigested food into the colon would contribute to diarrhea[187]; partially digested food exposed to bacterial degradation in the colon would result in gas production and increase the colonic osmotic load.

The myoelectric correlate of the GMC is a brief burst of ERA at the beginning of the contraction. Sometimes the GMC has phasic contractions superimposed on the down-stroke of the contraction. When this occurs, the electrical recording is followed by one or two ERA bursts during the down-stroke.[185] The velocity of GMCs is not bound by the normal constraints of ECA. These contractions require the enteric nervous system for propagation and for generation of the descending inhibition associated with them. Interestingly, ascending inhibition associated with GMCs requires neural input extrinsic to the bowel wall.[153]

The small intestine produces a large number of different contractions in various spatial and temporal patterns that promote efficient digestion, absorption, and propulsion of ingested material. The small intestine also serves a protective role through the use of special-situation contractions that rapidly propel enteric contents into the stomach or colon, from which they may be expelled. Contractile activity of the small intestine is coordinated by the interplay of myogenic, neural, and chemical control.

INTESTINAL NEUROENDOCRINE FUNCTION

The small intestine is a major source of peptides that regulate various aspects of gut function and influence events in the body as a whole. Since the discovery of secretin by Bayliss and Starling in 1902,[189] an increasing number of regulatory peptides have been identified from the gut. These substances are released by local, luminal, or neural stimuli and elicit biologic actions by binding to membrane receptor proteins. Some of the peptides act locally in a paracrine fashion, whereas others work at distant sites in an endocrine fashion as circulating hormones. Many of the receptors for these peptides belong to the superfamily of G protein–coupled receptors. Examples include receptors for secretin, VIP, and pituitary adenylate cyclase activating peptide (PACAP).[190] Some

---

Box 67–2   Human Gastrointestinal Peptides

Gastrin-Cholecystokinin Family

Gastrin

Cholecystokinin (CCK)

Secretin-Glucagon-VIP Family

Secretin

Glucagon

Gastric inhibitory peptide (GIP)

Vasoactive intestinal peptide (VIP)

Glucagon-like peptide 1 (GLP1)

Glucagon-like peptide 2 (GLP2)

Pituitary adenylate cyclase activating peptide (PACAP)

Tachykinin-Bombesin Family

Substance P (SP)

Gastrin-releasing peptide (GRP)

Insulin Family

Insulin

Insulin-like growth factor 1

Somatostatin Family

Somatostatin

Other Peptides

Motilin

Neurotensin

---

representative gastrointestinal peptides are categorized in Box 67–2.

Secretin and Related Peptides

Secretin is a 27–amino acid peptide released from the enteroendocrine cells of duodenal mucosa in response to luminal acid, bile salts, and fat. Its main function is to facilitate digestion by stimulating pancreatic and biliary bicarbonate and water secretion and, to a certain extent, pancreatic exocrine enzyme secretion.[191] At high concentrations, secretin inhibits gastrin release, gastric acid secretion, and postprandial gastric emptying and stimulates secretion of bicarbonate and epidermal growth factor from Brunner's glands.[192,193] Intravenous infusion of secretin stimulates rather than inhibits gastrin release in patients with Zollinger-Ellison syndrome and forms the basis of the diagnostic test for this condition.[194]

VIP is one of the major inhibitory neurotransmitters in the gut and induces relaxation of smooth muscle. Its receptor, a G protein–coupled receptor, elevates intracellular cAMP by means of adenylate cyclase. It is localized, along with PACAP, to the nerve terminals in humans[195] and is released as a neurotransmitter to act on smooth muscle cells to regenerate nitric oxide.[196] It relaxes many sphincter muscles, including the sphincter of Oddi, and mediates relaxation of the peristaltic reflex.[197] VIP also stimulates intestinal epithelial chloride secretion, as well as pancreatic bicarbonate, water, and enzyme secretion.[198-200] More recently, VIP has been shown to affect normal and neoplastic cell growth. It stimulates the growth of astrocytes and certain non–small cell lung cancer cells and inhibits the growth of colonic adenocarcinoma cell lines, probably by virtue of elevated intracellular cAMP.[201]

PACAP was isolated from bovine hypothalamus[202] and shares 68% sequence homology with VIP. PACAP activates both exocrine and endocrine pancreatic secretion in mammals.[203,204] More recently, PACAP activation of pancreatic fluid, bicarbonate, and protein secretion in rats was shown to involve release of secretin and CCK independent of cholinergic stimulation.[205]

Other members of the secretin family, including glucagon, gastric inhibitory polypeptide (GIP), glucagon-like peptide 1 (GLP1), and enteroglucagon, share substantial sequence homology and bind similar G protein–coupled receptors.[206-208] GIP is a 43–amino acid polypeptide released primarily from enterochromaffin cells of the jejunum when stimulated postprandially by carbohydrates and fat, and it subsequently elevates the serum insulin level. Enteroglucagon is primarily released in the distal portion of the small intestine on stimulation by carbohydrate and LCFA and inhibits intestinal motility. GLP1 may be the major hormonal factor responsible for gut adaptation and glucose homeostasis.[209]

Cholecystokinin

CCK is a 33–amino acid polypeptide released by specialized small intestinal mucosal cells in response to luminal amino acids and medium-chain to long-chain fatty acids, and its release is inhibited by intraluminal trypsin and bile salts.[210] The C-terminal tetrapeptides of CCK and gastrin are identical and possess the activity of both hormones. CCK enhances emptying of the gallbladder and bile flow by stimulating simultaneous contraction of the gallbladder and relaxation of the sphincter of Oddi, thus facilitating digestion by luminal mixing of bile with ingested food.[211] Additionally, CCK stimulates pancreatic enzyme secretion, intestinal mucosal cell growth, insulin release, and gut motility. The prostimulatory effect of CCK on gallbladder contraction is clinically used as a provocative test in patients with suspected acalculous biliary disease.[212,213]

Somatostatin

Somatostatin is a cyclic peptide consisting of 14 amino acids[214] and is released in various tissues, including the brain and gut. In the gastrointestinal tract and pancreas, somatostatin, released by specialized enteroendocrine and nerve cells, acts locally in an autocrine, paracrine, or neuronal regulatory manner to perform a wide variety of inhibitory functions.[215,216] It inhibits neurotransmission, smooth muscle contraction, intestinal and pancreaticobiliary secretion, the function of activated immune cells, and cell growth.[215-218] Synthetic analogues of somatostatin, such as octreotide, are used clinically in patients with enterocutaneous and pancreatic fistulas, as well as various hormone-secreting tumors.[218]

Motilin

Motilin, a peptide containing 22 amino acid residues, is released in the small intestine, primarily in the jejunum. Its major actions include local enhancement of smooth muscle contraction and acceleration of gastric emptying.[212] Its prokinetic activity is used clinically in the form of macrolide antibiotics such as erythromycin, a motilin receptor agonist. Erythromycin improves not only emptying of the stomach and gallbladder but also colonic motility.[219-221]

Guanylin and Uroguanylin

Guanylin and uroguanylin, peptides secreted in the intestine, are endogenous ligands for guanylate cyclase, the membrane receptor for the cGMP signaling pathway. Guanylin contains 15 amino acid residues, whereas bioactive uroguanylin exists as 13-, 14-, and 15-residue peptides.[222,223] Both guanylins are highly expressed in the small and large intestines as inactive propeptides that require enzymatic digestion to yield active peptides.[224,225] Heat-stable enterotoxin (Sta) from *Escherichia coli* causes traveler's diarrhea by means of the cGMP signaling pathway by binding the same guanylate cyclase receptor on the intestinal luminal surface.[222,226] Activation of guanylate cyclase by these ligands leads to stimulation of transepithelial secretion of Cl^- and HCO_3^- through the intracellular accumulation of cGMP and thereby results in enhanced fluid secretion and modulation of intraluminal pH.[222,227,228] In particular, uroguanylin, highly expressed in the proximal duodenum, appears to play an important role in neutralizing luminal acid by enhanced anion secretion at low pH.[227]

Other Peptides

Peptide YY is a 36–amino acid polypeptide released in the distal part of the small intestine. Its functions in the gastrointestinal tract are most inhibitory: it inhibits gastric acid secretion and decreases intestinal motility, pancreatic secretion, and release of various intestinal hormones.[229,230] Neurotensin is released from the ileum and enteric nerves and is thought to affect various gastrointestinal functions, such as gastric acid secretion, gastric emptying, and intestinal motility and secretion. Some of the peptides are released from enteric nerves and function primarily as neurotransmitters; such peptides include galanin, bombesin, neuropeptide Y, and substance P, among many others.[231,232] Although efforts to understand their precise physiologic roles are ongoing, these substances appear to influence multiple aspects of gut physiology, such as motility, local blood flow, and epithelial and exocrine secretion.

SUMMARY

The small intestine provides the largest interface with the outside world, provides immune integrity, allows the absorption of most nutrients required by our bodies, and functions largely independently of our perception. Our understanding of the complex mechanisms that allow these functions to occur is expanding.

ACKNOWLEDGMENT

The authors would like to acknowledge the authors of the previous chapters on small intestinal disorders in this textbook: Drs. Seth J. Karp, David I. Soybel, Edward C. Mun, and Jeffery B. Matthews. Their work formed the basis of the current revised chapter.

REFERENCES

1. Walker WA, Duie PR, Hamilton JR, et al: Pediatric Gastrointestinal Disease. St Louis, CV Mosby, 1996.
2. Gray SW, Skandalakis JE: Embryology for Surgeons: Embryological Basis for the Treatment of Congenital Defects. Philadelphia, WB Saunders, 1972.
3. Debas HT, Mulvihill SJ: Neuroendocrine design of the gut. Am J Surg 161:243-249, 1991.
4. Gannon BJ, Perry MA: Histoanatomy and ultrastructure of vasculature of alimentary tract. In Wood JD (ed): Handbook of Physiology: The Gastrointestinal System I, Motility and Circulation Part 2. Baltimore, Waverly, 1989, pp 1301-1334.
5. Granger DN, Kvietys PR, Korthuis RJ, et al: Microcirculation of the intestinal mucosa. In Wood JD (ed): Handbook of Physiology: The Gastrointestinal System I, Motility and Circulation Part 2. Baltimore, Waverly, 1989, pp 1405-1474.
6. Hatoum OA, Binion DG, Otterson MF, Gutterman DD: Acquired microvascular dysfunction in inflammatory bowel disease: Loss of nitric oxide–mediated vasodilation. Gastroenterology 125:58-69, 2003.
7. Hatoum OA, Binion DG, Phillips SA, et al: Radiation induced small bowel "web" formation is associated with acquired microvascular dysfunction. Gut 54:1797-1800, 2005.
8. Netter FH: Ciba Collection of Medical Illustrations. Summit NJ, RR Donnelley & Sons, 1979.
9. Feins NR, NS: Duplications of the alimentary tract. In Nimbkar S, Donnellan WL, Kimura K (eds): Abdominal Surgery of Infancy and Childhood. Newark, NJ, Harwood Academic Press, 1996, p 39/1-17.
10. Roberts DJ, Johnson RL, Burke AC, et al: Sonic hedgehog is an endodermal signal inducing Bmp-4 and Hox genes during induction and regionalization of the chick hindgut. Development 121:3163-3174, 1995.
11. Wesley JR: Pediatric abdomen. In Greenfield LJ (ed): Surgery. Philadelphia, Lippincott-Raven, 1997.
12. Ziegler MM: Abnormalities of intestinal rotation. In Rudolph AM (ed): Rudolph's Pediatrics. East Norwalk, CT, Appleton & Lange, 1996.
13. Wesson DE, Haddock G: The intestines, congenital abnormalities. In Walker WA, Duie PR, Hamilton JR, et al (eds): Pediatric Gastrointestinal Disease. St Louis, CV Mosby, 1996.

14. Merritt AJ, Potten CS, Kemp CJ, et al: The role of p53 in spontaneous and radiation-induced apoptosis in the gastrointestinal tract of normal and p53-deficient mice. Cancer Res 54:614-617, 1994.

15. Ouellette AJ: IV. Paneth cell antimicrobial peptides and the biology of the mucosal barrier. Am J Physiol 277:G257-G261, 1999.

16. Singh AK, Afink GB, Venglarik CJ, et al: Colonic Cl channel blockade by three classes of compounds. Am J Physiol 261:C51-C63, 1991.

17. Kockerling A, Fromm M: Origin of cAMP-dependent Cl⁻ secretion from both crypts and surface epithelia of rat intestine. Am J Physiol 264:C1294-C1301, 1993.

18. Anderson JM, Van Itallie CM: Tight junctions and the molecular basis for regulation of paracellular permeability. Am J Physiol 269:G467-G475, 1995.

19. Anderson JM, Fanning AS, Lapierre L, Van Itallie CM: Zonula occludens (ZO)-1 and ZO-2: Membrane-associated guanylate kinase homologues (MAGuKs) of the tight junction. Biochem Soc Trans 23:470-475, 1995.

20. Goodenough DA: Plugging the leaks. Proc Natl Acad Sci U S A 96:319-321, 1999.

21. Balda MS, Gonzalez-Mariscal L, Contreras RG, et al: Assembly and sealing of tight junctions: Possible participation of G-proteins, phospholipase C, protein kinase C and calmodulin. J Membr Biol 122:193-202, 1991.

22. Madara JL, Parkos C, Colgan S, et al: The movement of solutes and cells across tight junctions. Ann N Y Acad Sci 664:47-60, 1992.

23. Madara JL, Pappenheimer JR: Structural basis for physiological regulation of paracellular pathways in intestinal epithelia. J Membr Biol 100:149-164, 1987.

24. Pappenheimer JR: Physiological regulation of transepithelial impedance in the intestinal mucosa of rats and hamsters. J Membr Biol 100:137-148, 1987.

25. Atisook K, Carlson S, Madara JL: Effects of phlorizin and sodium on glucose-elicited alterations of cell junctions in intestinal epithelia. Am J Physiol 258:C77-C85, 1990.

26. Madara JL: Regulation of the movement of solutes across tight junctions. Annu Rev Physiol 60:143-159, 1998.

27. Hecht G, Pothoulakis C, LaMont JT, Madara JL: Clostridium difficile toxin A perturbs cytoskeletal structure and tight junction permeability of cultured human intestinal epithelial monolayers. J Clin Invest 82:1516-1524, 1988.

28. Fasano A, Fiorentini C, Donelli G, et al: Zonula occludens toxin modulates tight junctions through protein kinase C–dependent actin reorganization, in vitro. J Clin Invest 96:710-720, 1995.

29. Colgan SP, Parkos CA, Matthews JB, et al: Interferon-gamma induces a cell surface phenotype switch on T84 intestinal epithelial cells. Am J Physiol 267:C402-C410, 1994.

30. Taylor CT, Dzus AL, Colgan SP: Autocrine regulation of epithelial permeability by hypoxia: Role for polarized release of tumor necrosis factor alpha. Gastroenterology 114:657-668, 1998.

31. Meinild A, Klaerke DA, Loo DD, et al: The human Na⁺-glucose cotransporter is a molecular water pump. J Physiol 508:15-21, 1998.

32. King LS, Agre P: Pathophysiology of the aquaporin water channels. Annu Rev Physiol 58:619-648, 1996.

33. Brown D, Katsura T, Kawashima M, et al: Cellular distribution of the aquaporins: A family of water channel proteins. Histochem Cell Biol 104:1-9, 1995.

34. Agre P, Brown D, Nielsen S: Aquaporin water channels: Unanswered questions and unresolved controversies. Curr Opin Cell Biol 7:472-483, 1995.

35. Knepper MA: The aquaporin family of molecular water channels. Proc Natl Acad Sci U S A 91:6255-6258, 1994.

36. Ma T, Verkman AS: Aquaporin water channels in gastrointestinal physiology. J Physiol 517:317-326, 1999.

37. Koyama Y, Yamamoto T, Tani T, et al: Expression and localization of aquaporins in rat gastrointestinal tract. Am J Physiol 276:C621-C627, 1999.

38. Ma T, Song Y, Gillespie A, et al: Defective secretion of saliva in transgenic mice lacking aquaporin-5 water channels. J Biol Chem 274:20071-20074, 1999.

39. Ma T, Wang K, Yang B, et al: Defective dietary fat processing in transgenic mice lacking aquaporin-5 water channels [abstract]. Gastroenterology 116:A624, 1999.

40. Wang K, Ma T, Feliz F, et al: Involvement of aquaporin-4 in colonic water absorption and fecal dehydration [abstract]. Gastroenterology 116:A944, 1999.

41. Donowitz M, Khurana S, Tse CM, Yun CH: G protein–coupled receptors in gastrointestinal physiology. III. Asymmetry in plasma membrane signal transduction: Lessons from brush-border Na⁺/H⁺ exchangers. Am J Physiol 274:G971-G977, 1998.

42. Noel J, Pouyssegur J: Hormonal regulation, pharmacology, and membrane sorting of vertebrate Na⁺/H⁺ exchanger isoforms. Am J Physiol 268:C283-C296, 1995.

43. Orlowski J, Grinstein S: Na⁺/H⁺ exchangers of mammalian cells. J Biol Chem 272:22373-22376, 1997.

44. Hoogerwerf WA, Tsao SC, Devuyst O, et al: NHE2 and NHE3 are human and rabbit intestinal brush-border proteins. Am J Physiol 270:G29-G41, 1996.

45. Loo DD, Zeuthen T, Chandy G, Wright EM: Cotransport of water by the Na⁺/glucose cotransporter. Proc Natl Acad Sci U S A 93:13367-13370, 1996.

46. Burant CF, Takeda J, Brot-Laroche E, et al: Fructose transporter in human spermatozoa and small intestine is GLUT5. J Biol Chem 267:14523-14526, 1992.

47. Davidson NO, Hausman AM, Ifkovits CA, et al: Human intestinal glucose transporter expression and localization of GLUT5. Am J Physiol 262:C795-C800, 1992.

48. Shi X, Schedl HP, Summers RM, et al: Fructose transport mechanisms in humans. Gastroenterology 113:1171-1179, 1997.

49. Palacin M, Estevez R, Bertran J, Zorzano A: Molecular biology of mammalian plasma membrane amino acid transporters. Physiol Rev 78:969-1054, 1998.

50. Adibi SA: Glycyl-dipeptides: New substrates for protein nutrition. J Lab Clin Med 113:665-673, 1989.

51. Crampton RF, Gangolli SD, Matthews DM, Simson P: Rates of absorption from tryptic hydrolysates of proteins and the corresponding acid hydrolysates or amino acid mixtures. J Physiol 213:43P-44P, 1971.

52. Silk DB, Marrs TC, Addison JM, et al: Absorption of amino acids from an amino acid mixture simulating casein and a tryptic hydrolysate of casein in man. Clin Sci Mol Med 45:715-719, 1973.

53. Steinhardt HJ, Adibi SA: Kinetics and characteristics of absorption from an equimolar mixture of 12 glycyl-dipeptides in human jejunum. Gastroenterology 90:577-582, 1986.

54. Liang R, Fei YJ, Prasad PD, et al: Human intestinal H⁺/peptide cotransporter. Cloning, functional expression, and chromosomal localization. J Biol Chem 270:6456-6463, 1995.

55. Mackenzie B, Loo DD, Fei Y, et al: Mechanisms of the human intestinal H⁺-coupled oligopeptide transporter hPEPT1. J Biol Chem 271:5430-5437, 1996.

56. Adibi SA: The oligopeptide transporter (Pept-1) in human intestine: Biology and function. Gastroenterology 113:332-340, 1997.

57. Dantzig AH, Tabas LB, Bergin L: Cefaclor uptake by the proton-dependent dipeptide transport carrier of human intestinal Caco-2 cells and comparison to cephalexin uptake. Biochim Biophys Acta 1112:167-173, 1992.

58. Inui K, Yamamoto M, Saito H: Transepithelial transport of oral cephalosporins by monolayers of intestinal epithelial cell line Caco-2: Specific transport systems in apical and basolateral membranes. J Pharmacol Exp Ther 261:195-201, 1992.

59. Tobey N, Heizer W, Yeh R, et al: Human intestinal brush border peptidases. Gastroenterology 88:913-926, 1985.

60. Erickson RH, Bella AM Jr, Brophy EJ, et al: Purification and molecular characterization of rat intestinal brush border membrane dipeptidyl aminopeptidase IV. Biochim Biophys Acta 756:258-265, 1983.

61. Saito H, Inui K: Dipeptide transporters in apical and basolateral membranes of the human intestinal cell line Caco-2. Am J Physiol 265:G289-G294, 1993.

62. Thwaites DT, Brown CD, Hirst BH, Simmons NL: H(+)-coupled dipeptide (glycylsarcosine) transport across apical and basal borders of human intestinal Caco-2 cell monolayers display distinctive characteristics. Biochim Biophys Acta 1151:237-245, 1993.

63. Shiau YF: Mechanism of intestinal fatty acid uptake in the rat: The role of an acidic microclimate. J Physiol 421:463-474, 1990.

64. Strocchi A, Levitt MD: A reappraisal of the magnitude and implications of the intestinal unstirred layer. Gastroenterology 101:843-847, 1991.

65. Hirsch D, Stahl A, Lodish HF: A family of fatty acid transporters conserved from mycobacterium to man. Proc Natl Acad Sci U S A 95:8625-8629, 1998.
66. Schaffer JE, Lodish HF: Expression cloning and characterization of a novel adipocyte long chain fatty acid transport protein. Cell 79:427-436, 1994.
67. Stahl A, Hirsch DJ, Gimeno RE, et al: Identification of the major intestinal fatty acid transport protein. Mol Cell 4:299-308, 1999.
68. Kaikaus RM, Bass NM, Ockner RK: Functions of fatty acid binding proteins. Experientia 46:617-630, 1990.
69. Luxon BA: Inhibition of binding to fatty acid binding protein reduces the intracellular transport of fatty acids. Am J Physiol 271:G113-G120, 1996.
70. Luxon BA, Milliano MT: Cytoplasmic transport of fatty acids in rat enterocytes: Role of binding to fatty acid–binding protein. Am J Physiol 277:G361-G366, 1999.
71. Zierler K: Whole body glucose metabolism. Am J Physiol 276:E409-E426, 1999.
72. Samloff IM: Pepsins, peptic activity, and peptic inhibitors. J Clin Gastroenterol 3:91-94, 1981.
73. Nixon SE, Mawer GE: The digestion and absorption of protein in man. 2. The form in which digested protein is absorbed. Br J Nutr 24:241-258, 1970.
74. Turnberg L, Riley S: Digestion and absorption of nutrients and vitamins. In Sleisenger M, Fordtran J (eds): Gastrointestinal Disease. Philadelphia, WB Saunders, 1993.
75. Blow D: Enzymology. Lipases reach the surface. Nature 351:444-445, 1991.
76. Carey MC, Small DM: The characteristics of mixed micellar solutions with particular reference to bile. Am J Med 49:590-608, 1970.
77. Rigler MW, Honkanen RE, Patton JS: Visualization by freeze fracture, in vitro and in vivo, of the products of fat digestion. J Lipid Res 27:836-857, 1986.
78. Hernell O, Staggers JE, Carey MC: Physical-chemical behavior of dietary and biliary lipids during intestinal digestion and absorption. 2. Phase analysis and aggregation states of luminal lipids during duodenal fat digestion in healthy adult human beings. Biochemistry 29:2041-2056, 1990.
79. Davidson S, Passmore R, Brock J, et al: Human Nutrition and Dietetics. Edinburgh, Churchill Livingstone, 1979.
80. Siliprandi L, Vanni P, Kessler M, Semenza G: Na⁺-dependent, electroneutral L-ascorbate transport across brush border membrane vesicles from guinea pig small intestine. Biochim Biophys Acta 552:129-142, 1979.
81. Halsted CH: The intestinal absorption of dietary folates in health and disease. J Am Coll Nutr 8:650-658, 1989.
82. Naughton CA, Chandler CJ, Duplantier RB, Halsted CH: Folate absorption in alcoholic pigs: In vitro hydrolysis and transport at the intestinal brush border membrane. Am J Clin Nutr 50:1436-1441, 1989.
83. Reisenauer AM, Buffington CA, Villanueva JA, Halsted CH: Folate absorption in alcoholic pigs: In vivo intestinal perfusion studies. Am J Clin Nutr 50:1429-1435, 1989.
83a. Kolhouse JF, Allen RH: Absorption, plasma transport, and cellular retention of cobalamin analogues in the rabbit: Evidence for the existence of multiple mechanisms that prevent the absorption and tissue dissemination of naturally occurring cobalamin analogues. J Clin Invest 60:1381-1392, 1997.
83b. Kolhouse JF, Allen RH: Recognition of two intracellular cobalamin binding proteins and their identification as methylmalonyl-CoA mutase and methionine synthetase. Proc Natl Acad Sci USA 74:921-925, 1977.
84. Feher JJ: Facilitated calcium diffusion by intestinal calcium-binding protein. Am J Physiol 244:C303-C307, 1983.
85. Walters JR, Weiser MM: Calcium transport by rat duodenal villus and crypt basolateral membranes. Am J Physiol 252:G170-G177, 1987.
86. Karbach U, Rummel W: Cellular and paracellular magnesium transport across the terminal ileum of the rat and its interaction with the calcium transport. Gastroenterology 98:985-992, 1990.
87. Hollander D, Dadufalza VD, Fairchild PA: Intestinal absorption of aspirin. Influence of pH, taurocholate, ascorbate, and ethanol. J Lab Clin Med 98:591-598, 1981.
88. Rouault T, Klausner R: Regulation of iron metabolism in eukaryotes. Curr Top Cell Regul 35:1-19, 1997.
89. Addess KJ, Basilion JP, Klausner RD, et al: Structure and dynamics of the iron responsive element RNA: Implications for binding of the RNA by iron regulatory binding proteins. J Mol Biol 274:72-83, 1997.
90. Craddock AL, Love MW, Daniel RW, et al: Expression and transport properties of the human ileal and renal sodium-dependent bile acid transporter. Am J Physiol 274:G157-G169, 1998.
91. Christie DM, Dawson PA, Thevananther S, Shneider BL: Comparative analysis of the ontogeny of a sodium-dependent bile acid transporter in rat kidney and ileum. Am J Physiol 271:G377-G385, 1996.
92. Boyer JL, Hagenbuch B, Ananthanarayanan M, et al: Phylogenic and ontogenic expression of hepatocellular bile acid transport. Proc Natl Acad Sci U S A 90:435-438, 1993.
93. Hollander D: Vitamin K₁ absorption by everted intestinal sacs of the rat. Am J Physiol 225:360-364, 1973.
94. Hollander D, Rim E, Ruble PE Jr: Vitamin K₂ colonic and ileal in vivo absorption: Bile, fatty acids, and pH effects on transport. Am J Physiol 233:E124-E129, 1977.
95. Karbach U: Mechanism of intestinal calcium transport and clinical aspects of disturbed calcium absorption. Dig Dis 7:1-18, 1989.
96. Karbach U: Segmental heterogeneity of cellular and paracellular calcium transport across the rat duodenum and jejunum. Gastroenterology 100:47-58, 1991.
97. Bull PC, Cox DW: Wilson disease and Menkes disease: New handles on heavy-metal transport. Trends Genet 10:246-252, 1994.
98. Palmiter RD, Cole TB, Quaife CJ, Findley SD: ZnT-3, a putative transporter of zinc into synaptic vesicles. Proc Natl Acad Sci U S A 93:14934-14939, 1996.
99. Gunshin H, Mackenzie B, Berger UV, et al: Cloning and characterization of a mammalian proton-coupled metal-ion transporter. Nature 388:482-488, 1997.
100. Fleming MD, Trenor CC 3rd, Su MA, et al: Microcytic anaemia mice have a mutation in Nramp2, a candidate iron transporter gene. Nat Genet 16:383-386, 1997.
101. Fleming MD, Romano MA, Su MA, et al: Nramp2 is mutated in the anemic Belgrade (b) rat: Evidence of a role for Nramp2 in endosomal iron transport. Proc Natl Acad Sci U S A 95:1148-1153, 1998.
102. Andrews NC, Fleming MD, Gunshin H: Iron transport across biologic membranes. Nutr Rev 57:114-123, 1999.
103. Feder JN, Gnirke A, Thomas W, et al: A novel MHC class I–like gene is mutated in patients with hereditary haemochromatosis. Nat Genet 13:399-408, 1996.
104. Barrett KE: Bowditch lecture. Integrated regulation of intestinal epithelial transport: Intercellular and intracellular pathways. Am J Physiol 272:C1069-C1076, 1997.
105. Barrett KE: Positive and negative regulation of chloride secretion in T84 cells. Am J Physiol 265:C859-C868, 1993.
106. Dharmsathaphorn K, Pandol SJ: Mechanism of chloride secretion induced by carbachol in a colonic epithelial cell line. J Clin Invest 77:348-354, 1986.
107. Cartwright CA, McRoberts JA, Mandel KG, Dharmsathaphorn K: Synergistic action of cyclic adenosine monophosphate– and calcium-mediated chloride secretion in a colonic epithelial cell line. J Clin Invest 76:1837-1842, 1985.
108. Mun EC, Rangachari P, Song JC, et al: "Crosstalk" between intracellular signaling pathways: Regulation of basolateral K⁺ channels and intestinal Cl⁻ secretion. Surg Forum 48:229-230, 1997.
109. Matthews JB, Hassan I, Meng S, et al: Na-K-2Cl cotransporter gene expression and function during enterocyte differentiation. Modulation of Cl⁻ secretory capacity by butyrate. J Clin Invest 101:2072-2079, 1998.
110. Mayer L, Shlien R: Evidence for function of Ia molecules on gut epithelial cells in man. J Exp Med 166:1471-183, 1987.
111. Watanabe M, Ueno Y, Yajima T, et al: Interleukin 7 is produced by human intestinal epithelial cells and regulates the proliferation of intestinal mucosal lymphocytes. J Clin Invest 95:2945-2953, 1995.
112. Reinecker HC, Podolsky DK: Human intestinal epithelial cells express functional cytokine receptors sharing the common gamma c chain of the interleukin 2 receptor. Proc Natl Acad Sci U S A 92:8353-8357, 1995.
113. Madara JL: The chameleon within: Improving antigen delivery. Science 277:910-911, 1997.

114. Bland PW, Whiting CV: Antigen processing by isolated rat intestinal villus enterocytes. Immunology 68:497-502, 1989.

115. Hershberg RM, Framson PE, Cho DH, et al: Intestinal epithelial cells use two distinct pathways for HLA class II antigen processing. J Clin Invest 100:204-215, 1997.

116. Perdue MH, Masson S, Wershil BK, Galli SJ: Role of mast cells in ion transport abnormalities associated with intestinal anaphylaxis. Correction of the diminished secretory response in genetically mast cell–deficient W/W^v mice by bone marrow transplantation. J Clin Invest 87:687-693, 1991.

117. Castagliuolo I, Wershil BK, Karalis K, et al: Colonic mucin release in response to immobilization stress is mast cell dependent. Am J Physiol 274:G1094-G1100, 1998.

118. Thomsen L, Robinson TL, Lee JC, et al: Interstitial cells of Cajal generate a rhythmic pacemaker current. Nat Med 4:848-851, 1998.

119. Sanders KM: A case for interstitial cells of Cajal as pacemakers and mediators of neurotransmission in the gastrointestinal tract. Gastroenterology 111:492-515, 1996.

120. Lecoin L, Gabella G, Le Douarin N: Origin of the c-kit–positive interstitial cells in the avian bowel. Development 122:725-733, 1996.

121. Kluppel M, Huizinga JD, Malysz J, Bernstein A: Developmental origin and Kit-dependent development of the interstitial cells of Cajal in the mammalian small intestine. Dev Dyn 211:60-71, 1998.

122. Young HM, Ciampoli D, Southwell BR, Newgreen DF: Origin of interstitial cells of Cajal in the mouse intestine. Dev Biol 180:97-107, 1996.

123. Sarna SK: Gastrointestinal electrical activity: Terminology. Gastroenterology 68:1631-1635, 1975.

124. Sarna SK, Otterson MF: Small intestinal physiology and pathophysiology. Gastroenterol Clin North Am 18:375-404, 1989.

125. Szurszewski JH: A migrating electric complex of canine small intestine. Am J Physiol 217:1757-1763, 1969.

126. Weisbrodt NW: Patterns of intestinal motility. Annu Rev Physiol 43:21-31, 1981.

127. Hermon-Taylor J, Code CF: Localization of the duodenal pacemaker and its role in the organization of duodenal myoelectric activity. Gut 12:40-47, 1971.

128. Sarna SK, Daniel EE, Kingma YJ: Simulation of slow-wave electrical activity of small intestine. Am J Physiol 221:166-175, 1971.

129. Kerlin P, Zinsmeister A, Phillips S: Relationship of motility to flow of contents in the human small intestine. Gastroenterology 82:701-706, 1982.

130. Gidda JS, Goyal RK: Influence of vagus nerves on electrical activity of opossum small intestine. Am J Physiol 239:G406-G410, 1980.

131. Mir SS, Mason GR, Ormsbee HS 3rd: Vagal influence on duodenal motor activity. Am J Surg 135:97-101, 1978.

132. Evans DH, Murray JG: Histological and functional studies on the fibre composition of the vagus nerve of the rabbit. J Anat 88:330-337, 1954.

133. Euler C: Autonomic neuroeffector transmission. In Magoun H (ed): Handbook of Physiology, Section I: Neurophysiology. Washington, DC, American Physiology Society, 1959, pp 217-237.

134. Cooke HJ: Role of the "little brain" in the gut in water and electrolyte homeostasis. FASEB J 3:127-138, 1989.

135. Telford GL, Go VL, Szurszewski JH: Effect of central sympathectomy on gastric and small intestinal myoelectric activity and plasma motilin concentrations in the dog. Gastroenterology 89:989-999, 1985.

136. Furness JB, Costa M, Keast JR: Choline acetyltransferase- and peptide immunoreactivity of submucous neurons in the small intestine of the guinea-pig. Cell Tissue Res 237:329-336, 1984.

137. Gabella G: Ultrastructure of the nerve plexuses of the mammalian intestine: The enteric glial cells. Neuroscience 6:425-436, 1981.

138. Gershon MD: The enteric nervous system. Annu Rev Neurosci 4:227-272, 1981.

139. Boeckxstaens GE, Pelckmans PA, Bult H, et al: Non-adrenergic non-cholinergic relaxation mediated by nitric oxide in the canine ileocolonic junction. Eur J Pharmacol 190:239-246, 1990.

140. Boeckxstaens GE, Pelckmans PA, Rampart M, et al: GABA$_A$ receptor–mediated stimulation of non-adrenergic non-cholinergic neurones in the dog ileocolonic junction. Br J Pharmacol 101:460-464, 1990.

141. Boeckxstaens GE, Pelckmans PA, Ruytjens IF, et al: Bioassay of nitric oxide released upon stimulation of non-adrenergic non-cholinergic nerves in the canine ileocolonic junction. Br J Pharmacol 103:1085-1091, 1991.

142. Bult H, Boeckxstaens GE, Pelckmans PA, et al: Nitric oxide as an inhibitory non-adrenergic non-cholinergic neurotransmitter. Nature 345:346-347, 1990.

143. Stark ME, Szurszewski JH: Role of nitric oxide in gastrointestinal and hepatic function and disease. Gastroenterology 103:1928-1949, 1992.

144. Toda N, Baba H, Okamura T: Role of nitric oxide in non-adrenergic, non-cholinergic nerve-mediated relaxation in dog duodenal longitudinal muscle strips. Jpn J Pharmacol 53:281-284, 1990.

145. Fahrenkrug J, Haglund U, Jodal M, et al: Nervous release of vasoactive intestinal polypeptide in the gastrointestinal tract of cats: Possible physiological implications. J Physiol 284:291-305, 1978.

146. Furness JB, Costa M: Projections of intestinal neurons showing immunoreactivity for vasoactive intestinal polypeptide are consistent with these neurons being the enteric inhibitory neurons. Neurosci Lett 15:199-204, 1979.

147. Furness JB, Costa M: Types of nerves in the enteric nervous system. Neuroscience 5:1-20, 1980.

148. Larsson LI, Fahrenkrug J, Schaffalitzky De Muckadell O, et al: Localization of vasoactive intestinal polypeptide (VIP) to central and peripheral neurons. Proc Natl Acad Sci U S A 73:3197-3200, 1976.

149. Sarr MG, Kelly KA: Myoelectric activity of the autotransplanted canine jejunoileum. Gastroenterology 81:303-310, 1981.

150. Frantzides CT, Sarna SK, Matsumoto T, et al: An intrinsic neural pathway for long intestino-intestinal inhibitory reflexes. Gastroenterology 92:594-603, 1987.

151. Bayliss W, Starling E: The movements and innervation of the small intestine. J Physiol 24:100-143, 1899.

152. Miedema BW, Sarr MG, Hanson RB, Kelly KA: Electric and motor patterns associated with canine jejunal transit of liquids and solids. Am J Physiol 262:G962-G970, 1992.

153. Otterson MF, Sarna SK: Neural control of small intestinal giant migrating contractions. Am J Physiol 266:G576-G584, 1994.

154. Alizadeh H, Castro GA, Weems WA: Intrinsic jejunal propulsion in the guinea pig during parasitism with *Trichinella spiralis*. Gastroenterology 93:784-790, 1987.

155. Cowles VE, Sarna SK: Effect of *T. spiralis* infection on intestinal motor activity in the fasted state. Am J Physiol 259:G693-G701, 1990.

156. Nemeth PR, Ort CA, Wood JD: Intracellular study of effects of histamine on electrical behaviour of myenteric neurones in guinea-pig small intestine. J Physiol 355:411-425, 1984.

157. Palmer JM, Castro GA: Anamnestic stimulus-specific myoelectric responses associated with intestinal immunity in the rat. Am J Physiol 250:G266-G273, 1986.

158. Otterson MF, Sarna SK: Gastrointestinal motor effects of erythromycin. Am J Physiol 259:G355-G363, 1990.

159. Sarna SK: Cyclic motor activity migrating motor complex: 1985. Gastroenterology 89:894-913, 1985.

160. Code CF, Schlegel JF: The gastrointestinal interdigestive housekeeper motor correlates of the interdigestive myoelectric complex in the dog. In Proceedings of the Fourth International Symposium on GI Motility. Vancouver, Canada, Mitchell, 1973.

161. Berseth CL: Gestational evolution of small intestine motility in preterm and term infants. J Pediatr 115:646-651, 1989.

162. Bueno L, Ruckebusch Y: Perinatal development of intestinal myoelectrical activity in dogs and sheep. Am J Physiol 237:E61-E67, 1979.

163. Husebye E, Engedal K: The patterns of motility are maintained in the human small intestine throughout the process of aging. Scand J Gastroenterol 27:397-404, 1992.

164. Marik F, Code CF: Control of the interdigestive myoelectric activity in dogs by the vagus nerves and pentagastrin. Gastroenterology 69:387-395, 1975.

165. Thompson DG, Ritchie HD, Wingate DL: Patterns of small intestinal motility in duodenal ulcer patients before and after vagotomy. Gut 23:517-523, 1982.

166. Marlett JA, Code CF: Effects of celiac and superior mesenteric ganglionectomy on interdigestive myoelectric complex in dogs. Am J Physiol 237:E432-E443, 1979.

167. Dalton RR, Zinsmeister AR, Sarr MG: Vagus-dependent disruption of interdigestive canine motility by gastric distension. Am J Physiol 262:G1097-G1103, 1992.

168. McRae S, Younger K, Thompson DG, Wingate DL: Sustained mental stress alters human jejunal motor activity. Gut 23:404-409, 1982.

169. Thompson DG, Richelson E, Malagelada JR: Perturbation of gastric emptying and duodenal motility through the central nervous system. Gastroenterology 83:1200-1206, 1982.

170. Itoh Z, Takeuchi S, Aizawa I, et al: Changes in plasma motilin concentration and gastrointestinal contractile activity in conscious dogs. Am J Dig Dis 23:929-935, 1978.

171. Keane FB, DiMagno EP, Dozois RR, Go VL: Relationships among canine interdigestive exocrine pancreatic and biliary flow, duodenal motor activity, plasma pancreatic polypeptide, and motilin. Gastroenterology 78:310-316, 1980.

172. Lee KY, Chey WY, Tai HH, Yajima H: Radioimmunoassay of motilin. Validation and studies on the relationship between plasma motilin and interdigestive myoelectric activity of the duodenum of dog. Am J Dig Dis 23:789-795, 1978.

173. Wingate DL, Ruppin H, Thompson HH, et al: 13-Norleucine motilin versus pentagastrin: Contrasting and competitive effects on gastrointestinal myoelectrical activity in the conscious dog. Acta Hepatogastroenterol (Stuttg) 22:409-410, 1975.

174. Hall KE, Greenberg GR, El-Sharkawy TY, Diamant NE: Relationship between porcine motilin-induced migrating motor complex–like activity, vagal integrity, and endogenous motilin release in dogs. Gastroenterology 87:76-85, 1984.

175. Sarna S, Chey WY, Condon RE, et al: Cause-and-effect relationship between motilin and migrating myoelectric complexes. Am J Physiol 245:G277-G284, 1983.

176. Itoh Z, Nakaya M, Suzuki T: Neurohormonal control of gastrointestinal motor activity in conscious dogs. Peptides 2(Suppl 2):223-228, 1981.

177. Ormsbee HS 3rd, Telford GL, Suter CM, et al: Mechanism of propagation of canine migrating motor complex—a reappraisal. Am J Physiol 240:G141-G146, 1981.

178. Cowles VE, Sarna SK: Effect of cholera toxin on small intestinal motor activity in the fed state. Dig Dis Sci 35:353-359, 1990.

179. Kellow JE, Borody TJ, Phillips SF, et al: Human interdigestive motility: Variations in patterns from esophagus to colon. Gastroenterology 91:386-395, 1986.

180. Quigley EM, Phillips SF, Dent J: Distinctive patterns of interdigestive motility at the canine ileocolonic junction. Gastroenterology 87:836-844, 1984.

181. Summers RW, Anuras S, Green J: Jejunal manometry patterns in health, partial intestinal obstruction, and pseudoobstruction. Gastroenterology 85:1290-1300, 1983.

182. Kruis W, Azpiroz F, Phillips SF: Contractile patterns and transit of fluid in canine terminal ileum. Am J Physiol 249:G264-G270, 1985.

183. Lang IM, Sarna SK, Condon RE: Gastrointestinal motor correlates of vomiting in the dog: Quantification and characterization as an independent phenomenon. Gastroenterology 90:40-47, 1986.

184. Lang IM, Marvig J, Sarna SK: Comparison of gastrointestinal responses to CCK-8 and associated with vomiting in the dog. Am J Physiol 254:G254-G263, 1988.

185. Sarna SK: Giant migrating contractions and their myoelectric correlates in the small intestine. Am J Physiol 253:G697-G705, 1987.

186. Kamath PS, Hoepfner MT, Phillips SF: Short-chain fatty acids stimulate motility of the canine ileum. Am J Physiol 253:G427-G433, 1987.

187. Otterson MF, Sarna SK, Moulder JE: Effects of fractionated doses of ionizing radiation on small intestinal motor activity. Gastroenterology 95:1249-1257, 1988.

188. Kellow JE, Phillips SF: Altered small bowel motility in irritable bowel syndrome is correlated with symptoms. Gastroenterology 92:1885-1893, 1987.

189. Bayliss W, Starling E: On the causation of the so-called "peripheral reflex secretion" of the pancreas. Proc R Soc 69:352-353, 1902.

190. Ulrich CD 2nd, Holtmann M, Miller LJ: Secretin and vasoactive intestinal peptide receptors: Members of a unique family of G protein–coupled receptors. Gastroenterology 114:382-397, 1998.

191. Rausch U, Vasiloudes P, Rudiger K, Kern HF: In-vivo stimulation of rat pancreatic acinar cells by infusion of secretin. I. Changes in enzyme content, pancreatic fine structure and total rate of protein synthesis. Cell Tissue Res 242:633-639, 1985.

192. Waldum HL, Walde N, Burhol PG: The effect of secretin on gastric H^+ and pepsin secretion and on urinary electrolyte excretion in man. Scand J Gastroenterol 16:999-1004, 1981.

193. Lu Y, Owyang C: Secretin at physiological doses inhibits gastric motility via a vagal afferent pathway. Am J Physiol 268:G1012-G1016, 1995.

194. McGuigan JE, Wolfe MM: Secretin injection test in the diagnosis of gastrinoma. Gastroenterology 79:1324-1331, 1980.

195. Costa M, Furness JB: The origins, pathways and terminations of neurons with VIP-like immunoreactivity in the guinea-pig small intestine. Neuroscience 8:665-676, 1983.

196. Grider JR, Murthy KS, Jin JG, Makhlouf GM: Stimulation of nitric oxide from muscle cells by VIP: Prejunctional enhancement of VIP release. Am J Physiol 262:G774-G778, 1992.

197. Fahrenkrug J: Transmitter role of vasoactive intestinal peptide. Pharmacol Toxicol 72:354-363, 1993.

198. Holst JJ, Fahrenkrug J, Knuhtsen S, et al: Vasoactive intestinal polypeptide (VIP) in the pig pancreas: Role of VIPergic nerves in control of fluid and bicarbonate secretion. Regul Pept 8:245-259, 1984.

199. Robberecht P, Conlon TP, Gardner JD: Interaction of porcine vasoactive intestinal peptide with dispersed pancreatic acinar cells from the guinea pig. Structural requirements for effects of vasoactive intestinal peptide and secretin on cellular adenosine 3′:5′-monophosphate. J Biol Chem 251:4635-4639, 1976.

200. Krejs GJ, Fordtran JS, Fahrenkrug J, et al: Effect of VIP infusion in water and ion transport in the human jejunum. Gastroenterology 78:722-727, 1980.

201. Waschek JA: Vasoactive intestinal peptide: An important trophic factor and developmental regulator? Dev Neurosci 17:1-7, 1995.

202. Miyata A, Arimura A, Dahl RR, et al: Isolation of a novel 38 residue-hypothalamic polypeptide which stimulates adenylate cyclase in pituitary cells. Biochem Biophys Res Commun 164:567-574, 1989.

203. Lee KY, Lee YL, Kim CD, et al: Mechanism of action of insulin on pancreatic exocrine secretion in perfused rat pancreas. Am J Physiol 267:G207-G212, 1994.

204. Tornoe K, Hannibal J, Giezemann M, et al: PACAP 1-27 and 1-38 in the porcine pancreas: Occurrence, localization, and effects. Ann N Y Acad Sci 805:521-535, 1996.

205. Lee ST, Lee KY, Li P, et al: Pituitary adenylate cyclase–activating peptide stimulates rat pancreatic secretion via secretin and cholecystokinin releases. Gastroenterology 114:1054-1060, 1998.

206. Jelinek LJ, Lok S, Rosenberg GB, et al: Expression cloning and signaling properties of the rat glucagon receptor. Science 259:1614-1616, 1993.

207. Usdin TB, Mezey E, Button DC, et al: Gastric inhibitory polypeptide receptor, a member of the secretin–vasoactive intestinal peptide receptor family, is widely distributed in peripheral organs and the brain. Endocrinology 133:2861-2870, 1993.

208. Thorens B: Expression cloning of the pancreatic beta cell receptor for the gluco-incretin hormone glucagon-like peptide 1. Proc Natl Acad Sci U S A 89:8641-8645, 1992.

209. Drucker DJ: Glucagon-like peptides. Diabetes 47:159-169, 1998.

210. Liddle RA: Regulation of cholecystokinin secretion by intraluminal releasing factors. Am J Physiol 269:G319-G327, 1995.

211. Raybould HE, Lloyd KC: Integration of postprandial function in the proximal gastrointestinal tract. Role of CCK and sensory pathways. Ann N Y Acad Sci 713:143-156, 1994.

212. Geoghegan J, Pappas TN: Clinical uses of gut peptides. Ann Surg 225:145-154, 1997.

213. Sunderland GT, Carter DC: Clinical application of the cholecystokinin provocation test. Br J Surg 75:444-449, 1988.

214. Brazeau P, Vale W, Burgus R, et al: Hypothalamic polypeptide that inhibits the secretion of immunoreactive pituitary growth hormone. Science 179:77-79, 1973.

215. Reichlin S: Somatostatin. N Engl J Med 309:1495-1501, 1983.

216. Reichlin S: Somatostatin (second of two parts). N Engl J Med 309:1556-1563, 1983.

217. Reichlin S: Neuroendocrine-immune interactions. N Engl J Med 329:1246-1253, 1993.

218. Lamberts SW, van der Lely AJ, de Herder WW, Hofland LJ: Octreotide. N Engl J Med 334:246-254, 1996.

219. Yeo CJ, Barry MK, Sauter PK, et al: Erythromycin accelerates gastric emptying after pancreaticoduodenectomy. A prospective, randomized, placebo-controlled trial. Ann Surg 218:229-237, discussion 237-238, 1993.

220. Sharma SS, Bhargava N, Mathur SC: Effect of oral erythromycin on colonic transit in patients with idiopathic constipation. A pilot study. Dig Dis Sci 40:2446-2449, 1995.

221. Fiorucci S, Distrutti E, Gerli R, Morelli A: Effect of erythromycin on gastric and gallbladder emptying and gastrointestinal symptoms in scleroderma patients is maintained medium term. Am J Gastroenterol 89:550-555, 1994.

222. Currie MG, Fok KF, Kato J, et al: Guanylin: An endogenous activator of intestinal guanylate cyclase. Proc Natl Acad Sci U S A 89:947-951, 1992.

223. Hamra FK, Forte LR, Eber SL, et al: Uroguanylin: Structure and activity of a second endogenous peptide that stimulates intestinal guanylate cyclase. Proc Natl Acad Sci U S A 90:10464-1048, 1993.

224. Wiegand RC, Kato J, Huang MD, et al: Human guanylin: cDNA isolation, structure, and activity. FEBS Lett 311:150-154, 1992.

225. Fan X, Hamra FK, Freeman RH, et al: Uroguanylin: Cloning of preprouroguanylin cDNA, mRNA expression in the intestine and heart and isolation of uroguanylin and prouroguanylin from plasma. Biochem Biophys Res Commun 219:457-462, 1996.

226. Field M, Graf LH Jr, Laird WJ, Smith PL: Heat-stable enterotoxin of *Escherichia coli:* In vitro effects on guanylate cyclase activity, cyclic GMP concentration, and ion transport in small intestine. Proc Natl Acad Sci U S A 75:2800-2804, 1978.

227. Joo NS, London RM, Kim HD, et al: Regulation of intestinal Cl⁻ and HCO$_3^-$ secretion by uroguanylin. Am J Physiol 274:G633-G644, 1998.

228. Guba M, Kuhn M, Forssmann WG, et al: Guanylin strongly stimulates rat duodenal HCO$_3^-$ secretion: Proposed mechanism and comparison with other secretagogues. Gastroenterology 111:1558-1568, 1996.

229. Sheikh SP: Neuropeptide Y and peptide YY: Major modulators of gastrointestinal blood flow and function. Am J Physiol 261:G701-G715, 1991.

230. Hill FL, Zhang T, Gomez G, Greeley GH Jr: Peptide YY, a new gut hormone (a mini-review). Steroids 56:77-82, 1991.

231. Holzer P, Holzer-Petsche U: Tachykinins in the gut. Part II. Roles in neural excitation, secretion and inflammation. Pharmacol Ther 73:219-263, 1997.

232. Holzer P, Holzer-Petsche U: Tachykinins in the gut. Part I. Expression, release and motor function. Pharmacol Ther 73:173-217, 1997.

68

Small Bowel Obstruction

Soo Y. Kim · Jon B. Morris

Small bowel obstruction (SBO) is one of the most common admitting diagnoses in surgery, and yet these patients may be the most difficult to manage. They account for 12% to 16% of surgical admissions for acute abdominal complaints. Manifestations of SBO can range from a fairly good appearance with only slight abdominal discomfort and distention to a state of hypovolemic or septic shock (or both) requiring an emergency operation. The process of determining appropriate management can at times be extremely difficult. Despite our advances in the technology of diagnostic procedures, the decision to treat operatively or nonoperatively is still dependent on the surgeon's clinical experience and acumen. There has been some improvement in patient outcome over the years, however, with mortality from SBO declining from 50% in 1900 to less than 3% today. This reduced mortality may be due to multiple factors, including improved imaging techniques that prompt earlier operative intervention versus appropriate conservative management, as well as more advanced methods of resuscitation and intensive care in more severe cases.

CLASSIFICATION

Obstruction can be classified according to its mechanism. For instance, *mechanical* obstruction is the inability of contents to pass through an area because of physical blockage. It can be further divided into extrinsic or extraluminal (e.g., adhesions), intrinsic or mural (e.g., duodenal hematoma), and intraluminal (e.g., gallstone or intussusception) causes. Neoplastic processes may cause any of these mechanical obstructions by way of extrinsic compression of carcinomatosis, mural compression as a result of lymphoma or smooth muscle tumor, or mucosal tumor (Table 68–1).

In contrast, *functional* obstruction is caused by dysmotility of bowel without a physical obstacle to luminal flow. Neurogenic disturbances may contribute to this dysfunction of normal gut motility and peristalsis. Examples include ileus and pseudo-obstruction (Ogilvie's syndrome).

Obstruction can also be categorized as *partial* or *complete*. Partial obstruction may allow gas or liquid stool, or both, to pass the point of narrowing, whereas complete obstruction would not allow the passage of any substance at all. Similarly, obstruction may be labeled *low grade* or *high grade* to indicate the severity of obstruction as interpreted from radiology studies. This category is not to be confused with the designation *high* and *low* obstruction, which is used to stratify the location of pathology within the small bowel, that is, proximal versus distal.

MOTILITY

In the fasted state, migrating myoelectric complexes start in the duodenum and progress to the distal ileum. They occur every 90 to 150 minutes and normally last 90 minutes during their course through the small intestine.

In the case of early obstruction, these propulsive forces work aggressively to pass through the point of blockage and subsequently increase as intraluminal pressure increases. They subside and then recur episodically, alternating with quiescent periods. When the site of obstruction is high, or proximal, the duration of quiescence is shorter. In contrast, when the site is low, or distal, the duration is much longer. Bowel proximal to the site of obstruction becomes increasingly distended, and the distal bowel becomes increasingly inhibited.

In the case of partial obstruction, some intraluminal contents are able to pass through, whereas with complete obstruction, retrograde propulsion develops after bowel contents have accumulated.

PATHOPHYSIOLOGY OF OBSTRUCTION AND STRANGULATION

The clinical course of SBO is variable, depending on the site and severity of the obstruction, and it is even unpredictable. However, a common entity is volume depletion or *third spacing*. One method of fluid loss is net secretion into the lumen of the bowel. The small bowel secretes

Table 68–1	Classification of Small Bowel Obstruction

Extrinsic	Intrinsic	Intraluminal
Adhesions	Tumors of the bowel wall	Intussusception
Hernias	Carcinoid	Gallstones
External	Lymphoma	Bezoars
Inguinal	Leiomyosarcoma	Foreign body
Femoral	Inflammation	Mucosal tumors
Incisional	Crohn's disease	
Obturator	Tuberculosis	
Internal	Hematoma	
Paraduodenal	Endometriosis	
Epiploic foramen		
Diaphragmatic		
Transmesenteric		
Tumors		
Peritoneal metastasis		
Desmoid		
Abscess		
Diverticulitis		
Pelvic inflammatory disease		
Crohn's disease		

8.5 L of fluid daily, most of which is reabsorbed in the small intestine. The net flux of fluid in cases of SBO, however, results in fluid secretion into the lumen. The process is believed to be due to prostaglandin release as a response to bowel distention. It may be manifested in varying degrees of severity, from symptoms of thirst and dry mucous membranes to systemic consequences of renal failure and shock.[1]

Another route of fluid loss is into the wall of the bowel secondary to venous congestion and edema. This loss then results in ascites as the serosal layer of the bowel wall secretes fluid into the peritoneal cavity. The degree of wall edema corresponds to the duration of the obstruction process. In addition, bowel obstruction causes nausea and vomiting, which further contributes to the volume-depleted state of patients with SBO. Furthermore, if a nasogastric tube is placed to suction drainage, copious amounts of fluid, as well as electrolytes, may be lost via this route, and aggressive intravenous replacement may be required.

Early in the obstructive state, a patient is found to have isotonic volume depletion secondary to vomiting or nasogastric tube decompression, as well as third spacing of fluid. As the obstruction persists, hypokalemia occurs as a result of emesis, as well as hyperaldosteronism, which is a response to hypovolemia. In addition, bicarbonate is lost as it is expelled within pancreatic and enteric fluid.[2]

As more air and fluid accumulate within the obstructed bowel, the normal absorptive capabilities of the gut deteriorate and the distention is further exacerbated. In addition, bacterial colonization increases with protracted stasis of the bowel. As a result, more gas is produced by the bacteria, thereby worsening the luminal distention.[3] The risk for bacteremia, peritonitis, and subsequent bacterial translocation is also increased as more bacteria accumulate. If the obstruction is unresolved and the bowel lumen continues to enlarge, vascular compromise becomes more likely. As a result, strangulation occurs, with the later development of necrosis and, ultimately, perforation.[4] Examples include volvulus and mesenteric torsion, which may progress to strangulation, ischemia, and infarction. In these cases, fluid accumulation occurs as well as derangement of bowel motility. In addition, venous obstruction caused by strangulation results in bloody ascites and release of toxins from the bowel wall. Subsequently, toxic metabolic effects may lead to septic conditions and, ultimately, even circulatory collapse.

Closed-Loop Obstruction

Closed-loop obstruction is caused by obstruction of both the afferent and efferent limbs of the involved loop of bowel (Fig. 68–1). Such patients may not have the usual distended abdomen on physical examination because only a limited loop of bowel is usually affected and therefore dilated. Progression to strangulation may occur much sooner than with other forms of obstruction because of an inability to decompress proximally or distally, with subsequent vascular compromise. Causes of closed-loop SBO include mesenteric torsion, adhesive bands, and internal as well as abdominal and inguinal hernias. In the colon, any obstructing lesion may

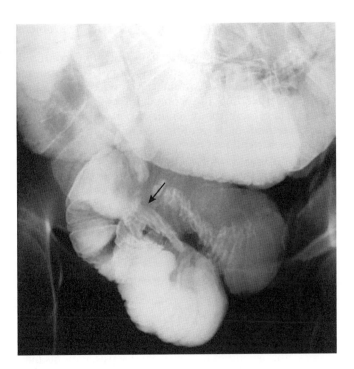

Figure 68–1.   Enteroclysis film showing closed-loop obstruction. Apposition of the entering and exiting limbs at the point of constriction is caused by an adhesive band *(arrow).*

cause a closed-loop phenomenon if the ileocecal valve is competent.

ETIOLOGY

The most common cause of SBO is peritoneal adhesions postoperatively, which constitutes about 75% of all cases of SBO.[5] Pelvic or lower abdominal procedures are blamed for adhesion formation more commonly than upper abdominal procedures are, although any abdominal operation can be responsible.

Hernias, particularly inguinal hernias, are considered the next most common cause of SBO (25%).[4] However, femoral hernias are thought to be more likely to cause incarceration and, possibly, strangulation. Internal hernias can also occur, such as obturator and paraduodenal hernias, as well as hernias through the foramen of Winslow.

Inflammatory processes may likewise cause obstruction by way of secondary angulation of bowel, such as diverticulitis and appendicitis. The remaining causes include Crohn's disease, ischemia, radiation, intussusception, volvulus, and mass lesions such as neoplasms, gallstones, and bezoars.[1]

Adhesions account for the majority of early postoperative obstructions that develop after violation of the peritoneum, reportedly occurring in up to 92% of patients requiring surgical treatment.[6] They result in an inflammatory cascade involving the activation of complement and coagulation. Fibrinogen is produced during this

response and is converted to fibrin by thrombin. If fibrin persists, it adheres to injured surfaces and initiates the formation of a matrix of collagen and fibroblasts, thereby forming *fibrous* adhesions from *fibrinous* adhesions. Fibrin degradation should then occur and allow the fibrinous adhesions to disintegrate and mesothelial regeneration to occur. An abdominal operation causing peritoneal injury dramatically inhibits this process of fibrin degradation by increasing levels of plasminogen activator inhibitors[7] and decreasing levels of tissue plasminogen activator.[8] Thereafter, adhesions are permitted to form and can be potential causes of bowel obstruction.

Another cause of postoperative SBO is internal herniation through defects created at the time of surgery. This category includes mesenteric or omental defects that occur after partial bowel resection. In addition, peritoneal defects that arise around a colostomy or enterostomy, as well as those that occur in the pelvic floor after abdominoperineal resection, can be sites of obstruction. In general, large defects do not seem to pose as much a threat as small defects do.[9] Therefore, controversy still exists regarding whether to close or leave mesenteric defects open after bowel resection or peritoneal defects after abdominoperineal resection.

Inflammatory processes can also cause bowel obstruction early in the postoperative period. Examples are abscesses after bowel surgery, which may form adhesions to nearby loops of bowel and thereby cause partial obstruction. Because of the time frame in which this situation may occur, differentiation between actual obstruction and postoperative ileus may be difficult.

Other consequences of bowel surgery include intramural bleeding with hematoma formation and intussusception. Postoperative anticoagulation can result in hemorrhage within the bowel wall or in the mesentery. Intussusception may occur with or without a lead point, particularly in pediatric patients. A well-described cause in this patient population is an inverted appendicular stump after appendectomy.[10] Another cause in adults is obstruction after retrocolic gastrojejunostomy for gastric bypass without concomitant gastrectomy when the jejunal limb intussuscepts into the gastric lumen.[11]

RISK FOR SMALL BOWEL OBSTRUCTION AFTER LAPAROSCOPY

With the advent of more and more laparoscopic procedures, surgeons are gaining increasing knowledge and experience with associated complications, as well as benefits. Less adhesion formation is one potential benefit of laparoscopy over laparotomy.

Theoretical advantages ensue from less abdominal wall injury as a result of smaller incisions, less use of foreign body materials (talc, gauze, lint from drapes), less tissue desiccation, and less tissue trauma and hemorrhage. However, because of the lack of uniform classification of adhesions in clinical and experimental studies, only suggestions rather than conclusions can be made.

Recent studies have compared adhesion formation after laparoscopy and laparotomy at various sites. With regard to adhesion formation at the operative site, more studies favored laparoscopy over laparotomy. As for adhesions at the incision site, studies consistently supported laparoscopy as causing less adhesion formation. Finally, there are few data assessing the adhesive effects of laparoscopy versus laparotomy at distant sites, such as within abdominal viscera or interenteric surfaces. Experimental studies, however, again favor laparoscopy over laparotomy.[12]

CLINICAL FINDINGS

The most common symptoms of SBO are nausea, vomiting, crampy abdominal pain, distention, and obstipation. Mechanical obstruction usually causes pain before the onset of nausea and emesis, whereas nonmechanical obstruction causes earlier emesis, perhaps followed by subsequent pain. In addition, the site of obstruction may be discernible by the pattern and type of symptoms. Proximal obstruction tends to cause early and more frequent nausea and vomiting, whereas distal obstruction causes crampy pain and obstipation with delayed nausea and vomiting.

Early in the process, the vomitus will represent partially digested food and light-colored liquid. However, later in the process, the vomitus becomes bilious and even feculent. As the luminal contents persist and conglomeration of intestinal bacteria takes place, the emesis becomes malodorous and more consistent with feces.

Abdominal distention develops as the bowel loops proximal to the site of obstruction accumulate gas and fluid. This is less likely in very proximal obstructions, such as those in the duodenum, and occurs more frequently in midgut obstructions. Because up to 10 L can be secreted and reabsorbed by the small intestine in normal situations, the bowel may become quite distended in the setting of obstruction in which routine absorption is hampered (Table 68–2).

Symptoms of obstipation may not be apparent initially because residual gas and stool in the bowel distal to the obstruction may continue to evacuate. In partial obstruction, patients may continue to pass flatus and feces, in conjunction with the other symptoms. However, in complete obstruction, nothing is able to traverse the problem area.

Symptoms of postoperative ileus are often confused with those of bowel obstruction, particularly after abdominal surgery. Extended hospital stay and associated complications, including nosocomial infections, arise as a result. Therefore, many clinicians have investigated various methods of preventing or diminishing the extent of postoperative ileus. One technique that has been published by various centers is gum chewing as an adjunct to postoperative care in which gastrointestinal motility is stimulated via *sham feeding*. This technique has been studied after laparoscopic colon surgery in the hope of further decreasing hospital stay in these patients. Interestingly, when patients were randomly assigned to gum chewing, earlier passage of flatus and feces than in the control group was reported by some authors.[13]

PHYSICAL EXAMINATION

Symptoms may range from minimal discomfort with few physical abnormalities to toxicity and sepsis. Patients may show signs and degrees of dehydration from poor skin turgor and dry mucous membranes to tachycardia, hypotension, oliguria, and mental status changes.

Abdominal examination may reveal distention of varying severity. Auscultation may reveal rushing or tinkling high-pitched bowel sounds or absent bowel sounds in more advanced stages.[14] The abdomen may be tympanitic to percussion if bowel loops are filled with gas, but it may be dull if filled with fluid. Palpation may elicit tenderness if strangulation is present or impending. Signs of guarding and peritonitis would also indicate strangulation and perhaps ischemia or perforation, and they are usually sufficient evidence for exploration. In addition, as part of the abdominal examination, previous surgical scars should be noted because they can be used to predict the location and degree of adhesions likely to be encountered at the time of exploration. When examining a patient with SBO, abdominal and inguinal hernias should always be sought as possible causes of the condition.

Table 68–2   Clinical Findings in Small Bowel Obstruction

Features	Proximal/High Obstruction	Distal/Low Obstruction
Onset of symptoms	Sudden	Gradual
Pain	Epigastric, intense, colicky, usually relieved by vomiting	Periumbilical, colicky
Vomiting	Early, bilious, voluminous, frequent	Later, infrequent, feculent
Tenderness	Epigastric or periumbilical, usually mild unless strangulated	Diffuse and progressive
Distention	Absent	Diffuse and progressive
Obstipation	Absent or mild	Mild or moderate
Radiologic findings	Distended proximal small bowel loops or gasless	Diffusely distended small bowel loops, air-fluid levels

Rectal examination should always be performed in these patients to search for rectal masses that could be obstructing. The finding of hematochezia is a possible indication of a more proximal mass, inflammation, or strangulation and infarction of bowel. Fecal impaction is not an uncommon finding in older patients and often mimics bowel obstruction. As an extension of the rectal examination, proctoscopy and sigmoidoscopy are helpful in the diagnosis and treatment of distal colonic volvulus.

LABORATORY TESTS

Patients with early or partial SBO who are initially seen soon after symptoms have started may have completely normal laboratory studies. However, evidence of dehydration may be evident in the form of abnormal electrolytes and elevated blood urea nitrogen, creatinine, and hematocrit levels. Hyponatremia and hypokalemia are also common abnormalities. Metabolic acidosis occurs as a result dehydration, starvation, ketosis, and loss of alkaline fluid by way of secretion. In the setting of severe vomiting, metabolic alkalosis can occasionally be seen secondary to vomiting of acidic juices.

Mild elevation in the white blood cell count can occur in patients with bowel obstruction, but severe leukocytosis and the presence of many immature polymorphonuclear cells suggest strangulation with possible ischemia. In the case of ischemia, hyperkalemia, lactic acidosis, and elevated amylase levels may be present. It is important, however, to keep in mind that bowel ischemia may be present despite normal laboratory studies and that clinical suspicion should prompt expeditious surgical intervention.

RADIOLOGIC INVESTIGATIONS

Plain Radiographs

Although the diagnosis of SBO may be made with only a thorough history and careful physical examination, diagnostic imaging is often used to verify, locate, and assess the severity. Plain radiographs in the form of an obstruction series, otherwise known as an abdominal series, are usually the initial study obtained in a patient with abdominal symptoms. Studies include an upright chest radiograph, a supine abdominal or kidney-ureter-bladder (KUB) film, and a left lateral decubitus abdominal radiograph. The goal of these films is to rule out free intra-abdominal air, delineate the severity of bowel distention, and possibly identify the location of obstruction.

Plain films are diagnostic in only 50% to 60% of cases of SBO and are only 66% sensitive in proven cases of SBO by experienced radiologists.[15] In addition, specificity has been reported to be low because both mechanical and functional large bowel obstructions may show similar findings on plain radiographs. Nevertheless, they remain a vital initial radiographic tool because of their low cost, availability, noninvasiveness, and value as a gauge of disease progression (Fig. 68–2).

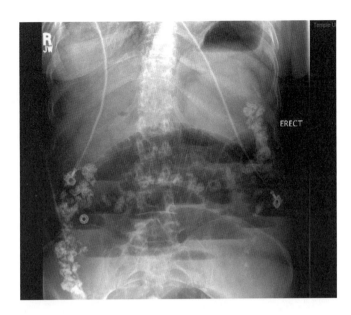

Figure 68–2. Upright abdominal radiograph showing multiple dilated small bowel loops with air-fluid levels.

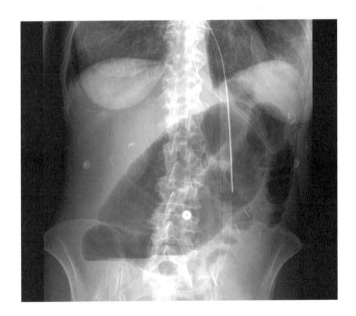

Figure 68–3. Plain abdominal radiograph showing extremely distended small bowel loops with very minimal air in the colon, representative of high-grade obstruction.

Patterns suggestive of SBO include multiple loops of small bowel filled with gas or fluid and a moderate amount of gas in the colon. The finding of colonic gas indicates partial SBO, early complete SBO, or ileus. This pattern is often nondiagnostic and may require further investigational studies such as computed tomography (CT). A more definitive diagnosis of SBO can be made when dilated gas- or fluid-filled small bowel loops are seen with minimal or no gas in the colon[16] (Fig. 68–3)

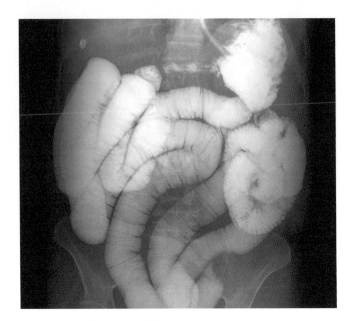

Figure 68–4. Small bowel follow-through film showing distention of multiple small bowel loops, representative of distal obstruction.

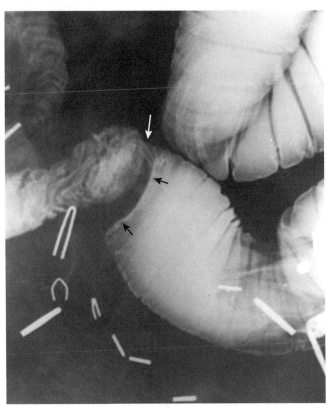

Figure 68–5. Partial small bowel obstruction with an adhesive band at the transition point *(white arrow)* between dilated proximal bowel and decompressed distal bowel. The *black arrows* point to the site of constriction caused by the band.

Contrast Radiographs

Barium films can be used for small bowel evaluation by either oral ingestion of contrast, as for **small bowel follow-through,** or as a retrograde study by way of an enema (Fig. 68–4). In the setting of high-grade SBO, these techniques have some limitations, such as dilution of barium as a result of fluid-filled dilated loops of bowel, which results in poor elucidation of mucosal detail. In addition, slow transit of contrast through the obstructed bowel may prohibit identification of sites of partial blockage or smaller lesions.[17]

Enteroclysis allows intubation of the jejunum and direct infusion of contrast boluses toward the site of obstruction regardless of the degree of peristalsis in the dilated proximal bowel. This technique has been shown to be extremely predictive of obstruction, as well as its absence, its site, and its cause. A positive diagnosis is made when a transition in luminal size is seen (Fig. 68–5). The upper limit of normal small bowel diameter by enteroclysis is 3 cm in the jejunum and 2.5 cm in the ileum.[17] This method can be especially helpful in discriminating between various causes of obstruction such as adhesions, tumors, and radiation.[18]

However, the use of enteroclysis is limited because of requirements for conscious sedation, nasojejunal tube placement, experienced staff, and extensive, time-consuming radiation exposure. In addition, once barium enteroclysis is performed to rule out obstruction, secondary imaging studies are obscured by the barium contrast. Therefore, small bowel follow-through with fluoroscopy is adequate is most situations.[19]

The therapeutic effect of water-soluble contrast is controversial. Some have shown that oral diatrizoate meglumine (Gastrografin) may have a therapeutic effect on SBO[20] and predict the need for early surgical intervention. It has been used as a mode of differentiating partial from complete SBO, thereby leading to operative intervention sooner when the latter situation is identified. After 24 hours, an operation is performed if Gastrografin is not found to have passed into the colon. In patients with partial SBO treated conservatively, hospital stay was found to be shorter and tolerance of a soft diet was noted to occur earlier. The incidence of surgery for SBO, however, was not found to be affected by Gastrografin administration.[21]

Computed Tomography

CT can be a valuable tool in the work-up for SBO. It is helpful in distinguishing SBO from other causes of bowel dilatation and can aid in the decision-making process between operative and nonoperative therapy. Although the sensitivity of CT may be as low as 48% in identifying low-grade obstruction, it is reported to be as high as 81% for high-grade obstruction.[22] CT is also very successful in delineating the cause of obstruction in greater than 90% of cases[19] and in diagnosing ischemic bowel, as well as its precipitating factors, including bowel volvulus, torsion, and intussusception (Fig. 68–6). Additionally, CT is a particularly helpful study for diagnosing external and internal hernias, such as an obturator hernia.

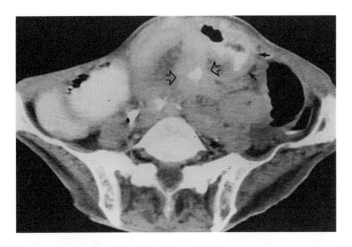

Figure 68–6. Computed tomography scan of the lower part of the abdomen. Dilated bowel loops surround a large mesenteric mass *(open arrows)*. In one bowel loop, wall thickening is demonstrated *(solid arrows)*.

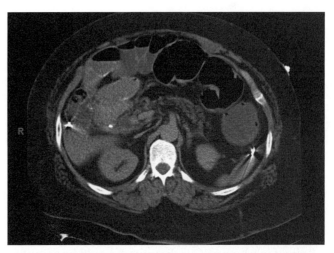

Figure 68–8. Computed tomography scan of the upper part of the abdomen showing high-grade or complete bowel obstruction with decompressed colon.

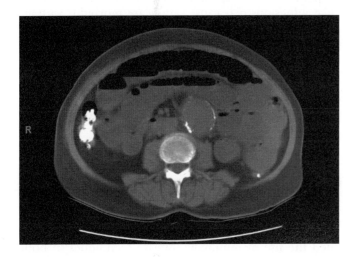

Figure 68–7. Computed tomography scan of the abdomen showing high-grade partial distal small bowel obstruction.

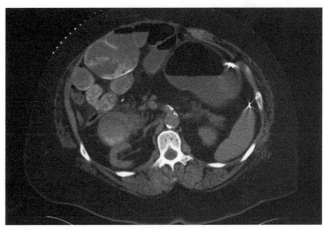

Figure 68–9. Computed tomography scan of the upper abdomen showing dilated loops of proximal small bowel with air-fluid levels adjacent to less dilated, more distal loops of small bowel.

Findings of partial SBO on CT include mildly dilated small bowel loops (>2.5 cm in diameter) with an ill-defined transition point and incompletely collapsed distal bowel in the setting of a moderate amount of gas and fluid in the colon (Figs. 68–7 to 68–9). To distinguish partial SBO from early high-grade SBO, oral contrast is expected to enter the colon within 6 hours, which may be confirmed by follow-up radiography or CT.[23]

For chronic, intermittent partial SBO, CT performed during the symptomatic period may be diagnostic. Alternatively, CT enteroclysis in this setting better delineates findings that may otherwise be missed, such as adhesions or small tumors, but still require surgical intervention. CT enteroclysis combines infusion of water-soluble contrast via a nasointestinal tube into the jejunum with CT imaging. This technique may also improve the low-yield results in cases of low-grade SBO by improving mucosal detail and the distensibility of the small bowel.

When high-grade obstruction, volvulus, torsion, intussusception, other causes of strangulation, or ischemia or infarction is not apparent on CT, conservative management with avoidance of an operation is reasonable. This strategy may prevent significant morbidity and mortality in patients who are at high risk for general anesthesia and abdominal surgery.

In cases of closed-loop obstruction, the involved segment of bowel is nearly completely filled with fluid, and the more proximal portion of the bowel is likely to contain air-fluid levels. The mesentery may also show a whorl sign, suggestive of twisted mesenteric vessels.[24] As for bowel strangulation, its findings are those of ischemic bowel, represented by ascites, a thickened wall, increased mural attenuation, and the target sign when intravenous contrast is administered. Additionally, pneumatosis, portal venous gas, mesenteric congestion, and hemorrhage may be seen in advanced ischemia.[19]

Another useful situation for CT imaging of SBO is in patients with preexisting pathology, such as abdominal malignancy or inflammatory processes. As a fairly noninvasive, reproducible, and readily available study, it serves a generally useful purpose as an early diagnostic study after initial plain radiographs are obtained. In addition, in the acute setting of evaluation for abdominal pain in the emergency department, CT is a reliable initial study to rule out other causes of pain.

MEDICAL TREATMENT

A patient in whom SBO is diagnosed should be admitted to the hospital, hydration instituted, electrolytes corrected, and a nasogastric tube placed. If the diagnosis is **partial** SBO with no evidence of complete obstruction, strangulation, or ischemia, conservative, nonoperative management may be instituted. Such management entails ensuring adequate intravenous hydration, close monitoring of urine output with or without a Foley catheter, nasogastric tube drainage, and frequent assessment of the patient's abdominal examination. A central venous pressure or pulmonary capillary wedge pressure monitor may also be necessary for fluid management in more complex cases. Approximately 80% to 90% of partial SBO cases resolve spontaneously with conservative measures.

In cases of postoperative SBO, long-tube decompression, such as with a Miller-Abbott tube, may be helpful. This topic is discussed further in the following section.

Long-Tube Decompression

Long-tube decompression has been used since the 1930s when Wangensteen reported advancing a long tube into the jejunum to the point of obstruction during explorative laparotomy. Recovery was seen in 80% of these patients with no other intervention.[25] Later, Abbott and Johnston passed the Miller-Abbott tube via the nose into the duodenum and inflated the distal balloon, which then allowed the tube to reach the point of obstruction by peristalsis. This technique was successful in relieving the obstruction in 80% of cases.[26] A major disadvantage was the time delay inconvenience caused by the dependence on peristalsis for advancement of the tube to the appropriate position.

In the 1970s and 1980s, endoscopic placement of long tubes into the small bowel was introduced and eliminated the need to wait for spontaneous migration of the tube. This technique was reported to take as little as 20 minutes for placement into the jejunum,[27] with immediate decompression. Success rates were reported to be as high as 90%.[28]

SURGICAL TREATMENT

Surgery is indicated early in the management of complete SBO or high-grade partial SBO. If there is any indication of bowel incarceration, strangulation, or ischemia,

an urgent operation should be performed after adequate resuscitation. Exceptions to early operative intervention may be cases of inflammatory bowel disease, radiation enteritis, and some cases of carcinomatosis in the absence of clinical signs of deterioration. These situations may best be managed conservatively in light of the limited benefits and potential high risks associated with operative management.

In cases of nonoperative management of partial SBO, factors prompting surgical intervention include (1) worsening abdominal pain and distention; (2) findings of peritonitis, fever, and leukocytosis; (3) failure of resolution of complete obstruction within 12 to 24 hours; and (4) failure of improvement of partial obstruction after 48 to 72 hours or progression to complete obstruction. Most cases of partial SBO secondary to adhesions resolve when managed conservatively, with only 10% to 20% requiring operative correction.

The decision to operate for SBO is not as straightforward in cases of early postoperative obstruction. Most surgeons initially manage these cases expectantly up to 4 weeks before operative intervention is performed. If reoperation is attempted before this time, dense and vascular adhesions may cause significant morbidity with an increased risk for enterotomy and bleeding. Pickleman and Lee reported resolution of postoperative obstruction in 96% of patients within 2 weeks, with the unlikelihood of resolution after 10 days.[29] Certainly, if symptoms or physical findings worsen during the waiting period, as well as the previously mentioned laboratory or radiologic abnormalities, surgical intervention should be implemented in timely fashion.

Laparoscopic Versus Open Adhesiolysis

Since laparoscopic cholecystectomy was introduced in the 1980s, increasing experience by surgeons has broadened the use of minimally invasive techniques in both elective and urgent situations. Laparoscopic adhesiolysis was first described in 1991,[30] and many other reports have been published ever since. Advantages over laparotomy include less postoperative pain, shorter time to return of bowel function, shorter hospital stay, shorter recovery time, fewer wound complications, and decreased adhesion formation. Although no prospective randomized trials comparing laparoscopic and open adhesiolysis for SBO are available at present, retrospective studies, albeit with short follow-up, indicate the safety of laparoscopy with the aforementioned benefits in the appropriate patient population.

Laparoscopy should be avoided in patients with peritonitis or free air requiring emergency exploration. Emergency laparoscopic adhesiolysis has been reported to result in a 36% conversion rate to laparotomy versus 7% when performed electively.[31] In addition, the degree of abdominal distention, bowel diameter (<4 cm),[32] and site of obstruction are important factors when considering laparoscopy. A correlation between the number of previous abdominal operations and successful laparoscopic adhesiolysis is controversial.[33]

Regardless of the method of surgery, adequate resuscitation of patients preoperatively is invaluable. Electrolytes should be corrected, urine output closely monitored, usually with a Foley catheter, and a nasogastric tube placed for decompression. Antibiotics should also be given approximately 1 hour before an incision is made.

Operative Treatment

The surgical approach depends on the suspected cause of obstruction, as well as the intra-operative findings. If adhesions are the presumed cause, laparoscopy or laparotomy is performed with careful and gentle handling of the inflamed, distended, and edematous bowel and friable mesentery. Once the point of obstruction is located and the adhesions released, the entire bowel should be inspected, and depending on the severity and comorbid conditions of the patient, placement of gastric or enteral draining tubes or feeding tubes (or both) should be considered. For example, when faced with a particularly lengthy or complex case, placement of a draining gastrostomy tube may allow early postoperative removal of the nasogastric tube and prevent its potential complications.

If an incarcerated or strangulated hernia is the culprit, the contents should be reduced after induction of general anesthesia if it can be accomplished without difficulty. Before repair of the defect, the visceral contents should be inspected to ensure viability, particularly in cases of suspected strangulation and ischemia.

When mass lesions are the cause of obstruction, partial bowel resection is performed with or without primary anastomosis, as determined on a case-by-case basis. In less common cases of obstruction from carcinomatosis or radiation, intestinal bypass may be warranted as a palliative measure. Obstruction secondary to Crohn's disease should be resected if minimal inflammation is present and fibrosis is the major component of this mostly isolated area of disease.

Prevention of Adhesion

Adhesions after abdominal surgery are the most common cause of SBO. In particular, colorectal surgery is noted to be one of the largest offenders, especially after proctocolectomy and ileal pouch–anal anastomosis. In addition to the morbidity and mortality caused by SBO and its treatment modalities, the financial burden is also noteworthy. In 1996, more than $3.2 billion was paid by Medicare for adhesion-related complications, and more than $1.3 billion was attributed to adhesiolysis costs in 1994 in the United States.[34] In fact, recurrent SBO developed in approximately a third of patients who underwent adhesiolysis for SBO, with most occurring in the first 5 years postoperatively. However, a quarter were found to have SBO complications more than 10 years later.

Various substances and methods have been used for the prevention of adhesions over the past 100 years. Technical efforts such as gentle tissue handling, minimal use of foreign materials, careful hemostatic measures,

and prevention of infection, ischemia, and desiccation have failed to achieve satisfactory results. Substances have also been used with minimal success, including amniotic fluid, bovine cecum, shark peritoneum, fish bladder, vitreous of calf's eye, lubricants, gels, polymers, and various physical barriers.

One notable form of physical barrier is a sodium hyaluronate–based bioresorbable membrane, Seprafilm, which persists in the abdomen for 5 to 7 days.[35] It has been studied in multiple large populations undergoing colorectal surgery. Studies showed decreased incidence, severity, and extent of adhesions after abdominopelvic procedures involving colorectal and gynecologic surgery at the locations of application.[36] In a large, prospective, randomized, multicenter, single-blind controlled study, it also was found to cause fewer cases of adhesive SBO requiring surgery. The number of cases of SBO, however, was not different from that of the control group.[37] Other anti-adhesive substances and techniques are also undergoing extensive research for safety and efficacy.

REFERENCES

1. Kahi CJ, Rex DK: Bowel obstruction and pseudo-obstruction. Gastroenterol Clin North Am 32:1229-1247, 2003.
2. Sakorafas GH, Poggio JL, Dervenis C, Sarr MG: Small bowel obstruction. In Zuidema GD, Yeo CJ (eds): Shackelford's Surgery of the Alimentary Tract, vol 5, 5th ed. Philadelphia, WB Saunders, 2001, pp 317-341.
3. Levitt MD: Volume and composition of human intestinal gas determined by means of an intestinal washout technique. N Engl J Med 284:1394-1398, 1971.
4. Mucha P Jr: Small intestinal obstruction. Surg Clin North Am 67:597-620, 1987.
5. Bizer LS, Liebline RW, Delany HM, Gliedman ML: Small bowel obstruction: The role of nonoperative treatment in simple intestinal obstruction and predictive criteria for strangulation obstruction. Surgery 89:407-413, 1981.
6. Parker MC, Ellis H, Moran BJ, et al: Postoperative adhesions: Ten-year follow-up of 12584 patients undergoing lower abdominal surgery. Dis Colon Rectum 44:822-830, 2001.
7. Raftery AT: Effect of peritoneal trauma on peritoneal fibrinolytic activity and intraperitoneal adhesion formation. An experimental study in the rat. Eur Surg Res 13:397-401, 1981.
8. Holmdahl L, Eriksson E, Eriksson BI, Risberg B: Depression of peritoneal fibrinolysis during operation is a local response to trauma. Surgery 123:539-544, 1998.
9. Sajja SBS, Schein M: Early postoperative small bowel obstruction. Br J Surg 91:683-691, 2004.
10. Holcomb GW III, Ross AJ III, O'Neill JA Jr: Postoperative intussusception: Increasing frequency or increasing awareness? South Med J 84:1334-1339, 1991.
11. Waits JO, Beart RW Jr, Charboneau JW: Jejunogastric intussusception. Arch Surg 115:1449-1452, 1980.
12. Gutt CN, Oniu T, Schemmer P, et al: Fewer adhesions induced by laparoscopic surgery? Surg Endosc 18:898-906, 2004.
13. Asao T, Nakamura J, Moringa N, et al: Gum chewing enhances early recovery from postoperative ileus after laparoscopic colectomy. J Am Coll Surg 195:30-32, 2002.
14. Turnage RT, Bergen P: Intestinal obstruction and ileus. In Feldman M, Friedman LS Sleisenger MH (eds): Gastrointestinal and Liver Disease, vol 2, 7th ed. Philadelphia, WB Saunders, 2002, pp 2113-2128.
15. Shrake PD, Rex DK, Lappas JC, et al: Radiographic evaluation of suspected small-bowel obstruction. Am J Gastroenterol 86:175-178, 1991.
16. Herlinger H, Maglinte DDT: Small bowel obstruction. In Herlinger H, Maglinte DDT (eds): Clinical Radiology of the Small Intestine. Philadelphia, WB Saunders, 1989, pp 479-507.

17. Maglinte DDT, Lappas JC, Kelvin FM, et al: Small bowel radiography: How, when, and why? Radiology 163:297-305, 1987.
18. Caroline DF, Herlinger H, Laufer J, et al: Small-bowel enema in the diagnosis of adhesive obstructions. AJR Am J Roentgenol 143:1133-1139, 1984.
19. Maglinte DDT, Heitkamp DE, Howard TJ, et al: Current concepts in imaging of small bowel obstruction. Radiol Clin North Am 41:263-283, 2003.
20. Assalia A, Schein M, Kopelman D, et al: Therapeutic effect of oral Gastrografin in adhesive, partial small-bowel obstruction: A prospective randomized trial. Surgery 115:433-437, 1994.
21. Biondo S, Pares D, Mora L, et al: Randomized clinical study of Gastrografin administration in patients with adhesive small bowel obstruction. Br J Surg 90:542-546, 2003.
22. Maglinte DDT, Gage SN, Harmon BH, et al: Obstruction of the small intestine: Accuracy and role of CT in diagnosis. Radiology 186:61-64, 1993.
23. Frager D: Intestinal obstruction: Role of CT. Gastroenterol Clin North Am 31:777-799, 2002.
24. Balthazar EJ: CT of the small-bowel obstruction. AJR Am J Roentgenol 162:255-261, 1994.
25. Wangensteen OH: Historical aspects of the management of acute intestinal obstruction. Surgery 65:363-383, 1969.
26. Abbott WO, Johnston CG: Intubation studies of the human small intestine. Surg Gynecol Obstet 66:691, 1938.
27. Gowen GF, DeLaurentis DA, Stefan NM: Immediate endoscopic placement of a long intestinal tube in partial small bowel obstruction. Surg Gynecol Obstet 165:456-457, 1987.
28. Gowen GF: Long tube decompression is successful in 90% of patients with adhesive small bowel obstruction. Am J Surg 185:512-515, 2003.
29. Pickleman J, Lee RM: The management of patients with suspected early post-operative small bowel obstruction. Ann Surg 210:216-219, 1989.
30. Bastug DF, Trammell SW, Boland JP, et al: Laparoscopic adhesiolysis for small bowel obstruction. Surg Laparosc Endosc Percutan Tech 1:259-262, 1991.
31. Chosidow D, Johanet H, Montario T, et al: Laparoscopy for acute small-bowel obstruction secondary to adhesions. J Laparoendosc Adv Surg Tech 10:155-159, 2000.
32. Suter M, Zermatten P, Halkic N, et al: Laparoscopic management of mechanical small bowel obstruction: Are there predictors of success or failure? Surg Endosc 14:478-483, 2000.
33. Nagle A, Ujiki M, Denham W, Murayama K: Laparoscopic adhesiolysis for small bowel obstruction. Am J Surg 187:464-470, 2004.
34. Ray NF, Denton WG, Thamer M, et al: Abdominal adhesiolysis: Inpatient care and expenditures in the United States in 1994. J Am Coll Surg 186:1-9, 1998.
35. Beck DE, Cohen Z, Fleshman JW, et al: A prospective, randomized, multicenter, controlled study of the safety of Seprafilm adhesion barrier in abdominopelvic surgery of the intestine. Dis Colon Rectum 46:1310-1319, 2003.
36. Becker JM, Dayton MT, Fazio VW, et al: Prevention of postoperative abdominal adhesions by a sodium hyaluronate–based bioresorbable membrane: A prospective, randomized, double-blind multicenter study. J Am Coll Surg 183:297-306, 1996.
37. Fazio VW, Cohen Z, Fleshman JW, et al: Reduction in adhesive small-bowel obstruction by Seprafilm adhesion barrier after intestinal resection. Dis Colon Rectum 49:1-11, 2006.

69

Volvulus of the Stomach and Small Bowel

Rebekah R. White ▪ Danny O. Jacobs

The term *volvulus* derives from the Latin word *volvere*, meaning to turn or roll. Clinically, *volvulus* refers to a greater than 180-degree twisting of a hollow organ about its mesentery and results in luminal obstruction, impaired venous return, and eventually ischemia. Though much less common than volvulus of the cecum and sigmoid colon (discussed elsewhere), small bowel volvulus and gastric volvulus are clinical problems that when not recognized promptly, can lead to necrosis of the involved organ with resultant high morbidity and mortality.

SMALL BOWEL VOLVULUS

Etiology

Small bowel volvulus is typically categorized as primary or secondary. Primary small bowel volvulus is relatively rare in the United States but is one of the most common causes of small bowel obstruction in many African and Asian populations. The reported annual incidence ranges from 1.7 to 5.7 per 100,000 population in Western countries as compared with 24 to 60 per 100,000 population in Africa and Asia.[1] Young adults are primarily affected, with a strong male preponderance. Small bowel volvulus is responsible for less than 5% of small bowel obstructions in Western series[2-4] and over half of small bowel obstructions in some African and Asian series.[5,6] The incidence of small bowel volvulus varies not only by country but also by region within certain countries and correlates with lower socioeconomic status.[7] These patterns have been attributed to the high-fiber, vegetarian diet consumed in these populations, as well as to the high proportion of laborers and farmers, who tend to eat infrequent, large meals.[7,8] An increased incidence of small bowel volvulus has been observed during Ramadan, when Muslims ingest large quantities of high-fiber food after prolonged fasting.[8] The incidence of small bowel volvulus is also higher in regions with endemic parasitism, which is known to increase bowel motility.[1] A particularly high incidence of small bowel volvulus was discovered in a Ugandan tribe that consumed a large amount of a beer rich in serotonin,[9] and laxative bowel preparation has been described as a precipitating factor.[10] In 80% of cases the intestinal torsion is clockwise, as it is for midgut volvulus associated with congenital malrotation.[11] However, although congenital malrotation can rarely be manifested in delayed fashion as midgut volvulus, only a minority of adolescent and adult patients with primary small bowel volvulus have an identified lack of mesenteric fixation. Anatomically, the small bowel in high-risk populations is longer and has a longer mesentery with a narrower insertion and a lack of mesenteric fat.[11] Interestingly, patients with small bowel volvulus are not usually emaciated but rather have firm, muscular abdomens, which theoretically might limit the mobility of bowel in the anterior-posterior plane.[5] Whether these observed differences are causative or merely correlative is unclear. Taken together, however, such observations support a popular theory that rapid filling of a segment of proximal intestine with high-bulk chyme pulls it down into the pelvis and displaces empty distal bowel upward, thereby initiating the torsion.

In contrast, secondary small bowel volvulus is much more common than primary small bowel volvulus in the United States. In secondary small bowel volvulus, the intestine is twisted around an underlying point of fixation; as the loop fills with fluid, peristalsis exacerbates the torsion. By far the most common point of fixation is a postoperative adhesion. Case reports have described a number of other causes, however, including internal hernias,[12] tumors,[13] mesenteric lymph nodes,[14] Meckel's diverticulum,[2] and pregnancy.[15] In the most recently published Western series, Roggo and Ottinger from Massachusetts General Hospital (MGH) reported 35 patients with small bowel volvulus; these patients represented 4% of all small bowel obstructions over the 10-year study

Table 69–1	Modern Series of Small Bowel Volvulus	
Author	Roggo	Ghebrat
Country	USA	Ethiopia
Study period	1980-1990	1995-1997
Number of patients	35	51
Male-female ratio	1:1.2	12:1
Average age	67	37
Primary small bowel volvulus	14%	92%
Gangrenous small bowel	46%	18%
Mortality overall	9%	12%
Mortality from gangrene	17%	NS

NS, not stated.

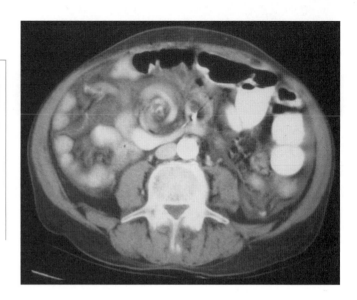

Figure 69–1. Abdominal computed tomography scan with a "whirl" sign in a patient with small bowel volvulus secondary to postoperative adhesions.

period (1980 to 1990).[2] In five patients (all men), the volvulus was primary. In 29 of the remaining 30 patients, the volvulus was secondary to postoperative adhesions. Unlike primary small bowel volvulus, secondary small bowel volvulus affected both sexes equally and mainly older adults. This study is compared with a contemporary series by Ghebrat et al. from Ethiopia[5] in Table 69–1, which illustrates some of the differences between primary and secondary small bowel volvulus.

Diagnosis

Clinically, the findings in patients with small bowel volvulus are nonspecific. Patients have signs and symptoms of small bowel obstruction that are usually sudden in onset. Central abdominal pain is almost always present.[1,2,5] In some cases, careful questioning may elicit a previous history of intermittent obstructive symptoms such as crampy epigastric or periumbilical abdominal pain. "Pain out of proportion" to the degree of obstruction should raise suspicion of vascular compromise, as should fever, tachycardia, peritoneal signs, acidosis, and leukocytosis. However, none of these signs alone are sensitive or specific enough to reliably rule bowel ischemia in or out. For example, in the MGH series, 9 of 35 patients (26%) with small bowel volvulus had peritoneal signs and two thirds of these patients had gangrenous bowel; 10 of the 26 patients without peritoneal signs had gangrenous bowel.[2]

Plain films are usually nonspecific and demonstrate dilated loops of bowel or air-fluid levels, or both. However, in a closed-loop obstruction such as volvulus, the loops may be filled with fluid and have little or no air. Thus, plain films may reveal a "gasless" abdomen or even be interpreted as normal.[16] In patients with gangrenous bowel, plain films may reveal pneumatosis or portal venous gas. However, these findings are notoriously insensitive and late signs. Gastrointestinal contrast studies may show a corkscrew pattern or an abrupt "bird beak" at the point of obstruction, and angiography may demonstrate a spiraling pattern of the mesenteric vessels.[14] However, these modalities have largely been replaced in the evaluation of acute small bowel obstruction by computed tomography (CT), which is rapid, noninvasive, and widely available. CT findings characteristic of a closed-loop obstruction include a radial distribution of dilated bowel loops converging toward a point of torsion or a C- or U-shaped loop of horizontally oriented, fluid-filled bowel.[17] The rotation of the mesentery may generate a "whirl" sign, which is virtually pathognomonic for small bowel volvulus (Fig. 69–1). Mesenteric thickening may be present as a result of previous intermittent, incomplete volvulus. Though not specific for volvulus, small bowel wall thickening, pneumatosis, portal venous gas, and free intraperitoneal fluid suggest small bowel ischemia.

Treatment

Evidence of ischemia mandates immediate exploration and resection of the involved, gangrenous small bowel. Suspicion of volvulus clinically or radiographically should also prompt immediate exploration because of the associated risk for ischemia. In Western series, up to 50% of patients with small bowel volvulus will require resection for gangrenous small bowel.[2] The rarity of small bowel volvulus in our society may lead to a delay in diagnosis and a higher incidence of gangrenous small bowel than in Asian and African series. Overall mortality in patients undergoing exploration for small bowel volvulus ranges from 10% to 35%,[1] which is considerably higher than that for small bowel obstruction in general. These overall mortality rates are attributable to the large proportion of patients with gangrenous bowel, in whom mortality rates are between 20% and 60% in most series.[1]

For patients without ischemic bowel, the optimal treatment is less clear. No prospective, randomized

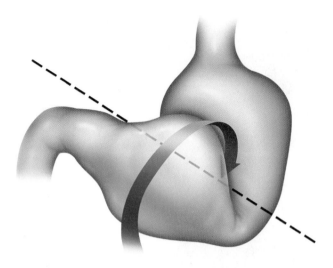

Figure 69–2. Organoaxial rotation occurs when the stomach rotates around a transverse line between the pylorus and gastroesophageal junction.

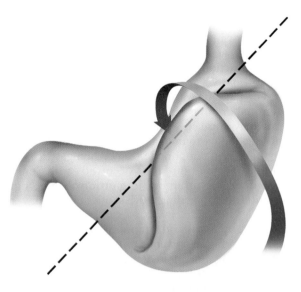

Figure 69–3. Mesenteroaxial rotation occurs when the stomach rotates around a longitudinal line parallel to the gastrohepatic omentum.

studies or even retrospective studies have addressed the issue of recurrence. Most studies describe simple detorsion without resection but rarely include long-term follow-up. The risk for recurrent volvulus is therefore not well established. Intestinopexy of a long segment of bowel is technically difficult and not recommended. In neonatal midgut volvulus caused by malrotation, intestinopexy is not routinely performed, and rates of recurrence are considered acceptably low. It is believed that the formation of intraperitoneal adhesions after laparotomy should prevent most recurrences. However, some authors have recommended resection of involved, nongangrenous intestine in order to prevent recurrent volvulus,[1] although the risk for short-gut syndrome prohibits this approach if a long segment of bowel is involved.

GASTRIC VOLVULUS

Etiology

Similar to small bowel volvulus, gastric volvulus occurs when the stomach or a portion of the stomach is rotated at least 180 degrees along its transverse or longitudinal axes. Gastric volvulus can be classified according to anatomy, etiology, or onset (acute or chronic). As defined by Singleton, organoaxial rotation is the most common (two thirds of cases) and occurs when the stomach rotates around a transverse line between the pylorus and the gastroesophageal junction (Fig. 69–2).[18] Mesenteroaxial rotation is less common (one third of cases), and the stomach rotates around a longitudinal line parallel to the gastrohepatic omentum (Fig. 69–3).

In 10% to 30% of cases the gastric volvulus is considered primary and results from laxity of the stomach's ligamentous attachments (gastrohepatic, gastrocolic, gastrolienal, and gastrophrenic).[19] Primary gastric volvulus has been seen in association with congenital asplenia

and with "wandering spleen."[20] Primary gastric volvulus is usually mesenteroaxial, with the pylorus rotating anteriorly (more common) or posteriorly from right to left.[21] Rarely, the fundus rotates around the same axis. As the stomach fills with fluid, the torsion is exacerbated. This type of volvulus is usually incomplete (less than 180 degrees) and is accompanied by chronic or intermittent symptoms.[19]

In the majority of cases, gastric volvulus is secondary to another anatomic abnormality, the most common of which is diaphragmatic hernia. Gastric volvulus is therefore commonly referred to as an intrathoracic "upside-down" stomach. Most cases of secondary gastric volvulus are organoaxial, with the greater curvature rotating up into the chest either anteriorly (more common) or posteriorly with respect to the fixed duodenum and esophagus.[19] Despite the rich blood supply of the stomach, strangulation can occur with torsion greater than 180 degrees and is much more common with organoaxial than with mesenteroaxial volvulus.[22] Paraesophageal hiatal hernia is the most common cause in adults as well as in children, whereas congenital diaphragmatic hernia (left-sided Bochdalek) is an additional common cause in children.[23] However, gastric volvulus has also been described in association with traumatic diaphragmatic hernia, diaphragmatic eventration,[24] and even Morgagni hernia.[25] Although secondary gastric volvulus is typically intrathoracic and occurs as a result of diaphragmatic hernia, secondary intra-abdominal gastric volvulus has also been reported to occur as a result of tumors[26] and after a variety of surgical procedures, including Nissen fundoplication[27] and gastric banding.[28]

Diagnosis

The clinical manifestation of acute gastric volvulus can be quite dramatic. In 1904, Borchardt described the triad of epigastric pain, retching with an inability to vomit, and difficulty or inability to pass a nasogastric tube. This triad describes acute organoaxial volvulus; the gastroesophageal junction is open in acute mesenteroaxial volvulus, and nasogastric tube placement should not be difficult. For patients with intrathoracic gastric volvulus, the abdominal findings may be minimal. Rather, the "gastrothorax" may cause chest pain, shortness of breath, and symptoms secondary to mediastinal compression, including arrhythmia and tamponade.[22,29,30] When gastric strangulation or perforation has occurred with either intra-abdominal or intrathoracic gastric volvulus, signs of gastrointestinal bleeding and septic shock may be evident.

In contrast, the signs and symptoms of chronic gastric volvulus may be vague and intermittent, or it may be an incidental finding on an imaging study. Symptoms of chronic primary gastric volvulus include upper abdominal discomfort, vomiting, early satiety, and dysphagia.[19,31] In addition to these obstructive symptoms, patients with chronic intrathoracic gastric volvulus may describe postprandial chest pain or shortness of breath. The differential diagnosis is broad and includes many much more common diseases, such as gastroesophageal reflux disease and peptic ulcer disease.

Radiographically, the diagnosis of primary gastric volvulus may be difficult to establish because the volvulus is often intermittent. Plain films may demonstrate a spherical stomach on supine views and a double air-fluid level on upright views. A retrocardiac air-fluid level on a lateral chest radiograph is highly suggestive of secondary gastric volvulus with an intrathoracic stomach. In the right clinical situation, further imaging studies may not be necessary. However, an upper gastrointestinal contrast study will confirm the diagnosis by demonstrating a contrast-filled stomach above a normally located gastroesophageal junction with narrowing at the site of the volvulus (Figs. 69–4 and 69–5).

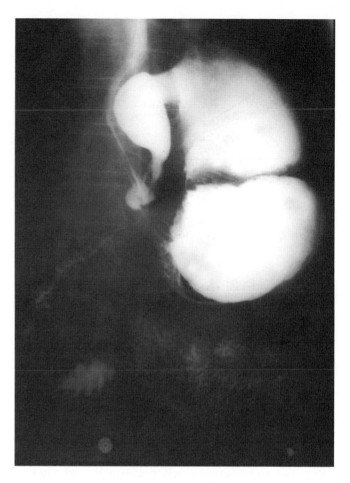

Figure 69–4. Upper gastrointestinal contrast study demonstrating a paraesophageal hernia with organoaxial volvulus. The greater curvature is intrathoracic, and the pylorus is in close proximity to the normally positioned gastroesophageal junction.

Treatment

For acute gastric volvulus, the traditional treatment is emergency laparotomy with reduction of the volvulus. Mortality rates as high as 30% to 50% have been reported for this condition, with the major cause of death being sepsis secondary to gastric strangulation.[19,22] Strangulation leads to gastric necrosis with or without perforation and requires resection by either local excision, subtotal gastrectomy, or even total gastrectomy. Other reported complications include ulceration, gastrointestinal hemorrhage, omental avulsion, splenic rupture, and pancreatic necrosis. Once the volvulus has been reduced and emergency conditions addressed, the goal of surgery is to prevent recurrence by fixing the stomach to the abdominal wall and correcting any predisposing conditions. Anterior gastropexy is easily accomplished by placement of a gastrostomy tube. The short gastric vessels should be preserved, if possible, both to retain their blood supply and to help anchor the greater curvature. In the case of gastric volvulus secondary to diaphragmatic hernia, the diaphragmatic defect should be repaired, although in septic or medically high-risk patients, reduc-

tion and gastropexy alone may be safer and sufficient, particularly in those with limited life expectancy. Otherwise, the best way to repair the diaphragmatic defect is debatable. Although retrospective data suggest that prosthetic mesh prevents recurrence, the risk for infection in the setting of gastric necrosis may be increased, and mesh should therefore be used selectively.[32]

For chronic gastric volvulus, the more important issues are whether and when to operate. It is difficult to know the percentage of patients with a diaphragmatic hernia and intrathoracic stomach who will progress to acute gastric strangulation. However, the high morbidity and mortality associated with such strangulation justify expeditious repair, even in asymptomatic patients. In contrast, chronic primary gastric volvulus is often intermittent and is much less likely to become strangulated. In the pediatric population, primary gastric volvulus has been successfully managed with nonoperative "postural" therapy and does not routinely require surgical intervention.[33]

More recently, endoscopic and laparoscopic approaches to both acute and chronic gastric volvulus have been popularized. In select cases of acute gastric

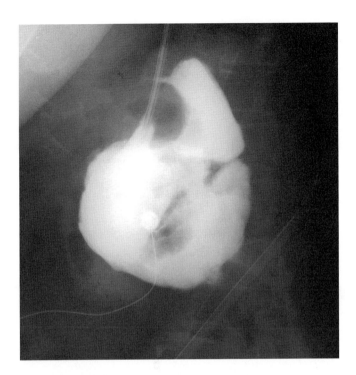

Figure 69–5. Upper gastrointestinal contrast study demonstrating a paraesophageal hernia with complete obstruction of the stomach because of volvulus. The patient was found to have gastric necrosis at exploration.

volvulus without gastric necrosis, gastric decompression—either by placement of a nasogastric tube or endoscopically—may convert an emergency to an urgent operation or even avoid an operation altogether. Endoscopic reduction of an intrathoracic stomach is relatively difficult. Various techniques have been described, including the use of two endoscopes[34] and expansion of an intragastric balloon.[35] Once the stomach has been reduced, gastropexy is relatively simple and is achieved by placement of a percutaneous endoscopic gastrostomy (PEG) tube. In the first description of endoscopic reduction, two PEG tubes were placed to help prevent recurrent volvulus.[36] Purely endoscopic techniques, however, are best reserved for high-risk patients because these techniques do not address the underlying pathology. In contrast, laparoscopic approaches[37] and combined laparoscopic and endoscopic approaches[38] have the potential to combine minimally invasive techniques with repair of the diaphragmatic defect. Although no randomized, controlled studies have been conducted, Teague et al. compared the results of open (13 patients) and laparoscopic (18 patients) repair in patients with acute or chronic gastric volvulus. Laparoscopic repair was technically difficult (three conversions to open procedures) but was safe and associated with a shorter hospital stay.[39]

SUMMARY

Small bowel volvulus and gastric volvulus are uncommon problems in this country and are often diagnosed in delayed fashion. Early recognition and treatment may help prevent the morbidity and mortality associated with small bowel and gastric ischemia.

ACKNOWLEDGMENT

The authors acknowledge William M. Thompson, MD, for providing the radiographic images of small bowel and gastric volvulus.

SUGGESTED READINGS

Iwuagwu O, Deans GT: Small bowel volvulus: A review. J R Coll Surg Edinb 44:150-155, 1999.

Teague WJ, Ackroyd R, Watson DI, Devitt PG: Changing patterns in the management of gastric volvulus over 14 years. Br J Surg 87:358-361, 2000.

Wasselle JA, Norman J: Acute gastric volvulus: Pathogenesis, diagnosis, and treatment. Am J Gastroenterol 88:1780-1784, 1993.

REFERENCES

1. Iwuagwu O, Deans GT: Small bowel volvulus: A review. J R Coll Surg Edinb 44:150-155, 1999.
2. Roggo A, Ottinger LW: Acute small bowel volvulus in adults. A sporadic form of strangulating intestinal obstruction. Ann Surg 216:135-141, 1992.
3. Frazee RC, Mucha P Jr, Farnell MB, et al: Volvulus of the small intestine. Ann Surg 208:565-568, 1988.
4. Welch GH, Anderson JR: Volvulus of the small intestine in adults. World J Surg 10:496-500, 1986.
5. Ghebrat K: Trend of small intestinal volvulus in northwestern Ethiopia. East Afr Med J 75:549-552, 1998.
6. Tegegne A: Small intestinal volvulus in adults of Gonder Region, northwestern Ethiopia. Ethiop Med J 30:111-117, 1992.
7. Gulati SM, Grover NK, Tagore NK, et al: Volvulus of the small intestine in India. Am J Surg 126:661-664, 1973.
8. Duke JH Jr, Yar MS: Primary small bowel volvulus: Cause and management. Arch Surg 112:685-688, 1977.
9. De Souza LJ: Volvulus of the small bowel. BMJ 1:1055-1056, 1955.
10. Kersting HW, Jahne J, Mai P: [Volvulus of the small intestine, a rare complication during laxative period before colonoscopy.] Dtsch Med Wochenschr 129:2711-2713, 2004.
11. Vaez-Zadeh K, Dutz W, Nowrooz-Zadeh M: Volvulus of the small intestine in adults: A study of predisposing factors. Ann Surg 169:265-271, 1969.
12. Catalano OA, Bencivenga A, Abbate M, et al: Internal hernia with volvulus and intussusception: Case report. Abdom Imaging 29:164-165, 2004.
13. Bissen L, Brasseur P, Sukkarieh F, et al: [Jejunal lipomatosis with intussusception and volvulus. A case report.] J Radiol 85:128-130, 2004.
14. Qayyum A, Cowling MG, Adam EJ: Small bowel volvulus related to a calcified mesenteric lymph node. Clin Radiol 55:483-485, 2000.
15. Wax JR, Christie TL: Complete small-bowel volvulus complicating the second trimester. Obstet Gynecol 82(Suppl):689-691, 1993.
16. Izes BA, Scholz FJ, Munson JL: Midgut volvulus in an elderly patient. Gastrointest Radiol 17:102-104, 1992.
17. Balthazar EJ, George W: Holmes Lecture. CT of small-bowel obstruction. AJR Am J Roentgenol 162:255-261, 1994.
18. Singleton AC: Chronic gastric volvulus. Radiology 34:53-61, 1940.
19. Wasselle JA, Norman J: Acute gastric volvulus: Pathogenesis, diagnosis, and treatment. Am J Gastroenterol 88:1780-1784, 1993.
20. Uc A, Kao SC, Sanders KD, et al: Gastric volvulus and wandering spleen. Am J Gastroenterol 93:1146-1148, 1998.

21. Ratan SK, Grover SB: Acute idiopathic mesenteroaxial gastric volvulus in a child. Trop Gastroenterol 21:133-134, 2000.
22. Carter R, Brewer LA 3rd, Hinshaw DB: Acute gastric volvulus. A study of 25 cases. Am J Surg 140:99-106, 1980.
23. Cameron AE, Howard ER: Gastric volvulus in childhood. J Pediatr Surg 22:944-947, 1987.
24. Oh A, Gulati G, Sherman ML, et al: Bilateral eventration of the diaphragm with perforated gastric volvulus in an adolescent. J Pediatr Surg 35:1824-1826, 1998.
25. Estevao-Costa J, Soares-Oliveira M, Correia-Pinto J, et al: Acute gastric volvulus secondary to a Morgagni hernia. Pediatr Surg Int 16:107-108, 2000.
26. Deevaguntla CR, Prabhakar B, Prasad GR, et al: Gastric leiomyoma presenting as gastric volvulus. Indian J Gastroenterol 22:230-231, 2003.
27. Baty V, Rocca P, Fontaumard E: Acute gastric volvulus related to adhesions after laparoscopic fundoplication. Surg Endosc 16:538, 2002.
28. Bortul M, Scaramucci M, Tonello C, et al: Gastric wall necrosis from organo-axial volvulus as a late complication of laparoscopic gastric banding. Obes Surg 14:285-287, 2004.
29. Shriki JE, Nguyen K, Rozo JC, et al: Rare chronic gastric volvulus associated with left atrial and mediastinal compression. Tex Heart Inst J 29:324-328, 2002.
30. Wolfgang R, Lee JG: Endoscopic treatment of acute gastric volvulus causing cardiac tamponade. J Clin Gastroenterol 32:336-339, 2001.
31. Cozart JC, Clouse RE: Gastric volvulus as a cause of intermittent dysphagia. Dig Dis Sci 43:1057-1060, 1998.
32. Targarona EM, Bendahan G, Balague C, et al: Mesh in the hiatus: A controversial issue. Arch Surg 139:1286-1296, 2004.
33. Elhalaby EA, Mashaly EM: Infants with radiologic diagnosis of gastric volvulus: Are they over-treated? Pediatr Surg Int 17:596-600, 2001.
34. Januschowski R: Endoscopic repositioning of the upside-down stomach and its fixation by percutaneous endoscopic gastrostomy. Dtsch Med Wochenschr 121:1261-1264, 1996.
35. Tabo T, Hayashi H, Umeyama S, et al: Balloon repositioning of intrathoracic upside-down stomach and fixation by percutaneous endoscopic gastrostomy. J Am Coll Surg 197:868-871, 2003.
36. Ghosh S, Palmer KR: Double percutaneous endoscopic gastrostomy fixation: An effective treatment for recurrent gastric volvulus. Am J Gastroenterol 88:1271-1272, 1993.
37. Katkhouda N, Mavor E, Achanta K, et al: Laparoscopic repair of chronic intrathoracic gastric volvulus. Surgery 128:784-790, 2000.
38. Beqiri A, VanderKolk WE, Scheeres D: Combined endoscopic and laparoscopic management of chronic gastric volvulus. Gastrointest Endosc 46:450-452, 1997.
39. Teague WJ, Ackroyd R, Watson DI, et al: Changing patterns in the management of gastric volvulus over 14 years. Br J Surg 87:358-361, 2000.

Crohn's Disease: General Considerations, Medical Management, and Surgical Treatment of Small Intestinal Disease

D. Wayne Overby ▪ Mark J. Koruda

GENERAL CONSIDERATIONS, MEDICAL THERAPY

Crohn's disease is a transmural inflammatory disease that can involve any part of the gastrointestinal tract from the mouth to the anus. Despite the large body of published literature and ongoing study dedicated to Crohn's disease, it remains an incurable disease of unknown etiology. Clinicians are faced with the difficulty of diagnosing and treating patients with a heterogeneous disease that has an array of features and manifestations.

Epidemiology

Wide variations in the incidence and prevalence of Crohn's disease have been reported. These differences may be due to diagnostic variations compounded by variations in reporting, or they may be due to real differences in genetic and environmental factors among geographically distinct populations.[1] Interestingly, these differences seem to follow political borders rather than natural boundaries. There have been studies showing increasing incidence at greater latitudes, but these results have not been universally observed.[1,2] Differences related to socioeconomic status have also been reported, with increasing affluence imparting increased risk, but this association has not been borne out in more recent studies. Moreover, it is useful to remember that with differences in affluence come differences in diet, hygiene, and population density,[2] all of which are the essence of cultural westernization.

The prevalence of Crohn's disease in North America has been estimated to be 26.0 to 198.5 cases per 100,000 people (recently, 144 to 198 cases per 100,000). Given the prevalence reported in the two most recent studies and given a population estimated to be 300 million, there are 400,000 to 600,000 cases of Crohn's disease in North America. Recent studies have demonstrated higher prevalence rates with relatively stable rates of incidence, thus suggesting that patients may be living longer with the disease. The incidence of Crohn's disease in recent studies has varied from 3.1 to 14.6 cases per 100,000 person-years. Again assuming a population of 300 million, Crohn's disease is diagnosed in 9000 to 44,000 people in North America yearly. There appears to be a slight female preponderance, with female prevalence ranging from 50% to 60% in most studies. The mean age at diagnosis in most North American cohorts is between 33 and 39 years, with the disease being diagnosed in the majority of patients in their second or third decade of life; a second peak was found in the sixth or seventh decade in roughly half of cohorts, which has given rise to the idea of bimodal distribution of disease with regard to age.[1] The second peak may be due to differences in environment leading to differences in disease expression or variations in diagnosis, or it may in fact represent a delay in diagnosis as the disease relapses.[1,2]

Natural History

The severity of disease observed in any group of patients with Crohn's disease will exist on a continuum from asymptomatic, to medical or surgical remission, to mild, moderate, or severe disease. There are European and North American cohorts that are probably the best-studied populations outside specialty referral centers. These studies indicate that among patients in their first year after diagnosis, 80% had high disease activity, 15% had low activity, and 5% were in remission.[3] At any point in time after the first year, examination of a group of patients with Crohn's disease will find a majority (approximately 65%) in remission, with another 25% experiencing low activity and 10% experiencing high activity; 13% will have chronically active disease. About 43% of cohort patients required steroids during the course of their disease, whereas 10% of patients in any given year required steroids and 30% of patients in any given year required sulfasalazine or 5-aminosalicylate products. Up to 57% of patients required at least one surgical resection. In most patients, Crohn's disease has a relapsing and remitting course, with relatively small numbers of patients experiencing prolonged remission or unremitting disease.[1] Mortality in patients with Crohn's disease is slightly increased in cohort studies with long-term follow-up; the absolute difference in survival at 20 years was 6% to 7%.[4-6] The most unfortunate aspect of Crohn's disease may be that it strikes the majority of patients in the prime of their lives, which increases the potential for early long-term or permanent disability, so aside from direct medical costs, there are indirect costs associated with decreased productivity.[7]

Risk Factors and Pathogenesis

Respected authors bemoan the lack of knowledge regarding the underlying causes of Crohn's disease. It is generally accepted that a combination of environmental and genetic factors are at work to produce altered mucosal integrity of the gastrointestinal tract and complex alterations in local and systemic immune response.

Environmental Factors

A number of environmental factors have been implicated in Crohn's disease, including microorganisms of both infectious and commensal varieties; smoking; various components of diet; medications, including antibiotics, nonsteroidal anti-inflammatory drugs, and oral contraceptives; and hygienic factors, with increasing hygiene imparting increased risk. It is generally accepted that cigarette smoking, though not a cause, makes Crohn's disease worse, but no other single environmental factor or combination of environmental factors has been convincingly implicated as causative. One widely held hypothesis suggests that Crohn's disease is manifested when genetically predisposed individuals are exposed to an environmental trigger or triggers.[8-11]

Genetic Factors

As for genetic predisposition, it has long been known that there exist familial aggregations of inflammatory bowel disease. The finding that disease concordance is much higher in monozygotic twins (44%) than dizygotic twins (3.8%)[12] adds weight to the argument that genetics plays a significant role in the development of inflammatory bowel disease while at the same time suggesting a potentially complex relationship between environmental factors, genetic susceptibility, and incomplete phenotypic penetrance.[13] Recent studies using DNA screening and linkage analysis of members in affected kindreds have identified nine genetic susceptibility loci for inflammatory bowel disease (IBD1 to IBD9). Mapping of the IBD loci led to the identification of a gene that increases susceptibility to Crohn's disease.[14]

Variants of a gene in the IBD1 locus (16q12), which was named NOD2 on discovery and later renamed CARD15 (for caspase activation and recruitment domain), cause susceptibility to ileal Crohn's disease; CARD15 polymorphisms are not linked to ulcerative colitis. The CARD15 gene product and the pathway in which it is involved have been studied extensively. After stimulation with lipopolysaccharide or proinflammatory cytokines such as tumor necrosis factor-α (TNF-α), the CARD15 gene is expressed in cells such as monocytes, macrophages, dendritic cells, and small intestinal Paneth cells (Paneth cells are most numerous in the terminal ileum). The CARD15 gene product is a cytoplasmic protein that probably acts as a pattern recognition receptor for a breakdown product of the peptidoglycan that is a cell wall component of gram-negative and gram-positive bacteria; the proteolysis occurs in phagocytes and the resulting substance is called muramyl dipeptide. Muramyl dipeptides are subsequently transported into the cytoplasm of cells, where they bind to the CARD15 protein, which in turn activates a signaling cascade that leads to translocation of nuclear factor κB (NF-κB) into the nucleus. Translocation is followed by activation of NF-κB responsive genes, which leads to the production of proinflammatory cytokines. In this way, CARD15 is a part of the innate immune system. It may be that the CARD15 polymorphisms found in patients with Crohn's disease lead to decreased cellular apoptosis, which could in turn cause the overexpression of NF-κB that is seen in Crohn's lesions. Although CARD15 variants increase susceptibility to Crohn's disease, the relationship is complex and not fully understood.[12-14]

The three common mutations that account for 82% of mutated alleles of the CARD15 gene can be found in up to 50% of patients with Crohn's disease, but they can also be found in 20% of normal individuals, so CARD15 mutations are neither necessary nor sufficient for expression of the disease; CARD15 variants account for only 20% of the genetic susceptibility to Crohn's disease in white individuals, whereas CARD15 variants are absent in Asian and sub-Saharan African populations. However, when compared with normal individuals, the odds ratio for the development of Crohn's disease in heterozygous carriers is 2 to 3, and for homozygous carriers it is 20 to 40. Questions about the benefit of genetic screening of

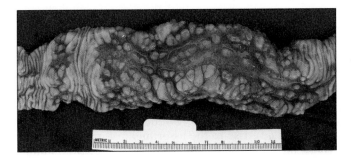

Figure 70–1. Segmental resection of small bowel showing cobblestoning ulceration in Crohn's disease. (From Hart J: Non-neoplastic diseases of the small and large intestine. In Silverberg SG, DeLellis RA, Frable WJ, et al [eds]: Silverberg's Principles and Practice of Surgical Pathology and Cytopathology, vol 2, 4th ed. Edinburgh, Churchill Livingstone, 2006, p 1391.)

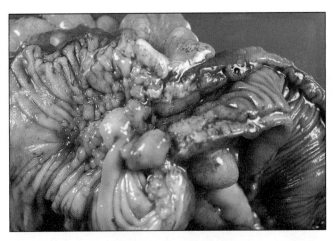

Figure 70–2. Crohn's ileitis with formation of a short stricture. (From Hart J: Non-neoplastic diseases of the small and large intestine. In Silverberg SG, DeLellis RA, Frable WJ, et al [eds]: Silverberg's Principles and Practice of Surgical Pathology and Cytopathology, vol 2, 4th ed. Edinburgh, Churchill Livingstone, 2006, p 1390.)

the general population or family members of carriers are sure to arise; detailed answers to such questions are beyond the scope of this text, but the bottom line answer is that there is no benefit.[13,14] For a more detailed understanding of the current work regarding genetic susceptibility to Crohn's disease, the authors recommend reading the references cited for this section.

Pathology

Crohn's disease is a transmural inflammatory disease with discontinuous lesions that can involve any part of the gastrointestinal tract from the mouth to the anus, but most commonly it involves the ileocecal region. The relapsing and remitting course of Crohn's disease is marked by pathologic changes that are manifested in the clinical course; as the disease flares and abates, the gross and microscopic findings change.

Gross Features

The active phase of the disease is marked initially by the formation of aphthous ulcers that can involve any part the gastrointestinal tract mucosa. The ulcers are small, flat, and soft with a whitish center and red border. As the inflammation continues, the ulcers deepen; eventually they become transmural, and in turn they may lead to deep fissures that can cause abscess formation, fistulization, and in rare cases, free perforation as penetration occurs. The ulcers are scattered at first, but as they progress, they coalesce; the islands of normal mucosa that remain give the mucosal surface a cobblestone appearance (Fig. 70–1). When the involved organ is intestine, continued inflammation causes thickening of the bowel wall with narrowing of the lumen, concomitant thickening of the adjacent mesentery, and wrapping of the outer surface by fat that creeps from the mesentery. The mesenteric involvement includes engorged lymphatic channels and enlarged lymph nodes. As the disease abates and heals, fibrosis and stricture of previously inflamed areas can occur (Fig. 70–2).[8,15,16]

Anatomically, the disease is discontinuous and segmental, which has given rise to the descriptive term *skip lesions;* 29% of patients have disease confined to the small intestine, in 27% it is confined to the colon, and 41% have disease involving both the colon and small intestine, so overall, 70% of patients with Crohn's disease have small bowel involvement.[17] Although the exact incidence and prevalence of upper gastrointestinal Crohn's disease is not known and such involvement is historically rare, it is thought that improvements in diagnostic techniques have led to an increasing incidence in recent reports. Careful examination and biopsy of the upper gastrointestinal tract in patients with known distal disease will reveal histologic evidence of proximal Crohn's disease in a significant number (in as many as 30% to 50% of patients in recent studies), although many will lack upper gastrointestinal symptoms. Upper gastrointestinal Crohn's disease has been most frequently found in the gastric antrum and duodenum, with only rare involvement of the esophagus and remainder of the stomach.[18]

Microscopic Features

The microscopic pathologic changes begin as inflammatory cells, including lymphocytes, macrophages, and neutrophils, aggregate; in the intestine, such aggregations are associated with intestinal crypts. These cellular aggregations represent microabscesses that underlie the superficially appearing aphthous ulcers and penetrate to form fissures (Fig. 70–3). Continued influx of inflammatory cells may lead to noncaseating granulomas with multinucleated giant cells, which is the lesion that is essentially pathognomonic for Crohn's disease (Fig. 70–4). However, the reported incidence of these granulomas varies widely, and they are absent in 50% or more of Crohn's patients, which means that finding granulomas

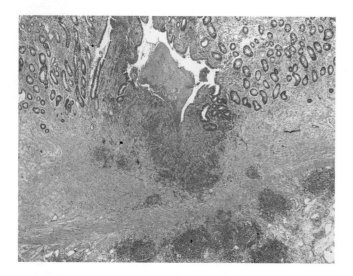

Figure 70–3. Fissuring ulceration extending into the submucosa with associated abundant chronic inflammation. This is a characteristic lesion of Crohn's disease and can progress to form a fistula (ileal resection, hematoxylin-eosin stain). (From Dilworth HP, Montgomery E, Iacobuzio-Donahue CA: Non-neoplastic and inflammatory disorders of the small intestine. In Iacobuzio-Donahue CA, Montgomery E [eds]: Gastrointestinal and Liver Pathology. Philadelphia, Churchill Livingstone, 2005, p 172.)

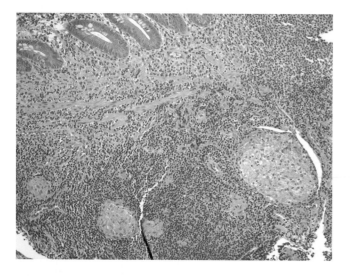

Figure 70–4. Multiple submucosal granulomas *(bottom)* embedded in a large lymphoid aggregate (ileal biopsy, hematoxylin-eosin stain). (From Dilworth HP, Montgomery E, Iacobuzio-Donahue CA: Non-neoplastic and inflammatory disorders of the small intestine. In Iacobuzio-Donahue CA, Montgomery E [eds]: Gastrointestinal and Liver Pathology. Philadelphia, Churchill Livingstone, 2005, p 170.)

helps rule the disease in but the absence of granulomas does not rule the disease out.[15,16,19]

Clinical Features

The variability that is evident in every aspect of Crohn's disease underlies the heterogeneity of its findings. The nature, location, and extensiveness of the gastrointestinal lesions give rise to the assortment of gastrointestinal symptoms while dictating the disease's severity and clinical course. Extraintestinal manifestations are a frequent accompaniment of the gastrointestinal disease.

Classification of Crohn's Disease

As it becomes obvious that Crohn's patients are a heterogeneous group, it follows that different subgroups will manifest their disease in different ways; these variations in the natural history and clinical features among subgroups will affect a clinician's interpretation of a patient's prognosis and the treatment decisions. In addition to aiding clinicians, a better understanding of the variables that create the different subgroups may lay the groundwork for understanding the relationship between the environmental and genetic factors that underlie Crohn's disease.[20] Attempts to develop a reasonably simple and objective method for categorizing patients with Crohn's disease led to the Vienna classification system, which groups patients on the basis of age (<40 or ≥40), disease location (terminal ileum, colon, ileocolon, upper gastrointestinal), and disease behavior (inflammatory, stricturing, penetrating).[21] Recent studies that used the Vienna classification system to examine Crohn's disease in a variety of settings have provided significant insight into its clinical findings.

Manifestations

Crohn's disease will be diagnosed in the majority of patients, on the order of 70%, within a year of becoming symptomatic; however, the time between symptom onset and diagnosis can be much longer, with 14% of patients having at least 5 years between symptom onset and diagnosis. Patients who are older at diagnosis tend to have a longer time between the onset of symptoms and diagnosis of their disease. Time to diagnosis will typically be shorter in younger patients, and there tends to be a higher proportion of patients with a young age at disease onset in referral centers.[22] As stated earlier, almost all patients (95%) will have active disease during the first year after diagnosis, whereas only 35% of patients will have active disease in any following year.[3] There are differences reported in the initial location of disease, although studies agree that the greatest proportion of patients will have disease involving the small intestine or a combination of the small and large intestine at diagnosis.[22,23] In a substantial number of patients (85%) the location of the diseased segment will be the most stable aspect of Crohn's disease over time; inflammation will tend to extend and regress within the involved segment and does not usually extend to other segments.[23] Most patients will have strictly inflammatory versus stricturing or penetrating disease,[23,24] although referral centers, which tend to see more complicated disease at initial contact, will have a greater proportion of patients with stricturing and penetrating disease at diagnosis.[22] In sharp contrast to anatomic location, which tends to remain stable over time, disease behavior in an individual patient tends to progress over time, with the majority of patients who initially have strictly inflammatory disease progressing to stricturing or penetrating disease over the course of their illness.[23,24] Studies have found that the initial location of disease correlates with later disease behavior; isolated small bowel disease is more likely to be associated with strictures, colonic and ileocolonic disease is more likely to be associated with penetration,[23-25] and in long-term (20 years) follow-up, complications develop in 94% of patients with terminal ileal disease versus 78% of patients with colonic disease.[24]

With the aforementioned findings in mind, there is a logical progression to the typical gastrointestinal and extraintestinal manifestations of Crohn's disease.

- Abdominal pain—The abdominal pain experienced by patients with Crohn's disease is usually obstructive in nature, which gives rise to intermittent, crampy pain. It is caused by the narrowing of the lumen of the gastrointestinal tract, usually small bowel, that develops as segments become inflamed and eventually stricture. It occurs as an initial symptom with similar frequency (approximately 60% to 70% of patients) across age groups and genders.[26-28]
- Diarrhea—Diarrhea may be caused by decreased absorption in inflamed segments; in particular, decreased absorption of bile acids and steatorrhea may be an underlying cause in patients with terminal ileal disease. Resection of the terminal ileum and ileocecal valve may be causative in surgically treated patients. As an initial symptom, it occurs with a frequency similar to abdominal pain (roughly 60% to 70% of patients).[26-28]
- Bleeding—Bleeding is not a constant feature of Crohn's disease, but it may still be the initial symptom in a significant number of patients (23.5% in one large series). The bleeding may be slight and detectable only with Hemoccult testing. Severe acute hemorrhage is rare (0.9% to 6%); in most studies it is more common in patients with colonic involvement, although it may emanate from any part of the gastrointestinal tract from the upper to the lower, which is why localization of the bleeding will be of extreme importance in treatment.[29,30]
- Weight loss—Weight loss and malnutrition obviously follow on the heels of abdominal pain, obstruction, and malabsorption. It is a part of the initial symptom complex in about 25% to 30% of adults. It is, significantly, almost twice as frequent in children.[26-28] The specifics of malnutrition in patients with Crohn's disease are covered later in the chapter.
- Fever—Fever may be due to ongoing inflammation of diseased segments, dysregulation of systemic immunity, or infection secondary to penetrating disease. It occurs as an initial symptom in approximately 15% of patients.[27,28]

- Fatigue/malaise—Malaise is probably caused by both malnutrition and dysregulation of the immune system, which changes the balance of immune cells and the inflammatory mediators that they release. It occurs in roughly 10% to 15% of patients.[27,28]
- Perianal disease—Although this chapter is focused on upper gastrointestinal and small bowel Crohn's disease, it is worth mentioning that perianal disease is frequently (about 10% of the time[27,28]) a part of the initial symptom complex, and in some (in as many as 5% of patients) it will be the sole indicator of Crohn's disease.[31]
- Extraintestinal manifestations—There are a number of chronic inflammatory disorders of unknown etiology that are diagnosed in patients with inflammatory bowel disease so frequently (in up to 50% of patients in some studies) that they are considered to be extraintestinal manifestations of the disease. Of those found in Crohn's disease, the most common are iritis/uveitis (0% to 6.4%), primary sclerosing cholangitis (0.4% to 1.2%), ankylosing spondylitis (excluding asymptomatic sacroiliitis, 1.2% to 8%), peripheral arthritis (12.8% to 23%), pyoderma gangrenosum (0.6% to 1.2%), and erythema nodosum (1.9% to 7.2%). There is some disagreement among recent studies regarding the overall (from 6% to 40%) and individual incidence of these disorders, which is due at least in part to different study populations and study methodologies. Many studies do attempt to separate and compare the rates of occurrence of the various extraintestinal manifestations of Crohn's disease versus ulcerative colitis, and the most constant difference is a higher rate of primary sclerosing cholangitis in ulcerative colitis than in Crohn's disease.[32-34]

Laboratory Findings

Traditionally, the diagnosis of inflammatory bowel disease has relied on clinical, endoscopic, histopathologic, and radiologic findings. Although it is true that the etiology and pathophysiology of inflammatory bowel diseases remain incompletely solved mysteries, it is becoming clear that a dysregulated immune response develops in genetically predisposed individuals exposed to one or more environmental factors. It is reasonable to expect quantifiable evidence of this dysregulation in the form of clinical laboratory abnormalities that are both generalized with respect to inflammation, such as leukocytosis, and specific to inflammatory bowel disease, such as the formation of unique serum antibodies that can be measured as markers in serologic tests.[35]

Nonspecific measures of inflammation include an elevated white blood cell count, platelet count, erythrocyte sedimentation rate, and C-reactive protein. Although these findings usually correlate with increased Crohn's disease activity,[36] their usefulness is limited, both in initial diagnosis and in monitoring of disease activity, because of their lack of specificity.

A number of antibodies to both self and non-self proteins that occur in patients with inflammatory bowel disease have been identified. The best studied antibodies by far are perinuclear antineutrophil cytoplasmic antibodies (pANCAs), which are found primarily in patients with ulcerative colitis (48% to 82% of patients) and less frequently in patients with Crohn's disease (5% to 20% of patients), and anti–*Saccharomyces cerevisiae* antibodies (ASCAs), which are found primarily in patients with Crohn's disease (48% to 69% of patients) and less frequently in patients with ulcerative colitis (5% to 15% of patients). A number of other antibodies have received attention, including antibodies to outer membrane porin C (anti-OmpC), which are antibodies to the *Escherichia coli* cell wall protein and are found in patients with Crohn's disease; antibodies to I2, which are antibodies to an antigen derived from the DNA of *Pseudomonas fluorescens* and are found inside macrophages from the intestinal mucosa of patients with Crohn's disease; and antibodies to pancreatic antigens, which are found in patients with Crohn's disease. To date, a single serologic test that discriminates patients with inflammatory bowel disease from those without it or that discriminates patients with Crohn's disease from those with ulcerative colitis and does so with high sensitivity and specificity has not been found.[35] There is evidence that using panels of serologic tests, for instance, combining pANCA plus ASCA or combining pANCA, ASCA, and anti-OmpC, will increase their specificity, but at the expense of decreased sensitivity. The specificity and sensitivity for diagnosing Crohn's disease and ulcerative colitis in adults when pANCA and ASCA are combined are on the order of 95% and 50%, respectively.[35,37-39] Studies of the utility of serologic testing in patients with inflammatory bowel disease are ongoing, and the degree of utility will probably be a moving target for years to come as new antigens are identified and compared with or combined with tests for other antigens and validated.

In addition to their potential usefulness in diagnostic testing, investigations that identify antibodies unique to patients with inflammatory bowel disease may lead to a better understanding of the underlying causes of the disease or to better immunomodulatory treatments directed more specifically at points of immune system dysregulation. Serologic testing has the potential to identify patients who are susceptible to the development of inflammatory bowel disease, to identify subgroups of patients who will have more or less aggressive forms of disease, and to predict or monitor response to therapy.[35,38] For a more detailed understanding of serologic testing in inflammatory bowel disease, the authors recommend reading the references cited for this section.

Radiographic Imaging

Gastrointestinal imaging continues to evolve on all fronts, including imaging of the small intestine. Various forms of contrast-enhanced axial imaging using computed tomography (CT) and magnetic resonance imaging (MRI) vie with better techniques in ultrasound to improve on the results that can be obtained with conventional barium studies of the small intestine. In the future, some combination of these modalities may eventually supplant barium studies of the small intestine for

the diagnosis of small bowel Crohn's disease in much the same way that push endoscopy has largely replaced barium studies for evaluation of the mucosa of the upper and lower gastrointestinal tract.

All endoscopic and radiographic imaging studies used in Crohn's disease attempt, with varying degrees of effectiveness, to accomplish one or more of the following goals: confirm the diagnosis; localize lesions while gauging their extent, severity, and degree of inflammatory activity; identify the presence of extraintestinal manifestations; and ultimately aid in medical and surgical decision making.[40]

Small Bowel Follow-Through and Enteroclysis

In many clinical situations, push endoscopy has replaced barium studies as the preferred method for evaluating the mucosa of the upper gastrointestinal tract and colon.[41] On the other hand, "conventional" radiographic studies using intraluminal contrast agents, either small bowel follow-through or small bowel enteroclysis (also known as small bowel enema), are still considered to be first-line studies for the evaluation of small bowel disease in general and Crohn's disease in particular.[42-45] Small bowel follow-through is performed after the oral administration of barium; the protocol for the examination is variable between operators and institutions, with some performing a few plain radiographs and others performing extensive fluoroscopic evaluations with multiple compression views to separate bowel loops in order to provide detailed anatomic information and assessment of motility. Enteroclysis is performed by introducing the barium suspension directly into the small intestine via a tube; when compared with small bowel follow-through, the technique for enteroclysis is more uniform between operators.[44,46] There is still debate about which conventional radiographic method is best when evaluating the small bowel to make or exclude the diagnosis of Crohn's disease, and there is literature to support both views; it is likely that the aforementioned operator and institutional variability accounts for some of the perceived difference and that preferences reflect local demands by clinicians and available expertise.[41] Although enteroclysis does not evaluate gastroduodenal disease and is considered to be more uncomfortable for the patient, it is generally accepted that it produces superior small bowel images with better mucosal detail.[42,46] That being said, a detailed, fluoroscopy-based small bowel follow-through, augmented to demonstrate the distal ileum if necessary, is adequate for the initial assessment of small bowel Crohn's disease. The sensitivity and specificity of small bowel enteroclysis for the diagnosis of Crohn's disease have been reported to be 93% to 100% and 97% to 98%, respectively.[41]

A number of possible radiologic findings can be seen on small bowel follow-through and enteroclysis in patients with Crohn's disease; given the heterogeneity of the disease, it follows that these findings can appear in combination and can vary significantly from patient to patient. Imaging of the terminal ileum is of particular importance because many patients have disease involving this part of the gastrointestinal tract and disease may be limited to the terminal ileum on initial evaluation. Findings seen on small bowel follow-through and enteroclysis (Figs. 70–5 and 70–6) include discrete ulcers, fissures or longitudinal ulcers, fistulas and sinus tracts, cobblestoning, thickened and distorted mucosal folds, wall thickening; enlargement of the ileocecal valve, short or long and single or multiple areas of luminal narrowing with pre-stenotic dilation, and skip lesions, which are areas of diseased bowel interspersed with areas of normal bowel or asymmetric involvement of a portion of bowel.[44]

Cross-Sectional Imaging in Crohn's Disease

Traditional push endoscopy, which is increasingly being supplemented with capsule endoscopy, and barium studies are currently the preferred methods for diagnosing the more subtle mucosal lesions associated with early Crohn's disease. However, when evaluating the transmural, extramural, or extraintestinal extent of disease, cross-sectional imaging, CT for the majority of providers and MRI for a growing number, has distinct advantages over intraluminal imaging modalities and can compensate for the limitations of conventional imaging. Moreover, as cross-sectional imaging technology continues to improve with faster image acquisition times and increased resolution, its role in imaging of Crohn's disease will probably grow.[40] In a comparison of spiral CT and conventional enteroclysis, the sensitivity and specificity of CT for the diagnosis of Crohn's disease were reported to be 94% and 95%, respectively, versus 96% and 98% for enteroclysis.[47] MRI has a similar profile. Both MRI and CT are probably less sensitive than conventional radiographic studies for early lesions.[40]

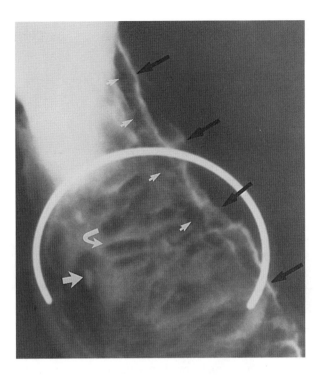

Figure 70–5. This image of the terminal ileum contains a long mesenteric border ulcer *(black arrows)* with a radiolucent line along its luminal aspect *(small white arrows)*. Interrupted, thickened folds *(curved arrow)* are present. Aphthoid ulcers have enlarged and deepened *(large white arrow)*. (From Herlinger H, Caroline DF: Crohn's disease of the small bowel. In Gore RM, Levine MS [eds]: Textbook of Gastrointestinal Radiology, vol 1, 2nd ed. Philadelphia, WB Saunders, 2000, p 732.)

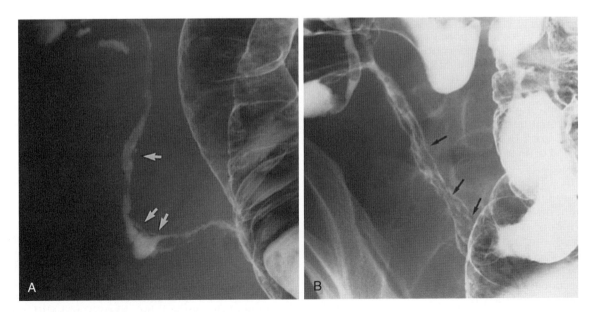

Figure 70–6. Narrowed terminal ileum in active Crohn's disease. **A,** There is marked narrowing of the terminal ileum with probable tiny ulcers *(arrows)*. **B,** Enteroclysis in double contrast widens the lumen to reveal an extensively fissured stenotic stage of advanced Crohn's disease *(arrows)*. (From Herlinger H, Caroline DF: Crohn's disease of the small bowel. In Gore RM, Levine MS [eds]: Textbook of Gastrointestinal Radiology, vol 1, 2nd ed. Philadelphia, WB Saunders, 2000, p 735.)

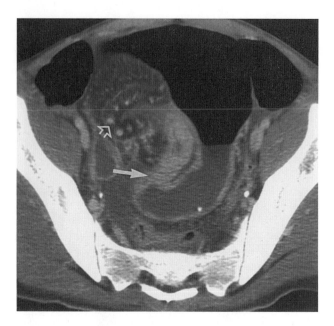

Figure 70–7. High-grade obstruction as a result of Crohn's disease. Computed tomography demonstrates a grossly dilated, gas-filled small bowel proximal to a narrowed, thick-walled, enhancing segment of Crohn's disease *(solid arrow)* that was causing obstruction. Dilated vessels are seen in the mesentery *(open arrow)*. (From Herlinger H, Caroline DF: Crohn's disease of the small bowel. In Gore RM, Levine MS [eds]: Textbook of Gastrointestinal Radiology, vol 1, 2nd ed. Philadelphia, WB Saunders, 2000, p 737.)

When using CT and MRI for Crohn's disease, a combination of intravascular and intraluminal contrast is generally used. The intraluminal contrast may be positive (high attenuation, e.g., diatrizoate meglumine [Gastrografin] in CT, iso-osmolar polyethylene glycol solution in MRI) or negative (low attenuation, e.g., methylcellulose in CT, dilute barium in MRI); the lumen must be clean and fully distended with contrast because undistended bowel loops can mimic abscesses, masses, enlarged lymph nodes, or a segment with wall thickening. Full luminal distention requires a large volume of contrast (1.5 to 2 L or more) given relatively rapidly (over a period of 45 to 90 minutes); it can be given orally or via a nasogastric/jejunal tube. Motion artifacts can be problematic, so antiperistaltic agents may be given before scanning, particularly with MRI. In addition, rapid distention with large volumes of intraluminal contrast can induce reflex atony, and faster multidetector scanners allow the acquisition of images during a single breath hold. Please see referenced material for descriptions of CT and MRI scanning protocols.[40,48]

Cross-sectional images (Figs. 70–7 and 70–8) should be analyzed for the following[40,49]:

- Length of involved segments.
- Skip lesions.
- Wall thickening—Normal wall thickness is 1 to 2 mm for distended small intestine and 3 mm for colon.

Bowel wall thickness exceeding 4 to 5 mm is considered abnormal. Bowel wall thickening is the most consistent feature of Crohn's disease on cross-sectional imaging. Adequate distention with intraluminal contrast is a necessity.

- Degree of enhancement and patterns of attenuation—After the administration of intravenous contrast, active lesions have increased enhancement, which is a marker of inflammation; alternating layers of mural enhancement and attenuation (double-halo or target sign) can also be seen in active lesions.
- Stenosis and pre-stenotic lesions—The small bowel lumen is normally 2.5 cm in diameter; luminal dilation proximal to areas of stenosis and luminal narrowing is easily identified on cross-sectional imaging. Adequate distention with intraluminal contrast is required because inadequate contrast beyond stenotic lesions may lead to underestimation of more distal disease.
- Abscess and fistula—A phlegmon or abscess is easily identified on cross-sectional imaging; however, CT and MRI are less sensitive in identifying fistulas and sinus tracts than conventional enteroclysis is.
- Fibrofatty proliferation—Also known as creeping mesenteric fat, it is seen adjacent to involved bowel segments as slightly increased attenuation on CT and slightly decreased attenuation on MRI.
- Increased vascularity of the vasa recta (comb sign).
- Mesenteric adenopathy—Abnormally large mesenteric lymph nodes from 3 to 8 mm can be identified; nodes larger than 10 mm should increase suspicion for carcinoma and lymphoma.
- Early-stage lesions—Small aphthous ulcers, subtle distortions of bowel folds, and slight enlargement of lymph follicles may not be appreciated on cross-sectional imaging because of limitations in spatial resolution.

Ultrasound

The idea that ultrasound is useful in the diagnosis of abdominal surgical diseases, particularly in those that involve transmural inflammation and wall thickening of hollow viscera, should not seem unusual given its usefulness in cholecystitis and appendicitis; it is no surprise that the use of ultrasound for the assessment of a variety of inflammatory disorders of the small and large intestine is gaining increasingly widespread acceptance. Although transabdominal ultrasound for the evaluation of Crohn's disease is well supported in the literature and is becoming more commonplace in Europe, it remains a rarity in the United States. The oft-cited advantages of ultrasound, including cost, availability, noninvasiveness, and lack of ionizing radiation, have been augmented by technologic advances that have improved resolution. These improvements not only allow good cross-sectional imaging of the gut wall but, like CT and MRI, also allow examination of the surrounding mesentery and abdominal cavity for evaluation of extramural disease manifestations. It is now possible to visualize, localize, and gauge the extent of transmural inflammation while

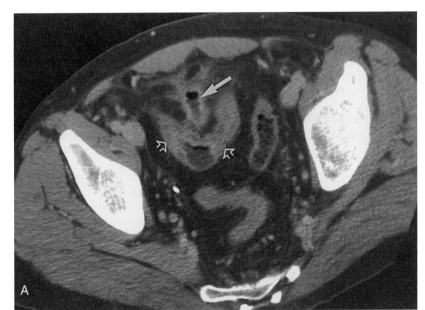

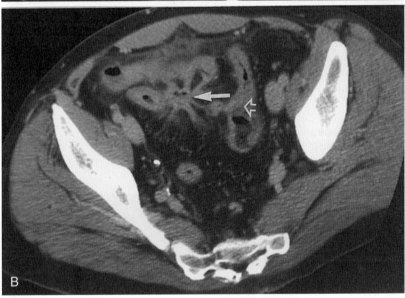

Figure 70–8. Ileal Crohn's disease with tracts and abscesses. **A,** A gas-containing mesenteric abscess *(solid arrow)* is close to transmural Crohn's disease of the terminal ileum *(open arrows).* **B,** Top of the abscess in the mesentery *(solid arrow)* with a fistula to the adjacent Crohn's disease–involved ileum *(open arrow).* Multiple tracts are related to the abscesses. (From Herlinger H, Caroline DF: Crohn's disease of the small bowel. In Gore RM, Levine MS [eds]: Textbook of Gastrointestinal Radiology, vol 1, 2nd ed. Philadelphia, WB Saunders, 2000, p 740.)

detecting extraintestinal complications such as strictures, abscesses, and fistulas. Techniques that use anechoic intraluminal contrast or intravenous contrast agents with Doppler ultrasound will probably improve ultrasound's diagnostic capabilities even more. As is so often the case with complex ultrasound studies, their advantages can be offset by the degree of expertise required of the ultrasound technologists and radiologists; this shortcoming can lead to concerns regarding intraoperator variability and can engender questions regarding the applicability of study results to widespread practice. In addition, like CT and MRI, ultrasound is not sensitive enough to detect the subtle mucosal lesions that may be the only radiographic sign of early disease. Furthermore, ultrasound has been found to be less effective in the imaging of Crohn's disease localized to the anorectum. Finally, patient characteristics that make transabdominal ultrasound technically difficult in other settings, such as

obesity or intraluminal gas, make transabdominal ultrasound in Crohn's disease more difficult as well. Even so, recent prospective studies comparing the accuracy of bowel ultrasound as the first imaging procedure in diagnosing Crohn's disease with the accuracy of endoscopy, radiologic studies, or surgical exploration followed by pathologic examination of the surgical specimens found sensitivities and specificities of 76% to 88% and 98% to 100%, respectively, results that support continued investigation.[50]

Endoscopy

Radiology and endoscopy have complementary roles in the diagnosis and subsequent management of Crohn's disease[51]; despite continued evolution in the state of the art for both, neither has gained primacy.

Push Endoscopy

The advantages afforded by push endoscopy, including colonoscopy with ileoscopy and esophagogastroduodenoscopy, in the diagnosis and management of Crohn's disease are many: the ability to detect subtle mucosal lesions, which in many cases are the only sign of early disease; the ability to obtain biopsy samples for histologic examination; and increasingly, the ability to perform intraluminal therapeutic interventions.

Patients with Crohn's disease most commonly have abdominal pain and chronic diarrhea as their initial complaints. The majority of patients with chronic diarrhea will undergo some type of endoscopy, and if the remainder of the antecedent clinical evaluation is suggestive of inflammatory bowel disease, colonoscopy with the addition of ileoscopy is a good first choice of diagnostic procedure[51] because it can help differentiate between Crohn's disease and ulcerative colitis on the basis of mucosal changes, disease distribution, and histology (multilevel biopsy specimens that include the terminal ileum, along with histologic examination, significantly increase the diagnostic sensitivity and specificity of endoscopy in inflammatory bowel disease[52]).

In the differentiation of Crohn's disease from ulcerative colitis, the most important colonoscopic findings are aphthous ulcers (Fig. 70–9), cobblestoning, and discontinuous lesions.[53] In addition, terminal ileal involvement and rectal sparing are strongly suggestive of Crohn's disease. Although there may be "backwash ileitis" on ileoscopy in patients with ulcerative colitis, this finding is observed in the setting of pan-colitis with continuous involvement of the colon from the rectum to the cecum[52,54]; in patients with inflammatory bowel disease and isolated terminal ileal involvement, the diagnosis of Crohn's disease is secure.[55,56] Because rectal involvement is essentially a prerequisite for the diagnosis of ulcerative colitis, rectal sparing, which occurs in about 40% of patients with Crohn's disease, is useful in differentiation between the two forms of inflammatory bowel disease, although there are caveats: the rectal mucosa may appear normal despite histologic evidence of pathology on biopsy, and rectal sparing can occur in up to 40% of medically treated patients with ulcerative colitis.[57]

Because Crohn's disease may involve the upper gastrointestinal tract, esophagogastroduodenoscopy plays a role in diagnosis and management. Indeed, because the frequency of upper gastrointestinal tract Crohn's involvement seems to be much higher than previously reported, the role that upper endoscopy plays will probably increase. For example, in patients with indeterminate colitis, involvement of the upper gastrointestinal tract provides strong evidence in favor of Crohn's disease; in patients with known Crohn's disease who have upper gastrointestinal symptoms, upper endoscopy can facilitate diagnosis of the underlying cause, whether it be Crohn's or some other disease; and it is certainly possible that patients might have Crohn's disease isolated to the upper gastrointestinal tract.[58,59]

The use of endoscopy in the clinical management of Crohn's disease subsequent to diagnosis is evolving. With regard to monitoring of disease activity after initiation of

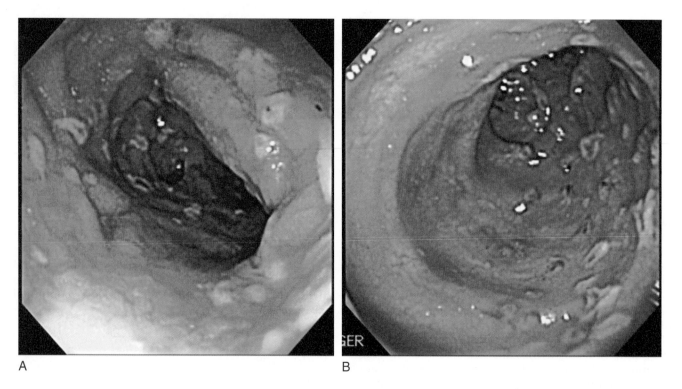

A   B

Figure 70–9. **A** and **B,** Multiple aphthous ulcers seen in recurrent Crohn's disease in the neoterminal ileum of the ileocolonic anastomosis 3 months after resection. (From Krok KL, Lichtenstein GR: Inflammatory bowel disease. In Ginsberg GG, Kochman ML, Norton ID, et al [eds]: Clinical Gastrointestinal Endoscopy. Philadelphia, WB Saunders, 2005, p 317.)

medical therapy, endoscopy does not have a firmly established role. Although endoscopic indices of disease activity have been developed and validated, with the most extensively studied being the Crohn's Disease Endoscopic Index of Severity (CDEIS) and the newest being the Simplified Endoscopic Activity Score for Crohn's Disease (SES-CD), they have not seen widespread use for a variety of reasons. Though reliable and reproducible, CDEIS is complex, which limits its use in clinical trials and day-to-day practice. The SES-CD is probably easier to use, but because of its recent development, it is has yet to be widely applied. Neither CDEIS nor SES-CD has been shown to correlate especially well with clinical disease activity, nor have studies shown that steroid-induced clinical remission is closely linked to mucosal healing. In contrast, studies of treatment with immune modulators such as infliximab and azathioprine have shown correlation between mucosal healing and clinical improvement, so evidence of healing on endoscopy is becoming an important therapeutic target.[60,61] When considering surveillance after curative resection, endoscopic severity evaluated with the Rutgeerts' score predicts the likelihood of symptomatic recurrence.[61] Endoscopy also has an important role in cancer surveillance in patients with long-standing colonic Crohn's disease.[62] From an interventional perspective, endoscopic balloon dilation with or without steroid injection may offer an alternative to surgical therapy for primary and postsurgical Crohn's strictures, although randomized controlled trials are needed for comparisons of safety and efficacy with more standard therapies.[63]

Wireless Video Capsule Endoscopy

Wireless video capsule endoscopy requires a system made up of several components. There is a single-use capsule 26 mm long by 11 mm in diameter that contains a color camera chip, lens, light source from a light-emitting diode, radiofrequency transmitter, antenna, and batteries. Two images are acquired every second, for a total of about 50,000 in an 8-hour study. The images are sent to a belt-worn receiver with a 5-gigabyte hard drive. Images are then downloaded to a computer workstation and viewed as continuous video, with viewing and interpretation typically requiring 1 to 2 hours. Study length is dictated by the capsule's battery life, so the belt is worn for approximately 8 hours after ingestion of the capsule, during which time patients are able to continue their normal daily activities. The capsule's movement is completely passive and relies on peristalsis to progress distally, and it is designed to be passed spontaneously.[64,65] Studies report complete evaluation of the small intestine in as few as 50% and as many as 85% of cases, with most studies reporting 65% to 80% success rates.[66]

Before the introduction of wireless capsule endoscopy in the year 2000, a majority of the small intestine's length was essentially inaccessible to endoscopy performed in the nonsurgical setting. A subsequent pilot study in 2002 reported the use of capsule endoscopy for obscure gastrointestinal tract bleeding, and it has rapidly become the test of choice for obscure small bowel bleeding.[64]

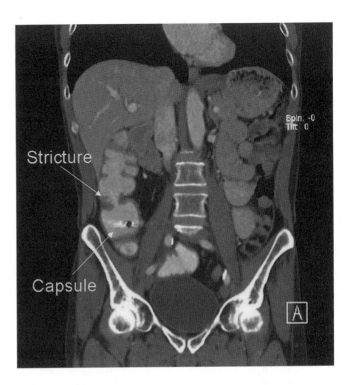

Figure 70–10. Abdominal computed tomography scan illustrating Crohn's stricture of an ileocolonic anastomosis trapping a video endoscopy capsule.

Because 70% of patients with Crohn's disease have involvement of the small intestine[25] and subtle mucosal lesions may be the only signs of early disease, it follows that capsule endoscopy could be extremely useful in the diagnosis and subsequent management of Crohn's disease. Early investigators were understandably reluctant to use the capsule in Crohn's patients; given the capsule's size and the propensity for stricture formation in Crohn's disease, the fear of capsule-induced mechanical obstruction must have loomed large.[67] The rate of "non-natural excretion," that is, capsules requiring endoscopy or surgery for removal, has been reported to be as low as 0% and as high as 15%, depending on study indications and patient populations.[66,68] Even so, a number of studies have been completed in which the diagnostic utility of capsule endoscopy was evaluated in patients with Crohn's disease.[68] Capsules that do not pass spontaneously in patients with Crohn's disease are usually due to strictures (Fig. 70–10), with many of these patients having undergone radiographic studies before ingestion that showed no evidence of stenosis. To reduce the likelihood of retained capsules and possibly obviate the need for radiographic studies before capsule ingestion, a similarly sized, dissolvable "patency capsule" has been developed. When they are retained, wireless endoscopy capsules do not usually cause acute small bowel obstruction; instead, the diagnosis is typically made several days after ingestion based on patient suspicion and intermittent obstructive symptoms. Separate from concerns about obstruction caused by capsules, other problems inherent in the interpretation of these studies in patients with Crohn's disease still remain[64,68]:

- Study results from institutions with special expertise in capsule endoscopy may not be generalizable to everyday practice.
- Prospective studies to determine the sensitivity, specificity, accuracy, and positive and negative predictive values have not been completed for want of a clear nonsurgical gold standard for diagnosis and for want of a group of prospective patients with long-term follow-up.
- Capsule endoscopy gives information about mucosal lesions and possibly stenosis, leaving aside information about wall thickening or any extraluminal findings.
- The commonality and importance of scattered mucosal breaks, aphthous ulcers, or erosions in various groups of patients, from asymptomatic volunteers to those with suspected or known Crohn's disease, need to be determined, and diagnostic standards need to be created and validated.

Despite these problems, capsule endoscopy is destined to become an important part of the armamentarium for the diagnosis and management of Crohn's disease.

Medical Therapy

All modes of therapy for Crohn's disease have similar goals, which are to reduce symptoms while maintaining or improving patient quality of life. As previously stated, patients with Crohn's disease are usually initially seen with active disease, so typically, a sequential approach to therapy is used in which remission is first induced and then maintained. Current medical regimens require careful consideration of disease location and the level of disease activity (mild, moderate, or severe). Therapy should be individualized according to the patient's disease activity, as well as response to and tolerance of the medical intervention (Fig. 70–11).[20]

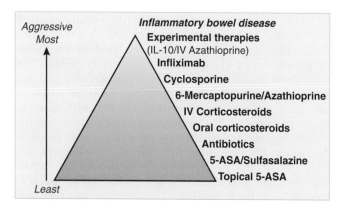

Figure 70–11. Therapeutic pyramid for escalation of medical therapy for Crohn's disease. ASA, acetylsalicylic acid. (From Johns Hopkins University Crohn's Disease Resource Web Page. Copyright Johns Hopkins 2000.)

Inducing Remission in Patients with Active Disease

Corticosteroids have long been used to induce remission in patients with Crohn's disease, and randomized controlled trials have proved the effectiveness of conventional steroids such as prednisone in patients with mild or moderate disease. However, the benefits of conventional steroid treatment may be offset by serious adverse effects in some patients (giving rise to steroid-intolerant patients), little or no improvement in others (steroid-resistant patients), and disease flares during or shortly after tapering (steroid-dependent patients). More than 35% of patients treated acutely with conventional steroids will become steroid dependent or steroid resistant. Budesonide is a corticosteroid with extensive first-pass liver metabolism that results in low systemic bioavailability, which gives it the potential to reduce side effects; the oral version for use in Crohn's disease (inhaled versions are used for the treatment of allergic rhinitis and asthma) is an enteric-coated, controlled-release formulation. Unfortunately, budesonide is effective in a limited number of patients: 30% to 40% of patients will not respond, and studies show that it is useful in patients with ileal and right-sided colonic disease, but not in those with left-sided colonic disease.[20,69] Steroids are not useful in maintaining remission.[70]

Aminosalicylates, including 5-aminosalicylic acid (mesalamine and the controlled-release forms Asacol and Pentasa) and sulfasalazine (a sulfonamide antibiotic, sulfapyridine, linked to mesalamine), can be used selectively to induce remission. Sulfasalazine has been proved effective for inducing remission in patients with colitis or ileocolitis and mildly to moderately active Crohn's disease; it is not useful in maintaining remission. The studies evaluating mesalamine, including Asacol and Pentasa, in active Crohn's disease have been mixed, and experts disagree with regard to their usefulness in inducing and maintaining remission, although they are still considered to be first-line therapy at many centers.[20,69,71]

Antibiotics, including metronidazole and ciprofloxacin, are currently used clinically and have been studied singly, together, and in combination with budesonide for induction of remission (although not for maintaining remission) in mild to moderately active Crohn's disease. Metronidazole has not been proved to be superior to placebo for inducing remission, although one Scandinavian crossover trial found it to be as effective as sulfasalazine.[69,72] The data for ciprofloxacin in Crohn's disease are mixed; controlled trials have shown the superiority of ciprofloxacin over placebo for inducing remission, but another showed that in combination with metronidazole, it is less effective than prednisone. Combinations with budesonide and prednisolone have not been demonstrated to be more effective than monotherapy with these agents.[71,72] Besides inconsistently proven efficacy, significant side effects can occur with the long-term use of either drug, and the development of antibiotic-resistant organisms is a justifiable concern.[20]

For patients with mild to moderate disease that fails to respond to first-line treatment with steroids (including budesonide) or sulfasalazine or for patients with more severe disease, treatment with immunomodulators is appropriate.[69] *Azathioprine* is the prodrug of 6-mercaptopurine, which is a precursor to intracellular purine antimetabolites that have an antiproliferative effect on mitotically active lymphocyte populations. Multiple randomized studies and a meta-analysis of these studies support the use of azathioprine and 6-mercaptopurine in the treatment of active Crohn's disease, although it may take 4 to 8 weeks for them to begin to take effect.[69,73] Side effects include pancreatitis, bone marrow suppression, allergic reactions, and increased rates of infection.[73]

Methotrexate is a folic acid structural analogue that competitively inhibits the binding of dihydrofolic acid to the enzyme dihydrofolate reductase, which is involved in purine and pyrimidine synthesis; thus, the drugs impair DNA synthesis. The relevant mechanism of action in inflammatory bowel disease, however, has not been fully elucidated.[73] Methotrexate has been shown in randomized controlled trials to be more effective than placebo in treating active Crohn's disease and will induce remission in a significant proportion of patients with corticosteroid- and azathioprine/6-mercaptopurine–resistant disease; it usually requires at least 4 to 6 weeks to take effect.[69,73,74] Liver toxicity is the most serious potential side effect in patients taking methotrexate, and nausea is a common complaint. In addition, methotrexate is teratogenic and an abortifacient.[73]

Infliximab is a chimeric mouse-human monoclonal antibody against TNF-α. In a study that established the use of infliximab in Crohn's disease, a single infusion allowed 33% of patients to enter remission as compared with a placebo rate of 4%, it improved disease in 81% as compared with 17% of controls, and response to infliximab can be seen in as little as 1 to 2 weeks.[69] The effectiveness of infliximab has led to the development of a number of new biologic agents for the treatment of Crohn's disease, including a variety of antibodies with TNF-α as their target, as well as antibodies to interleukins, interferon-γ, and leukocyte adhesion molecules, all of which are in various phases of clinical trials.[75]

Maintaining Remission

A vitally important goal of therapy for Crohn's disease is maintenance of remission. Daily azathioprine and 6-mercaptopurine have been proved in randomized controlled trials to be more effective than placebo in maintaining remission after medical induction; a retrospective study suggests that azathioprine may prevent recurrence after surgery as well.[74] Because of their side effects, potential for significant toxicity, and toxicity-monitoring requirements, important questions remain concerning the discontinuation of azathioprine and 6-mercaptopurine therapy. A recent study of patients with Crohn's disease in remission for at least 42 months found that withdrawal of azathioprine led to an 18-month relapse rate of 21% versus 8% in the group randomized to continue treatment.[69] Another study found that the efficacy of azathioprine is maintained over a period of at least 5 years.[74] Weekly methotrexate has a proven role in

maintaining remission of Crohn's disease, with its use generally preceded by methotrexate induction; the optimum duration of therapy has yet to be confirmed, although it is suggested that it could be effective for 3 to 4 years. Given methotrexate's primary adverse effects, it is best avoided in patients with risk factors for liver disease or established liver disease and in those desiring to conceive.[69,74] Infliximab infusions given every 8 weeks have been shown to be effective in maintaining remission in those who respond to the initial infusion. Patients may form antibodies to infliximab, and these antibodies are responsible for acute and delayed hypersensitivity reactions, as well as loss of responsiveness in those who responded previously; this has led to the use of concomitant immunosuppression in Crohn's patients receiving infliximab.[69,74,75] Steroids are not effective in maintaining remission of Crohn's disease, although budesonide can prolong the time to relapse. The use of 5-aminosalicylates for maintaining remission is controversial, with current evidence not supportive of their use in medically induced patients, although they do show some promise in maintaining remission in surgically treated patients.[69,74]

Because most patients will relapse after medical induction, a reasonable approach to maintenance would include azathioprine, 6-mercaptopurine, methotrexate, or infliximab and, in select cases, budesonide (in patients with distal small intestinal or right-sided colonic disease, with the understanding that the treatment effect will probably last less than a year).[69] Infliximab is very expensive (the average third-party reimbursement per dose administered to a 70-kg patient is more than $5200),[76] so it should probably be reserved for patients refractory to other agents, thus leaving azathioprine, 6-mercaptopurine, and methotrexate for most patients. Given the toxicity profiles of infliximab and the immunosuppressive agents, it is reasonable to give patients at least one trial free of maintenance therapy; if symptoms recur within 6 to 12 months, repeat induction should be followed by maintenance therapy with the aforementioned agents indefinitely as patient tolerance allows.[69,71]

Nutrition

Nutrition is an important consideration in the care of patients with Crohn's disease, both in terms of supportive care, which is directed at correcting malnutrition, and potentially as an alternative means of treatment.[77]

Malnutrition

Deficiencies in macronutrients (protein, energy) and micronutrients (vitamins, minerals, and electrolytes) are common in patients with Crohn's disease.[78] The degree of malnutrition depends on disease location, extent, and activity. The long-term malnutrition seen in patients with Crohn's disease may have a multitude of consequences, including growth failure and pubertal delay in children, bone loss, delayed healing of fistulas, poor wound healing after surgery, and increased susceptibility to infection.[79] Assessment of nutritional status includes a history, physical examination, and laboratory studies focusing on intake, body mass index, serial body weight, muscle wasting, edema, serum albumin, and iron studies; more detailed assessment may include anthropometry and the use of scoring systems such as the Subjective Global Assessment.[77] Factors that contribute to malnutrition in patients with Crohn's disease include the following[78]:

- Anorexia—Decreased appetite is probably due to the high levels of inflammatory cytokines, such as TNF-α, that result from dysregulation of systemic immunity.
- Bowel obstruction—Caused by stricture or abscess.
- Abdominal pain—Caused by inflammation or obstruction.
- Malabsorption—Caused by altered or reduced absorption as a result of inflammation, postinflammatory changes, or surgical resection.
- Losses from the gut—Protein-losing enteropathy may develop in patients with mucosal injury; components of serum, including proteins, iron, lipids, and trace elements, are lost intraluminally because of leaky capillaries in inflamed areas of bowel.
- Direct drug effects and drug-nutrient interactions.
- Increased metabolic requirements, particularly in the setting of complicated disease.
- Prescription of restricted diets.

Specific nutrient deficiencies include the following:

- Vitamin B_{12} (cobalamin)—Deficiency is secondary to decreased absorption of the vitamin B_{12}–intrinsic factor complex in diseased or resected ileum. Vitamin B_{12} deficiency may contribute to anemia in Crohn's patients, and it is a cofactor in homocysteine metabolism (for more detail, see discussion of folate later).[78]
- Calcium—Patients with Crohn's disease do have malabsorption of calcium as a result of complexes formed with unabsorbed intraluminal fats and decreased absorption of vitamin D (a fat-soluble vitamin), although serum calcium levels are maintained by the action of parathyroid hormone, potentially at the expense of bone density. Osteopenia is common in patients with Crohn's disease, with steroid use, along with patient factors such as genetics, contributing to the problem.[77,78,80]
- Fat-soluble vitamins—The adequacy of vitamins A, E, D, and K may be affected as a result of fat malabsorption secondary to disease affecting any part of the small intestine and as a result of alterations in bile acid metabolism, particularly with terminal ileal disease or resection.[81]
- Folate—Folate deficiency is common in patients with Crohn's disease; it is caused by dietary deficiency, increased utilization, and drug treatments, including sulfasalazine, which can bind folate and thereby make it unavailable for absorption, and methotrexate, which is a folic acid antagonist. Inadequate levels of folate may play a role in development of anemia in patients with Crohn's disease. Increased levels of folate may have a protective effect

with regard to the development of dysplasia and colorectal cancer, so decreased levels may be another factor in the increased cancer risk seen in Crohn's patients. Folate is a cofactor in homocysteine metabolism, and deficiency may lead to elevated plasma homocysteine levels, which may induce a hypercoagulable state and increase the incidence of thromboembolic events in patients with inflammatory bowel disease.[77]

- Iron—Deficiencies may result from loss secondary to intraluminal bleeding, from decreased absorption because of small bowel disease or resection, and from dietary restrictions, all of which can contribute to the anemia seen in Crohn's disease.[82]
- Selenium—A number of studies have demonstrated decreased selenium concentrations in Crohn's disease patients with a concomitant decrease in glutathione peroxidase activity; the catalytic action of this enzyme protects cells from oxidative damage by lipid peroxides.[80,83]
- Zinc—Deficiencies are difficult to assess because serum levels correlate poorly with total-body zinc stores, but deficiencies are thought to be fairly common in patients with Crohn's disease as a result of decreased absorption or increased loss because the diets of adults with Crohn's disease typically contain a similar amount of zinc as the diets of control subjects. In addition to detrimental effects on wound healing, severe zinc deficiency leads to clinical features of acrodermatitis, such as alopecia, anorexia, diarrhea, dermatitis, poor growth, and impaired immune function.[84]

Supportive nutritional therapy is aimed at improving the nutritional status of the malnourished patient, and unless absolutely contraindicated, the enteral route is preferred. Oral or tube feeding supplementation with protein, calories, and micronutrients can be implemented with any number of commercially available formulas; the decision about which oral or tube feeding formula to use should be based on cost, palatability, and patient tolerance. Initial electrolyte monitoring and replacement are important in severely malnourished patients to prevent the refeeding syndrome. Given its cost and potential for complications, total parenteral nutrition (TPN) as a means of nutritional supportive care should be limited to short-term use in those with bowel obstruction or fistulas, with long-term use reserved for those with short-gut syndrome; there is some, albeit limited, evidence to support the use of TPN in severely malnourished Crohn's disease patients in preparation for surgery.[77]

Nutrition as Primary Therapy

There is evidence to support the use of restricted diets based on enteral nutrition formulas as therapy to induce remission of Crohn's disease, and although potential mechanisms of action such as decreased antigenic presentation have been postulated, the physiology underlying the treatment effect is unknown. There are three meta-analyses and a Cochrane review of randomized control trials involving enteral therapy as primary treatment of Crohn's disease.[77] They have found that elemental formulations do not have greater efficacy than nonelemental formulations do in induction of remission and that enteral nutrition is not as effective as steroids for induction of remission.[85] Although enteral nutrition has not been compared with placebo, the response rates in studies to date have been greater than one would expect from placebo.[77] Given the side effects associated with steroid treatment and the benign nature of nutritional therapy, there is continued interest in enteral nutrition as primary therapy for Crohn's disease.[77,85]

SURGICAL THERAPY

In addition to general considerations and medical therapy for Crohn's disease, this chapter focuses on surgical therapy for Crohn's disease involving the small intestine. Studies that have monitored patients with Crohn's disease after diagnosis have found variable rates for the requirement for intestinal surgery, but the rates are consistently high[86]; 57% of patients studied in a population-based American cohort required at least one surgical resection,[1] whereas 78% of patients in the National Cooperative Crohn's Disease Study required surgery by 20 years after symptom onset.[87] Because the majority of patients with Crohn's disease have small bowel involvement, a discussion focused on the surgical management of small bowel Crohn's disease is of particular importance. However, surgical management of Crohn's disease can be made complicated by the potential for involvement of any part of the gastrointestinal tract, the segmental nature of involvement, the likelihood of recurrence requiring multiple procedures, penetrating disease causing abscesses and fistulas, adhesions, malnutrition, and medical therapy with immunosuppressive agents. Indications for surgical therapy and subsequent decisions with regard to technique must be carefully considered.

Indications

Surgical therapy for diseased segments does not cure Crohn's disease; therefore, it should be used only to treat complications that are not amenable to medical therapy, and with the potential for recurrence and the need for reoperation in mind, all procedures should be performed with consideration for the conservation of small intestinal length. Indications for operative intervention are directly related to the site of intestinal involvement (Box 70–1)[88]:

- Failure of medical therapy—Medical therapy has failed when maximal medical therapy proves inadequate, successful medical induction is followed by failure of maintenance therapy, and significant complications related to medical treatment develop. As medical therapies improve, definitions for failure of medical therapy will continue to evolve.
- Penetrating disease—Patients with a penetrating pattern of disease may also require surgical therapy.

Box 70–1   Indications for Surgery in Patients with Crohn's Disease

Failure of medical treatment
- Persistence of symptoms despite corticosteroid therapy for longer than 6 months
- Recurrence of symptoms when high-dose corticosteroids are tapered
- Worsening symptoms or new onset of complications with maximal medical therapy
- Occurrence of steroid-induced complications (cushingoid features, cataracts, glaucoma, systemic hypertension, aseptic necrosis of the head of the femur, myopathy, or vertebral body fractures)

Obstruction
- Intestinal obstruction (partial or complete)

Penetrating disease
- Fistula if
  - Drainage causes personal embarrassment (e.g., enterocutaneous fistula, enterovaginal fistula, fistula in ano)
  - Fistula communicating with the genitourinary system (e.g., enterovesical or colovesical fistula)
  - Fistula producing functional or anatomic bypass of a major segment of intestine with consequent malabsorption and/or profuse diarrhea (e.g., duodenocolic or enterorectosigmoid fistula)
- Inflammatory mass or abscess (intra-abdominal, pelvic, perineal)
- Free perforation

Hemorrhage

Carcinoma

Fulminant colitis with or without toxic megacolon

Growth retardation

Adapted from Sartor RB, Sanborn WJ (eds): Kirsner's Inflammatory Bowel Diseases. Philadelphia, WB Saunders, 2004:597.

Although penetrating disease is not always an absolute indication, it may require operative intervention if complicated (see Box 70–1). If feasible, abscesses may be treated by percutaneous drainage and systemic antibiotics, thereby delaying definitive surgery until it can be safely performed.
- Free perforation—Although a rare complication, perforation requires immediate surgical intervention.
- Obstruction—Obstruction as a result of single or multiple, sometimes lengthy strictures may require stricturoplasty or resection; patients should be decompressed and resuscitated before surgery.

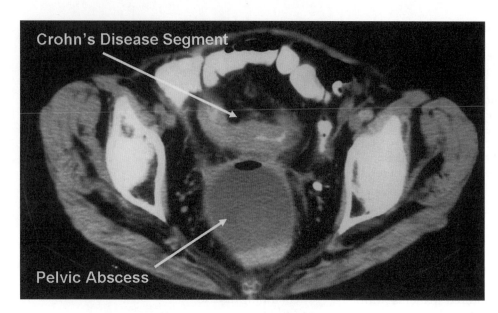

Figure 70–12. Pelvic abscess associated with diseased ileum.

- Other less frequent complications such as massive gastrointestinal hemorrhage, cancer, toxic megacolon, and growth retardation are also indications for surgery.

Preoperative Evaluation and Preparation

Proper preparation of a patient with Crohn's disease for surgery cannot be overemphasized. Every effort should be made to optimize the patient's medical status before surgery, including identifying and mitigating any medical comorbid conditions. If infectious complications secondary to penetrating disease are suspected, cross-sectional imaging is essential because it allows identification of potential abscesses. To minimize the risk for anastomotic leak and the need for diversion, any abscesses that are found should be drained, with percutaneous techniques if possible, before embarking on operations that may require resection (Fig. 70–12). In some instances, complete evaluation of the entire gastrointestinal tract should be undertaken preoperatively to localize areas affected by disease; such evaluation can be accomplished with a combination of endoscopy, contrast studies, cross-sectional imaging, and capsule endoscopy. Complete evaluation of the gastrointestinal tract may not be possible when emergencies arise, which leaves intraoperative evaluation as the primary means of diagnosis. When urgent or emergency intervention is required, patients should not be denied appropriate resuscitation, antibiotics for treatment or surgical prophylaxis, or thromboembolism prophylaxis.

Any patient in whom construction of an intestinal stoma is even a remote possibility should be adequately prepared for the eventuality. Preparation should include preoperative consultation with an enterostomal therapist and, at the very least, marking of an appropriate site or sites for the potential stoma. Blind intraoperative selection of an intestinal stoma site frequently leads to inappropriate placement; a location that is too close to an incision, in a body crease, or in a belt line can make postoperative stoma management difficult.

When operative therapy can or must be delayed, attention should be paid to assessing and correcting malnutrition and metabolic abnormalities. If patients have lost more than 5% of their baseline weight in the preceding 3 months or if they have an albumin concentration that is less than 3.0 g/dl, their nutritional status puts them at increased risk for perioperative complications, and if possible, they should be considered for nutritional intervention before surgery. The enteral route is always preferred if it can be tolerated and when disease complications allow. There is limited evidence to support the use of TPN in the preoperative setting, although a severely malnourished patient may benefit.[88]

With regard to mechanical bowel preparation, a number of randomized controlled trials and meta-analyses have concluded that it is not beneficial and potentially harmful in colorectal surgery[89]; it should certainly be avoided in small bowel procedures.

Patients with suppressed adrenal function because of treatment with corticosteroids should continue steroid treatment in the perioperative period, and although the use of superphysiologic so-called stress-dose steroids in patients who are not critically ill is of unproven benefit, it is still recommended by some experts,[88,90] which should not be confused with steroid use in critically ill patients with hypotension requiring vasopressors, in whom current and mounting evidence suggests that testing for adrenocortical insufficiency and treatment with stress-dose steroids may be beneficial.[91]

Operative Strategies and Techniques

Abdominal Incision

In patients with Crohn's disease who are undergoing abdominal operations, the importance of selection and placement of incisions cannot be overemphasized. Many of these patients will require multiple abdominal operations during the course of their disease. Some will

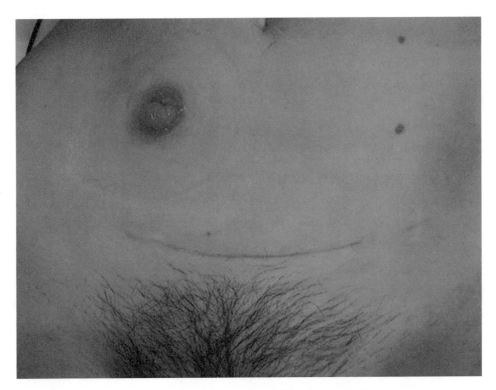

Figure 70–13. Pfannenstiel incision and diverting ileostomy.

require a stoma, if not at the time of their initial procedure, then in the future, so the placement of scars may potentially have long-term consequences. Transverse incisions or incisions off the midline for either open or laparoscopic surgery should be avoided because scars at these sites may preclude their use for future stoma placement; moreover, because future laparotomies may require an incision that is entirely different from the initial transverse incision, the patient may be put at increased risk for hernia formation.

In our practice, a low, transverse Pfannenstiel incision has been used in more than 300 Crohn's disease patients with excellent results. It is a useful approach for procedures involving the small intestine, the lower part of the abdomen, and the pelvis, and with the use of mechanical retractor systems and headlights, access to the upper part of the abdomen may be achieved. The incision yields excellent cosmetic results with a negligible rate of hernia in our hands, and the literature reports similarly low hernia rates (0% to 3.7% versus as high as 42% with midline incisions).[92,93] It allows ample room to pack away the abdominal contents, and it facilitates stoma placement (Fig. 70–13). We use a retractor consisting of two elastic rings connected by a clear plastic sleeve to facilitate exposure through these smaller incisions (Alexis Wound Retractor, Applied Medical, Rancho Santa Margarita, CA, 92688) (Fig. 70–14).

Abdominal Exploration and Identification of Diseased Segments

Complete exploration of the abdomen with a focus on identifying diseased segments of the gastrointestinal tract should be performed. Crohn's involvement may be

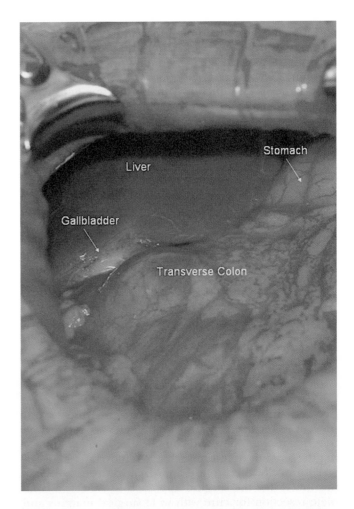

Figure 70–14. Exposure afforded by a Pfannenstiel incision.

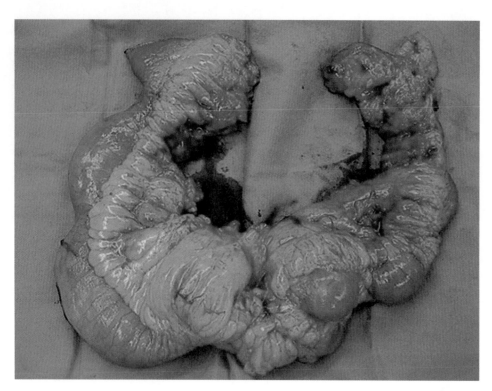

Figure 70–15. Specimen from ileocecectomy for Crohn's disease depicting serosal hyperemia and extension of mesenteric fat onto the serosal surface, which is commonly referred to as "fat wrapping" or "creeping fat."

obvious with thickened bowel wall and adjacent mesentery, serosal hyperemia, and extension of mesenteric fat onto the serosal surface, commonly referred to as "fat wrapping" or "creeping fat" (Fig. 70–15). If the mesenteric border is examined by visual inspection and palpation, more subtle disease may be identified at sites where the bowel wall becomes indistinguishable from the mesentery.[94] Another method for identifying clinically significant obstructing disease that we use infrequently involves the use of a Foley catheter; after creating an enterotomy over a known area of disease or stenosis that is to be resected or is to undergo stricturoplasty, an 18-French Foley catheter on an introducer is placed in the lumen, and the small bowel is telescoped onto the Foley catheter until the duodenum or ileocecal valve is reached. After inflating the balloon to 2 to 2.5 cm in diameter, it is gently pulled through the small intestine; strictures are identified when passage of the balloon is arrested.[95]

Bowel Resection Versus Stricturoplasty

Surgical techniques for the treatment of small intestinal Crohn's disease can be broadly classified into two groups: those that involve bowel resection and those that do not. Because surgery does not cure Crohn's disease nor prevent its recurrence, surgical strategies are focused on relieving its symptoms and complications while minimizing the amount of intestine that is removed.

Historically, the surgical approach to Crohn's disease was much like the surgical approach to cancer; a complete resection for cure with wide surgical margins and even intraoperative frozen sections to identify microscopic involvement seemed logical and was widely practiced. However, significant recurrence rates were seen even after extensive resections. It has since been established that recurrence is not negatively affected by disease at the surgical margins or positively affected by increased length of resection. This understanding, as well as the fear of iatrogenic short-bowel syndrome, has led to a bowel-sparing approach to surgical therapy for Crohn's disease that has made short-bowel syndrome in modern centers very rare[86] (one study of 464 patients with Crohn's disease undergoing surgery found that 21 [5%] had residual intestine <180 cm with just 7 of them requiring home TPN[96]). The bowel-sparing approach to surgical therapy for Crohn's disease has evolved to include techniques that avoid resection altogether. The application of stricturoplasty to small bowel stenoses caused by Crohn's disease is a relatively recent innovation, with the first report being published in 1982 by Lee and colleagues.[97] Since then, multiple studies have shown it to be safe and effective without an increased risk for recurrence.[86,95]

Indications for stricturoplasty include single or multiple fibrotic strictures within diffusely involved segments of small bowel, previous extensive (>100 cm) resections of small bowel, short-bowel syndrome, rapid recurrence of disease with obstruction (within 12 months), duodenal strictures, and strictures at previous anastomotic sites. Contraindications to stricturoplasty include perforation of the small bowel with or without peritonitis; phlegmonous inflammation, abscess, or fistula at the intended stricturoplasty site; likelihood of tension on closure of the stricturoplasty; and location of the intended stricturoplasty site in close proximity to a segment requiring resection.[95]

Given the contraindications to stricturoplasty, it is obvious that resection continues to be an important part of the surgical armamentarium in the treatment of Crohn's disease. A common indication for resection continues to be small bowel obstruction, and in many cases of obstruction, resection may be the treatment of choice, particularly in those with septic complications or those that involve the terminal ileum. Other indications for resection include penetrating disease with or without sepsis, major hemorrhage, and carcinoma.

Stricturoplasty Techniques

There are two main types of stricturoplasty: the Heineke-Mikulicz technique and its variations and those involving some form of side-to-side anastomosis. Stricture length is perhaps the most important consideration when choosing the type of stricturoplasty to be performed. Short strictures, or those less than 10 cm in length, may be treated with the Heineke-Mikulicz technique. Longer strictures or many short strictures close together require side-to-side techniques; the Finney stricturoplasty can be used with strictures that are 10 to 25 cm long,[95] and Michelassi and Upadhyay report using side-to-side isoperistaltic stricturoplasty in diseased segments averaging 51 cm and as long as 109 cm.[98]

The Heineke-Mikulicz stricturoplasty is performed by opening the antimesenteric wall of the strictured bowel longitudinally through all layers and reorienting the incision so that it is closed transversely with seromuscular interrupted or running absorbable suture (Fig. 70–16). Variations include the following[95,99]:

- Judd stricturoplasty, which allows longitudinal elliptical resection of a small portion of bowel wall, followed by transverse closure in situations in which there is a small area of penetration or damaged wall within a short stricture (Fig. 70–17).
- Moskel-Walske-Neumayer stricturoplasty, which uses a Y-shaped enterotomy rather than a longitudinal one, followed by transverse closure, which helps avoid undue suture line tension when performing stricturoplasty in segments with mismatched diameters, such as those with pre-stenotic dilation (Fig. 70–18).

Techniques for longer strictures that involve the use of side-to-side anastomosis include the following[95,99]:

- Finney stricturoplasty, which is performed by creating a longitudinal antimesenteric enterotomy, which is then oriented in side-to-side fashion by creating a U-shaped bend, followed by closure with absorbable suture in running fashion beginning on the posterior wall (Fig. 70–19).
- Jaboulay stricturoplasty, which is similar to the Finney technique in many respects in that it orients the intestine in a U shape, but instead of a single antimesenteric enterotomy, two separate enterotomies are made with the most strictured portion left unopened; subsequent closure creates a side-to-side enteroenterostomy (Fig. 70–20).

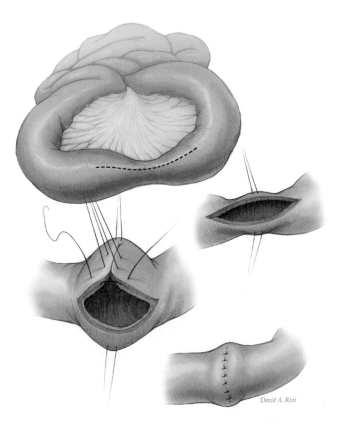

Figure 70–16. Heineke-Mikulicz stricturoplasty using an interrupted Gambee stitch. A longitudinal enterotomy over the stricture is followed by transverse closure. (From Talamini M: Stricturoplasty in Crohn's disease. In Cameron JL [ed]: Current Surgical Therapy, 8th ed. Philadelphia, CV Mosby, 2004, p 117.)

- Side-to-side isoperistaltic stricturoplasty, which is begun by dividing the small bowel mesentery at the midpoint of the affected segment, followed by division of the bowel itself between atraumatic bowel clamps; the proximal loop is then placed over the distal loop, antimesenteric enterotomies are made, the ends of the small bowel are tapered to avoid any blind pouches that could result after closure, and a running two-layer closure results in a long enteroenterostomy (Fig. 70–21).[95,98,99]

Bowel Resection and Anastomotic Techniques

After gaining safe entry into the abdomen, mobilizing diseased segments as required, and identifying the extent of diseased segments as described earlier, the proximal and distal margins may be divided with a linear cutting gastrointestinal stapler. If there is significant obstruction with dilated, fluid-filled loops, it may be necessary to decompress the intestine before stapling by milking the small bowel contents proximally or distally, followed by the application of atraumatic bowel clamps or umbilical tape, or by careful enterotomy and suction. The mesentery may be taken just beneath the small bowel; because it is often thickened, shortened, and hyperemic, this can present a technical challenge.

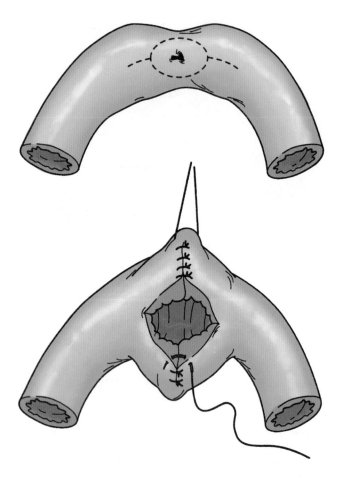

Figure 70–17. Judd stricturoplasty. The fistulous site is resected as part of the longitudinal enterotomy, which is then closed transversely. (From Michelassi F, Hurst RD: Stricturoplasty in Crohn's disease. In Cameron JL [ed]: Current Surgical Therapy, 7th ed. St Louis, CV Mosby, 2001, p 134.)

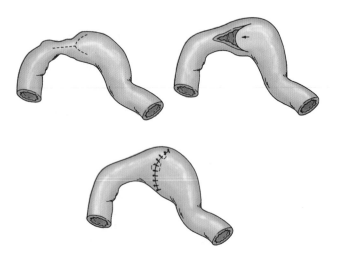

Figure 70–18. Moskel-Walske-Neumayer stricturoplasty. A Y-shaped enterotomy is performed before transverse closure. The Y-shaped enterotomy facilitates tailoring the large lumen of the proximal intestinal loop into the small lumen of the distal loop. (From Michelassi F, Hurst RD: Stricturoplasty in Crohn's disease. In Cameron JL [ed]: Current Surgical Therapy, 7th ed. St Louis, CV Mosby, 2001, p 134.)

After resection, the decision to perform a primary reanastomosis, a primary reanastomosis with a proximally placed loop stoma for diversion, or resection with an end stoma depends on factors such as urgency or emergency, stability of the patient in the operating room, patient nutritional status, the degree and temporality of steroid use, the condition of the bowel undergoing resection and anastomosis, and the condition of the abdomen in general, with septic complications such as abscess being of particular concern.[88] As in any bowel anastomosis, close attention must be paid to all technical details, including the blood supply to the bowel undergoing anastomosis, ensuring a tension-free anastomosis, consideration of proximal and distal bowel diameter, and avoidance of any distal obstruction. Although resection and anastomosis may be performed in areas of active disease and small ulcers should not place the anastomosis at risk, wherever possible, large longitudinal ulcers should not be incorporated into the anastomosis.[100]

With regard to recurrence and the need for reoperation, there is some evidence to support the superiority of a functional end-to-end stapled anastomosis over other stapled or hand-sewn techniques. Moreover, complication rates are low, the technique is quick and easy to perform, and it lends itself well to anastomosis of bowel with different calibers.[65] We typically use a 75-mm linear cutting stapler to create the common channel and close the remaining defect with a noncutting linear stapler.

A summary of salient issues regarding resections in patients with Crohn's disease includes the following points:

- Resection of gross disease is appropriate.
- Wide margins and frozen sections are unnecessary.
- The available evidence does not absolutely compel the use of any appropriate stapled or sewn anastomotic technique.

Stoma Formation

All patients undergoing operative therapy for Crohn's disease should be reasonably prepared, including mental preparation and stoma site marking, for the possibility of stoma creation to the extent dictated by clinical circumstances. Although permanent stomas are rarely required in the treatment of small bowel Crohn's disease, a poorly placed or constructed stoma, even if temporary, is at best a daily inconvenience and at worst a source of major morbidity.[101]

Selection of the stoma site is the first step in stoma construction; ideally, site selection occurs before surgery. Consultation with a certified enterostomal therapist can facilitate all aspects of patient preparation and stoma management, including ideal site selection. In general, stomas should be located within the rectus muscle. A scar-free portion of the abdominal wall should be chosen to allow good appliance seal. Care should be taken to avoid bony prominences such as ribs or the iliac crest. Evaluation of the stoma site should be performed by taking into account the proposed incision and using a template of the stoma appliance with the patient lying, sitting, and standing, especially in obese individuals,

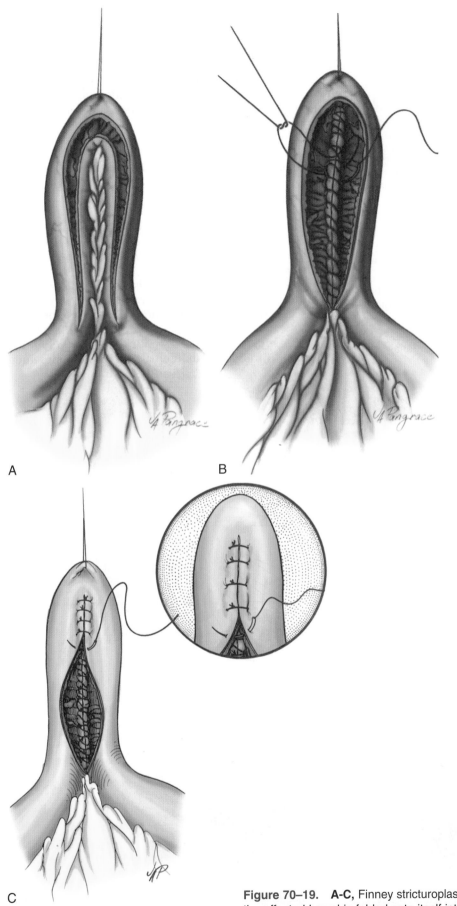

Figure 70–19. **A-C,** Finney stricturoplasty. Enteroenterostomy is performed after the affected bowel is folded onto itself into a U-shape. (From Talamini M: Stricturoplasty in Crohn's disease. In Cameron JL [ed]: Current Surgical Therapy, 8th ed. Philadelphia, CV Mosby, 2004, pp 118-119.)

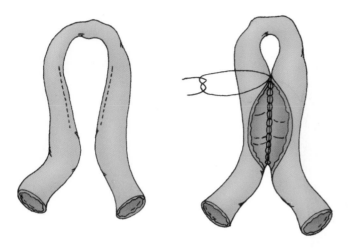

Figure 70–20. Jaboulay stricturoplasty. Two separate enterotomies are made, with the most strictured portion left unopened. Subsequent closure creates a side-to-side enteroenterostomy. (Adapted from Tichansky D, Cagir B, Yoo E, et al: Strictureplasty for Crohn's disease: Meta-analysis. Dis Colon Rectum 43:911, 2000.)

because shifting of the abdominal wall can reveal creases or protrusions that can interfere with appliance seal and the patient's ability to see or reach the stoma site. If the patient has a history of multiple abdominal operations, abdominal sepsis, the potential for a shortened mesentery, or other factors that could interfere with the bowel reaching a proposed stoma site, several alternative sites should be chosen and marked. Marking should be done with indelible ink, and the marking should be reinforced in the operating room immediately before surgery by re-inking or lightly scratching the skin so that the mark can be found after preparing the abdomen.[101]

Standard techniques are used to create and mature the end or loop stoma (we do not use bars in the creation of our loop stomas): a 2-cm disk of skin is sharply excised, the subcutaneous fat is opened to the level of the rectus fascia, a cruciate incision is made with electrocautery in the anterior rectus sheath, the rectus muscle is spread in the direction of its fibers, the posterior sheath and peritoneum are opened with a cruciate incision, the tract is dilated with two fingers, the bowel is brought through the abdominal wall with the mesentery

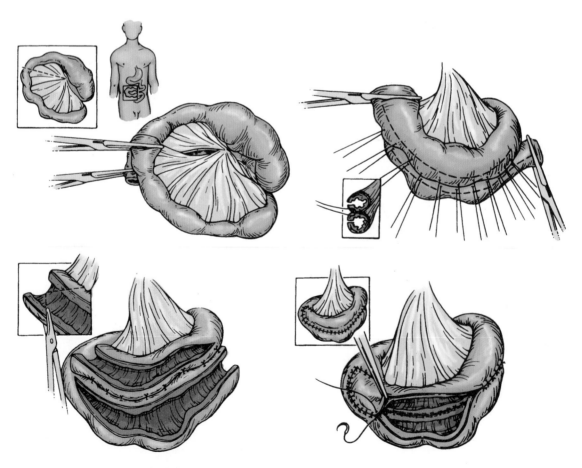

Figure 70–21.   Side-to-side isoperistaltic stricturoplasty. A long side-to-side isoperistaltic enteroenterostomy is performed after dividing the diseased intestinal segment and moving the proximal loop over the distal loop in a side-to-side fashion. (From Michelassi F, Hurst RD: Stricturoplasty in Crohn's disease. In Cameron JL [ed]: Current Surgical Therapy, 7th ed. St Louis, CV Mosby, 2001, p 136.)

cephalad to ensure that the dependent portion of the stoma is well formed, the abdominal incision is closed, the bowel is opened, and the stoma is matured so that 2 to 3 cm of everted bowel projects from the abdominal wall.[101] It is important to pull the fascia to the midline with a midline incision or caudad with a Pfannenstiel incision before creating the abdominal wall defect to ensure that all openings are aligned, thus preventing kinking of the bowel, which can lead to obstruction or ischemia of the stoma.

Bypass Procedures

Intestinal bypass or exclusion procedures are rarely, if ever indicated in the treatment of Crohn's disease that involves the jejunum and ileum. However, treatment of Crohn's disease of the duodenum may require bypass procedures such as gastrojejunostomy or duodenojejunostomy.[94]

Laparoscopic Surgery in Crohn's Disease

Crohn's disease presents an array of challenges to surgeons approaching treatment of the disease laparoscopically, including multiple previous abdominal operations, intense inflammation, mesenteric thickening, penetrating disease, and segmental involvement. Patients, many of whom are acutely aware of the high likelihood that they will require surgical therapy at some point in the course of their disease, are eager to pursue laparoscopic approaches that promise better cosmetic outcomes and reduced recovery time. The laparoscopic, laparoscopically assisted, or hand-assisted approach in Crohn's disease may lend itself to diagnosis in cases in which previous attempts at work-up have been nondiagnostic; to diversion in the treatment of more distal disease, particularly in complicated disease; and to resection using primarily hand-assisted techniques and the endoscopic Ligasure (10-mm Ligasure Atlas or 5-mm Ligasure V), which allows safe laparoscopic division of the thickened mesentery. Although the overwhelming majority of evidence to date supporting the benefits of laparoscopy over open approaches has not come from prospective randomized controlled trials, there do seem to be advantages in terms of blood loss, postoperative pulmonary function, duration of postoperative ileus, and length of hospital stay. Characterization of the long-term results after laparoscopic surgery for Crohn's disease awaits adequate numbers of patients with long-term follow-up.[102]

Indications for laparoscopic surgery are essentially the same as those for open surgery. Contraindications to a laparoscopic approach include the following[102]:

- Diffuse peritonitis
- Acute obstruction with distention accompanied by dilated of loops of intestine
- A history of multiple previous laparotomies or known dense intra-abdominal adhesions
- Coagulopathy not correctable at the time of surgery
- Portal hypertension with known intra-abdominal varices

Management of Complicated Small Bowel Crohn's Disease

The Vienna classification system groups Crohn's disease patients on the basis of age (<40 or ≥40), disease location (terminal ileum, colon, ileocolon, upper gastrointestinal), and disease behavior (inflammatory, stricturing, penetrating).[21] Because surgical therapy does not cure Crohn's disease, it is used only to treat complications that are not amenable to medical therapy.[88] Although any of the three types of disease behavior may require surgical therapy, the most common indications involve stricturing or penetrating types of disease behavior.

Stricturing Disease

Patients with Crohn's disease and a primarily stricturing pattern of disease behavior may have an array of symptoms with a wide range of severity reflecting the degree of underlying obstruction, from chronic and low-grade to acute and high-grade or complete. Patients may have abdominal pain, nausea, vomiting, distention, and even obstipation leading to food avoidance, weight loss, failure to thrive, malnourishment, or hospital admission for medical or surgical therapy. Patients with obstructive symptoms caused by stricturing disease who require admission should be initially treated with nonoperative therapy, including bowel rest, nasogastric suction, and resuscitation. If patients have evidence of active disease on colonoscopy or contrast radiography, it is reasonable to treat them with aggressive medical therapy because inflammation may contribute to the partial obstruction. A low-residue diet may reduce the incidence of subsequent episodes of partial bowel obstruction. Patients with recurrent bouts of partial obstruction, those who fail to respond to nonoperative therapy, and patients with complete bowel obstruction require surgery.[103] It bears mentioning again that to the extent possible dictated by the urgency of their operation, patients should always be resuscitated and decompressed before their arrival in the operating room.

The decision to treat strictures with resection or stricturoplasty will be influenced by a variety of factors, including the surgeon's comfort and experience with stricturoplasty techniques for strictures of various length; patient factors such as malnutrition, steroid use, or sepsis; concomitant penetrating disease with phlegmon, abscess, fistula, or free perforation; and the condition of the bowel to be treated. Many authors advocate stricturoplasty as the first choice for patients with almost any type of stricturing disease, including complicated strictures or anastomotic strictures, whereas others argue that resection should generally be the first choice, with stricturoplasty being reserved for patients with short-bowel syndrome or those with multiple recurrences. Depending on the clinical scenario, patients may be served best by a combination of resection and stricturoplasty.

Enteric Fistulas

Patients with Crohn's disease and a primarily penetrating pattern of disease behavior are subject to the formation of fistulas, which are abnormal passages from a normal cavity or hollow organ to a free surface (external fistulas) or to another cavity or hollow organ (internal fistulas). Fistulas involving the small intestine are discussed in this chapter. Examples include small intestine to small intestine (enteroenteric); small intestine to colon (enterocolonic); small intestine to any part of the urogenital tract, including the bladder (enterovesical), ureters (enteroureteral), and vagina (enterovaginal); and small intestine to skin (enterocutaneous fistula). The transmural nature of Crohn's disease leads to fistula formation, and although downstream obstruction or stricture is not a prerequisite for fistula formation, obstruction may contribute to fistula formation or decrease the likelihood that a fistula will heal. In a recent population-based study, fistulas developed in 35% of patients with Crohn's disease, with 20% of the fistulas being perianal (which is considered in another chapter).[104,105] A prospective study of the features, indications, and surgical treatment in 513 consecutive patients affected by Crohn's disease from 1985 to 1996 found that although fistulas were present in nearly a third of patients, they were rarely the primary indication for operative therapy.[96] This indicates that many of the fistulas found in patients with Crohn's disease, particularly those between loops of small bowel, will be asymptomatic and found incidentally on radiographs or during surgical exploration for treatment of septic complications or obstruction. However, small bowel fistulas may cause complications requiring surgery when long segments of bowel are bypassed, thereby leading to diarrhea or malabsorption; when the genitourinary or biliopancreatic systems are involved; or when the fistula results in external drainage.[100] Medical therapy has shown little promise in the treatment of Crohn's disease–induced enteric fistulas until recently; immunomodulator therapy for enteric fistulas, particularly with infliximab, has been modestly successful in the treatment of enteric fistulas, although the majority of patients in studies to date had perianal disease. It is probably justifiable to give patients who are otherwise reasonably well a trial of medical therapy, but not at the exclusion of indicated surgical therapy.[106]

Enteroenteric Fistulas

Crohn's disease–induced fistulas from one loop of small bowel to another are usually, in and of themselves, of little clinical consequence, although the active disease and inflammation that are the underlying cause typically require treatment. A simple enteroenteric fistula that encompasses a short length of bowel between connections may be found incidentally on radiographs, on abdominal exploration, or in a resected specimen and does not require further surgical intervention. An enteroenteric fistula can be symptomatic and require surgical therapy if a long section of small bowel is bypassed. Short-segment fistulas that are in close proximity should not be separated, but taken en bloc. Long-segment fistulas in which en bloc resection would sacrifice significant bowel length should be separated close to bowel that will undergo resection while leaving the possibility

of primary repair for the healthy segment. Most ileocecal fistulas behave clinically like enteroenteric fistulas and are treated similarly.[88,104]

Ileosigmoid Fistulas

Ileosigmoid fistulas occur in up to 6% of all Crohn's disease patients and in 16% to 26% of Crohn's disease patients with internal fistulas. They are generally the result of penetration from the small intestine into the sigmoid, and the sigmoid is not usually affected primarily by Crohn's disease. As with enteroenteric fistulas, ileosigmoid fistulas are frequently asymptomatic, but they can be associated with abdominal pain, diarrhea, and malabsorption. Commonly, they are not detected with endoscopic or contrast studies. These fistulas can generally be treated without sigmoid resection by taking down the fistula and, after débridement of the sigmoid, closing the colon primarily. Sigmoid resection is reasonable if colonic Crohn's disease is present or if technical difficulties prevent easy primary closure, such as local inflammation with rigidity and thickening of the colonic wall, a large defect after débridement, or involvement of the colon wall close to the mesentery. If sigmoid resection is required, primary reanastomosis for restoration of intestinal continuity can usually be performed; temporary proximal diversion may be necessary in patients with long-term steroid use or extensive inflammation that precludes safe primary closure of the fistula defect.[88,100,104]

Enterovesical and Enteroureteral Fistulas

The reported incidence of fistulas from the gastrointestinal tract to the genitourinary system in patients with Crohn's disease has been 1% to 8%.[107] They originate most commonly from the ileum, colon, or rectum; they may also result from anastomotic leak after resection.[104] Although they may be the initial complaint in patients with Crohn's disease, they typically occur in patients with established disease. Common symptoms include dysuria, urinary urgency, urinary frequency, suprapubic discomfort, pneumaturia, and fecaluria. Chronic or recurrent urinary tract infections and urogenital tract infections such as prostatitis or epididymitis may give rise to fever and hematuria.[107] The diagnosis should be suspected in a patient with history, physical examination, and laboratory findings that are typical. The diagnosis can be confirmed and the lesion localized with the aid of cystoscopy, plain radiography, including small bowel follow-through or small bowel enteroclysis, or axial imaging with CT or MRI.[104] The fistulas rarely close spontaneously, and although medical therapy may be mitigating, definitive treatment generally requires surgical therapy. The dome of the bladder is most commonly involved and the trigone is usually spared, thus allowing a relatively straightforward approach. The basic operative steps are division of the fistula, resection of the involved portion of bowel, and débridement and primary closure of the bladder with postoperative Foley catheter drainage.[88,100]

Enterocutaneous Fistulas

Most enterocutaneous fistulas in patients with Crohn's disease occur in the postoperative setting; the involved bowel is essentially normal, and the fistulas, which tend to drain through surgical scars, are the result of anastomotic leak after resection or unrecognized bowel injury. Although reported numbers vary, it seems that spontaneous enterocutaneous fistulas that are the direct result of penetration from a diseased segment of small bowel to the exterior are relatively rare. *Even though it may be difficult to definitively say which is more common, it is worth considering that spontaneous enterocutaneous fistulas that occur before a patient has undergone surgery or after a patient is far removed from surgery are probably the result of penetrating Crohn's disease and that those that occur in the postoperative setting are probably the result of surgical misadventure.* These observations necessarily have an impact on decision making with regard to treatment of enterocutaneous fistulas because postoperative fistulas involving bowel not affected by Crohn's disease will behave differently from spontaneous fistulas that are the result of penetration from bowel affected by Crohn's disease. Fistulas that are not a direct result of Crohn's disease should respond to conventional treatment in a fairly predictable fashion; long, low-output fistulas have an increased probability of closing with nonoperative therapy such as bowel rest, strategies to decrease the output of the gastrointestinal tract, and TPN support, whereas short, high-output fistulas are more likely to require operative therapy. In contrast, spontaneous fistulas that are the direct result of penetrating Crohn's disease rarely close without operative therapy, although as mentioned earlier, newer medical therapies with immunomodulators such as infliximab may be of benefit. Of course, operative therapy should not be delayed when there is distal obstruction, if fistula output or wound care becomes difficult to manage, or if medical treatment has obviously failed. Operative therapy relies on division of the fistula, resection of the involved bowel, débridement of the entire fistulous tract, and safe repair of the ensuing bowel defects.[88,106]

Enterogenital Fistulas

Fistulas from the rectum to the vagina are common in women with Crohn's disease (9% of all fistulas observed in a recently published, population-based study[105]), and although fistulas from the small intestine to the female genital tract, including enterovaginal, enterosalpingeal, and enterouterine, do occur, they are less common. Symptoms of an enterovaginal fistula include malodorous vaginal discharge and passage of air from the vagina; enterosalpingeal and enterouterine fistulas may be difficult to identify preoperatively, with diagnosis occurring at the time of abdominal exploration. The common themes continue, including division of the fistulous tract with resection of involved bowel and débridement of the victim organ, although effort should be made to preserve reproductive, endocrine, and sexual function, especially in women of childbearing age.[94]

Abscesses

Abscesses in patients with Crohn's disease are common (reports indicate that 10% to 30% of patients with Crohn's disease will have an abscess at some point in their illness[108]); they can be an intermediate step in the formation of fistulas, and like fistulas, they may be the result of penetrating disease from a segment of bowel affected by Crohn's disease, or they may be the result of surgical misadventure (see Fig. 70–12). Patients may have few, if any symptoms because the abscesses are frequently contained in loops of bowel, between leaves of mesentery, by abdominal viscera, in the retroperitoneum, or in the pelvis; symptoms may also be quelled by medical therapies such as steroids or immunomodulators. If patients do have signs and symptoms, they are those typical of intra-abdominal infections, including fever, ileus or obstruction, abdominal pain, tenderness, or a palpable mass. Diagnosis and localization are aided most by axial imaging. Classically, treatment was strictly operative, with abscess drainage as a first stage followed by bowel resection as a second stage. With the advance of radiographically guided percutaneous techniques, abscesses can be effectively drained outside the operating room; concomitant medical therapy for any active Crohn's disease, along with resuscitation, antibiotics for systemic infection, nutritional support, and bowel rest as indicated, can be administered. If the abscess cavities collapse and the patient's Crohn's disease is controlled, no further therapy may be needed. If operative therapy is required, the patient will benefit in terms of physiologic preparedness and technical ease, which may make the operation less extensive, preserve bowel length, and allow restoration of bowel continuity without diversion in a single stage.[30,108]

Ureteral Obstruction

The majority of cases of ureteral obstruction in patients with Crohn's disease are not caused by stones, with 50% to 73% of cases of ureteral obstruction in patients with Crohn's disease being acalculous. Acalculous ureteral obstruction was seen in 4.7% to 14.3% of Crohn's patients who had diagnostic intravenous pyelography studies performed; in contrast, intravenous pyelograms performed on asymptomatic Crohn's patients reveal acalculous ureteral obstruction in 18% to 50% of those tested, which suggests that acalculous obstruction in these patients is a more prevalent problem that probably goes unrecognized fairly frequently. When symptoms do occur, they can be nonspecific, with patients reporting urinary frequency and urgency, flank pain, and fever and, on examination, a palpable abdominal mass is possible. The results of urinalysis and culture are often normal. The diagnosis is most often confirmed with axial imaging. The inflammation associated with ileocecal disease is usually the cause of acalculous ureteral obstruction, so it occurs more commonly on the right and less commonly on the left or bilaterally. Current recommendations advocate a staged approach to treatment consisting of medical control of active Crohn's disease, ureteral stenting for significant obstruction, and percutaneous drainage of any associated abscess, followed by resection of diseased bowel and ureterolysis as required if nonoperative therapy fails.[107]

Free Perforation

Free perforation in patients with Crohn's disease is rare; as alluded to in the sections on abscess and fistula, the adhesions that are a result of the transmural inflammatory nature of Crohn's disease create an environment around affected segments that does not favor free perforation. Free perforation usually occurs in Crohn's patients with toxic colitis, distal obstruction, or cancer and after endoscopy or surgery. Perforation in patients with prodromal signs and symptoms will generally be heralded by a sudden worsening in their clinical course; as usual, such assumptions are dangerous in patients treated with steroids and immunomodulators, in whom a high index of suspicion is required for diagnosis. Plain films showing free air confirm the diagnosis, and in cases in which the diagnosis goes unsuspected, CT scans will show the same. It should go without saying that emergency exploration is required when free perforation is suspected; while the operating room is being prepared, the patient should be resuscitated, treated prophylactically with broad-spectrum antibiotics, receive stress-dose steroids if appropriate, have laboratory tests performed, including blood type and crossmatch, and be marked for stoma placement. Débridement and primary repair of gastroduodenal perforation or resection with primary anastomosis after jejunoileal perforation is often possible, and proximal diversion with a loop or end stoma should be considered if conditions are unfavorable.[30]

Crohn's Disease of the Duodenum

As stated previously, the exact incidence and prevalence of upper gastrointestinal Crohn's disease are not known, and even though it is historically rare, the incidence has increased in recent reports. Careful examination and biopsy of the upper gastrointestinal tract in those with Crohn's disease will reveal histologic evidence of disease in as many as 30% to 50% of patients, although many will lack upper gastrointestinal symptoms. The duodenum can be primarily affected by Crohn's disease, or it can be secondarily affected as the victim organ of penetrating disease (Fig. 70–22). Symptoms of duodenal involvement include dyspepsia or epigastric pain, anorexia, and proximal obstructive symptoms such as early satiety, nausea, vomiting, and weight loss. Complications of proximal Crohn's disease are similar to those found with more distal disease; inflammation, strictures, and fistulas (almost all of which are the result of penetration into a normal duodenum) occur along with an increased risk for cancer in areas of long-standing disease. Because the majority of patients with upper gastrointestinal disease have concomitant lower gastrointestinal disease and because medical therapy for proximal Crohn's disease has not been well studied, the course of medical treatment is typically determined by the clinical course of the distal disease. Many of the principles of surgical

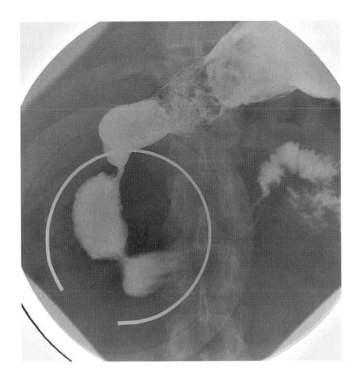

Figure 70–22. Upper gastrointestinal series demonstrating multifocal Crohn's disease of the duodenum.

management discussed in previous sections apply to complicated duodenal disease: after medical therapy has been instituted for active Crohn's disease, the patient should receive nutritional support with preference given to the enteral route; frank abscesses that are accessible should be percutaneously drained; fistulas should be divided and the bowel segments from which they arose should be resected; minimal débridement of the duodenum may allow primary closure with the Heineke-Mikulicz technique, although more extensive débridement may require a duodenojejunostomy, gastrojejunostomy, or Roux-en-Y anastomosis for reconstruction; and strictures can be treated with a stricturoplasty when technically feasible or may require a duodenojejunostomy, gastrojejunostomy or Roux-en-Y anastomosis for reconstruction.[109]

Postoperative Care

In most respects, the postoperative care of patients who have undergone surgery for Crohn's disease is not different from that in patients who have undergone any other type of gastrointestinal surgery. Routine use of postoperative nasogastric suction is not required for distal procedures, but it may be considered for procedures involving the upper gastrointestinal tract. If stress-dose steroids were required, they can be tapered quickly if the patient is not critically ill.[94]

Recurrence of Crohn's disease after resection, which usually occurs at the site of surgical anastomosis, is seen in almost all patients when they are monitored long-term. First, there is endoscopic recurrence, which in a significant number of patients is followed by symptomatic recurrence. One study found endoscopic evidence of Crohn's disease recurrence in 73% of patients 1 year after surgery, with only 20% of patients having symptoms; when observations were repeated 3 years after surgery, the endoscopic recurrence rate had increased to 85%, and symptoms were present in 34%. Perhaps the most important measure of recurrence is the need for reoperation, with about half of patients undergoing ileocolonic resection requiring reoperation within approximately 10 years of surgery.[86]

There is evidence to support the use of some types of medical therapy to prevent both endoscopic and symptomatic recurrence of Crohn's disease after surgery. Besides being inappropriate for maintenance therapy in nonsurgical Crohn's patients, steroids have proved ineffective for prophylaxis against disease recurrence in the postoperative setting. Sulfasalazine has not been shown to be consistently helpful in preventing postoperative recurrence. Although there is evidence to support the efficacy of other 5-acetylsalicylate preparations in the maintenance of postsurgical remission in Crohn's disease, the overall beneficial effect of mesalamine is small. Only a modest benefit has been shown with azathioprine and 6-mercaptopurine in the postoperative setting, but because there is much stronger evidence supporting their use in maintenance therapy after medically induced remission, they are probably justified in high-risk postoperative patients.[65,86]

Finally, smoking cessation is advised in all postoperative Crohn's disease patients; smokers have double the rate of recurrence, and smokers who quit have decreased rates of recurrence.[65]

REFERENCES

1. Loftus EV Jr, Schoenfeld P, Sandborn WJ: The epidemiology and natural history of Crohn's disease in population-based patient cohorts from North America: A systematic review. Aliment Pharmacol Ther 16:51-60, 2002.
2. Ekbom A: The epidemiology of IBD: A lot of data but little knowledge. How shall we proceed? Inflamm Bowel Dis 10(Suppl 1):S32-S34, 2004.
3. Munkholm P, Langholz E, Davidsen M, Binder V: Disease activity courses in a regional cohort of Crohn's disease patients. Scand J Gastroenterol 30:699-706, 1995.
4. Wolters FL, Russel MG, Stockbrugger RW: Systematic review: Has disease outcome in Crohn's disease changed during the last four decades? Aliment Pharmacol Ther 20:483-496, 2004.
5. Loftus EV Jr, Silverstein MD, Sandborn WJ, et al: Crohn's disease in Olmsted County, Minnesota, 1940-1993: Incidence, prevalence, and survival. Gastroenterology 114:1161-1168, 1998.
6. Jess T, Winther KV, Munkholm P, et al: Mortality and causes of death in Crohn's disease: Follow-up of a population-based cohort in Copenhagen County, Denmark. Gastroenterology 122:1808-1814, 2002.
7. Bodger K: Cost of illness of Crohn's disease. Pharmacoeconomics 20:639-652, 2002.
8. Sanders DS: Mucosal integrity and barrier function in the pathogenesis of early lesions in Crohn's disease. J Clin Pathol 58:568-572, 2005.
9. Korzenik JR: Past and current theories of etiology of IBD: Toothpaste, worms, and refrigerators. J Clin Gastroenterol 39(4 Suppl 2):S59-S65, 2005.
10. Ekbom A, Montgomery SM: Environmental risk factors (excluding tobacco and microorganisms): Critical analysis of old and new hypotheses. Best Pract Res Clin Gastroenterol 18:497-508, 2004.
11. Birrenbach T, Bocker U: Inflammatory bowel disease and smoking: A review of epidemiology, pathophysiology, and therapeutic implications. Inflamm Bowel Dis 10:848-859, 2004.
12. Hume G, Radford-Smith GL: The pathogenesis of Crohn's disease in the 21st century. Pathology 34:561-567, 2002.
13. Gasche C, Grundtner P: Genotypes and phenotypes in Crohn's disease: Do they help in clinical management? Gut 54:162-167, 2005.
14. Newman B, Siminovitch KA: Recent advances in the genetics of inflammatory bowel disease. Curr Opin Gastroenterol 21:401-407, 2005.
15. Sabiston DC, Lyerly HK (eds): Textbook of Surgery, the Biological Basis of Modern Surgical Practice, 15th ed. Philadelphia, WB Saunders, 1997.
16. Greenfield LJ (ed): Surgery, Scientific Principles and Practice, 2nd ed. Philadelphia, Lippincott-Raven, 1997.
17. Farmer RG, Hawk WA, Turnbull RB Jr: Indications for surgery in Crohn's disease: Analysis of 500 cases. Gastroenterology 71:245-250, 1976.
18. van Hogezand RA, Witte AM, Veenendaal RA, et al: Proximal Crohn's disease: Review of the clinicopathologic features and therapy. Inflamm Bowel Dis 7:328-337, 2001.
19. Heresbach D, Alexandre JL, Branger B, et al: Frequency and significance of granulomas in a cohort of incident cases of Crohn's disease. Gut 54:215-222, 2005.
20. Lichtenstein GR, Hanauer SB, Kane SV, Present DH: Crohn's is not a 6-week disease: Lifelong management of mild to moderate Crohn's disease. Inflamm Bowel Dis 10(Suppl 2):S2-S10, 2004.
21. Gasche C, Scholmerich J, Brynskov J, et al: A simple classification of Crohn's disease: Report of the Working Party for the World Congresses of Gastroenterology, Vienna 1998. Inflamm Bowel Dis 6:8-15, 2000.
22. Zankel E, Rogler G, Andus T, et al: Crohn's disease patient characteristics in a tertiary referral center: Comparison with patients from a population-based cohort. Eur J Gastroenterol Hepatol 17:395-401, 2005.
23. Louis E, Collard A, Oger AF, et al: Behaviour of Crohn's disease according to the Vienna classification: Changing pattern over the course of the disease. Gut 49:777-782, 2001.
24. Cosnes J, Cattan S, Blain A, et al: Long-term evolution of disease behavior of Crohn's disease. Inflamm Bowel Dis 8:244-250, 2002.
25. Farmer RG, Hawk WA, Turnbull RB Jr: Clinical patterns in Crohn's disease: A statistical study of 615 cases. Gastroenterology 68:627-635, 1975.
26. Sawczenko A, Sandhu BK: Presenting features of inflammatory bowel disease in great Britain and Ireland. Arch Dis Child 88:995-1000, 2003.
27. Wagtmans MJ, Verspaget HW, Lamers CB, van Hogezand RA: Crohn's disease in the elderly: A comparison with young adults. J Clin Gastroenterol 27:129-133, 1998.
28. Wagtmans MJ, Verspaget HW, Lamers CB, van Hogezand RA: Gender-related differences in the clinical course of Crohn's disease. Am J Gastroenterol 96:1541-1546, 2001.
29. Belaiche J, Louis E, D'Haens G, et al: Acute lower gastrointestinal bleeding in Crohn's disease: Characteristics of a unique series of 34 patients. Belgian IBD Research Group. Am J Gastroenterol 94:2177-2181, 1999.
30. Berg DF, Bahadursingh AM, Kaminski DL, Longo WE: Acute surgical emergencies in inflammatory bowel disease. Am J Surg 184:45-51, 2002.
31. Schwartz DA, Pemberton JH, Sandborn WJ: Diagnosis and treatment of perianal fistulas in Crohn disease. Ann Intern Med 135:906-918, 2001.
32. Bernstein CN, Blanchard JF, Rawsthorne P, Yu N: The prevalence of extraintestinal diseases in inflammatory bowel disease: A population-based study. Am J Gastroenterol 96:1116-1122, 2001.
33. Ricart E, Panaccione R, Loftus EV Jr, et al: Autoimmune disorders and extraintestinal manifestations in first-degree familial and sporadic inflammatory bowel disease: A case-control study. Inflamm Bowel Dis 10:207-214, 2004.
34. Turkcapar N, Toruner M, Soykan I, et al: The prevalence of extraintestinal manifestations and HLA association in patients with inflammatory bowel disease. Rheumatol Int 1-6, 2005.
35. Beaven SW, Abreu MT: Biomarkers in inflammatory bowel disease. Curr Opin Gastroenterol 20:318-327, 2004.

36. Nielsen OH, Vainer B, Madsen SM, et al: Established and emerging biological activity markers of inflammatory bowel disease. Am J Gastroenterol 95:359-367, 2000.

37. Plevy S: Do serological markers and cytokines determine the indeterminate? J Clin Gastroenterol 38(5 Suppl):S51-S56, 2004.

38. Reumaux D, Sendid B, Poulain D, et al: Serological markers in inflammatory bowel diseases. Best Pract Res Clin Gastroenterol 17:19-35, 2003.

39. Zholudev A, Zurakowski D, Young W, et al: Serologic testing with ANCA, ASCA, and anti-OmpC in children and young adults with Crohn's disease and ulcerative colitis: Diagnostic value and correlation with disease phenotype. Am J Gastroenterol 99:2235-2241, 2004.

40. Furukawa A, Saotome T, Yamasaki M, et al: Cross-sectional imaging in Crohn disease. Radiographics 24:689-702, 2004.

41. Maglinte DD, Kelvin FM, O'Connor K, et al: Current status of small bowel radiography. Abdom Imaging 21:247-257, 1996.

42. Cirillo LC, Camera L, Della Noce M, et al: Accuracy of enteroclysis in Crohn's disease of the small bowel: A retrospective study. Eur Radiol 10:1894-1898, 2000.

43. Low RN, Sebrechts CP, Politoske DA, et al: Crohn disease with endoscopic correlation: Single-shot fast spin-echo and gadolinium-enhanced fat-suppressed spoiled gradient-echo MR imaging. Radiology 222:652-660, 2002.

44. Nolan DJ: Enteroclysis of non-neoplastic disorders of the small intestine. Eur Radiol 10:342-353, 2000.

45. Parente F, Greco S, Molteni M, et al: Oral contrast enhanced bowel ultrasonography in the assessment of small intestine Crohn's disease. A prospective comparison with conventional ultrasound, x ray studies, and ileocolonoscopy. Gut 53:1652-1657, 2004.

46. Toms AP, Barltrop A, Freeman AH: A prospective randomised study comparing enteroclysis with small bowel follow-through examinations in 244 patients. Eur Radiol 11:1155-1160, 2001.

47. Mako EK, Mester AR, Tarjan Z, et al: Enteroclysis and spiral CT examination in diagnosis and evaluation of small bowel Crohn's disease. Eur J Radiol 35:168-175, 2000.

48. Rollandi GA, Curone PF, Biscaldi E, et al: Spiral CT of the abdomen after distention of small bowel loops with transparent enema in patients with Crohn's disease. Abdom Imaging 24:544-549, 1999.

49. Del Campo L, Arribas I, Valbuena M, et al: Spiral CT findings in active and remission phases in patients with Crohn disease. J Comput Assist Tomogr 25:792-797, 2001.

50. Parente F, Greco S, Molteni M, et al: Modern imaging of Crohn's disease using bowel ultrasound. Inflamm Bowel Dis 10:452-461, 2004.

51. Marshall JK, Cawdron R, Zealley I, et al: Prospective comparison of small bowel meal with pneumocolon versus ileo-colonoscopy for the diagnosis of ileal Crohn's disease. Am J Gastroenterol 99:1321-1329, 2004.

52. Coremans G, Rutgeerts P, Geboes K, et al: The value of ileoscopy with biopsy in the diagnosis of intestinal Crohn's disease. Gastrointest Endosc 30:167-172, 1984.

53. Pera A, Bellando P, Caldera D, et al: Colonoscopy in inflammatory bowel disease. Diagnostic accuracy and proposal of an endoscopic score. Gastroenterology 92:181-185, 1987.

54. Odze R: Diagnostic problems and advances in inflammatory bowel disease. Mod Pathol 16:347-358, 2003.

55. Geboes K, Ectors N, D'Haens G, Rutgeerts P: Is ileoscopy with biopsy worthwhile in patients presenting with symptoms of inflammatory bowel disease? Am J Gastroenterol 93:201-206, 1998.

56. Cherian S, Singh P: Is routine ileoscopy useful? An observational study of procedure times, diagnostic yield, and learning curve. Am J Gastroenterol 99:2324-2329, 2004.

57. Robert ME, Skacel M, Ullman T, et al: Patterns of colonic involvement at initial presentation in ulcerative colitis: A retrospective study of 46 newly diagnosed cases. Am J Clin Pathol 122:94-99, 2004.

58. Abdullah BA, Gupta SK, Croffie JM, et al: The role of esophagogastroduodenoscopy in the initial evaluation of childhood inflammatory bowel disease: A 7-year study. J Pediatr Gastroenterol Nutr 35:636-640, 2002.

59. Wright CL, Riddell RH: Histology of the stomach and duodenum in Crohn's disease. Am J Surg Pathol 22:383-390, 1998.

60. Daperno M, D'Haens G, Van Assche G, et al: Development and validation of a new, simplified endoscopic activity score for Crohn's disease: The SES-CD. Gastrointest Endosc 60:505-512, 2004.

61. Sostegni R, Daperno M, Scaglione N, et al: Review article: Crohn's disease: Monitoring disease activity. Aliment Pharmacol Ther 17(Suppl 2):11-17, 2003.

62. Mpofu C, Watson AJ, Rhodes JM: Strategies for detecting colon cancer and/or dysplasia in patients with inflammatory bowel disease. Cochrane Database Syst Rev (2):CD000279, 2004.

63. Singh VV, Draganov P, Valentine J: Efficacy and safety of endoscopic balloon dilation of symptomatic upper and lower gastrointestinal Crohn's disease strictures. J Clin Gastroenterol 39:284-290, 2005.

64. Kornbluth A, Legnani P, Lewis BS: Video capsule endoscopy in inflammatory bowel disease: Past, present, and future. Inflamm Bowel Dis 10:278-285, 2004.

65. Yamamoto T: Factors affecting recurrence after surgery for Crohn's disease. World J Gastroenterol 11:3971-3979, 2005.

66. Napierkowski JJ, Maydonovitch CL, Belle LS, et al: Wireless capsule endoscopy in a community gastroenterology practice. J Clin Gastroenterol 39:36-41, 2005.

67. Swain P: Wireless capsule endoscopy and Crohn's disease. Gut 54:323-326, 2005.

68. Legnani P, Kornbluth A: Video capsule endoscopy in inflammatory bowel disease 2005. Curr Opin Gastroenterol 21:438-442, 2005.

69. Egan LJ, Sandborn WJ: Advances in the treatment of Crohn's disease. Gastroenterology 126:1574-1581, 2004.

70. Steinhart AH, Ewe K, Griffiths AM, et al: Corticosteroids for maintenance of remission in Crohn's disease. Cochrane Database Syst Rev (4):CD000301, 2003.

71. Sandborn WJ: Evidence-based treatment algorithm for mild to moderate Crohn's disease. Am J Gastroenterol 98(12 Suppl):S1-S5, 2003.

72. Guslandi M: Antibiotics for inflammatory bowel disease: Do they work? Eur J Gastroenterol Hepatol 17:145-147, 2005.

73. Siegel CA, Sands BE: Review article: Practical management of inflammatory bowel disease patients taking immunomodulators. Aliment Pharmacol Ther 22:1-16, 2005.

74. Brookes MJ, Green JR: Maintenance of remission in Crohn's disease: Current and emerging therapeutic options. Drugs 64:1069-1089, 2004.

75. Van Assche G, Vermeire S, Rutgeerts P: Medical treatment of inflammatory bowel diseases. Curr Opin Gastroenterol 21:443-447, 2005.

76. Podolsky DK: Inflammatory bowel disease. N Engl J Med 347:417-429, 2002.

77. Goh J, O'Morain CA: Review article: Nutrition and adult inflammatory bowel disease. Aliment Pharmacol Ther 17:307-320, 2003.

78. Jeejeebhoy KN: Clinical nutrition: 6. Management of nutritional problems of patients with Crohn's disease. CMAJ 166:913-918, 2002.

79. Gassull MA, Cabre E: Nutrition in inflammatory bowel disease. Curr Opin Clin Nutr Metab Care 4:561-569, 2001.

80. Geerling BJ, Badart-Smook A, Stockbrugger RW, Brummer RJ: Comprehensive nutritional status in patients with long-standing Crohn disease currently in remission. Am J Clin Nutr 67:919-926, 1998.

81. Duggan P, O'Brien M, Kiely M, et al: Vitamin K status in patients with Crohn's disease and relationship to bone turnover. Am J Gastroenterol 99:2178-2185, 2004.

82. de Silva AD, Mylonaki M, Rampton DS: Oral iron therapy in inflammatory bowel disease: Usage, tolerance, and efficacy. Inflamm Bowel Dis 9:316-320, 2003.

83. Hatanaka N, Nakaden H, Yamamoto Y, et al: Selenium kinetics and changes in glutathione peroxidase activities in patients receiving long-term parenteral nutrition and effects of supplementation with selenite. Nutrition 16:22-26, 2000.

84. Griffin IJ, Kim SC, Hicks PD, et al: Zinc metabolism in adolescents with Crohn's disease. Pediatr Res 56:235-239, 2004.

85. Zachos M, Tondeur M, Griffiths AM: Enteral nutritional therapy for inducing remission of Crohn's disease. Cochrane Database Syst Rev (3):CD000542, 2001.

86. Penner RM, Madsen KL, Fedorak RN: Postoperative Crohn's disease. Inflamm Bowel Dis 11:765-777, 2005.
87. Mekhjian HS, Switz DM, Watts HD, et al: National Cooperative Crohn's Disease Study: Factors determining recurrence of Crohn's disease after surgery. Gastroenterology 77:907-913, 1979.
88. Sartor RB, Sandborn WJ (eds): Kirsner's Inflammatory Bowel Diseases, 6th ed. Philadelphia, WB Saunders, 2004.
89. Wille-Jorgensen P, Guenaga KF, Matos D, Castro AA: Pre-operative mechanical bowel cleansing or not? An updated meta-analysis. Colorectal Dis 7:304-310, 2005.
90. Brown CJ, Buie WD: Perioperative stress dose steroids: Do they make a difference? J Am Coll Surg 193:678-686, 2001.
91. Beilman GJ: New strategies to improve outcomes in the surgical intensive care unit. Surg Infect (Larchmt) 5:289-300, 2004.
92. Kisielinski K, Conze J, Murken AH, et al: The Pfannenstiel or so called "bikini cut": Still effective more than 100 years after first description. Hernia 8:177-181, 2004.
93. Luijendijk RW, Jeekel J, Storm RK, et al: The low transverse Pfannenstiel incision and the prevalence of incisional hernia and nerve entrapment. Ann Surg 225:365-369, 1997.
94. Zuideman G, Yeo C (eds): Shackelford's Surgery of the Alimentary Tract, 5th ed. Philadelphia, WB Saunders, 2001.
95. Roy P, Kumar D: Strictureplasty. Br J Surg 91:1428-1437, 2004.
96. Hurst RD, Molinari M, Chung TP, et al: Prospective study of the features, indications, and surgical treatment in 513 consecutive patients affected by Crohn's disease. Surgery 122:661-667, discussion 667-668, 1997.
97. Lee EC, Papaioannou N: Minimal surgery for chronic obstruction in patients with extensive or universal Crohn's disease. Ann R Coll Surg Engl 64:229-233, 1982.
98. Michelassi F, Upadhyay GA: Side-to-side isoperistaltic strictureplasty in the treatment of extensive Crohn's disease. J Surg Res 117:71-78, 2004.
99. Tichansky D, Cagir B, Yoo E, et al: Strictureplasty for Crohn's disease: Meta-analysis. Dis Colon Rectum 43:911-919, 2000.
100. Michelassi F, Milsom JW (eds): Operative Strategies in Inflammatory Bowel Disease. New York, Springer-Verlag, 1999.
101. Beck DE (ed): Handbook of Colorectal Surgery. St Louis, Quality Medical, 1997.
102. Milsom JW: Laparoscopic surgery in the treatment of Crohn's disease. Surg Clin North Am 85:25-34, vii, 2005.
103. Friedman SL (ed): Current Diagnosis & Treatment in Gastroenterology, 2nd ed. New York, McGraw-Hill, 2003.
104. Levy C, Tremaine WJ: Management of internal fistulas in Crohn's disease. Inflamm Bowel Dis 8:106-111, 2002.
105. Schwartz DA, Loftus EV Jr, Tremaine WJ, et al: The natural history of fistulizing Crohn's disease in Olmsted County, Minnesota. Gastroenterology 122:875-880, 2002.
106. Poritz LS, Gagliano GA, McLeod RS, et al: Surgical management of entero and colocutaneous fistulae in Crohn's disease: 17 year's experience. Int J Colorectal Dis 19:481-485, discussion 486, 2004.
107. Pardi DS, Tremaine WJ, Sandborn WJ, McCarthy JT: Renal and urologic complications of inflammatory bowel disease. Am J Gastroenterol 93:504-514, 1998.
108. Jawhari A, Kamm MA, Ong C, et al: Intra-abdominal and pelvic abscess in Crohn's disease: Results of noninvasive and surgical management. Br J Surg 85:367-371, 1998.
109. van Hogezand RA, Witte AM, Veenendaal RA, et al: Proximal Crohn's disease: Review of the clinicopathologic features and therapy. Inflamm Bowel Dis 7:328-337, 2001.

71

Ileostomy

Riaz Cassim • David W. McFadden

HISTORICAL PERSPECTIVES

An ileostomy is a communication constructed between the distal part of the small intestine and the abdominal wall. It may be temporary or permanent and is classified according to the anatomic configuration upon creation. When performed after removal of the entire colon and rectum, it takes the form of a permanent end ileostomy. With the growing popularity and success of restorative proctocolectomy for ulcerative colitis, familial adenomatous polyposis, and low rectal cancer, the number of permanent ileostomies being performed has shown a downward trend.[1] Protection of these low-lying anastomoses has brought about the need for temporary diversion of the intestinal contents. This has been accomplished with the use of a temporary loop ileostomy.

The first recorded case of creation of an ileostomy is credited to Baum in 1879 for relieving an obstruction secondary to cancer of the ascending colon.[2-4] During the early half of the 20th century the ileum was simply brought out several inches through the abdominal wall for subsequent drainage.[5] Initially, the ileum was exteriorized via the inferior portion of the abdominal incision. It was not until the 1930s that the ileostomy was created through a separate right lower quadrant incision.[2] Healing was achieved by the formation of scar tissue between the serosa of the small bowel and the abdominal wall. This led to inflammation of the exposed serosa and ultimately resulted in stricture formation at the ileostomy exit site and subsequent intestinal obstruction with signs of abdominal cramping, voluminous ileostomy output, and hypovolemia. This condition was termed *ileostomy dysfunction* and was described by Warren and McKittrick in 1951.[6] In an effort to expedite healing and prevent irritation of the abdominal wall, Dragstedt in 1941 started covering the ileostomy with a skin graft, which led to a long and unsightly stoma.[4]

Ileostomy, as we know it today, has been around only for past 50 years. Dr. Bryan N. Brooke described it in 1952 when he inverted the end of the ileum before maturing the stoma in the operating room, and it has thus come to bear his name.[2,7,8] In 1953 Turnbull advised a similar technique whereby the seromuscular layer of the distal half of the exteriorized small bowel was removed and the mucosal tube was everted over the proximal half, thereby covering the exposed serosa.[2,8,9]

Significant advances were made by the development of a practical ileostomy appliance in 1936. Strauss, a Chicago surgeon, Koenig, his patient, and Rutzen, who made it commercially available, share the credit.[2,8,10] In addition, a major step in ileostomy care was establishment of the first ileostomy club by Turnbull at the Mount Sinai Hospital in New York.[2,10,11] As of 2001 there are over 450 chapters in the United Ostomy Association with 25,000 members. Turnbull also initiated the training program for enterostomal therapists in 1961 at the Cleveland Clinic.[2,9,10]

INDICATIONS

Total proctocolectomy with a permanent end Brooke ileostomy still remains the gold standard operation for patients with ulcerative colitis and familial polyposis. An end ileostomy may be potentially reversible if it is deemed that an ileoanal anastomosis may be hazardous, such as in patients with severe malnutrition, peritoneal contamination, or vascular compromise. A total abdominal colectomy with end ileostomy can then be performed, with completion proctectomy and ileoanal pouch anastomosis done as a second-staged precedure.[1]

Many conditions require temporary decompression and diversion after colorectal surgery. Few studies have compared the morbidity and mortality associated with diverting loop colostomy and loop ileostomy for protection of a colorectal anastomosis, and the results have been divided.[12-16] Rullier et al. have shown that the morbidity after loop ileostomy construction and closure, including the risk for reoperation, is significantly lower for loop ileostomy than for loop colostomy.[16] Other studies have also shown excellent results with loop ileostomy.[17,18] Quality of life, although altered in all patients with stomas, is less impaired after a loop ileostomy because the effluent is odorless and the stoma is less bulky and less prone to prolapse.[13,19-21]

A temporary loop ileostomy may be warranted for the following conditions[15,22,23]:

Anastomotic factors
  Protecting a complicated anastomosis, such as coloanal and ileoanal anastomoses
  Proven anastomotic leakage at surgery
  Technical difficulties, such as incomplete staple rings and tension
  Anastomosis in an irradiated field
  Anastomosis in the presence of mild peritonitis or contamination
  Multiple distal anastomoses
Crohn's disease
Carcinomatosis with distal obstruction
Abdominal trauma
Congenital anomalies

PHYSIOLOGY

An ileostomy starts to function 48 to 72 hours after construction. A mature ileostomy produces between 400 and 700 mL of effluent per day. This volume remains relatively constant for an individual. The contents are weakly acidic (pH 6.1 to 6.5). Sodium excretion is 60 to 120 mEq/day, which is two to three times higher than in normal feces. Equilibrium is established by renal conservation of salt and water.[24] If the ileostomy output is excessive and leads to dehydration, the urine becomes concentrated and acidic. This may result in the formation of uric acid calculi, which have been reported in 3% to 13% of ileostomates.[11,25]

Cholelithiasis after permanent ileostomy has been reported in up to 30% of patients.[25,26] Patients older than 50 years and females are at a slightly higher risk for unknown reasons.[26] Cholesterol stones are precipitated by disruption of the enterohepatic circulation of bile acids by removal or inflammation of the terminal ileum.[27]

PREOPERATIVE PREPARATION

The thought of a stoma, whether permanent or temporary, is frightful and anxiety provoking for most patients. It is important to relieve patient fear about living with a stoma. Providing patients with literature on their disease and the proposed surgery is often helpful. Getting a patient in touch with ostomy support groups, especially with an individual of similar age, gender, and socioeconomic status, will aid the patient in realizing that a normal life is possible with an ileostomy.

Proper positioning of the stoma and meticulous surgical technique are the two most important factors that ensure success with a well-functioning ileostomy. A preoperative visit with the enterostomal therapist is essential. The latter can provide important preoperative counseling and perform proper marking of the stoma site, which has a direct bearing on the subsequent outcome of the ileostomy and management.[28,29] Ileostomy effluent is liquid, corrosive to the skin, and voluminous. An ileostomy that is properly located will often prevent complications such as leakage resulting in skin breakdown, prolapse, and peristomal hernia.[29,30]

Typically, the ileostomy is positioned in the right lower portion of the abdomen through the rectus abdominis muscle. This point usually corresponds to a third of the distance on an imaginary line stretching from the umbilicus to the right anterior superior iliac spine. The stoma should lie on the bulge of the infraumbilical skin fold.[21] Another way to determine the location is to draw a vertical line through the umbilicus and another horizontal line through the inferior margin of the umbilicus. The faceplate of the appliance is positioned in the right lower quadrant so that it abuts against the two imaginary lines. The opening of the faceplate usually corresponds to the outer half of the rectus muscle.[22]

Previous scars, bony prominences, the waistline, the beltline, the inguinal crease, the costal margin, the umbilicus, and skin folds should be avoided if at all possible. These sites interfere with proper placement and management of the ileostomy appliance and thus lead to poor clinical outcomes. The faceplate of the ileostomy appliance should be placed on the patient and its appropriateness confirmed by having the patient bend, stand, sit, and lay down. In patients who are obese, it should be placed at the level of the umbilicus or higher for ease of management. Ostomates have to be able to visualize the stoma if they are to participate effectively in stoma care. Once the ideal stoma site has been determined, it is marked with a permanent marking pen or preferably by intradermal injection of methylene blue dye.

TECHNIQUES

For an optimal outcome one must focus on potential complications and postoperative care while constructing an ileostomy. Adhering to the basic surgical principles of gentle tissue handling, good hemostasis, and prevention of tension will ensure good results. Placing the ileostomy in the main incision should be condemned because this prevents the placement of a well-fitting appliance and leads to a higher incidence of wound infection, dehiscence, and incisional hernia.[28]

END ILEOSTOMY

The patient is placed in the supine or the perineolithotomy position, depending on the resection being performed (Fig. 71–1). A hypodermic needle is used to scratch a mark at the preoperatively marked stoma site in the right lower part of the abdomen because if the site is marked with a pen, it will be erased with vigorous surgical preparation. For most operations, a midline approach passing to the left of the umbilicus is preferable to help minimize scars and preserve the remaining quadrants of the abdomen should revision or relocation of the ileostomy be required in the future. Such an approach is particularly important in patients with Crohn's disease.

Preparation of the terminal or distal ileum is an important aspect of the procedure. The ileocolic artery is divided as part of the right colectomy, but the

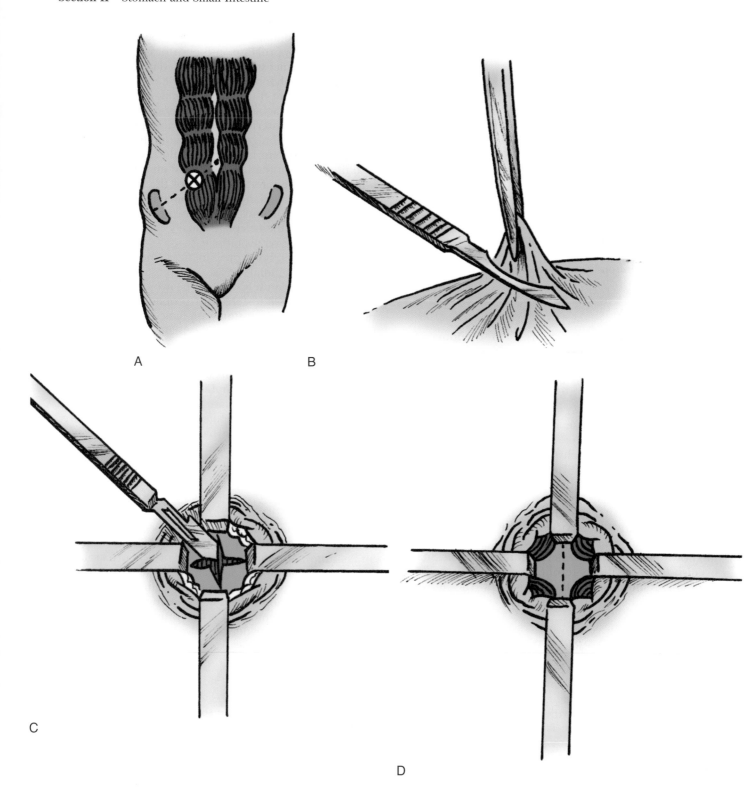

A

B

C

D

Figure 71–1.   Technique of end ileostomy (Brooke) construction. **A,** Ileostomy site marked preoperatively in the right lower quadrant (a third of the way between the umbilicus and the anterior superior iliac spine, overlying the rectus muscle). **B,** Two-centimeter disk of skin excised with a scalpel. **C,** Anterior fascia divided via a cruciate incision. **D,** Posterior rectus sheath divided longitudinally after spreading the rectus muscle.

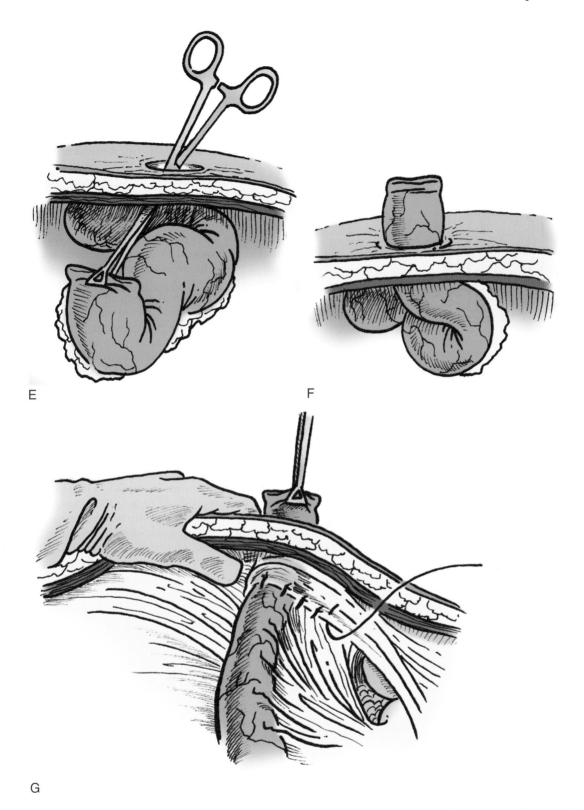

E

F

G

Figure 71–1, cont'd. **E,** Ileum delivered through the ileostomy site with a Babcock clamp. **F,** Ileum protruding 2 to 3 cm above the anterior abdominal wall without tension. **G,** Intraperitoneal fixation of the ileum and its mesentery.

Continued

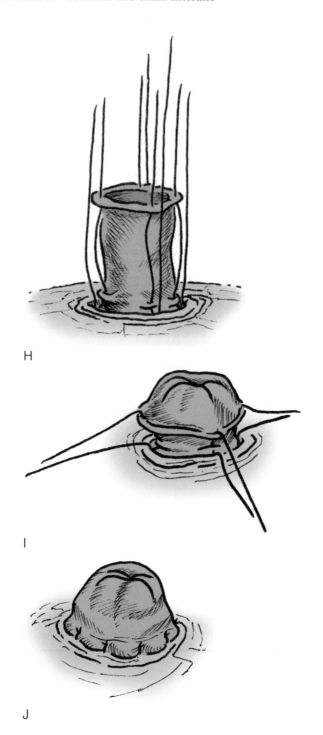

Figure 71–1, cont'd. H and **I,** Placement of three-point sutures in each of the four quadrants helps evert the ileal mucosa. **J,** Matured ileostomy.

remaining small bowel mesentery and vascular arcades are preserved. The mesentery of the distal small bowel is mobilized along the right posterior abdominal wall all the way to the duodenum to ensure adequate mobilization and construction of a tension-free stoma. Once the ileum is exteriorized, it should lay there without any mechanical effort.

After the appropriate resection has been performed, the ileum is divided with a GIA stapler or between clamps. It is important to preserve as much terminal ileum as possible, especially in patients with benign disease.[1] The bowel is divided 2 to 3 cm proximal to the ileocecal valve and should be free of any visible inflammatory changes, which is important in patients with Crohn's disease. The distal 2 to 3 cm of ileum to be exteriorized is cleansed of its mesentery so that eversion can take place without difficulty.

Before making a skin incision at the stoma site, all layers of the abdominal wall are apposed to reduce the shearing effect of the layers of the abdominal wall on the stoma. Such shearing predisposes to stenosis. Apposition is achieved by placing clamps on the cut edge of the fascia, peritoneum, and dermis of the skin and applying traction to keep the layers at the same level. A 2-cm disk of skin is removed at the previously marked stoma site and can be effectively accomplished by grasping and elevating the skin with a Kocher clamp and removing the skin with a horizontal sweep of the knife. The subcutaneous fatty tissue is divided and not excised to help provide support for the ileostomy, as well as the appliance.[1] In obese patients, a cylinder of subcutaneous fatty tissue may be excised to provide room for the bulky exteriorized bowel. With good retraction the anterior rectus sheath is easily identified and incised in a cruciate fashion. The rectus muscle is separated in the direction of its fibers with scissors or a blunt clamp. The posterior rectus sheath is identified and made prominent by pushing it through the separated rectus muscle fibers with the index and middle fingers introduced through the midline abdominal wound. A vertical incision is made in the posterior sheath. The newly constructed stoma opening should permit the passage of two fingers.

Babcock clamps are introduced into the peritoneal cavity through the stoma opening and used to grasp and deliver the end of the ileum out onto the abdominal surface. About 4 cm of ileum should be exteriorized and should lie without tension. Greater lengths of ileum need not be exteriorized because the everted ileostomy does not have to be more than 2 cm in height. Care is taken to ensure that the mesentery of the distal portion of the small bowel is not twisted, the divided edge of the mesentery points cephalad, and the proximal portion of the small bowel occupies the left side of the abdomen.

If the ileostomy is to be permanent, intraperitoneal fixation of the bowel and mesentery to the posterior rectus sheath is performed. Such fixation helps distribute the tension evenly around the stoma. Three or four interrupted sutures with fine (4-0) absorbable material are used. Seromuscular bites are taken through the ileum and secured to the parietal peritoneum. This step is omitted in patients with Crohn's disease because inadvertent full-thickness bites through the bowel may lead to the development of fistulas. The right lateral aspect of the abdomen is left open. However, closure may be accomplished by suturing the mesentery of the distal ileum to the anterior abdominal wall. This maneuver is believed to prevent herniation of the small bowel around the intra-abdominal portion of the ileostomy. Superiorly, the mesentery may be sutured to the falciform ligament to ensure complete closure. It is important to completely obliterate this space. If there is any tension on the mesentery, it is better to leave the defect wide open. Alternatively, performing an extraperitoneal ileostomy can close this defect.[29] Closure of the lateral abdominal space has not been shown to decrease the subsequent development of small bowel obstruction.[31,32]

Once it is deemed that the ileostomy is viable and there is no twist in the small bowel mesentery, the midline incision is closed. The skin is approximated and the incision is covered so that it is protected from coming in contact with the intestinal contents, which would increase the risk for wound infection.

The staple line is divided with a knife or electrocautery. Fresh bleeding from the mucosal edges ensures viability of the ileostomy. Maturation is begun by placing a three-point stitch in each of the four quadrants.[1] Fine (3-0 or 4-0) absorbable sutures are used for incorporating full-thickness bites of the open end of the ileum, a seromuscular bite just proximal to the anterior fascia, and finally a bite through the dermis of the skin. By placing traction on these sutures the ileum is easily everted. Before tying down the sutures, one or two further sutures are placed in each quadrant. These are simple sutures that incorporate full-thickness bites of the edge of the open bowel and the dermis of the skin. Tying down all the sutures should result in a "rosebud" or spigot formation. Sutures through the full thickness of the skin should be avoided because scarring will prevent the application of a watertight appliance seal. The ileostomy should be protruding 1 to 2 cm above the abdominal wall to allow the placement of a well-fitting appliance. This is extremely important because the ileal effluent is very irritating and, if allowed to bathe the peristomal skin, will result in skin breakdown.

The skin surrounding the stoma is painted with skin adhesive, and a transparent ileostomy appliance is placed and allowed to hang to the right side of the patient. This facilitates emptying of the appliance in the immediate postoperative period, as well as inspection of the stoma without having to remove the ileostomy bag. The opening in the faceplate should be 2 mm wider than the stoma to allow for postoperative edema. The appliance is usually changed after the second postoperative day once the midline dressing is removed. If there is leakage around the appliance at any time, the device should be changed immediately.

LOOP ILEOSTOMY

A loop ileostomy is also located in the right lower quadrant (Fig. 71–2). The site is chosen preoperatively just as for an end ileostomy. At the completion of the appropriate procedure a loop of bowel is chosen for creation of the diverting ileostomy. It should be as distal as possible in the small intestine at a point where the bowel can be brought up onto the abdominal wall without tension. The proximal or distal limb should be marked with a suture so that orientation is maintained before maturation of the stoma.

A small opening is created in an avascular part of the mesentery at the apex of the loop. A ¼-inch Penrose drain is placed through this opening to help place trac-

tion and deliver the bowel to the anterior abdominal wall. The skin incision for the stoma site is made exactly as for an end ileostomy. Subcutaneous fat may have to be removed to accommodate the two loops of bowel along with its mesentery.

Some authors prefer to position the proximal limb in the dependent inferior position, but such positioning requires twisting the mesentery of the small bowel. Although placing the functional proximal end inferiorly theoretically achieves complete diversion and drainage, this is easily and very well achieved by maturing the stoma with the proximal end more prominent as described.

Because the stoma will be temporary, there is no need to anchor it to the posterior sheath. The Penrose drain is substituted for a commercially produced plastic ileostomy bridge, which is available in different lengths. This rod is anchored to the skin with nonabsorbable sutures and should protrude just beyond the stoma so that it does not interfere with proper placement of the ileostomy appliance. After ensuring that the bowel is oriented properly, the abdominal incision is approximated and protected. The small bowel is opened by making an incision two thirds of the way along the antimesenteric wall of the distal loop just above the skin surface. Three-point anchoring sutures are placed toward the proximal limb as described for the Brooke ileostomy. Three such sutures are placed, one on each side of the mesentery and the third bisecting these. The remaining bowel wall, including the distal limb, is matured by using simple fine absorbable sutures that incorporate full-thickness bites of the cut end of the bowel and the dermis of the skin, which should result in an accentuated proximal limb and a recessive crescent-shaped distal limb flush with the skin. A watertight ileostomy appliance is placed in the operating room. The ileostomy bridge is removed after about a week when the edema has partially subsided and the ileostomy is functioning.

DIVIDED-LOOP ILEOSTOMY

In 1984, Abcarian and Prasad described their experience in constructing a modified loop ileostomy (Fig. 71–3). The segment to be exteriorized is identified and the ileum is divided near the apex of the loop with a GIA stapler. The proximal end is pulled through the right lower quadrant stoma opening, and 5 cm is exteriorized. The antimesenteric staple line of the distal limb is brought up through the same opening and positioned cephalad to the proximal limb. The entire staple line of the proximal limb is removed and the stoma constructed as for an end Brooke ileostomy. One corner of the recessive limb staple line is excised, and it is matured as a mucous fistula flush with the skin, thus allowing for distal decompression. Two transitional sutures are placed between the adjoining walls of the two limbs to create a completely diverting, perfectly circular stoma, which allows for a better appliance fit.[25,33]

END-LOOP ILEOSTOMY

This rarely performed procedure should be in the armamentarium of all abdominal surgeons because it can be

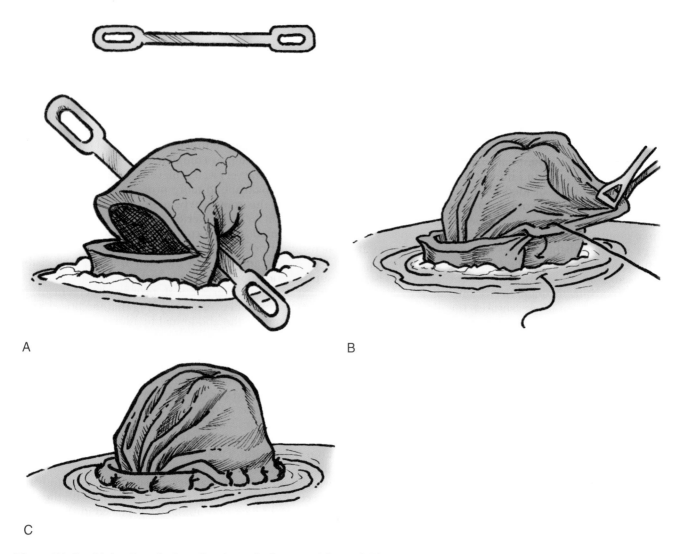

Figure 71–2. Maturation of a loop ileostomy. **A,** Commercially available plastic rod (shown separately) supporting the ileal loop. A transverse incision is made along the distal limb at the level of the skin. **B,** Eversion of the prominent proximal limb with three-point sutures. **C,** Fully matured loop ileostomy (shown without the plastic rod).

of great benefit when tension on the mesentery of the small intestine precludes construction of a viable end Brooke ileostomy (Fig. 71–4). This circumstance can be seen in patients with Crohn's disease who possess a thick short mesentery, in morbidly obese patients with thick anterior abdominal walls,[1] or in abdominal catastrophes in which edema and circulatory deficiencies prevent safe construction of an end ileostomy.

The distal part of the small bowel is transected as for an end ileostomy. The staple line may be oversewn and reinforced with absorbable seromuscular suture. A segment of bowel proximal to the closed end is chosen so that it can be exteriorized through the stoma opening on the right lower abdominal wall without tension. The construction then proceeds exactly as it would for a loop ileostomy. If the stoma is to be permanent, the bowel and its mesentery are anchored to the peritoneum and the posterior sheath with fine absorbable sutures.[22,25]

CLOSURE OF A LOOP ILEOSTOMY

Closure can be accomplished in most cases by a local procedure, thus eliminating performance of a formal celiotomy (Fig. 71–5). Closure is undertaken once it is ascertained that the distal anastomosis has healed completely and its integrity has been confirmed by contrast studies. In most cases the loop is closed a minimum of 6 weeks after the initial procedure to allow adequate tissue healing and softening of intra-abdominal adhesions. In a nonrandomized prospective study, Menegaux et al. have shown that temporary small bowel stomas may be closed safely on postoperative day 10 in healthy patients.[34]

The patient is positioned supine and a circumferential skin incision is made close to the mucocutaneous junction. Allis clamps can be used for vertical traction on the ileostomy. Circumferential subcutaneous dissection is carried out with electrocautery or scissors to reach the

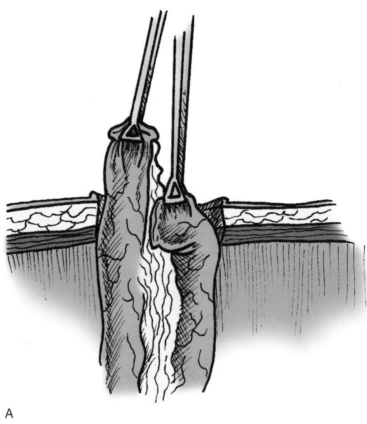

Figure 71–3. Divided-loop ileostomy. **A,** Proximal limb of the divided ileum delivered as for an end ileostomy. Only the antimesenteric border of the distal limb is brought up to the skin surface. **B,** On maturation it appears as an end ileostomy.

A

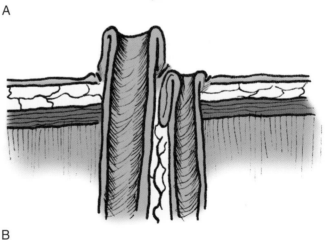

B

base of the ileostomy and identify the anterior fascia. Care is taken to prevent injury to the small intestinal wall or mesentery. The anterior sheath is incised close to the bowel wall to gain access to the peritoneal cavity. The intestine is circumferentially freed from peritoneal attachments by sharp dissection. The excess scar and skin are trimmed away from the bowel wall. The closure can be accomplished in various ways. The enterotomy can be closed transversely via a two-layer hand-sewn technique with an inner full-thickness layer and an outer seromuscular layer. Fine absorbable sutures are used for both layers. Alternatively, a linear stapler can be used to accomplish the same transverse closure.

If there is any concern about luminal narrowing, a linear cutting stapler is used to form a stapled side-to-side

functional end-to-end anastomosis. The antimesenteric walls are aligned, and a GIA stapler is deployed to create the anastomosis. With a second GIA stapler placed transversely, the excess skin and ostomy opening are transected to complete the anastomosis.[1,29] No major difference in morbidity has been demonstrated between stapled and sutured closure, although stapled closure can be accomplished faster.[35] Hasegawa et al. have shown that postoperative bowel obstruction is less common after staple than after suture closure.[36]

The small bowel is returned to the peritoneal cavity and the fascia approximated with nonabsorbable suture. The subcutaneous space is thoroughly irrigated. The skin can be packed open or loosely approximated with staples and intervening Telfa wicks to drain the subcutaneous

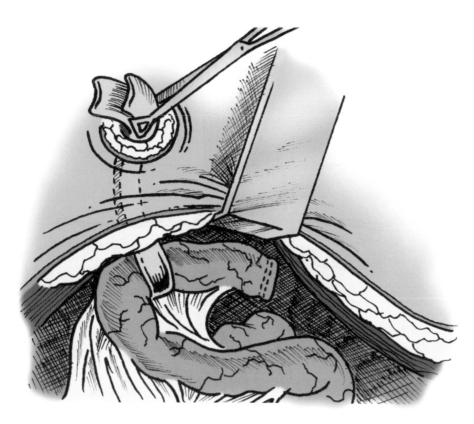

Figure 71–4. End-loop ileostomy. A loop of ileum proximal to the stapled end is delivered through the stoma site. Maturation takes place as for a loop ileostomy.

space. They can be removed after 48 to 72 hours. Sutton et al.[37] propose closing the skin with circular subcuticular nonabsorbable suture. The suture is tightened to draw the wound edges together while leaving a small 5- to 10-mm central defect, which allows the subcutaneous space to drain and heal by secondary intention. The suture is removed around the 14th postoperative day. They performed such a closure in 51 patients, with wound infections developing in none of them.

COMPLICATIONS OF ILEOSTOMY

Meticulous surgical technique and proper location of the stoma can minimize complications attributable to ileostomy construction and closure. The reported complication rates vary from 7% to 76%.[17,18,38-45]

Stoma Necrosis

Stoma ischemia with necrosis has been reported in 1% to 5% of patients undergoing construction of an ileostomy.[17,18,21,31,32,46] It is more often seen in the obese and after emergency procedures.[46] The most common cause is devascularization secondary to overzealous skeletonization of the terminal ileum for eversion. The viability of the stoma should be ascertained in the operating room. If the mucosa appears dusky, the ileostomy should be revised before leaving the operating suite. If discovered postoperatively (usually within 48 hours), one must determine the depth of viability, which can be accomplished by placing a test tube through the stoma opening

and illuminating the lumen with a flashlight. If the ischemia is limited to the subcutaneous space and above the fascia, the patient can be treated by observation with revision performed later if stenosis develops. If the necrosis extends below the peritoneum, immediate revision is required.

Bowel Obstruction

Small bowel obstruction can occur after creation or closure of the ileostomy. It is important to differentiate between mechanical blockage because of food indiscretion (high-fiber foods), which occurs more distally at the stoma site just below the fascial level, and more proximal obstruction from intra-abdominal disease, such as adhesions, internal herniations, and recurrent strictures secondary to Crohn's disease. Bowel obstruction may also be caused by skin-level stoma stenosis as a result of ischemia. The clinical signs and symptoms are the same regardless of the cause and include cessation of ileostomy output, abdominal distention, crampy abdominal pain, nausea, vomiting, and dehydration. Patients with partial obstruction may have increased output. Treatment begins by instituting aggressive resuscitation, intravenous hydration, and nasogastric decompression. Kodner[22] proposed a logical algorithm to deal with this complication. A Foley catheter (24 French) is inserted into the stoma and held in place by partially inflating the balloon. Irrigation is performed with 50 ml of warm water. If there is return of food particles, the irrigation is carried out slowly until the return is clear and the mechanical food obstruction is relieved. If the initial fluid return is clear, one can

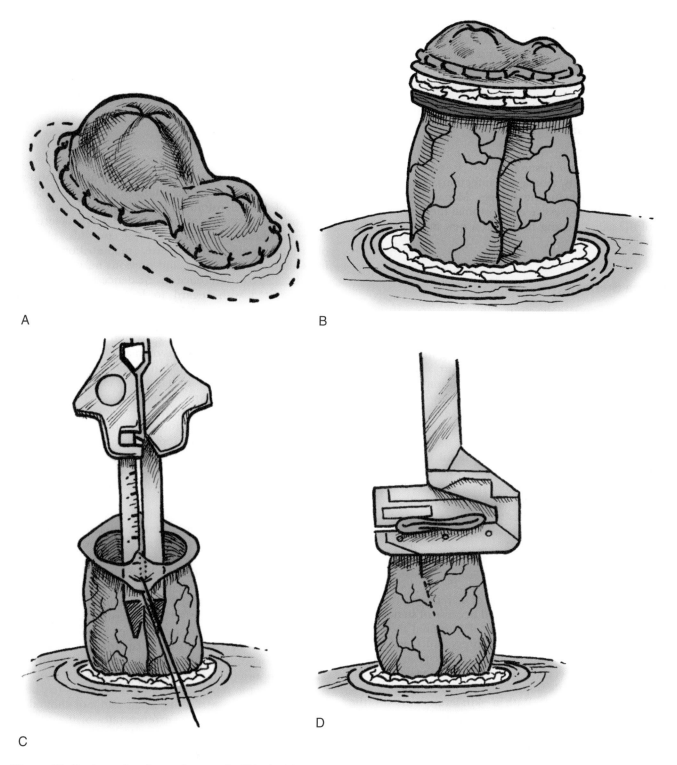

A

B

C

D

Figure 71–5. Loop ileostomy closure. **A,** Skin incision made around the ileostomy close to the mucocutaneous junction. **B,** Stoma and small bowel elevated after the intraperitoneal adhesions are divided. **C** and **D,** Stapled side-to-side anastomosis.

assume a proximal obstruction and perform a water-soluble contrast study to delineate the site of obstruction. This may be therapeutic if the obstruction is due to food particles. Patients should show signs of rapid improvement within 24 to 48 hours after conservative therapy. If any signs of impending bowel ischemia are present, early surgery is the prudent course.

Bowel obstruction has been reported in 3% to 17% of patients with ileostomies.[42,43,47-50] Feinberg et al.[42] had an 11% incidence of bowel obstruction after creation of a loop ileostomy. Senapati et al.[43] reported a bowel obstruction rate of 11.4% after ileostomy closure; two thirds of these obstructions were treated conservatively, whereas 11 (4.2% of all ileostomy closures) patients required operative intervention. In Feinberg and colleagues' study, no patient had bowel obstruction after resection with anastomosis, and such treatment was better than a hand-sewn anastomosis or simple closure, although it did not reach statistical significance.

Mucocutaneous Separation

The newly matured stoma may separate from the surrounding skin if the tissue is friable, as in patients taking high-dose steroids, stoma site infections, and excessive tension on the maturing sutures. Management is conservative, with aggressive enterostomal therapy provided until the skin opening heals and a new mucocutaneous junction forms.[1]

Stoma Stenosis

Stomal stenosis develops in 2% to 10% of ileostomies.[21,31,32] It may occur if the fascial opening is made too small. The surgeon's middle and index fingers should pass through the stoma opening in the abdominal wall to ensure an adequate aperture size. Skin-level stenosis develops as a result of stomal ischemia or subcutaneous infection. Initial management is gentle dilation, which can be accomplished with Hegar dilators. If there is no relief from obstructive symptoms, surgical revision is undertaken. The stenosis may be corrected with a local procedure by taking down the mucocutaneous junction, dissecting down to the fascia, and making the opening larger with re-creation of the stoma. Laparotomy may be necessary if exteriorization of the bowel was initially inadequate.

Stoma Retraction

Retraction has been reported in 3% to 17% of all ileostomies.[17,18,21,31,36,46] Goldblatt et al. reported that 30% of their revisions were performed because of stenosis and retraction.[51] Tension on the small intestinal mesentery and lack of fixation of the mesentery and bowel to the peritoneum may result in this complication. A flush stoma may also occur as a result of weight gain and is seen in morbidly obese patients, who have a higher rate of stoma retraction.[52] With a skin-level ileostomy the effluent leaks onto the surrounding skin, causes breakdown, and prevents secure application of the appliance. It may be managed with skilled enterostomal therapy, but many patients require revision of the stoma.

Stoma Prolapse

Ileostomy prolapse has been reported in 0% to 11% of patients.[13,17,21,31,32,53,54] Causes include too large an abdominal wall fascial opening, lack of fixation of the mesentery to the abdominal wall, and placement of the ileostomy outside the rectus muscle or in previous incisions. It is usually associated with a parastomal hernia.[54] The prolapse may be intermittent or fixed. If the appliance can still be applied without leakage and the prolapse is stable and not bothersome to the patient, it need not be corrected. Repair is accomplished by a local approach that involves resecting the excess ileum and re-creating a Brooke ileostomy. Laparotomy for intraperitoneal fixation may be needed to preserve bowel length.

Parastomal Hernia

Parastomal hernia is seen less frequently after ileostomy than after colostomy construction.[53-55] It affects 1.8% to 28.3% of end ileostomies and 0% to 6.2% of loop ileostomies.[55] Patients with poor tissue characteristics, such as obesity, use of high-dose steroids, chronic obstructive pulmonary disease, malnutrition, raised intra-abdominal pressure, and previous herniations, are at risk.[53,54,56] No difference in incidence rates has been demonstrated with regard to location of the stoma through the rectus muscle, fascial fixation, or closure of the lateral space.[55-58]

The majority of patients are asymptomatic. Operative indications include symptoms of small bowel obstruction, localized discomfort, an enlarging mass, and poor appliance fit that may result in leakage of effluent and peristomal skin breakdown. About 30% of patients with peri-ileostomy hernias require operative repair.[59]

Repair may be accomplished by direct fascial approximation, prosthetic mesh repair, and relocation of the stoma to new site. Although fascial reapproximation is the simplest option because it avoids a formal laparotomy, it carries with it an unacceptably high rate of hernia recurrence (46% to 100%).[55,59,60] The prosthetic mesh may be placed intraperitoneally or as a fascial onlay. There is a small risk of mesh infection and erosion into the bowel (3%).[59] Recurrence rates after mesh repair are reported to be between 0% and 39%.[55,59,60] Reiger et al., in their series of 41 patients who underwent 51 repairs, showed that the lowest recurrence rates were seen after stoma relocation (24%).[60] The reported rates vary between 0% and 76%.[55,59,60] If the hernia defect is large, the ileostomy can be relocated via the paraileostomy incision and thereby avoid a formal laparotomy. No clinical trials have compared the aforementioned procedures, and the reported numbers are small.[55]

Laparoscopic repair of paraostomy hernias has been reported, but the series are small and not limited to paraileostomy hernias. Recurrence rates of 0% to 44% are reported.[61-63] Safadi reviewed 11 studies with a total of 37 patients and added 9 of his own. He described a recurrence rate of 44.4% within 6 months of the operation.[61] As experienced is gained and techniques are refined, the results may improve. The advantage of this approach is that it avoids stoma relocation and reduces postoperative pain and wound complications.

Peri-ileostomy Fistula

The incidence of peri-ileostomy fistula is unknown. Older studies reported rates of 24% to 40%.[51,64] A fistula may result from recurrent Crohn's disease, operative injury when an anchoring stitch incorporates the full thickness of the bowel wall, ischemic injury to the stoma, or ill-fitting appliances.[65] Greenstein et al.[66] reported a series of 214 patients with an ileostomy constructed for Crohn's disease. Parastomal fistulas developed in 14 patients (6.5%), and all cases were a consequence of recurrent Crohn's disease.

Because fistulas pose a difficult proposition of maintaining a secure ostomy appliance, treatment consists of reconstruction of the ileostomy either at the same location or at a new one, depending on the complexity of the fistula.[66] Medical therapy has not been successful in treating these fistulas, although infliximab may be of benefit.

Hemorrhage and Peri-ileostomy Varices

Trauma to the stoma from ill-fitting appliances may cause mucosal tears or shallow ulcers that result in troublesome bleeding. These lesions heal spontaneously with proper stomal care and enterostomal therapy.

Sclerosing cholangitis leading to cirrhosis is seen in patients with inflammatory bowel disease. These patients may manifest parastomal varices in addition to anorectal and esophageal varices. Local treatment with sclerosing agents or variceal ligation provides temporary control. Definitive treatment consists of portosystemic shunting or selective splenorenal shunting.[67,68]

Peri-ileostomy Skin Problems

Peristomal skin irritation has been reported in 15% to 79% of patients with an ileostomy.[42,53,54,69] It commonly accompanies flush or retracted stomas, which result in poor appliance fit and leakage of effluent. Skin problems are seen more frequently after emergency procedures because preoperative stoma positioning is not usually possible.[52] The peristomal skin may secondarily become infected with bacterial or fungal organisms (11%), most commonly *Candida albicans*.[30] Treatment consists of local antifungal powder and enterostomal therapy.

Paraileostomy skin ulceration can be secondary to recurrent Crohn's disease or be a manifestation of pyoderma gangrenosum. The latter is due to underlying active inflammatory disease and resolves after removing the diseased segment of bowel. Aggressive enterostomal therapy is needed in the interim.[69]

Ileostomy Diarrhea

Increased ileostomy output may be seen with gastroenteritis, partial small bowel obstruction, radiation enteritis, short-bowel syndrome, and Crohn's disease.[54] Ileostomy effluent totaling greater than 1000 ml/day may lead to dehydration and sodium depletion requiring hospitalization and intravenous fluid replacement. In the first month after construction of a new ileostomy, dehydration secondary to stomal water and electrolyte loss is common. Treatment includes intravenous fluid resuscitation, dietary manipulation, antidiarrheal agents, and fiber. The risk of dehydration requiring hospitalization

from a loop ileostomy can be as high as 20%.[42,54] Chronic dehydration leads to acidic urine and predisposes to the formation of uric acid calculi.[54]

CONCLUSION

Living with an ileostomy is a major life-altering event for patients. With thorough preoperative preparation, patient education, meticulous surgical technique, and patient access to enterostomal therapy, complications can be prevented and the patient's quality of life improved.

SUGGESTED READINGS

Corman ML (ed): Intestinal Stomas. Colon and Rectal Surgery. Philadelphia, Lippincott-Raven, 1998, pp 1264-1319.

Gordon PH, Rolstad BS, Bubrick MP: Intestinal stomas. In Gordon PH, Nivatvongs S (eds): Principles and Practice of Surgery for the Colon, Rectum and Anus. St Louis, Quality Medical, 1999, pp 1117-1180.

Shellito PC: Complications of abdominal stoma surgery. Dis Colon Rectum 41:1562-1572, 1998.

REFERENCES

1. Gordon PH, Rolstad BS, Bubrick MP: Intestinal stomas. In Gordon PH, Nivatvongs S (eds): Principles and Practice of Surgery for the Colon, Rectum and Anus. St Louis, Quality Medical, 1999, pp 1117-1180.
2. McGarity WC: The evolution of continence following total colectomy. Am Surg 58:1-16, 1992.
3. Turnbull RB Jr: Management of the ileostomy. Am J Surg 86:617-624, 1953.
4. Dragstedt LR, Dack GM, Kirsner JB: Chronic ulcerative colitis: Summary of evidence implicating *Bacterium necrophorum* as an etiologic agent. Ann Surg 114:653-662, 1941.
5. Cattell RB: A new type of ileostomy for chronic ulcerative colitis. Surg Clin North Am 19:629, 1939.
6. Warren R, McKittrick LS: Ileostomy for ulcerative colitis. Technique, complications and management. Surg Gynecol Obstet 93:555-567, 1951.
7. Brooke BN: The management of an ileostomy including its complications. Lancet 2:102-104, 1952.
8. Cataldo PA: Intestinal stomas: 200 years of digging. Dis Colon Rectum 42:137-142, 1999.
9. Turnbull RB: Management of the ileostomy. Am J Surg 86:617-624, 1953.
10. Brooke BN: Conventional ileostomy: Historical perspectives. In Dozois RR (ed): Alternatives to Conventional Ileostomy. Chicago, Year Book, 1985, pp 19-28.
11. Abrams JS (ed): Abdominal Stomas. Bristol, England, John Wright, 1984.
12. Fasth S, Hulten L, Palselius I: Loop ileostomy: An attractive alternative to a temporary transverse colostomy. Acta Chir Scand 146:203-207, 1980.
13. Williams NS, Nasmyth DG, Jones D, Smith AH: De-functioning stomas: A prospective controlled trial comparing loop ileostomy with loop transverse colostomy. Br J Surg 73:566-570, 1986.
14. Rutegard J, Dahlgren S: Transverse colostomy or loop ileostomy as diverting stoma in colorectal surgery. Acta Chir Scand 153:229-232, 1987.
15. Gooszen AW, Geelkerken RH, Hermans J, et al: Temporary decompression after colorectal surgery: Randomized comparison of loop ileostomy and loop colostomy. Br J Surg 85:76-79, 1998.

16. Rullier E, Le Toux N, Laurent C, et al: Loop ileostomy versus loop colostomy for defunctioning low anastomoses during rectal cancer surgery. World J Surg 25:274-277, 2001.

17. Wexner SD, Taranow DA, Johansen OB, et al: Loop ileostomy is a safe option for fecal diversion. Dis Colon Rectum 36:349-354, 1993.

18. Khoo REH, Cohen MM, Chapman GM, et al: Loop ileostomy for temporary fecal diversion. Am J Surg 167:519-522, 1994.

19. Gooszen AW, Geelkerken RH, Hermans J, et al: Quality of life with a temporary stoma: Ileostomy vs. colostomy. Dis Colon Rectum 43:650-655, 2000.

20. Silva MA, Ratnayake G, Deen KI: Quality of life of stoma patients: Temporary ileostomy versus colostomy. World J Surg 27:421-424, 2003.

21. Shellito PC: Complications of abdominal stoma surgery. Dis Colon Rectum 41:1562-1572, 1998.

22. Kodner IJ, Intestinal stomas. In Zinner JM, Schwartz SI, Ellis H (eds): Maingot's Abdominal Operations. Stamford, CT, Appleton & Lange, 1997, pp 427-460.

23. Shirley F, Kodner IJ, Fry RD: Loop ileostomy: Techniques and indications. Dis Colon Rectum 27:382-386, 1984.

24. Gallagher ND, Harrison DD, Skyring AP: Fluid and electrolyte disturbances in patients with long-established ileostomies. Gut 3:219-223, 1962.

25. Abcarian H, Pearl RK: Stomas. Surg Clin North Am 68:1295-1305, 1988.

26. Bluth EI, Merritt CR, Sullivan MA, et al: Inflammatory bowel disease and cholelithiasis: The association in patients with an ileostomy. South Med J 77: 690-692, 1984.

27. Hill GL: Physiology of conventional ileostomy. In Dozois RR (ed): Alternatives to Conventional Ileostomy. Chicago, Year Book, 1985, pp 29-39.

28. Kretschmer PK (ed): The Intestinal Stoma. Philadelphia, WB Saunders, 1978.

29. Corman ML (ed): Intestinal Stomas. Colon and Rectal Surgery. Philadelphia, Lippincott-Raven, 1998, pp 1264-1319.

30. Hellman J, Lago CP: Dermatologic complications in colostomy and ileostomy patients. Int J Dermatol 29:129-133, 1990.

31. Leong AP, Londono-Schimmer EE, Phillips RK: Life table analysis of stomal complications following ileostomy. Br J Surg 81:727-729, 1994.

32. Carlsen E, Bergan A: Technical aspects and complications of end-ileostomies. World J Surg 19:632-636, 1995.

33. Prasad ML, Pearl RK, Orsay CP, et al: Rodless ileostomy: A modified loop ileostomy. Dis Colon Rectum 27:270-271, 1984.

34. Menegaux F, Jordi-Galais P, Turrin N, Chigot JP: Closure of small bowel stomas on postoperative day 10. Eur J Surg 168:713-715, 2002.

35. Hull TL, Kobe I, Fazio VW: Comparison of handsewn with stapled loop ileostomy closures. Dis Colon Rectum 39:1086-1089, 1996.

36. Hasegawa H, Radley S, Morton DG, Keighley MR: Stapled versus sutured closure of loop ileostomy: A randomized controlled trial. Ann Surg 231:202-204, 2000.

37. Sutton CD, Williams N, Marshall LJ, et al: A technique for wound closure that minimizes sepsis after stoma closure. Aust N Z J Surg 72:766-767, 2002.

38. Corman ML, Veidenheimer MC, Coller JA: Complications of ileostomy: Prevention and treatment. Contemp Surg 8:36-41, 1976.

39. Carlstedt A, Fasth S, Hulton L, et al: Long-term ileostomy complications in patients with ulcerative colitis and Crohn's disease. Int J Colorectal Dis 2:22-25, 1987.

40. Stothert JC Jr, Brubacher L, Simonowitz DA: Complications of emergency stoma formation. Arch Surg 117:307-309, 1982.

41. Grobler SP, Hosie KB, Keighley MR: Randomized trial of loop ileostomy in restorative proctocolectomy. Br J Surg 79:903-906, 1992.

42. Feinberg SM, McLeod RS, Cohen Z: Complications of loop ileostomy. Am J Surg 153:102-107, 1987.

43. Senapati A, Nicholls RJ, Ritchie JK, et al: Temporary loop ileostomy for restorative proctocolectomy. Br J Surg 80:628-630, 1993.

44. Babcock G, Bivins BA, Sachatello CR: Technical complications of ileostomy. South Med J 73:329-331, 1980.

45. Duchesne JC, Wang Y, Weintraub SL, et al: Stoma complications: A multivariate analysis. Am Surg 68:961-966, 2002.

46. Leenen LP, Kuypers JH: Some factors influencing the outcome of stoma surgery. Dis Colon Rectum 32:500-504, 1989.

47. Fasth S, Hulton L: Loop-ileostomy: A superior diverting stoma in colorectal surgery. World J Surg 8:401-407, 1984.

48. Hughes ESR, McDermott FT, Masterton JP: Intestinal obstruction following operation for inflammatory disease of bowel. Dis Colon Rectum 22:469-471, 1979.

49. Bubrick MP, Jacobs DM, Levy M: Experience with the endorectal pull-through and S-pouch for ulcerative colitis and familial polyposis in adults. Surgery 98:689-699, 1985.

50. Francois Y, Dozois RR, Kelly KA, et al: Small intestinal obstruction complicating ileal pouch–anal anastomosis. Ann Surg 209:46-50, 1989.

51. Goldblatt MS, Corman ML, Haggitt RC, et al: Ileostomy complications requiring revision: Lahey Clinic experience, 1964-1973. Dis Colon Rectum 20:209-214, 1977.

52. Arumugam PJ, Bevan L, Macdonald L, et al: A prospective audit of stomas: Analysis of risk factors and complications and their management. Colorectal Dis 5:49-52, 2003.

53. Flehman JW: Ostomies. In Hicks TC, Beck DE, Opelka FG, Timmcke AE (eds): Complications of Colon & Rectal Surgery. Baltimore, Williams & Wilkins, 1996, pp 357-381.

54. Fleshman JW: Prevention and management of stoma complications. In Fazio VW, Church JM, Delaney CP (eds): Current Therapy in Colon and Rectal Surgery. Philadelphia, Elsevier, 2005, pp 549-555.

55. Carne PW, Robertson G, Frizelle FA: Parastomal hernia. Br J Surg 90:784-793, 2003.

56. Londono-Schimmer EE, Leong APK, Phillips RKS: Life table analysis of stomal complications following colostomy. Dis Colon Rectum 37:916-920, 1994.

57. Williams JG, Etherington R, Hayward MWJ, et al: Paraileostomy hernia: A clinical and radiological study. Br J Surg 77:1355-1357, 1990.

58. Ortiz H, Sara MJ, Armendariz P, et al: Does the frequency of paracolostomy hernias depend on the position of the colostomy in the abdominal wall? Int J Colorectal Dis 9:65-67, 1994.

59. Steele SR, Lee P, Martin MJ, et al: Is parastomal hernia repair with polypropylene mesh safe? Am J Surg 185:436-440, 2003.

60. Reiger N, Moore J, Hewett P, et al: Parastomal hernia repair. Colorectal Dis 6:203-205, 2004.

61. Safadi B: Laparoscopic repair of parastomal hernias: Early results. Surg Endosc 18:676-680, 2004.

62. LeBlanc KA, Bellanger DE: Laparoscopic repair of paraostomy hernias: Early results. J Am Coll Surg 194:232-239, 2002.

63. Berger DB, Bientzle MB, Muller AM: Technique and results of the laparoscopic repair of parastomal hernias. Surg Endosc 17(Suppl):S3, 2003.

64. Roy PH, Saver WG, Beahrs OH, Farrow GM: Experience with ileostomies. Evaluation of long-term rehabilitation in 497 patients. Am J Surg 119:77-86, 1970.

65. Block GE, Giuliano A: Complications of the surgical treatment of ulcerative colitis and Crohn's disease. In Kirsner JB, Shorter RG (eds): Inflammatory Bowel Disease. Philadelphia, Lea & Febiger, 1980, pp 577-604.

66. Greenstein AJ, Dicker A, Meyers S, Aufses AH: Periileostomy fistulae in Crohn's disease. Ann Surg 197:179-182, 1983.

67. Conte JV, Arcomano TA, Naficy MA, Holt RW: Treatment of bleeding stomal varices. Report of a case and review of the literature. Dis Colon Rectum 33:308-314, 1990.

68. Roberts PL, Martin FM, Schoetz DJ Jr, et al: Bleeding stomal varices. The role of local treatment. Dis Colon Rectum 33:547-549, 1990.

69. Tjandra JJ, Hughes LE: Parastomal pyoderma gangrenosum in inflammatory bowel disease. Dis Colon Rectum 37:938-942, 1994.

72

Suturing, Stapling, and Tissue Adhesives

John Migaly · Rolando Rolandelli

The healing of a bowel anastomosis proceeds in a stepwise, time-dependent fashion. At the time of transection of the bowel, there is an immediate inflammatory response elicited by activation of the clotting cascade, recruitment of platelets, and perpetuation of the inflammatory cascade via the elaboration of inflammatory mediators stored in platelet granules. Neutrophils are subsequently recruited into the wound. During these first 3 to 5 days, termed the inflammatory phase of wound healing, the collagen matrix undergoes degradation by metalloproteinases. It is in this initial phase that the integrity of the anastomosis depends almost entirely on technical factors, suture materials, or the integrity of stapled margins of bowel.[1]

Around the fifth postoperative day there is a crucial switch from collagen degradation to collagen deposition, which corresponds to the transition from the inflammatory phase to the fibroplasia phase (Fig. 72–1). The fibroplasia phase reaches its maximal level at day 7.[2] Any delay or impairment of the fibroplasia phase can result in the potentially catastrophic consequence of anastomotic dehiscence.[3] Indeed, it is at the end of the first postoperative week that anastomotic dehiscence usually occurs and becomes clinically evident.

Although it may seem that surgical stapling devices have completely supplanted hand-sewn suturing of bowel anastomoses, hand suturing remains a crucial skill in every surgeon's armamentarium. Certain situations are not amenable to surgical stapling, and it is in these situations that the surgeon's facility with suturing techniques can vastly affect the outcome of an intestinal anastomosis.

Hand suturing uniformly invokes an inflammatory response from dragging the suture material through the bowel. The choice of suture material used by surgeons is not based on a strong preponderance of scientific evidence. Everting and inverting anastomoses have come in and out of favor over the last 2 centuries, as have many anastomotic techniques.

SURGICAL SUTURING AND TECHNIQUE

Suture Material

All sutures produce some degree of inflammation as they are dragged through tissues. The degree of inflammation corresponds to the amount of collagenases and metalloproteinases produced in the local wound environment and the subsequent loss of tensile strength in both the wound and the suture material itself.[4]

The ideal suture material should elicit minimal tissue reaction and be easy to handle and tie without fraying. It should also be relatively easy to sterilize while maintaining all of the ideal characteristics after sterilization.[5]

The type of suture used has traditionally been tailored to the particular layer of the intestinal tract that the suture material is being used to approximate. Chromic catgut is the most commonly used as an inner layer of suture in a two-layer intestinal anastomosis.

In the 1950s, Madsen studied 12 different suture materials and concluded that absorbable suture materials display a marked tissue reaction with delay of collagen formation.[6-8] Because chromic catgut is reabsorbed between 18 and 21 days, it is not the material of choice for single-layer applications such as bilioenteric anastomoses.[9] The absorbable synthetic sutures of polydioxanone (PDS) and polyglyconate (Maxon) are the commonly used sutures in these anastomoses because of their longer retention time in wounds and sustained breaking strength.

The absorbable synthetic suture materials polyglactin (Vicryl) and polyglycolic acid (Dexon) are used interchangeably with chromic catgut but have the added benefits of decreased inflammatory response and increased strength. The downside of these sutures is that they are braided and produce more drag across the intestinal wall.

Silk suture is still the traditional nonabsorbable suture most commonly used for intestinal anastomoses, and it

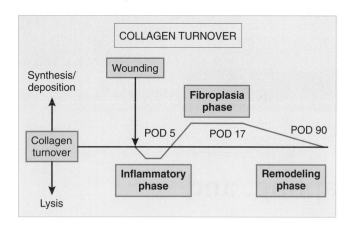

Figure 72–1. Collagen deposition and lysis as a function of time in intestinal healing. POD, postoperative day. (From Migaly J, Lieberman J, Long W, et al: Effect of adenoviral-mediated transfer of transforming growth factor-beta1 on colonic anastomotic healing. Dis Colon Rectum 47:1703, 2004.)

was lauded as the most reliable suture by Halstead as far back as 1913.[10] Silk is used most often as the outer layer of a two-layer anastomosis and is most commonly used as an interrupted seromuscular stitch.

In conclusion, in two-layer anastomoses, the inner layer is usually an absorbable suture such as chromic catgut, Dexon, or Vicryl, with the outer seromuscular stitch being silk. If a one-layer anastomosis is to be performed, a nonabsorbable suture such as silk is used. Bilioenteric anastomoses are commonly performed as one-layer anastomoses with more durable absorbable synthetics such as PDS or Maxon.

Suture Material and Infection

As in the case of any implantable foreign body, suture material can potentiate bacterial infection in an intestinal anastomosis. The particular properties of a suture determine its ability to thwart or encourage bacterial infection. Bacterial adherence is variable among the various suture types.

Chu and Williams examined 10 types of suture ranging from absorbable to nonabsorbable, monofilament to braided, and synthetic to natural origins and quantitatively determined the adhesion of radiolabeled bacteria to these various sutures. They found that PDS sutures exhibited the lowest affinity to the adherence of *Escherichia coli* and *Staphylococcus aureus*. Dexon sutures exhibited the highest affinity to these species.[11]

Katz et al. confirmed these results and, furthermore, demonstrated via an in vivo model of wound infection that suture materials potentiate bacterial growth and cause infection in mice. They injected suspensions of staphylococci into subcutaneous pockets in mice and found that 10^9 bacteria were necessary to cause wound infection in mice in the absence of suture whereas only 10^5 were necessary to elicit significant wound infection in the presence of suture. They also found that the inflammatory response and infectivity scores correlated nicely with the adherence indices of the various types of suture. The fastest removal of bacteria was from nylon, and the slowest was from silk.[12] Consideration should be given to the type of suture used in the event of gross fecal soilage.

Suture Material and Tumor Cell Adherence

Both in vitro and animal data support the theory that certain suture materials support the growth of tumor cells more than others do.[13] Using a rodent model, Reinbach demonstrated that radiolabeled tumor cells adhere more avidly to silk suture used to close enterotomies of the colon than they did to PDS sutures.[14] Further investigation is obviously warranted before deciding which suture truly conveys an oncologic advantage in bowel anastomoses.

Methods of Suturing

Suture lines can be created either in a simple or interrupted fashion or in a continuous or running manner. The advantage of a continuous suture is that the suture line is more watertight, with the disadvantage being that the integrity of the entire suture line is based on one stitch. Hemostasis is also improved with a continuous suture, with the converse effect being that continuous suturing may constrict anastomotic blood flow more than interrupted suturing does.

Regardless of whether the suture is run in continuous or interrupted fashion, a bowel anastomosis must adhere to the following principles. The anastomosis must be watertight and must have mucosal apposition. The submucosa, which supplies much of the strength to a bowel anastomosis, must be incorporated into the closure. Care must be taken to not strangulate the edges of the bowel during closure in order to avoid stricture or necrosis and subsequent anastomotic leakage.

Lembert Suture

Lembert suture is the most commonly used suture in gastrointestinal surgery (Fig. 72–2). It is used as the outer layer of a two-layer bowel anastomosis and is also used to repair seromuscular tears in the bowel wall. The stitch is started approximately 3 to 4 mm lateral to the incision and placed at a right angle to the long axis of the incision. It incorporates only the seromuscular layer; care must be taken to not incorporate the full thickness of the bowel wall. The tip of the needle is brought out close to the edge of the incision and is then reinserted in the apposing wound edge and brought out 3 to 4 mm lateral to the wound edge. The suture is then tied down to a tension that approximates the tissue, but not tight enough to tear the tissue. The most commonly used material for a Lembert suture is either silk or PDS suture. This stitch can be performed in an interrupted or continuous manner.

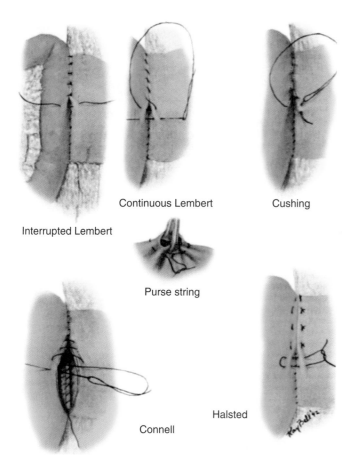

Continuous Lembert   Cushing

Interrupted Lembert

Purse string

Connell   Halsted

Figure 72–2. Common methods of intestinal suturing. (From Orr TG: Operations of General Surgery, 2nd ed. Philadelphia, WB Saunders, 1949.)

Horizontal Mattress Suture (Halsted Suture)

A horizontal mattress suture, or Halsted suture, is predominantly used for seromuscular apposition in multilayer bowel anastomoses (see Fig. 72–2). The suture is passed through the seromuscular layer 2 to 3 mm lateral to the wound edge and brought out at the wound edge; the needle is then passed through the opposing edge of the wound and brought out 2 to 3 mm lateral. On that same side of the wound approximately 2 mm distal, the suture is passed through both edges of the wound to create two free ends of the suture on one side of the wound edge with the loop of the suture on the other side. This stitch is particularly useful in damaged, inflamed, or abnormal tissue where a Lembert suture pulls through the tissue. Because the horizontal mattress stitch distributes tension in a plane perpendicular to that of a Lembert suture, it allows for apposition of tissues with less crushing effect on them.

Purse-String Suture

A purse-string suture is used to invert appendiceal stumps or to secure feeding tubes or drainage tubes in place. It is basically a circular continuous Lembert suture

about a fixed point or opening in the gastrointestinal tract. It is most commonly performed with nonabsorbable suture (see Fig. 72–2).

Connell Suture

The Connell suture is a full-thickness, usually continuous suture that allows for the mucosa to be inverted into the lumen of a bowel anastomosis (see Fig. 71–2). The suture is started at the edge of the anastomosis and brought, full thickness, from inside to out on one side and then outside to in on the opposite side. The suture is tied so that the knot is inside the lumen. The suture is then passed through the tissues from inside to out on one side to begin the Connell stitch. On the other limb of the anastomosis the suture is driven through the tissues, full thickness, from outside to in. On the inside of the bowel lumen the stitch is advanced 2 to 3 mm along the wall and then driven through the bowel wall from inside to out on the *same* side. With the suture now on the outside of the bowel, the next throw is performed on the opposite side in an identical manner. This creates a U-shaped, full-thickness, running inverted suture line. It usually serves as an inner layer of a two-layer anastomosis. Absorbable sutures such as chromic or Vicryl are generally used for these applications.

Inverted Versus Everted Intestinal Anastomosis

The concept of inverting versus everting intestinal anastomoses has long been debated. The overwhelming majority of hand-sewn anastomoses are currently performed in an inverting fashion in either one or two layers.

Gambee and associates, in 1956, published a 156-patient series of various large bowel anastomoses in which they used a single-layer, full-thickness, interrupted, inverting technique with silk suture (Fig. 72–3).[15] They reported five deaths as a result of anastomotic leaks with a mortality of 3%. The incidence of all anastomotic complications was 8.6%, with the majority being radiographic leaks that were not clinically evident.

In 1966, Getzen published a clinical series of 136 everted gastrointestinal anastomoses in which only one leak occurred (resulting in death).[16] Getzen compared inverting and everting bowel anastomoses in a canine model. In 293 anastomoses in dogs, there was no evidence of mucocele or fistula formation. Anastomotic edema was more pronounced in the everted group up to 21 days after surgery. The tensile strength of the inverted anastomosis was two thirds that of the everted group up to 21 days after surgery. Anastomotic strength was comparable in the two groups after 21 days. There were no deaths attributable to everted mucosa.[17]

As with any other wound, the ideal form of intestinal healing is by primary intention. This is accomplished when the individual layers of the intestine reconnect at each side of the anastomosis. Of all layers, the submucosa is particularly important because it harbors fibroblasts, which will produce the collagen that ultimately holds the anastomosis together. Inversion of the anastomosis presents the ends of mucosa to the lumen, where

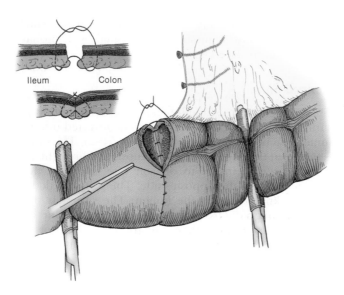

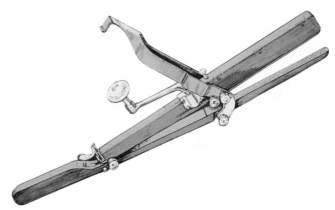

Figure 72–4. Depiction of the Hültl stapler. (From Feil W, Lippert H, Lozac'h P, et al: Atlas of Surgical Stapling. Heidelberg, Germany, Johann Ambrosius Barth, 2000.)

Figure 72–3. The Gambee method of intestinal suturing involving the use of interrupted, inverting sutures. (From Gambee LP, Garnjobst W, Hardwick CE: Ten years' experience with a single layer anastomosis in colon surgery. Am J Surg 92:222, 1956.)

they are further degraded until the submucosa of one side is apposed to the submucosa on the other side. In an inverted anastomosis, the exposed submucosa tends to become adherent to any surrounding structure, thereby eliciting adhesions and delaying healing into a secondary-intention process. It is from this experience that most surgeons have adopted the inverting method for intestinal anastomosis.

STAPLERS AND STAPLING TECHNIQUES

Surgical staplers have become the standard for the creation of bowel anastomoses. In 1826, Henroz first described a device made from two rings that would approximate two open ends of bowel. He successfully tested the device on dogs.

One of the first stapling devices used in humans was the Hültl stapler (Fig. 72–4). This stapler was used to close the stomach during gastrectomies. The array of staplers now available has virtually eliminated the need for hand-sewn anastomoses and has subsequently reduced operative times drastically.

Modern-day staplers deliver staples of either fixed or variable staple height. Linear staplers deliver staples of fixed height, whereas circular staplers can be adjusted to variable heights. A vascular stapler has a closed staple length of 1.0 mm. Tissue staplers have "blue" cartridges and "green" cartridges, which are used for thin tissues and thick tissues, respectively. The closed staple length of a "blue" stapler is 1.5 mm, and it is used for standard tissues such as the small bowel, colon, and esophagus. The closed staple length of a "green" stapler is 2.0 mm. These staplers are used for thicker tissues such as the stomach or rectum. Variable-length staplers are discussed later.

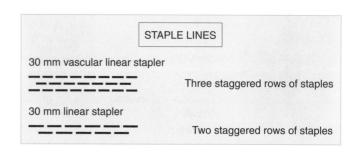

Figure 72–5. Vascular staple lines versus intestinal staple lines. (From Feil W, Lippert H, Lozac'h P, et al: Atlas of Surgical Stapling. Heidelberg, Germany, Johann Ambrosius Barth, 2000.)

Tissue staplers deliver two staggered rows of staples, whereas vascular staplers are used to divide large-caliber vessels while maintaining hemostasis. Vascular staplers deliver three staggered rows of staples (Fig. 72–5).

Types of Staplers

Linear staplers (TA staplers) deliver a double staggered row of staples. They are used in a wide variety of situations, including closure of a hollow viscus, such as the common enterotomy in a side-to-side bowel anastomosis, closure of gastrotomies, and division of large vessels (Fig. 72–6). They can be of variable staple length or fixed staple length, and they can be articulating and nonarticulating.

Linear cutters (GIA staplers) both transect and resect tissues by delivering two double staggered rows of staple lines and deploying a knife to divide the tissue between the staple lines (Figs. 72–7 and 72–8). They are used for a variety of gastrointestinal procedures, such as the formation of enteroenterostomies and gastroenterostomies and the resection of solid organs such as the liver or pancreas.

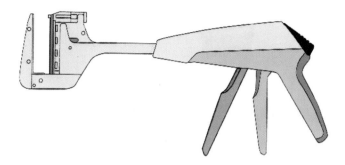

Figure 72–6. Depiction of a TA stapler. (From Feil W, Lippert H, Lozac'h P, et al: Atlas of Surgical Stapling. Heidelberg, Germany, Johann Ambrosius Barth, 2000.)

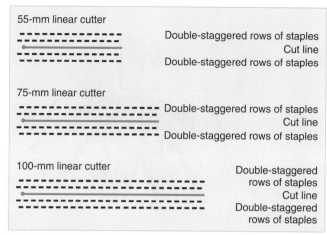

Figure 72–8. Configuration of the staple lines of linear cutting staplers in relation to the knife. (From Feil W, Lippert H, Lozac'h P, et al: Atlas of Surgical Stapling. Heidelberg, Germany, Johann Ambrosius Barth, 2000.)

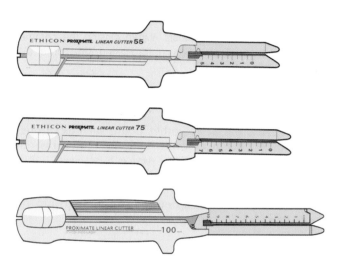

Figure 72–7. Various sizes of linear cutting staplers. (From Feil W, Lippert H, Lozac'h P, et al: Atlas of Surgical Stapling. Heidelberg, Germany, Johann Ambrosius Barth, 2000.)

Circular staplers (EEA, ILS, PPH staplers) are used for inverted end-to-end and end-to-side anastomoses. These staplers usually have a detachable head and lay down a circular, double staggered row of staples. The staples can be variably tightened to a closed length of 2.5 to 1.0 mm, depending on the thickness of the tissue. Circular staplers with nondetachable shafts are used to suspend and excise prolapsed hemorrhoidal tissue.

Techniques/Pitfalls in Surgical Stapling

Functional End-to-End Anastomosis

A functional end-to-end anastomosis (Fig. 72–9), first described in the 1960s, involves apposing the antimesenteric surfaces of two segments of bowel and placing each arm of the GIA stapler in each lumen and firing the stapler to create a common lumen.[18] The lumen is examined and the staples are checked for hemostasis; bleeding points along the staple line in the lumen may be

controlled with 3-0 PDS figure-of-eight sutures. Application of cautery above the staple lines should be discouraged because the current is transmitted along both sides of the staple line and thus can subsequently harm otherwise healthy tissue below the staple line. The common enterotomy is grasped, full thickness, at its edges with Allis clamps to ensure that the serosa and muscularis do not slip under the staple after the stapler is approximated. A single firing of the TA stapler is used to close the common enterotomy. Before firing the TA across the common enterotomy, an important technical point is to ensure that the anterior termination and posterior termination of the GIA staple line are staggered to avoid the crossing of three staple lines.[19] When multiple staple lines cross at the same point, the staples may not close properly, which could lead to anastomotic leakage (see Fig. 72–9).

Stapled End-to-End Anastomosis

This type of anastomosis is performed with a circular stapler (EEA) and is commonly used for the creation of a coloproctostomy but also for esophagostomies and gastroenterostomies. In the case of a colorectal anastomosis, the proximal end of the two ends to be anastomosed is opened, and EEA sizers are placed into the lumen to assess the size of the stapler to be used. Optimal size for these anastomoses should be either 29 or 31 mm. Care should be taken to not create serosal or muscular tears in the colon. Muscular tears of the colon may not always be evident because they might be hidden by the mesentery. The anvil for the EEA is then placed into the open end of the colon, and a Prolene purse-string suture is placed around the rod of the anvil and tied tightly around the rod. If there are any gaps in the purse-string suture, the staple line might be incomplete and a leak could ensue. A mattress suture may be placed around the

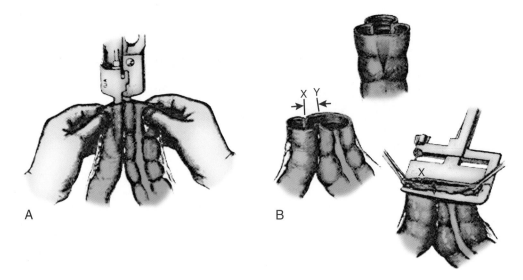

Figure 72–9. Example of a side-to-side, functional end-to-end stapled intestinal anastomosis. When closing the common enterotomy, care must be taken to stagger the anterior and posterior staple lines. (From Chassin JL, Rifkind KM, Turner JW: Errors and pitfalls in stapling gastrointestinal tract anastomoses. Surg Clin North Am 64:447, 1984.)

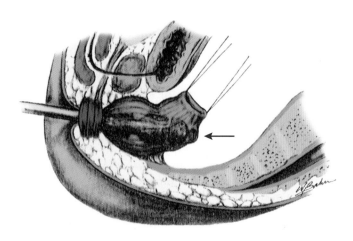

Figure 72–10. When passing a circular stapler for a coloproctostomy, care must be taken to follow the contour of the rectum and sacrum to avoid inadvertently pushing the stapler through the back of the rectum. (From Chassin JL, Rifkind KM, Turner JW: Errors and pitfalls in stapling gastrointestinal tract anastomoses. Surg Clin North Am 64:451, 1984.)

rod to reinforce the purse-string suture. Care must be taken to ensure that the both ends of the bowel are freed up because any fat incorporated into the staple lines may predispose the anastomosis to leakage. The blood supply should also not be too close to the ends for fear of intraluminal bleeding after the stapler is fired.

The stapling device is inserted into the rectum transanally. Care must be taken to follow the contour of the rectum and sacrum to avoid perforating the back wall of the rectum (Fig. 72–10). At the top of the rectum, the stapler should be positioned so that the pin of the EEA comes out right in the middle of the staple line at the portion of rectum that has been cleaned rather than

advancing the pin at any other point, such as through the mesorectum. Once the pin is advanced, the anvil and stapler are engaged and the device is screwed tightly. Before firing the EEA, the stapler should be gently rotated to ensure that no other tissue, such as vagina or bladder, has been inadvertently incorporated into the staple line.

Hand-Sewn Versus Stapled Bowel Anastomoses

Beart and Kelly randomized 80 patients to hand-sewn versus stapled coloproctostomies and found no differences in postoperative complications.[20]

In a prospective multicenter randomized study, Docherty et al. compared manually constructed and stapled colorectal anastomoses in 732 patients.[21] Despite a significant increase in radiologic leak rates in the sutured group (14% versus 5%), there was no difference in clinical anastomotic leak rates, morbidity, and postoperative mortality. Univariate analysis correcting for tumor stage demonstrated that the rate of tumor recurrence and cancer-specific mortality was higher in the sutured patients (7.5% and 6.5%, respectively) and in patients with anastomotic leaks.

A meta-analysis of 13 studies that examined manual versus stapled colon and rectal anastomoses found no differences in leak rate, morbidity, mortality, and cancer recurrence. It did, however, demonstrate a higher rate of intraoperative technical problems and a higher rate of anastomotic strictures after stapled anastomoses.[22] This higher rate of stricture in stapled anastomoses is contraintuitive based on the fact that in animal models, the blood flow rate through stapled anastomoses is significantly higher than the flow rate through the standard two-layer and the Gambee anastomoses.[23]

Another observation in experimental animals is that stapled anastomoses tend to heal by secondary intention as compared with hand-sewn anastomoses, which heal by primary intention.[24] This is most noticeable in the functional end-to-end type. Leakage from this anastomosis tends to take place at its closure with the TA stapler and often occurs weeks after being created rather than in the typical first week. During reoperation, the anastomosis is found to be attached by the TA line to some raw surfaces of the laparotomy.

TISSUE ADHESIVES

Ever since the first use of fibrin powder for hemostasis in 1909, the utility of fibrin and fibrin glue products has rapidly increased in a wide spectrum of different areas of surgery.[25,26] Though more commonly used for hemostasis, skin grafting, bone sealing, and other straightforward tissue repairs, its use in the formation of sutureless anastomoses or in the reinforcement of bowel anastomoses is controversial.

Fibrin glue promotes the coagulation of blood by accelerating the conversion of fibrinogen to fibrin. Fibrin glue contains fibrinogen, plasma proteins, factor VIII, aprotinin, and calcium chloride. It is generally packaged as two separate vials that need to be mixed before use. The first vial usually contains fibrinogen, factor VIII, and plasma proteins. The second usually contains thrombin, calcium chloride, and aprotinin. As the two components are mixed, factor VIII is activated and fibrin is subsequently cross-linked, which results in the hemostatic effect and more importantly has effects of varying degree on wound-breaking strength and tissue adhesion.

Data on fibrin glue reinforcement of surgical anastomoses are inconsistent but seem to point to a detrimental effect on bowel anastomoses. In a rat model of intestinal anastomosis, sutureless anastomoses performed with fibrin glue were associated with a higher leak rate than traditional sutured anastomoses were. Furthermore, the bursting pressure of the fibrin glue anastomoses, when compared with sutured anastomoses, was lower at 4 and 7 days postoperatively, which is the critical period in intestinal healing and is also the period associated with anastomotic leakage.[27]

Reinforcement of intestinal anastomoses with fibrin sealant also has a detrimental effect on anastomotic strength. Van der Ham demonstrated in a rat model that reinforcement of the suture lines in intestinal anastomoses had a detrimental effect on anastomotic strength, bursting pressure, and hydroxyproline content. Thus, these anastomoses were both physiologically and biologically inferior.[28,29] These results were duplicated by Byrne, who showed quite clearly not only the negative effects on bursting pressure but also impressive rates of perianastomotic adhesions, toxic sepsis, and death in rats.[30]

Microscopically, there is an intense perianastomotic inflammatory reaction, and levels of hydroxyproline and subsequently collagen are significantly lower in the fibrin glue anastomoses.[28-30] More importantly, high levels of fibrin have been found to inhibit macrophage migration.[31] Fibrin has also been shown to predispose to residual abscess formation in rat peritonitis models. Fibrin inhibits neutrophil phagocytosis of radiolabeled bacteria through a reversible, but dose-dependent mechanism.[32] Thus, fibrin not only acts as an inhibitor to macrophage migration but also inhibits neutrophil function and thus can be a potential nidus for bacterial infection.

In conclusion, the routine use of tissue adhesives for the reinforcement of bowel anastomoses cannot be recommended.

Octyl-2-cyanoacrylate (Dermabond), commonly used for superficial lacerations, was evaluated in a rat model of high-risk and uncomplicated intestinal anastomoses. The results confirmed that there was no significant advantage to the use of octyl-2-cyanoacrylate over the use of traditional intestinal anastomoses in either uncomplicated or high-risk anastomoses. No appreciable difference was noted in gross perianastomotic appearance, adhesions, or hydroxyproline concentrations in rats with and without the use of octyl-2-cyanoacrylate. There was, however, a marked reduction in postoperative day 7 anastomotic bursting pressure in the rats that received octyl-2-cyanoacrylate.[33] This is, of course, significant because it coincides with the fibroplasia phase of anastomotic healing and thus the period for anastomotic leakage should wound healing be altered. The use of octyl-2-cyanoacrylate cannot be recommended at this time.

SUTURELESS INTESTINAL ANASTOMOSES

Biofragmentable Anastomosis Ring

In 1985, Thomas G. Hardy, Jr. described a biofragmentable anastomosis ring (Valtrac) intended to facilitate sutureless intestinal anastomosis.[34] The device consists of two identical circular rings composed of Dexon and 12% barium sulfate. Prolene sutures are used to create purse-string stitches at the two cut ends of the bowel, and the sutures are tightened around the rings after the rings are placed inside the bowel lumens (Fig. 72–11). The device is closed by applying pressure to both sides of the anastomosis. An audible or palpable click of the device signifies proper closure of the device. The device is broken down and passed in stool at some later time.

Hardy et al. validated the feasibility and safety of this device in a dog model.[34] The safety and efficacy of the Vatrac device for human use was examined in a prospective, randomized, multicenter clinical study involving 438 patients. The patients were randomized to sutured or stapled intestinal anastomoses versus use of the biofragmentable anastomotic ring. There were no significant differences in age, gender, or comorbidity. The overwhelming majority of patients underwent oncologic resections. In 13% of the patients, a technical complication such as a serosal tear or inability to fit the device into the lumen of the bowel precluded use of the device. No difference was found in the postoperative complications of anastomotic leak, fistula, hemorrhage, wound infection, ileus, or small bowel obstruction between groups. There was no advantage or difference in length of stay,

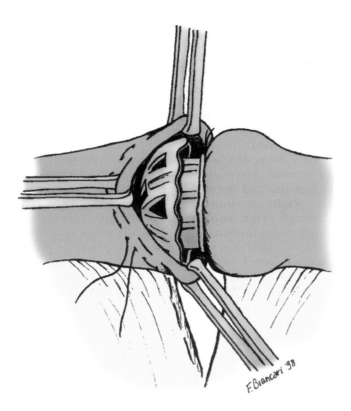

F.Biancari '98

Figure 72–11. Example of the biofragmentable anastomosis ring. (From Di Castro A, Biancari A, Brocato R, et al: Intestinal anastomosis with the biofragmentable anastomosis ring. Am J Surg 176:473, 1998.)

diet, or return to bowel function.[35] Therefore, the biofragmentable anastomosis ring was found to be at least as efficacious as traditional sutured or stapled anastomoses. Di Castro et al. published similar results in a retrospective series of 453 patients with anastomoses created by the biofragmentable anastomosis ring in both elective and emergency situations.[36] They reported a 3% anastomotic leak rate with a 1% rate of reoperation. There were no postoperative intestinal obstructions, but late anastomotic strictures requiring endoscopic dilatation developed in four patients.

The use of biofragmentable anastomosis rings is not superior to traditional suturing or stapling; it does, however, offer a slightly quicker method of anastomosis and allows uniformity of bowel anastomoses throughout the small and large bowel.

CONCLUSION

At the present time, it is not possible to categorically state which is the ideal method of intestinal anastomosis that will work well in every patient. Therefore, it is up to the surgeon to decide in the course of an operation which method is most appropriate. Much of this decision-making process is based on well-established scientific principles. However, part of the decision is also based on the surgeon's skill and experience. Our current inability to scientifically test these factors places them in the realm of art. As in many other biologic processes, further technologic progress will enable us to apply scientific principles even to what is now considered the art of surgery.

REFERENCES

1. Migaly J, Lieberman J, Long W, et al: Effect of adenoviral-mediated transfer of transforming growth factor-beta1 on colonic anastomotic healing. Dis Colon Rectum 47:1699-1705, 2004.
2. Buckmire M, Parquet G, Greenway S, Rolandelli RH: Temporal expression of TGF-beta 1, EGF, and PDGF-BB in a model of colonic wound healing. J Surg Res 80:52-57, 1998.
3. Fukuchi SG, Seeburger JL, Parquet G, Rolandelli RH: Influence of 5-fluorouracil on colonic healing and expression of transforming growth factor-beta 1. J Surg Res 84:121-126, 1999.
4. Ballantyne GH: The experimental basis of intestinal suturing. Effect of surgical technique, inflammation, and infection on enteric wound healing. Dis Colon Rectum 27:61-71, 1984.
5. Postlethwait RW, Schauble D, Dillon ML, et al: Wound healing. II. An evaluation of surgical suture material. Surg Gynecol Obstet 108:555-566, 1959.
6. Madsen ET: An experimental and clinical evaluation of surgical suture materials. Surg Gynecol Obstet 97:73-80, 1953.
7. Madsen ET: An experimental and clinical evaluation of surgical suture materials: II. Surg Gynecol Obstet 97:439-444, 1953.
8. Madsen ET: An experimental and clinical evaluation of surgical suture materials: III. Surg Gynecol Obstet 106:216-224, 1958.
9. Postlethwait RW, Willigan DA, Ulin LW: Human tissue reaction to sutures. Ann Surg 181:144-150, 1975.
10. Halstead HW: Ligature and suture material. The employment of fine silk in preference to catgut and the advantage of transfixion of tissues and vessels in the control of hemorrhage. JAMA 60:1119-1126, 1913.
11. Chu CC, Williams DF: Effects of physical configuration and chemical structure of suture materials on bacterial adhesion. A possible link to wound infection. Am J Surg 147:197-204, 1984.
12. Katz S, Izhar M, Mirelman D: Bacterial adherence to surgical sutures. A possible factor in suture induced infection. Ann Surg 194:35-41, 1981.
13. O'Dwyer P: Serum dependent variability in the adherence of tumour cells to surgical sutures. Br J Surg 72:466-469, 1985.
14. Reinbach D, McGregor JR, O'Dwyer PJ: Effect of suture material on tumour cell adherence at sites of colonic injury. Br J Surg 80:774-776, 1993.
15. Gambee LP, Garnjobst W, Hardwick CE: Ten years' experience with a single layer anastomosis in colon surgery. Am J Surg 92:222-227, 1956.
16. Getzen LC: Clinical use of everted intestinal anastomoses. Surg Gynecol Obstet 123:1027-1036, 1966.
17. Getzen LC, Roe RD, Holloway CK: Comparative study of intestinal anastomotic healing in inverted and everted closures. Surg Gynecol Obstet 123:1219-1227, 1966.
18. Steichen FM: The use of staplers in anatomical side-to-side and functional end-to-end enteroanastomoses. Surgery 64:948-953, 1968.
19. Chassin JL, Rifkind KM, Turner JW: Errors and pitfalls in stapling gastrointestinal tract anastomoses. Surg Clin North Am 64:441-459, 1984.
20. Beart RW, Kelly KA: Randomized prospective evaluation of the EEA stapler for colorectal anastomoses. Am J Surg 141:143-147, 1991.
21. Docherty JG, McGregor JR, Akyol M, et al: Comparison of manually constructed and stapled anastomoses in colorectal surgery. Ann Surg 221:176-184, 1995.
22. MacRae HM, McLeod RS: Handsewn vs stapled anastomoses in colon and rectal surgery: A meta-analysis. Dis Colon Rectum 41:180-189, 1998.
23. Wheeless CR, Smith JJ: A comparison of the flow of iodine 125 through three different intestinal anastomoses: Standard, Gambee, and stapler. Obstet Gynecol 62:513-518, 1983.
24. Caporossi C, Cecconello I, Aguilar-Nascimento JE, et al: Hand-sewn and stapled esophageal anastomosis: Experimental study in dogs. Acta Cir Bras [serial online] 19(4), 2004.

25. Bergel S: Ueber Wirkungen des Fibrins. Dtsch Med Wochenschr 35:663-665, 1909.

26. Detweiler MB: Sutureless and reduced suture anastomosis of hollow vessels with fibrin glue: A review. J Invest Surg 12:245-262, 1999.

27. Haukipuro KA, Hulkko OA, Alavaikko MJ, et al: Sutureless colon anastomosis with fibrin glue in the rat. Dis Colon Rectum 31:601-604, 1988.

28. Van der Ham KA, Kort WJ, Weijma IM, et al: Effect of fibrin sealant on the healing colonic anastomosis in the rat. Br J Surg 78:49-53, 1991.

29. Van der Ham KA, Kort WJ, Weijma IM, et al: Healing of colonic anastomoses: Fibrin sealant does not improve wound healing. Dis Colon Rectum 35:884-891, 1992.

30. Byrne DJ: Adverse influence of fibrin sealant on the healing of high-risk sutured colonic anastomoses. J R Coll Surg Edinb 37:394-398, 1992.

31. Ciano PS, Colvin RB, Dvorak AM, et al: Macrophage migration in fibrin gel matrices. Lab Invest 54:62-70, 1986.

32. Rotstein OD, Pruett TL, Simmons RL: Fibrin in peritonitis: V. Fibrin inhibits phagocytic killing of *Escherichia coli* by human polymorphonuclear leukocytes. Ann Surg 203:413-419, 1986.

33. Nursal TZ, Anarat R, Bircan S, et al: The effect of tissue adhesive, octyl-cyanoacrylate, on the healing of experimental high-risk and normal colonic anastomoses. Am J Surg 187:28-32, 2004.

34. Hardy TG, Pace WG, Maney JW, et al: A biofragmentable ring for sutureless anastomosis: An experimental study. Dis Colon Rectum 28:484-490, 1985.

35. Corman ML, Prager ED, Hardy TG, et al: Comparison of the Valtrac biofragmentable anastomosis ring with conventional suture and stapled anastomosis in colon surgery. Dis Colon Rectum 32:183-187, 1989.

36. Di Castro A, Biancari A, Brocato R, et al: Intestinal anastomosis with the biofragmentable anastomosis ring. Am J Surg 176:472-474, 1998.

73

Gastric, Duodenal, and Small Intestinal Fistulas

Michael S. Nussbaum • David R. Fischer

The word *fistula* comes from the Latin meaning "pipe" or "flute" and is defined as an abnormal communication between two epithelialized surfaces. Gastrointestinal fistulas continue to cause significant morbidity and mortality, even though many factors important in their management are known. Over the past 35 to 40 years, the mortality associated with gastrointestinal fistulas has diminished from approximately 40% to 60% to about 15% to 20%.[1] This improvement in prognosis is attributable to general advances in fluid and electrolyte/acid-base therapy, blood administration, critical care, ventilatory management, antibiotic regimens, and nutritional management. Formerly, malnutrition and electrolyte imbalance were the causes of death in the majority of these patients. In the present era of fistula treatment, mortality is largely attributable to uncontrolled sepsis and sepsis-associated malnutrition.

The mechanism of fistula formation is varied. Congenital fistulas are caused by errors in development. Acquired fistulas may occur as a result of inflammatory disease, abdominal trauma, surgical complications, radiation, and benign or malignant neoplasm. Spontaneous causes account for 15% to 25% of gastrointestinal fistulas and include radiation, inflammatory bowel disease, diverticular disease, appendicitis, ischemic bowel, perforation of gastric and duodenal ulcers, pancreatic and gynecologic malignancies, and intestinal actinomycosis or tuberculosis. The remaining 75% to 85% of gastrointestinal fistulas are of iatrogenic origin and occur as a result of technical complications of surgical procedures and trauma. Such complications include dehiscence of anastomoses, mechanical injury to the gastrointestinal tract during dissection, cautery injury, retractor injury, indwelling tubes, and misplacement of a suture through the bowel during abdominal closure. Other technical complications resulting in fistulas are those that occur at delayed periods after surgery, such as intraperitoneal bleeding and abscess formation with or without suture line dehiscence. Fistulas may also develop after drainage of a percutaneous abscess, with a connection created between the intestine and abdominal wall.

Treatment of patients with gastrointestinal fistulas requires an understanding of metabolic and anatomic derangements. For patient mortality to be minimized, nutrition, volume, and electrolyte derangements must be promptly corrected. Additionally, ongoing losses must be anticipated and prevented. Malnutrition is easier to prevent than correct. Once established, malnutrition is difficult to correct, especially in the face of continuing sepsis. After the initial stabilization period, including control of sepsis and establishment of nutritional support, management can be divided into phases, starting with determination of the anatomy of the fistula and the likelihood of spontaneous closure. This may then be followed by definitive surgical therapy for a fistula that does not close spontaneously, but a waiting period of at least 6 weeks is usually required. The final process is healing. The critical points in successful management of gastrointestinal fistulas are recognition of the fistula, control of infection and further contamination, restoration of fluid and electrolyte losses, and re-establishment of a positive nutritional balance before undertaking major definitive corrective procedures.

GENERAL CONSIDERATIONS

Gastrointestinal fistulas result from perforations that communicate with adjacent organs or intestine (internal fistulas) or communicate externally with the abdominal wall (enterocutaneous fistulas). Although they may resolve spontaneously, specific intervention or operative therapy may be needed. The small intestine's length, as well as its unique convoluted anatomy, predisposes it to involvement in a variety of diseases, and almost any surgical procedure involving the abdomen can result in iatrogenic injury to the small intestine and subsequent fistula formation. The development of a fistula between the small intestine and an internal structure can be a life-threatening event, as with exsanguination from an aortoenteric fistula or cholangitis from communication with the intestine and subsequent bacterial contamination of the biliary tree. Other fistulas, particularly internal fistulas between loops of small intestine, may be asymptomatic. Enterocutaneous fistulas are the most common form of small intestinal fistula. Though not usually lethal, an enterocutaneous fistula mandates careful and multitiered management to avoid further complicating the well-being of the patient.

Multiple factors make a gastrointestinal fistula a complex and potentially lethal condition. First, the patients in whom such fistulas develop are usually systemically ill. Sepsis is a recognized antecedent risk factor for the development of a gastrointestinal fistula, and the high metabolic requirement of the septic state can preclude spontaneous closure of the fistula. In fact, sepsis is often secondary to the factor leading to the fistula itself. Malnutrition is also a common occurrence that results both from the hypermetabolic state of the septic, postoperative patient and from the large volume of protein-rich fluid produced, and subsequently lost, by the small intestine. Fluid and electrolyte abnormalities, including hypovolemia, hypokalemia, hypomagnesemia, and metabolic acidosis, are common and result from the continued loss of intestinal fluid. Such losses are not limited to fistulas communicating externally because internal fistulas, such as enterocolic fistulas, can bypass the normal intestinal continuity and overwhelm the absorptive capacity of the recipient organ. Malabsorption and malnutrition from bacterial overgrowth may complicate gastrocolic or enterocolic fistulas. Finally, local wound excoriation and discomfort from the enzymatically active intestinal effluent can complicate potential abdominal wall reconstruction and recovery after surgical attempts to repair a fistula. Furthermore, operating on a fistula before control of sepsis and nutritional optimization can lead to increased mortality and often further fistula formation.

ETIOLOGY

Gastric and Duodenal Fistulas

The vast majority of gastric and duodenal fistulas still occur after surgical, endoscopic, or interventional procedures. Postoperative anastomotic or suture line leaks account for 80% to 85% of all fistulas. Basic general surgical principles of adequate blood supply, lack of tension, no distal obstruction, and uncompromised technique are essential. External fistulas that occur in conjunction with large abdominal wall defects are particularly difficult to treat and often require multiple staged operations, with mortality rates of 20% to 60%.[2] Before 1950, greater than 60% mortality was observed in patients with gastric and duodenal fistulas, but as of 1975, with improved perioperative care and the advent of total parenteral nutrition (TPN), the mortality rate had decreased to just below 25%.[3] The gastric and duodenal fistula rate of just 0.6% at this time was ascribed in part to the liberal use of

catheter duodenostomies after gastrectomy.[3] Around 1990, Schein and Decker noted a 17% mortality rate for gastric and duodenal fistulas, with a 13% mortality rate for duodenal stump fistulas.[2] Reconstruction of the common bile duct uncommonly results in duodenal injury and fistula. Numerous comparisons of sutured versus stapled anastomoses show comparable results, without an obvious superiority of either. The ease of stapler use does not compensate for edematous or inflamed tissues, for which better tissue approximation may be achieved with hand-sewn techniques, although anastomoses in these types of tissue may be doomed to failure no matter which technique is used. Postoperative leaks from gastric staple or suture lines after ulcer surgery have accounted for most perforations in the past. However, the decline in gastric resection for ulcer disease, along with the broad application of new endoscopic and laparoscopic techniques for other diseases, accounts for many other newer causes of perforation.

Gastric operations for morbid obesity include vertical banded gastroplasty, Roux-en-Y gastric bypass, gastric banding with adjustable prosthetics, and the duodenal switch procedure. Gastric staple line disruption may develop in the early postoperative period or can occur many months after surgery. Importantly, early anastomotic leaks after gastrojejunostomy in this patient population are highly morbid and often lethal. A high index of suspicion is required to detect these leaks, and they should be controlled early in the process. Mortality may occur even before the development of a fistula. Internal gastric fistulas after gastric stapling are well known, with subsequent weight gain after a fistula has formed between the proximal gastric pouch and the distal part of the stomach. For gastric bypasses, the 10% to 30% incidence rate of internal fistula formation after simple stapling has been reduced to 3% to 6% by either gastric division after stapling or up to three applications of the stapler without division.[4,5]

In a series of 318 partial gastrectomies, Pickleman et al. reported a 1.3% anastomotic leak rate, all from gastrojejunostomy and without any duodenal stump leaks. After total gastrectomy with Roux-en-Y esophagojejunostomy, anastomotic leaks occurred in 4.8%.[6] A perforation rate of 1.5% has been reported after vertical banded gastroplasty for morbid obesity,[7] and a rate as high as 6% has been reported after divided gastric bypass, again from the gastrojejunostomy.[8] Gastric perforation is also a risk in patients who have undergone splenectomy as a result of greater curvature partial-thickness ligatures with devascularization. The incidence of eventual perforation at stapled gastric closures may be increased with the use of cautery to control bleeding at the stapled edge, intersecting staple lines within an anastomosis, and the use of a stapler on a thickened, edematous gastric wall, which causes overcompression, tearing, and devascularization at the line of closure. In such tissue, a hand-sewn closure more adequately approximates tissue without excessive tension.

Duodenal stump leakage has been long feared, although the overall incidence has declined, in part because of the decreased use of antrectomy for ulcer disease and the increased use of reliable staplers for duodenal division and closure. Duodenal stump leakage is more common after difficult gastric resections, for example, after antrectomy for giant duodenal ulcer disease.[9] Reports indicate a very low incidence of stump leakage after gastric resection. In a high-risk patient, morbidity and mortality can be decreased and possibly prevented by placement of a duodenostomy tube along with closed suction drains external to the duodenum. Duodenal diverticulectomy or lateral duodenotomy for periampullary procedures may result in leakage in edematous or inflamed tissue or with poor hand-sewn technique. Biliary tract surgery is not usually associated with duodenal injury, with the exception of dissection of a markedly inflamed or chronically fibrotic gallbladder, an adherent choledochal cyst, or an unsuspected duodenal diverticulum.

Gastrojejunocolic internal fistula, a rare complication after distal gastrectomy with gastrojejunostomy, is due to marginal ulceration causing perforation at the gastrojejunostomy and a fistula to the adjacent transverse colon. Typical symptoms include diarrhea, pain, gastrointestinal bleeding, and weight loss. Neoplastic causes of internal fistulas are uncommon. Gastrocolic fistulas have resulted from gastric ulcer erosion and invasion of the transverse colon by gastric adenocarcinoma or lymphoma. Primary hepatic flexure or transverse colon adenocarcinoma may in rare instances invade and create a fistula to the duodenum or stomach.

The ongoing extension of laparoscopic techniques to gastric surgery has not eliminated the risk of perforation. Veress needle insertion for establishing pneumoperitoneum may result in the perforation of any intraabdominal organ, as can the other varied techniques of abdominal access for laparoscopy, especially in a reoperative abdomen. Laparoscopic fundoplication and laparoscopic Heller myotomy are now widely used for the surgical management of gastroesophageal reflux disease and achalasia, respectively. Although morbidity rates are low, the esophagus or stomach may be perforated during the procedures, with the majority occurring in the first 10 to 25 fundoplications or myotomies performed by the surgeon. The incidence of esophageal or gastric perforation during fundoplication ranges from 0.3% to 1.9%,[10-12] with a large retrospective review of 2453 procedures by Perdikis et al. showing an overall incidence of 1.0%.[13] These perforations are acquired in at least four ways:

1. During retroesophageal dissection, the gastric fundus that is adherent to the left crus of the diaphragm may be lacerated during the right-to-left dissection through fatty tissue.
2. Direct injury can be inflicted on the anterior aspect of the stomach with graspers while retracting in a caudad and anterior direction. These graspers are often temporarily out of the laparoscopic field of view. The fundus may also be lacerated as a result of excessive tension while maneuvering it behind the esophagus.
3. Esophageal bougie insertion can cause perforation at the gastroesophageal junction or along the greater curvature.
4. Full-thickness suture placement while securing the fundoplication, with eventual tearing of the gastric wall, may result in delayed recognition of the perforation.

Laparoscopic fundoplication may also result in delayed gastric perforation along the greater curvature from inadvertent thermal or cautery injury during division of the short gastric artery. If the diaphragmatic crura are not approximated adequately, the fundoplication can herniate into the chest during postoperative straining, vomiting, or heavy lifting, with subsequent gastric ischemia and perforation. Laparoscopic revision of a previous fundoplication requires more gastric traction and division of adhesions, with a 3% risk for gastric laceration.[14] Other laparoscopic procedures that have caused perforation include diaphragmatic hernia repair, paraesophageal hernia repair (perforation in 6%), Heller myotomy, splenectomy, pyloromyotomy, and gastrostomy tube placement. The laparoscopically placed adjustable silicone gastric band, positioned around the proximal part of the stomach for the treatment of morbid obesity, has also resulted in gastric perforation in less than 1% of patients.[15,16]

Laparoscopic cholecystectomy may produce duodenal injury if the duodenum and gallbladder are densely adherent to one another as a result of either direct cutting action or cautery and thermal injury. Laparoscopic cholecystectomy may also result in colonic injury by the same mechanisms. In addition, improperly insulated instruments may cause electrical arcing to the duodenum, small bowel, or colon with resultant perforation. These injuries may not be immediately apparent. Coincident bile spillage from the gallbladder may also mask a duodenal injury. Likewise, duodenal perforation and bile duct injury may coexist. Laparoscopic bile duct exploration usually risks cystic duct or common bile duct injuries more than injuries to the duodenum. However, advanced procedures such as antegrade sphincterotomy and antegrade stent insertion may also result in duodenal injury.

Crohn's disease is a rare cause of gastrocolic, duodenocolic, or duodenocutaneous fistulas. Primary gastric or duodenal involvement is reported in less than 1% of patients with Crohn's disease; duodenocutaneous fistulas may develop from the first or second portion of the duodenum. However, most gastric or duodenal fistulas are internal and result from involvement of primary Crohn's disease of the transverse colon or, more commonly, from recurrence at the ileocolic anastomosis after previous resection. Those with gastrocolic fistulas have a 40% incidence of vomiting, which may be feculent; duodenocolic fistulas are often asymptomatic, with only a 4% incidence of vomiting, which is not usually feculent.[17]

Inflammatory fistula formation can result from gallstone erosion through the gallbladder and migration into the contiguous second portion of the duodenum, which causes a persistent cholecystoduodenal fistula. It may remain asymptomatic (as should a similar surgically created cholecystojejunostomy) but should be suspected in patients with the uncommon finding of gallstone ileus with distal small bowel obstruction because of the stone. Renogastric fistula has been reported secondary to a staghorn calculus.[18] Duodenal hematomas may also lead to fistula formation. Severe necrotizing pancreatitis requiring necrosectomy, with subsequent open packing or closed drainage, has resulted in both gastric and duodenal fistulas. These fistulas may already exist at the time of initial laparotomy, or they may develop as late as 1 to 3 months later, either from the inflammatory process or from an iatrogenic cause. Although they may be more frequent after open packing, spontaneous closure is common (up to 54%).[19,20]

The capacity and compliance of the stomach make endoscopic examination routine, with a low incidence of injury. However, endoscopic polypectomy or attempts at tumor removal with a snare and cautery may cause either immediate full-thickness perforation or deep penetration with thermal injury to the remaining tissue and subsequent delayed perforation. Similar injury may occur with the use of thermal contact methods (heater probe, multipolar electrocoagulation, laser) or dilute epinephrine injections into bleeding ulcers and arteriovenous malformations, with exacerbation of the injury by successive treatments. Esophageal dilatation performed with a semirigid dilator over a wire has caused gastric perforation from the end of the wire. Percutaneous endoscopic gastrostomy tube placement, though often routine, has also resulted in perforation, either from dislodgment of the tube before complete gastric adhesion to the abdominal wall or from trauma during placement. Lack of adhesion to the abdominal wall may be more common in immunosuppressed patients taking steroids, for instance. Gastric necrosis may also occur as a result of ischemia and subsequent gastric leakage from a tube that is pulled too tight. Improper tube placement along the posterior wall below the greater curvature, while the stomach is distended, can result in excessive tension on the posterior gastric wall when traction is applied, with subsequent leakage into the lesser sac. Tube placement that is too proximal in the stomach has also caused perforation because of excessive gastric wall tension and eventual tube dislodgment through the wall. In addition, tube insertion may perforate the adjacent jejunum or transverse colon and result in a persistent gastrojejunal or gastrocolic fistula, even after the gastrostomy tube has been removal. This complication may also require early laparotomy to address peritonitis and sepsis. A percutaneously placed gastrostomy tube results in a thin fibrous cylinder connecting the stomach to the anterior abdominal wall; manual replacement of the gastrostomy tube can perforate this cylinder and give liquid feeding solutions direct access to the peritoneal cavity, with resultant peritonitis. Gastrostomy tube placement may cause a persistent gastrocutaneous fistula that enlarges through erosion or infection of fascia and skin. These fistulas may be difficult to control, with continued drainage of gastric fluid onto the surrounding skin. The substitution of a larger gastrostomy tube will not control the leakage and usually results in enlargement of the opening. Persistent drainage may require either tube removal or placement of a smaller tube, along with direct or nasogastric suction until the tract contracts down around the tube. Surgical closure is required for a persistent gastrocutaneous fistula that does not respond to such measures.

Because many endoscopic duodenal procedures involve the second portion of the duodenum, perforation is usually retroperitoneal. Failure to recognize an injury or a delay in treatment markedly increases morbidity and mortality. Perforation after endoscopic retrograde cholangiopancreatography (ERCP) with ampullary sphincterotomy for stone extraction or biliary stent placement is one of the more frequent postendoscopic indications for urgent surgical intervention. Repair of the distal bile duct, as well as repair of the duodenum, may be required. Controlled leaks confined to the retroperitoneum can often be monitored with very close clinical observation in stable patients. Retroperitoneal perforation is more common during therapeutic ERCP, with an incidence of 0.6% to 1.8% and a mortality rate of up to 25%.[21,22] Delayed duodenal perforation from the biliary stent itself may be caused by partial extrusion and impingement of the end of the stent on the distal second or proximal third portion of the duodenum, with eventual erosion and perforation. Proximal stent migration into the common bile duct may cause a choledochoduodenal fistula to subsequently form if the stent reenters the duodenum away from the papilla. Similarly, pancreatic duct stents may produce a pancreaticogastric fistula with proximal migration of the stent into the gastric antrum. Other procedures at risk for the development of duodenal perforation include endoscopic polyp or tumor removal, push enteroscopy, endoscopic ultrasound with transduodenal biopsy, and endoscopically assisted transgastric jejunal feeding tube placement.

An aortoduodenal fistula involving the third portion of the duodenum must be suspected in any patient with a previous abdominal aortic graft and upper gastrointestinal bleeding or a patient with graft infection without gastrointestinal bleeding. An aortogastric fistula may occur intra-abdominally in a patient with a ruptured abdominal aortic aneurysm without previous aortic surgery,[23] as well as intrathoracically after esophagectomy at the esophagogastric suture line (treated successfully by direct repair and endovascular graft placement).[24] Reconstruction of the inferior vena cava with a stented polytetrafluoroethylene (Teflon) graft has also resulted in a fistula to the adjacent duodenum.[25]

Percutaneous transhepatic wire and biliary stent placement may lead to duodenal perforation. However, a transhepatic biliary drain also provides effective duodenal decompression if subsequent operative repair is needed. Because of the proximity of the duodenum and inferior vena cava, caval filter placement has resulted in duodenal penetration from the filter hooks. Percutaneous drainage of upper abdominal abscesses uncommonly results in duodenal injury. Swallowed foreign bodies that are small enough to traverse the pylorus may not escape the duodenum; typically, toothpicks and fish bones may penetrate the duodenum and form a phlegmon or an abscess. Stiff feeding tubes or nasogastric tubes passing through the pylorus have also resulted in duodenal perforation.

Nonoperative causes of perforation include strangulated paraesophageal hernia, foreign body ingestion, and esophageal intubation with gastric overpressure. Gastric adenocarcinoma may uncommonly result in perforation. Treatment of gastric lymphoma with chemotherapy or radiation (or both) has caused perforation along with cytoreduction. Mycotic infection with eventual gastric perforation has been reported in immunosuppressed heart, lung, and liver transplant recipients.[26]

Small Intestinal Fistula

Small intestinal fistulas can form in a number of ways. External small intestinal fistulas (enterocutaneous fistulas) are by far the most frequent type of small intestinal fistula. Enterocutaneous fistulas most commonly follow postoperative complications and are often the result of technical errors at the time of an abdominal procedure. Of 35 fistulas originating in the jejunum or ileum reported by MacFadyen and associates, 75% drained externally.[27] The ileum is the most common site of origin of an enterocutaneous fistula. Reber and colleagues found that of 120 small intestinal enterocutaneous fistulas, 72 originated from the ileum and 48 from the jejunum.[28] Enterocutaneous fistulas can be classified according to the daily volume of drainage. A high-output fistula drains 500 ml/day or more of fluid. In most instances, a high-output fistula is associated with greater morbidity and mortality and a decreased likelihood of spontaneous closure. Soeters and associates found that patients with high-output fistulas had a greater incidence of malnutrition and fluid and electrolyte disturbances.[3] Mortality increased, and the rate of fistula closure was low. In contrast, excellent results with high-output fistulas were reported in Graham's series, in which 35 of 39 consecutive patients underwent spontaneous fistula closure with a 3% mortality rate.[29] In general, high-output fistulas usually originate from a proximal portion of the small intestine. Conditions that are independent of the surgical technique, such as previous intestinal irradiation, intra-abdominal sepsis, or the presence of diseased or ischemic intestine, can also give rise to external fistulas. Enteroenteric or enterocolic fistulas develop almost exclusively from the transmural inflammation associated with Crohn's disease.

Webster and Carey proposed five general mechanisms for fistula formation[30]:

Congenital A rare form of congenital small intestinal fistula involves complete failure of the vitellointestinal duct to obliterate, which results in an enterocutaneous fistula to the umbilicus. When incomplete obliteration of the duct occurs, the enteric portion of the duct is the usual portion that persists and forms a Meckel diverticulum. Rarely, the entire omphalomesenteric duct remains patent and forms an external fistula. The diagnosis should be suggested by the appearance of fecal material at the umbilicus after postnatal slough of the umbilical cord.

Trauma Traumatic injury to the small intestine that results in fistula formation usually occurs from an internal source, such as a swallowed fish bone, toothpick, or metallic object. Erosion of these objects into an adjacent loop of small intestine results in an internal enteroenteric fistula. Major penetrating trauma, such as knife or bullet wounds, rarely results in fistula formation because these cases are usually explored surgically and the intestinal injuries repaired. Locally unexplored knife wounds, however, have resulted in the development of an enterocutaneous fistula when minor intestinal injuries were not diagnosed in timely fashion.

Infection An abscess or invasive intestinal infection may erode through the intestine and create a fistula. Amebiasis, coccidiomycosis, tuberculosis, cryptosporidiosis, actinomycosis, and salmonellosis have all been implicated in the development of intestinal fistulas. Intestinal perforation at the ileum from tuberculosis and typhoid fever is still occasionally seen, especially in countries where these diseases are endemic. *Actinomyces* is a common cause of enterocutaneous fistulas after appendectomy. Fistulas may also result from the proximity of the small intestine to an abscess involving a solid organ, such as when rupture of a perinephric abscess results in a nephroenteric fistula.

Perforation or Injury with Abscess Perforation of the intestinal wall by tumor, inflammation, or operative injury may result in the local formation of an abscess. A fistula may develop if this abscess subsequently erodes into an adjacent structure. Most enterocutaneous fistulas develop as a result of injury to the small intestine during surgery or from exposure of the bowel to a large abdominal defect or prosthetic mesh used to repair such defects. An enterocutaneous fistula rarely develops spontaneously. In fact, most develop after an abdominal surgical procedure. In most large series, 60% to more than 90% of enterocutaneous fistulas were caused by operative complications. Faulty operative technique involving injury to the intestine during handling, lysis of adhesions, or abdominal fascial closure often results in fistulas. In addition, enterocutaneous fistulas may be caused by leakage from an intestinal anastomosis or enterotomy closure. Fistulas may also develop as a result of percutaneous drainage of an intra-abdominal abscess. After perforation, an abscess may develop at the site of injury and then drain either internally into another loop of intestine or externally through the abdominal wall or wound. Commonly, a fistula has been found to have feculent drainage from the wound after the wound is opened for a presumed wound infection.

Inflammation, Irradiation, or Tumor The small intestine and an adjacent structure can become densely adherent from chronic inflammatory conditions, abdominal radiation injury, or tumor erosion. Subsequent degeneration of the common wall results in fistula formation. Inflammatory bowel disease, particularly Crohn's disease, is well known to create enteroenteric, enterocolic, perineal, enterocutaneous, and other fistulas in this fashion. In Crohn's disease, the diseased intestine makes fistula formation after anastomosis more likely. Although a spontaneous external fistula can develop as a direct result of Crohn's disease, most occur only after a previous operation has caused the diseased intestine to adhere to the abdominal wall. Postoperative fistulas in the setting of Crohn's disease are just as likely to develop after simple exploration, bypass, or appendectomy as after primary resection. Fistula formation after laparotomy is usually an early complication, especially when arising from an anastomosis, whereas a late fistula generally indicates recurrent Crohn's disease. Erosion of the intestine by a foreign body such as swallowed objects or polypropylene mesh, abdominal wall dehiscence with evisceration, and strangulation of a hernia with infarction and perforation of the intestine have all been implicated in the development of external fistulas. Enlarging carcinomas of the stomach or colon may adhere to and erode into adjacent small intestine with some frequency. Fistula formation is particularly apt to occur after irradiation of a pelvic malignant lesion. Fistulas that arise secondary to radiation injury rarely, if ever close spontaneously.

DIAGNOSIS OF PERFORATIONS AND FISTULAS

Acute intraoperative perforations are best handled by maintaining a strong index of suspicion for technical errors, recognizing the injury before the end of the procedure, and immediately repairing, suturing, or reinforcing weakened tissues. Especially during prolonged laparoscopic procedures, the tendency for potential injuries must be recognized and overcome. Serosal injuries should be carefully examined and sutured. Intraluminal instillation of methylene blue and saline or direct endoscopic examination can demonstrate a small perforation or provide reassurance that an area of concern is not a full-thickness injury.

Postoperatively, unrecognized perforations caused during surgery or leaks that develop at suture or staple lines are manifested as instability or failure to improve as expected. A gastrointestinal fistula can be obvious in some patients and extremely difficult to identify in others. Fistula formation is frequently heralded by fever and abdominal pain until gastrointestinal contents discharge through an abdominal incision or the umbilicus. Spontaneous fistulas from neoplasm or inflammatory disease usually develop in a more indolent manner. Enterocutaneous fistulas often have intestinal contents or gas exiting from a drain site or through the abdominal incision after an operation. The drainage fluid is usually typical of intestinal contents, with obvious bile staining, and intestinal gas may accompany the effluent. At times the initial fistula drainage may initially appear clear rather than yellow or green, and the fistula may be misdiagnosed as a seroma or wound infection. At other times a heavy purulent component may also mask the enteric communication and instead suggest a wound infection. If the drainage persists and the diagnosis is uncertain, the patient may be given activated charcoal or indigo carmine by mouth and the drainage inspected for these substances.

Endoscopic gastroduodenal perforations are suspected when fever, tachycardia, or abdominal tenderness is present after the procedure. Initial chest and abdominal radiographic films may demonstrate free intraperitoneal air or retroperitoneal air outlining the duodenal wall. Unexplained fever, ongoing or new tachycardia, hypotension, worsening leukocytosis, new or continuing abdominal pain, persistent ileus, and persistent oliguria all raise suspicion for a pathologic intra-abdominal process.

STAGING/CLASSIFICATION

Gastrointestinal fistulas can be classified by their anatomic characteristics, and they are either internal or external (enterocutaneous). The actual anatomic course of the fistula should be defined. Typically, the name of a fistula is derived from the involved and connected organs or structures. Examples include gastrocolic, jejunoileal, and aortoenteric fistulas. In general, the anatomy of a fistula will suggest the cause and help predict whether spontaneous closure will occur.[31,32] Fistulas can be classified physiologically in terms of output over a 24-hour period. They can be classified as low (less than 200 ml/day), moderate (200 to 500 ml/day), and high (greater than 500 ml/day).[3,31] An accurate measure of fistula output, as well as the chemical make-up of the effluent, can provide assistance in preventing and treating metabolic deficits and correcting ongoing fluid, electrolyte, and protein losses. The anatomic and etiologic factors are much more important in predicting spontaneous closure than the actual output of the fistula. The underlying disease process will help in prognisticating both the closure rate and mortality.

External or enterocutaneous fistulas are by far the most common type of small intestinal fistula and are usually readily recognizable. In contrast, internal fistulas that communicate between the intestine and another hollow viscus or structure may not be suspected for some time because the symptoms may be minimal or may mimic the underlying disease process. Relatively rare, such fistulas have been reported between adjacent segments of the gastrointestinal tract, as well as between the small intestine and the biliary tree, genitourinary system, and arterial and venous trees.

COMPLICATIONS

The loss of gastrointestinal contents either prematurely by diversion to the body surface or by "short-circuiting" within the gastrointestinal tract may result in profound fluid and electrolyte deficits, the specific nature of which depends on the portion of the gastrointestinal tract whose contents are lost. Malabsorption with severe nutritional and vitamin deficiencies may also ensue. Fistulas are commonly associated with one or more abscesses, which often drain incompletely with fistulization. Therefore, persistent sepsis may occur as a result of contamination of a normally sterile space or organ system by gastrointestinal flora traversing the fistula. Gastrointestinal hemorrhage, intestinal obstruction, and excoriation and erosion of the skin by gastrointestinal secretions may also complicate the course of a patient with a fistula. These problems may be superimposed on other abnormalities inherent to the underlying disease that produced the fistula.

Fluid and Electrolyte Abnormalities

Fluid and electrolyte disturbances occur commonly in patients with enterocutaneous fistulas. Secretions from the salivary glands, stomach, duodenum, pancreas, liver, and small intestine amount to 8 to 10 L/day, and this fluid is rich in sodium, potassium, chloride, and bicarbonate. The degree of volume depletion and electrolyte imbalance depends on the anatomic location of the fistula and can vary from 50 to 3000 ml/day.[27] Duodenal fistulas are particularly prone to volume and electrolyte loss, and aggressive fluid management is necessary for patients with such high-output fistulas. A distal fistula, such as one arising from the terminal ileum in a patient with Crohn's disease, is usually associated with less fluid loss because considerable absorption occurs in the proximal part of the gut.

Fluid and electrolyte imbalances were noted in 35 of 128 patients with gastrointestinal fistulas reported by Soeters and associates from 1970 to 1975.[3] The most common abnormalities were hypovolemia, hypokalemia, and metabolic acidosis. Hypokalemia occurs primarily from potassium loss in the fistula effluent, although hypovolemia also contributes by causing renal retention of sodium in exchange for potassium secretion. Sepsis contributes to the hypovolemic state by altering the metabolic rate and increasing insensible water loss through fever. Metabolic acidosis is generally caused by the loss of pancreatic juice rich in bicarbonate and is thus more common with proximal intestinal fistulas. Gastric fistulas, especially in conjunction with gastric outlet obstruction, will cause a hypokalemic, hypochloremic metabolic alkalosis secondary to the loss of a large volume of hydrochloric acid.

Patients with fistulas causing fluid and electrolyte abnormalities have a higher mortality rate.[33] Advances in critical care, invasive monitoring, and aggressive fluid and electrolyte management can reduce this early mortality considerably, as evidenced by data from the Massachusetts General Hospital. Before 1960, nearly all patients at this institution died when an electrolyte deficit complicated a fistula involving the small intestine. Improvements in therapy and control of sepsis have resulted in a substantial decrease in the mortality rate.[3]

Malnutrition

The small intestine contains fluid rich in ingested nutrients and endogenous proteins, such as enzymes and albumin. Thus, malnutrition develops in almost all patients with a small intestinal fistula if the absorptive surface area is bypassed or the enteric contents are lost externally. Nutritional deficiency may be exacerbated by the extra metabolic demands of sepsis or additional surgery. Soeters and associates reported moderate to severe malnutrition in 86 of 128 patients.[3] Before the introduction of TPN, 74% of patients with intestinal fistulas exhibited malnutrition, and 59% of these patients died.

Sepsis

With advances in fluid replacement, management of electrolyte deficits, and nutritional support, sepsis remains the major determinant of mortality in patients with fistulas of the small intestine. Most fistulas develop after contamination of a sterile space by gastrointestinal bacteria. Abscesses not only cause but can also complicate fistulas of the intestine. Uncontrolled abdominal sepsis can lead to bacteremia, local and distant infection, and multisystem organ failure. Local extension usually results in wound infection. Distant bacterial seeding may cause splenic and hepatic abscess or endocarditis. Large defects in the abdominal wall predispose the patient to repeated episodes of sepsis and consequently a high mortality rate. In a large series by Schein and Decker, the overall mortality rate associated with fistulas of the small bowel was 33%.[34] However, when a large abdominal wall defect accompanied the fistula, the mortality rate rose to 60%, with the main cause of death cited as infection.

Abdominal Wall and Wound Abnormalities

Skin erosion and excoriation commonly occur from an externally draining gastrointestinal fistula. The local digestive action of the gastrointestinal secretions, particularly pancreatic enzymes, can result in considerable discomfort to the patient. The degree of local skin excoriation depends on the output and contents of the fistula effluent and is most severe with proximal intestinal fistulas. Malnutrition contributes to this process by delaying the formation of scar or granulation tissue.

Other Complications

Other complications of small intestinal fistulas occur with less frequency. Massive gastrointestinal hemorrhage can result from the formation of a fistula between the small intestine and a blood vessel. One or more "herald bleeds" may be a prelude to exsanguinating hemorrhage. More commonly, anemia develops chronically and is associated with slow blood loss from a friable fistula tract. Colonization and overgrowth of the small intestine by colonic bacteria can occur with enterocolic fistulas and may result in malabsorption and severe, malodorous diarrhea. Distal obstruction of the fistula tract from adhesions or other disease can develop and result in an increase in fistula output or failure of the proximal tract to close. Finally, carcinoma has been reported in chronic fistulas, especially those associated with Crohn's disease. It is believed that chronic irritation of the epithelium promotes the development of such malignancies.[35]

MANAGEMENT

Management of a gastrointestinal fistula is a difficult and complex process. However, if one uses a systematic approach in dealing with these difficult problems, their treatment becomes manageable and potentially rewarding. In general, management can be compartmentalized into five stages: stabilization, investigation, decision, definitive therapy, and healing.[36]

The ultimate goal when treating gastrointestinal fistulas is restoring continuity of the gastrointestinal tract. However, most fistulas are not treated simply by taking the patient back to the operating room. Rather, many weeks and perhaps months of care is often required to manage most patients successfully. As just outlined, management of patients with such fistulas can be conceptualized as a series of steps to control life-threatening abnormalities rapidly and to intervene in a timely and controlled manner with convalescent or surgical care. Although these steps address the physical well-being of the patient, one should not underestimate the impact of a fistula on mental and emotional health. A gastrointestinal fistula places a great deal of stress on a patient's self-esteem. Therefore, family members, social workers, and mental health professionals can play a vital role during the prolonged convalescence that is typical with this disease process.

The present approach and understanding of fistula management have developed significantly over the past 40 years. In their classic paper in 1960, Edmunds, Williams, and Welch called attention to the serious nature and the high mortality of such fistulas and pointed out the relationship between infection, malnutrition, fistula output, and mortality.[33] In addition, they advocated earlier surgical intervention for all high-output fistulas and recommended total resection of the fistula with end-to-end anastomosis or complete bypass of the fistula when resection was not possible. With early correction of fistulas, malnutrition and its attendant complications were thereby less likely to develop. The overall mortality in their series was 44%.[33] Modern fistula management has evolved significantly and mortality has decreased substantially. Urgent surgery in a debilitated, malnourished patient is rarely necessary nowadays.

Stabilization

As outlined earlier, the first step in the management of any intestinal fistula is stabilization of the patient, which is usually accomplished within the first 24 to 48 hours of management. These patients are typically in a vulnerable state of health. They may be febrile and septic from what was thought to be a wound infection that was treated by opening the wound. The wound drainage contains succus entericus and the patient may be deteriorating. Alternatively, they may be immunocompromised secondary to ongoing therapy (e.g., cancer radiation treatment, chemotherapy) or additional infectious processes. Therefore, the most important priority is to stabilize the patient. Patients typically require correction of obligate third-space losses, as well as emesis, fistula output, urine output, or a combination of these and other causes. Initial efforts should be directed toward intravenous fluid resuscitation, control of infection, ongoing measurement of fistulous and urine output, and protection of the surrounding skin. The incision should be examined for fascial integrity, and any remaining subcutaneous collections should be drained. Thereafter, attention is shifted to identification of the fistulous source, the nature of the tract, and associated fluid collections or abscesses.

Resuscitation

Restoration of a normal circulating blood volume and correction of electrolyte and acid-base imbalances are top priority. Rehydration usually requires isotonic fluid until the patient is euvolemic again. Depending on the site of the fistula, replacement of fistula output varies. High-output fistulas, those exceeding 500 ml/day, continue to result in the highest mortality rate, up to 35%, because of malnutrition, electrolyte imbalance, and sepsis. Moderate-output fistulas range from an output of 200 to 500 ml/day, whereas low-output fistulas produce less than 200 ml/day and are associated with low mortality rates and high spontaneous closure rates. Small bowel, pancreatic, and biliary losses are isotonic. Colonic losses may be hypotonic, and gastric fistulas may be associated with the classic hypokalemic, hypochloremic metabolic alkalosis. Although certain patterns can be predicted, electrolyte levels in an aliquot of the fistula output, as well as electrolyte levels in the patient's serum, should be measured and corrected appropriately according to the particular electrolyte profile. Because most patients require considerable volume replacement, close monitoring of the patient's physiologic parameters is essential to ensure the safety and efficacy of therapy.

The natural course of an improperly managed high-output fistula is dehydration, electrolyte abnormalities, malnutrition, infection and sepsis, renal failure, and death. Initial management should address any existing hypovolemia; anemia; hypoalbuminemia; sodium, chloride, or potassium depletion; and acid-base disorders. Strict intake and output measurements are essential, and central venous pressure monitoring and urinary catheterization are especially helpful with high-output fistulas. Invasive monitoring is often necessary because it is usually difficult to estimate antecedent fluid deficits accurately. A central venous catheter can be extremely useful in this capacity and provides the additional benefit of supplying access for parenteral nutrition. The patient's urine output should be restored to greater than 30 ml/hr, assuming that renal function has not been impaired. In patients with cardiovascular impairment or evidence of shock, a pulmonary artery catheter may be needed to guide ongoing fluid repletion after initial fluid boluses have not resulted in adequate urinary output.

Ongoing fluid losses should be fully replaced, and potassium, calcium, phosphorus, and magnesium deficits should be corrected. These electrolyte deficits may take time to correct because the measured serum levels reflect only a small percentage of what can be a massive depletion of intracellular ions. Sodium bicarbonate administration may be required to correct the metabolic acidosis that usually develops with a high-output or proximal fistula. Because the deficit in circulating blood volume is caused primarily by extracellular fluid losses, replacement should be in the form of an isotonic solution. Normal saline or lactated Ringer's solution is most appropriate for this purpose. However, specific parenteral fluids may be selected on the basis of the initial electrolyte levels. Transfusion of red blood cells may be necessary because of chronic blood loss and anemia of chronic disease. To optimize the patient's hemodynamic status, blood transfusion may be required. There is no specific hemoglobin or hematocrit level that requires transfusion; rather, transfusion should be based on the patient's overall hemodynamic status, oxygen-carrying capacity, and oxygen delivery.

Often, these patients are in a severe catabolic state and have extremely low protein and albumin levels. This is important for several reasons. First, patients will have low capillary oncotic pressure, which may contribute to profound edema, especially after resuscitation has begun. Severe hypoalbuminemia will take weeks to correct through nutritional repletion alone. Supplemental intravenous salt-poor albumin administration for a limited period will help increase oncotic pressure and minimize edema and may improve wound healing.[37] More importantly, however, the patient is in a state of nutritional emergency. For this patient to be stabilized and to potentially heal the fistula, positive nitrogen balance must be achieved. If nutritional therapy is not started early, these patients are at great risk for multisystem organ failure, infection, and other complications of severe malnutrition that could lead to death. An initial infusion of albumin will not correct these problems, and nutritional repletion will take weeks to accomplish.

Nutrition

Ongoing nutritional assessment and institution of nutritional support have improved the overall outcome in patients with small intestinal fistulas. The signal study in 1964 by Chapman et al. emphasized that the key to successful management was to "get control of fistula," combat sepsis, and from the very beginning maintain adequate nutritional support.[38] They stressed the vital role of nutrition and reported a decreased mortality rate of 14% in patients treated with an excess of 3000 calories per day via a combination of intravenous (peripheral administration of protein hydrolysates) and tube feedings and 55% mortality in patients receiving a suboptimal nutritional regimen. They also emphasized that supportive and surgical treatment go hand in hand; the two are not mutually exclusive. Their indications for operative closure of the fistula included the presence of distal intestinal obstruction, continued massive loss of fluid from the fistula despite control of the infection and an adequate nutritional regimen, and persistence of the fistula even without high losses over a prolonged period. In a follow-up report in 1971, Sheldon et al. documented the success of such a treatment regimen and noted that most patients could be given adequate nutrition by standard methods such as tube and enterostomy feedings. At the time of their report, TPN was a new technique that had been used only in a select few patients.[39] Roback and Nicholoff reported closure of

73% of enteric fistulas in patients with adequate caloric supplementation, but only 19% healed when nutritional support was inadequate.[40]

Provision of sufficient calories and protein is necessary to minimize further skeletal muscle breakdown and organ dysfunction. Fluid, electrolyte, and trace element losses must be repleted. With the widespread advent of parenteral nutrition in the 1970s, the overall reduction in mortality to a range of 15% to 20% was achieved consistently in a variety of reports. In their reviews of large series of patients, Reber et al. in 1978 (786 patients) and Soeters and associates in 1979 (404 patients) reported that the addition of parenteral nutrition in large scale to the treatment of gastrointestinal fistulas improved the spontaneous closure rate.[3,28] Parenteral nutrition, however, had no impact on fistula mortality; maintenance of adequate nutrition with more conventional methods was equally effective.[3,28] Nevertheless, parenteral nutrition has greatly simplified the nutritional management of patients with gastrointestinal fistulas. Once a patient is both malnourished and septic, it becomes quite difficult to replete such a patient. Even though these patients often have abdominal abscesses and bacteremia, parenteral nutrition is safe and the overall incidence of septic complications from the central line or parenteral nutrition is no greater than that in other clinical situations.

It is much better to begin to provide nutritional support as soon as the patient is stabilized. Full caloric and nitrogen replacement can be provided within a few days of instituting nutritional support.[37] Nutrition can be given by several routes. Frequently, these patients may be too ill to eat, or they cannot consume enough calories even if they can take some oral nutrition. Usually, either enteral tube feeding or parenteral nutrition will be required. The choice of which to use depends on the fistula anatomy. It is advantageous to provide at least a portion of the calories through the enteral route because the gastrointestinal tract is a much more efficacious way of providing nutrition, maintaining the intestinal mucosal barrier and immunologic integrity, and stimulating hepatic protein synthesis, which has been found to be of critical value in determination of the outcome in fistula patients.[41] Thus, whenever possible, enteral nutrition is preferable to parenteral nutrition and probably decreases the incidence of multisystem organ failure and sepsis if administered appropriately.

Enteral nutrition is not without complications, however, and the process should be closely monitored. Complications such as diarrhea, aspiration, and bowel ischemia are not uncommon without careful clinical monitoring. Enteral nutrition can be given for upper gastrointestinal fistulas, especially when the feeding tube can be placed beyond the fistula (for instance, a feeding tube placed beyond the ligament of Treitz for a gastric, duodenal, or pancreatic fistula). In general, feeding tubes should be placed when possible beyond the ligament of Treitz to decrease the potential risk for aspiration. Enteral feeding should also be used for distal fistulas (e.g., a colonic fistula), as long as feedings do not significantly increase fistula output. On the other hand, parenteral nutrition can be a valuable tool in the treatment of fistulas as well. Patients with small bowel fistulas may not be able to tolerate enteral nutrition without increasing fistula output. In these cases and in others in which patients cannot tolerate enteral feeding, parenteral nutrition is indicated. In patients with a persistent adynamic ileus and before the fistula tract is well established, parenteral nutrition is very useful. Parenteral nutrition techniques and advantages are well known, although complications also occur with some frequency. In the Reber et al. study of 91 patients with gastrointestinal fistulas managed with TPN, 28% had complications, with catheter-related sepsis and subclavian vein thrombosis occurring most frequently.[28] Hyperglycemia is common when initiating TPN in patients with gastrointestinal fistulas. New-onset hyperglycemia in a patient with an established TPN regimen should alert the treating physician to the possibility of new or ongoing sepsis (e.g., intra-abdominal abscess, wound infection, line sepsis, pneumonia).

The presence of a gastric or duodenal fistula will not usually permit oral alimentation, unless it is of low output and eating does not markedly worsen losses. If a feeding tube beyond the ligament of Treitz or a tube jejunostomy is in place, enteral nutrition should be started; with normal small and large intestinal function, all nutritional needs can be met. However, the presence of distention or diarrhea will limit the rate of tube feeding and may necessitate parenteral nutrition and fluid repletion. TPN via central venous access enables the delivery of full caloric and fluid requirements, unless poorly controlled hyperglycemia or hypercapnia limits caloric delivery. Those with low-output fistulas require 30 to 35 kcal/kg/day, with 1.0 to 2.0 g protein per kilogram body weight per day. Those with high-output fistulas require more calories—up to 1.5 to 2.0 times normal energy expenditure, with a protein supply of 1.5 to 2.5 g/kg/day.[37] This is especially the case with duodenal fistulas because of the loss of gastric, duodenal, biliary, and pancreatic exocrine protein-rich secretions. Short-turnover protein (prealbumin, retinol-binding protein, transferrin) levels should be measured at least weekly to assess the adequacy of protein delivery. An ongoing catabolic state will adversely affect short-turnover protein levels, even with maximal protein delivery. Those with high-output fistulas may benefit from twice the recommended daily allowance of vitamins, trace elements, and zinc and up to 5 to 10 times the daily requirement for vitamin C.[37] The daily delivered volume should include both maintenance fluids and ongoing fistulous losses.

Historically, high output from a fistula was a relative contraindication to enteral nutrition. Both human and animal data, however, suggest that even these complicated fistulas can be adequately managed with enteral nutrition, although the parenteral route may still succeed in further reducing fistula output. Enteral nutrition, both orally and by tube feeding, has been used increasingly when treating small intestinal fistulas because of its trophic effect on the intestine. The overall success with nutritional supplementation by the enteric route rivals that of parenteral nutrition. Indications for enteral supplementation depend on the site of the fistula and the extent of the remaining small intestine that can be used for absorption. By using a combination of enteral nutrition techniques along with parenteral nutrition, adequate caloric and nitrogen intake should be achieved rapidly. As little as 20% to 25% of the nutrition supplied enterally is usually sufficient to provide the advantages of enteral nutrition, and the remainder can be supplied via parenteral nutrition. Conversely, the decreased fistula output that usually accompanies the institution of parenteral nutrition can greatly simplify the management of high-output fistulas. In addition to this adjunctive role in conjunction with parenteral nutrition, tube feeding continues to be an important measure in the complete nutritional management of some fistula patients with distal and low-output fistulas, when the fistulas are nearly healed, or when parenteral nutrition is difficult or impossible to institute. The ability to provide TPN may also be limited by recurrent line infections, which can lead to endocarditis, or the lack of adequate access sites secondary to thrombosis in patients maintained on long-term TPN. A single-lumen catheter dedicated solely to TPN is preferable and may decrease infectious and thrombotic complications.

Because both enteric and parenteral feeding has advantages and disadvantages, the source of nutritional supplementation should depend on the individual patient and the surgeon's preference and experience. In most cases, parenteral nutrition should be instituted as soon as possible. Thereafter, steps to localize the fistula and control infection can be taken. Normal intestinal motility and function generally return once abdominal sepsis is controlled and fluid and electrolyte imbalances are corrected. If the fistula location is such that enteric access and alimentation are possible, enteral nutrition can be instituted and parenteral nutrition phased out. By using a combination of approaches, adequate nutrition can be maintained throughout the patient's course.

Control of Sepsis

Uncontrolled sepsis remains the major factor contributing to mortality in patients with small intestinal fistulas. Aggressive management of all ongoing infections and careful surveillance for new septic foci are thus absolutely necessary for successful management. Tachycardia, persistent fever, and leukocytosis usually portend inadequate control of the fistula or abscess formation. Frequent physical examination and judicious use of ultrasonography and computed tomography (CT) are mandatory.

Advances in patient monitoring, correction of fluid, electrolyte, and acid/base imbalances, and the use of parenteral nutrition have largely alleviated electrolyte disturbances secondary to high-output fistulas and malnutrition. In the present era, mortality is mostly determined by uncontrolled sepsis and sepsis-associated malnutrition. Malnutrition in the presence of uncontrolled sepsis cannot be treated without effective surgical drainage of the septic source. As long as uncontrolled sepsis persists, the patient's condition will continue to deteriorate. The stabilization phase often involves control of a septic source. Typically, drainage of an intra-abdominal abscess is required, which is ideally accomplished in an image-guided, percutaneous fashion. In addition, fistula drainage must be controlled and the skin of the abdominal wall protected. Local control is an extremely important component of the early management of a fistula. Discontinuation of oral intake and initiation of parenteral nutrition are important steps. Placement of a nasogastric tube or a nasoenteric tube positioned proximal to the fistula may be helpful with enteric fistulas involving the duodenum or proximal jejunum. Egress of the fistula output from the abdominal cavity must be facilitated with an immature enterocutaneous fistula because inadequate external drainage results in internal loculation, abscess formation, or peritonitis. It is extremely important to prevent the severe local skin excoriation that frequently develops around the site of an enterocutaneous fistula. Fistulas that have been controlled with a tube should cause minimal injury to fascia, subcutaneous tissue, and skin. Such injuries typically include perforations with abscesses that have been percutaneously drained or have been converted at surgery to a controlled fistula with an indwelling tube or an adjacent drain.

Drainage should be collected to measure the output and provide a gauge for fluid and electrolyte replacement. The method of controlling fistula drainage must be individualized for each patient. Precautionary steps should be instituted early because once excoriation is present, healing is difficult in the presence of ongoing drainage. A fistula should be exteriorized on a flat portion of the abdominal wall with avoidance of bony prominences and skin folds. This permits secure application of an ostomy bag or other device to collect and monitor fluids and protect the skin. Specialized nursing assistance by an enterostomal therapist or wound care specialist is frequently necessary and can be quite helpful in the management of these often complex wounds. Drainage with a single catheter placed into the site generally fails because the catheter becomes occluded or the volume of fluid expelled with peristalsis exceeds the capacity of the catheter. In some instances, a sump suction catheter can be placed through the external opening and gentle continuous suction applied to control fistula drainage (a sump catheter can be constructed by inserting a soft rubber catheter in the wound with an angiocatheter placed in the side of the rubber catheter to create a sump system by applying low continuous wall suction through the catheter). A surrounding ostomy appliance can then be placed around the tube to collect any excess drainage. When fistula drainage has been controlled, the sump catheter should be gradually withdrawn or progressively replaced with smaller-caliber tubes. This allows the tract to contract and close. Sump suction can eventually be replaced by gravity drainage in most patients. D'Harcour and associates reported an 81% overall closure rate with this method in 147 patients with both high-output (93 patients) and low-output (54 patients) fistulas.[42]

One useful modification of fistula wound management has been described by Suripaya and Anderson (Fig. 73–1). A disposable ileostomy bag with adhesive backing is fitted to the fistula site.[43] The opening in the ileostomy bag is cut to fit the fistula as exactly as possible. Two 18-French or larger catheters with multiple side perforations are tied together and passed into the fistula through the open end of the bag. All perforations are placed within the fistula below skin level. A third 18-French catheter with multiple perforations is placed in the ileostomy bag, and the open end of the bag is tied securely around all three catheters. One of the two catheters within the fistula and the catheter lying free in the bag are set for continuous suction at a minimum of 40 mm Hg of negative pressure. The adjacent catheter in the fistula serves as an air vent. When functioning, the bag is completely collapsed, and fluid leaking from the tract is immediately aspirated away. The surrounding skin must be protected from excoriation and erosion because skin breakdown can cause discomfort and also increase metabolic requirements. Protection can best be accomplished by attaching a disposable ostomy appliance with either a Stomahesive or a karaya ring around the fistula. The surrounding skin can be protected with Stomahesive paste, karaya gum powder, aluminum paste, tincture of benzoin, or zinc oxide/menthol cream.

Alternatively, a wound vacuum (V.A.C. [vacuum-assisted closure] device) drainage system works very well to control fistula drainage and protect the skin (Fig. 73–2). With negative pressure application to the wound, the V.A.C. apparatus allows for excellent control of drainage, minimizes the size of the abdominal wound, simplifies management by decreasing the frequency of dressing changes, and may actually promote healing of the fistula.[44,45] By simplifying wound care and control of output, patients can be discharged from the hospital sooner and the V.A.C. can easily be managed in a home care or extended care setting. For the majority of enterocutaneous fistulas, this has become our method of choice for controlling fistula drainage and protecting the surrounding skin.

The therapeutic use of appropriate antibiotics for intra-abdominal abscess and sepsis should be carefully reserved for septicemia and cholangitis, as well as in preparation for surgery. Once signs of intra-abdominal sepsis have occurred, the use of antibiotics does not obviate the necessity of treating the process surgically or via percutaneous drainage. Adequate drainage of an abscess cavity must be accomplished. If possible, general anesthesia and major surgical procedures should be avoided or postponed until the patient's condition has stabilized. Although drainage of the abscess must be complete, it is important to choose the least traumatic procedure that is consistent with this goal. Ultrasound and CT are most often used to search for peritonitis or an intra-abdominal abscess. These two modalities not only localize such processes but also permit guided percutaneous drainage, an invaluable procedure in a critically ill patient who may not tolerate an operative procedure (Fig. 73–3). Abdominal exploration may be required in septic patients who are losing ground, even if diagnostic studies have not pinpointed an abscess. If exploratory laparotomy is required for drainage, it is best to avoid definitive operative repair of the fistula because such attempts are usually unsuccessful in the setting of adjacent sepsis. Failure of repair may make subsequent attempts more difficult and possibly result in spread of

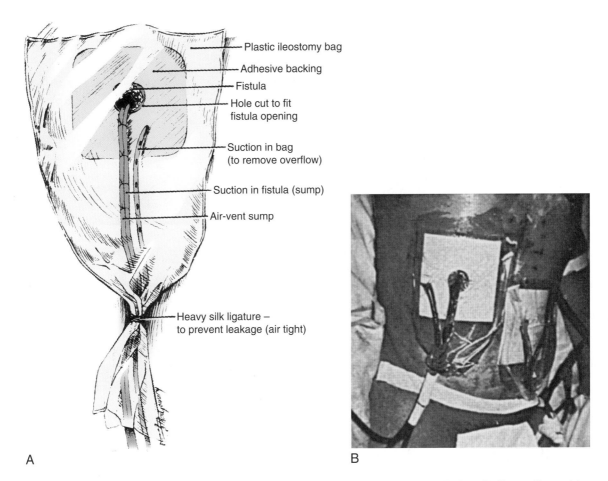

A   **B**

Figure 73–1.   Enterocutaneous fistula drainage device. **A,** Components of the suction device. **B,** Bag collapsed by negative suction. (From Suriyapa C, Anderson MC: A simple device to control drainage from enterocutaneous fistulas. Surgery 70:456, 1971.)

infection to previously uninvolved areas of the abdomen. Control of the fistula should be established during the operation by allowing complete drainage to the skin surface or by actually exteriorizing the fistula.

The fistula effluent should be cultured for both bacteria and fungi. Sputum, urine, wound, and blood cultures, including those from central venous lines, should also be obtained. Wound or drain site collections should be evacuated. The wound should be débrided of all grossly infected and necrotic tissue. Culture results and the eventual patient systemic response should modify subsequent antibiotic therapy, particularly if *Enterococcus,* resistant gram-negative bacteria, or fungus is cultured. Percutaneous drainage can often temporize the situation until the patient's condition stabilizes and may, in some cases, lead to eradication of the fistula.

Once sepsis is controlled or when no sepsis is present, parenteral/enteral nutrition should result in improved nutritional status and allow skin lesions to heal and the future operative field to become quiescent. Early operative intervention in the presence of malnutrition is not necessary and may be detrimental. Even if the regimen of bowel rest in conjunction with intravenous and enteral nutrition does not lead to successful spontaneous fistula

closure, the patient is generally in better nutritional and metabolic condition to withstand an operation to correct the fistula.

Pharmacologic Support

Use of the long-acting somatostatin analogue octreotide for decreasing pancreatic and enterocutaneous fistulous output has been popularized during the 1990s. An inhibitory effect on gastric, biliary, and pancreatic secretions is generally observed in clinical use. With typical subcutaneous dosages of 100 to 250 µg every 8 hours, fistulous output is reduced by 40% to 60% after the first day regardless of fistula site or volume of output.[46] Side effects are not usually severe and include hyperglycemia, decreased bowel motility, and elevated cholesterol levels. Placebo-controlled studies indicate that octreotide decreases fistula-related complications, reduces fistulous output, and decreases fistula healing time and the time required for TPN.[47] Octreotide has been shown to promote fistula closure within a significantly shorter time than TPN alone does, even with malignant enterocutaneous disease, and is particularly helpful in decreasing secretions in high-output fistulas to a manageable

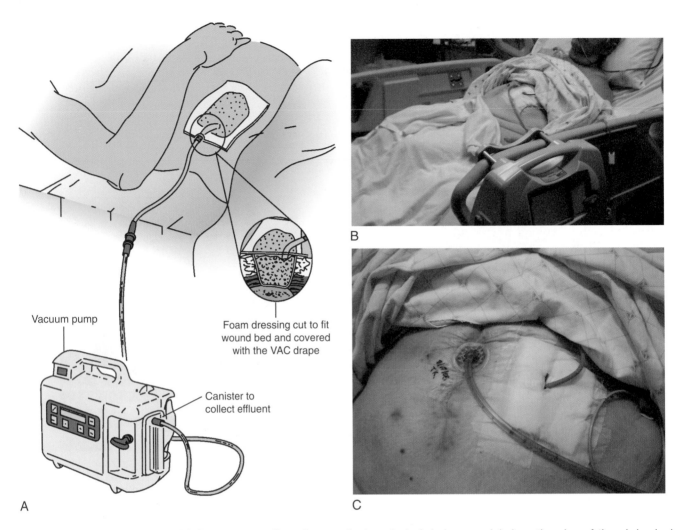

Vacuum pump

Foam dressing cut to fit
wound bed and covered
with the VAC drape

Canister to
collect effluent

A

B

C

Figure 73–2. A, The wound V.A.C. apparatus allows for excellent control of drainage, minimizes the size of the abdominal wound, and simplifies management. (From Cro C, George KJ, Donnelly J, et al: Vacuum assisted closure system in the management of enterocutaneous fistulae. Postgrad Med J 78:364, 2002.) **B,** Wound V.A.C. on a patient with a gastrocutaneous fistula (see Fig. 73–3). **C,** Control of gastrocutaneous fistula with the wound V.A.C. apparatus.

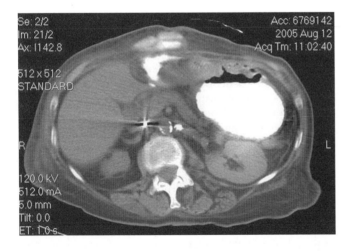

```
Se: 2/2                          Acc: 6769142
Im: 21/2                         2005 Aug 12
Ax: I142.8                       Acq Tm: 11:02:40
512x512
STANDARD



R                                            L




120.0 kV
512.0 mA
5.0 mm
Tilt: 0.0
ET: 1.0 s
```

Figure 73–3. Computed tomography scan demonstrating free air and contrast extravasation from the stomach into an anterior intra-abdominal abscess after vagotomy, antrectomy, and Billroth II gastrojejunostomy for a giant duodenal ulcer.

level.[48-50] However, the mortality rate, hospitalization time, and overall fistula closure rate were not improved, although even in the fistulas that eventually required operative closure, octreotide in general both reduced their output and simplified management.

Proton pump inhibitors or histamine H_2 receptor antagonists are advisable both to reduce gastric acid production and to reduce gastric secretions. These medications may be useful in decreasing fistula output, particularly with proximal fistulas or when the amount of gastric secretions is high. Patients with refractory fistulas related to Crohn's disease have been successfully treated with short courses of cyclosporine. In five patients with a total of 12 fistulas, Hanauer and Smith used an infusion of 4 mg/kg/day for 6 to 10 days, followed by oral dosing at 8 mg/kg/day adjusted to maintain serum cyclosporine levels of 100 to 200 ng/ml.[51] All fistulas responded to cyclosporine infusion with decreased drainage and improvement in both local inflammation and patient comfort. Complete resolution occurred in 10 of the 12 fistulas after a mean of 8 days. Therapy was continued for a mean of 6 months, with five recurrences, two of which were related to inadequate cyclosporine serum levels. Similar results with cyclosporine were reported by Present and Lichtiger.[52] Side effects consisted of infectious complications, mild hypertension, paresthesias, and hirsutism. Although useful for short-term treatment, long-term administration of cyclosporine is generally avoided because of the potentially septic complications of immunosuppression, as well as hypertension and nephrotoxicity. In addition, the use of immunosuppressive drugs such as cyclosporine may theoretically impair healing of the fistula.

Azathioprine and 6-mercaptopurine are both effective in treating active Crohn's disease and in maintaining remission, with the cumulative dose being the primary factor in predicting response. Associated small bowel fistulas may also improve with such treatment. Adverse reactions such as leukopenia, pancreatitis, and nausea may preclude therapy with these agents. Combination therapy with tacrolimus and either azathioprine or 6-mercaptopurine may be useful when treating perineal fistulas related to Crohn's disease. In one study involving 11 patients, 7 had a complete response and 4 had a partial response.[53] The most common side effects with such combination therapy are nausea, paresthesias, nephrotoxicity, and tremor.

More recently, infliximab (Remicade), a chimeric monoclonal antibody to tumor necrosis factor-α, was developed as treatment of Crohn's disease. Infliximab is effective in closing fistulas in patients with Crohn's disease. In a randomized, multicenter trial investigating infliximab administered intravenously at 0, 2, and 6 weeks and dosed at 5 mg/kg for the treatment of 94 adult Crohn's patients with chronic fistulas, partial resolution of multiple lesions occurred in 68% and complete closure occurred in 55% of patients.[54] Other studies also support the efficacy of infliximab in treating Crohn's disease–related small bowel fistulas.[55,56] In 282 patients with fistulizing Crohn's disease, infliximab, 5 mg/kg every 8 weeks, significantly reduced hospitalizations, surgeries, and procedures in comparison to placebo.[57] Complications of this therapy occur in more than 60% of patients and include headache, abscess, upper respiratory tract infection, and fatigue.

Investigation

The next phase of management is investigation. After stabilization is accomplished in the first 24 to 48 hours, investigation usually takes place over the next 7 to 10 days. Investigation implies a thorough evaluation of the gastrointestinal tract, definition of the anatomy of the fistula, and identification of any complicating features such as abscess, stricture, or distal obstruction.[31,32] Investigative studies should be designed to not only determine the presence and location of the fistula but also provide information regarding its cause. This objective can be accomplished by several investigational methods. Oral administration of indigo carmine or charcoal can be used to demonstrate the presence of a connection

between the gastrointestinal tract and the abdominal wall or urinary bladder. These tests, however, prove only the presence of a fistula and do not identify its site or source. Probably the most important first test is a fistulogram, which will define the length and width of the fistula, as well as its anatomic location. A fistulogram can be performed by inserting a small catheter through the drainage site into the fistula tract and then slowly injecting water-soluble contrast under fluoroscopy (Fig. 73–4). It is best performed by the responsible surgeon in collaboration with the radiologist. The value of the procedure is enhanced by close involvement of the surgeon

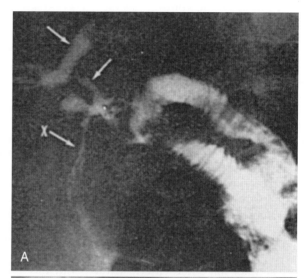

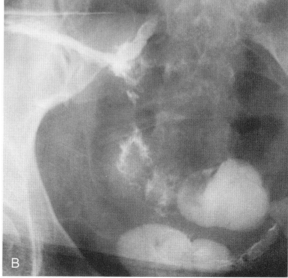

Figure 73–4. **A,** Fistulogram. Injection of a cutaneous fistula demonstrates several tracts *(arrows)* leading to the ileum. Crohn's disease is present in one loop *(arrow with X).* **B,** Fistulogram demonstrating an enterocutaneous fistula in a patient after appendectomy for acute perforated appendicitis. **(A,** From Goldfarb WB, Monafo W, McAlister WH: Clinical value of fistulography. Am J Surg 108:902, 1964.)

and the radiologist as the study is performed. The procedure is safe and can be performed even in seriously ill patients.[58,59]

Fistulography performed early in the course of the disease will help determine (1) the site of the fistula, (2) intestinal continuity with the fistula, (3) the presence or absence of distal intestinal obstruction, (4) the nature of the intestine immediately adjacent to the fistula, and possibly (5) the presence or absence of an intra-abdominal abscess. Other tests such as an upper gastrointestinal series with small bowel follow-through and barium enema are helpful in further elucidating the exact anatomy and location of the fistula. Performing the fistulogram first is prudent because contrast from an upper gastrointestinal series, contrast enema, or even CT may make it difficult, if not impossible to interpret a fistulogram until all of the contrast has passed. Fistulography should be followed by a complete contrast study of the gastrointestinal tract either orally or through existing intraluminal tubes. Such study is valuable both for identifying the internal source of the fistula and for defining its size and complicating factors such as distal obstruction. The fistulogram should always be performed before the complete contrast study because the latter will not usually define the fistula and may decrease visualization or make fistulography impossible. Internal fistulas may be more difficult to evaluate. Patients with enteroenteric fistulas often suffer a delay in diagnosis because of a lack of symptoms or symptoms that mimic the primary disease or event creating the fistula. An internal small intestinal fistula may be asymptomatic, particularly if the amount of absorptive area bypassed by the fistula is small. Other internal fistulas may not be readily recognized because the symptoms may mimic those of the primary disease. For example, an enteroenteric fistula, which is most often secondary to Crohn's disease, is frequently accompanied by abdominal pain, diarrhea, weight loss, or fever. These symptoms are similar to those accompanying an acute exacerbation of Crohn's disease itself. Thus, at times the diagnosis is not made until surgery in these patients. If the colon is involved with the fistula, a fluoroscopic water-soluble or barium enema will assist in definition of both the fistula and any associated colonic disease.

Additional useful tests in the early stage of investigation are CT and ultrasonography. These tests can further define the anatomy of the vicinity of the fistula and evaluate for any ongoing or unrecognized intra-abdominal processes or abscesses, as well as distal obstruction. A CT scan will be required in almost all patients for these reasons, especially to rule out any undrained collections. CT scanning with oral and intravenous contrast media is highly sensitive and specific for intra-abdominal free air and will assist in locating the fistula and identifying adjacent fluid collections and concomitant bowel obstruction. The use of CT, however, within the first week after surgery is associated with the expected presence of postoperative air within the abdominal cavity and thus may be difficult to interpret. Obviously, extravasation of intraluminal contrast on CT examination is diagnostic of perforation. CT and ultrasound are useful adjuncts when an intra-abdominal abscess is suspected (Fig. 73–5). Significant fluid collections should be drained, preferably under CT or ultrasound guidance via a percutaneous route, and an indwelling catheter left in the cavity. This then permits subsequent examination of the cavity under fluoroscopy with water-soluble contrast to assist in delineation of the fistula tract. Although the site of perforation may not be identified on initial injection because of inflammation, subsequent examinations after several days of drainage will often show the site of the fistula. CT scanning is highly recommended for suspected duodenal perforations; no other imaging modality is currently better at demonstrating gas in the retroperitoneum surrounding the duodenum, which is a diagnostic sign of perforation. An elevated serum amylase level may accompany duodenal perforation after ERCP and give the impression of pancreatitis, thus leading to a delay in diagnosis with an increase in the mortality rate.[22]

Intravenous pyelography and retrograde pyelography may be helpful in defining a nephroenteric fistula, whereas cystoscopy is usually a more accurate method for determining the presence of an enterovesical fistula. In general, CT is the most sensitive study for identifying a colovesical or enterovesical fistula. ^{99m}Tc-labeled hepatoiminodiacetic acid (HIDA) scanning or ^{111}In-labeled leukocyte scintigraphy may have an advantage over conventional radiography in certain proximal enterocutaneous or biliary-enteric fistulas.

Endoscopic evaluation, including colonoscopy, esophagogastroduodenoscopy, and ERCP, may be helpful in certain specific clinical situations. However, endoscopy is not usually advisable if an acute perforation is suspected and should generally be delayed until the acute inflammatory process has resolved. Endoscopic examination of the stomach and duodenum may occasionally be used to identify a fistulous source and to take biopsy samples of adjacent tissue for exclusion of malignancy. Billroth II anatomy will usually preclude duodenal examination, although enteroscopy through the afferent jejunal limb is possible by highly skilled endoscopists. ERCP will allow the diagnosis of fistulas connecting the gallbladder or biliary tract to the duodenum or stomach. For suspected gastrocolic or duodenocolic fistulas, colonoscopy may identify the involved site and enable a biopsy to be performed to diagnose inflammatory bowel disease or malignancy. The fistulous output may be analyzed for electrolytes and cultured to determine drug sensitivities, as well as assayed for bilirubin and amylase for comparison with serum values.

In the rare circumstance when perforation has not been excluded by noninvasive tests and the patient's condition is not improving or is worsening, diagnostic laparotomy should be considered. Morbidity and mortality rates are only increased by a delay under these circumstances. Diagnostic laparoscopy may be useful to rule out perforation after a previous laparoscopic procedure or after an endoscopic procedure. It is not usually appropriate in a septic, hypotensive patient and does not enable a satisfactory examination of the retroperitoneal duodenum. As mentioned previously, early laparoscopy for tachycardia or unexplained fever is essential to prevent mortality from an anastomotic leak after gastric bypass surgery.

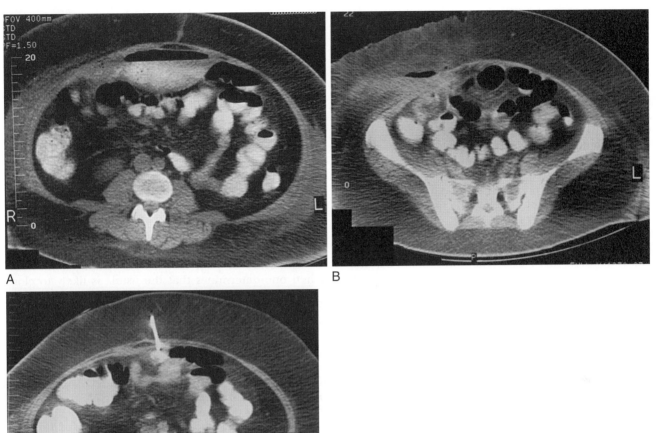

Figure 73–5. Computed tomography scans obtained in the patient whose fistulogram is demonstrated in Figure 73–4B. **A,** Intra-abdominal air-fluid collection containing contrast just below the abdominal wall in the midline. **B,** Lower cuts showing the inflammatory response and subcutaneous air representing the early stages of fistula development. **C,** Computed tomography scan demonstrating resolution of an intra-abdominal abscess after percutaneous catheter drainage.

Decision

The next step in fistula management is a decision on management and the timing of such management. When one is making these decisions, the likelihood of spontaneous closure must be determined. The likelihood of closure depends on several factors. The first is anatomic location. In general, anatomic locations that are favorable for closure are the oropharynx, esophagus, duodenal stump, pancreas, biliary tree, and jejunum. Alternatively, unfavorable locations include the stomach, lateral duodenum, ligament of Treitz, and the ileum. As mentioned previously, nutritional status is very important. Patients with poor nutritional status, as measured by overall assessment, albumin, short-turnover proteins (serum transferrin, thyroxin-binding prealbumin, retinol-binding protein), injected skin antigens, and other factors, are much less likely to close a fistula no matter what the anatomic location.[41] More importantly, if a patient's nutritional status is poor, the mortality rate is higher. Another important factor is the presence or absence of sepsis. The absence of sepsis has a positive

predictive value for closure, whereas the converse is true in the presence of sepsis. Elimination of sepsis should be considered a necessity for spontaneous closure. The cause of the fistula is also predictive of closure. Postoperative fistulas and fistulas secondary to appendicitis or diverticulitis are likely to close. Fistulas associated with active Crohn's disease are unlikely to close until the Crohn's disease is quiescent. Fistulas associated with cancer will usually require excision of the tumor along with the fistula. In addition, the presence of a foreign body will prevent closure of the fistula without operative intervention.

After sepsis has been controlled and diagnostic studies have been completed, management of a fistula should follow a conservative course. An opportunity for spontaneous healing should be permitted. It is important to provide adequate nutritional support and to aggressively investigate any new onset of signs of sepsis during this convalescent period. The duration of conservative treatment must be individualized. If a positive nitrogen balance is maintained, fistula output decreases, and no septic complications develop, nonoperative management may be continued. The spontaneous closure rate of enterocutaneous fistulas in several large series ranged from 32% to 80%.[27,28] Reber and associates reported that more than 90% of small intestinal fistulas that closed did so within a month.[28] Less than 10% closed after 2 months, and none closed spontaneously after 3 months. Thus, a reasonable management plan may consist of at least 1 month of nonoperative management, with reasonable extensions should the fistula show signs of slow but continued healing. Delaying surgery allows peritoneal reaction and inflammation to subside, thus making a definitive surgical procedure easier and safer. Delaying repair also permits nutritional optimization, thereby decreasing the likelihood of postoperative wound complications. A postoperative enterocutaneous fistula usually extends hospitalization by 2 to 3 months, but this period may shorten somewhat with refinements in TPN, administration of somatostatin analogue, and wider availability of outpatient nursing care. In fact, many patients are candidates for discharge home or to a skilled nursing facility during the convalescent period because of the availability of these agents in such settings.

The condition of the bowel or other organ involved in the fistula is also important. Healthy adjacent tissue is a favorable factor. Other favorable factors include a small fistula, quiescent disease, and the absence of an abscess. On the other hand, total disruption of the bowel negates closure, as does distal obstruction, abscess, malignancy or irradiation (or both), epithelialization of the fistula tract, and active disease. Typically, a long fistula tract (longer than 2 cm) is more likely to close than a short fistula tract. Similarly, a thin, narrow tract is a favorable prognostic indicator (i.e., less than 1 cm^2). Therefore, short, wide tracts are unlikely to close spontaneously.[31,32] Nutrition has been mentioned as an important factor in stabilization and spontaneous closure. The short-turnover proteins can provide prognostic information. Specifically, a serum transferrin level less than 200 mg/dl predicts a low likelihood of spontaneous closure.[41]

Failure of an enterocutaneous fistula to close spontaneously is associated with a number of factors (represented by the acronym *FRIENDS*): the presence of a *foreign body* within the tract or adjacent to it, previous *radiation* exposure of the site, ongoing *inflammation* (most commonly from Crohn's disease) *or infection* that contributes to a catabolic state, *epithelialization* of the fistula tract (particularly if the fistula tract is less than 2 cm long), *neoplasm, distal intestinal obstruction,* and pharmacologic doses of *steroids.* Fistulas associated with a concurrent pancreatic fistula also have a low rate of spontaneous closure, as do those occurring in the presence of malnutrition or adjacent infection. As mentioned, the loss of intestinal continuity or the presence of abdominal wall defects makes operative correction more likely. Vigorous attempts to identify each of these confounding factors and to modify their influence may increase the success of nonoperative strategies, but operative intervention is generally necessary when they are present.

Campos et al. analyzed prognostic factors for closure of external duodenal fistulas and found that the odds of spontaneous closure were (1) three times greater with

low-output fistulas than with high-output fistulas, (2) five times greater with postoperative fistulas than with fistulas associated with inflammatory bowel disease or trauma, and (3) two times greater with duodenal fistulas than with jejunoileal fistulas.[60] For duodenal fistulas, spontaneous closure was observed in 33%, with an overall mortality rate of 36%. Williams et al. found that even high-output lateral duodenal fistulas spontaneously closed in 63% with TPN and eradication of sepsis.[61] Their median output was 1480 ml/day, with a median time to closure of 29 days and an overall mortality rate of 15%. Kuvshinoff et al. found that seven of eight gastric fistulas closed spontaneously but only one of four duodenal fistulas did so; approximately 50 days was required for closure.[41]

After considering all the aforementioned factors, one determines whether to observe the fistula for spontaneous closure or plan early surgery after stabilization. When one determines that the fistula is likely to close and does not operate, if the fistula has not closed after 4 to 5 weeks without sepsis, an operation will probably be required. General wisdom holds that a fistula that has not closed by 4 to 6 weeks is unlikely to do so and surgery is indicated. The decision to operate is tempered by the patient's condition and the state of the abdomen. In particular, when faced with a firm, indurated abdomen, it is better to stabilize the infection, nutrition, and fluid balance in this circumstance and wait until the abdomen is soft, without significant induration, to maximize the chance for operative success and minimize the risk of creating new enterocutaneous fistulas. In certain cases then, the period of waiting may be greater than 6 weeks.

Definitive Therapy

The next important decision is to determine whether definitive operative therapy is necessary and the timing of such therapy. In situations that are favorable, between 80% and 90% of fistulas that are going to close spontaneously will close within 4 to 5 weeks. When spontaneous closure is unlikely or has not occurred within 4 to 5 weeks, an operation will be required. When operative therapy has been chosen, the operation must be carefully planned. Whenever possible, the operation should not take place until the patient is stable, not septic, and in an adequate nutritional state. The most favorable time to reoperate on patients is either within 10 days of diagnosis or after 4 months.[32]

Gastric and Duodenal Perforations and Fistulas

Endoscopically produced gastroduodenal perforations are appropriately referred for surgical management when a free perforation is recognized by the presence of intra-abdominal air on radiographic films. However, retroperitoneal duodenal perforations that occur during ERCP and sphincterotomy have been treated both medically and surgically, depending on the size of the perforation and the patient's response. Loperfido et al. reported 12 retroperitoneal perforations in a series of 2769 ERCP procedures; 6 were treated nonoperatively, with one death.[21] From a surgical standpoint, Bell et al.[22] warned that patients with perforations diagnosed within 24 hours of surgery had a mortality rate of 13% whereas delay beyond 24 hours increased mortality rates to 43% because of sepsis or multiorgan failure. If medical therapy is undertaken for a small, contained perforation, close monitoring should be performed, with surgical exploration initiated within 24 hours for perforations that do not improve or that worsen.

Acute intraoperative gastric or duodenal perforations should be repaired during the course of the operation. This simple principle presupposes both that the perforation is recognized and its repair is possible. In particular, laparoscopic surgical procedures may produce perforations that are not recognized at that time. Frequently, if recognized, such injuries can be repaired with laparoscopic suturing techniques. However, in some situations laparoscopic repair of gastric or duodenal lacerations may be quite difficult to perform, particularly if the surgeon is not expert in advanced laparoscopic maneuvers. Conversion to laparotomy in these circumstances to ensure a safe repair reflects good surgical judgment rather than failure. Initial complications tend to breed subsequent complications, which are minimized by prompt and thorough treatment of the initial problem.

Gastric perforation occurring during a surgical procedure can usually be primarily repaired with an inner layer of continuous absorbable suture and an outer layer of interrupted silk suture. Alternatively, a stapler may be used if the anatomy is appropriate and the tissues are not inflamed or markedly edematous. During laparoscopic procedures, serosal lacerations are often visible; methylene blue instillation via a nasogastric tube will reveal extravasation. Intraoperative endoscopy with air insufflation and distal occlusion under saline irrigation may be even more accurate in identifying a leak. Manual distal occlusion and removal of the insufflated air by suction at the conclusion of the test are essential because air insufflation of the intestine can make the remainder of the procedure very difficult. Serosal lacerations may be sutured laparoscopically if amenable, but laparotomy is appropriate for difficult anatomy or poor exposure.

Usually, patients with perforations that are recognized in the immediate postoperative period should be returned to the operating room for repair. For initial laparoscopic procedures, repeat laparoscopy may be appropriate to diagnose the perforation and to close it, if possible. Laparotomy will often be required for satisfactory identification, washout, and closure. With both laparoscopic and open procedures, anastomotic leaks will frequently occur later, about 1 week after surgery. The decision to operate will be influenced by the ability to drain associated abscesses percutaneously and the presence of peritonitis. Focal collections that are adequately drained, with a good systemic response and only local tenderness, may continue to be observed for eventual closure. Ongoing sepsis, poorly drained collections, or generalized peritoneal signs should mandate re-exploration, débridement, drainage, and management of the perforation.

Surgical options for gastric perforation include simple closure, partial gastric excision with reclosure, or partial gastrectomy. An indurated stomach with extensive inflammation will make resection hazardous; in this situation, an omental patch of the perforation should be considered. Placement of a drain or sump in the area may convert the perforation to a controlled fistula if the repair or patch leaks again. Placement of a gastrostomy tube, if possible, will permit gastric decompression and avoid the prolonged use of a nasogastric tube with its risk for sinusitis. Placement of the gastrostomy tube through the area of perforation may be optional if closure or excision cannot be safely accomplished. Consideration should be given to placement of a feeding jejunostomy tube (or a combined gastrostomy-jejunostomy tube). A leaking gastroduodenostomy may be treated by distal gastric resection with conversion to a Billroth II gastrojejunostomy.

Perforations that are recognized in the first several days postoperatively should usually be treated by reoperation and closure or by anastomotic revision. More typically, nearly 1 week after surgery, the onset of fever, tachycardia, respiratory failure, and acidosis with ileus and pain will suggest a leak or abscess. After CT-guided percutaneous drainage, with appropriate antibiotic therapy, the perforation will often heal. Failure to resolve shifts the focus to management of a fistula. An early leak after gastric bypass surgery should be recognized and repaired as soon as possible to prevent significant morbidity and mortality. This complication usually requires revision of the anastomosis and drainage.

Repair of ERCP-induced duodenal perforations should be performed as soon as possible after diagnosis and hemodynamic and respiratory stabilization. Delay increases the friability and edema of the duodenum and increases retroperitoneal contamination and the possibility of damage to the small and large intestine and mesentery. A midline laparotomy is advised to allow access to all of the small bowel and mesentery. Wide kocherization of the second portion of the duodenum, with mobilization of the hepatic flexure if needed, allows close inspection of the second and third retroperitoneal portions. In most cases with an early diagnosis, local débridement of the wound edges with suture closure will close the duodenal defect. If the perforation occurred during sphincterotomy, the location of the bile duct must be determined before suture closure. If the duct location is uncertain, cholecystectomy may be performed, and a small catheter can be passed through the cystic duct stump into the distal common bile duct and duodenum. For a significant ampullary injury, proximal bile drainage with either a T-tube or a tube cholecystostomy should be considered. Proximal decompression is accomplished with a gastrostomy tube. Internal duodenal decompression can be achieved with either a retrograde tube duodenostomy (placed through the proximal jejunum) or a combination gastrostomy-jejunostomy tube, with the distal end cut short appropriate to a duodenal tip location. The duodenal repair is reinforced with omentum, if possible, and a local closed suction drain will, in many cases, facilitate evacuation of the fluid. It also serves to convert any subsequent leakage to a controlled fistula. A feeding jejunostomy should be created for postoperative enteral nutrition. With a delay in the diagnosis of duodenal perforation, there may be widespread inflammation or necrosis in the retroperitoneum that extends under the transverse mesocolon and small bowel mesentery. Much of this can be accessed by hepatic flexure mobilization, but a counterincision beside or below the small bowel mesentery may be needed to adequately débride and drain the areas of necrosis. Sump drain placement under the small bowel mesentery and near the duodenum generally permits good drainage; the sumps may be gradually withdrawn later after tube checks and CT scans demonstrate healing.

Pyloric exclusion has been used successfully in trauma patients with extensive duodenal injury, with diagnosis delayed more than 24 hours after injury, and after initial primary duodenal repair with subsequent breakdown and a high-output lateral fistula. Closure of the pylorus, gastrojejunostomy, gastrostomy, and feeding jejunostomy without vagotomy are performed in the expectation that the pylorus will reopen within 3 to 6 weeks, although subsequent intra-abdominal abscesses may require drainage. This technique may be most suitable for nontrauma patients with a delayed diagnosis of duodenal perforation in which the bowel wall is markedly thickened, friable, and inflamed and where other options, such as closure, serosal patching, or tube duodenostomy, are not thought to be adequate (see Chapter 53 on duodenal trauma).

Gastroduodenal fistulas that develop in association with necrotizing pancreatitis and necrosectomy may be treated during laparotomy or by subsequent percutaneous drainage. Tsiotos et al. treated two gastrocutaneous fistulas 1 month after necrosectomy by percutaneous drainage, with eventual closure.[19] Duodenal fistulas were treated by tube duodenostomy or Roux-en-Y duodenojejunostomy; late-developing duodenal fistulas were treated by percutaneous drainage. Ho and Frey used primary closure and delayed external drainage for gastric fistulas after necrosectomy and treated duodenal fistulas with pyloric exclusion or external drainage.[20]

If the gastric or duodenal defect is too large to allow primary closure or the fistula originates in conjunction with the ampulla and pancreatic duct, a Roux-en-Y gastrojejunostomy or duodenojejunostomy is a flexible and valuable technique for dealing with such difficult gastric or duodenal fistulas. It is best used in the absence of ongoing infection, when sufficient time has been allowed, and the jejunum is pliable and not edematous. Although mucosa-to-mucosa apposition is best, hand sewing the end of the Roux limb even with the chronically thickened tissue around a fistula usually results in healing. A feeding jejunostomy distal to the enteroenterostomy should always be considered.

Treatment of a duodenal stump fistula is based on the condition of the stump and surrounding tissue and the surgeon's judgment. Options include primary suture closure, mobilization of the stump with resuture or stapling, lateral tube duodenostomy for duodenal decompression, direct tube drainage through the fistula, a serosal patch, or the use of a Roux jejunal limb. Duode-

nal fistulas that are associated with recurrence of Crohn's disease at an ileocolic anastomosis are managed by resection of the recurrent disease with reanastomosis. The duodenal end of the fistula is débrided and primarily closed, and omentum is interposed to separate it from the new anastomosis. Difficult duodenal closure has been managed by either a jejunal serosal patch or duodenojejunostomy. Primary colonic Crohn's disease with either a gastric or duodenal fistula is similarly treated by resection of the primary source and closure of the fistula, with duodenojejunostomy reserved for large residual defects.

Internal gastrocolic or duodenocolic fistulas from colon carcinoma are generally managed by partial colon resection, as well as resection of the involved stomach or duodenum, along with primary closure. Large duodenal defects require a patch or duodenojejunostomy. A gastrojejunocolic fistula is treated by a partial gastrectomy that includes the anastomosis and by excision of the involved jejunum and colon. Reconstruction may be performed by either reanastomosis of the jejunum with a more distal loop gastrojejunostomy (to include truncal vagotomy if ulcer related) or conversion to a Roux-en-Y gastrojejunostomy. The colon may be anastomosed, or a proximal colostomy may be performed if extensive local inflammation is present.

For repair of both perforations and fistulas, the use of fibrin sealant as an adjunct should be considered. It has been used successfully in the transthoracic repair of esophageal perforations to anchor a pleural flap over the sutured repair. Bardaxoglou et al. also reported successful use of fibrin sealant for esophageal perforations, combined with absorbable mesh.[62] Lau et al. compared sutured repair and fibrin sealant with a gelatin sponge for the treatment of perforated ulcers and also compared laparoscopic and open techniques.[63] They did not find any significant differences between sutured and fibrin sealant repair. These results, combined with successful reports of nonoperative fistula closure with the use of fibrin sealant, suggest a broader role in operative management.

Enterocutaneous Fistulas

Many enterocutaneous fistulas close spontaneously if infection is controlled, nutrition is adequate, and distal obstruction is not present. Definitive operative correction remains the final step in the management of nonhealing small intestinal fistulas. As with the duration of medical management, the surgical procedure needs to be individualized. Direct suture closure of the fistula is associated with a high incidence of breakdown and fistula recurrence.[28] This operation is rarely useful except as a last resort in patients with dense abdominal adhesions from previous surgeries or in medically moribund patients. In most cases, the preferred operation is resection of the involved segment of intestine and primary end-to-end anastomosis. This technique was successful in 57 of 66 patients reported by Reber and colleagues.[28] In the setting of extensive sepsis, primary anastomosis may not be appropriate. In these circumstances, exteriorization of both the proximal and distal ends of the intestine may be performed. It is critical that the proximal end be constructed as a standard everted Brooke stoma so that a proper appliance can be fitted and the subsequent effluent adequately managed.

If the fistula is not deemed appropriate for resection, such as when it develops as a complication of a deep pelvic procedure, staged approaches involving bypass should be considered. A simple side-to-side anastomosis proximal and distal to the fistula is inadequate, as is unilateral (proximal or distal) exclusion of the involved segment. Bilateral exclusion with isolation of *both* the proximal and distal portions of the involved intestine is necessary for effective defunctionalization of the fistula. In a staged procedure, the fistulous segment is left in situ, or the ends are exteriorized as mucous fistulas; the afferent and efferent bowel loops are anastomosed to restore intestinal continuity. Alternatively, if the efferent loop cannot be mobilized, the intestine proximal to a distal ileal fistula can be divided and anastomosed to the transverse colon. The fistulous segment is again returned to the pelvis or exteriorized as a mucous fistula. This technique is not as satisfactory as complete exclusion but works reasonably well if the ileocecal valve is competent. Optimally, the staged procedure is completed when the fistula segment is removed at a later date, although this is not always possible.

Gastrointestinal fistulas associated with large abdominal defects are not only the most difficult to manage surgically but also the most likely to result in mortality. The wound V.A.C. works well to keep these wounds smaller and easier to manage and frequently closes even large abdominal wall defects. Musculocutaneous flaps and the application of abdominal wall reconstruction techniques involving component separation and prosthetic materials may be required to obtain adequate coverage.

Enteroenteric Fistulas

An internal fistula refers to a communication between the small intestine and some other organ or structure within the peritoneal cavity. An enteroenteric fistula occurs when the small intestine joins with either another segment of small intestine or the colon. Most enteroenteric fistulas are caused by Crohn's disease, although colonic diverticulitis and colon cancer can also be antecedent events. Fistulas develop in direct proportion to the length of the involved intestine. Fistula formation in Crohn's disease begins with serosal cohesion of healthy small or large bowel to the diseased intestinal segment. The process is usually gradual and results in internal perforation and subsequent fistula formation as the ulcer penetrates through the newly formed common wall. Free perforation and generalized peritonitis are unusual. Ileocecal fistulas are most common because of the high percentage of patients with Crohn's disease who have chronic inflammation of the terminal ileum. The jejunum and duodenum are involved less frequently.

Careful evaluation is needed to diagnose an enteroenteric fistula because abnormalities may be subtle, reported as generalized complaints, or even absent. Symptoms such as diarrhea, abdominal pain, weight loss, and fever are not specific and are frequently caused by

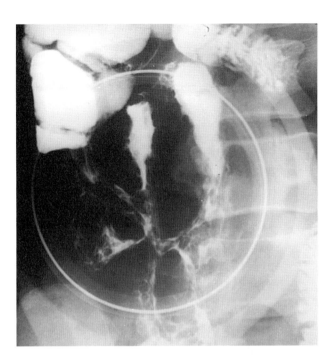

Figure 73–6. Small bowel series demonstrating a complex "starburst" enteroenteric fistula.

the underlying disease process, as well as the fistula. Abdominal tenderness or a mass may be noted on physical examination. In some patients there may be evidence of obstruction. Enteroenteric fistulas are often serendipitously diagnosed on a small bowel series or barium enema obtained for evaluating vague abdominal discomfort or dysfunction (Fig. 73–6). Sometimes the fistula is not discovered until laparotomy. In others with Crohn's disease, long-term parenteral nutrition, bowel rest, and the use of pharmacologic therapy that includes 6-mercaptopurine, cyclosporine, or infliximab has been successful in resolving certain types of fistulas.[51-57] This outcome contrasts greatly with the natural history of these fistulas before such pharmacologic innovation. For instance, a 1974 study involving 63 patients with Crohn's disease and enteroenteric fistulas found that 52 ultimately required surgery.[64] However, surgical intervention is still necessary in many patients because of refractory disease or intolerance to medications and their side effects.

When surgical intervention is warranted, the operative procedure of choice is en bloc resection of the diseased intestine in continuity with the fistula tract. If inflammation or an abscess is present, primary resection may be unwise. In such a situation, proximal diversion or percutaneous drainage of any associated abscess cavity is prudent. Resection of the diseased intestine and fistula should be delayed for 6 weeks, if possible, to allow the inflammatory process to subside. Nutritional support during this time is essential.

Any resection, whether primary or as part of a staged procedure, should be confined to the involved segment of intestine to conserve overall bowel length. Extensive resection does not appear to protect against further

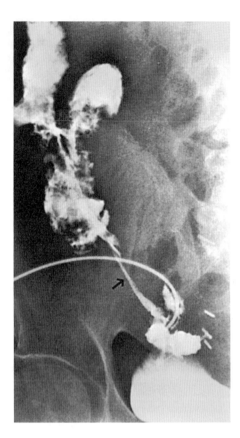

Figure 73–7. Fistulogram demonstrating an enterovesical fistula in a patient with long-standing ileal Crohn's disease (the *arrow* indicates a fistula tract). (From Tassiopoulos AK, Baum G, Halverson ID: Small bowel fistulas. Surg Clin North Am 76:1175, 1996.)

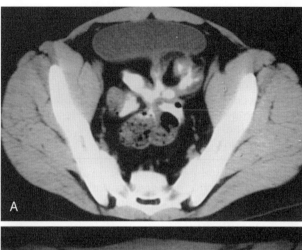

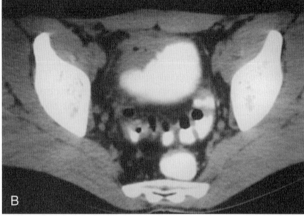

Figure 73–8. Computed tomographic scans in patients with enterovesical fistulas **A,** Complex enteroenteric and enterovesical fistula. **B,** A loop of small intestine is adherent and causing significant inflammation on the wall of the bladder with subsequent fistula formation.

complications and only increases the likelihood of subsequent malabsorption. This is particularly true in Crohn's disease, in which repeat laparotomy, intestinal resection, and subsequent absorptive loss are common and could result in short-gut syndrome.

Enterovesical Fistulas

Although a colonic communication with the urinary bladder caused by diverticulitis or colon cancer is seen with some frequency, fistula formation between the small intestine and the bladder is rare. More than half of all enterovesical fistulas occur as a complication of Crohn's disease; however, radiation injury to the small bowel can also result in their formation. An ileovesical fistula develops in 2% to 4% of patients with regional enteritis, usually as a late manifestation of their disease. Such fistulas tend to be long, narrow, and tortuous (Fig. 73–7). Many seem to maintain patency only intermittently. The fistula frequently tracks downward from the ileum in the right iliac fossa. The uterus does not function as an anatomic barrier to such fistula tracts as it does with the short, localized fistulas resulting from diverticulitis or rectosigmoid cancer. Thus, enterovesical fistulas have an even distribution among the sexes.

More than 80% of patients with enterovesical fistulas have urinary symptoms such as fecaluria or pneumaturia.[65] Evidence of bladder irritability and subsequent dysuria are common. In a few patients fulminant sepsis may develop because of contamination of the urine with intestinal organisms. The presence of an internal fistula involving the urinary tract can be confirmed by the appearance of charcoal or indigo carmine in the urine after administration. Cystoscopy is helpful in establishing or confirming the diagnosis. The most consistent finding is an area of bullous edema, usually on the posterior-lateral wall or the fundus of the bladder. In some patients, the fistula opening can be directly visualized. Biopsy should be performed to evaluate for unusual causal processes such as tuberculosis or cancer.

CT is the most accurate and efficient radiographic means for diagnosing an enterovesical fistula (Fig. 73–8). Barium contrast studies of the gastrointestinal tract often do not demonstrate the fistula but are invaluable in determining the nature of the underlying disease process and assessing its extent. Intravenous pyelography and cystography are rarely useful in evaluation of the fistula itself. They may be important as a means of demonstrating bilateral renal function and evaluating abnormalities of the upper urinary tract.

In the absence of obstruction, inflammation, or abscess, the preferred treatment of an enterovesical fistula is resection of the diseased intestine and involved portion of the bladder. Removal of the fistula is particularly important to prevent continued contamination of the urinary tract. A primary anastomosis is used to restore intestinal continuity, and the bladder wall is closed. As with other fistulas, if an inflamed intestine or mass makes resection unsafe, transection plus cutaneous diversion of the proximal and distal intestinal segments is recommended.

Nephroenteric Fistulas

Fistulas between the gastrointestinal system and the upper urinary tract are rare. Primary renal disease causes most nephrogenic fistulas. As with bladder fistulas, the colon is more frequently involved than the small intestine. When a small bowel fistula is present, anatomic proximity appears to be the prime determinant of the affected segment of intestine. Therefore, the duodenum is most often involved, whereas nephrojejunal fistulas are rare.

Bissada and associates analyzed a group of 43 patients with nephroenteric fistulas identified over a period of several decades. Before 1945, fulminant infections were responsible for fistula formation in 21 of 26 patients.[66] Renal tuberculosis and bacterial infections were equally responsible, whereas obstructing renal calculous disease was a rare finding. With the advent of effective antimicrobial agents, however, tuberculosis has become a rare cause of fistulization. Bacterial infections are still an important antecedent event but are now almost always associated with secondary staghorn calculi. Since 1945, renal trauma has become the second most common cause of nephroenteric fistulas, and it accounted for 35% of the cases reported in this series. Penetrating, blunt, and iatrogenic types of trauma have all been reported to result in the formation of a fistula. Rarely, fistulas arise spontaneously from the alimentary tract, primarily in association with diverticulitis.

The symptom complex associated with a nephroenteric fistula is determined by the nature of the underlying renal disease, the rapidity with which the fistula forms, and the presence of associated conditions such as diverticulitis or perinephric abscess. Often, development of the fistula is insidious. The patient appears chronically ill and debilitated. There are invariably manifestations of a chronic urinary tract infection with chills and fever, and fulminant sepsis is not uncommon. Flank pain, tenderness to palpation, or a mass may be present. Pneumaturia, fecaluria, nausea and vomiting, and watery purulent diarrhea are frequent symptoms. Dehydration and uremia develop in the more advanced stages of the disease. Hyperchloremic acidosis may occur as urine electrolytes are reabsorbed in the gastrointestinal tract.

As with enterovesical fistulas, oral administration of charcoal or indigo carmine can confirm a suspected fistula between the intestine and the urinary tract.

Barium contrast studies are usually ineffective in demonstrating nephroenteric fistulas.[66] An intravenous pyelogram can be helpful, but only if the involved kidney remains functional, which is uncommon. Invasive pyelography, both retrograde and antegrade, is sensitive in diagnosing nephroenteric fistulas, with dye often passing into the intestine, especially if the fistula is large. Retrograde pyelography combined with cinefluorography is most commonly performed. When obstruction precludes a retrograde approach, percutaneous access to the renal pelvis followed by antegrade pyelography is useful. CT remains an important radiographic adjuvant to the evaluation and management of nephrogenic fistulas by diagnosing associated perinephric abscesses and thus should always be performed.

Treatment of a nephrogenic fistula is initiated by correcting fluid and electrolyte imbalances and anemia, along with administering broad-spectrum antibiotics. Nutritional support should begin by the parenteral route to help correct further debilitation. Urinary obstruction, if present, should be relieved either by retrograde placement of a ureteral catheter or by a temporary nephrostomy tube. A perinephric abscess must be drained if present.

Medical management alone rarely results in closure of the fistula. The involved kidney is often dysfunctional or nonfunctional and thus continues to be a nidus for ongoing infection and inflammation. The affected intestine generally has extensive inflammatory changes. In most cases, therefore, nephrectomy with intestinal resection is the procedure of choice. Primary intestinal anastomosis can be carried out, depending on the severity of disease.

Procedures conserving the involved renal parenchyma are reserved for nephrogenic fistulas detected before severe renal functional impairment has occurred. Conservation is more likely to be appropriate for fistulas of traumatic origin. If the contralateral kidney has adequate function, the outcomes associated with surgical intervention are good, with perioperative mortality occurring in less than 10% of patients.

Enterovaginal Fistulas

Fistulas from the small intestine to the vagina are rare. As with colovaginal fistulas, enterovaginal fistulas are more likely to occur in women who have undergone a hysterectomy. Enterovaginal fistulas are usually caused by regional enteritis, radiation enteritis, granulomatous disease, or rarely, malignant tumors.

Most patients have a purulent or feculent vaginal discharge. Gas may also be intermittently expelled from the vagina. Associated intra-abdominal sepsis is common and may cause fever, chills, and abdominal pain. Enterovaginal fistulas can lead to hypovolemia and severe fluid and electrolyte abnormalities, particularly when the drainage is profuse. Speculum examination generally confirms the diagnosis by revealing vaginal erosion and drainage of intestinal contents. CT scanning, as well as contrast studies of the small intestine or vagina, may also be diagnostic. In more subtle cases, a suspected fistula between the intestine and the vagina may be identified by placing a tampon in the vagina before the oral administration of charcoal or indigo carmine.

Management of an enterovaginal fistula is similar to that for an enterocutaneous fistula. Local drainage through sump drains placed through the vagina may allow adequate control of sepsis and fistula output. If sepsis is eradicated, fistula output is low, and adequate nutrition is provided, an enterovaginal fistula may close without an operation. Spontaneous closure of a fistula associated with Crohn's disease, however, is rare. Resection of a cuff of vaginal tissue along with the fistula and involved intestine is the preferred surgical approach. A primary intestinal anastomosis should be performed if the surrounding inflammation permits. The vaginal defect may be left open to allow external drainage of the pelvis postoperatively.

Enterouterine, Enterocervical, and Enterofallopian Fistulas

On rare occasion, a fistula forms between the intestine and the uterus, cervix, or fallopian tube. Enterouterine fistulas have been reported to occur secondary to various pelvic malignancies or as an unusual sequela to a long-standing ectopic pregnancy. The thick muscular wall of the uterus makes the development of such fistulas unusual. Appropriate treatment of the underlying disease together with a hysterectomy is usually indicated.

Fistulas to the cervix generally develop secondary to radiation therapy to the cervical stump and occur only when a previous supracervical hysterectomy has been performed. Fistulas from the intestine to the fallopian tube can result from endometriosis, tuberculosis, and lymphogranuloma venereum. Rarely, an ectopic pregnancy can rupture into the intestine and cause lower gastrointestinal bleeding.[67]

Aortoenteric Fistulas

The most common fistula between the arterial tree and the small intestine arises from the aorta. Complications of aortic aneurysms and their repair are by far the most frequent cause of this entity, although such fistulas have occurred after other abdominal procedures. Spontaneous or primary aortoenteric fistulas usually occur when the plaque of an atherosclerotic aortic aneurysm ruptures into the intestine. On rare occasion, mycotic, tubercular, or traumatic aneurysms may also rupture into the small bowel. The duodenum is most often involved when a spontaneous fistula develops. Reckless and associates reviewed 131 spontaneous aortoenteric fistulas and found that rupture into the third portion of the duodenum occurred in 57.6% of cases whereas the remainder of the small intestine was involved in only 8%.[68]

Secondary aortoenteric fistulas complicate 2% to 4% of all aortic reconstructions and generally involve aortoiliac or aortofemoral prosthetic grafts. The fistulas usually occur at the level of the proximal aortic anastomosis, and most rupture into the duodenum. If the fistula occurs at the anastomosis between the prosthesis and the iliac arteries, the ileum is the most commonly involved segment of intestine.

Two processes can cause secondary aortoenteric fistulas and result in different clinical manifestations. A direct communication between the intestine and the arterial lumen ultimately leads to massive gastrointestinal hemorrhage. Initially, bleeding is intermittent and is rarely exsanguinating. Such episodic bleeding, known as *herald* or *sentinel* bleeding, is generally painless and may cause chronic anemia. Melena or hematemesis in any patient with an aortic prosthesis should be assumed to be from an aortoenteric fistula until proved otherwise. Several months may elapse between the initial bleeding episode and the inevitable massive hemorrhage. The second form of secondary fistula is known as a *paraprosthetic-enteric* fistula. In this type of aortoenteric fistula, the intestine communicates with a perigraft abscess or aneurysm and not directly with the arterial lumen. Most of these patients have manifestations of sepsis. In a group of 21 patients with such fistulas, O'Mara and Imbembo noted 14 with sepsis, 4 with gastrointestinal hemorrhage, and 3 with abdominal pain.[69] Although a distinct clinical entity, a paraprosthetic fistula ultimately leads to a direct communication with the arterial lumen and subsequent hemorrhage if untreated.

The mechanism by which aortoenteric fistulas develop is controversial. A combination of mechanical and infectious factors probably contributes in most instances. Mechanical injury to the intestine can occur from the trauma of the adjacent arterial pulsation. This is more apt to transpire when the intestine has become fixed to the area of anastomosis, which may be avoided by separating the intestine from the aorta with interposed omentum or surrounding tissues. After the intestine has been sufficiently traumatized, leakage of intestinal contents occurs, with subsequent infection and enzymatic digestion at the suture line. The localized septic process ultimately leads to suture line disruption. Other methods of fistula formation have been hypothesized, including aneurysmal degeneration of the graft with subsequent mechanical erosion into the intestinal wall. Occasionally, a false aneurysm develops at the suture line and ultimately ruptures into the intestine. False aneurysms are usually a consequence of technical errors during the graft anastomosis, but they can also result from infected grafts.

Although the presence of an aortoenteric fistula may be suspected clinically, extensive evaluation and confirmation may not be possible if severe hemorrhage is present. In such instances, immediate laparotomy and proximal control of the aorta are priorities. Fortunately, most aortoenteric fistulas are associated with multiple episodes of limited gastrointestinal bleeding. These patients should be prepared for an urgent operation, but there is generally enough time to perform further diagnostic investigation. Upper gastrointestinal endoscopy should be performed initially to exclude common causes of hemorrhage, such as peptic ulcer disease or esophageal varices. The actual erosion into the intestinal wall can often be seen if the endoscopist is instructed to examine the distal end of the duodenum. Biopsy of such an erosion is absolutely contraindicated. CT is sensitive in evaluating the retroperitoneum for suspected aortoenteric fistulas. CT has the advantages of rapid imaging

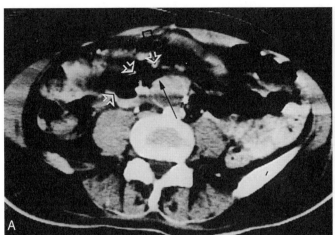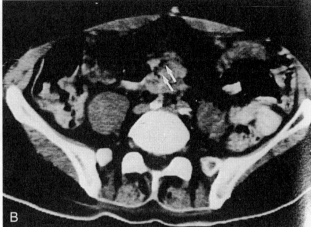

Figure 73–9. Computed tomographic scan of aortoenteric erosion. **A,** Apparent erosion of an aortic graft *(black arrow)* into the overlying duodenum *(open arrows).* **B,** Perigraft air *(arrows).* (From Bernhard VM: Aortoenteric fistulas. In Rutherford RB [ed]: Vascular Surgery. Philadelphia, WB Saunders, 1989, p 530.)

and wide availability (Fig. 73–9). Because it is a noninvasive study, CT does not require technical expertise and does not cause patient discomfort, thereby avoiding the potentially disastrous consequences of raising the patient's blood pressure. CT may demonstrate loss of the normal fatty plane between the aortic graft and the duodenum, a finding indicative of a probable fistula. It may also reveal a false aneurysm at the anastomosis or the presence of a periaortic gas or fluid collection.

When the diagnosis remains elusive, aortography should be performed. Aortography is particularly useful if there is active hemorrhage or if a false aneurysm is suspected. Extravasation of contrast material into the intestine or retroperitoneum confirms the diagnosis. If endoscopy, CT, and aortography fail to find the suspected fistula, upper and lower gastrointestinal barium contrast studies can be performed. Barium evaluation should be postponed until after endoscopy, CT, and aortography, however, because residual barium decreases the sensitivity of these procedures. Barium studies may demonstrate a sinus tract from the intestine. The presence of an intestinal diverticulum or ulcer may result in a false-negative evaluation. If the patient is febrile or a perigraft infection is suspected, blood for culture should be drawn from both upper and lower extremity veins. Positive blood cultures, particularly if limited to the lower extremities, are predictive of a poor clinical outcome.[70]

Management of an aortoenteric fistula, once confirmed, consists of early and aggressive operative intervention. Removal of the prosthesis and extra-anatomic bypass should be coupled with broad-spectrum antibiotics appropriate for the multiple enteric organisms usually present. Conventional wisdom holds that the presence of infection at the prosthetic site precludes less involved procedures such as local closure of the fistula or replacement of the prosthesis. In a series reported by O'Mara and associates, a recurrent aortoenteric fistula developed in all four of the patients treated by initial repair of the fistula, but without extra-anatomic bypass.[71]

By contrast, five of the seven patients who had the prosthesis removed, followed by an axillobifemoral bypass, lived and did well. However, there have been successful reports of in situ repair of the aorta with prosthetic grafts or cryopreserved aortic homografts. Walker and colleagues reported excellent overall results with in situ replacement of the abdominal graft and primary closure of the duodenal fistula in 20 patients. Of the 18 survivors, 15 had no further complications.[72] Vogt and associates reported a similar low operative mortality rate and no complications of reinfection when in situ cryopreserved aortic homografts were used to replace the infected aortic prosthesis.[73] The intestinal defect can be débrided and primarily closed in most cases, but bowel resection and end-to-end anastomosis may be necessary or technically easier in some patients.

The survival rate in patients with aortoenteric fistulas is poor, often because of exsanguinating hemorrhage or associated cardiovascular or renal impairment. The mortality rate has been reported to be as high as 50%. A multicenter retrospective study of 98 patients found an improved mortality rate of 24% in patients with aortoenteric fistula or infection treated by axillobifemoral bypass and aortic exclusion. Bypass patency rates at 2 and 5 years were reported to be 82% and 65%, respectively, and limb salvage was achieved in 90% and 82% of patients, respectively, over the same time course.[74]

General Considerations

When planning the operation for fistula patients, the surgeon should allow adequate time for a difficult and prolonged procedure. Depending on the complexity of the abdominal wound, component release and other reconstructive maneuvers may be required to achieve closure of the abdominal wall. It is frequently helpful to enlist the expertise of a plastic surgeon for closure of the abdominal wound (Fig. 73–10A). The component separation release technique is useful for the reconstruction

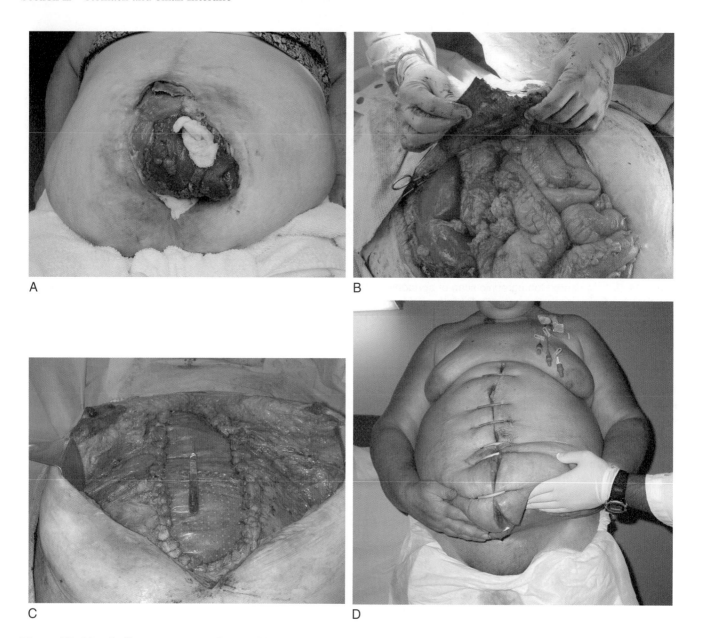

Figure 73–10. **A,** Enterocutaneous fistula with epithelialization of the tract and a large abdominal wall defect. **B,** The entire intestinal tract has been mobilized and complete enterolysis performed. **C,** The large abdominal wall defect is closed with a combination of abdominal wall and small intestinal submucosa (Surgisis Gold). **D,** Completed resection of the fistula and abdominal wall closure with loose closure of the skin and the use of retention sutures.

of large abdominal wall defects, especially when contaminated conditions exist in which the use of prosthetic material may be contraindicated. Thus, preoperative consultation and evaluation by the plastic and reconstructive surgery team should be considered. Preoperative preparation should include a mechanical bowel preparation whenever feasible, preoperative abdominal wall preparation with antiseptic (e.g., chlorhexidine) scrubs beginning at least 24 hours in advance, and perioperative antibiotics directed toward bowel and skin flora, as well as any specific organisms identified by recent culture and sensitivity information.

Whenever possible, a new incision or extension of the previous incision over "virgin" abdominal wall will make

reentry into the abdominal cavity easier and safer. Once the peritoneal cavity is entered, the entire intestinal tract should be mobilized, and complete enterolysis should be performed if possible, especially is there is any question of distal obstruction (see Fig. 73–10B). A useful adjunct during this portion of the operation is to use laparotomy pads soaked in saline solution to "rehydrate" the adhesions before attempting adhesiolysis. By using a combination of gentle compression and palpation with one hand and sharp dissection with either scissors or a scalpel in conjunction with the use of copious amounts of saline-soaked sponges, one can usually carry out complete mobilization of the involved intestine. In general, an intestinal fistula cannot be repaired primarily; such repair usually results in recurrence. Fistulas require complete resection back to healthy tissue with enteroenterostomy. If the anastomosis is performed on healthy bowel, the choice between a stapled or hand-sewn anastomosis does not matter. More importantly, the anastomosis should be under no tension, there must be adequate blood supply, and distal obstruction cannot be present. A feeding jejunostomy or nasoenteric tube should be placed. Ongoing nutritional repletion is an extremely important constituent of a successful outcome, and most patients will not be able to take enough calories by mouth during the postoperative recovery period. A gastrostomy tube may also be a useful adjunct in the postoperative period. Depending on the state of the intestinal tract, the extent of enterolysis required, and the underlying process that led to fistula formation, prolonged postoperative ileus will commonly occur, and decompression via a gastrostomy tube, while downstream enteral nutrition is given, may be very beneficial. Because of the usual extensive nature of the dissection during such operations, the formation of intra-abdominal adhesions is likely. Methods for decreasing intra-abdominal adhesions, such as the use of hyaluronic acid–carboxymethylcellulose membrane (Seprafilm), may be beneficial in preventing postoperative complications.[75] Finally, abdominal wall closure is extremely important to allow the best chance for success and to prevent recurrent fistulization. It is essential that the abdominal wall be closed with autologous tissue (using component separation or musculocutaneous flaps) or an absorbable prosthesis consisting of either small intestinal submucosa (Surgisis Gold) (see Fig. 73–10C) or dermis (AlloDerm) or with a permanent prosthesis that is resistant to infection such as titanium mesh (TiMesh). Assistance by surgeons with specific skills in abdominal reconstruction (plastic and reconstructive surgery) is often quite helpful in these situations, and their advice and consultation should be readily sought (see Fig. 73–10D).

Healing

Most postoperative fistula patients are in a profoundly catabolic state in the early postoperative period and are at risk for nutritional complications. Again, optimal nutrition is as important postoperatively as preoperatively. Supplemental nutrition via enteral, parenteral, or a combination is frequently required, and with time, the patient can be transitioned to complete intake by mouth. Even when a patient cannot tolerate full caloric intake via the enteral route, providing a portion of the nutrition enterally remains an important objective. It may be useful to cycle tube feeding at night once the patient is eating in an attempt to stimulate appetite. Meals from home also occasionally help with appetite stimulation. A dietitian consultation can be very helpful as well. A period of home tube feeding or, if necessary, home parenteral nutrition is not unreasonable in these patients because re-establishing normal eating habits may be a long process. The final phase of the treatment of fistulas, then, is healing, and this phase is highly dependent on good nutrition after a well-performed operation. If the patient cannot tolerate at least 1500 kcal/day enterally, parenteral nutrition should be continued until this goal is achieved. Once enteral intake approaches this range, the parenteral nutrition can be weaned.

The overall mortality rate if one includes all fistulas is approximately 20%. Mortality with a postoperative fistula is not as high. Postoperative fistulas are associated with less than 2% mortality and approximately 12% morbidity. Delayed complications may include short-bowel syndrome, depending on the extent of the intestinal resection, previous resections, and the underlying disease state (i.e., Crohn's disease). In patients with a marginal amount of bowel remaining, some intestinal adaptation may occur, and with time, weaning of parenteral nutrition may be possible. As a general guide, approximately 90 cm of small intestine with an intact ileocecal valve may be adequate to prevent short-bowel syndrome, whereas 150 cm may be necessary when the ileocecal valve has been resected. The surgeon must be vigilant for recurrent fistulas postoperatively. These patients are also highly susceptible to adhesive small bowel obstruction. It is generally prudent to manage early postoperative small bowel obstruction in these patients with long-tube decompression and TPN rather than risk further complications with another operation in the early postoperative period.

SUMMARY

Management of intestinal fistulas provides a surgeon with multiple challenges. Careful attention must be paid to the physiologic, metabolic, and immunologic derangements in these patients. An organized and tolerant approach to the stabilization, investigation, planning and implementation of medical and surgical therapy, and healing phase should allow for a successful outcome in the majority of patients.

SUGGESTED READINGS

Edmunds LH, Williams GH, Welch CE: External fistulas arising from the gastrointestinal tract. Ann Surg 152:445, 1960.

Fazio VW, Coutsoftides T, Steiger E: Factors influencing the outcome of treatment of small bowel cutaneous fistula. World J Surg 7:481, 1983.

Fischer JE: The pathophysiology of enterocutaneous fistulas. World J Surg 7:446, 1983.

Kuvshinoff BW, Brodish RJ, McFadden DW, Fischer JE: Serum transferrin as a prognostic indicator of spontaneous closure and mortality in gastrointestinal cutaneous fistulas. Ann Surg 217:615, 1993.

Lichtenstein GR, Yan S, Bala M, et al: Infliximab maintenance treatment reduces hospitalizations, surgeries, and procedures in fistulizing Crohn's disease. Gastroenterology 128:862, 2005.

Reber HA, Roberts C, Way LW, Dunphy JE: Management of external gastrointestinal fistulas. Ann Surg 188:460, 1978.

Soeters PB, Ebeid AM, Fischer JE: Review of 404 patients with gastrointestinal fistulas: Impact of parenteral nutrition. Ann Surg 180:393, 1979.

REFERENCES

1. Berry SM, Fischer JE: Enterocutaneous fistulas. Curr Probl Surg 31:469, 1994.
2. Schein M, Decker GA: Postoperative external alimentary tract fistulas. Am J Surg 161:435, 1991.
3. Soeters PB, Ebeid AM, Fischer JE: Review of 404 patients with gastrointestinal fistulas: Impact of parenteral nutrition. Ann Surg 180:393, 1979.
4. MacLean LD, Rhode BM, Nohr C, et al: Stomal ulcer after gastric bypass. J Am Coll Surg 185:1, 1997.
5. Cucchi SG, Pories WJ, MacDonald KG, et al: Gastrogastric fistulas: A complication of divided gastric bypass surgery. Ann Surg 221:387, 1995.
6. Pickleman J, Watson W, Cunningham J, et al: The failed gastrointestinal anastomosis: An inevitable catastrophe? J Am Coll Surg 188:473, 1999.
7. Papakonstantinou A, Alfaras P, Komessidou V, et al: Gastrointestinal complications after vertical banded gastroplasty. Obes Surg 8:215, 1998.
8. Kirkpatrick JR, Zapas JL: Divided gastric bypass: A fifteen-year experience. Am Surg 64:62, 1998.
9. Nussbaum MS, Schusterman MA: Management of giant duodenal ulcer. Am J Surg 199:357, 1985.
10. Coelho JCU, Wiederkehr JC, Campos ACL, et al: Conversions and complications of laparoscopic treatment of gastroesophageal reflux disease. J Am Coll Surg 189:356, 1999.
11. Schauer PR, Meyers WC, Eubanks S, et al: Mechanisms of gastric and esophageal perforations during laparoscopic Nissen fundoplication. Ann Surg 223:43, 1996.
12. Eshragi N, Farahmand M, Soot SJ, et al: Comparison of outcomes of open versus laparoscopic Nissen fundoplication performed in a single practice. Am J Surg 175:371, 1998.
13. Perdikis G, Hinder RA, Lund RJ, et al: Laparoscopic Nissen fundoplication: Where do we stand? Surg Laparosc Endosc 7:17, 1997.
14. Hunter JG, Smith CD, Branum GD, et al: Laparoscopic fundoplication failures: Patterns of failure and response to fundoplication revision. Ann Surg 230:595, 1999.
15. Chelala E, Cadiere GB, Favretti F, et al: Conversions and complications in 185 laparoscopic adjustable silicone gastric banding cases. Surg Endosc 11:268, 1997.
16. Watkins BM, Montgomery KF, Ahroni JH: Laparoscopic adjustable gastric banding: Early experience in 400 consecutive patients in the USA. Obes Surg 15:82, 2005.
17. Spirt M, Sachar DB, Greenstein AJ: Symptomatic differentiation of duodenal from gastric fistulas in Crohn's disease. Am J Gastroenterol 85:455, 1990.
18. Curtis M, Ney C, Dave M, et al: Renogastric fistula secondary to a staghorn calculus. J Urol 156:1434, 1996.
19. Tsiotos GG, Smith CD, Sarr MG: Incidence and management of pancreatic and enteric fistulas after surgical management of severe necrotizing pancreatitis. Arch Surg 130:48, 1995.
20. Ho HS, Frey CF: Gastrointestinal and pancreatic complications associated with severe pancreatitis. Arch Surg 130:817, 1995.
21. Loperfido S, Angelini G, Benedetti G, et al: Major early complications from diagnostic and therapeutic ERCP: A prospective multicenter study. Gastrointest Endosc 48:1, 1998.
22. Bell RCW, Stiegman GV, Goff J, et al: Decision for surgical management of perforation following endoscopic sphincterotomy. Am Surg 57:237, 1991.
23. Lorimer JW, Goobie P, Rasuli P, et al: Primary aortogastric fistula: A complication of ruptured aortic aneurysm. J Cardiovasc Surg 37:363, 1996.
24. Sato O, Miyata T, Matsubara T, et al: Successful surgical treatment of aortogastric fistula after an esophagectomy and subsequent endovascular graft placement: Report of a case. Surg Today 29:431, 1999.
25. San Nicolo M, Achammer T, Flora G: Duodenal fistula after reconstruction of the inferior vena cava with an externally stented PTFE graft. J Cardiovasc Surg 31:382, 1990.
26. Knoop C, Antoine M, Vachiery JL, et al: Gastric perforation because of mucormycosis after heart-lung and heart transplantation. Transplantation 66:932, 1998.
27. MacFadyen BV, Dudrick SJ, Ruberg RL: Management of gastrointestinal fistulas with parenteral hyperalimentation. Surgery 74:100, 1973.
28. Reber HA, Roberts C, Way LW, Dunphy JE: Management of external gastrointestinal fistulas. Ann Surg 188:460, 1978.
29. Graham JA: Conservative treatment of gastrointestinal fistulas. Surg Gynecol Obstet 144:512, 1977.
30. Webster NW, Carey LC: Fistulae of the Intestinal Tract, vol 13, No 6. Chicago, Year Book, 1976.
31. Fischer JE: The pathophysiology of enterocutaneous fistulas. World J Surg 7:446, 1983.
32. Fazio VW, Coutsoftides T, Steiger E: Factors influencing the outcome of treatment of small bowel cutaneous fistula. World J Surg 7:481, 1983.
33. Edmunds LH, Williams GH, Welch CE: External fistulas arising from the gastrointestinal tract. Ann Surg 152:445, 1960.
34. Schein M, Decker GA: Gastrointestinal fistula associated with large abdominal wall defects: Experience with 43 patients. Br J Surg 77:97, 1990.
35. Church JM, Weakley FL, Fazio VW, et al: The relationship between fistulas in Crohn's disease and associated carcinoma: Report of four cases and review of the literature. Dis Colon Rectum 28:361, 1985.
36. Pritts TA, Fischer DR, Fischer JE: Postoperative enterocutaneous fistula. In Holzheimer RG, Mannick JA (eds): Surgical Treatment—Evidence-Based and Problem-Oriented. New York, W Zucksschwerdt Verlag, 2001, pp 134-139.
37. Dudrick SJ, Maharaj AR, McKelvey AA: Artificial nutritional support in patients with gastrointestinal fistulas. World J Surg 23:570, 1999.
38. Chapman R, Foran R, Dunphy JE: Management of intestinal fistulas. Am J Surg 108:157, 1964.
39. Sheldon GF, Gardiner BN, Way LW, Dunphy JE: Management of gastrointestinal fistulas. Surg Gynecol Obstet 133:385, 1971.
40. Roback SA, Nicholoff DM: High output enterocutaneous fistulas of the small bowel. Am J Surg 123:317, 1972.
41. Kuvshinoff BW, Brodish RJ, McFadden DW, Fischer JE: Serum transferrin as a prognostic indicator of spontaneous closure and mortality in gastrointestinal cutaneous fistulas. Ann Surg 217:615, 1993.
42. D'Harcour JB, Boverie JH, Dondelinger RF: Percutaneous management of enterocutaneous fistulas. AJR Am J Roentgenol 167:33, 1996.
43. Suriyapa C, Anderson MC: A simple device to control drainage from enterocutaneous fistulas. Surgery 70:456, 1971.
44. Alvarez AA, Maxwell GL, Rodriguez GC: Vacuum-assisted closure for cutaneous gastrointestinal fistula management. Gynecol Oncol 80:413, 2001.
45. Cro C, George KJ, Donnelly J, et al: Vacuum assisted closure system in the management of enterocutaneous fistulae. Postgrad Med J 78:364, 2002.
46. Paran H, Neufeld D, Kaplan O, et al: Octreotide for treatment of postoperative alimentary tract fistulas. World J Surg 19:430, 1995.
47. Dorta G: Role of octreotide and somatostatin in the treatment of intestinal fistulas. Digestion 60(Suppl 2):53, 1999.
48. Ayache S, Wadleigh RG: Treatment of a malignant enterocutaneous fistula with octreotide acetate. Cancer Invest 17:320, 1999.
49. Spiliotis J, Briand D, Gouttebel MC, et al: Treatment of fistulas of the gastrointestinal tract with total parenteral nutrition and octreotide in patients with carcinoma. Surg Gynecol Obstet 176:575, 1993.
50. Torres AJ, Landa JI, Moreno-Azcoita M, et al: Somatostatin in the management of gastrointestinal fistulas: A multicenter trial. Arch Surg 127:97, 1992.
51. Hanauer SB, Smith MB: Rapid closure of Crohn's disease fistulas with continuous intravenous cyclosporin A. Am J Gastroenterol 88:646, 1993.
52. Present DH, Lichtiger S: Efficacy of cyclosporine in treatment of fistula of Crohn's disease. Dig Dis Sci 39:374, 1994.

53. Lowry PW, Weaver AL, Tremaine WJ, Sandborn WJ: Combination therapy with oral tacrolimus (FK506) and azathioprine or 6-mercaptopurine for treatment-refractory Crohn's disease perianal fistulae. Inflamm Bowel Dis 5:239, 1999.

54. Present DH, Rutgeerts P, Targan S, et al: Infliximab for the treatment of fistulas in patients with Crohn's disease. N Engl J Med 340:1398, 1999.

55. Lofberg R: Treatment of fistulas in Crohn's disease with infliximab. Gut 45:642, 1999.

56. Ricart E, Sandborn WJ: Infliximab for the treatment of fistulas in patients with Crohn's disease. Gastroenterology 117:1247, 1999.

57. Lichtenstein GR, Yan S, Bala M, et al: Infliximab maintenance treatment reduces hospitalizations, surgeries, and procedures in fistulizing Crohn's disease. Gastroenterology 128:862, 2005.

58. Aguirre A, Fischer JE, Welch CE: The role of surgery and hyperalimentation in the therapy of gastrointestinal-cutaneous fistulae. Ann Surg 180:393, 1974.

59. Goldfarb WB, Monafo W, McAlister WH: Clinical value of fistulography. Am J Surg 108:902, 1964.

60. Campos ACL, Andrade DF, Campos GMR, et al: A multivariate model to determine prognostic factors in gastrointestinal fistulas. J Am Coll Surg 188:483, 1999.

61. Williams NM, Scott NA, Irving MH: Successful management of external duodenal fistula in a specialized unit. Am J Surg 173:240, 1997.

62. Bardaxoglou E, Manganas D, Meunier B, et al: New approach to surgical management of early esophageal thoracic perforation: Primary suture repair reinforced with absorbable mesh and fibrin glue. World J Surg 21:618, 1997.

63. Lau WY, Leung KL, Kwong KH, et al: A randomized study comparing laparoscopic versus open repair of perforated peptic ulcer using suture or sutureless technique. Ann Surg 224:131, 1996.

64. Greenstein AJ, Kark AE, Drieling DA: Crohn's disease of the colon. Am J Gastroenterol 62:419, 1974.

65. Kirsh GM, Hampel N, Shuck JM, Resnick MI: Diagnosis and management of vesicoenteric fistulas. Surg Gynecol Obstet 173:91, 1991.

66. Bissada N, Cole AT, Fried FA: Reno-alimentary fistula: An unusual urological problem. J Urol 110:273, 1973.

67. Bigg RL, Jarolim C, Kram DD, Bessinger HE: Ruptured intestinal pregnancy causing massive rectal bleeding. Arch Surg 91:1021, 1965.

68. Reckless JPD, McColl I, Taylor GW: Aortoenteric fistulas: An uncommon complication of abdominal aortic aneurysms. Br J Surg 59:458, 1972.

69. O'Mara CS, Imbembo AL: Paraprosthetic-enteric fistula. Surgery 81:556, 1977.

70. Peck JJ, Eidemiller JR: Aortoenteric fistulas. Arch Surg 127:1191, 1992.

71. O'Mara CS, Williams GM, Ernst CB: Secondary aortoenteric fistula. Am J Surg 142:203, 1981.

72. Walker WE, Cooley DA, Duncan JM, et al: The management of aortoduodenal fistula by in situ replacement of the infected abdominal aortic graft. Ann Surg 205:727, 1987.

73. Vogt PR, Pfammatter T, Schlumpf R, et al: In situ repair of aortobronchial, aortoesophageal, and aortoenteric fistulae with cryopreserved aortic homografts. J Vasc Surg 26:11, 1997.

74. Bacourt F, Koskas F: Axillobifemoral bypass and aortic exclusion for vascular septic lesions: A multicenter retrospective study of 98 cases. French University Association for Research in Surgery. Ann Vasc Surg 6:119, 1992.

75. Vrijland WW, Tseng LN, Eijkman HJ, et al: Fewer intraperitoneal adhesions with use of hyaluronic acid–carboxymethylcellulose membrane: A randomized clinical trial. Ann Surg 235:193, 2002.

Internal Hernias— Congenital and Acquired

Mohammad K. Jamal · Eric J. DeMaria

Small bowel obstruction (SBO) is a common surgical emergency that accounts for nearly 20% of acute surgical admissions and often requires definitive operative treatment. The diagnosis of SBO is relatively straightforward in most instances and is based on a history of nausea, vomiting, and abdominal pain. Physical examination in most cases reveals vital signs suggestive of hypovolemia and a distended abdomen with high-pitched bowel sounds. The diagnosis of SBO is confirmed with plain radiographic films and in some instances computed tomography (CT) scans of the abdomen, which typically show air- and fluid-filled distended small bowel loops with or without a transition zone—denoting a complete or partial bowel obstruction.

Initial treatment of SBO involves nasogastric tube decompression, aggressive replacement of fluids, and correction of electrolyte imbalance. Surgical exploration should not be delayed because bowel incarceration or strangulation can occur. Strangulated obstructions are surgical emergencies and, if not diagnosed and properly treated, lead to vascular compromise resulting in bowel ischemia and further morbidity and mortality. Because as many as 40% of patients have strangulated obstructions, differentiating the characteristics and causes of obstruction is critical to proper patient treatment. The leading causes of SBO include adhesive disease (50% to 75%), malignancies (20%), abdominal wall hernias (10%), and inflammatory bowel disease (10%).

Internal hernias, either congenital or acquired, account for a small percentage of SBO cases (0.6% to 5.8%).[1-5] This condition involves herniation of a viscus, usually small bowel, through a normal or abnormal aperture within the peritoneal cavity. This herniation may be intermittent or persistent and may pose a diagnostic challenge given the rare nature of its occurrence. Only rarely is an internal hernia accurately diagnosed preoperatively. Because of the risk for strangulation of the hernia contents, even small internal hernias are dangerous and may be lethal. However, as a result of their rarity, discovery of an internal hernia at laparotomy may be confusing to an unsuspecting surgeon who is not familiar with this abnormality, and thus appropriate management may be compromised.

CONGENITAL INTERNAL HERNIAS

Congenital internal hernias are the result of malformation of the peritoneum and, in some instances, malrotation of the midgut during the embryonic period. A paraduodenal hernia (PDH) is the most common variety of congenital internal hernia, followed by the transmesenteric and transomental varieties. Others, including Foramen of Winslow and paracecal hernias, are extremely rare and are briefly discussed at the end of the section.

Paraduodenal Hernia

Also known as a paramesocolic hernia, PDH accounts for nearly 53% of the 500 published series of all internal hernias and was first described by Neubaur in 1786.[6-10] One hundred years later, Treitz and Waldeyer additionally described *hernia retroperitonealis*—several peritoneal folds and fossae through which small bowel could potentially herniate. The pathogenesis of PDH is controversial, but two theories regarding its origin appear to be most popular.[11] In a report by Moynihan in 1889, it was proposed that paraduodenal fossae were congenital and the hernia was acquired by gradual enlargement of an existing fossa. In 1923, Andrews disputed this theory and proposed that PDH forms as a result of a congenital anomaly in development of the peritoneum that arises during midgut rotation. As a consequence, small bowel becomes invaginated into an avascular, and therefore unsupported, segment of the left mesocolon. The resulting small bowel thus becomes trapped between the posterior abdominal wall, with the mesocolon and inferior

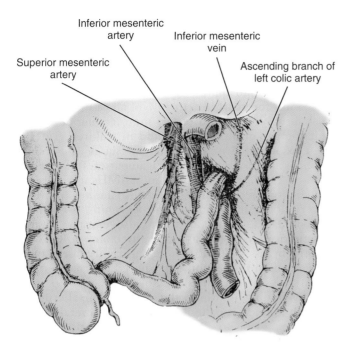

Figure 74–1. Left paraduodenal hernia. The opening of the hernia sac lies above the ascending branch of the left colic artery and the inferior mesenteric vein. The sac lies behind the left mesocolon. (From Newsom BD, Kukora JS: Congenital and acquired internal hernias: Unusual causes of small bowel obstruction. Am J Surg 152:279-285, 1986.)

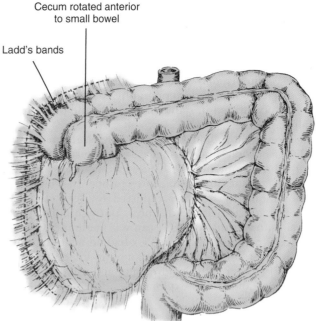

Figure 74–2. Right paraduodenal hernia. This hernia is caused by failure of the small bowel to rotate to the left with the right colon continuing to rotate anterior to it. This results in trapping of the small bowel behind the right mesocolon when fusion with the retroperitoneum occurs. The *dotted line* represents the plane opened to mobilize the right colon and reduce the hernia. (From Newsom BD, Kukora JS: Congenital and acquired internal hernias: Unusual causes of small bowel obstruction. Am J Surg 152:279-285, 1986.)

mesenteric vein (IMV) forming the anterior wall of the hernia sac.

Of the published cases of PDH, nearly 75% were left sided with a male-to-female ratio of 3:1.[11] The average age at diagnosis is reported to be between the third and fourth decades of life. A left PDH contains most of the small bowel, with the afferent limb being the fourth part of the duodenum and the efferent limb being the terminal ileum (Fig. 74–1). The small bowel invaginates into the fossa of Landzert, which lies to the left of the fourth portion of the duodenum. After formation of the hernia, the colon usually retains its normal position. Several other possibilities exist—the colon can undergo malrotation, the left colon can lie on the right side of the hernia, or if it is on a long mesentery, there is the potential for colonic volvulus.[12-14]

A right PDH similarly originates from abnormalities arising during the second phase of embryonic intestinal rotation; it results in arrest of further rotation of the pre-arterial segment of the gut in the right side of the abdomen (Fig. 74–2). Continued rotation of the postarterial segment leads to entrapment of small bowel behind the right colonic mesentery, with the superior mesenteric artery forming the anterior edge of the hernia sac.[15]

Clinical Findings

PDH may be asymptomatic and be discovered incidentally at laparotomy, at autopsy, or during radiologic studies for other unrelated causes.[11,16,17] More commonly, PDH is manifested as acute SBO on a background of recurrent chronic, vague abdominal pain. The abdominal pain associated with a left PDH is typically left sided but can be variable in location and sometimes even right sided.[18] The pain is often exacerbated by eating and postural changes and relieved by lying supine. It is postulated that the pain arises from recurrent incarceration of the hernia contents and is relieved by spontaneous reduction of the hernia.[5] Weight loss is variable and may be severe if symptoms are present for a long time. In its most malignant form, PDH may be associated with bowel strangulation with a resultant increase in death. On occasion, a tender left-sided abdominal mass may be palpable during an acute episode.

Diagnosis

The diagnosis of PDH generally requires a high index of suspicion and is usually made by upper gastrointestinal barium contrast study. The small bowel is found clustered to the left of the midline with a well-circumscribed edge that corresponds to the hernia sac.[5,11,19-21] Passage of contrast may be delayed with a change in position of the patient. There is usually a mass effect causing displacement of the posterior wall of the stomach, duodenojejunal flexure, and transverse colon. In some instances, a CT scan may detect a PDH by showing a similar clustering of small bowel loops in the retroperitoneum.[8,22] Upward displacement of the IMV by the hernia contents may also be noted on intravenously enhanced CT scans or arteriography.[5,22] A barium enema may be performed in stable patients to rule out colonic malrotation.

However, all radiologic studies may be normal, especially in chronic intermittent cases because the hernia may reduce spontaneously. These investigations are most often diagnostic during an acute episode. In a literature review of nearly 32 cases reported by Tong and colleagues,[22] a preoperative diagnosis through either small bowel follow-through or CT scan was made in 23 (72%) of the 32 patients, but 14 (61%) had an acute manifestation. Given the rarity of symptoms, an incidental diagnosis of PDH is relatively infrequent and usually made at the time of abdominal exploration.

Treatment

The lifetime risk for bowel incarceration associated with PDH is around 50%. Incarceration can result in increased morbidity and mortality, and therefore these hernias should be treated if found incidentally.[11,15,20,23] Treatment of PDH follows the basic principles of hernia surgery—reduction of the contents, resection of the hernia sac, restoration of normal bowel anatomy, and repair of the hernia defect. Initial exploration of the abdomen will often reveal the classic empty abdomen sign, with only a segment of the ileum present in the abdominal cavity and the remainder encased in the hernia sac to the left of the midline. The small bowel may be manually reduced if the hernia orifice is large enough and the defect can be closed with nonabsorbable suture.[11,23] If the small bowel is edematous, the hernia orifice is tight, or adhesions within the sac prevent manual reduction of the contents, the hernia orifice can be widened by excising the avascular plane to the right of the IMV. Care should be taken to avoid damage to this structure and the left colic artery, both of which lie in close proximity to the anterior edge of the orifice.[24]

If the hernia orifice cannot be widened, the sac should be opened along the anterior wall and the contents reduced. A decompressive enterotomy is sometimes beneficial to evacuate the contents of the incarcerated bowel, thus allowing easy reduction. The sac should then be excised from the left of the IMV toward the left colon while taking care to preserve the marginal artery of Drummond. In cases of obvious bowel strangulation, the appropriate length of small bowel should be resected and a decision made regarding reanastomosis or creation of an end ostomy, depending on the hemodynamic stability of the patient and the overall condition of the involved bowel segments.

More recently, several authors have reported laparoscopic repair of both right and left PDH.[19,25,26] However, the role of laparoscopy in the diagnosis and treatment of PDH is relatively recent, and to date, experience with this modality is limited.

Transmesenteric Hernia

A transmesenteric hernia (TMH) is an intraperitoneal hernia that may be either congenital or acquired. As the name suggests, TMH consists of protrusion of a loop of bowel through an aperture in the mesentery (Fig. 74–3). It accounts for nearly 5% to 10% of all cases of congenital internal hernia and occurs more commonly in the pediatric age group. When found in children, TMH is often associated with intestinal atresia or mesenteric ischemia and occurs near the ligament of Treitz or the ileocecal valve.[15,27] In contrast, most TMHs in adults are related to predisposing factors, including previous surgery, abdominal trauma, and peritonitis. A common type of TMH occurs after an iatrogenically created mesenteric defect, such as after gastrectomy or Roux-en-Y gastric bypass (RYGBP). These hernias are discussed in more detail in the section on acquired internal hernias.

TMH was first reported by Rokitansky in 1836 as an autopsy finding in which the cecum alone herniated through a hole near the ileocolic angle. Several others, including Loebl in 1844 and then Turel in 1932, described variations of TMH through the transverse mesocolon and sigmoid colon, respectively.[28] Several etiologic hypotheses for the occurrence of idiopathic mesenteric defects causing TMH have been proposed in the surgical literature, three of which have gained relative acceptance. Federschmidt in 1920 stated that these defects represented partial regression of the dorsal mesentery in humans. Menegaux, on the other hand, postulated the presence of fenestrations during developmental enlargement of an inadequately vascularized

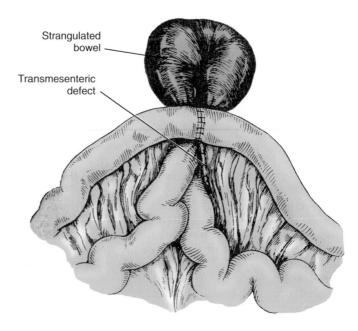

Strangulated bowel

Transmesenteric defect

Figure 74–3. Transmesenteric hernia caused by herniation of a loop of small bowel through an unclosed mesenteric defect after small bowel resection. (From Newsom BD, Kukora JS: Congenital and acquired internal hernias: Unusual causes of small bowel obstruction. Am J Surg 152:279-285, 1986.)

area as a cause of TMH. Judd, Kiebel, and Mall believed that because the greater part of the gut is displaced from the abdominal cavity into the umbilical cord in fetal life, considerable pressure might displace the colon along the path of least resistance and gradually force it through the delicate mesentery. Another theory by Macklin assumes that when two epithelial layers are apposed with a deficient intervening supportive stroma of connective tissue, coalescence inevitably takes place, with development of a space or defect.

There is no sex and age predominance in the occurrence of TMH. In a collective review by Janin et al., nearly 70% of reported TMHs occurred through defects in the small bowel mesentery.[28] Ileocecal defects accounted for 53% of these and 37% of the entire group of TMHs. These ileocolic defects are typically circular or oval, lie in the area of the mesentery between the ileocolic artery and the last ileal branch of the superior mesenteric artery, and range in size from 2 to 3 cm. Transverse mesocolic defects, on the other hand, are bound by the vascular arch formed by the middle and left colic arteries, whereas defects of the sigmoid mesocolon are usually circular and lie immediately above the superior rectal vessels.

Clinical Findings

The clinical manifestations of TMH are similar to those of any other case of SBO—crampy abdominal pain, nausea, vomiting, and abdominal distention. These patients most frequently have right-sided abdominal tenderness but, occasionally, diffuse pain accompanied by various degrees of abdominal distention is noted. Patients typically appear to be severely ill and may rapidly progress to a shock-like state concurrent with mesenteric ischemia and bowel necrosis. A palpable abdominal mass is sometimes present, usually sausage shaped and tympanitic, and a localized succession splash may be elicited over it.

Because most mesenteric defects are small and there is no limiting hernia sac, a large portion of the small bowel can herniate through a tight opening. The resulting pressure of the herniated bowel and its thickened mesentery compresses the vessels in the free margins of the mesenteric defect and results in early incarceration and strangulation of the loop forming the margin of the defect. This may explain why the latter may be found to be gangrenous whereas the herniated bowel may not even be strangulated. Furthermore, the herniated segment of bowel or a redundant sigmoid can freely undergo volvulus, a condition more commonly seen in TMH than in other types of internal hernias.

Diagnosis

TMHs are more difficult to diagnose than other internal hernias. Based on a history of bowel obstruction, a CT scan may show a cluster of small bowel loops, SBO, and central or posterior displacement of the colon. Mesenteric vessels may be stretched, crowded, and engorged and have a *whorl sign*. Furthermore, the major mesenteric trunk may be displaced by herniated small bowel loops. Signs of volvulus or mesenteric ischemia, including

bowel wall thickening, twisting of the mesenteric vessels (the whorl sign), engorged blood vessels, and mesenteric ascites, may be the predominant CT findings and denote a delayed diagnosis.[29,30] In patients with acquired TMH after gastrectomy or RYGBP, a retro-anastomotic TMH can be detected on CT scan as an abnormal position of an efferent loop of the gastrojejunostomy, an obstructed afferent or efferent loop (or both), or clumped and fixed jejunal loops in the left upper portion of the abdomen. Rarely, small bowel herniation occurs through a peritoneal defect in the pouch of Douglas as a result of previous hysterectomy.[29]

Treatment

Nasogastric decompression, aggressive preoperative fluid replacement, and correction of electrolyte disturbances are essential before surgical exploration. Laparotomy is mandated in all cases of TMH given the high incidence of incarceration and strangulation. Treatment is dependent on viability of the bowel—if the herniated loops are gangrenous, resection is mandatory, with or without primary anastomosis. If the bowel is viable, reduction of the incarcerated loops plus repair of the defect with interrupted nonabsorbable suture is recommended. Furthermore, if a mesenteric defect is discovered during laparotomy for an unrelated cause, it is imperative that it be closed with a similar technique.

Transomental Hernia

Transomental hernias typically represent less than 5% of all internal hernias. Only a handful of cases have been reported in the surgical literature.[15] As the name suggests, internal herniation of a viscus, typically small bowel, occurs through an opening in the gastrocolic omentum (Fig. 74–4). The actual cause of the omental rent is unknown, but inflammatory, traumatic, circulatory, and congenital mechanisms have all been implicated. A variant of this hernia, the *internal double omental hernia,* has been reported by some authors and denotes herniation of the small bowel through an opening in the gastrocolic omentum and exit through the gastrohepatic omentum.[31,32]

Management consists of simply releasing the constricting ring of omentum, which typically tends to be stiff and fibrous, and resecting or reducing the bowel, depending on its viability.[33,34]

Miscellaneous Congenital Internal Hernias

Foramen of Winslow hernias are rarely encountered. Only 117 cases have been reported in the world literature through 1977[35] (Fig. 74–5). In cases reported since 1966, the cecum was the most commonly herniated viscus, followed by the small bowel.[36] Preoperative diagnosis of a Foramen of Winslow hernia is generally established in less than 10% of cases. In some instances, an epigastric mass and radiographic evidence of a retrogastric mass containing air are suggestive of this entity.[9] Management involves manual reduction of the hernia

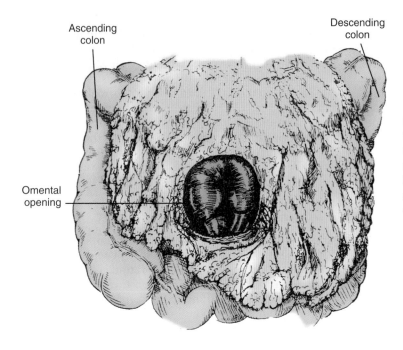

Ascending colon

Descending colon

Omental opening

Figure 74–4. Transomental hernia with strangulation of a loop of bowel through the transomental hernia defect. Management consists of simply cutting the constricting ring around the bowel and resection of involved bowel. (From Newsom BD, Kukora JS: Congenital and acquired internal hernias: Unusual causes of small bowel obstruction. Am J Surg 152:279-285, 1986.)

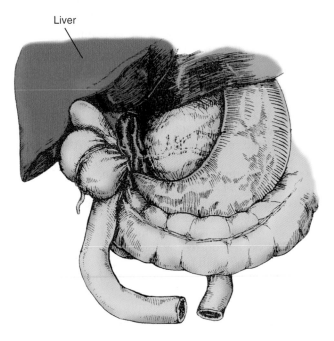

Liver

Figure 74–5. Foramen of Winslow hernia. The mobile right colon has been shown to be incarcerated through the opening into the lesser sac. The neck of the sac contains vital structures that must be preserved when repairing these hernias. (From Newsom BD, Kukora JS: Congenital and acquired internal hernias: Unusual causes of small bowel obstruction. Am J Surg 152:279-285, 1986.)

contents, which sometimes requires opening of the lesser sac for counterpressure or decompressive enterotomy. A wide Kocher maneuver may at times be necessary to enlarge the hernia opening. Attempts at closure of the opening are not generally recommended, although fixation of a mobile cecum is advised.[35,37-39]

Paracecal hernias, as well as herniation into fossae of the sigmoid mesentery, account for a small percentage of internal hernias. Others, including herniation through fossae or defects in the broad ligament and foramina in the falciform ligament, are extremely rare varieties of internal hernia.[40-43]

ACQUIRED INTERNAL HERNIAS

Acquired internal hernia (AIH) refers to herniation of a viscus, most commonly small intestine, through iatrogenically created defects in the peritoneum after major abdominal surgery, including Roux-en-Y reconstructions after gastrectomy, gastric bypass, esophageal replacement, and pancreatic and hepatobiliary surgery. With the recent increase in the number of certain bariatric surgical procedures performed in the United States, especially RYGBP, the incidence of AIH has risen in recent years. Therefore, herniation after gastric bypass will be discussed in this section as a representative AIH.

Nearly 150,000 bariatric surgical procedures are performed in the United States each year, the majority of which involve RYGBP. With the advent of minimally invasive techniques, the associated morbidity with this relatively high-risk procedure has decreased somewhat. When compared with the open procedure, there has been a reduction in incision-related complications such as wound infections and incisional hernias after laparoscopic gastric bypass; other complications, including the risk for anastomotic leak and SBO, have remained essentially unchanged or have increased in certain series. SBO is a known complication of gastric bypass surgery, with an incidence varying anywhere from 1.3% to 5% in several series of experienced bariatric surgeons using the open technique.[44-48] The incidence of bowel obstruction

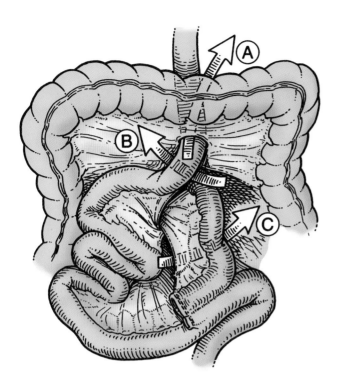

Figure 74–6. Internal hernia after a retrocolic Roux-en-Y gastric bypass. Potential sites of internal herniation of small bowel include the mesocolic mesenteric defect (A), the Petersen defect (B), and the jejunojejunostomy mesenteric defect (C). (From Schweitzer MA, DeMaria EJ, Broderick TH, Sugerman HJ: Laparoscopic closure of mesenteric defects after Roux-en-Y gastric bypass. J Laparoendosc Adv Surg Tech A 10:173-175, 2000.)

appears to be similar in earlier series of laparoscopic gastric bypass—anywhere from 1.5% to 3.5%, with most obstructions caused by internal hernias.[49,50] Other unrelated causes of SBO in gastric bypass patients include adhesions, incarcerated ventral hernias, and rarely, intussusception of the jejunojejunostomy.

The technique of laparoscopic gastric bypass has not been standardized, and there are several variations in the technique. The laparoscopic approach may involve the use of a circular stapler, linear stapler, or a hand-sewn technique for the two anastomoses; the Roux limb may be placed in antecolic or retrocolic fashion, with or without closure of the mesenteric defect; the enterotomies may be closed by suture or staples; and finally, the trocar sites may or may not be closed. It is closure of the several different mesenteric defects that may prevent internal herniation of small bowel in these patients. Internal herniation in gastric bypass patients can occur through any of the two mesenteric defects when an antecolic approach is used and through any of the three defects when a retrocolic approach is used. These potential hernia defects occur at the jejunojejunostomy, the mesocolic window, and Petersen's space (Fig. 74–6).

An enteroenterostomy mesenteric defect is created as a standard step in essentially all variations of gastric bypass, and in our practice, it is closed with a running absorbable suture. If an antecolic approach is used, an opening is created in the gastrocolic omentum, and the Roux limb is brought over in an antecolic and antegastric fashion. If the greater omentum is especially thin, the Roux limb can be passed anterior to it without a window. In the retrocolic approach, a window is created in the transverse mesocolon, and the Roux limb is brought through the lesser sac in retrogastric fashion to the transected pouch. Mesenteric defects are again routinely closed in our practice with running absorbable suture, beginning at the medial edge of the mesocolic window and running superiorly over the Roux limb, with incorporation of the bowel serosa and closure of the base of the Petersen defect.

The debate between proponents of antecolic and retrocolic gastric bypass continues among bariatric surgeons. Several authors have reported a higher incidence of internal hernia after laparoscopic RYGBP—this difference is probably explained by the absence of adhesion formation after a minimally invasive approach.[51-53] In the series reported by Champion and Williams, the incidence of SBO from all causes was 4.5% in the retrocolic group and 0.43% in the antecolic group.[51] Seventy-one percent of the obstructions in this group of 711 patients were caused by internal hernias. Furthermore, the incidence of bowel obstruction in the group with sutured mesenteric defects was slightly lower (4.1%) than in those with an unsutured mesenteric defect (4.5%). In another report by Higa et al., the incidence of SBO from an internal hernia was 3.1% in a group of 63 patients undergoing retrocolic RYGBP.[52] The site of internal hernias varied—they occurred at the mesocolon (70%), jejunal mesentery (22%), and Petersen's space (8%) in that order. Although most patients were symptomatic, 5% of internal hernias were incidental findings at the time of another surgical procedure.

Clinical Findings

The diagnosis of AIH is difficult, and radiologic evaluation is often nondiagnostic. The presence of colicky, postprandial left upper quadrant abdominal pain after gastric bypass should raise suspicion of an obstruction. The location of the abdominal pain generally correlates with the side of internal herniation, with left upper quadrant pain occurring when the small bowel herniates through the defect to the patient's left side and right upper quadrant pain typically being seen when the small bowel herniates to the right side of the defect. Other symptoms may include nausea, emesis, and abdominal distention. Although similar symptoms may be seen in other pathologic conditions, including a marginal ulcer or SBO from other causes, persistence of such symptoms, even in the absence of radiologic findings, generally mandates exploration.

Diagnosis

Patients with acute intermittent abdominal pain should be evaluated initially with plain films. An obstructed bowel gas pattern with air-fluid levels is sometimes enough evidence of an internal hernia that urgent exploration is required. Others with vague abdominal pain can be investigated with contrast-enhanced upper gastrointestinal series with small bowel follow-through or CT, or with both. A high index of suspicion is required for proper diagnosis and management of these patients. In a series reported by Blachar et al., 463 patients were investigated for complications after RYGBP.[54] The incidence of internal hernia after gastric bypass was 3%, whereas SBO from other causes developed in nine patients.

Several important features diagnostic of internal hernia that are found on upper gastrointestinal series include a cluster of small bowel loops seen in the mid or left upper portion of the abdomen.[54] This cluster is relatively fixed and remains high on erect radiographs, which reveal stasis and delay in passage of contrast material. The CT appearance of internal hernias often depends on their location, although clustering of dilated small bowel loops with crowding and congestion of the mesenteric vessels is seen in all instances. In cases of herniation through the transverse mesocolon, the herniated cluster of bowel is located posterior relative to the stomach and may exert a mass effect on its posterior wall. Furthermore, herniations through the small bowel mesentery cause the clustered bowel to press against the abdominal wall with no overlying omental fat and thereby result in central displacement of the colon. A Peterson-type hernia is difficult to diagnose because it has neither a confining sac nor a characteristic location, and the only clues to its presence may be engorgement and crowding of the mesenteric vessels and evidence of SBO.

Treatment

On diagnosis of AIH, exploration is mandatory and can be performed laparoscopically by experienced surgeons with minimal morbidity and complications.[51,52,55,56] The biliopancreatic limb and the common channel should be run from the ligament of Treitz to the ileocecal valve. The Roux limb should be identified and the entire length run from the gastrojejunostomy to the enteric anastomosis. Any herniated segment of small bowel should be reduced, and any mesocolic and jejunojejunostomy mesenteric defects should be closed with nonabsorbable running suture. Controversy exists regarding closure of Petersen's defect, with some authors recommending interrupted closure of this mesenteric defect to prevent internal herniation postoperatively.

REFERENCES

1. Blachar A, Federle MP, Brancatelli G, et al: Radiologist performance in the diagnosis of internal hernia by using specific CT findings with emphasis on transmesenteric hernia. Radiology 221:422-428, 2001.
2. Leffall LD Jr, Quander J, Syphax B: Strangulation intestinal obstruction. Arch Surg 91:592-596, 1965.
3. Bizer LS, Liebling RW, Delany HM, Gliedman ML: Small bowel obstruction: The role of nonoperative treatment in simple intestinal obstruction and predictive criteria for strangulation obstruction. Surgery 89:407-413, 1981.
4. Passas V, Karavias D, Grilias D, Birbas A: Computed tomography of left paraduodenal hernia. J Comput Assist Tomogr 10:542-543, 1986.
5. Meyers MA: Paraduodenal hernias. Radiologic and arteriographic diagnosis. Radiology 95:29-37, 1970.
6. Miller PA, Mezwa DG, Feczko PJ, et al: Imaging of abdominal hernias. Radiographics 15:333-347, 1995.
7. Warshauer DM, Mauro MA: CT diagnosis of paraduodenal hernia. Gastrointest Radiol 17:13-15, 1992.
8. Day DL, Drake DG, Leonard AS, Letourneau JG: CT findings in left paraduodenal herniae. Gastrointest Radiol 13:27-29, 1988.
9. Harbin WP: Computed tomographic diagnosis of internal hernia. Radiology 143:736, 1982.
10. Bell-Thomson J, Vieta JO, Yiavasis AA: Paraduodenal hernias. Am J Gastroenterol 68:254-259, 1977.
11. Berardi RS: Paraduodenal hernias. Surg Gynecol Obstet 152:99-110, 1981.
12. Hirasaki S, Koide N, Shima Y, et al: Unusual variant of left paraduodenal hernia herniated into the mesocolic fossa leading to jejunal strangulation. J Gastroenterol 33:734-738, 1998.
13. Luosto R, Ketonen P: Left paraduodenal hernia with chronic abdominal symptoms. Acta Chir Scand 144:263-265, 1978.
14. Bartlett MK, Wang C, Williams WH: The surgical management of paraduodenal hernia. Ann Surg 168:249-254, 1968.
15. Newsom BD, Kukora JS: Congenital and acquired internal hernias: Unusual causes of small bowel obstruction. Am J Surg 152:279-285, 1986.
16. Osadchy A, Keidar A, Zissin R: Small bowel obstruction due to a paracecal hernia: Computerized tomography diagnosis. Emerg Radiol 11:239-241, 2005.
17. Patti R, Arcara M, Davi V, et al: Paraduodenal hernia: An uncommon cause of recurrent abdominal pain. G Chir 25:183-186, 2004.
18. Tong RS, Sengupta S, Tjandra JJ: Left paraduodenal hernia: Case report and review of the literature. Aust N Z J Surg 72:69-71, 2002.
19. Uematsu T, Kitamura H, Iwase M, et al: Laparoscopic repair of a paraduodenal hernia. Surg Endosc 12:50-52, 1998.
20. Brigham RA, Fallon WF, Saunders JR, et al: Paraduodenal hernia: Diagnosis and surgical management. Surgery 96:498-502, 1984.
21. Patil R, Smith C, Brown MD: Paraduodenal hernia presenting as unexplained recurrent abdominal pain. Am J Gastroenterol 94:3614-3615, 1999.
22. Schaffler GJ, Groell R, Kammerhuber F, et al: Anterior and upward displacement of the inferior mesenteric vein: A new diagnostic clue to left paraduodenal hernias? Abdom Imaging 24:29-31, 1999.
23. Davis R: Surgery of left paraduodenal hernia. Am J Surg 129:570-573, 1975.
24. Campanale RP, Cavanagh MJ: Left paraduodenal hernia. Am J Surg 91:436-440, 1956.
25. Antedomenico E, Singh NN, Zagorski SM, et al: Laparoscopic repair of a right paraduodenal hernia. Surg Endosc 18:165-166, 2004.
26. Rollins MD, Glasgow RE: Left paraduodenal hernia. J Am Coll Surg 198:492-493, 2004.
27. Zarvan NP, Lee FT Jr, Yandow DR, Unger JS: Abdominal hernias: CT findings. AJR Am J Roentgenol 164:1391-1395, 1995.
28. Janin Y, Stone AM, Wise L: Mesenteric hernia. Surg Gynecol Obstet 150:747-754, 1980.
29. Inoue Y, Shibata T, Ishida T: CT of internal hernia through a peritoneal defect of the pouch of Douglas. AJR Am J Roentgenol 179:1305-1306, 2002.
30. Blachar A, Federle MP, Dodson SF: Internal hernia: Clinical and imaging findings in 17 patients with emphasis on CT criteria. Radiology 218:68-74, 2001.
31. Talebpour M, Habibi GR, Bandarian F: Laparoscopic management of an internal double omental hernia: A rare cause of intestinal obstruction. Hernia 9:195-197, 2005.
32. See JY, Ong AW, Iau PT, Chan ST: Double omental hernia—case report on a very rare cause of intestinal obstruction. Ann Acad Med Singapore 31:799-801, 2002.
33. Leissner KH: Transomental strangulation. A rare case of an internal hernia. Acta Chir Scand 142:483-485, 1976.
34. Iuchtman M, Berant M, Assa J: Transomental strangulation. J Pediatr Surg 13:439-440, 1978.

35. Ohkuma R, Miyazaki K: Hernia through the foramen of Winslow. Jpn J Surg 7:151-157, 1977.

36. Richardson JB, Anastopoulos HA: Hernia through the foramen of Winslow. Md State Med J 30(11):56-59, 1981.

37. Cohen DJ, Schoolnik ML: Herniation through the foramen of Winslow. Dis Colon Rectum 25:820-822, 1982.

38. Sorin B, Paineau J, Heloury Y, et al: Hernia through the foramen of Winslow. Report of a cecal hernia. Ann Radiol (Paris) 25:217-221, 1982.

39. Erskine JM: Hernia through the foramen of Winslow. A case report of the cecum incarcerated in the lesser omental cavity. Am J Surg 114:941-947, 1967.

40. Chapman VM, Rhea JT, Novelline RA: Internal hernia through a defect in the broad ligament: A rare cause of intestinal obstruction. Emerg Radiol 10:94-95, 2003.

41. Andren-Sandberg A, Ihse I: False hernias through parametric defects. A report of two cases. Acta Chir Scand 147:381-382, 1981.

42. Blunt A, Rich GF: Intestinal strangulation through an aperture in the falciform ligament. Aust N Z J Surg 37:310, 1968.

43. Miller BJ: Falciform ligament aperture causing intestinal strangulation. Can J Surg 24:401-402, 1981.

44. Fobi MA, Lee H, Holness R, Cabinda D: Gastric bypass operation for obesity. World J Surg 22:925-935, 1998.

45. Fernandez AZ Jr, DeMaria EJ, Tichansky DS, et al: Experience with over 3,000 open and laparoscopic bariatric procedures: Multivariate analysis of factors related to leak and resultant mortality. Surg Endosc 18:193-197, 2004.

46. DeMaria EJ, Jamal MK: Surgical options for obesity. Gastroenterol Clin North Am 34:127-142, 2005.

47. MacLean LD, Rhode BM, Nohr CW: Late outcome of isolated gastric bypass. Ann Surg 231:524-528, 2000.

48. Halverson JD, Zuckerman GR, Koehler RE, et al: Gastric bypass for morbid obesity: A medical-surgical assessment. Ann Surg 194:152-160, 1981.

49. Higa KD, Boone KB, Ho T, Davies OG: Laparoscopic Roux-en-Y gastric bypass for morbid obesity: Technique and preliminary results of our first 400 patients. Arch Surg 135:1029-1033, 2000.

50. Schauer PR, Ikramuddin S, Gourash W, et al: Outcomes after laparoscopic Roux-en-Y gastric bypass for morbid obesity. Ann Surg 232:515-529, 2000.

51. Champion JK, Williams M: Small bowel obstruction and internal hernias after laparoscopic Roux-en-Y gastric bypass. Obes Surg 13:596-600, 2003.

52. Higa KD, Ho T, Boone KB: Internal hernias after laparoscopic Roux-en-Y gastric bypass: Incidence, treatment and prevention. Obes Surg 13:350-354, 2003.

53. Garza E Jr, Kuhn J, Arnold D, et al: Internal hernias after laparoscopic Roux-en-Y gastric bypass. Am J Surg 188:796-800, 2004.

54. Blachar A, Federle MP, Pealer KM, et al: Gastrointestinal complications of laparoscopic Roux-en-Y gastric bypass surgery: Clinical and imaging findings. Radiology 223:625-632, 2002.

55. Quebbemann BB, Dallal RM: The orientation of the antecolic Roux limb markedly affects the incidence of internal hernias after laparoscopic gastric bypass. Obes Surg 15:766-770, 2005.

56. Cho M, Carrodeguas L, Pinto D, et al: Diagnosis and management of partial small bowel obstruction after laparoscopic antecolic antegastric Roux-en-Y gastric bypass for morbid obesity. J Am Coll Surg 202:262-268, 2006.

75

Mesenteric Arterial Trauma

Rao R. Ivatury

EPIDEMIOLOGY

Injuries to the mesenteric arteries are rare and occur in less than 1% of all trauma admissions. No mesenteric arterial injuries were found in a collective review of 3705 arterial injuries from World War II, the Korean War, and the Vietnam War, as reported by DeBakey and Simeone, Hughes, and Rich and associates.[1-3] This rarity is also substantiated by civilian series reported by several authors.[4-16] In a recent multi-institutional study, Asensio and colleagues[16] could collect only 250 patients with these injuries over a period of 10 years from 34 participating trauma centers. It is evident that even an established trauma surgeon may not have a large experience dealing with these difficult lesions.

SURGICAL ANATOMY

The superior mesenteric artery (SMA) originates about 1.5 cm below the celiac axis and is the second branch of the abdominal aorta; it is located at approximately the level of L1. Surrounded by the portal vein, pancreas, and duodenum, the SMA soon disappears under the neck of the pancreas. The zones of the artery as described by Fullen and associates[7] in 1972 were based on the collateral circulation and the extent of ischemia resulting from injury or ligation of the different portions of the artery (Fig. 75–1). Zone I extends from the origin of the artery at the aorta to the first major branch (inferior pancreaticoduodenal artery). Loss of this portion of the artery leads to maximal ischemia. Zone II extends from the inferior pancreaticoduodenal artery to the origin of the middle colic artery. Injuries in this area lead to severe ischemia. Zone III extends distal to the origin of the middle colic artery to the origin of the segmental branches. Zone IV is the region of the artery termed by segmental names: ileocolic, right colic, and so forth. The collateral circulation of the SMA is not as well developed as that of the celiac axis and the inferior mesenteric artery (IMA). Superior and inferior pancreaticoduodenal branches of the celiac axis and the SMA and the marginal artery of Drummond between the SMA and IMA are the usual collateral channels. These vessels, however, are inconstant and variable, thus making the SMA essentially an end artery.

OPERATIVE EXPOSURE AND MANAGEMENT DECISIONS

Operative exposure of the SMA is very difficult because of its high location and a dense celiac plexus and lymphatics around the origin of the artery. Active bleeding from the region behind the pancreas may be an indication of SMA injury in zone I. This zone is best approached by dividing the pancreas at its neck anterior to the mesenteric vessels. Further exposure is facilitated by medial visceral rotation (Figs. 75–2 and 75–3). Rotation is commenced by incising the avascular line of Toldt on the left colon, dividing the lienosplenic ligament, and rotating the left colon, spleen, tail and body of the pancreas, and stomach toward the midline. The left kidney may also be mobilized and reflected medially (Mattox maneuver) to gain access to the proximal infradiaphragmatic aorta and its first two branches (the celiac axis and SMA). Transection of the dense celiac and peripancreatic venous plexus is also required. This medial visceral rotation, especially when the left kidney is included, does take time and experience to perform. Potential pitfalls are damage to the spleen, kidney, and renal pedicle during the maneuver. In addition, the resulting altered anatomy may prove confusing to an inexperienced operator.

Injuries with hematoma below the transverse mesocolon can be approached by several methods. Dividing the mesocolon and performing an extended Kocher maneuver with extension along the third portion of the duodenum allow one to palpate the SMA. The Cattell-Braasch maneuver, in which the root of the small bowel mesentery is dissected in a diagonal line to the junction of the third and fourth portions of the duodenum and reflected cephalad, also exposes the SMA pulsations for dissection and isolation. Injuries to the distal zones of the

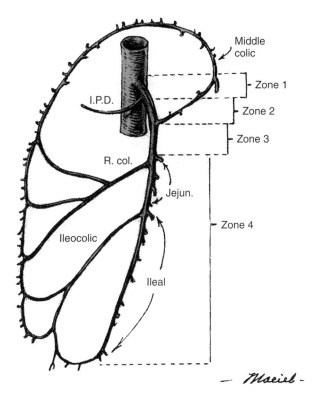

Figure 75–1. Fullen's anatomic classification of injuries to the superior mesenteric artery based on the location of the injury in relation to the main arterial branches. I.P.D., inferior pancreaticoduodenal artery; R. col., right colic artery. (From Fullen WD, Hunt J, Altemeier WA: The clinical spectrum of penetrating injury to the superior mesenteric arterial circulation. J Trauma 12:656-663, 1972.)

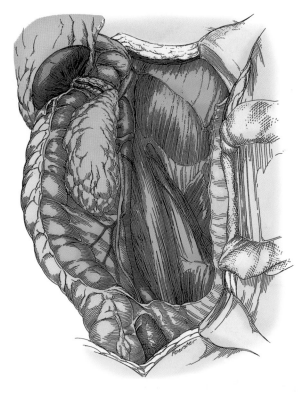

Figure 75–2. Left medial visceral rotation. The descending colon, left kidney, spleen, and distal pancreas are mobilized en bloc to expose the suprarenal aorta in the retroperitoneum. (From Rutherford RB: Atlas of Vascular Surgery—Basic Techniques and Exposures. Philadelphia, WB Saunders, 1993.)

SMA can be approached directly. The frequent presence of associated injuries to other abdominal vessels and intra-abdominal organs and the severe associated hypotension may make it necessary to compress the aorta under the diaphragm while the patient is resuscitated with transfusions. Aortic compression can be performed initially with a sponge stick or the assistant's fingers. Longer periods of compression may necessitate enlargement of the aortic isthmus in the diaphragm, mobilization of the aorta, and the application of a Satinsky clamp (Fig. 75–4). The dense celiac plexus of nerves and lymphatics and the long hiatal fibers of the diaphragm make the dissection difficult and time-consuming. One useful technique is to divide the left crus of the diaphragm at the 2-o'clock position, widen the aortic isthmus, bluntly dissect the distal portion of the thoracic aorta, and then apply a clamp on the suprarenal aorta.[5] A left anterolateral thoracotomy and occlusion of the descending aorta may be faster and easier.

Frequently, these patients will have major associated injuries causing extensive blood loss and hemodynamic instability. Onset of the critical "triad of death," namely, hypothermia, acidosis, and coagulopathy, is often the rule rather than the exception and is precipitated by associated abdominal injuries, multiple transfusions, the need for aortic compression, and dilutional coagulop-

athy. In these circumstances, it is prudent to institute "damage control" principles.[17] Rapid termination of the laparotomy is the goal. Ligation of the SMA is usually reserved as a means to control life-threatening hemorrhage or exsanguination in these circumstances. The morbidity associated with SMA ligation is high, but because the patient may not tolerate a prolonged vascular replacement at this time of physiologic exhaustion, placement of a temporary arterial shunt between the ends of the divided SMA is the preferred approach.[18] Javed shunts or any vascular shunt available in the operating room will serve the purpose. If none is immediately available, intravenous infusion tubing will be a good substitute. This will maintain SMA flow distally and avoid mesenteric ischemia. These shunts are well tolerated for at least 24 hours. A heparin-bonded shunt, if available, is another option. Control of contamination is achieved by rapid closure of bowel perforations. In these patients the abdomen is usually left "open" by the placement of a "Vac-Pac" dressing. The patient is transferred to the intensive care unit (ICU) for resuscitation. This ICU phase of "damage control" will focus on correction of the hypothermia, acidosis, and coagulopathy. Acidosis is reversed by aggressive blood and fluid resuscitation. It must be remembered that ligation of the SMA and superior mesenteric vein (SMV) may cause profound bowel

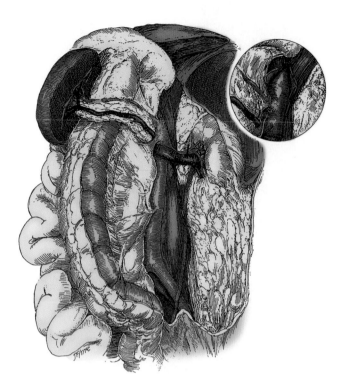

Figure 75–3.   Modified left medial visceral rotation. The left kidney is left in situ in the retroperitoneum while the rest of the viscera are mobilized. With division of the left crus of the diaphragm *(inset),* this maneuver gives better exposure of the proximal celiac axis and superior mesenteric artery. (From Rutherford RB: Atlas of Vascular Surgery—Basic Techniques and Exposures. Philadelphia, WB Saunders, 1993.)

Table 75–1	Survival After Superior Mesenteric Artery Injury	
Author	**No. of Patients**	**No. of Survivors (%)**
Fullen, 1972	8	5 (62.5%)
Graham, 1978	45	27 (60.6%)
Lucas, 1981	15	10 (66.7%)
Kashuk, 1982	6	4 (66.7%)
Sirinek, 1983	20	14 (70%)
Accola, 1986	22	7 (31.8%)
Asensio, 2000	28	13 (46.4%)
Davis, 2001	15	8 (53.3%)
Tyburski, 2001	41	20 (48.8%)
Asensio, 2001	250	153 (61.2%)
Total	*450*	*261 (58%)*

Adapted from Feliciano DV: Injury to abdominal aorta and visceral arteries. In Rich NM, Mattox KL, Hirshberg A (eds): Vascular Trauma, 2nd ed. Philadelphia, Elsevier, 2004, pp 219-314.

edema and increase the need for massive volume replenishment. Intra-abdominal hypertension and abdominal compartment syndrome are common complications in these circumstances and must be carefully watched for by frequent measurement of bladder pressure as a surrogate for intra-abdominal pressure.[19] It is our practice to perform decompressive laparotomy if bladder pressure is greater than 20 mm Hg with organ dysfunction.

More definitive SMA repair is usually undertaken at the second laparotomy, when the patient is in a better physiologic state. Injuries to zone III and beyond the middle colic branch and those at the origin of zone IV before the origin of the enteric branches should be repaired primarily. Distal zone IV injuries involving segmental branches to the small and large bowel may be ligated. Only occasionally it is possible to perform lateral arteriorrhaphy of the SMA. Bypass grafting to the proximal SMA is ideally performed as a short graft taken directly off the infrarenal aorta. SMA bypass may be performed safely with a synthetic graft, even in the face of a contaminated field,[5] unless the injury involves a high-velocity missile. This graft is routed through the root of the mesentery of the small bowel to anastomose with the mid or distal part of the SMA.[5] It is imperative that the aortic suture line be protected from adjacent bowel by omentum or a retroperitoneal flap to prevent an aortoenteric fistula in the future.[5] After successful mesenteric revascularization, bowel viability must be critically assessed. There is no single good test to determine bowel viability after revascularization. Ballard and associates[20] found that in patients who were revascularized for acute mesenteric ischemia, the overall accuracy of clinical judgment, intravenous fluorescein, and intraoperative Doppler was 50%, 56%, and 0%, respectively. Bulkley and colleagues[21] also found fluorescein to be the best tool to assess viability. A recent study reported that clinical judgment alone had an overall accuracy of 87% and a predictive value of only 69% versus 100% overall accuracy, sensitivity, and predictive value for laser Doppler flow measurements of the bowel mucosa.[22] There should be a low threshold for second-look or third-look laparotomy, especially if the patient fails to improve in the early postoperative period.

RESULTS

As indicated earlier, SMA injury is rare and the majority of series in the literature included less than 25 patients per report (Table 75–1). A recent study of these injuries, conducted under the auspices of the multi-institutional trials committee of the American Association for the Surgery of Trauma, was published by Asensio and coauthors. This is the largest series yet reported, and 250 patients were analyzed during a 10-year period from 34 participating centers. The majority of SMA injuries occurred as a result of penetrating trauma (52%) and were predominantly in Fullen zone IV (112). Zone I, II, and III injuries totaled 51, 35, and 42, respectively. Twenty-two percent of patients underwent primary repair, and 16 (7%) underwent interposition grafts consisting of 10 (4%) autogenous reverse saphenous vein grafts and 6 (2%) polytetrafluoroethylene grafts. Forty-four of 206 patients (21%) underwent planned second-look procedures, and 9 died during their hospitalization.

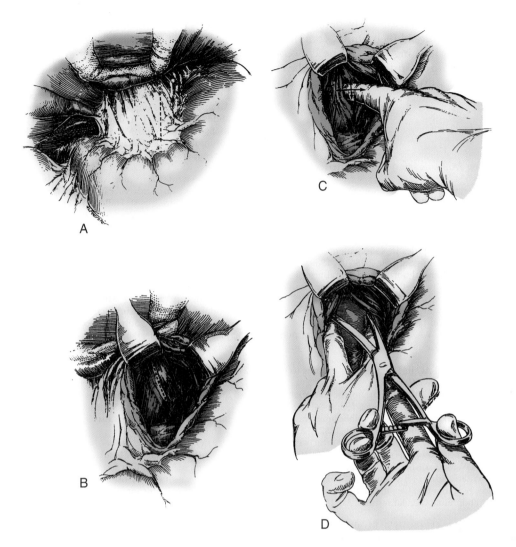

Figure 75–4.   Sequential maneuvers for rapid exposure of the supraceliac aorta. **A,** Longitudinal opening in the lesser omentum. **B,** Blunt dissection of the left crural fibers. **C,** Freeing of the aorta from the surrounding loose areolar tissue with a finger. **D,** Guiding the occluding vascular clamp in over two fingers until its tips "touch bottom" on the vertebral body behind the aorta. (From Rutherford RB: Atlas of Vascular Surgery—Basic Techniques and Exposures. Philadelphia, WB Saunders, 1993.)

Overall mortality was 39% (97 of 250); of these patients, 69 (71%) died in the operating room or within the first 24 hours of admission, either from exsanguination or injury-related causes; the other 28 patients (29%) succumbed as a result of complications in the postoperative period. As might be expected, Fullen zone I injuries had the highest mortality (76.5%). This report should be carefully studied for its detailed account of the outcome after these injuries.

Interesting case reports describe some sequelae from injury to the superior mesenteric vessels.[23-28] Radonic et al.[23] described two cases of SMA-SMV fistula from penetrating trauma that were diagnosed by angiography and treated operatively. Deitrick et al.[26] reported a proximal SMA–portal vein fistula that was embolized by angiographic methods. Miglietta et al.[27] presented a case of traumatic SMA–duodenal fistula from a gunshot wound of the abdomen. At the initial laparotomy a hematoma around the SMA was not explored. One month later the

patient experienced massive upper gastrointestinal hemorrhage. Immediate exploratory laparotomy revealed a large fistula between the SMA and the duodenum, but the patient could not be resuscitated after an intraoperative cardiac arrest. These cases illustrate the importance of careful exploration of the SMA and its surrounding hematoma at the initial laparotomy.

In summary, injuries to the mesenteric arteries are associated with high mortality. Most result from penetrating trauma, but blunt injury, usually to the SMA, does occur. Proximal injuries to the celiac artery or SMA are manifested as intraperitoneal bleeding or a central retroperitoneal hematoma. All central retroperitoneal hematomas should be explored so that major vascular injuries are not missed. In cases of extreme blood loss with accompanying coagulopathy, acidosis, and hypothermia, damage control principles yield the best results, with temporary intravascular shunting of the SMA being the preferred approach. Planned second- and third-look laparotomy is crucial for early detection of bowel nonviability. Interventional techniques, combined with improved abdominal imaging, can also be effective in avoiding laparotomy entirely and dealing with delayed complications such as arteriovenous fistulas and pseudoaneurysms.

REFERENCES

1. DeBakey ME, Simeone FA: Battle injuries of the arteries in World War II. Ann Surg 123:534-579, 1946.
2. Hughes CW: Arterial repair during the Korean War. Ann Surg 147:555-561, 1958.
3. Rich NM, Baugh JH, Hughes CW: Acute arterial injuries in Vietnam: 1,000 cases. J Trauma 10:359-369, 1970.
4. Mattox KL, Feliciano DV, Burch J, et al: Five thousand seven hundred sixty cardiovascular injuries in 4459 patients: Epidemiologic evolution 1958 to 1987. Ann Surg 209:698-705, 1989.
5. Feliciano DV: Injury to abdominal aorta and visceral arteries. In Rich NM, Mattox KL, Hirshberg A (eds): Vascular Trauma, 2nd ed. Philadelphia, Elsevier, 2004, pp 219-314.
6. Asensio JA, Berne JD, Chahwan S, et al: Traumatic injury to the superior mesenteric artery. Am J Surg 178:235-239, 1999.
7. Fullen WD, Hunt J, Altemeier WA: The clinical spectrum of penetrating injury to the superior mesenteric artery circulation. J Trauma 12:656-664, 1972.
8. Graham JM, Mattox KL, Beall AC Jr, DeBakey ME: Injuries to the visceral arteries. Surgery 84:835-839, 1978.
9. Lucas AE, Richardson JD, Flint LM, et al: Traumatic injury of the proximal superior mesenteric artery. Ann Surg 193:30-34, 1981.
10. Kashuk JL, Moore EE, Millikan JS, et al: Major abdominal vascular trauma: A unified approach. J Trauma 22:672-679, 1982.
11. Sirinek KR, Gaskill HV 3rd, Root HD, et al: Truncal vascular injury—factors influencing survival. J Trauma 23:372-377, 1983.
12. Accola KD, Feliciano DV, Mattox KL, et al: Management of injuries to the superior mesenteric artery. J Trauma 26:313-319, 1986.
13. Asensio JA, Chahwan S, Hanpeter D, et al: Operative management and outcome of 302 abdominal vascular injuries. Am J Surg 80:528-533, 2000.
14. Davis TP, Feliciano DV, Rozycki GS, et al: Results with abdominal vascular trauma in the modern era. Am Surg 67:565-570, 2001.
15. Tyburski JG, Wilson RF, Dente C, et al: Factors affecting mortality rates in patients with abdominal vascular injuries. J Trauma 50:1020-1026, 2001.
16. Asensio JA, Britt LD, Borzotta A, et al: Multiinstitutional experience with the management of superior mesenteric artery injuries. J Am Coll Surg 193:354-366, 2001.
17. Rotondo MF, Schwab CW, McGonigal MD, et al: "Damage control": An approach for improved survival in exsanguinating penetrating abdominal injury. J Trauma 35:375-382, discussion 382-383, 1993.
18. Reilly PM, Rotondo MF, Carpenter JP, et al: Temporary vascular continuity during damage control: Intraluminal shunting for proximal superior mesenteric artery injury. J Trauma 39:757-760, 1995.
19. Ivatury RR, Cheatham M, Malbrain M, Sugrue M: Abdominal compartment syndrome. Available at http://www.eurekah.com/categories.php?catid=83&category=SURGERY.
20. Ballard JL, Stone WM, Hallett JW, et al: A critical analysis of adjuvant techniques used to assess bowel viability in acute mesenteric ischemia. Am Surg 59:309-311, 1993.
21. Bulkley GB, Zuidema GD, Hamilton SR, et al: Intraoperative determination of small intestinal viability following ischemic injury: A prospective, controlled trial of two adjuvant methods (Doppler and fluorescein) compared with standard clinical judgment. Ann Surg 193:628-637, 1981.
22. Redaelli CA, Schilling MK, Buchler MW: Intraoperative laser Doppler flowmetry: A predictor of ischemic injury in acute mesenteric infarction Dig Surg 15:55-59, 1998.
23. Radonic V, Baric D, Petrucevic A, et al: Advances in diagnostics and successful repair of proximal posttraumatic superior mesenteric arteriovenous fistula. J Trauma 38:305-312, 1995.
24. Reed JK, McGiin RF, Gorman JF, Thomford NR: Traumatic mesenteric arteriovenous fistula presenting as the superior mesenteric artery syndrome. Arch Surg 121:1209, 1986.
25. Saunders MS, Riberi A, Massullo EA: Delayed traumatic superior mesenteric arteriovenous fistula after a stab wound: Case report. J Trauma 32:101-106, 1992.
26. Deitrick J, McNeill P, Posner MP, et al: Traumatic superior mesenteric artery–portal vein fistula. Ann Vasc Surg 4:72-76, 1990.
27. Miglietta MA, Tanquilut EM, Madlinger RV, et al: Superior mesenteric artery–duodenal fistula presenting as a late complication of an abdominal gunshot wound. J Trauma 52:554-555, 2002.
28. Chiriano J, Abou-Zamzam AM Jr, Teruya TH, et al: Delayed development of a traumatic superior mesenteric arteriovenous fistula following multiple gunshot wounds to the abdomen. Ann Vasc Surg 19:470-473, 2005.

76

Reoperative Surgery of the Stomach and Duodenum

Bruce Schirmer ▪ C. Joe Northup

Reoperative surgery of any type is always more difficult than operating on virgin tissue. Scarring from previous surgery means, at best, additional time and dissection to establish appropriate tissue planes to perform the operation. At worst, it predisposes the patient to more serious consequences, including significant intraoperative bleeding, leading to transfusion and increasing the risk of postoperative infection. Damage to organs in the dissection process through such scar tissue may leave the patient with unrecognized perforations or organ injury that may result in disastrous postoperative complications, such as leak, abscess, fistulas, sepsis, and death.

Although clinical circumstances may force the performance of a reoperation on an emergent or urgent basis, when reoperative surgery is elective, the surgeon must take into consideration the need to avoid severe intraoperative scarring as much as possible. The most important rule to follow to minimize the consequences of scarring from previous surgery is *waiting an adequate period of time* since the last laparotomy to perform further abdominal surgery.

This chapter examines the aspects of reoperative surgery of the stomach and duodenum that the authors believe are particularly important for optimizing the outcomes of such procedures. In some situations, the procedures are performed only as a last resort when medical therapy has failed. In other situations, reoperative surgery has a stronger and more effective track record for success. This chapter focuses on elective reoperative surgery or surgery for longer term complications or failures of previous upper digestive system operations. Emergent reoperation of the stomach and duodenum may be required for immediate complications of recently performed surgery. These types of operations are not dealt with for the most part in this chapter because they essentially constitute immediate complications and treatment of complications of the initial operation. These complications are discussed in most circumstances in the various chapters covering the index operation. The focus in the present chapter is on reoperations that are done at a later date after the original operation. For the most part, these are elective procedures, but semiurgent ones for commonly occurring late problems of previous gastroduodenal surgery also are discussed as appropriate.

The types of reoperations are grouped according to the disease type for which they are being performed. These categories include peptic disease, gastroparesis and motility disorders, gastroesophageal reflux disease, bile reflux gastritis, cancer, bariatric surgery, and obstructive processes of the distal duodenum or segments of intestine draining a gastrojejunostomy.

GENERAL PRINCIPLES OF REOPERATIVE SURGERY

Although the individual operation planned as a reoperative procedure has varying degrees of success, and indications are based on previous outcomes data, the success of most reoperative operations depends on adhering to certain basic principles (Box 76–1). Most reoperative procedures are performed based on background knowledge of the likelihood of success of a repeat operative procedure achieving the intended goal. As with any operative procedure, reoperations have a higher degree of success the more severe the symptoms and the more likely the cause of the symptoms can be correlated with a clearly definable anatomic abnormality or pathology. Procedures that have variable success, particularly when the goal is eradication of nonspecific symptoms, should be avoided or performed only when a good benefit-to-risk ratio can be established.

Information Acquisition and Preparation

Preparation for reoperative surgery should always include obtaining as complete as possible records from

Box 76–1   **Basic Principles of Reoperative Surgery**

Potential benefits must outweigh risks or likely outcome without intervention.

Confirm that there is an anatomic and not a functional problem.

Obtain all possible information regarding previous operations.

Define the anatomy by radiographic, functional, and endoscopic studies as indicated.

Allow an adequate amount of time to pass to minimize previous operative scarring, which can prevent ease of operation and increase complications.

Be certain of blood supply to remaining tissues, especially anastomoses.

Do not leave sections of the upper gastrointestinal tract without adequate drainage of luminal contents.

Provide for a fail-safe mechanism of nutrition should postoperative complications occur.

Assess the success of a reoperative procedure constantly as it is in progress. Do not hesitate to stop if more harm than good is being done. Do not leave the patient worse off than before.

Anticipate that complications, such as leaks, may occur, and prepare for their possibility intraoperatively.

earlier operative procedures. Recent complete nonsurgical medical records also must be obtained. Attention to the details of which, if any, major blood vessels were divided during previous surgery may prove helpful in planning the appropriate reoperative approach. Knowledge of the relative location of Roux limbs and afferent and efferent intestinal limbs relative to other abdominal organs enables the initial dissection process to proceed with confidence based on such information.

Preoperative assessment of the current gastroduodenal anatomy is essential before embarking on any reoperative procedure of the upper gastrointestinal system. Such assessment often requires radiographic studies, endoscopy, or both. The surgeon should be certain he or she has a firm grasp on the existing anatomy of the stomach and duodenum, to as great an extent as possible, before embarking on an elective reoperation.

Assessment and Counseling

The patient and his or her current condition must be assessed carefully by a thorough history, physical examination, and review of the records and imaging studies. It is important for the surgeon to make a recommendation for reoperative surgery when there is a clear anatomic indication for the operation. In several areas of reoperative upper digestive surgery, such as bariatric surgery and antireflux surgery (see later), relying solely on symptoms or a patient's desire for further improvement of their symptoms as a basis for performing reoperative surgery may lead to a poor ultimate outcome from the reoperation. If a previously well-constructed operation remains intact, there is little reason to think that revising it would likely improve the situation.

After a thorough review of all pertinent information, the surgeon must make an assessment and recommendation as to whether reoperation is indicated. A thorough counseling session by the surgeon with the patient is necessary to discuss the relative merits or lack of merits of reoperative surgery. Such counseling sessions can be multiple if the initial encounter occurs at a time when appropriate and needed imaging studies or other laboratory evaluations are still pending.

Because reoperative surgery carries increased risks for complications, it must be entered into with significant planning and with careful contemplation on the part of the surgeon as to the risks and potential benefits of the procedure. The potential benefits are often less likely to be as good as the original procedure, if a revision is planned. Similarly, the risks are almost always increased. This combination puts the burden of proof on the surgeon to counsel the patient appropriately as to these parameters and to advise reoperation only when the likelihood of success is clear, and the danger of life-threatening complications is mitigated as much as possible.

Technical Aspects of Performing Reoperative Surgery

Open Surgery

The multiply-operated abdomen presents a challenge for all surgeons. Adhesion formation and subsequent obstruction is a frequent indication for surgical intervention. A careful approach must be undertaken to enter a previously operated abdomen. The typical approach is first to identify an area that would tend to have fewer adhesions or an unoperated area. Typically, the most superior aspect of the midline adhesion is often the best place to approach the adhesions associated with a previous scar. Inadvertent injury to the liver is generally less of a problem than injury to a piece of small intestine or colon. We advocate the use of sharply entering the abdomen to avoid any risk of thermal injury from cautery. When the fascia has been identified, Kocher clamps can be placed on the fascia with gentle traction by an assistant. The surgeon should apply gentle countertraction on the bowel and sharply take down adhesions from the abdominal wall. Adhesiolysis should be completed to the point where the operative goals can be accomplished. There is no benefit in taking down unnecessary adhesions.

Historically, attempts have been made to reduce the development of obstruction from intraoperative adhesions, including bowel plication and long intestinal tubes. Careful surgical technique remains the most effective method of adhesion prevention. Removal of foreign material, careful handling of tissues, adequate hemostasis, and avoidance of unnecessary dissection are the most efficient methods to prevent adhesions.[1,2]

Newer, bioresorbable materials have been shown to provide some benefit in reducing the severity or formation of adhesions. Cohen et al.[3] prospectively showed a reduction in adhesion formation and a decrease in severity using a hyaluronate-based barrier. In another prospective trial, Becker et al.[4] also showed a significant decrease in incidence, extent, and severity of postoperative adhesions with a similar product. Pharmacologic agents, such as anticoagulants and anti-inflammatory agents, have not reliably decreased adhesion formation.

When a surgeon performs an operation in which there is a high likelihood of returning, consideration must be given to adhesion prevention. Surgeons may want to consider using a hyaluronate-based barrier in these situations. Future advances in bioresorbable materials may improve their benefit in adhesion prevention further and possibly result in a decrease in the risk of postoperative bowel obstruction.

Laparoscopic Surgery

Since the advent of the laparoscopic era of performing general surgery operations, there is no question that a laparoscopic approach results in considerably less intra-abdominal adhesions than a celiotomy. Laparoscopy is currently the best approach a gastrointestinal surgeon can use to prevent significant and difficult postoperative adhesion formation. Not all operations described in this chapter are amenable to a laparoscopic approach, however, unless the surgeon has considerable expertise in laparoscopic surgery. Each individual operation must be assessed for the potential to apply a laparoscopic technique if possible, and such a decision must be based on the patient's previous operations, reports of the intra-abdominal condition at the time of those procedures, and the skill of the surgeon in performing laparoscopic surgery. Although most primary upper gastrointestinal operations are routinely performed laparoscopically by skilled laparoscopic gastrointestinal surgeons, reoperative surgery is approached more often using a celiotomy because of the time element and extreme technical difficulty encountered in using laparoscopy for revisional surgery of the foregut. Nevertheless, for bariatric and antireflux operations, there is a considerable body of published experience with successful use of a laparoscopic approach for revisional operations.

Laparoscopic Technique With the increasing use of laparoscopy, one of the most challenging barriers remains the previously operated abdomen. The initial difficulty is the approach to obtaining intra-abdominal access. The surgeon may choose a closed (Veress needle) or open (Hasson trocar) approach. An open versus closed approach has not shown any significant differences in the ease of use or the complication rate when entering the abdomen.[5,6] The open approach to laparoscopy is often thought to be safer with better visualization of the tissues. The open approach tends to be more complicated, however, when a trocar is inserted away from the midline. Also, in an overweight or morbidly obese patient, the open approach results in several technical problems, including the fact that the incision needs to be larger to allow for safe entry into the peritoneal cavity. The larger incision is subsequently more prone to leak gas from the pneumoperitoneum.

Our approach of choice is to use the Veress needle in an unoperated field or area of the abdomen. Optimal areas for safe entry to the reoperated abdomen are the right or left upper quadrants, 1 to 2 cm below the costal margin. Through a small incision, a tracheotomy hook is used to elevate the fascia, and the Veress needle is inserted. Initial aspiration should be performed to evaluate for any potential organ violation. Aspiration of gross blood or enteric contents should prompt a change in entry location or a conversion to an open procedure, and the damaged organ should be repaired. Structures underlying any site of attempted peritoneal access always must be given special attention on reentering the abdomen.

When adequate pneumoperitoneum has been achieved, a bladeless trocar is inserted. After the initial trocar is placed, a telescope is inserted to confirm intra-abdominal placement. The bowel should be carefully inspected directly below and surrounding the initial entry site to identify any possible injury.

After entry, the extent of adhesion formation must be assessed. The first priority is the placement of an additional operating port. An area of the anterior abdominal wall must be identified that is free of adhesions and safe for placement of an operating trocar. If no space is readily apparent, consideration must be given to converting to an open procedure. After a second operating port is placed, a careful adhesiolysis is begun. We prefer first to free enough space to be able to place a third trochar an adequate distance from the first operating port, preferably on the opposite side of the abdomen. This allows for a grasper to apply gentle, downward traction, while bluntly and sharply dividing adhesions to the anterior abdominal wall.

We use 5-mm ports and a 5-mm 30- to 45-degree angled laparoscope. An angled scope allows for visualization of the adhesions at different perspectives and decreases the chance of injury to adherent intestine. Additionally, using a 5-mm telescope allows for movement of the camera from port to port to inspect adhesions and organs from a different viewpoint.

Adhesiolysis should be continued until the surgical objective can be accomplished. Excessive adhesiolysis places the patient at greater risk for a bowel injury. Little benefit is gained by doing a total abdominal adhesiolysis, and this only lengthens the procedure time. Omental adhesions to the anterior abdominal wall are commonplace in the previously operated abdomen and relatively easy to divide. Bowel adhesions may be more difficult, and care should be taken to avoid an enterotomy at all costs because recognition of enterotomy with a laparoscopic approach may be more difficult than with open surgery. We sometimes divide the peritoneum to dissect the bowel down off the abdominal wall still densely adherent to the peritoneum if this would prevent injury. Small bowel interloop adhesions also are a technical challenge and must be divided carefully. Probably the most difficult situation technically in reoperative laparoscopic enterolysis involves an area of the abdominal wall where previously placed mesh exists that was used to repair an incisional or ventral hernia. In such situations, bowel can be so tightly stuck to the mesh as to preclude its safe enterolysis using a laparoscopic approach, and conversion to an open approach is necessary.

Bowel Injury During Laparoscopic Enterolysis   Management of a bowel injury during laparoscopy varies depending on the procedure being performed. Any enterotomy that occurs can be repaired with primary repair with interrupted sutures. Any large tear in the intestine must be evaluated carefully for resection. Typically, an enterotomy of greater than or equal to 50% of the lumen should be resected. A colon injury also can be managed with primary closure with laparoscopy.

In patients undergoing laparoscopy with multiple previous operations, we require patients to have a bowel preparation before surgery. Bowel preparation allows for decreased contamination if an injury occurs and decreases bowel "bulk" to allow for increased intraoperative space.

A missed bowel or gastric injury during laparoscopic enterolysis is a major complication that usually results in significant morbidity for the patient. The patient often presents with severe abdominal pain and peritonitis. Sepsis also may be a complicating accompanying problem. The patient should be re-explored immediately and undergo resection or primary repair of the injury, placement of drains if indicated by tissue quality, and diversion of the gastrointestinal stream if needed for severe injuries.

Nutritional Issues and Access

A final note is needed for reoperative surgery of the upper gastrointestinal system. Because nutritional intake is based on food or nutrients passing through these organs if an oral route of postoperative nutrition is expected (as it usually is), the operation must be highly likely to guarantee that eventuality in the relatively immediate postoperative period. If there is a significant likelihood that oral feeding may be precluded by a typical and common postoperative complication resulting from the reoperation, the burden is also on the surgeon to make provisions for a reliable enteral feeding access to be placed at the time of the operation for postoperative use. This access is usually an operatively placed gastrostomy or jejunostomy tube, depending on the operation performed.

PEPTIC DISEASE

Gastric Outlet Obstruction After Pyloric or Duodenal Ulcer Surgery

Gastric outlet obstruction after a previous operation for obstructing peptic ulcer may occur as a result of technical problems with the anastomosis, postoperative scarring, recurrence of the peptic disease with ulceration resulting in anastomotic scarring, or functional disorders of gastric emptying, the most common of which is postvagotomy syndrome with poor gastric emptying. Patients typically present with nausea, vomiting, early satiety, and postprandial pain. Patients can be extremely miserable if the nausea and vomiting are severe. Secondary dehydration and abnormalities in electrolytes, such as hypokalemia, also may develop. Malnutrition may be present. Gastric outlet obstruction at the level of the anastomosis may present as vomiting of clear gastric juice with undigested food contents. Obstruction at a level beyond the anastomosis, or of the efferent limb of a gastrojejunostomy, manifests more typically as bilious vomiting.

The diagnosis is strongly suggested by the clinical picture and secondarily reinforced by plain radiographs showing a distended gastric remnant. Definitive diagnosis is confirmed by contrast upper gastrointestinal series. Unless perforation is suspected, barium is the oral contrast medium of choice for improved visualization in perhaps a large reservoir of gastric secretions and as a less dangerous material if any aspiration of vomitus were to occur. Upper endoscopy may be helpful in determining the degree and level of obstruction of an anastomosis, although it often can be inaccurate in determining emptying ability of the anastomosis.

For more chronic situations, in which poor gastric emptying is intermittent and of varying severity, solid and liquid radionuclide gastric emptying studies should be performed to assess the emptying capacity of the stomach. Patients who present with delayed gastric emptying by radionuclide studies, but who have a patent anastomosis confirmed by upper gastrointestinal series, must be presumed to have primarily a functional gastric emptying disorder rather than an anatomic outlet obstruction. These patients should be managed medically whenever possible, with prokinetic agents being the mainstay of therapy. The reader is directed to the subsequent section on gastroparesis for further details.

In a situation in which a pyloroplasty or Billroth I procedure has been performed, and in which the pyloric channel has become re-obstructed, conservative measures of eliminating any potential causes of recurrent ulcer, such as smoking, nonsteroidal anti-inflammatory drugs, and steroids, and treatment for existing *Helicobacter pylori* in the stomach, must precede reoperation and be given an adequate trial to determine if they alone may provide adequate relief of the obstructive process. Balloon dilation of a scarred pylorus may provide satisfactory relief in some situations, particularly when the recurrent ulcer disease or cause has been eliminated or successfully treated. Balloon dilation may be done endoscopically or fluoroscopically.

When conservative measures at reopening the pyloric region have failed, the operative procedure of choice for relieving this obstruction is a gastrojejunostomy. *Trying to resect the stenotic and scarred pylorus is difficult, dangerous, and contraindicated for benign disease.* Adding a vagotomy is indicated only if recurrent peptic ulceration has occurred at the pyloric channel area, contributing to the re-stenosis. Often, adding a vagotomy is detrimental to the overall result of the operation because it greatly inhibits gastric emptying through the newly created gastrojejunostomy. Patients should be tested and treated for the presence of *H. pylori* before undergoing reoperation, even if other causes for the recurrent ulcer exist. Eradication of the bacteria must be confirmed by hydrogen breath testing.

Operative Technique

Gastrojejunostomy for an obstructed pyloric outflow must emphasize several principles:

1. The anastomosis must be adequately large. We prefer to use a 60-cm length linear stapler to perform the anastomosis or duplicate sequential firings of a 45-cm length stapler. This creates an anastomosis of at least 4 to 5 cm in length.
2. The location of the anastomosis should be dependent to allow maximum gravitational drainage. This means creation of the gastrojejunostomy on the posterior surface of the stomach, with a retrocolic location of the jejunal limb (Fig. 76–1).

3. The critical outflow to the stomach is not the anastomosis size itself, but the patency of the efferent limb of a gastrojejunostomy. To ensure that the lumen of the efferent limb is open to drainage, the bowel should be tacked to the posterior surface of the stomach 1 to 2 cm beyond the anastomosis to prevent kinking downward of the efferent limb and limiting the surface area for drainage. The tacking stitches should serve to stent open the lumen of the efferent limb.
4. A smooth and unobstructed passageway of the afferent and efferent limbs of the gastrojejunostomy through the mesentery of the transverse colon should be assured. Similarly, the mesenteric opening needs to be sutured to the sides of the bowel to prevent herniation of other loops of bowel superior to the level of the colon mesentery.

Gastric Outlet Obstruction at the Site of a Surgical Gastrojejunostomy

In a patient with a previous antrectomy or subtotal gastrectomy of some portion and a gastrojejunostomy, reobstruction at the site of the anastomosis may occur immediately after surgery or later. Immediate postoperative issues involve technical problems, anastomotic edema, distal efferent loop obstruction, or other kinking or obstruction of the efferent limb of intestine draining the stomach. These complications are discussed elsewhere. Chronic causes of gastric outlet obstruction after a previous gastrojejunostomy include efferent limb obstruction, marginal ulcer at the anastomosis with scarring, and simply stenosis of the anastomosis.

Patient presentation with this anatomic problem is similar to that of gastric outlet obstruction after stenotic pyloroplasty, but vomitus is bilious if the anastomosis is patent to the afferent limb of the gastrojejunostomy. This most often is true. Diagnosis is by upper gastrointestinal series or by endoscopy. The upper gastrointestinal series gives a better anatomic picture of the situation and a better analysis of gastric emptying. Passage of an endoscope through an anastomosis may suggest patency, but functional emptying may be seriously compromised despite the ability to pass an endoscope through the anastomosis. This is especially true if there is an element of obstruction of the efferent intestinal drainage limb, not appreciated by endoscoping the anastomotic area alone.

Initial measures to improve stenotic gastrojejunostomy involve medical therapy to treat and eliminate any marginal ulcer present. Endoscopy with anastomotic dilation is often helpful to relieve symptoms while medical therapy has a chance to reverse the obstructing ulcer process. Eradication of *H. pylori* also is important in this situation, as are other measures to eliminate causes of recurrent ulcer of the stomach (mentioned previously).

Stenosis of the anastomosis is unusual without accompanying reulceration. It may occur on the basis of foreign body reaction to anastomotic staples or sutures, however, or on the basis of chronic ischemia. These causes can

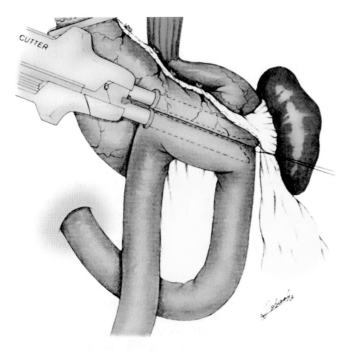

Figure 76–1. Stapled gastrojejunostomy. Creation of a stapled Billroth II anastomosis. Note the preferred method of placing the staple line in a posterior position to improve gastric emptying. (From Feil W, Lippert H, Lozac'H P, et al [eds]: Atlas of Surgical Stapling, New York, Thieme Medical Publisher, 2000, p 132.)

produce a progressive stenosis of the anastomosis, which is usually amenable to treatment with multiple dilations.

Marginal ulcer may cause obstruction at the site of a previous gastrojejunostomy. Diagnosis is usually by endoscopy because contrast studies often do not clearly identify the presence of a marginal ulcer. The site of the ulcer is normally at or just beyond the anastomosis, and this must be confirmed on endoscopy as well. Endoscopic dilation and fluoroscopic dilation may prove successful in treating these obstructions.[7] The presence of a marginal ulcer and a more chronic pattern of stenosis are factors that decrease the likelihood of success using balloon dilation alone. If dilations have failed, and a marginal ulcer persists, a barium radiograph should be performed before reoperation to confirm the marginal ulcer has not fistulized to surrounding structures, such as the transverse colon. This situation is rare, but important to determine if present preoperatively. At times, such a fistula is small and difficult to visualize on the contrast study. Severe scarring in the area of the anastomosis and adherence of an adjacent organ to the area may suggest the presence of such a fistula, even if it is not seen clearly on the contrast study. Such fistulas represent an indication for reoperation because conservative measures are not likely to result in healing.[8]

A minimally invasive approach that has been used in treating fistulas elsewhere in the gastrointestinal tract, but that is currently little proved as a definitive treatment for marginal ulcer fistulas at a gastrojejunostomy site, is fibrin glue injection of the fistula tract to produce occlusion of it. Fibrin glue has been shown to be effective in closing some enterocutaneous fistulas,[9] but its role in treating marginal ulcer fistulas is as yet unproven.

Confirmatory determination of the obstruction site to be at the area of the anastomosis is done with the upper gastrointestinal series, but also may be accomplished with endoscopy. Obstruction of the efferent limb of the gastrojejunostomy may result from stenosis and kinking of the bowel as it exits through the transverse colon mesentery or may be on the basis of postoperative intra-abdominal adhesions, internal hernia, or other less common causes that produce bowel obstruction. Operative treatment of this condition is much more likely, and balloon dilation usually has little role if the obstruction is much beyond the anastomosis.

Operative Technique

Operative treatment of an obstruction at a previous gastrojejunostomy site includes adherence to the following general principles:

1. If a vagotomy was not performed at the initial gastrojejunostomy, a completion vagotomy is indicated in the setting of marginal ulceration. Most incomplete vagotomies result from inaccurate identification of the posterior vagus nerve, which may lie considerably away from the posterior esophageal surface, coursing over the top of the diaphragmatic crura. Dissection further up the right side of the esophagus in the mediastinum often allows the surgeon to find, identify clearly, and follow the posterior vagus trunk. Intraoperative frozen section confirming neural tissue and skeletonization of the distal 5 cm of esophagus are crucial components of completion vagotomy.

2. The area of the previous anastomosis is usually best resected, to eliminate the scarred and obstructed portion of the stomach containing the previous anastomosis. The more proximal stomach is used for creation of the gastrojejunostomy. If resection is substantial, the surgeon may wish to perform a Roux-en-Y drainage of the stomach because this allows a greater length of intestine to reach the more proximal stomach. In addition, resection that includes the jejunal portion of the gastrojejunostomy predisposes to the use of a Roux limb for drainage because the bowel already is divided. Another factor in favor of using a Roux limb for any resection beyond the mid body of the stomach is to prevent potential bile reflux esophagitis.

3. Either the Roux limb or the gastrojejunostomy must be created without any tension on the anastomosis.

4. The efferent limb of the gastrojejunostomy or the Roux limb itself must lie in a position such that the outlet pathway of the bowel is not kinked or in any way obstructed.

5. Orienting the gastrojejunostomy in an isoperistaltic fashion is favorable, but not essential, to good emptying. Either retroperistaltic or isoperistaltic orientation to the stomach functions as long as the efferent limb is widely patent.

6. The bowel must be sutured to the transverse colon mesentery as it passes through it, to prevent postoperative internal hernias of other loops of bowel through the defect. Excessive suturing, especially running permanent suture lengths, may result in stenosis at this site, however.

Postgastrectomy Dumping and Diarrhea

Postgastrectomy dumping is a manifestation of the loss of pyloric control of gastric emptying and is present, to a greater or lesser extent, after any gastric resection with gastrojejunostomy or pyloroplasty. Rapid emptying of food into the jejunum results in the release of vasoactive amines and peptides, including insulin.[10] The vasoactive amines cause early dumping, which occurs within 30 to 60 minutes of eating and consists of physical manifestations including tachycardia, mild hypotension, and symptoms of nausea, abdominal pain and fullness, weakness, dizziness, and a sick feeling after meals with a high osmotic content. The major offending types of foods are calorically dense ones, such as sweets. Eating and drinking at the same time exacerbates symptoms. Late dumping occurs 2 to 4 hours after eating and is characterized by diaphoresis, tachycardia, light-headedness, and confusion. Hypoglycemia often, but not always, is present. Glucagon-like polypeptide (GLP-1) has been implicated as a vasoactive amine contributing to early and late dumping syndrome.[11]

Treatment for postgastrectomy dumping is nonoperative. In almost all situations, the patient can adjust food intake and speed to ameliorate symptoms. Separating eating from drinking, avoiding high-calorie foods and concentrated sweets, and eating slowly prevent most severe symptoms of dumping. If dumping proves still refractory even with these measures, subcutaneous octreotide is effective in reversing the symptoms of dumping.[12] Longer acting intramuscular dosing of the drug has been shown to prevent the need for subcutaneous injections three to four times a day[13] with equal efficacy. Usually patients experience a decrease in dumping severity as time passes after surgery. Similarly, patients usually can be tapered off octreotide after a several-month course of treatment. For severe cases, the drug is effective long-term, but side effects, which often lead to its discontinuation, include diarrhea and gallstone formation.[14]

Postgastrectomy diarrhea is a sequela of the postprandial dumping that follows the loss of pyloric-controlled gastric emptying after gastric resection. It may be exacerbated further by vagotomy. Diarrhea typically follows mild to more severe dumping symptoms by about 30 minutes and can be as debilitating as the dumping. Following the same approach of alteration of eating pattern that is used to treat dumping often improves the diarrhea as well. Octreotide is less useful for diarrhea alone, whereas antidiarrheal agents are usually of some symptomatic benefit. Adaptation and time usually also are helpful for this condition.

Operative treatments of reversing short segments (10 to 15 cm) of intestine, previously advocated in past decades as a treatment for postprandial dumping (proximal segment of bowel reversal) or diarrhea (more distal small bowel reversal), are no longer generally advocated for the treatment of these conditions and are now rarely used by surgeons working on the upper gastrointestinal tract.[15] Nonoperative therapy usually results in enough improvement of symptoms to satisfy most patients. The conditions usually improve with time, and the ability to obtain an adequate experience in such procedures is so rare as to preclude most surgeons from obtaining expertise in them. Despite the occasional reports of success with such operations, many surgeons have found that these operations often are associated with a high incidence of bowel obstruction, stenosis, and not appreciably greater improvement in symptoms than less aggressive nonoperative measures. One relatively recent report described elimination of dumping when an isoperistaltic 10- to 12-cm segment of jejunum was placed as an interposition graft as an alternative to Billroth I reconstruction after distal gastrectomy for gastric cancer.[16]

The amount of nonbariatric gastric surgery that is done for benign gastric disease, such as peptic disease, has decreased greatly over the past several decades. Medical therapy is often adequate to relieve many of the symptoms of peptic ulcer and cure the disease without surgical therapy. Patients who still require surgery for benign gastric disease, although less numerous, still may manifest the same severe complications and symptoms that made gastric surgery difficult in the past. For those patients, appreciating the experience of past decades helps in planning any needed reoperative surgery.

GASTROPARESIS AND GASTRIC EMPTYING OR MOTILITY PROBLEMS

Gastroparesis

Gastroparesis is defined as poor intrinsic gastric emptying resulting from a lack of peristaltic activity. Most patients with gastroparesis have this condition secondary to another medical condition, such as diabetes, vagotomy, collagen vascular disease, viral illness, medications, Parkinson's disease, hypothyroidism, or amyloidosis. Rarely, patients have primary gastroparesis, and this is part of an overall neural or smooth muscle disease of the gut that manifests itself as overall pseudo-obstruction or ileus, rather than isolated gastroparesis. Gastroparesis is often idiopathic as well.

Patients with gastroparesis present with early satiety, vomiting of undigested food, abdominal pain, nausea, and food intolerance and aversion. Patients with idiopathic cases, believed sometimes to result from a viral illness, may develop sudden severe symptoms. Other secondary causes are usually more insidious in onset except for postvagotomy patients. These patients have perhaps the most profound symptoms and are perhaps the one subgroup of patients with gastroparesis for whom reoperative surgery may be indicated for severe symptoms.

The diagnosis of gastroparesis is made by the clinical syndrome and symptoms accompanied by a documentation of solid food and liquid food delayed emptying using radionuclide gastric emptying studies. Such studies are considered the gold standard for confirming the presence of delayed gastric emptying of solids and liquids. Gastroparesis can be mistaken for rapid gastric emptying, and gastric emptying studies are necessary sometimes to define clearly the cause of patient symptoms.[17]

Gastroparesis is mentioned here largely as a warning to surgeons that the primary and best therapy for such patients is *medical*. Prokinetic agents, either erythromycin or metoclopramide, are the medications of choice for treating gastroparesis. Erythromycin, a macrolide antibiotic, has a chemical structure similar to the gastrointestinal regulatory peptide motilin. Erythromycin exerts gastric-specific contractile stimulation and assists in gastric emptying. It has been shown to be effective for short-term and long-term use. Side effects include cramping. Metoclopramide is a procainamide derivative that acts to stimulate the entire gastrointestinal tract by antagonism of peripheral dopamine receptors and increasing acetylcholine release from the myenteric plexus. It is the most commonly prescribed prokinetic agent available in the United States today and is effective for gastroparesis. The side effects of long-term metoclopramide use are its major detraction; these include extrapyramidal side effects and nightmares particularly in elderly patients, dystonic reactions in young patients, and hyperprolactinemia.

Reoperative surgery for causes of gastroparesis is uncommon and generally limited to cases of severe postvagotomy gastroparesis.[18] Diabetic gastroparesis is usually treated adequately with medical therapy. Nutritional compromise occasionally may occur, however, secondary to the disease. In such situations, placement of enteral access is needed for management of the disease. Such enteral access must be a *jejunal* feeding tube, not a gastrostomy. Placement of nutrients directly into the stomach not only does not guarantee they will reach the intestine before being vomited but also exacerbates symptoms of the gastroparesis. Surgeons are urged to use a conservative approach to patients with idiopathic gastroparesis because these individuals may resolve their disease spontaneously over months to years and should not be subjected to irreversible gastric resection, which could compound subsequent upper gastrointestinal symptoms.

Patients with severe persistent symptoms of gastroparesis, who have had the disease for a long time, who have a known cause for the disease, who have experienced nutritional compromise, and who have a poor quality of life secondary to the problem occasionally may be considered candidates for surgical therapy. Most individuals who fit this description have postvagotomy gastroparesis, and so reoperative surgery is the norm. In such patients, removal of most of the stomach, leaving only a small gastric reservoir that cannot serve as a large atonic pouch to store food, is indicated. The operation resembles the Roux-en-Y gastric bypass (RYGB) that currently is the most frequent operation performed for morbid obesity except that the distal stomach is resected. Near-total gastrectomy with Roux-en-Y gastric drainage is relatively successful in relieving symptoms in this patient population. One study by Echauser et al.[19] showed nearly 80% relief of symptoms for patients undergoing near-total gastrectomy for postvagotomy motor disorders of the stomach. Even this radical surgical approach to gastroparesis is not guaranteed to restore a good quality of life to the patient, but it remains the only surgical option for the most severely affected patients.

Reports have arisen regarding the use of gastric electrical stimulation for the treatment of gastroparesis. Although symptomatic relief has been achieved in patients, data showing pacing produces an increase in gastric emptying by radionuclide testing are still lacking.[20] This treatment modality still must be considered an experimental procedure.

Roux Limb Syndrome

The Roux limb syndrome, described previously in the surgical literature, is manifested by symptoms of early satiety, bloating, upper abdominal pain, and vomiting after eating. Patients who have this syndrome have had previous gastric resection with vagotomy and often had a second operation to convert the gastric drainage from a loop gastrojejunostomy to a Roux-en-Y drainage. The cause of the Roux syndrome was attributed to a primary motor disorder of the Roux limb by some authorities. Other authors, including us, believe the vagotomy itself was the primary reason for the symptoms and the dysfunction.[21] Evidence to support this position derives from the fact that patients who did have Roux syndrome, and who underwent subsequent near-total gastrectomy with

Roux-en-Y drainage, usually were relieved of symptoms with the same frequency as patients with gastroparesis. As a result of improvements in medical treatment for peptic ulcer disease, the performance of gastric resection with vagotomy has decreased markedly over the past 3 decades, and this situation is now rarely encountered in clinical practice. The numerous morbidly obese patients who have undergone RYGB, without vagotomy, without producing a large number of patients with the Roux syndrome, lends further evidence to the fact that the vagotomy and gastroparesis were likely the underlying cause of the symptoms experienced in the past by patients given the diagnosis of the Roux limb syndrome. If such patients are encountered today, they should be managed in a similar fashion as patients with gastroparesis, reserving surgical therapy for patients refractory to medical management, and using near-total gastrectomy as the surgical procedure of choice if reoperation is performed.

GASTROINTESTINAL NEOPLASMS

Adenocarcinoma of a Gastric Remnant

Patients who have undergone previous distal gastrectomy for benign peptic ulcer disease are at risk for cancer of the remaining gastric remnant. This risk has been well documented in the surgical literature.[22] The occurrence of tumors is on average several decades after the original operation, however. Routine screening endoscopy for all such patients is recommended starting 20 years after surgery. Should a suspicious lesion be found on gastroscopy in this setting, multiple biopsy specimens of the lesion should be obtained. The highest likelihood for yield of a correct diagnosis is when biopsy specimens are taken at the edge of the ulcerated lesion, not in the often necrotic central portion of a tumor ulcer. Completion gastrectomy is the surgical treatment of choice and is curative in nearly all cases that are diagnosed by endoscopic screening.

Patients who have had previous gastric resection for adenocarcinoma are at risk for local recurrence. Surveillance endoscopy in this patient population is performed on a 6- to 12-month basis, until several years of disease-free interval have passed. Then endoscopic frequency is decreased. If a recurrent cancer is diagnosed, reoperative surgery with total gastrectomy and en bloc radical resection including an R2 nodal dissection as indicated is the procedure of choice. Achievement of an R0 status is the goal of resection. Roux-en-Y esophagojejunostomy is indicated for reconstruction, and a feeding jejunostomy is placed for assurance of enteral access and feeding capability should any problems arise at the esophagojejunostomy anastomosis. Results of resection for recurrent gastric adenocarcinoma show a high incidence of ultimate death from recurrent cancer.[23] If recurrent gastric cancer has progressed beyond the realm of feasible curative resection, options for palliation of the problem include laparoscopic gastrojejunostomy[24] and endoscopic placement of metallic stents.[25]

Recurrent Stromal Cell Tumor

Gastrointestinal stromal cell tumors, known in the past as leiomyomas of the gastrointestinal tract, have variable malignant potential. Their tumor biology behavior mimics sarcomas, in the sense that local recurrence is the most common manifestation of recurrent neoplastic disease. If such a situation occurs for a previously resected gastric stromal tumor, radical re-resection is indicated to cure the condition. A 5-cm proximal and distal margin of resection is optimal, if possible. Intraoperative frozen section of the margins of the resected specimen is appropriate to help confirm the adequacy of surgical excision of the recurrent tumor. Neither radiation nor chemotherapy has much efficacy in this disease; surgery remains the only chance for complete cure. If the tumor has extended into surrounding structures, en bloc resection including the spleen, distal pancreas, and colon or wedge resection of the left hepatic lobe may be necessary. Reconstruction usually is achieved with a Roux-en-Y gastrojejunostomy or esophagojejunostomy. Recurrent stromal cell tumors have a penchant for repeat recurrence, and the potential for cure is markedly diminished over that of initial resection.[26]

Recurrent Desmoid Tumors

Desmoid tumors, which are commonly associated with patients with familial colon polyposis and Gardner's syndrome, are a difficult surgical problem. They are generally slow-growing tumors and manifest themselves by creating symptoms of obstruction or pain. They tend to occur in the mesentery of the small bowel.

Diagnosis is usually by suggestive clinical picture and computed tomography. A mass in the mesentery of the small bowel is diagnostic. Desmoids most commonly involve the bowel distal to the duodenum, but may occur in the area of the celiac axis or duodenum. In such cases, they tend to be difficult tumors to remove completely because they often present at a stage where perivascular invasion of major mesenteric arteries, such as the superior mesenteric artery or branches of the celiac axis, is involved. Radical excision with vascular reconstruction is occasionally possible, but often tumor extent and invasion preclude this option as well. Debulking of the tumor has some benefit, but offers only palliative therapy.[27] Because desmoid tumors are so difficult to cure, a high index of suspicion for their presence must be maintained in patients at risk for the disease.

GASTROESOPHAGEAL REFLUX DISEASE

Reoperation for failed antireflux surgery is becoming increasingly commonplace, especially at major referral centers for complex gastrointestinal problems. During the mid-1990s, the incidence of fundoplication performed in the United States dramatically increased with the availability of a laparoscopic option for the procedure. The number of procedures increased by approximately 800% between 1989 and 1999.[28] Foregut surgeons now are seeing an increasing number of patients who have developed problems from their initial operation and present as potential candidates for revisional surgery. Patients who develop recurrent symptoms after previous antireflux surgery do so because the operation may have failed for the following reasons:

1. Recurrent diaphragmatic herniation with migration of the wrap to an intrathoracic location
2. Slippage of the wrap with recurrent gastroesophageal reflux
3. Inadequacy of the wrap or disruption of the wrap with recurrent gastroesophageal reflux
4. Inadequate length of abdominal esophagus at the original operation, with the wrap placed around the proximal stomach, preventing adequate increase in lower esophageal sphincter pressure and resulting in subsequent recurrence of gastroesophageal reflux
5. Stenosis of the wrap area with persistent postoperative dysphagia

The symptoms that generally occur after failure of antireflux surgery differ. Symptoms should be a guide to suspicion of one of the above-listed failures of the previous fundoplication. Symptoms alone are notoriously unreliable for confirming the presence of a failed previous fundoplication, however, and the surgeon must confirm the presence of recurrent disease and the anatomic problem with the fundoplication before offering reoperation to the patient. Only with such information can a rational plan for reoperation be constructed and the appropriate counseling occur regarding the likelihood of success of the revisional operation.

Recurrent and persistent epigastric pain after a previous fundoplication should raise the suspicion that recurrent herniation of the wrap through the diaphragm and into the mediastinum has occurred. This is the classic symptom of recurrent diaphragmatic herniation. An upper gastrointestinal series is usually diagnostic and may be the only test needed in this setting before reoperation is recommended. Recurrent herniation of the wrap into the chest does not always manifest with significant symptoms. Hashemi et al.[29] reviewed the University of Southern California series of repairs of large paraesophageal hernias by obtaining a routine upper gastrointestinal series an average of 27 months postoperatively for patients undergoing repair of type III hiatal hernias with fundoplication. Patients who had a previous laparoscopic repair had a 42% incidence of recurrent hernia, and more than half had few, if any, symptoms.

Reoperation for recurrent diaphragmatic herniation can be performed through the abdomen or through the chest. If multiple previous upper abdominal operations have been performed, the latter approach may allow a technically easier repair. Left thoracotomy, reduction of the herniated wrap back into the abdomen, and crural diaphragm repair are indicated in this setting. Use of reinforcing mesh is still controversial, but may be considered if the diaphragm tissue is of poor quality. Mesh must be placed so as to avoid potential erosion into the esophagus. Materials that have a smooth surface (e.g., Gore-Tex or composite meshes) are preferred to materials with an open weave configuration (e.g., Prolene or Marlex).

Repair of the reherniation also can be accomplished with high likelihood of success through the abdomen. Our experience has been that performance of this recurrent surgery may require an open incision, depending on the severity of scarring at the diaphragmatic hiatus. A previous operation done via celiotomy usually requires another open approach. If the previous antireflux operation was done laparoscopically, however, and scarring in the area of the diaphragm is not excessive, we have repaired the recurrent herniation successfully with a laparoscopic approach. The same consideration must be entertained for the use of a nonadherent mesh material to reinforce the crural repair through the abdomen and when a laparoscopic approach is used. Mesh should be securely fixed with sutures, not stapled or tacked to the diaphragm.

Patients who present with symptoms resembling recurrent gastroesophageal reflux after a previous fundoplication should be assessed carefully to determine that recurrent reflux is present. Patients are often restarted on proton pump inhibitor therapy for presumed recurrent reflux after surgery when vague or nonspecific symptoms that could be reflux are voiced to the patient's internist or gastroenterologist. Lord et al.[30] showed that at a mean time of 28 months after fundoplication, 43% of symptomatic patients were taking acid suppression medications, and only 24% of patients taking acid suppression medications had abnormal 24-hour pH studies.

If a patient complains of symptoms of recurrent reflux, full evaluation of the patient and the previous operation is indicated. Minimum tests include an upper gastrointestinal series to assess for potential disruption of the wrap, herniation of the wrap into the chest, or gross reflux on contrast agent ingestion. If the upper gastrointestinal study shows a clear problem with the wrap, some surgeons proceed to reoperation. A pH test is the gold standard for documenting recurrent reflux in this setting. Upper endoscopy should be liberally performed, especially if considerable time has passed since the first operation, or if there is any concern that Barrett's esophagitis may have developed in the interim. Upper endoscopy also gives good information regarding the current position of the wrap and further enhancing information regarding diaphragmatic herniation. Lord et al.[30] reported that endoscopic assessment of the fundoplication was the most significant factor associated with an abnormal pH test, documenting the accuracy of endoscopy to assess a disrupted wrap.

Our general recommended approach to the re-evaluation of patients with a failed antireflux operation is to obtain an upper gastrointestinal series and upper endoscopy and proceed with pH testing if those studies do not show gross herniation of the wrap into the chest. Adding a repeat esophageal manometry in this setting is controversial and should be based on the patient's symptoms. Any symptoms that suggest atypical pain, esophageal spasm, or dysphagia are indications for a preoperative manometry study before reoperative surgery.

The outcomes of reoperation for failed antireflux operations are generally good. The largest series in the literature was reported by the group from Emory.[31] In their series of 1892 patients who underwent fundoplication at Emory, 2.8% required reoperation. Most reoperations occurred within 2 years of the initial procedure. Transdiaphragmatic wrap herniation was the most common reason (61% of cases) for reoperation in that group. A group of 231 patients had fundoplication done elsewhere, and in that group transdiaphragmatic herniation was the problem in 47% of cases. Slipped or disrupted wraps were found in 19% and 18% of the two groups and were the second most common reason for failure. Most of the reoperations were done laparoscopically (70%). Mortality for the series was 0.3%. Intraoperative perforation occurred in 17% of the laparoscopic cases and 29% of the open cases. Postoperative complication rates were 11.7% for the laparoscopic cases and 40.3% for the open cases. Relief of postoperative symptoms to the mild or absent category was achieved in 73% to 89% of patients. Failure of the reoperations requiring a second reoperation was reported in 8% of patients, with transdiaphragmatic herniation again being the leading cause of failure.

Other reports of reoperative surgery for failed fundoplication also have shown relatively good results, although never as good as the initial operation. Neuhauser and Hinder[32] reported results of 100 consecutive patients undergoing reoperative surgery for failed fundoplication. Only 52% of the patients had a previous laparoscopic operation. These authors performed reoperative laparoscopic fundoplication in 83% of cases. There was a 30% perioperative or postoperative complication rate, however, and the authors cautioned that such reoperative surgery is a major surgical technical challenge. Byrne et al.[33] described their experience with 118 patients undergoing reoperative antireflux surgery, with 101 of the 118 being able to be done laparoscopically. Heartburn was relieved or minimal in 84%, and regurgitation was relieved or minimal in 87% of patients. Patients having preoperative dysphagia were improved in 25 of 32 cases. Rosemurgy et al.[34] reoperated on 64 patients: 28% owing to hiatal failure, 19% owing to wrap failure, and 33% owing to failure of both. Most (76%) reoperations were done laparoscopically. Improvement in dysphagia was observed in 100% of symptomatic patients, improvement of reflux was seen in 79%, and improvement of both when both were present was seen in 74% of patients. Heniford et al.[35] reoperated on 55 patients. They did 37 of the procedures laparoscopically and had a 12.7% complication rate and an average hospitalization of 4.6 days; greater than 90% of patients experienced good to excellent symptom relief. Dutta et al.[36] reported a series of 28 redo fundoplications, most for symptoms of gastroesophageal reflux disease. All but two were done laparoscopically, with an average operating room time of less than 1 hour. Three patients required reoperation for reherniation of the wrap.

Reoperation for failed fundoplication can be performed with good symptomatic and overall outcomes. Patients must be cautioned that the reoperations have a higher complication rate and a slightly lower symptomatic improvement rate than the initial operation.

Success at performing reoperations laparoscopically depends on the severity of previous scarring and the surgeon's skill and persistence. These reoperations should be performed by surgeons with extensive laparoscopic and antireflux surgical experience.

Technical Aspects of Revisional Antireflux Surgery

Revisional antireflux surgery poses a significant technical challenge. The following are recommendations for successful laparoscopic performance of the operation:

1. The initial approach should be as for all previously operated abdomens, with care being taken to avoid organ injury on accessing the abdomen.

2. The most difficult initial organ dissection plane is the one between the inferior surface of the left lobe of the liver and the anterior proximal stomach. Dissection of the liver off the stomach without excessive violation of Glisson's capsule and significant bleeding is important. If liver parenchymal violation occurs, often the liver retractor can be positioned to place direct pressure on the area of the injury, tamponading any bleeding and achieving hemostasis as the operation progresses. Significant liver laceration warrants the placement of a closed-suction drain in the area at the completion of the operation to drain any potential bile leak. Liver surface hemostasis, if difficult, can be enhanced by high-energy electrocautery applied 1 to 2 mm off the surface of the liver to seal the tissue. The argon beam coagulator is even more effective if significant areas of capsular disruption have occurred. If one uses this instrument during laparoscopic surgery, the abdomen must be vented while the energy source is turned on.

3. The fundoplication position and the relationship to the diaphragmatic crura must be assessed. Usually is it evident if the problem is wrap herniation through the diaphragm, wrap disruption, or wrap misplacement.

4. Sutures used to create the wrap should be identified and cut, loosening the wrap.

5. The fundoplication should be taken down carefully and completely. Tissue planes should be confirmed. If any question exists as to the location and edge of the esophagus, an intraoperative endoscope or lighted bougie can facilitate location of its borders. Nonlighted bougies also are helpful if neither an intraoperative endoscope nor lighted bougie is available.

6. Conversion to an open incision should be performed if the tissue planes of the gastric fundus, the borders of the esophagus, or the borders of the diaphragmatic crura are not clearly seen. It is hoped that this decreases the incidence of intraoperative organ injury.

7. The fundus must be redissected to achieve good mobilization, and the retroesophageal area must be maximized for adequate room to pass the wrap.

8. Abdominal esophageal length must be 2 cm at rest. Mobilization of the esophagus to achieve this length must be performed. An esophageal lengthening procedure rarely is necessary. If so, we have successfully used a circular then linear stapler laparoscopically, similar to a laparoscopic vertical banded gastroplasty (VBG) being done for morbid obesity.

9. Re-repair of the crura is almost always necessary. Poor tissue quality of the crura should raise the consideration of placement of a soft mesh across the lower crura, not in contact with the esophagus, for reinforcement of the closure.

10. The wrap must be constructed over a dilator, preferably one No. 54 to 60 French size.

11. Any concerns for injury to the esophagus or stomach should be tested by air insufflation using an endoscope intraoperatively.

12. The wrap, when reconstructed, should be placed as high as possible on the esophagus and fixed to the crura of the diaphragm in revisional surgery. This placement should help prevent a second hiatal failure.

13. If a hiatal failure is still of concern, anterior gastropexy may help prevent gastric migration upward into the mediastinum.

The most important of these principles are summarized in Box 76–2.

BARIATRIC SURGERY

Revisional bariatric surgery should be performed only by an experienced bariatric surgeon. Laparoscopic revisional bariatric surgery requires extremely advanced laparoscopic skills, significant bariatric surgical experience and skill, and an efficient and supportive operating room team that is well equipped for such a surgically challenging operation. A skilled laparoscopic first assistant is a necessity for all bariatric surgery, but particularly revisional surgery.

Box 76–2   Major Principles of Reoperative Antireflux Surgery

Expect the plane between the undersurface of the left lobe of the liver and the stomach to be difficult to dissect cleanly.

Identify the source of the failure—wrap slippage, disruption, diaphragmatic hernia, or combination.

Clearly identify the esophagus.

Take down the wrap.

Confirm adequate length of abdominal esophagus.

Reconstruct the operation, and test for leaks or organ injury.

Patient Selection

Based on supply, demand, and public health concerns, one can make a strong case that revisional bariatric surgery is rarely indicated. Currently more than 23 million people in the United States are candidates for bariatric surgery, and less than 1% of them receive surgical therapy annually. There is a shortage of well-trained bariatric surgeons, especially those who perform the operation laparoscopically, for the patient demand. Use of surgeon time and medical facility resources for revisional bariatric surgery is, in light of these facts, of debatable merit. The practice of medicine and surgery holds care of the individual patient as the paramount concern, however, and as such, revisional surgery may be appropriate at times.

All bariatric operations have some failures. A figure of approximately 10% is often used in discussions regarding the "failure rate" of various well-established bariatric operations. The reasons for failure may vary. These reasons must be assessed carefully and understood before reoperative surgery is entertained or offered. If the failure is *primarily of the operation,* consideration for reoperation is appropriate. If the failure is *primarily of the patient and the patient's eating habits and compliance,* reoperation has little likelihood of succeeding any more than the initial failed operation. Surgical ego, compassion for a noncompliant patient who is upset with his or her current condition, and the incentive to perform a technically challenging operation all should be avoided in such situations and should not lead the surgeon to offer reoperation to a patient who has failed a previous bariatric operation because of behavioral and eating issues.

Reoperation should be considered in a situation where the operation has failed. The surgeon must define this anatomic failure. Reoperation is based on correcting the previous failure or safely revising the first operation to another bariatric procedure appropriate for the patient and his or her needs, expectations, and eating patterns. It is wise to have several counseling sessions with patients who request reoperative surgery. A dietary history not only from the patient, but also from the patient's family is appropriate in this setting. The patient needs to have demonstrated the appropriate behavior after the initial failed operation.

Any patient who is a candidate for reoperative surgery, if the surgery is to produce further weight loss, must meet the National Institutes of Health criteria for qualifying for weight loss surgery. The patient must have a body mass index (BMI) of greater than 40kg/m^2 without weight-related comorbid medical problems or a BMI greater than 35kg/m^2 with a comorbid problem. Psychological stability, motivation, documentation of previous appropriate behavior after the initial operation, and no medical conditions making the reoperation of excessively high risk are criteria that we mandate before reoperative bariatric surgery.

Failed Vertical Banded Gastroplasty

The VBG was the most popular bariatric operation performed in the 1980s. By 1990, it had fallen out of favor largely because of the poor long-term weight loss record of the operation[37] and because a considerable percentage of patients also develop progressive stenosis of the gastric outlet,[38] prompting conversion to a high-calorie liquid diet.[39] Multiple reports exist in the bariatric surgical literature documenting the ability to convert patients with previously failed VBG operations successfully to RYGB. Jones[40] reported only a 13% complication rate for a series of 141 patients undergoing reoperative surgery to convert from failed bariatric procedures to RYGB. Sugerman et al.[41] performed conversion of 53 VBG procedures with complications to RYGB, achieving 67% excess weight loss. The complication rate was high—about 50% for the series, including 20 marginal ulcers. Cariani et al.[42] also reported a high incidence of complications after reoperative surgery for VBG or failed RYGB, totaling greater than 55% between early and late complications. Reoperative surgery, especially bariatric surgery, carries increased risk for infection, wound complications, pulmonary complications, and intraabdominal crises from leaks above that seen for initial operations.

Most reoperative surgery for failed VBG has been done using a celiotomy approach. Some surgeons have performed this operation laparoscopically, however. Gagner et al.[43] reported laparoscopically converting 27 patients with failed open or laparoscopic gastroplasty, adjustable gastric banding, or RYGB to a new or revised RYGB. The average BMI for these patients decreased from 43kg/m^2 to 36kg/m^2, and the complication rate was 22%. There are increasing reports of small experiences in the bariatric surgical literature where surgeons have used a laparoscopic approach successfully to convert a failed previous bariatric operation to a RYGB. These failed procedures are most often VBG or laparoscopic adjustable gastric banding (LAGB). Technical considerations when performing a conversion of a VBG to a RYGB, whether laparoscopic or open, are as follows:

1. Dissection of the left lobe of the liver off the area of the band, on the lesser curvature of the stomach, is usually the most difficult tissue plane encountered.
2. The proximal gastric pouch must be clearly identified.
3. The new gastric pouch must be made above the level of the band. This is not usually difficult because the existing pouch above the band is usually distended and of more than adequate size to divide and still have an adequate proximal gastric pouch.
4. A decision to resect or leave the distal portion of the existing proximal pouch above the band must be made. If it is left in place, the opening through the band must be adequate to drain this isolated gastric segment. If it is resected, the band and the section must be completely resected, with the distal resection line below any previous staple lines.

The failed fixed banding procedure of the VBG also has been successfully revised to placement of an adjustable gastric band. The adjustable gastric banding procedure is the most common bariatric operation performed throughout the world outside the United States and is gaining popularity in this country. O'Brien et al.[44] placed an adjustable band to revise failed gastroplasty and other procedures for 50 patients. The 3-year weight loss was 47% of excess weight. The early complication rate of placement of these bands, done via a celiotomy, was considerably increased versus band placement as a primary operation (17% versus 1.1%), always done laparoscopically. Late (2% versus 18%) complication rates were lower for the revision series than for initial LAGB.

Failed Laparoscopic Adjustable Gastric Banding

Reports in the literature that have described reoperation for failed LAGB have usually taken the approach of using only one other alternative operation for this problem. Conversion of a failed LAGB to a laparoscopic RYGB was performed by Mognol et al.[45] for 70 patients. They reported a conversion rate of only 4.3%, an operative time of 4 hours, hospital stay of 7 days, complication rate of 14.3% early and 8.6% late, and no deaths. Excess weight loss averaged 70%, and more than 60% of patients achieved a BMI less than 33kg/m^2. These results are excellent and are similar to the results reported by Calmes et al.[46] for a series of 49 patients converted from LAGB or VBG to laparoscopic RYGB. They had no conversions, operating room time was 3.25 hours, morbidity was 20%, and nearly 75% of patients achieved a BMI less than 35kg/m^2.

The use of a laparoscopic biliopancreatic diversion to treat patients with failed weight loss after LAGB was reported by Fielding.[47] Having performed a large series of LAGB procedures, surgeons reoperated on 5.4% of the initial LAGB group who had their bands removed for a variety of reasons. They performed the biliopancreatic diversion 38 times laparoscopically and 20 times via celiotomy. They also performed a laparoscopic duodenal switch procedure for 21 patients. In this entire group, excellent weight loss of 40% excess weight was achieved with only a 6.3% complication rate and no mortality.

Failed Roux-en-Y Gastric Bypass

RYGB may fail for several reasons. If the surgeon does not divide the stomach in creating the proximal gastric pouch, there is a significant incidence of disruption of the gastric staple line with regain of weight and associated development of marginal ulceration at the site of the gastrojejunostomy. MacLean et al.[48] reported the incidence of such staple line disruption in 29% of cases followed up to 8 years. Our own experience with not dividing the stomach in the first few years of performing RYGB was a 5% incidence of staple breakdown per year, which accumulated to 25% by 5 years' follow-up. It is now commonly accepted in bariatric surgery that dividing the stomach to create the proximal gastric pouch results in fewer long-term complications from staple line breakdown.

If staple line breakdown is the reason for the failure of the RYGB, reoperation is indicated to redivide the stomach at or above the original staple line. Care must be taken by the surgeon not to leave an isolated undrained closed section of stomach between staple lines. If staple line identification intraoperatively is difficult, we have used upper endoscopy to help define the proximal edge of the staple line. If confirmation of a preexisting staple line can be done only from the distal stomach, we have no concerns about creating a small gastrotomy in the distal stomach during revisional gastric surgery to identify with absolute certainty the level of the previous staple line. This maneuver is useful for all types of reoperative gastric surgery, not just bariatric. The gastrotomy is easily closed later.

Failed RYGB has been treated by adding a malabsorptive component to the original procedure by Fobi et al.[49] and Sugerman et al.[50] Fobi's group[49] performed a distal RYGB, decreasing the absorptive length of the alimentary tract in half. They reported an excessive protein malnutrition incidence of 23% in the 65 patients for whom this was done. Weight loss was from a BMI of 42kg/m^2 to 35kg/m^2. Sugerman's group[50] similarly found adding malabsorption to significant restriction can be problematic when they created a distal RYGB with only a 50-cm common channel after failed gastric bypass. All five reported patients developed protein-calorie malnutrition, and two died of hepatic failure. Creation of a 150-cm common channel in 22 patients resulted in only 3 developing protein-calorie malnutrition and reoperation to lengthen the common channel. Bariatric surgeons must be aware of the *significant* potential morbidity that may result from adding a malabsorptive operation on to an already present restrictive one.

There is a trend in the bariatric field, especially by bariatric surgeons or their colleagues who perform advanced intraluminal endoscopic surgery, to consider reoperating on patients after RYGB who have regained weight or failed to lose adequate weight and who have a larger than 1-cm gastrojejunostomy. The reasoning is that the enlarged anastomosis has allowed excess food intake and weight regain. Initiatives of performing endoscopic intraluminal suturing to narrow the gastrojejunostomy anastomotic opening have begun in several centers.[51] Endoscopists use the same endoscopic tissue suturing device that has been used to treat gastroesophageal reflux disease endoscopically for several years in some centers. The latter experience has been less than satisfying and does not compare in efficacy with laparoscopic antireflux surgery. The major concern with this reoperative procedure is that to date there is *no direct evidence* anywhere in the bariatric literature that a smaller anastomosis produces improved weight loss after RYGB. The experience with failed VBG should have taught bariatric surgeons that a small anastomosis does not guarantee good prolonged weight loss. Similarly, no study has been published showing that reoperation to narrow the anastomosis has any efficacy. Endoscopists who venture into this arena should be aware of the lack of evidence substantiating these procedures. Until proved effective (including lack of placebo and associated diet and exercise effects), these procedures must be considered experimental.

Failed Malabsorptive Procedure

Few reports of reoperative surgery for biliopancreatic diversion or duodenal switch operations exist. This is largely because the operation usually produces satisfactory weight loss. The reoperations that do occur usually are due to the consequence of protein-calorie malnutrition and the need for repeated episodes of parenteral nutrition and persistent hypoalbuminemia. This situation is corrected by revision to increase the length of the common channel. Surgeons usually revise the operation to make a considerably longer common channel, but there are no clear guidelines for the amount or percentage that the surgeon must increase the common channel to avoid residual protein-calorie malnutrition and still preserve some degree of weight loss. Cases must be individualized, and the surgeon does well to err on the side of safety in restoring adequate digestive function in these situations.

All bariatric operations may fail for a variety of reasons. The success with reoperation, as noted earlier for many of the reported series, is usually only modest. It is typical for the reoperative candidate to have a BMI in the low to mid 40s and to have some additional weight loss to achieve a BMI near $35 \, kg/m^2$. Achieving a BMI less than $30 \, kg/m^2$ is unusual based on most reported experiences. Many reoperations are done via an open celiotomy approach. Performance of laparoscopic reoperation should be restricted to only surgeons with significant advanced laparoscopic experience in bariatric surgery. Overall, the complication rates of reoperative bariatric surgery are considerably higher than the rates reported for initial procedures. Because of this combination of facts, the bariatric surgeon is cautioned to be particularly selective in offering reoperative surgery for failed previous bariatric operations. The concerns elaborated earlier regarding patient rather than operation failure always must be heeded when assessing a patient for reoperative bariatric surgery.

BILE REFLUX GASTRITIS

Enterogastric reflux is within the normal pattern of gastrointestinal physiology. The gastric mucosa is relatively resistant to modest amounts of bile, and gastritis normally does not occur with such quantities of bile. If bile reflux is excessive, however, bile gastritis may occur. Patients with this problem typically have epigastric abdominal pain, nausea, and bilious vomiting. The diagnosis of bile reflux gastritis requires first that no concurrent obstructive process is present. Such problems include afferent limb syndrome, efferent limb obstruction after gastrojejunostomy, more distal bowel obstruction, and gastroparesis, particularly postvagotomy gastroparesis. Upper gastrointestinal series, endoscopy with careful examination and biopsy of the gastric mucosa, gastric emptying studies, and quantitative assessment of the amount of enterogastric reflux all should be

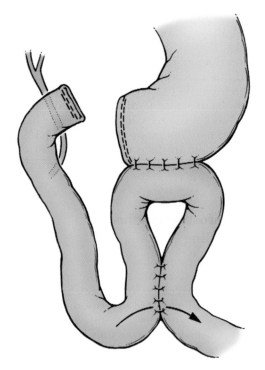

Figure 76–2. Braun's enteroenterostomy. Anastomosis between afferent and efferent limbs for surgical management of bile reflux gastritis. (From Madura JA: Postgastrectomy problems: Remedial operations and therapy. In Cameron JL [ed]: Current Surgical Therapy, 7th ed. Philadelphia, Mosby, 2001, p 92.)

performed in patients suspected to have bile reflux gastritis. Radionuclide scintigraphy of the biliary tree is helpful in quantitating the amount of bile reflux. In most cases, an underlying cause for the patient's symptoms can be found after such a battery of tests. Often the problem is not true bile reflux. The surgeon must *avoid* operating on patients for this condition without a complete evaluation. Performing reoperative surgery for presumptive bile reflux when the true cause of the problem is gastroparesis leads to poor outcomes and persistently symptomatic patients.

Treatment of a patient with true bile reflux gastritis is based on the existing anatomy. If the patient has a gastrojejunostomy, the options include conversion to a Roux-en-Y drainage or creation of a Braun enteroenterostomy between the afferent and efferent limbs of bowel. This is performed by simply creating a side-to-side anastomosis between the afferent and efferent limbs draining the stomach (Fig. 76–2). Typically, the distance is 30 cm away from the gastrojejunostomy. Vogel et al.[52] reported excellent reversal of alkaline reflux gastritis by use of the Braun enteroenterostomy in a group of 30 patients.

The duodenal switch operation, first described by DeMeester et al.[53] for the treatment of this condition, treats bile reflux gastritis when there is no gastrojejunostomy or previous gastric resection. The duodenal switch is performed by dividing the duodenum 2 to 3 cm distal to the pylorus, then performing an anastomosis of the duodenal stump to a Roux-en-Y loop of jejunum (Fig.

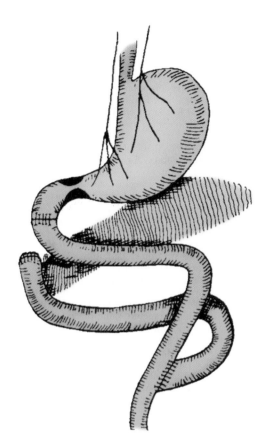

Figure 76–3.   Duodenal switch procedure. The duodenum is transected 2 to 3 cm distal to the pylorus and anastomosed to a Roux-en-Y limb.

76–3). The enteroenterostomy of the Roux limb is typically at least 75 cm downstream to avoid any potential for bile reflux under normal circumstances. Marginal ulceration is a common problem after this operation, and consideration should be given to long-term proton pump inhibitor therapy postoperatively.

AFFERENT LIMB SYNDROME

Afferent limb syndrome is the term used to describe the partial obstruction of the afferent limb of a gastrojejunostomy after previous gastric resection and Billroth II gastrojejunostomy. The afferent limb contains the biliary and pancreatic secretions carried from the duodenum. Obstruction to drainage of the afferent limb may arise as a result of any obstructive process, benign or neoplastic. Early obstruction after a recent operation is usually the result of technical error in creating the gastrojejunostomy, with resulting kinking of the efferent limb. More chronic obstruction may result from progressive scarring of the afferent limb as it passes through the transverse colon mesentery; adhesion formation with stricture, chronic volvulus, or internal hernia; or any other chronic obstructive process.

Symptoms of the afferent limb syndrome commonly include postprandial epigastric and right upper quadrant pain, followed by bilious vomiting with simultaneous relief of the pain. The pain occurs as a result of the increased biliary secretions causing distention of the duodenum and afferent limb. When the limb pressure is sufficient to decompress into the stomach, bilious vomiting results. Because the syndrome is usually slowly progressive, it may cause enough partial obstruction of the drainage of the bile and pancreatic juice to elevate bilirubin and amylase. Chronic obstruction in the afferent limb also may result in a chronic diarrhea syndrome from bacterial overgrowth. Pancreatitis also has been reported.[54] Diagnosis of the afferent limb syndrome is often a clinical one. Radiographic studies, including upper gastrointestinal series or computed tomography with oral contrast administraton, often clearly delineate the problem and are usually diagnostic.

Treatment of afferent limb syndrome is reoperative, and the operative findings should dictate the procedure performed. If simple adhesiolysis resolves the problem, and the intestine is not chronically scarred and narrowed, that is all that is indicated. If the afferent limb is chronically scarred near the gastrojejunostomy, however, which is usually the case, surgical treatment is division of the bowel just proximal to the obstruction point and creation of a Roux-en-Y drainage of the stomach by reanastomosing the proximal end of the divided afferent limb to the jejunum 50 to 75 cm beyond the gastrojejunostomy. Closure of the mesenteric defect completes the procedure.

HOSTILE ABDOMEN

A taxing challenge a surgeon faces is the *hostile abdomen*. This term is used to describe an abdomen in which tissue planes are obscured, and bowel mobility is limited or absent. Severe scarring and carcinomatosis are the most common reasons for such an abdomen. Bowel obstruction is a common occurrence with abdominal or pelvic cancer. Patients develop an obstruction with a prevalence of 5.5% to 42% with ovarian cancer and 10% to 28.4% with colorectal cancer.[55] A complete obstruction requires operative intervention regardless of the patient's history. Most operative management of this situation would not involve reoperation on the stomach or duodenum, but often a gastrostomy tube is placed at the time of such procedures to help decompress the stomach; this may be the only option for patient palliation in the presence of an abdomen filled with carcinomatosis. Indications for placement of a gastrostomy tube are listed in Box 76–3. This is not a comprehensive list, but includes the most frequent indications for gastrostomy.

Gastrostomy tube placement is generally a straightforward procedure. Care must be taken to choose an area of the stomach that most easily reaches the anterior abdominal wall; this is usually the greater curvature area in the proximal body area of the stomach. The traditional Stamm gastrostomy serves adequately in almost all cases. Janeway gastrostomies, created from a greater curvature tube of stomach anastomosed to the skin, are indicated only as a permanent feeding access.

When encountering diffuse carcinomatosis in the setting of an obstructed gastrointestinal tract, the surgeon is wise to do as little as necessary and feasible to

Box 76–3   Indications for Gastrostomy

As an alternative to nasogastric intubation during operations in which a prolonged postoperative ileus is expected

As a means of long-term enteral access for patients who cannot eat without assistance

For patients with obstructing lesions of the hypopharynx or esophagus

As a reliable means of decompressing the stomach and giving enteral nutrition after esophageal and bariatric surgery

Palliative decompression for distal obstructing lesions in which resection or bypass is not technically feasible or medically indicated

improve the patient's remaining time. Bowel obstruction in patients with metastatic cancer is often considered a relatively terminal event, with median survival following being 3 months.[56] Patients with terminal cancer who are unfit for an operation may benefit from nonoperative management of a malignant obstruction. Analgesics, antiemetics, and antisecretory medications have been shown to provide an alternative management of a chronic obstruction.[57] Surgery is an appropriate option in low-risk to moderate-risk patients. Only 30% of patients with malignant bowel obstruction have prolonged postoperative symptom relief after surgical intervention.[58]

When a lysis of adhesions is attempted in a patient with multiple previous operations, the patient is at great risk for multiple enterotomies. In contrast to an enterotomy during a standard dissection, an enterotomy in a "frozen abdomen" is much more hazardous. The bowel injury may be extremely difficult to close if the intestine cannot be safely mobilized to allow for adequate closure. Also, there is a slightly greater risk for luminal narrowing from a repair of a bowel injury that is poorly visualized and mobilized. When multiple enterotomies have been made, or no progress is being safely made, consideration must be given to backing out of the operation. This is a difficult decision for any surgeon to make. Although the original operative goals may not have been accomplished, consideration must be given to avoiding causing further morbidity to the patient.

REFERENCES

1. Ellis H: The cause and prevention of postoperative intraperitoneal adhesions. Surg Gynecol Obstet 133:497-511, 1971.
2. Ellis H, Moran BJ, Thompson JN, et al: Adhesion-related hospital readmissions after abdominal and pelvic surgery: A retrospective cohort study. Lancet 353:1456-1457, 1999.
3. Cohen Z, Cohen Z, Senagore AJ, et al: Prevention of postoperative abdominal adhesions by a novel, glycerol/sodium hyaluronate/carboxymethylcellulose-based bioresorbable membrane: A prospective, randomized, evaluator-blinded multicenter study. Dis Colon Rectum 48:1130-1139, 2005.
4. Becker JM, Dayton MT, Fazio VW, et al: Prevention of postoperative abdominal adhesions by a sodium hyaluronate-based bioresorbable membrane: A prospective, randomized, double-blind multicenter study. J Am Coll Surg 183:406-407, 1996.
5. Catarci M, Carlini M, Gentileschi P, Santoro E: Major and minor injuries during the creation of pneumoperitoneum: A multicenter study on 12,919 cases. Surg Endosc 15:566-569, 2001.
6. Schwartz ML, Drew RL, Andersen JN: Induction of pneumoperitoneum in morbidly obese patients. Obes Surg 13:601-604, discussion 604, 2003.
7. Vance PL, de Lange EE, Shaffer HA Jr, Schirmer B: Gastric outlet obstruction following surgery for morbid obesity: Effect of fluoroscopically guided balloon dilation. Radiology 222:70-72, 2002.
8. Capella JF, Capella RF: Gastro-gastric fistulas and marginal ulcers in gastric bypass procedures for weight reduction. Obes Surg 9:22-27, 1999.
9. Huang CS, Hess DT, Lichtenstein DR: Successful endoscopic management of postoperative GI fistula with fibrin glue injection: Report of two cases. Gastrointest Endosc 60:460-463, 2004.
10. Ukleja A: Dumping syndrome: Pathophysiology and treatment. Nutr Clin Pract 20:517-525, 2005.
11. Yamamoto H, Mori T, Tsuchihashi H, et al: A possible role of GLP-1 in the pathophysiology of early dumping syndrome. Dig Dis Sci 50:2263-2267, 2005.
12. Li-Ling J, Irving M: Therapeutic value of octreotide for patients with severe dumping syndrome—a review of randomized controlled trials. Postgrad Med 77:441-442, 2001.
13. Penning C, Vecht J, Masclee AA: Efficacy of depot long-acting release octreotide therapy in severe dumping syndrome. Aliment Pharmacol Therap 22:963-969, 2005.
14. Vecht J, Lamers CBHW, Masclee AAM: Long-term results of octreotide-therapy in severe dumping syndrome. Clin Endocrinol 51:619-624, 1999.
15. Behrns KE, Sarr MG: Diagnosis and management of gastric emptying disorders. Adv Surg 27:233-255, 1994.
16. Morii Y, Arita T, Shimoda K, et al: Jejunal interposition to prevent postgastrectomy syndromes. Br J Surg 87:1576-1579, 2000.
17. Singh A, Gull H, Sing RJ: Clinical significance of rapid (accelerated) gastric emptying. Clin Nucl Med 28:658-662, 2003.
18. Bouras E, Scolapio JS: Gastric motility disorders: Management that optimizes nutritional status. J Clin Gastroenterol 38:549-557, 2004.
19. Echauser FE, Conrad M, Knol JA, et al: Safety and long-term durability of completion gastrectomy in 81 patients with postsurgical gastroparesis syndrome. Am Surg 64:711-716, 1998.
20. Abell T, McCallum R, Hocking M, et al: Gastric electrical stimulation for medically refractory gastroparesis. Gastroenterology 125:421-428, 2003.
21. Schirmer BD: Gastric atony and the roux syndrome. Gastroenterol Clin North Am 23:327-343, 1994.
22. Greene FL: Management of gastric remnant carcinoma based on the results of a 15-year endoscopic screening program. Ann Surg 223:701-706, 1996.
23. Takeyoshi I, Ohwada S, Ogawa T, et al: The resection of non-hepatic intraabdominal recurrence of gastric cancer. Hepatogastroenterology 47:1479-1481, 2000.
24. Cogliandolo A, Scarmozzino G, Pidoto RR, et al: Laparoscopic palliative gastrojejunostomy for advanced recurrent gastric cancer after Billroth I resection. J Laparoendosc Adv Surg Tech A 14:43-46, 2004.
25. Wai CT, Ho KY, Yeoh KG, Lim SG: Palliation of malignant gastric outlet obstruction caused by gastric cancer with self-expandable metal stents. Surg Laparosc Endosc Percutan Tech 11:161-164, 2001.
26. Lai IR, Hu RH, Chang KJ: Is imatinib justified as an adjuvant chemotherapy for patients with recurrent gastrointestinal stromal tumors. Hepatogastroenterology 52:826-828, 2005.
27. Tulchinsky H, Keidar A, Strul H, et al: Extracolonic manifestations of familial adenomatous polyposis after proctocolectomy. Arch Surg 140:159-163, 2005.
28. Morton J, Lucktong T, Behrns K, et al: National trends in fundoplication utilization and outcomes from 1989 and 1999. J Am Coll Surg 195:S55, 2002.
29. Hashemi M, Peters JH, DeMeester TR, et al: Laparoscopic repair of large type III hiatal hernia: Objective followup reveals high recurrence rate. J Am Coll Surg 190:553-560, 2000.

30. Lord RV, Kaminski A, Oberg S, et al: Absence of gastroesophageal reflux disease in a majority of patients taking acid suppression medications after Nissen fundoplication. J Gastrointest Surg 6:3-9, 2002.

31. Smith DC, McClusky DA, Rajad MA, et al: When fundoplication fails: Redo? Ann Surg 241:861-871, 2005.

32. Neuhauser B, Hinder RA: Laparoscopic reoperation after failed antireflux surgery. Semin Laparosc Surg 8:281-286, 2001.

33. Byrne JP, Smithers BM, Nathanson LK, et al: Symptomatic and functional outcome after laparoscopic reoperation for failed antireflux surgery. Br J Surg 92:996-1001, 2005.

34. Rosemurgy AS, Arnaoutakis DJ, Thometz DP, et al: Reoperative fundoplications are effective treatment for dysphagia and recurrent gastroesophageal reflux. Am Surgeon 70:1061-1067, 2004.

35. Heniford BT, Matthews BD, Kercher KW, et al: Surgical experience in fifty-five consecutive reoperative fundoplications. Am Surgeon 68:949-954, 2002.

36. Dutta S, Bamehriz F, Boghossian T, et al: Outcome of laparoscopic redo fundoplication. Surg Endosc 18:440-443, 2004.

37. Balsinger BM, Poggio JL, Mai J, et al: Ten and more years after vertical banded gastroplasty as primary operation for morbid obesity. J Gastrointest Surg 4:598-605, 2000.

38. Schirmer B, Erenoglu C, Miller A: Flexible endoscopy in the management of patients undergoing Roux-en-Y gastric bypass. Obes Surg 12:634-638, 2002.

39. Brolin RE, Robertson LB, Kenler HA, et al: Weight loss and dietary intake after vertical banded gastroplasty and Roux-en-Y gastric bypass. Ann Surg 220:782-790, 1994.

40. Jones KB Jr: Revisional bariatric surgery—safe and effective. Obes Surg 11:183-189, 2001.

41. Sugerman HJ, Kellum, JM, DeMaria EJ: Conversion of failed or complicated vertical banded gastroplasty to gastric bypass in morbid obesity. Am J Surg 171:263-269, 1996.

42. Cariani S, Nottola D, Grani S, et al: Complications after gastroplasty and gastric bypass as a primary operation and as a reoperation. Obes Surg 11:487-490, 2001.

43. Gagner M, Gentileschi P, deCsepel J, et al: Laparoscopic reoperative bariatric surgery: Experience from 27 consecutive patients. Obes Surg 12:254-260, 2002.

44. O'Brien P, Brown W, Dixon J: Revisional surgery for morbid obesity—conversion to the Lap-Band system. Obes Surg 10:557-563, 2000.

45. Mognol P, Chosidow D, Marmuse JP: Laparoscopic conversion of laparoscopic gastric banding to Roux-en-Y gastric bypass: A review of 70 patients. Obes Surg 14:1349-1353, 2004.

46. Calmes JM, Guisti V, Suter M: Reoperative laparoscopic Roux-en-Y gastric bypass: An experience with 49 cases. Obes Surg 15:316-322, 2005.

47. Fielding GA: Laparoscopic biliopancreatic diversion with or without duodenal switch as revision for failed lapband. Surg Endosc 17(Suppl):S187, 2003.

48. MacLean LD, Rhode BM, Nohr C, et al: Stomal ulcer after gastric bypass. J Am Coll Surg 185:87-88, 1997.

49. Fobi MAL, Lee H, Igew D Jr, et al: Revision of failed gastric bypass to distal Roux-en-Y gastric bypass: A review of 65 cases. Obes Surg 11:190-195, 2001.

50. Sugerman HJ, Kellum JM, DeMaria EJ: Conversion of proximal to distal gastric bypass for failed gastric bypass for superobesity. J Gastrointest Surg 1:517-525, 1997.

51. Thompson C: Endoscopy and the bariatric patient. Presented at the Sixth Minimally Invasive Surgery Symposium, Vail, CO, February 25, 2006.

52. Vogel SB, Drane WE, Woodward ER: Clinical and radionuclide evaluation of bile diversion by Braun enteroenterostomy: Prevention and treatment of alkaline reflux gastritis: An alternative to Roux-en-Y diversion. Ann Surg 219:458-465, 1994.

53. DeMeester TR, Fuchs KH, Ball CS, et al: Experimental and clinical results with proximal end-to-end duodenojejunostomy for pathological duodenogastric reflux. Ann Surg 206:414-424, 1987.

54. Kaya E, Senyurek G, Dervisoglu A, et al: Acute pancreatitis caused by afferent loop herniation after Billroth II gastrectomy: Report of a case and review of the literature. Hepatogastroenterology 51:606-608, 2004.

55. Ripamonti C, De Conno F, Ventafridda V, et al: Management of bowel obstruction in advanced and terminal cancer patients. Ann Oncol 4:15-21, 1993.

56. Blair SL, Chu DZ, Schwarz RE: Outcome of palliative operations for malignant bowel obstruction in patients with peritoneal carcinomatosis from nongynecological cancer. Ann Surg Oncol 8:632-637, 2001.

57. Mystakidou K, Tsilika E, Kalaidopoulou O, et al: Comparison of octreotide administration vs conservative treatment in the management of inoperable bowel obstruction in patients with far advanced cancer: A randomized, double-blind, controlled clinical trial. Anticancer Res 22:1187-1192, 2002.

58. Pameijer CR, Mahvi DM, Stewart JA, Weber SM: Bowel obstruction in patients with metastatic cancer: Does intervention influence outcome? Int J Gastrointest Cancer 35:127-133, 2005.

77

Radiation Enteritis

Rainer K. Saetzler · Thomas Wiegel · Doris Henne-Bruns

Radiation therapy or combined chemoradiation therapy is a widely accepted adjuvant or neoadjuvant treatment modality for various tumors. Despite steady technical improvements in irradiation techniques, the major drawback is the unnecessary irradiation of normal tissue in close vicinity to the tumor, which can result in radiation toxicity such as radiation enteritis, an entity that can occur in an acute or chronic form.

This chapter attempts to shed some light on the pathogenesis of radiation-induced toxicities or complications and discusses possible future treatments for patients suffering from this condition. Moreover, new technical developments in radiation oncology and radiochemotherapy that will improve the protection of nonmalignant tissue and hence decrease the complication rate of radiation therapy without compromising the tumor-killing activity of these methods are discussed as well.

BACKGROUND

Radiation is a common adjuvant and, more recently, a neoadjuvant therapy in the multimodality approach to the treatment of various abdominal and pelvic cancers and has been proved in multiple studies to be an important tool for destroying cancer cells. Besides these beneficial effects, radiation also affects normal and healthy tissue surrounding the targeted tumor, such as the small and large intestine, liver, kidney, and lung.[1-9]

Radiation enteritis is one of the most feared complications of abdominal and pelvic irradiation. The mucosa and submucosal vasculature of the intestine are most sensitive to radiation and might sustain severe acute or chronic damage leading to malabsorption, strictures, and fistulas, with considerable impact on the patient's quality of life.[10]

The amount of radiation required to produce clinical signs of enteritis varies with the treatment regimen and from patient to patient. Because of the current trend of combined chemotherapy and radiation therapy, the incidence of radiation enteritis is increasing.[11]

Clinicians are usually confronted with the sequelae of early and late complications of radiation enteritis and therefore need a detailed understanding of the mechanisms leading to early and late radiation enteritis.

INCIDENCE

Radiation enteritis is a relentless disease process reflecting widespread bowel involvement. The first patient with radiation-induced enteropathy was described by Walsh in 1897, only 2 years after Roentgen's description of ionizing radiation.[12,13]

According to the literature, the exact incidence of radiation enteropathy is not known. However, since the 1980s, the incidence of acute enteritis appears to have increased because more than 50% of patients with cancer receive radiotherapy as a component of their treatment.[14-18]

The incidence of *acute* radiation enteritis shows great variation and has been reported in the literature as being between 20% and 80%.[19,20]

The exact incidence of *chronic* radiation enteritis remains controversial and ranges from 0.5% to 36% with an average of 5%.[16,21-23] However, the prevalence seems to be underestimated in the literature because of losing track of patients, patient death as a result of malignancies, and differences in treatment regimens.[12,15,22] Moreover, one has to bear in mind that this wide variation is also due to different factors such as radiation dose per fraction and total dose of radiation and to patient-related predisposing factors such as location and size of the treatment volume, hypertension, diabetes mellitus, and pre-existing vascular or pelvic inflammatory disease.[16,24]

A total radiation dose of less than 4000 cGy (4000 rad) rarely causes deleterious effects on bowel mucosa and hence radiation enteritis (1 Gy is equivalent to 100 cGy or 100 rad).[15,16] If the dose does exceed 5000 cGy, the complication rate increases significantly. Doses of radiation producing clinical damage in up to 5% or in up to 50% of patients within 5 years are termed $TD_{5/5}$ or $TD_{50/5}$, respectively, depending on the volume of irradiated tissue. The range is 60 to 75 Gy for the esophagus, 45 to 50 Gy for the stomach, 45 to 65 Gy for the small bowel and colon, and 55 to 80 Gy for the rectum.[25]

In addition, the use of certain adjuvant chemotherapeutic agents such as 5-fluorouracil (5-FU), doxorubicin, actinomycin D, and methotrexate increase the likelihood of enteritis secondary to radiation therapy. A history of laparotomy and previous abdominal operations also increases the risk for enteritis, probably because of adhesions that tether portions of the small bowel into the irradiated field.

ETIOLOGY

Roentgen rays have their most destructive effect on rapidly dividing cells such as bowel epithelium, and as a consequence many of these epithelial cells die during radiotherapy. Cells in other tissues are sublethally damaged and die off later when entering the mitosis phase.

The pathophysiologic effect behind radiation-induced cell death is the deposition of energy in the anatomic structure of the chemical constituents of cells.[16] Disruption of the DNA helix or abnormal reconstitution of the genetic code will result in cell death or cell dysfunction. Radiation injury will subsequently occur in the mucosa, submucosa, muscularis propria, and serosa as a function of cell turnover in these tissue layers.

Therefore, three distinct phases of radiation effects have been identified:

1. *Acute phase:* primarily affecting the mucosa
2. *Subacute phase:* predominantly affecting the submucosa
3. *Chronic phase:* affecting all layers of the bowel wall

During radiation therapy, adjacent healthy tissues are invariably located within the irradiated field and therefore represent the main dose-limiting factor of radiation therapy. The small bowel appears to be one of the most radiosensitive organs of the abdomen because of the high number of proliferating cells, the extensive vascular network, and important metabolic activities.[16] However, its mobility seems to be somewhat protective. The most sensitive cells of the bowel wall are those of the crypt of Langerhans in the small intestine.

Late radiation injuries more frequently involve the immobile and fixed terminal ileum. Because the jejunum, except for its upper portion and the proximal ileum, is relatively protected by its mobility, repeated exposure of selected small bowel segment is avoided.[16,22]

Predisposing Risk Factors

Many factors are thought to predispose to radiation injury. Dose-escalating techniques in radiation oncology, combined with chemotherapy and thin-built patients, are associated with a higher risk of sustaining small bowel injury.[26,27] Thin patients, especially females, and the elderly have an increased amount of small bowel in the pelvic cul-de-sac.[12,26,28,29] They also have a decreased amount of subcutaneous tissue, which would allow greater depth of penetration of ionizing radiation.

Any previous operation or pelvic infection may cause intra-abdominal fixation of the small bowel and thereby expose the same segment of bowel to the radiation field.

This situation is predominantly seen after rectal surgery because of the development of more adhesions as a result of a high level of physical injury to the gut serosa and increasing microbial leakage through the intestinal wall into the peritoneum, unsuccessful reperitonealization, and the impaired vasculature of small bowel loops in the sacral cavity.[30] Low splanchnic blood flow as seen in congestive heart failure or conditions associated with vascular occlusion or narrowing predisposes to radiation-induced injury. Moreover, DeCosse et al. demonstrated a significant association between hypertension, diabetes, and cardiovascular disease and the subsequent development of radiation enteritis.[31,32]

PATHOPHYSIOLOGY AND HISTOPATHOLOGIC FEATURES

The gut wall is damaged by ionizing radiation either directly or indirectly. The direct effect of intestinal irradiation is loss of regenerating cells within the crypts of the intestinal epithelium.[16,22,30,33] Indirectly, damage to the fine vasculature of the intestine may progress to obliterative vasculitis and cause ischemia of the bowel many years after radiation therapy.

Early Histologic Findings

The first 2 weeks after radiation therapy is characterized by four early histologic findings. The first is *mucosal ulceration.* In early stages these ulcers are small and shallow but get bigger and deeper in the later stages and thereby lead to perforation and fistulization. The second histologic feature consists of *epithelial atypia.* Radiation-induced fine mutation is the single important factor involved in malignant transformation of intestinal epithelium in humans. The third finding is termed *ileitis cystica profunda,* which is defined by the presence of cystic glandular structures in the intestinal wall below the muscularis mucosae. Its mechanism remains controversial, but it has been suggested that fragmentation of the muscularis mucosae leads to herniation of epithelium into deeper layers of the intestinal wall. Moreover, mucosal trapping during the re-epithelialization phase of deep ulcers has been proposed as a potential explanation. The fourth characteristic is *serosal thickening.* This finding reflects an increased amount of fibrous connective tissue and edema. Its pathogenesis, however, is controversial. It is believed that radiation-induced vascular permeability is followed by edema, intestinal protein deposition, and subsequent fibrosis. These histopathologic findings decrease gradually and remain constant for 20 weeks on. Other features such as vascular sclerosis, intestinal fibrosis, and lymph congestion are virtually absent at 2 weeks but with time increase and reach a constant level 8 to 14 weeks after irradiation.

Late Histologic Findings

Late histologic features include three distinct entities. The first is characterized by vascular sclerosis. The structural and functional alterations in blood vessels consist of three stages: *early* (hours to days after irradiation), *intermediate* (4 weeks after irradiation), and *late* (4 to 6 months after irradiation). During the *early stage* an inflammatory reaction takes place with deletion of capillaries secondary to substances released by the damaged endothelial cells. The *intermediate phase* is characterized by destruction and obliteration of capillaries, sloughing of endothelial cells, and the formation of focal thrombi. Plasma proteins accumulate in the extravascular space and possibly lead to hyalinization, which is also seen histologically. In the *late phase* several histologic entities are observed, such as necrosis of the vessel wall, ulcerations, and thrombosis. Thickening of the vessels and media necrosis induce total vascular occlusion and disruption. The second late histologic finding is *intestinal wall fibrosis* as a result of deposition of collagen in the intestinal wall. Several pathophysiologic mechanisms have been discussed and are briefly outlined. Radiation has a direct effect on collagen and components of the extracellular matrix such as glycosaminoglycans. Cell injury or cell death involved in the production or degradation of collagen leads to fibrosis. Moreover, vascular and lymphatic damage contributes to the ongoing fibrosis. Some authors suspect nonspecific inflammatory or autoimmune processes. The third characteristic is *lymph congestion.* Loss of the epithelial barrier of the bowel leads to exposure of deeper layers of the bowel wall to intraluminal contents, which induces a severe inflammatory reaction. In late radiation enteropathy, fibrotic constriction of lymph vessels, rather than their direct damage, is the cause of obstructed lymph flow and consequent dilation.

MOLECULAR BIOLOGY OF RADIATION ENTERITIS AND MICROCIRCULATION

Recent progress in molecular biology has led to new concepts of the pathogenesis of radiation enteritis. The first concept involves *apoptosis,* which is defined as an active mode of cell death characterized by chromatin and cytoplasmic condensation as a result of the activation of DNA endonucleases and transglutaminases. It is controlled by regulatory genes such as *p53, bcl-2, ced-3, ced-4,* and *ced-9.* Under normal physiologic conditions, both small intestinal and colonic epithelia undergo a low rate of spontaneous apoptosis.

Animal experiments have shown that exposure to low-dose radiation leads to an increase in the rate of apoptosis of intestinal crypt cells, especially stem cells of the crypts. The rate of apoptosis was dose dependent and depended on the expression of tumor suppressor genes in stem cells.[34-36]

Paris et al. demonstrated in mouse models that microvascular endothelial cell apoptosis is the primary lesion leading to stem cell dysfunction.[37]

Garcia-Barros et al. provided evidence that tissue and tumor response to radiation is also determined by microvascular sensitivity to radiation. Their studies indicated that microvascular damage in response to radiation occurs at clinically relevant dose ranges.[27] Another concept comprises the pathogenesis of fibrosis. Herskind et al. investigated the role of cytokines in radiation enteritis.[38] They found that transforming growth factor β (TGF-β) is of particular importance in extracellular matrix deposition and development of tissue fibrosis.

Ionizing radiation activates translation of the gene coding for TGF-β. Radiation induces the formation of hydroxyl radicals that stimulate the production of TGF-β_1. This cytokine remains elevated even at 26 weeks after radiation, especially in vascular endothelial cells, fibroblasts, and smooth muscle cells and is mainly implicated in the pathogenesis of fibrosis.[39,40] Immunohistochemical studies of bowel mucosa showed that TGF-β_1 is primarily located in intestinal villi or at the top of colonic crypts.[41-43] Animal experiments demonstrated increased TGF-β immunoreactivity in the small intestine. It acts as a potent fibrogenic and proinflammatory cytokine that leads to connective tissue hyperplasia and increased leukocyte migration and activation in the intestinal wall.[44] The molecular or chemical inhibition of TGF-β_1 caused less structural injury and significantly decreased intestinal wall fibrosis when exposed to high doses of radiation.[44] Further studies have demonstrated a prominent role of TGF-β in the pathogenesis of not only radiation-induced enteritis but also radiation-induced organ dysfunction and fibrosis.[1-9] These radiation-induced processes are strikingly similar to the pathogenesis of known clinical entities characterized by an excess of fibrosis, such as scleroderma,[45-47] idiopathic pulmonary fibrosis,[48-50] diabetic nephropathy,[51] and membranous glomerulonephritis.[52]

RADIATION AND THE MICROCIRCULATION

Recent evidence showed that radiation is leading to significant microcirculatory perturbations, eventually causing microvascular dysfunction and organ damage. It was demonstrated that irradiation causes an increase in leukocyte–endothelium interaction and vascular permeability, a similar process seen during inflammation or ischemia/reperfusion injury.[45,53-62] This finding was also substantiated in histologic studies in which irradiated intestinal tissue showed a significant interstitial accumulation of polymorphonuclear leukocytes.[63] The inhibition of leukocyte adhesion to endothelial cells through the administration of antibodies directed toward specific adhesion molecules resulted in a significant reduction in radiation-induced tissue damage.[45,53-58,62,64] This radiation-induced intestinal inflammatory process at the microcirculatory level was also inhibited by the application of oxygen–free radical scavengers such as SOD.[65]

NATURAL HISTORY AND CLINICAL FEATURES

According to the aforementioned pathologic changes, radiation enteritis is manifested as acute radiation enteritis or late radiation enteropathy with early and late symptoms, respectively.

The *acute phase* occurs during the course of irradiation and results from direct radiation-induced depletion of the actively proliferating intestinal crypt cells with concomitant inflammation of the lamina propria. The clinical symptoms of acute radiation enteritis consist mainly of diarrhea, abdominal pain, anorexia, malaise, and vomiting, all of which are usually self-limited. These symptoms disappear after 2 to 6 weeks and require only symptomatic treatment. They are dependent on the rate and duration of time over which radiation is applied rather than on the total dose. This stage frequently remains subclinical despite marked mucosal damage.

The symptoms of *late radiation enteropathy* occur after a variable latency period averaging 2 to 3 years with a range of 6 months to 20 years. The symptoms are the result of progressive occlusive vasculitis and diffuse collagen deposition and fibrosis.

Symptoms of late radiation enteritis consist of abdominal pain as a result of obstruction secondary to radiation-induced strictures or perforation and necrosis. The onset of symptoms is often insidious, and they are mostly due to changes in intestinal transit and include intermittent diarrhea and constipation. Fistulization between the bowel and pelvic organs, such as the bladder, vagina, or other bowel segments, causes pneumaturia, feculent vaginal discharge, and rapid passage of undigested food in stool, respectively. Moreover, intestinal malabsorption, bile salt malabsorption, anemia, and hypoalbuminemia have been observed. Multiple segments of small bowel can be involved simultaneously.[14]

Abscesses can occur as well, usually in the pelvis, and may cause signs of sepsis. Intestinal perforation may cause acute peritonitis, but this complication is uncommon. Significant intestinal bleeding occurs rarely as a result of ileal ulcerations, but rectal bleeding from radiation proctitis is relatively common.[66]

A four-point injury scale from 0 to 4 has been introduced by O'Brian et al.[30] for the classification of radiation-induced bowel injury: *0*, no complaints; *1*, mild diarrhea (controlled by diet and reassurance); *2*, marked diarrhea and rectal pain, which are relieved by antidiarrheal pain medications or antibiotics; and *3*, severe complications, including fistula formation, perforation, or stricture. The Radiation Therapy Oncology Group (RTOG) introduced a gastrointestinal morbidity scoring system with five grades: *0*, no symptoms; *1*, mild diarrhea, cramping, bowel movements five times daily, slight rectal discharge; *2*, moderate diarrhea and colic, bowel movements more than five times daily, excessive rectal mucus or intermittent bleeding; *3*, obstruction or bleeding requiring surgery; and *4*, necrosis, fistula, or perforation.

It is important to stress that radiation can lead to the development of secondary radiation-induced malignancies, synchronous radiation lesions, or recurrent malignant disease.[67-77] The pathophysiologic mechanisms of radiation-related carcinogenesis and malignant transformation have been studied intensively.[78,79] In a series of 51 patients, Galland and Spencer reported that 47% remained symptom-free at a median follow-up of 1 year. In the remainder, new radiation-related GI problems developed. In none of the patients who were initially seen with bleeding did new problems develop. In comparison, 33% of the patients with strictures and 89% of those with perforation or fistula formation went on to manifest new lesions. Patients whose initial manifestation was fistulas also appeared to be at increased risk of having synchronous radiation lesions at the time of diagnosis. These patients were at increased risk of dying as a result of recurrent malignant disease within a relatively short period.[26-29,80]

Associated collateral radiation damage, frequently underestimated, has been described in the urinary tract system, specifically in the bladder. Other injuries include radiation myelitis, osteitis pubis, pathologic fractures, and atheromatous changes in blood vessels within the radiation field.[32]

Most deaths are due to recurrent disease or the effects of radiation on the gut. Galland and Spencer reported in their study that radiation enteritis was responsible either directly or indirectly for the death of 23 of the 37 patients who died. Nine of these patients died with no evidence of their original tumor.[26,27]

DIAGNOSIS

Establishing the diagnosis of radiation enteritis can be challenging and should include a detailed history and physical examination, followed by laboratory tests and radiologic imaging studies.

The clinical findings in a patient suffering from radiation enteritis can range from subtle symptoms to malabsorption and bowel perforation, as described earlier in the section on natural history. The physician should be guided by a high index of suspicion and eliminate all possible differential diagnoses.

A complete blood count should be obtained when patients are bleeding or suffering from malabsorption. Moreover, a metabolic panel is essential for patients with vomiting or diarrhea. To establish the cause of diarrhea, stool cultures should be obtained, as well as stool volume and stool fat studies. Measurement of bile acid absorption by synthetic gamma-labeled bile acid might be useful.[81] Its absorption and enterohepatic circulation are identical with that of taurine-conjugated bile acids; however, it cannot be deconjugated. Therefore, its absorption is sensitive and specific for terminal ileal function. However, this test is cumbersome to perform and not usually available for clinical use on a routine basis. Measurements of changes in intestinal permeability may be useful in the diagnosis of chronic intestinal damage. Intestinal permeability to large molecules such as chromium-ethylenediaminetetraacetic acid is increased in acute radiation enteritis, but there have been no reports on chronic radiation enteritis.[82]

An acute abdominal series is needed to evaluate for obstruction and ileus. Barium contrast studies provide better mucosal detail and can identify areas of stricture, as well as fistulas. Mendelson and Nolan and Sellink and Miller described the radiologic findings after a single-contrast barium infusion technique, enteroclysis.[83,84] This method seems to be more sensitive and specific for radiation-induced changes and has been shown to be superior to the conventional follow-through examination in demonstrating stenotic segments and mucosal pathology because of optimal bowel distention.[20,83] In addition, information regarding GI motility can be obtained. However, with the advancement of modern technology, these small bowel imaging studies have been partially replaced by MRI-enteroclysis, multislice CT-enteroclysis, and sono-enteroclysis.[63,85-87]

Abdominal and pelvic CT scans are the best studies to confirm obstruction and perforation and to exclude extraintestinal processes, including possible abscesses.

Endoscopy allows mucosal biopsy, which can reveal classic histologic changes consistent with radiation injury, as described earlier.

Many studies have addressed the radiologic features of chronic radiation enteritis in an attempt to identify specific radiologic signs.[19,88,89] Many of them used barium follow-through techniques, whereas others used enteroclysis as the preferred method.

A pathologic fold pattern in the ileum as a result of submucosal edema was observed in 71% of patients.[19] Approximately 50% of patients had no fold pattern at all because of mucosal atrophy. Mural thickening and stenosis were also found. More than 70% of patients showed delayed intestinal transit with dilatation of the jejunum and proximal ileum. These findings were associated with hypoperistalsis of the affected ileal loops. More than half of the patients showed dilatation of the proximal ileum with a maximum diameter of 60 mm. In more than two thirds of all cases an associated dilatation of the jejunum was noted. Radiologic features reflecting the presence of adhesions are known as fixed bowel loops that can be displaced only by deep palpation or as mucosal tacking associated with focal adhesions.

Puddling of barium in the terminal ileum or a segmental saw-toothed appearance of the small bowel is commonly seen. Kinking of bowel loops was attributed to by some authors to mesenteric shortening or adhesions and wall thickening.[83,88,89]

Multiple studies, however, have shown that the extent of the disease is clearly underestimated by radiologic methods when the radiographic results are compared with data obtained during laparotomy. Nonetheless, there is good correlation between intraoperative and radiologic findings with regard to the presence and site of strictures and adhesions.[83] Poor correlation was observed for peritoneal metastases extrinsic to the bowel wall.[20]

PROGNOSIS

It is generally believed that radiation enteritis is a progressive disease. The median latent period between radiation therapy and intestinal symptoms is usually 6 to 24 months with a range between 1 month and 37 years.[27-29,45,90]

Gilinsky et al. reviewed patients with radiation-induced proctosigmoiditis and found that those who had not received blood transfusions had a higher rate of spontaneous remission. In contrast, patients whose symptoms were so severe that transfusions were required rarely experienced remissions and were more likely to undergo surgery.[91] Galland and Spencer reported new radiation-induced GI problems in 39% of patients (20 of 51). Ten patients underwent surgery, 5 of whom died.[16]

No new problems developed in patients whose initial manifestation was bleeding, as opposed to 33% of patients with strictures and 89% of patients with perforation or fistula formation as their initial symptom.[27] Harling and Balslev found cumulative 10-year survival rates of 37% and 64% in patients with perforation or fistula versus bleeding or stricture.[27]

Hatcher et al. made similar observations that patients whose initial manifestation was fistulas appear to be at increased risk of having synchronous radiation lesions at the time of diagnosis, as well as at increased risk of dying.[80] They estimated that additional complications become apparent in about half of those surviving the initial lesion. Harling and Balslev found in their study that during an observation period of 14 years (from 1972 to 1986), 23% of all deaths (13 of a total of 75 deaths) were related to radiation complications and 47% were due to recurrent malignant disease.[90] The cumulative 10-year survival rates were 58% for the entire series of 136 patients, not including those who died from radiation enteritis.[90] However, the 10-year survival rate of patients presenting with bowel perforation or fistulae compared to those presenting with bleeding or stricture was 37% and 64%, respectively.[90]

All investigative groups have confirmed that the risk for new radiation-induced lesions is greater in patients who initially have perforation or fistula than in patients with initial bleeding or stricture. Moreover, life expectancy was poorer in patients with fistulas. The presence of a fistula seems to imply wider dissemination of the destructive process and an excessive rate of recurrent disease.[26,80] However, Perez et al. did not support this finding.[92]

Galland and Spencer and Harling and Balslev reported a 40% to 60% 5-year survival rate.[26,90] Galland and Spencer showed that radiation enteritis was responsible either directly or indirectly for the death of 23 of 37 patients. Nine of these patients had no evidence of their original tumor.[26] It has also been reported that small bowel injuries carry more than four times the mortality than colorectal injuries do[93]; however, this observation was not confirmed by others.[94]

Regimbeau et al. estimated that approximately one third of all patients suffering from chronic radiation enteritis will need to undergo surgery at one point.[23] Furthermore, they found that reoperation was more common in the conservative surgical group of patients who did not undergo bowel resection (50%) compared to those patients who underwent bowel resection (34%).[23] Reoperations were associated with a higher mortality rate overall.[23]

Libotte et al. reviewed the clinical and survival data of 108 patients with radiation enteritis at a median follow-up of 11 years. The median time of occurrence of severe radiation-induced lesions (obstruction, perforation) after radiotherapy was 18 months, 9 months for rectal bleeding and 10.5 months for mild symptoms.[95] They showed that patients with rectal bleeding had a poorer prognosis than did those with mild symptoms but an equivalent prognosis to patients with severe complications.[95]

The development of radiation-induced malignancy is a pivotal factor in the patient's prognosis. It has been shown experimentally that colonic adenocarcinoma will develop in 47% of rats after having been exposed to 4500 rad.[96] Galland and his group examined colonic resection specimens from 26 patients with radiation-induced colitis and found a significant increase in the prevalence of dysplasia and other premalignant changes.[27,97] The relative risk for the development of colonic carcinoma after radiotherapy has been calculated as being 2 to 3.6 in women who undergo irradiation for gynecologic cancer.[98]

MANAGEMENT OF RADIATION ENTERITIS

Methods of Prevention

Prophylactic measures that help reduce the incidence of radiation enteritis include methods to exclude the small bowel from the pelvis, such as reperitonealization, omental transposition, or placement of absorbable mesh slings.[99-101] The small bowel is a mobile structure that can be altered by a variety of positions and techniques, including the prone, Trendelenburg, and decubitus positions.[14] Das et al. studied the efficacy of a belly board device that resulted in a 70% reduction in small bowel volume within the irradiated pelvic field.[102] Ferguson described the use of omental pedicle grafts.[103]

The use of radioprotectant chemicals during radiotherapy is an evolving strategy of clinical importance. Amifostine was the first cytoprotectant approved by the Food and Drug Administration for ovarian cancer patients receiving cisplatin-based chemotherapy and for the prevention of xerostomia in patients undergoing radiation therapy for head and neck cancer.[104-106] The protection of normal cells is believed to occur predominantly by scavenging of free radicals. Active metabolites of amifostine react with free radicals in competition with oxygen.[107] Pretreatment with amifostine in clinical trials reduced the frequency of cyclophosphamide-induced neutropenia and nephrotoxicity and the neurotoxicity of platin compounds.[108] Halberg et al. reported that the intraluminal administration of amifostine during intraoperative radiation therapy produced localized radioprotection and reduced duodenal damage.[109] Despite all these promising results, there is still controversy regarding the selectivity of amifostine because some studies have shown variable degrees of tumor protection as well.[110,111] A few phase I and II studies suggest that amifostine could be beneficial in limiting the radiation damage.[112] Superoxide dismutase, a free radical scavenger, has been used successfully to reduce radiation-induced complications.[65]

Numerous pharmacologic interventions have been reported to reduce the symptoms of radiation enteritis. Diarrhea associated with abdominal irradiation has been positively affected by sucralfate. A randomized, placebo-controlled trial of 70 patients who were treated by pelvic irradiation for bladder and prostate cancer showed that patients who received sucralfate during radiation therapy had statistically significant reductions in both the acute and chronic symptoms of radiation enteritis when compared with patients who received placebo.[113,114]

Glutamine-enriched enteral formulas, as well as hormones such as bombesin, growth hormone, glucagon-like peptide 2, and insulin-like growth factor 1, have proved useful in preventing symptoms of acute radiation enteritis.[115-117]

Novel Techniques in Radiotherapy and Combined Radiotherapy/Chemotherapy

The goal of all new technologic changes in the field of radiation oncology is to allow safe administration of greater radiation doses to the tumor and achieve an increased rate of cure with acceptable normal tissue toxicity. The irradiation technique must prevent unnecessary irradiation of tissues outside the tumor-containing areas.

Radiation enteritis can be minimized by using special ports to deliver optimal treatment specifically to the tumor and not to the surrounding tissues. Radiopaque markers such as titanium clips could be placed during laparotomy to further delineate and identify the area of interest for future, more targeted radiation therapy.

Frykholm et al. have found that technically, a two-field radiation approach cannot spare the surrounding tissues to the same extent as three or four fields can,[118] and hence two types of conformal radiation therapy have evolved and been introduced into clinical practice: *three-dimensional conformal radiation (3DCRT)* and *intensity-modulated radiation therapy (IMRT)*.

Traditional radiation therapy techniques, including 3DCRT with uniform radiation intensity or with simple beam fluence–modifying devices such as wedges, do not provide a method for sparing critical structures that push into the target or that are partially or fully surrounded by a target or combination of targets. True 3DCRT dose distributions are now possible, in large part because of continuing advances in computer technology that have led to the development of sophisticated *three-dimensional radiation treatment planning (3DRTP)* systems with inverse planning capabilities and computer-controlled radiation therapy delivery systems equipped with a multileaf collimator. Such planning and delivery systems have made the implementation of 3DCRT with modulated radiation fluence practical. The ultimate goal of 3DCRT is to conform the spatial distribution of the prescribed dose to the three-dimensional target volume (cancerous cells plus a margin for spatial uncertainties) while at the same time minimizing the dose to surrounding normal structures (RTOG, The National Cancer Institute Guidelines for the Use of Intensity-Modulated Radiation Therapy in Clinical Trials).

IMRT represents a new paradigm in radiation therapy that requires knowledge of patient immobilization, multimodality imaging, setup uncertainties and internal organ motion, tumor control probabilities, normal tissue complication probabilities, three-dimensional dose calculation and optimization, and dynamic beam delivery of nonuniform beam intensities. This new process of planning and treatment delivery shows significant potential for further improving the therapeutic ratio and reducing toxicity. The radiation beam is broken into beamlets for which the intensity can be adjusted individually. Up to now, however, it is not clear whether IMRT will fulfill the expectations that it has raised,[119,120] and hence further studies need to be conducted and evaluated.

Adjuvant (postoperative) and *neoadjuvant* (preoperative) radiotherapy for resectable rectal cancer, for example, has been studied extensively.[17,121-125] In terms of neoadjuvant therapy, a meta-analysis of 4000 patients found that both a *short-term course* (25 Gy in 5 fractions, common approach in Europe) and a *long-term course* (45 Gy in 25 fractions, commonly applied in the United States) of radiation therapy were equally effective in reducing local recurrence.[126,127] Neoadjuvant radiation therapy using 25 Gy with daily fractions of 5 Gy, administered within 1 week followed by surgery the next week, is a widely used treatment for patients with resectable rectal cancer.[18,121,128,129] Nevertheless, the high dose per daily fraction (5 Gy) led to significant impairment of bowel function.[130]

This regimen was changed to 2.5 Gy per fraction twice daily for 5 days preoperatively and provided excellent results in terms of local tumor control without marked late morbidity. This modification was called non–downstaging *hyperfractionation* and was thought to be safe for the treatment of selected patients. Hypofractionation with greater doses per fraction led to an increase in the occurrence of radiation-induced damage.[131]

Kupelian et al. reported a clinical trial of 166 patients with early-stage prostate cancer who were treated with hypofractionated intensity–modulated radiotherapy delivering 2.5 Gy/fraction (total of 70 Gy) in comparison to 116 patients who were treated with 3DCRT delivering 2.0 Gy/fraction (total of 78 Gy). Rectal toxicity was observed in only 5% of patients treated with IMRT as compared with 12% in a group of patients treated with 3DCRT.[132]

The German Rectal Cancer Study Group trial published by Sauer et al. provided evidence that preoperative or neoadjuvant chemoradiation has numerous potential advantages over postoperative chemoradiation, such as less toxicity, a lower incidence of radiation enteritis, a lower rate of local recurrence, and a lower rate of anastomotic stricture after surgery.[17,133] It was suggested that this should be the preferred treatment for patients with locally advanced and low-lying rectal cancer. The theoretical background for the advantage of preoperative radiotherapy in comparison to postoperative treatment has been discussed in various publications.[121,122] Despite all positive aspects of preoperative chemoradiotherapy in the treatment of rectal cancer, Sauer et al., for example, pointed out the possibility of overtreating early-stage tumors (TNM stage I). Despite the use of endorectal ultrasound, approximately 18% of the patients (stage I) had been over-staged during the initial evaluation and received unnecessary postoperative chemoradiotherapy.[17,134] The percentage of unnecessary postoperative chemoradiation was even higher if those patients with stage IV disease (7%) and those with unknown TNM stage (6%) were included. This important issue illustrates the importance of correct preoperative clinical staging, which might improve with the additional use of MRI, leading to better patient selection.[135]

Preoperative combined-modality treatment with conventional radiation doses and fractionation plus concurrent 5-FU–based chemotherapy has yielded better results than preoperative radiation therapy has alone.[17,18,133] Patients with clinical T3 rectal tumors or positive lymph nodes, or both, are commonly treated with combined-modality treatment, followed by surgery and four cycles of postoperative chemotherapy.[136,137] This concept, however, is not completely accepted and is being currently investigated as part of the European Organization for Research and Treatment of Cancer (EORTC) trial.[104,138-140]

Other studies have investigated the effect of conventional fractionation, hypofractionation, accelerated and hyperfractionated regimens, and radiation dose escalation techniques and found that with concurrent chemoradiotherapy, either the dose of the chemotherapeutic drug or the radiation dose needs to be reduced to avoid significant GI complications such as ulceration or hemorrhage without affecting the tumoricidal effects of both radiation therapy and chemotherapy.[119,141-145]

New drug-radiation combinations with such drugs as *capecitabine, raltitrexed, oxaliplatin,* and *irinotecan* are currently being investigated in several trials.[145,146] In addition to these cytotoxic drugs, novel targeted biologic agents, including *epidermal growth factor inhibitors* and *vascular endothelial growth factor inhibitors,* have been shown to enhance the antitumor effect of both radiation therapy and chemotherapy.[146]

The time interval between the completion of radiation therapy and definitive surgery turned out to be a pivotal factor for achieving maximal tumor response to radiation in order to achieve R0 resections or perform sphincter-sparing operations.[147,148] Grann et al. recommended a minimum of 4 weeks.[147] This was supported by the Lyon R90-01 randomized trial.[149] Beets-Tan and coworkers determined the applicability of MRI in predicting tumor-free resectability of the primary lesion.[150]

Because pancreatic cancer is only moderately sensitive to radiation, doses of 50 to 50.4 Gy can be applied safely in combination with chemotherapy. Early experimental trials initially stated that doses of 70 Gy and higher can be administered to patients with pancreatic cancer when given without chemotherapy.[145,151] However, at these high doses, the radiosensitivity of adjacent organs considerably limited the option of percutaneous radiation therapy. A significant number of radiation-induced toxicities occurred.[151] Moreover, radiotherapy alone did not improve the overall survival rate. *Intraoperative radiation therapy (IORT)* using fast electrons allows the application of high radiation doses to the tumor and tumor bed while protecting adjacent organs and tissues.[152] However, such treatment did not translate into improved overall survival rates. Nevertheless, IORT might help reduce the percutaneous radiation dose to 40 to 50 Gy, thereby significantly reducing the frequency of radiation-induced toxicity.[152]

Treatment Options

Conservative/Symptomatic Management

Treatment of acute radiation enteritis is directed toward controlling the symptoms.[81] Antispasmodics and analgesics, including opiates, may alleviate the abdominal pain and cramping. The use of steroids is of uncertain value. Conservative measures such as the administration of intravenous fluids, bowel rest, and antidiarrheal drugs are indicated.[30,153] Dietary manipulation, including oral elemental diets, has been advocated to ameliorate the symptoms of radiation enteritis. Diets low in milk, fat, and lactose had beneficial effects in patients with acute radiation enteritis.[12] Loiudice and Lang showed that administration of total parenteral nutrition (TPN) to patients with chronic small bowel problems was superior to a low-residue diet in clinical improvement and immunologic and radiologic parameters.[154] The addition of methylprednisolone appeared to enhance the effects of TPN.[12,154-156] In contrast, Silvain and co-workers found that TPN alone was not superior to surgical management, with clinical radiation enteritis recurrence rates of 34% and 47% at 1 and 2 years, respectively.[157] Although TPN corrected nutritional deficits effectively and deferred surgery in some patients, radiation enteritis remains an unpredictable progressive disease.[157]

Acute enterocolitis may be mediated by prostaglandin, at least in part. In a small prospective study, Mennie et al. found that aspirin as an inhibitor of prostaglandin E synthesis caused a significant decrease in diarrhea and abdominal pain.[158] Cholestyramine (4 to 12 g/day), which binds bile salts, has also been found to be effective.[159] Kilic et al. reported that sulfasalazine (2 g/day) was effective in reducing the symptoms of acute radiation enteritis.[160] Probiotics have been found to be effective in preventing various gastrointestinal diseases, especially radiation-induced enteritis.[161]

In the acute phase of radiation proctitis, hydrophilic stool softeners may help control mucous diarrhea, whereas sitz baths and perineal compresses have been used in an attempt to ease tenesmus if analgesics fail. Steroid retention enemas are helpful for both acute and chronic radiation proctitis. Jacobs et al. found that the administration of oral or rectal Salazopyrin alleviated the symptoms of acute and chronic radiation proctitis in 37 of 40 patients.[162] Moreover, hemorrhagic radiation proctitis can be alleviated by the topical application of formalin. If the bleeding is refractory to local formalin treatment, argon plasma coagulation has been shown to be an effective and safe treatment.[163-165] In addition, bipolar electrocoagulation or endoscopic laser coagulation has been described for the management of hemorrhagic radiation injury or radiation-induced mucosal vascular lesions.[166,167]

Surgical Management

Before definitive surgical treatment is considered, it is important that the extent of both the original malignancy and the radiation damage be established and any sepsis, malnutrition, or biochemical abnormalities be corrected.[35]

Radiation enteritis is one of the most challenging problems in GI surgery. The operations are complex and prone to complications.[168]

Operative interventions may be required in only a subgroup of patients with chronic effects of radiation enteritis. This subgroup of patients represents just a small percentage (2% to 3%) of the total number of patients who have undergone abdominal or pelvic irradiation.[153]

Indications for surgery include obstruction, fistula formation, perforation, and bleeding. Complete bowel obstruction as a result of strictures is the most common

indication for surgery. Surgeons are frequently confronted with dense adhesions, unexpected problems, and fragile irradiated tissues that are difficult to handle and poor to heal.[153]

Caution must be exercised when operating on patients with previously irradiated bowel because the vascular injury may be widespread and not readily recognizable by gross inspection of the intestine. The risk for dehiscence of the anastomosis, however, is not negligible. Extensive adhesiolysis should be avoided if possible. Perforation should be treated by resection and anastomosis. When the anastomosis is thought to be unsafe, ostomies should be created. The utility of frozen section or laser Doppler flowmetry for assessment of blood flow at the anastomosis site is of limited value.[169]

Bowel perfusion at the resection borders is usually assessed by gross examination, color, capillary refill, and bleeding tendency, depending on the surgeon's experience.

If resection and anastomosis are planned, at least one end of the anastomosis should be from intestine outside the irradiated field. An incidence of anastomotic breakdown as high as 50% has been reported after resection and anastomosis involving diseased segments of bowel because of the poor healing properties of irradiated tissue.[28,29]

In a retrospective analysis from 1970 to 1982, Wobbes et al. showed 27 patients who were operated on for stenosis, perforation, fistulization, and chronic blood loss of the small bowel after radiotherapy for malignant disease.[170] Bypass procedures in the form of ileotransversostomies were performed on 20 patients who presented with either obstruction or fistulization. Two patients died postoperatively. In contrast, 4 of 7 patients who underwent bowel resection for perforation, fistulization, or obstruction died of intra-abdominal sepsis. The researchers concluded that a bypass procedure should be performed if possible. In case of resection, the anastomosis should be done during a second operation. Obstruction caused by rigid and fixed pelvis incorporating small intestinal loops is best treated by bypass procedures.

Regimbeau et al. retrospectively studied 109 patients, from 1984 to 1994, who were operated on for radiation enteritis. Of these patients, 68% had been irradiated for gynecologic carcinoma, 28% for digestive cancer (24 colorectal cancer and 4 anal cancer), 7% for urologic carcinoma, and 4% for Hodgkin's disease, cutaneous neoplasia, and soft tissue carcinoma.[23] The operative mortality was approximately 5%. Thirty-three patients (30%) experienced postoperative complications, including anastomotic leak in 11 patients. Overall survival, after a mean follow-up of 40 months in patients without cancer recurrence, was 85% at 1 year and 69% at 5 years after surgery. Overall survival was influenced by the nature of the treatment, with 51% and 71% 5-year survival after conservative and resection treatment, respectively. Despite high initial mortality and morbidity rates, life expectancy in patients who underwent bowel resection was superior to conservative surgical treatment.[23] They and other investigators said that bypass procedures are associated with a higher relative risk of radiation-induced cancer in the irradiated bowel that is not resected but left in place.[27,98] However, the bypass operation is a valid surgical alternative for patients with high risk of short-gut syndrome and poor medical condition.[23] Regimbeau et al. mentioned in their publication that reoperation after the first surgical procedure was mandatory for approximately 40% of their patients because of recurrence of gastrointestinal symptoms. The mortality and morbidity rate was higher for those patients. They also found a higher reoperation rate among patients who were treated conservatively without resection of small bowel.[23] Onodera et al. retrospectively analyzed 48 patients who underwent small bowel resection for intestinal obstruction and pull-through reconstruction for proctitis. They postulated that generous small bowel resection of affected bowel is a safe procedure for small bowel injury, whereas rectal resection is best dealt with by restorative proctectomy.[171]

Multiple resections and bypass of large segments of intestine will eventually place the patient at risk for short-bowel syndrome, as well as dependence on TPN. The use of TPN has been described as a life-prolonging measure; however, the long-term outcome of patients who have radiation enteritis and receive home TPN is dismal, with 5-year survival rates of only 36%.[157] Most of these patients died because of complications due to radiation therapy. The others had cancer recurrences.

In a retrospective study, Scolapio et al. reviewed 225 patients requiring home TPN for various diseases; 32 patients suffered from radiation enteritis. The overall 5-year survival probability was 60%, irrespective of age and underlying disease. The 5-year survival of patients with home TPN suffering from radiation enteritis was only 54%.[172] Therefore, efforts to preserve the remaining intestinal length may be warranted in an attempt to avoid the metabolic and nutritional consequences of further major resections or bypass procedures. Dietz and co-workers presented the use of strictureplasty for the management of patients with obstructing complications of radiation enteritis.[172] Three patients presented with small bowel obstruction and enterocutaneous fistula, two patients with chronic small bowel obstruction and rectovaginal fistula. Four patients required home TPN. Strictureplasty was successfully performed on all patients. All patients who were dependent on home TPN were eventually weaned from TPN. The authors pointed out that strictureplasty procedures should not be recommended as a primary surgical procedure for the treatment of perforation, hemorrhage, or fistula. It may be considered a useful option if resection would be likely to induce short-bowel syndrome.[173]

SUMMARY

Radiation enteritis is a serious complication of abdominal or pelvic irradiation and should be understood as a progressive and chronic disease with early and late clinical symptoms. The clinical manifestations range from mild diarrhea to severe complications such as bowel obstruction, fistula formation, and hollow viscus perforation. Management of this relentless disease varies from supportive care to surgical intervention, depending on the initial clinical symptoms. New molecular and microcirculatory insights into the pathomechanism of radiation enteritis can lead to novel therapeutic concepts for preventing rather than treating this relentless disease.

Improved long-term survival after radiotherapy should be achieved primarily by better tumor control. The use of novel techniques in radiation oncology, such as IMRT combined with new cytotoxic and biologic agents, might lead to improved protection of nonmalignant tissue without compromising the tumor-killing activity of these methods. Other methods such as hypofractionation, accelerated and hyperfractionated regimens, concurrent chemoradiotherapy, and neoadjuvant and adjuvant chemotherapy might help reduce GI complications without affecting the tumoricidal effects of the therapy.

REFERENCES

1. Bai YH, Wang DW, Cui XM, et al: Expression of transforming growth factor beta in radiation interstitial pneumonitis. J Environm Pathol Toxicol Oncol 16:15-20, 1997.
2. Datta PK, Moulder JE, Fish BL, et al: TGF-β1 production in radiation nephropathy: role of angiotensin II. Int J Radiat Oncol Biol Phys 4:473-479, 1999.
3. Geraci JP, Mariano MS: Radiation hepatology of the rat: Parenchymal and non-parenchymal cell injury. Radiat Res 136:205-213, 1993.
4. Gottlober P, Steinert M, Bahren W, et al: Interferon-gamma in 5 patients with cutaneous radiation syndrome after radiation therapy. Int J Radiat Oncol Biol Phys 50:159-166, 2001.
5. Jagels MA, Hugli TE: Mixed effects of TGF-β on human airway epithelial-cell chemokine responses. Immunopharmacology 48:17-26, 2000.
6. Lewin K, Millis RR: Human radiation hepatitis: A morphological study with emphasis on the late changes. Arch Pathol 96:21-26, 1973.
7. Peter RU, Gottlober P, Nadeshina N, et al: Interferon gamma in survivors of the Chernobyl power plant accident: new therapeutic option for radiation-induced fibrosis. Int J Radiat Oncol Biol Phys 45:147-152, 1999.
8. Rube CE, Uthe D, Schmid KW, et al: Dose-dependent induction of transforming growth factor β in the lung tissue of fibrosis-prone mice after thoracic irradiation. Int J Radiat Oncol Biol Phys 47:1033-1042, 2000.
9. Seong J, Kim SH, Chung EJ, et al: Early alteration in TGF-β mRNA expression in irradiated rat liver. Int J Radiat Oncol Biol Phys 46:639-643, 2000.
10. Mann WJ: Surgical management of radiation entseropathy. Surg Clin North Am 71:977-990, 1991.
11. Ooi BS, Tjandra JJ, Green MD: Morbidities of adjuvant chemotherapy and radiotherapy for resectable rectal cancer. An overview. Dis Col Rectum 42:403-418, 1999.
12. Sher ME, Bauer J: Radiation-induced enteropathy. Am J Gastroenterol 85:121-128, 1990.
13. Walsh D: Deep tissue traumatism from roentgen ray exposure. Br Med J 2:272-273, 1897.
14. Bismar MM, Sinicrope FA: Radiation enteritis. Curr Gastroenterol Reports 4:361-365, 2002.
15. Kinsella TJ, Bloomer WD: Tolerance of the intestine to radiation therapy. Surg Gynec Obstet 151:273-284, 1980.
16. Rodier JF: Radiation enteropathy—incidence, aetiology, risk factors, pathology and symptoms. Tumori Supplement 81:122-125, 1995.
17. Sauer R, Becker H, Hohenberger W, et al, for the German Rectal Cancer Study Group: Preoperative versus postoperative chemoradiotherapy for rectal cancer. N Engl J Med 351:1731-1740, 2004.
18. Swedish Rectal Cancer Trial: Improved survival with preoperative radiotherapy in resectable rectal cancer. N Engl J Med 336:980-987, 1997.
19. Weijers RE, van der Jagt EJ, Jansen W: Radiation enteritis: An overview. Fortschr Röntgenstr 152:453-459, 1990.
20. Wittich G, Salomonowitz E, Szepesi T, et al: Small bowel double-contrast enema in stage III ovarian cancer. Am J Roentgenol 142:299-304, 1984.
21. Fenner MN, Sheehan P, Nanavati PJ, et al: Chronic radiation enteritis: a community hospital experience. J Surg Oncol 41:246-249, 1989.

22. Hauer-Jensen M: Late radiation injury of the small intestine clinical, pathophysiologic and radiobiologic aspects. A review. Acta Oncologica 29:401-415, 1990.

23. Regimbeau JM, Panis Y, Gouzi JL, et al: Operative and long term results after surgery for chronic radiation enteritis. Am J Surg 182:237-242, 2001; erratum in Am J Surg 182:752, 2001.

24. Letschert JGJ, Lebesque JV, De Boer RW, et al: Dose-volume correlation in radiation-related small bowel complications: A clinical study. Radiother Oncol 18:307-320, 1990.

25. Rubin P, Casarett G: A direction for clinical radiation pathology: The tolerance dose. In Vaeth JM, ed: Frontiers of Radiation Therapy and Oncology, vol 16. Baltimore, University Park Press, 1972, 1-16.

26. Galland RB, Spencer J: The natural history of clinically established radiation enteritis. Lancet 1(8440):1257-1258, 1985.

27. Galland RB, Spencer J: Natural history and surgical management of radiation enteritis. Br J Surg 74:742-747, 1987.

28. Galland RB, Spencer J: Surgical management of radiation enteritis. Surgery 99:133-139, 1986.

29. Galland RB, Spencer J: Radiation-induced gastrointestinal fistulae. Ann R Coll Surg Engl 68:5-7, 1986.

30. O'Brian PH, Jenrette JMI, Garvin AJ: Radiation enteritis. Am Surg 53:501-504, 1987.

31. De Cosse JJ, Rhodes RS, Wentz WB, et al: The natural history and management of radiation induced injury of the gastrointestinal tract. Ann Surg 170:369-384, 1969.

32. De Cosse JJ: Radiation injury to the intestine. In Sabistan DC, ed.: Textbook of Surgery. Philadelphia, WB Saunders, 1986, 962-966.

33. Berthrong M, Fajardo LF: Radiation injury in surgical pathology. Part II: Alimentary tract. Am J Surg Path 5:153-178, 1981.

34. Clarke AR, Gledhill S, Hooper ML, et al: P53 dependence of early apoptotic and proliferative responses within the mouse intestinal epithelium following gamma-irradiation. Oncogene 9:1767-1773, 1994.

35. Nguyen NP, Antoine JE, Dutta S, et al: Current concepts in radiation enteritis and implications for future clinical trials. Cancer 95:1151-1163, 2002.

36. Potten CS, Grant HK: The relationship between ionizing radiation-induced apoptosis and stem cells in the small and large intestine. Br J Cancer 78:993-1003, 1998.

37. Paris F, Fuks Z, Kang A, et al: Endothelial apoptosis as the primary lesion initiating intestinal radiation damage in mice. Science 293:293-297, 2001.

38. Herskind C, Bamberg M, Rodermann HP: The role of cytokines in the development of normal-tissue reactions after radiotherapy. Strahlenther Onkol 174:12-15, 1998.

39. Wang J, Zheng H, Sung CC, et al: Cellular sources of transforming growth factor-beta isoforms in early and chronic radiation enteropathy. Am J Pathol 153:1531-1540, 1998.

40. Wang J, Richter KK, Sung CC, et al: Upregulation and spatial shift in the localization of the mannose 6-phosphate/insulin-like growth factor II receptor during radiation enteropathy development in the rat. Radiother Oncol 50:205-213, 1999.

41. Langberg CW, Hauer-Jensen M, Sung CC, et al: Expression of fibrogenic cytokines in rat small intestines after fractionated irradiation. Radiother Oncol 32:29-36, 1994.

42. Roberts AB, Sporn MB: Transforming growth factor β. Adv Cancer Res 51:107-145, 1988.

43. Thompson JS, Saxena SK, Sharp J: Regulation of intestinal regeneration: New insights. Microsc Res Tech 51:129-137, 2000.

44. Richter KK, Langberg CW, Sung CC, et al: Increased transforming growth factor beta immunoreactivity is independently associated with chronic injury in both sequential and primary radiation enteropathy. Int J Radiat Oncol Biol Phys 39:187-195, 1997.

45. Hallahan D, Kuchibhotla J, Wyble C: Cell adhesion molecules mediate radiation-induced leukocyte adhesion to the vascular endothelium. Cancer Res 56:5150-5155, 1996.

46. Krieg T, Meurer M: Systemic scleroderma. Clinical and pathological aspects. J Am Acad Dermatol 18:457-481, 1988.

47. Querfeld C, Eckes B, Huerkamp C, et al: Expression of TGF-beta 1, -beta 2 and -beta 3 in localized and systemic scleroderma. J Dermatol Sci 21:13-22, 1999.

48. Katzenstein ALA, Myers JL: Idiopathic pulmonary fibrosis. Clinical relevance of pathologic classification. Am J Respir Crit Care Med 157:1301-1315, 1998.

49. Ramos C, Montano M, Garcia-Alvarez J, et al: Fibroblasts from idiopathic pulmonary fibrosis and normal lungs differ in growth rate, apoptosis and tissue inhibitor of metalloproteinases expression. Am J Respir Cell Mod Biol 24:591-598, 2001.

50. Ziesche R, Hofbauer E, Wittmann K, et al: A preliminary study of long-term treatment with interferon gamma-1b and low dose prednisolone in patients with idiopathic pulmonary fibrosis. N Engl J Med 341:1264-1269, 1999.

51. Lane PH, Steffes MW, Fioretto P, et al: Renal interstitial expansion insulin-dependent diabetes mellitus. Kidney Int 43:661-667, 1993.

52. Mezzano SA, Droguett MA, Burgos ME, et al: Overexpression of chemokines, fibrogenic cytokines, and myofibroblasts in human membranous nephropathy. Kidney Int 57:147-158, 2000.

53. Behrends U, Peter RU, Hintermeier-Knabe R, et al: Ionizing radiation induces human intercellular adhesion molecule 1 in vitro. J Invest Dermatol 103:726-730, 1994.

54. Gaugler MH, Squiban C, van der Meeren A, et al: Late and persistent up-regulation of intercellular adhesion molecule 1 (ICAM-1) expression by ionizing radiation in human endothelial cells in vitro. Int J Radiat Biol 72:201-209, 1977.

55. Hallahan DE, Kuchibhotla J, Wyble C: Sialyl Lewis X mimetics attenuate E-selectin-mediated adhesion of leukocytes to irradiated human endothelial cells. Radiat Res 147:41-47, 1997.

56. Hallahan D, Clark ET, Kuchibhotla J, et al: E-selectin gene induction by ionizing radiation is independent of cytokine induction. Biochem Biophys Res Commun 217:784-795, 1995.

57. Krutmann J, Czech W, Parlow F, et al: Ultraviolet radiation effects on human keratinocyte ICAM-1 expression: UV-induced inhibition of cytokine-induced ICAM-1 mRNA expression is transient, differentially restored for IFN-γ versus TNF-α and followed by ICAM-1 induction via a TNF-α-like pathway. J Invest Dermatol 98:923-928, 1992.

58. Molla M, Gironella M, Miquel R, et al: Relative roles of ICAM-1 and VCAM-1 in the pathogenesis of experimental radiation-induced intestinal inflammation. Int J Radiat Oncol Biol Phys 57:264-273, 2003.

59. Molla M, Gironella M, Salas A, et al: Role of P-selectin in radiation-induced intestinal inflammatory damage. Int J Cancer 96:99-109, 2001.

60. Molla M, Panes J, Casadevall M, et al: Influence of dose-rate on inflammatory damage and adhesion molecule expression after abdominal radiation in the rat. Int J Radiat Oncol Biol Phys 45:1011-1018, 1999.

61. Panés J, Molla M, Casadevall M, et al: Tepoxalin inhibits inflammation and microvascular dysfunction induced by abdominal irradiation in rats. Aliment Pharmacol Ther 14:841-850, 2000.

62. Panés J, Anderson DC, Miyasaka M, et al: Role of leukocyte endothelial cell adhesion in radiation-induced microvascular dysfunction in rats. Gastroenterology 108:1761-1769, 1995.

63. Nagi B, Rana SS, Kochhar R, et al: Sonoenteroclysis: A new technique for the diagnosis of small bowel diseases. Abdom Imaging Jan 30 2006 [Epub ahead of print].

64. Gironella M, Molla M, Salas A, et al: The role of P-selectin in experimental colitis as determined by antibody immunoblockade and genetically deficient mice. J Leukoc Biol 72:56-64, 2002.

65. Molla M, Gironella M, Salas A, et al: Protective effect of superoxide dismutase in radiation-induced intestinal inflammation. Int J Radiat Oncol Biol Phys 61:1159-1166, 2005.

66. Babb RR: Radiation proctitis: A review. Am J Gastroenterol 36:450-456, 1996.

67. Baxter NN, Tepper JE, Durham SB, et al: Increased risk of rectal cancer after prostate radiation: a population-based study. Gastroenterology 128:819-824, 2005.

68. Duhrsen U: Therapy-induced leukemia: an underestimated complication of antineoplastic chemotherapy? Zentralbl Gynakol 127:235-241, 2005.

69. Greten TF, Manns MP, Reinisch I, et al: Hepatocellular carcinoma occurring after successful treatment of childhood cancer with high dose chemotherapy and radiation. Gut 54:732, 2005.

70. Kawaguchi T, Matsumura A, Iuchi K, et al: Second primary cancers in patients with stage III non-small cell lung cancer successfully treated with chemo-radiotherapy. Jpn J Clin Oncol 36:7-11, 2006.

71. Ohno T, Kakinuma S, Kato S, et al: Risk of second cancers after radiotherapy for cervical cancer. Expert Rev Anticancer Ther 6:49-57, 2006.

72. Rubino C, Shamsaldin A, Le MG, et al: Radiation dose and risk of soft tissue and bone sarcoma after breast cancer treatment. Breast Cancer Res Treat 89:277-288, 2005.

73. Thijssens KM, van Ginkel RJ, Suurmeijer AJ, et al: Radiation-induced sarcoma: a challenge for the surgeon. Ann Surg Oncol 12:237-245, 2005.

74. Travis LB, Hill D, Dores GM, Gospodarowicz M, et al: Cumulative absolute breast cancer risk for young women treated for Hodgkin lymphoma. J Natl Cancer Inst 97:1394-1395, 2005.

75. West JG, Qureshi A, West JE, et al: Risk of angiosarcoma following breast conservation: a clinical alert. Breast J 11:115-123, 2005.

76. Brenn T, Fletcher CD: Radiation-associated cutaneous atypical vascular lesions and angiosarcoma: Clinicopathologic analysis of 42 cases. Am J Surg Pathol 29:983-996, 2005.

77. Brenner DJ, Hall EJ, Curtis RE, Ron E: Prostate radiotherapy is associated with second cancers in many organs, not just the colorectum. Gastroenterology 129:773-774, 2005.

78. Allan JM, Travis LB: Mechanisms of therapy-related carcinogenesis. Nat Rev Cancer 5:943-955, 2005.

79. Barcellos-Hoff MH, Park C, Wright EG: Radiation and the microenvironment—tumorigenesis and therapy. Nat Rev Cancer 5:867-875, 2005.

80. Hatcher PA, Thomson HJ, Ludgate SN, et al: Surgical aspects of intestinal injury due to pelvic radiotherapy. Ann Surg 201:470-475, 1985.

81. Yeoh EK, Horowitz M: Radiation enteritis. Surg Gynecol Obstet 165:373-379, 1987.

82. Ruppin H, Hotze A, During A, et al: Reversible functional disorders of the intestinal tract caused by abdominal radiotherapy. Z Gastroenterol 25:261-269, 1987.

83. Mendelson RM, Nolan DJ: The radiologic features of chronic radiation enteritis. Clin Radiol 36:141-148, 1985.

84. Sellink JL, Miller RE: Radiology of the Small Bowel: Technique and Atlas. Nijhoff, The Hague, 1982.

85. Maglinte DD: Small bowel imaging—a rapidly changing field and a challenge to radiology. Eur Radiol 16:967-971, 2006.

86. Rajesh A, Maglinte DD: Multislice CT enteroclysis: technique and clinical applications. Clin Radiol 61:31-39, 2006.

87. Schneider G, Reimer P, Mamann A, et al: Contrast agents in abdominal imaging current and future directions. Top Magn Reson Imaging 16:107-124, 2005.

88. Mason GR, Dietrich P, Friedland GW, et al: The radiological findings in radiation–induced enteritis and colitis. A review of 30 cases. Clin Radiol 21:232-247, 1970.

89. Rogers LF, Goldstein HM: Roentgen manifestations of radiation injury of the gastrointestinal tract. Gastrointest Radiol 2:281-291, 1977.

90. Harling H, Balslev I: Long-term prognosis of patients with severe radiation enteritis. Am J Surg 155:517-519, 1988.

91. Gilinsky NH, Burns DG, Barbezat GO, et al: The natural history of radiation-induced proctosigmoiditis: an analysis of 88 patients. Q J Medicine 205:40-53, 1983.

92. Perez CA, Breaux S, Bedwinek JM, et al: Radiation therapy alone in the treatment of carcinoma of the uterine cervix. II. Analysis of complications. Cancer 54:235-246, 1984.

93. Russell JC, Welch JP: Operative management of radiation injuries to the intestinal tract. Am J Surg 137:166-172, 1979.

94. Harling H, Balslev I: Radical surgical approach to radiation injury of the small bowel. Dis Colon Rectum 29:371-373, 1986.

95. Libotte F, Autier P, Delmelle M, et al: Survival of patients with radiation enteritis of the small and the large intestine. Acta Chir Belg 95(4 Suppl):190-194, 1995.

96. Denman D, Kirchner F, Osborne J: Induction of colonic adenocarcinoma in the rat by X-irradiation. Cancer Res 38:1899-1905, 1978.

97. Dawson PM, Galland RB, Rees HC, et al: Mucin abnormalities in the radiation-damaged colon. Dig Surg 4:19-21, 1987.

98. Sandler RS, Sandler DP: Radiation-induced cancer of the colon and rectum. Assessing the risk. Gastroenterology 84:51-57, 1983.

99. Choi HJ, Lee HS: Effect of omental pedicle hammock in protection against radiation-induced enteropathy in patients with rectal cancer. Dis Colon Rectum 38:276-280, 1995.

100. Deutsch AA, Stern HS: Technique of insertion of pelvic Vicryl mesh sling to avoid postradiation enteritis. Dis Colon Rectum 32:628-630, 1989.

101. Rodier JF, Janser JC, Rodier D, et al: Prevention of radiation enteritis by an absorbable polyglycolic acid mesh sling: A 60 case multicenter study. Cancer 68:2545-2549, 1991.

102. Das IJ, Lanciano R, Movasas B, et al: Efficacy of a belly board device with CT-stimulation in reducing small bowel volume within pelvic irradiation fields. Int J Radiat Oncol Biol Phys 39:67-76, 1997.

103. Ferguson CM: Use of omental pedicle grafts in abdominoperineal resection. Am Surg 56:310-312, 1990.

104. Bosset JF, Calais G, Daban A, et al, EORTC Radiotherapy Group: Preoperative chemoradiotherapy versus preoperative radiotherapy in rectal cancer patients: Assessment of acute toxicity and treatment compliance. Report of the 22921 randomised trial conducted by the EORTC Radiotherapy Group. Eur J Cancer 40:219-224, 2004.

105. Kemp G, Rose P, Lurain J, et al: Amifostine pretreatment for protection against cyclophosphamide-induced toxicities: results of a randomized trial in patients with ovarian cancer. J Clin Oncol 14:2101-2112, 1996.

106. Brizel DM, Wasserman TH, Henke M, et al: Phase III randomized trial of amifostine as a radioprotector in head and neck cancer. J Clin Oncol 18:3339-3345, 2000.

107. Lindegaard J, Grau C: Has the outlook improved for amifostine as a clinical radioprotector? Radiother Oncol 57:113-118, 2000.

108. Capizzi R, Oster W: Chemoprotective and radioprotective effects of amifostine: an update of clinical trials. Int J Hematol 72:425-435, 2000.

109. Halberg FE, LaRue SM, Rayner AA, et al: Intraoperative radiotherapy with localized radioprotection: Diminished duodenal toxicity with intraluminal WR2721. Int J Radiat Oncol Biol Physics 29:1241-1246, 1991.

110. Block KI, Gyllenhaal C: The pharmacological antioxidant amifostine—implications of recent research for integrative cancer care [commentary]. Integr Cancer Ther 4:329-351, 2005.

111. Denekamp J, Stewart FA, Rojas A: Is the outlook gray for WR-2721 as a clinical radioprotector? Int J Radiat Oncol Biol Physics 9:595-598, 1983.

112. Abbasakoor F, Vaizey CJ, Boulos PB: Improving the morbidity of anorectal injury from pelvic radiotherapy. Colorectal Dis 81:2-10, 2006.

113. Grigsby PW, Plipich MV, Parsons CL: Preliminary results of a phase I/II study of sodium pentosanpolysulfate in the treatment of chronic radiation-induced proctitis. Am J Clin Oncol 13:28-31, 1990.

114. Henrikson R, Franzen L, Lithbrood B: Effect of sucralfate on acute and late bowel discomfort following radiotherapy of pelvic cancer. J Clin Oncol 10:969-975, 1992.

115. Alexandrides T, Spiliotis J, Mylonas P, et al: Effects of growth hormone and insulin-like growth factor-1 on radiation enteritis: A comparative study. Eur Surg Res 30:305-311, 1998.

116. Chu KU, Higashide S, Evers BM, et al: Bombesin improves survival from methotrexate-induced enterocolitis. Ann Surg 220:570-577, 1994.

117. Klimberg VS, Souba WW, Dolson DJ, et al: Prophylactic glutamine protects the intestinal mucosa from radiation injury. Cancer 66:62-68, 1990.

118. Frykholm GJ, Isacsson U, Nygard K, et al: Preoperative radiotherapy in rectal carcinoma—aspects of acute adverse effects and radiation technique. Int J Radiat Oncol Biol Phys 35:1039-1048, 1996.

119. Crane CH, Antolak JA, Rosen II, et al: Phase I Study of concomitant gemcitabine and IMRT for patients with unresectable adenocarinoma of the pancreatic head. Int J Gastrointest Cancer 30:123-132, 2001.

120. Landry JC, Yang GY, Ting JY, et al: Treatment of pancreatic cancer tumors with intensity-modulated radiation therapy (IMRT) using the volume at risk approach (VARA): Employing dose-volume histogram (DVH) and normal tissue complication probability (NTCP) to evaluate small bowel toxicity. Med Dosim 27:121-129, 2002.

121. Glimelius B: Radiotherapy in rectal cancer. Br Med Bull 64:141-157, 2002.

122. Glimelius B, Isacsson U, Jung B, et al: Radiotherapy in addition to radical surgery in rectal cancer: evidence for a dose response effect favoring preoperative treatment. Int J Radiat Oncol Biol Phys 37:281-287, 1997.

123. Mermershtain W, Gluzman A, Gusakova I, et al: Preoperative radio-chemotherapy treatment in locally advanced rectal carcinoma. Results of 8-year follow-up. Onkologie 28:267-269, 2005.

124. Rödel C, Sauer R: Neoadjuvant radiotherapy and radiochemotherapy for rectal cancer. Recent Results in Cancer Research 165:221-230, 2005.

125. Widder J, Herbst F, Dobrowsky W, et al: Preoperative short-term radiation therapy (25Gy, 2.5Gy twice daily) for primary resectable rectal cancer (phase II). Br J Cancer 92:1209-1214, 2005.

126. Camma C, Guinta M, Fiorica F, et al: Preoperative radiotherapy for resectable rectal cancer: A meta-analysis. JAMA 284:1008-1015, 2000.

127. Madoff RD: Chemoradiotherapy for rectal cancer—when, why and how? N Engl J Med 351:1790-1792, 2004.

128. Birgisson H, Pahlman L, Gumnarsson U, et al, Swedish Rectal Cancer Trial Group: Adverse effects of preoperative radiation therapy for rectal cancer: Long-term follow-up of the Swedish Rectal Cancer Trial. J Clin Oncol 23:8697-8705, 2005.

129. Stockholm Rectal Cancer Study Group: Preoperative short-term radiation therapy in operable rectal carcinoma: a prospective randomized trial. Cancer 66:49-55, 1990.

130. Dahlberg M, Glimelius B, Graf W, et al: Preoperative irradiation affects functional results after surgery rectal cancer: results from a randomized study. Dis Colon Rectum 41:543-549, 1998.

131. Michalski JM, Winter K, Purdy JA, et al: Toxicity after three-dimensional radiotherapy for prostate cancer on RTOG 9406 dose level V. Int J Radiation Oncol Biol Phys 62:706-713, 2005.

132. Kupelian PA, Reddy CA, Carlson TP, et al: Preliminary observations on biochemical relapse-free survival rates after short-course intensity-modulated radiotherapy (70 Gy at 2.5 Gy/fraction) for localized prostate cancer. Int J Radiat Oncol Biol Phys 53:904-912, 2002.

133. Ngan SYK, Fisher R, Burmeister BH, et al: Promising results of cooperative group phase II trial of preoperative chemoradiation for locally advanced rectal cancer (TROG 9801). Dis Colon Rectum 48:1389-1396, 2005.

134. Hühnerbein M: Endorectal ultrasound in rectal cancer. Colorectal Dis 5:402-405, 2003.

135. Beets-Tan RG, Beets GL, Vliegen RF, et al: Accuracy of magnetic resonance imaging in prediction of tumour-free resection margin in rectal cancer surgery. Lancet 357:497-504, 2001.

136. Minsky BD: Adjuvant therapy of rectal cancer. Semin Oncol 26:540-544, 1999.

137. Minsky BD, Cohen AM, Kemeny N, et al: Combined modality therapy of rectal cancer: decreased acute toxicity with preoperative approach. J Clin Oncol 10:1218-1224, 1992.

138. Bosset JF, Calais G, Daban A, et al, EORTC Radiotherapy Group: Does the addition of chemotherapy to preoperative radiation therapy increase acute toxicity in patients with rectal cancer: report of 22921 EORTC phase III trial. Proc ASCO 22:249, 2003.

139. Cionini L, Cartei F, Manfredi B, et al: Randomized study of preoperative chemoradiation (CT-RT) in locally advanced rectal cancer. Preliminary results. Int J Radiat Oncol Biol Phys 45(3 Suppl):178, 1999.

140. Gérard A, Buyse M, Nordlinger B, et al: Preoperative radiotherapy as adjuvant treatment in rectal cancer: Final results of a randomized study of the European Organization for Research and Treatment of Cancer (EORTC). Ann Surg 208:606-614, 1988.

141. Ashamalla H, Zaki B, Mokhtar B, et al: Hyperfractionated radiotherapy and paclitaxel for locally advanced/unresectable pancreatic cancer. Int J Radiat Oncol Biol Phys 55:679-687, 2003.

142. Crane CH, Abbruzzese JL, Evans DB, et al: Is the therapeutic index better with gemcitabine-based chemoradiation than with 5-fluorouracil-based chemoradiation in locally advanced pancreatic cancer? Int J Radiat Oncol Biol Phys 52:1293-1302, 2002.

143. De Lange SM, van Groeningen CJ, Meijer OW, et al: Gemcitabine-radiotherapy in patients with locally advanced pancreatic cancer. Eur J Cancer 28:1212-1217, 2002.

144. McGinn CJ, Zalupski MM, Shureiqi I, et al: Phase I trial of radiation dose escalation with concurrent weekly full-dose gemcitabine in patients with advanced pancreatic cancer. J Clin Oncol 19:4202-4208, 2001.

145. Wilkowski R, Thoma M, Weingrandt H, et al: Chemoradiation for ductal pancreatic carcinoma: Principles of combining chemotherapy with radiation, definition of target volume and radiation dose. JOP 6:216-230, 2005.

146. De Paoli A, Innocente R, Buonadonna A, et al: Neoadjuvant therapy of rectal cancer. New treatment perspectives. Tumori 90:373-378, 2004.

147. Grann A, Feng C, Wong D, et al: Preoperative combined modality therapy for clinically resectable UT3 rectal adenocarcinoma. Int J Radiat Oncol Biol Phys 49:987-995, 2001.

148. Kapiteijn E, Marijnen CAM, Nagtegaal ID, et al, for the Dutch Colorectal Cancer Group: Preoperative radiotherapy combined with total mesorectal excision for resectable rectal cancer. N Engl J Med 345:638-646, 2001.

149. Francois Y, Nemoz CJ, Baulieux J, et al: Influence of the interval between preoperative radiation therapy and surgery on down-staging and on the rate of sphincter-sparing surgery for rectal cancer: The Lyon R90-01 randomized trial. J Clin Oncol 17:2396-2402, 1999.

150. Beets-Tan RGH: MRI in rectal cancer: The T-stage and circumferential resection margin. Colorectal Dis 5:392-295, 2003.

151. Dobelbower PR Jr: The radiotherapy of pancreatic cancer. Semin Oncol 6:378-389, 1979.

152. Tepper JE, Noyes D, Krall JM, et al: Intraoperative radiation therapy of pancreatic carcinoma: A report of RTOG-8505. Radiation Therapy Oncology Group. Int J Radiat Oncol Biol Phys 21:1145-1149, 1991.

153. Cross MJ, Frazee RC: Surgical treatment of radiation enteritis. Am Surg 58:132-135, 1992.

154. Loiudice TA, Lang JA: Treatment of radiation enteritis: A comparison study. Am J Gastroenterol 78:481-487, 1983.

155. Beer WH, Fan A, Halstead CH: Clinical and nutritional implications of radiation enteritis. Am J Clin Nutr 41:85-91, 1985.

156. Perino LE, Schuffler MD, Mehta SJ, et al: Radiation-induced intestinal pseudo-obstruction. Gastroenterology 91:994-998, 1986.

157. Silvain C, Besson I, Ingrand P, et al: Long-term outcome of severe radiation enteritis treated by total parenteral nutrition. Dig Dis Sciences 37:1065-1071, 1992.

158. Mennie AT, Dalley VM, Dinneen LC, et al: Treatment of radiation-induced gastrointestinal distress with acetylsalicylate. Lancet 2(7942):942-943, 1975.

159. Heusinkveld RS, Manning MR, Aristizabal SA: Control of radiation-induced diarrhea with cholestryamine. Int J Radiation Oncology Biol Phys 4:487-490, 1978.

160. Kilic D, Ozenirler S, Egehan I, et al: Sulfasalazine decreases acute gastrointestinal complications due to pelvic radiotherapy. Ann Pharmacother 1:942-943, 2001.

161. Matarese LE, Seidner DL, Steiger E: The role of probiotics in gastrointestinal disease. Nutr Clin Pract 18:507-516, 2003.

162. Jacobs H, Rindt W, Schmid N: Beitrag zur Behandlung der Strahlenproktitis. Geburtsh Frauenheilk 31:1114-1117, 1971.

163. Isomoto H, Hazama H, Shikuwa S, et al: A case of haemorrhagic radiation proctitis: successful treatment with argon plasma coagulation. Eur J Gastroenterol Hepatol 14:901-904, 2002.

164. Taieb S, Rolachon A, Cenni JC, et al: Effective use of argon plasma coagulation in the treatment of severe radiation proctitis. Dis Colon Rectum 44:1766-1771, 2001.

165. Tjandra JJ, Sengupta S: Argon plasma coagulation is an effective treatment for refractory hemorrhagic radiation proctitis. Gastrointest Endosc 56:779-781, 2002.

166. Maunoury V, Brundetaud JM, Cortot A: Bipolar electrocoagulation treatment for hemorrhagic radiation injury of the lower digestive tract. Gastrointest Endosc 37:492-493, 1991.

167. Zighelboim J, Viggiano TR, Ahlquist DA, et al: Endoscopic laser coagulation of radiation-induced mucosal vascular lesions in the upper gastrointestinal tract and proximal colon. Am J Gastroenterol 88:1224-1227, 1993.

168. Krook JE, Moertel CG, Gunderson LL, et al: Effective surgical adjuvant therapy for high-risk rectal carcinoma. N Engl J Med 324:709-715, 1991.

169. Boyle NH, Manifold D, Jordan MH, et al: Intraoperative assessment of colonic perfusion using scanning laser Doppler flowmetry during colonic resection. J Am Coll Surg 191:504-510, 2000.

170. Wobbes T, Verschueren RC, Lubbers EJ, et al: Surgical aspects of radiation enteritis of the small bowel. Dis Colon Rectum 27:89-92, 1984.

171. Onodera H, Nagayama S, Mori A, et al: Reappraisal of surgical treatment for radiation enteritis. World J Surg 29:459-463, 2005.

172. Scolapio JS, Fleming CR, Kelly DG, et al: Survival on home parenteral nutrition-treated patients: 20 years of experience at the Mayo Clinic. Mayo Clin Proc 74:217-222, 1999.

173. Dietz DW, Remzi FH, Fazio VW: Stricutreplasty for obstructing small-bowel lesions in diffuse radiation enteritis—Successful outcome in five patients. Dis Colon Rectum 44:1772-1777, 2001.

78

Short-Bowel Syndrome

Jon S. Thompson · Alan N. Langnas

Intestinal failure refers to a condition that results in inadequate digestion or absorption of nutrients, or both, so that an individual becomes malnourished and requires specialized medical and nutritional support.[1] Short-bowel syndrome is a type of intestinal failure caused by a shortened remnant after intestinal resection. The pathophysiologic changes that occur in short-bowel syndrome relate primarily to the loss of intestinal absorptive surface and more rapid intestinal transit (Box 78–1). The consequences of malabsorption of nutrients include malnutrition, diarrhea, steatorrhea, specific nutrient deficiencies, and fluid and electrolyte abnormalities. These patients are at risk for other specific complications, including an increased incidence of nephrolithiasis, cholelithiasis, and gastric hypersecretion. The clinical manifestations of short-bowel syndrome vary greatly among patients and depend on intestinal remnant length, location, and function; the status of the remaining digestive organs; the presence or absence of the ileocecal valve; and the adaptive capacity of the intestinal remnant. Thus, short-bowel syndrome is not entirely dependent on a given length of remaining intestine.

The prevalence of short-bowel syndrome is 3 to 4 per million, and thousands of patients are now surviving with short-bowel syndrome.[1] This condition occurs in about 15% of adult patients who undergo intestinal resection, with three fourths of these cases resulting from massive intestinal resection and one fourth from multiple sequential resections.[2] Massive intestinal resection continues to be associated with significant morbidity and mortality, primarily related to the underlying diseases necessitating resection.[2,3] About 70% of patients in whom short-bowel syndrome develops are discharged from the hospital, and a similar percentage are alive 1 year later.[4] This improved survival rate has been achieved primarily by the ability to deliver long-term nutritional support. The long-term outcome of these patients is often determined not only by their age and underlying disease but also by complications related to the management of short-bowel syndrome.

FACTORS INFLUENCING OUTCOME

Intestinal remnant length is the primary determinant of outcome in patients with short-bowel syndrome. The length of the small intestine in adults varies between 12 and 20 ft (360 to 600 cm), depending on how it is measured and the height and sex of the individual. The duodenum measures 10 to 12 inches (25 to 30 cm). The length of the small intestine from the ligament of Treitz to the ileocecal junction is about 16 ft (480 cm), with the proximal two fifths being jejunum and the distal three fifths being ileum. Resection of up to half of the small intestine is generally well tolerated. Although short-bowel syndrome may develop in patients with less than 180 cm of small intestine, or about a third the normal length, permanent parenteral nutrition (PN) support is likely to be needed in patients with less than 120 cm of intestine remaining without colon in continuity and less than 60 cm remaining with colonic continuity (Table 78–1).[4,5]

The site of resection is also an important factor. Patients with an ileal remnant generally fare better than those with a jejunal remnant. The ileum has specialized absorptive properties for bile salts and vitamin B_{12}, unique motor properties, a hormone profile different from that of the jejunum, and a greater capacity for intestinal adaptation.[6,7] The presence of the ileocecal junction improves the functional capacity of the intestinal remnant.[7] Although previously this had been attributed to a barrier function and transit-prolonging property of the ileocecal valve, this advantage may actually be related to the specialized property of the terminal ileum itself.

The status of the other digestive organs also contributes to outcome. The stomach influences oral intake, mixing of nutrients, transit time, pancreatic secretion, and protein absorption. Pancreatic enzymes are important in the digestive process and particularly influence fat absorption. The colon absorbs fluid and electrolytes, slows transit, and participates in the absorption of energy from malabsorbed carbohydrates. When compared with

Box 78–1 Pathophysiologic Consequences of Massive Resection

General

Malnutrition and weight loss

Diarrhea and steatorrhea

Vitamin and mineral deficiencies

Fluid and electrolyte abnormalities

Specific

Cholelithiasis

Gastric hypersecretion

Liver disease

Nephrolithiasis

Table 78–2 Causes of Short-Bowel Syndrome

Postoperative	52 (25%)
Irradiation/cancer	51 (24%)
Mesenteric vascular disease	46 (22%)
Crohn's disease	34 (16%)
Other benign causes	27 (13%)
Total	210

From Thompson JS, DiBaise JK, Iver KR, et al: Short bowel syndrome as a postoperative complication. J Am Coll Surg 201:85, 2005.

Table 78–1 Intestinal Length and Nutritional Prognosis

Intestinal Anatomy	Intestinal Length to Avoid Permanent Parenteral Nutrition
End-jejunostomy (type 1)	100 cm
Jejunocolic anastomosis (type 2)	65 cm
Jejunoileocolic anastomosis (type 3)	30 cm

Adapted from Messing B, Crenn P, Beau P, et al: Long term survival and parenteral nutrition dependence in adult patients with the short bowel syndrome. Gastroenterology 117:1043, 1999.

an end-jejunostomy (type 1 anatomy), a jejunoileal anastomosis with an intact colon (type 3 anatomy) is equivalent to 60 cm of additional small intestine, and a jejunocolic anastomosis (type 2 anatomy) is equivalent to about 30 cm of small intestine.[5]

A variety of conditions requiring intestinal resection lead to short-bowel syndrome (Table 78–2).[8] Patients with underlying inflammatory disease may have impaired intestinal function. The cause of resection will also influence the outcome because of the effect on other digestive organs. Long-term treatment and survival are influenced by the patient's age and other morbid conditions. Underlying disease will also influence these parameters.

INTESTINAL ADAPTATION

The small intestine is able to adapt to compensate for the reduction in absorptive surface area caused by intestinal resection.[9-11] This process occurs within the first year or two after resection and improves intestinal absorptive capacity (Fig. 78–1).[11] Whether the adaptive response can be significantly accelerated or augmented is not clear. The overall intestinal adaptive response results from changes in intestinal structure, function, and motility.

Structural adaptation after intestinal resection involves all layers of the intestine.[9,10] Mucosal DNA and protein synthesis and crypt cell proliferation are increased within hours after resection. Both the total number of cells and the proportion of proliferating cells are increased in the crypt. Enterocytes migrate at a faster rate along the villus. Villus lengthening occurs by an overall increased number of cells. Rates of apoptosis, or programmed cell death, increase in both crypt and villus enterocytes after resection. However, the proliferative stimulus dominates, so adaptation occurs. The ratio of crypts to villi may also increase. Microvilli along the epithelial surface increase as well. Overall, mucosal weight increases.

The thickness and length of the muscle layers also increase after resection, primarily as a result of hyperplasia rather than hypertrophy of the muscle cells.[9] Muscle adaptation, however, occurs at a later time than mucosal adaptation and only after more extensive resection. These changes in the components of the intestinal wall result in marked thickening of the intestinal wall, as well as increased intestinal circumference and length. Thus, there is an overall increase in mucosal surface area because of both villus hypertrophy and the increases in length and circumference of the remnant.

Intestinal motor activity is also altered by intestinal resection.[6] The canine small intestine demonstrates a biphasic motor response to varying degrees of distal resection. There is initial disruption of motor activity, followed by adaptation. In the distal segment of the intestinal remnant after limited resection and more generally after 75% resection, motility recordings are initially dominated by recurring bursts of clustered contractions.[12] With extensive resection, these clusters are prolonged and associated with baseline tonic changes. With limited resection, there is evidence of progressive motor adaptation with eventual slowing of transit and return of migrating motor complex (MMC) cycling. This adaptation is less apparent after massive resection. Motor adaptation

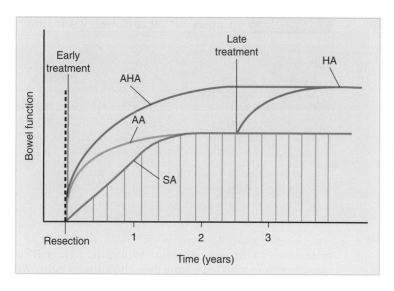

Figure 78–1. Schematic presentation of intestinal adaptation. AA, accelerated adaptation; AHA, accelerated hyperadaptation; HA, hyperadaptation; SA, spontaneous adaptation. (From Jeppesen PB: Clinical significance of GLP-2 in short bowel syndrome. J Nutr 133:3721, 2003.)

is more prominent in the jejunum than in the ileum. These changes are accompanied by modest alterations in smooth muscle contractility. Clinical reports also demonstrate a biphasic adaptive motor response during the first year after resection. There is disrupted motor activity in the first few months after resection, but these changes occur only after extensive resection (remnant shorter than 100 cm). Long-term human studies demonstrate a shorter duration of the MMC cycle and fed pattern after resection.[13]

Functional adaptation has been well documented after resection,[1,5,14,15] and structural adaptation increases intestinal absorptive surface area. Both structural adaptation and motor adaptation lead to prolonged transit time. Although the formerly accepted theory of improved absorption by individual enterocytes was discounted, more recent studies suggest that certain transport capabilities do improve. Within months of resection, diarrhea diminishes and nutritional status improves.

The mechanism of intestinal adaptation has been studied extensively but is still not entirely understood. The degree of structural adaptation is related to the extent and site of resection.[9,10] Adaptation is greater with more extensive resection, and the ileum has a greater adaptive capacity than the jejunum does. Subsequent resection elicits a further adaptive response. Luminal nutrients and secretions and growth factors are important for achieving the maximal response but are not essential for adaptation to occur (Box 78–2).[9,10] The early molecular events associated with this hyperplastic response are being investigated.[16,17] Intestinal resection results in increased levels of a variety of gene products in enterocytes within hours. There is an immediate increase in genes that encode transcription factors, not only genes that influence cell proliferation but also those that augment nutrient trafficking, as well as heat shock genes, which maintain normal cellular function. Many of these are novel genes not normally present in intestinal epithelium. The specific triggers for these events are not clear, and there are obviously many candidates. Currently,

Box 78–2   Factors Influencing Intestinal Adaptation

Gastrointestinal regulatory peptides
Luminal contents
   Nutrients
   Secretions
Systemic factors
   Growth factors
   Hormones
   Cytokines
Tissue Factors
   Immune system
   Mesenchymal factors
   Mesenteric blood flow
   Neural influences

there is clinical interest in manipulating the adaptive response pharmacologically.

MEDICAL MANAGEMENT

The early management of a patient with short-bowel syndrome is that of a critically ill surgical patient who has recently undergone intestinal resection and other concomitant procedures. Thus, control of sepsis, maintenance of fluid and electrolyte balance, and initiation of nutritional support are important in the early management of these patients. For patients who have survived this early phase, the primary goals of management are to maintain adequate nutritional status, maximize the absorptive capacity of the remaining intestine, and prevent the development of complications related to both the underlying pathophysiology and the nutritional therapy.

Maintain Nutritional Status

The most important therapeutic objective in the management of short-bowel syndrome is to maintain the patient's nutritional status. This usually requires PN support in the early period after surgery. Fluid and electrolyte losses from the gastrointestinal tract may be great during the early postoperative period and must be monitored and replaced as soon as possible. Enteral nutritional support should be started as soon as possible when the ileus has resolved. With time, an increasing amount of nutrients are absorbed by the enteral route. This is important for maximizing intestinal adaptation and preventing complications related to PN. As their condition improves and intestinal adaptation occurs, many patients can absorb the necessary nutrients entirely by the enteral route. The length of the intestinal remnant and the status of the colon have important prognostic implications in this regard (see Table 78–1).

The ability of patients with short-bowel syndrome to maintain adequate caloric intake enterally is determined by a variety of factors, including intestinal remnant length and location, any underlying intestinal disease, and the status of the remaining digestive organs.[15,18] Whether there is continuity in the intestinal tract or a stoma is also an important consideration. Diarrhea and perianal complications may markedly diminish oral intake. Patients with stomas are more likely to have a greater percentage of their calories taken enterally. Hyperphagia develops in many patients with short-bowel syndrome to overcome inefficient absorption.[19]

Many patients with short-bowel syndrome require long-term PN for survival, and this therapy has considerable expense and morbidity. Patients without malignancy have 1-, 3-, and 5-year survival rates of about 90%, 70%, and 60%, respectively.[4] One third of deaths are related to the underlying disease, 50% to other supervening disease, and 10% to 15% to PN therapy. Sepsis and liver disease related to PN are important factors in long-term survival.

The incidence of sepsis varies from 0.1 to 0.3 episodes per patient year of PN. Sepsis may be associated with catheter thrombosis. The need for prolonged therapy makes vascular access a long-term problem, and catheters may eventually need to be placed in the azygos, hepatic, or inferior vena cava veins.

End-stage liver disease develops in about 15% of long-term adult PN patients and is associated with a survival time of about 1 year without liver transplantation.[20,21] Although the etiology of the liver disease is not completely understood, it appears to be a multifactorial process that is initially reversible but ultimately leads to severe steatosis, cholestasis, and cirrhosis. Liver disease occurs more frequently in children than adults. Provision of enteral nutrients may prevent this problem, but overfeeding is a predisposing factor. Control of sepsis and bacterial overgrowth is important to minimize this liver disease. Patients with abnormal liver function test results while receiving PN should undergo abdominal ultrasound for evaluation of the gallbladder and bile ducts and should have a liver biopsy performed as appropriate.

Maximize Enteral Nutrient Absorption

Because the morbidity associated with nutritional support in patients with short-bowel syndrome is related primarily to PN, maximizing enteral absorption of nutrients is important for long-term survival. Furthermore, diarrhea and stomal fluid losses can also be important clinical problems that affect the patient's quality of life. Thus, it is beneficial to ensure that the patient's intestinal remnant is functioning optimally and absorbing nutrients and fluid.

The optimal diet for patients with short-bowel syndrome remains controversial. Provision of nutrients in their simplest form to minimize digestion has been one strategic approach. Simple sugars and dipeptides and tripeptides are rapidly absorbed from the intestinal tract. However, partially hydrolyzed diets appear to be just as effective and are less expensive. Complex carbohydrates reduce the osmotic load, but concentrated sugars, such as fruit juices, should be avoided because they generate a high osmotic load. Whether the diet should have a high-fat or low-fat content is another issue. There appears to be increasing agreement that patients with colon should have a low-fat (20% to 30% of calories), high-carbohydrate (50% to 60% of calories) diet but that patients with an end-enterostomy do not require fat restriction (30% to 40% of calories). Fat absorption obviously requires more digestion unless the fat is supplied in the form of medium-chain triglycerides. The ability to absorb these nutrients improves with time, so the diet may need to be continually modified. Specific problems such as lactase deficiency are often present, and the diet should be altered appropriately. Ingestion of a glucose-electrolyte oral rehydration solution with a sodium concentration of at least 90 mmol/L will optimize water and sodium absorption in the proximal jejunum and prevent secretion into the lumen.

Minimizing gastrointestinal secretions and controlling diarrhea are also important goals for maximizing absorption. Both histamine H_2 receptor antagonists and proton pump inhibitors are effective in controlling gastric hypersecretion, correcting malabsorption, and improving nutritional status in patients with short-bowel syndrome. Furthermore, cimetidine may also increase intestinal adaptation. Somatostatin and its long-acting analogue octreotide have been investigated for the management of severe refractory diarrhea in short-bowel syndrome. They improve diarrhea by prolonging small intestinal transit time and reducing salt and water excretion. Part of the beneficial effect may also be related to a reduction in gastric hypersecretion. Although these therapeutic agents are beneficial in the short term, it is not clear whether they continue to be effective after a few months, and they may have some potential deleterious effects. Somatostatin may exacerbate steatorrhea because of impaired pancreatic exocrine function. Other potential adverse effects of octreotide are inhibition of intestinal adaptation and the development of cholelithiasis. Recent evidence supports the use of ox bile and cholylsarcosine, a synthetic conjugated bile acid, as replacement therapy because they improve fat absorption without exacerbating diarrhea.

Box 78–3 **Restoration of Intestinal Continuity**

Advantages

Absorptive capacity increased

Energy absorbed from short-chain fatty acids

Infectious complications reduced

Transit time prolonged

Stoma avoided

Disadvantages

Bile acid diarrhea

Dietary restrictions

Nephrolithiasis increased

Perianal complications

From Thompson JS: Intestinal resection and the short bowel syndrome. In Quigley EMM, Sorrell MF (eds): Medical Management of the Gastrointestinal Surgery Patient. Baltimore, Williams & Wilkins, 1994, p 327.

Another important aspect of dietary management is to provide a diet that will maximize the intestinal adaptive response.[9,10,18] Provision of fat and dietary fiber may be particularly important in this regard. Long-chain and short-chain fatty acids appear to have a greater trophic effect on the intestine than medium-chain fatty acids do. Although these nutrients directly stimulate intestinal adaptation, nutrients also stimulate intestinal adaptation through endocrine and paracrine effects.

Pharmacologic therapy for short-bowel syndrome is a rapidly expanding area of investigation. Recent evidence suggests that provision of the appropriate diet, nutritional supplements such as glutamine, and growth factors such as growth hormone improves intestinal absorption and perhaps modifies the adaptive response in patients with established short-bowel syndrome.[22] However, which of these components is actually responsible for improved absorption is controversial. Growth hormone and glutamine do not have a consistent beneficial effect.[23,24] Currently, glucagon-like peptide-2 appears to have the most promise for promoting absorption and adaptation.[11] Epidermal growth factor also stimulates intestinal adaptation and may soon be studied in clinical trials.[25]

An important clinical issue is whether to establish intestinal continuity in patients who have a colonic remnant. There are both advantages and disadvantages to restoring continuity (Box 78–3). The colon may improve intestinal absorption by increasing the absorptive surface area, deriving energy from short-chain fatty acids, and prolonging transit time, particularly if the ileocecal valve is intact. Avoiding a stoma also improves quality of life. However, the response of the colon to luminal contents is somewhat unpredictable. Bile acids may cause a secretory diarrhea. Perianal problems can be

quite disabling and decrease the patient's oral intake. Oxalate is absorbed primarily in the colon, and restoring continuity places the patient at increased risk for the formation of calcium oxalate stones. Serum and intestinal fluid markers have been investigated as a means of predicting the response of the individual patient to restoring continuity, but none is generally available and useful. Distal reinfusion of enteral contents into a mucus fistula to assess the functional outcome has some usefulness, but it is cumbersome. Not all patients who initially have a stoma created eventually have continuity restored with a satisfactory outcome.[26] This decision should be considered on an individual basis and depends on the length of the intestinal remnant, the status of the ileocecal valve and the colon, and the patient's overall condition. Generally, at least 3 ft of small intestine is required to prevent severe diarrhea and perianal complications. Restoring continuity, however, should always be given strong consideration because of possible improvement in absorption.

Prevent Complications

Metabolic complications are common in patients with short-bowel syndrome because of their tremendous fluid and electrolyte losses and the need to replace these losses with specialized solutions. Intravascular volume has to be maintained to prevent dehydration and renal dysfunction. Hypocalcemia is a common problem related to poor absorption and binding by intraluminal fat. Maintaining adequate calcium and magnesium levels and vitamin D supplementation are important to minimize bone disease. Hyperglycemia and hypoglycemia are frequent complications of patients receiving a large amount of their calories parenterally. Both metabolic acidosis and metabolic alkalosis can occur. A specific problem is D-lactic acidosis, which results from bacterial fermentation of unabsorbed nutrients, particularly simple sugars. Lactate reduces colon pH, thereby permitting the growth of acid-resistant anaerobes capable of producing D-lactate. Impaired metabolism of D-lactic acid may also contribute to elevated serum D-lactic acid levels. This diagnosis is suggested by an unexplained metabolic acidosis and associated neurologic symptoms, such as confusion and somnolence. D-Lactic acid is not measured by standard laboratory techniques for lactic acid determination. Thus, an increased anion gap but normal lactate level in the appropriate clinical setting mandates measurement of D-lactic acid. D-Lactic acidosis is treated by minimizing overall caloric intake or by instituting a low-carbohydrate diet. Administration of intestinal antibiotics may be appropriate, but the optimal duration of such treatment is unclear, and recurrence rates are significant.

Specific nutrient deficiencies need to be prevented and monitored closely, including iron and vitamin deficiencies, as well as deficiencies in micronutrients such as selenium, zinc, and copper. Because fat is poorly absorbed, fatty acid deficiency can also occur. Although medium-chain fatty acids can supplement the diet enterally, parenteral lipids are required in patients who depend primarily on that route. Serum free fatty acid levels and triene-to-tetraene ratios may need to be monitored periodically to determine the need for supplementation and response to treatment. In general, enteral intake must greatly exceed the absorptive needs to ensure that these needs are being met.

Catheter-related sepsis is an important problem that often necessitates rehospitalization and replacement of catheters. Attention to technique and meticulous patient education are important to prevent this complication. Most infections are due to *Staphylococcus* species, but gram-negative bacteria and fungi are also associated with line sepsis. An attempt at line sterilization before removal is appropriate when infections are caused by coagulase-negative staphylococci and gram-negative bacteria. Repeated placement of catheters can lead to catheter thrombosis, which is the other common problem. In patients who require PN permanently, this may become an important factor in the patient's survival because vascular access may not be achievable indefinitely.

PN-induced liver disease is another potential long-term problem.[20,21] It can be minimized by providing as large a portion of the calories as possible enterally, avoiding overfeeding, using mixed fuels (less than 30% fat), and preventing specific nutrient deficiencies. Treating bacterial growth and preventing recurrent sepsis are also important. Ursodeoxycholic acid administration may likewise be beneficial.

Bacterial overgrowth is another long-term complication associated with both intestinal disease and resection. It may result from impaired motility or stasis caused by obstructive lesions (Fig. 78–2). Achlorhydria is also a contributing factor. Bacterial deconjugation of luminal bile salts impairs bile salt reabsorption. Bacteria also metabolize intraluminal vitamin B_{12}. Depending on the bacterial species present, secretory diarrhea may occur as well. Bacterial overgrowth requires a high degree of suspicion to make the diagnosis. This complication should be suspected when a patient's absorptive capacity and stool habits change acutely. It may result from a mechanical obstruction or a blind loop, which can be relieved by surgery. However, it is often a primary motor abnormality and requires intermittent therapy with antibiotics. Colonization of the lumen with acidophilus or other nonpathogenic organisms is another potential therapy.[27]

Cholelithiasis occurs in 30% to 40% of patients with intestinal insufficiency.[28,29] Factors that predispose these patients to gallstone formation include altered hepatic bile metabolism and secretion, gallbladder stasis, and malabsorption of bile acids. Depending on the dominant mechanism, either mixed pigment stones or cholesterol stones may occur. Long-term PN is an important contributing factor causing altered hepatic bile metabolism and gallbladder stasis. Patients receiving PN are susceptible to the development of cholelithiasis and hepatocellular dysfunction and thus require careful clinical evaluation.[28,29] Biliary sludge forms within a few weeks of initiating PN if there is no enteral intake, but it rapidly disappears when enteral nutrition is resumed. Intestinal mucosal disease and resection, particularly of the ileum, cause bile acid malabsorption, which leads to lithogenic

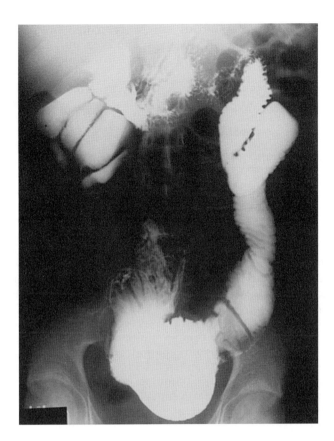

Figure 78–2. Contrast study of a patient with short-bowel syndrome. The shortened remnant lies primarily in the left side of the abdomen with a large dilated segment in the pelvis. Contrast has passed into the right colon beyond this area.

bile and the formation of cholesterol stones. The risk for cholelithiasis is significantly increased if less than 120 cm of intestine remains after resection, the terminal ileum has been resected, and PN is required. The incidence of cholelithiasis can be minimized by providing nutrients enterally whenever possible. Patients totally dependent on PN may be treated with intermittent cholecystokinin injections to prevent stasis and the formation of sludge. Administration of intravenous lipids also stimulates gallbladder emptying. Cholelithiasis may lead to complications in a higher number of patients with short-bowel syndrome than in the general population and also requires more complicated surgical treatment. Thus, several authors now recommend prophylactic cholecystectomy in these patients when laparotomy is being undertaken for other reasons.[29]

Nephrolithiasis also occurs with some frequency. Calcium oxalate stones form as a result of increased oxalate absorption from the colon.[29] Oxalate is normally bound to calcium in the intestinal lumen and is not absorbed. Decreased availability of calcium secondary to reduced intake or binding by intraluminal fat leaves free oxalate in the lumen. Thus, the oxalate is absorbed in the colon and forms calcium oxalate in the urine. Nephrolithiasis is unusual in patients after intestinal resection and jejunostomy but occurred in a fourth of such patients with an intact colon within 2 years of resection. Nephrolithiasis can be prevented by maintaining a diet low in oxalate, minimizing intraluminal fat, supplementing the diet with calcium orally, and maintaining a high urinary volume. Foods with high oxalate content include chocolate, tea, cola, spinach, celery, carrots, and other fruits and vegetables. Cholestyramine, which binds oxalic acid in the colon, is another potential treatment.

Gastric hypersecretion is a potential problem in patients with short-bowel syndrome. Massive intestinal resection can cause gastric hypersecretion as a result of parietal cell hyperplasia and hypergastrinemia. This phenomenon is usually transient and lasts several months. The etiology has not been elucidated but may involve loss of an inhibitor from the resected intestine. The associated hyperacidity exacerbates malabsorption and diarrhea. Clinical development of peptic ulcer disease may also occur and is seen in about a fourth of patients undergoing massive resection.[26] Treatment of gastric acid secretion may improve absorption but also prevents peptic ulcer disease. Control of acid secretion by H_2 receptor antagonists or proton pump inhibitors should be initiated in the perioperative period after resection and maintained until the increased acid production resolves. Some patients, however, continue to have symptoms of peptic ulcer disease that eventually require surgical intervention. Gastric resection therapy should be avoided when possible. A highly selective vagotomy may be the most desirable procedure if feasible.

SURGICAL MANAGEMENT

The primary goal of surgical therapy for short-bowel syndrome is to increase intestinal absorptive capacity, which can be achieved either by improving absorption by existing intestine or by increasing the area of absorption (Box 78–4). Recruiting additional intestine into continuity, relieving obstruction, or slowing intestinal transit will often improve absorption. The intestinal lengthening procedure is feasible in selected patients. The most significant increase in length, however, is potentially achieved by intestinal transplantation. The choice of surgical therapy for short-bowel syndrome is influenced by intestinal remnant length and caliber and the clinical condition of the patient (Table 78–3).[3]

Preserve and Maximize the Intestinal Remnant

An abdominal reoperation is required in about half the patients with short-bowel syndrome after discharge from the hospital.[26] Intestinal problems are the most common indication. An important goal with any reoperation in patients with short-bowel syndrome is to preserve the length of the intestinal remnant. Several strategies can be used when further intestinal disease requires surgery.[30] Resection can often be avoided by intestinal tapering to improve the function of dilated segments, performing stricturoplasty for benign strictures, and using serosal patching for certain strictures and chronic

---

Box 78–4 **Surgical Strategies for Short-Bowel Syndrome**

Preserve and maximize remnant
  Avoid resection
  Restore continuity
  Recruit additional intestine
Improve intestinal function
  Relieve obstruction
  Taper dilated bowel
  Slow intestinal transit
Increase absorptive area
  Intestinal lengthening
  Intestinal transplantation

Table 78–3 Surgical Approach to Short-Bowel Syndrome

Intestinal Remnant	Clinical Condition	Surgical Options
Adequate length with normal diameter	Enteral nutrition (remnant >120 cm in adults, >60 cm in children)	Optimize intestinal function, recruit additional length
Adequate length with dilated bowel	Bacterial overgrowth, stasis	Treat obstruction, intestinal tapering
Marginal length with normal diameter (remnant 60-120 cm in adults, 30-60 cm in children)	Rapid transit, need for parenteral nutrition	Recruit additional length, reversed intestinal segment, artificial valve, colon interposition
Short length with normal diameter (remnant <60 cm in adults, <30 cm in children)	Need for parenteral nutrition	Optimize intestinal function
Short length with dilated bowel	Need for parenteral nutrition	Intestinal lengthening
Short length	Complications of parenteral nutrition	Intestinal transplantation

From Thompson JS: Surgical approach to the short bowel syndrome: Procedures to slow intestinal transit. Eur J Pediatr Surg 9:263, 1999.

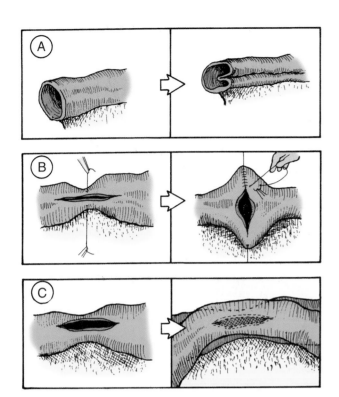

Figure 78–3. Techniques for preserving intestinal length include tapering of dilated segments rather than resection **(A)**, stricturoplasty for strictures **(B)**, and serosal patches for strictures and perforation **(C)**. (From Thompson JS: Recent advances in the surgical treatment of the short bowel syndrome. Surg Ann 22:110, 1990.)

perforations (Fig. 78–3). Resections should be limited in extent when they cannot be avoided. An end-to-end anastomosis is favored both to prevent blind loops and to maximize functional length of the intestine. Depending on the previous operations performed, patients occasionally have intestinal segments that can be recruited into continuity at the time of reoperation. This should always be given careful consideration. The length, location, and characteristics of the remnant should be carefully documented at the time of any operation.

Stricturoplasty is most often performed in the fashion of a Heineke-Mikulicz pyloroplasty. The stricture is incised longitudinally and closed transversely. The incision extends at least 1 cm proximal and distal to the stricture, but larger incisions may be required to achieve a satisfactory orifice. The enterotomy can be repaired with either a single-layer or a two-layer anastomosis. Longer strictures or multiple closely associated strictures can be opened with a side-to-side stapled anastomosis. Blind loops should be avoided, however.

Serosal patching is performed by apposition of an adjacent serosal surface, usually either small intestine or colon, to a nonhealing fistula, stricture, or other focal defect. A single-layer seromuscular-to-seromuscular anastomosis is created in either an interrupted or continuous fashion. The serosal patch becomes covered by normal mucosa from adjacent tissue. This technique is most

applicable to smaller defects because contraction of the patch does occur and could lead to a stenotic segment.

Improve Intestinal Function

Improve Motility

Patients with short-bowel syndrome have a propensity for the development of dilated intestine secondary to chronic obstruction or intestinal adaptation. Dilated intestine may lead to stasis and bacterial overgrowth, which can further aggravate the malabsorption associated with the short remnant. Mechanical obstruction at an anastomosis or from adhesions or strictures related to the underlying disease process should always be sought in these patients and corrected with the techniques mentioned previously. These dilated segments, however, are often not associated with distal obstruction. Tapering dilated segments improves motility by permitting closure of the lumen during contraction of the wall, which improves peristalsis. Simple imbrication of the redundant bowel is the preferred method, although longitudinal transection plus removal of intestine along the antimesenteric border has also been performed. A continuous nonabsorbable suture line is usually most expeditious, particularly for lengthy segments. Excisional techniques are easily performed with stapling devices but can also be performed with bowel clamps. Tapering enteroplasty improves intestinal function in patients with short-bowel syndrome.[3] Blind loops should be sought and eliminated, preferably by revision of the anastomosis rather than resection.

Prolong Intestinal Transit

Procedures designed to prolong intestinal transit time have been evaluated experimentally and performed clinically, but their efficacy remains questionable (Fig. 78–4).[31,32] Most of the reports are anecdotal. These adjunctive procedures are often performed during the adaptive phase; hence, it is difficult to determine whether the improvement in nutritional status and absorption was due to the surgical procedure or the normal adaptive process. Three procedures have been attempted in sufficient numbers to be considered, including reversed intestinal segments, colon interposition, and artificial sphincters (Table 78–4).

Reversed Intestinal Segments Reversing segments of intestine to slow intestinal transit is the surgical procedure that has been reported most extensively. The antiperistaltic segment functions by inducing retrograde peristalsis distally and disrupting the motility of the proximal part of the intestine. In addition, disruption of the intrinsic nerve plexus slows myoelectrical activity in the distal remnant. Reversed segments also alter the hormonal milieu after resection.

Most experimental studies of antiperistaltic segments demonstrate slowed intestinal transit, improved absorption, reduced weight loss, and prolonged survival after intestinal resection, but some reports do not show a

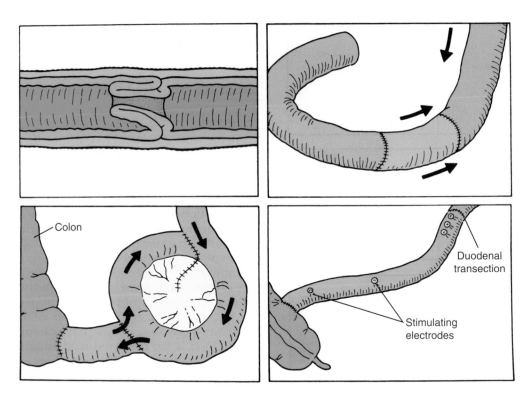

Figure 78–4. Techniques for slowing intestinal transit: intestinal valve *(upper left)*, antiperistaltic segment *(upper right)*, recirculating loop *(lower left)*, and intestinal pacing *(lower right)*. (From Thompson JS, Rikkers JS: Surgical alternatives for the short bowel syndrome. Am J Gastroenterol 82:97, 1987.)

Table 78–4 Clinical Experience with Procedures to Prolong Transit for Short-Bowel Syndrome

Procedure	Number of Patients	Number of Children (%)	Number of Patients with Clinical Improvement (%)
Reversed segment	55	6 (11)	45 (81)
Intestinal valve	12 (6)*	1 (16)	4 (67)
Colon interposition	12	11 (92)	6 (50)
Pouch or loop	4	1 (25)	1 (25)
Intestinal pacing	1	0 (0)	0 (0)

*Six procedures performed as a staged approach for intestinal lengthening.
From Thompson JS: Surgical approach to the short bowel syndrome: Procedures to slow intestinal transit. Eur J Pediatr Surg 9:263, 1999.

beneficial effect.[33,34] The variable outcomes may be explained by several factors, including variation in the extent of resection, timing of the procedure, and the use of different lengths of antiperistaltic segments. Reversed segments performed simultaneously with 75% resection in canines blunted the normal adaptive response, which may be related to the altered hormonal response.[35]

The ideal antiperistaltic segment slows transit without causing complete obstruction. Several technical details are important. The optimal length of the reversed segment would appear to be about 10 cm or less in adults and 3 cm in children. The reversed segment should be created as distal in the small intestinal remnant as feasible. Care must be taken to avoid complete rotation of the mesentery to prevent intestinal ischemia.

Antiperistaltic segments have been reported clinically in more than 50 patients, about 90% of whom were adults.[31] In these anecdotal reports, clinical improvement with slowed intestinal transit and increased absorption has been reported in 80% of patients. Transient obstructive symptoms and anastomotic leak are potential problems. The length of the segment has varied from 5 to 15 cm in these reports. Performance of this procedure in patients with Crohn's disease does not appear to influence recurrence rates. Long-term function has been demonstrated.

Intestinal Valves The effect of valves and sphincters on intestinal motility involves several different mechanisms. They create a partial mechanical obstruction, disrupt the normal motor pattern of the small intestine, and prevent retrograde reflux of colonic contents.[31] In experimental studies, intestinal valves and sphincters have been shown to prolong transit time, increase absorptive capacity, and extend survival, although the results have been inconsistent. Effective valves usually result in some dilation of the proximal part of the intestine and may cause, at least transiently, obstructive symptoms. Potential complications include necrosis of the valve, complete obstruction, and intussusception. Durability of the sphincter function of valves has been questioned.

Several different techniques for creating intestinal valves and sphincters to replace the ileocecal valve have been reported, including external constriction of the intestine, segmental denervation, and intussusception of intestinal segments to increase intraluminal pressure, with the latter being used most frequently. Intussuscepted valves should be 2 cm in length if retrograde and 4 cm if the intussuscepted valve is prolapsed antegrade. We have generally created a retrograde sphincter similar to that used in the continent ileostomy procedure, but it is only 2 cm in length.[3]

The reported clinical experience with intestinal valves and sphincters is less extensive than that with reversed segments. Nipple valves were recently used in six infants to cause dilation of the intestine so that subsequent intestinal lengthening could be performed.[33] Intussuscepted valves were reported as primary treatment in five adults and one infant with short-bowel syndrome.[31] Four patients improved markedly, one had questionable benefit, and takedown of the valve was required in the other. Ileocolic nipple valves were lost in a third of patients monitored for more than 5 years in one study, again raising the issue of durability.

Colon Interposition Interposing a colonic segment in the small intestinal remnant in either an isoperistaltic or antiperistaltic fashion retards intestinal transit. Isoperistaltic interposition is performed proximally and functions by slowing down the rate at which nutrients are delivered to the distal portion of the small intestine.[31] The antiperistaltic colon interposition is placed distally, similar to the reversed small intestinal segment. Interposed colonic segments absorb water, electrolytes, and nutrients, in addition to their effect on intestinal transit. Although it has been suggested that interposed colon might develop structural and functional similarities to the small intestine, this has not been substantiated.

In experimental studies, isoperistaltic colon interposition generally resulted in slower transit time, less weight loss, and improved survival after resection. Results with antiperistaltic colon interposition, however, have been less consistent. The length of colon interposed seems to be less critical than with reversed segments.

The use of colon interposition has been reported in 12 patients, 11 of whom underwent isoperistaltic interposition.[32] All but one of the patients were infants younger than 1 year. The interposed colon segment varied between 8 and 24 cm in length. All patients were PN dependent preoperatively. Six (50%) patients demonstrated sustained clinical improvement; the other six, including the one with the antiperistaltic colon, did not improve and subsequently died of sepsis or hepatic failure. Colonic stasis with bacterial overgrowth may have contributed. This experience suggests that isoperistaltic colon interposition may have some merit.

Other Approaches Intestinal pouches and recirculating loops would theoretically prolong transit time by permitting prolonged exposure of luminal nutrients to the intestinal absorptive surface. In experimental studies, however, these procedures have not improved absorption or survival rates after massive resection. Four clinical reports involving recirculating loops have been disappointing as well.

Intestinal pacing in a retrograde fashion has also been investigated as a means of prolonging transit time. Retrograde electrical pacing promotes peristalsis in a reverse direction but also alters proximal intestinal motility, possibly through a hormonal mechanism. Postprandial retrograde pacing in canines improved absorption and intestinal status. In the one reported attempt to achieve retrograde pacing in a patient with short-bowel syndrome, the pacemaker failed to stimulate the intestine.

Choice of Procedure Procedures designed to slow intestinal transit should be applied cautiously in patients with nearly adequate remnant length and demonstrated rapid transit. They should be considered only after maximal adaptation has occurred. Reversed intestinal segments and artificial valves have the greatest appeal as procedures to slow intestinal transit. Antiperistaltic segments should be used in patients with longer remnants. The 10-cm segment still leaves sufficient remnant for absorption. Valves should be considered in patients with shorter remnants because less bowel is used. In one experimental study, an intestinal valve was more effective than an antiperistaltic segment in prolonging transit time after resection. The efficacy of these procedures remains questionable, however, and other approaches have been even less encouraging. Furthermore, these procedures are applicable to only a small proportion of patients with short-bowel syndrome.

Increase Absorptive Area

Dilated intestinal segments may be amenable to an intestinal tapering and lengthening procedure. Theoretically, such a procedure has the advantage of not only improving motility and reducing stasis but also improving intestinal absorption by the increased absorptive area. The primary technique was initially described by Bianchi[34] (Fig. 78–5). More recently, an alternative technique called serial transverse enteroplasty (STEP) has been reported[36,37] (Fig. 78–6). In these approaches the

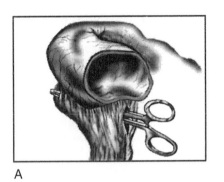

A

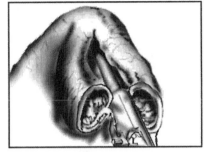

B

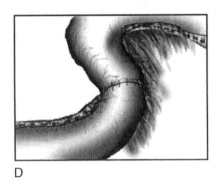

C

D

Figure 78–5. The Bianchi procedure. Longitudinal dissection between the blood vessels on the mesenteric border **(A)** permits the use of staples to divide the intestine longitudinally **(B** and **C)**. The two parallel segments are then anastomosed end to end **(D)**. (From Thompson JS: Surgical rehabilitation of the intestine in short bowel syndrome. Surgery 135:465, 2004.)

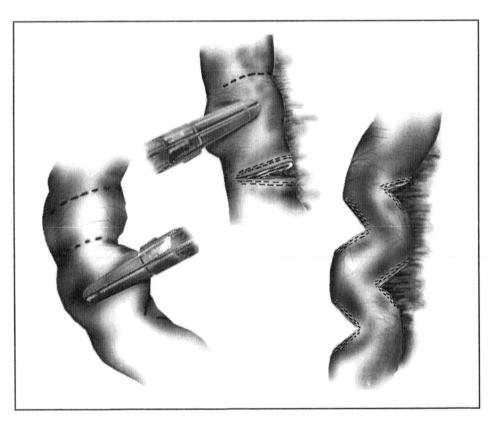

Figure 78–6. The STEP procedure. Several transverse applications of a linear stapler from opposite directions on the bowel wall allow the intestine to lengthen with reduced diameter. (From Thompson JS: Surgical rehabilitation of the intestine in short bowel syndrome. Surgery 135:465, 2004.)

dilated segments are tapered, and the redundant intestine is preserved and restored into continuity for additional length.

In experimental studies, intestinal lengthening by the Bianchi procedure prolongs transit time but does not clearly improve absorption in the short term.[38] Intestinal lengthening causes motor disruption in the proximal portion of the intestine and alters the hormonal response to resection. The jejunum may yield better results than lengthening of ileum. Improved nutrition has been demonstrated in an animal model after the STEP procedure.[36]

The Bianchi procedure is performed by transecting distal to the dilated segment to be tapered. Dissection is performed longitudinally for about 5 cm on the mesenteric edge of the bowel between the terminal branching vessels to create a space that permits longitudinal division of the bowel with a stapler. A hand-sewn anastomosis can also be used. If the diameter of the bowel permits, the staple line can be imbricated as well. This procedure is repeated until the desired length is achieved. The two parallel longitudinal segments can then be anastomosed end to end to halve the diameter and double the length of the segment. Intestinal lengthening of segments from 5 to 90 cm has been reported. Obviously, longer segments are at greater risk for complications.

The STEP procedure involves serial transverse applications of a linear stapler from alternating directions to divide the bowel perpendicular to the long axis of the intestine. The length and spacing of the transverse division are determined by the diameter of the intestine. Multiple stapler applications are required. The net result is an increase in length and a reduction in diameter. This procedure is less complicated than the Bianchi procedure because it avoids the extensive mesenteric dissection and the additional anastomosis. It is feasible for very short segments and those near the ligament of Treitz.

Intestinal lengthening, primarily the Bianchi procedure, has now been reported in more than 100 patients.[34,37,39,40] After an initial prolonged ileus, significant improvement in absorptive capacity and nutritional status has been reported in 90% of these patients in the short term. Potential complications, however, such as necrosis of divided segments, anastomotic leak, and obstruction develop in up to 20% of patients. Gastrostomy tubes are often placed because of the prolonged dysmotility that occurs. Although short-term results have been encouraging, emerging long-term results suggest that about half the patients undergoing this procedure have a sustained benefit for up to 10 years.[39] The initial experience with the STEP procedure has been favorable.[37,40] Initial short-term results in 10 patients have demonstrated the feasibility and safety of the technique in the clinical setting. The outcome of these procedures is heavily influenced by patient selection in terms of age, remnant length, hepatic function, and requirement for PN. Thus, these procedures should be applied cautiously.

One of the limitations of lengthening procedures is that they can be applied only to a fairly select group of patients. Obviously, the procedures should be considered only if bacterial overgrowth or other signs of malabsorption are identified that appear to be related to the dilated segment. The intestinal diameter should be at least 4 cm to provide an adequate lumen size after tapering. Sequential operations, first using a procedure such as an artificial valve to produce intestinal dilation and then performing the lengthening at a later time, have been used to expand the applicability of this technique. The vascular anatomy must be favorable for the Bianchi procedure. Effort is also being directed at recruiting additional vascular supply to permit further lengthening. The STEP procedure should markedly increase the applicability of intestinal lengthening.

INTESTINAL TRANSPLANTATION

The development of intestinal transplantation must be placed in the context of patients and physicians faced with catastrophic clinical circumstances in the absence of reliable alternatives. The mortality rate of patients requiring PN for benign disease has been estimated at 5% to 25% per year, or about 15% at 3 years.[41] For infants, the risk for PN-induced liver disease is especially great. It is estimated that half the deaths in children receiving PN are due to liver failure.[42] Currently, intestinal transplantation is applied as rescue therapy for patients with life-threatening complications of intestinal failure. In 2001 the U.S. federal government through the Centers for Medicare and Medicaid Services (CMS) approved payment for intestinal transplantation at select centers.

Indications

Indications for intestinal transplantation are restricted to life-threatening complications of intestinal failure, with the most common complication being the development of liver disease. It is important to determine whether the liver disease is reversible. If the liver disease is found to be irreversible, based on either biopsy findings or clinical features such as massive splenomegaly, ascites, encephalopathy, or gastrointestinal bleeding, the patient should undergo combined liver–small bowel transplantation. Greater emphasis has recently been placed on considering isolated small bowel transplantation for patients with potentially reversible PN-induced liver disease. Regardless of the type of transplant required, early referral and listing are important to ensure the patient the greatest opportunity to obtain a transplant.

The other common indications for intestinal transplantation are an irreversible permanent PN requirement along with episodes of sepsis or loss of venous access. Septic episodes that would prompt consideration for intestinal transplantation are typically catheter related. Patients who have undergone multiple hospitalizations related to catheter sepsis, often requiring intensive unit care with the need for vasopressors, fall in this category. Other indications for intestinal transplantation are multiantibiotic-resistant bacteremia or metastatic infection in sites such as the tricuspid valve or brain. Loss of venous access typically implies an inability to place a catheter in the subclavian or intrajugular veins and the use of extemporaneous sites such as the hepatic veins or the inferior vena cava. A transplant evaluation is strongly recommended in patients with known poor survival on PN, such as those with microvillus inclusion disease, intestinal aganglionosis, or desmoid tumors that have previously been eviscerated. Today, with improved outcomes and large numbers of patients dying on the waiting list, greater responsibility is being placed on the treating physician to make earlier referral to a transplant center.

The transplantation evaluation process for patients with intestinal failure requires a multidisciplinary group of health care professionals, including surgeons, gastroenterologists, dietitians, social workers, and nurse specialists. The evaluation process also incorporates an assessment of the feeding program that the patient is currently receiving. Contrast studies of the small and large bowel are frequently performed. A liver biopsy is performed in patients with evidence of liver dysfunction to help select the appropriate type of transplantation procedure. During the evaluation process, other problems are addressed, including worsening liver failure, sepsis, difficult vascular access, and septic episodes. After being identified as a potential candidate, the patient is placed on an active transplantation waiting list.

Operative Procedure

The donor operation begins similarly regardless of the organs being removed. Potential organ donors are matched with recipients according to blood type, size, and medical necessity. Most patients with short-bowel syndrome have a loss of peritoneal domain, thus requiring the donor to be about 50% smaller than the potential recipient. Recent success with reduced-size intestinal transplants has challenged these donor size guidelines. Donors should be ABO blood group identical, although exceptions to this rule have been reported.[43] Human leukocyte antigen matching and a negative T-cell crossmatch may be beneficial, particularly for recipients of isolated small bowel allograft. Donor logistics often prevent this type of testing from being performed prospectively.

Removal of the intestine for isolated small bowel transplantation involves removal of the liver and small bowel together, after which they are separated on the back table.[44] The donor operation for a future liver–small bowel transplantation is relatively similar, but no hilar dissection is performed. The colon and stomach are mobilized out of the field, and the liver–small bowel composite is removed en bloc, with care taken to remove as much aorta proximal to the celiac axis as possible.[44]

Back-table preparation for an isolated small bowel graft involves removing the duodenum–head of the pancreas from the portal vein and superior mesenteric artery. For liver and small bowel grafting procedures, the preparation involves removal of the distal pancreas and spleen. The numerous intercostal arteries are ligated, and the distal end of the aorta is oversewn. Critical for a liver–small bowel graft is that no hepatic hilar dissection take place so that the hepatobiliary-duodenal complex remains undisturbed.[44]

The recipient operation typically makes use of previous incisions. For isolated small bowel transplantation, the infrarenal aorta is isolated, and the arterial anastomosis for the small bowel graft is typically performed between the donor superior mesenteric artery and the infrarenal aorta.[44] Venous drainage can be systemic or portal, but systemic drainage is preferred whenever liver disease is present. An enterostomy is created to decompress the small bowel and to facilitate biopsy. A loop

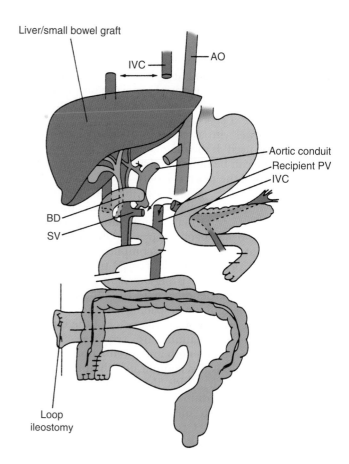

Figure 78–7. Diagram of a liver–small bowel allograft. This diagram demonstrates the intact hepatobiliary duodenal complex. AO, aorta; BD, bile duct; IVC, inferior vena cava; PV, portal vein; SV, splenic vein. (From Deroover A, Langnas A: Surgical methods of small bowel transplantation and liver-bowel transplantation. Curr Opin Organ Transplant 4:335, 1999.)

ileostomy is the most common type of stoma created for both liver–small bowel and isolated small bowel transplantation.

The liver–small bowel transplantation surgical technique leaves the donor hepatic hilar structures undisturbed and the hepatic-duodenal-biliary system intact (Fig. 78–7). The advantage of this approach is that it limits the necessary back-table dissection, prevents any torsion around the portal vein after implantation, and virtually eliminates any possible biliary tract complications after transplantation. The liver–small bowel composite allograft is implanted orthotopically. Arterial inflow is through the donor aortic conduit, and a native portacaval shunt is created to decompress the recipient's viscera. Under certain circumstances, particularly when the native foregut is diseased or dysfunctional, complete abdominal evisceration is performed before implantation of the donor organs. With evisceration of the native foregut the operation is often referred to as a multivisceral transplant. The proximal gastrointestinal anastomosis is frequently performed between the remnant proximal part of the stomach and the donor jejunum.

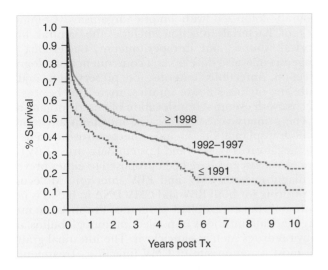

Figure 78–8. Graft survival rates after intestinal transplantation have improved over time. (From Grant D, Abu-Elmagd K, Reyes J, et al: 2003 Report of the intestine transplant registry: A new era has dawned. Ann Surg 241:607, 2005.)

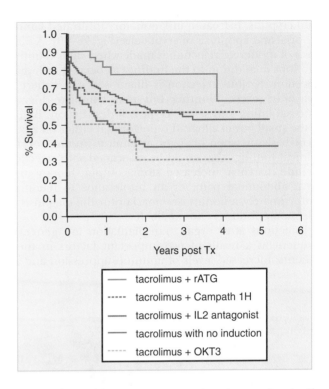

Figure 78–9. Graft-survival rates plotted according to the type of immunosuppressive protocol with particular reference to induction therapy. ATG, antithymocyte globulin; IL2, interleukin-2. (From Grant D, Abu-Elmagd K, Reyes J, et al: 2003 Report of the intestine transplant registry: A new era has dawned. Ann Surgery 241:607, 2005.)

After transplantation, the cornerstone of immunosuppressive management is the administration of tacrolimus and steroids. The majority of intestinal transplant programs now make use of some form of induction therapy, either with biologic agents such as Thymoglobulin or with interleukin-2 receptor blocking agents.[45-47] Reports have been made of other drugs being administered, including sirolimus, alemtuzumab (Campath 1H), and mycophenolate.[48] Numerous other agents are given as prophylaxis for infection, in particular, broad-spectrum antibiotics, antifungal agents, and antiviral drugs.

Outcome

Worldwide, based on published data from the 2003 Intestinal Transplant Registry (ITR) contributed by 61 programs in 10 countries, 989 transplants have been performed in 923 patients.[49] According to ITR data, isolated intestinal transplantation was performed 433 times and an intestinal allograft transplanted with a liver 556 times. Thirty-two grafts were obtained from living donors, including an identical twin and a triplet. In 2001 the CMS approved intestinal transplantation as therapy for patients with life-threatening complications of intestinal failure.

A total of 484 of the 923 patients reported in the ITR who underwent any type of intestinal transplantation are alive. The longest survivor has been on an enteral diet for over 14 years. Patient and graft survival has also steadily increased over time (Fig. 78–8). The ITR results also demonstrated factors important in improving patient and graft survival.[49] In a log-logistic model, factors associated with improved patient and graft survival included transplantation of a patient coming from home and the use of induction therapy (Fig. 78–9). As expected, programs that have performed at least 10 transplantations have better patient survival rates than do programs that have performed less than 10 transplantations. Patients who are called in from home have much higher survival rates, which should encourage physicians to refer patients earlier. Clinical experience remains confined to a small number of programs, with 83% of the cases performed at 10 institutions. The most common causes of death after intestinal transplantation included sepsis, multiorgan system failure, graft thrombosis, rejection, and post-transplantation lymphoma.

Rejection episodes continue to be a major problem in small bowel transplantation, even with tacrolimus-based immunosuppression combined with some form of induction therapy. The incidence of transplant rejection remains variable. According to the ITR, graft rejection rates were 57% for intestine grafts, 39% for combined intestine and liver grafts, and 48% for multivisceral grafts.[49] Contemporary single-center reports demonstrate even further reductions in rejection rates. At the University of Pittsburgh, Thymoglobulin induction combined with tacrolimus has resulted in a 44% rejection rate in the first month, whereas patients receiving interleukin-2 receptor blocking agents combined with tacrolimus at the University of Nebraska had a rate of about 5%.[45,47] These rates of rejection are now similar to those seen in recipients of heart, liver, and kidney transplants. The diagnosis of rejection is based on histologic findings. Mild rejection is diagnosed by the findings of mild cryptitis, increased inflammatory infiltrated lamina propria, and apoptosis of crypt cells (Fig. 78–10). A diagnosis of moderate rejection is made when villus blunting develops in addition to the findings associated with mild rejection. Serious rejection is diagnosed when there is not only severe blunting but also complete loss of mucosal lining and severe crypt cell destruction. Biopsy of the small bowel allograft is performed either on a protocol basis or when changes in clinical findings occur. Clinical findings that could be associated with rejection include diarrhea, increased stoma output, bloody diarrhea, abdominal pain, or an intolerance to feedings. Unfortunately, a noninvasive marker for the diagnosis of rejection episodes is not available.

Infections after organ transplantation are generally frequent as a result of two important factors in these patients: increased levels of immunosuppression and an allograft colonized with enteric organisms. Common sites of bacterial infection include the central line, surgical wound, and intraperitoneum. Bacteremia or fungemia may also develop as a consequence of allograft rejection, infectious enteritis, or preservation injury. With any of these bowel injuries, there can be loss of mucosa with eventual translocation of enteric organisms.

The primary viruses that cause infections after intestinal transplantation include herpesviruses such as cytomegalovirus (CMV) and Epstein-Barr virus (EBV). A variety of strategies have been proposed to either prevent or diagnose both CMV and EBV infection. Molecular monitoring for both EBV and CMV DNA in blood is now routine in most transplant programs. Prophylactic measures include infusions of pooled immunoglobulins and antiviral drugs such as ganciclovir. The intestinal graft is the most common site of CMV infection. Treatment is based on the use of antiviral drugs such as ganciclovir or foscarnet.

Post-transplant lymphoproliferative disease (PTLD) is an EBV-associated process that occurs after all solid organ transplantations. Intestinal transplant recipients appear to be at higher risk for PTLD than do recipients of other organ transplants, probably in part because of the high level of immunosuppression needed to control rejection, as well as the relatively young age of recipients. The reported incidence of PTLD after intestinal transplantation is between 7% and 29%.[45-47,49] Treatment of PTLD often involves lowering of immunosuppression and the use of antiviral agents as a first line of therapy. Newer treatments being proposed include the use of a low-dose cyclophosphamide (Cytoxan) regimen to control PTLD without the side effects of more traditional chemotherapeutic regimens.[50] Rituximab, a monoclonal antibody directed at CD20-positive B cells, is now being used to treat PTLD. Recently, the use of blood tests to measure qualitative and quantitative amounts of EBV DNA in the peripheral blood of transplant recipients has been advocated.[51] Measurements of EBV DNA are used

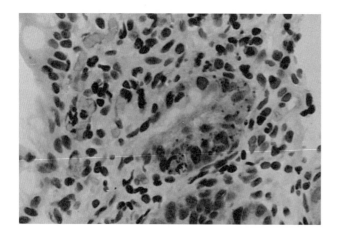

Figure 78–10. Photomicrograph of intestinal rejection in a transplanted intestinal graft. Apoptosis is a prominent feature. A single crypt is seen in the center with multiple apoptotic cells.

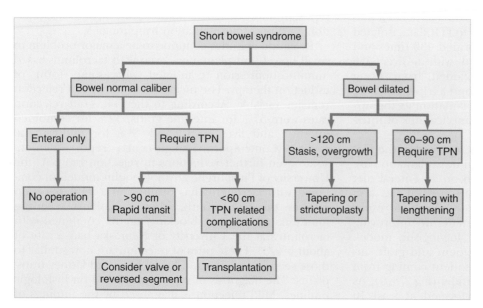

Figure 78–11. Surgical management of short-bowel syndrome. TPN, total parenteral nutrition. (From Thompson JS, Langnas AN, Pinch LW, et al: Surgical approach to the short bowel syndrome: Experience in a population of 160 patients. Ann Surg 22:600, 1995.)

in the hope of identifying PTLD before it becomes clinically evident so that less toxic preemptive therapy can be administered.

Graft-versus-host disease has been a relatively uncommon clinical event after intestinal transplantation. Its incidence was 7% in one series.[45] The diagnosis is based on traditional histopathologic criteria of skin, native gastrointestinal tract, or mucosa. Treatment of graft-versus-host disease is based primarily on increases in immunosuppression.

The functional status of the small bowel allograft is the foremost factor in determining the long-term quality of life for recipients. According to the ITR, enteral autonomy develops in 81% of recipients. Data also demonstrate that intestinal transplantation becomes cost-effective in comparison to PN at 2 years.[52]

The increasing experience and improved outcome of intestinal transplantation support the clinical use of this treatment modality. Although the potential morbidity of transplantation is greater than that of nontransplant surgical procedures, so too is the benefit. Intestinal transplantation is potentially applicable to a greater number of patients with short-bowel syndrome than nontransplant procedures are. All these procedures should be performed only in carefully selected patients (Fig. 78–11).

SUGGESTED READINGS

DiBaise JK, Young RJ, Vanderhoof JA: Intestinal rehabilitation and the short bowel syndrome: Part I. Am J Gastroenterol 99:1386, 2004.

DiBaise JK, Young RJ, Vanderhoof JA: Intestinal rehabilitation and the short bowel syndrome: Part 2. Am J Gastroenterol 99:1823, 2004.

Grant P, Abu-Elmagd K, Reyes J, et al: 2003 Report of the intestine transplant registry: A new era has dawned. Ann Surg 241:607, 2005.

Messing B, Crenn P, Beau P, et al: Long term survival and parenteral nutrition dependence in adult patients with the short bowel syndrome. Gastroenterology 117:1043, 1999.

Sudan D, DiBaise J, Torres C, et al: A multidisciplinary approach to the treatment of intestinal failure. J Gastrointest Surg 9:165, 2005.

Thompson JS, Langnas AN: Surgical approaches to improving intestinal function in short bowel syndrome Arch Surg 134:706, 1999.

REFERENCES

1. DiBaise JK, Young RJ, Vanderhoof JA: Intestinal rehabilitation and the short bowel syndrome: Part I. Am J Gastroenterol 99:1386, 2004.
2. Thompson JS: Comparison of massive versus repeated resection leading to the short bowel syndrome. J Gastrointest Surg 4:101, 2000.
3. Thompson JS, Langnas AN, Pinch LW, et al: Surgical approach to the short bowel syndrome: Experience in a population of 160 patients. Ann Surg 222:600, 1995.
4. Messing B, Crenn P, Beau P, et al: Long term survival and parenteral nutrition dependence in adult patients with the short bowel syndrome. Gastroenterology 117:1043, 1999.
5. Carbonnel F, Cosnes J, Chevret S, et al: The role of anatomic factors in nutritional autonomy after extensive small bowel resection. JPEN J Parenter Enteral Nutr 20:275, 1996.
6. Thompson JS, Quigley EMM, Adrian TE: Factors affecting outcome following proximal and distal intestinal resection in the dog. Dig Dis Sci 44:63, 1999.
7. Cosnes J, Gendre JP, LeQuintrec Y: Role of the ileocecal valve and site of intestinal resection in malabsorption after extensive small bowel resection. Digestion 18:329, 1998.
8. Thompson JS, DiBaise JK, Iver KR, et al: Short bowel syndrome as a postoperative complication. J Am Coll Surg 201:85, 2005.
9. Thompson JS : Intestinal adaptation: Nutritional and metabolic implications. In Latifi R, Dudrick SJ (eds): Current Surgical Nutrition. Austin, TX, RG Landes, 1996, p 147.
10. Wilmore DW, Byrne TA, Persinger RL: Short bowel syndrome: New therapeutic approaches. Curr Probl Surg 34:389, 1997.
11. Jeppesen PB: Clinical significance of GLP-2 in short bowel syndrome J Nutr 133:3721, 2003.
12. Quigley EMM, Thompson JS: The motor response to intestinal resection: Motor activity in the canine small intestine following distal resection. Gastroenterology 105:791, 1993.
13. Schmidt T, Pfeiffer A, Hackelsberger N, et al: Effect of intestinal resection on human small bowel motility. Gut 38:859, 1996.
14. Cosnes J, Carbonnel F, Beaugerie L, et al: Functional adaptation after extensive small bowel resection in humans. Eur J Gastroenterol Hepatol 6:197, 1994.
15. AGA Technical Review on short bowel syndrome and intestinal transplantation. Gastroenterology 124:1111, 2003.
16. Ehrenfried JA, Townsend CM, Thompson JC, Evers BM: Increases in nup 475 and c-jun are early molecular events that precede the adaptive hyperplastic response after small bowel resection. Ann Surg 225:51, 1995.
17. Rubin DC: Enterocyte gene expression in intestinal adaptation: Evidence for a specific cellular response. Am J Physiol 270:G143, 1996.
18. DiBaise JK, Young RJ, Vanderhoof JA: Intestinal rehabilitation and the short bowel syndrome: Part 2. Am J Gastroenterol 99:1823, 2004.
19. Cosnes J, Lamy P, Beaugerie L, et al: Adaptive hyperphagia in patients with post surgical malabsorption. Gastroenterology 99:1814, 1990.
20. Chan S, McCowen KC, Bistrian BR, et al: Incidence, prognosis and etiology of end stage liver disease in patients receiving home total parenteral nutrition. Surgery 126:28, 1999.
21. Cavicchi M, Beau P, Crenn P, et al: Prevalence of liver disease and contributing factors in patients receiving home parenteral nutrition for permanent intestinal failure. Ann Intern Med 132:525, 2000.
22. Wilmore T, Lacey JM, Soultanakis RP, et al: Factors predicting a successful outcome after pharmacologic bowel compensation. Ann Surg 226:228, 1997.
23. Skudlarek J, Jeppesen PB, Mortensen PB: Effect of high dose growth hormone with glutamine and no change in diet or intestinal absorption in short bowel patients: A randomized, double blind, crossover, placebo controlled trial. Gut 47:199, 2000.
24. Scolapio JS, Camilleri M, Fleming CR, et al: Effect of growth hormone, glutamine and diet on adaptation in short bowel syndrome: A randomized, controlled study. Gastroenterology 113:1074, 1997.
25. Thompson JS: EGF and the short bowel syndrome. JPEN J Parenter Enteral Nutr 23:S113, 1999.
26. Thompson JS, Langnas AN: Surgical approaches to improving intestinal function in short bowel syndrome Arch Surg 134:706, 1999.
27. Vanderhoof JA, Young RJ, Murray N, et al: Treatment strategies for small bowel bacterial overgrowth in short bowel syndrome. J Pediatr Gastroenterol Nutr 27:155, 1998.
28. Thompson JS: The role of prophylactic cholecystectomy in the short bowel syndrome. Arch Surg 131:556, 1996.
29. Nightingale JMD, Lennard-Jones JE, Gerner DJ, et al: Colonic preservation reduces need of parenteral therapy, increases incidence of renal stones, but does not change high prevalence of gallstones in patients with a short bowel. Gut 33:1493, 1992.

30. Thompson JS: Strategies for preserving intestinal length in the short bowel syndrome. Dis Colon Rectum 30:208, 1987.

31. Thompson JS: Surgical approach to the short bowel syndrome: Procedures to slow intestinal transit. Eur J Pediatr Surg 9:263, 1999.

32. Panis Y, Messing B, Rivet P, et al: Segment reversal of the small bowel as an alternative to intestinal transplantation in patients with short bowel syndrome. Ann Surg 225:401, 1997.

33. Georgeson K, Halpin D, Figuera R, et al: Sequential intestinal lengthening procedures for refractory short bowel syndrome. J Pediatr Surg 29:316, 1994.

34. Bianchi A: Longitudinal intestinal lengthening and tailoring: Results in 20 children. J R Soc Med 90:429, 1997.

35. Thompson JS, Quigley EMM, Adrian TE: Effect of reversed intestinal segments on intestinal structure and function. J Surg Res 58:19, 1995.

36. Kim HB, Fanza D, Garfad T, et al: Serial transverse enteroplasty (STEP): A novel bowel lengthening procedure. J Pediatr Surg 38:425, 2003.

37. Javid PJ, Kim HB, Duggan CP, et al: Serial transverse enteroplasty is associated with successful short term outcome in infants with the short bowel syndrome. J Pediatr Surg 40:1019, 2005.

38. Thompson JS, Quigley EMM, Adrian TE: Effect of intestinal tapering and lengthening on intestinal structure and function. Am J Surg 169:111, 1995.

39. Thompson JS, Pinch LW, Young R, Vanderhoof JA: Long term outcome of intestinal lengthening. Transplant Proc 32:1242, 2000.

40. Sudan D, DiBaise J, Torres C, et al: A multidisciplinary approach to the treatment of intestinal failure. J Gastrointest Surg 9:165, 2005.

41. Howard L, Malone M: Current status of home parenteral nutrition in the United States. Transplant Proc 28:2691, 1996.

42. Kelly D: Liver complications of pediatric parenteral nutrition: Epidemiology. Nutrition 14:153, 1998.

43. Sindhi R, Landmark J, Shaw B Jr, et al: Combined liver/small bowel transplantation using a blood group compatible but nonidentical donor. Transplantation 61:1782, 1996.

44. Grant W, Langnas AN: Pediatric small bowel transplantation: Techniques and outcomes. Curr Opin Organ Transplant 7:2020, 2002.

45. Reyes J, Mazariegos GV, Abu-Elmagd K, et al: Intestinal transplantation under tacrolimus monotherapy after perioperative lymphoid depletion with rabbit anti-thymocyte globulin (Thymoglobulin). Am J Transplant 5:1430, 2005.

46. Kato T, Gaynor JJ, Selvaggi G, et al: Intestinal transplantation in children: A summary of clinical outcomes and prognostic factors in 108 patients from a single center. J Gastrointest Surg 9:75, discussion 89, 2005.

47. Grant WJ, Botha JF, Sudan DL, et al: Improved survival after intestinal transplantation with lower immunosuppression. Paper presented at the Ninth International Small Bowel Transplantation Symposium, June 30-July 2, 2005, Brussels.

48. Farmer DG: Clinical immunosuppression for intestinal transplantation. Curr Opin Organ Transplant 9:214, 2004.

49. Grant D, Abu-Elmagd K, Reyes J, et al: 2003 Report of the intestine transplant registry: A new era has dawned. Ann Surg 241:607, 2005.

50. Gross T, Hinrichs S, Winner J, et al: Treatment of post-transplant lymphoproliferative disease (PTLD) following solid organ-transplantation with low-dose chemotherapy. Ann Oncol 9:339, 1998.

51. Berney T, Delis S, Kato T, et al: Successful treatment of posttransplant lymphoproliferative disease with prolonged rituximab treatment in intestinal transplant recipients. Transplantation 74:1000, 2002.

52. Sudan D: Cost and quality of life after intestinal transplantation. Gastroenterology 130(suppl):S158, 2006.

79

Gastrointestinal Carcinoid Tumors

Cletus A. Arciero · Elin R. Sigurdson

Lubarsch first described carcinoid tumors in 1888.[1] Oberndorfer used the term "karzinoide" in 1907 to describe a tumor that was more indolent behaving than adenocarcinoma.[2] Since these early discoveries, carcinoid neoplasms have been described in most organs in the body. Carcinoid neoplasms are neuroendocrine tumors that span the realm from benign to malignant. They are derived from enterochromaffin cells, or secretory cells found within respiratory and gastrointestinal epithelial tissues. These cells, which belong to the amine precursor uptake decarboxylase (APUD) system, are often argentaffinic (silver staining), are usually argyrophilic (silver staining only with the addition of a reducing agent), and produce a wide array of biogenic amines, neuropeptides, and peptide hormones. Although gastrointestinal neuroendocrine tumors are rare, carcinoid tumors are the most common of them.

INCIDENCE AND EPIDEMIOLOGY

The incidence of gastrointestinal carcinoids in the United States is estimated to be 2.47 to 2.58 per 100,000, with similar rates noted in Europe and Japan.[3] The incidence of carcinoid tumors is higher in African Americans, who have rates of 3.98 to 4.48 per 100,000. Necroscopy studies have shown that upward of 0.65% to 1.2% of all patients examined exhibit evidence of a small intestine carcinoid.[4] However, because of their often indolent course, far fewer diagnoses are made. The tumor occurs most commonly in the fifth to sixth decade of life with a slight predilection for females (55 : 44 female-to-male ratio). Sixty-seven percent of all carcinoids arise in the gastrointestinal tract, with the majority (25.3%) of the remaining occurring in the tracheobronchial tree.[3]

Gastrointestinal carcinoids are distributed via embryologic origins: foregut, midgut, and hindgut. Foregut carcinoids account for approximately 7% of all carcinoids, whereas midgut and hindgut carcinoids represent 62% and 30% of all carcinoids, respectively. Because of the preponderance of APUD cells within the ileum and appendix, the most common sites are the appendix (35%) and small intestine (23%), followed by the rectosigmoid (12%) and colon (6%). The majority of the small intestine carcinoids occur within 2 ft of the ileocecal valve. Both foregut and midgut carcinoids are associated with a second, synchronous primary carcinoid tumor of similar embryologic origin in 25% of cases. Non-neuroendocrine, synchronous cancers are discovered in 17% to 53% of patients with carcinoid tumors.[5]

Some patients have a genetic predisposition to carcinoid tumors. First-degree relatives of patients with carcinoid have an increased relative risk (RR = 3.6) for development of a carcinoid tumor.[5] There is also a notably increased risk for carcinoid tumors in those who have a well-educated social background (RR = 2.8) and reside in a major metropolitan region (RR = 1.39).[5]

PATHOLOGY

Carcinoid tumors are composed of enterochromaffin cells (which are cells that stain with chromaffin). Grossly, these tumors are well-circumscribed, round, submucosal lesions that reveal a yellow coloration when sectioned because of the high lipid content of the tumors (Fig. 79–1). They are typically small (<2 cm) and multicentric. Microscopically, carcinoid tumors are pathologically categorized by the presence of small, uniform cells in orderly bands or ribbons (Fig. 79–2). They have benign cytologic features with rare mitotic figures. The cytoplasm is marked by the abundant presence of neurosecretory granules, and immunohistochemical staining reveals numerous peptides. The exact microscopic features of carcinoid neoplasms vary according to their origin. Foregut tumors are mostly argyrophilic, whereas midgut tumors are mostly argentaffinic. Hindgut tumors appear to be a mix, with 60% to 70% being argyrophilic, 8% to 16% being argentaffinic, and the rest having no

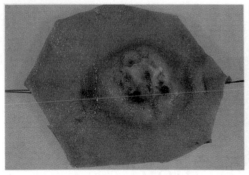

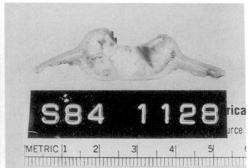

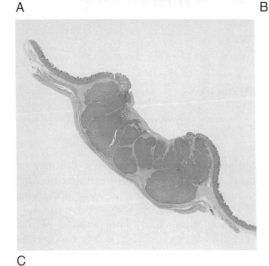

Figure 79–1. Gastric carcinoid tumor. **A,** Large, ulcerated tumor (gross). **B,** Fixed specimen (gross). **C,** Low-power histologic study showing a large tumor with mucosal ulceration but confined to the wall of the stomach. (Courtesy of Edward Lee, M.D. From Koh TJ, Wang TC: Tumors of the Stomach. In Feldman M, Friedman LS, Sleisenger MH [eds]: Sleisenger & Fordtran's Gastrointestinal and Liver Disease, 7th ed. Philadelphia, WB Saunders, 2002, p 847.)

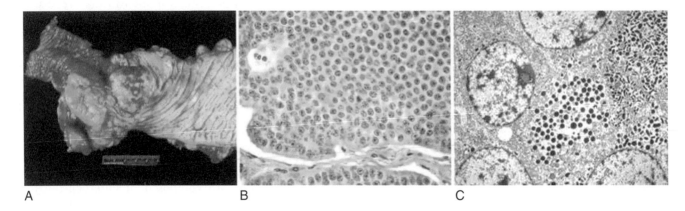

Figure 79–2. Carcinoid tumor. **A,** Multiple protruding tumors are present at the ileocecal junction. **B,** The tumor cells exhibit a monotonous morphology, with a delicate intervening fibrovascular stroma. **C,** Electron micrograph showing dense core bodies in the cytoplasm (From Liu C, Crawford JM: The gastrointestinal tract. In Kumar V, Abbas A, Fausto N [eds]: Robbins and Cotran: Pathologic Basis of Disease, 7th ed. Philadelphia, Elsevier, 2005, p 867.)

evidence of any silver staining. Carcinoid tumors have five histologic patterns: insular, trabecular, glandular, undifferentiated, and mixed.[6]

Although pathologic examination of the primary tumor cannot clearly define malignant versus benign without evidence of metastasis, certain features indicate increased aggressiveness. These more aggressive-appearing carcinoids are termed atypical/anaplastic carcinoid and have features of increased cellular atypia,

high mitotic rate/activity, or necrosis. Immunohisto-chemical staining to detect increased levels of p21 or MIB-1, or both, can aid in determining the increased aggressiveness of a tumor.[7,8]

CLINICAL FEATURES

Carcinoid tumors are marked by their relatively slow growth and often dearth of symptoms. The median duration of symptoms is 2 years before diagnosis. Eighty percent to 90% of patients who do have symptoms at initial evaluation are found to have metastatic or advanced disease.

The behavior of carcinoid neoplasms is dependent on the embryologic origin of the tumor. Foregut carcinoids consist of gastric and duodenal tumors. Duodenal carcinoids may cause gastrointestinal obstruction, biliary obstruction, or duodenal ulcers, although they are often discovered incidentally during endoscopy. Gastric carcinoids, 0.3% of all stomach neoplasms, can be associated with a myriad of symptoms, including abdominal pain, bleeding, and rarely, atypical carcinoid syndrome. Gastric carcinoids arise from enterochromaffin-like cells and are classified into three groups. Type I consists of gastric carcinoids associated with chronic atrophic gastritis type A. This group represents 75% of all gastric carcinoids and is marked by a lack of parietal cells, achlorhydria, and hypergastrinemia. The tumors are often less than 1 cm in diameter, diffusely involve the stomach, and metastasize in 10% of all cases, with an overall 5-year survival rate approaching 100%. The present theory is that these carcinoid tumors arise secondary to chronic stimulation by high gastrin levels and possibly mutations of the RegI alpha gene.[9] Animal models have shown a direct relationship between hypergastrinemia and carcinoid tumor formation, therefore raising the issue of the safety of using chronic proton pump inhibitors and whether antrectomy might lead to tumor regression. Patients with type I gastric carcinoid are often 70 to 80 years of age and female with symptoms of abdominal pain. Carcinoid syndrome is not seen, and these tumors usually follow an indolent course.

Type II gastric carcinoid tumors are associated with Zollinger-Ellison syndrome and familial multiple endocrine neoplasia type I syndrome. Patients in this group, 5% of those with gastric carcinoids, are younger (in their sixth decade of life), exhibit no evidence of carcinoid syndrome, and have a tumor size less than 1.5 cm with an equal gender distribution. Although metastases develop in up to 25%, the clinical course is usually indolent.

The last group of gastric carcinoids (type III) consists of sporadic carcinoid tumors. Patients in this group have larger tumors, and hepatic metastases develop in more than 65%. This group of patients (15% to 25% of those with gastric carcinoids) is associated with the development of an atypical carcinoid syndrome and have a 5-year survival rate near 50%. Indicators of tumor aggressiveness include angiolymphatic invasion, clinicopathologic type, mitotic index, Ki-67 grade, and tumor size.[10]

Midgut carcinoid tumors are the most common and include neoplasms arising from the ileum, jejunum, appendix, and proximal part of the colon. The tumors can lead to obstruction, abdominal pain, diarrhea, and gastrointestinal bleeding. Small intestinal carcinoids are also well known to cause intense fibrosing reactions leading to obstruction, ischemia, and strangulation of the small bowel and ureters (Fig. 79–3). Although carcinoid syndrome develops in only 5% to 7% of patients with midgut carcinoid, these patients represent 90% of all patients in whom carcinoid syndrome develops.

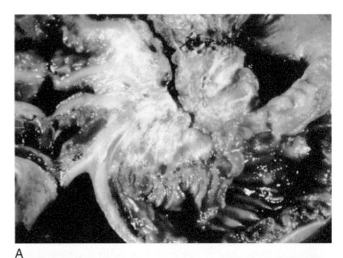

A

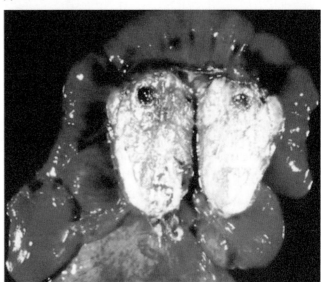

B

Figure 79–3. Gross pathologic characteristics of carcinoid tumor. **A,** Carcinoid tumor of the distal ileum demonstrating intense desmoplastic reaction and fibrosis of the bowel wall. **B,** Mesenteric metastases from a carcinoid tumor of the small bowel. (Adapted from Evers BM, Townsend CM Jr, Thompson JC: Small intestine. In Schwartz SI [ed]: Principles of Surgery, 7th ed. New York, McGraw-Hill, 1999, p 1245, with permission of The McGraw-Hill Companies.)

Abdominal pain is the initial complaint in 40% of patients with midgut carcinoid. This pain can be multifactorial and be due to bulky lymphadenopathy, mesenteric vascular invasion/occlusion, microvascular metastasis, hepatic metastases, or the vasoactive effects of serotonin. Patients can also have obstruction as a result of mesenteric kinking from the desmoplastic response. The fibrosis associated with midgut carcinoids can be quite extensive. Not only can intestinal obstruction occur, but retroperitoneal fibrosis can also develop and lead to ureteral obstruction and even Peyronie's disease (inflammation and scarring of the tunica albuginea).

Appendiceal carcinoid tumor is one of the most common forms of carcinoid disease and accounts for 50% of all diagnosed carcinoids. Ninety percent of appendiceal carcinoids are found via pathologic examination in patients undergoing incidental appendectomy. Another 10% undergo appendectomy for appendicitis, with two thirds of these patients having an incidental finding of a carcinoid tumor, usually located at the tip of the appendix. In general, less than 1% of all appendiceal carcinoid tumors have carcinoid syndrome as the initial clinical manifestation.

Hindgut carcinoids arise from the distal end of the colon and rectum. These nonsecretory carcinoid tumors are most often asymptomatic and discovered during colonoscopy for screening or evaluation of unrelated complaints. If symptoms are present, they are usually due to the increased size of the tumor, and these patients will often have symptoms similar to those with colorectal adenocarcinoma (bleeding, changes in bowel habits, or obstruction).

Carcinoid Syndrome

Malignant carcinoid syndrome is a clinical entity marked by flushing, diarrhea, abdominal cramping, wheezing, heart valve dysfunction, and pellagra. Although classically described as the hallmark of a carcinoid tumor, carcinoid syndrome occurs relatively infrequently. It is found in 10% to 18% of all patients with carcinoid tumors, but the incidence increases to 40% to 50% in patients with advanced disease.[11]

Carcinoid syndrome is based on the biochemical behavior of the tumors involved. Carcinoid tumors are neoplasms of peptide- and amine-producing cells, the enterochromaffin or Kulchitsky cells. These cells produce a large number of substances, including serotonin, tachykinins, and histamine. Ultimately, it is the metabolism of tryptophan that leads to the development of carcinoid syndrome. In carcinoid tumors that produce large amounts of serotonin, dietary tryptophan is diverted for this purpose. It is the actions of serotonin that lead to many of the manifestations of carcinoid syndrome. The syndrome develops in the presence of hepatic metastasis, which precludes hepatic inactivation of the active metabolites of serotonin.

The development of carcinoid syndrome is related to the embryologic origin of the original tumor. Midgut carcinoids are the most common source of carcinoid syndrome because these tumors produce high levels of serotonin. More than 90% of all patients suffering from carcinoid syndrome have a midgut primary. Foregut carcinoids, on the other hand, lack the aromatic amino acid decarboxylase required to convert 5-hydroxytryptamine (5-HT) to serotonin and therefore cannot produce the classic carcinoid syndrome. Hindgut carcinoids also lack the ability to convert tryptophan to serotonin, and thus even if metastatic lesions are present, carcinoid syndrome will not develop.

The symptoms associated with carcinoid syndrome include cutaneous flushing, which occurs in 85% of affected patients. This flushing, which has diverse patterns, including diffuse erythematous, violaceous, prolonged, and bright red patches, is possibly caused by the release of various kinins. The flushing lasts 2 to 10 minutes in patients with facial flushing and can last 2 to 3 days in those whose flushing occurs throughout their body. There may also be an associated tachycardia and hypotension. This rash can increase in duration as the disease progresses. Onset of the rash has been linked to eating, alcohol intake, defecation, emotion, palpation of the liver, and induction of anesthesia. General anesthesia can induce a carcinoid crisis marked by the sudden release of catecholamines from the tumor, acute hypotension, flushing, and bronchospasm. Pretreatment with octreotide can help avoid this anesthetic complication.

The diarrhea associated with carcinoid syndrome is directly related to serum serotonin levels; serotonin stimulates secretin release, which results in an increase in intestinal motility and decreased intestinal absorption. This watery, nonbloody diarrhea affects 80% of patients with carcinoid syndrome and is the symptom described by patients as the most debilitating. It is associated with abdominal cramping, and the number of daily bowel movements ranges from a few to more than 30.

Bronchospasm develops in 10% to 20% of patients with carcinoid syndrome. This wheezing/dyspnea often occurs during flushing episodes. However, treatment with β-adrenergic agonists can worsen the situation by triggering an intense, prolonged symptomatic vasodilation.

The valvular disease associated with carcinoid syndrome is a result of valvular fibrosis secondary to high concentrations of circulating amines. Serotonin is thought to be a major cause of the fibrosing reaction via stimulation of fibroblasts and fibrogenesis. Fibrous plaques develop on the endocardium of the valvular cusps, cardiac chambers, and occasionally, the intima of the pulmonary arteries or aorta (or both). The right side of the heart is the most commonly affected because of pulmonary inactivation of the humoral substances before exposure to the left side of the heart.

Other symptoms that can develop include venous telangiectasia, pellagra as a result of diversion of dietary tryptophan, and muscle wasting secondary to protein malnutrition.

Atypical or variant carcinoid syndrome is a syndrome that occurs in patients with gastric carcinoid tumors. These patients experience cutaneous flushes that are patchy and highly pruritic. Diarrhea, bronchospasm, and cardiac lesions are rare. It is thought that the syndrome is secondary to large release of histamine from the tumor rather than serotonin.

DIAGNOSIS

Laboratory Studies

Biochemical testing can often be the cornerstone of diagnosing a carcinoid tumor preoperatively. The 24-hour urinary excretion of 5-hydroxyindoleacetic acid (5-HIAA) is a helpful laboratory study. This test has a sensitivity of 75% to 100%, with the greatest sensitivity in patients with midgut carcinoids. Consumption of a large amount of tryptophan-containing food before urine specimen collection can confound the test results. Therefore, dietary intake must be controlled for accurate measurements. The sensitivity is decreased somewhat in patients with foregut and hindgut tumors. Foregut tumors generally lack aromatic amino acid decarboxylase; therefore 5-HIAA secretion is relatively unhelpful. However, 5-HT urinary secretion is increased and, with foregut tumor, has a sensitivity of 60%.[12,13]

The serum chromogranin level is another biochemical assay that parallels urinary 5-HIAA. Although the sensitivity and specificity are not well supported for all gastrointestinal carcinoids, studies indicate that chromogranin A is 100%, chromogranin B is 85%, and chromogranin C is 5% specific for carcinoid tumor.[14] Chromogranin A and an associated protein neurokinin A have also been used as a prognostic indicator, with increasing levels correlating with decreased survival.[13]

Although serum serotonin levels are increased in patients with carcinoid tumors, its specificity is low. Other markers such as substance P, neurotensin, human chorionic gonadotropin, and neuropeptides K and PP have not been useful.

Several provocative tests have historically been used to aid in the diagnosis of carcinoid. An epinephrine provocation test involves the use of escalating doses of epinephrine to produce carcinoid syndrome. A pentagastrin provocation test similarly involves the use of pentagastrin to stimulate a flushing response. Neither of the tests is commonly used.

Imaging Studies

Radiographic imaging of primary carcinoid tumors is difficult because of the small size of most tumors and their common submucosal location. A large proportion of these tumors are also located within the small bowel, which is historically difficult to image. Common approaches to the diagnosis of carcinoid tumors are based on the features of the tumors themselves. Gastric and rectal carcinoids are often asymptomatic and are thus most commonly imaged on screening or diagnostic endoscopy. The advent of endoscopic ultrasound has aided in the characterization of these tumors.

Barium studies, including small bowel series and enteroclysis, have shown good success in the diagnosis of larger carcinoid tumors of the small bowel (Fig. 79–4). The submucosal location of carcinoid tumors actually lends itself to more accurate localization with contrast studies, especially enteroclysis, than with conventional sectional imaging, such as computed tomography (CT).[15] Barium studies can also display the characteristics of a carcinoid tumor, including target signs of ulcerated tumors and angulation or narrowing from fibrosis. These characteristics, however, are shared by many other small bowel tumors, thus decreasing the specificity of barium studies.

The most commonly used radiologic examination in patients with a carcinoid neoplasm is CT. Primary tumor

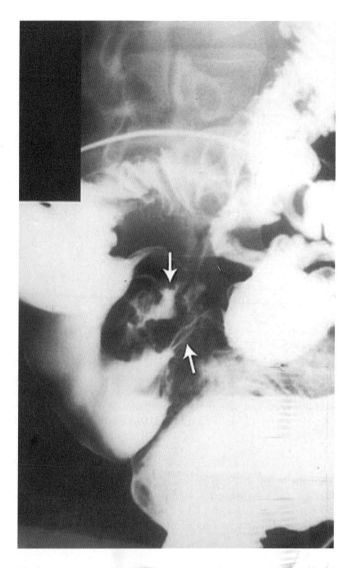

Figure 79–4. A barium radiograph of a carcinoid tumor of the terminal ileum demonstrates fibrosis with multiple filling defects and high-grade partial obstruction *(arrows)*. (Courtesy of Melvyn H. Schreiber, M.D., The University of Texas Medical Branch.)

localization is rare with CT because of its submucosal location and often small size. CT is effective at identifying the mesenteric stranding/fibrosis that often accompanies carcinoid tumors, as well as mesenteric nodal involvement. The desmoplastic response can also cause changes in the mesenteric vasculature that can be identified with CT-angiography. The advent of three-dimensional CT imaging/reconstruction has likewise aided in the radiographic identification of small bowel tumors, including carcinoids.[16] CT is most effective for identifying hepatic metastasis, with sensitivity greater than 85%.[17,18] Metastatic carcinoid tumors are highly vascular and hence display bright enhancement during arterial-phase imaging.

The role of magnetic resonance imaging (MRI) in the diagnosis of a primary carcinoid tumor is limited, and it

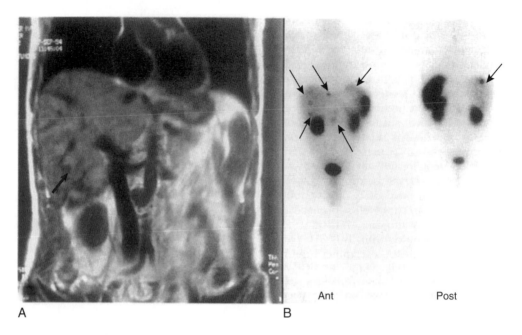

Figure 79–5. A, Magnetic resonance image showing a single focus of metastatic disease *(arrow)* in the right lobe of the liver in a patient with a carcinoid tumor and elevated 5-hydroxyindoleacetic acid. **B,** A ^{111}In-labeled pentetreotide scan of the same patient shows multiple hepatic lesions and two involved para-aortic lymph nodes. These findings were confirmed at laparotomy. Radionuclide activity in the kidneys, spleen, and bladder is evident. (From Anthony T, Kim L: Gastrointestinal carcinoid tumors and the carcinoid syndrome. In Feldman M, Friedman LS, Sleisenger MH [eds]: Sleisenger & Fordtran's Gastrointestinal and Liver Disease, 7th ed. Philadelphia, WB Saunders, 2002, p 2160.)

adds little or no information above that provided by CT. In the assessment of hepatic metastases, MRI has recently been shown to be more effective than either CT or somatostatin receptor–based scintigraphy (SRS) (Fig. 79–5).[19]

SRS has been used to image carcinoid tumors. Based on ^{111}In-labeled diethylenetriamine pentaacetic acid (DPTA)-D-Phe1-octreotide, Octreoscan uses a somatostatin analogue to obtain 80% to 90% sensitivity and specificity in identifying carcinoid neoplasms (see Fig. 79–5).[20] Various ligands have been used, including octreotide, pentetreotide, and lanreotide, with octreotide showing the greatest sensitivity for carcinoid tumors.[21] The technology is most effective in somatostatin receptor–positive carcinoid tumors, thus limiting its use in tumors that are nonfunctional. The technology is also limited in patients who do not exhibit carcinoid syndrome, for whom the sensitivity is only 60% for identification of the primary tumor.[22] The addition of single-photon emission computed tomography (SPECT) has increased the sensitivity of SRS in the detection of abdominal carcinoid.[23,24] SRS technology is also well suited to monitor response to treatment and progression of disease.

Positron emission tomography (PET) has had mixed results in imaging carcinoid tumors.[25] 2-Deoxy-2-[^{18}F]fluoro-D-glucose (FDG)-PET appears to be sensitive and specific in identifying carcinoid tumors that exhibit high proliferative activity or are poorly differentiated. However, for tumors that have low proliferative activity and are well differentiated, somatostatin-based imaging is much more sensitive and specific.[26] FDG-PET has shown some utility in identifying the retroperitoneal fibrosis that may develop in patients with carcinoid neoplasms.[27] FDG-PET should be used in patients with suspected or known carcinoid who have negative somatostatin receptor imaging.[21,28] A newer modality that has found improved success with PET technology is 5-HT–PET. 5-HT–PET has shown improved accuracy in comparison to both FDG-PET and conventional CT.[29] In a direct comparison of FDG-PET, 5-HT–PET, Octreoscan, and conventional imaging (CT/MRI), researchers report that conventional imaging is the most sensitive technique.

Another modality that has been tested for the evaluation of patients with carcinoid tumors is ^{131}I-metaiodobenzylguanidine (MIBG) scans. Limited studies have shown results roughly equivalent to those of CT, with a sensitivity of 55% to 70% and a specificity of 95%.[22,30] This scan may be especially helpful in patients who are being maintained on long-term octreotide therapy or who have had previously unrevealing Octreoscan findings.

TREATMENT AND OUTCOME

Surgery is the only cure currently available for patients with carcinoid tumors. The extent of resection is based on the location of the tumor within the gastrointestinal tract, the size of the tumor, the presence/absence of metastatic disease, and the presence/absence of symptoms. The embryologic origin also determines not only the surgical approach but also the overall prognosis. Patients with foregut carcinoids can expect 5-year survival rates of 74%, 40%, and 18% for locoregional, nodal, and metastatic disease, respectively. The 5-year survival rates with midgut (80%, 75%, 35%) and hindgut carcinoids (76%, 46%, 19%) reveal the differences.[3]

Locoregional Disease

Duodenal carcinoid tumors are extremely rare, and therefore there is no standard surgical approach. Duodenal carcinoid tumors smaller than 1 cm should be treated by endoscopic or local resection. Although tumors 1 to 2 cm in diameter can be removed endoscopically, it is recommended that transduodenal resection be performed.[31] In tumors larger than 2 cm, more aggressive resection should be undertaken, which may entail segmental resection or pancreaticoduodenectomy with en bloc lymph node dissection. The overall 5-year survival rate for patients with duodenal carcinoids is 60%, but patients with tumors larger than 2 cm have a much higher rate of recurrence and lower survival than those with smaller tumors.[31,32]

Resection of gastric carcinoids is based on the type of tumor. Type I and II gastric carcinoids small than 1 cm in diameter can be treated by local excision or endoscopic removal, followed by endoscopic surveillance every 6 to 12 months. Therapy for lesions 1 to 2 cm in diameter is variable. Some report using antrectomy to remove gastrin stimulation along with local excision of the tumor or tumors, whereas others approach all tumors larger than 1 cm in diameter with resection via gastrectomy, partial or total.[22,33,34] However, the success of this approach is still unknown. Tumors 2 cm or larger in diameter should be resected via partial or total gastrectomy, depending on their location. The prognosis for patients with type I and II gastric carcinoids is excellent, with a nearly 100% 5-year survival rate.

Type III gastric carcinoids are much more aggressive. These tumors should be treated by partial/total gastrectomy and lymph node dissection.[22,33] Despite this aggressive surgical approach, 5-year survival rates are closer to 50%, in part because of the large percentage of patients initially seen with metastatic disease.

Carcinoid tumors of the jejunum and ileum should be treated by segmental resection and en bloc lymphadenectomy. This approach should be undertaken even in patients with metastatic disease in an attempt to avoid the fibrotic complications that are often associated with primary small bowel carcinoids.[35] Patients with localized disease have a 5-year survival rate of 75%, which drops to 59% to 65% for nodal disease and to less than 36% for metastatic disease.[34] Patients with recurrent disease may live many years.

Treatment of carcinoid tumor of the appendix is largely based on its excellent prognosis and the likelihood of metastatic disease. Tumors that are smaller than 2 cm and do not involve the base can be safely removed via appendectomy alone. If the base is involved in an otherwise low-risk tumor, cecectomy can be performed.

Tumors that are 2 cm or larger in diameter or have mesoappendiceal invasion should be treated by right colectomy.[36] Overall, the rate of lymphatic spread of appendiceal carcinoid is very low, and such spread is rare in tumors smaller than 2 cm in diameter.[36] Five-year survival rates are 94% for patients with localized disease, 85% for nodal disease, and 34% for metastatic disease.[3,37]

Carcinoid tumors of the colon should be managed in the same manner as colonic adenocarcinoma. Therefore, all tumors of the colon should be treated by segmental colectomy and resection of the accompanying lymph nodes.[38] Five-year survival rates for colonic carcinoid range from 71% in patients with locoregional disease to 20% in those with metastatic disease.[3]

Rectal carcinoids that are smaller than 1 cm in diameter can be treated by local excision, often endoscopically. Tumors larger than 2 cm in diameter should be treated by radical resection, either low anterior resection or abdominoperineal resection. The role of the more radical resection has been questioned because of the lack of a survival benefit over local excision.[39] Overall, 5-year survival rates are 81% for patients with locoregional disease, 47% for nodal disease, and 18% for metastatic disease.[3] Management of rectal carcinoid tumors that are 1 to 2 cm in diameter is more controversial. Researchers have proposed that poor prognostic markers such as muscular invasion, ulceration, or symptoms at diagnosis should lead to radical resection rather than local excision.[34]

These guidelines for resection of carcinoid tumors are not absolute; individual clinical scenarios must be considered when deciding on the treatment plan and extent of resection.

Metastatic Disease

Surgical Therapy

The approach to the treatment of patients with metastatic disease is based on symptoms. Patients whose only symptoms are mild diarrhea may be successfully treated with oral codeine. However, the role of surgical intervention for metastatic disease has increased in modern times. The biologic activity of carcinoid neoplasms lends itself to aggressive treatment of metastatic disease.

Most patients with carcinoid tumors should undergo resection of the primary tumor regardless of metastasis. Such resection aids in avoiding complications from growth of the primary tumor in terms of bleeding, obstruction, and abdominal pain, especially with midgut carcinoids because of their propensity to cause intense fibrosing reactions. Even large tumors that are locally advanced with nodal disease are usually amenable to surgical resection.[40]

Patients with hepatic metastases may also benefit from surgical intervention. By using a resection or ablative approach to hepatic metastases, the patient can be palliated and even enjoy a long-term survival benefit. Surgical therapy for metastatic carcinoid tumors is aimed at removing more than 90% of the tumor burden via either anatomic or wedge resections, with acceptable morbidity and mortality rates of 15% and 1.2%, respectively.[40] By using this cytoreductive approach, symptoms from metastatic carcinoid are reduced in 95% of patients, with a median symptom-free duration of 45 months. Five-year survival rates improve from 40% to 50% in patients who do not undergo surgery to 60% to 82% in patients after hepatic resection of their metastatic disease.[41,42]

Patients whose tumor is unresectable or in whom reduction of greater than 90% of the tumor burden is not feasible may be palliated with techniques of hepatic therapy. Palliation methods include radiofrequency ablation (RFA), cryotherapy, hepatic arterial occlusion, embolization, and chemoembolization.

RFA has found success as an ablative technique for colorectal metastases. Its application to metastatic carcinoid has also been shown to be effective in patients with unresectable hepatic disease or as an adjunct to resection. In one study, the use of RFA for metastatic carcinoid provided symptomatic relief in greater than 80% of patients, and 41% showed no progression of disease during a short follow-up period.[43] Cryotherapy has also provided good symptomatic relief for up to 100% of patients with metastatic carcinoid.[44] Both modalities have relatively short-term response rates, but they can be successfully used on multiple occasions in patients with recurrent disease.

Ablative techniques that are based on vascular occlusion or embolization have also been studied. Their ability to induce tumor necrosis has largely been unsuccessful because of the rich collateral circulation within the liver. Hepatic arterial vascular occlusive therapy produces biochemical and tumor response rates of 37%. Embolization, often with gelatin, has shown slightly better results. Chemoembolization combines inflow disruption with the local administration of chemotherapeutic agents. This technique has led to a reduction of symptoms in 60% to 100% of patients with carcinoid syndrome and a biochemical response in 57% to 91%.[45] However, the results of these therapies have been mostly symptomatic and short lived. Patients undergoing either of these therapies are also subject to complications after occlusion/embolization, including abdominal pain, fever, fatigue, and even carcinoid crises as a result of the sudden release of hormones from the targeted lesion or lesions.

Orthotopic liver transplantation has also been performed in patients with metastatic carcinoid; however, its true role in the treatment of patients with metastatic carcinoid remains unclear. There have been limited attempts at liver transplantation in this patient population, but with significant morbidity and mortality and high rates of recurrence. Recently, researchers have attempted to define a more select group of patients for transplantation. Patients who appear to have the greatest survival rates are those with well-differentiated tumors that exhibit low proliferative activity. In this select group, orthotopic liver transplantation can yield a 5-year survival rate of up to 69%.[46]

Medical Therapy

Systemic treatment of patients with advanced carcinoid tumors has focused mainly on relief of the symptoms of carcinoid syndrome. The most commonly used therapy for such patients is somatostatin receptor–mediated hormonal therapy. The somatostatin receptors are blocked with a somatostatin analogue, thereby relieving the flushing, diarrhea, and other symptoms of carcinoid syndrome. The most commonly prescribed agent has been octreotide. Octreotide administration leads to resolution or a reduction in symptoms, including flushing (53% complete response, 32% partial response) and diarrhea (25% complete response, 49% partial response). However, the short half-life (2 to 4 minutes) of octreotide necessitates continuous infusion or twice-daily subcutaneous injections.

Newer analogues with longer half-lives have recently been developed with similar response rates. Lanreotide is administered every 10 to 14 days, whereas depot octreotide is given just once monthly. Side effects of the treatment include sinus bradycardia, arrhythmias, gallbladder stones, steatorrhea, hypothyroidism, and hypoglycemia.

Although designed to reduce the symptoms of carcinoid syndrome, there has been some objective tumor responses noted with somatostatin analogues. A biochemical response is seen in 27% to 72% of patients with carcinoid treated with somatostatin analogues; however, the actual tumor response is only 2%. Tumor stabilization has been noted in nearly 50%, but over a relatively short follow-up period of 5 months.[22]

Systemic treatment with interferon has been examined as possible systemic therapy for patients with advanced carcinoid disease. The mechanism that has been proposed is interferon's ability to inhibit cellular proliferation, inhibit angiogenesis, and enhance immune cell–mediated cytotoxicity. Trials including interferon alfa and gamma and human leukocyte interferon have been performed. Treatment with either human leukocyte interferon or interferon alfa has resulted in biochemical responses but little tumor response. The results were less favorable for combination therapy consisting of interferon alfa and gamma, for which no response was noted. The combination of interferon alfa and octreotide led to a reduced risk for tumor progression, without any survival benefit.[47]

Various studies have examined the effects of systemic chemotherapy, both single agent and combination, in patients with metastatic carcinoid with little success. A more recent phase II trial examined docetaxel as a potential therapeutic agent.[48] Although the therapy was well tolerated, there was minimal tumor response, and only a small proportion of patients experienced even a biochemical response. To date, systemic chemotherapy has failed to have a role in the treatment of metastatic carcinoid disease.

Biologic therapies are currently being examined for a potential role in the treatment of metastatic carcinoid tumors. Epidermal growth factor receptor (EGFR)-based therapy has shown success in solid tumors such as lung, breast, colon, and head and neck cancers. Recent basic science research has shown that gefitinib, which targets EGFR, induces apoptosis, growth inhibition, and cell cycle arrest.[49] These findings indicate that EGFR-based treatments may be an effective therapy in the future.

Case reports and small series have reported the use of hormone receptor–mediated radiation therapy for metastatic carcinoid tumors. Peptide-targeted therapies include ^{131}I-MIBG–octreotide; [177]Lu-, [111]In-, and ^{90}Y-labeled somatostatin analogues; and more recently, bombesin and neuropeptide Y (Y1) analogues. Research to date has shown some success with these therapies, although the success is often noted to be equivalent to that of treatment with nonradiolabeled somatostatin analogues. Most reports show short-term stabilization of disease, with greater than half of all treated patients reporting some symptomatic relief.[50,51] However, tumor response rates (complete and/or partial) have been low, 23% to 30%. Combined peptide approaches are being used in an attempt to improve tumor and patient response to therapy.[51]

External beam radiotherapy has had some limited role in the treatment of advanced carcinoid disease. As a palliative procedure for bulky disease, brain metastasis, spinal cord compression, and bony metastasis, radiation therapy has shown some benefit.

FUTURE DIRECTIONS

Gastrointestinal carcinoid tumors have varied manifestations and clinical courses. Advances in molecular biology will continue to aid the clinician in determining what clinical course a particular tumor will take. The application of high-throughput genomic and proteomic analysis to the pathologic examination of tumors, as well as the application of this technology to the serum of patients with carcinoid disease, will possibly enable a more accurate prognosis.

Advances in peptide receptor–aided imaging will enable more accurate and earlier diagnosis of carcinoid tumors. Possibly, the use of multiple markers in a single radionuclide-based scan will permit the localization of small carcinoid tumors that currently remain unrecognized and undiagnosed.

The emerging field of biologic therapies may also aid in the treatment of patients with advanced or metastatic disease, or both. Phase III trials of EGFR-targeted therapies are hoped to produce exciting results. There are numerous other potential biologic therapies that have yet to be discovered and examined.

Overall, gastrointestinal carcinoid is a variable disease process because of its varied embryologic origin. Surgical resection is the only chance for cure. As the expansion of molecular biology and biologic therapy continues, treatment options for this disease will improve.

SUGGESTED READINGS

Kulke MH, Mayer RJ: Carcinoid tumors. N Engl J Med 340:858-868, 1999.

Modlin IM, Lye KD, Kidd M: A 5-decade analysis of 13,715 carcinoid tumors. Cancer 97:934-959, 2003.

Norton JA, Warren RS, Kelly MG, et al: Aggressive surgery for metastatic liver neuroendocrine tumors. Surgery 134:1057-1063, 2003.

REFERENCES

1. Lubarsch O: Ueber den primaren Krebs des ileum, nebst Bemerkungen uber das gleichzeitige Vorkommen von Krebs und Tuberkolos. Virchows Arch 11:280-317, 1888.
2. Oberndorfer S: Karzinoide: Tumoren des dunndarms. Frankf Z Pathol 1:426-429, 1907.
3. Modlin IM, Lye KD, Kidd M: A 5-decade analysis of 13,715 carcinoid tumors. Cancer 97:934-959, 2003.
4. Moertel CG, Sauer WG, Docherty MB, Baggenstoss AH: Life history of the carcinoid tumor of the small intestine. Cancer 14:291-293, 1961.
5. Hemminki K, Li X: Incidence trends and risk factors of carcinoid tumors. Cancer 92:2204-2210, 2001.
6. Soga J, Tazawa K: Pathologic analysis of carcinoids. Histologic reevaluation of 62 cases. Cancer 28:990-998, 1971.
7. Kawahara M, Kammori M, Kanauchi H, et al: Immunohistochemical prognostic indicators of gastrointestinal carcinoid tumors. Eur J Surg Oncol 28:140-146, 2002.
8. Amarapurkar AD, Davies A, Ramage JK, et al: Proliferation of antigen MIB-1 in metastatic carcinoid tumours removed at liver transplantation: Relevance to prognosis. Eur J Gastroenterol Hepatol 15:139-143, 2003.
9. Higham AD, Bishop LA, Dimaline R, et al: Mutations of RegI alpha are associated with enterochromaffin-like cell tumor development in patients with hypergastrinemia. Gastroenterology 116:1310-1318, 1999.
10. Rindi G, Azzoni C, La Rosa S, et al: ECL cell tumor and poorly differentiated endocrine carcinoma of the stomach: Prognostic evaluation by pathologic analysis. Gastroenterology 116:532-542, 1999.
11. Caplin ME, Buscombe JR, Hilson AJ, et al: Carcinoid tumor. Lancet 352:799-805, 1998.
12. Feldman JM: Urinary serotonin in the diagnosis of carcinoid syndrome. Clin Chem 32:840-844, 1986.
13. Gough DB, Thompson GB, Crotty TB, et al: Diverse clinical and pathologic features of gastric carcinoid and the relevance of hypergastrinemia. World J Surg 18:473-479, discussion 479-480, 1994.
14. Stridsburg M, Oberg K, Li Q, et al: Measurements of chromogranin A, chromogranin B (secretogranin I), chromogranin C (secretogranin II) and pancreastatin in plasma and urine from patients with carcinoid tumors and endocrine pancreatic tumors. J Endocrinol 144:49-59, 1995.
15. Bessette JR, Maglinte DD, Kelvin FM, Chernish SM: Primary malignant tumors in the small bowel: A comparison of the small-bowel enema and conventional follow-through examination. AJR Am J Roentgenol 153:741-744, 1989.
16. Horton KM, Kamel I, Hofmann L, Fishman EK: Carcinoid tumors of the small bowel: A multitechnique imaging approach. AJR Am J Roentgenol 182:559-567, 2004.
17. Dudiak KM, Johnson CD, Stephens DH: Primary tumors of the small intestine: CT evaluation. AJR Am J Roentgenol 152:995-998, 1989.
18. Cockey BM, Fishman EK, Jones B, Siegelman SS: Computed tomography of abdominal carcinoid tumor. J Comput Assist Tomogr 9:38-42, 1985.
19. Dromain C, de Baere T, Lumroso J, et al: Detection of liver metastases from endocrine tumors: A prospective comparison of somatostatin receptor scintigraphy, computed tomography and magnetic resonance imaging. J Clin Oncol 23:70-78, 2005.
20. Krenning EP, Kwekkeboom DJ, Oei HY, et al: Somatostatin-receptor scintigraphy in gastroenteropancreatic tumors. An overview of European results. Ann N Y Acad Sci 733:416-424, 1994.
21. Virgolini I, Patri P, Novotny C, et al: Comparative somatostatin receptor scintigraphy using In-111-DOTA-lanreotide and in-111-DOTA-Tyr3-octreotide versus F-18-FDG-PET for evaluation of somatostatin receptor–mediated radionuclide therapy. Ann Oncol 12(Suppl 2):S41-S45, 2001.
22. Schnirer II, Yao JC, Ajani JA: Carcinoid: A comprehensive review. Acta Oncol 42:672-692, 2003.
23. Schillaci O, Scopinaro F, Danieli R, et al: Single photon emission computerized tomography increases the sensitivity of indium-111-pentetreotide scintigraphy in detecting abdominal carcinoids. Anticancer Res 17(3B):1753-1756, 1997.

24. Krausz Y, Keidar Z, Kogan I, et al: SPECT/CT hybrid imaging with ^{111}In-pentetreotide in assessment of neuroendocrine tumours. Clin Endocrinol (Oxf) 59:565-573, 2003.

25. Sundin A, Eriksson B, Bergstrom M, et al: PET in the diagnosis of neuroendocrine tumors. Ann N Y Acad Sci 1014:246-257, 2004.

26. Adams S, Baum R, Rink T, et al: Limited value of fluorine-18 fluorodeoxyglucose positron emission tomography for the imaging of neuroendocrine tumors. Eur J Nucl Med 25:79-83, 1998.

27. Chander S, Ergun EL, Chugani HT, et al: High 2-deoxy-2-[^{18}F]fluoro-D-glucose accumulation in a case of retroperitoneal fibrosis following resection of carcinoid tumor. Mol Imaging Biol 4:363-368, 2002.

28. Belhocine T, Foidart J, Rigo P, et al: Fluorodeoxyglucose positron emission tomography and somatostatin receptor scintigraphy for diagnosing and staging carcinoid tumours: Correlations with the pathological indexes p53 and Ki-67. Nucl Med Commun 23:727-734, 2002.

29. Hoegerle S, Altehoefer C, Ghanem N, et al: Whole-body ^{18}F dopa PET for detection of gastrointestinal carcinoid tumors. Radiology 220:373-380, 2001.

30. Adolph JM, Kimmig BN, Georgi P, zum Winkel K: Carcinoid tumors: CT and I-131 meta-iodo-benzylguanidine scintigraphy. Radiology 164:199-203, 1987.

31. Zyromski NJ, Kendrick ML, Nagorney DM, et al: Duodenal carcinoid tumors: How aggressive should we be? J Gastrointest Surg 5:588-593, 2001.

32. Zar N, Garmo H, Holmberg L, et al: Long-term survival of patients with small intestinal carcinoid tumors. World J Surg 28:1163-1168, 2004.

33. Modlin IM, Lye KD, Kidd M: Carcinoid tumors of the stomach. Surg Oncol 12:153-172, 2003.

34. Kulke MH, Mayer RJ: Carcinoid tumors. N Engl J Med 340:858-868, 1999.

35. Sutton R, Doran HE, Williams EM, et al: Surgery for midgut carcinoid. Endocr Relat Cancer 10:469-481, 2003.

36. Goede AC, Caplin ME, Winslet MC: Carcinoid tumour of the appendix. Br J Surg 90:1317-1322, 2003.

37. Sandor A, Modlin IM: A retrospective analysis of 1570 appendiceal carcinoids. Am J Gastroenterology 93:422-428, 1998.

38. Goede AC, Winslet MC: Surgery for carcinoid tumors of the lower gastrointestinal tract. Colorectal Dis 5:123-128, 2003.

39. Koura AN, Giacco GG, Curley SA, et al: Carcinoid tumors of the rectum: Effect of size, histopathology, and surgical treatment on metastasis free survival. Cancer 79:1294-1298, 1997.

40. Ohrvall U, Eriksson B, Juhlin C, et al: Method for dissection of mesenteric metastases in mid-gut carcinoid tumors. World J Surg 24:1402-1408, 2000.

41. Sarmiento JM, Que FG: Hepatic surgery for metastases from neuroendocrine tumors. Surg Oncol Clin N Am 12:231-242, 2003.

42. Norton JA, Warren RS, Kelly MG, et al: Aggressive surgery for metastatic liver neuroendocrine tumors. Surgery 134:1057-1063, 2003.

43. Berber E, Flesher N, Siperstein AE: Laparoscopic radiofrequency ablation of neuroendocrine liver metastases. World J Surg 26:985-990, 2002.

44. Bilchik AJ, Sarantou T, Foshag LJ, et al: Cryosurgical palliation of metastatic neuroendocrine tumors resistant to conventional therapy. Surgery 122:1040-1047, 1997.

45. O'Toole D, Maire F, Ruszniewsi P: Ablative therapies for liver metastases of digestive endocrine tumours. Endocr Relat Cancer 10:463-468, 2003.

46. Le Treut YP, Delpero JR, Dousset B, et al: Results of liver transplantation in the treatment of metastatic neuroendocrine tumors. A 31-case French multicentric report. Ann Surg 225:355-364, 1997.

47. Kolby L, Persson G, Franzen S, Ahren B: Randomized clinical trial of the effect of interferon alpha on survival in patients with disseminated midgut carcinoid. Br J Surg 90:687-693, 2003.

48. Kulke MH, Kim H, Stuart K, et al: A phase II study of docetaxel in patients with metastatic carcinoid tumors. Cancer Invest 22:353-359, 2004.

49. Hopfner M, Sutter AP, Gerst B, et al: A novel approach in the treatment of neuroendocrine gastrointestinal tumours. Targeting the epidermal growth factor receptor by gefitinib (ZD1839). Br J Cancer 89:1766-1775, 2003.

50. Lewington VJ: Targeted radionuclide therapy for neuroendocrine tumors. Endocr Relat Cancer 10:497-501, 2003.

51. Krenning EP, Kwekkeboom DJ, Valkema R, et al: Peptide receptor radionuclide therapy. Ann N Y Acad Sci 1014:234-245, 2004.

Gastrointestinal Stromal Tumors

Burton L. Eisenberg ▪ Kari M. Rosenkranz

Although rare, gastrointestinal stromal tumors (GISTs) are the most common mesenchymal neoplasms of the gastrointestinal (GI) tract. Understanding and treatment of these tumors have improved dramatically over the last several years. Enhanced diagnostic specificity and recognition of the pathophysiology and natural history of this previously poorly defined clinical entity have resulted in novel treatment approaches. Initially managed as a surgical disease with a relatively poor prognosis, a greater understanding of GIST pathobiology has transformed therapeutic options and led to an improved prognosis for patients with advanced disease. The present management of this GI tumor could potentially serve as a paradigm for the combined surgical management of a solid tumor with molecularly specific, targeted therapeutics enhanced by optimal pharmacologic and pharmacodynamic properties.

HISTORICAL PERSPECTIVE AND NATURAL HISTORY

The true incidence of GIST has been somewhat obscured by the fact that until recently this clinical entity was ill defined. It is now recognized as the most common mesenchymal tumor of the GI tract, with an estimated annual incidence of approximately 6000 cases per year. Previous reported series of GI sarcomas, particularly those compiled before the year 2000, were dominated by the defining nomenclature of smooth muscle tumors (leiomyosarcoma and leiomyoblastoma). It is now recognized that many of these tumors that were previously reported as smooth muscle neoplasms have distinctive pathologic features and could be retrospectively reclassified as GIST. As suggested by Mazur and Clark, who first introduced the term stromal tumor,[1] these neoplasms are probably not derived from a direct smooth muscle cell lineage. Further advances in the defining pathology of GIST indicated that GIST cells originate from the same precursor cell as the interstitial cells of Cajal (ICC), the GI myenteric plexus pacemaker cell, and therefore have characteristics of both smooth muscle and neural differentiation, as evidenced by morphology and immunophenotype.[2]

Strict criteria for recognition of GIST have now enabled retrospective studies to be performed to evaluate the prognosis and natural history relevant to clinical care. A variety of different tumor-related variables have been assessed by both univariate and multivariate analysis to determine their importance in outcome prediction, as well as malignant potential. The most significant prognostic features of the primary tumor are size and mitotic index (Table 80–1).[3] These two primary tumor categories allow reliable risk assessment, although other tumor features that are surrogates of proliferation, such as Ki67 expression, have also been found to be helpful in risk modeling. These patient risk profiles suggest that greater than 50% of high-risk tumors will recur within 10 years after initial diagnosis, the majority within 3 years. In contrast, low-risk/very-low-risk tumors have a less than 5% probability of recurrence, with the intermediate-risk category being less predictable and therefore necessitating very close follow-up. At the time of diagnosis approximately a third to a half of all clinically detected GISTs are either overtly malignant by virtue of demonstrated metastatic disease or high risk for malignant behavior, and approximately two thirds will have pathologic features suggestive of potential malignant behavior, such as larger size or increased mitotic index.[4,5] For this reason, classification of GIST into benign versus malignant is often problematic, and therefore GIST in aggregate represents a biologic continuum, with even small contained tumors historically noted to recur 15 to 20 years after initial diagnosis. Obviously, this risk stratification strategy provides important guidelines for the necessity of

Table 80–1	Gastrointestinal Stromal Tumor Risk Assessment	

Risk of Recurrence	Tumor Size (cm)	Mitotic Index (50 HPF)
Very low	<2	<5
Low	2-5	<5
Intermediate	<5	10-16
	5-10	<5
High	>5	>5
	>10	Any
	Any	>10

HPF, high-power field.

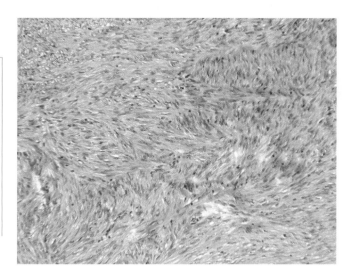

Figure 80–1. Spindled GIST. Although the histologic patterns of GIST vary, many demonstrate short interlacing fascicles of spindled cells with indistinct cytoplasm, uniform nuclei, and a variable degree of matrix production.

long-term patient follow-up and radiologic surveillance, as well as consideration of more aggressive primary tumor management directed toward high- and intermediate-risk groups.

Tumor location has also been linked to prognosis, with primary gastric GISTs seeming to fare better than those of small bowel or rectal origin.[6] The rare GIST of the retroperitoneum, mesentery, or omentum will similarly generally display a malignant aggressive course when compared with those of primary gastric origin.

PATHOLOGY

Elucidation of the pathology of GIST has been closely paralleled by therapeutic advancements. As the specific diagnosis of GIST has been defined by morphology, ultrastructure, and immunohistochemistry, the true incidence and prevalence of this tumor are now more accurately reflected in population studies.[7] The annual incidence of GIST is approximately 5000 to 6000 cases in the United States yearly. The incidence statistics are more reliable at this time because in the past many of these tumors were reported as GI smooth muscle tumors. It is now evident that through ultrastructural studies and lineage-specific immunomarkers, GIST cells have features in common with ICC, with both GIST and ICC staining positive for KIT (CD117).[8] Although approximately 95% of GIST cells stain positive for KIT, a variety of other immunomarkers can also be demonstrated, including BCL-2 (80%), CD34 (70%), muscle-specific actin (50%), smooth muscle actin (35%), S-100 (10%), and desmin (5%).[9] The differential diagnosis of GIST includes a number of different mesenchymal tumors such as schwannomas, leiomyomas, and leiomyosarcomas; however, morphology and KIT staining will generally establish the diagnosis.

The majority of GISTs are composed of a uniform population of spindle cells (approximately 70% of cases), with epithelioid cells (20% of cases) and a mixed variety (10% of cases) accounting for the rest (Figs. 80–1 to 80–3). The spindle cells are generally arranged in short fascicles but can align in a schwannian pattern. Most

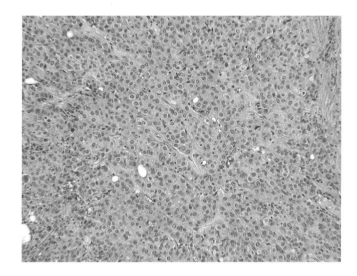

Figure 80–2. Epithelioid GIST. In contrast to spindle cell GIST, the epithelioid variant is composed of polygonal cells with abundant eosinophilic cytoplasm and well-defined cytoplasmic borders.

GISTs have a uniform cytology, and marked cytologic pleomorphism is uncommon. Approximately 5% of cases can have a prominent myxoid stroma. Nuclear atypia is more common in epithelioid GISTs and often represents a malignant phenotype. The use of KIT immunostaining has been helpful in the diagnosis of GIST; however, it is possible that because of technical issues, such as overstaining with inappropriately titered KIT antibodies, there may be instances of false-positive reporting. The possibility of overstaining is important to consider because KIT-negative, desmin-positive tumors, such as desmoid tumors or leiomyosarcoma, may have similar

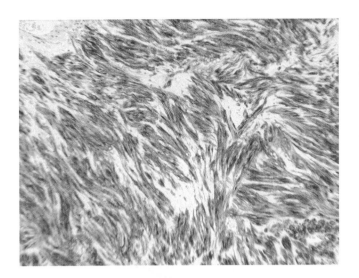

Figure 80–3. CD117 immunohistochemistry. GIST stains uniformly with CD117.

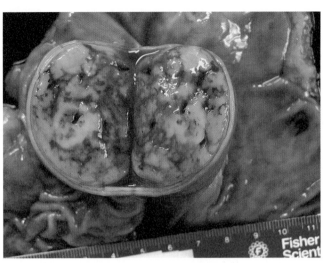

Figure 80–4. Photograph of a small submucosal gastric GIST after partial gastric resection.

spindle cell morphology. It is also important to note that the overall intensity of KIT staining, which may be cytoplasmic, membranous, or paranuclear, is not related to either prognosis or response to therapeutic KIT-specific inhibition.

As with most spindle cell neoplasms, adequate tissue is essential for making an accurate diagnosis. In the case of a primary GIST that is surgically resectable, it is not recommended that an immediate transabdominal tissue biopsy be performed because tumor cell exfoliation after biopsy manipulation can lead to tumor recurrence. Tissue can, however, be safely obtained by endoscopic core biopsy when necessary.

When assessing malignant potential, the pathology of GIST is somewhat unreliable in that malignant potential is more closely related to risk stratification (see the section on natural history and Table 80–1), which is based mainly on mitotic index and tumor size rather than tumor morphology and pleomorphism. However, cytogenetic analyses of GIST have provided some clues with regard to the malignant phenotype. Karyotypes from two thirds of GISTs demonstrate either monosomy 14 or partial loss of 14q, with at least two regions of 14q deletions appearing to be hot spots and representing probable areas of tumor suppressor genes.[10] In addition, loss of the long arm of chromosome 22 is present in 50% of GISTs and is often associated with progression to a borderline or malignant lesion. Losses on chromosomes 1p, 9p, and 11p are more significantly found in malignant GISTs. Common pathways for the genetic changes that have been observed in the development and progression of GIST are KIT or platelet-derived growth factor receptor-α (PDGFR-α) mutation → 14q deletion → 22q deletion → 1p deletion → 8p gain → 11p deletion → 9p deletion → 17q gain.[10]

Approximately 5% of GISTs will be KIT negative by immunostaining, yet by all other morphologic/clinical criteria these tumors can be classified as GISTs. They are generally a rather heterogeneous group of tumors consisting mostly of tumors containing mutations in PDGFR. This small subset of GISTs characterized by negative KIT staining is more likely to be of epithelioid histology, be nongastric in location, and have activating PDGFR-α mutations. A few of these weakly positive or non–KIT-staining GISTs will have evidence of KIT mutations on genotyping, and in rare instances there will be no discernible mutations in either PDGFR-α or KIT, thus suggesting that a KIT-negative GIST can arise through alternative oncogenic mechanisms.[11] An adequate tumor sample in the clinical instance of KIT negativity should be evaluated by genotyping because a mutation in KIT or PDGFR-α can be diagnostic and has important therapeutic implications. In addition, new tumor markers of GIST, such as DOG1 (discovered on GIST-1) and protein kinase C-θ, can be helpful in the differential diagnosis in difficult cases.[12,13]

CLINICAL EVALUATION

GIST is most commonly diagnosed in adults 50 to 80 years of age, with a mean age of 60. The male-to-female ratio is approximately 1:1. The majority of patients with GIST are symptomatic, with the most common symptoms being abdominal pain, early satiety, and bloating related to the presence of a space-occupying mass. GI bleeding and anemia are frequently noted and are due to erosion of mucosa by the tumor, even though GISTs originate within the muscular layer of the bowel wall and are often manifested by evidence of an extrinsic mass. The most common location is the stomach (60% to 70%), followed by the small bowel (20% to 25%), colorectum (5%), and esophagus (5%). Rarely, cases of GIST originating within the retroperitoneum, omentum, appendix, gallbladder, pancreas, and mesentery have been described. Approximately 20% of GISTs are asymptomatic and discovered incidentally by radiographic imaging or endoscopy, or they may be an unexpected surgical finding (Fig. 80–4). These incidental tumors are often asymptomatic, noncystic submucosal masses most commonly found during endoscopy. Recommendations for management of an asymptomatic incidental GIST with regard to biopsy or resection are not based on large cohort follow-up studies. However, in general, even a subcentimeter, submucosal suspected GIST should undergo biopsy or be removed, or both, if the clinical situation allows because of the necessity for long-term observation and the potential for malignant clinical progression based on the defined risk profile.

The clinical work-up for a suspected GIST should follow the pattern for evaluation of any patient with an undiagnosed intra-abdominal mass. Although some GISTs are small submucosal solid tumors found incidentally, the majority are larger than 5 cm and are symptomatic because they are a space-occupying abdominal mass. GI bleeding and the insidious anemia of chronic blood loss are not uncommon with large necrotic GISTs. The initial work-up should consist of a history and physical examination, which may reveal the presence of a palpable abdominal mass, followed by a cross-sectional abdominal imaging study, usually a contrast-enhanced computed tomography (CT) scan. Routine chest radiographs and blood work, including liver function tests, are indicated. Endoscopy, endoscopic ultrasound, and possibly endoscopic biopsy can be recommended if the clinical situation warrants because the majority of GISTs are of gastric origin. Early surgical involvement should address the potential for complete resection, and in patients with locally advanced or metastatic disease, consultation with medical oncology, evaluation for systemic therapy with imatinib mesylate, and close surgical follow-up should be considered. Close surgical follow-up is especially important for patients with large GISTs involving bowel mucosa, which may subsequently bleed either intra-abdominally or intraluminally as a manifestation of rapid tumor response after the initiation of systemic therapy.

Percutaneous core or intraoperative biopsy of a suspected GIST that is localized and presumed to be resectable is not necessary. These tumors tend to be soft, well vascularized, and friable, and tumor spill or spontaneous rupture portends a poor prognosis and compounds the difficulty of treatment decisions. Conversely, it is relatively safe to biopsy the tumor by endoscopic means, either by direct visualization of a mucosal component or by endoscopic ultrasound guidance. Image-guided percutaneous tumor biopsy is considered as part of the work-up, however, for a metastatic tumor or a primary tumor that is marginally resectable. Additionally, careful biopsy and tissue diagnosis can be considered when immediate tumor resection could lead to considerable morbidity or functional disability. In this instance the possibility of tumor down-staging with a preoperative neoadjuvant targeted therapy regimen should be considered. Although data regarding the efficacy of this combined neoadjuvant approach are insufficient, it has the theoretical benefit of organ preservation and function-sparing management of some GISTs, such as those originating in the rectum or the pancreas.

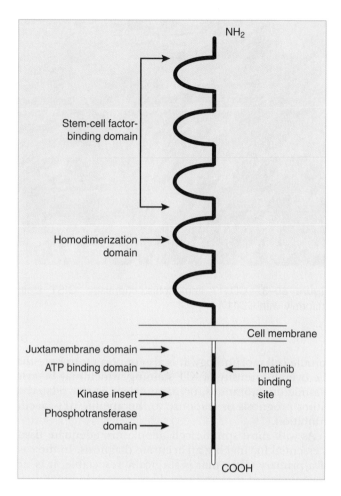

Figure 80–5. The structure of the transmembrane KIT receptor tyrosine kinase. (From Joensuu H, Fletcher C, Dimitrijevic S, et al: Management of malignant gastrointestinal stromal tumors. Lancet Oncol 3:655-664, 2002.)

MOLECULAR BIOLOGY OF GASTROINTESTINAL STROMAL TUMORS

Greater insight into the pathogenesis and subsequently the pathobiology of GIST has altered the diagnostic parameters and therapeutic implications for this mesenchymal tumor. These tumors are nearly universally characterized by the expression of KIT, a transmembrane receptor tyrosine kinase encoded by the c-kit proto-oncogene and recognized by the immunohistochemical stain for CD117, an antigen to an epitope on the extramembranous portion of the KIT molecule (Fig. 80–5).[14]

The c-kit gene is a cellular homologue of the v-kit oncogene found in the genome of the feline sarcoma virus.[15] Stem cell factor is the natural ligand for KIT, and under normal physiologic conditions, two molecules of KIT form a dimer by binding to two molecules of the ligand, with the resulting dimerization leading to activation of the intracellular tyrosine kinase. Ligand-independent activation of the KIT kinase leads to signal transduction abnormalities favoring proliferation and enhancement of cell survival mechanisms.[16] Structurally, the KIT molecule has an extracellular domain of five immunoglobulin-like repeats and a tyrosine kinase domain split by a variable kinase insert that separates the adenosine triphosphate binding site and the phosphotransferase regions, thus placing this receptor kinase in the same category as similar type 3 tyrosine kinase receptors such as macrophage colony-stimulating factor and PDGF.[17]

A seminal event in the definition of GIST initially reported by Hirota et al. and subsequently verified by a number of investigators was identification of a c-kit gain-of-function mutation by gene sequencing in the majority of these tumors.[18] These in-frame mutations are noted early in GIST tumorigenesis and are important drivers of the malignant phenotype. The gain-of-function kinase activity results in ligand-independent KIT autophosphorylation and constitutive activation and is probably a hyperproliferative transforming event. The mutations are often physically located within 11 amino acids (Lys-550 to Val-560) in the juxtamembrane domain (exon 11) and can be characterized as either deletions, point mutations, or insertions. In the unusual event that these mutations occur in a germ cell line, the family lineage is characterized by instances of multiple GISTs.[19] Further compelling evidence for KIT mutation in the pathogenesis of GIST has been substantiated by transfection experiments of mutated KIT leading to cellular clonal transformation of the transfectant.[20] In addition, there is a transgenic mouse model of a KIT mutation leading to spontaneous GISTs that are morphologically similar to the human counterpart.[21]

The reported frequency of KIT mutations in GIST is variable and depends on the methodology used, but a mutational event probably occurs in 85% to 90% of malignant GISTs.[22] In addition, these mutations generally occur in exonic hot spots: 11 (intracellular juxtamembrane region), 9 (extracellular domain), and rarely 13 or 17 (both found in the intracellular portion of the receptor).[23] It is also notable that KIT mutations were found in 85% of a series of morphologically benign GISTs found incidentally, and these tumors ranged in size from 4 to 10 mm.[24] This suggests that mutated KIT is an early sign of genomic instability and may not be prognostically important in predicting the extent of malignant behavior. KIT mutations are distinctive, however, and have not been found in morphologically similar tumors, such as leiomyomas or leiomyosarcomas, thus making this mutation pathognomonic for GIST.[25]

TARGETED THERAPY

Enhanced appreciation of the pathobiology of this mesenchymal tumor, particularly with regard to autonomous kinase activation, has prompted clinical trials involving pharmacologic exploitation of the dysregulated KIT receptor tyrosine kinase.[26] Imatinib mesylate (Gleevec), a rationally designed small-molecule oral drug that is a selective inhibitor of type 3 tyrosine kinases, showed remarkable efficacy in preclinical studies against the KIT oncoprotein. This activity was manifested by antiproliferative effects and a measurable decrease in the tyrosine phosphorylation of KIT in KIT-expressing malignant cell lines.[27] These compelling preclinical data fostered interest in conducting the first clinical application of imatinib mesylate in a solid tumor, which resulted in a dramatic response in a patient with inoperable bulky metastatic GIST.[28] This report was followed by multi-institutional proof of the principal trial of imatinib mesylate in previously treated, unresectable patients with confirmed and measurable recurrent metastatic GIST. The study resulted in 147 patients being treated; 54%, 28%, and 14% demonstrated partial and durable responses, stable disease, and progressive disease, respectively.[29] It is important to note that all these patients had KIT expression confirmed by CD117 staining, thus emphasizing the important selectivity of this drug.[30] This clinical benefit has continued to be durable after a median follow-up of 3 years, with approximately 85% of patients still taking the drug. This study served as the basis for a registration study leading to Food and Drug Administration approval of imatinib mesylate for GIST patients with metastatic or recurrent disease.

Because the GIST clinical trial experience serves as a paradigm as one of the first in human trials to demonstrate efficacy for a designed small-molecule molecularly targeted therapeutic agent, evaluation of its pharmacodynamics and resistance patterns has potential applicability to other drugs of this classification. One interesting and clinically relevant response factor resides within the c-kit gene itself. The majority of GISTs sampled from patients in the initial metastatic disease trials with imatinib mesylate were found to harbor KIT mutations, with exon 11 being the most common site detected. The response to imatinib mesylate, as well as event-free and overall survival, was adversely affected by the presence of either an exon 9 mutation (extracellular portion of KIT) or wild-type KIT (Fig. 80–6).[31] The presence of wild-type KIT in approximately 10% of the patients in this series of KIT genomic mutational analyses was perplexing because the dysregulated KIT oncoprotein was initially thought to be the sole kinase driver of the transformed proliferative phenotype. A partial explanation for the GIST malignant phenotype without KIT mutant protein may be found in the recent identification of PDGFR-α gain-of-function mutations in GIST samples.[32] It appears that PDGFR-α mutations and KIT mutations are mutually exclusive, and in a series of GIST genotyping, 4.7% of patient samples were noted to have PDGFR-α mutations involving domains homologous to those often mutated in KIT (Fig. 80–7).[31] The uncommon patient with a PDGFR-α mutation can have a GIST that is morphologically and clinically identical to those with a KIT mutation. Some of these patients have a documented response to imatinib mesylate, thus implying that this drug can be clinically useful in inhibiting two different kinases. A small percentage of GISTs do not demonstrate a mutation in either KIT or PDGFR. The mechanism of malignant transformation and expression of the malignant phenotype is probably multifactorial in these GISTs and may be related to increased kinase activity downstream of the KIT receptor or amplification of the KIT gene or the KIT gene product. Knowledge of the GIST genotype can also have therapeutic implications because

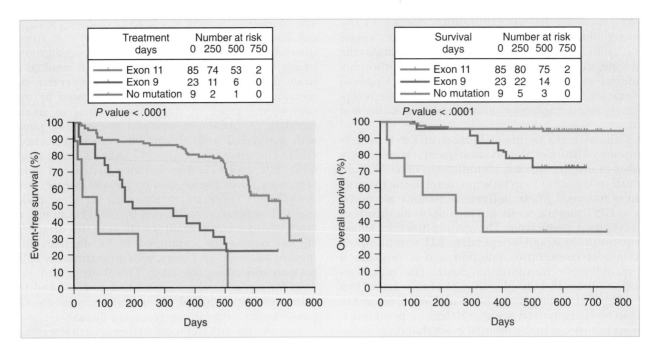

Figure 80–6. The GIST kinase genotype correlates with event-free and overall survival, as demonstrated by the Kaplan-Meier estimate of the probability of event-free and overall survival for patients with KIT exon 11 mutation, KIT exon 9 mutation, or no mutation of KIT or PDGFR. (From Heinrich M, Corless C, Demetri G, et al: Kinase mutations and imatinib response in patients with metastatic gastrointestinal stromal tumors. J Clin Oncol 21:4347, 2003.)

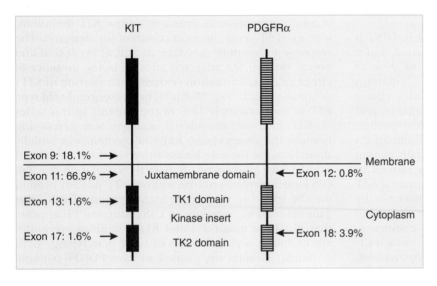

Figure 80–7. Structure of KIT and PDGFR-α. The locations of GIST kinase mutations are shown in relationship to the structural features of the proteins. GIST from 9 (7.1%) of 127 patients had no detectable KIT or PDGFR-α mutation. (From Heinrich M, Corless C, Demetri G, et al: Kinase mutations and imatinib response in patients with metastatic gastrointestinal stromal tumors. J Clin Oncol 21:4343, 2003.)

GIST patients harboring a KIT mutation outside of exon 11 are less likely to respond to imatinib mesylate. They may therefore be candidates for alternative therapies as they become available. It is especially important, however, to emphasize that approximately 5% of GISTs will be KIT "negative" by CD117 immunostaining. These KIT-negative GISTs, when compared with KIT-positive GISTs, are more likely to have epithelioid morphology, arise in the omentum/peritoneal surface, and contain PDGFR mutations. These GISTs may contain imatinib mesylate–sensitive clones, and therefore patients with morphologically and clinically confirmed KIT-negative GIST should not be denied a trial of imatinib mesylate therapy.[5,11] Because of the success of imatinib mesylate therapy in the management of GIST, the present recommendations in the work-up of a KIT-negative GI mesenchymal tumor with histopathology suggesting a spindle, epithelioid, or mixed variant of GIST are to evaluate tumor tissue for KIT or PDGFR-α mutations. Thus, genotype screening in this particular patient population may provide clinically actionable information.[33] Investigations into the molecular mechanisms of GIST response are ongoing with broad-based implications for specific targeted therapeutics in other solid tumor models. Data

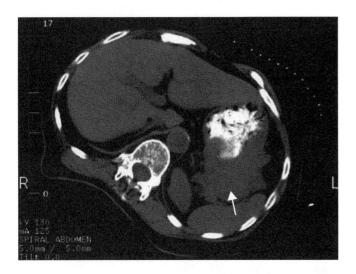

Figure 80–8. Computed tomographic scan of a primary gastric GIST (*arrow*). Note the extrinsic mass effect on the stomach.

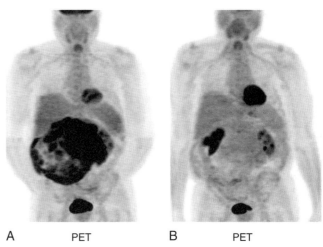

A   PET   B   PET

Figure 80–9. ^{18}F-fluorodeoxyglucose (FDG)–positron emission tomographic (PET) scan indicating a large bulky primary GIST before **(A)** and after **(B)** imatinib mesylate administration. The decreased FDG concentration in the tumor was noted within several weeks after initiation of drug therapy.

generated from evaluation of downstream signal transduction pathways suggest differential expression of signaling intermediates depending on the type of KIT mutation, and robust genomic-based platform arrays have identified differential-response gene expression signatures associated with GIST cells sensitive to imatinib mesylate. It is conceivable that future evaluations will provide enough data so that GIST patients can be phenotyped by tumor biopsy before and just after administration of imatinib mesylate to determine whether they will respond to single-drug therapy or whether alternative or combination therapies will be necessary to optimize their outcome.

IMAGING

Cross-sectional imaging, particularly in the initial work-up of a patient with suspected primary or recurrent GIST, is the diagnostic procedure of choice. A contrast-enhanced (oral and intravenous) CT scan is recommended and generally allows assessment of the extent of the primary, as well as the potential presence of metastatic disease. The typical primary GIST will be manifested as an intestinal-based mass with the bulk of the tumor extrinsic to the bowel, thus often providing an opportunity for complete resection, even in patients with a large primary tumor (Fig. 80–8). In many instances the primary tumor, although large, may be pedunculated, particularly if originating from the stomach. Guidelines for follow-up after successful GIST surgical resection, as recommended by the National Comprehensive Cancer Network, are as follows: CT of the abdomen/pelvis performed every 3 to 6 months for 3 to 5 years and annually thereafter, except in patients with very-low-risk primary GIST, in which case less frequent follow-up is required.[33] The frequency of metastasis of GIST to the lung is quite low, and therefore routine screening chest CT is not necessary.

Standard image-based response criteria are being re-evaluated in light of the information available for GIST patients treated with imatinib mesylate. These characteristic CT scan changes in GIST, consistent with a favorable response to a molecularly targeted agent, include a change in density of the measurable tumor to a more myxoid or hypodense appearance rather than a definitive decrease in size. This response can take place within a month of initiation of therapy and can be quantitated by measurement of Hounsfield units. Within 2 months of therapy a decrease in tumor size, usually confirmed by comparing the sum of the longest diameters of all target measurable lesions or a 15% decrease in density, can be considered predictive of a beneficial response, although a maximal decrease in tumor size may take 6 months or longer. Conversely, drug resistance may be manifested as the appearance of a small intratumoral nodule without a change in overall density or size of the tumor mass. Lessons learned about the clinical usefulness of these measurable response criteria may have more universal applicability to assessment of specific targeted therapy for other solid tumors as increasing numbers of these agents become clinically available.

Functional imaging with ^{18}F-fluorodeoxyglucose (FDG)–positron emission tomography (PET) can be an important adjunct to standard CT by assessing early changes in metabolic activity in GIST. FDG-PET can provide an immediate and sensitive measure of response in GISTs, which are generally PET avid tumors.[34] Imatinib mesylate may have a dramatic effect on abrogation of GIST cell glycolysis, and these measurable decreases in glucose uptake by the tumor can be visualized within hours of initiation of therapy and can be predictive of long-term response by comparison to the standard uptake value. This may be particularly helpful in the assessment of neoadjuvant treatment (Fig. 80–9). If FDG-PET is being considered as a diagnostic modality to monitor continued response, detect recurrence, or complement an ambiguous CT scan, a baseline PET scan should be obtained before initiation of therapy.

SURGICAL MANAGEMENT

Surgical management of GIST is based on sound oncologic principles, and before the introduction of imatinib mesylate as an effective systemic therapy, surgical resection was the only viable therapeutic option. However, approximately 50% of all GIST patients will have evidence of overt malignant disease at initial evaluation, and survival after surgical management of these patients has historically been quite poor. Because of the low incidence of GIST there is a paucity of information regarding the results of surgical resection from retrospective data. In several reported series, optimal patients with primary tumors predominantly gastric in origin and treated by complete tumor resection still had a relatively poor reported 5-year survival rate of approximately 50%.[35,36] Tumor size is a predominant factor in surgical resection series for primary GIST, and patients with tumors larger than 10 cm have reported survival rates in the 20% range at 5 years. There continues to be attrition in resected GISTs during prospective follow-up, with one series reporting only 10% of resected patients being free of disease after a median follow-up of 68 months.[37] The median time to recurrence after resection of a primary GIST is 2 years, but in subsets with small tumor size or slowly proliferating GIST, metastases can develop more than 10 years after diagnosis, and therefore all these patients require life-long follow-up.

Of patients with primary disease at initial diagnosis, approximately 75% will undergo complete resection. The most common sites of disease failure after complete resection are the peritoneal cavity and the liver. The finding of an extra-abdominal site is quite uncommon. Approximately half to two thirds of GIST primaries will have disease failure within the liver, and nearly 40% of patients will have the liver as the only site of failure. Generally, hepatic involvement is multifocal; however, one series of 34 patients reported a 5-year survival rate of 30% after hepatic resection.[38] Surgical resection for recurrent GIST has found limited use with rare long-term success, even after complete tumor removal or ablation. Palliative surgery for bleeding or obstruction can be entertained as a viable alternative in a patient with limited disease and a good performance status.

The goal of surgery in the management of primary GIST is complete gross resection with an intact pseudocapsule. At laparotomy the abdomen should be carefully explored for any evidence of metastatic disease on the peritoneal surfaces or in the liver. GISTs should be handled gently and with care to avoid rupture. GISTs are generally exophytic, tend to displace adjacent structures, and despite the CT appearance, can often be lifted away from surrounding organs. En bloc resection is infrequently necessary and only when there is evidence of dense adherence to adjacent organs. Segmental resection of the stomach or intestine can be performed with the intent of negative margins. Partial or wedge gastrectomy is a viable option because GIST cells do not manifest submucosal spread, as is common with adenocarcinoma. Lymphadenectomy is unnecessary because lymph node metastases are rare. The value of microscopically negative resection margins, especially in a large tumor, is questionable since margin status does not appear to be a prognostic indicator for recurrence when it has been evaluated as a meaningful risk factor. This may be because these large extrinsic tumors tend to shed cells into the peritoneal cavity, so local/regional recurrence is predicted more by tumor size than by resection margin. The value of reoperative surgery for microscopically positive margins is unproven and should depend on many factors, such as tumor size, potential morbidity, and the availability of adjuvant therapy. Laparoscopic wedge resection may be used for small GISTs (<2 cm) when the risk for rupture is minimal, but data on this approach are lacking.

Surgical considerations for the management of GIST have recently undergone considerable change. Although surgical resection remains the standard form of treatment of primary GIST, the efficacy of the KIT-targeted oral agent imatinib mesylate has transformed therapeutic considerations into a multimodality paradigm. There is increasing awareness that GIST needs to be managed with the combined expertise of pathology, surgery, medical oncology, and imaging in the initial evaluation and subsequent management. It is reasonable, then, to evaluate surgical considerations and outcomes with respect to pre–imatinib mesylate and post–imatinib mesylate time frames. Traditional sarcoma-based polychemotherapy and irradiation have historically been ineffective in the treatment of GIST, and surgical management in general has been associated with disappointing results in terms of recurrence-free and overall survival for high-risk GIST patients, particularly for large and highly proliferative tumors. Imatinib mesylate is a rationally based therapeutic agent that was developed as an antagonist to the KIT receptor on GIST cells and has shown remarkable effectiveness against metastatic and unresectable GIST.[39] Addition of this drug to surgical management decisions in GIST leads to the possibility of effective adjuvant therapy for improving long-term outcomes. Furthermore, surgical debulking of slowly responding, stable, or partially responding large primary or recurrent GISTs after "neoadjuvant" administration and assessment of response to imatinib mesylate may enhance long-term disease control in GIST patients with large tumor burdens. Advantages of this combined approach could also lead to organ preservation, an important consideration for GIST patients with primary tumor location in the proximal stomach, rectum, or duodenum. The results of ongoing clinical trials will probably provide more concrete recommendations for the surgical management of GIST and become part of the care standard in the future.

ADJUVANT THERAPY

Surgery is the primary initial treatment of resectable GIST, but it is seldom curative in patients with a high risk for recurrent disease. Surgery is even less effective in patients with locally recurrent or metastatic disease. Before the availability of imatinib mesylate the only treatment of GIST, other than surgical resection, was conventional chemotherapy and radiotherapy. However, lack of efficacy has been a constant in studies evaluating these modalities in the management of GIST patients.[40] The recent availability of an effective systemic therapy raises the issue of its potential use as adjuvant or neoadjuvant treatment in conjunction with surgical tumor resection with the objective of either cytoreduction of disease before surgery or improvement in long-term survival after successful resection. Other than anecdotal experience, data on the combined use of imatinib mesylate and surgical resection are lacking. Clearly, patient selection factors for adjuvant trial design are critical. Patients typically at high risk for recurrence, such as those with tumors larger than 10 cm or tumors with greater than five mitoses per 50 high-powered fields, are obvious candidates for such a trial. Patients with other risk factors, such as tumor perforation or rupture or a known specific drug-sensitive genotype, might also be considered for clinical trial participation. Presently, three national cooperative group trials are evaluating imatinib mesylate as adjuvant or neoadjuvant therapy.[39] One is already completed with the results pending for a phase II trial design of postoperative imatinib mesylate in high-risk patients, another is an ongoing phase II randomized postoperative trial for high- and intermediate-risk patients with comparison to placebo, and the third is an ongoing neoadjuvant design for patients with bulky primary or resectable recurrent/metastatic GIST. The possibility of pharmacologic debulking with imatinib mesylate, followed by surgical resection, may be a rational strategy for organ preservation, in vivo drug sensitivity testing, optimization of therapy for focal metastatic disease, and abrogation of emerging drug-resistant clones. Short follow-up clinical experience has suggested the usefulness of limited surgery in some patients with multiple-site recurrent disease whose tumor demonstrated a mixed pattern of response to imatinib mesylate and in whom resection or ablation was successful in removing unresponsive sites while the bulk quiescent residual disease was managed successfully with continued imatinib mesylate therapy. At this time the optimal dose plus duration of imatinib in the surgical adjuvant or neoadjuvant strategy has not been defined, and this combination in treating GIST in standard actual practice awaits elucidation in clinical trials.

SUGGESTED READINGS

Demetri G, von Mehren M, Blanke C, et al: Efficacy and safety of imatinib mesylate in advanced gastrointestinal stromal tumors. N Engl J Med 347:472-480, 2002.

Heinrich M, Corless C, Duensing A, et al: PDGFRA activating mutations in gastrointestinal stromal tumors. Science 299:708-710, 2003.

Hirota S, Isozaki K, Moriyama Y, et al: Gain of function mutations of C-KIT in human gastrointestinal stromal tumors. Science 279:577-580, 1998.

REFERENCES

1. Mazur MT, Clark HB: Gastric stromal tumors: Reappraisal of histogenesis. Am J Surg Pathol 7:507-519, 1983.
2. Miettinen M, Lasota J: Gastrointestinal stromal tumors—definition, clinical, histologic, immunohistochemical, and molecular genetic features and differential diagnosis. Virchows Arch 438:1-12, 2001.
3. Fletcher CD, Berman JJ, Corless C, et al: Diagnoses of gastrointestinal tumors: A consensus approach. Hum Pathol 33:459-465, 2002.
4. Miettinen M, el-Rifai W, Sobin L, et al: Evaluation of malignancy and prognosis of gastrointestinal stromal tumors. A review. Hum Pathol 33:478-483, 2002.
5. Corless C, Fletcher J, Heinrich M: Biology of gastrointestinal stromal tumors. J Clin Oncol 22:3813-3825, 2004.
6. Emory TS, Sobin HH, Lukes L, et al: Prognosis of gastrointestinal smooth muscle tumors: Dependence on anatomic site. Am J Surg Pathol 23:82-87, 1999.
7. Kindblom LG, Meis-Kindblom J, Bumming P, et al: Incidence, prevalence, phenotype and biological spectrum of gastrointestinal stromal tumors (GIST)—a population based study of 600 cases. Ann Oncol 13(Suppl 5):157, 2003.
8. Perez-Atayde AR, Shamberger RC, Kozakewich HW: Neuroectodermal differentiation of the gastrointestinal tumors in the Carney triad. An ultrastructural and immunohistochemical study. Am J Surg Pathol 17:706-714, 1993.
9. Miettinen M, Sobin LH, Sarlomo-Rikala M: Immunohistochemical spectrum of GISTs at different sites and their differential diagnosis with a reference to CD117 (KIT). Mod Pathol 13:1134-1142, 2000.
10. Heinrich MC, Rubin BP, Longley BJ, et al: Biology and genetic aspects of gastrointestinal stromal tumors: KIT activation and cytogenetic alterations. Hum Pathol 33:486-495, 2002.
11. Medeiros F, Corless C, Duensing A, et al: KIT-negative gastrointestinal stromal tumors: Proof of concept and therapeutic implications. Am J Surg Pathol 28:889-894, 2004.
12. West R, Corless C, Chen X, et al: The novel marker, DOG1, is expressed ubiquitously in gastrointestinal stromal tumor irrespective of KIT or PDGFRA mutation status. Am J Pathol 165:107-113, 2004.
13. Blay P, Astudillo A, Buesa J, et al: Protein kinase C theta is highly expressed in gastrointestinal stromal tumors but not in other mesenchymal neoplasias. Clin Cancer Res 10:4089-4095, 2004.
14. Savage D, Antman K: Imatinib mesylate—a new oral targeted therapy. N Engl J Med 346:683-693, 2002.
15. Besmer P, Murphy JE, George PC, et al: A new acute transforming feline retrovirus and relationship of its oncogene V-KIT with the protein kinase family. Nature 320:415-421, 1986.
16. Williams DE, Eisenman J, Baird A, et al: Identification of a ligand for the C-KIT proto-oncogene. Cell 63:185-194, 1990.
17. Hirota S: Gastrointestinal stromal tumors: Their origin and cause. Int J Clin Oncol 6:1-5, 2001.
18. Hirota S, Isozaki K, Moriyama Y, et al: Gain of function mutations of C-Kit in human gastrointestinal stromal tumors. Science 279:577-580, 1998.
19. Nishida T, Hirota S, Taniguchi M, et al: Familial gastrointestinal stromal tumors with germline mutations of the KIT gene. Nat Genet 19:323-324, 1998.
20. Nakahara M, Koji I, Hirota S, et al: A novel gain of function mutation of C-KIT gene in gastrointestinal stromal tumors. Gastroenterology 115:1090-1095, 1998.
21. Sommer G, Agosti V, Ehlers I, et al: Gastrointestinal stromal tumors in a mouse model by targeted mutation of the KIT receptor tyrosine kinase. Proc Natl Acad Sci U S A 100:6706-6711, 2003.
22. Lux M, Rubin B, Biase T, et al: KIT extracellular and kinase domain mutations in gastrointestinal stromal tumors. Am J Pathol 156:791-795, 2000.
23. Rubin BP, Singer S, Tsao C, et al: KIT activation is a ubiquitous feature of gastrointestinal stromal tumors. Cancer Res 61:8118-8121, 2001.
24. Corless CL, McGreevey L, Haley A, et al: KIT mutations are common in incidental gastrointestinal stromal tumors one centimeter or less in size. Am J Pathol 160:1567-1572, 2002.
25. Lasota J, Jasinski M, Sarlomo-Rikala M, et al: Mutations in exon 11 of C-Kit occur preferentially in malignant versus benign

gastrointestinal stromal tumors and do not occur in leiomyomas or leiomyosarcomas. Am J Pathol 154:53-60, 1999.

26. Heinrich M, Griffith D, Druker B, et al: Inhibition of C-Kit receptor tyrosine kinase activity by STI 571, a selective tyrosine kinase inhibitor. Blood 96:925-932, 2000.

27. Tuveson D, Willis N, Jacks T, et al: STI571 inactivation of the gastrointestinal stromal tumor C-KIT oncoprotein, biological and clinical implications. Oncogene 20:5054-5058, 2001.

28. Joensuu H, Roberts P, Sarlomo-Rikala M, et al: Effect of the tyrosine kinase inhibitor STI 571 in a patient with metastatic gastrointestinal stromal tumor. N Engl J Med 344:1052-1056, 2001.

29. Demetri G, von Mehren M, Blanke C, et al: Efficacy and safety of imatinib mesylate in advanced gastrointestinal stromal tumors. N Engl J Med 347:472-480, 2002.

30. Eisenberg B: Imatinib mesylate—a molecularly targeted therapy for gastrointestinal stromal tumors. Oncology 17:1615-1620, 2003.

31. Heinrich M, Corless C, Demetri G, et al: Kinase mutations and imatinib response in patients with metastatic gastrointestinal stromal tumors. J Clin Oncol 21:4342-4349, 2003.

32. Heinrich M, Corless C, Duensing A, et al: PDGFRA activating mutations in gastrointestinal stromal tumors. Science 299:708-710, 2003.

33. Demetri G, Benjamin R, Blanke C, et al: NCCN task force report: Optimal management of patients with gastrointestinal stromal

34. Von den Abbeele A, Badawi R: Use of positron emission tomography in oncology and its potential role to assess response to imatinib mesylate therapy in gastrointestinal stromal tumors (GISTs). Eur J Cancer 38(Suppl 5):560-565, 2002.

35. DeMatteo RP, Lewis JJ, Leung D, et al: Two hundred gastrointestinal stromal tumors: Recurrence pattern and prognostic factors for survival. Ann Surg 231:51-58, 2000.

36. DeMatteo RP, Heinrich M, El-Rifai WM, et al: Clinical management of gastrointestinal stromal tumors: Before and after STI-571. Hum Pathol 33:466-477, 2002.

37. Ng EH, Pollack RE, Romsdahl MM: Prognostic implications of patterns of failure for gastrointestinal leiomyosarcomas. Cancer 69:1334-1341, 1992.

38. DeMatteo RP, Shah A, Fong Y, et al: Results of hepatic resection for sarcoma metastatic to liver. Ann Surg 234:540-548, 2001.

39. Eisenberg B, Judson I: Surgery and imatinib in the management of GIST: Emerging approaches to adjuvant and neoadjuvant therapy. Ann Surg Oncol 11:465-475, 2004.

40. DePas T, Casali P, Toma S, et al: Gastrointestinal stromal tumors: Should they be treated with the same systemic chemotherapy as other soft tissue sarcomas? Oncology 64:186-188, 2003.

tumor (GIST)—expansion and update of NCCN clinical practice guidelines. J Natl Comp Cancer Network 2(Suppl 1):51-526, 2004.

81

Gastrointestinal Lymphomas

Lindsey N. Jackson ▪ B. Mark Evers

Despite recent advances in the diagnosis and treatment of non-Hodgkin's lymphoma (NHL), this disease remains the sixth leading cause of cancer-related deaths in the United States, with an approximate 5-year survival rate of 56%.[1] An estimated 56,000 cases of NHL will occur in the United States in 2005, and approximately 19,000 will die of the disease.[1] The incidence of NHL has increased rapidly, almost doubling, since the early 1970s, probably because of an increased incidence of human immunodeficiency virus (HIV) infection and environmental and toxic exposure.[1,2] However, the incidence stabilized in the 1990s, primarily as a result of a decline in acquired immunodeficiency syndrome–related malignancy.[1]

NHL classically originates in lymph node basins, but it may occur as extranodal lymphoma or lymphoma arising within a solid organ in up to 30% of cases.[3] The gastrointestinal (GI) tract is the most common site of extranodal disease and accounts for approximately 20% of all NHL and approximately half of extranodal NHL.[2,4] Requirements for the diagnosis of primary GI lymphoma include absence of palpable lymphadenopathy, normal bone marrow biopsy and peripheral blood smear, absence of mediastinal lymphadenopathy on chest radiographs, disease grossly confined to the affected viscus, and absence of hepatic or splenic involvement unless via direct extension of the primary tumor.[5] This chapter focuses on lymphomas occurring in the stomach and small intestine, the two most commonly affected organs of the digestive tract worldwide.

INCIDENCE AND EPIDEMIOLOGY

GI tract lymphomas may occur in any part of the digestive tract from the oral cavity to the rectum, and the incidence appears to depend on geographic location.[2] In Western and Middle Eastern regions, the stomach is the most commonly affected site, followed by the small intestine, colon, pancreas, and all other sites; however, in other parts of the world such as India, Africa, and the South Pacific, intestinal lymphoma is the predominant form, followed by the stomach, colon, and other organs (Table 81–1).[2,6]

Gastric Lymphoma

In the United States the stomach is the most common site of GI lymphoma and accounts for more than half of the lymphomas of the GI tract. Yet it is relatively uncommon and accounts for less than 15% of primary gastric neoplasms and 2% of all lymphomas.[6-8] Gastric lymphomas tend to occur in patients older than 50 years, with a peak incidence in the sixth and seventh decades, and they are two to three times more common in men.[6,7] However, recent studies have demonstrated that the disease is occurring more commonly in an increasingly younger age group, predominantly because of increased incidence in HIV-infected patients.[6] Gastric lymphomas most frequently occur in the gastric antrum or distal body, but they may arise from any portion of the stomach.[7,9]

Small Intestinal Lymphoma

Lymphoma of the small intestine is the second most common extranodal lymphoma of the GI tract in the United States. It is the third most common primary neoplasm of the small bowel and accounts for 15% to 20% of malignant small bowel tumors, 5% of all lymphomas, 4% to 12% of all NHLs, and 20% to 30% of primary GI lymphomas.[7,10,11] Small intestinal lymphomas, like gastric lymphomas, tend to occur in patients older than 50 years; however, it is the most common intestinal neoplasm in children younger than 10 years, thus resulting in a bimodal distribution.[7,11] Small bowel lymphoma is most commonly located in the ileum, the site of the highest concentration of gut-associated lymphoid tissue.[7]

CLINICAL FEATURES

The typical signs and symptoms of GI lymphoma are often nonspecific and commonly mimic other abdomi-

Table 81–1	Frequency and Sites of Extranodal Lymphomas in Series from Different Countries

	USA (1972)	The Netherlands (1989)	Denmark (1991)	Canada (1992)	Hong Kong (1984)	Pakistan (1992)	Egypt (1994)	Switzerland (1997)
Stomach	24	23	19	24*	39	10	10	36
Small intestine	8	5	9	—	24	17	5	11
Colon and rectum	5	7	2	—	—	10	6	4
Head and neck	21	23	8†	34	22	18	23	19
Orbit	2	3	1	4	1	<1	<1	5
Central nervous system	2	6	7	10	—	2	1	1
Lung, pleura	4	5	5	1	—	—	—	1
Bone	5	3	9	4	4	2	11	3
Soft tissue	9	2	3	5	3	—	—	1
Breast	2	2	1	2	—	—	—	3
Skin (except mycosis fungoides)	8	2	11	4	3	8	4	6
Genitourinary tract	3	4	6	5	8	12	6	5

*Including all gastrointestinal sites.
†Waldeyer's ring and tonsils not included.
From Zucca E, Roggero E, Bertoni F, Cavalli F: Primary extranodal non-Hodgkin's lymphomas. Part 1: Gastrointestinal, cutaneous and genitourinary lymphomas. Ann Oncol 8:727-737, 1997.

nal pathologies, such as gastritis, peptic ulcer disease, and pancreatic or gallbladder disorders, as well as other neoplasms.[6] The most common initial symptom of both gastric and intestinal lymphomas is abdominal pain; additional symptoms may include early satiety or abdominal fullness, fatigue, diarrhea, nausea, vomiting, and indigestion (Table 81–2).[8,12] Lymphoma of the small intestine is more likely to cause intussusception, obstruction, or perforation than gastric lymphoma is. In fact, approximately 30% to 50% of patients will have an abdominal emergency, with perforation present in up to 25% of cases.[2,5] Over half of patients with GI lymphoma will exhibit anemia secondary to chronic occult blood loss; overt bleeding is uncommon.[7] Constitutional B symptoms, which include fever, weight loss, and night sweats, are rare (less than 12% of patients) unless systemic disease is present.[8] Because of the insidious onset and nonspecific nature of many of these symptoms, it is often months or years before the diagnosis is made.[4] Physical examination is normal in approximately 55% to 60% of patients, with abdominal tenderness encountered in 20% to 35% and a palpable mass in 17% to 25%.[6] Other physical findings may include fever, lymphadenopathy, jaundice, hepatomegaly, and splenomegaly.[6]

PATHOLOGY

Appropriate management of GI lymphomas requires determination of the stage and subtype of the lymphoma,

as well as consideration of morphology, genetic alterations, and immunophenotype.[2] There are several classification systems for GI lymphomas (Table 81–3). In the World Health Organization (WHO) classification, the most common NHL arising in the GI tract is diffuse large B-cell lymphoma (DLBCL) (55%), followed in frequency by extranodal marginal cell lymphoma of mucosa-associated lymphoid tissue (MALT lymphoma) (40%), Burkitt's lymphoma (3%), and follicular, mantle cell, and enteropathy-type T-cell lymphomas (<1% each) (Table 81–4).[2]

Diffuse Large B-Cell Lymphoma

DLBCL is the most common type of NHL, extranodal lymphoma, and GI lymphoma. It may occur as de novo disease, but it may also arise from or coexist in a background of low-grade MALT lymphoma, chronic lymphocytic leukemia, small lymphocytic lymphoma, or follicular lymphoma (Fig. 81–1).[2,13] DLBCL is often manifested as a tumor mass replacing the normal architecture of its tissue of origin and is most commonly located in the stomach or ileocecal region (Fig. 81–2).[2] There are several morphologic variants of DLBCL that are distinguished by histologic, cytogenetic, and molecular genetic features; patterns of gene expression dictate the prognosis.[14,15] A Bcl-2 gene mutation, commonly involved in a (14;18)(q32;q21) translocation, is present in 10% to 40% of DLBCLs, and a Bcl-6 gene mutation with a (14;3)(q32;q27) rearrangement may occur in

Table 81–2 Symptoms at Diagnosis in Patients with Primary Gastrointestinal Non-Hodgkin's Lymphoma*

Symptom[†]	Stomach (N = 277)		Small Bowel (N = 32)		Ileocecal Region (N = 26)		Multiple GI Sites (N = 24)	
	No. of Patients	%	No. of Patients	%	No. of Patients	%	No. of Patients	%
Pain	216	78.0	24	75.0	20	76.9	14	58.3
Loss of appetite	131	47.3	13	40.6	6	23.1	14	58.3
Loss of weight[‡]	68	24.5	11	34.4	4	15.4	6	25.0
Bleeding	50	18.8	2	6.3	3	11.5	2	8.3
Vomiting	52	18.1	10	31.3	2	7.7	5	20.8
Night sweats	31	11.2	4	12.5	5	19.2	11	45.8
None	10	3.6	—	—	—	—	—	—
Diarrhea	10	3.6	4	12.5	5	19.2	7	29.2
Constipation	9	3.2	8	25.0	6	23.1	3	12.5
Fever	6	2.2	2	6.3	2	7.7	1	4.2
Perforation	5	1.8	3	9.4	—	—	—	—
Ileus	—	—	12	37.5	5	19.2	1	4.2
B symptoms (fever, night sweats)	33	11.9	5	15.6	3	11.5	6	25.0
Median time to diagnosis (days)	93		135		76		142	

*Major sites only.
[†]More than one possible.
[‡]Not considered a B symptom but caused by non-Hodgkin's lymphoma.
From Koch P, del Valle F, Berdel WE, et al: Primary gastrointestinal non-Hodgkin's lymphoma: I. Anatomic and histologic distribution, clinical features, and survival data of 371 patients registered in the German Multicenter Study GIT NHL. J Clin Oncol 19:3861-3871, 2001.

Table 81–3 Comparison of Gastrointestinal Lymphoma Classifications

WHO	REAL	Working	Lukes-Collins	Kiel	Rappaport
Extranodal marginal zone lymphoma (MALT)		Small cleaved cell type	Small cleaved cell type	Immunocytoma	Well-differentiated lymphocytic
Follicular lymphoma	Follicular center lymphoma	Small cleaved cell type	Small cleaved cell type	Centroblastic/centrocytic, follicular and diffuse	Nodular poorly differentiated lymphocytic
Mantle cell lymphoma				Centrocytic	Intermediately or poorly differentiated lymphocytic, diffuse or nodular
Diffuse large B-cell lymphoma	Diffuse large B-cell lymphoma	Large cleaved follicular center cell	Large cleaved follicular center cell	Centroblastic, B-immunoblastic	Diffuse mixed lymphocytic and histiocytic
Burkitt's lymphoma	Burkitt's lymphoma	Small noncleaved cell, follicular center cell	Small noncleaved follicular center cell	Burkitt's lymphoma with intracytoplasmic immunoglobulin	Undifferentiated lymphoma, Burkitt's type

MALT, mucosa-associated lymphoid tissue; REAL, Revised European-American Lymphoma; WHO, World Health Organization.
From Mercer DW, Robinson EK: Stomach. In Townsend CM (ed): Sabiston's Textbook of Surgery: The Biological Basis of Modern Surgical Practice. Philadelphia, Elsevier, 2004, pp 1265-1321.

Table 81–4   Frequency of Organ Involvement

Gastrointestinal Lymphoma	Stomach	Small Intestine	Colon*	Pancreas*
Diffuse large cell lymphoma	55	55	60	60
MALT lymphoma	40	20	15	
Burkitt's lymphoma	3	5	15	15
Peripheral T-cell lymphoma	0	15	10	5
Mantle cell lymphoma	<1	0	1	10
Follicular lymphoma	<1	0	1	10

*Relative frequency of particular malignancies estimated from small case series in the literature.
MALT, mucosa-associated lymphoid tissue.
Adapted from Koniaris LG, Drugas G, Katzman PJ, et al: Management of gastrointestinal lymphoma. J Am Coll Surg 197:127-141, 2003.

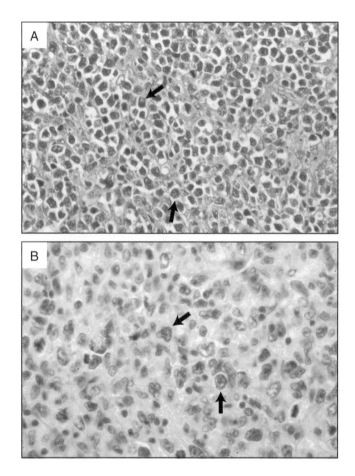

Figure 81–1.   Diffuse large B-cell lymphoma of the stomach showing a monotonous high-grade infiltrate of large centroblast-like cells *(arrows)* under low **(A)** and high-power **(B)** magnification. (Courtesy of Mary R. Schwartz, M.D., Baylor College of Medicine.)

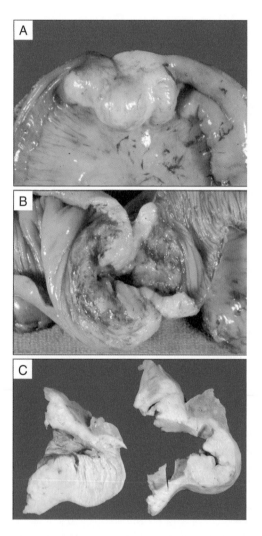

Figure 81–2.   Diffuse large B-cell lymphoma of the jejunum demonstrating the external aspect **(A),** the mucosal aspect **(B),** and cross sections showing transmural involvement and expansion of the wall by lymphoma **(C).** (Courtesy of Mary R. Schwartz, M.D., Baylor College of Medicine.)

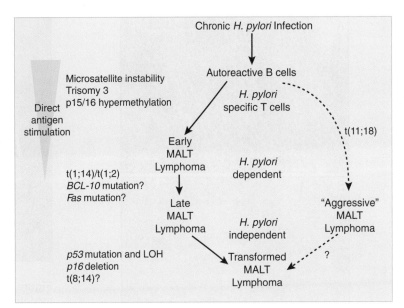

Figure 81–3. Schematic presentation of the pathogenesis of MALT lymphoma. LOH, loss of heterozygosity. (From Du M, Isaccson PG: Gastric MALT lymphoma: From aetiology to treatment. Lancet Oncol 3:97-104, 2002.)

approximately 30% to 40% of cases; variabilities in survivin expression and p53 mutations have also been described.[14-16] The Bcl-2 protein is involved in the prevention of apoptosis, and recent evidence suggests that overexpression of it is associated with decreased overall, disease-free, and relapse-free survival.[15] In contrast, overexpression of the Bcl-6 protein, which normally regulates T-cell–dependent antigen responses, is associated with increased overall survival.[14]

MALT Lymphoma

MALT lymphomas were first described in 1983 and have since been reclassified as extranodal marginal zone lymphomas of the MALT type.[17] The stomach, which is paradoxically devoid of organized lymphoid tissue, is the site most frequently affected by MALT lymphomas.[18] These gastric tumors are thought to arise from MALT acquired as a result of chronic inflammation, most commonly gastritis associated with *Helicobacter pylori* because more than 90% of patients with gastric MALT lymphoma are infected with this bacterium.[4] Chronic activation of tumor-infiltrating T-cells is responsible for B-cell activation, with subsequent oligoclonal and monoclonal proliferation in an *H. pylori* strain–specific manner.[17] Once an active, proliferating monoclonal B-cell population develops, reactive oxygen species released at the site of inflammation contribute to an accumulation of oxidative stress and resultant genetic abnormalities.[9]

Genetically, two predominant translocations, t(11;18)(q21;q21) and t(1;14)(p22;q32), are implicated in the development of MALT lymphoma.[19] The t(11;18)(q21;q21) translocation, which fuses the inhibitor of apoptosis *(IAP2)* gene to the MALT 1 *(MLT)* gene, is detected in approximately 21% to 60% of gastric MALT lymphomas.[20] The resultant IAP2-MLT fusion protein is associated with nuclear localization of Bcl-10, a protein with transforming and proapoptotic functions

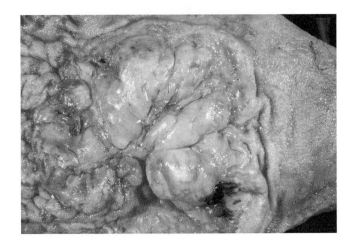

Figure 81–4. Gastric MALT lymphoma, gross photograph. (Courtesy of Mary R. Schwartz, M.D., Baylor College of Medicine.)

normally localized in the cytoplasm, as well as activation of the nuclear factor kappa B (NF-κB) pathway, which results in antigen-independent growth and disease dissemination.[17] This translocation is associated with resistance to *H. pylori* eradication, lymphoma regression, and more aggressive, advanced stages of disease.[7,17] The t(1;14)(p22;q32) translocation, which occurs in less than 5% of gastric MALT lymphomas, transfers the Bcl-10 gene to the immunoglobulin heavy chain promoter region and thereby results in a similar pattern of Bcl-10 overexpression and nuclear localization, activation of the NF-κB pathway, and an association with more advanced stages of disease.[20] Mutations leading to the formation of MALT lymphoma are summarized in Figure 81–3.

Gastric MALT lymphoma is often multifocal, with most tumors located in the antrum or distal body of the stomach (Fig. 81–4).[9] Histologically, there is diffuse

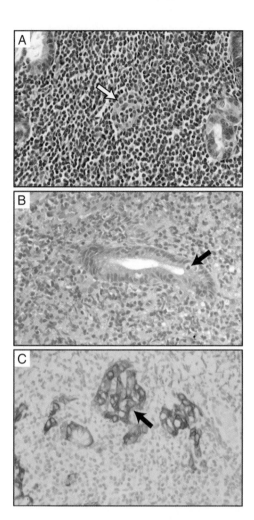

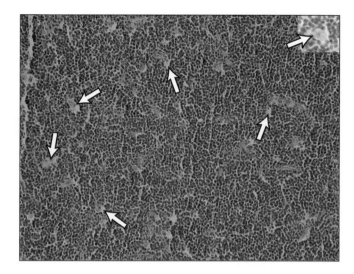

Figure 81–6. Low-power view of Burkitt's lymphoma with monotonous lymphocytic infiltrate and scattered clear spaces (starry sky appearance) *(arrows).* Clear spaces are actually large histiocytes *(inset).* (Courtesy of Suimin Qiu, M.D., The University of Texas Medical Branch.)

Figure 81–5. Histopathologic characteristics of MALT lymphoma. **A,** Monocytoid, lymphocytic infiltrate with lymphocytes infiltrating the epithelial component (lymphoepithelial lesion) *(arrow).* (Courtesy of Suimin Qiu, M.D., The University of Texas Medical Branch.) **B,** Low-grade MALT lymphoma of the stomach demonstrating lymphoepithelial lesions *(arrow),* and **C,** keratin immunohistochemical stain demonstrating lymphoepithelial lesions with infiltration and partial destruction of glandular structures by lymphocytes *(arrow).* (Courtesy of Mary R. Schwartz, M.D., Baylor College of Medicine.)

permeation of the lamina propria with germinal centers; neoplastic cells infiltrate the marginal zone around reactive lymphoid follicles and invade gastric glands, with the formation of characteristic lymphoepithelial lesions (Fig. 81–5).[9,13] The neoplastic MALT lymphoma cells generally express B-cell markers, including CD20, CD22, and CD79a, but they lack markers expressed by other B-cell neoplasms, such as CD5, CD10, CD23, and Bcl-6.[13,19]

Burkitt's Lymphoma

Burkitt's lymphoma is an aggressive lymphoma that may occur as endemic (in equatorial Africa) or sporadic disease.[2] It has a well-established association with Epstein-Barr virus infection.[7] Burkitt's lymphoma generally affects younger populations than other types of gastric lymphoma do and is typically located in the cardia or body of the stomach or the terminal ileum.[7,13] Apoptosis and mitosis are common within the tumor, which attracts circulating macrophages and thereby results in the classic "starry sky" appearance (Fig. 81–6).[13] Burkitt's lymphoma generally expresses CD10, CD20, CD79a, and Bcl-6 but lacks Bcl-2. Rearrangement of the *c-myc* oncogene is typical of this lymphoma.[21]

Follicular Lymphoma

Follicular lymphoma is most commonly a systemic disease, but it may rarely be manifested as localized GI tract involvement.[13] There is an apparent predilection for the duodenum, and differentiation from MALT lymphoma is often difficult because of the lymphoepithelial lesions common to both.[13] Transformation of follicular lymphoma to diffuse large B-cell disease may occur in as many as 32% of patients and carries a poor prognosis.[22] The most useful markers for the diagnosis of follicular lymphoma are CD10, Bcl-6, and Bcl-12.[13] Additionally, up to 85% of tumors will demonstrate a t(14;18)(q32;q21) translocation leading to Bcl-2 overexpression.[23]

Mantle Cell Lymphoma

Mantle cell lymphoma, in contrast to other forms of GI lymphoma, tends to be manifested as polyposis predominantly involving the small bowel (Fig. 81–7).[24] There is an infiltrate of small or medium-sized cells with irregular nuclei and little cytoplasm, and lymphoepithelial lesions are rare (Fig. 81–8).[13] Unlike other lymphomas, the tumor cells tend to compress rather than infiltrate.[13] Typical tumor markers include CD5, CD20, CD79a, and cyclin D1.[13,24]

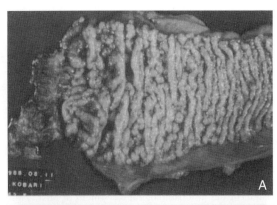

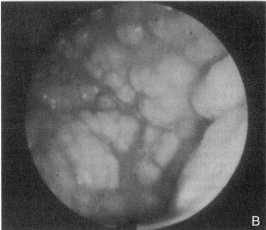

Figure 81–7. Growth manifestations of multiple lymphomatous polyposis. **A,** A surgically resected rectum shows a myriad of confluent polyps and the formation of giant folds. **B,** Endoscopic examination of the duodenum shows numerous polyps that were densely present with the same lesions extending throughout from the esophagus to the rectum. (From Hashimoto S, Nakamura N, Kuze T, et al: Multiple lymphomatous polyposis of the gastrointestinal tract is a heterogenous group that includes mantle cell lymphoma and follicular lymphoma: Analysis of somatic mutation of immunoglobulin heavy chain gene variable region. Hum Pathol 30:581-587, 1999.)

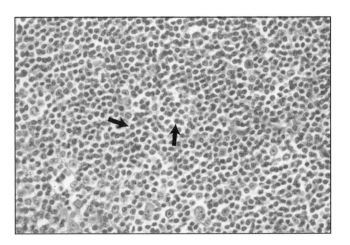

Figure 81–8. Mantle cell lymphoma of the stomach demonstrating the characteristic diffuse infiltration of small- to medium-sized cells with little cytoplasm *(arrows)*. (Courtesy of Mary R. Schwartz, M.D., Baylor College of Medicine.)

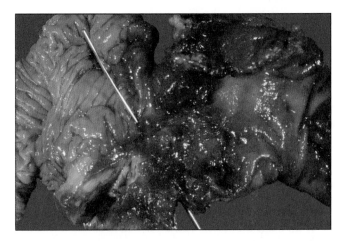

Figure 81–9. Duodenal T-cell lymphoma with circumferential ulceration extending from the pylorus to the ampulla. (Courtesy of Mary R. Schwartz, M.D., Baylor College of Medicine.)

Enteropathy-Type T-Cell Lymphoma

Enteropathy-type T-cell lymphoma (ETL) is an unusual lymphoma variant most commonly localized to the jejunum and ileum.[25,26] A well-defined relationship exists between celiac disease and the development of ETL, and compliance with a gluten-free diet reduces the risk for lymphoma in these patients.[25,27] Perforation is a frequent complication of ETL.[28] Circumferential ulceration of the mucosa is common with this lymphoma, and a heavy eosinophilic and histiocytic infiltrate may obscure tumor cells, which are generally blastic with prominent nucleoli (Fig. 81–9).[29] Adjacent normal bowel generally demonstrates villus atrophy and crypt hyperplasia.[30] ETL exhibits variable tumor markers, which may include CD3, CD4, CD8, and TIA-1.[29] A summary of the immunophenotypes characteristic of various GI lymphomas is shown in Table 81–5.

GRADING

Grading GI lymphomas is important for determination of the prognosis and proper treatment strategy for the disease. GI lymphomas are considered to be low-grade, indolent NHL or high-grade, aggressive NHL by the new WHO classification.[8] Low-grade lymphomas are almost always a derivative of MALT and are thus termed low-grade MALT lymphomas. High-grade lymphomas contain low-grade MALT components in about a third of cases and represent progression of disease; in the remaining two thirds of high-grade tumors, the disease may have progressed from low-grade lesions or may have arisen as a de novo high-grade tumor.[8] Low-grade lymphomas are generally composed of a diffuse infiltrate of small- to medium-sized lymphocytes demonstrating monoclonality. In contrast, high-grade lymphomas appear histologically as large numbers of transformed blasts that

Table 81–5   Common Immunophenotypes of Gastrointestinal Lymphomas

Lymphoma	CD3	CD4	CD5	CD8	CD10	CD20	Bcl-2	Cyclin D1
Diffuse large B-cell lymphoma	–	–	–	–	±	+	±	–
MALT lymphoma	–	–	–	–	–	+	+	–
Mantle cell lymphoma	–	–	+	–	–	+	+	+
Follicular lymphoma	–	–	–	–	+	+	±	–
Burkitt's lymphoma	–	–	–	–	+	+	–	–
Enteropathy-type T-cell lymphoma	+	+	–	+	–	–	–	–

Adapted from El-Zimaity HM, Wotherspoon A, de Jong D: Interobserver variation in the histopathological assessment of MALT/MALT lymphoma: Towards a consensus. Blood Cells Mol Dis 34:6-16, 2005.

Box 81–1   TNM Classification of Gastric Lymphoma

Primary Tumor (T)

TX   Primary tumor cannot be assessed
T0   No evidence of primary tumor
Tis   Carcinoma in situ
T1   Tumor invades the lamina propria or submucosa
T2   Tumor invades the muscularis propria or subserosa
T3   Tumor penetrates the serosa (visceral peritoneum) without invasion of adjacent structures
T4   Tumor invades adjacent structures

Lymph Node (N)

NX   Regional lymph node(s) cannot be assessed
N0   No regional lymph node metastasis
N1   Metastasis in perigastric lymph node(s) within 3 cm of the edge of primary tumors
N2   Metastasis in perigastric lymph node(s) more than 3 cm from the edge of the primary tumor or in lymph nodes along the left gastric, common hepatic, splenic, or celiac arteries

Distant Metastasis

MX   Presence of distant metastasis cannot be assessed
M0   No distant metastasis
M1   Distant metastasis

Adapted from Green FL, Page DL, Fleming ID, et al: AJCC Cancer Staging Manual, 6th ed. New York, Springer-Verlag, 2001.

Box 81–2   Ann Arbor Classification System for Primary Lymphomas

Stage	Definition
I	Involvement of a single extranodal site or a single lymph node region or structure
II	Involvement of two or more lymph node regions or lymph structures on the same side of the diaphragm
III	Involvement of lymph node regions or lymph node structures on both sides of the diaphragm
IV	Diffuse or disseminated involvement of one or more extranodal organs or tissues with or without associated lymph node involvement

Adapted from Koniaris LG, Drugas G, Katzman PJ, et al: Management of gastrointestinal lymphoma. J Am Coll Surg 197:127-141, 2003.

may coalesce in clusters or sheets, ultimately effacing the residual low-grade elements.[8]

STAGING

No consensus has been reached on the optimal system for staging GI lymphoma, but the TNM staging system (as proposed for gastric carcinoma, Box 81–1) is commonly used in surgical applications.[7] The Ann Arbor classification system (Box 81–2) was modified by Musshoff[5] for staging of GI lymphomas (Box 81–3), and both are still commonly applied. Accurate staging often requires evaluation by endoscopy, ultrasonography, chest radiography, bone marrow biopsy, and computed tomography (CT).[6]

DIAGNOSIS

A high index of suspicion is required to make the diagnosis of GI lymphoma because the clinical and radiologic

Musshoff's Criteria for Staging of Gastric Lymphomas

Stage	Definition
IE	Lymphoma restricted to the GI tract on one side of the diaphragm
IE$_1$	Infiltration limited to the mucosa and submucosa
IE$_2$	Lymphoma extending beyond the submucosa
IIE	Lymphoma additionally infiltrating lymph nodes on the same side of the diaphragm
IIE$_1$	Infiltration of regional lymph nodes
IIE$_2$	Infiltration of lymph nodes beyond the regional nodes
IIIE	Lymphoma infiltrating the GI tract and/or the lymph nodes on both sides of the diaphragm
IVE	Localized infiltration of associated lymph nodes together with diffuse or disseminated involvement of extra-GI organs

Adapted from Ahmad A, Govil Y, Frank BB: Gastric mucosa-associated lymphoid tissue lymphoma. Am J Gastroenterol 98:975-986, 2003.

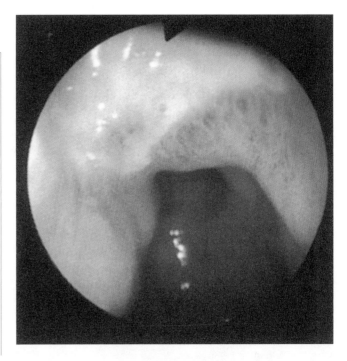

Figure 81–10. Gastric lymphoma manifested as gastric ulceration with atypical erythematous surrounding mucosa. (From Tytgat GNJ: Upper gastrointestinal endoscopy. In Yamada T [ed]: Atlas of Gastroenterology. Philadelphia, Lippincott, Williams & Wilkins, 2003, pp 823-840.)

Figure 81–11. A and **B,** Endoscopic appearances of MALT lymphoma, exophytic type. A large friable, nodular mass with evidence of bleeding is located in the antrum of the stomach. This lesion proved to be a MALT lymphoma. (From Ahmad A, Govil Y, Frank BB: Gastric mucosa-associated lymphoid tissue lymphoma. Am J Gastroenterol 87:975-986, 2003.)

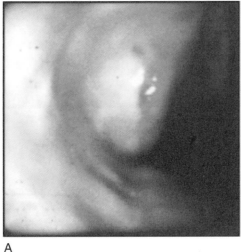

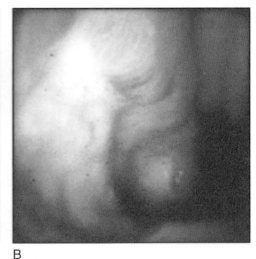

A

B

features are often vague. A careful physical examination should include palpation of all lymph node regions and evaluation of the abdomen for palpable masses or hepatosplenomegaly.[8] Laboratory evaluation should include a complete blood count with differential, routine biochemical assays, lactate dehydrogenase level, and serum protein electrophoresis.[8] Once the diagnosis of GI lymphoma is established, evidence of metastatic disease should be sought by performing an upper airway examination, bone marrow biopsy, and CT of the chest and abdomen to evaluate for lymphadenopathy; any enlarged lymph nodes should be biopsied.[7]

Gastric Lymphoma

The diagnosis of gastric lymphoma is generally made by upper endoscopy and biopsy, with a diagnostic yield of approximately 90%.[31] The most frequent endoscopic finding is ulceration in both low-grade and high-grade lesions (Fig. 81–10). Diffuse infiltration and polypoid masses are also common findings (Fig. 81–11).[31] Such appearances are mistaken for benign conditions such as gastritis or peptic ulcer disease in approximately 50% of patients with low-grade disease and 25% of patients with high-grade disease, thus reinforcing the importance of

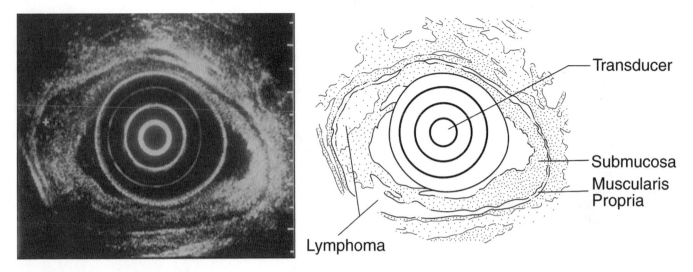

Figure 81–12.   A radial ultrasound image obtained at 12 MHz shows an advanced gastric lymphoma producing diffuse gastric wall thickening involving all layers of the stomach. (From Kimmey MB, Vilmann P: Endoscopic ultrasonography. In Yamada T [ed]: Atlas of Gastroenterology. Philadelphia, Lippincott, Williams & Wilkins, 2003, pp 1042-1054.)

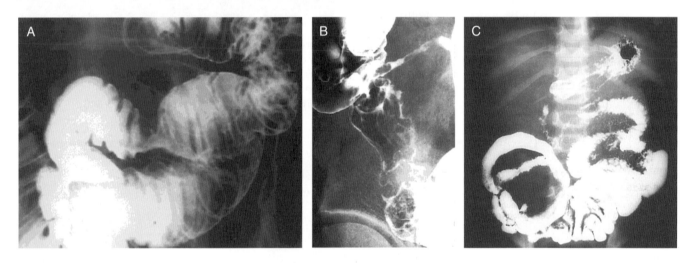

Figure 81–13.   The utility of contrast imaging of gastrointestinal lymphomas. **A,** Double-contrast radiography showing a severely constricted lesion in the ileum that was subsequently diagnosed as MALT lymphoma. **B,** Double-contrast radiography revealing an ulcerative lesion with mucosal destruction in the terminal ileum, later diagnosed as diffuse large B-cell lymphoma. **C,** Small bowel lymphoma complicating celiac disease with a mass in the right iliac fossa. (**A** and **B,** From Nakamura S, Matsumoto T, Takeshita M, et al: A clinicopathologic study of primary small intestine lymphoma: Prognostic significance of mucosa-associated lymphoid tissue–derived lymphoma. Cancer 88:286-294, 2000; **C,** from Ciclitira PJ: Celiac disease. In Yamada T [ed]: Atlas of Gastroenterology. Philadelphia, Lippincott, Williams & Wilkins, 2003, pp 331-340.)

biopsy for tissue diagnosis.[31,32] Endoscopic ultrasound is an important adjunct for detecting intramural tumor infiltration and determining tumor stage and is considered to be more reliable than routine CT scanning (Fig. 81–12). The sensitivity of lymph node detection is more variable, with 45% to 90% accuracy.[31] *H. pylori* testing should be performed on biopsy samples and, if negative, confirmed by serology.[7]

Intestinal Lymphoma

In approximately 30% to 50% of patients, the initial manifestation of small bowel lymphoma is an abdominal emergency.[2] As many as 90% of small bowel lymphomas

are diagnosed intraoperatively, either as part of a treatment plan or to establish a diagnosis.[33] Commonly used preoperative imaging modalities include CT of the abdomen and pelvis, lymphangiography, gallium scanning, upper GI series, barium enema, upper endoscopy, and colonoscopy; the appropriate work-up depends on the suspected location of the tumor, and decisions should be made on an individual basis (Fig. 81–13).[33]

TREATMENT

Initial treatment of both gastric and intestinal lymphomas should take into account *H. pylori* status because approximately 70% to 80% of MALT lymphomas and a variable

| Table 81–6 | *Helicobacter pylori* Treatment |

Regimen 1	Regimen 2	Regimen 3
Omeprazole (20 mg, twice a day)	Omeprazole (20 mg, twice a day)	Omeprazole (20 mg, twice a day)
Amoxicillin (1 g, twice a day)	Metronidazole (500 mg, twice a day)	Tetracycline (500 mg, 4 times a day)
Clarithromycin (500 mg, twice a day)	Clarithromycin (500 mg, twice a day)	Metronidazole (500 mg, 4 times a day)
		Bismuth (525 mg, 4 times a day)

Treatment duration is 10 to 14 days. Regimen 1 is the treatment of choice. Regimen 2 is for penicillin-allergic patients. Other proton pump inhibitors may be substituted at equivalent dosages. Eradication rates exceed 85% with all three regimens.
From Kahl BS: Update: Gastric MALT lymphoma. Curr Opin Oncol 15: 347-352, 2003.

number of DLBCLs regress after *H. pylori* eradication in patients harboring the bacterium.[34] Currently, management of gastric lymphoma takes a predominantly conservative, nonsurgical approach, whereas treatment of many intestinal lymphomas involves a multidisciplinary approach with surgical management being a key component of therapy.

Gastric Lymphoma

Optimal treatment of gastric lymphoma depends on *H. pylori* status, disease stage, degree of large cell transformation, and the presence of genetic mutations such as t(1;14), t(11;18), or Bcl-10 overexpression.[16] The indolent nature of low-grade MALT lymphomas lends itself to conservative treatment, with antibiotic therapy being the sole initial agent, given that the patient can be monitored closely.[35] Approximately 77% of patients with gastric MALT lymphoma will experience complete remission after *H. pylori* eradication.[9] Remission is generally achieved within 12 months of therapy, but a latent period of up to 45 months may occur, with a relapse rate of less than 10%.[9] Current *H. pylori* eradication therapy should include a 2-week regimen of either (1) omeprazole or lansoprazole, clarithromycin, and amoxicillin; (2) omeprazole or lansoprazole, metronidazole, and clarithromycin; or (3) omeprazole or lansoprazole, bismuth, metronidazole, and tetracycline (Table 81–6). Strict endoscopic surveillance with biopsy is recommended 2 months after treatment and at least twice per year for 2 years to monitor for regression.[35] Indicators of possible failure of *H. pylori* eradication include lymphomas of stage IIE and above, stage IE₂ cases that involve the muscularis propria or serosa, lymphomas demonstrating t(11;18)(q21;q21) or t(1;14)(p22;q32) translocations or nuclear expression of Bcl-10, or lymphomas associated with underlying autoimmune disorders.[9] However, eradication should still be pursued in these patients. An algorithm for the management of MALT lymphoma is presented in Figure 81–14.

There are no treatment guidelines for the management of patients who experience antibiotic failure. Surgical therapy is highly curative for localized tumors, but many gastric lymphomas disseminate widely within the mucosa, with frequent tumor relapse in the gastric stump and eventual need for total gastrectomy, which has a significant impact on quality of life.[9] Thus, a multimodal approach consisting of any combination of chemotherapy, radiation therapy, and surgery is common.[4] Chemotherapy with a single alkylating agent, such as cyclophosphamide or chlorambucil, is useful either alone or as an adjunct to surgical resection for *H. pylori* eradication–resistant MALT lymphomas.[9,35] Combination chemotherapy with CHOP (cyclophosphamide, hydroxydaunomycin, Oncovin [vincristine], and prednisone), with the possible addition of rituximab (a chimeric monoclonal antibody against the CD20 B-cell antigen), is preferred for the treatment of high-grade MALT lymphoma or DLBCL.[35-37] MALT lymphomas are also highly radiosensitive, and the use of low-dose localized radiation alone is highly effective in the management of lymphomas unresponsive to *H. pylori* eradication, with a 5-year survival rate of greater than 90%.[9] The combination of surgery and radiotherapy has been advocated for management of low-grade disease, with the addition of chemotherapy for high-grade disease, but no consensus has been reached.[4,36]

Intestinal Lymphoma

Patients with lymphoma of the intestine who are *H. pylori* positive benefit from eradication therapy, as with gastric lymphoma.[11] Initial management of stage I or II small bowel lymphoma should otherwise include segmental surgical resection with regional lymph node excision, regardless of patient age or lymphoma type, given the increased risk for perforation and obstruction associated with these tumors (Fig. 81–15).[2] An aggressive multimodal therapeutic approach combining both surgical resection and polychemotherapy can improve the outcome in patients with all intestinal lymphoma variants, but decisions on the appropriate course of therapy must be made on an individual basis.[11,38] The most commonly applied chemotherapy regimen for patients with intestinal DLBCL or MALT lymphoma is CHOP, with the addition of rituximab in those with mantle cell or follicular variants.[2,11] Treatment of Burkitt's lymphoma is similar to CHOP, with the substitution of methotrexate for prednisone.[2] T-cell lymphomas are notoriously chemotherapy resistant; the best chance for cure in this patient population is achieved by enrollment in clinical trials.[2] Radiotherapy is infrequently used in the treatment of intestinal lymphomas because of a high risk of late complications.[38]

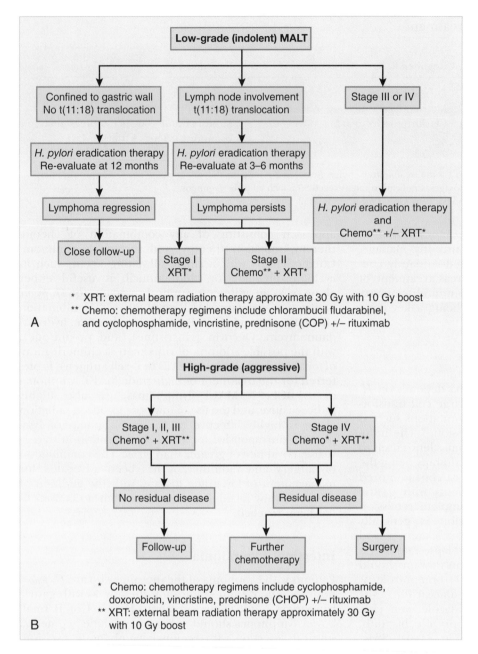

Figure 81–14. Algorithm for the management of primary gastric lymphoma. **A,** Low grade; **B,** high grade. (From Yoon S, Coit DG, Portlock CS, et al: The diminishing role of surgery in the treatment of gastric lymphoma. Ann Surg 240:28-37, 2004.)

PROGNOSIS

Factors affecting prognosis in patients with GI lymphoma include lymphoma type, grade, stage, location, molecular markers, genetic rearrangements, and age of the patient. MALT and MALT-derived lymphomas have the best overall prognosis, regardless of location.[2,11] Gastric lymphomas have a better overall prognosis than intestinal lymphomas do; 5-year survival rates for tumors localized to the stomach are approximately 91% for low-grade, 73% for secondary high-grade, and 56% for primary high-grade tumors, whereas the 5-year survival rate for aggressive small intestinal lymphomas is approximately 25% to 30%.[5,6,39] Intestinal B-cell lymphomas are associated with a better prognosis than those of T-cell origin, with average 5-year survival rates of 75% and 25%, respectively.[5,40]

SUMMARY

GI lymphomas are a diverse group of neoplasms that are often associated with vague symptoms that imitate common intra-abdominal pathologies; a high degree of suspicion is frequently required to make the diagnosis. Many advances have been made in the diagnosis and management of GI lymphomas over the past decade. The importance of *H. pylori* infection to the development of lymphomas has only recently been realized, and this realization has revolutionized treatment of the disease. Gastric lymphoma, once a surgical disease, is now managed conservatively, with *H. pylori* eradication being central to treatment. Although surgery remains the mainstay of treatment of small intestinal lymphoma, *H. pylori* eradication has proved to be a useful adjunct in its management as well.

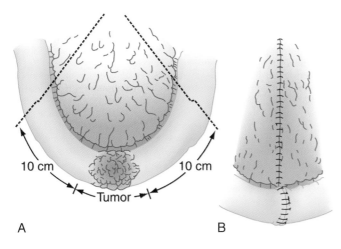

Figure 81–15. Segmental surgical resection of the small intestine. **A,** Malignant tumors should be resected with a wide margin of normal bowel and a wedge of mesentery to remove the immediate draining lymph nodes. **B,** End-to-end anastomosis of the small bowel and repair of the mesentery. (Adapted from Thompson JC: Atlas of Surgery of the Stomach, Duodenum and Small Bowel. St Louis, Mosby–Year Book, 1992, p 299.)

SUGGESTED READINGS

Du MQ, Isaccson PG: Gastric MALT lymphoma: From aetiology to treatment. Lancet Oncol 3:97-104, 2002.

Koniaris LG, Drugas G, Katzman PJ, et al: Management of gastrointestinal lymphoma. J Am Coll Surg 197:127-141, 2003.

Nakamura S, Matsumoto T, Takeshita M, et al: A clinicopathologic study of primary small intestine lymphoma: Prognostic significance of mucosa-associated lymphoid tissue–derived lymphoma. Cancer 88:286-294, 2000.

Rooney N, Dogan A: Gastrointestinal lymphoma. Curr Diagn Pathol 10:69-87, 2004.

Yoon SS, Coit DG, Portlock CS, et al: The diminishing role of surgery in the treatment of gastric lymphoma. Ann Surg 240:28-37, 2004.

REFERENCES

1. Cancer Facts and Figures 2005. American Cancer Society, Atlanta.
2. Koniaris LG, Drugas G, Katzman PJ, et al: Management of gastrointestinal lymphoma. J Am Coll Surg 197:127-141, 2003.
3. Pandey M, Wadhwa MK, Patel HP, et al: Malignant lymphoma of the gastrointestinal tract. Eur J Surg Oncol 25:164-167, 1999.
4. Ahmad A, Govil Y, Frank BB: Gastric mucosa-associated lymphoid tissue lymphoma. Am J Gastroenterol 98:975-986, 2003.
5. Gill SS, Heuman DM, Mihas AA: Small intestinal neoplasms. J Clin Gastroenterol 33:267-282, 2001.
6. Al-Akwaa AM, Siddiqui N, Al-Mofleh IA: Primary gastric lymphoma. World J Gastroenterol 10:5-11, 2004.
7. Mercer DW, Robinson EK: Stomach. In Townsend CM (ed): Sabiston's Textbook of Surgery: The Biological Basis of Modern Surgical Practice. Philadelphia, Elsevier, 2004, pp 1265-1321.
8. Yoon SS, Coit DG, Portlock CS, et al: The diminishing role of surgery in the treatment of gastric lymphoma. Ann Surg 240:28-37, 2004.
9. Du MQ, Isaccson PG: Gastric MALT lymphoma: From aetiology to treatment. Lancet Oncol 3:97-104, 2002.
10. Horton KM, Fishman EK: Multidetector-row computed tomography and 3-dimensional computed tomography imaging of small bowel neoplasms: Current concept in diagnosis. J Comput Assist Tomogr 28:106-116, 2004.
11. Nakamura S, Matsumoto T, Takeshita M, et al: A clinicopathologic study of primary small intestine lymphoma: Prognostic significance of mucosa-associated lymphoid tissue–derived lymphoma. Cancer 88:286-294, 2000.
12. Koch P, del Valle F, Berdel WE, et al: Primary gastrointestinal non-Hodgkin's lymphoma: I. Anatomic and histologic distribution, clinical features, and survival data of 371 patients registered in the German Multicenter Study GIT NHL 01/92. J Clin Oncol 19:3861-3873, 2001.
13. Rooney N, Dogan A: Gastrointestinal lymphoma. Curr Diagn Pathol 10:69-78, 2004.
14. Lossos IS, Jones CD, Warnke R, et al: Expression of a single gene, BCL-6, strongly predicts survival in patients with diffuse large B-cell lymphoma. Blood 98:945-951, 2001.
15. Gascoyne RD, Krajewska M, Krajewski S, et al: Prognostic significance of Bax protein expression in diffuse aggressive non-Hodgkin's lymphoma. Blood 90:3173-3178, 1997.
16. Skinnider BF, Horsman DE, Dupuis B, et al: Bcl-6 and Bcl-2 protein expression in diffuse large B-cell lymphoma and follicular lymphoma: Correlation with 3q27 and 18q21 chromosomal abnormalities. Hum Pathol 30:803-808, 1999.
17. Kahl BS: Update: Gastric MALT lymphoma. Curr Opin Oncol 15:347-352, 2003.
18. Correa P: Gastric neoplasia. Curr Gastroenterol Rep 4:463-470, 2002.
19. El-Zimaity HM, Wotherspoon A, de Jong D: Interobserver variation in the histopathological assessment of MALT/MALT lymphoma: Towards a consensus. Blood Cells Mol Dis 34:6-16, 2005.
20. Nardone G, Morgner A: *Helicobacter pylori* and gastric malignancies. Helicobacter 8(Suppl 1):44-52, 2003.
21. Pienkowska-Grela B, Witkowska A, Grygalewicz B, et al: Frequent aberrations of chromosome 8 in aggressive B-cell non-Hodgkin lymphoma. Cancer Genet Cytogenet 156:114-121, 2005.
22. Rohatiner AZ, Lister TA: The clinical course of follicular lymphoma. Best Pract Res Clin Haematol 18:1-10, 2005.
23. Bentley G, Palutke M, Mohamed AN: Variant t(14;18) in malignant lymphoma: A report of seven cases. Cancer Genet Cytogenet 157:12-17, 2005.
24. Hashimoto Y, Nakamura N, Kuze T, et al: Multiple lymphomatous polyposis of the gastrointestinal tract is a heterogenous group that includes mantle cell lymphoma and follicular lymphoma: Analysis of somatic mutation of immunoglobulin heavy chain gene variable region. Hum Pathol 30:581-587, 1999.
25. Catassi C, Fabiani E, Corrao G, et al: Risk of non-Hodgkin lymphoma in celiac disease. JAMA 287:1413-1419, 2002.
26. Daum S, Ullrich R, Heise W, et al: Intestinal non-Hodgkin's lymphoma: A multicenter prospective clinical study from the German Study Group on Intestinal non-Hodgkin's Lymphoma. J Clin Oncol 21:2740-2746, 2003.
27. Howdle PD, Jalal PK, Holmes GK, et al: Primary small-bowel malignancy in the UK and its association with coeliac disease. QJM 96:345-353, 2003.
28. Kataoka I, Arima F, Nishimoto J, et al: Enteropathy-type T-cell lymphoma showing repeated small bowel rupture and refractoriness to chemotherapy: A case report. Jpn J Clin Oncol 32:546-549, 2002.
29. Gale J, Simmonds PD, Mead GM, et al: Enteropathy-type intestinal T-cell lymphoma: Clinical features and treatment of 31 patients in a single center. J Clin Oncol 18:795-803, 2000.
30. Daum S, Weiss D, Hummel M, et al: Frequency of clonal intraepithelial T lymphocyte proliferations in enteropathy-type intestinal T cell lymphoma, coeliac disease, and refractory sprue. Gut 49:804-812, 2001.
31. Boot H, de Jong D: Gastric lymphoma: The revolution of the past decade. Scand J Gastroenterol Suppl 236:27-36, 2002.
32. Ernst M, Stein H, Ludwig D, et al: Surgical therapy of gastrointestinal non-Hodgkin's lymphomas. Eur J Surg Oncol 22:177-181, 1996.
33. Ha CS, Cho MJ, Allen PK, et al: Primary non-Hodgkin lymphoma of the small bowel. Radiology 211:183-187, 1999.

34. Sepulveda AR, Coelho LG: *Helicobacter pylori* and gastric malignancies. Helicobacter 7(Suppl 1):37-42, 2002.

35. Zucca E, Conconi A, Cavalli F: Treatment of extranodal lymphomas. Best Pract Res Clin Haematol 15:533-547, 2002.

36. Couderc B, Dujols JP, Mokhtari F, et al: The management of adult aggressive non-Hodgkin's lymphomas. Crit Rev Oncol Hematol 35:33-48, 2000.

37. Coiffier B, Lepage E, Briere J, et al: CHOP chemotherapy plus rituximab compared with CHOP alone in elderly patients with diffuse large-B-cell lymphoma. N Engl J Med 346:235-242, 2002.

38. Geara F: Radiotherapy for gastrointestinal lymphomas: Indications and techniques. Cancer Radiother 3:141-148, 1999.

39. Kocher M, Muller RP, Ross D, et al: Radiotherapy for treatment of localized gastrointestinal non-Hodgkin's lymphoma. Radiother Oncol 42:37-41, 1997.

40. Rodriguez J, Munsell M, Yazji S, et al: Impact of high-dose chemotherapy on peripheral T-cell lymphomas. J Clin Oncol 19:3766-3770, 2001.

82

Surgical Conditions of the Small Intestine in Infants and Children

Marshall Z. Schwartz • Ahmed Mami

Conditions of the small intestine in infants and children can be categorized into congenital abnormalities and acquired abnormalities. These two categories combined represent the majority of abdominal surgical emergencies in infants and young children. They are also the major cause of mortality. The advent of new and better imagining technologies has led to more precise and earlier diagnosis. For example, detailed fetal ultrasonography and fetal magnetic resonance imaging are more precise than they were 5 to 10 years ago. In addition, new minimally invasive surgical approaches have allowed for more rapid recovery.

Congenital abnormalities refer to developmental anomalies such as malrotation. Acquired abnormalities are entities that evolve after birth.

Congenital abnormalities covered in this chapter include malrotation, intestinal atresia, duplications, meconium obstruction, and omphalomesenteric duct remnants. Acquired lesions include necrotizing enterocolitis and intussusception.

Over the past 8 to 10 years two significant changes have occurred in the evaluation and treatment of many of the conditions discussed in this chapter. Imaging technology and techniques have continued to improve, which allows for more precise diagnosis. Although it could be stated that the usual approach to surgical problems in children is minimally invasive (i.e., through very small incisions), the use of laparoscopic techniques with very small ports (3 mm) and instruments has become common in pediatric surgery.

MALROTATION

The term *malrotation* refers to incomplete midgut rotation and fixation during in utero development. Thus, a more appropriate term would be *incomplete rotation*. The midgut, which is supplied by the superior mesenteric vessels and extends from the duodenojejunal junction to the midtransverse colon, remains unfixed and suspended on a narrow mesentery. This abnormal anatomy predisposes the midgut to life-threatening volvulus. Although this condition was first described by Mall in 1898,[1] it was William Ladd who described the currently used principles of malrotation repair in 1936.[2]

The primitive gut is recognized as a straight tube in the fourth week of embryologic development (Fig. 82–1). Rapid growth plus elongation of the midgut starting in the fifth week leads to herniation of the midgut with the superior mesenteric vessels as its stalk. This results in the formation of a physiologic umbilical hernia at the base of the umbilical cord. The midgut undergoes 270-degree counterclockwise rotation around the superior mesenteric vessels. This initial rotation results in the normal position of the duodenojejunal flexure in the left upper quadrant at the level of the gastric antrum. The duodenojejunal flexure becomes fixed to the posterior abdominal wall by the ligament of Treitz. As a result of this rotation and fixation, the third portion of the duodenum lies posterior to the superior mesenteric artery (SMA). In the 10th week the herniated intestinal loop begins to return to the abdominal cavity. The cecocolic loop undergoes another 270-degree counterclockwise rotation around the SMA, which leads to the normal position of the cecum in the right lower quadrant. Subsequently, the ascending colon and descending colon become fixed to the posterior abdominal wall. During the fourth and fifth weeks of gestation, the small intestine mesentery attaches itself to the posterior abdominal wall in a broad base extending diagonally from the duodenojejunal flexure to the cecum.

There are several degrees of rotational abnormality. Nonrotation is characterized by failure of counterclockwise rotation after return of the midgut to the

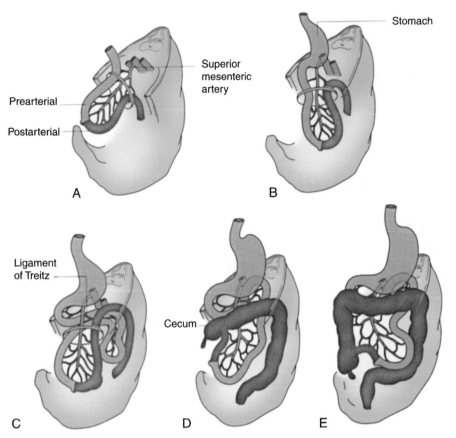

Prearterial

Postarterial

Superior mesenteric artery

A

Stomach

B

Ligament of Treitz

Cecum

C

D

E

Figure 82–1. Normal midgut rotation is shown beginning in the 5th gestational week **(A)** through completion of the process in the 12th week **(E)**. (From Ashcraft KW, Holder TM [eds]: Pediatric Surgery. Philadelphia, WB Saunders, 1999.)

abdominal cavity (Fig. 82–2A). In incomplete rotation, the counterclockwise rotation is arrested at around 180 degrees. These are the most common forms of malrotation. The small intestine lies on the right side with the duodenojejunal flexure to the right of the vertebral column, and the duodenum has a corkscrew configuration. The large intestine lies on the left side with the cecum at abnormal locations, usually in the midline. Other forms of fixation anomalies may be due to failure of fixation of the ascending colon in the right hypochondrium. Associated with this abnormal fixation is a narrow intestinal mesentery and Ladd's bands. Ladd's bands represent the retroperitoneal attachments that normally fix the cecum and ascending colon to the posterior abdominal wall. Because the right colon is more medial, the bands extend across the duodenum from the right upper quadrant to the cecum and ascending colon. In reverse rotation, part of the rotation occurs in a clockwise direction around the SMA (see Fig. 82–2D). The duodenum assumes an anterior position and the colon lies posterior to the duodenum and the SMA. If the counterclockwise rotation extends beyond 270 degrees, the cecum comes to rest in the left hypochondrium position (see Fig. 82–2E). This rare form is called hyper-rotation. Other forms of fixation anomalies may be due to failure of fixation of the ascending or descending colon to the posterior abdominal wall. In this condition, the small intestine is at risk of entrapment in the potential space between the mesocolon and the posterior abdominal wall and is referred to as a mesocolic or paraduodenal

hernia (see Fig. 82–2F). Lesser degrees of malrotation may affect only the cecocolic loop. Although the duodenum may lie in a normal position, the cecum remains unfixed and in an abnormal position with Ladd's bands. These patients are at risk for duodenal obstruction and cecal volvulus.

Patients with malrotation have a 30% to 62% risk of having associated anomalies, and most involve the gastrointestinal tract.[3] Five percent to 26% are associated with duodenal or other small intestinal atresias. Other less common anomalies include imperforate anus, cardiac anomalies, duodenal web, Meckel's diverticulum, and trisomy 21. Rare associations include biliary atresia, esophageal atresia, mesenteric cyst, Hirschsprung's disease, and craniosynostosis. Malrotation is always present in infants with congenital diaphragmatic hernia, omphalocele, and gastroschisis.

Malrotation is documented in 0.5% of autopsy studies,[4] although the incidence of clinically symptomatic malrotation is estimated to be 1 in 6000 live births.[5] Malrotation may initially be recognized at any age, but in approximately 90% of patients symptoms develop before 1 year of age, with 50% to 75% appearing within the first month of life.[6-8]

Malrotation can be totally asymptomatic and discovered only during work-up for an unrelated condition or during an autopsy examination. The initial symptoms depend on the cause. Neonates typically have bilious emesis, which may be the only initial symptom of midgut volvulus. If the diagnosis is delayed and the bowel

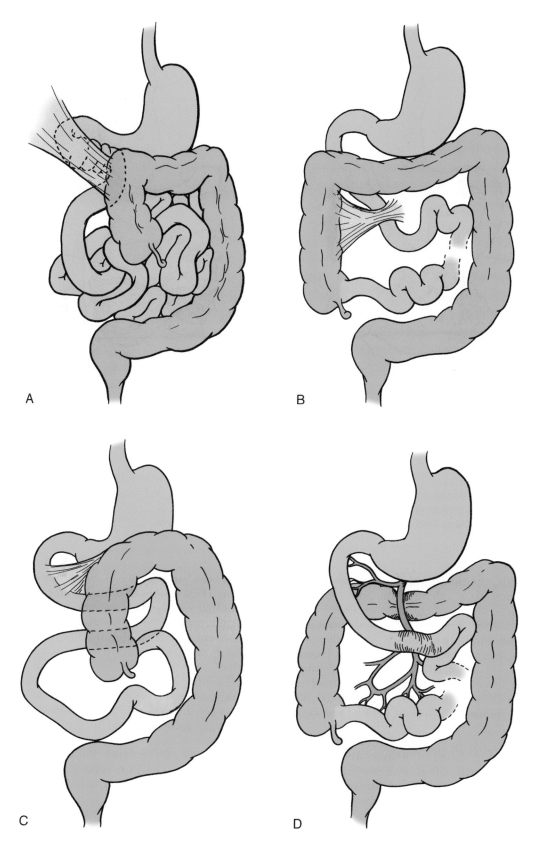

Figure 82–2. **A,** Complete nonrotation of the midgut. Neither the duodenojejunal junction nor the cecum has rotated around the superior mesenteric artery (SMA). All of the small bowel lies to the right of the SMA, and all of the colon lies to the left. This anomaly is the most frequent type of malrotation, and the risk for midgut volvulus is ever present. **B,** Nonrotation of the duodenojejunal junction with normal rotation of the cecum. This abnormality may be manifested clinically as duodenal obstruction as a result of abnormal mesenteric (Ladd's) bands from the colon across the anterior duodenum. **C,** Normal rotation of the duodenojejunal junction with nonrotation of the cecum. These patients are at risk for midgut volvulus. **D,** Reverse rotation of the duodenojejunal junction passing ventral rather than dorsal to the SMA, followed by reverse rotation of the colon (the cecum rotating dorsal rather than ventral to the SMA). This abnormality may be manifested clinically as obstruction of the transverse colon.

Continued

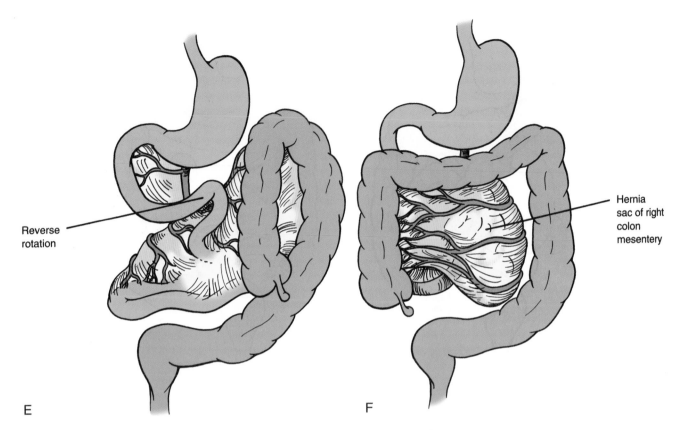

Reverse
rotation

Hernia
sac of right
colon
mesentery

E

F

Figure 82–2, cont'd.   E, Reverse rotation of the duodenojejunal junction (passing ventral rather than dorsal to the SMA), followed by normal rotation of the colon. **F,** A paraduodenal hernia sac is created by the mesentery of the colon as the cecum passes over the small intestine to lie in the right lower quadrant. (From Oldham KT, Colombani PM, Foglia RP [eds]: Surgery of Infants and Children: Scientific Principles and Practice. Philadelphia, Lippincott-Raven, 1997.)

becomes ischemic, the infant will demonstrate systemic signs such as increasing lethargy with poor perfusion, temperature instability, cardiopulmonary compromise, and low urine output. The patient may deteriorate to septic shock and multiorgan failure with other signs such as melena, hematemesis, and peritonitis. Hematologic studies may show metabolic acidosis, thrombocytopenia, and leukopenia. Malrotation without volvulus may be manifested as chronic, vague abdominal pain, with or without intermittent bilious emesis, and failure to thrive.

Successful treatment of malrotation depends on early diagnosis. The acute onset of bilious vomiting in a neonate is a sign of malrotation until proved otherwise. It demands immediate radiologic evaluation. The gold standard test for the diagnosis of malrotation is an upper gastrointestinal contrast study. Malrotation is diagnosed by an abnormal position of the ligament of Treitz. The normal location is typically to the left of the vertebral column and posterior to the stomach. In the absence of a ligament of Treitz, the duodenum remains to the right of the spine. Another possibility is that the duodenojejunal flexure crosses to the left of the vertebral column but lies below the level of the gastric antrum. Volvulus can be diagnosed by contrast-enhanced upper gastrointestinal series showing a corkscrew configuration of the upper portion of the small intestine (Fig. 82–3) or a

"bird's beak" appearance at the third portion of the duodenum (Fig. 82–4). It must be emphasized that plain abdominal radiographs are not helpful in ruling in or out midgut volvulus.[4] The abdominal radiograph may show a wide range of abnormalities, including a dilated stomach and proximal duodenum, similar to a "double-bubble" sign, a paucity of abdominal gas, or dilated bowel loops with multiple air-fluid levels, or the radiograph may appear normal. A contrast enema study is not part of the work-up for malrotation. The presence of a normally located cecum in the right lower quadrant does not rule out malrotation. Abdominal ultrasonography may be used to study the position of the superior mesenteric vein (SMV) in relation to the SMA. Normally, the SMV lies to the right of the SMA. An abnormal position of the SMV in relation to the SMA may indicate the presence of malrotation with volvulus.

Children who are acutely ill with peritonitis need emergency surgery without radiologic studies. Patients who are symptomatic from volvulus as a result of malrotation should undergo nasogastric decompression, be resuscitated with intravenous fluid, and receive broad-spectrum antibiotics. Blood samples should be sent for laboratory analysis, including a complete blood count and type and crossmatching. The patient should be taken to the operating room urgently. Unnecessary delay may further compromise the bowel and lead to infarction.

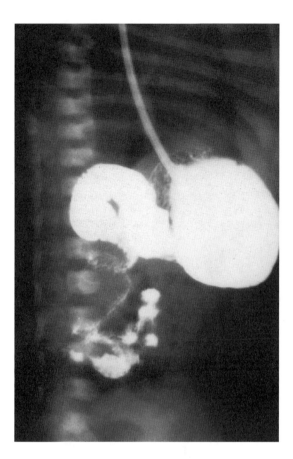

Figure 82–3. Midgut volvulus. A spot film from an upper gastrointestinal series demonstrates a distended, contrast-filled stomach with corkscrew configuration of the proximal part of the small bowel. (Courtesy of A. B. Campbell, MD, St. Christopher's Hospital for Children.)

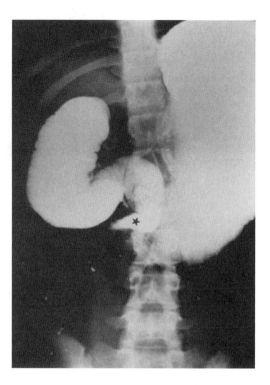

Figure 82–4. This upper gastrointestinal contrast study shows malrotation with volvulus. The "beak" is illustrated by the *asterisk*. Note the malposition of the distal duodenum as well. (From Oldham KT: Pediatric abdomen. In Greenfield LJ, Mulholland M, Oldham KT, et al [eds]: Surgery: Scientific Principles and Practice. Philadelphia, Lippincott-Raven, 1997.)

Children with vague chronic symptoms or children who are symptom-free should undergo elective correction.

The standard approach to correction of malrotation has been via a right upper quadrant transverse incision. However, a Ladd procedure in the absence of volvulus can be performed laparoscopically as long as there is no question of bowel compromise. The entire small intestine is eviscerated and carefully examined for the presence of volvulus (Fig. 82–5). If volvulus is present, it should be reduced by counterclockwise rotation as necessary because volvulus usually occurs in a clockwise direction. The bowel is assessed for viability. Mild to moderately ischemic bowel resumes its normal color after reduction of the volvulus. Bowel with uncertain viability should be wrapped with warm moist gauze sponges for at least 15 minutes. Frankly gangrenous bowel should be resected and a stoma or stomas fashioned. Bowel with marginal viability should be left in continuity if possible with a view to perform a second-look operation 24 to 36 hours later. At the second operation any necrotic bowel should become obvious, and further resections may be necessary. After reducing the volvulus if it is present, Ladd's bands, which represent the posterior peritoneal attachments of the right colon that cross over the duodenum, should be divided on the lateral aspect of the duodenum (Fig. 82–6). Widening of the mesenteric base is necessary, and the duodenum is mobilized and straightened by dividing the abnormal ligament of Treitz and Ladd's bands. The duodenum is carefully examined for intrinsic obstruction. If there is any doubt, a balloon catheter can be passed transorally and manipulated into the upper jejunum. An inability to pass the catheter or to pull the catheter back with the balloon inflated indicates the presence of intrinsic obstruction. Incidental appendectomy should be performed to avoid diagnostic confusion in the future because the cecum will be placed in the left lower quadrant. The intestine is returned to the abdominal cavity, starting with the duodenum and proximal jejunum, which are placed on the right side, and ending with the terminal ileum and cecum, which are placed in the left hypochondrium.

Postoperative care of these patients includes nasogastric decompression and intravenous fluid until return of bowel function. Prolonged ileus is not unusual postoperatively, especially if volvulus was present. Postoperative complications include bleeding and recurrent volvulus. The latter is rare if the initial operation is technically complete. The most serious complication is short-gut syndrome as a result of volvulus and bowel necrosis requiring extensive small bowel resection.

The operative mortality of Ladd's procedure ranges from 3% to 9%,[3] with the higher mortality being

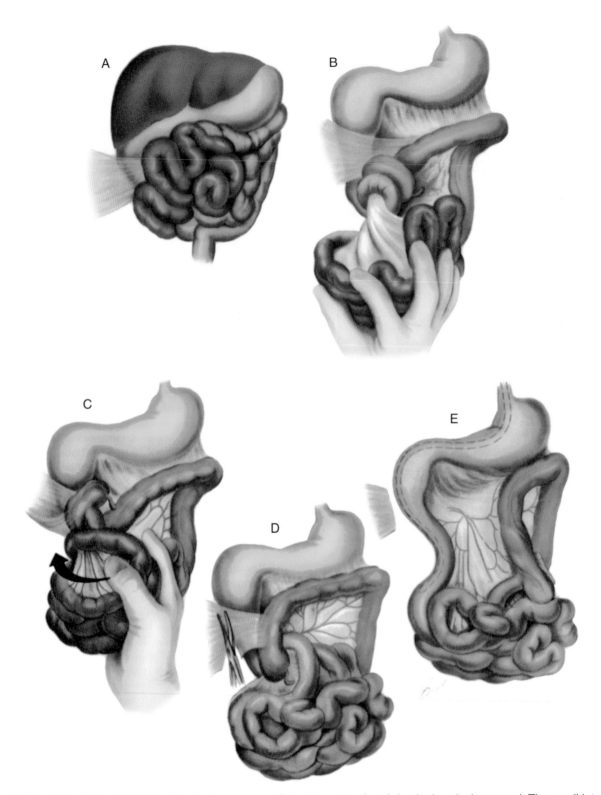

Figure 82–5. Malrotation of the intestine. **A,** Appearance of the viscera as the abdominal cavity is opened. The small intestines are seen at once and seem to hide the colon. Vascular compromise of the intestine may be obvious. **B,** The entire intestinal mass is delivered out of the wound and drawn downward to reveal the base of the mesentery. Coils of intestine or ascending colon are wrapped around the root of an incompletely anchored mesentery. The volvulus has taken place in a clockwise direction. The descending duodenum is dilated because of extrinsic pressure from Ladd's bands or peritoneal folds that cross it. **C,** The volvulus is reduced by taking the entire intestinal mass in the hand and rotating it counterclockwise (in most cases). **D,** With reduction of the volvulus, the cecum lies in the right paravertebral gutter. The peritoneal folds from the cecum obstruct the duodenum. The folds are incised close to the lateral serosal border of the duodenum. The underlying superior mesenteric pedicle is identified and carefully preserved. **E,** Appearance of the intestines and ascending colon at the end of surgery. The duodenum descends along the right gutter. The small intestines lie on the right side of the abdomen, and the cecum and ascending colon are in the midline or left side of the abdomen. The superior mesenteric artery and its branches are left exposed as shown. A nasogastric tube has been passed into the jejunum to exclude intrinsic obstruction. (From O'Neill JA Jr, Rowe MI, Grosfeld JL, et al [eds]: Pediatric Surgery. St Louis, Mosby–Year Book, 1998.)

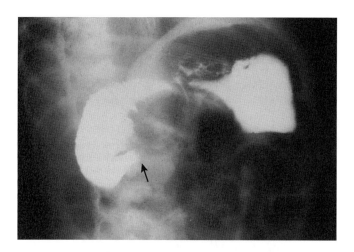

Figure 82–6. Ladd's bands. This upper gastrointestinal contrast study demonstrates the site of Ladd's bands. Cutoff of contrast is marked by an *arrow*.

associated with complete small intestinal necrosis, prematurity, or other serious congenital abnormalities.[9]

ATRESIA AND STENOSIS

Atresia and stenosis are among the most common causes of neonatal intestinal obstruction.[10] The reported incidence of jejunoileal atresia is about 1 in 1000 live births with a range of 1 in 300 to 1500 live births.[11-15] The most widely accepted cause of these defects is a localized intrauterine vascular accident leading to necrosis and resorption of the affected segments.[13] The vascular event can be thrombosis, embolism, intussusception, or volvulus. The general acceptance of this etiology is based in part on animal studies in which in utero occlusion of mesenteric vessels led to atresia.[13,16] The association of atresia with certain disease states such as gastroschisis and midgut volvulus adds weight to the ischemia/necrosis theory.[17]

The gender ratio is equal. Jejunal atresia is slightly more common than ileal atresia. In 80% to 90% of cases the atresia is isolated. However, in up to 20% of cases atresias are multiple.[10,18] Hence, it is important to evaluate the whole intestine for other atresias. In one study, about a third of patients had associated anomalies, predominantly gastrointestinal.[19] An important comorbid condition that can be overlooked in infants with jejunoileal atresia is cystic fibrosis. The reported incidence is 10% to 20%.[18-21] White infants with jejunoileal atresia have more than 210 times the risk for cystic fibrosis than white infants in the general population do.[22] These children should be screened routinely for cystic fibrosis.[20,23]

Small intestine atresias have been classified into four types (Fig. 82–7), and the outcome can vary significantly depending on the type. Intestinal atresia is being diagnosed more frequently with prenatal ultrasonography.[19] The more proximal small bowel atresias can be associated with maternal polyhydramnios as a result of

decreased fetal intestinal absorption of amniotic fluid.[24] Ultrasonography may show dilated, fluid-filled intestinal loops. Antenatal diagnosis permits earlier recognition, which allows for more effective parental counseling and appropriate preparation for surgical intervention postnatally.[25] At the time of delivery, bile staining of amniotic fluid is associated with intestinal obstruction.[26]

Infants with atresia or stenosis usually have bilious vomiting on the first day of life. However, in about 20% of cases, the vomiting may be delayed for 24 hours.[13,27] The higher the obstruction, the earlier the vomiting. Abdominal distention is more pronounced with distal obstruction. More than 60% of these infants fail to pass meconium in the first day of life.[10,13] They may have grayish mucoid contents in the rectal vault. Other associated symptoms and signs include fever, dehydration, aspiration pneumonia, and unconjugated hyperbilirubinemia. The latter may be due to impairment of the enterohepatic circulation.[18] Examination of the abdomen may also reveal signs of peritonitis or ischemia, such as tenderness, edema, and erythema of the abdominal wall. The clinical manifestations of intestinal stenosis are more subtle, with intermittent partial bowel obstruction, malnutrition, and failure to thrive. The initial findings in infants with intestinal stenosis may be unremarkable, but higher-grade bowel obstruction ultimately develops and requires surgical intervention.

Abdominal radiographs show gas- and fluid-filled bowel loops with absence of gas distally (Fig. 82–8A). In proximal obstruction, there are fewer distended bowel loops. Distal ileal atresia may be difficult to differentiate from meconium ileus or colonic obstruction. In patients with atresia or meconium ileus, a contrast enema will show a microcolon and small, unused distal ileum (see Fig. 82–8B). In meconium ileus, some of the contrast may outline the impacted stool and thus make the diagnosis. In colonic atresia, contrast will not demonstrate the cecum or ileocecal valve. Ten percent of patients with atresia have meconium peritonitis from in utero bowel perforation.[10,18]

Management of infants with atresia includes intravenous fluid, decompression of the stomach, withholding of enteral feeding, and administration of antibiotics. After resuscitation the infant is taken to the operating room for exploratory laparotomy. The goals of the operation are to restore intestinal continuity after resection of the atretic segment while preserving intestinal length. Through a right upper or lower quadrant transverse incision, the small bowel is eviscerated. A transition point is usually identified. Normal saline is injected distal to the transition point and milked more distally to rule out other obstructions. If the proximal dilated bowel appears ischemic and nonviable, it should be resected. Resection of massively dilated proximal bowel may expedite bowel recovery postoperatively. A tapering procedure may be performed in the proximal bowel segment. It is important to note that in atresia the proximal blind end is dilated and hypertrophied with ineffective peristaltic activity.[28] It is also deficient in mucosal enzymes and muscular adenosine triphosphate.[29] Although dysmotility resolves after removal of the obstruction, recovery may take longer in patients with very dilated bowel loops. The

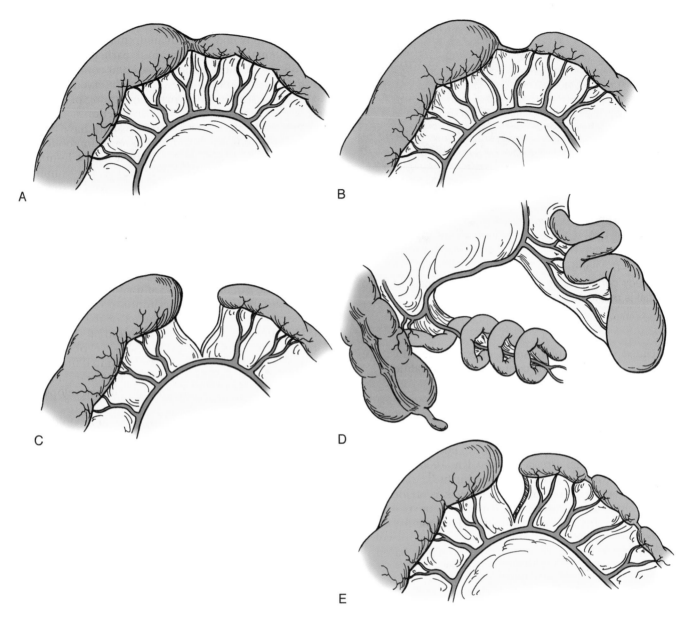

Figure 82–7. Classification of intestinal atresia. **A,** Type I, membranous atresia with intact bowel and mesentery. **B,** Type II, blind ends separated by a fibrous cord. **C,** Type IIIa, blind ends separated by a V-shaped mesenteric defect. **D,** Type IIIb, "apple peel" atresia. **E,** Type IV, multiple atresias ("string of sausages"). (From Oldham KT, Colombani PM, Foglia RP [eds]: Surgery of Infants and Children: Scientific Principles and Practice. Philadelphia, Lippincott-Raven, 1997.)

tapering procedure can be performed by resecting a part of the antimesenteric side of the bowel with a stapling device. Another technique to reduce the caliber of the proximal part of the bowel is imbrication of the antimesenteric side with running suture. Studies suggest that bowel plication may prevent disturbed intestinal transit postoperatively.[30] Continuity of the bowel is achieved by an end-to-oblique anastomosis after opening the distal part of the bowel and making a longitudinal antimesenteric incision to accommodate the difference in size between the proximal and distal bowel loops. Simple atresias of the small intestine can be managed with "laparoscopic assistance" by identifying the anatomy laparoscopically, bringing the atretic ends out through an enlarged umbilical port incision, performing the anastomosis extraperitoneally, and replacing it back through the umbilicus.

Infants with gastroschisis and intestinal atresia present a special problem. Atresia may be missed initially because of thick peel obscuring the bowel. It is preferred that the gastroschisis defect be repaired initially and the atresias be addressed after a period of bowel decompression and parenteral nutrition to give the peritoneal and bowel inflammation time to resolve. However, early enterostomy may be needed, especially in patients with complicated distal atresia.[31,32]

Postoperatively, parenteral nutrition is started pending return of bowel function. Proximal atresias tend

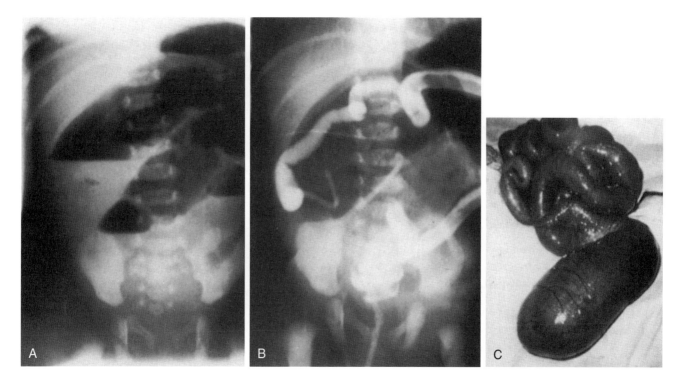

Figure 82–8. Ileal atresia. **A,** Erect abdominal radiograph showing distended intestinal loops with air-fluid levels. **B,** Contrast enema demonstrating a microcolon (unused), suggestive of small bowel obstruction. **C,** Atresia of the ileum (type IIIa) at laparotomy. (From O'Neill JA Jr, Rowe MI, Grosfeld IL, et al [eds]: Pediatric Surgery. St Louis, Mosby-Year Book, 1998.)

to take a longer time before return of bowel motility. Enteral feeding is started when the infant shows signs of return of bowel function. Passing of gas and stool together with decreasing and clearing of the gastric aspirate is a good indicator of return of bowel function.

The prognosis in these patients is excellent, with survival rates of 90%, as opposed to a mortality rate of 90% before 1952.[13] The reduction in mortality is probably due to improvements in neonatal care, nutrition, and surgical techniques. Anastomotic leak or stricture requiring surgical intervention develops in 10% to 15% of infants.[33] These patients are also at risk for adhesive bowel obstruction and necrotizing enterocolitis (NEC); however, these complications are infrequent. Extensive resection of the bowel can lead to short-bowel syndrome. Adaptation and recovery of bowel motility take 12 to 24 months in these patients.

DUPLICATIONS AND CYSTS OF THE SMALL INTESTINE

Three forms of cystic structures can be associated with the small intestine. Abnormalities that are in direct contact with the small intestinal wall are referred to as duplications because they contain all three layers of bowel. Two forms of duplication can occur. The most common is a spherical structure referred to as a *cystic duplication* (Fig. 82–9). These lesions do not have communication with the lumen of the normal small intestine.

Another form of duplication is a *tubular duplication* (Fig. 82–10).

These duplications parallel the normal bowel lumen and share a common wall and blood supply with the adjacent bowel. They have a higher incidence of communication with the existing lumen of the small intestine and have a significant incidence of ectopic gastric mucosa.[34]

The second category of cystic structures consists of cysts that arise in the mesentery of the bowel, whereas the third category includes cysts that involve the omentum. Several theories have been proposed to explain the origin of these structures, but because of the numerous types of cysts in and around the small intestine, there is no common theory that best explains all of them.

The small intestine is the most common location for enteric duplications and accounts for more than half of such anomalies.[35] Twenty percent of the remaining duplications occur in the thorax and 5% are found at the junction of the thorax and abdomen. Seventy-five percent of enteric cysts do not communicate with the lumen of the bowel.[36] It is important to emphasize that both tubular and cystic duplications of the bowel share a common wall and a common blood supply with the adjacent normal intestine. It is also relevant that 25% of duplications contain ectopic tissue.[37] The most common ectopic tissue is gastric mucosa.

The clinical findings vary significantly, depending on the size and site of the duplication or cyst. Cystic duplications of the bowel are typically manifested as partial small bowel obstruction as a result of the cyst gradually

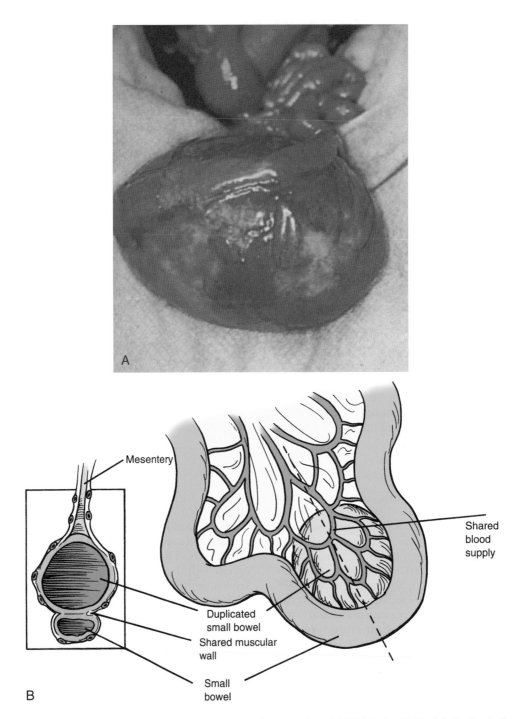

Figure 82–9. A, Large cystic duplication of the small intestine. (From Ashcraft KW, Holder TM [eds]: Pediatric Surgery. Philadelphia, WB Saunders, 1999.) **B,** Small bowel duplication in cross section demonstrating the common wall, shared blood supply, and intramesenteric location. (From Oldham KT, Colombani PM, Foglia RP [eds]: Surgery of Infants and Children: Scientific Principles and Practice. Philadelphia, Lippincott-Raven, 1997.)

enlarging and compressing the adjacent lumen. Tubular duplications of the bowel may likewise cause bowel obstruction. However, bleeding is also a common manifestation because of the high incidence of ectopic gastric mucosa with secondary ulcer formation. Very large mesenteric or omental cysts can be manifested as a palpable mass producing vague abdominal symptoms or pain.

Treatment of duplications of the small intestine depends on the specific findings and circumstances. Cystic duplications of the small intestine usually require resection of the adjacent bowel because of the shared common wall and blood supply. Tubular duplications that are relatively short (under 20 cm) can be resected along with the adjacent intestine. If the tubular duplication is extensive, which would result in major loss of

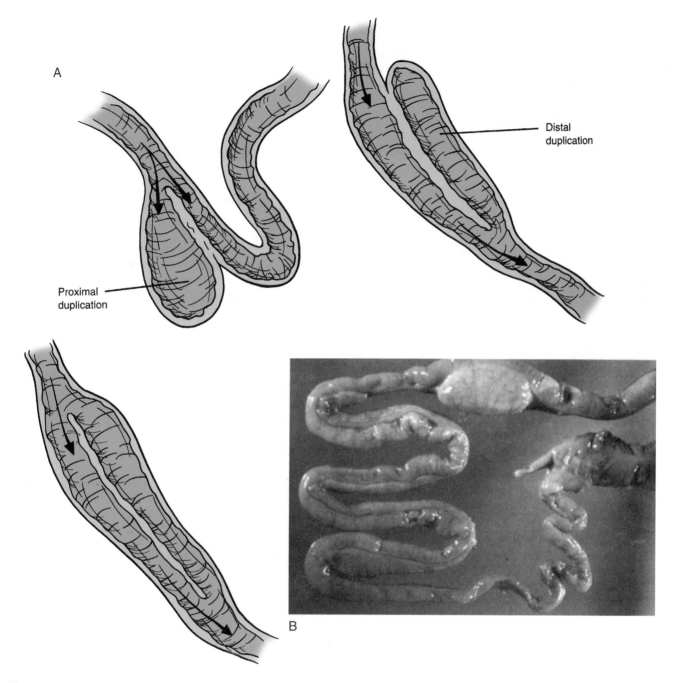

Figure 82–10. **A,** Schematic depiction of the various forms of communicating tubular duplications: duplication communicating proximally and forming a bulbous mass, duplication communicating distally and remaining clinically asymptomatic, and duplication communicating proximally and distally. **B,** Autopsy specimen showing a tubular small bowel duplication involving a portion of the ileum and much of the jejunum. (From Oldham KT, Colombani PM, Foglia RP [eds]: Surgery of Infants and Children: Scientific Principles and Practice. Philadelphia, Lippincott-Raven, 1997.)

normal small intestine, the duplication can be opened along its longitudinal direction and the mucosa of the duplication excised. Any communication with the adjacent normal small intestine would have to be closed.

Omental cysts can readily be removed by excising the adjacent omentum. Very large cysts can be decompressed by aspiration of fluid and therefore require less of an abdominal incision for removal. Treatment of cysts within the mesentery of the small intestine can be difficult if they are extensive and large. Every effort should

be made to carefully dissect a mesenteric cyst to achieve complete removal. However, such dissection may not be safe because of extensive involvement of the blood supply to the small bowel. In these circumstances it may be necessary to leave some of the cyst behind.

The overall outcome of treatment of these cysts should be excellent. Recurrence is likely only in large mesenteric cysts, where complete excision might compromise the blood supply to the normal small intestine, and extensive tubular small intestinal duplications.

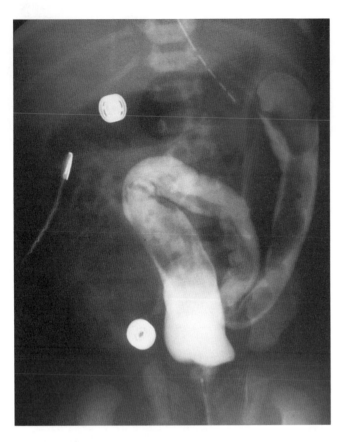

Figure 82–11. Image from a water-soluble contrast enema demonstrating an intraluminal meconium plug extending from the transverse colon to the rectum, as well as a small left colon. (Courtesy of A. B. Campbell, MD, St. Christopher's Hospital for Children.)

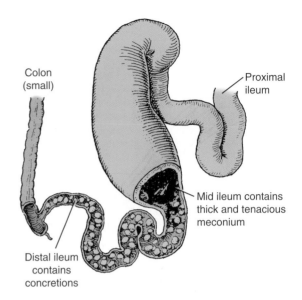

Figure 82–12. Schematic of meconium ileus. (From Lloyd DA: Meconium ileus. In Welch KJ [ed]: Pediatric Surgery, Chicago, Year Book Medical Publishers, 1986.)

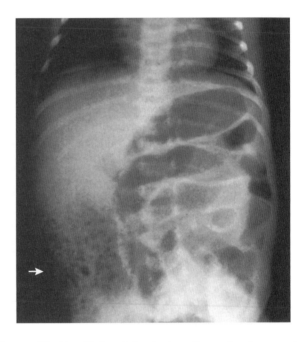

Figure 82–13. Plain abdominal radiograph of meconium ileus with distended loops of bowel and a mass of meconium *(arrow)* with a "ground glass" appearance from mixed air and stool. (From Ashcraft KW, Holder TM [eds]: Pediatric Surgery. Philadelphia, WB Saunders, 1999.)

MECONIUM SYNDROMES

Intestinal obstruction secondary to meconium impaction occurs frequently. In a newborn infant, entities such as meconium plug syndrome and small left colon syndrome can develop. These conditions involve meconium impaction in the descending and rectosigmoid colon. A water-soluble contrast enema is performed for diagnosis and treatment (Fig. 82–11). Passage of the meconium plug generally resolves the problem, with recurrence being uncommon.

Meconium ileus is a much more complicated entity characterized by meconium impaction beginning at the terminal ileum and extending proximally for various distances (Fig. 82–12). It can involve up to a third to half of the small intestine. Almost all infants with meconium ileus have cystic fibrosis with secondary pancreatic exocrine enzyme deficiency, which leads to thick, tenacious meconium. Cystic fibrosis, an autosomal recessive disease, results in chloride transport abnormalities produced by a defect in chromosome 7. The thickened secretions also affect the biliary tract, pancreas, and most commonly, the respiratory tract. Approximately 10% to 20% of cystic fibrosis patients will have meconium ileus.[38]

Meconium ileus is usually manifested at birth as abdominal distention and bilious vomiting. Plain abdom-inal radiographs demonstrate dilated bowel loops with a "ground glass" appearance in the right lower quadrant (Fig. 82–13).[39] These infants require resuscitation with intravenous fluids, bowel decompression, and broad-spectrum antibiotics. If there is no evidence of complicated meconium ileus, a water-soluble contrast enema should be performed. This study may be therapeutic as well as diagnostic. If meconium ileus is present, the goal of the study is to reflux the contrast past the obstructing meconium and free it from adherence to the mucosa. A more hypertonic solution or a mucolytic substance (e.g., 4% Mucomyst) may enhance the effectiveness of the procedure. The success rate is 50%, but it is dependent on the length of bowel impacted with meconium.[40] Failure to relieve the obstruction after a few attempts is an indication for exploratory laparotomy.

A subset of these patients have complicated meconium ileus, which refers to evidence of perforation with free air, a meconium cyst, or atresia secondary to in utero perforation. The findings on the first day of life are indicative of bowel perforation, meconium peritonitis, volvulus, or atresia. Abdominal radiographs may show free air, free fluid, or calcifications in addition to bowel obstruction. A contrast study may be contraindicated in patients with complicated meconium ileus, or it may be performed for diagnosis only. If laparotomy is necessary, the usual approach is to irrigate the obstructing meconium with 4% acetylcysteine solution, which can be performed via a proximal enterotomy. The inspissated meconium may be gently milked out through the enterotomy or into the colon. Only a small subset of patients may require bowel resection and primary anastomosis. It would be unusual, but if the distal part of the bowel cannot be cleared of the obstructing meconium, an ostomy and mucous fistula should be created. The mucous fistula can be used to irrigate the bowel distally. Infants with complicated meconium ileus are managed operatively, with resection of atretic or necrotic bowel and exteriorization enterostomies possibly being required. The most complicated form is a meconium cyst secondary to in utero perforation (Fig. 82–14). In this sit-

uation the perforation does not close, and a large cyst that often fills the entire peritoneal cavity can develop. In such circumstances, finding the two ends of the bowel in the setting of generalized inflammation may be difficult.

Spontaneous prenatal bowel perforation may lead to a condition known as meconium peritonitis. Postnatally, an abdominal radiograph may show scattered areas of calcification in the peritoneal cavity. In many cases the perforation seals and heals in utero and does not result in any postnatal bowel sequelae. The presence of pneumoperitoneum, intestinal obstruction, or clinical deterioration mandates surgical intervention, which usually involves resection of atretic or necrotic bowel with exteriorization.

MECKEL'S DIVERTICULUM AND OTHER OMPHALOMESENTERIC DUCT REMNANTS

The omphalomesenteric, or vitelline, duct is a remnant of the embryonic yolk sac. Remnants of these structures are the most common postnatal anomalies of the gastrointestinal tract (Fig. 82–15). The most frequently occurring residual of the yolk sac is a diverticulum arising from the antimesenteric border of the distal ileum, which has come to be known as *Meckel's diverticulum.* Knowledge of these omphalomesenteric duct remnants is important because complications related to these structures are numerous and may be life-threatening. It is estimated that a remnant of an embryonic yolk sac is present in 1% to 4% of all infants.[41] Although the incidence of omphalomesenteric duct remnants (especially Meckel's diverticulum) is high, the risk for development of symptoms from these anomalies is relatively low. The apparent risk of a complication developing as a result of Meckel's diverticulum is approximately 4%, with 80% of these patients initially being seen at younger than 10 years of age.[42]

Partial or complete failure of involution of the omphalomesenteric duct results in various residual structures, depending on the stage in which this process fails to progress.[41] The portion of the omphalomesenteric duct that does not become atretic will persist and develop along with the remainder of the gastrointestinal tract. Persistent patency of the omphalomesenteric duct can be determined by the 10th week of gestation.

There are many abnormalities that result from remnants of the embryonic yolk sac, and the various abnormalities can generally be categorized as either a patent omphalomesenteric (vitelline) duct, Meckel's diverticulum, omphalomesenteric cyst, omphalomesenteric duct remnants at the umbilicus, omphalomesenteric band, or vitelline blood vessel remnants.

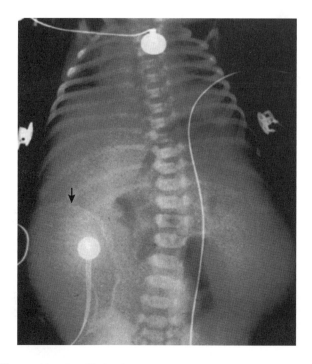

Figure 82–14. Abdominal radiograph of meconium peritonitis with a giant pseudocyst demonstrating calcification *(arrow)* in the cyst wall. (From Ashcraft KW, Holder TM [eds]: Pediatric Surgery. Philadelphia, WB Saunders, 1999.)

Patent Omphalomesenteric (Vitelline) Duct

This structure represents a persistent connection between the distal ileum and the umbilicus and accounts for approximately 2.5% to 6% of the spectrum of

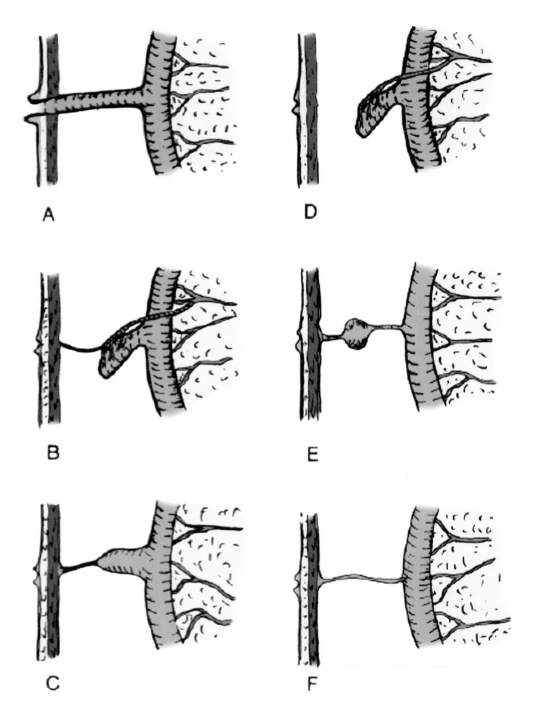

Figure 82–15.   Illustrated are some of the more common residual congenital abnormalities that result from the embryonic yolk sac. **A,** Patent omphalomesenteric duct representing a communication from the terminal ileum to the umbilicus. **B,** Meckel's diverticulum with a patent right vitelline artery illustrated as a cord to the undersurface of the umbilicus. **C,** Meckel's diverticulum with a cord connecting the tip of the diverticulum to the undersurface of the umbilicus. The cord (band) represents the distal residual of the omphalomesenteric duct. **D,** Typical appearance of Meckel's diverticulum with persistence of the vitelline artery. **E,** Involution of the proximal and distal ends of the omphalomesenteric duct with a residual cord or band and central preservation of the omphalomesenteric duct resulting in a mucosa-lined cyst. **F,** Intraperitoneal band from the ileum to the undersurface of the umbilicus representing involution without resolution of the omphalomesenteric duct. (From Wyllie R, Hyams J [eds]: Pediatric Gastrointestinal Disease. Philadelphia, WB Saunders, 1999.)

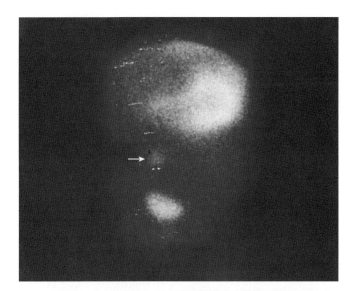

Figure 82–16. Typical appearance of a positive Meckel scan with an area of increased uptake above the area of the bladder in the lower midportion of the abdomen *(arrow)*.

omphalomesenteric duct remnants. Of interest is that males predominate by a ratio of 5 to 1.[43] Ectopic gastric mucosa is identified in approximately a third of patients with a complete fistula. Clinical manifestations of the anomaly usually appear in the first 2 weeks of life. After separation of the umbilical cord, drainage from the umbilicus (which has the appearance of intestinal contents) occurs. Once a diagnosis is made, resection of the entire omphalomesenteric duct is indicated.

Meckel's Diverticulum

This congenital abnormality is the most common of the embryonic yolk sac remnants and represents at least 80% of all of these anomalies. Meckel's diverticulum contains all three layers of the intestinal wall and is typically located within 40 to 50 cm of the ileocecal valve. However, this distance is related to age. The diverticulum originates from the antimesenteric border and is typically 3 to 6 cm in length. Of considerable significance is the presence of ectopic tissue within Meckel's diverticulum. This tissue can include gastric, duodenal, or colonic mucosa, as well as pancreatic tissue.[44] In the majority of patients who become symptomatic as a result of Meckel's diverticulum, the symptoms are caused by this ectopic tissue. A bleeding Meckel's diverticulum is diagnosed with a technetium 99 pertechnetate uptake scan ("Meckel's scan"), which identifies gastric mucosa (Fig. 82–16).

Treatment of Meckel's diverticulum depends on symptoms or anatomic findings at the time of incidental identification. Patients who have symptoms from Meckel's diverticulum such as bleeding or obstruction require resection of the diverticulum. With the presence of gastric mucosa or other ectopic mucosa or tissue, complete resection may require a sleeve resection of the attached small intestine. If the ectopic tissue is contained

in the tip of the Meckel diverticulum, amputation at the antimesenteric border of the bowel will result in complete resection. In patients who are asymptomatic or in whom Meckel's diverticulum is incidentally identified at the time of abdominal exploration, removal is indicated if ectopic tissue can be palpated within the diverticulum or if there is a very narrow base, which would be associated with a high potential for obstruction.

Omphalomesenteric Cyst

Involution of the omphalomesenteric duct at the umbilicus and at the ileal end of the duct results in a mucosa-lined cyst. The cyst can be located in the intraperitoneal or preperitoneal space and may become quite large. Most often they are associated with secondary infection, which requires initial drainage and subsequent excision.

Omphalomesenteric Duct Remnants at the Umbilicus

These remnants are uncommon but, when present, are identified within the first 1 to 2 weeks of life. Identification occurs when the umbilical stalk falls off and a polypoid mass covered by mucosa is present at the umbilicus. If an omphalomesenteric duct remnant is identified at the umbilicus, it should be excised.

Omphalomesenteric Band

This abnormality results from involution of the omphalomesenteric duct without disappearance of the tissue. As a result, a solid cord connecting the ileum to the undersurface of the umbilicus is present. This abnormality generally becomes evident as the cause of intestinal obstruction.

Vitelline Blood Vessel Remnants

Occlusion but failure of involution of this structure also results in a fibrous cord within the peritoneal cavity. This remnant becomes clinically evident by producing intestinal obstruction as a result of twisting of a segment of small intestine around the band.

In general, treatment of symptomatic omphalomesenteric duct remnants is resection; however, symptoms from these remnants can be vague and difficult to diagnosis. Radiographic and clinical evidence of bowel obstruction in the absence of previous surgery or other clear-cut etiology suggests the presence of remnants of the omphalomesenteric duct as the cause of the bowel obstruction. If a symptomatic Meckel's diverticulum is identified and there is no evidence of perforation, the current approach is to remove the diverticulum laparoscopically.

NECROTIZING ENTEROCOLITIS

NEC is the most common and the most lethal surgical emergency affecting the gastrointestinal tract in premature infants. This entity was first described in 1967[45] and became more common as neonatal intensive care units

(NICUs) became more advanced in supporting premature infants. NEC produces various degrees of ischemic necrosis affecting the large and small intestine and usually involves the watershed areas of the bowel, namely, the terminal ileum and the cecum. The degree of involvement may be limited to the mucosa, or it can be more extensive and lead to total intestinal necrosis. NEC tends to be patchy and can affect both the large and small intestine in 44% of cases.[46] The most severe form of the disease leading to pan-necrosis develops in 20% of patients. The mortality rate of this disease is 13 per 100,000 live births, with a case fatality rate ranging from 20% to 40%.[47] Although more than 90% of affected patients are born prematurely, the disease can also affect full-term infants. It is estimated that NEC develops in up to 10% of premature infants weighing less than 1500 g.[48] Despite the high incidence of this disease, the pathogenesis remains elusive. Prematurity, low birth weight, and excessive feeding are known risk factors. These infants are usually stressed and may have had poor intestinal perfusion as a result of a number of causes, such as asphyxia, patent ductus arteriosus, exchange transfusion, catheterization of the umbilical artery or vein, anemia, systemic infection, and cardiac anomalies. Premature infants have an immature intestinal mucosal barrier that predisposes them to bacterial translocation.[49] In addition, they have an immature immune system with a reduction in both specific and nonspecific immune defense mechanisms.[50] Premature infants also have impaired gut motility and higher gastric pH, which puts them at risk for bacterial colonization.[51] Moreover, many of them are colonized with nosocomial bacteria from their stay in the NICU. Enteral feeding also provides the substrate for bacterial overgrowth. Formulas increase the risk for development of NEC 20-fold in comparison to breast milk. Formulas lack immunoglobulins, lactoferrin, macrophages or platelet-activating factor, acetylhydrolase, and numerous other peptides that are present in breast milk.[52] However, studies have shown the efficacy of hypocaloric feeding in reducing the risk for NEC in premature infants by "conditioning" the immature gut.[53]

Patients usually have nonspecific signs such as apnea, bradycardia, hemodynamic and temperature instability, hypoglycemia, and lethargy.[54] Initial gastrointestinal signs include abdominal distention, increased gastric residuals, vomiting, and Hemoccult-positive stools, which may become frank blood as the disease progresses. In infants with more advanced disease, signs of peritonitis develop as a result of bowel necrosis and perforation. There may be discoloration, edema, and tenderness of the abdominal wall, and a mass may be palpable. Multiorgan failure with hypotension, poor urinary output, and worsening respiratory status may develop. Metabolic acidosis and falling platelet counts are ominous signs. Abdominal radiographs may demonstrate pneumatosis intestinalis (Fig. 82–17), which is the hallmark of NEC.[55] However, absence of pneumatosis intestinalis does not rule out the diagnosis because it is usually a transient finding.

Other radiologic findings include dilated bowel loops, which may be persistent and fixed, diminished bowel gas, portal venous gas, and ascites. Fixed, dilated bowel loops and ascites may be signs of intestinal necrosis. Abdomi-

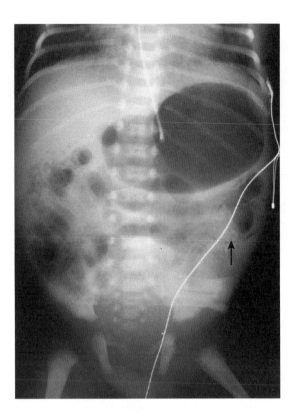

Figure 82–17.   Patterns of intestinal pneumatosis. A supine abdominal radiograph in a neonate with necrotizing enterocolitis demonstrates submucosal (right hemiabdomen) and linear intramural pneumatosis *(arrow)*. (Courtesy of A. B. Campbell, MD, St. Christopher's Hospital for Children.)

nal radiographs may show free intraperitoneal air, indicative of bowel perforation (Fig. 82–18). This sign is best demonstrated on a left lateral decubitus radiograph as air between the liver and the lateral abdominal wall.

When NEC is diagnosed or suspected, medical therapy is initiated and includes discontinuation of enteral feeding, placement of an orogastric tube for intestinal decompression, intravenous fluids, and broad-spectrum antibiotics. It is necessary to obtain serial abdominal radiographs, a complete blood count, and platelet counts (typically every 6 to 8 hours) to monitor the infant's status and look for free intra-abdominal air as an indicator for surgical intervention. Sixty percent to 70% of infants improve with medical management. However, infants who fail to improve with maximal medical management or continue to deteriorate with persistent metabolic acidosis, significant thrombocytopenia, and hemodynamic instability may need surgical exploration. Currently, the only absolute indication for surgical intervention is free intra-abdominal air as an indication of bowel perforation. Other "relative" indications are persistent metabolic acidosis, profound thrombocytopenia, a palpable abdominal mass, abdominal wall erythema, and portal venous gas. However, none of these signs, by themselves, are indications for surgery. The objectives of surgery are to resect nonviable bowel while preserving as much viable bowel as possible to avoid

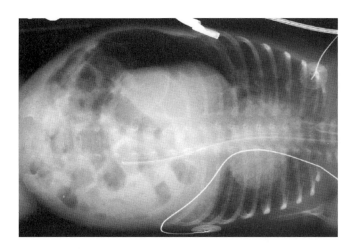

Figure 82–18. Pneumoperitoneum in necrotizing enterocolitis. An abdominal radiograph in the left lateral decubitus position demonstrates a large amount of free intraperitoneal air and extensive intestinal pneumatosis. (Courtesy of A. B. Campbell, MD, St. Christopher's Hospital for Children.)

creating short-bowel syndrome. Exploratory laparotomy is generally performed through a right supraumbilical or infraumbilical transverse incision. The entire gastrointestinal tract is inspected. Infants with the most severe form of the disease have their entire bowel affected (NEC totalis), which may result in an "open and close" procedure. If more than one area of nonviable bowel is present, multiple resections with primary anastomosis and proximal diversion at the point of the first bowel resection may be required. If multiple affected areas are of questionable viability but not frankly necrotic, a proximal diverting enterostomy may be indicated, followed by a "second look" 24 to 48 hours later. A technique described by Lessin et al. to treat multiple bowel involvement involves multiple resections of nonviable segments and lining up the remaining viable segments of the intestine over a feeding tube without anastomosis.[56] Contrast studies have shown that the segments undergo auto-anastomosis. This technique avoids multiple stoma-related complications and further loss of intestinal length with closure and may help avoid a reoperation.[56] If only a single bowel segment is affected, this area is resected with the formation of a proximal ostomy and distal mucus fistula. The ostomy is usually brought through the lateral aspect of the incision. Another important technique is placement of peritoneal drains, which was first reported in 1975.[57] Although this technique was originally described as a temporizing procedure for very-low-birth-weight premature infants, subsequent reports have described it as the primary and sole operative intervention.[58,59] With more experience in using this approach, it appears to be more beneficial in infants with pneumoperitoneum who weigh less than 1000 g. It involves placing one or two Penrose drains at the bedside through a small incision in the lower abdominal quadrants. Bowel continuity is evaluated later with contrast studies. Azarow et al. compared the survival rate of neonates with NEC who weighed less than 1000 g

and were treated by either laparotomy or percutaneous peritoneal drains. The survival rate in the peritoneal drainage group was 69% as opposed to only 22% in the laparotomy group.[60] Placement of peritoneal drains for increasing ventilatory requirements because of severe abdominal distention in the absence of free peritoneal air offers rapid stabilization. However, the mortality remains high in this group of critically ill patients.[61] A major sequela of NEC is the formation of stenosis or strictures of the small and large bowel. Strictures develop in 29% to 35% of infants after NEC. After recovery from NEC, all infants require a contrast enema or a distal colostogram before stoma take-down. Strictures are resected at the time of reversal of the ostomy. Recurrence of NEC is seen in less than 6% of patients.[62] The mortality associated with NEC has improved because of advances in neonatal and surgical care. It is estimated that 50% of premature infants weighing less than 1000 g and 75% weighing less than 1500 g survive an episode of NEC.[63] The long-term outcome after NEC treated at one tertiary NICU was favorable, with 83% of infants subsequently attending school full-time and only 14.3% suffering from developmental delay.[64]

INTUSSUSCEPTION

Intussusception is a process whereby the intestine telescopes into itself. The telescoping bowel segment is referred to as the intussusceptum. Although it was first described by Paul Barbette of Amsterdam in 1674,[65] it was not until nearly 200 years later that the first successful operation for intussusception (in a toddler) was performed.[66] The incidence of intussusception is highest between 4 and 10 months of age, and 80% to 90% of cases occur between 3 and 36 months.[67] Nearly all intussusceptions in infants and toddlers are idiopathic. That is, there is no clear etiology. In addition, most are ileocolic or ileoileocolic. Upper respiratory tract infections or gastroenteritis (adenovirus and rotavirus have been implicated) have been thought to be contributory to the development of "idiopathic" intussusception.[68] Hypertrophy of Peyer's patches can be seen at surgery, but no single etiologic factor predominates. Approximately 5% to 10% of cases have a true pathologic lead point.[69] The older the toddler, the more likely there will be a lead point.[70] The most common lead point is Meckel's diverticulum. Other lead points include polyps, the appendix, intestinal duplication, foreign bodies, and tumors such as hamartomas associated with Peutz-Jeghers syndrome. Children with Henoch-Schönlein purpura may have intussusception with submucosal hemorrhage acting as a lead point. Patients with cystic fibrosis may be at risk for recurrent intussusception, and these children tend to be older than the usual age at which it occurs.[68]

The typical history is that of sudden, short-duration, cyclic crampy abdominal pain. During these episodes the infant cries inconsolably with the knees drawn up. Between episodes the infant is asymptomatic. After the development of intussusception, lymphatic and venous obstruction of the intussusceptum occurs and leads to congestion (Fig. 82–19). Subsequently, swelling develops

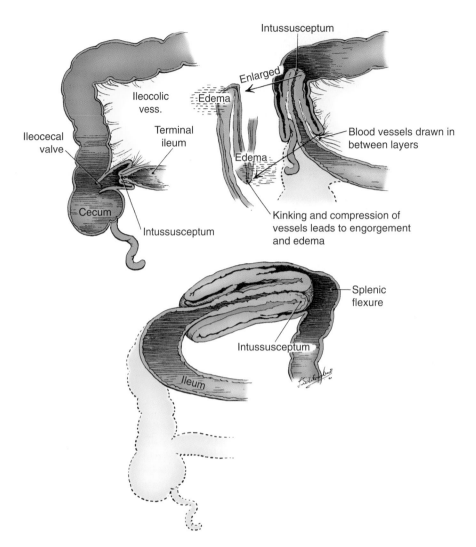

Figure 82–19. Development of an intussusception. Most intussusceptions in infants and children are of the kind shown here. The intussusception begins at or near the ileocecal valve without an obvious local anatomic lesion to cause it. From the first moment there is simultaneous interference with patency of the alimentary canal and with the vascular supply of the intussusceptum. The drawings indicate the manner in which the mesenteric vessels are drawn between the layers of the intussusception and compressed. The slight interference with lymphatic and venous drainage that occurs almost immediately results in edema and an increase in tissue pressure. This further increases resistance to the return of venous blood, the venules and capillaries become enormously engorged, and bloody edema fluid drips into the lumen. The mucosal cells swell into goblet cells and discharge mucus, which after mixing in the lumen with the bloody transudate, forms a "currant jelly" stool. Edema increases until venous inflow is completely obstructed. As arterial blood continues to pump in, tissue pressure rises until it is higher than arterial pressure, and gangrene ensues. The drawings indicate the sharp U-shaped turns of the intestine and mesenteric vessels at either end of the intussusceptum. The outer coat of the intussusceptum (middle layer of the intussusception) is isolated between the two sharp bends and understandably is the first to become gangrenous. Gangrene appears in this coat near the tip of the intussusception and progresses back toward the neck of the intussusceptum. Rarely, the intussuscipiens is damaged. (From Ravitch MM, Welch KJ, Benson CD, et al [eds]: Pediatric Surgery, 3rd ed. Chicago, Year Book, 1979.)

and results in impairment of arterial flow and mucosal necrosis. This produces the classic "currant jelly" stool. On examination the child may show signs of dehydration or lethargy, depending on the length of time that has passed and whether bowel necrosis is present. A sausage-shaped mass may be palpable in the right upper quadrant. The presence of peritoneal signs is ominous and mandates operative intervention. In 60% to 90% of cases, rectal examination demonstrates either occult or gross blood.[71]

Abdominal radiographs may be normal or show a paucity of gas in the colon and dilated small bowel loops (Fig. 82–20). Ultrasonography has been used more frequently to diagnose intussusception. It may show a kidney-shaped mass in the longitudinal view or a target sign in the transverse view (Fig. 82–21). A barium contrast enema was the "gold standard" for diagnosis, and in over 50% of cases, hydrostatic pressure was successful in reducing the intussusception (Fig. 82–22). However, this treatment strategy changed in 1990 as a result of a report

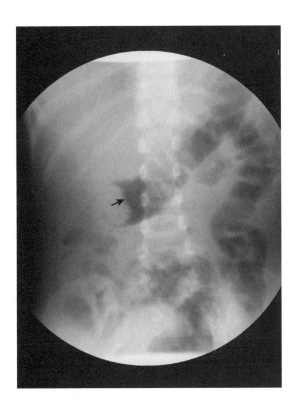

Figure 82–20. Ileocolic intussusception. A scout film for a contrast enema demonstrates a rounded soft tissue mass in the right upper quadrant with central radiolucency along the inferior margin of the liver. This pseudotumor suggests the presence of intussusception. (Courtesy of A. B. Campbell, MD, St. Christopher's Hospital for Children.)

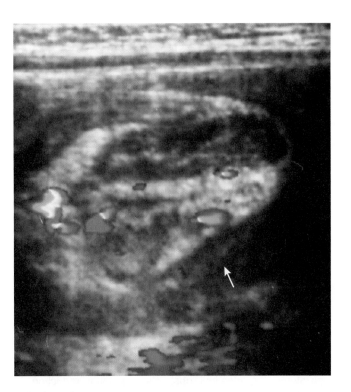

Figure 82–21. Intussusception, color Doppler imaging. A cross-sectional color Doppler ultrasound image of intussusception demonstrates the typical target appearance with compression of an eccentric small bowel segment, a hypoechoic peripheral colon wall *(arrow)*, echogenic mesenteric fat, and incidental mesenteric lymph nodes. Brisk flow is noted within the mesenteric vessels centrally. (Courtesy of A. B. Campbell, MD, St. Christopher's Hospital for Children.)

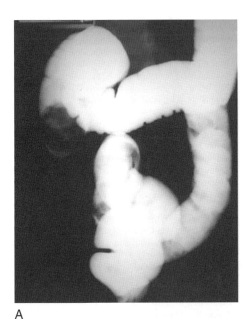

A

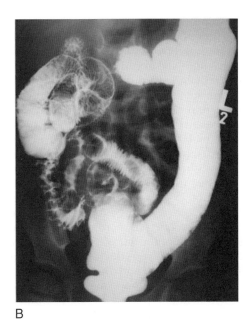

B

Figure 82–22. Barium enema reduction of intussusception. **A,** A filling defect in the ascending colon is shown. **B,** The intussusception is successfully reduced with reflux of contrast into the small bowel. (Courtesy of A. B. Campbell, MD, St. Christopher's Hospital for Children.)

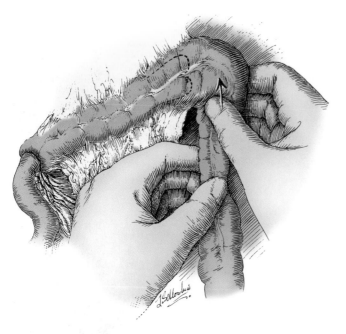

Figure 82–23. Manual reduction of intussusception. If a barium enema fails or intussusception is encountered during laparotomy for intestinal obstruction, manual reduction is required. The intestine is occluded immediately distal to the intussusception with the fingers of one hand and stripped proximally with the fingers of the other. In effect, this maneuver increases intraluminal pressure just as an enema does. The intestine should not be pulled. If reduction is not readily achieved, resection and anastomosis should be performed. (From Ravitch MM, Welch KJ, Benson CD, et al [eds]: Pediatric Surgery, 3rd ed. Chicago, Year Book, 1979.)

from a Chinese group describing air-contrast enema as a diagnostic and therapeutic tool.[72] The intussusception is reduced under fluoroscopic guidance. The patient receives intravenous fluid and antibiotics before the procedure. Successful reduction is confirmed by reflux of air (or barium) into the small bowel. The success rate with air or barium reduction should exceed 70%. Failure of reduction or the presence of peritonitis mandates operative intervention, which can be performed laparoscopically or by a standard approach. If done laparoscopically, reduction is accomplished by gently pulling the intussusceptum from the intussuscipiens. In the open approach an infraumbilical transverse incision is made. The intussusception is reduced by applying gentle pressure retrogradely in a distal-to-proximal direction and milking the intussusceptum out of the intussuscipiens (Fig. 82–23). After operative reduction the bowel is carefully inspected for viability and the presence of a "lead point." The intussuscepted bowel may be congested and edematous. Observation over a 10- to 20-minute period may be necessary to assess viability. If the lead point was Meckel's diverticulum or a polyp, it should be resected. Intussusception may recur in 5% to 10% of cases after successful hydrostatic reduction.[68] In contrast, the reported recurrence rate after operative reduction is

1% to 4%.[68,73] Recurrence is usually managed by hydrostatic reduction. Repeated episodes of intussusception mandate operative intervention to look for a lead point. Bowel perforation is a serious complication that occurs in 0.2% of cases treated by hydrostatic reduction and requires emergency surgery. If there is necrosis of the intussuscepted bowel or operative reduction is impossible, resection is necessary. Usually, an end-to-end anastomosis can be safely performed.

SUGGESTED READINGS

Grosfeld JL: The small intestine. In Ravitch MM, Welch KJ, Benson CD, et al (eds): Pediatric Surgery. Chicago, Year Book, 1986, p 838.

Oldham KT, Colombani PM, Foglia RP (eds): Surgery of Infants and Children: Scientific Principles and Practice. Philadelphia. Lippincott-Raven, 1997.

Skandalakis JE, Gray SW, Ricketts R, et al: The small intestines. In Skandalakis JE, Gray SW (eds): Embryology for Surgeons, 2nd ed. Baltimore, Williams & Wilkins, 1994, p 184.

Taeusch HW, Ballard RA, Avery ME (eds): Schaffer and Avery's Diseases of the Newborn, 6th ed. Philadelphia, WB Saunders, 1991, p 685.

REFERENCES

1. Mall FP: Development of the human intestine and its position in the adult. Bull John Hopkins Hosp 9:197, 1898.
2. Ladd WE: Surgical diseases of the alimentary tract in infants. N Engl J Med 215:705, 1936.
3. Warner BW: Malrotation. In Oldham KT, Colombani PM, Foglia RP (eds): Surgery of Infants and Children: Scientific Principles and Practice. Philadelphia, Lippincott-Raven, 1997, p 1229.
4. Skandalakis JE, Gray SW, Ricketts R, et al: The small intestines. In Skandalakis JE, Gray SW (eds): Embryology for Surgeons, 2nd ed. Baltimore, Williams & Wilkins, 1994, p 184.
5. Bryne WJ: Disorders of the intestines and pancreas. In Taeusch HW, Ballard RA, Avery ME (eds): Schaffer and Avery's Diseases of the Newborn, 6th ed. Philadelphia, WB Saunders, 1991, p 685.
6. Seashore JH, Touloukian RJ: Midgut volvulus: An ever present threat. Arch Pediatr Adolesc Med 148:43, 1994.
7. Spigland N, Brandt ML, Yazbeck S: Malrotation presenting beyond the neonatal period. J Pediatr Surg 25:1139, 1990.
8. Gross RE: Malrotation of the intestine and colon. In The Surgery of Infancy and Childhood. Philadelphia, WB Saunders, 1953, p 192.
9. Rescorla FJ, Shedd FJ, Grosfeld JL, et al: Anomalies of intestinal rotation in childhood: Analysis of 447 cases. Surgery 108:710, 1990.
10. Grosfeld JL: Jejunoileal atresia and stenosis, section 3: The small intestine. In Ravitch MM, Welch KJ, Benson CD, et al (eds): Pediatric Surgery. Chicago, Year Book, 1986, p 838.
11. Grosfeld JL, Ballantine TVN, Shoemaker R: Operative management of intestinal atresia and stenosis based on pathologic findings. J Pediatr Surg 14:368, 1979.
12. Hays DM: Intestinal atresia and stenosis. In Ravitch M (ed): Current Problems in Surgery. Chicago, Year Book, 1969, p 3.
13. Louw JH, Barnard CN: Congenital intestinal atresia: Observation on its origin. Lancet 2:1065, 1955.
14. Louw JH: Congenital intestinal atresia and severe stenosis in the newborn. S Afr J Sci 3:109, 1952.
15. Touloukian RJ: Diagnosis and treatment of jejuno-ileal atresia. World J Surg 17:310, 1993.
16. Evans GH: Atresias of the gastrointestinal tract. Int Abstr Surg 92:1, 1951.

17. Gornall P: Management of intestinal atresia complicating gastroschisis. J Pediatr Surg 24:522, 1989.

18. De Lorimier AA, Fonkalsrud EW, Hays DM: Congenital atresia and stenosis of the jejunum and ileum. Surgery 65:819, 1969.

19. Kumaran N, Shanker KR, Lloyd DA, Losty PD: Trends in the management and outcome of jejuno-ileal atresia. Eur J Pediatr Surg 12:163, 2002.

20. Kimble RM, Harding J, Kolbe A: Additional congenital anomalies in babies with gut atresia or stenosis: When to investigate, and which investigation. Pediatr Surg Int 12:565, 1997.

21. Nixon HH, Tawes R: Etiology and treatment of small intestinal atresia: Analysis of a series of 127 jejunoileal atresias and comparison with 62 duodenal atresias. Surgery 69:41, 1971.

22. Rickham PP, Karplus M: Familial and hereditary intestinal atresia. Helv Paediatr Acta 26:561, 1971.

23. Takahashi A, Suzuki N, Ikeda H, et al: Results of bowel plication in addition to primary anastomosis in patients with jejunal atresia. J Pediatr Surg 36:1752, 2001.

24. Patrapinyokul S, Brereton RJ, Spitz L, et al: Small-bowel atresia and stenosis. Pediatr Surg Int 4:390, 1989.

25. Snyder CL, Miller KA, Sharp RJ, et al: Management of intestinal atresia in patients with gastroschisis. J Pediatr Surg 36:1542, 2001.

26. Deleze G, Sidiropoulus D, Paumgartner G: Determination of bile acid concentration in human amniotic fluid for prenatal diagnosis of intestinal obstruction. Pediatrics 59:647, 1977.

27. Adeyemi D: Neonatal intestinal obstruction in a developing tropical country: Patterns, problems, and prognosis. J Trop Pediatr 35:66, 1989.

28. Doolin J, Ormsbee HS, Hill JL: Motility abnormality in intestinal atresia. J Pediatr Surg 22:320, 1987.

29. Phelps S, Fisher R, Partington A, Dykes E: Prenatal ultrasound diagnosis of gastrointestinal malformations. J Pediatr Surg 32:438, 1997.

30. Stoll C, Alembik Y, Dott B, Roth MP: Evaluation of prenatal diagnosis of congenital gastro-intestinal atresias. Eur J Epidemiol 12:611, 1996.

31. Fleet MS, de la Hunt MN: Intestinal atresia with gastroschisis: A selective approach to management. J Pediatr Surg 35:1323, 2000.

32. Roberts HE, Cragan JD, Cono J, et al: Increased frequency of cystic fibrosis among infants with jejunoileal atresia. Am J Med Genet 78:446, 1998.

33. Pickard LR, Santoro S, Wyllie RG, et al: Histochemical studies of experimental fetal intestinal obstruction. J Pediatr Surg 16:256, 1981.

34. Wrenn EL: Alimentary tract duplications. In Ashcraft KW, Holder TM (eds): Pediatric Surgery, 2nd ed. Philadelphia, WB Saunders, 1993, p 421.

35. Holcomb GW III, Gheissari A, O'Neill JA: Surgical management of alimentary tract duplications. Ann Surg 209:167, 1989.

36. Kurtz RJ, Heimann TM, Holt J, Beck AR: Mesenteric and retroperitoneal cysts. Ann Surg 203:109, 1986.

37. Hebra A, Brown MF, McGeehin KM, Ross AJ 3rd: Mesenteric, omental, and retroperitoneal cysts in children: A clinical study of 22 cases. South Med J 86:173, 1993.

38. Welsh MJ, Tsui LC, Boat TF, et al: Cystic fibrosis. In Scriver CR, Beaudet AL, Sly WE, et al (eds): The Metabolic and Molecular Bases of Inherited Disease, 7th ed. New York, McGraw-Hill, 1994.

39. Hussain SM, Meradji M, Robbin SGF, et al: Plain film diagnosis in meconium plug syndrome, meconium ileus and neonatal Hirschsprung's disease. Pediatr Radiol 21:556, 1991.

40. Kao SCS, Franken EA Jr: Nonoperative treatment of simple meconium ileus: A survey of the Society for Pediatric Radiology. Pediatr Radiol 25:97, 1995.

41. Gray SW, Skandalakis JE: Embryology for Surgeons. Philadelphia WB Saunders, 1972, p 156.

42. Soltero MJ, Bill AH: The natural history of Meckel's diverticulum and its relations to incidental removal. Am J Surg 132:168, 1976.

43. Soderlund S: Meckel's diverticulum, a clinical and histologic study. Acta Chir Scand Suppl 118:1, 1959.

44. Yammaguchi M, Takeuchi S, Awazu S: Meckel's diverticulum: Investigation of 600 patients in Japanese literature. Am J Surg 136:247, 1978.

45. Touloukian RJ, Berdon WE, Amoury RA, et al: Surgical experience with necrotizing enterocolitis in the infant. J Pediatr Surg 2:389, 1967.

46. Kliegman RM, Fanaroff AA: Necrotizing enterocolitis. N Engl J Med 310:1093, 1984.

47. Kosloske AM: Epidemiology of necrotizing enterocolitis. Acta Paediatr Suppl 396:2, 1994.

48. Uauy RD, Fanaroff AA, Korones SB, et al: Necrotizing enterocolitis in very low birth weight infants: Biodemographic and clinical correlates. National Institute of Child Health and Human Development Neonatal Research Network. J Pediatr 119:630, 1991.

49. Wells CL, Maddaus MA, Simmons RL: Proposed mechanism for the translocation of intestinal bacteria. Rev Infect Dis 10:958, 1988.

50. Udall JN Jr: Gastrointestinal host defense and necrotizing enterocolitis: An update. J Pediatr 117:S33, 1990.

51. Hyman PE, Clarke KK, Everett SL, et al: Gastric acid secretory function in preterm infants. J Pediatr 106:467, 1985.

52. Lucas A, Cole TJ: Breast milk and neonatal necrotizing enterocolitis. Lancet 336:1519, 1990.

53. Gross SJ, Slagle TA: Feeding the low birth weight infant. Clin Perinatol 20:19, 1993.

54. Kanto WP Jr, Hunter JE, Stoll BJ: Recognition and medical management of necrotizing enterocolitis. Clin Perinatol 21:335, 1994.

55. Kliegman RM, Fanaroff AA: Neonatal necrotizing enterocolitis in the absence of pneumatosis. Am J Dis Child 136:618, 1982.

56. Lessin MS, Schwartz DL, Wesselhoeft CW Jr: Multiple spontaneous small bowel anastomosis in premature infants with multisegmental necrotizing enterocolitis. J Pediatr Surg 35:170, 2000.

57. Ein SH, Shandling B, Wesson D, et al: A 13-year experience with peritoneal drainage under local anesthesia for necrotizing enterocolitis perforation. J Pediatr Surg 25:1034, 1990.

58. Morgan LJ, Shochat SJ, Hartman GE: Peritoneal drainage as primary management of perforated NEC in the very low birth weight infant. J Pediatr Surg 29:30, 1994.

59. Gollin G, Abardanell A, Baerg JE: Peritoneal drainage as definitive management of intestinal perforation in extremely low-birth-weight infants. J Pediatr Surg 38:1814, 2003.

60. Azarow KS, Ein SH, Shandling B, et al: Laparotomy or drain for perforated necrotizing enterocolitis: Who gets what and why. Pediatr Surg Int 12:137, 1997.

61. Dzakovic A, Notrica DM, Smith EO, et al: Primary peritoneal drainage for increasing ventilatory requirements in critically ill neonates with necrotizing enterocolitis. J Pediatr Surg 36:730, 2001.

62. Stringer MD, Bereton RJ, Drake DP, et al: Recurrent necrotizing enterocolitis. J Pediatr Surg 28:979, 1993.

63. Ricketts RR, Jerles ML: Neonatal necrotizing enterocolitis: Experience with 100 consecutive surgical patients. World J Surg 14:600, 1990.

64. Stanford A, Upperman JS, Boyle P, et al: Long-term follow-up of patients with necrotizing enterocolitis. J Pediatr Surg 37:1048, 2002.

65. Barbette P: Oeuvres Chirugiques et Anatomiques. Geneva, François Miege, 1674, p 522.

66. Hutchinson J: A successful case of abdominal section for intussusception. Proc R Med Chir Doc 7:195-198, 1873.

67. Beasley SW, Auldist AW, Stokes KB: Recurrent intussusception: Barium or surgery? Aust N Z J Surg 57:11, 1987.

68. Stringer MD, Pablot SM, Bereton FJ: Paediatric intussusception. Br J Surg 46:484, 1992.

69. Meier DE, Coln CE, Rescorla FJ, et al: Intussusception in children: International perspective. World J Surg 20:1035, 1996.

70. Ong NT, Beasley SW: The leadpoint in intussusception. J Pediatr Surg 25:640, 1990.

71. Losek JD, Fiete RL: Intussusception and the diagnostic value of testing stool for occult blood. Am J Emerg Med 9:1, 2001.

72. Guo JZ, Ma XY, Zhow QH: Results of air pressure enema reduction of intussusception: 6,396 cases in 13 years. J Pediatr Surg 21:1201, 1986.

73. Liu KW, MacCarthy J, Guiney EJ, et al: Intussusception: Current trends in management. Arch Dis Child 61:5, 1986.

83

Anatomy and Physiology of the Mesenteric Circulation

Steven B. Goldin · Alexander Rosemurgy

This chapter discusses the anatomy of the mesenteric arterial circulation, including common normal arterial variations.[1] Collateral pathways between the major arterial vessels and their clinical significance are also discussed. Reviewing embryonic developmental anatomy[2] simplifies understanding of the arterial anatomy. Venous anatomy is detailed elsewhere in this text. The intestine serves a variety of functions, including digestion, absorption of fluids and nutrients, secretion of fluids and hormones, and propulsion of enteric contents, and it forms a barrier that contributes to host defense mechanisms. This chapter also concentrates on regulation of mesenteric blood flow. Detailed understanding of the physiologic factors that augment blood flow to and from the intestinal circulation requires a closer look at the arteriolar, capillary, venule, and venous anatomy. For purposes of this discussion, the mesenteric circulation designates blood flow only to the intestinal circulation, and the splanchnic circulation refers to blood flow to any of the gastrointestinal organs or structures within the peritoneal cavity as seen in Figure 83–1.

EMBRYOLOGY

The foregut structures of the digestive tract, including the esophagus, stomach, duodenum, liver, gallbladder, and pancreas, develop when the embryo is approximately 4 weeks old. These structures receive blood flow from the celiac artery, which begins at the proximal ends of the vitelline arteries near the seventh cervical vertebra. With growth of the embryo, the celiac artery migrates caudally to T12. The midgut begins just distal to the entrance of the ampulla of Vater and extends to the proximal two thirds of the transverse colon. The midgut's vascular supply is from the superior mesenteric artery (SMA). The midgut develops from two limbs called the cephalic and caudal limbs. During development of the midgut, there is rapid elongation of these limbs and its mesentery, as well as counterclockwise rota-

tion of approximately 270 degrees around the SMA, as seen in Figure 83–2A. This rotation occurs just after the SMA has given off its duodenal branches. Therefore, the proximal SMA branches to the small bowel originate on the right side of the SMA, whereas distally, branches to the small bowel originate on the left side of the SMA. Likewise, the colonic branches of the SMA, which branch off distally from the SMA, originate from the right side of the SMA, as shown in Figure 83–2B. The hindgut gives rise to the distal third of the transverse colon, extends to the upper part of the anal canal, and terminates in the cloaca. The blood supply to the hindgut is via the inferior mesenteric artery (IMA). The cloaca is divided into an anterior portion, called the primitive urogenital sinus, and a posterior portion, called the anorectal canal, by the urorectal septum, as seen in Figure 83–3. Descent of the urorectal septum to the cloacal membrane results in formation of the perineum, as well as a posterior anal membrane and an anterior urogenital membrane. The anal membrane contacts the anal pit, or proctodeum, which has an ectodermal origin. Therefore, the upper portion of the anal canal has an endodermal origin, whereas the lower portion is of ectodermal origin. Accordingly, the upper portion of the anal canal is supplied by the IMA, with the lower portion being supplied by the systemic circulation.

ANATOMY

The small intestine, or small bowel, extends from the pylorus in the right upper quadrant to the cecum in the right lower quadrant. A large fold of peritoneum that extends from the posterior abdominal wall suspends the small bowel within the peritoneal cavity and prevents significant rotation. This fold of peritoneum is called the mesentery and contains arteries, veins, nerves, lymphatic vessels, lymph nodes, and fat. The small bowel mesentery begins at its base, just to the left of the second lumbar vertebral body, and extends inferiorly and obliquely to

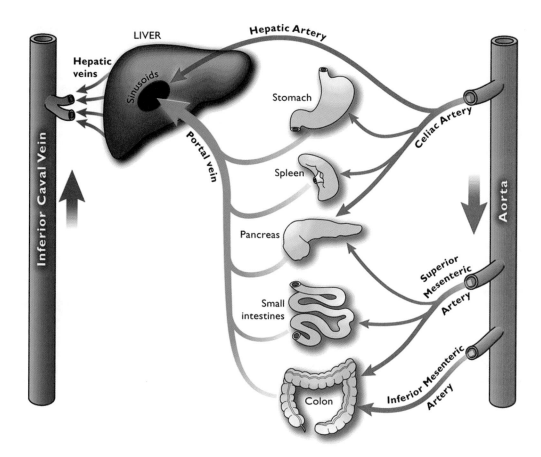

Figure 83–1. Schematic representation of the splanchnic circulation. (From Gelmen S, Mushlin PS: Catecholamine-induced changes in the splanchnic circulation affecting systemic hemodynamics. Anesthesiology 100:434-439, 2004.)

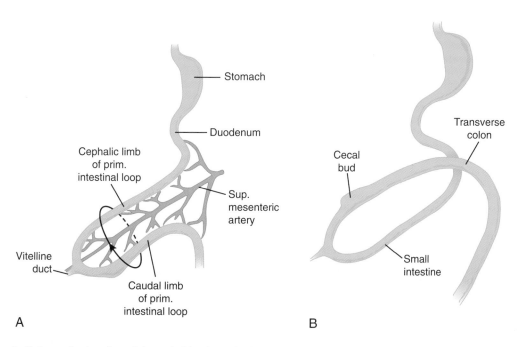

Figure 83–2. **A,** Schematic drawing of the primitive intestinal loop before rotation (lateral view). The superior mesenteric artery forms the axis of the loop. The *arrow* indicates the direction of the counterclockwise rotation. **B,** Similar view as in **A,** but showing the primitive intestinal loop after 180-degree counterclockwise rotation. Note that the transverse colon passes in front of the duodenum. (From Sadler TW: Langman's Medical Embryology, 7th ed. Baltimore, Williams & Wilkins, 1995.)

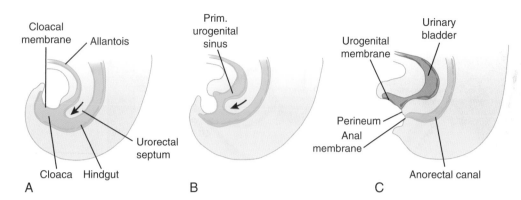

Figure 83–3. A-C, Drawings of the cloacal region in embryos at successive stages of development. The *arrows* indicate the route of descent followed by the urorectal septum. Note the anorectal canal and perineum. (From Sadler TW: Langman's Medical Embryology, 7th ed. Baltimore, Williams & Wilkins, 1995.)

the right toward the iliac fossa. The mesentery attaches in a fan-like pattern to the entire length of the small bowel along one side termed the *mesenteric border of the small bowel*. In humans, the total length of the duodenum is approximately 20 cm, and that of the jejunum and ileum is 260 cm. The duodenum begins at the pylorus and extends in a C-loop fashion to the duodenojejunal junction, which is located just to the left of the second lumbar vertebra and is supported by the ligament of Treitz. The jejunum makes up approximately two fifths of the length of the small bowel, with the remaining three fifths constituting the ileum. There is no clear anatomic demarcation between the jejunum and ileum.

The colon, which begins in the right lower quadrant and extends in a question mark pattern throughout the abdominal cavity to reach the rectum, also has mesenteric attachments composed of similar elements. The length of the human colon is approximately 110 cm. The cecum is the first portion of the colon and begins at the ileocecal valve. It is approximately 6.3 to 7.5 cm long and 7.5 cm wide. Like the small bowel, it is completely covered by peritoneum, but it differs from the small intestine by not having a mesentery. The vermiform appendix is attached to the cecum 2.5 cm below the ileocecal valve and may vary in length from 2.5 to 23 cm. The appendix may be located in a variety of locations, including the pelvis and retrocecal area, or it may be directed superiorly and to the left. The appendix is completely covered with peritoneum and has a mesentery, which furnishes its blood supply. The ascending colon is continuous with the cecum and located on the right side of the abdomen. It ascends toward the inferior surface of the liver, where it turns medially to make the hepatic flexure. The ascending colon and hepatic flexure are retroperitoneal structures. The transverse colon begins at the hepatic flexure and crosses the peritoneal cavity. It is an intraperitoneal structure and has a mesentery, which makes its location and relationship to other structures variable. The transverse colon ends at the splenic flexure, which is usually higher than the hepatic flexure. It is also a retroperitoneal structure. The descending colon begins at the distal end of the splenic flexure, where it courses retroperitoneally and inferiorly on the left side of the abdomen until it reaches the left iliac fossa and becomes the sigmoid colon. The sigmoid colon is intraperitoneal and has a mesentery. It is S-shaped, starts in the left iliac fossa, and continues to the rectum. The

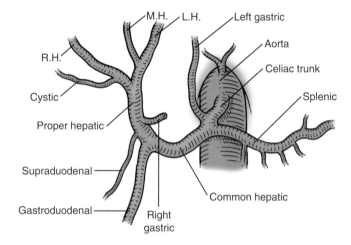

Figure 83–4. Major branches of the celiac trunk. L.H., left hepatic artery; M.H., middle hepatic artery; R.H., right hepatic artery. (From Blumgart LH, Hann LE: Surgery of the liver and biliary tract. In Blumgart LH, Fong Y [eds]: Surgical and Radiologic Anatomy of the Liver and Biliary Tract, 3rd ed. London, WB Saunders, 2000.)

rectum is approximately 15 cm long and begins at the midsacral area. It then follows the curve of the sacrum and coccyx into the pelvic cavity.

Mesenteric attachments, as mentioned, contain all the blood vessels going to the viscera. Clinically understanding the relationship of the vasculature, mesentery, and bowel is extremely important. Resectional strategies are based entirely on the blood supply. The mesentery contains a large number of collateral blood flow pathways, which also have extremely important clinical implications that will be described in subsequent sections.

Celiac Axis

The celiac artery is the largest branch of the abdominal aorta and it supplies the embryologic foregut. It leaves the aorta at a 90-degree angle between T12 and L1 just after the aorta has penetrated the diaphragm. There is considerable variability in both the celiac artery and the SMA, as described later. Classically, the celiac artery trifurcates into the left gastric, splenic, and common hepatic arteries, as seen in Figure 83–4. Multiple

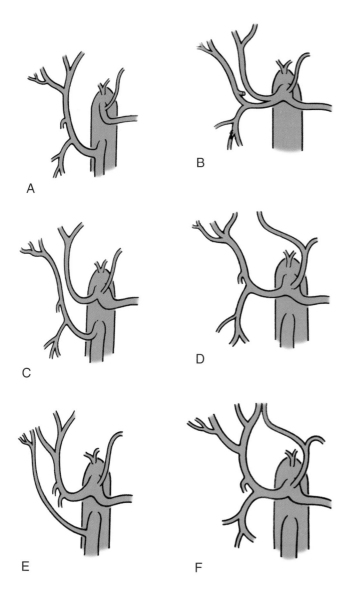

A

B

C

D

E

F

Figure 83–5. Hepatic artery variation. In 25%, the right hepatic artery arises partially or completely from the superior mesenteric as seen in **A, C,** and **E.** A similar proportion of individuals have a variation in the left hepatic artery, with flow arising from the left gastric artery as seen in **D** and **F.** Rarely, the right or left hepatic arteries originate independently from the celiac trunk or a branch after a very short common hepatic artery origin from the celiac as seen in **B** and **C.** The gastroduodenal artery may originate from the right hepatic artery as seen in **B** and **C.** (From Blumgart LH, Hann LE: Surgery of the liver and biliary tract. In Blumgart LH, Fong Y [eds]: Surgical and Radiologic Anatomy of the Liver and Biliary Tract, 3rd ed. London, WB Saunders, 2000.)

anatomic variations of the celiac artery and SMA branches are common and are shown in Figure 83–5. Within the lesser omentum, the left gastric artery first sends branches to supply the distal portion of the esophagus. It then follows a course along the lesser curvature of the stomach and anastomoses with the right gastric artery, which is a branch off the common hepatic artery. The common hepatic artery is also visualized and first

gives off a variable number of branches to the pancreas before the branching of the right gastric artery and the gastroduodenal artery. The common hepatic artery then becomes the proper hepatic artery, which subsequently divides into the right and left hepatic arteries supplying the liver. Before dividing, the proper hepatic artery often gives off branches to the duodenum, including a retroduodenal artery that follows the common bile duct. In approximately 75% of individuals, the cystic artery originates from the right hepatic artery. In approximately 20%, the right hepatic artery may not originate from the proper hepatic artery or is lacking. In the majority of these individuals, the blood supply to the right lobe of the liver originates from the SMA and is called a *replaced right hepatic artery.* If both a right hepatic artery and a supply vessel from the SMA are present, the latter vessel is termed a *recurrent* or *accessory right hepatic artery.* The replaced and accessory right hepatic arteries usually run just posterior, inferior, and lateral to the bile duct and can be injured during pancreaticoduodenectomy and other procedures that involve the porta hepatis if care is not taken to assess their presence. Another 20% of individuals will also have an aberrant left hepatic artery. In this case, some of the blood supply to the left lobe of the liver originates from the left gastric artery and runs with the hepatic branch of the vagus nerve through the lesser omentum to the left lobe of the liver. Rarely, the entire arterial supply to the liver originates from the SMA. The right gastric artery, as mentioned, courses on the lesser curvature of the stomach to anastomose with the left gastric artery. The gastroduodenal artery courses posterior to the duodenum and usually divides into the superior pancreaticoduodenal and right gastroepiploic arteries. The superior pancreaticoduodenal artery divides into duodenal and pancreatic branches. The duodenal branch courses between the pancreas and duodenum anteriorly and continues caudally to anastomose with a branch of the inferior pancreaticoduodenal artery. The superior pancreaticoduodenal artery runs on the posterior surface of the head of the pancreas. The right gastroepiploic artery runs along the greater curvature of the stomach in the greater omentum and eventually communicates with the left gastroepiploic artery. The last branch of the celiac artery is the splenic artery. It courses toward the spleen and lies on the cephalad boarder of the pancreas, which it also supplies. Just before reaching the spleen, the splenic artery gives off multiple short gastric branches to supply the stomach, as well as the left gastroepiploic artery, which courses along the greater curvature of the stomach inferiorly to anastomose with the right gastroepiploic artery.

Superior Mesenteric Artery

The SMA supplies the entire embryologic midgut and is the second largest intra-abdominal branch of the aorta. It branches off the aorta 0.5 to 1.5 cm caudal to the celiac artery. In approximately 1% of individuals, the SMA and celiac arteries arise from a common trunk. The SMA and celiac vessels may also communicate by the artery of Buhler if this embryologic remnant has not been

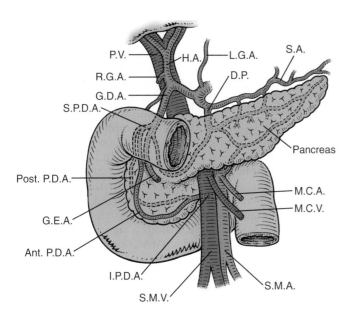

sends branches to the ascending colon and the ileum. The branch to the ileum supplies the cecum and appendix, with the appendiceal artery usually passing posterior to the ileum and entering the mesoappendix, or the mesentery of the appendix. The ascending branches of the ileocolic artery join the right colic artery, which again divides into ascending and descending branches that anastomose with the ileocolic vessels as mentioned and the middle colic artery. The middle colic artery is usually the second branch of the SMA and supplies the transverse colon. It forms collateral anastomoses to the right and left colic arteries. The right colic artery, as mentioned, is a branch of the SMA, but the left colic branches are derived from the IMA. The middle colic artery arises as a common right-middle colic vessel in approximately 50% of people. In approximately 40%, the right colic comes directly off the SMA. The ileocolic artery may originate directly from the SMA or arise as a common vessel with the right colic artery.

Inferior Mesenteric Artery

The IMA, like the celiac artery and SMA, arises from the anterior surface of the aorta; it is located approximately 3.8 cm proximal to the bifurcation of the aorta into the common iliac arteries at L3. The IMA supplies the embryologic hindgut. It courses approximately 3.5 cm before branching and is approximately 0.5 cm in diameter. It supplies the distal third of the transverse colon, the splenic flexure, the descending colon, the sigmoid colon, and the proximal part of the rectum. Its branches include the left colic, three or four vessels to the sigmoid colon, and the superior rectal vessels. The left colic artery branches ascend on the descending colon and anastomose with branches of the middle colic artery from the SMA at the splenic flexure. The sigmoidal branches form arcades that anastomose with the left colic artery and the superior rectal artery. The superior rectal artery supplies blood to the wall of the upper two thirds of the rectum and to the mucosa of the lower third of the rectum.

Figure 83–6. Arterial vascular arcades supplying the duodenum and pancreas. Ant. P.D.A., anterior pancreaticoduodenal artery; D.P., dorsal pancreatic artery; G.D.A., gastroduodenal artery; G.E.A., right gastroepiploic artery; H.A., hepatic artery; I.P.D.A., inferior pancreaticoduodenal artery; L.G.A., left gastric artery; M.C.A., middle colic artery; M.C.V., middle colic vein; Post. P.D.A., posterior pancreaticoduodenal artery; P.V., portal vein; R.G.A., right gastric artery; S.A., splenic artery; S.M.A., superior mesenteric artery; S.M.V., superior mesenteric vein; S.P.D.A., superior pancreaticoduodenal artery. (From Blumgart LH, Hann LE: Surgery of the liver and biliary tract. In Blumgart LH, Fong Y [eds]: Surgical and Radiologic Anatomy of the Liver and Biliary Tract, 3rd ed. London, WB Saunders, 2000.)

Celiac Axis–Superior Mesenteric Arterial Communications/Collaterals

Approximately 20% of individuals will have greater than 50% stenosis of the celiac artery at the time of death.[3] The majority of these patients are asymptomatic[4] because of the presence of rich collateral vessels from the SMA. The network of collaterals between the celiac artery, SMA, and IMA is demonstrated in Figure 83–7. The most common collateral pathways surrounding the duodenum and pancreas are shown in Figure 83–6 and involve the pancreaticoduodenal vessels and the dorsal pancreatic artery.[5] The pancreaticoduodenal arcades course anterior and posterior through the head of the pancreas, which they supply along with the duodenum.[6,7] Both the anterior and the posterior pancreaticoduodenal arcades are fed by the gastroduodenal artery from the cephalad direction. These arcades communicate with the SMA via separate inferior pancreaticoduodenal arteries from the

obliterated. The SMA leaves the aorta at a 20- to 30-degree angle posterior to the body of the pancreas at L1. The artery then passes inferiorly and just medial and anterior to a small portion of the uncinate process of the pancreas, where it gives off its first branch, the inferior pancreaticoduodenal artery, as seen in Figure 83–6. This vessel usually arises on the right side because of a relative lack of rotation of this part of the vessel during development. The artery then passes anterior to the third portion of the duodenum, where it divides into anterior and posterior branches that anastomose with pancreaticoduodenal branches of the superior pancreaticoduodenal artery previously described. After passing the duodenum, the SMA enters the root of the mesentery. Other major SMA branches seen in the majority of patients include multiple jejunal and ileal branches and the ileocolic, right colic, and middle colic vessels. There are approximately 12 to 20 jejunal and ileal branches. They run in the mesentery and form a series of arcades before reaching the intestines. The mesentery is longer in the ileum, and there are more arcades in this area. The last ileal artery also forms arcades with the branch supplying the cecum and thus forms a collateral circulation with the ileocolic artery. The ileocolic artery often has a common takeoff with the right colic artery and

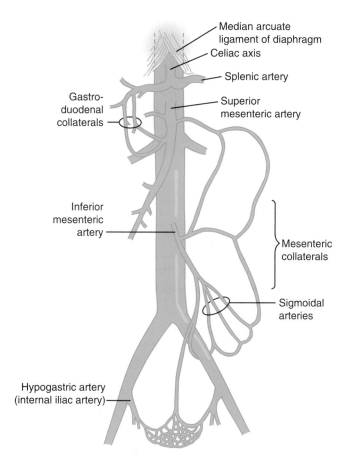

Figure 83–7. Schematic depiction of the major visceral vessels and collateral pathways. (Adapted from Hanson KJ: Mesenteric ischemia syndromes. In Dean RH, Yao JST, Brewster DC [eds]: Current Diagnosis and Treatment in Vascular Surgery. Englewood Cliffs, NJ, Appleton & Lange/ Prentice Hall, 1995, p 264.)

SMA. The dorsal pancreatic artery may arise from a variety of sites, including the splenic artery (39%), the right hepatic artery (12%), the SMA (14%), the celiac artery (22%), or another vessel (13%).[8] This artery has numerous connections between the celiac artery and SMA. The dorsal pancreatic artery also divides into two right and one left branch, with one of the right branches joining the pancreaticoduodenal arcades. The other right branch supplies the uncinate process of the pancreas. The left branch becomes the transverse pancreatic artery, which communicates with caudal pancreatic vessels supplied by the splenic artery. A fourth branch of the dorsal pancreatic artery runs below the inferior border of the pancreas and communicates with the SMA or with branches from the SMA. The collaterals that form may be extensive and a variety of unusual pathways may exist in light of the large variety of hepatic arterial anatomic variants that exist.[5]

Superior Mesenteric–Inferior Mesenteric Arterial Communications

As for the celiac axis, it is not uncommon for the SMA (30%) and IMA (30%) to be stenotic at the time of death.[3,9] Collateral circulation therefore plays a large role in maintaining visceral health. Besides the communicating arcades just described for these vessels, there are a variety of other important vascular communications between the SMA and IMA. The marginal artery of Drummond is located peripherally in the mesentery of the colon. It is usually a continuous arterial pathway along the colon. An anastomosis between the middle and left colic arteries is present in 95% of people and occurs at the splenic flexure of the colon. The location of these anastomoses is designated Griffiths' point. This artery may also be lacking in the proximal portion of the descending colon just beyond the splenic flexure in 5%, in the sigmoid colon in 20%, and at the rectosigmoid junction in an even larger number. Likewise, there is a critical point of Sudeck that occurs between the last sigmoidal branch and the superior rectal artery. When undertaking colonic resection, it is important to ensure adequate blood supply to both ends of the bowel, and rectal resections should include a portion of the sigmoid colon taken above this potential critical point to ensure adequate vascular supply at the anastomosis. Other important vascular communications include the meandering mesenteric artery (MMA), which is its preferred name. The MMA is present in approximately two thirds of the population. It has also been called the central anastomotic artery of the colon, the accessory middle colic artery, the mesomesenteric artery, the middle-left colic collateral, the arch of Riolan, the arch of Treves, and the artery of Drummond (not the marginal artery of Drummond). The MMA is a communication between a branch leaving the SMA just proximal to the middle colic artery and a branch of the ascending left colic artery.

Inferior Mesenteric–Hypogastric Communications

The rectum receives three main sources of blood flow. The superior rectal arteries arise from the IMA and have been described. The two other vessels are the middle and inferior rectal vessels, as seen in Figure 83–8. The superior rectal artery is largely responsible for supplying the upper two thirds of the rectum, but its branches course submucosally and anastomose with branches from the inferior rectal artery in the anal columns. The middle rectal arteries are branches of the internal iliac arteries and supply the muscular layer of the lower third of the rectum. The inferior rectal arteries are branches of the internal pudendal arteries and supply the lower end of the anal canal, where they anastomose with the superior rectal vessels. The mesenteric circulation is therefore in communication with the systemic circulation via these vessels, which can provide a route of collateral circulation.

Rare Communicating Vessels

Occasionally, other collateral pathways also play significant roles. The splenic artery may supply a branch to the left colic artery, and the iliolumbar branches and superior and inferior epigastric vessels may provide important collaterals via the circumflex iliac and femoral arteries. Parietovisceral communications may also exist.

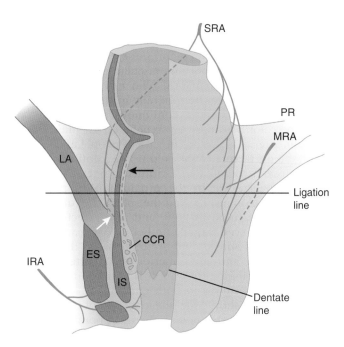

Figure 83–8. Schematic illustration of the rectum and anal canal. The rectal wall has been removed on the right side to demonstrate the transmural course of the branches of the superior rectal artery (SRA). The middle rectal artery (MRA), inferior rectal artery (IRA), corpus cavernosum recti (CCR), levator ani muscle (LA), internal sphincter muscle (IS), external sphincter muscle (ES), and peritoneal reflection (PR) are shown. The *black arrow* indicates longitudinal submucosal branches; the *white arrow* indicates transmural "piercing" branches of the SRA. (From Aigner F, Bodner G, Conrad F, et al: The superior rectal artery and its branching pattern with regard to its clinical influence on ligation techniques for internal hemorrhoids. Am J Surg 187:102-108, 2004.)

CLINICAL CORRELATIONS

Understanding the mesenteric collateral circulation is fundamental to comprehending a variety of disease processes and the compensatory issues that occur in individuals. Chronic blockage of any single mesenteric vessel is usually inconsequential if the collateral pathways are functional. Blockage of the celiac artery usually results in blood flow being routed through the SMA via the pancreaticoduodenal arcades and the dorsal pancreatic vessels that communicate with the gastroduodenal and left gastroepiploic arteries to supply the liver, stomach, pancreas, duodenum, and spleen. Likewise, blockage of the SMA will usually result in blood being routed via the same vessels, as well as the MMA and IMA, to supply the small bowel and right colon. Blockage of the IMA is usually compensated for by blood flow through the MMA, marginal artery of Drummond, and collateral vessels from the inferior and superior rectal arteries.

Acutely, the hypogastric or internal iliac arterial collateral circulation plays an insignificant role. Critical ischemia from acute occlusion can result from single-vessel disease in the absence of adequate collateral

circulation or when multiple vessels are involved. The individual is also much more apt to compensate appropriately when the blood flow disturbance occurs slowly or chronically than when blood flow through a major mesenteric vessel is abruptly or acutely stopped. Likewise, it is important for an operating surgeon to be cognizant of the locations of the anastomosing systems. As mentioned, these communicating systems may be lacking and compounded by disease processes in the native vessels. Segmental colectomy may interrupt critical anastomotic networks between the SMA and IMA and result in acute ischemia in patients with severe mesenteric occlusive disease. Similarly, a Whipple operation in a patient with chronic celiac occlusion can cause hepatic ischemia by interrupting collateral arterial flow from the SMA through the pancreaticoduodenal arcades.

The mesenteric artery most frequently occluded by chronic vascular disease is the IMA. Abdominal aortic aneurysm repair usually results in sacrifice of the IMA. Understanding the collateral circulation is imperative to prevent the development of ischemic colitis in these patients. Likewise, if the SMA is severely diseased and the midgut is receiving a large proportion of blood from the MMA, sacrificing this vessel during aneurysm repair can result in infarction of the small bowel and right colon.

PHYSIOLOGY OF THE MESENTERIC CIRCULATION

The major arterial vessels to the splanchnic system include the celiac axis, SMA, and IMA. In the resting or unfed state, these vessels receive approximately 20% to 25% of cardiac output.[10,11] Approximately 25% of the splanchnic circulation flows directly to the liver, with the remaining 75% of blood flow reaching the liver via the portal system. The splanchnic circulation contains approximately a third of the total blood volume, which makes it the circulatory system's largest reservoir. Branches of the celiac artery, SMA, and IMA penetrate the bowel wall and continue to divide into smaller vessels that result in a vascular plexus within the submucosa.[12] At rest, approximately 70% to 80% of the blood flow is distributed to the mucosa, 15% to 25% is directed to the muscular and serosal layers, and the remaining 5% is distributed to the submucosal layer.[13,14] Sixty percent of the blood flow to the mucosa supplies the epithelial cells in the terminal villi, with the remaining 40% supplying the crypts and goblet cells.[13]

Arterioles are arteries approximately 25 μm in diameter. They are the main resistance vessels to the intestine and are composed of three layers, including an outer tunica adventitia, the tunica media, and an inner tunica intima. The adventitia contains nerve cells that are capable of augmenting the tone of the media, which is composed of a thick layer of smooth muscle. This muscle responds to a variety of neurohumoral stimulatory signals, as described later in this chapter. The intima contains endothelial cells.

Arterioles continue to divide, and at approximately the third-order division they become vessels that supply the tips of the mucosal villi and feed a capillary system.

The capillaries, or exchange vessels, allow for the transfer of particles less than 3 nm in size, such as fluid, electrolytes, nutrients, and oxygen, between cells and the bloodstream. A valve-like mechanism located between arterioles and capillaries controls the entry of blood into capillaries. These valves control blood flow into nutrient beds where exchange takes place, but they have no significant effect on vascular resistance. These valves are, however, responsible for physiologic shunting whereby blood flow is redistributed between nutrient beds. The capillaries coalesce to form venules located in the center of each villus and course along the arterial pathways in reverse.

Venules and veins serve as capacitance vessels and contain the majority of blood in the mesenteric circulation. The small bowel venous system contains approximately 300 to 400 ml of blood that can be readily diverted into the systemic circulation. The walls of capacitance vessels are much thinner than the walls of resistance vessels. These walls, however, do contain smooth muscle, which can significantly affect vessel tone and blood volume within these vessels.

Resistance vessels (arterioles) and capacitance vessels (venules) have different sensitivities to various stimuli, including sympathetic, baroreceptor, and chemoreceptor stimulation.[15-17] These vessels are also innervated by entirely separate sympathetic neurons, which allows for differential control.[18] An increase in venous sympathetic activity results in increased tone within this system and the shifting of a large quantity of blood from the mesenteric circulation to the general circulation. This increased venous tone is also reflected on the capillary bed and results in increased hydrostatic pressure causing an influx of fluid from the capillaries into the bowel, which may be manifested as bowel wall edema.

CONTROL MECHANISMS

Multiple control mechanisms of splanchnic blood flow exist, with some degree of interdependency between them. Control mechanisms may be either extrinsic or intrinsic. Extrinsic mechanisms are systemic, whereas intrinsic mechanism function locally. Both mechanisms affect mesenteric blood flow by altering arteriolar smooth muscle vascular tone.[19]

Extrinsic Control of Splanchnic Blood Flow

Extrinsic control begins with hemodynamic parameters, including cardiac output, blood pressure, and blood volume. Inadequate perfusion results in reduction of blood flow to the intestine. Extrinsic mechanisms may also be neuronal, humoral, or combinations of both. Neuronal control mechanisms include the autonomic reflexes. The intestine is directly innervated by both the sympathetic and parasympathetic nervous systems. Stimulation of the sympathetic and parasympathetic nervous systems results in vasoconstriction and vasodilatation, respectively. Sympathetic activity is the most important single determinant of intestinal blood flow and consists of both adrenergic fibers and nonadrenergic, non-cholinergic fibers that result in vasoconstriction and vasodilatation, respectively. These fibers originate in the brainstem or medulla. Afferent fibers also arise in the intestine and regulate blood flow by releasing neurohumoral substances. These substances are released by a variety of stimuli, including heat, ischemia, and hypoxia. These fibers also connect to the medulla via the vagus nerve and provide feedback to the sympathetic nervous system.[20]

The sympathetic nervous system tonically innervates small arteries, submucosal arterioles, and the myenteric and submucosal plexuses in the small intestine. Norepinephrine, adenosine triphosphate, and neuropeptide Y are the neurotransmitters released from synaptic vesicles in these nerves. Activation of nicotinic or muscarinic receptors by various drugs augments or diminishes the release of norepinephrine.

Functionally, the parasympathetic nervous system does not play a significant role in augmenting blood flow, although three types of parasympathetic nerves exist and travel with the vagus nerves. The parasympathetic nervous system's main role involves intestinal motility. The neurotransmitter in all three parasympathetic pathways is acetylcholine,[21] which does causes vasodilation. The receptors are located on the endothelium, and activation of these receptors results in the release of nitric oxide from the endothelium. Nitric oxide then diffuses to the vascular smooth muscle, where it results in vasodilation. Vasoactive intestinal polypeptide (VIP) may also play a role as a second messenger to acetylcholine.

Intrinsic Control of Splanchnic Blood Flow

Intrinsic regulation involves the intramural nervous system, endothelial signal transduction, and paracrine secretion of vasoactive substances. The response depends on the receptor status of the tissue in the region of the vasoactive material. Mucosal perfusion is largely regulated by products of the endothelium, mainly the vasodilators prostaglandin I_2 and nitric oxide and the vasoconstrictor endothelin. The intrinsic sympathetic tone is mediated by norepinephrine.[22] The resultant blood flow is determined by contributions from the aforementioned factors.

Intrinsic control involves both metabolic and myogenic mechanisms. Metabolic control links the available blood supply to the nutritional needs of the tissue. Cellular by-products and oxygen depletion result in vasodilation and an increase in tissue perfusion. Myogenic control mechanisms are related to transmural pressure. Increased vascular transmural pressure results in diminished blood flow because of increased vascular resistance and arteriolar vasoconstriction, whereas decreased vascular transmural pressure results in increased blood flow because of diminished vascular resistance and arteriolar vasodilation. The metabolic and myogenic control mechanisms therefore exist to ensure autoregulation of blood flow to the intestine, which remains constant between perfusion pressures of 30 and 100 mm Hg.

Direct intraluminal contact of a variety of agents and intramural neurotransmitters (Box 83–1) also affects

Box 83–1   Agents That Alter or Possibly Alter Mesenteric Blood Flow*

Vasoconstriction

Increased sympathetic tone (adrenergic), decreased parasympathetic tone (cholinergic), catecholamines (except in liver and muscle), angiotensin I, II, and III, antidiuretic hormones, calcium, dopamine (high dose), endothelin-1, epinephrine, leukotrienes, motilin, neuromedin U, neuropeptide Y, norepinephrine (high dose), oxytocin, peptide YY, vasopressin, phenylephrine, potassium, prostaglandin B_2, D, F_1, $F_{2\alpha}$, H_2, serotonin (high dose), somatostatin, thromboxane A_2, vasopressin, methoxamine, metaraminol, propranolol, digoxin, ergotamine, platelet-activating factor, increased PO_2, decreased PCO_2, increased pH, decreased metabolites (K^+, lactate, adenosine, etc.)

Vasodilation

Decreased sympathetic tone, increased parasympathetic tone, acetylcholine, adenosine, adenosine diphosphate, adenosine triphosphate, bradykinin, calcitonin gene–related peptide, carbon dioxide, cholecystokinin, dopamine (low dose), gastric inhibitory peptide, gastrin, glucagon, glucocorticoids, glucose-dependent insulinotropic peptide, histamine, hydrogen, insulin, kallikrein, magnesium, neuromedin N, neurotensin, endothelium-derived relaxing factor, nitric oxide, endothelium-derived hyperpolarizing factor, nitroglycerin, norepinephrine (low dose), catecholamines (only in liver and muscle), opiates (enkephalins), pituitary adenylate cyclase–activating polypeptide, prostacyclin, prostaglandin E and I, secretin, serotonin (low dose), substance P, thrombin, thyrotropin-releasing hormone, uridine triphosphate, vasoactive intestinal polypeptide, xenin, adrenomedullin, xenopsin, phentolamine, isoproterenol, pentagastrin, tolazoline (Priscoline), papaverine, nitroprusside, caffeine, sodium nitrite, aminophylline, decreased PO_2, increased PCO_2, decreased pH, increased metabolites

Unknown or Variable Effects

Bombesin, chromogranin A, chromogranin B, cryptins, cholecystokinin, duodenal cholecystokinin-releasing peptide, duodenal secretin-releasing peptide, enteroglucagon, galanin, gastrin-releasing polypeptide, glucagon, glucagon-like peptides, guanylin, incretins, monitor peptides, neuromedin B, neuromedin C, pancreastatin, pancreatic polypeptide, sorbin, trefoil peptides

*Vasoconstriction diminishes blood flow, whereas vasodilation increases blood flow.

mucosal blood flow.[23,24] The actual role that these agents have in vivo in the local regulation of blood flow is largely uncertain. Increased blood flow occurs with local vasodilation in the submucosal vascular network and can be triggered by a variety of substances that work through both cholinergic and noncholinergic pathways.[25] The observed vasodilation is a result of inhibition of sympathetic activity by VIP-containing sensory neurons.

RESTING STATE

Vascular tone is mediated by a variety of mechanisms, including neural mediators, circulating humoral mediators, paracrine and autocrine mediators, and metabolic vasodilators. Neural and humoral mediators have their largest effect on the heart and large vessels and less effect on the microvasculature in the intestine. Paracrine and metabolic mediators have their greatest effect on the microvasculature and significantly less effect on larger vessels. Metabolic autoregulation plays a significant role in modulating vascular tone in the resting state.

DIGESTION

During digestion, blood flow to the gastrointestinal organs increases and is called postprandial intestinal hyperemia. This increased flow is probably required to maintain intestinal function and integrity.[26-28] The intestinal response to a meal includes an increase in blood flow to the submucosal arterioles.[29] This increase in flow may be up to 200% of the resting state flow.

There are two phases of the response to food: the anticipatory phase and the postprandial phase.[10,26] During the anticipatory phase, mesenteric vascular resistance is increased in response to higher sympathetic activity.[30,31] The increased sympathetic activity causes an increase in cardiac output, blood pressure, heart rate, and splanchnic and renal vascular resistance. The postprandial phase begins as the stomach fills with food.

Postprandially, the mesenteric vasculature dilates and blood flow in the SMA increases within 5 minutes by as much as 60%.[32,33] This increase in mesenteric blood flow occurs as a result of redistribution from the extremities.[34] Peak flow occurs 30 to 90 minutes after ingestion and then declines over a period of 2 to 3 hours.[35] The major increase in blood flow is largely to the mucosal layer and is determined by both neurohumoral and paracrine agents released secondary to chemical and mechanical stimuli,[10,25,26,36-38] as well as digested food (protein, lipid, carbohydrates), bile, and chime.[25] Lipids in combination with bile salts produce the greatest net increase in blood flow, whereas the response to carbohydrates occurs quickest.[35] Distention of the bowel lumen does not affect blood flow.[38,39] Various peptides and hormones, including cholecystokinin, secretin, gastrin, serotonin, and bradykinin, may also contribute to postprandial hyperemia.

Postprandial hyperemia cannot occur simultaneously in the entire gastrointestinal tract. Vasodilation of the entire mesenteric circulation would result in the capacity to accommodate a blood flow of 4 to 5 L/min (majority of cardiac output). Therefore, blood flow to the mesentery increases in a sequential manner, with areas containing food receiving the majority of flow.[38,40] According to some reports, hyperemia occurs in the segment containing food,[25,41,42] and once the chyme passes a particular region in the intestinal tract, blood flow returns to baseline.[30,43]

AUTOREGULATORY ESCAPE

Blood flow is maintained at normal levels during a variety of physiologic conditions, including those with elevated sympathetic activity and catecholamine levels. This process is called splanchnic autoregulation and acts via multiple mechanisms as described earlier. As long as mean blood pressure remains higher than 70 mm Hg, intestinal blood flow is not dependent on blood pressure. Blood flow may initially decrease under the vasoconstrictor effects, but then it gradually returns toward normal. Resumption of blood flow is most likely a result of local metabolic factors that result in vasodilation, including ischemia. Blood flow, under such circumstances, is preferentially increased to the submucosa over the mucosa, which probably explains why the mucosa may sustain ischemic damage with the bowel still remaining viable if flow is restored. When blood pressure drops below 70 mm Hg, intestinal perfusion will have a linear relationship to blood pressure. Below a pressure of 40 mm Hg, the bowel will become ischemic and sustain injury.[44]

DOPAMINE

Administration of low-dose dopamine (<5 µg/kg/min) produces preferential dopaminergic and β-adrenergic effects over α-adrenergic effects. Activation of these receptors results in dilation of the splanchnic circulation and a net increase in splanchnic blood flow.[45,46] This blood flow, however, is redistributed away from the gut mucosa,[47] and although net splanchnic flow increases, mucosal ischemia worsens. Mucosal ischemia results in increased translocation of microorganisms and endotoxins into the portal circulation. Dopamine also increases hepatic ischemia, which results in decreased clearance of proinflammatory cytokines. To conclude, low-dose dopamine probably worsens mesenteric ischemia.[48-50] Besides being harmful to the gastrointestinal tract, recent evidence also suggests that dopamine is not useful in the treatment or prevention of renal dysfunction and is harmful to the endocrine, immunologic, and respiratory systems in critically ill patients.[51] The long upheld practice of administering low-dose dopamine to improve renal function and mesenteric perfusion should be abandoned.

CATECHOLAMINES

Sympathetic stimulation is a major determinant of tone in both the arterial resistance vessels and venous capacitance vessels. Table 83–1 lists some commonly used intra-

Table 83–1 Commonly Used Intravenous Agents That Augment Mesenteric Vascular Blood Flow*

Agent	Mechanism of Action in Normovolemic Patients
Amrinone	Direct inhibition of phosphodiesterase results in increased cAMP and vasodilation
Dobutamine	Mild β₂ stimulation
Dopamine	Dopaminergic effects at 1 µg/kg/min†
	Predominately β effects between 3 and 10 µg/kg/min
	Combined α and β between 10 and 20 µg/kg/min
	Predominately α at >20 µg/kg/min
Epinephrine	Renal vasoconstriction at less than 1 µg/min
	Cardiac β stimulation between 1 and 4 µg/min
	Increasing α stimulation between 5 and 20 µg/min
	Predominantly α at >20 µg/min
Isoproterenol	Pure β-agonist
Nitroglycerin	Directly relaxes arteries and veins
	Venodilation predominates at doses <50 µg/min
	Arterial vasodilation predominates at doses >200 µg/min
Nitroprusside	Directly dilates arteries and veins
Norepinephrine	Predominately α effects
Papaverine	Blocks angiotensin II– and vasopressin-mediated vasoconstriction
Phenylephrine	Pure α-agonist

*Generally, vasoconstriction occurs with stimulation of α-receptors, which diminishes mesenteric blood flow, whereas vasodilation occurs with stimulation of β-receptors, which increases mesenteric blood flow. These effects, however, are dependent on the location of the receptors, which is shown in Figure 83–9; the density of receptors in the mesenteric arterial and venous circulation, which is shown in Table 83–2; the affinity of the agent for the receptor subtype; the plasma concentration of other agents; the preexisting tone of the mesenteric vessels; and the volume of blood in the circulation. The effects of catecholamines administered during hypovolemia depend on the blood volume in the splanchnic reservoir.

†See text specific to dopamine action on mesenteric vascular flow.

cAMP, cyclic adenosine monophosphate.

venous agents, including catecholamines, that augment mesenteric vascular blood flow. Vascular tone is largely dependent on the type of receptors stimulated. Receptor stimulation depends on the type of catecholamine and its concentration at the receptors. Understanding the effects of catecholamines on mesenteric blood flow requires a full understanding of catecholamine actions on the entire splanchnic circulation.[11] The receptors located on various splanchnic beds are detailed in Table 83–2 and shown in Figure 83–9. The hepatic arterial vascular bed contains mainly α_1-, a smaller quantity of α_2-, and an intermediate number of β_2-receptors.[52] The hepatic capacitance vessels, including the sinusoids, have α-adrenergic receptors, and the hepatic veins have both α- and β_2-adrenergic receptors. Activation of α-receptors results in vasoconstriction, whereas activation of β_2-receptors results in vasodilation. The intestinal resistance (arterial) vessels have roughly equal numbers of α_1- and β_2-receptors and a lesser number of α_2-receptors. The mesenteric venous system contains largely α_1-, a smaller number of α_2-, and a questionable number of β_2-receptors. Activation of α-receptors results in venoconstriction and a decrease in venous capacitance, whereas activation of β_2-receptors results in venodilation and an increase in venous capacitance.

Sympathetic activity causes a variety of hemodynamic consequences, including an increase in cardiac output. This increased output is dependent on an increase in blood volume, which largely comes from the splanchnic circulation. When arterial flow decreases, pressure within the venous capacitance vessels also decreases. The decrease in venous pressure is minimized by elastic recoil in the veins, which maintains a pressure adequate to force the splanchnic vascular volume into the systemic circulation. This phenomenon of elastic recoil can function even as arterial inflow is decreased. These two methods of venoconstriction are also responsible for the decreased splanchnic flow and shift of blood volume from the splanchnic circulation to the systemic circulation with exercise or hemorrhage. With mild exercise, there is a 35% decrease in splanchnic blood volume. In cases of moderate hemorrhage, approximately 65% of the total splanchnic blood volume can be directed into the systemic circulation.[53]

SUMMARY

Nature has developed a mesenteric circulatory system that is rich in collateral circulation. A significant survival advantage is probably held by animals and people who foster a rich blood supply to their mesenteric circulation. Understanding the blood supply to the mesenteric circulation is critical for clinicians and especially surgeons, for all resectional and other procedures performed within the abdomen have the potential to result in

| Table 83–2 | Vascular Bed Receptor Subtypes |

Vascular Bed	Receptor Subtype		
	α_1	α_2	β_2
Mesenteric arterial	+++	++	----
Hepatic arterial	+++	+	--
Mesenteric venous	+++	+	-?

From Gelman S, Mushlin PS: Catecholamine-induced changes in the splanchnic circulation affecting systemic hemodynamics. Anesthesiology 100:434-439, 2004.

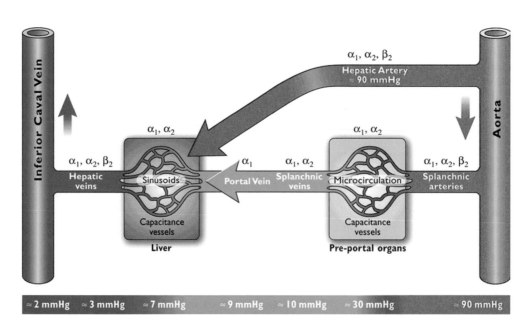

Figure 83–9. Diagrammatic representation of the splanchnic vasculature. Splanchnic arteries represent all arterial vessels of the preportal organs; splanchnic veins represent the pooled venous blood from all these organs. The distribution of adrenoceptor subtypes (α_2, β_2) and approximate intravascular pressures are shown for corresponding segments of the splanchnic vasculature. (From Gelmen S, Mushlin PS: Catecholamine-induced changes in the splanchnic circulation affecting systemic hemodynamics. Anesthesiology 100:434-439, 2004.)

ischemia of the mesenteric organs if done without attention to their vascular supply. The complexity of the situation grows exponentially when dealing with the multitude of pathologic states that can affect vessel patency, as well as the variety of anatomic variations, including the presence of collateral vessels.

Regulation of mesenteric blood flow is an extremely complex process that involves a variety of control mechanisms operating at multiple levels. Adding to the complexity, these control mechanisms directly influence and augment each other. Changes that occur within humans after ingestion of a meal further complicates the scenario. Clinically, it is essential to understand where various receptors are located and their function when stimulated. It is also crucial to understand the effects of various pressor agents on both the systemic and mesenteric systems and realize that progress is still being made in understanding the effects of these agents. The best example of this continues to be dopamine. Low-dose dopamine was once touted as being a drug that improves both renal and mucosal blood flow. Recent studies have now shown that it is actually harmful and should not be used for this indication. With the extremely large number of chemicals and hormones that directly affect the mesenteric circulation and the large number of disease states that affect patients, there will probably be further important changes in the manner in which we practice medicine in the future.

REFERENCES

1. Crafts RC: A Textbook of Human Anatomy, 3rd ed. New York, Wiley, 1985.
2. Langman J, Sadler TW: Langman's Medical Embryology, 5th ed. Baltimore, Williams & Wilkins, 1985.
3. Derrick JR, Pollard HS, Moore RM: The pattern of arteriosclerotic narrowing of the celiac and superior mesenteric arteries. Ann Surg 149:684-689, 1959.
4. Valentine RJ, Martin JD, Myers SI, et al: Asymptomatic celiac and superior mesenteric artery stenoses are more prevalent among patients with unsuspected renal artery stenoses. J Vasc Surg 14:195-199, 1991.
5. Song SY, Chung JW, Kwon JW, et al: Collateral pathways in patients with celiac axis stenosis: Angiographic–spiral CT correlation. Radiographics 22:881-893, 2002.
6. Kornblith PL, Boley SJ, Whitehouse BS: Anatomy of the splanchnic circulation. Surg Clin North Am 72:1-30, 1992.
7. Ruzicka FF Jr, Rossi P: Normal vascular anatomy of the abdominal viscera. Radiol Clin North Am 8:3-29, 1970.
8. Michels NA: Blood supply of the pancreas and the duodenum. In Michels NA (ed): Blood Supply and Anatomy of the Upper Abdominal Organs, with a Descriptive Atlas. Philadelphia, JB Lippincott, 1955, pp 236-247.
9. Reiner L, Jimenez FA, Rodriguez FL: Atherosclerosis in the mesenteric circulation: Observations and correlations with aortic and coronary atherosclerosis. Am Heart J 66:200-209, 1963.
10. Chou CC: Splanchnic and overall cardiovascular hemodynamics during eating and digestion. Fed Proc 42:1658-1661, 1983.
11. Gelman S, Mushlin PS: Catecholamine-induced changes in the splanchnic circulation affecting systemic hemodynamics. Anesthesiology 100:434-439, 2004.
12. Gannon BJ, Perry MA: Vascular organization of alimentary tract. In Schultz SG, Rauner BB, Wood JD (eds): Handbook of Physiology. The Gastrointestinal System. Bethesda, Md, American Physiological Society, distributed by Oxford University Press, 1989, pp 1301-1334.
13. Chou CC: Intestinal blood flow regulation. In Dulbecco R (ed): Encyclopedia of Human Biology, vol 4. San Diego, Calif, Academic Press, 1991, pp 547-556.
14. Hirst GDS: Neuromuscular transmission in intramural blood vessels. In Schultz SG, Rauner BB, Wood JD (eds): Handbook of Physiology. The Gastrointestinal System. Bethesda, Md, American Physiological Society, distributed by Oxford University Press, 1989, pp 1635-1665.
15. Karim F, Hainsworth R: Responses of abdominal vascular capacitance to stimulation of splanchnic nerves. Am J Physiol 231:434-440, 1976.
16. Hainsworth R, Karim F: Responses of abdominal vascular capacitance in the anaesthetized dog to changes in carotid sinus pressure. J Physiol 262:659-677, 1976.
17. Ford R, Hainsworth R, Rankin AJ, Soladoye AO: Abdominal vascular responses to changes in carbon dioxide tension in the cephalic circulation of anaesthetized dogs. J Physiol 358:417-431, 1985.
18. Zheng ZL, Travagli RA, Kreulen DL: Patterns of innervation of sympathetic vascular neurons by peptide-containing primary sensory fibers. Brain Res 827:113-121, 1999.
19. Horowitz A, Menice CB, Laporte R, Morgan KG: Mechanisms of smooth muscle contraction. Physiol Rev 76:967-1003, 1996.
20. Guyton AC: Textbook of Medical Physiology, 8th ed. Philadelphia, WB Saunders, 1991.
21. Jodal M, Lundgren O: Neurohormonal control of gastrointestinal blood flow. In Schultz SG, Rauner BB, Wood JD (eds): Handbook of Physiology. The Gastrointestinal System. Bethesda, Md, American Physiological Society, distributed by Oxford University Press, 1989, pp 1667-1711.
22. Salzman AL: Nitric oxide in the gut. New Horizons 3:352-364, 1995.
23. Hansen MB, Dresner LS, Wait RB: Profile of neurohumoral agents on mesenteric and intestinal blood flow in health and disease. Physiol Res 47:307-327, 1998.
24. Matheson PJ, Wilson MA, Garrison RN: Regulation of intestinal blood flow. J Surg Res 93:182-196, 2000.
25. Chou CC, Alemayehu A: Peptidergic regulation of gastrointestinal blood flow. In Alemayehu A, Brown DR (eds): Gastrointestinal Regulatory Peptides. New York, Springer-Verlag, 1993, pp 325-342.
26. Chou CC, Coatney RW: Nutrient-induced changes in intestinal blood flow in the dog. Br Vet J 150:423-437, 1994.
27. Pawlik WW, Fondacaro JD, Jacobson ED: Metabolic hyperemia in canine gut. Am J Physiol 239:G12-G17, 1980.
28. Shepherd AP: Intestinal capillary blood flow during metabolic hyperemia. Am J Physiol 237:E548-E554, 1979.
29. Vanner S, Jiang MM, Surprenant A: Mucosal stimulation evokes vasodilation in submucosal arterioles by neuronal and nonneuronal mechanisms. Am J Physiol 264:G202-G212, 1993.
30. Vatner SF, Franklin D, Van Citters RL: Coronary and visceral vasoactivity associated with eating and digestion in the conscious dog. Am J Physiol 219:1380-1385, 1970.
31. Burns GP, Schenk WG Jr: Effect of digestion and exercise on intestinal blood flow and cardiac output. An experimental study in the conscious dog. Arch Surg 98:790-794, 1969.
32. Norryd C, Denker H, Lunderquist A, et al: Superior mesenteric blood flow during digestion in man. Acta Chir Scand 141:197-202, 1975.
33. Fronek K, Stahlgren LH: Systemic and regional hemodynamic changes during food intake and digestion in nonanesthetized dogs. Circ Res 23:687-692, 1968.
34. Vatner SF, Patrick TA, Higgins CB, Franklin D: Regional circulatory adjustments to eating and digestion in conscious unrestrained primates. J Appl Physiol 36:524-529, 1974.
35. Granger ND, Kvietys PR, Korthuis RJ, Premen AJ: Microcirculation of the intestinal mucosa. In Schultz SG, Rauner BB, Wood JD (eds): Handbook of Physiology. The Gastrointestinal System. Bethesda, Md, American Physiological Society, distributed by Oxford University Press, 1989, pp 1405-1474.
36. Gallavan RH Jr, Chou CC: Possible mechanisms for the initiation and maintenance of postprandial intestinal hyperemia. Am J Physiol 249:G301-G308, 1985.
37. Gallavan RH Jr, Chou CC, Kvietys PR, Sit SP: Regional blood flow during digestion in the conscious dog. Am J Physiol 238:H220-H225, 1980.

38. Chou CC, Hsieh CP, Yu YM, et al: Localization of mesenteric hyperemia during digestion in dogs. Am J Physiol 230:583-589, 1976.

39. Chou CC, Kvietys P, Post J, Sit SP: Constituents of chyme responsible for postprandial intestinal hyperemia. Am J Physiol 235:H677-H682, 1978.

40. Kato M, Naruse S, Takagi T, Shionoya S: Postprandial gastric blood flow in conscious dogs. Am J Physiol 257:G111-G117, 1989.

41. Bond JH, Prentiss RA, Levitt MD: The effects of feeding on blood flow to the stomach, small bowel, and colon of the conscious dog. J Lab Clin Med 93:594-599, 1979.

42. Fara JW, Rubinstein EH, Sonnenschein RR: Intestinal hormones in mesenteric vasodilation after intraduodenal agents. Am J Physiol 223:1058-1067, 1972.

43. Vatner SF, Franklin D, Van Citters RL: Mesenteric vasoactivity associated with eating and digestion in the conscious dog. Am J Physiol 219:170-174, 1970.

44. Bradbury AW, Brittenden J, McBride K, Ruckley CV: Mesenteric ischaemia: A multidisciplinary approach. Br J Surg 82:1446-1459, 1995.

45. Kullmann R, Breull WR, Reinsberg J, et al: Dopamine produces vasodilation in specific regions and layers of the rabbit gastrointestinal tract. Life Sci 32:2115-2122, 1983.

46. Ruokonen E, Takala J, Kari A, et al: Regional blood flow and oxygen transport in septic shock. Crit Care Med 21:1296-1303, 1993.

47. Giraud GD, MacCannell KL: Decreased nutrient blood flow during dopamine- and epinephrine-induced intestinal vasodilation. J Pharmacol Exp Ther 230:214-220, 1984.

48. Segal JM, Phang PT, Walley KR: Low-dose dopamine hastens onset of gut ischemia in a porcine model of hemorrhagic shock. J Appl Physiol 73:1159-1164, 1992.

49. Marik PE, Mohedin M: The contrasting effects of dopamine and norepinephrine on systemic and splanchnic oxygen utilization in hyperdynamic sepsis. JAMA 272:1354-1357, 1994.

50. Neviere R, Mathieu D, Chagnon JL, et al: The contrasting effects of dobutamine and dopamine on gastric mucosal perfusion in septic patients. Am J Respir Crit Care Med 154:1684-1688, 1996.

51. Holmes CL, Walley KR: Bad medicine: Low-dose dopamine in the ICU. Chest 123:1266-1275, 2003.

52. Richardson PD, Withrington PG: Physiological regulation of the hepatic circulation. Annu Rev Physiol 44:57-69, 1982.

53. Brooksby GA, Donald DE: Dynamic changes in splanchnic blood flow and blood volume in dogs during activation of sympathetic nerves. Circ Res 29:227-238, 1971.

Mesenteric Ischemia

Anthony J. Comerota · Matthew Todd Miller

Mesenteric ischemia is a frequently lethal condition resulting from critically reduced perfusion to the gastrointestinal tract. It has acute and chronic forms that involve both the arterial and venous sides of the circulation. Common to all forms of mesenteric ischemia are the diagnostic difficulties and challenging management decisions accompanying these patients. First described in the 1500s, diagnosis and management of mesenteric ischemia consisted of abdominal exploration with resection of the involved bowel, but the diagnosis was often made too late to save the patient. In 1950, using the newly delineated principles of vascular surgery, Klass[1] performed an early abdominal exploration with superior mesenteric artery (SMA) embolectomy in a patient with acute mesenteric ischemia. Although the patient died of acute heart failure during the postoperative period, the significant advance of visceral revascularization was apparent when normal bowel was observed at autopsy. In the years that followed, numerous cases of successful mesenteric embolectomy with patient survival were reported, and operations were developed for revascularization of patients with acute and chronic mesenteric ischemia.[2] It is conceptually important that physicians involved in the care of patients with mesenteric ischemia, especially acute mesenteric ischemia, recognize that the major advances in care and the improved survival of these patients have been achieved as a result of revascularization of the ischemic bowel.

Despite the remarkable advances in vascular surgical technique, vascular imaging, percutaneous intervention, and surgical critical care, mesenteric ischemia remains a complex and often disheartening disease. Acute mesenteric ischemia is a life-threatening vascular emergency that requires a high degree of clinical suspicion and early intervention to avoid a poor outcome. Unfortunately, recent reports indicate that its incidence is on the rise.[3,4] Mesenteric ischemia accounts for 0.1% of hospital admissions and 1% to 2% of admissions for abdominal pain.[5] One population-based study showed the incidence of mesenteric ischemia to be 9 per 100,000 person-years; however, as anticipated, the incidence increases substantially with age.[6] The reported mortality ranges from 24% to a high of 96%, with an average of 69%.[7]

The mesenteric arterial circulation comprises three major aortic branches with multiple collaterals: the celiac axis, the SMA, and the inferior mesenteric artery (IMA). The celiac axis consists of three major branch vessels to the foregut: the common hepatic, left gastric, and splenic arteries. The SMA supplies blood flow to the majority of the small intestine and the right colon and a portion of the transverse colon. Finally, the IMA is responsible for blood flow to the remaining transverse, descending, and sigmoid colon. The arterial collaterals with their anastomotic arcades often allow for compensatory intestinal blood flow when one or more of the major visceral arteries becomes diseased or occluded, most commonly as a result of chronic disease. Therefore, patients with acute or, more often, chronic disease may be protected from intestinal ischemia because of their collateral circulation (Fig. 84–1). It is commonly observed that in patients with chronic mesenteric ischemia, two of the three major visceral arteries are diseased, and these patients have symptoms of intestinal ischemia. However, patients with acute arterial occlusion of one major artery, usually the SMA, experience severe symptoms because the compensatory collateral circulation is inadequate.

The splanchnic circulation receives approximately 25% of the resting and 35% of the postprandial cardiac output.[8-10] Seventy percent of the mesenteric blood flow is directed to the mucosal and submucosal layers of the bowel, with the remainder supplying the muscularis and serosal layers.

Not surprisingly, the mucosal layer of the bowel wall is the most severely affected by acute mesenteric ischemia, and abnormalities have been observed as early as 10 minutes after arterial occlusion in experimental models.[11] Mucosal integrity is compromised early, and bowel wall edema, loss of capillary integrity leading to bacterial translocation and endotoxemia, and exudation of fluid into the bowel lumen ensue. The mucosa sloughs, with ulcerations left in the bowel wall. Up to this point the intestine remains viable; however, if the

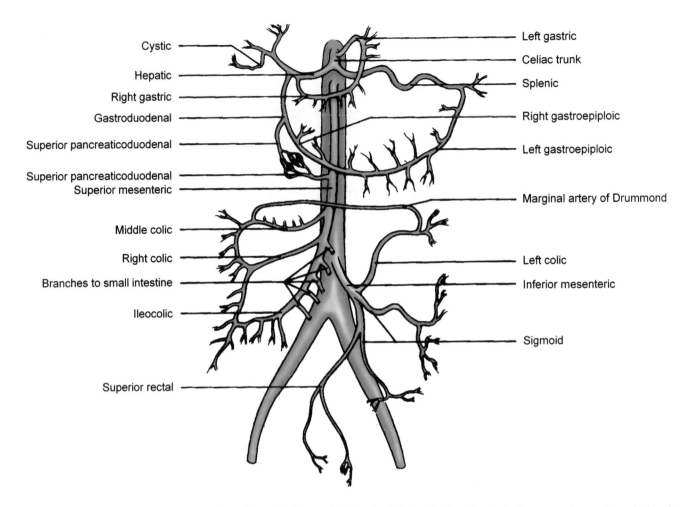

Cystic
Hepatic
Right gastric
Gastroduodenal
Superior pancreaticoduodenal
Superior pancreaticoduodenal
Superior mesenteric
Middle colic
Right colic
Branches to small intestine
Ileocolic
Superior rectal

Left gastric
Celiac trunk
Splenic
Right gastroepiploic
Left gastroepiploic
Marginal artery of Drummond
Left colic
Inferior mesenteric
Sigmoid

Figure 84–1.   The mesenteric circulation. (From Schwartz LB, Davis RD Jr, Heinle JS, et al: The vascular system. In Lyerly HK, Gaynor JW Jr [eds]: The Handbook of Surgical Intensive Care, 3rd ed. St Louis: Mosby–Year Book, 1992, p 287.)

ischemia progresses, there is ongoing necrosis of the muscularis and serosal layers of the bowel wall, at which point the involved segment is no longer salvageable.

Although acute mesenteric ischemia results in profound illness, correcting the ischemia and reperfusing the ischemic bowel can cause further deterioration because of myocardial depression and a generalized systemic inflammatory response. Escape of oxygen free radicals, myocardial depressant factor, and other products of tissue injury into the circulation contributes to the reperfusion phenomenon, which can lead to disseminated intravascular coagulation and multiorgan system dysfunction. This is mentioned not to discourage mesenteric revascularization, but to emphasize the importance of expedient diagnosis and reversal of the ischemia. Hypoxia disrupts bowel wall metabolism and thereby causes cellular damage leading to profound vasoconstriction, which further compromises tissue perfusion, even after large-vessel revascularization. Early intraarterial infusion of vasodilators has improved mesenteric revascularization and resulted in more favorable outcomes.[2,8,12,13] A limited experience with infusion of superoxide free radical scavengers has shown benefit in reducing mesenteric reperfusion complications[14];

however, the benefit of superoxide free radical scavengers remains under investigation.

ACUTE ARTERIAL MESENTERIC ISCHEMIA

Unfortunately, the prognosis of patients with acute mesenteric ischemia is poor and, in most communities, has not changed during the past 30 or more years. This is true despite the surgical, technical, endovascular, and pharmacologic advances that have occurred during the same time frame. This state of affairs should cause one to reflect on the disease process, appreciate the benefit of revascularization, and recognize that delay in diagnosis is costly and that traditional approaches to these difficult patients require modifications to improve outcomes.

Insight can be gained by reviewing advances in the management of mesenteric ischemia and putting them into the perspective of personal and clinical experience. Personal observation has revealed that patients who undergo emergency exploratory laparotomy without a definitive diagnosis preoperatively have a prohibitively high mortality rate. A common scenario in these patients is resection of ischemic bowel without mesenteric revascularization. Absent a preoperative diagnosis and knowledge of patients' underlying anatomy and pathophysiologic contributors to their mesenteric ischemia, attempts at revascularization are often unsuccessful and are generally ill advised. On the other hand, in patients in whom the diagnosis is made preoperatively and who undergo hemodynamically guided aggressive resuscitation with appropriately planned revascularization that addresses the anatomic and pathophysiologic causes of the mesenteric ischemia, the likelihood of survival is maximized.

These clinical observations are supported by a number of animal experiments performed by Boley and colleagues.[15-17] They demonstrated that when mesenteric blood flow is reduced, either from a systemic cause or from mesenteric obstruction, vascular resistance increases within several hours as a result of mesenteric vasoconstriction. If normal mesenteric blood flow could be promptly restored, the vasoconstriction was immediately reversible. If, however, vasoconstriction was present for several hours, it remained even after large-artery mesenteric occlusion was corrected because of the profound vasospasm. These experiments were followed by others demonstrating that small-vessel mesenteric vasoconstriction was relieved by the intra-arterial infusion of papaverine into the SMA; therefore, a method of treating the vasoconstriction was proposed.

These experimental observations ultimately led to an aggressive diagnostic and revascularization approach to acute mesenteric ischemia. The improved outcomes with precise diagnosis and revascularization and the recent literature demonstrating the benefit of percutaneous techniques form the basis for the recommendations outlined in Figure 84–2. Early diagnosis is essential and is most often achieved by having a low threshold for arteriography and placement of a catheter for the infusion of papaverine. Using this approach of early arteriographic diagnosis with catheter-directed papaverine infusion, Boley et al.[2] and Clark and Gallant[18] reduced the mortality to less than 50% in patients with acute intestinal ischemia. Even in the subset of patients with acute SMA embolism in whom the diagnosis was made promptly (≤12 hours), Boley et al.[19] reported a 33% mortality rate. Though high, this is considered a substantial improvement over what had traditionally been reported.

Embolic Occlusion

Embolic occlusion of the SMA accounts for 40% to 50% of cases of acute mesenteric ischemia.[3,12] Most emboli originate in the heart and are secondary to myocardial infarction, cardiac arrhythmia, endocarditis, cardiomyopathy, ventricular aneurysm, valvular disorders, or depressed left ventricular function as a result of ischemic heart disease (Box 84–1). Rarely, a paradoxical embolus traveling through a patent foramen ovale from a thrombus in the venous system is the cause. Most mesenteric emboli lodge in the SMA because it branches from the aorta at an oblique angle, as opposed to the celiac artery,

---

> **Box 84–1**   **Etiology and Distribution of Mesenteric Ischemia**
>
> **Acute Mesenteric Ischemia**
>
> Emboli (50%)
>   Arrhythmia
>   Valvular disease
>   Myocardial infarction
>   Hypokinetic ventricular wall
>   Cardiac aneurysm
>   Aortic atherosclerotic disease
>   Iatrogenic
>
> Thrombosis (25%)
>   Atherosclerotic disease
>
> Nonocclusive (5% to 15%)
>   Pancreatitis
>   Heart failure
>   Sepsis
>   Cardiac bypass
>   Burns
>   Renal failure
>   Medications
>
> Venous occlusion
>   Hypercoagulable state
>   Sepsis
>   Compression
>   Pregnancy
>   Portal hypertension
>   Malignancy
>
> **Chronic Mesenteric Ischemia**
>
> Atherosclerotic disease
>
> Arterial hyperplasia/dysplasia
>
> Inflammatory disease

---

which is nearly perpendicular to the axis of the aorta. More than 50% of emboli lodge in the mid to distal segment of the SMA. The SMA tapers after major branch points, and emboli are commonly found distal to the middle colic artery. Less than 15% of emboli occlude the SMA at its origin.

The point of occlusion affects the magnitude and distribution of the ischemia that it produces. Occlusion at the origin of the SMA causes intestinal ischemia extending from the ligament of Treitz to the transverse colon, whereas occlusion distal to the middle colic artery preserves the right colon and proximal part of the small bowel. As emphasized earlier, the key to successful management of patients with acute mesenteric ischemia is a high index of suspicion leading to early diagnosis, aggressive resuscitation, and early mesenteric revascularization.

Patients with acute SMA embolism usually have sudden and dramatic symptoms that reflect the abruptness of the occlusion and the severity of ischemia distal to the embolus because of the absence of collateral circulation. As with all forms of acute mesenteric ischemia in patients who are evaluated early after the onset of occlusion, their complaints of severe abdominal pain contrast markedly with the absence of physical findings. Rectal examination is not generally helpful because the presence of occult blood is typically a late occurrence. Early on the pain may be colicky in nature, but it then becomes constant. Nausea and vomiting may occur in some patients and, less commonly, diarrhea, which may lead to diagnostic confusion.

Thrombotic Occlusion

Acute thrombotic occlusion generally occurs in conjunction with chronically diseased vessels and may have a somewhat more insidious onset because of previously developed collateral circulation. These patients account for 25% to 35% of cases of acute mesenteric ischemia. A history of general abdominal discomfort, anorexia, and perhaps symptoms of postprandial abdominal pain, weight loss, and food aversion before their acute episode assists an astute clinician in differentiating between acute thrombotic versus acute embolic occlusion in some patients. Unfortunately, such a history is not found consistently because many patients with acute thrombotic occlusion have no symptoms until the occlusive event. This may be due to rupture of a previously noncritical atherosclerotic plaque that abruptly occludes the vessel, a pathophysiologic catastrophe similar to embolic occlusion because the patient may not have had significant stenosis before the acute event.

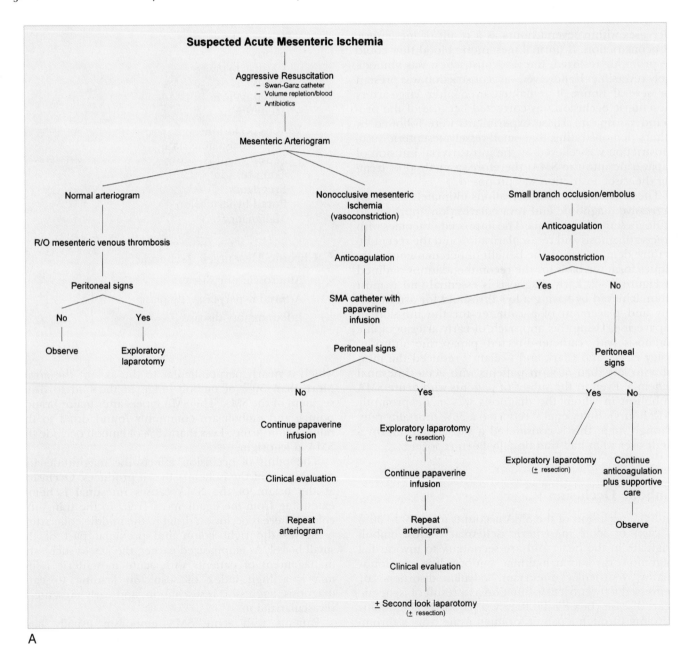

A

Figure 84–2. **A** and **B,** Recommended treatment of acute mesenteric ischemia. R/O, rule out; SMA, superior mesenteric artery.

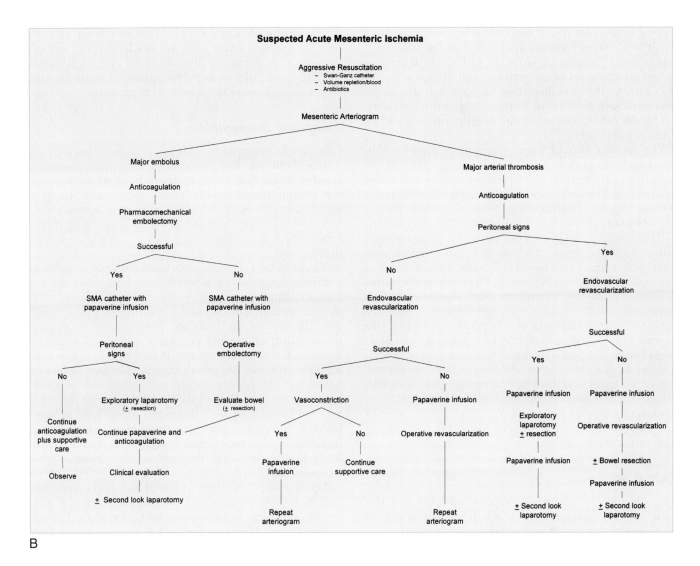

Figure 84–2, cont'd.

Nonocclusive Mesenteric Ischemia

Nonocclusive mesenteric ischemia, which accounts for approximately 20% of all cases of acute mesenteric ischemia, has manifestations similar to those of mesenteric arterial thrombosis, but it occurs with patent mesenteric arteries. Splanchnic vasoconstriction is the underlying pathophysiologic process and is precipitated by hypoperfusion from medications, depressed cardiac output, or renal or hepatic disease.[13] When blood pressure in the bowel falls below a critical pressure of 40 mm Hg, ischemia develops and eventually leads to infarction and bowel necrosis.

Diagnosis of nonocclusive mesenteric ischemia can be especially difficult in hospitalized patients, who are often critically ill and unable to complain because of either ongoing sedation or intubation. The diagnosis is often delayed because their clinical manifestations may be wrongfully attributed to their underlying critical illness. Older patients who have acute myocardial infarction, congestive heart failure, dysrhythmia, sepsis, or hypovolemia or use splanchnic vasoconstrictors are at increased risk for nonocclusive mesenteric ischemia. Other patient populations at particularly high risk are hemodialysis patients and those with a recent history of cardiopulmonary bypass, major abdominal surgery, pancreatitis, aortic dissection, or burns.[20,21]

Diagnosis

Early diagnosis is the key to successful management of most diseases and is especially true for acute mesenteric ischemia. Acute arterial mesenteric ischemia results from a number of causes (see Box 84–1), which if uncorrected often lead to intestinal infarction. Recognition of acute mesenteric ischemia can be difficult because most patients have nonspecific symptoms of abdominal pain. *Abdominal pain out of proportion to the findings on physical examination and persisting beyond 2 to 3 hours* is the classic picture. Diarrhea, nausea, vomiting, and anorexia can also be part of the initial symptom complex. Fifteen percent of patients report melena or hematochezia, and occult fecal blood is found in at least half the patients.[22] Leukocytosis is common. However, with delay in diagnosis and progression of ischemia to full-thickness bowel wall injury, the manifestation is one of an acute abdomen, with findings of distention, guarding, rigidity, and hypotension, consistent with overt peritonitis and its septic consequences.

The patient should have intravenous access established with blood drawn and sent for a complete blood count with differential, electrolytes, evaluation of renal and hepatic function, blood urea nitrogen, creatinine, amylase, lipase, prothrombin time, activated partial thromboplastin time, and cardiac enzymes. Frequently, the laboratory findings are consistent with hemoconcentration resulting from the patient's hypovolemia and dehydration. The white blood cell count is often elevated and metabolic acidosis is present. Hyperamylasemia and elevations in lactate dehydrogenase, aspartate aminotransferase, and creatine phosphokinase levels are common. If hyperkalemia and hyperphosphatemia are present, bowel infarction should be suspected.[23] An electrocardiogram is performed and the patient placed on a monitor to evaluate cardiac rhythm. Depending on the history and physical findings, a nasogastric tube can reduce further abdominal distention and vomiting. Patients with cardiac disease who are hypovolemic should have a Swan-Ganz catheter placed to assist in monitoring their resuscitation.

Plain Films

Plain films of the abdomen (supine, upright) and the chest (anteroposterior) are obtained, predominantly to exclude other processes such as bowel obstruction or free air as a result of perforation. Up to 25% are normal in appearance. Portal venous gas is an advanced finding that suggests intestinal necrosis. Suspicious findings on plain films include a nonspecific ileus pattern with dilated, fluid-filled loops of bowel, thumbprinting, separation of bowel loops (edematous mesentery), intramural gas, and free air. In the majority of cases, however, plain films are nondiagnostic.[24,25]

Ultrasonography

Although duplex ultrasonography can be helpful in patients with chronic mesenteric ischemia, its utility in patients with acute mesenteric ischemia is limited. Even when requested for elective evaluation of patients with chronic ischemia, up to 40% cannot be adequately assessed because of body habitus or bowel gas.[26] These limitations are magnified when ultrasonography is attempted in patients with acute mesenteric ischemia. Abnormalities such as calcification, thrombus, and arterial stenosis or occlusion can occasionally be identified in the acute setting, assuming that the patient can cooperate, does not have dilated bowel that interferes with sound wave penetration, and has a favorable body habitus. Though able to evaluate the proximal mesenteric circulation, duplex evaluation of peripheral mesenteric perfusion is indirect and based on the velocity profile of the proximal artery.[27] Duplex sonography may have its greatest utility after revascularization[28] because patients with persistent abnormalities face high mortality with graft failure; therefore, planned reintervention to preserve mesenteric perfusion is prudent.

Computed Tomography

Computed tomography (CT) has rapidly become the initial diagnostic test for most patients with abdominal disease. It is a quick (approximately 19 seconds to scan the abdomen and pelvis), noninvasive, easily tolerated test that can show the indirect findings of arterial bowel ischemia and may show the arterial occlusion or mesenteric venous thrombus. Moreover, it is available in most institutions.

Findings on CT scans associated with bowel ischemia include dilation of the bowel lumen, bowel wall thickening, abnormal bowel wall enhancement, arterial occlusion, venous thrombosis, and intramural or portal venous gas. Dilation of an ischemic bowel segment suggests interruption of normal peristaltic activity. Symmetrical bowel wall thickening greater than 3 mm in a distended segment of bowel suggests ischemia. Greater degrees of bowel wall thickening should raise suspicion of mesenteric venous thrombosis (MVT). Oral contrast should be avoided in patients with suspected mesenteric ischemia because it may obscure subsequent arteriographic imaging of the mesenteric vasculature, which usually leads to the definitive diagnosis. Intravenous contrast is useful in demonstrating the heterogeneity of the ischemic bowel wall (lack of bowel wall enhancement)[29] and may show occlusion of mesenteric arteries if given by rapid bolus administration. Correlation between ischemia and CT scan findings is delineated in Table 84–1.[30]

Taourel et al.[31] reported a sensitivity of 64% and specificity of 92% for the CT diagnosis of acute arterial mesenteric ischemia. However, CT is the diagnostic technique

Table 84–1   Correlation Between Pathologic Damage and Computed Tomography Findings

Pathologic Damage	CT Findings
Vasoconstriction	Wall hyperdensity
	Absence of wall enhancement
Increased capillary permeability	Wall thickening
	Bowel dilation
Mucosal cellular necrosis	Pneumatosis
	Gas in mesenteric vein branches
	Gas in portal vein branches
Transmural bowel necrosis	Pneumoperitoneum
	Retropneumoperitoneum
	Ascites

From Angelelli G, Scardapane A, Memeo M, et al: Acute bowel ischemia: CT findings. Eur J Radiol 50:37-47, 2004.

of choice for acute MVT, with a sensitivity exceeding 90%.[32,33] As CT scan technology has advanced, three-dimensional reconstructions of the aorta and its branches show additional detail, which has improved the sensitivity and specificity to 94% to 96%.[31,34] As the technology continues to evolve, newer-generation scanners will further improve diagnostic capability. The limitations and risks of CT angiography center around patients with renal insufficiency or contrast allergies, limitations of contrast volume, and metal artifacts obscuring the area of interest.

Magnetic Resonance Angiography

When compared with catheter arteriography, current contrast-enhanced (gadolinium) three-dimensional magnetic resonance angiography (MRA) performs favorably in the common and proper hepatic arteries, the splenic artery, the SMA, and the portal, superior mesenteric, and splenic veins. Agreement is poor, however, for evaluation of the intrahepatic arteries, the SMA branches, and frequently the IMA, and catheter-directed arteriography remains necessary for detailed evaluation of these branch vessels.[35] However, because of the compromised clinical status of many patients and the need for urgent diagnosis, MRA is not often the procedure of choice.

MRA is frequently used for the evaluation of patients suspected of having chronic mesenteric ischemia since it can provide both anatomic and functional information regarding mesenteric perfusion. Because deoxyhemoglobin is paramagnetic and oxyhemoglobin is not, an increase in deoxyhemoglobin reduces the T2 of blood. By using this effect, patients with chronic mesenteric ischemia have been shown to have a decrease in the percentage of oxygenated blood in the superior mesenteric vein.[36] MRA spares patients the side effects of ionizing radiation and contrast toxicity.[27]

Arteriography

Catheter-directed contrast arteriography has been and remains the method of definitive diagnosis for acute and chronic mesenteric ischemia. Through the arteriographic access, catheter-based interventions are being performed with increased frequency in both patients with acute disease and those with chronic disease. Arteriograms establish the diagnosis; assist in differentiating between acute embolic, thrombotic, or nonocclusive mesenteric ischemia as the cause; and allow proper planning of the revascularization procedure. Anteroposterior (AP) and lateral views of the aorta and the mesenteric branches are required for proper arteriographic evaluation. The lateral view is particularly important to examine the proximal celiac artery and SMA, which overlap the aortic contrast column on AP views.

Acute embolic occlusion of the SMA is characterized arteriographically by abrupt occlusion of the artery, usually at a branch point where the vessel tends to narrow (Fig. 84–3). If imaged acutely, a meniscus sign (crescent) is often observed. If secondary thrombosis occurs proximal to the embolus, the classic meniscus sign of embolic

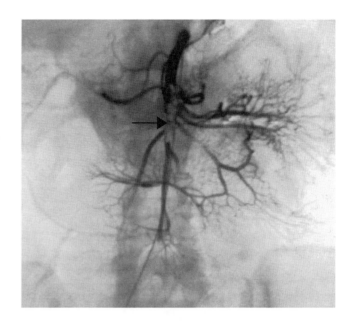

Figure 84–3. Acute embolus (*arrow*) occluding the superior mesenteric artery. (From Hladík P, Raupach J, Lojík M, et al: Treatment of acute mesenteric thrombosis/ischemia by transcatheter thromboaspiration. Surgery 137:122-123, 2005.)

occlusion will be obscured. The specific location of the occlusion depends on the size of the embolus, with the most common location being just distal to the middle colic artery, at which point the SMA rapidly narrows. Because these patients generally have a cardiac source for the embolus and peripheral atherosclerosis is not etiologically related to their mesenteric ischemia, the aorta and other arteries may show little atherosclerotic disease. Emboli rarely lodge in the proximal SMA (<15%).

Acute thrombotic occlusion usually occurs in an artery with significant underlying atherosclerosis. Atherosclerotic plaque most frequently develops at branch points of arteries from the aorta, most commonly at the origin of the celiac artery, SMA, and IMA. When segmental occlusion occurs as the result of chronic disease, the chronicity of the process is suggested by the development of collateral circulation to the distal branches. Delayed arteriographic imaging is often required to properly opacify the distal vessels. Patients with mesenteric arterial thrombosis frequently have more advanced atherosclerotic disease in their abdominal aorta and its branches than do those with acute embolic occlusion.

The diagnosis of nonocclusive mesenteric ischemia is typified by diffuse spasm of the SMA branches with intermittent areas of narrowing and dilation. Perfusion is markedly compromised because the intense distal vasospasm causes high peripheral resistance, with frequent reflux of contrast into the aorta. The distal mesenteric arterial arcades are not usually visualized. Patients with acute critical illness, those taking vasopressors, and those who are hypovolemic can demonstrate these arteriographic findings as a result of the body's physiologic response to hypovolemia. Additionally, acute proximal mesenteric arterial occlusion is often followed by distal

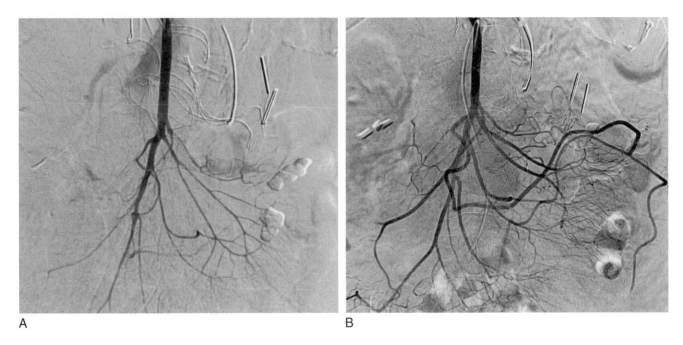

A   B

Figure 84–4. Arteriogram of a patient with typical nonocclusive mesenteric ischemia. **A,** Characteristic distal pruning of the mesenteric arcades. **B,** Repeat arteriogram after 24 hours of papaverine infusion demonstrating improved (normal) distal perfusion.

vasospasm, thus compounding the severity of the intestinal ischemia. This underscores the need for rapid and effective resuscitation of these patients, performed most efficiently while monitoring their cardiopulmonary hemodynamics. Aggressive rehydration reduces the compensatory mesenteric vasoconstriction and decreases the nephrotoxic effects of the contrast agent.

Patient Management

Effective management of patients with mesenteric ischemia is linked to (1) early diagnosis, (2) aggressive resuscitation, (3) early revascularization, and (4) ongoing supportive care. Resuscitative efforts should begin immediately on suspicion of the diagnosis because these patients often have multiple medical comorbid conditions and associated cardiac disease. Early and aggressive resuscitation is aimed at correcting the patient's hypovolemia and low cardiac output. A Swan-Ganz catheter is frequently required to gauge the patient's response. Because the mucosal layer of the bowel wall is the most sensitive to ischemia, bacterial translocation should be anticipated and intravenous antibiotics used to treat the associated bacteremia. Catheter-directed papaverine to reverse the often severe mesenteric vasospasm is initiated early after arteriography. Anticoagulation is given to prevent propagation of mesenteric thrombus. The most expedient evaluation of patients with acute arterial mesenteric ischemia is mesenteric arteriography. Further delay caused by relatively insensitive or nonspecific diagnostic testing puts the patient at greater risk for a poor outcome. Once the nature of the mesenteric ischemia is delineated, a

specific plan for revascularization can be initiated. A treatment-specific algorithm is summarized in Figure 84–2.

A normal arteriogram should include its venous phase and be followed by a CT scan, if not already performed, to exclude the diagnosis of MVT. If the diagnosis of MVT is excluded, the patient should be aggressively supported and observed. If peritoneal signs are present, exploratory laparotomy should be performed.

Approximately 20% of patients with acute mesenteric ischemia will have a nonocclusive mesenteric vasospastic phenomenon alone. This is generally associated with low cardiac output or a history or present condition of congestive heart failure and treatment with a digitalis preparation. Associated hypovolemia in patients receiving vasopressors and those undergoing operative coronary revascularization who were on cardiopulmonary bypass round out this clinical scenario. The arteriogram generally shows diffuse vasospasm with marked narrowing of the major branches of the SMA (Fig. 84–4), often with the "string of lakes" appearance. Because of the high outflow resistance in the SMA, reflux of contrast into the aorta is common. In addition to aggressively correcting the low cardiac output, terminating vasoconstrictor use, and discontinuing digitalis preparations, intra-arterial papaverine infusion at 30 to 60 mg/hr is the treatment of choice. In the absence of peritonitis, supportive care with anticoagulation and continued papaverine infusion is recommended. The arteriogram is repeated at 12- to 24-hour intervals, and the papaverine infusion is discontinued once the vasospasm has resolved.

Ideally, patients who demonstrate evidence of peritonitis should undergo exploratory laparotomy, with appropriately conservative resection of necrotic bowel during the papaverine infusion. Postoperatively, the infusion is continued and repeat arteriography is performed. Depending on the patient's clinical evaluation, a second-look laparotomy is considered. In the event that abdominal surgery has been performed without arteriography, clearly necrotic bowel is expeditiously resected, and then arteriography with papaverine infusion is performed. Second-look laparotomy is considered.

Patients who have embolic occlusion of a small branch are also treated with anticoagulation to avoid additional thromboemboli. Associated vasoconstriction is treated with catheter-directed papaverine. In the absence of peritonitis, patients can be observed. In the presence of peritoneal signs, exploratory laparotomy is performed.

During the past several years, remarkable technologic advances have been made with percutaneous interventions. Patients who have major embolic occlusion or major thrombotic occlusion of their visceral vessels can often be approached with a percutaneous, pharmacomechanical method to dissolve or extract the embolus or thrombus and correct an underlying stenosis, if found.[37-41] Combining plasminogen activators with mechanical thrombus disruption and suction extraction can often restore perfusion more quickly and potentially with less morbidity than is the case with standard operative techniques. Because vasospasm is frequently associated with acute mesenteric occlusion, SMA catheter infusion of papaverine should be used to relieve the vasospasm. In the presence of peritonitis, exploratory laparotomy with appropriate resection is performed. The papaverine infusion is continued to relieve ongoing vasospasm and improve bowel perfusion, and anticoagulation is continued to avoid additional embolic or thrombotic events. A second-look laparotomy is planned if the condition of the bowel wall is tenuous at the time that the abdomen is closed. If a second-look laparotomy has been planned and the patient is clinically improving, the repeat laparotomy should be delayed to allow maximal improvement.

If catheter-based pharmacomechanical techniques are unsuccessful in the management of an acute SMA embolus, the catheter should be left in the proximal SMA and papaverine infusion initiated, followed by an expedient operative thromboembolectomy. After perfusion is restored to the bowel, it should be carefully examined for areas of irreversible ischemia. Areas of necrosis should be resected. If there is no irreversible ischemia and blood flow is restored, it can be anticipated that bowel wall perfusion will improve, with good prospects for ultimate bowel viability. Papaverine infusion is continued postoperatively and a repeat arteriogram performed to assess reperfusion and the degree of ongoing vasospasm.

In patients with major arterial thrombosis, anticoagulation should be initiated to minimize progressive thrombotic occlusion of branch vessels. Endovascular revascularization is recommended, including balloon angioplasty and stenting (if necessary) of the celiac artery, SMA, or IMA, or any combination of these arteries. Intra-arterial lytic therapy can be used to clear the acute thrombus[37,38] and unmask an underlying lesion, which should be corrected with adjunctive angioplasty and stenting.[39,42] If the endovascular approach is suc-cessful, the completion arteriogram is evaluated for mesenteric vasoconstriction. If present, a catheter is left in place and papaverine infusion continued with subsequent repeat arteriography. In the absence of vasoconstriction, continued supportive care is offered. If endovascular revascularization is unsuccessful, the catheter is left in the SMA for intra-arterial papaverine infusion if a portion of the artery is available for catheter positioning. The patient is then taken to the operating room for operative revascularization. A repeat arteriogram is performed postoperatively and the catheter appropriately repositioned if continued papaverine infusion is indicated.

Patients with peritoneal signs require exploratory laparotomy. Before operating, however, endovascular reconstruction is attempted. If successful, a papaverine infusion is initiated before exploratory laparotomy. Postoperatively, the papaverine infusion is continued and a second-look laparotomy performed, if appropriate.

In the absence of successful endovascular reconstruction, the patient is taken to the operating room for operative revascularization while papaverine is being infused into the SMA. Bowel infarction is often more extensive with arterial thrombosis than with embolic occlusion and has been observed from the duodenum to the transverse colon. Performing an adequate thrombectomy of a diseased visceral artery is difficult and not usually successful as an isolated procedure. Antegrade or retrograde bypass of the diseased artery is generally warranted to restore perfusion. Autologous vein grafts are preferred if bowel resection is required; however, synthetic grafts have fewer problems with compression and kinking,[43] although their use is discouraged in patients with questionable bowel viability. McMillan et al.[44] reported 3-year patency rates of 93% for antegrade grafts, 95% for retrograde grafts, 95% for saphenous vein grafts, and 89% for synthetic grafts. Outcomes were not as favorable in the experience of Cho et al.,[45] who reported 5- and 10-year patency rates of 57% and 46%, respectively, for all grafts. When the SMA beyond an occlusion is an adequate target for revascularization, it appears that a single bypass is all that is required in the majority of cases.[46] After operative revascularization, the bowel is inspected for areas of necrosis and appropriate resection performed. The papaverine infusion should be continued through the new conduit, with subsequent arteriography and a second-look laparotomy performed if indicated.

ACUTE MESENTERIC VENOUS THROMBOSIS

MVT accounts for 5% to 15% of patients with mesenteric ischemia.[47] The superior mesenteric vein is most commonly involved, frequently with extension of thrombus into the portal vein. Interestingly, the inferior mesenteric vein is most often spared.[48] The patient's clinical findings depend largely on the extent of thrombosis, the mesenteric veins involved, and the degree of bowel wall ischemia. Unfortunately, the mortality rate in these patients remains high, up to 50% in some reports.

Although patients with acute MVT have a more abrupt symptom onset than do patients with subacute and chronic mesenteric venous occlusion, the diagnosis remains difficult. Most commonly, patients complain of midabdominal colicky pain, which suggests small bowel involvement. Because of the diffuse and nondescript nature of their symptoms, most patients delay seeking medical care for 2 or more days after symptom onset.[49] Nausea, vomiting, diarrhea, and anorexia frequently accompany their abdominal discomfort. Although findings of occult blood in the stool are present in half of the patients,[50] gross bleeding such as hematemesis, hematochezia, or melena occurs in approximately 15%.[51]

Because of the generalized nature of the patient's symptoms and the relative infrequency of MVT, the definitive diagnosis is often delayed. The past medical history or family history is often informative because venous thromboembolism is part of the history in half of the patients.[48-50]

Physical findings are frequently similar to those in patients with early arterial mesenteric ischemia. Their abdomen is soft, without tenderness or peritoneal signs, and in the early stage the abdominal examination is often unimpressive save for some abdominal distention. Fever, muscular guarding, and rebound tenderness are indicators of more advanced disease progression and bowel infarction leading to peritonitis. Bowel infarction ultimately develops in 30% to 60% of patients with acute MVT.

Because of fluid sequestration within the bowel wall and lumen and the development of ascites, hypotension with hemodynamic instability is often part of the clinical picture. Patients first seen in this advanced clinical condition have a poor prognosis.[51,52]

Blood tests are obtained but are not generally helpful. Elevation of the white blood count with a shift toward immature white cells can be found in 50% to 65% of patients.[51] Serum amylase is usually normal, and serum lactate is elevated only in patients with advanced bowel ischemia and suggests necrosis.

Plain abdominal films are often the initial diagnostic test and are generally of little value. Although abnormalities can be found in 50% of patients,[47] the findings are nonspecific. Thumbprinting, when seen, is indicative of the mucosal edema resulting from venous congestion. Pneumatosis intestinalis, portal vein gas, and free air in the abdomen usually represent bowel infarction.[52]

CT of the abdomen with intravenous contrast is the diagnostic test of choice for patients with suspected acute MVT. A definitive diagnosis can be made in more than 90% of patients. Harward et al.[50] reported 90% sensitivity of abdominal CT with observation of a luminal venous thrombus. However, if one includes other characteristic findings of the bowel wall, such as thickening, pneumatosis, or streaking of the mesentery, CT sensitivity increases to nearly 100%.[33,52] Magnetic resonance venography is used less commonly, but when properly performed, it is highly sensitive.

Depending on the timing of the examination, color duplex ultrasound of the mesenteric veins can be helpful. If performed early, before significant bowel dis-

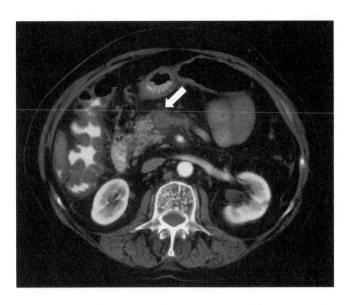

Figure 84–5. Computed tomographic scan of a patient with mesenteric venous thrombosis showing a thrombosed superior mesenteric vein at the splenic vein junction *(arrow)*, streaking of the mesentery, and bowel wall thickening.

tention, a sensitivity of 80% or greater can be anticipated.[53]

Selective mesenteric arteriography is not frequently used to establish the diagnosis of MVT, although it may be helpful in the management of these patients. Findings such as incomplete filling of the mesenteric veins, prolonged opacification of the arterial arcades, and the presence of thrombus or nonfilling of the superior mesenteric, splenic, or portal vein (Fig. 84–5) are seen in these patients. Most report a sensitivity of 70% to 80%.[54,55]

Treatment is generally directed at limiting progressive venous thrombosis, reducing the risk for bowel necrosis, and performing timely resection in those with irreversible bowel ischemia. Unfortunately, because of delay in diagnosis, the diffuse nature of the thrombosis, and the rarity of this condition, treatment directed at restoring patency to the thrombosed veins is unusual. In light of the rapid technologic advances in percutaneous interventions, which incorporate pharmacologic and mechanical methods of thrombus dissolution/extraction, it appears reasonable, if not advisable to initiate a strategy of thrombus dissolution/extraction to restore venous drainage because with the traditional care of anticoagulation alone, these patients continue to face a mortality rate ranging from 15% to 50%.[48,50,55,56] The diagnosis of MVT should trigger a search for an underlying thrombophilia. Such an evaluation includes factor V Leiden, prothrombin gene mutation, antiphospholipid/anticardiolipin antibodies, antithrombin III, protein C, protein S, factor VIII levels, hyperhomocysteinemia, paroxysmal nocturnal hemoglobinuria, and assessment for an underlying myeloproliferative disorder.

Rapid initiation of systemic anticoagulation is important. In patients with localized or diffuse peritoneal irritation, exploratory laparotomy is indicated. Laparoscopy should be avoided in these patients because the increased abdominal pressure associated with the pneumoperitoneum further diminishes mesenteric blood flow.

On entering the abdomen, the superior mesenteric and portal veins should be assessed to determine the relative age of the thrombus. If the large veins appear to have an acute thrombus within them, thrombectomy is recommended, followed by bolus infusion of a recombinant tissue plasminogen activator (rt-PA) solution. The authors use a high-volume, low-dose solution of rt-PA, typically diluting 2 mg in 50 ml and infusing the entire 2-mg dose. Necrotic bowel is conservatively resected with preservation of viable intestine. The patient is treated with heparin intraoperatively and anticoagulation is continued postoperatively.

Associated arterial vasospasm should be evaluated by arteriography and treated with catheter-directed papaverine into the SMA, which improves perfusion to the ischemic bowel and reduces the necessity for additional resection. Patients treated for MVT have a high risk of recurrence (35% to 70%),[49] most frequently within 30 days, thus emphasizing the need for early and persistent anticoagulation.

Patients surviving the acute episode of MVT face chronic mesenteric venous hypertension with a subsequent risk for varices. This post-thrombotic venous hypertension occurs most commonly in patients with persistent large-vein mesenteric thrombosis, which further supports a strategy to remove the thrombus in patients with acute large-vein MVT. Some have reported success with transhepatic portography and instillation of a plasminogen activator directly into the thrombus.[57,58] Unfortunately, thrombolytic agents have been used infrequently in these patients because of the perceived risk for hemorrhage. The success of thrombolysis is often compromised by the delay in diagnosis. Intrathrombus thrombolytic therapy and, alternatively, intra-arterial thrombolytic therapy via the SMA should be considered in patients with thrombosis of large mesenteric veins when the potential benefit outweighs the risk of bleeding.

CHRONIC MESENTERIC ISCHEMIA

Chronic mesenteric ischemia is most commonly the result of advanced atherosclerotic disease of multiple mesenteric arteries. Because of the good collateral circulatory network that exists between the mesenteric vessels, symptomatic chronic mesenteric ischemia is rare. Risk factors for its development are the same as those for atherosclerotic disease in general: a positive family history, smoking, hypertension, and hypercholesterolemia. Generally, when symptomatic disease does occur, there is a female preponderance. Nonatherosclerotic causes of chronic mesenteric ischemia are less frequent and include inflammatory arterial disease, middle aortic syndrome, celiac artery compression (median arcuate ligament syndrome), chronic aortic dissection, aortic coarctation, fibromuscular dysplasia, and neurofibromatosis.

The finding of mesenteric artery atherosclerotic disease does not necessarily indicate intestinal ischemia. Significant atherosclerotic obstruction of the mesenteric arteries has been observed in 6% to 10% of individuals at autopsy.[59] In patients who undergo abdominal aortography, which is a select group of patients who are more likely to have occlusive disease, obliterative disease of the celiac or mesenteric artery has been found in 14% to 24%.[60] Although visceral artery stenosis is frequent, symptoms resulting from visceral arterial occlusive disease are uncommon because of the extensive collateral circulation.

As imaging techniques are becoming more common and stenosed visceral arteries detected more frequently, a temptation exists to correct "asymptomatic" visceral arterial stenosis. This approach is not prudent in light of the natural history study of asymptomatic intestinal arterial occlusive disease performed by Thomas and colleagues.[61] They identified 60 patients with significant mesenteric artery occlusive disease and monitored these patients for a mean of 2.6 years. In none of the 45 patients with one- or two-vessel mesenteric arterial occlusive disease did signs or symptoms of intestinal ischemia develop. Fifteen patients had severe three-vessel disease. During follow-up, fatal intestinal infarction developed in one patient and symptoms of intestinal angina in three.

The natural history of asymptomatic mesenteric occlusive disease appears to be reasonably documented. It has been our experience, which is supported by the literature, that few if any of these patients require mesenteric revascularization.

Clinical Features and Diagnosis

The classic picture of patients with chronic mesenteric ischemia is postprandial abdominal pain leading to an aversion to food and resulting in weight loss. The pain has been characterized as intestinal angina or, in the authors' parlance, intestinal claudication. The pain is characteristically diffuse and often midabdominal, midepigastric, and crampy in nature. The pain generally develops within 15 to 45 minutes after eating, with the severity frequently related to the size of the meal ingested. The authors have observed early-onset pain with foregut (celiac artery distribution) ischemia, with later-onset pain occurring with more diffuse ischemic disease. Because of the association of abdominal pain with food ingestion, fear of eating develops and leads to the characteristic weight loss and subsequent malnutrition.

Other symptoms of nausea, vomiting, and diarrhea have accompanied chronic mesenteric ischemia. Bloating has also been observed. Symptoms of constipation and findings of occult blood in the stool and ischemic colitis represent hindgut ischemia. Because none of these symptoms or signs is specific for chronic mesenteric ischemia, the majority of these patients will have been subjected to an extensive diagnostic evaluation before referral to a vascular surgeon. If a complete evaluation has not been performed, conditions that produce abdominal pain and weight loss more commonly than visceral ischemic disease does should be excluded before plans for revascularization.

Evaluation of the mesenteric arteries frequently begins with a noninvasive mesenteric duplex scan. This should be performed with the patient in a fasted state because mesenteric outflow resistance changes with food intake and increases in bowel gas.

The most frequent criterion used to identify celiac artery stenosis is a peak systolic velocity of 200 cm/sec or higher, which has been reported to have a sensitivity of 75% and a specificity of 89%.[62] The same investigators reported that a peak systolic velocity of 275 cm/sec or higher predicted 70% to 99% stenosis of the SMA with a sensitivity of 89% and a specificity of 92%. The absence of a Doppler signal in the SMA represents occlusion. Others have reported an end-diastolic velocity of 45 cm/sec or higher to be the best indicator of 50% or greater stenosis of the SMA, with a sensitivity of 100% and specificity of 92%.[63] Retrograde flow in the common hepatic artery is a reliable indicator of severe proximal celiac artery occlusive disease.[64]

Aortography with AP and lateral views has been the diagnostic technique of choice. Lateral aortograms are important for evaluation of the origin of the mesenteric vessels. CT angiography is rapidly becoming the preferred technique for contrast visualization of the aorta and its branches. Contrast-enhanced (gadolinium) MRA is useful in patients with dye allergy and renal compromise.

Laboratory tests to evaluate the malabsorption that may accompany intestinal ischemia, such as stool fat content, D-xylose tolerance, and vitamin B_{12} absorption, may yield positive results; however, they are nonspecific and not generally useful in the overall management of these patients.

Mesenteric Revascularization

Although it is generally true that patients with symptomatic chronic mesenteric ischemia have at least two, if not three intestinal vessels diseased, this is not always the case. Patients with single-vessel occlusive disease who do not have adequate collateral circulation from other mesenteric arteries will suffer chronic mesenteric ischemia. The authors have successfully revascularized a single celiac artery, and others have reported similar findings.[65]

As with all vascular reconstruction, patient selection and the physician's judgment, combined with operative skill, play an important role in overall success. Dogma should be replaced by intelligent decision making based on knowledge of the disease process, awareness of the current options for revascularization, both endovascularly and operatively, and the patient's inherent risk.

Surgical Revascularization

Because chronic symptomatic mesenteric ischemia is relatively unusual in the majority of vascular practices, few physicians have broad-based experience with surgical mesenteric revascularization. There is a wide range of operative techniques, and the one chosen should be based on the patient's anatomy, disease distribution, and associated comorbid conditions and the surgeon's comfort and expertise with the available technique.

Mesenteric Artery Endarterectomy

Endarterectomy of the SMA and the celiac artery was initially performed in retrograde fashion, often attempting a "blind endarterectomy" through a distal arteriotomy.[66] The technique served its purpose during the formative years of vascular surgery. Though occasionally successful, this approach is often complicated by failure, and blind endarterectomy is no longer acceptable in any area of the vascular tree. An improved technique popularized by Wylie et al.[67] advocates complete exposure of the aorta from below the renal arteries to the supraceliac aorta. Such exposure is most reliably accomplished through an extended retroperitoneal approach. A "trapdoor" aortic incision is made from above the celiac artery and extended laterally and then medially below the SMA. The atherosclerotic plaque of the aorta and the orifices of the celiac artery and SMA is then removed by the technique of endarterectomy. Because the plaque in the SMA often extends beyond the orifice of this vessel, subsequent SMA arteriotomy, endarterectomy, and patch angioplasty are frequently required (Fig. 84–6). Although good results are reported by those experienced in this technique, most vascular surgeons are not comfortable with this exposure and extensive dissection and are more likely to encounter complications. The risks associated with suprarenal aortic clamping during visceral endarterectomy include cholesterol embolization, renal failure, and paraplegia, as well as higher pulmonary and cardiac risk.

Aortomesenteric Bypass

On the basis of previous reports, many vascular surgeons favor multivessel revascularization for chronic mesenteric ischemia.[67-71] There seems to be an intuitive advantage to multivessel revascularization; however, others have convincingly argued that the single most important artery is the SMA and that successful bypass to the SMA will provide durable relief with outcomes equivalent to those of multivessel repair.[46,72] Furthermore, the controversy regarding antegrade versus retrograde bypass continues. The correct answer to these important questions for any given patient lies in the judgment of the treating physician. Success is likely for those who make appropriate judgments based on the distribution of disease, the patient's anatomy, and other clinical factors. For example, isolated revascularization of the IMA has been shown to be successful in properly selected patients. The degree of benefit from single-vessel revascularization is related to the number and quality of collateral channels to other portions of the ischemic gut.

Even the proponents of isolated SMA bypass recommend multivessel revascularization in patients in whom (1) the SMA is diffusely diseased, (2) there is a question of durability with a single bypass, and (3) a previous

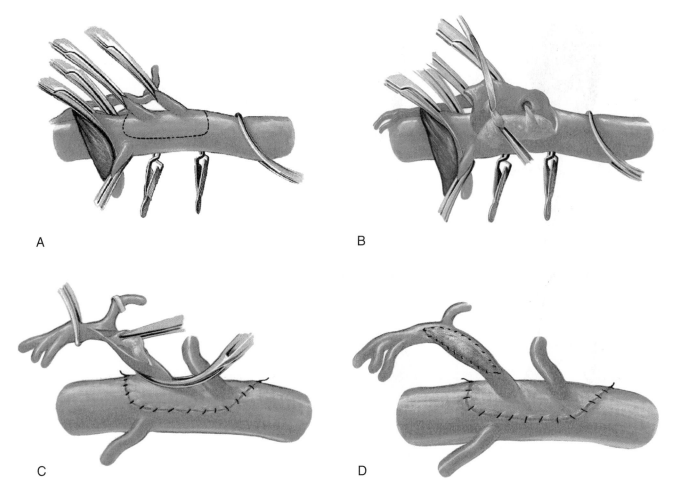

A

B

C

D

Figure 84–6. Transaortic endarterectomy for celiac and superior mesenteric stenosis. Exposure is obtained through a left thoracoabdominal retroperitoneal approach. **A,** Trapdoor aortotomy. **B,** Removal of orifice lesions from branches. **C,** After completion of transaortic endarterectomy, superior mesenteric artery (SMA) endarterectomy is completed through a separate incision (if needed). **D,** Vein patch closure of SMA. (From Wylie EJ, Stoney RJ, Ehrenfeld WK: Manual of Vascular Surgery, vol 1. New York, Springer-Verlag, 1980, pp 215-217.)

abdominal operation (especially gastrectomy and colectomy) has potentially interrupted the normal collateral connections between the superior mesenteric and celiac vascular beds.[65]

The antegrade aorta-to-celiac or aorta-to-SMA bypass is usually performed through a transperitoneal approach. The supraceliac aorta is generally soft and has much less atherosclerotic disease than the infrarenal aorta does. It is exposed by retracting the left lobe of the liver to the right after division of the triangular ligament. The gastrohepatic ligament is divided, and after entry into the lesser sac, the esophagus (which has a nasogastric tube coursing through it) is mobilized, encircled with a 1-inch Penrose drain, and retracted to the left. The diaphragmatic crura and median arcuate ligament are divided to expose a generous portion of the supraceliac aorta. The proximal celiac artery is also exposed during the course of this dissection, usually during transection of the median arcuate ligament.

The SMA is exposed through an incision at the base of the transverse mesocolon. Occasionally, the duode-

num can be mobilized to aid exposure as the SMA exits from beneath the pancreas. A variety of techniques have been used, including anastomosing a 12×6 or 14×7 aortic bifurcation graft. The celiac and SMA anastomoses have been variously performed in an end-to-end or end-to-side fashion. Most frequently, the celiac revascularization is accomplished with an end-to-side anastomosis to the right hepatic artery and the SMA revascularization with an end-to-side anastomosis to the infrapancreatic SMA. Many surgeons tunnel the SMA bypass behind the pancreas, but anterior to the renal vein. A useful technique is sequential mesenteric revascularization with a single 8-mm graft, which revascularizes the celiac artery with a side-to-side anastomosis and the SMA with an end-to-side anastomosis.[69]

Mesenteric bypass from the mid infrarenal aorta to the SMA (Fig. 84–7) should be avoided because of the likelihood of kinking once the viscera are replaced after the procedure. The concept of the shortest graft being the best does not necessarily hold for mesenteric bypasses. The choice of graft material is often debated among

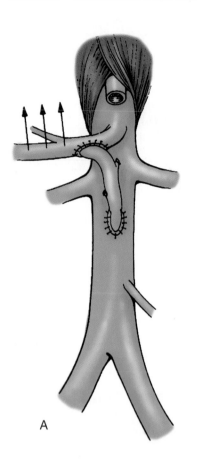

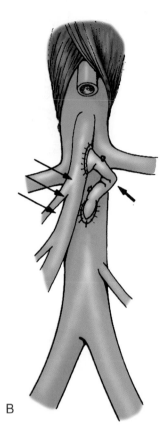

Figure 84–7. Illustration of the potential for kinking when using short saphenous vein grafts from the infrarenal aorta to the superior mesenteric artery. (From Taylor LM, Moneta GL, Porter JM: Treatment of chronic visceral ischemia. In Rutherford RB [ed]: Vascular Surgery, 5th ed. Philadelphia, WB Saunders, 2000, p 1536.)

surgeons. Although autogenous grafts are inherently more attractive from an infection and thrombogenicity perspective, they are subject to kinking and compression and may not be of adequate size to carry the blood flow required for the intestines. Normal SMA blood flow usually exceeds 750 ml/min,[73] and saphenous vein grafts of average size (<6 mm in diameter) rarely carry more than 500 ml/min.

Retrograde Bypass

Visceral bypass grafts originating from the distal infrarenal aorta or the iliac arteries offer the advantage of anatomic familiarity to all vascular surgeons and limit the amount of dissection required to achieve revascularization. Several authors have suggested that retrograde bypasses are not as durable as antegrade revascularization; however, avoidance of the common pitfalls leading to graft kinking and improvement in patient selection may eliminate many of these disadvantages.[74,75] Even proponents of antegrade bypass recognize that in certain clinical conditions retrograde bypasses are indicated: (1) emergency revascularization in patients undergoing laparotomy for acute mesenteric ischemia (an autogenous vein should be the conduit), (2) an inaccessible supraceliac aorta because of previous surgery or inflammation, (3) severe cardiac disease with contraindications to supraceliac aortic clamping, and (4) the need for simultaneous infrarenal aortic and mesenteric revascularization.[76]

Selection of the section of distal infrarenal aorta or iliac artery should be based on the distribution of atherosclerotic disease. If the infrarenal aorta and iliac artery are severely diseased, they should be replaced, with the mesenteric graft originating from the aortic prosthesis.

The most proximal suitable segment of the SMA as it passes from beneath the pancreas should be used. This maximizes the outflow bed and minimizes the likelihood of graft kinking.

The SMA anastomosis is performed first. If the conduit is autogenous vein, the viscera are returned to the abdomen and the graft placed under mild tension while constructing the aortic or iliac anastomosis (Fig. 84–8). If a prosthetic is used, it is configured in a gentle curve with the goal being to reduce the risk for graft kinking. The right hepatic artery is often a good target for celiac revascularization. Mobilization of the duodenum with a Kocher maneuver to expose the right hepatic artery or the use of a retropancreatic tunnel with the graft approaching the right hepatic artery from the left side of the abdomen provides a proper configuration that reduces the chance of graft kinking and maximizes technical success (Fig. 84–9).

Endovascular Revascularization

Operative reconstruction for mesenteric ischemia is a large operation that is usually performed on a patient with multiple risk factors who is often malnourished.

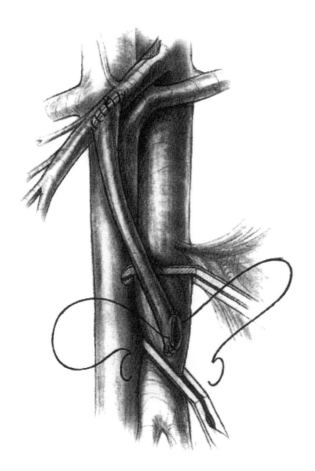

Figure 84–8. Retrograde infrarenal aorta–superior mesenteric artery bypass with autologous vein. (From Zarins CK, Gewertz BL: Atlas of Vascular Surgery. New York, Churchill Livingstone, 1989, p 107.)

Percutaneous techniques of mesenteric revascularization are intuitively attractive if they can be performed successfully with low complication rates. Tables 84–2 and 84–3 review operative and endovascular revascularization procedures for chronic mesenteric ischemia. In most operative reports, there appears to be nearly uniform early patency. However, early patency in operated patients is not usually based on objective imaging, but rather on operative observation and clinical follow-up. In contrast, endovascular procedures are always accompanied by completion arteriography, which offers more objective assessment of technical success and patency.

Procedure-related morbidity is considerably less with the endovascular approach, although it may not be readily apparent by a review of selected literature. This difference in significant morbidity may be hidden by the definition of procedure-related complications. As an example, the brachial artery approach is associated with a frequent need to repair the brachial puncture site, typically performed under local anesthesia. The authors plan to perform brachial artery repair in all patients undergoing this approach. However, when reviewing procedure-related complications, the need for a brachial artery repair is often considered numerically equivalent to renal failure, a respiratory complication, or acute myocardial infarction.

Balloon dilation of the SMA was first reported in 1980 by Furrer et al.[98] Early results have been encouraging, with technical success reported in up to 80% of patients along with symptomatic relief and improvement of nutritional status.[87,88,99,100] Current results of endovascular techniques have improved (see Table 84–3) as the technology has advanced and low-profile balloons and stents and better pharmacotherapy have become available. The high brachial approach is preferred by some because it offers a mechanical advantage in advancing balloon catheters and stents (if necessary) into the mesenteric arteries, especially the SMA. The celiac artery is externally surrounded by the dense fibers of the arcuate ligament and the crus of the diaphragm. Therefore, angioplasty alone is less likely to be effective and stenting is required more frequently. Generally, balloon angioplasty is all that is recommended, assuming that an arteriographically good result is observed. Indications for mesenteric artery stenting include (1) residual stenosis of 30% or greater, (2) an obstructing dissection or flap after percutaneous transluminal angioplasty, and (3) recurrent stenosis within 12 months of balloon dilation.[94] When these guidelines have been observed, technical success rates of 96% to 100% have been reported.[94,96] Procedure-related mortality is low and has been reported as 0% in most series. The hospital stay is short for most patients, and an increasing number are being treated as outpatients. Few, if any, require intensive care monitoring.

Figure 84–10A and B shows an arteriogram of a patient with postprandial abdominal pain and an associated 30-lb weight loss. High-grade celiac artery and SMA stenosis is apparent, and the IMA is occluded. The patient had minimal improvement of the celiac stenosis with angioplasty alone, but an excellent anatomic result of angioplasty and stenting of the SMA. The completion arteriogram in the AP view (see Fig. 84–10C and D) shows excellent collaterals to the celiac branches via the pancreatic duodenal and gastroduodenal arteries. After the procedure, the patient became asymptomatic.

The important end point is improvement in symptoms and long-term clinical success. This has been observed in approximately 85% with a mean follow-up of about 26 months (see Table 84–3). Repeat angioplasty and stenting (if necessary) for recurrent disease can generally be performed with equally low complication rates and has been associated with good technical and clinical success.

Text continued on p. 1266

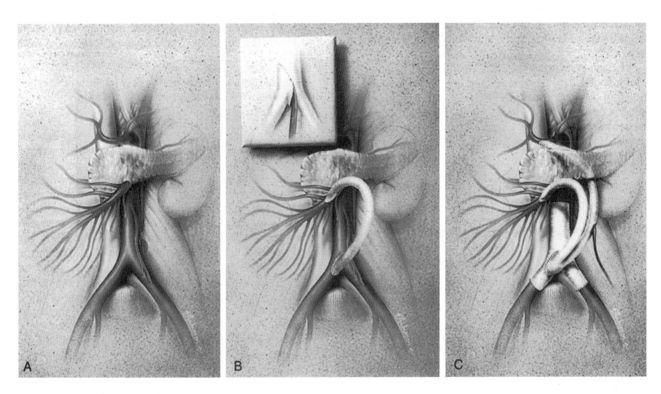

Figure 84–9. **A,** Exposure of the infrarenal aorta and the superior mesenteric and celiac arteries. **B,** Method of infrarenal aorta–superior mesenteric artery (SMA) bypass. *Inset,* method of forming the graft origin from an aortic bifurcation graft. **C,** Method of infrarenal aortic graft placement with bypass to the SMA and hepatic artery. Note the reimplantation of the inferior mesenteric artery. (From Taylor LM, Porter JM: Treatment of chronic intestinal ischemia. Semin Vasc Surg 3:193, 1990.)

Table 84–2 Literature Review of Surgical Revascularization in Patients with Chronic Mesenteric Ischemia

Author	Year	N	Vessels Revascularized	Immediate Clinical Success	Follow-up (mo)	Long-Term Clinical Success	Operative Complications	Operative Mortality	Long-Term Patency
Kieny R, et al.[72]	1990	53	62	NA	102	91% (48)	4% (2)	2% (1)	NA
Cormier JM, et al.[77]	1991	91	131	NA	69	NA	9% (8)	3% (3)	91% (83)
Cunningham CG, et al.[78]	1991	74	140	88% (65)	71	86% (64)	35% (26)	12% (9)	NA
McAfee MK, et al.[79]	1992	56	116	89% (50)	60	90% (50)	41% (23)	10% (5)	90% (50)
Calderon M, et al.[80]	1992	20	36	100% (20)	36	100%	20% (4)	0	100% (20)
Christensen MG, et al.[81]	1994	65	65	NA	55	68% (44)	NA	2% (1)	NA
Gentile AT, et al.[46]	1994	24	24	100% (24)	40	89% (21)	NA	0	89% (21)
Johnston KW, et al.[75]	1995	21	37	NA	120	NA	19% (4)	0	86% (18)
McMillan WD, et al.[44]	1995	16	24	92% (15)	35	97% (15)	31% (5)	6% (1)	89% (14)
Moawad J, et al.[68]	1997	24	38	96% (23)	29	78% (19)	46% (11)	4% (1)	78% (19)
Mateo RB, et al.[82]	1999	85	NA	92% (78)	57	81% (69)	45% (38)	8% (7)	81% (69)
Kihara TK, et al.[83]	1999	42	66	NA	36	96% (40)	30% (13)	10% (4)	65% (27)
Foley MI, et al.[84]	2000	29	29	97% (28)	44	NA	NA	3% (1)	79% (23)
Park WM, et al.[85]	2002	98	179	93% (91)	60	92% (90)	21% (21)	5% (5)	NA
English WP, et al.[86]	2004	34	NA	NA	42	94% (32)	NA	9% (3)	89% (30)
TOTAL		732	947	394	44,271	512	155	41	374
MEAN				93%	61	87%	27%	6%	85%

NA, not available.

Table 84–3   Literature Review of Endovascular Revascularization of Patients with Chronic Mesenteric Ischemia

Author	Year	N	Vessels Revascularized	Technical Success	Immediate Clinical Success	Follow-up (mo)	Long-Term Clinical Success	Complications	Mortality Rate	Long-Term Patency
Sniderman KW[87]	1994	13	20	91% (12)	85% (11)	NA	82% (11)	8% (1)	0	NA
Hallisey MJ, et al.[88]	1995	15	23	93% (14)	88% (13)	28	75% (11)	0%	0	75% (11)
Allen RC, et al.[89]	1996	19	24	95% (13)	79% (15)	39	86% (16)	11% (2)	5% (1)	NA
Maspes F, et al.[90]	1998	23	41	90% (21)	77% (18)	27	88% (20)	9% (2)	0	NA
Nyman U, et al.[42]	1998	5	6	83% (4)	100% (5)	21	80% (4)	40% (2)	0	40% (2)
Sheeran SR, et al.[91]	1999	6	13	83% (5)	92% (5)	16	75% (4)	0	8% (1)	83% (5)
Kasirajan K, et al.[92]	2001	28	32	89% (25)	NA	36	66% (18)	18% (5)	11% (3)	73% (20)
Pietura R, et al.[93]	2002	6	9	100% (6)	100% (6)	12	100% (6)	NA	0	100% (6)
Matsumoto AH, et al.[94]	2002	33	47	87% (29)	88% (29)	38	97% (32)	13% (4)	0	97% (32)
Steinmetz E, et al.[95]	2002	19	19	100% (19)	93% (18)	31	94% (18)	16% (3)	0	100% (19)
Sharafuddin MJ, et al.[96]	2003	25	26	96% (24)	88% (22)	11	92% (23)	12% (3)	0	92% (23)
Chahid T, et al.[97]	2004	14	17	100% (14)	100% (14)	29	93% (13)	14% (2)	0	NA
TOTAL		206	277	186	156	5587	176	24	5	118
MEAN				90%	88%	29	85%	12%	2%	86%

NA, not available.

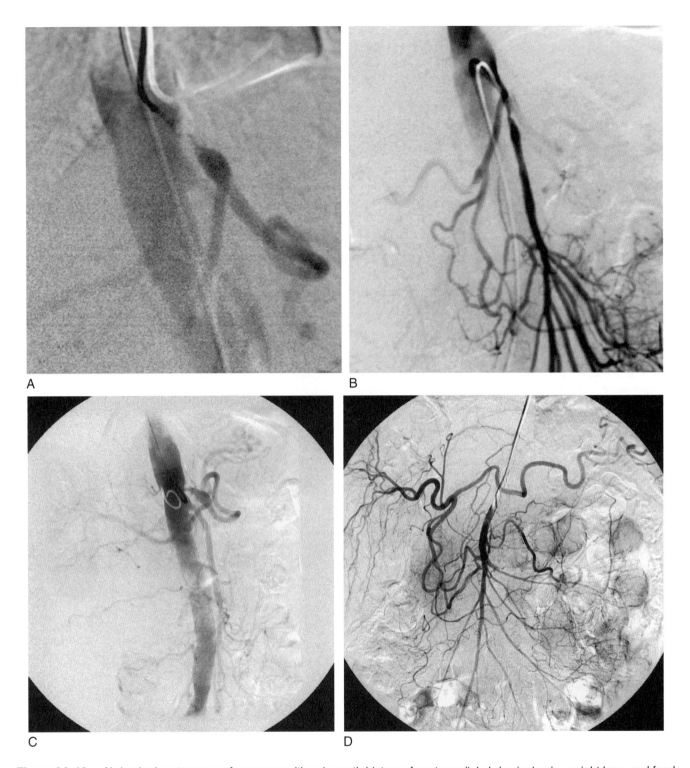

Figure 84–10. Abdominal aortograms of a woman with a 4-month history of postprandial abdominal pain, weight loss, and food avoidance. **A,** Lateral aortogram demonstrating high-grade stenosis of the origin of the celiac artery. **B,** Lateral aortogram demonstrating stenosis of the superior mesenteric artery (SMA) and no visualization of the inferior mesenteric artery. **C,** Lateral aortogram after percutaneous intervention with angioplasty of the celiac artery and angioplasty and stenting of the SMA. Note the residual stenosis of the celiac artery but good technical result of the SMA. **D,** Anteroposterior arteriogram after SMA angioplasty and stenting showing excellent filling of the celiac branches via collaterals (pancreaticoduodenal and gastroduodenal arteries). The patient remains asymptomatic 1 year after the procedure.

ACKNOWLEDGMENTS

The authors express their appreciation to Marilyn Gravett for her expert editorial assistance and to Victor Cantu for his graphics expertise during the writing of this manuscript.

SUGGESTED READINGS

Cho J-S, Carr JA, Jacobsen G, et al: Long-term outcome after mesenteric artery reconstruction: A 37-year experience. J Vasc Surg 35:453-460, 2002.

Foley MI, Moneta GL, Abou-Zamzam AM, et al: Revascularization of the superior mesenteric artery alone for treatment of intestinal ischemia. J Vasc Surg 32:37-47, 2000.

Kim AH, Ha KH: Evaluation of suspected mesenteric ischemia: Efficacy of radiologic studies. Radiol Clin North Am 41:327-342, 2003.

Martinez JP, Hogan GJ: Mesenteric ischemia. Emerg Med Clin North Am 22:909-928, 2004.

Park WM, Gloviczki P, Cherry KJ, et al: Contemporary management of acute mesenteric ischemia: Factors associated with survival. J Vasc Surg 35:445-452, 2002.

REFERENCES

1. Klass AA: Embolectomy in acute mesenteric occlusion. Ann Surg 134:913-917, 1951.
2. Boley SJ, Brandt LJ, Sammartano RJ: History of mesenteric ischemia. The evolution of a diagnosis and management. Surg Clin North Am 77:275-288, 1997.
3. Bradbury AW, Brittenden J, McBride K, Ruckley CV: Mesenteric ischaemia: A multidisciplinary approach. Br J Surg 82:1446-1459, 1995.
4. McKinsey JF, Gewertz BL: Acute mesenteric ischemia. Surg Clin North Am 77:307-318, 1997.
5. Martinez JP, Hogan GJ: Mesenteric ischemia. Emerg Med Clin North Am 22:909-928, 2004.
6. Acosta S, Ogren M, Sternby NH, et al: Incidence of acute thrombo-embolic occlusion of the superior mesenteric artery—a population-based study. Eur J Vasc Endovasc Surg 27:145-150, 2004.
7. Park WM, Gloviczki P, Cherry KJ Jr, et al: Contemporary management of acute mesenteric ischemia: Factors associated with survival. J Vasc Surg 35:445-452, 2002.
8. Oldenburg WA, Lau LL, Rodenberg TJ, et al: Acute mesenteric ischemia: A clinical review. Arch Intern Med 164:1054-1062, 2004.
9. McFadden DW, Rongione AJ: Intestinal circulation and vascular disorders. In Miller TA (ed): Modern Surgical Critical Care: Physiologic Foundation and Clinical Application, 2nd ed. St Louis, Quality Medical, 1998, pp 443-463.
10. Granger DN, Richardson PD, Kvietys PR, Mortillaro NA: Intestinal blood flow. Gastroenterology 78:837-863, 1980.
11. Brown RA, Chiu CJ, Scott HJ, Gurd FN: Ultrastructural changes in the canine ileal mucosal cell after mesenteric arterial occlusion. Arch Surg 101:290-297, 1970.
12. Edwards MS, Cherr GS, Craven TE, et al: Acute occlusive mesenteric ischemia: Surgical management and outcomes. Ann Vasc Surg 17:72-79, 2003.
13. Trompeter M, Brazda T, Remy CT, et al: Non-occlusive mesenteric ischemia: Etiology, diagnosis, and interventional therapy. Eur Radiol 12:1179-1187, 2002.
14. Buyukgebiz O, Aktan AO, Yegen C, et al: Captopril increases endothelin serum concentrations and preserves intestinal mucosa after mesenteric ischemia-reperfusion injury. Res Exp Med (Berl) 194:339-348, 1994.
15. Boley SJ, Regan JA, Tunick PA: Persistent vasoconstriction—a major factor in nonocclusive mesenteric ischemia. Curr Top Surg Res 3:425-434, 1971.
16. Boley SJ, Freiber W, Winslow PR: Circulatory responses to acute reduction of superior mesenteric arterial flow. Physiologist 12:180, 1969.
17. Everhard ME, Regan JA, Veith FJ: Mesenteric vasomotor response to reduced mesenteric blood flow. Physiologist 13:191, 1970.
18. Clark RA, Gallant TE: Acute mesenteric ischemia: Angiographic spectrum. AJR Am J Roentgenol 142:555-562, 1984.
19. Boley SJ, Feinstein FR, Sammartano R, et al: New concepts in the management of emboli of the superior mesenteric artery. Surg Gynecol Obstet 153:561-569, 1981.
20. Howard TJ, Plaskon LA, Wiebke EA, et al: Nonocclusive mesenteric ischemia remains a diagnostic dilemma. Am J Surg 171:405-408, 1996.
21. Neri E, Sassi C, Massetti M, et al: Nonocclusive intestinal ischemia in patients with acute aortic dissection. J Vasc Surg 36:738-745, 2002.
22. Boley SJ, Sprayregen S, Veith FJ, Siegelman SS: An aggressive roentgenologic and surgical approach to acute mesenteric ischemia. Surg Annu 5:355-378, 1973.
23. May LD, Berenson MM: Value of serum inorganic phosphate in the diagnosis of ischemic bowel disease. Am J Surg 146:266-268, 1983.
24. Klein HM, Lensing R, Klosterhalfen B, et al: Diagnostic imaging of mesenteric infarction. Radiology 197:79-82, 1995.
25. Smerud MJ, Johnson CD, Stephens DH: Diagnosis of bowel infarction: A comparison of plain films and CT scans in 23 cases. AJR Am J Roentgenol 154:99-103, 1990.
26. Hermsen K, Chong WK: Ultrasound evaluation of abdominal aortic and iliac aneurysms and mesenteric ischemia. Radiol Clin North Am 42:365-381, 2004.
27. Kim AY, Ha HK: Evaluation of suspected mesenteric ischemia: Efficacy of radiologic studies. Radiol Clin North Am 41:327-342, 2003.
28. Oderich GS, Panneton JM, Macedo TA, et al: Intraoperative duplex ultrasound of visceral revascularizations: Optimizing technical success and outcome. J Vasc Surg 38:684-691, 2003.
29. Lee R, Tung HK, Tung PH, et al: CT in acute mesenteric ischaemia. Clin Radiol 58:279-287, 2003.
30. Angelelli G, Scardapane A, Memeo M, et al: Acute bowel ischemia: CT findings. Eur J Radiol 50:37-47, 2004.
31. Taourel PG, Deneuville M, Pradel JA, et al: Acute mesenteric ischemia: Diagnosis with contrast-enhanced CT. Radiology 199:632-636, 1996.
32. Desai SR, Cox MR, Martin CJ: Superior mesenteric vein thrombosis: Computed tomography diagnosis. Aust N Z J Surg 68:811-812, 1998.
33. Vogelzang RL, Gore RM, Anschuetz SL, Blei AT: Thrombosis of the splanchnic veins: CT diagnosis. AJR Am J Roentgenol 150:93-96, 1988.
34. Kirkpatrick ID, Kroeker MA, Greenberg HM: Biphasic CT with mesenteric CT angiography in the evaluation of acute mesenteric ischemia: Initial experience. Radiology 229:91-98, 2003.
35. Hagspiel KD, Leung DA, Angle JF, et al: MR angiography of the mesenteric vasculature. Radiol Clin North Am 40:867-886, 2002.
36. Li KC, Dalman RL, Ch'en IY, et al: Chronic mesenteric ischemia: Use of in vivo MR imaging measurements of blood oxygen saturation in the superior mesenteric vein for diagnosis. Radiology 204:71-77, 1997.
37. Gallego AM, Ramirez P, Rodriguez JM, et al: Role of urokinase in the superior mesenteric artery embolism. Surgery 120:111-113, 1996.
38. McBride KD, Gaines PA: Thrombolysis of a partially occluding superior mesenteric artery thromboembolus by infusion of streptokinase. Cardiovasc Intervent Radiol 17:164-166, 1994.
39. VanDeinse WH, Zawacki JK, Phillips D: Treatment of acute mesenteric ischemia by percutaneous transluminal angioplasty. Gastroenterology 91:475-478, 1986.
40. Hladik P, Raupach J, Lojík M, et al: Treatment of acute mesenteric thrombosis/ischemia by transcatheter thromboaspiration. Surgery 137:122-123, 2005.

41. Ogihara S, Yamamura S, Tomono H, et al: Superior mesenteric arterial embolism: Treatment by trans-catheter thrombo-aspiration. J Gastroenterol 38:272-277, 2003.
42. Nyman U, Ivancev K, Lindh M, Uher P: Endovascular treatment of chronic mesenteric ischemia: Report of five cases. Cardiovasc Intervent Radiol 21:305-313, 1998.
43. Mansour MA: Management of acute mesenteric ischemia. Arch Surg 134:328-330, 1999.
44. McMillan WD, McCarthy WJ, Bresticker MR, et al: Mesenteric artery bypass: Objective patency determination. J Vasc Surg 21:729-740, 1995.
45. Cho JS, Carr JA, Jacobsen G, et al: Long-term outcome after mesenteric artery reconstruction: A 37-year experience. J Vasc Surg 35:453-460, 2002.
46. Gentile AT, Moneta GL, Taylor LM Jr, et al: Isolated bypass to the superior mesenteric artery for intestinal ischemia. Arch Surg 129:926-931, 1994.
47. Grendell JH, Ockner RK: Mesenteric venous thrombosis. Gastroenterology 82:358-372, 1982.
48. Naitove A, Weismann RE: Primary mesenteric venous thrombosis. Ann Surg 161:516-523, 1965.
49. Rhee RY, Gloviczki P, Mendonca CT, et al: Mesenteric venous thrombosis: Still a lethal disease in the 1990s. J Vasc Surg 20:688-697, 1994.
50. Harward TR, Green D, Bergan JJ, et al: Mesenteric venous thrombosis. J Vasc Surg 9:328-333, 1989.
51. Boley SJ, Kaleya RN, Brandt LJ: Mesenteric venous thrombosis. Surg Clin North Am 72:183-201, 1992.
52. Tomchik FS, Wittenberg J, Ottinger LW: The roentgenographic spectrum of bowel infarction. Radiology 96:249-260, 1970.
53. Miller VE, Berland LL: Pulsed Doppler duplex sonography and CT of portal vein thrombosis. AJR Am J Roentgenol 145:73-76, 1985.
54. Rhee RY, Gloviczki P: Mesenteric venous thrombosis. Surg Clin North Am 77:327-338, 1997.
55. Grieshop RJ, Dalsing MC, Cikrit DF, et al: Acute mesenteric venous thrombosis. Revisited in a time of diagnostic clarity. Am Surg 57:573-577, 1991.
56. Abdu RA, Zakhour BJ, Dallis DJ: Mesenteric venous thrombosis—1911 to 1984. Surgery 101:383-388, 1987.
57. Bilbao JI, Rodriguez-Cabello J, Longo J, et al: Portal thrombosis: Percutaneous transhepatic treatment with urokinase—a case report. Gastrointest Radiol 14:326-328, 1989.
58. Robin P, Gruel Y, Lang M, et al: Complete thrombolysis of mesenteric vein occlusion with recombinant tissue-type plasminogen activator. Lancet 1:1391, 1988.
59. Croft RJ, Menon GP, Marston A: Does 'intestinal angina' exist? A critical study of obstructed visceral arteries. Br J Surg 68:316-318, 1981.
60. Moneta GL, Lee RW, Yeager RA, et al: Mesenteric duplex scanning: A blinded prospective study. J Vasc Surg 17:79-84, 1993.
61. Thomas JH, Blake K, Pierce GE, et al: The clinical course of asymptomatic mesenteric arterial stenosis. J Vasc Surg 27:840-844, 1998.
62. Moneta GL, Yeager RA, Dalman R, et al: Duplex ultrasound criteria for diagnosis of splanchnic artery stenosis or occlusion. J Vasc Surg 14:511-518, 1991.
63. Bowersox JC, Zwolak RM, Walsh DB, et al: Duplex ultrasonography in the diagnosis of celiac and mesenteric artery occlusive disease. J Vasc Surg 14:780-786, 1991.
64. LaBombard FE, Musson A, Bowersox JC, Zwolak RM: Hepatic artery duplex as an adjunct in the evaluation of chronic mesenteric ischemia. J Vasc Tech 16:7-11, 1992.
65. Taylor LM, Moneta GL, Porter JM: Treatment of chronic visceral ischemia. In Rutherford RB (ed): Vascular Surgery, 5th ed. Philadelphia, WB Saunders, 2000.
66. Shaw RS, Maynard EP III: Acute and chronic thrombosis of the mesenteric arteries associated with malabsorption: A report of two cases successfully treated by thromboendarterectomy. N Engl J Med 258:874-878, 1958.
67. Wylie EJ, Stoney RJ, Ehrenfeld WK: Visceral atherosclerosis. In Manual of Vascular Surgery. New York, Springer-Verlag, 1980, p 211.
68. Moawad J, McKinsey JF, Wyble CW, et al: Current results of surgical therapy for chronic mesenteric ischemia. Arch Surg 132:613-618, 1997.
69. Wolf YG, Berlatzky Y, Gewertz BL: Sequential configuration for aorto-celiac-mesenteric bypass. Ann Vasc Surg 11:640-642, 1997.
70. Geroulakos G, Tober JC, Anderson L, Smead WL: Antegrade visceral revascularisation via a thoracoabdominal approach for chronic mesenteric ischaemia. Eur J Vasc Endovasc Surg 17:56-59, 1999.
71. Cooley DA, Wukasch DC: Techniques in Vascular Surgery. Philadelphia, WB Saunders, 1979.
72. Kieny R, Batellier J, Kretz JG: Aortic reimplantation of the superior mesenteric artery for atherosclerotic lesions of the visceral arteries: Sixty cases. Ann Vasc Surg 4:122-125, 1990.
73. Bergan JJ, Yao JS: Chronic intestinal ischemia. In Rutherford RB (ed): Vascular Surgery, 3rd ed. Philadelphia, WB Saunders, 1989, pp 1097-1103.
74. Rapp JH, Reilly LM, Qvarfordt PG, et al: Durability of endarterectomy and antegrade grafts in the treatment of chronic visceral ischemia. J Vasc Surg 3:799-806, 1986.
75. Johnston KW, Lindsay TF, Walker PM, Kalman PG: Mesenteric arterial bypass grafts: Early and late results and suggested surgical approach for chronic and acute mesenteric ischemia. Surgery 118:1-7, 1995.
76. Schwartz LB, McKinsey JF, Gewertz BL: Visceral ischemic syndromes. In Moore WS (ed): Vascular Surgery: A Comprehensive Review, 6th ed. Philadelphia, WB Saunders, 2002, pp 570-584.
77. Cormier JM, Fichelle JM, Vennin J, et al: Atherosclerotic occlusive disease of the superior mesenteric artery: Late results of reconstructive surgery. Ann Vasc Surg 5:510-518, 1991.
78. Cunningham CG, Reilly LM, Rapp JH, et al: Chronic visceral ischemia. Three decades of progress. Ann Surg 214:276-287, 1991.
79. McAfee MK, Cherry KJ Jr, Naessens JM, et al: Influence of complete revascularization on chronic mesenteric ischemia. Am J Surg 164:220-224, 1992.
80. Calderon M, Reul GJ, Gregoric ID, et al: Long-term results of the surgical management of symptomatic chronic intestinal ischemia. J Cardiovasc Surg (Torino) 33:723-728, 1992.
81. Christensen MG, Lorentzen JE, Schroeder TV: Revascularisation of atherosclerotic mesenteric arteries: Experience in 90 consecutive patients. Eur J Vasc Surg 8:297-302, 1994.
82. Mateo RB, O'Hara PJ, Hertzer NR, et al: Elective surgical treatment of symptomatic chronic mesenteric occlusive disease: Early results and late outcomes. J Vasc Surg 29:821-831, 1999.
83. Kihara TK, Blebea J, Anderson KM, et al: Risk factors and outcomes following revascularization for chronic mesenteric ischemia. Ann Vasc Surg 13:37-44, 1999.
84. Foley MI, Moneta GL, Abou-Zamzam AM Jr, et al: Revascularization of the superior mesenteric artery alone for treatment of intestinal ischemia. J Vasc Surg 32:37-47, 2000.
85. Park WM, Cherry KJ Jr, Chua HK, et al: Current results of open revascularization for chronic mesenteric ischemia: A standard for comparison. J Vasc Surg 35:853-859, 2002.
86. English WP, Pearce JD, Craven TE, et al: Chronic visceral ischemia: Symptom-free survival after open surgical repair. Vasc Endovasc Surg 38:493-503, 2004.
87. Sniderman KW: Transluminal angioplasty in the management of chronic intestinal ischemia. In Strandness D, van Breda A (eds): Vascular Diseases: Surgical and Interventional Therapy. New York, Churchill Livingstone, 1994, pp 803-809.
88. Hallisey MJ, Deschaine J, Illescas FF, et al: Angioplasty for the treatment of visceral ischemia. J Vasc Interv Radiol 6:785-791, 1995.
89. Allen RC, Martin GH, Rees CR, et al: Mesenteric angioplasty in the treatment of chronic intestinal ischemia. J Vasc Surg 24:415-421, 1996.
90. Maspes F, Mazzetti di Pietralata G, Gandini R, et al: Percutaneous transluminal angioplasty in the treatment of chronic mesenteric ischemia: Results and 3 years of follow-up in 23 patients. Abdom Imaging 23:358-363, 1998.
91. Sheeran SR, Murphy TP, Khwaja A, et al: Stent placement for treatment of mesenteric artery stenoses or occlusions. J Vasc Interv Radiol 10:861-867, 1999.
92. Kasirajan K, O'Hara PJ, Gray BH, et al: Chronic mesenteric ischemia: Open surgery versus percutaneous angioplasty and stenting. J Vasc Surg 33:63-71, 2001.
93. Pietura R, Szymanska A, El FM, et al: Chronic mesenteric ischemia: Diagnosis and treatment with balloon angioplasty and stenting. Med Sci Monit 8:R8-R12, 2002.

94. Matsumoto AH, Angle JF, Spinosa DJ, et al: Percutaneous transluminal angioplasty and stenting in the treatment of chronic mesenteric ischemia: Results and long-term followup. J Am Coll Surg 194:S22-S31, 2002.

95. Steinmetz E, Tatou E, Favier-Blavoux C, et al: Endovascular treatment as first choice in chronic intestinal ischemia. Ann Vasc Surg 16:693-699, 2002.

96. Sharafuddin MJ, Olson CH, Sun S, et al: Endovascular treatment of celiac and mesenteric arteries stenoses: Applications and results. J Vasc Surg 38:692-698, 2003.

97. Chahid T, Alfidja AT, Biard M, et al: Endovascular treatment of chronic mesenteric ischemia: Results in 14 patients. Cardiovasc Intervent Radiol 27:637-642, 2004.

98. Furrer J, Gruntzig A, Kugelmeier J, Goebel N: Treatment of abdominal angina with percutaneous dilatation of an arteria mesenterica superior stenosis. Preliminary communication. Cardiovasc Intervent Radiol 3:43-44, 1980.

99. Wilms G, Baert AL: Transluminal angioplasty of superior mesenteric artery and celiac trunk. Ann Radiol (Paris) 29:535-538, 1986.

100. Matsumoto AH, Tegtmeyer CJ, Fitzcharles EK, et al: Percutaneous transluminal angioplasty of visceral arterial stenoses: Results and long-term clinical follow-up. J Vasc Interv Radiol 6:165-174, 1995.

85

Aortoenteric Fistula and Visceral Artery Aneurysms

John Blebea · Rashad Choudry

AORTOENTERIC FISTULA

Aortoenteric fistula (AEF) remains an uncommon, but potentially lethal problem that typically arises from the progressive growth of an abdominal aortic aneurysm (AAA) or, more commonly, as a complication of aortic reconstructive surgery. Early recognition and diagnosis rest on a high index of suspicion, although timely and accurate diagnosis remains difficult despite improvements in diagnostic technology. Prompt treatment can be lifesaving and prevents severe enteric hemorrhage, multisystem organ failure, or limb amputation. Recent advances in surgical and endovascular techniques, as well as perioperative care, continue to improve both the morbidity and mortality associated with AEF.

Classification

An AEF is an abnormal communication between the aorta and any gastrointestinal lumen. The classification of AEFs is based on the underlying pathophysiology, and they are categorized into either *primary* or *secondary* types. Primary AEF reflects erosion of an AAA or, in unusual circumstances, erosion of an atherosclerotic aorta into an overlying segment of intestine. Foregut, midgut, and hindgut fistulas have all been reported in the literature. The third and fourth segments of the duodenum are most commonly involved (70%) because of their close approximation to the infrarenal aorta and their fixed immobile position in the retroperitoneum.[1] Although the true incidence of primary AEF is not known, autopsy studies have found them to be present in 0.04% to 0.07% of specimens involving an atherosclerotic aorta, whereas 0.69% to 2.36% have been discovered in the presence of native aortic aneurysms.[2,3] *Secondary* AEFs are more frequently observed clinically, with an overall incidence of between 0.36% and 1.6%.[4] They typically occur after surgery on the aorta, particularly graft replacement for

an AAA or atherosclerotic occlusive disease, endarterectomy, and renal or visceral artery bypass procedures. Two different types of *secondary* fistulas may develop. The first is a *graft-enteric fistula,* which originates from partial disruption of the proximal graft-aortic anastomosis. The other is a *graft-enteric erosion,* in which the bypass prosthesis directly erodes into the adjacent enteric wall. It is believed that despite a low overall incidence in the published literature, the actual occurrence of AEFs may be higher than reported. *Secondary* AEF is more commonly seen than *primary* types because of the number of aortic reconstructions performed. Recently, AEF has also been associated with endovascular aortic graft placement.[5]

Pathogenesis

Aortic wall pathology accounts for over three quarters of all *primary* fistulas and usually develops from the pulsatile enlargement of an AAA. In addition to atherosclerotic aneurysmal disease, enlargement secondary to an underlying aortic dissection can lead to AEF. More worrisome are inflammatory arteritides and infective mycotic aneurysms, tuberculosis, and syphilis, which can be initiating events of aorta-to-enteric fistulas.[2] The remainder of *primary* AEFs are thought to begin with gastrointestinal rather than aortic disease processes, including penetrating peptic ulcers, bowel wall ischemia, infection, foreign body erosion, trauma, operative injury, neoplasia, pancreatic pseudocyst, gallstones, and radiation therapy.[2,6,7]

Secondary AEFs involve a more complicated series of events ultimately leading to a similar result. Two specific mechanisms help explain the pathogenesis of these AEFs. The first involves degeneration of a proximal aortic suture line to a prosthetic graft. The etiology of such a breakdown of this anastomosis can be multifactorial, including a technical error with an insufficient amount of healthy tissue incorporated in the suture line, aneurysmal enlargement above the anastomosis when the original graft replacement was too distal from the renal arteries, suture failure, although this is quite infrequent today, or pseudoaneurysm formation secondary to infection. All of these processes lead to localized arterial disruption and, with a progressive increase in size, can erode into nearby enteric structures and result in a *graft-enteric fistula*, which accounts for three quarters of all AEFs.[8] Because pseudoaneurysm formation after graft insertion may be the initiating event for AEF formation, yearly postoperative ultrasound scans of prosthetic aortic grafts is performed by many clinicians.

A second mechanism of AEF development involves postoperative direct erosion of a prosthetic graft into overlying adherent bowel. Long-standing contact between bowel and pulsatile prosthetic material eventually leads to thinning of the overlying bowel wall, ischemic degeneration, and enteric wall perforation and ultimately results in soilage of the underlying vascular graft. Gastrointestinal proteolytic and bacterial enzymes then erode more surface area along the graft with extension to the proximal suture line. Although the prosthetic graft itself is quite resistant to bacterial and lytic breakdown, the native aortic tissue at the anastomosis is not nearly as hardy. Eventually, a small disruption of the aorta at the anastomosis takes place and leads to bleeding from the aorta along the outside of the prosthesis and into the enteral opening with associated gastrointestinal bleeding. This process is known as *graft-enteric erosion*. The development of a *secondary* AEF without graft placement, for instance, after non–graft-related aortic reconstruction such as endarterectomy, is seen in only about 2% of patients.[8]

Surgical intervention for a ruptured AAA and for aortic atherosclerotic occlusive disease results in higher rates of secondary AEF development,[9] most likely because of the lack of an aneurysmal wall to cover the prosthetic graft in the latter circumstance and a large retroperitoneal hematoma and possible visceral wall ischemia in the former.

Several important principles can be used to prevent secondary AEF formation after aortic surgery. It is clear that direct contact between prosthetic grafts and enteric structures is key to the development of AEFs. Therefore, every effort should be made to place viable, healthy, autologous tissue between these two structures, and several options are available at the time of surgery to do so. Most commonly, in the case of AAA, the native aneurysmal wall is sufficient to cover the graft material, although this can be challenging at its most proximal point where the aortic anastomosis is located. This area, however, is usually just above the duodenum and the beginning portions of the jejunum. Although there may not be sufficient aneurysmal wall for coverage, this area should still be covered by reattaching the posterior layer of peritoneum. A greater challenge involves the placement of an aortofemoral or aortoiliac graft for occlusive disease when there is no aneurysmal wall at all to cover the prosthetic graft. This situation is especially problematic when a proximal end-to-side anastomosis is performed and more of the graft is extending anteriorly into the peritoneal cavity. In such circumstances, when insufficient retroperitoneal fat and posterior peritoneum are available to cover the graft, an omental flap can be mobilized and interposed between the graft and overlying bowel. It should cover all of the graft and be sutured in place to maintain its protective position. Correct length of the graft during insertion for any aortic procedure should be ensured so that there is no redundancy and angulation, which can also be associated with graft erosion.

Occasionally, in a hostile abdomen that has undergone previous laparotomies or has endured radiation therapy, incidental enterotomies may occur during aortic dissection. They characteristically involve the small bowel, and if they are small and without extensive spillage, aortic reconstruction can proceed safely. Similarly, associated open cholecystectomy can be performed for symptomatic cholelithiasis after the aortic procedure is completed.[10]

Perioperative administration of prophylactic antibiotics effective against gram-positive organisms, such as a first-generation cephalosporin, is routine clinical practice. Similarly, antibiotic irrigation of the abdominal cavity before closure is routinely performed. Although most primary graft infections are thought to result from prosthetic contamination at the time of placement, infection as a result of transient bacteremia from other sources may also develop, especially infection by anaerobic or gram-negative organisms.[11]

Clinical Findings

One of the most challenging aspects about AEFs is the difficulty of making a correct and timely diagnosis, which remains critical to effective resuscitation and successful treatment. Indeed, only a third of all AEFs are correctly diagnosed before surgical intervention.[4] The timing of the clinical manifestations of an AEF is quite variable and ranges from a few weeks to several years after the initial aortic reconstructive surgery.[12] Probably because of gender differences in the prevalence of AAAs, men with AEFs outnumber women by a ratio of 4:1.[13] The diagnosis of AEF is most often considered during evaluation for gastrointestinal bleeding because up to 64% of patients are seen in this manner.[2,14] Conversely, however, AEF is a rare cause of the bleeding inasmuch as less than 5% of patients with previous aortic surgery and gastrointestinal bleeding have an AEF as the underlying cause.[15] In those who do, an initial herald bleeding event is considered characteristic of AEF.[3] This may be manifested in a number of ways but commonly involves brisk upper and lower gastrointestinal bleeding. Rarely is this initial episode life-threatening, and some time is available to arrange for an endoscopic evaluation.[15] Although the initial event may be self-limited, subsequent uncontrolled fatal hemorrhage will occur if a correct diagnosis is not made and the cause left untreated.

More frequently seen is gastrointestinal hemorrhage with signs and symptoms of systemic infection. Hematemesis and fever are the two most common initial symptoms associated with a graft-enteric fistula, whereas melena and fever (sepsis) are more often seen with graft-enteric erosions.[8] Along with fever and leukocytosis, infection as an initial manifestation of AEF may be found in 25% of patients. When present, sepsis with AEF is usually more severe than prosthetic graft infection alone. Seen less often than bleeding is abdominal pain. Primary AEF patients may complain of insidious abdominal pain, possibly related to an underlying cause such as peptic ulcer disease or neoplasia. Physical examination of patients with primary AEF reveals a palpable abdominal aneurysm in only 30%. Uncommonly, septic embolization to the lower extremities may occur and result in ischemic changes. Rarely do patients have the classic triad of gastrointestinal bleeding, abdominal pain, and a pulsatile abdominal mass.[16]

Aortoesophageal fistulas have been considered a separate pathologic entity. Like AEFs in other enteric sites, underlying aortic pathology and aortic surgery account for a large percentage of cases. Unique to esophageal fistulas, lesions of the esophagus and foreign body erosion constitute an equally prevalent number of cases. The typical site of aortic involvement in these circumstances is the thoracic aorta. Aortoesophageal fistulas remain rare, with a large proportion of cases being found at autopsy. The classic constellation of symptoms, or *Chiari's triad* (midthoracic pain, sentinel arterial hemorrhage, and subsequent exsanguination), is ascribed to this type of fistula. Like other types, upper gastrointestinal bleeding is the most common initial symptom, followed by chest pain and dysphagia.

Diagnosis

Diagnosis of an AEF may be difficult and depends on a high index of suspicion because the clinical findings may be subtle.[17] In any patient with a surgical history of bowel or aortic reconstruction and gastrointestinal hemorrhage, AEF should be considered. Attention to the patient's hemodynamic stability should take highest precedence, with unstable patients requiring immediate aggressive resuscitation followed by operative exploration of the abdomen. Patients with intermittent or self-limited bleeding can safely undergo a short preoperative work-up to assist in planning for corrective AEF surgery. Despite the spontaneous initial cessation of bleeding from many AEFs, early rebleeding occurs in 40% of patients, thus limiting the time available to arrive at an accurate diagnosis. It should be remembered that the only test that has 100% diagnostic accuracy is exploratory laparotomy.[8]

Esophagogastroduodenoscopy (EGD) remains the first and most frequently performed test in patients suspected of having an AEF.[18] EGD may best be conducted in the operating room with a qualified vascular surgeon present for patients with a high suspicion of AEF because manipulation of a quiescent AEF can lead to brisk and life-threatening bleeding. Essential to complete EGD is visualization of the fourth portion of the duodenum because it overlies the aorta and previously placed prosthetic grafts. Findings on EGD may range from mucosal surface changes to complete bowel perforation with visible prosthetic graft and active arterial bleeding. There are no therapeutic options during endoscopy to stop the bleeding. It serves only as a diagnostic procedure.

Unless other definitive gastrointestinal pathology is found on EGD to explain the gastrointestinal bleeding, an indeterminate EGD cannot exclude an AEF in patients with prosthetic aortic grafts or those with aneurysmal aortas.

After EGD, computed tomography (CT) is the next most used tool (50%) in the work-up of AEF, and it has both high sensitivity (94%) and high specificity (85%).[18,19] CT scans are helpful because of their ability to image not only the aorta but also the entire retroperitoneum and bowel wall, as well as spatial relationships between the two. In patients who have previously undergone aortic reconstruction, abnormal perigraft findings may include air bubbles, fluid, obliteration of soft tissue planes, and a pseudoaneurysm. Considerable overlap does exist between CT findings in aortic infection and AEF.[19,20] Though pathognomonic, oral or intravenous contrast leak is a rare finding. Perigraft air or fluid more than a few weeks after an aortic operation is strong evidence of an AEF.[21]

Angiography is best used for preoperative planning before necessary vascular reconstruction. It rarely reveals a graft-enteric erosion or specific vascular defect, which is usually covered with thrombus, and is rarely diagnostic.[22] Angiography may document other graft characteristics that can cause overlying bowel erosion, such as a pseudoaneurysm or kink in the prosthesis.[23] The use of magnetic resonance imaging may be helpful for prosthetic graft infection; however, few convincing data have been published regarding its efficacy in the diagnosis of fistulas, and its utility in critically ill patients is also likely to be limited.

Nuclear imaging, including technetium 99m and indium 111 scans, offer high sensitivity for the diagnosis of AEF, but the associated false-positive rate may be unacceptably high for routine use (Fig. 85–1). Their applicability may be of benefit by using red blood cells to suggest the location of active gastrointestinal bleeding or in differentiating aortic graft infection with radiolabeled white blood cells.[24,25] Limited experience with ^{18}F-2-deoxy-D-glucose positron emission tomography (FDG-PET)

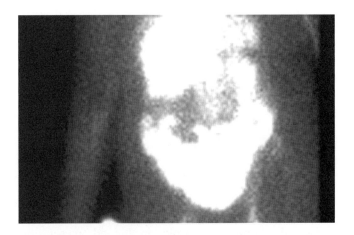

Figure 85–1. Red blood cell–labeled nuclear scan demonstrating diffuse blood in the small bowel without localization of the source of arterial bleeding.

scanning for AEF has been reported in patients with subtle signs of graft compromise.[26]

Ultrasound evaluation of the aorta and periaortic structures may be useful to screen for an aneurysm or pseudoaneurysm after surgery; however, its use in detection of AEFs is limited and therefore not recommended. Other modalities for bowel imaging, such as plain films and barium swallow, are seldom helpful for diagnosis or localization of fistulas and may interfere with other imaging because of barium artifacts.[11]

Surgical Treatment

The initial approach to patients suspected of having an AEF or those with an established diagnosis begins with an appreciation of the patient's cardiovascular status and underlying comorbid conditions. Central to planning of treatment is an appraisal of the survivability of these gravely ill patients after another major operation. Placement in an intensive care unit before and after surgery, central venous access, intra-arterial pressure monitoring, appropriate fluid resuscitation, correction of electrolyte abnormalities, and blood transfusions as needed should be undertaken. Antibiotic coverage is typically empirical until tissue culture results are available; however, appropriate coverage for gram-negative organisms, enteric bacterial species, and *Staphylococcus aureus* should be initiated.

The present standard of treatment of both primary and secondary AEFs remains surgery. Without surgery, a patient harboring an AEF will ultimately succumb to bleeding or sepsis. The primary aim of operative intervention is to stop active bleeding and prevent potential life-threatening hemorrhage. After successful vascular control, the surgeon can then address the enteric defect, infection control, and vascular reconstruction with preservation of distal blood flow.

Patients with any degree of hemodynamic instability should be resuscitated quickly and taken to the operating room without delay or extensive work-up. The initial approach should be through a midline laparotomy from the xiphoid to the pubis symphysis. Retroperitoneal exposure is an alternative approach to a diseased aorta and to avoid a hostile abdomen. However, limited visualization of the right iliac artery or graft limb and involved bowel make it a less than ideal choice for a patient in extremis. The first priority on abdominal entry should be proximal vascular control, which will in most cases best be accomplished through supraceliac aortic exposure and control. After proximal control, if the patient is hemodynamically stable, distal aortic or iliac artery control can be established. In unstable patients, distal control can be achieved through placement of occlusion balloon catheters, either through the open aorta or via a transfemoral approach. Once proximal and distal control is established, infrarenal dissection is undertaken and aortic cross-clamping performed in the infrarenal position to avoid prolonged mesenteric and renal ischemia. If hemostasis is present, systemic heparinization is induced before cross-clamping to prevent distal arterial thrombosis.

If there is no active bleeding, examination of the gastrointestinal tract should be performed. Beginning with the stomach and looking for evidence of peptic ulcer disease, a methodical running of the bowel should continue distally with particular attention paid to the area at the ligament of Treitz. Dissection of the bowel directly overlying the aorta should be performed sharply. Once the dense adhesions are freed, the AEF should be isolated and bowel repair or resection carried out as necessary. Because there is no definitive method of restoring bowel continuity, the operative anatomy should dictate the method selected. Enteric spillage into the operative field should be minimized by either clamping or oversewing any obvious defects. Small defects may be amenable to a transverse, two-layered repair, whereas segmental resection to healthy tissue is needed in other patients. Serosal patch placement and end-to-end, end-to-side, or Roux-en-Y anastomosis may be required for fistulated bowel.

Management of the aortic portion of the AEF should begin with extensive débridement of any infected retroperitoneal soft tissue. Intraoperative tissue Gram stain and culture will help in identifying the degree of infection and bacterial pathogens. Once clear tissue margins are ensured, full exposure through meticulous sharp dissection of the native aorta for primary AEF or the prosthetic graft for secondary AEF is performed. It is essential that dissection along the length of the aorta or graft be extended to well-incorporated healthy and uninfected tissue. The type of AEF will guide the manner in which the aorta is handled and the definitive reconstruction performed. If an AEF is not discovered at the usual location near the ligament of Treitz, the entire small bowel and colon should be assessed to look for other unsuspected pathology.

Primary Aortoenteric Fistula

Treatment of a primary AEF, once vascular and enteric control is established, rests on the degree of infection found at surgery. With more proximal AEFs involving structures such as the duodenum, it is possible for the bacterial inoculum to be lower than for AEFs involving more distal structures such as the colon. Nevertheless, historical studies report that up to 30% of primary AEFs may harbor infection.[27] In most cases, primary AEFs can be attributed to the progressive evolution of an aneurysmal aorta. Primary AEFs, as a result of either an aneurysmal or gastrointestinal etiology, may be repaired by either in situ graft placement or extra-anatomic bypass (EAB). Patients' medical comorbid conditions and cardiovascular instability usually dictate the use of a prosthetic graft. The use of antibiotic (rifampin)-impregnated grafts may lower the risk for infection. Alternatively, in stable patients, autologous aortoiliac bypass with superficial femoral veins is an available option.[28] In an operative field in which gross contamination or purulence is encountered, EAB is the safer alternative, although it prolongs the operative time. The key tenet in repair remains adequate débridement of all infected tissue and placement of healthy tissue between the aortic reconstruction and overlying bowel.

Secondary Aortoenteric Fistula

Of the *secondary* AEFs, aortoenteric erosions are the easier to treat. As in *primary* AEFs, the involved bowel is treated by either repair or resection. Because the aortic graft is only secondarily contaminated, excision of this segment of graft plus in situ replacement of it with another prosthetic graft is usually satisfactory. Treatment of *secondary* AEFs caused by associated aortic anastomotic disruption can be significantly more complicated because they generally involve more extensive prosthetic infection and less normal aortic tissue. Traditionally, a single operation addressing both graft excision and creation of an EAB has been associated with a high level of morbidity and mortality. In an effort to lower complications secondary to the long cross-clamp times required to perform both phases of the operation, a reversed staging approach has been adopted by some, with favorable results reported in the literature.[4] Reversed staging begins with placement of an EAB, followed by excision of the infected graft 1 to several days later.[4,9] Use of the reversed staging approach, however, depends on patient stability. Those with active bleeding or profound sepsis cannot undergo this sequence and require urgent graft excision. When possible, staging allows for decreased intraoperative blood loss, as well as avoidance of the metabolic and hemodynamic consequences of prolonged interruption of perfusion to the lower extremities. Though performed in two separate operations, each stage remains a challenging step in full reconstruction. The typical EAB includes an axillofemoral and femorofemoral bypass with preservation of pelvic blood flow in a retrograde manner from the common femoral arteries. Patients with previous bifemoral grafting and extension of infection into the groin present much more of a challenge because of the need to excise the existing anastomoses and then select new sites for distal graft placement, usually tunneled lateral to and downstream from the previous reconstruction. Once the EAB is completed, the patient is returned to the intensive care unit, where resuscitation and antibiotic coverage are continued. One to several days later, the patient is returned to the operating room for removal of the infected prosthetic graft and repair of the enteric defect.

Before graft excision, the enteric defect should be repaired or resected and gastrointestinal continuity reestablished. After complete exposure of the prosthetic graft and proximal and distal aorta, excision of the involved graft and radical débridement of infected perigraft tissue are performed. Complete removal of aortic tissue at the proximal suture line is required. If necessary to obtain viable aortic tissue because of infectious involvement extending to the renal arteries, separate revascularization with antegrade bypasses to the renal arteries can be performed. Fortunately, this is a rare occurrence. Insufficient débridement of the proximal aorta adjacent to the anastomosis has been associated with later aortic stump blowout and death from recurrent bleeding.[29] Recent studies, however, show a reduction in this complication with meticulous closure technique and the onlay of healthy autologous tissue. The stump and area of excised graft are optimally covered with an omental flap. The distal end of the aorta, after graft excision, is oversewn with monofilament polypropylene suture to prevent disruption. Thorough irrigation of the entire abdomen is required before abdominal closure. Specimens of all prosthetic and perigraft tissue should be taken for culture to help in tailoring the selection of postoperative antibiotics.

In situ reconstruction remains an important option for patients in whom EAB is not possible. Recent advances in replacement graft options have renewed interest in this type of repair, with a greater than 22% survival benefit over extra-anatomic repair.[2,30] The risk for aortic stump blowout after EAB is reported to be as high as 16% and can be avoided by using this approach.[2] Additionally, the amputation rate is 14% lower with in situ revascularization.[18] Currently, several choices of replacement conduit are available for reconstruction. Autologous tissue is ideal when reconstruction takes place in a known infected field. One useful type of autologous tissue is the superficial femoral vein used to reconstruct the aortoiliac system. An advantage over other venous tissue is its larger diameter. However, proper vein harvesting and construction of the bifurcation may be time-consuming and can lead to longer lower extremity ischemic times.[28] Saphenous vein, when sewn into a larger-diameter conduit through panel or spiral techniques, may be suitable, even for aortic replacement. Arterial allografts are seldom used because of the known risk for late aneurysmal degeneration. The use of cryopreserved homografts has been successfully reported in the literature, albeit with limited clinical experience. Authors using homografts as replacement conduits cite the inherent infection-fighting ability of this conduit, as well as its ability to function as a temporizing conduit, with definitive reconstruction performed in a delayed manner after the infection has cleared.[31] Rifampinimpregnated Dacron prosthetic grafts have demonstrated better protection against reinfection when used during in situ reconstruction.[32,33] Newer manufacturing techniques of antibiotic bonding with collagen or gelatin allow for longer antibiotic availability at the in situ site.[34]

Occasionally, in patients in whom aortic grafting was performed for occlusive disease or in patients with bilateral lower extremity amputations, graft excision without revascularization may be possible. In such circumstances, preoperative noninvasive vascular studies and arteriography can be helpful in determining the degree of available collateral circulation. Cases in which an end-to-side graft was initially placed may be handled by graft excision with aortic endarterectomy and patch closure, provided that thorough débridement of infected aortic tissue has been performed.

Endovascular Therapy

Endovascular therapies for AAA have not prevented the later development of an AEF. Such techniques, however, may also provide new options for interventions in the treatment of AEF. Despite the less invasive nature of endovascular surgery, AEF after stent deployment has been reported in the literature.[35-37] Specific aneurysmal characteristics that may lend to the later development of an AEF after stent placement include the ongoing presence of an AAA under endotension, treatment of inflammatory aneurysms, the choice of stent, migration or kinking of endovascular devices, and unrecognized occult *primary* AEF.[37]

The therapeutic use of endovascular devices for AEF may be most helpful in the setting of acute, life-threatening hemorrhage, where timely operative control may be hindered by extensive adhesions and a hostile abdomen. Successful use of balloon control of aortic hemorrhage in a situation involving traumatic AEF has been reported.[38,39] Temporizing the bleeding from an AEF may also be accomplished through transcatheter coil embolization before operative intervention and open repair.[40] The use of endovascular repair in the presence of known aortic infection or AEF should be individualized to the patient because there is no current consensus on treatment in these circumstances. Successful stent placement in the presence of an AEF has been reported; however, recurrence of infection and fistula hemorrhage continue to be clear risks.[41-44] Stent repair of AEF is not definitive therapy because débridement and removal of associated retroperitoneal infection are not possible.[45] The use of more novel techniques, including the combined application of an aortic stent and endoscopic injection of fibrin sealant, has also been reported.[46,47] In the future, stent placement in patients with a known AEF may possibly be indicated as a bridge to definitive open repair once the acute, life-threatening circumstances are controlled or for palliative reasons.[48,49]

Results

The natural, untreated clinical course of *primary* AEF remains eventual death from gastrointestinal hemorrhage. Surgical approaches short of closure of the enteric defect, removal of infection, and vascular reconstruction, such as local patch repair or aneurysmorrhaphy, are complicated by reinfection and increased mortality.[50]

Secondary AEF follows a similar course if left untreated. Several options are currently available to handle this type of AEF, including the traditional method of fistula takedown and bowel repair, followed by graft excision, débridement, and EAB. The reversed staging technique still maintains these surgical principles but allows for reduced lower extremity ischemia times by EAB construction before intra-abdominal decontamination and repair. This method has produced improved results over the traditional technique, with an AEF cure rate of 70% (>3 years postoperatively) and 18% mortality.[4] Graft excision may be performed without revascularization, as potentially indicated for patients with occlusive disease, but it still carries a high mortality rate. More recently, renewed interest in in situ graft replacement has emerged, with investigators reporting improved surgical outcomes with appropriate patient selection and a range of bypass graft choices. A 20% reduction in mortality has been reported with in situ replacement versus EAB.[2]

Reinfection, graft occlusion, amputation, aortic stump blowout, and need for revision surgery are still seen. In a meta-analysis of *secondary* AEF by Pipinos et al., a third of patients undergoing AEF surgery suffered complications.[8] In another subset group, revision of graft placement was required in 40%, and recurrent *secondary* AEFs developed in 34%. Aortic stump rupture and anastomotic rupture occurred in 19% and 7%, respectively.[8] Amputation complicating AEF ranges from 6% after in situ repair, to 8% with lower extremity revascularization before graft excision, to 20% after EAB.[18]

Despite improvements in surgical technique and perioperative care, AEF remains a rare complication that is difficult to diagnose and treat. The majority of published data regarding AEF are in the form of small-volume, retrospective analyses or case reports, with multiple different practice standards applied. Definitive conclusions regarding any single method or technique are more difficult because of this lack of data. Death after AEF occurs in 30% to 40% of patients. Thirty-day survival rates after surgical treatment range from 13% to 86%, with an average of 33%. Overall, morbidity and mortality rates have been relatively unchanged and remain higher than seen with prosthetic graft infection. Quality of life after AEF and reconstruction has not been studied in the current literature.

VISCERAL ARTERY ANEURYSMS

Visceral artery aneurysms are relatively rare lesions. However, they are clinically important because of the potential for rupture and life-threatening hemorrhage. An increased frequency of abdominal imaging has brought to attention more visceral aneurysms than has previously been reported.[51,52] Although there is a paucity of prospective natural history data on which to base treatment recommendations, general guidelines for intervention have been developed. Newer techniques for treatment have expanded the available options for patients with visceral artery aneurysms.

Splenic Artery Aneurysms

Incidence

Splenic artery aneurysms (SAAs) are the most common visceral artery aneurysms found intra-abdominally. Only aortic and iliac artery aneurysms are more frequent. It is difficult to define the exact incidence of SAAs, with postmortem studies suggesting an incidence ranging from 0.1% to 10%. An average prevalence of 0.8% is suggested, with SAAs developing more commonly in multiparous women.[53,54] Improved and more frequently used radiographic imaging modalities are likely to increase the frequency of diagnosis of such aneurysms.

Pathogenesis

The exact etiology of SAA is not completely understood. Multiple underlying disorders are thought to be associated or directly responsible for SAA formation. Abbas et al. reported the presence of hypertension (50%), obesity (28%), smoking (28%), and hypercholesterolemia (22%) in 217 patients with SAAs.[55] Historically, the most commonly implicated condition is arteriosclerosis. More recently, however, it has been suggested that the arteriosclerotic changes are secondary alterations in the composition of the vascular wall that are possibly associated with abnormal hemodynamic flow patterns.[56] Commonly seen in patients with SAAs is the presence of arterial fibrodysplasia, thus supporting a causative role of medial layer degeneration in the formation of these aneurysms.[54,57] Portal hypertension, cirrhosis, and splenomegaly are linked to the development of SAAs because of their contribution to elevated portal pressure and an increased diameter of the splenic artery. Accordingly, orthotopic liver transplantation has also resulted in an increased incidence of SAAs, probably because of the same mechanism. Other pathologic conditions that can lead to the development of SAAs include connective tissue disorders such as Marfan's syndrome, inflammatory states, and infection. Pseudoaneurysms can occur after traumatic injury to the abdomen, whereas chronic pancreatitis with pseudocysts leads to a 10% incidence of false aneurysms of the splenic artery.

A history of multiple pregnancies is common in women with SAAs. A recent analysis showed an average of 3.5 pregnancies in women with SAAs.[55] No single cause has explained the relationship between pregnancy and aneurysm development. Molecular and physiologic data suggest a predilection of the splenic artery to respond to changes of pregnancy, including hormonal effects and blood flow changes.[53]

Most SAAs appear saccular and may occur anywhere along the vessel. Typically, they are found along the main trunk or branch points, with multiple aneurysms occurring in up to 20% of patients. Smaller SAAs, such as those associated with systemic disease, may be found within the spleen itself. SAAs may vary in size considerably but largely fall between 2 and 3 cm. Calcification of the aneurysms occurs commonly and is found in up to 90% of splenic aneurysms.[55]

Clinical Findings

The majority of patients with SAAs are asymptomatic at the time of diagnosis. Those who do have symptoms at diagnosis are often found to have another cause for their complaints. Typical symptoms that may raise suspicion for SAA include vague, radiating left upper quadrant or epigastric pain that is exacerbated by positional changes. Episodic abdominal discomfort may be related to distal embolization of thrombus resulting in splenic infarction. SAAs are usually found incidentally by plain film radiography, CT, or arteriography for unrelated reasons. Calcification outlining the aneurysm sac tends to appear curvilinear and at the expected location of the splenic artery in the left upper quadrant.

The lifetime risk for SAA rupture may be as high as 10%, although some series have reported mortality rates as high as 25%.[58,59] Patients at increased risk for rupture include pregnant, multiparous women during the third trimester, cirrhotic patients, and those with connective

tissue diseases. Symptomatic SAAs are typically due to intraperitoneal rupture. The phenomenon of *double rupture* refers to temporary lesser sac containment of a bleeding aneurysm resulting in transient symptoms, followed by breakthrough exsanguination into the rest of the abdominal cavity leading to hemodynamic collapse. SAAs may rarely rupture into adjacent structures such as the bowel, biliary tract, and splenic vein and result in occult bleeding. Symptomatic SAAs found in pregnant women have ruptured. The correct diagnosis, however, is difficult to make and can be confused with other obstetric, gynecologic, and general surgical conditions, thereby delaying emergency treatment. Mortality in pregnant women after ruptured SAAs has historically been reported to be as high as 70%, with fetal salvage being rare.[53,60]

Diagnosis

Diagnosis of a symptomatic SAA rests on clinical suspicion. The initial clinical findings may lead to an evaluation for other intra-abdominal conditions first, with incidental identification of an SAA on radiographic studies. Plain abdominal radiographs may identify concentric calcifications in the left upper quadrant that suggest the presence of an aneurysm. CT scans, CT angiography, and duplex ultrasound will also be useful in the identification and diagnosis of an SAA (Fig. 85–2). Arteriography is not usually needed for identification of an aneurysm but can be helpful for operative planning before elective surgical repair. In patients in whom other modalities do not clearly define the precise vessel of origin, selective arteriography can provide the definitive diagnosis.

Treatment

The indications for treatment of an SAA have become better defined. Although definitive management of asymptomatic SAAs does not involve a fixed size cutoff for operative intervention, in good-risk patients, intervention is appropriate when the diameter of the aneurysm exceeds 2 cm. Lesions in young patients or women of childbearing age or aneurysms with progressive enlargement should be repaired electively. SAAs that are found during pregnancy are best treated at diagnosis because of the high mortality in the mother and fetus if rupture occurs. Symptomatic aneurysms should be repaired on an emergency basis.

Surgical treatment of SAAs may be individualized for each patient because several approaches are available for repair. Surgical techniques include aneurysm ligation, resection, and resection with splenectomy when the aneurysm is close to the hilum of the spleen. Because of the abundant collateral blood supply to the spleen via short gastric arteries, arterial reconstruction is not necessary. Aneurysm exclusion, accomplished through proximal and distal artery ligation, is all that is required and the preferred approach in most circumstances. Aneurysmorrhaphy, or opening of the aneurysm and oversewing the inflow and outflow vessel, is performed when adequate exposure of the proximal or distal splenic artery is

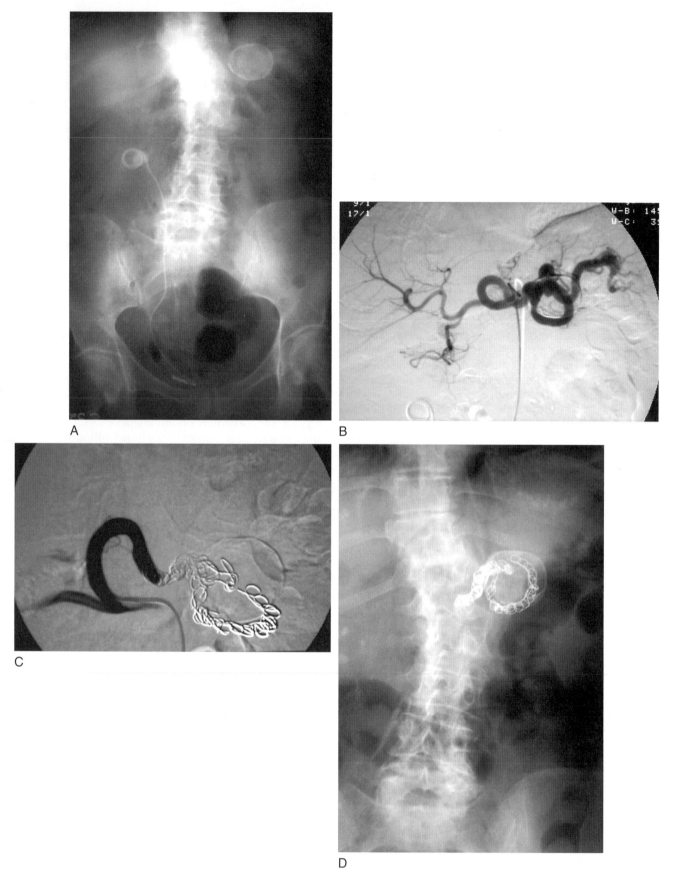

Figure 85–2. **A,** A plain abdominal radiograph shows a large calcified aneurysm in the left upper quadrant. **B,** Selective angiography of the celiac artery identifies signet-ring opacification of a splenic artery aneurysm. Thrombus on the inside of the aneurysm induces flow of contrast within the outer edges of the aneurysm. **C,** Coil embolization within the splenic aneurysm induces thrombosis of the aneurysm and occlusion of the mid and distal splenic artery. **D,** An abdominal roentgenogram illustrates the coils within the curvilinear structure of the splenic aneurysm.

not possible as a result of surrounding inflammation. Proximal ligation alone is not recommended because retrograde blood flow can potentially continue to enlarge an SAA. Splenectomy may be needed in cases in which an SAA is near the hilum or is encroaching on the parenchyma and might make exclusion hazardous. Splenectomy is not generally recommended, however, because of loss of splenic function and host resistance. A laparoscopic approach using any of these methods has been performed successfully.[61]

The characteristics of the SAA also define the manner in which exposure and subsequent aneurysm treatment are carried out. Ruptured aneurysms, patients with previous abdominal surgery and extensive adhesions, or those with severe inflammation from recent pancreatitis may make the operative approach technically challenging. SAAs are usually best approached surgically through the lesser sac with exposure and control of the proximal splenic artery. Patients with rupture and instability because of blood loss may benefit from proximal control of the splenic artery at its takeoff from the celiac trunk, after which evacuation of the contained hematoma in the lesser sac will allow easier dissection and identification of the aneurysm. Pregnancy can complicate surgery further, with the gravid uterus displacing the abdominal viscera superiorly. Cesarean delivery may be required before definitive therapy because the majority of SAAs rupture during the third trimester.

SAA embolization is an alternative endovascular technique for repair with a high reported success rate of 85%.[62] This method may be ideal for patients who are unfavorable candidates for either open or laparoscopic repair. Postembolization risks are real, however, and consist of incomplete aneurysm obliteration, coil migration, end-organ ischemia, and pain from splenic infarction.[63] Recently, stent graft exclusion of SAAs has been reported in carefully selected, high-risk patients who would benefit long-term from spleen salvage.[63-65] Endovascular stent graft placement requires sufficient normal proximal and distal splenic artery anatomy for graft anchoring. Additionally, feeding vessels to the aneurysm sac may not allow for complete endovascular exclusion and thus may contribute to a persistent endoleak.

The results of SAA treatment remain favorable, with low mortality rates in elective patients. Complications after surgery relate specifically to the performance of splenectomy when required. Recurrence after repair is rare and contingent on the technique used. Earlier diagnosis of SAA, continuing improvements in minimally invasive surgery, and endovascular stent graft placement should reduce the number and complexity of emergency aneurysm repairs in the future.

Hepatic Artery Aneurysms

Incidence

Hepatic artery aneurysms (HAAs) have historically been rare, with an incidence of approximately 0.4%.[66] They account for up to 20% of all splanchnic artery aneurysms.[67] The recent application of percutaneous procedures for biliary disease and the increased use of radiologic procedures performed for other reasons have increased the number of identified HAAs. Such aneurysms have the potential for rupture and continue to pose a threat for major hemorrhage and possible death.

Pathogenesis

Multiple different causes are responsible for the development of HAAs. Previously, an infectious cause was largely responsible for the formation of most HAAs. This incidence has decreased significantly, with only 10% presently related to infection, typically as a result of intravenous drug use or endocarditis.[68] Improvements in antimicrobial therapy have most likely also reduced this number. A significant number of HAAs found are false aneurysms, probably related to operative or percutaneous instrumentation and traumatic injury. Systemic inflammatory arterial diseases, infection, pancreatitis, liver transplantation, pregnancy, and portal hypertension have been associated with aneurysm formation. Medial degeneration and arteriosclerosis are factors in a significant number of HAAs.

Approximately 80% of HAAs are extrahepatic, with the common hepatic artery accounting for 63%. The remainder are most often seen to involve the intraparenchymal, right hepatic artery.[68] One third of HAAs are associated with aneurysms of other visceral arteries.[55] Hepatic aneurysms are usually solitary, with multiple aneurysms more frequently seen in patients with inflammatory arteriopathies, such as polyarteritis nodosa. Larger aneurysms tend to be saccular, whereas smaller ones are more fusiform in shape.

Clinical Findings

HAAs are seen twice as frequently in men as women. Both extremes of age are affected; however, patients average between 50 and 60 years of age at diagnosis. Traumatic causes may affect a younger population. Because a larger number of HAAs probably exist without being diagnosed, the majority of aneurysms are asymptomatic. Patients who do report complaints and are later found to have lesions typically have vague, right upper quadrant abdominal pain suggestive of other causes. The extreme manifestation of symptomatic HAA occurs after rupture, where peritonitis and hemodynamic compromise are usually seen. Other less common manifestations include jaundice and biliary colic secondary to extrahepatic biliary compression and obstruction. Aneurysms may also erode or rupture into adjacent organs or biliary ducts and cause massive gastrointestinal hemorrhage and hematobilia. Most often, hematobilia results from rupture of false aneurysms related to trauma. Fever is commonly seen with hematobilia. Physical examination rarely yields specific findings, and abdominal bruits are seldom found. Patients with long-standing fistulas from aneurysm rupture may have signs of chronic anemia. Quincke's triad of jaundice, abdominal pain, and hematobilia is not seen with any regularity.[69]

Diagnosis

Unless ruptured, most HAAs are not correctly diagnosed initially because other factors account for the symptoms and the HAA is an incidental finding. Some radiographic signs may indicate the presence of an HAA. Calcification of the aneurysm sac may be seen on plain films or CT. Compression of adjacent structures, such as bowel lumen or biliary ducts, can also be identified radiographically.

There are no accepted screening tests for HAA. Duplex ultrasonography and CT remain the primary methods of investigation when an aneurysm is suspected. Arteriography will effectively diagnose an HAA, but its role should most often be limited to preoperative evaluation of hepatic artery perfusion and surgical planning.

Treatment

Although aneurysm size has not been definitively correlated with the potential for rupture, HAAs carry the highest risk for rupture (44%) of any visceral aneurysm, and the mortality associated with rupture is greater than 35%.[70,71] Accordingly, aneurysm repair is recommended for all medically fit patients.

Operative planning is aided by arteriography in elective patients. Most importantly, the location of the aneurysm along the hepatic artery determines the approach. A subcostal incision or midline laparotomy is appropriate for most HAAs. Early proximal vascular control of the common hepatic artery should be carried out. Realizing the relationship of the foregut collateral vessels to an extraparenchymal aneurysm allows for determination of the need for revascularization of blood flow to the liver. Aneurysms proximal to the gastroduodenal artery takeoff may be treated by exclusionary ligation on both sides of the aneurysm with or without excision of the aneurysm.[66] An exception to this recommendation is the rare occluded superior mesenteric artery (SMA), which would limit collateral flow through the gastroduodenal artery.[66] HAAs found distal to the gastroduodenal artery involve more careful operative planning. The risk for liver necrosis after proper hepatic artery ligation can be avoided by arterial reconstruction. Arterial revascularization in such circumstances is required. A useful way to test for potential postligation liver ischemia is temporary intraoperative artery occlusion and parenchymal assessment. Multiple strategies to reconstruct the hepatic artery are available and include the use of primary end-to-end anastomosis with an autologous vein interposition graft, splenohepatic or aortohepatic bypass, and prosthetic graft placement.[71-73] Right or left hepatic artery aneurysm repair should be approached in a similar reconstructive manner. If ligation is required, adjunctive cholecystectomy is advocated to avoid postoperative necrosis of the gallbladder. Rarely, partial liver resection may be required to treat HAAs.

Advanced experience with endovascular stent graft placement makes it an attractive option in some patients. Its application may be particularly useful for intrahepatic aneurysms, small aneurysms, hostile abdomens, and patients who cannot tolerate open procedures. Percutaneous transcatheter embolization has also been used successfully in the management of HAAs but carries its own inherent risks, including parenchymal necrosis and hepatic abscess.[74] This option appears less appealing than graft placement.

Superior Mesenteric Artery Aneurysms

Incidence

Superior mesenteric artery aneurysms (SMAAs) are the third most frequent visceral aneurysms, after SAAs and HAAs. Aneurysms of the SMA and its branches have an incidence of less than 0.01%.[75] An increase in the number of reported aneurysms is likely to be seen as routine CT scans are increasingly being performed for a variety of other reasons. SMAAs are important because of their potential for rupture and the risk that they pose to small and large bowel supplied by the SMA.

Pathogenesis

Unlike other aneurysms, trauma and atherosclerosis do not account for the majority of SMAAs. Interestingly, the SMA is associated with an infectious etiology more frequently than any other muscular artery. Historically, an infectious cause was thought to be responsible for up to half of these aneurysms; however, recent reports do not support this high number of mycotic aneurysms. When infection is the underlying cause, *Streptococcus* is most commonly involved and may be related to left-sided bacterial endocarditis. Collagen vascular disorders and systemic syndromes affecting the arterial vasculature may also contribute to SMAA development in selected patients. Atherosclerosis has not been accepted as the primary cause of SMAA development; however, its presence is seen in a number of aneurysms.[76]

Clinical Findings

Similar to other visceral aneurysms, vague, intermittent abdominal pain is the leading complaint in patients found to have an SMAA. Unlike the silent nature of other abdominal aneurysms, SMAAs typically produce symptoms. Oftentimes, the symptoms may be similar to an episode of acute mesenteric ischemia. A pulsatile, mobile, epigastric mass may be found in a significant number of patients. The ability to displace the mass manually helps distinguish it from AAAs. A strong clinical suspicion should be present for patients with this type of manifestation and documented bacterial endocarditis. Ruptured SMAAs will probably cause cardiovascular collapse unless they are temporarily contained. Rupture into gastrointestinal structures does not occur routinely.

Diagnosis

Unlike other visceral aneurysms, calcification of SMAAs is not routinely seen and thus limits the usefulness of plain abdominal radiographs. Cross-sectional imaging is the preferred method of diagnosing these aneurysms, with CT scanning or duplex ultrasound yielding the most accurate results. The role of arteriography is limited to preoperative planning and specific delineation of the celiac artery, inferior mesenteric artery, and surrounding collateral vessels.

Treatment

Operative repair of SMAAs is indicated in all patients because of the significant risk for rupture. Aneurysmorrhaphy and simple ligation are both acceptable surgical approaches. In cases in which appreciable collateral circulation has developed in response to a progressively diseased SMA, ligation proximal and distal to the aneurysm can be performed without enteric blood flow compromise. If, however, sufficient collateral flow has not developed because of stenosis in either the celiac or inferior mesenteric artery, reconstruction should be performed. Autologous vein and prosthetic routes are both acceptable and may be bypassed from the infrarenal or supraceliac aorta. In some cases, concomitant bowel resection may be required despite adequate resection and reconstruction.

Transcatheter embolization may be applied to a select group of patients who are at high risk for complications during open surgical repair. These patients should have excellent collateral flow on arteriography, and postprocedural clinical monitoring for bowel viability is warranted. Limited reports of successful embolization and stent graft placement in high-risk patients are available. There will probably be increased application of these techniques in the future.

Celiac Artery Aneurysms

Incidence

Celiac artery aneurysms (CAAs) are not well studied in the current literature, presumably because of a low overall incidence in the population. A prevalence of 5.9% has been reported, with two thirds of aneurysms found in men.[77] As with other visceral aneurysms, better and more frequent cross-sectional imaging should increase the radiographic identification of asymptomatic patients with CAAs. The importance of a CAA is related to its potential rupture and subsequent risk for death.

Pathogenesis

Unlike SAAs and HAAs, exposure to traumatic injury is uncommon in the development of CAAs. Historically, infection was thought to be a common cause of their development; however, atherosclerosis is currently the most common precursor. Other factors in the development of CAAs may include celiac axis instrumentation and medial degeneration. The frequency of associated aneurysms in other arteries may be as high as 38%.[78]

Clinical Findings

Demographically, CAAs are similar to other visceral artery aneurysms. Most aneurysms are asymptomatic

before diagnosis, but epigastric pain seems to occur in a significant number of patients. Other common findings may include abdominal bruits or pulsatile masses.[79] Previously, a high incidence of CAA rupture was reported; however, a recent reappraisal does not seem to support this finding. Stone et al. reported a 6% rupture rate in a series of 18 patients, which is significantly lower than historical reports.[77] The risk for rupture has not been attributable to known risk factors. When ruptured, CAAs typically have symptoms similar to other visceral aneurysms. Intra-abdominal bleeding with hemodynamic compromise is likely to occur rapidly. The initial manifestation of a CAA may include acute mesenteric ischemia secondary to embolization of a mural thrombus within the aneurysm sac.[80]

Diagnosis

Incidental diagnosis during work-up for other disease most commonly identifies CAAs. Calcifications may be present in a small percentage of CAAs and helps in its diagnosis through plain roentgenographic studies. Ultrasound can also be useful for diagnosis. CT scanning was shown to identify 67% of CAAs in one series and is the preferred noninvasive imaging modality for CAAs.[77] Previously, arteriography was considered essential for work-up; however, its utility is effectively limited to preoperative planning.

Treatment

Not much data are available on which to base management recommendations for asymptomatic CAAs. The risk for rupture is difficult to measure in these patients, with recent reviews yielding a low overall rupture rate. The influence of aneurysm size on rupture is not clearly defined, but a size of 2 cm or greater in diameter has been recommended as a cutoff for operative treatment.[77] However, given the potential for mortality if rupture occurs (up to 40%), patients with CAAs should undergo operative intervention if they are medically fit.[78] A ruptured CAA is handled similar to other visceral aneurysms in the abdomen. Emergency surgery with early ligation of the CAA controls hemorrhage without significant ischemic threat to the liver or bowel. After proximal control is achieved, antegrade bypass revascularization from the aorta to the common hepatic and splenic artery should be attempted if the patient is hemodynamically stable.

Patients eligible for elective aneurysm resection should undergo revascularization. Reconstruction of the celiac trunk may be performed through several techniques. Either aortoceliac bypass after aneurysmectomy or aortohepatic/aortosplenic bypass should be performed. Autologous saphenous vein and prosthetic conduit are reasonable alternatives, especially with a short celiac artery. Some have suggested that prosthetic grafting may have better long-term patency than saphenous vein grafts.[77]

The use of endovascular stent grafts and embolization is currently not well reported. The short length of the celiac artery and acute angulation at its bifurcation may limit the use of stent grafts in the near future for this indication.

Inferior Mesenteric Artery Aneurysms

Inferior mesenteric artery aneurysms are quite rare, and there are no recent reports of an increased incidence in the current literature. They will probably continue to be identified as incidental findings on cross-sectional imaging with CT or arteriography. Symptoms of these aneurysms are similar to those of other visceral aneurysms. Colonic ischemia as a result of embolization or rupture is possible, but rare. Aneurysmectomy with ligation of the inferior mesenteric artery is probably adequate treatment. The relative ease of access to this vessel would appear to make treatment recommended for all identified aneurysms. Future application of transcatheter embolization or stent grafting remains to be seen.

Mesenteric Artery Branch Aneurysms

Gastroduodenal, Pancreaticoduodenal, and Pancreatic Artery Aneurysms

Aneurysms of arteries providing collateral flow between the celiac and superior mesenteric systems are rare. Pancreaticoduodenal artery aneurysms account for only 2% to 3% of all splanchnic artery aneurysms.[81] When present, epidemiologic factors are similar to those for aneurysms found at other sites, including a gender propensity for development in men. The risk for rupture associated with these branch aneurysms is quite high (50% to 80%), and the resultant mortality exceeds 50%.[82,83]

Multiple causes exist for the development of these aneurysms; however, localized inflammation from pancreatitis is the most commonly theorized underlying cause. Pancreatitis is present in up to 60% of patients with gastroduodenal artery aneurysms and 30% of those with pancreaticoduodenal aneurysms.[79] The presence of a pancreatic pseudocyst may contribute to the arteriosclerosis leading to aneurysm formation.

The rarity and asymptomatic or nonspecific symptomatic nature of these aneurysms present a challenge for timely diagnosis and intervention. Most of them are small and nonpalpable. Physical examination alone is therefore rarely of diagnostic value before the aneurysm becomes quite large or has ruptured.[84] When calcified, the diagnosis may be suggested by its presence on an abdominal roentgenogram. Abdominal ultrasonography performed for ill-defined abdominal pain may identify the unsuspected vascular lesion (Fig. 85–3). Similarly, an abdominal CT scan can both identify these mesenteric branch aneurysms and provide an accurate measurement of their size (Fig. 85–4). In other circumstances, the diagnosis is mostly dependent on appropriate clinical suspicion and more objective subsequent evaluation. Mesenteric angiography is the definitive diagnostic modality because it not only confirms the diagnosis but also provides a necessary road map with which an appropriate therapeutic decision can be made. With

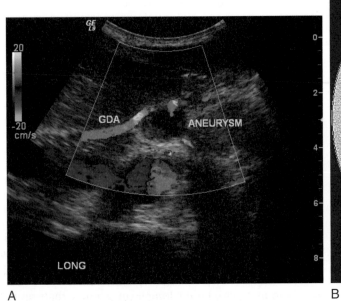
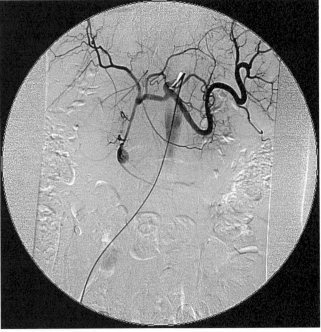

A   B

Figure 85–3. **A,** A longitudinal abdominal color duplex ultrasound demonstrates an aneurysm of the gastroduodenal artery (GDA) and an echogenic thrombus within it. **B,** Selective angiography of the celiac trunk shows the aneurysm with retained contrast in the distal portion of the gastroduodenal artery.

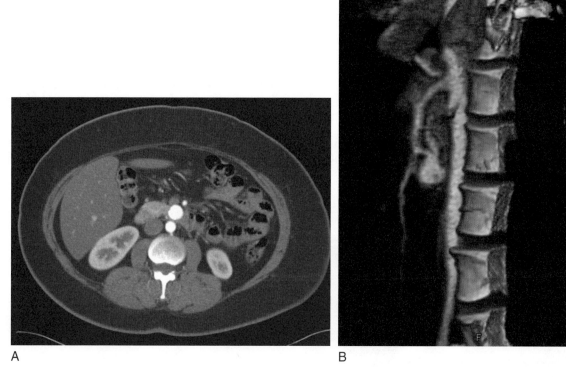

Figure 85–4. **A,** An abdominal computed tomography (CT) scan of the midabdomen with intravenous contrast identifies an aneurysm of the inferior pancreaticoduodenal artery lying between the underlying aorta and the smaller superior mesenteric artery above it. **B,** A sagittal three-dimensional reconstruction CT angiogram illustrates the inferior pancreaticoduodenal artery aneurysm arising posterior to the superior mesenteric artery.

improvements in technology, magnetic resonance angiography is also a useful noninvasive alternative to arteriography. Patients with hypotension and an evident surgical abdomen may require surgical intervention without the opportunity for a definitive preoperative diagnostic evaluation.

Most aneurysms are associated with nonspecific symptoms before the final correct diagnosis is made. Epigastric pain is the most common complaint, and it may initially appear clinically as pancreatitis. Rupture occurs with hemorrhage typically into the stomach or duodenum. Intra-abdominal cavity rupture is unusual. Rarely, obstructive jaundice may result from compression of the biliary ductal system by the expanding aneurysm. Preoperative diagnosis is rarely correctly made without a high index of suspicion. Typically, this group of ruptured aneurysms is identified at laparotomy for refractory gastrointestinal hemorrhage.

As with most visceral aneurysms, intervention is indicated when the risk for rupture and exsanguinating hemorrhage is thought to be greater than the potential risks associated with surgical or other interventional procedures. The risk for rupture of aneurysms is believed to be proportional to the size of the aneurysm.[81] Interestingly, Neville et al. found that 37% of ruptured pancreaticoduodenal aneurysms were less than 1.0 cm and there were no differences in size between ruptured and

unruptured aneurysms.[85] Once such an aneurysm is diagnosed, surgical excision with or without vascular reconstruction or embolization is recommended because of the unpredictability of rupture of these aneurysms. Surgical excision is the treatment of choice. Surgical treatment of this group of aneurysms may be more difficult, however, because of the enteric erosion found in most cases and their location within the parenchyma of structures such as the pancreas. Additionally, the presence of pancreatic pathology, including pseudocysts, must be addressed at the time of surgery. A Kocher maneuver will usually be necessary for adequate exposure to ligate the aneurysm. Dissection of the aneurysm sac may be tedious and hazardous in the presence of pancreatitis. In such a situation, ligation of the feeding vessels to the aneurysm sac should suffice as treatment. In only rare cases will pancreatic resection be required. Surgical resection with revascularization is recommended in patients with significant celiac axis occlusion in order to prevent intestinal ischemia and death. If celiac or superior mesenteric artery stenosis is not an issue or if the collateral circulation is adequate, excision or ligation without vascular repair would be appropriate and is less technically demanding.

Transcatheter embolization can be used in unstable patients, those with high operative risk because of comorbid conditions, and those with unfavorable anatomy. The presence of significant collateral circulation in this region may contribute to ineffective treatment with resultant rebleeding or rupture. The use of endovascular stent occlusion with embolization and thrombin injection has also been reported to be successful for these aneurysms.[86] Additional studies are needed to assess outcomes with these techniques.

Gastric and Gastroepiploic Artery Aneurysms

Aneurysms of these branch vessels occur with similar rarity as other branch aneurysms. Their origins may be related to a variety of initiating events, and no single cause is identified. Trauma, infection, congenital predisposition, medial degeneration, and other causes are plausible for their development.

Typical symptoms include epigastric pain and gastrointestinal complaints related to irritation or compression. Intraluminal rupture of an aneurysm may result in profound hematemesis in a significant number of patients.[87] Up to 30% of patients may have an abdominal rupture requiring laparotomy for control of bleeding.[88] Significant mortality is associated with rupture of these branch aneurysms.[83] Operative treatment includes ligation of the involved vessel and the aneurysm when technically possible. Aneurysms within the wall of the stomach may require partial gastric resection.

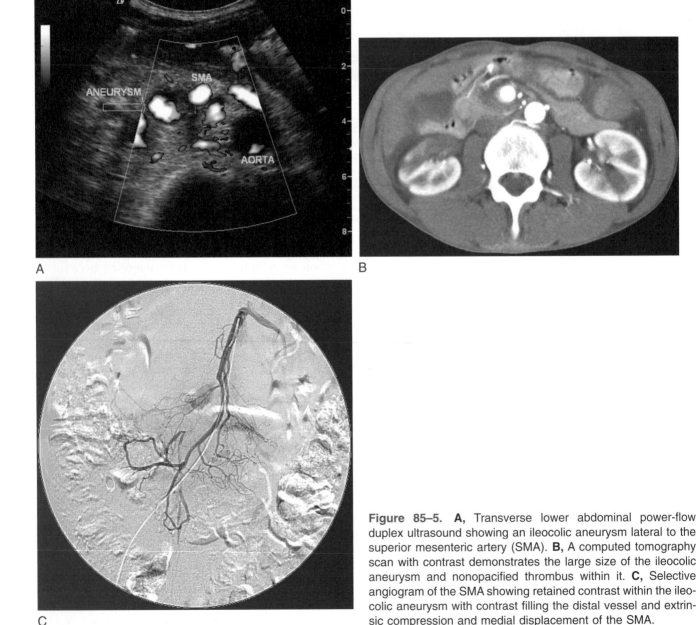

Figure 85–5. **A,** Transverse lower abdominal power-flow duplex ultrasound showing an ileocolic aneurysm lateral to the superior mesenteric artery (SMA). **B,** A computed tomography scan with contrast demonstrates the large size of the ileocolic aneurysm and nonopacified thrombus within it. **C,** Selective angiogram of the SMA showing retained contrast within the ileocolic aneurysm with contrast filling the distal vessel and extrinsic compression and medial displacement of the SMA.

Jejunal, Ileal, and Colic Artery Aneurysms

This group of aneurysms is rare and typically seen as small, solitary lesions. Multiple lesions in a single patient may be found with systemic vasculitides, including polyarteritis nodosa.[89] There remains no single cause for the presence of these lesions, and congenital as well as degenerative arterial disease probably contributes to their progression. Most aneurysms remain relatively silent clinically and may be found initially at surgery for other disease. As with other aneurysms, cross-sectional imaging, including CT, duplex ultrasonography, and arteriography, can help in the diagnosis (Fig. 85–5). Arteriography may be particularly important in identifying the presence of multiple aneurysms before treatment. Rupture is difficult to predict; however, aneurysms of colic arteries are thought to rupture more commonly than those associated with the small bowel.[90,91]

REFERENCES

1. Voorhoeve R, Moll FL, de Letter JAM, et al: Primary aortoenteric fistula: Report of eight new cases and review of the literature. Ann Vasc Surg 10:40-48, 1996.
2. Busuttil SJ, Goldstone J: Diagnosis and management of aortoenteric fistulas. Semin Vasc Surg 14:302-311, 2001.
3. Barry PA, Molland JG, Falk GL: Primary aortoduodenal fistula. Aust N Z J Surg 68:243-244, 1998.
4. Kuestner LM, Reilly LM, Jicha DL, et al: Secondary aortoenteric fistula: Contemporary outcome with use of extraanatomic bypass and infected graft excision. J Vasc Surg 21:184-196, 1995.
5. Kahle V, Brossmann J, Klomp HJ: Lethal hemorrhage caused by aortoenteric fistula following endovascular stent implantation. Cardiovasc Intervent Radiol 25:205-207, 2002.
6. Hansen KS, Sheley RC: Aortoenteric fistula in advanced germ cell tumor: A rare lethal complication. J Urol 167:2131, 2002.
7. Moore RD, Tittley JG: Laparoscopic aortic injury leading to delayed aortoenteric fistula: An alternative technique for repair. Ann Vasc Surg 13:586-588, 1999.
8. Pipinos II, Carr JA, Haithcock BE, et al: Secondary aortoenteric fistula. Ann Vasc Surg 14:688-696, 2000.
9. Menawat SS, Gloviczki P, Serry RD, et al: Management of aortic graft-enteric fistulae. Eur J Vasc Endovasc Surg 14(Suppl A):74-81, 1997.
10. Ouriel K, Ricotta JJ, Adams JT, Deweese JA: Management of cholelithiasis in patients with abdominal aortic aneurysms. Ann Surg 198:717-719, 1983.
11. Montgomery RS, Wilson SE: The surgical management of aortoenteric fistulas. Surg Clin North Am 76:1147-1157, 1996.
12. Antinori CH, Andrew CT, Santaspirt JS, et al: The many faces of aortoenteric fistulas. Am Surg 62:344-349, 1996.
13. Tareen AH, Schroeder TV: Primary aortoenteric fistula: Two new case reports and a review of 44 previously reported cases. Eur J Vasc Surg 12:5-10, 1996.
14. Sweeny MS, Gadacz TR: Primary aortoduodenal fistula: Management, diagnosis, and treatment. Surgery 96:492-497, 1984.
15. Pabst TS 3rd, Bernhard VM, McIntyre KE Jr, Malone JM: Gastrointestinal bleeding after aortic surgery. The role of laparotomy to rule out aortoenteric fistula. J Vasc Surg 8:280-285, 1988.
16. Mirarchi FL, Scheatzle MD, Mitre RJ: Primary aortoenteric fistula in the emergency department. J Emerg Med 20:25-27, 2001.
17. Embil JM, Koulack J, Greenberg H: Aortoenteric fistula. Am J Surg 182:75-76, 2001.
18. Lawlor DK, DeRose G, Harris KA, Forbes TL: Primary aorto/iliac-enteric fistula: Report of 6 new cases. Vasc Endovasc Surg 38:281-286, 2004.
19. Low RN, Wall SD, Jeffrey RB Jr, et al: Aortoenteric fistula and perigraft infection: Evaluation with CT. Radiology 175:157-162, 1990.
20. Perks FJ, Gillespie I, Patel D: Multidetector computed tomography imaging of aortoenteric fistula. J Comput Assist Tomogr 28:343-347, 2004.
21. Peirce RM, Jenkins RH, MacEneaney P: Paraprosthetic extravasation of enteric contrast: A rare and direct sign of secondary aortoenteric fistula. AJR Am J Roentgenol 184:S73-S74, 2005.
22. Lemos DW, Raffetto JD, Moore C, Menzoian JO: Primary aortoduodenal fistula: A case report and review of the literature. J Vasc Surg 37:686-689, 2003.
23. O'Mara CS, Williams GM, Ernst CB: Secondary aortoenteric fistula: A 20 year experience. Am J Surg 142:203-209, 1981.
24. Ganatra RH, Haniffa MA, Hawthorne AB, Rees JIS: Aortoenteric fistula complicating an infected aortic graft. Clin Nucl Med 26:800-801, 2001.
25. Thomson S: Aortoenteric fistula. J R Soc Med 92:440, 1999.
26. Krupnick AS, Lombardi JV, Engels FH, et al: 18-Fluorodeoxyglucose position emission tomography as a novel imaging tool for the diagnosis of aortoenteric fistula and aortic graft infection. Vasc Endovasc Surg 37:363-366, 2003.
27. Trout HH III, Kozloff L, Giordano JM: Priority of revascularization in patients with graft enteric fistulas, infected arteries, or infected arterial prostheses. Ann Surg 199:669-683, 1984.
28. Clagett GP, Bowers BL, Lopez-Viego MA, et al: Creation of a neo-aortoiliac system from lower extremity deep and superficial veins. Ann Surg 210:239-248, discussion 248-249, 1993.
29. England DW, Simms MH: Recurrent aorto-duodenal fistula: A final solution? Eur J Vasc Surg 4:427-429, 1990.
30. van Baalen JM, Kluit AB, Maas J, et al: Diagnosis and therapy of aortic prosthetic fistulas: Trends over a 30-year experience. Br J Surg 83:1729-1734, 1996.
31. Vogt PR, Pfammatter T, Schlumpf R, et al: In situ repair of aortobronchial, aortoesophageal, and aortoenteric fistulae with cryopreserved aortic homografts. J Vasc Surg 26:11-17, 1997.
32. Young RM, Cherry KJ, Davis PM, et al: The results of in situ prosthetic replacement for infected aortic grafts. Am J Surg 178:136-140, 1999.
33. Nasim A, Hayes P, London N, et al: In situ replacement of infected aortic grafts with rifampin-bonded prostheses. Br J Surg 86:690-711, 1999.
34. Hayes PD, Nasim A, London NJM, et al: In situ replacement of infected aortic grafts with rifampin-bonded prostheses: The Leicester experience (1992 to 1998). J Vasc Surg 30:92-98, 1999.
35. Abou-Zamzam AM, Bianchi C, Mazraany W, et al: Aortoenteric fistula development following endovascular abdominal aortic aneurysm repair: A case report. Ann Vasc Surg 17:119-122, 2003.
36. d'Othee BJ, Soula P, Otal P, et al: Aortoduodenal fistula after endovascular stent graft of an abdominal aortic aneurysm. J Vasc Surg 31:190-195, 2001.
37. Parry DJ, Waterworth A, Kessel D, et al: Endovascular repair of an inflammatory abdominal aortic aneurysm complicated by aortoduodenal fistulation with an unusual presentation. J Vasc Surg 33:874-879, 2001.
38. Schwab W, McMahon DJ, Phillips G, Pentecost MJ: Aortic balloon control of a traumatic aortoenteric fistula after damage control laparotomy: A case report. J Trauma 40:1021-1023, 1996.
39. Loftus IM, Thompson MM, Fishwick G, et al: Technique for rapid control of bleeding from an aortoenteric fistula. Br J Surg 84:1114, 1997.
40. Karkos CD, Vlachou PA, Hayes PD, et al: Temporary endovascular control of a bleeding aortoenteric fistula by transcatheter coil embolization. J Vasc Interv Radiol 16:867-871, 2005.
41. Deshpande A, Lovelock M, Mossop P, et al: Endovascular repair of an aortoenteric fistula in a high-risk patient. J Endovasc Surg 6:379-384, 1999.
42. Eskandari MK, Makaroun MS, Abu-Elmagd KM, Billar TR: Endovascular repair of an aortoduodenal fistula. J Endovasc Ther 7:328-332, 2000.
43. Schlensak C, Doenst T, Spillner G, et al: Palliative treatment of a secondary aortoduodenal fistula by stent-graft placement. Thorac Cardiovasc Surg 48:41-42, 2000.
44. Chuter TAM, Lukaszeicz GC, Reilly LM, et al: Endovascular repair of a presumed aortoenteric fistula: Late failure due to recurrent infection. J Endovasc Ther 7:240-244, 2000.
45. Burks JA, Faries PL, Gravereaux EC, et al: Endovascular repair of bleeding aortoenteric fistulas: A 5-year experience. J Vasc Surg 34:1055-1059, 2001.

46. Mok VWK, Ting ACW, Law S, et al: Combined endovascular stent grafting and endoscopic injection of fibrin sealant for aortoenteric fistula complicating esophagectomy. J Vasc Surg 40:1234-1237, 2004.

47. Finch L, Heathcock RB, Quigley T, et al: Emergent treatment of a primary aortoenteric fistula with N-butyl 2-cyanoacrylate and endovascular stent. J Vasc Interv Radiol 13:841-843, 2002.

48. Gonzalez-Fajardo JA, Gutierrez V, Martin-Pedrosa M, et al: Endovascular repair in the presence of aortic infection. Ann Vasc Surg 19:94-98, 2005.

49. Allen RC, Sebastian MG: The role of endovascular techniques in aortoesophageal fistula repair. J Endovasc Surg 8:602-603, 2001.

50. Bunt TJ: Synthetic vascular graft infections: II. Graft-enteric erosions and graft-enteric fistulas. Surgery 94:1-9, 1983.

51. Moore SW, Guida PM, Schumacher HW: Splenic artery aneurysm. Bull Soc Int Chir 29:210-218, 1970.

52. Bedford PD, Lodge B: Aneurysm of the splenic artery. Gut 1:312-320, 1960.

53. Hallett JW: Splenic artery aneurysms. Semin Vasc Surg 8:321-326, 1995.

54. Stanley JC, Fry WJ: Pathogenesis and clinical significance of splenic artery aneurysms. Surgery 76:898-909, 1974.

55. Abbas MA, Stone WM, Fowl RJ, et al: Splenic artery aneurysms: Two decades experience at Mayo Clinic. Ann Vasc Surg 16:442-449, 2002.

56. Bergner LH, Bentivegna SS: Aneurysm of the splenic artery. Ann Surg 166:767-772, 1967.

57. Stanley JC, Gewertz BL, Bove EL, et al: Arterial fibrodysplasia: Histopathologic character and current etiologic concepts. Arch Surg 110:561-566, 1975.

58. Mattar SG, Lumsden AB: The management of splenic artery aneurysm: Experience with 23 cases. Am J Surg 169:580-584, 1995.

59. Carr JA, Cho J-S, Shepard AD, et al: Visceral pseudoaneurysms due to pancreatic pseudocysts: Rare but lethal complications of pancreatitis. J Vasc Surg 32:722-730, 2000.

60. Angelakis EJ, Bair WE, Barone JE, Lincer RM: Splenic artery aneurysm during pregnancy. Obstet Gynecol Surg 48:145-148, 1993.

61. de Csepel J, Quinn T, Gagner M: Laparoscopic exclusion of a splenic artery aneurysm using a lateral approach permits preservation of the spleen. Surg Laparosc Endosc Percutan Tech 11:221-224, 2001.

62. McDermott VG, Shlansky-Goldberg R, Cope C: Endovascular management of splenic artery aneurysms and pseudoaneurysms. Cardiovasc Intervent Radiol 17:179-184, 1994.

63. Larson RA, Solomon J, Carpenter JP: Stent graft repair of visceral artery aneurysms. J Vasc Surg 36:1260-1263, 2002.

64. Saltzberg SS, Maldonado TS, Laparello PJ, et al: Is endovascular therapy the preferred treatment for all visceral artery aneurysms. Ann Vasc Surg 19:1-9, 2005.

65. Arepally A, Dagli M, Hofmann LV, et al: Treatment of splenic artery aneurysm with use of stent-graft. J Vasc Interv Radiol 13:631-633, 2002.

66. Arneson MA, Smith RS: Ruptured hepatic artery aneurysm: Case report and review of literature. Ann Vasc Surg 19:1-6, 2005.

67. Lumsden AB, Mattar SG, Allen RC, Bacha EA: Hepatic artery aneurysms: The management of 22 patients. J Surg Res 60:345-350, 1996.

68. Schroeyers P, Lismonde M, Vermonden J, Six C: Management of hepatic artery aneurysm. Case report and literature review. Acta Chir Belg 95:89-91, 1995.

69. Ibach EG, O'Halloran MJ, Prendergast FJ: Hepatic artery aneurysm: Two case reports and review of the literature. Aust N Z J Surg 67:143-147, 1997.

70. Busuttil RW, Brin BJ: The diagnosis and management of visceral artery aneurysms. Surgery 88:619-624, 1980.

71. Zachary K, Geier S, Pellecchia C, Irwin G: Jaundice secondary to hepatic artery aneurysm: Radiologic appearance and clinical features. Am J Gastroenterol 81:295-298, 1986.

72. Salo JA, Salmenkivi K, Tenhunen A, Kivilaakso EO: Rupture of splanchnic artery aneurysms. World J Surg 10:123-127, 1986.

73. Psathakis D, Muller G, Noah M, et al: Present management of hepatic artery aneurysms. Symptomatic left hepatic artery aneurysm; right hepatic artery aneurysm with erosion into the gallbladder and simultaneous colocholecystic fistula—a report of two unusual cases and the current state of etiology, diagnosis, histology, and treatment. Vasa 21:210-215, 1992.

74. Messina LM, Shanley CJ: Visceral artery aneurysms. Surg Clin North Am 77:425-442, 1997.

75. Grech P, Rowlands P, Crofton M: Aneurysm of the inferior pancreaticoduodenal artery diagnosed by real-time ultrasound and pulsed Doppler. Br J Radiol 62:753-755, 1989.

76. Stone WM, Abbas MA, Cherry KJ, et al: Superior mesenteric artery aneurysms: Is presence an indication for intervention? J Vasc Surg 36:234-237, 2002.

77. Stone WM, Abbas MA, Glovicki P, et al: Celiac arterial aneurysms: A critical reappraisal of a rare entity. Arch Surg 137:670-674, 2002.

78. Graham LM, Stanley JC, Whithouse WM Jr, et al: Coeliac artery aneurysms: Historic (1745-1949) versus contemporary (1950-1984) differences in etiology and clinical importance. J Vasc Surg 2:757-764, 1985.

79. Eckhauser FE, Stanley JC, Zelenock GB, et al: Gastroduodenal and pancreaticoduodenal artery aneurysms: A complication of pancreatitis causing spontaneous gastrointestinal hemorrhage. Surgery 88:335-344, 1980.

80. Carr SC, Mahvi DM, Hoch JR, et al: Visceral artery aneurysm rupture. J Vasc Surg 33:806-811, 2001.

81. Iyomasa S, Matsuzaki Y, Hiei K, et al: Pancreaticoduodenal artery aneurysm: A case report and review of the literature. J Vasc Surg 22:161-166, 1995.

82. Schlefan M, Kadir S, Athanasoulis CA, Hedberg SE: Pancreaticoduodenal artery aneurysm simulating carcinoma of the head of the pancreas. Arch Surg 112:1201-1203, 1977.

83. Stanley JC, Thompson NW, Fry WJ: Splanchnic artery aneurysms. Arch Surg 101:689-697, 1970.

84. Chiou AC, Josephs LG, Menzoian JO: Inferior pancreaticoduodenal artery aneurysm: Report of a case and review of the literature. J Vasc Surg 17:784-789, 1993.

85. Neville P, Garces D, Martinez R, Castellani L: Rupture of pancreaticoduodenal artery aneurysm in duodenum. Report of a case. J Cardiovasc Surg (Torino) 35:537-539, 1994.

86. Nyman U, Svendsen P, Jivegard L, et al: Multiple pancreaticoduodenal aneurysms: Treatment with superior mesenteric artery stent–graft placement and distal embolization. J Vasc Interv Radiol 11:1201-1205, 2000.

87. Mandelbaum I, Kaiser GD, Lempke RE: Gastric intramural aneurysm as a cause for massive gastrointestinal hemorrhage. Ann Surg 155:199-203, 1962.

88. Thomford NR, Yurko JE, Smith EJ: Aneurysm of gastric arteries as a cause of intraperitoneal hemorrhage: Review of literature. Ann Surg 168:294-297, 1968.

89. Sellke FM, William GB, Donovan DL, Clarke RE: Management of intra-abdominal aneurysms associated with periarteritis nodosa. J Vasc Surg 4:294-298, 1986.

90. Diettrich NA, Cacioppo JC, Ying DPW: Massive gastrointestinal hemorrhage caused by rupture of a jejunal branch artery aneurysm. J Vasc Surg 8:187-189, 1988.

91. Tessier DJ, Abbas MA, Fowl RJ, et al: Management of rare mesenteric arterial branch aneurysms. Ann Vasc Surg 16:586-590, 2002.

Index

Note: Page numbers followed by b refer to boxed material; those followed by f refer to figures; those followed by t refer to tables.

A

Abdomen
  anatomy of, 16
  "frozen," 1148
  hostile, 1147–1148, 1148b
Abdominal abscesses, percutaneous
  drainage of, duodenal perforation due
  to, 1095
Abdominal aortic surgery, colonic ischemia
  complicating, management of, 2006,
  2008f, 2008–2009, 2009f
Abdominal distention
  differential diagnosis of, 1884
  in small bowel obstruction, 1028
Abdominal examination, for small bowel
  obstruction, 1028
Abdominal exploration, in Crohn's disease,
  1057–1058, 1058f
Abdominal incisions, for Crohn's disease,
  1056–1057, 1057f
Abdominal masses, in appendicitis, 2142
Abdominal pain
  in appendicitis, 2141–2142
  in Crohn's disease, 1045
  differential diagnosis of, 1884
  in mesenteric ischemia, chronic,
    1257
  with pancreatic pseudocysts, 1330
  in pancreatitis, chronic, 1344–1345
  in small bowel obstruction, 1028
Abdominal plain films
  with colon, rectal, and anal disorders,
    1891
  in colonic volvulus, 1981
  in duodenal injury, 765
  with hepatic abscesses
    amebic, 1654
    pyogenic, 1646
  in mesenteric ischemia, 1252
  in mesenteric venous thrombosis, 1256
  of obturator hernias, 693, 694f
  in small bowel obstruction, 1029, 1029f
  in small bowel volvulus, 1036
  in small intestinal atresia, 1219, 1221f
Abdominal trauma, in pediatric patients,
  evaluation of, 1806–1808, 1807f, 1808t,
  1809f, 1810f, 1811t
Abdominal wall
  abnormalities of, with gastrointestinal
    fistulas, 1098
  anterior, anatomy of, 636–640, 640f

Abdominal wall *(Continued)*
    of muscles, ligaments, and
      aponeurosis, 636–639, 637f–639f
    of skin, fascia, vessels, and nerves,
      636
  innervation of, 641–642
  vasculature of, 642, 642f
Abdominoperineal approach, for
  retrorectal tumors, 2307–2309, 2308f
Abdominoperineal resection, of rectum.
  See Rectum, abdominoperineal resection
  of.
Abhandlung von den Bruchen (Richter), 632
Ablative therapies
  cryoablation as
    for Barrett's esophagus, 371
    hepatic, external biliary fistulas
      following, etiology and
      prevention of, 1540
    for hepatocellular carcinoma, 1738
    for metastatic colorectal cancer, 2283
  laser, for Barrett's esophagus, 370–371
  radiofrequency
    circumferential balloon-based, for
      Barrett's esophagus, 367–370,
      368f, 369f
    for hepatocellular carcinoma,
      1737–1738, 1738
    transarterial, hepatic abscesses
      following, pyogenic, 1642
Abscesses
  abdominal, percutaneous drainage of,
    duodenal perforation due to,
    1095
  anastomotic cuff, following ileal pouch–
    anal anastomosis, 2111
  anorectal. *See* Anorectal abscesses.
  in Crohn's disease, 1065
  hepatic. *See* Liver abscesses.
  intra-abdominal
    with appendicitis, 2150
    following ileal pouch–anal
      anastomosis, 2111
    management of, 1101–1103, 1103f,
      1104f
  liver. *See* Liver abscesses.
  pancreatic, 1329
    definition of, 1296
    with pancreatic pseudocysts,
      1342–1343, 1343f
    with trauma, 1405
  pelvic, with appendicitis, 2150

Abscesses *(Continued)*
  perianal, in Crohn's disease, surgical
    treatment of, 2135, 2136f
  periappendiceal, 2148–2149
  pericolic, in colonic diverticular disease,
    2016–2017
  pilonidal. *See* Pilonidal disease.
  splenic, 1818–1820
    characteristics of, 1819
    diagnosis of, 1818, 1819f
    image-guided interventional therapy
      for, 1795, 1795f
    management of, 1820
    presenting signs and symptoms of,
      1818
    splenectomy for, 1833
  subphrenic, with appendicitis, 2150
Absorption
  duodenal, 978–980
    of calcium, 979
    of iron, 979–980, 980f
  of energy, in ultrasonography, 111
  enteral, of nutrients, maximizing in
    short-bowel syndrome, 1165–1166,
    1166b
  by gallbladder, 1456, 1457f, 1458
  small intestinal. *See* Small intestinal
    epithelium, digestion and absorption
    and.
Acarbose, for dumping syndrome, 871
Accessory hemiazygos vein, 22
Acetaminophen
  fulminant liver failure due to,
    1703
  hepatotoxicity of, 1720
Acetic acid, for hepatocellular carcinoma,
  1738
Achalasia, 405–409, 411–417
  Chagas' disease and, 406–407
  classic, imaging in, 71–72, 72f
  clinical features of, 407
  complications of, 409
  cricopharyngeal, 427. *See also* Zenker's
    diverticulum.
  diagnosis of, 407, 408f, 408t, 411–412,
    412f
  dilation therapy for, esophageal
    perforation following, 538
  early (mild), imaging in, 72
  endoscopic ultrasonography in, 124–125
  epidemiology of, 405, 406f
  esophageal carcinoma and, 466

Index

Achalasia *(Continued)*
esophageal replacement for, 294f, 294–296, 295f
esophagomyotomy for, complications of, 619–620
Heller myotomy with, 416
historical background of, 411
imaging in, 71–74, 72f
medical therapy for, 412
botulinum toxin for, 412
pharmacologic, 412
pneumatic dilatation for, 412
pathogenesis of, 136, 405–407, 406f
secondary, 407–409
radiographic appearance of, 76, 77f
surgical therapy for, 413–417. *See also* Heller myotomy, laparoscopic.
early development of, 5
vigorous, imaging in, 72, 73f
Acid ingestion, gastric injury due to, 762
Acid perfusion test, esophageal, 164, 165t
for esophageal motility disorders, 159–160
Acid reflux test, standard, 164, 165t
Acid secretion, basal, in esophageal disease, 195
Acidosis, metabolic, in short-bowel syndrome, 1166
Acinar cell(s), 1291, 1291f
injury of, 1296–1297
Acinar cell carcinoma, 1432, 1433f, 1434
Acoustic impedance, in ultrasonography, 111
Acquired immunodeficiency syndrome. *See also* Human immunodeficiency virus infection.
anal fissures in, 2038
immunosuppression due to, 2376–2377
surgical risk assessment in, 2380–2381
Acute Physiology and Chronic Health Evaluation-II scoring system, for pancreatitis, acute, 1300, 1301b, 1302
Adalimumab
for inflammatory bowel disease, 2093
mechanism of action of, 2377t
Adenocarcinoma. *See specific site, e.g.* Esophageal adenocarcinoma.
Adenoma(s)
bile duct, 1526, 1729
flat
gastric, 885
small intestinal, in hereditary flat adenoma syndrome polyposis, 894t, 896
gastric, 884
hepatic, 1729
diagnosis of, 1729, 1730f
drug-induced, 1723
etiology of, 1729
treatment of, 1729, 1730f
pancreatic. *See* Mucinous cystic neoplasms, pancreatic; Serous cystic neoplasms, pancreatic.
papillary, gastric, 885
tubular, small intestinal, 891–892
villous, small intestinal, 892–893
Adenoma-carcinoma cascade, 2183
Adenomatosis, 1729

Adenomatous polyps
colorectal. *See* Colorectal polyps, adenomatous.
endoscopic appearance of, 740, 741f
Adenomyomas, gastric, 884
Adhesiolysis, for small bowel obstruction, open vs. laparoscopic, 1032–1033
Adhesions
with laparoscopic surgery, 1135
lysis of
with hostile abdomen, 1148
with ventral herniorrhaphy, 681
prevention of, 1033
reoperative surgery and, 1135
small bowel obstruction due to, 1027
Advancement flaps
for anal stenosis, 2063, 2063f
anorectal, for anorectal fistulas, 2056, 2056f
mucosal, for anal stenosis, 2063
sleeve, for rectovaginal fistulas, 1951, 1951f
Y-V, for anal stenosis, 2063, 2063f
Aerophagia, partial fundoplication for, 279
Afferent loop obstruction
following gastrectomy, 809, 877–879, 879f
reoperative surgery for, 1147
Age. *See also* Elderly people; Pediatric patients.
Barrett's esophagus and, 342
drug-induced liver disease and, 1717
esophageal cancer and, 442, 442f
ileal pouch–anal anastomosis outcome and, 2118
AIDS. *See also* Human immunodeficiency virus infection.
anal fissures in, 2038
immunosuppression due to, 2376–2377
surgical risk assessment in, 2380–2381
Alagille's syndrome, 1546
diagnosis of, 1546
Alanine aminotransferase, elevated, 1611b, 1611–1612
Albumin, elevated, patient approach for, 1615–1616
Alcohol ingestion
abuse and
esophageal motility disorders in, 140
pancreatitis and, acute, 1298
esophageal cancer and, 444, 466
pruritus ani associated with, 2069
Alcohol sclerotherapy
for esophageal cancer, 488, 489t
for hepatocellular carcinoma, 1737
Alcoholic liver disease
end-stage liver disease due to, 1687
hepatic laboratory tests in, 1612
Alemtuzumab, for islet transplantation, 1428
Alfa-fetoprotein, in hepatocellular carcinoma, 1734
Alkaline phosphatase, elevated, patient approach for, 1614–1615
Alkaline reflux gastritis. *See* Bile reflux gastritis.
Alkalosis, metabolic, in short-bowel syndrome, 1166

Allergic dermatitis, pruritus ani associated with, 2069
Allis forceps, 633
Allison, Phillip, 5, 6
Allison repair, 228
Allison's membrane. *See* Phrenoesophageal membrane.
AlloDerm, for ventral herniorrhaphy, 676
Altemeier procedure, for rectal prolapse, 1962, 1964t
Amanita mushrooms, hepatotoxicity of, 1720
Amebiasis. *See* Liver abscesses, amebic.
Amifostine, for radiation enteritis prevention, 1155
Amiloride, for ascites, 1764
5-Aminosalicylates, for Crohn's disease, 1052, 1053
Amiodarone, hepatotoxicity of, 1720
Amoxicillin
hepatotoxicity of, 1723
for lymphoma, 1209t
Ampullary balloon dilation, 1484–1485, 1485f
Amrinone, mesenteric blood flow and, 1243t
Amsterdam Criteria, for hereditary nonpolyposis colorectal cancer, 2171, 2171b, 2188
Amsterdam Criteria II, for hereditary nonpolyposis colorectal cancer, 2171, 2171b
Amylase, serum
in pancreatic trauma, 1401
in pancreatitis, 1299, 1300b
Amyloidosis
esophageal motility disorders in, 140
splenectomy for, 1835
Anabolic steroids, hepatotoxicity of, 1723
Anal adenocarcinoma, 2296
Anal anastomosis, colopouch, for rectal radiation injury, 2324
Anal canal
lesions of, in Crohn's disease, 2088
neoplasms of, 1912–1913, 1913f, 1913t
ultrasound of. *See* Endoanal ultrasound.
Anal carcinoma
adenocarcinoma as, 2296
squamous cell, 2291–2294
clinical features of, 2291
physical examination of, 2291
staging of, 2291, 2292f
therapy of, 2291–2294
combined chemotherapy and radiation therapy for, 2292–2293, 2293t
salvage surgery as, 2293–2294, 2294f
surgical, primary, 2291–2292
Anal disorders
diagnosis of, 1883–1897
examination for, 1885–1888
with anorectal pain or swelling, 1887
for bleeding, 1887
for constipation, 1888
general principles of, 1885–1886

Anal disorders (Continued)
inspection and palpation in,
1886–1887
positioning for, 1886, 1886f
for urgency and incontinence,
1888
history in, 1883
investigation for, 1888–1897
blood and stool testing in,
1888–1889
endoscopy in, 1889f, 1889–1891,
1890f
radiologic tests in, 1891f,
1891–1897, 1892f, 1894f–1897f
symptoms in, 1883–1885
abdominal pain and distention
as, 1884
anorectal pain, itching and
swelling as, 1884
bleeding as, 1883–1884
constipation as, 1884–1885
diarrhea as, 1885
urgency and incontinence as,
1885
ultrasound in. See Endoanal ultrasound.
Anal encirclement, 1923
for rectal prolapse, 1964f, 1964t,
1964–1965
Anal fissures, 2038–2043, 2039f
diagnosis of, 2039, 2039f
etiology of, 2038–2039
examination for, 1887
nonsurgical management of, 2039–2040
botulinum toxin for, 2040
calcium-channel blockers for, 2040
general approaches for, 2039–2040
topical nitroglycerin for, 2040
surgical treatment of, 2041, 2041f,
2042f, 2042t
treatment algorithm for, 2042f, 2043
Anal fistulas
chronic, malignant transformation in,
2058
classification of, 2045, 2047f, 2048t
in Crohn's disease, 2057–2058, 2088
diagnosis of, 2049–2051
colonoscopy in, 2049
computed tomography in, 2051
fistulography in, 2049
fistuloscopy in, 2051
history in, 2049
magnetic resonance imaging in, 2051
manometry in, 2051
physical examination in, 2049, 2050f
sigmoidoscopy in, 2049
ultrasonography in, 2049–2051,
2050f–2052f
endoanal ultrasound in, 1911–1912,
1912f
etiology of, 2045
in infancy, 2058
recurrent, 2057
treatment of
anorectal advancement flaps for,
2056, 2056f
complications of, 2057
fibrin glue for, 2056–2057
fistulotomy for, 2055

Anal fistulas (Continued)
postoperative care for, 2057
seton management for, 2055f,
2055–2056
Anal infections, in immunocompromised
patients, 2383, 2383t
Anal neoplasms, 2288–2296
adenocarcinoma as, 2296
anal intraepithelial neoplasia as,
2289–2291, 2290f
anatomy and, 2288
basal cell carcinoma as, 2295–2296
histology of, 2288–2289
in immunocompromised patients, 2384
incidence of, 2289
inguinal and pelvic lymph node
metastasis and, 2294, 2295f
melanoma as, 2295
in Paget's disease, 2294–2295
Anal sphincter, artificial, 1924, 1924f
Anal sphincter defects, endoanal ultrasound
in, 1910–1911, 1911f
Anal sphincter reconstruction, 1922f,
1922–1923
Anal sphincterotomy
internal, partial, for anal fissures, 2041,
2041f, 2042f
lateral, for anal fissures, 2041, 2042t
Anal stenosis, 2062–2065
medical therapy for, 2062
surgical therapy for, 2062–2065
advancement flaps as, 2063, 2063f
island flaps as, 2063f, 2063–2064,
2064f
rotational flaps as, 2064–2065, 2065f
Anal wipes, pruritus ani associated with,
2069
Analgesia
for pancreatitis
acute, mild, 1302
severe, necrotizing, 1303
patient controlled, following bariatric
surgery, 937
Anastomotic complications, of
esophagectomy, 481
Anastomotic cuff abscesses, following ileal
pouch–anal anastomosis, 2111
Anastomotic leaks
with esophageal and tracheoesophageal
atresia repair, 569–570
esophagogastric, following esophageal
surgery, 599
following esophageal resection with
visceral esophageal substitution,
611–613, 612f
Anastomotic stricture
with esophageal and tracheoesophageal
atresia repair, 570
following esophageal resection with
visceral esophageal substitution,
613
Androgen(s), hepatotoxicity of, 1722,
1723
Androgenic metabolic steroids,
hepatotoxicity of, 1724
Anemia
following gastrectomy, 873
with gastrointestinal fistulas, 1098

Anemia (Continued)
iron deficiency
in Crohn's disease, 1054
following gastrectomy, 873
splenectomy for hematologic disorders
causing, 1825–1827
hemolytic, acquired anemia and,
1826–1827
hereditary anemia and, 1825–1826
Anesthesia
in biliary disease, 1626
for groin hernia surgery, 646
in liver disease, 1626
Anesthesiologists, on portal hypertension
multidisciplinary team, 1767
Aneurysm(s). See also Pseudoaneurysms.
celiac artery, 1279–1280
clinical findings in, 1279
diagnosis of, 1279
incidence of, 1279
pathogenesis of, 1279
treatment of, 1279–1280
colic artery, 1282f, 1283
gastric artery, 1282
gastroduodenal artery, 1280f, 1280–1282
gastroepiploic artery, 1282
hepatic artery, 1277–1278, 1711–1712,
1712f
arteriography in, 1278
clinical findings in, 1278
diagnosis of, 1278
false, 1277
incidence of, 1277
pathogenesis of, 1277
treatment of, 1278
ileal artery, 1282f, 1283
inferior mesenteric artery, 1280
pancreatic artery, 1280–1282
pancreaticoduodenal artery, 1280–1282,
1281f
splenic artery, 1274–1277
clinical findings in, 1275
diagnosis of, 1275, 1276f
incidence of, 1274
pathogenesis of, 1274–1275
splenectomy for, 1833–1834
treatment of, 1275, 1277
superior mesenteric artery, 1278–1279
clinical findings in, 1278
diagnosis of, 1278–1279
incidence of, 1278
pathogenesis of, 1278
treatment of, 1279
Aneurysmorrhaphy
for splenic artery aneurysms, 1275, 1277
for superior mesenteric artery
aneurysms, 1279
Angiodysplasia
gastric, 887
endoscopic appearance of, 739
signs and symptoms of, 887
treatment of, 887
small intestinal, 898
Angiography
in aortoenteric fistulas, 1271
calcium, for insulinoma localization,
1378
with colonic vascular ectasias, 1993

Angiography (Continued)
with duodenal diverticula, 779, 780f
mesenteric, with colon, rectal, and anal
disorders, 1896–1897, 1897f
Angiomyolipomas, hepatic, 1730
Angiosarcomas, hepatic, 1747–1748, 1748f
drug-induced, 1724
end-stage liver disease due to, 1687
Angiozyme, for colorectal cancer
metastases, 2271
Anismus, surgical treatment of, 1936–1938,
1939f, 1940f, 1941t
Ann Arbor staging system with Cotswold
modification, 1827, 1828t
Annular pancreas, 1407–1408, 1408f
Anocutaneous reflex, 1918
Anoplasty
cutback, for low imperforate anus,
2394f, 2395–2396
Martin, for anal stenosis, 2063
transplant, for low imperforate anus,
2396, 2397f
Anorectal abscesses
classification of, 2045, 2046f, 2048t
diagnosis of, 2045, 2048–2049
history in, 2045, 2048
magnetic resonance imaging in,
2051
physical examination in, 2048–2049
ultrasonography in, 2049–2051,
2050f–2052f
etiology of, 2045
horseshoe extension and
diagnosis of, 2049
treatment of, 2053–2054, 2054f
in human immunodeficiency virus
disease, 2058
intersphincteric
diagnosis of, 2048
treatment of, 2053
ischiorectal
diagnosis of, 2048
treatment of, 2053
in leukemia, 2058
management of, 2057–2058
perianal
diagnosis of, 2048
treatment of, 2052–2053, 2053f
postanal
diagnosis of, 2049
treatment of, 2053–2054, 2054f
submucosal
diagnosis of, 2048
treatment of, 2053
supralevator
diagnosis of, 2048–2049
treatment of, 2053, 2053f
treatment of, 2051–2055
complications of, 2057
for horseshoe extension, 2053–2054,
2054f
for intersphincteric abscesses, 2053
for ischiorectal abscesses, 2053
for perianal abscesses, 2052–2053,
2053f
for postanal abscesses, 2053–2054,
2054f
postoperative care for, 2057

Anorectal abscesses (Continued)
primary versus delayed fistulotomy
for, 2054–2055
for submucosal abscesses, 2053
for supralevator abscesses, 2053,
2053f
Anorectal advancement flaps, for anorectal
fistulas, 2056, 2056f
Anorectal anomalies, 2387–2406
associations among, 2390–2391
genitourinary types of, 2390
sacral and spinal types of, 2390
classification of, 2388t, 2388–2390,
2389t, 2390f–2393f
embryology of, 2387–2388
initial management of newborn with,
2394–2395
in all infants, 2395
in female infant, 2394–2395
in male infant, 2394, 2394f
operative technique for, 2395
pelvic muscular anatomy and physiology
of continence and, 2391–2394
surgical management of, 2395–2406
functional results of, 2403–2406,
2404f
with cloacal surgery, 2406
constipation as, 2405
continence and, 2404
genitourinary, 2405–2406
with high imperforate anus,
2404–2405
treatment of incontinence and,
2405
for high imperforate anus, 2396,
2398–2402, 2399f
with cloacal malformation, 2402,
2403f
colostomy construction and,
2396, 2398f
minimally invasive repair as,
2400–2402, 2401f, 2402f
neonatal pull-through procedures
for, 2400
for low imperforate anus, 2395–2396
anterior perineal anorectoplasty
as, 2396, 2397f
cutback anoplasty as, 2395f,
2395–2396
transplant anoplasty as, 2396,
2397f
postoperative complications of,
2402–2403
reoperative surgery for, 2403
Anorectal disorders. See also specific disorders.
abscesses as. See Anorectal abscesses.
congenital. See Anorectal anomalies.
in Crohn's disease
abscesses as, 2057–2058
fistulas as, 2057
surgical treatment of, 2135
itching as, differential diagnosis of,
1884
swelling as
differential diagnosis of, 1884
examination for, 1887
ultrasound in. See Endoanal ultrasound;
Endorectal ultrasound.

Anorectal injury, 1977–1978
Anorectal mucosectomy, with muscular
plication, for rectal prolapse, 1962,
1962f–1964f, 1964, 1964t
Anorectal pain
differential diagnosis of, 1884
examination for, 1887
Anorectal pull-through
for high or intermediate imperforate
anus, 2400
laparoscopically assisted, for high
imperforate anus, 2400–2402, 2401f,
2402f
Anorectal ring, 2220
Anorectoplasty
perineal, anterior, for low imperforate
anus, 2396
sagittal, posterior, 2387, 2398, 2399f,
2400
Anorexia, in appendicitis, 2142
Anoscopy, 1889, 1889f
Anovaginal fistulas, 1946
Antacids, for gastroesophageal reflux
disease, 253
Antibiotics
for asplenia, in pediatric patients,
1811
for cholangitis prophylaxis, 1550t
for cholangitis treatment, with primary
sclerosing cholangitis, 1588
for hepatic abscesses, pyogenic,
1648–1649
for inflammatory bowel disease, 1052,
2090–2091, 2128
for intra-abdominal abscesses, 1102
for pancreatitis
acute, mild, 1302
severe, necrotizing, 1303, 1304t
preoperative
for colorectal surgery, 2328–2329
oral, 2328
parenteral, 2328–2329
prophylactic
for cholangitis, 1550t
for overwhelming postsplenectomy
infection, 1838
prophylactic vs. therapeutic use of,
2329
for splenic abscesses, 1820
Antibodies
anti-Saccharomyces cerevisae, in Crohn's
disease, 1046
cytoplasmic, perinuclear antineutrophil,
in Crohn's disease, 1046
hOKT3-γ1-ala-ala, for islet
transplantation, 1428
for pancreas transplantation, 1419
Anticoagulation
for mesenteric ischemia, 1255
for mesenteric venous thrombosis,
1256–1257
Antidiarrheal agents, for fecal incontinence,
1921
Antiemetic agents, for gastroparesis, 921
Antiestrogens, for desmoids, in familial
adenomatous polyposis, 2161, 2162
Antifungals, hepatotoxicity of, 1722
Antihistamines, for gastroparesis, 921

Anti-inflammatory drugs, nonsteroidal
  for Barrett's esophagus, 258
  for desmoids, in familial adenomatous
    polyposis, 2161, 2162
  esophageal cancer and, 445
Anti-interleukin-12, mechanism of action of,
  2377t
Antilymphocyte globulin, mechanism of
  action of, 2377t
Antireflux procedures. *See also specific
  procedures.*
  for Barrett's esophagus, 354–363
    dysplastic
      high-grade, 361–363, 362f
      low-grade, 360–361, 361b
      impact on metaplasia-dysplasia-
        carcinoma sequence, 358–359
      regression of Barrett's esophagus
        and, 358–359, 359f, 360f
      outcome of, 355–357
        choice of operation and, 356
        objective measures of reflux
          control and, 357
        symptomatic, 356–357, 357f
      rationale for, 354–355, 355t, 356t
    chylothorax following, 609
    contraindications to, in severe
      gastroesophageal reflux disease, 267
    early development of, 6–7
    endoscopic, 306–331
      endoluminal gastroplasty as, 309–314
        physiologic/anatomic
          mechanisms of, 328–329,
          330f
      Enteryx for, 320–323
        physiologic/anatomic
          mechanisms of, 330–331
      Gatekeeper for, 323–325, 326t, 327t
        physiologic/anatomic
          mechanisms of, 330–331
      historical background of, 307–308,
        308b
      NDO plicator for, 308b, 314–316
        complications of, 316
        efficacy of, 315–316, 316t
        physiologic/anatomic
          mechanisms of, 329–330,
          330f
        procedure for, 314f, 314–315,
          315f
      physiologic/anatomic mechanisms
        of, 326, 328–331
        for endoluminal gastroplasty,
          328–329, 330f
        for Enteryx, 330–331
        for Gatekeeper, 330–331
        for NDO plicator, 329–330, 330f
        for Stretta procedure, 330–331
      Plexiglas for, 325
      reflux pathophysiology and, 306–307
      selection criteria for, 308f, 308–309
      Stretta procedure for, 317–320, 325,
        326t, 327t
        physiologic/anatomic
          mechanisms of, 330–331
      Syntheon device for, 316f, 316–317
    endoscopic evaluation following, 106,
      108, 108f

Antireflux procedures *(Continued)*
  esophageal imaging following, 85, 86f
  with esophagomyotomy, controversy
    about, 620
  failure of
    barium examination for, 70
    reoperative surgery for, 1141–1143
      technical aspects of, 1143, 1143b
  with Heller myotomy, for achalasia,
    416
  hemorrhage following, 609–610
  with intraoperative stricture dilatation
    for esophageal strictures, 241–248
  laparoscopic, complications of, 610–611
  predischarge barium swallow study for,
    610, 610f
  retrosternal dysphagia following, low,
    609
Anti-*Saccharomyces cerevisae* antibodies, in
  Crohn's disease, 1046
Antiserotoninergics, for gastroparesis, 921
Antithymocyte globulin
  for islet transplantation, 1428
  mechanism of action of, 2377t
Antral hypomotility, detection by
  antroduodenal manometry, 188
Antral webs, endoscopic appearance of,
  738
Antrectomy
  for caustic injury, gastric, 763
  with long-limb Roux-en-Y gastric bypass,
    for Barrett's esophagus, 303–304
  with vagotomy
    for duodenal ulcers, 796, 798t
    for gastric outlet obstruction, in
      peptic ulcer disease, 826
Antroduodenal manometry, delayed gastric
  emptying and, 186–188, 188f, 188t, 189f,
  190, 190t
Anus
  coloanal anastomosis and. *See* Coloanal
    anastomosis.
  imperforate. *See* Anorectal anomalies;
    Imperforate anus.
Anxiety, with levator spasm, 2075
Aortoduodenal fistulas, 1095
Aortoenteric fistulas, 1269–1274
  classification of, 1269
  clinical features of, 1270–1271
  diagnosis of, 1271f, 1271–1272
  graft-enteric erosion and, 1269, 1270
  graft-enteric fistula and, 1269, 1270
  pathogenesis of, 1269–1270
  treatment of, 1114
    endovascular, 1273–1274
    results with, 1274
    surgical, 1272–1273
      for primary aortoenteric fistula,
        1272
      for secondary aortoenteric fistula,
        1273
Aortography
  with aortoenteric fistulas, 1115
  in mesenteric ischemia, chronic, 1258
Aortomesenteric bypass, for mesenteric
  revascularization, 1258–1260, 1260f
APACHE-II scoring system, for pancreatitis,
  acute, 1300, 1301b, 1302

APC gene
  familial adenomatous polyposis and,
    2163
  screening for mutations in, 2164
Aphthous ulcers, in Crohn's disease, 1043
Aponeurotic arch, 638, 638f
Appendiceal distention, with mucinous
  cystadenoma and cystadenocarcinoma,
  2150
Appendiceal orifice, on colonoscopy,
  1867
Appendiceal tumors, 2150–2151
  carcinoid, 1182
    treatment of, 1185
Appendices epiploicae, 1845
Appendicitis
  acute, 2141–2150
    differential diagnosis of, 2144–2145
    in elderly people, 2144
    in immunocompromised patients,
      2381
    in infants and young children,
      2143–2144
    laboratory tests in, 2142–2143
    pathophysiology of, 2141
    physical examination in, 2142
    during pregnancy, 2144
    radiographic examination in, 2143
    symptoms of, 2141–2142
    treatment of, 2145–2150
      complications of, 2150
      examination under anesthesia
        and, 2145
      laparoscopic appendectomy for,
        2147, 2149f
      for normal appendix when
        appendicitis is suspected,
        2150
      for perforated appendicitis with
        diffuse peritonitis, 2149
      for perforated appendicitis with
        localized abscess formation,
        2148–2149
      for perforated or gangrenous
        appendicitis with a
        periappendiceal mass,
        2147–2148
      preoperative preparation for,
        2145
      for uncomplicated appendicitis
        without a palpable mass,
        2145–2147, 2146f–2148f
    in young women, 2144
    chronic and recurrent, 2150
Aprepitant, for gastroparesis, 921
Arch of Riolan, 1239
Arch of Treves, 1239
Argon beam coagulation, for esophageal
  cancer, 489t, 492
Argon plasma coagulation
  for Barrett's esophagus, 371
  for gastric bleeding, 741–742, 742f
  for watermelon stomach, 740
Aristotle, 632, 1813
Arrhythmias, with inguinal herniorrhaphy,
  laparoscopic, 667
Arsenic, hepatotoxicity of, 1723, 1724
Arteries. *See specific arteries.*

Arteriography
  with diverticular hemorrhage, 2016,
    2017f
  for esophageal reconstruction, 581–582,
    582f
  in hepatic artery aneurysms, 1278
  mesenteric, preoperative, for esophageal
    replacement, 287–288, 288f
  in mesenteric ischemia, 1253f,
    1253–1254, 1254f
  in mesenteric venous thrombosis, 1256,
    1256f
  in portal hypertension, 1757
Arterioles, mesenteric, 1240, 1241
Arteriomesenteric duodenal
  ileus/compression, 974–975, 975f, 976f
Arterioportal shunts, hepatic, 1713f,
  1713–1714
Arteriovenous malformations
  colonic, congenital, 1997, 1998f
  gastric
    congenital, 740, 740f, 886–887
      symptoms and diagnosis of, 887
      treatment of, 887
    endoscopic appearance of, 739, 739f
  small bowel, capsule endoscopy of, 746f
Arteriovenous shunts, hepatic, 1713f,
  1713–1714
Artery of Drummond, 1239
Artificial anal sphincter, 1924, 1924f
Artificial liver support systems, 1704–1708
  biologic, 1706–1707, 1707f
  future of, 1707–1708, 1708f
  need for, 1705
  nonbiologic, 1705–1706
Ascites, 1751, 1755–1756
  in cirrhosis, 1624–1625
  pancreatic, 1349–1352, 1350f–1352f
    in chronic pancreatitis, 1312
  in portal hypertension, 1755–1756,
    1763–1765
    diagnosis of, 1764
    management of, 1764–1765, 1765f
    pathophysiology of, 1763–1764, 1764f
  refractory, 1765
Ascorbic acid, small intestinal absorption of,
  1006, 1007t
Aspartate aminotransferase, elevated, 1611,
  1611b
Aspergillus, splenic abscess due to, 1819
Aspiration
  in achalasia, 407
  closed, for hepatic abscesses, pyogenic,
    1649
  following esophageal surgery, 599
  of hepatic cysts, in polycystic liver
    disease, 1634–1635
  percutaneous, of pancreatic pseudocysts,
    1333
Asplenia, prophylaxis for, in pediatric
  patients, 1811–1812
Asthma, gastroesophageal reflux disease
  associated with
    diagnosis of, 171, 172f
    medical therapy for, 258, 259f, 260f
Atheroembolism, peripheral, following
  esophageal resection with visceral
  esophageal substitution, 615

Atherosclerosis
  celiac artery aneurysms due to, 1278
  superior mesenteric artery aneurysms
    due to, 1278
Atlanta Classification, 1296
Atopic eczema, pruritus ani associated with,
  2070
Attenuated familial adenomatous polyposis,
  small intestinal, 894t, 896
Attenuation, in ultrasonography, 112
Auerbach's plexus, 26, 720
Aureobasidum pullulans, splenic abscess due
  to, 1819
Autoimmune hepatitis, hepatic laboratory
  tests in, 1613
Autoimmune neutropenia, splenectomy for,
  1827
Autonomic nerve plexuses, pelvic, total
  mesorectal excision with autonomic
  nerve preservation and, 2237–2238,
  2238f
Autoregulation, splanchnic, 1243
Azathioprine
  for Crohn's disease, 1053, 2128
  for gastrointestinal fistulas, 1105
  hepatotoxicity of, 1723
  for inflammatory bowel disease,
    2091–2092
  mechanism of action of, 2377t
Azygos vein, 15f, 22

B

Baker tubes, 750, 751f
Balloon catheters
  for bile duct stone removal, 1494, 1495f
  biliary, 1484
Balloon dilation
  of bile duct strictures, 1588
  of biliary sphincter, for stone removal,
    1496–1497
  of superior mesenteric artery, 1261,
    1264t
Balloon expulsion, in obstructed
  defecation, 1879b
Balsalazide, for inflammatory bowel disease,
  2090
Band ligation, endoscopic, for gastric
  bleeding, 743, 743f
Bannayan-Zonana (Bannayan-Riley-
  Ruvalcaba) syndrome, 894t, 897, 2159t,
  2176
Barbette, Paul, 1229
Barcelona Chronic Liver Cancer staging
  system, 1735
Bariatric surgery
  amelioration of obesity-related diseases
    and, 938–939
  biliopancreatic diversion for, 936, 936f
  dietary management following, 938
  fistulas following, 1093
  follow-up for, 938
  gastric banding for, 934–935, 935f
  gastric restrictive operations for,
    930–931, 931f
  indications for, 929–930
  jejunoileal bypass for, 930, 930f

Bariatric surgery (Continued)
  perioperative care for, 937–938
  revision operations and, 936–937,
    1143–1146
    for failed laparoscopic adjustable
      gastric banding, 1145
    for failed malabsorptive procedures,
      1146
    for failed Roux-en-Y gastric bypass,
      1145–1146
    for failed vertical banded
      gastroplasty, 1144–1145
    patient selection for, 1144
  Roux-en-Y gastric bypass for, 931–934,
    932f, 933t
Barium burger studies, radiographic, for
  gastric emptying assessment, 190
Barium examination
  barium enema as
    in appendicitis, 2142–2143
    with colon, rectal, and anal
      disorders, 1891–1892, 1892f
    in colonic volvulus, 1981, 1982f
    in constipation, 1929–1930, 1931f
    double-contrast
      with colon, rectal, and anal
        disorders, 1892f, 1892–1893
      screening for adenomatous
        polyps with, 2157
    in small bowel obstruction, 1030,
      1030f
  barium swallow as
    in achalasia, 411, 412f
    in epiphrenic diverticulum, 432f,
      433f, 433–434
    with paraesophageal hernia, 552,
      553f
    for staging of esophageal cancer,
      455, 456f
  with carcinoid tumors, 1183, 1183f
  esophageal, 64
    air-contrast technique for, 64, 64f,
      65f
    in esophageal carcinoma, 75f–79f,
      75–76
      for staging, 77
    in esophageal motility disorders, 68,
      71
    esophagography as, 164, 165t
      in esophageal carcinoma, 469,
        469f
      for esophageal reconstruction,
        582
    esophagoscopy as, with leiomyoma,
      517, 517f
    full-column technique for, 64, 65f,
      66f
    in gastroesophageal reflux disease,
      68–70
      to detect esophageal injury,
        68–69, 69f, 70f
      to detect gastroesophageal reflux,
        68
      to evaluate esophageal clearance,
        68
      to exclude motility disorder, 68
      for postoperative complication
        evaluation, 70

Barium examination (*Continued*)
    for preoperative planning, 70, 71f
    single- or double-contrast technique
      for, in esophageal carcinoma, 75
  with varices, 95, 97f
Barostat system, 1874
Barostat test, in esophageal disease, 195
Barrett, Norman, 5, 7, 336f, 336–337, 341
Barrett's esophagus, 341–351
  ablation therapy for, 360, 361, 362
    endoscopic, 365–372
      argon plasma coagulation for, 371
      cryotherapy for, 371
      laser, 370–371
      mucosal resection for, 370
      multipolar electrocoagulation for,
        371
      photodynamic, 370
      radiofrequency, circumferential
        balloon-based, 367–370, 368f,
        369f
      rationale for, 367
  adenocarcinoma and, 445
    invasive, 219, 219f
  bile acid injury to esophageal mucosa
    and, 232
  classification systems for, 103–104
  columnar epithelium in, detection of,
    barium examination for, 69, 70f
  definition of, 334, 341–342
  diagnosis of, 215f, 218f, 218–219, 219f
    endoscopic
      conventional, 102–104, 103f, 104f
      specialized techniques for, 104,
        105f
  duodenogastroesophageal reflux
    associated with, 190
  dysplastic, 347–348, 349t, 359–363, 360t,
    361t
    high-grade, 219, 219f
      surgical treatment of, 361–363,
        362f
    low-grade, surgical treatment of,
      360–361, 361b
  endoscopic examination in, 108, 109f
  epidemiology of, 342
  gastroesophageal reflux disease and,
    200, 203
  goblet cells in, 215f, 218
  hiatal hernia and, 60
  historical background of, 334–338, 336f,
    338f
  ideal end point of treatment for, 60
  length of, 335, 341
  long-segment, 335, 346
  malignant transformation in, 347–348,
    349t
  medical treatment of, 60–61, 257–258
  microscopic stage of, 218, 218f, 219f
  natural history of, 348, 350
  nondysplastic, risk of progression to
    dysplasia and adenocarcinoma, 365,
    366t
  pathophysiology of, 343–347
    intestinalization of cardiac mucosa
      and, 345f, 345–347
    metastatic columnarization with
      cardiac mucosa and, 343–345

Barrett's esophagus (*Continued*)
  patient approach for, 60–61
  prevention of, 358–359, 360f
  progression to colorectal cancer, risk of,
    366
  refluxate in, 60
  regression of, after antireflux
    procedures, 358–359, 359f, 360f
  reversibility of, 358
  risk for, 348
    biomarkers for stratifying, 348
    risk factors and, 342–343
  screening for, 350
  short-segment, 335, 346
  surgical treatment of, 354–363
    for dysplastic Barrett's esophagus
      high-grade, 361–363, 362f
      low-grade, 360–361, 361b
    esophagectomy as, 248
    impact on metaplasia-dysplasia-
      carcinoma sequence, 358–359
      regression of Barrett's esophagus
        and, 358–359, 359f, 360f
    outcome of, 355–357
      choice of operation and, 356
      objective measures of reflux
        control and, 357
      symptomatic, 356–357, 357f
    rationale for, 354–355, 355t, 356t
  surveillance for, 350–351
  treatment goals for, 354
  ultrashort, 335
  vagotomy and antrectomy for, with long-
    limb Roux-en-Y gastric bypass, 303–304
Barrett's mucosa, esophageal
  adenocarcinoma and, 468, 468f
Basal cell carcinoma, anal, 2295–2296
Basiliximab, mechanism of action of, 2377t
Baskets, for bile duct stone removal, 1494
Bassini, Edoardo, 632–633
Bassini hernia repair, 648
Bear claw defect, 1660
Beck, Claude, 4
Beger procedure, for pancreatitis, chronic,
  1314, 1315
Belching, gastroesophageal reflux disease
  and, 227–228
Bell, Charles, 5
Belsey, Ronald, 6
Belsey fundoplication, for esophageal
  strictures, 241–242
Belsey Mark IV procedure, 276, 277f
  Collis gastroplasty with, for esophageal
    strictures, 242, 243f
  early development of, 6
  for esophageal strictures, 241
  imaging following, 85
  recurrent reflux following, 598
  results with, 283, 283t
  transthoracic, 282f, 282–283
Benzimidazoles, substituted, gastric acid
  secretion and, 727
Bernstein test, 164, 165t
Bethanechol, for gastroesophageal reflux
  disease, 253, 254
Bethesda Guidelines, for hereditary
  nonpolyposis colorectal cancer, 2171,
  2172b

Bevacizumab
  for metastatic colorectal cancer, 2202,
    2270–2271
  palliative, for esophageal cancer, 496
Bezoars, 943–945, 944t
  clinical features and diagnosis of, in
    pediatric patients, 959
  definition and types of, in pediatric
    patients, 959
  diagnosis of, 944f, 944–945, 945f
  management of, 945
    in pediatric patients, 959–960, 960f
  in pediatric patients, 959–960
    clinical features and diagnosis of, 959
    definition and types of, 959
    management of, 959–960, 960f
  signs and symptoms of, 944
  types of, 943–944, 944t
Bianchi procedure, for short-bowel
  syndrome, 1171, 1172f, 1173
Bicarbonate, gastric secretion of, 728–729
Bilayer hernia repair, 653
Bile
  bilirubin metabolism and, 1454
  cholesterol in, 1452–1453, 1455f, 1456f
  composition of, 1455, 1455t
  enterohepatic circulation and,
    1453–1454, 1457f
  flow of, 1454–1455
  formation of, 1451–1452, 1608
Bile acids
  Barrett's esophagus and, 346
  esophageal mucosal injury due to,
    mechanism of, 231–232
Bile duct(s). *See also* Biliary *entries;* Common
  bile duct; Cystic duct; Hepatic ducts.
  adenomas of, 1526, 1729
  cancer of, after cyst excision, 1556
    staging of, 1529b
  common. *See* Common bile duct.
  cysts of, classification of, 1552
  extrahepatic, anatomy and embryology
    of, 1441, 1442f, 1443
  intrahepatic, anatomy and embryology
    of, 1440–1441, 1442f
  obstruction of, malignant, biliary
    drainage procedures for, 1505–1508,
    1506f
  perforation of, spontaneous, with
    choledochal cysts, 1554
Bile duct stones. *See* Biliary stones.
Bile duct strictures. *See* Biliary strictures.
Bile leaks, liver transplantation and, 1698
Bile reflux gastritis
  following gastrectomy, 875–877, 876f–878f
  reoperative surgery for, 1146f,
    1146–1147, 1147f
Bile salts, small intestinal absorption of,
  1007t, 1008
Biliary atresia, 1545
  classification of, 1546, 1547f
  diagnosis of, 1545
  etiology of, 1546
  management of
    liver transplantation for, 1550–1551
    operative, 1546, 1548, 1549f
    outcome of, 1550
    postoperative care and, 1550, 1550t

Biliary balloon catheters, 1484

Biliary bypass, for pancreatitis, chronic, with bile duct stricture, 1347–1348

Biliary cystadenocarcinoma, end-stage liver disease due to, 1687

Biliary cystadenomas, 1526, 1636

Biliary decompression, for cholangiocarcinoma, 1531

Biliary disease. *See also specific conditions.*
anesthesia in, 1626
with duodenal diverticula, 780–781
hepatic abscesses due to, pyogenic, 1641–1642
operative considerations in, 1626–1627
perioperative management for, 1622
postoperative management in, 1627–1628

Biliary drainage, 1500–1509
for benign biliary strictures, 1500–1503
distal, secondary to chronic pancreatitis, 1501, 1502f, 1502t, 1503
postoperative, 1500f, 1500–1501
for biliary fistulas, 1504–1505
for choledochal cysts and anomalous pancreaticobiliary union, 1508–1509
for malignant bile duct obstruction, 1505–1508, 1506f
tissue sampling at endoscopic retrograde cholangiopancreatography and, 1507–1508
for primary sclerosing cholangitis, 1503f, 1503–1504
for sump syndrome, 1508

Biliary fistulas
biliary drainage procedures for, 1504–1505
drainage procedures for, 1504–1505
external, 1537–1543
clinical presentation of, 1541, 1541f
diagnosis of, 1541–1542
etiology and prevention of, 1537–1541
of fistulas after gastrectomy, 1540
of fistulas after invasive radiologic procedures, 1540–1541
of fistulas after liver injury, 1539, 1539f
of fistulas after liver surgery, 1539–1540
of fistulas after liver transplantation, 1540
of fistulas following biliary-intestinal anastomosis, 1538–1539
of fistulas following cholecystectomy, 1537, 1538, 1539f
of fistulas following common duct exploration, 1537–1538
hydatid disease of liver and, 1540, 1540f
pathophysiologic consequences of, 1541
treatment of, 1542–1543
initial, 1542

Biliary hamartomas, 1729–1730, 1730f

Biliary hypoplasia, 1545
diagnosis of, 1545
etiology of, 1546

Biliary neoplasms. *See also specific neoplasms.*
benign, 1526
malignant, percutaneous image-guided therapy of, 1466–1468

Biliary obstruction, with pancreatic pseudocysts, 1344

Biliary reconstruction
liver transplantation and, 1696–1697
for primary sclerosing cholangitis, 1568–1569

Biliary stents, percutaneous, duodenal perforation due to, 1095

Biliary stones, 1494–1500
cholangitis and, acute, 1499–1500
endoscopic retrograde cholangiopancreatography/laparo-scopic cholecystectomy interface and, 1497, 1498f
extraction of, 1494–1497
dissolution therapy for, 1495–1496
endoscopic balloon dilation for, 1496–1497
lithotripsy techniques for, 1494–1495
standard method for, 1494, 1495f
stents and nasobiliary tubes for, 1496, 1496f
gallstone pancreatitis and, acute, 1497–1499
percutaneous management of, 1466

Biliary strictures
benign
biliary drainage procedures for, 1500–1503
for distal common bile duct strictures secondary to chronic pancreatitis, 1501, 1502f, 1502t, 1503
for postoperative strictures, 1500f, 1500–1501
dilation of, technique of, 1464–1466
dominant, with primary sclerosing cholangitis, 1565
treatment of, 1567
liver transplantation and, 1698
postoperative, 1573–1579
clinical presentation of, 1577f, 1577–1578
imaging of, 1578f, 1578–1579, 1579f
laboratory studies with, 1578
pathogenesis of, 1573–1574, 1575f–1577f, 1576–1577
surgical management of, 1579–1585
elective repair for, 1580, 1581f, 1582f, 1582–1583
immediate repair for, 1579–1580, 1580f
long-term results with, 1583t, 1583–1585, 1584f, 1584t, 1585f
nonsurgical repair compared with, 1585–1586
postoperative complications and death and, 1583

Biliary surgery. *See also specific procedures.*
transfusion therapy with, 1619–1620

Biliary tract, 1659, 1661f. *See also* Bile duct *entries;* Hepatobiliary *entries.*
anatomy and embryology of, 1440–1447, 1441f
of extrahepatic ducts, 1441, 1442f, 1443
of gallbladder and cystic duct, 1443f, 1443–1444, 1444f
of intrahepatic ducts, 1440–1441, 1442f
lymphatic, 1446–1447
neural, 1447, 1447f
of sphincter of Oddi, 1444–1445, 1445f
vascular, 1445f, 1445–1446, 1446f
anomalies of, 1447–1451
of biliary ducts, 1447–1448, 1448f, 1449f
of gallbladder, 1448–1451, 1449b, 1451f–1453f
vascular, 1451, 1454f
imaging modalities for, 1460–1462
computed tomography as, 1461f, 1461–1462
magnetic resonance imaging as, 1462, 1462f
nuclear medicine as, 1462, 1463f
ultrasonography as, 1460–1461, 1461f
interventional radiology for, 1462–1469
for benign biliary disease, 1468
complications of, 1468–1469
image-guided therapy of malignant biliary disease and, 1466–1468
percutaneous transhepatic cholangiography and percutaneous biliary drainage and, 1464–1466
radiologist's role in, 1462–1464, 1463f–1465f
for stone management, 1466
physiology of, 1451–1459
bile composition and, 1455, 1455t
bile flow and, 1454–1455
bile production and, 1451–1454
gallbladder function and, 1455–1458
of sphincter of Oddi, 1458f, 1458–1459
trauma to. *See* Hepatobiliary trauma.

Biliary-enteric bypass, pancreatic ductal drainage with, with common bile duct strictures, 1348

Biliary-intestinal anastomosis, external biliary fistulas following, etiology and prevention of, 1538–1539

Biliopancreatic diversion
failed, revision surgery for, 1146
for obesity, 936, 936f

Bilirubin
in bile, 1452
metabolism of, 1454
serum, elevated, patient approach for, 1613–1614, 1614f
24-hour ambulatory detection of, 168–169
Bilitec probe for, 168–169, 169f
clinical use of, 169–173
test performance and, 169, 170b, 170f

Bilirubin (Continued)
24-hour monitoring of, for duodenogastroesophageal reflux, 193–195, 194f, 194t
Bilitec probe, 168–169, 169f, 193
Billroth I gastroduodenostomy
for caustic injury, gastric, 763
for duodenal ulcers, 795, 796, 796f, 797f
following gastrectomy, 911
Billroth II gastrojejunostomy
bile reflux gastritis following. See Bile reflux gastritis.
for caustic injury, gastric, 763
for duodenal ulcers, 795, 796, 796f, 797f
following gastrectomy, 911
gastroparesis following, 923
revision of, for bile reflux gastritis, 877, 878f
Bioartificial liver support system, 1706, 1707
Biofeedback
for constipation, 1938
for fecal incontinence, 1921–1922
for perineal pain syndromes, 2074–2075
Biofragmentable anastomosis ring, 1089–1090, 1090f
Biologic therapies
for carcinoid tumors, 1186, 1187
for colorectal cancer metastases, 2270–2271
for inflammatory bowel disease, 2092–2093
Biomaterials, injectable, for fecal incontinence, 1925–1926
Biotin, small intestinal absorption of, 1006, 1007t
Bipolar electrocoagulation, for esophageal cancer, 489t, 492
"Bird's beak" appearance
in colonic volvulus, 1981, 1982f
in malrotation, 1216, 1217f
Bismuth, for lymphoma, 1209t
Bladder
identification of, 2413
injury of
with hernia repair, 654
with inguinal herniorrhaphy, laparoscopic, 666
Blastomyces dermatitidis, splenic abscess due to, 1819
Bleeding. See also Hemorrhage.
control of, with reoperative pelvic surgery, 2414–2415
in Crohn's disease, 1045
ectasias and, colonic. See Colon, vascular ectasias of.
with esophageal stricture dilatation, 240–241
in fulminant hepatic failure, management of, 1704
gastric, endoscopic management of, 741–745, 742f–744f
with hepatobiliary trauma, control of, 1664f, 1664–1665
herald (sentinel), with aortoenteric fistulas, 1114
lower gastrointestinal, in diverticular disease, surgical treatment of, 2026–2027

Bleeding (Continued)
with Nissen fundoplication, 274
with paraesophageal hernia, 552
rectal, 1883–1884
examination for, 1887
in ulcerative colitis, 2085
with reoperative pelvic surgery, anticipation of, 2410
of ulcers
emergency surgery for, 802t, 802–804, 803f, 804f
for gastric ulcers, 804
in pediatric patients, 962
vagotomy and drainage for, 824–825, 825f
variceal. See Esophageal varices, bleeding.
Bleeding scans, with diverticular hemorrhage, 2016, 2017f
Blind probe(s), radial mechanical, 113, 113f
Blood loss
control of
in biliary disease, 1627
in liver disease, 1627
intraoperative, with splenic vein thrombosis, 1353
Bloodless fold of Treves, 1862
Blue rubber bleb syndrome, colonic hemangiomas in, 1997
Blumer's shelf nodes, 906, 1361
B-mode ultrasonography, 112
Bochdalek, foramen of, 36
Bochdalek hernias, 561
"Body packers," 943, 943f
Body position, in gastroesophageal reflux disease, 252–253
Boerhaave, Hermann, 528
Boerhaave's syndrome, 91, 93, 528, 529, 530f, 530–531. See also Esophageal perforation.
Bone
colorectal cancer metastases to, 2270
disease of, following gastrectomy, 873
hepatic osteodystrophy and
in end-stage liver disease, 1693
with primary sclerosing cholangitis, treatment of, 1568
retrorectal osseous lesions and, 2306
Borrke ileostomy, 1070
Botulinum toxin
for achalasia, 412
for anal fissures, 2040
for constipation, 1938–1939
for gastric bleeding, 743
for gastroparesis, 921
for perineal pain syndromes, 2075
Bougienage, for esophageal cancer, 488–489, 489t
Bougies, for esophageal stricture dilatation, 237, 238f, 239f, 240
Bowditch, Henry Ingersoll, 6
Bowel activity, return of, following laparoscopic colorectal surgery, 2343
Bowel injury
with hernia repair, 654
with inguinal herniorrhaphy, laparoscopic, 665–666
during laparoscopic enteroclysis, 1136

Bowel preparation
for abdominoperineal resection of rectum, 2235
antibiotics with, 2328–2329
for gastric resection and reconstruction, 831
for low anterior colorectal resection, 2222
mannitol for, 2328
mechanical, 2328
polyethylene glycol for, 831, 2328
Bowel resection. See also Colon resection; Colorectal resection.
for Crohn's disease, stricturoplasty vs., 1058–1059
duodenal, for duodenal adenocarcinoma, 915
ileal, diarrhea following, 1880
for mesenteric ischemia, 1254–1255
short-bowel syndrome following. See Short-bowel syndrome.
of small bowel
for Crohn's disease, 2132, 2133f
for intestinal dysmotility, 927
Bowen's disease
anorectal, 1887
colorectal, 2318
pruritus ani and, 2068
Brain, colorectal cancer metastases to, 2270
Braun enteroenterostomy, for bile reflux gastritis, 877, 878f, 1146, 1146f
Bravo probe, 167–168, 168f, 266
Breath hydrogen test, in constipation, 1932
Bricker-Johnston technique, 2323
Bronchial artery, 20, 20f
Bronchogenic carcinoma, esophageal endoscopic ultrasonography in, 125
Bronchogenic cysts, esophageal, 525, 525f
Bronchoscopy
in esophageal carcinoma, 471
for staging of esophageal cancer, 456
Bronchospasm, in carcinoid syndrome, 1182
Brooke, Bryan N., 1070
Brunner's gland polyps, 884
Brush cytology, in malignant bile duct obstruction, 1507–1508
Budd-Chiari syndrome, 1714f, 1714–1715, 1757
Budesonide
for Crohn's disease, 1052, 2128
for inflammatory bowel disease, 2090
Burchardt's triad, 550–551
Burkitt's lymphoma, pathology of, 1204, 1204f
Burns, immunosuppression due to, 2376
Buschke-Lowenstein tumors, colorectal, 2318
Busulfan, hepatotoxicity of, 1723
Button batteries, ingested, 942–943

C

"C and M" classification system, for Barrett's esophagus, 104
^{13}C breathing test, for delayed gastric emptying, 185–186

CA 19-9
  in pancreatic and periampullary
      adenocarcinomas, 1361
  pancreatic pseudocysts and, 1332
CA-125, pancreatic pseudocysts and,
      1331–1332
"-Caines," pruritus ani associated with, 2069
Calcium
  deficiency of, in Crohn's disease, 1054
  duodenal absorption of, 979
  small intestinal absorption of, 1007t,
      1008
Calcium angiography, for insulinoma
      localization, 1378
Calcium-channel blockers
  for anal fissures, 2040
  hepatotoxicity of, 1721
Calot's triangle, 1444, 1444f, 1473, 1474
Camper's fascia, 636
Cancer. See Malignancies; Metastases; specific
      cancers.
Cancer antigen 125, pancreatic pseudocysts
      and, 1331–1332
Cancer of the Liver Italian Program, 1736
Candida infection
  pruritus ani associated with, 2070
  splenic abscess due to, 1819
Cantlie's line, 1673, 1673f
Cantor tubes, 750, 751f
Capecitabine, for metastatic colorectal
      cancer, 2202
Capillaries, mesenteric, 1241
Capsule endoscopy
  in Crohn's disease, 1051f, 1051–1052
  of small bowel, 745–746, 746f
Carbohydrate(s)
  duodenal absorption of, 980
  small intestinal absorption of, 1002,
      1002f, 1003f, 1003t
Carbohydrate antigen 19-9
  in pancreatic and periampullary
      adenocarcinomas, 1361
  pancreatic pseudocysts and, 1332
Carbon monoxide, gastric innervation and,
      720
Carbon tetrachloride, hepatotoxicity of,
      1719
Carcinoembryonic antigen
  colorectal cancer and, 1888, 2200, 2201
  to detect tumor relapse, of colorectal
      cancer, 2259
  in pancreatic and periampullary
      adenocarcinomas, 1361
  pancreatic pseudocysts and, 1331t,
      1331–1332
Carcinoid syndrome, 1182
  atypical (variant), 1182
  diarrhea in, 1880
Carcinoid tumors, 1179–1187
  appendiceal, 1182
      treatment of, 1185
  appendiceal distention by, 2150
  clinical features of, 1180–1182, 1181f
  colonic, 2312
      treatment of, 1185
  diagnosis of, 1182–1184
      imaging in, 1183f, 1183–1184, 1184f
      laboratory studies in, 1182–1183

Carcinoid tumors (Continued)
  duodenal, 1181
      treatment of, 1185
  epidemiology of, 1179
  future directions for, 1187
  gastric, 1181
      treatment of, 1185
  ileal, treatment of, 1185
  incidence of, 1179
  jejunal, treatment of, 1185
  midgut, 1181, 1181f
  pathology of, 1179–1180, 1180f
  rectal, 2313
      treatment of, 1185
  treatment and outcome with, 1184–1187
      for locoregional disease, 1185
      for metastatic disease, 1185–1187
          medical therapy and, 1186–1187
          surgical therapy and, 1185–1186
Carcinomatosis, with hostile abdomen,
      1147–1148
Cardia
  anchorage of, 12–14, 14f
  prenatal development of, 34, 34f
  spastic, surgery for, early development
      of, 5
Cardiac complications, of esophagectomy,
      480
Cardiac mucosa, 335–336
  development of, 229, 344
  distal extent of, 207–210, 209f, 210b,
      210f
  esophageal, 213–215, 215f
  etiology of, 41–42
  goblet cell acquisition by, 347
  with intestinal metaplasia, 335
  intestinalization of, 345f, 345–347
Cardiologists, on portal hypertension
      multidisciplinary team, 1767
Cardiomyotomy, esophageal imaging
      following, 85, 86f
Cardioplasty, early development of, 5
Cardiopulmonary assessment, preoperative,
      for esophageal replacement, 287
Cardiopulmonary disorders, in cirrhosis,
      1623–1624
Cardiovascular disorders
  with immunosuppressive therapy,
      following liver transplantation, 1700
  with inguinal herniorrhaphy,
      laparoscopic, 667
  obesity and, bariatric surgery and, 938
Carditis, reflux, 213f, 213–215. See also
      Cardiac mucosa.
  evolution of, 215, 215f
Carmustine, hepatotoxicity of, 1723
Caroli's disease, 1546, 1557–1558, 1558f
Carrell patch, 2008
Cast syndrome, 974–975, 975f, 976f
Catecholamines, splanchnic circulation and,
      1243t, 1243–1244, 1244f, 1244t
Catgut, chromic, for bowel anastomoses,
      1083, 1084
Cattell-Braasch maneuver, in duodenal
      injury, 766, 767f
Caustic ingestions
  esophageal injury due to, 540–547
      in children, 540

Caustic ingestions (Continued)
      clinical features of, 541
      endoscopic assessment of, 542, 542b
      esophageal carcinoma and, 466
      historical background of, 540
      imaging of, 91
      long-term consequences of, 547
      management of
          chronic dilation for, 544
          in chronic phase, 544–547
          emergency department, 542
          esophageal substitutes for, 545
          in-patient, 543–544
          for intractable strictures, 544–545
          for oropharyngeal strictures, 546f,
              546–547
          principles of, 541–542
          for strictures in cervical
              esophagus and below,
              545–546, 546f
      pathophysiology of, 540–541
          pH and, 541
          phases of injury and, 541
  gastric injury due to, 762
      diagnosis of, 763
      treatment of, 763
Cavernous hemangiomas, rectal, 1996
CEA. See Carcinoembryonic antigen.
Cecal volvulus, 1984–1985
  etiology and pathophysiology of, 1984
  treatment of, 1984–1985
      outcomes following, 1985
Cecorectal anastomosis, for colonic inertia,
      1934
Cecum
  anatomy of, 1845–1846, 1862
  diverticulitis of, 2019, 2020f
Celiac artery, 1292, 1293f
  anatomy of, 1236f, 1236–1237, 1237f
  aneurysms of, 1279–1280
      clinical findings in, 1279
      diagnosis of, 1279
      incidence of, 1279
      pathogenesis of, 1279
      treatment of, 1279–1280
  stenosis of, identification of, 1258
Celiac axis
  anatomy of, 1236f, 1236–1237, 1237f
  in mesenteric ischemia, 1247, 1248f. See
      also Mesenteric ischemia.
  superior mesenteric artery
      communications with, 1238–1239,
      1239f
Celiac nerve, alcohol block of, for pain
      palliation, in pancreatic and
      periampullary carcinoma, 1367, 1367f
Celiac plexus, 1447, 1447f
  anatomy of, 720
Cell membrane, pancreatic, function of,
      1292
Certolizumab, for inflammatory bowel
      disease, 2093
Cetuximab, for metastatic colorectal cancer,
      2202, 2203, 2203f, 2271
Chagas' disease
  achalasia and, 406–407
  esophageal motility disorders in, 140
      imaging in, 74

Change agent, as clinical nurse specialist role, in palliative treatment, for esophageal cancer, 498

Charcoal hemoperfusion, for liver failure, acute, 1706

CHARGE association, with esophageal and tracheoesophageal atresia, 564

Chauliac, Guy de, 623

Chemoradiotherapy
  for colorectal cancer, 2199–2200
  for esophageal cancer
    in multimodality therapy, 505–508
      as definitive therapy, 505t, 505–506
      postoperative, 509
      preoperative, 506–508, 507t
    neoadjuvant, 482–483
    palliative, 495
  for gastric adenocarcinoma
    adjuvant, 912
    neoadjuvant, 913–914
  for pancreatic and periampullary carcinoma, 1372
  radiation enteritis and, 1156

Chemotherapy. *See also* Chemoradiotherapy.
  for anal squamous cell carcinoma, 2292–2293, 2293t
  for carcinoid tumors, 1186
  for colorectal cancer
    adjuvant, 2198–2199
    locally recurrent, preoperative, 2262–2263
    metastases of, 2270
  for desmoids, in familial adenomatous polyposis, 2161
  for esophageal cancer
    in multimodality therapy, 502–505
      postoperative, 504t, 504–505
      preoperative, 502–504, 503t
    palliative, 495–496
      combination therapy for, 495–496
      new agents for, 496
      patient selection for, 495
      response to, 495
      single-agent therapy for, 495
  for gallbladder cancer, 1524
  for gastric adenocarcinoma
    adjuvant, 912
    neoadjuvant, 913
    palliative, 914
  for hepatocellular carcinoma, 1736
  immunosuppression due to, 2376
  for lymphoma, 1209
  for pancreatic and periampullary carcinoma, 1372
    palliative, 1372–1373

Chest, anatomy of, 15f, 15–16

Chest pain
  in achalasia, 407
  in esophageal disease, 57
  in esophageal motility disorders, 71
  gastroesophageal reflux disease associated with, diagnosis of, 171

Chest radiography
  with colon, rectal, and anal disorders, 1891, 1891f
  in colonic volvulus, 1981, 1982f
  in esophageal carcinoma, 469

Chest radiography *(Continued)*
  in esophageal perforation, 93, 95f, 531
  with hepatic abscesses, pyogenic, 1646
  with liver abscesses, amebic, 1654
  with paraesophageal hernia, 552, 553f
  postoperative, following esophageal surgery, 83
  with splenic abscesses, 1818

Chiari's triad, with aortoenteric fistulas, 1271

Child-Pugh score, 1674, 1674t
  in portal hypertension, 1758, 1758t

Children. *See* Pediatric patients.

Child-Turcotte-Pugh system, 1691, 1691t

Chlamydia proctitis, in immunocompromised patients, 2383t

Chloride
  colonic absorption of, 1872
  small intestinal secretion of, 1008–1009, 1010f

Chlorpromazine, hepatotoxicity of, 1722–1723

Cholangiocarcinoma, 1526–1534
  adjuvant therapy for, 1531
  diagnosis of, 1527–1528
    of distal cholangiocarcinoma, 1528
    of hilar cholangiocarcinoma, 1528, 1528f
    of intrahepatic cholangiocarcinoma, 1527–1528, 1528f
  distal
    diagnosis of, 1528
    practical management of, 1531–1532
    surgical treatment of, 1530
  epidemiology of, 1526–1527
  hepatocellular carcinoma and, 1534
  hilar
    diagnosis of, 1528, 1528f
    practical management of, 1531–1532
      surgical technique for, 1532, 1533f–1534f, 1534
    surgical treatment of, 1529–1530
  intrahepatic, 1743–1745, 1745f
    diagnosis of, 1527–1528, 1528f
    practical management of, 1531
    surgical treatment of, 1529
  palliation for, 1531
  pathology of, 1527
  practical management of, 1531–1532
    for distal cholangiocarcinoma, 1531–1532
    for hilar cholangiocarcinoma, 1531–1532
      surgical technique for, 1532, 1533f–1534f, 1534
    for intrahepatic cholangiocarcinoma, 1531
  presentation of, 1527
  with primary sclerosing cholangitis, 1565–1566
    treatment of, 1570
  in primary sclerosing cholangitis, treatment of, 1588
  staging of, 1529, 1529t, 1530t
  surgical treatment of, 1529–1531
    for distal cholangiocarcinoma, 1530
    for hilar cholangiocarcinoma, 1529–1530, 1532, 1533f–1534f, 1534

Cholangiocarcinoma *(Continued)*
  for intrahepatic cholangiocarcinoma, 1529
  liver transplantation as, 1530–1531

Cholangiography, 1493, 1493f
  in biliary atresia, 1548
  with biliary strictures, benign, 1500, 1500f
  with hepatic abscesses, pyogenic, 1646, 1646f
  operative, with bile duct strictures, 1576
  in pancreatitis
    acute, mild, 1302
    chronic, 1347
  retrograde, endoscopic, with biliary fistulas, 1542
  transhepatic, percutaneous
    with bile duct strictures, 1578–1579
    with biliary fistulas, 1542
    complications of, 1468–1469
    indications for, 1463–1464
    in periampullary carcinoma, 1363, 1364f
    technique of, 1464–1466
  tube, with biliary fistulas, 1542

Cholangiohepatocellular carcinoma, mixed, 1745–1746, 1746f

Cholangiopancreatography. *See also* Endoscopic retrograde cholangiopancreatography.
  with bile duct strictures, 1578f

Cholangiopathy, human immunodeficiency virus, 1615

Cholangitis
  acute, treatment of, 1499–1500
  fibro-obliterative, in primary sclerosing cholangitis, 1562
  liver transplantation and, 1694
  in pancreatitis, chronic, 1347
  postoperative, prevention of, 1550, 1550t
  primary sclerosing. *See* Primary sclerosing cholangitis.
  recurrent, bacterial, with primary sclerosing cholangitis, treatment of, 1567

Cholecystectomy
  anatomic considerations for, 1473f, 1473–1474
  external biliary fistulas following, etiology and prevention of, 1537
  for gallbladder cancer, 1521, 1523f, 1523–1524
  gastroparesis following, 923
  hepatectomy and, 1678
  indications for, 1471, 1472b
  laparoscopic
    for bile duct strictures, 1574, 1575f, 1576
    duodenal injury due to, 1094
    endoscopic retrograde cholangiopancreatography, 1497, 1498f
    external biliary fistulas following, etiology and prevention of, 1538, 1539f
    gallbladder cancer diagnosed incidentally after, 1525

Cholecystectomy (Continued)
  minicholecystectomy as, 1477
  morbidity and mortality with, 1479f,
    1479–1480
  open
    external biliary fistulas following,
      etiology and prevention of, 1537
    technique for, 1474–1477
      fundus-down approach and,
        1476–1477, 1477f, 1478f
      neck-toward-fundus approach
        and, 1474f–1476f, 1474–1475
  for pancreatitis
    acute, mild, 1302
    severe, necrotizing, 1303
  partial, 1477–1478, 1478f
  prophylactic, 1471, 1472b
  timing of, 1473
Cholecystectomy triangle, 1444, 1444f,
  1473, 1474
Cholecystitis, 1472–1473
  cholecystostomy for, 1478–1479, 1479f
Cholecystokinin
  duodenal function and, 980–981, 981t
  pancreatic cell function and, 1292
  small intestinal neuroendocrine
    function and, 1018
Cholecystostomy, 1478–1479, 1479f
Choledochal cysts, 1545, 1552–1556, 1553f
  classification of, 1546, 1547f
  complications of, 1554, 1554f
  diagnosis of, 1545–1546, 1553–1554
  etiology of, 1546
  signs and symptoms of, 1553
  surgical treatment of, 1508–1509, 1548,
    1554–1556
    operative technique for, 1555, 1555f,
      1556f
    outcome of, 1550
    postoperative care and, 1550
    postoperative complications of,
      1555–1556
    preoperative care for, 1554–1555
Choledochocele, 1556–1557, 1557f
Choledochoduodenostomy
  external biliary fistulas following,
    etiology and prevention of,
    1538–1539
  for pancreatitis, chronic, with bile duct
    stricture, 1348
  side-to-side, sump syndrome as
    complication of, 1508
Choledochoenterostomy, for common bile
  duct stones, 1594
Choledochojejunostomy
  external biliary fistulas following,
    etiology and prevention of,
    1538–1539
  with liver transplantation, 1551
  for pancreatitis, chronic, with bile duct
    stricture, 1348
  Roux-en-Y, for duodenal diverticula,
    782–783, 784f
Choledocholithiasis, 1590–1594, 1591f
  common bile duct exploration and
    laparoscopic, 1590, 1592–1593, 1593f
    open, 1594
  detection of, 1590

Choledocholithiasis (Continued)
  endoscopic therapy for
    postoperative, 1590, 1593–1594
    preoperative, 1590–1591
  intraoperative diagnosis and treatment
    of, 1591–1592
  laparoscopic management of, 1482–1488
    ampullary balloon dilation as,
      1484–1485, 1485f
    antegrade sphincterotomy as, 1485
    biliary balloon catheter as, 1484
    choledochoscopy for, 1482–1484,
      1483f, 1484f, 1484t
    choledochotomy as, 1485–1487,
      1486f, 1487f, 1487t, 1488t
    cystic duct catheter technique as, 1485
    fluoroscopic wire basket stone
      retrieval as, 1484
    transcystic common bile duct
      exploration or choledochotomy
      for, 1482, 1483t
  in pancreatitis, acute, mild, 1302
  with primary sclerosing cholangitis, 1565
    treatment of, 1567
Choledochoscopy, 1482–1484, 1483f, 1484f,
  1484t
  with choledochal cysts, 1555
Choledochotomy
  indications for, 1482, 1483t
  laparoscopic, 1485–1487, 1486f, 1487f,
    1487t, 1488t
Cholelithiasis, 1471–1480
  asymptomatic, 1471–1472, 1472b
  cholecystectomy for. See
    Cholecystectomy.
  cholecystitis secondary to, 1472–1473
  with choledochal cysts, 1554
  following gastrectomy, 875
  following ileostomy, 1071
  with primary sclerosing cholangitis,
    1565
    treatment of, 1567
  in short-bowel syndrome, 1167
  stone erosion and, fistulas due to,
    1094–1095
Cholestasis
  canalicular, in primary sclerosing
    cholangitis, 1562
  drug-induced, 1722–1723
    canalicular, 1722
    hepatocanalicular, 1722–1723
Cholestatic liver disease. See Primary
  biliary cirrhosis; Primary sclerosing
  cholangitis.
Cholesterol, 1452–1453, 1455f, 1456f
  small intestinal absorption of,
    1004–1006, 1005f, 1006f
Cholestyramine
  hepatotoxicity of, 1722
  for pruritus
    in primary sclerosing cholangitis,
      1567, 1588
  for steatorrhea, following ileal resection,
    1880
Chordomas, sacrococcygeal, 2304,
  2304f–2306f
Chromoendoscopy, in Barrett's esophagus,
  104

Chromogranin, carcinoid tumors and, 1183
Chronic lymphocytic leukemia, splenectomy
  for, 1830t, 1830–1831, 1831t
Chronic myelogenous leukemia,
  splenectomy for, 1831
Chylomicrons, 1005, 1006f
Chylothorax
  after antireflux procedures, 609
  following esophageal resection with
    visceral esophageal substitution,
    614–615
Cicatricial pemphigoid, esophageal
  strictures in, 89, 92f
Cigarette smoking
  cessation of, for gastroesophageal reflux
    disease, 253
  esophageal cancer and, 444, 466
  pancreatic adenocarcinoma and, 1359
Cimetidine, 255. See also Histamine$_2$
  receptor antagonists.
  for peptic ulcer disease, 870
Cinedefecography
  in perineal pain syndromes, 2074
  in rectal prolapse, 1959
Ciprofloxacin, for inflammatory bowel
  disease, 1052, 2091, 2128
Circular staplers, 1087
Cirrhosis, 1623f, 1623–1626
  ascites in, 1624–1625
  cardiopulmonary disorders in,
    1623–1624
  coagulopathy in, 1625–1626
  decompensated, with primary sclerosing
    cholangitis, treatment of, 1568
  drug-induced, 1719t, 1720–1721
  gastrointestinal disorders in, 1625
  hemodynamics in, 1623, 1692–1693
  hepatic encephalopathy in, 1625
  hepatocellular carcinoma and, 1732,
    1733f
  infectious diseases in, 1626
  metabolic abnormalities in, 1625
  pathophysiology of, 1618–1619
  portal hypertension in, 1624, 1624t
  pulmonary disorders in, 1693, 1693b
  pyogenic hepatic abscesses associated
    with, 1643
  renal dysfunction in, 1625
Cisapride. See also Prokinetic agents.
  for gastroesophageal reflux disease, 253
  for gastroparesis, 921
Clarithromycin, for lymphoma, 1209t
Claudication, esophageal, 138–139
Claudins, 999
Clavulanic acid, hepatotoxicity of, 1723
Clean-contaminated cases, 2327
Cleft lip technique, for pilonidal disease,
  1969, 1970f
Clinical expert, as clinical nurse specialist
  role, in palliative treatment, for
  esophageal cancer, 497–498
Clinical nurse specialist, role of, in palliative
  treatment, for esophageal cancer,
  497–498
Cloaca, 2390, 2393f
  malformation of, surgical treatment of,
    2402, 2403f
Cloacal membrane, 2387

Cloacal surgery, outcome of, 2406
Clonidine, for diarrhea, in diabetic
neuropathy, 1880
Cloquet's node, 641
Clostridium difficile colitis
antibiotics and, 2329
in immunocompromised patients, 2382
Coagulation testing
in biliary tract disease, 1620
in liver disease, 1620
Coagulopathy, in cirrhosis, 1625–1626
Cobalamin. *See* Vitamin B$_{12}$.
Coccygectomy, for benign tumors, 2309
Coccygodynia, 2071, 2072
idiopathic, 2074
Coelom, development of, 31
Coiled spring sign, 765–766
Colchicine, pruritus ani associated with,
2069
Colectomy
with ileorectal anastomosis
for familial adenomatous polyposis,
2165, 2165t, 2166t, 2166–2167,
2168
for ulcerative colitis, 2122
with ileorectostomy, for intractable
constipation, 1880
laparoscopic, 2345
subtotal, with ileorectal anastomosis, for
colonic inertia, 1934, 1935t, 1936
Colic arteries, 1849–1850, 1851f, 1852f
anatomy of, 1867–1868
variations in, 1868–1869
aneurysms of, 1282f, 1283
middle, accessory, 1239
middle-left collateral, 1239
Colitis
Clostridium difficile (pseudomembranous)
antibiotics and, 2329
in immunocompromised patients,
2382
granulomatous. *See* Crohn's disease.
indeterminate, 2086
infectious, in immunocompromised
patients, 2381–2382
ulcerative. *See* Ulcerative colitis.
universal, fulminating, colonic ischemia
complicating, management of, 2009
Colitis cystica profunda, 2075–2076
diagnosis of, 2075–2076, 2076f
endoanal ultrasound in, 1913–1914, 1914f
treatment of, 2075–2076
Collagen vascular disorders, superior
mesenteric artery aneurysms due to,
1278
Colles' fascia, 636
Collis, Lee, 6–7
Collis gastropexy, 599
Collis gastroplasty
with Belsey repair, for esophageal
strictures, 242, 243f
laparoscopic, for esophageal strictures,
247f, 247–248, 248f
with Nissen fundoplication, for
esophageal strictures, 244f, 244–245,
246f–248f, 247–248
for short esophagus, acquired, 272f,
272–273, 273f

Coloanal anastomosis, 2245–2253
functional results with, 2253, 2253t
oncologic results with, 2252t, 2252–2253
operative technique for, 2245–2252
for hand-sewn colonic pouch-anal
anastomosis, 2247–2250
anastomosis and, 2249, 2249f,
2250f
colon preparation and division
for, 2247–2248
colonic pouch construction for,
2248, 2249f
drainage, loop stoma, and
postoperative care for,
2249–2250
mucosectomy of rectal stump
and, 2247, 2247f, 2248f
non-mucosectomy technique for,
2247, 2248f
incision and abdominal exploration
and, 2245
inferior mesenteric vessel division
and colon mobilization and,
2245–2246, 2246f
laparoscopy and, 2252
preoperative preparation and,
2245
for stapled colonic pouch-anal
anastomosis, 2250–2252
anastomosis and, 2251, 2251f
pouch construction for, 2251,
2251f
section of rectum for, 2250, 2250f
transverse coloplasty and,
2251–2252, 2252f
total mesorectal excision and, 2246
type of anastomosis and, 2246–2247,
2247f
for rectal radiation injury, 2323–2324
for rectovaginal fistulas, 1952, 1954
Colocolostomy, for colorectal cancer, 2331
Colocutaneous fistulas, in colonic
diverticular disease, 2018
Colon
anatomy of, 1236, 1845–1856, 1846f,
1861–1870, 1863f, 1864f, 1871–1872
arterial, 1849–1851, 1850f–1853f,
1867–1868
variations in, 1868–1869
of ascending colon, 1846–1847,
1848f, 1863, 1865f
of cecum, 1845–1846, 1862
on colonoscopy, 1866–1867
of descending colon, 1848–1849,
1866
of ileocecal valve, 1846
lymphatic, 1854f, 1854–1855, 1869,
1869f
neural, 1855f, 1855–1856,
1869–1870, 1870f, 1871–1872
of sigmoid colon, 1849, 1866, 1867f,
1868f
surface, 1845, 1847f
of transverse colon, 1847–1848,
1848f, 1849f, 1864, 1866, 1866f
venous, 1851, 1853f, 1854, 1869
of vermiform appendix, 1846, 1863,
1864f

Colon (*Continued*)
arteriovenous malformations of,
congenital, 1997, 1998f
ascending, anatomy of, 1846–1847,
1848f, 1863, 1865f
cancer of. *See* Colon carcinoma;
Colorectal adenocarcinoma;
Colorectal cancer; Colorectal
carcinoma.
Crohn's disease in, surgical treatment
of, 2130, 2133, 2135
descending, anatomy of, 1848–1849,
1866
duplication of, 1858, 1860–1861, 1862f
embryology of, 1857–1861, 1858f–1860f
as esophageal substitute, 579
esophagocoloplasty and, 588b,
588–592
abdominal team and, 589–591,
590f
cervical team and, 591
operative technique for, 589–591
preoperative preparation for, 589
results with, 591t, 591–592, 592t
short-segment colon interposition
and, 596–597
results of, 596t, 596–597
fixation of, anomalies of, 1858, 1861f
function of, 1872–1881
colonic metabolism and, 1873
colonic sensation as, 1876–1878,
1877f, 1877t
defecation as, 1876, 1876f
fluid and electrolyte transport as,
1872
motor, 1873–1876
perturbation of, in disease states,
1878–1880
regional heterogeneity in, 1872
surgical implications of, 1880–1881
intussusception of, 1980, 1981f
juvenile polyposis syndrome in, 2173
in Klippel-Trénaunay-Weber syndrome,
1999
left, vascular supply to, 2223, 2224f
lymphatics of, regional, 2194–2195,
2195f, 2196f
motor response of, to eating, 1875
sigmoid
anatomy of, 1849, 1866, 1867f, 1868f
mobilization of, for low anterior
resection, 2225f, 2225–2226
torsion of, 1983
telangiectasias of, 1997, 1999
transverse, anatomy of, 1847–1848,
1848f, 1849f, 1864, 1866, 1866f
varices of, 1997
vascular ectasias of, 1987–1995
clinical aspects of, 1988–1989
diagnosis of, 1989, 1991, 1992f,
1993–1995
with active major bleeding, 1993,
1994f
with major bleeding, 1991, 1993
with major bleeding that has
ceased, 1993–1994
with nonmajor bleeding,
1994–1995

Colon *(Continued)*
   incidence and pathophysiology of, 1987–1988, 1989f–1991f
   treatment of, 1995
      for control of acute hemorrhage, 1995
      definitive, 1995
Colon carcinoma. *See also* Colorectal adenocarcinoma; Colorectal carcinoma.
   colitis associated with, in colonic ischemia, management of, 2010
   lesions mimicking, in colonic ischemia, management of, 2009–2010
   locally recurrent, trimodality therapy for, results with, 2269
   ulcerative colitis with, surgical management of, restorative proctocolectomy for, 2335
Colon diversion, for colorectal cancer, 2330–2331
Colon interposition
   for caustic ingestions, 545
   for foregut reconstruction for benign disease, 295, 295f, 296–299, 297f–299f
   short-segment, 596–597
   results of, 596t, 596–597
Colon resection
   for colorectal cancer, 2331
   with end sigmoid stoma, for colonic obstruction, 2330
   extent of, 2329–2330
   laparoscopic, 2338
   right, steps for, 2349b, 2349f, 2350f
Colonic atresia, 1858
Colonic carcinoid tumors, treatment of, 1185
Colonic circulation, 1999–2000
Colonic disorders. *See also specific disorders.*
   diagnosis of, 1883–1897
      examination for, 1885–1888
         with anorectal pain or swelling, 1887
         for bleeding, 1887
         for constipation, 1888
         general principles of, 1885–1886
         inspection and palpation in, 1886–1887
         positioning for, 1886, 1886f
         for urgency and incontinence, 1888
      history in, 1883
      investigation for, 1888–1897
         blood and stool testing in, 1888–1889
         endoscopy in, 1889f, 1889–1891, 1890f
         radiologic tests in, 1891f, 1891–1897, 1892f, 1894f–1897f
      symptoms in, 1883–1885
         abdominal pain and distention as, 1884
         anorectal pain, itching and swelling as, 1884
         bleeding as, 1883–1884
         constipation as, 1884–1885
         diarrhea as, 1885
         urgency and incontinence as, 1885

Colonic hemangiomas, 1995–1997, 1996f
   in blue rubber bleb syndrome, 1997
   cavernous, rectal, 1996
   in diffuse intestinal hemangiomatosis, 1997
Colonic inertia, surgical treatment of, 1934, 1935t, 1936
Colonic interposition, gastroparesis following, 923
Colonic ischemia, 1999–2010, 2000f
   colonic circulation and, 1999–2000
   demographics of, 2001
   diagnosis of, 2003, 2004f
   distribution of, 2001f, 2001–2002
   management of, 2003, 2005–2010
      with abdominal aortic surgery, 2006, 2008f, 2008–2009, 2009f
      in acute mesenteric ischemia, 2010
      of colitis associated with colon carcinoma, 2010
      in fulminating universal colitis, 2009
      general principles of, 2003, 2005
      of irreversible lesions, 2005
      of ischemic strictures, 2006, 2007f
      of late manifestations, 2005–2007, 2006f
      of lesions mimicking colon carcinoma, 2009–2010
      of reversible lesions, 2005
   natural history of, 2002, 2002f
   pathophysiology of, 2000, 2000b
   symptoms of, 2001
Colonic J pouch, 2104–2105, 2334
Colonic lavage, intraoperative, for colonic obstruction, 2330
Colonic motility, 1873–1876
   assessment of, 1873–1874
      radiopaque marker methods for, 1873, 1873f
      recording techniques for, 1874, 1874f
      scintigraphic techniques for, 1873f, 1873–1874
   cellular basis for, 1875, 1875f
   normal, 1875–1876, 1876f
   peristalsis and, 1874f, 1874–1875
Colonic obstruction
   in colonic diverticulitis, 2018–2019
   in diverticular disease, surgical treatment of, 2025–2026, 2026f
   as emergency surgical indication, 2102
   left-sided, 2330
   right-sided, 2330
   treatment of, 2330
Colonic pain, referral of, 1856
Colonic perforation
   as emergency surgical indication, 2102
   in immunocompromised patients, 2381
Colonic pseudo-obstruction, acute, 1879
Colonic sensation, 1876–1878, 1877f, 1877t
Colonic strictures, ischemic, management of, 2006, 2007f
Colonic transit
   in constipation, 1931–1932, 1932f
   in rectal prolapse, 1959

Colonic volvulus, 1980–1985, 1982f, 1983f
   cecal, 1984–1985
      etiology and pathophysiology of, 1984
      outcomes following treatment of, 1985
      treatment of, 1984–1985
   ileosigmoid knot and, 1984
   sigmoid, 1981, 1983–1984
      etiology and pathophysiology of, 1981, 1983
      outcomes following treatment of, 1984
      treatment of, 1983–1984
   transverse colon and splenic flexure, 1985
      etiology and pathophysiology of, 1985
      outcomes following treatment of, 1985
      treatment of, 1985
Colonoscopic polypectomy, 2157
   complications of, 2157
   for malignant polyps, 2156f, 2156–2157
   for pedunculated polyps, 2155–2156
   for sessile polyps, 2156
Colonoscopy, 1890–1891
   with anorectal fistulas, 2049
   colonic anatomy and, 1866–1867
   with colonic vascular ectasias, 1993
   in constipation, 1929–1930
   in Crohn's disease, 2088
   with diverticular hemorrhage, 2016, 2016f
   preoperative, for esophageal replacement, 287
   risks of, 1891
   screening with
      for adenomatous polyps, 2153–2155, 2154t
      for colorectal carcinoma, 1888, 2189–2192
         goals of, 2189–2190, 2190t, 2191t
         with high risk, 2190
         with low and average risk, 2190
         with previous colorectal cancer and family history of colorectal cancer, 2190–2192
   stent positioning using, 2331
   surveillance, for adenomatous polyps, 2157
   total, with small intestinal tumors, benign, 890
Coloplasty
   for rectal radiation injury, 2324
   transverse, 2251–2252, 2252f
Colopouch anal anastomosis, for rectal radiation injury, 2324
Colorectal adenocarcinoma, 2183–2204
   chemotherapy for, 2198–2200
      adjuvant, for stages II and III disease, 2198–2199
      combined chemoradiation therapy and, 2199–2200
      survival and, 2200, 2200f, 2201f
   genetic pathways to, 2183, 2186, 2186f
   incidence and epidemiology of, 2183, 2183f–2185f

Colorectal adenocarcinoma (Continued)
  metastatic, treatment of, 2201–2204,
    2203f
    chemotherapy for, 2201–2202, 2203f
    surgical, 2203–2204
  risk factors for, 2186–2189
    age as, 2186–2187
    familial adenomatous polyposis as,
      2188
    familial colorectal cancer as, 2187f,
      2187–2188
    familial juvenile polyposis as,
      2188–2189
    hereditary nonpolyposis colorectal
      cancer as, 2188, 2188b
    inflammatory bowel disease as, 2187
    Peutz-Jeghers syndrome as,
      2188–2189
  screening for, 2189–2192
    goals of, 2189–2190, 2190t, 2191t
    high risk and, 2190
    low and average risk and, 2190
    previous colorectal cancer and family
      history of colorectal cancer and,
      2190–2192
  staging of, 2192b, 2192–2194, 2193f,
    2193t, 2194b
  surgical treatment of
    of hereditary bowel cancer, 2197
    local excision of rectal cancer and,
      2197–2198
    for malignant polyps, 2197
    for metastatic cancer, 2203–2204
    minimally invasive, 2198
    postresection follow-up for, 2200
    for primary cancers, 2194–2195,
      2195f–2197f, 2197
  surveillance for, 2200–2201
  tumor markers for, 2200–2201
Colorectal cancer, 2312–2318. See also Colon
  carcinoma; Colorectal adenocarcinoma;
  Colorectal carcinoma; Rectal cancer.
  adenoma to carcinoma sequence and,
    2153
  in Bowen's disease, 2318
  Buschke-Lowenstein tumors as, 2318
  carcinoid tumors as, 2312–2313
    colonic, 2312
    rectal, 2313
  in Crohn's disease, 2089
  gastrointestinal stromal tumors as,
    2314–2317
    epidemiology of, 2314
    investigation of, 2315, 2315f
    management of, 2315–2316
    pathophysiology and pathology of,
      2314f, 2314–2315, 2315f
    presentation of, 2315
    prognosis of, 2316
  laparoscopic surgery for. See
    Laparoscopic colorectal surgery, for
    cancer.
  leiomyomas as, 2316–2317
  leiomyosarcomas as, 2316f, 2316–2317
  liposarcoma as, 2317
  lymphoma as, 2314
  malignant fibrous histiocytoma as, 2317
  melanoma as, 2317–2318, 2318f

Colorectal cancer (Continued)
  metastases of
    to bone, 2270
    to brain, 2270
    diffuse, 2270–2271
      biologic response modifiers for,
        2270–2271
      chemotherapy for, 2270
      palliative treatments for, 2271
    hepatic. See Hepatic metastases, of
      colorectal cancer.
    ovarian, 2270
    pulmonary, management of,
      2269–2270
      patient selection for, 2269
      pulmonary resection results and,
        2269–2270
    systemic, treatment of, 2201–2204,
      2203f
  neuroendocrine carcinomas as, 2313
  nonpolyposis, hereditary, 2159t,
    2169–2173
    clinical considerations in, 2169
    as colorectal cancer risk factor, 2188,
      2188b
    diagnosis of, 2171, 2171b, 2172b
    extracolonic cancers and, 2169
    genetic testing and counseling and,
      2171–2172
    genetics of, 2169–2171, 2170f
    surgical treatment of, 2172–2173
  recurrent, 2255–2269
    detection of, 2256–2259
      carcinoembryonic antigen for,
        2259
      endoscopy for, 2258–2259
      history and physical examination
        for, 2257
      laboratory and imaging studies
        for, 2258
      positron-emission tomography
        for, 2259
      surveillance for, 2256–2259, 2258f
    incidence of, 2255, 2256f
    locoregional, 2259–2269
      preoperative evaluation and
        patient selection for,
        2260–2262, 2261f, 2262b
      trimodality therapy for,
        2262–2269
    risk factors for, 2255–2256, 2257b
      technical, 2256
      tumor-related, 2255–2256
    trimodality therapy for, 2262–2269
      with fixed-resectable, anterior
        lesions, 2265
      with fixed-resectable, posterior
        lesions, 2265, 2266f, 2267f
      intraoperative delivery of electron
        beam radiation therapy and,
        2265–2267, 2268f
      with nonfixed lesions, 2265
      operative procedures for, 2263f,
        2263–2265, 2264f
      perineal wound closure and, 2267
      preoperative irradiation therapy
        and chemotherapy and,
        2262–2263

Colorectal cancer (Continued)
    results for locally recurrent
      disease, 2267–2269
  rhabdomyosarcoma as, 2317
  squamous cell carcinoma as, 2313
  surgical treatment of, 2330–2331
    low anterior resection for. See
      Colorectal resection, low anterior.
  in ulcerative colitis, 2082–2084
Colorectal carcinoma. See also Colon
  carcinoma; Colorectal adenocarcinoma;
  Colorectal cancer.
  blood and stool testing for, 1888–1889
  prevention of, 366–367
  risk of, in Barrett's esophagus, 366
  surgical intervention for, 366
Colorectal polyps, 2152–2158. See also
  Polyposis syndromes; specific polyposis
  syndromes.
  adenomatous, 2152–2157, 2153f
    adenoma to carcinoma sequence
      and, 2153
    follow-up surveillance for, 2157
    initial management of, 2155–2157
      complications of therapeutic
        colonoscopy and, 2157
      for malignant polyps, 2156f,
        2156–2157
      for pedunculated polyps,
        2155–2156
      for sessile polyps, 2156
      for small polyps, 2155
    screening for, 2153–2155, 2154t
  definitions and classification of, 2152,
    2153t
  hamartomatous, 2157f, 2157–2158, 2158f
  hyperplastic, 2158, 2158f
  inflammatory, 2158, 2159f
  laparoscopic surgery for
    outcomes of, 2353
    technical points for, 2353
  malignant, surgical treatment of, 2197
  pedunculated, 2152
  retention, 2157
Colorectal reconstruction, 2230–2231, 2231f
Colorectal resection
  low anterior, 2218–2233, 2219t
    anterior, 2228–2229
      in men, 2228–2229, 2229f
      in women, 2228, 2228f
    bowel division and distal traction for,
      2226–2227
    bowel preparation for, 2222
    colorectal reconstruction and,
      2230–2231, 2231f
    defining and dividing lateral
      attachments for, 2229, 2229f
    distal bowel management technique
      for, 2230, 2230f
    distal mural margins and extent of,
      2221
      distal mesorectal margin and, 2221
      lateral mesorectal margins and,
        2221
      lateral pelvic lymph nodes and,
        2221
      proximal vascular ligation and,
        2221

Colorectal resection (Continued)
  double-staple technique for, 2231–2232, 2232f
  extent of, 2221
  goals and terminology for, 2219–2220
  initial exploration for, 2222
  initial posterior dissection for, 2227, 2227f
  left colon mobilization for, 2226, 2226f
  level of distal transection for, 2230
  for obstructing cancer, 2220–2221
  open vs. laparoscopic, 2222
  patient position for, 2222–2223, 2223f
  patient selection for, 2220
  pelvic anatomy relevant for, 2222
  pelvic dissection for, 2222
  postoperative management with, 2232–2233
  preoperative radiation therapy with, 2220
  for rectal radiation injury, 2323
  retrosacral fascia division for, 2227–2228, 2228f
  sagittal anatomy and, 2223, 2223f
  sigmoid mobilization for, 2225–2226
    from left, 2225, 2225f
    from right, 2225f, 2225–2226
  steps for, 2351b, 2351f–2353f
  sympathetic nerves and, 2223, 2225
  synchronous organ resection and, 2221–2222
  transverse midpelvic anatomy and, 2223, 2224f
  vascular supply to rectum and left colon and, 2223, 2224f
  for rectal prolapse, 1961, 1964t
  with rectopexy, for rectal prolapse, 1961, 1961f, 1964t
Colorectal surgery. See also specific procedures.
  colonic physiology and, 1880–1881
  laparoscopic. See Laparoscopic colorectal surgery.
Colorectal trauma, 1972–1977, 1973t, 1974t
  diagnosis of, special problems in, 1975
  foreign bodies causing, 1977
  iatrogenic, 1976–1977
  initial resuscitation and assessment of, 1973–1975
  intraoperative management of, 1976, 1977f, 1977t
  postoperative complications of, 1978, 1978t
  preoperative management of, 1975–1976, 1976t
Colostomy
  abdominoperineal resection and, 2242–2243
  decompressing, for colonic obstruction, 2330
  end, 2364–2365
  end-loop, 2367
  following colorectal trauma, 1978, 1978t
  for high imperforate anus, 2396, 2398
  loop, 2366
  permanent, indications for, 2362, 2363b

Colovesical fistulas, in colonic diverticular disease, 2017–2018, 2018f
Columnar transformation, esophageal
  Barrett's esophagus and, 343–345
  gastroesophageal reflux and, 212, 212f, 230
  short esophagus and, 234
Combination tubes, 756–757
Comfrey, hepatotoxicity of, 1723
Common bile duct, 1442f, 1444
  anomalies of, 1448
  cysts of
    classification of, 1552
    congenital. See Choledochal cysts.
  diverticulum of, congenital, 1556, 1556f
  obstruction of, in pancreatitis, chronic, 1345–1348, 1346f
  stenosis of, in pancreatitis, chronic, 1311
  strictures of, in pancreatitis, chronic, 1345–1347, 1346f
    distal, biliary drainage procedures for, 1501, 1502f, 1502t, 1503
Common bile duct exploration
  external biliary fistulas following, etiology and prevention of, 1537–1538
  transcystic
    choledochoscopic, 1482–1484, 1483f, 1484f, 1484t
    laparoscopic techniques of, contraindications to, 1482, 1483t
Common bile duct stones. See Choledocholithiasis.
Compartments, esophageal, anatomy of, 11–12
Components separation techniques, for hernia repair, 682–683, 683f
Composite mesh, for ventral herniorrhaphy, 676
Computed tomography
  in abdominal trauma, in pediatric patients, 1807, 1807f
  with aortoenteric fistulas, 1114–1115, 1115f
  in appendicitis, 2142–2143
  of carcinoid tumors, 1183
  with choledochal cysts, 1553–1554
  with colon, rectal, and anal disorders, 1893–1894, 1894f
  in colorectal trauma, 1974
  in Crohn's disease, 1047–1048, 1048f, 1049f
  in diverticular disease, colonic, 2014b, 2014f, 2014–2015
  in duodenal injury, 766, 766f
  of echinococcal cysts, 1637, 1638f
  in esophageal cancer
    abdominal imaging and, 471
    chest imaging and, 471
    for staging, 77, 80f, 457, 457f
      therapy monitoring and, 461
  in esophageal perforation, 93–94, 531, 532f
  following esophageal surgery, 84
  in gastric adenocarcinoma, 907
  in gastric blunt trauma, 762
  in gastroduodenal artery aneurysms, 1280, 1280f

Computed tomography (Continued)
  of gastrointestinal stromal tumors, 1195
  of hepatic abscesses, pyogenic, 1646–1647, 1647f
  of hepatic cysts, solitary, 1630–1631
  in hepatocellular carcinoma, 1734–1735, 1735f
  for insulinoma localization, 1377, 1377f
  with intra-abdominal abscesses, 1102, 1104f
  in jaundice, obstructive, 1461f, 1461–1462
  with liver abscesses, amebic, 1654
  in mesenteric ischemia, 1252t, 1252–1253
  in mesenteric venous thrombosis, 1256
  of obturator hernias, 693, 693f
  in pancreatic and periampullary carcinoma, for preoperative staging, 1365
  with pancreatic cystic neoplasms, 1393f–1395f, 1393–1394
  with pancreatic pseudocysts, 1332–1333
  in pancreatic trauma, 1401, 1401f
  in pancreaticoduodenal artery aneurysms, 1280, 1281f
  in pancreatitis
    acute, 1299–1300, 1300f, 1302f
    chronic, 1347
  with paraesophageal hernia, 552, 553f
  in periampullary carcinoma, 1361–1362, 1362f
  in perineal pain syndromes, 2074
  in portal hypertension, 1757
  with retrorectal tumors, 2301
  in small bowel injury, 771–772, 772f
  in small bowel obstruction, 1030–1032, 1031f
  in small bowel volvulus, 1036, 1036f
  with splenic abscesses, 1818, 1819f
  in splenic artery aneurysms, 1275, 1276f
  in splenic trauma, 1799
  in Zollinger-Ellison syndrome, 863
Computed tomography enteroclysis, in small bowel obstruction, 1031
Computed tomography enterography, 1894, 1895f
Condylomata acuminata, pruritus ani associated with, 2070
Congenital diaphragmatic hernias, 36–37
Congenital disorders. See also specific disorders.
  esophageal, 32–33
  gastric, 35
  in pediatric patients. See Anorectal anomalies; Pediatric patients, congenital disorders in.
Congenital membranous web/diaphragm, 573
Conjoint tendon, 638, 638f
Connell suture, 1085
Constipation, 1878, 1878f, 1884–1885, 1929–1941
  in appendicitis, 2142
  botulinum toxin for, 1938–1939
  etiology of, 1929, 1930b
  evaluation of, 1929–1934
    clinical approach and, 1930–1931, 1931b

Constipation (Continued)
  diagnostic studies in, 1929–1930
  history and physical examination in, 1929
  Minnesota Multiphasic Personality Inventory in, 1934
  physiologic studies in, 1931–1934
    of colonic transit, 1931–1932, 1932f
    defecography as, 1933
    electromyography and pudendal nerve terminal motor latency as, 1933–1934
    manometry as, 1932–1933
    of small bowel transit, 1932
  results of, interpretation of, 1934
  examination for, 1888
  following surgery for anorectal anomalies, 2405
  rectal prolapse due to, 1958
  treatment of, 1934–1939
    pelvic floor retraining and biofeedback for, 1938–1939
    surgical, 1934–1938
      for colonic inertia, 1934, 1935t, 1936
      for paradoxical puborectalis contraction, 1936–1938, 1939f, 1940f, 1941t
      for pelvic outlet obstruction, 1936, 1937f, 1938f
Contact dermatitis, pruritus ani associated with, 2069
Contaminated cases, 2327
Continence. See Fecal continence; Fecal incontinence.
Cooper, Astley, 632
Cooper's ligament, 636
Copper salts, hepatotoxicity of, 1724
Corkscrew configuration, of small intestine, 1216, 1217f
"Corkscrew" esophagus, 419, 420f
Corticosteroids
  altered hormonal response to stress and, 2378
  for Crohn's disease, 1052, 2128
  in immunocompromised patients, 2377–2379
  immunosuppression induced by, 2377–2378
  impaired wound healing associated with, 2378
  for inflammatory bowel disease, 2090
  mechanism of action of, 2377t
  stress-dose, 2378–2379, 2379b, 2379t
Corticotropin-producing tumor, 1382–1383
  diagnosis of, 1383
  therapy for, 1383
Corynebacterium minutissimum infection, pruritus ani associated with, 2070
Costs, of obesity-related treatments, 929
Cough
  chronic, in gastroesophageal reflux disease, medical therapy for, 258–259
  gastroesophageal reflux disease associated with, diagnosis of, 171, 172f
  in tracheomalacia, 570

Counseling, for reoperative surgery, 1134
Courvoisier's sign, 1361
Cowden's disease, 894t, 897, 2159t, 2175–2176
COX-2
  bile acid injury to esophageal mucosa and, 232
  cancer and, 348
  esophageal cancer and, 445
COX-2 inhibitors
  for Barrett's esophagus, 258
  for esophageal cancer, 509–510
Cranial nerves, prenatal development of, 44
"Creeping fat," in Crohn's disease, 1058, 1058f
Cricopharyngeal achalasia, 427. See also Zenker's diverticulum.
Cricopharyngeal dysfunction, swallowing disorders caused by, 134
Cricopharyngeal myotomy. See Myotomy, cricopharyngeal.
Critical care physicians, on portal hypertension multidisciplinary team, 1767
Critical illness, gastric dysmotility in, 730
Crohn's disease, 1041–1067. See also Inflammatory bowel disease.
  abscesses in, 1065
    anorectal, 2057–2058
  anal fissures in, 2038
  anorectal, surgical treatment of, 2135
  capsule endoscopy of, 746f
  chronic, cancer risk in, 2191
  classification of, 1044
  clinical features of, 1044–1045, 2087–2088
  colonic, surgical treatment of, 2133, 2135
  colorectal cancer and, 2089
  diagnosis of, 2088f, 2088–2089
  diverticulitis vs., 2015
  duodenal, 1066, 1066f
  epidemiology of, 1041, 2085–2086
  esophageal, 91, 94f
  etiopathogenesis of, 2085–2086
  fistulas in, 1063–1065, 1094
    anorectal, 2057
    endoanal ultrasound in, 1912
    enterocutaneous, 1065
    enteroenteric, 1064
    enterogenital, 1065
    enterovesical and enteroureteral, 1064
    ileosigmoid, 1064
    treatment of, 1104–1105, 1110, 1111
  free perforation in, 1066
  ileal pouch–anal anastomosis failure in, 2121–2122
  imaging in, 1046–1049
    cross-sectional, 1047–1048, 1048f, 1049f
    endoscopy as, 1049–1052
    small bowel follow-through and enteroclysis as, 1046–1047, 1047f
    ultrasound, 1048–1049

Crohn's disease (Continued)
  laboratory findings in, 1045–1046
  laparoscopic surgery for
    outcomes of, 2354, 2356, 2356t
    technical points for, 2356
  medical treatment of, 1052f–1055, 2089–2093, 2127–2128
    5-aminosalicylic acid compounds in, 2089–2090
    antibiotics in, 2090–2091
    biological therapies in, 2092–2093
    corticosteroids in, 2090
    immunosuppressive agents in, 2091–2092
    to induce remission of active disease, 1052–1053
    to maintain remission, 1053
    nutrition in, 1053–1055
    sulfasalazine in, 2089
  natural history of, 1042
  pathology of, 1043–1044, 2086f, 2086–2087, 2087f
    gross features and, 1043, 1043f
    microscopic features and, 1043–1044, 1044f
  perianal, 2087–2088
  quality of life in, 2096
  risk factors and pathogenesis of, 1042–1043
    environmental factors in, 1042
    genetic factors in, 1042–1043
  of small bowel
    complicated, treatment of, 1063
    treatment of, 2132
  surgical treatment of, 1055–1067, 2094–2096, 2127, 2128–2138
    abdominal exploration and disease segment identification in, 1057–1058, 1058f
    abdominal incision for, 1056–1057, 1057f
    for anorectal disease, 2135
    bowel resection and anastomotic techniques for, 1059–1060
    bowel resection vs. strictureplasty for, 1058–1059
    bypass procedures for, 1063
    for colonic disease, 2130, 2133, 2135
    for fistulas, 2135–2136, 2137f–2138f
    ileal pouch–anal anastomosis for, 2130, 2132
    indications for, 1055b, 1055–1056, 2127
    laparoscopic, 1063
    laparoscopy-assisted, 2132
    operative concerns for, 2128–2130
      anastomotic technique as, 2129
      recurrence as, 2129
      resection margin as, 2129–2130
    for perianal abscesses, 2135, 2136f
    postoperative care for, 1066–1067
    preoperative evaluation and preparation for, 1056, 1056f, 2128
    for rectovaginal fistulas, 2136, 2138
    resection as, 2132, 2133f
    for small bowel, 2132
    stoma formation and, 1060, 1062–1063

Crohn's disease *(Continued)*
    stricturoplasty as, 2132, 2134f–2135f
        techniques for, 1059, 1059f–1062f
    ulcerative colitis differentiated from, 1050, 1050f
    ureteral obstruction in, 1065–1066
Crohn's Disease Endoscopic Index of Severity, 1051
Cronkhite-Canada syndrome, 884, 2159t, 2176
    small intestinal, 894t, 898
Crural repair, anterior, for gastric volvulus, 950
Cryoablation
    for Barrett's esophagus, 371
    hepatic, external biliary fistulas following, etiology and prevention of, 1540
    for hepatocellular carcinoma, 1738
    for metastatic colorectal cancer, 2283
Cryptococcus neoformans, splenic abscess due to, 1819
Cryptosporidiosis, diarrhea due to, in immunocompromised patients, 2382
Cullen's sign, 1299
Curling's ulcers, in pediatric patients, 961
"Cushing ulcers," in pediatric patients, 961
Cutaneous flushing, in carcinoid syndrome, 1182
Cyclooxygenase-2
    bile acid injury to esophageal mucosa and, 232
    cancer and, 348
    esophageal cancer and, 445
Cyclooxygenase-2 inhibitors
    for Barrett's esophagus, 258
    for esophageal cancer, 509–510
Cyclophosphamide, hepatotoxicity of, 1723
Cyclosporine
    for gastrointestinal fistulas, 1104–1105
    hepatotoxicity of, 1722
    for inflammatory bowel disease, 2092
    mechanism of action of, 2377t
Cyst(s)
    bronchogenic, esophageal, 525, 525f
    choledochal. *See* Choledochal cysts.
    dermoid, retrorectal, 2302, 2302t
    duplication
        esophageal, 570–572
            evaluation of, 572, 572f
            imaging of, 82–83
            treatment of, 572, 573f
        gastric, 888
        small intestinal, 901, 1221–1223, 1222f
    enterogenous, retrorectal, 2302, 2302t
    epidermoid, retrorectal, 2302, 2302t
    esophageal, 524b, 524–525, 525f
        endoscopic ultrasonography in, 123–124, 124f
    gastric, esophageal, 525, 525f
    glandular, gastric, 884
    hepatic, 1630–1638
        cystic neoplasms and, 1636, 1636f, 1637f
        echinococcal, 1636–1638, 1638f
        in polycystic liver disease, 1634–1635, 1635f
        solitary, 1630–1633, 1631f–1634f

Cyst(s) *(Continued)*
    inclusion, esophageal, 525
    mesenteric, 1860
    neuroenteric, esophageal, 525
    pancreatic. *See* Pancreatic cystic neoplasms.
    small intestinal, in pediatric patients, 1221–1223, 1222f, 1223f
    splenic, 1813–1815
        nonparasitic
            congenital, 1814
            secondary (false), 1813, 1814
        parasitic, 1813–1814
        true, 1813
    tailgut, retrorectal, 2302t, 2302–2304, 2303f
Cyst fenestration, for hepatic cysts
    in polycystic liver disease, 1635
    solitary, 1632–1633
Cystadenocarcinoma
    biliary, 1534, 1636
        end-stage liver disease due to, 1687
    mucinous, 1391
        appendiceal distention by, 2150–2151
Cystadenomas
    biliary, 1526, 1636, 1636f, 1637f
    mucinous, 1390
        appendiceal distention by, 2150
Cystic artery, 1445, 1445f, 1446, 1446f
Cystic duct
    anatomy and embryology of, 1443, 1444
    anomalies of, 1448
Cystic duct artery, 1445
Cystic duct catheter technique, 1485
Cystic fibrosis, jejunoileal atresia associated with, 1219
Cystic veins, 1603
Cystoduodenostomy
    for choledochal cysts, 1554
    for pancreatic pseudocysts, 1339, 1342f
Cystoenterostomy, for choledochal cysts, 1554
Cystogastrostomy
    for pancreatic ductal disruption, 1352
    for pancreatic pseudocysts, 1335, 1339, 1340f–1341f
Cystohepatic ducts, 1603
Cystojejunostomy
    laparoscopic, 1339, 1342f
    for pancreatic pseudocysts, 1335, 1335f–1339f
Cytologic analysis, in gastric adenocarcinoma, 908
Cytomegalovirus infection, colitis due to, in immunocompromised patients, 2382

D

Daclizumab
    for islet transplantation, 1424
    mechanism of action of, 2377t
Dallemagne, Bernard, 7
Danazol, hepatotoxicity of, 1723
Dantrolene, hepatotoxicity of, 1722
Débridement, with hepatobiliary trauma, 1666

Decompression, long-tube, for small bowel obstruction, 1032
Deep vein thrombosis, with inguinal herniorrhaphy, laparoscopic, 667
Defecation, 1876, 1876f
    obstructed, 1879, 1879b
Defecography
    with colon, rectal, and anal disorders, 1893
    in constipation, 1933
    in fecal incontinence, 1920
    in obstructed defecation, 1879b
Deglutitive inhibition, 52–53, 54f
Deglutitive lower esophageal sphincter relaxation, 54
DeLorme procedure
    for rectal prolapse, 1962, 1962f–1964f, 1964, 1964t
    for solitary rectal ulcer syndrome, 2076
Delta agents. *See* Hepatitis D.
Denk, Wolfgang, 4
Dental caries, gastroesophageal reflux disease associated with, diagnosis of, 171
Depression, with levator spasm, 2075
Dermatitis, pruritus ani associated with, 2069
Dermatologic conditions, pruritus ani associated with, 2069–2070
Dermatomyositis, esophageal motility disorders in, 140
Dermoid cysts, retrorectal, 2302, 2302t
Deroofing, of hepatic cysts, in polycystic liver disease, 1635
Desmoid(s)
    in familial adenomatous polyposis, 2161
    recurrent, reoperative surgery for, 1141
Desmoid precursor lesions, 2161
Desmoid reaction, 2161
Devascularization procedures, for bleeding varices, 1763
Dextropropoxyphene, hepatotoxicity of, 1723
DGER. *See* Duodenogastroesophageal reflux.
Diabetes mellitus
    esophageal motility disorders in, 140
    islet transplantation for. *See* Islet transplantation.
    obesity and, bariatric surgery and, 938
    in pancreatitis, chronic, 1345
    type 1, pancreas transplantation for. *See* Pancreas transplantation.
Diabetic neuropathy, diarrhea in, 1880
Diagnostic peritoneal lavage
    in abdominal trauma, in pediatric patients, 1807–1808
    in colorectal trauma, 1974
    in gastric trauma, 762–763
Diamond-shaped island flaps, for anal stenosis, 2064, 2064f
Diaphragm
    dysfunction of, with inguinal herniorrhaphy, laparoscopic, 667
    pelvic, perineal pain and, 2072
    prenatal development of, 35–36, 37f

Diaphragmatic hernias, 549–561
  congenital, 36–37, 560–561
    Bochdalek, 561
    Morgagni, 560
  paraesophageal. *See* Paraesophageal
    hernias.
  parahiatal, 560
  postoperative, 560
  recurrent, reoperative surgery for,
    1141–1142
  traumatic, 560
Diaphragmatic hiatus, 100
Diarrhea, 1885
  in afferent loop syndrome, 878
  in appendicitis, 2142
  in carcinoid syndrome, 1182
  in Crohn's disease, 1045
  following gastrectomy, 873–874, 874f
    reoperative surgery for, 1138–1139
  following vagotomy, 809
  functional, 1879–1880
  with gastrointestinal fistulas, 1098
  with ileostomy, 1081
  in pancreatitis, chronic, 1345
  pruritus ani and, 2068
  in short-bowel syndrome, controlling,
    1165
Diathermy, bipolar, for hemorrhoids, 2031,
  2031f, 2033
Diazepam, for endoscopic retrograde
  cholangiopancreatography, 1491
Diclofenac, hepatotoxicity of, 1722
Didanosine, hepatotoxicity of, 1720
Diet. *See also* Nutrition.
  Barrett's esophagus and, 343
  esophageal cancer and, 443, 445
  for fecal incontinence, 1921
  following bariatric surgery, 938
  gastroesophageal reflux disease and,
    200, 252
  pancreatic adenocarcinoma and, 1359
  pruritus ani and, 2068
  resumption of, following laparoscopic
    colorectal surgery, 2343
Dieulafoy's lesions, 886–887
  endoscopic appearance of, 740, 740f
  symptoms and diagnosis of, 887
  treatment of, 887
Diffuse esophageal spasm, 139–140,
  419–421
  examinations in, 419–421
  historical background of, 419
  imaging in, 73, 73f
  manometric features of, 419–420, 420t,
    421f
  treatment of, 421
Diffuse gastrointestinal hemangiomatosis,
  887
Diffuse large B-cell lymphoma, pathology
  of, 1200, 1202f, 1203
Digestion
  duodenal, 978–980
  mesenteric circulation and, 1242–1243
  small intestinal. *See* Small intestinal
    epithelium, digestion and absorption
    and.
Digestive system, embryonic development
  of, 31, 32f

Dilators, for esophageal stricture dilatation,
  237, 238f, 239f
Diloxanide furoate, for liver abscesses,
  amebic, 1655
Dissolution therapy, for bile duct stones,
  1495–1496
Distal splenorenal shunt, for bleeding
  varices, 1762–1763
  follow-up for, 1762–1763
  management of, 1762
  procedure for, 1762, 1762f
Disulfiram, hepatotoxicity of, 1721
Diverticula. *See also* Diverticulitis;
  Diverticulosis.
  cervical, lateral (Killian-Jamison), 95
  colonic, 2012, 2013f
    giant, 2019–2020, 2021f
  of common bile duct, congenital, 1556,
    1556f
  epiphrenic, 433–437
    diagnosis of, 433f, 433–434
    pathophysiology of, 433
    symptoms of, 433
    treatment of, 434–435
      surgical, methods and results of,
        434f–437f, 435–437
  esophageal
    imaging of, 94–95, 96f
    midesophageal, 437–438, 438f,
      439f
    pulsion, 94, 96f
    Zenker's, 94–95, 96f
  of gallbladder, 1449–1450, 1451f
  periampullary, 780
  pharyngoesophageal. *See* Zenker's
    diverticulum.
  small bowel. *See* Duodenal diverticula;
    Jejunoileal diverticula; Meckel's
    diverticula.
  "tenting" of, 94, 96f
  Zenker's. *See* Zenker's diverticulum.
Diverticular disease. *See also* Diverticula;
  Diverticulitis; Diverticulosis.
  colonic, 2012–2027
    clinical features of, 2015–2021
      atypical, 2021, 2021t
      in cecal diverticulitis, 2019,
        2020f
      diseases confused with
        diverticulitis and, 2015f,
        2015–2016
      with diverticular hemorrhage,
        2016, 2016f, 2017f
      diverticulitis and, 2015
      with fistulas, 2017–2018, 2018f
      with generalized peritonitis, 2018,
        2019f
      with giant diverticula, 2019–2020,
        2021f
      in immunocompromised patients,
        2020
      with intestinal obstruction,
        2018–2019
      with pericolic abscess, 2016–2017
      in subacute diverticulitis, 2016
      in young patients, 2021
    diagnostic modalities for, 2012–2015,
      2013f, 2014b, 2014f, 2014t

Diverticular disease *(Continued)*
    laparoscopic surgery for
      outcomes of, 2353–2354, 2355t
      technical points for, 2354
    medical management of, 2022
    pathophysiology and epidemiology
      of, 2012, 2013f
    surgical management of, 2022–2027
      with bleeding, 2026–2027
      elective resection as, 2022–2024,
        2023f, 2024f
      emergency surgery for,
        2024–2025, 2025f
      for obstruction, 2025–2026, 2026f
      for postresection diverticulitis,
        2027
  in immunocompromised patients, 2381
Diverticular hemorrhage, colonic, 2016,
  2016f, 2017f
Diverticular resection
  colonic, postresection diverticulitis
    following, 2027
  elective, for colonic diverticular disease,
    2022–2023, 2023f, 2024f
Diverticulectomy
  early development of, 5–6
  epiphrenic, for epiphrenic diverticulum,
    435, 435f, 436f
  esophageal, complications of, 618f,
    618–619, 619f
  with esophagomyotomy, for epiphrenic
    diverticulum, 435
  incidental, for Meckel's diverticulum, 787
  for Meckel's diverticulum, 788–789
  pharyngoesophageal, for Zenker's
    diverticulum, methods and results of,
    430–431
  for Zenker's diverticulum, 396
Diverticulitis. *See also* Diverticula.
  colonic
    clinical features of, 2015
    Crohn's disease vs., 2015
    diseases confused with, 2015f,
      2015–2016
    postresection, surgical treatment of,
      2027
    subacute (persistent), 2016
  Meckel's, 787, 789f
Diverticulization, duodenal, 768
Diverticulopexy
  early development of, 6
  for Zenker's diverticulum, 396
Diverticulosis. *See also* Diverticula.
  colonic, 1880
  painful, 2016
Diverticulum hepatis, 1598
Diverting stomas, 2365
Dobbhoff tube, 750, 751f
Dobutamine, mesenteric blood flow and,
  1243t
Domperidone
  for gastroesophageal reflux disease, 253
  for gastroparesis, 921
Dopamine, mesenteric blood flow and,
  1243, 1243t
Dor fundoplication, 276, 277f
  for achalasia, 416
  for esophageal perforation, 417

Dor fundoplication (Continued)
  laparoscopic
    for epiphrenic diverticulum,
      435–437, 437f
    surgical technique for, 282
  results with, 283
"Downhill" varices, 95, 97f
Doxorubicin, esophageal malformations
  due to, 564
Drainage
  external, of pancreatic pseudocysts,
    1341–1342
  internal, of pancreatic pseudocysts,
    1335, 1335f–1342f, 1339
    laparoscopic, 1339, 1342f
  laparoscopic, for splenic abscesses, 1820
  for pancreatitis, chronic, 1314–1315
    "extended" procedures for, rationale
      for, 1314–1315, 1315f–1317f
    indications for, 1316–1317, 1318f
    rationale for, 1314
  percutaneous
    for hepatic abscesses, pyogenic, 1649
    for liver abscesses, amebic, 1656
    of pancreatic pseudocysts, 1333–1334
    for splenic abscesses, 1820
  surgical
    for hepatic abscesses, pyogenic,
      1649–1650
    for liver abscesses, amebic, 1656
Droperidol, for endoscopic retrograde
  cholangiopancreatography, 1491
Drug(s), illicit, ingested packages of, 943,
  943f
Drug therapy. See also specific drugs and drug
  types.
  for bleeding varices, 1624
  immunosuppression due to, 2375–2376,
    2377t
  pancreatitis due to, 1299
  pharmacobezoars and, 943, 944, 944t
  pruritus ani associated with, 2069
Drug-induced liver disease, 1717–1724
  alternative remedies and, 1724
  conditions associated with, 1719–1724
    cholestasis as, 1722–1723
    cirrhosis as, 1719t, 1720–1721
    hepatic tumors as, 1719t, 1723–1724
    hepatitis as, 1719t, 1720–1721
      acute, 1721
      chronic, 1722
    hepatocellular zone 1 necrosis as,
      1719t, 1720
    hepatocellular zone 3 necrosis as,
      1719t, 1719–1720
    immunoallergy as, 1721
    metabolic idiosyncrasy and, 1722
    mitochondrial cytopathies as, 1719t,
      1720
    steatohepatitis as, 1719t, 1720–1721
    vascular toxicity as, 1723
  diagnosis and treatment of, 1718,
    1719t
  environmental agents and, 1724
  epidemiology of, 1717
  fulminant liver failure as, 1703
  hepatotoxic reactions to, 1615
  mechanisms of liver injury and, 1718

Drug-induced liver disease (Continued)
  pathophysiology of, 1717–1718
  recreational drugs and, 1724
Drummond, artery of, 1239
DualMesh, for ventral herniorrhaphy, 676,
  676f
Ductal epithelial cells, pancreatic, 1290f,
  1290–1291, 1291f
Ducts of Luschka, 1444
Ductus venosus, 1598
Dumping syndrome
  following gastrectomy, 809, 870–873, 872f
  following gastric bypass, 934
  reoperative surgery for, 1138–1139
Duodenal adenocarcinoma, 915–916
Duodenal cap, 964, 966f
Duodenal carcinoids, 1181
  treatment of, 1185
Duodenal diverticula, 775–783, 776f, 777f,
  977
  complications of, 779–781
    biliary-pancreatic, 780–781
    hemorrhage as, 780
    obstruction as, 779
    perforation as, 779
  diagnosis of, 777–779, 778f–780f
  disease associated with, 776–777
  management of, 781–783
    nonoperative, 781
    operative, 781f–784f, 781–783
  pathogenesis of, 775–776
  symptoms of, 777
Duodenal fistulas
  with duodenal injuries, 768
  etiology of, 1093–1096
  treatment of, 1110
Duodenal function, gastrin and, 985
Duodenal injury, 764–770
  anatomy and, 764
  with biliary stent placement, 1095
  diagnosis of, 765–766, 766f
  historical background of, 764
  with laparoscopic cholecystectomy, 1094
  management of, 766, 767f, 768–770,
    769f
  mechanisms of, 765
  morbidity and mortality with, 770
  with percutaneous transhepatic wire
    placement, 1095
  physiology and, 764–765
Duodenal motility, intrinsic and extrinsic
  control of, 985
Duodenal obstruction
  with duodenal diverticula, 779
  in pancreatic and periampullary
    carcinoma
    nonoperative palliation of,
      1365–1366
    operative palliation of, 1366–1367
  with pancreatic pseudocysts, 1344
  in pancreatitis, chronic, 1311,
    1348–1349, 1349f
  in pediatric patients, 952–954
    clinical features and diagnosis of,
      953, 953f, 954f
    embryology and etiology of, 952
    incidence and epidemiology of, 952
    management of, 953–954, 955f

Duodenal perforation
  with duodenal diverticula, 779
  treatment of, 1108–1110
Duodenal reflux, esophageal mucosal injury
  and, 230–232
  animal studies of, 230
  human studies of, 230–231
  mechanism of, 231–232
Duodenal resection, for duodenal
  adenocarcinoma, 915
Duodenal stump fistulas, treatment of,
  1110
Duodenal stump leakage, 1093–1094
Duodenal switch operation
  for bile reflux gastritis, 1146–1147,
    1147f
  failed, revision surgery for, 1146
Duodenal ulcers
  intractable, elective surgery for, 792–798
    choice of operation for, 796–798,
      798f, 798t
    drainage procedures as, 794–795
    gastric resection procedures as,
      795–796, 796f–798f
    laparoscopic, 798, 799f
    for recurrent ulcers, 798
    vagotomy as, 792–794
  pathogenesis of, 811–812
  perforated, emergency surgery for, 805,
    806f, 807f
  surgery for, gastric outlet obstruction
    following, reoperation for,
    1136–1137
Duodenocolic fistulas, in Crohn's disease,
  1094
Duodenocolic ligament, 1863
Duodenocutaneous fistulas, in Crohn's
  disease, 1094
Duodenoduodenostomy, for annular
  pancreas, 1407–1408, 1408f
Duodenogastric reflux, 185
Duodenogastroesophageal reflux, 185,
  190–195
  assessment of, 191–195
    Barostat test for, 195
    basal acid secretion for, 195
    electrogastrography for, 195
    gastric acid secretion for, 195
    impedance measurement for, 195
    24-hour bilirubin monitoring for,
      193–195, 194f, 194t
    24-hour gastric pH monitoring for,
      191f–193f, 191–193, 192t
  with Barrett's esophagus, 190
  diagnosis of, 168–169
  with gastroesophageal reflux disease,
    194
  with postgastrectomy syndrome, 190
Duodenojejunostomy
  for duodenal injury, 768
  Roux-en-Y
    for duodenal diverticula, 782, 783f
    for gastroduodenal fistulas, 1110
    for superior mesenteric artery
      syndrome, 975, 975f
Duodenostomy
  for gastroduodenal fistulas, 1110
  tube, for duodenal stump fistulas, 1110

Duodenotomy
    for bleeding ulcers, 824–825, 825f
    with inversion and mucosal excision, for
        duodenal diverticula, 781
    in Zollinger-Ellison syndrome, 865, 865f,
        868
Duodenum. *See also* Small intestine.
    anatomy of, 964, 965f–967f, 968, 969f,
        970f, 971–977
        adult abnormalities of, 971, 974–977
        arterial, 968, 971f
        histology and, 971, 973f
        innervation and, 971, 974f
        lymphatic, 968
        venous, 968, 972f
    Crohn's disease of, 1066, 1066f
    embryology of, 947
    pathophysiologic aspects of, in
        esophageal disease, 184–185
    physiology of, 977–985
        absorption and digestion and,
            978–980
            of calcium, 979
            of iron, 979–980, 980f
            of macronutrients, 980
        endocrine, 980–985, 981t
            cholecystokinin and, 980–981,
                981t
            endorphins and, 984
            enkephalins and, 984
            gastric inhibitory polypeptide
                and, 981t, 981–982
            gastrin and, 981t, 985
            gastrin-releasing peptide and,
                981t, 984
            ghrelin and, 981t, 984
            melatonin and, 981t, 985
            motilin and, 981t, 982
            neuropeptide Y and, 981t
            neurotensin and, 981t, 983
            nitric oxide and, 981t, 983
            opioids and, 981t
            pancreatic polypeptide and, 981t,
                984
            peptide YY and, 981t, 984–985
            secretin and, 980, 981t
            serotonin and, 981t, 982–983
            somatostatin and, 981t, 982
            substance P and, 981t, 983–984
            vasoactive intestinal peptide and,
                981t, 983
        in esophageal disease, 184–185
        exocrine, 977–978, 978f, 979f
    prenatal development of, 34
Duplications
    cystic
        esophageal, 570–572
            evaluation of, 572, 572f
            imaging of, 82–83
            treatment of, 572, 573f
        gastric, 888
        small intestinal, 901, 1221–1223,
            1222f
    esophageal, 524b, 524–525, 525f
    small intestinal, in pediatric patients,
        1221–1223, 1222f, 1223f
    tubular, of small intestine, 1221, 1223f
Duval procedure, in pediatric patients, 1410

Dynamic myoplasty, for fecal incontinence,
    1923–1924
Dysejaculation syndrome, following hernia
    surgery, 654
Dysphagia
    in achalasia, 407, 411
    with epiphrenic diverticulum, 433
    in esophageal cancer, 61
    esophageal carcinoma and, 468, 469t
    in esophageal disease, 57
    in esophageal motility disorders, 71
    following esophagomyotomy, for
        achalasia, 620
    following fundoplication, 611
    following Heller myotomy, 417
    imaging in, gastric, 66
    myogenic, cricopharyngeal myotomy for,
        384, 386, 386f, 387f, 388
    neurologic, cricopharyngeal myotomy
        for, 382, 384, 385f–386f
    oropharyngeal, 374
        assessment of, 377–378, 378t
        causes of, 374, 375b
        surgical management of, 378–390
            cricopharyngeal myotomy for,
                379–384
            for idiopathic upper esophageal
                sphincter dysfunction, 388,
                389f
            indications for, 378–379
            for myogenic dysphagia, 384, 386,
                386f, 387f, 388
            after neck surgery, 388, 390
            operative technique for,
                379f–382f, 379–380
    partial fundoplication for, 278–279
    patient approach for, 61
    retrosternal, low, after antireflux
        procedures, 609
Dysplasia
    Barrett's esophagus and
        ablation of, rationale for, 367
        classification of, 359
        development of, incidence of, 360
        grading of, 347–348
        high-grade, 219, 219f
            adenocarcinoma distinguished
                from, 359–360
            prevention of, 366–367
            risk of, 366
            surgical management of,
                361–363, 362f
        low-grade
            prevalence of, 360, 361t
            surgical management of,
                360–361, 361b
        high-grade
            Barrett's esophagus and, 219, 219f
                adenocarcinoma distinguished
                    from, 359–360
                prevention of, 366–367
                risk of, 366
                surgical management of,
                    361–363, 362f
            colorectal cancer and, 2192
            prevention of, 366–367
        low-grade, Barrett's esophagus and
            prevalence of, 360, 361t

Dysplasia *(Continued)*
        surgical management of, 360–361,
            361b
    in residual rectal mucosa, following ileal
        pouch–anal anastomosis, 2112
    ulcerative colitis with, 2082–2084
        surgical management of, restorative
            proctocolectomy for, 2335
Dysrhythmias, with inguinal herniorrhaphy,
    laparoscopic, 667

E

Eating, colonic motor response to, 1875
Echinococcal cysts
    hepatic, 1636–1638, 1638f
    splenic, 1832
Echoendoscopes, electronic, curvilinear,
    113–114, 115f
Ectopic rests, congenital, esophageal, 522
Ectopic tissue polyps, small intestinal,
    892–893
Ectropion, 2062
Eczema, atopic, pruritus ani associated with,
    2070
Edmonton Protocol, 1426, 1427
Edrophonium test, for esophageal motility
    disorders, 160
Educator, as clinical nurse specialist role, in
    palliative treatment, for esophageal
    cancer, 497
EEA staplers, 1087
Efferent loop obstruction, following
    gastrectomy, 809, 877, 878
Elderly people, appendicitis in, 2144
Electrical hazard zone, 639–640
Electrocoagulation, bipolar, for esophageal
    cancer, 489t, 492
Electrogalvanic muscle stimulation, for
    perineal pain syndromes, 2074
Electrogastrography, in esophageal disease,
    195
Electrohydraulic lithotripsy, for bile duct
    stones, 1495
Electromyography
    anal sphincter, in obstructed defecation,
        1879b
    in constipation, 1933
    in perineal pain syndromes, 2074
Embolization
    for celiac artery aneurysms, 1278–1279
    radiographic, of injured spleens, in
        pediatric patients, 1808, 1810f
    for splenic artery aneurysms, 1277
    transarterial, hepatic abscesses following,
        pyogenic, 1642
    transcatheter
        for mesenteric artery branch
            aneurysms, 1281–1282
        for superior mesenteric artery
            aneurysms, 1279
Emphysema
    preperitoneal, with inguinal
        herniorrhaphy, laparoscopic, 667
    subcutaneous, with inguinal
        herniorrhaphy, laparoscopic,
        667

Index

En bloc esophagectomy, for localized esophageal cancer, 477–478

Encephalopathy, hepatic
  in end-stage liver disease, 1694, 1694b
  portal hypertension, 1756

Endarterectomy, mesenteric artery, 1258, 1259f

End-loop stomas, 2366–2368
  colostomy and, 2367
  ileocolostomy and, 2367–2368, 2369f
  ileostomy and, 2367, 2368f

Endoanal ultrasound, 1909–1914
  with anal canal neoplasms, 1912–1913, 1913f, 1913t
    with retrorectal tumors, 1913, 1914f
  with anal sphincter defects and fecal incontinence, 1910–1911, 1911f
  in fecal incontinence, 1920, 1920f
  normal anatomy on, 1909–1910, 1910f
  in perianal sepsis and fistula-in-ano, 1911–1912, 1912f
  with rectovaginal fistulas, 1912
  in solitary rectal ulcer syndrome and colitis cystica profunda, 1913–1914, 1914f

Endobiliary forceps biopsy, in malignant bile duct obstruction, 1508

EndoCinch therapy. See Gastroplasty, endoluminal.

Endocrine disorders, intestinal motility and, 926

Endometriosis, small intestinal, 893

Endorectal magnetic resonance imaging, in rectal cancer, 2209

Endorectal ultrasound, 1899–1909
  with colon, rectal, and anal disorders, 1893, 1894f
  limitations of, 1907
  after neoadjuvant therapy, accuracy of, 1908
  normal anatomy on, 1900, 1901f
  for postoperative follow-up, 1908–1909, 1909f
  in rectal cancer, 1900–1909, 2209
    staging and
      accuracy for, 1900–1903, 1903t
      depth of invasion and, 1904t, 1904–1906
      modification of staging system and, 1907, 1907t
      nodal involvement and, 1906f, 1906–1907
      uT0 lesions and, 1904, 1904f
      uT1 lesions and, 1904, 1905f
      uT2 lesions and, 1905, 1905f
      uT3 lesions and, 1905f, 1905–1906
      uT4 lesions and, 1906, 1906f
  technique of, 1899–1900, 1900f
  three-dimensional, 1909

Endorphins, duodenal function and, 981t, 984

Endoscopes
  electronic, 113–114, 115f
  standard, for endoscopic ultrasonography, 113, 113f
  ultrasound, radial mechanical, 112f, 112–113

Endoscopic balloon dilation, for gastric bleeding, 743

Endoscopic band ligation, for gastric bleeding, 743, 743f

Endoscopic clips, for gastric bleeding, 743, 743f

Endoscopic examination. See also specific techniques, e.g. Colonoscopy.
  in achalasia, 407, 411–412
  anorectal, 1889–1891
  capsule
    in Crohn's disease, 1051f, 1051–1052
    of small bowel, 745–746, 746f
  in caustic ingestions, 542, 542b
  chromoendoscopy as, in Barrett's esophagus, 104
  with colonic vascular ectasias, 1991
  complications of, esophageal perforation as, 529
  in Crohn's disease, 1049–1052
    capsule endoscopy as, 1051f, 1051–1052
    push endoscopy as, 1050f, 1050–1051
  to detect tumor relapse, of colorectal cancer, 2258–2259
  with duodenal diverticula, 779, 779f
  esophageal, 100–109
    in Barrett's esophagus
      conventional technique for, 102–104, 103f, 104f
      specialized techniques for, 104, 105f
    in esophageal cancer, 108–109, 109f
    in esophageal carcinoma, 469–470
    esophageal perforation due to, 529
    for esophageal reconstruction, 581
    in esophageal spasm, 419
    following antireflux surgery, 106, 108, 108f
    of gastroesophageal junction, 100–102, 101f, 102f
    in gastroesophageal reflux disease, 59–60
    normal appearance on, 100, 101f, 207–210, 208b, 208f–210f, 210b
    in nutcracker esophagus, 422
    in reflux esophagitis, 105–106, 106t, 107f
    for staging of esophageal cancer, 455–456
    for structural abnormality detection, 143
    surveillance, for Barrett's esophagus, 350
    of swallowing, 378
  gastric, 733–741
    in gastric adenocarcinoma, 907
    indications for, 733
    instrumentation for, 733–734
    pathology on, 736–741, 737f–741f
    patient preparation for, 734
    technique for, 734f–736f, 734–736
  with gastrointestinal fistulas, 1106
  with leiomyoma, 517, 518f
  magnification, in Barrett's esophagus, 104, 105f
  with pancreatic tumors, unusual, 1432
  with paraesophageal hernia, 552

Endoscopic examination (Continued)
  in periampullary carcinoma, 1363
  in portal hypertension, 1757
  push, in Crohn's disease, 1050f, 1050–1051
  screening, for Barrett's esophagus, 350
  of small bowel, 745f–747f, 745–747
    with benign tumors, 890
    double-balloon, 747

Endoscopic gastrostomy, percutaneous, in pediatric patients, 960

Endoscopic mucosal resection, for Barrett's esophagus, 370

Endoscopic polypectomy, fistulas due to, 1095

Endoscopic retrograde cholangiography
  with bile duct strictures, 1578, 1578f
  with biliary fistulas, 1542

Endoscopic retrograde cholangiopancreatography, 1490–1513
  with alkaline phosphatase elevation, 1615
  cannulation success rates with, 1494
  cholangiography and, 1493, 1493f
  in cholangitis, acute, 1499–1500
  cholecystectomy and, laparoscopic, 1497, 1498f
  with choledochal cysts, 1553
    anomalous pancreaticobiliary union and, 1508–1509
  complications of, 1494
    fistulas as, 1095
    gastroduodenal perforations as, 1108–1110
  in gallstone pancreatitis, acute, 1497–1499, 1498–1499
  indications for, 1463, 1490
  laparoscopic cholecystectomy and, 1497, 1498f
  in malignant bile duct obstruction, tissue sampling and, 1507–1508
  with pancreatic cystic neoplasms, 1394, 1395f
  with pancreatic pseudocysts, 1332, 1332f
  with pancreaticoduodenal injury, 769
  in pancreatitis
    acute, 1300
      mild, 1302
    chronic, 1347
    severe, necrotizing, 1303
  pancreatitis following, 1298
  pancreatography and, 1493, 1493f
  in pediatric patients, 1412–1413
  in periampullary carcinoma, 1362–1363, 1363f
  preparation for, 1490–1491, 1492t
  in primary sclerosing cholangitis, 1503, 1503f, 1503–1504, 1504, 1561, 1562f
  technique for, 1491–1493

Endoscopic sphincterotomy, 1493
  complications of, 1494

Endoscopic therapy. See also specific procedures.
  for achalasia, 409
  for bezoars, 945
  for bleeding, gastric, 741–745, 742f–744f
  for bleeding varices, 1624

Endoscopic therapy (Continued)
for chronic pancreatitis, 1321–1327,
1322f, 1322t
results after endotherapy for stones,
1324, 1324f
results after endotherapy for
stricture without stones, 1323
results after head resection with
pylorus-preserving
pancreaticoduodenectomy,
1325–1327
surgical resection techniques and,
1324, 1325f, 1326f
techniques for, 1323
for common bile duct stones
postoperative, 1593–1594
preoperative, 1590–1591
for duodenal diverticula, 781
for gastric cancer, 744–745
palliative, 914
for gastric volvulus, 1038–1039
mucosal reconstruction as, for gastric
adenocarcinoma, 909
transgastric surgery as, 745
for variceal bleeding, 1759, 1760f
for Zenker's diverticulum, 397–398,
398f, 429
methods and results of, 431–433, 432f
Endoscopic transgastric surgery, 745
Endoscopic ultrasonography
esophageal, 111–125
in achalasia, 124–125
of benign tumors, 122–123, 123t
of cysts, 123–124, 124f
of esophageal carcinoma, 116–122,
117b, 470f, 470–471
during clinical stage, 117–121,
118f–122f
during re-treatment stage,
121–122
esophageal wall and, 114–116, 115f,
116f
instruments and techniques for,
112–114, 112f–115f
in paraesophageal diseases, 125
for staging of esophageal cancer,
457–458, 458f
therapy monitoring and, 461
for structural abnormality detection,
143
ultrasonography fundamentals and,
111–112
of varices, 124, 125f
in gastric adenocarcinoma, 907
for insulinoma localization, 1378, 1378f
with leiomyoma, 517–519, 518f, 518t
in pancreatic and periampullary
carcinoma, for preoperative staging,
1365
in pancreatic carcinoma, 1354
with pancreatic cystic neoplasms, 1396
in periampullary carcinoma, 1363, 1364f
with small intestinal tumors, benign, 890
in Zollinger-Ellison syndrome, 864–865
Endoscopists, on portal hypertension
multidisciplinary team, 1767
Endovascular mesenteric revascularization,
1260–1261, 1263t, 1264t, 1265f

Endovascular therapy
for aortoenteric fistulas, 1273–1274
for celiac artery aneurysms, 1278–1279
for hepatic artery aneurysms, 1278
Enkephalins, duodenal function and, 984
Entamoeba infection, liver abscesses due to.
See Liver abscesses, amebic.
Enteral nutrition
for biliary surgery, 1622
for liver surgery, 1622
Enteric feeding, 753–755, 754f
gastric access for, 754–755
Enteric fistulas, 1096
congenital, 1096
in Crohn's disease, 1063–1065
enterocutaneous, 1065
enteroenteric, 1064
enterogenital, 1065
enterovesical and enteroureteral,
1064
ileosigmoid, 1064
treatment of, 1104–1105, 1110, 1111
infection causing, 1096
inflammatory causes of, 1096–1097
radiation-induced, 1097
traumatic, 1096
tumors causing, 1097
Enteritis
ischemic, on push enteroscopy, 745f
neutropenic, in immunocompromised
patients, 2382–2383
radiation. See Radiation enteritis.
Enterobius vermicularis infection, pruritus ani
associated with, 2070
Enterocervical fistulas, treatment of, 1114
Enterochromaffin cells, 1179, 1182
Enteroclysis
computed tomography, in small bowel
obstruction, 1031
laparoscopic, bowel injury during, 1136
small bowel, in Crohn's disease,
1046–1047, 1047f
in small bowel obstruction, 1030, 1030f
Enterocolitis, necrotizing, in premature
infants, 1227–1229, 1228f, 1229f
Enterocutaneous fistulas
in Crohn's disease, 1065
failure to close spontaneously, 1108
following ileal pouch–anal anastomosis,
2112
small intestinal, 1096
treatment of, 1110–1111
Enteroendocrine cells, small intestinal, 998
Enteroenteric fistulas
in Crohn's disease, 1064
treatment of, 1111f, 1111–1112
Enteroenterostomy, Braun, for bile reflux
gastritis, 877, 878f, 1146, 1146f
Enterofallopian fistulas, treatment of, 1114
Enterogenital fistulas, in Crohn's disease,
1065
Enterogenous cysts, retrorectal, 2302, 2302t
Enteroglucagon, small intestinal
neuroendocrine function and, 1018
Enterohepatic circulation, 1453–1454, 1457f
Enteropathy, neutropenic, in
immunocompromised patients,
2382–2383

Enteropathy-type T-cell lymphoma,
pathology of, 1205, 1205f, 1206t
Enteroscopy
intraoperative, 746–747
push, 745, 745f
with small intestinal tumors, benign,
890
sonde, push, with small intestinal
tumors, 890
Enterotomy, longitudinal, for gastric outlet
obstruction, 952
Enteroureteral fistulas, in Crohn's disease,
1064
Enterouterine fistulas, treatment of, 1114
Enterovaginal fistulas, treatment of,
1113–1114
Enterovesical fistulas
in Crohn's disease, 1064
treatment of, 1112f, 1112–1113
Enterra stimulator, 921–923, 922f
Enteryx, for endoscopic antireflux
procedures, 320–323, 325, 326t,
327t
complications of, 323
efficacy of, 321–323, 322t, 323f
histologic changes and, 321
patient selection for, 320
physiologic/anatomic mechanisms of,
330–331
precautions recommended with, 323
procedure with, 320–321, 321f
results with, 325, 326t, 327t
Eosinophilic esophagitis, esophageal
strictures in, 90, 93f
Epidermal growth factor receptors, for
esophageal cancer, 510
Epidermoid cysts, retrorectal, 2302, 2302t
Epidermolysis bullosa, esophageal strictures
in, 89
Epidermophyton infection, pruritus ani
associated with, 2070
Epigastric artery
inferior, 657, 659f, 673
superior, 673
Epinephrine, mesenteric blood flow and,
1243t
Epiphrenic diverticulum, 433–437
diagnosis of, 433f, 433–434
pathophysiology of, 433
symptoms of, 433
treatment of, 434–435
surgical, methods and results of,
434f–437f, 435–437
Epithelial cells, ductal, pancreatic, 1290f,
1290–1291, 1291f
Epithelioid hemangioendotheliomas,
hepatic, 1748–1749
Epithelium. See Esophageal epithelium;
Small intestinal epithelium.
Erasistratus, 632
Erlotinib, for colorectal cancer metastases,
2271
Erythrasma, pruritus ani associated with,
2070
Erythromycin
for bowel preparation, 831
for gastroparesis, 921
hepatotoxicity of, 1723

Erythromycin (Continued)
  for intestinal dysmotility, 926
  preoperative, 2328
Escherichia coli
  hepatic abscesses and, 1644
  overwhelming postsplenectomy infection
    and, 1782
  splenic abscess due to, 1819
Esomeprazole. See also Proton pump
  inhibitors.
  gastric acid secretion and, 727
Esophageal adenocarcinoma
  endoscopic examination in, 108–109,
    109f
  epidemiology of, 441, 442f
    age, sex, and race distribution and,
      442f, 442–443
    risk factors and, 443–446
      alcohol as, 443
      Barrett's esophagus as, 445
      diet and nutrition as, 443, 445
      gastroesophageal reflux disease
        as, 445
      Helicobacter pylori infection as,
        445–446
      lower sphincter-relaxing
        medications as, 445
      nonsteroidal anti-inflammatory
        drugs as, 445
      obesity as, 443, 443t, 444f
      tobacco as, 443
  high-grade dysplasia distinguished from,
    359–360
  invasive, in Barrett's esophagus, 219,
    219f
  prevention of, 366–367
  resection for, extent of, 475–477
  risk of nondysplastic Barrett's esophagus
    progression to, 365, 366t
Esophageal ampulla, radiographic
  appearance of, 66–67, 67f
Esophageal anastomosis, for short-segment
  esophagectomy, 291
Esophageal anatomy, 9–27
  of esophageal body, muscular, 16, 17f–19f
  of innervation, 23, 25–27
    extramural, 25–26, 26f, 27f
    intramural, 26
  lymphatic, 22–23, 24f
  macroscopic, 9–16
    abdominal anatomy and, 16
    anchorage and
      of cardia, 12–14, 14f
      of esophageal body, 12, 13f
      in neck, 12, 13f
    chest anatomy and, 15f, 15–16
    of compartments, 11–12
    diameter of esophagus and, 10–11
    of fascial planes, 11
    general aspects of, 9–10, 10f, 11f
    length of esophagus and, 10
    length of orthotopic bypass and, 10
    neck anatomy and, 14–15, 15f
    of periesophageal tissue, 11
  of sphincters, 17–18, 19f
  of tissues, 16f, 16–19
    tela submucosa as, 16f, 18
    tunica adventitia as, 16, 16f

Esophageal anatomy (Continued)
    tunica mucosa as, 16f, 18–19
    tunica muscularis as, 16f, 16–19,
      17f–19f
  vascular, 20–22
    arterial, 20, 20f, 21f
    venous, 20–22, 22f, 23f
Esophageal arteries, 20
Esophageal atresia, 563–571
  abnormalities associated with, 564,
    565f
  classification of, 564, 565f
  clinical findings and diagnostic
    evaluation of, 565, 566f
  development and, 563–564
  development of, 32–33
  historical background of, 563
  management of, 565–566
    complications of, 569–571, 571f
    operative, 566–569, 567f–570f
    pure, 568–569, 569f, 570f
Esophageal balloon distention, for
  esophageal motility disorders, 160–161
Esophageal biopsy, mucosal, 165t
Esophageal body
  anatomy of, 16f, 16–17
    muscle types and, 17, 19f
    muscular arrangement and, 17,
      17f–19f
  "corkscrew" appearance of, 73, 73f
  disorganized contractions of, 138–139
  motor disorders of, primary, 135–140,
    136b, 137t, 138f–140f
  "rosary-bead" appearance of, 73, 73f
  swallowing and, 129–132, 132f
Esophageal bolus clearance, tests to
  evaluate, 154–159
  ambulatory esophageal impedance and
    pH monitoring as, 158–159, 159f,
    160f
  esophageal transit scintigraphy as,
    154–155
  impedance testing as, 155–156, 157f,
    158, 158f
  multichannel intraluminal impedance
    as, 175–183
    combined with manometry, 175–176,
      178f, 179, 179f
    combined with pH monitoring,
      180f–183f, 180–181
    principles of, 175, 176f–178f
  videocineroentgenography as, 154, 155f,
    156f
Esophageal bypass, for strictures,
  intractable, 544–545
Esophageal cancer, 465–483. See also specific
  cancers.
  clinical features of, 446, 468, 469t
  diagnosis of, 469
  epidemiology of, 441–446, 442f, 466
    age, sex, and race distribution and,
      442f, 442–443
    changing, reasons for, 446
    mortality/prognosis and, 441–442
    risk factors and, 443–445
      alcohol as, 443
      Barrett's esophagus as, 445
      diet and nutrition as, 443, 445

Esophageal cancer (Continued)
    gastroesophageal reflux disease
      as, 445
    Helicobacter pylori infection as,
      445–446
    lower sphincter-relaxing
      medications as, 445
    nonsteroidal anti-inflammatory
      drugs as, 445
    obesity as, 443, 443t, 444f
    tobacco as, 443
  esophageal perforation associated with,
    538
  etiology of, 466t, 466–467
    of adenocarcinoma, 467
    of squamous cell carcinoma, 466
  evaluation of, 74–81, 469–472
    barium esophagography in, 469, 469f
    bronchoscopy in, 471
    chest radiography in, 469
    computed tomography in, 471
    endoscopic, 108–109, 109f
    endoscopic ultrasonography in, 470f,
      470–471
    for metastasis detection, 471–472
    minimally invasive surgery for staging
      and, 472
    radiologic appearance and, 74–76,
      75f–79f
    for recurrent esophageal cancer
      assessment, 79, 81
    for staging, 76–78
    for treatment evaluation, 79
    upper gastrointestinal endoscopy in,
      469–470
  historical background of, 465–466
  localized, en bloc esophagectomy for,
    477–478
  management of, 474–483
  multimodality treatment of, 499–510
    chemoradiation in, 505–508
      definitive therapy using, 505t,
        505–506
      preoperative, 506–508, 507t
    chemotherapy in, 502–505
      postoperative, 504t, 504–505
      preoperative, 502–504, 503t
    meta-analyses of, 508–509
      of postoperative chemoradiation,
        509
    radiation therapy in, 499–502
      postoperative, 501t, 501–502
      preoperative, 499–501, 500t
    rationale for, 499
  neoadjuvant therapy for, 482–483
  new treatment modalities for, 509–510
    cyclooxygenase-2 inhibitors as,
      509–510
    epidermal growth factor receptors as,
      510
    tumor necrosis factor as, 510
  palliative treatment of, 487–498
    endoscopic methods for, 488–493
      alcohol sclerotherapy as, 488,
        489t
      bougienage as, 488–489, 489t
      esophageal prostheses as, 489t,
        489–492

Esophageal cancer (*Continued*)
  photodynamic, 489t, 493
  thermal, 489t, 492–493
  oncologic management in, 493–497
    chemoradiation for, 495
    chemotherapy for, 495–496
    options for, 493
    with prominent local symptoms, 496, 496f
    radiotherapy for, 493–495
    with systemic symptoms, 496–497
  patient assessment for, 487–488, 488b, 489t
  surgical, 497
  for terminal patients, 497
  upper gastrointestinal clinical nurse specialist's role in, 497–498
  pathology of, 467b, 467–468
    of adenocarcinoma, 468, 468f
    of squamous cell carcinoma, 467–468, 468f
  patient approach for, 61, 61f
  recurrent, assessment of, 79, 81
  squamous cell, association with achalasia, 409
  stage-directed treatment of, 461–462
  staging methods for, 455–461
    barium contrast study as, 455, 456f
    bronchoscopy as, 456
    computed tomography as, 457, 457f
    endoscopic examination as, 455–456
    endoscopic ultrasonography as, 457–459, 458f
    laparoscopy as, 460
    minimally invasive surgery as, 472
    percutaneous ultrasonography as, 457
    positron-emission tomography as, 459f, 459–460
    therapy monitoring and, 460–461
    thoracoscopy as, 460
  staging systems for, 448–455, 472–474
    anatomic subsites and, 448–449, 449f
    cancer around gastroesophageal junction and, 450–451, 452f
    choice of, 451–455
    inadequacies in, 473–474, 474t
    nodal metastases and (N stage), 449b, 449–450, 450t, 451f, 452f, 453t–455t
    TNM, 472t, 472–473, 473t
    TNM residual tumor classification and, 455
    tumor infiltration depth and (T stage), 449
  surgical treatment of, 475–482
    complications of, 480t, 480–481
    extent of resection for early adenocarcinoma and, 475–477
    extent of resection for localized cancer and, 477t, 477–478
    historical background of, 3–5
    patient assessment for, 475, 476f
    postoperative care for, 480
    reconstruction and, 478–479
    results with, 481t, 481–482
    transhiatal esophagectomy as, 479–480

Esophageal cancer (*Continued*)
  TNM classification of, endoscopic ultrasonography for, 116–122, 117b
    in clinical state, 117–121, 118f–122f
    in re-treatment stage, 121–122
Esophageal claudication, 138–139
Esophageal clearance, evaluation of, barium examination for, 68
Esophageal compression, vascular, 573–574, 574f
Esophageal contraction abnormalities, tests to detect, 143–154
  ambulatory 24-hour esophageal manometry as, 152–154
  stationary esophageal manometry as, 144–146, 145f–155f, 145t, 150, 152
Esophageal cysts, 524b, 524–525, 525f
Esophageal dilatation
  for caustic ingestions, 544
  for esophageal strictures, 237, 238f, 239f, 240
  fistulas due to, 1095
Esophageal disorders. *See also specific conditions.*
  Barrett's esophagus as. *See Barrett's esophagus.*
  benign, end-stage
    clinical manifestations of, 286b, 286t, 286–287, 287t
    esophageal replacement for. *See Esophageal replacement, for end-stage benign esophageal disease.*
  congenital, 563–574. *See also specific disorders.*
    embryology and anatomic considerations in, 563, 564f
  delayed gastric emptying in, 185–190
    antroduodenal manometry and, 186–188, 188f, 188t, 189f, 190, 190t
    barium burger studies and, 190
    ^{13}C breathing test for, 185–186
    gastric emptying scintigraphy and, 185, 186f, 187f
  duodenum in, physiologic and pathophysiologic aspects of, 184–185
  gastric function tests in, 184–195
  malignant. *See Esophageal cancer.*
  motor. *See Dysphagia; Esophageal dysmotility.*
  reflux as. *See Gastroesophageal reflux disease.*
  stomach in, physiologic and pathophysiologic aspects of, 184–185
  symptoms of, 56–57, 57b
    mechanisms of, 57–58, 58f
Esophageal diverticula, surgery for, early development of, 5–6
Esophageal duplication cysts, 570–572
  evaluation of, 572, 572f
  imaging of, 82–83
  treatment of, 572, 573f
Esophageal duplications, 524b, 524–525, 525f
Esophageal dysmotility, 134–161. *See also specific disorders.*
  barium examination for, 68

Esophageal dysmotility (*Continued*)
  esophageal perforation associated with, 538
  imaging in, 71–74
  nonspecific, 71, 74
  partial fundoplication for, 278
  pathophysiology of, 134–142
    gastroesophageal reflux disease and, 140–142, 141f
    obesity and, 142, 142t
    of pharyngoesophageal swallowing disorders, 134–135, 135f, 136f
    of primary disorders of esophageal body and lower esophageal sphincter, 135–140, 136b, 137t, 138f–140f
    of secondary disorders, 140
  patient approach for, 61
  primary. *See also* Achalasia; Diffuse esophageal spasm; Nutcracker esophagus.
    imaging in, 71–74, 72f, 73f
  secondary, imaging in, 74
  surgery for, early development of, 5
  symptoms of, 71
  tests for assessment of, 142–161
    for esophageal bolus clearance evaluation, 154–159
      ambulatory esophageal impedance and pH monitoring as, 158–159, 159f, 160f
      esophageal transit scintigraphy as, 154–155
      impedance as, 155–156, 157f, 158, 158f
      videocineroentgenography as, 154, 155f, 156f
    for esophageal contraction abnormality detection, 143–154
      ambulatory 24-hour esophageal manometry as, 152–154
      stationary esophageal manometry as, 144–146, 145f–155f, 145t, 150, 152
    for esophageal structural abnormality detection, 143
    esophageal symptom provocation, 159–161
      acid perfusion test as, 159–160
      edrophonium test as, 160
      esophageal balloon distention as, 160–161
    for increased esophageal exposure to gastric and duodenal juice detection, 24-hour esophageal pH monitoring as, 161
Esophageal epithelium
  columnar
    ciliated, prenatal development of, 40–41, 41f
    detection of, barium examination for, 69, 70f
  squamous, stratified, prenatal development of, 41
  vacuolization of, 39–40, 40f
Esophageal impedance, measurement of, in esophageal disease, 195

Esophageal injury, detection of, barium examination for, 68–69, 69f, 70f
Esophageal leiomyosarcoma, imaging in, 81
Esophageal lumen, prenatal development of, 42, 43f
Esophageal lymphoma, imaging in, 81
Esophageal manometry
    combined with multichannel intraluminal impedance, 175–176, 178f, 179, 179f
    24-hour
        ambulatory, 152–154
        stationary, 144–146, 145f–155f, 145t, 150, 152
Esophageal melanoma, imaging in, 81
Esophageal motility
    disorders of. See Esophageal dysmotility.
    physiology of, 128–134
        esophageal body and, 129–132, 132f
        lower esophageal high-pressure zone and, 132–134, 133f
        upper esophageal sphincter and, 129, 129f–131f
    preoperative studies of, for Nissen fundoplication, 266
Esophageal mucosal injury, duodenal reflux and, 230–232
    animal studies of, 230
    human studies of, 230–231
    mechanism of, 231–232
Esophageal neoplasms. See also specific neoplasms.
    benign, 513–522
        classification of, 514b, 514–515
        endoscopic ultrasonography in, 122–123, 123t
        historical background of, 514
        imaging of, 81–83, 83f
        incidence of, 513
        intraluminal/mucosal, 522–524
            fibrovascular polyps as, 522–523, 523t
            squamous papillomas as, 523–524, 524f
        intramural/extramucosal
            congenital ectopic rests as, 522
            gastrointestinal stromal tumor as, 520
            granular cell, 520–521, 521f
            hemangioma as, 521–522
            inflammatory pseudotumors as, 522
            leiomyoma as, 515–520, 516f–519f, 516t, 518t
            lipomas as, 522
            mesenchymal, 515t, 515–520
            rhabdomyomas as, 522
            schwannoma as, 520
        surgical treatment of, 514
        symptoms of, 513–514
Esophageal obstruction
    following fundoplication, 85
    following gastric banding, 935
Esophageal perforation, 528–538
    clinical findings in, 529–531, 530f
    diagnosis of, 531, 531f, 532f
    with dilatation, 240f, 240–241
        management of, 532–537, 533f

Esophageal perforation (Continued)
    with dysmotility, 532–537, 533f
    with esophageal cancer, 532–537, 533f
    in esophageal disease, 537–538
    with esophageal strictures, intractable, 532–537, 533f
    during esophageal surgery, 600f, 600–602, 601b
        diagnosis of, 601, 602f
        treatment of, 601–602, 603f–605f
    etiology of, 528–529, 529t
    with gastroesophageal reflux, end-stage, 532–537, 533f
    with Heller myotomy, 417
    historical background of, 528
    imaging of, 91, 93–94, 95f
    management of, 532–537, 533f
        after dilation therapy for achalasia, 532–537, 533f
        nonoperative, 532
        surgical
            of cervical perforation, 533
            of intrathoracic and intra-abdominal perforations, 533–537
    with Nissen fundoplication, 273
    operative, 1094
    spontaneous (Boerhaave's syndrome), 91, 93
Esophageal pH monitoring. See pH monitoring, esophageal.
Esophageal propulsive force, 53
Esophageal prostheses, for esophageal cancer, 489–492
Esophageal reconstruction, 578–597
    conduits for, 249, 578–579
        guidelines for choosing, 581
        studies useful for decision making about, 581–582
    for esophageal strictures, 248–249, 249f
    esophagocoloplasty for, 588b, 588–592
        operative technique for, 589–591
            abdominal team and, 589–591, 590f
            cervical team and, 591
        postoperative care for, 591
        preoperative preparation for, 589
        results with, 591t, 591–592, 592t
    esophagogastrostomy for, 582–588
        anastomosis for, 586–587, 587f, 588
        drainage of stomach for, 584–585, 585f
        functional results with, 588
        lengthening of stomach for, 584, 584f
        mobilization of stomach for, 582–584, 583f
        transposition of stomach for, 585, 586f
    esophagojejunoplasty for, 592–596
        free transfer and, 595f, 595–596
        interposition and, 593f, 593–594, 594f
        results of, 596t, 596–597
        Roux-en-Y limb and, 594f, 594–595
    for esophageal cancer, 478–479
    historical background of, 578
    incision placement for, 579–580, 580f

Esophageal reconstruction (Continued)
    level of anastomosis for, 580–581
    route of replacement for, 580
    short-segment colon interposition for, 596–597
    results of, 596t, 596–597
Esophageal replacement
    for end-stage benign esophageal disease, 285–304, 286b
        clinical manifestations of disease and, 286b, 286t, 286–287, 287t
        conduits for, 289, 289b, 289f, 296–299, 297f–300f
        esophagectomy as primary therapy and, 299, 301b, 301–302, 302t
        long- vs. short-segment esophagectomy for, 289–291, 290f
        operative approach for esophagectomy and foregut reconstruction for, 291–294, 292f–294f
        preoperative evaluation for, 287–289, 288f
        proximal gastrectomy or gastric bypass for, 302–304, 303f
        vagal-sparing vs. standard esophagectomy for, 294f, 294–296, 295f
    substernal, complications of, 615, 616f
Esophageal resection
    for esophageal cancer. See Esophageal cancer, surgical treatment of.
    esophageal imaging following, 86, 87f, 88f
    for esophageal strictures, 248–249, 249f
    for leiomyoma, 519f, 519–520
    for strictures, intractable, 544–545
    with visceral esophageal substitution, complications of, 611–618
        anastomotic leak as, 611–613, 612f
        anastomotic stricture as, 613
        of bypassing or excluding native esophagus, 616, 617f, 618
        chylothorax as, 614–615
        diaphragmatic hiatal obstruction or herniation as, 614, 615f
        gastric outlet obstruction as, 613–614, 614f
        pancreatitis as, 615
        peripheral atheroembolism as, 615
        pulmonary, 613
        splenic injury as, 615
        of substernal esophageal replacement, 615, 616f
Esophageal rings, imaging of, 88f, 88–89, 90f, 91f
Esophageal shortening
    evaluation of, barium examination for, 70, 71f
    with paraesophageal hernia, 558–559
Esophageal spasm
    diffuse and segmental, 419–421
        examinations in, 419–421
        historical background of, 419
        treatment of, 421
    esophagomyotomy for, complications of, 619–620

Esophageal squamous cell carcinoma, epidemiology of
  age, sex, and race distribution and, 443
  risk factors and, 443–445
    alcohol as, 443
    diet and nutrition as, 443, 445
    nonsteroidal anti-inflammatory drugs as, 445
    obesity as, 443, 443t, 444f
    tobacco as, 443
Esophageal squamous epithelium
  acid-induced damage to, 210–212, 211f
  cardiac mucosa and, 213f, 213–215, 215f
  columnar transformation in, 212, 212f, 230
  normal appearance of, 208–210, 209f, 210b, 210f
Esophageal stenosis, congenital, 572–573
  esophageal strictures in, 90, 90f
Esophageal strictures
  anastomotic, following esophageal resection, 86, 88f
  in caustic ingestions, development of, 541
  in cicatricial pemphigoid, 89, 92f
  in congenital esophageal stenosis, 90, 90f
  detection of, barium examination for, 69, 69f
  in eosinophilic esophagitis, 90, 93f
  in epidermolysis bullosa, 89
  gastroesophageal reflux causing, 234–249
    anatomic variation of, 235, 235f, 236f
    classification of, 236–237
    evaluation of, 235–236, 236f, 237
    medical therapy for, 256–257
    short esophagus and, 234. See also Short esophagus.
    treatment of, 237–249
      antireflux surgery with intraoperative stricture dilatation for, 241–248
      esophageal resection and reconstruction for, 248–249, 249f
      nonoperative, 237, 238f–240f, 240–241
  imaging of, 89–91, 92f–94f
  intractable
    with caustic ingestions, management of, 544–545
    esophageal perforation associated with, 538
  in lichen planus, 89–90, 92f
  midesophageal, 90, 93f
  nasogastric intubation causing, 90
  oropharyngeal, 546f, 546–547
  recurrence of, 241
Esophageal stripping, transhiatal, vagal-sparing, for Barrett's esophagus, 362–363
Esophageal surgeons, 7–8
Esophageal surgery. See also specific procedures.
  complications of, 598–620
    anatomic and physiologic considerations in, 598–599, 599f, 600f

Esophageal surgery (Continued)
    of esophageal diverticulectomy, 618f, 618–619, 619f
    esophageal perforation as, 600f, 600–602, 601b
      diagnosis of, 601, 602f
      treatment of, 601–602, 603f–605f
    of esophageal resection and visceral esophageal substitution, 611–618
    of esophagomyotomy, 619–620
    of esophagoscopy, 598, 602–604, 606, 606f
    of hiatal hernia repair, 606b, 606–607, 607f, 608f, 609–610, 610f
    of laparoscopic antireflux/hiatal hernia surgery, 610–611
  historical background of, 3–8
Esophageal transit scintigraphy, 154–155
Esophageal varices
  bleeding, 1755, 1758–1763
    acute, 1759, 1759f, 1760f
    in cirrhosis, 1693
    decompression for, 1761–1763
      distant splenorenal shunt for, 1752f, 1762
      surgical stents for, 1762
      transjugular intrahepatic portocaval shunt procedures for, 1693, 1761f, 1761–1762
    prophylaxis of, 1758f, 1758–1759
    recurrent, prevention of, 1759–1760, 1760f
    treatment of, 1624, 1624t
      decompression for, 1761–1763
      devascularization procedures for, 1763
      primary therapy for, 1760–1761
  "downhill," 95, 97f
  endoscopic ultrasonography in, 124, 125f
  imaging of, 95, 97f
  in pancreatitis, chronic, 1352–1353
  "uphill," 95, 97f
Esophageal wall, anatomy of, ultrasound, 114–116, 115f, 116f
Esophageal webs
  cervical, imaging of, 89, 91f
  esophageal imaging of, 88f, 88–89, 90f, 91f
Esophagectomy
  for Barrett's esophagus, 362
    mortality and, 363
  cervical, esophagogastric anastomotic strictures following, 292, 292f
  complications of, 480t, 480–481
    atheroembolism as, 615
    chylothorax as, 614
    pancreatitis as, 615
    splenic injury as, 615
  conduit for, route of passage for, 292–294, 293f, 294f
  early development of, 4
  en bloc, for localized esophageal cancer, 477–478
  for esophageal cancer, results with, 481–482
  for esophageal perforation, 536, 536f

Esophagectomy (Continued)
  for esophageal strictures, 248–249, 249f
  for foregut reconstruction for benign disease
    long- vs. short-segment, 289–291, 290f
    operative approach to, 291–294, 292f–294f
    as primary therapy, 299, 301b, 301–302, 302t
    vagal-sparing, 294f, 294–296, 295f
  gastroparesis following, 923
  imaging following, 86
  operative approach to, for foregut reconstruction for benign disease, 291–294, 292f–294f
  partial, incision for, 579
  postoperative care for, 480
  short-segment
    advantages of, 290
    clinical experience with, 291, 291t
    esophageal anastomosis with, 291
    gastroesophageal reflux following, 290
    limitations of, 290–291
  thoracic, total, with cervical esophagogastric anastomosis, 249
  transhiatal, 291–292, 292f, 479–480, 579–580, 580f
    technique of, 479–480
  vagal-sparing, 249, 249f
    for adenocarcinoma, 477
    for foregut reconstruction for benign disease, 294f, 294–296, 295f
  with vein stripper, for caustic ingestions, 544
Esophagitis
  achalasia and, 409
  caustic, imaging in, 91
  classification of, 236
  detection of, barium examination for, 69, 69f
  eosinophilic, esophageal strictures in, 90, 93f
  erosive
    natural history of gastroesophageal reflux disease and, 202
    prevention prevalence of, 199–200, 200t
  in gastroesophageal reflux disease, medical therapy for, 255–256, 256f
Esophagocoloplasty, 588b, 588–592
  operative technique for, 589–591
    abdominal team and, 589–591, 590f
    cervical team and, 591
  postoperative care for, 591
  preoperative preparation for, 589
  results with, 591t, 591–592, 592t
Esophagogastric anastomosis
  cervical, for esophageal structure, 249
  early development of, 4
  intrathoracic, for esophageal structure, 249
Esophagogastric junction, wall structure at, 16f
Esophagogastroduodenoscopy, 165t
  for aortoenteric fistulas, 1271
  esophageal perforation due to, 529

Esophagogastrostomy, 582–588
  anastomosis for, 586–587, 587f, 588
  drainage of stomach for, 584–585,
    585f
  functional results with, 588
  imaging following, 86, 87f
  intrathoracic
    for Barrett's esophagus, 362
    early development of, 4
  lengthening of stomach for, 584, 584f
  mobilization of stomach for, 582–584,
    583f
  transposition of stomach for, 585, 586f
Esophagography
  in achalasia, 407
  barium, 164, 165t
    in esophageal carcinoma, 469, 469f
    for esophageal reconstruction, 582
  in esophageal perforation, 93, 95f
  postoperative, 83–86
    contrast materials for, 84, 84t
    following antireflux procedures, 85,
      86f
    following cardiomyotomy, 85, 86f
    following cricopharyngeal myotomy,
      84–85, 85f
Esophagojejunoplasty, 592–596
  free transfer and, 595f, 595–596
  interposition and, 593f, 593–594, 594f
  results of, 596t, 596–597
  Roux-en-Y limb and, 594f, 594–595
Esophagomyotomy
  for achalasia or esophageal spasm,
    complications of, 619–620
  concomitant antireflux procedure with,
    controversy about, 620
  with diverticulectomy, for epiphrenic
    diverticulum, 434f, 435
Esophagoscopy
  barium, with leiomyoma, 517, 517f
  complications of, 598, 602–604, 606,
    606f
    esophageal perforation as, 602–604,
      606, 606f
  in esophageal perforation, 531, 532f,
    601, 602f
  with gastric tumors, in pediatric
    patients, 959, 959f
  stricture dilation using, 237, 240, 240f
Esophagus
  body of, anchorage of, 12, 13f
  caustic injury of. See Caustic ingestions.
  columnar-lined. See Barrett's esophagus.
  compression of, with paraesophageal
    hernia, 551–552
  "corkscrew," 419, 420f
  Crohn's disease involving, 91, 94f
  diameter of, 10–11
  endoscopic examination of. See
    Endoscopic examination,
    esophageal.
  exposure to gastric juice, increased,
    causes of, 141f, 141–142
  feline, radiographic appearance of, 67,
    67f
  function of, 63
  imaging of. See Imaging, esophageal;
    specific imaging modalities.

Esophagus (Continued)
  irradiation of, esophageal carcinoma
    and, 466
  length of, 10
  metastatic disease to, imaging in, 81, 82f
  minor deviations along, 9–10, 10f
  native, bypassing or excluding,
    complications of, 616, 617f, 618
  nutcracker, 74, 421–423
    examinations in, 422f, 422–423, 423f
    manometric features of, 420t, 422f,
      422–423, 423f
    treatment of, 423
  rosary-bead, 419, 420f
  scarring of, detection of, barium
    examination for, 69, 70f
  segmental narrowing of, barium
    examination for, 69
  sigmoid shaped, Heller myotomy with,
    416
  structural abnormalities of, tests to
    detect, 143
  submucosa of, benign tumors of,
    endoscopic ultrasonography in, 123
  swallowing and. See Swallowing.
  tears of, hiatal herniorrhaphy and, 607,
    607f, 608f
  "trachealization" of, 90, 93f
Estrogens
  hepatotoxicity of, 1722, 1723
  synthetic, hepatotoxicity of, 1721
Etanercept, for inflammatory bowel disease,
  2093
Ethanol injection
  for esophageal cancer, 488, 489t
  percutaneous, for hepatocellular
    carcinoma, 1737, 1738
Ethnicity
  Barrett's esophagus and, 342–343
  esophageal cancer and, 442–443
Etoposide, hepatotoxicity of, 1723
Etretinate, hepatotoxicity of, 1721, 1722
Evans's syndrome, splenectomy for, 1827
External oblique muscle, anatomy of, 636,
  637f
Extracellular matrix, groin hernias and, 635
Extracorporeal liver assist device, 1706
Extracorporeal shock-wave lithotripsy
  for bile duct stones, 1494, 1495
  for pancreatic duct stones, 1510–1511
Extrahepatic portal hypertension, in
  pancreatitis, chronic, 1312–1313

F

Falciform ligament, 1598
Familial adenomatous polyposis, 2159t,
  2159–2169
  attenuated, 2168
    small intestinal, 894t, 896
  clinical features of, 2159–2160, 2160f
  as colorectal cancer risk factor, 2187f,
    2187–2188
  diagnosis of, 2164
  extracolonic manifestations of,
    2160–2163
    desmoids as, 2161–2162

Familial adenomatous polyposis (Continued)
  upper gastrointestinal neoplasia as,
    2162t, 2162–2163
  genetic testing and counseling for,
    2164–2165
  genetics of, 2163–2164
    APC gene and, 2163
    APG genotype-FAP phenotype
      correlation and, 2163f,
      2163–2164
    MYH polyposis and, 2168–2169
  small intestinal, 893f, 893–895, 894t
    symptoms and diagnosis of, 894–895
    treatment of, 895
  surgical management of, 2165–2168
    issues modifying, 2167–2168
    restorative proctocolectomy for, 2335
    surgical options for, 2165t,
      2165–2167, 2166t
Famotidine, 255. See also Histamine₂
  receptor antagonists.
  gastric acid secretion and, 727
  for gastroesophageal reflux disease, 254
Fascial planes, esophageal, anatomy of, 11
FAST. See Focused abdominal sonography
  for trauma.
"Fat wrapping," in Crohn's disease, 1058,
  1058f
Fatigue
  in Crohn's disease, 1045
  with primary sclerosing cholangitis, 1566
Fatty liver
  nonalcoholic, hepatic laboratory tests in,
    1612–1613
  of pregnancy, acute, 1703
Fecal continence. See also Fecal
  incontinence.
  following surgery for anorectal
    anomalies, 2404
  pelvic muscular anatomy and,
    2391–2394
Fecal diversion
  for fecal incontinence, 1926
  for rectovaginal fistulas, 1954
Fecal fistulas, with appendicitis, 2150
Fecal incontinence, 1885, 1917–1926
  after anorectal surgery, 2057
  endoanal ultrasound in, 1910–1911,
    1911f
  evaluation of, 1917–1921, 1918b
    history in, 1917–1918
    laboratory assessment in, 1919–1921
      benefits and limitations of,
        1920–1921
      defecography for, 1920
      endoanal ultrasound for, 1920,
        1920f
      manometry for, 1919
      pudendal nerve terminal motor
        latency for, 1919–1920
    physical examination in, 1918–1919
  examination for, 1888
  following surgery for anorectal
    anomalies, treatment of, 2405
  treatment of, 1921–1926
    biofeedback for, 1921–1922
    following surgery for anorectal
      anomalies, 2405

Fecal incontinence *(Continued)*
  medical, 1921
  surgical, 1922–1926
    artificial anal sphincter and, 1924, 1924f
    dynamic myoplasty as, 1923–1924
    fecal diversion as, 1926
    injectable biomaterials and, 1925–1926
    sacral nerve stimulation and, 1925, 1925f
    salvage therapy as, 1923
    sphincter reconstruction as, 1922f, 1922–1923
Fecal occult blood testing, 1888–1889
Fecal urgency, 1885
  examination for, 1888
Feces, pruritus ani due to, 2066–2067
Feline esophagus, radiographic appearance of, 67, 67f
Felty's syndrome, splenectomy for, 1827
Females
  anorectal anomalies in, 2394, 2394f
    initial management of newborn with, 2394–2395
  fertility in, following ileal pouch–anal anastomosis, 2117, 2167–2168
  groin hernias in, 643
  low anterior resection in, 2228, 2228f
  pregnancy and
    acute fatty liver of, 1703
    appendicitis during, 2144
    gastroesophageal reflux disease and, 200
  young, appendicitis in, 2144
Femoral hernias, 623–630, 643, 644
  anatomy and, 623, 624f, 625f
  in children, 712
  diagnosis of, 626
  etiology of, 626
  historical background of, 623–626
  treatment of, 626–629, 627f–629f
    femoral approach for, 626–627, 627f
    inguinal approach for, 624–625, 627, 627f, 628f
    laparoscopic approach for, 625–626, 628–629, 629f
    preperitoneal approach for, 625, 627–628, 628f
    results with, 629, 629t
Femoral nerve, 657, 658f
Ferguson hemorrhoidectomy, 2033
Fertility, female, following ileal pouch–anal anastomosis, 2117, 2167–2168
Fever, in Crohn's disease, 1045
Fibrin glue
  for anorectal fistulas, 2056–2057
  autologous, for rectovaginal fistulas, 1952
  for bowel anastomoses, 1089
Fibroid polyps, inflammatory, gastric, 884
Fibromas
  esophageal, endoscopic ultrasonography in, 123
  gastric, 887–888, 888
  small intestinal, 901
Fibromuscular hypertrophy, idiopathic, 572
Fibromuscular stenosis, idiopathic, 572

Fibrosarcomas, hepatic, 1747, 1747f
Fibrosis, drug-induced, 1719t, 1720–1721
Fibrovascular polyps, esophageal, 522–523, 523t
Fine-needle aspiration
  endoscopic ultrasonography, in bronchogenic carcinoma, 125
  with pancreatic cystic neoplasms, 1396
  with pancreatic tumors, unusual, 1432
Finney pyloroplasty, 5, 816, 818, 819f
  for duodenal ulcers, 795
  technique for, 842f
Finney stricturoplasty, for Crohn's disease, 1059, 1061f
Fissure-in-ano. *See* Anal fissures.
Fistulas, 1092–1117
  anal. *See* Anal fistulas.
  anovaginal, 1946
  aortoduodenal, 1095
  aortoenteric. *See* Aortoenteric fistulas.
  biliary. *See* Biliary fistulas.
  colocutaneous, in colonic diverticular disease, 2018
  colovesical, in colonic diverticular disease, 2017–2018, 2018f
  complications of, 1097–1098
  in Crohn's disease, 1063–1065, 1094
    enterocutaneous, 1065
    enteroenteric, 1064
    enterogenital, 1065
    enterovesical and enteroureteral, 1064
    ileosigmoid, 1064
    treatment of, 1104–1105, 2135–2136, 2137f–2138f
  diagnosis of, 1097
  duodenal
    with duodenal injuries, 768, 770
    etiology of, 1093–1096
    treatment of, 1110
  duodenal stump, treatment of, 1110
  duodenocolic, in Crohn's disease, 1094
  duodenocutaneous, in Crohn's disease, 1094
  enterocervical, treatment of, 1114
  enterocutaneous
    in Crohn's disease, 1065
    failure to close spontaneously, 1108
    following ileal pouch–anal anastomosis, 2112
    small intestinal, 1096
    treatment of, 1110–1111
  enteroenteric
    in Crohn's disease, 1064
    treatment of, 1111f, 1111–1112
  enterofallopian, treatment of, 1114
  enterogenital, in Crohn's disease, 1065
  enteroureteral, in Crohn's disease, 1064
  enterouterine, treatment of, 1114
  enterovaginal, treatment of, 1113–1114
  enterovesical, treatment of, 1112f, 1112–1113, 1115
  etiology of, 1093–1097
    of gastric and duodenal fistulas, 1093–1096
    of small intestinal fistulas, 1096–1097
  fecal, with appendicitis, 2150
  gastric, etiology of, 1093–1096

Fistulas *(Continued)*
  gastrocolic, in Crohn's disease, 1094
  gastroduodenal, treatment of, 1110
  gastrojejunocolic, internal, 1094
  ileosigmoid, in Crohn's disease, 1064
  intestinal. *See also* Enteric fistulas; *specific sites, e.g.* Anal fistulas.
    in Crohn's disease, surgical treatment of, 2095
  intra-abdominal, in colonic diverticular disease, 2021
  management of, 1098–1117
    definitive therapy for, 1108–1117
      for aortoenteric fistulas, 1114–1115, 1115f
      for enterocervical fistulas, 1114
      for enterocutaneous fistulas, 1110–1111
      for enteroenteric fistulas, 1111f, 1111–1112
      for enterofallopian fistulas, 1114
      for enterouterine fistulas, 1114
      for enterovaginal fistulas, 1113–1114
      for enterovesical fistulas, 1112f, 1112–1113
      for gastric and duodenal perforations and fistulas, 1108–1110
      general considerations for, 1115–1117, 1116f
      healing and, 1117
      for nephroenteric fistulas, 1113
    investigation in, 1105f, 1105–1106, 1107f
    stabilization for, 1099–1105
      control of sepsis and, 1101–1103, 1103f, 1104f
      nutrition and, 1100–1101
      pharmacologic support and, 1103–1105
      resuscitation and, 1099–1100
    treatment decisions and, 1107–1108
  nephroenteric, treatment of, 1113
  pancreatic
    external, 1352
    internal, in pancreatitis, chronic, 1311
    management of, 1307–1308
    pancreatic drainage procedures for, 1511f, 1511–1513, 1512f
    with trauma, 1404
  paraprosthetic-enteric, 1114
  peri-ileostomy, 1080–1081
  pouch-vaginal, following ileal pouch–anal anastomosis, 2112–2113, 2114f
  rectourethral, 1954–1955
    meconium in urine and, 2394, 2394f
  rectovaginal. *See* Rectovaginal fistulas.
  renogastric, 1095
  small intestinal, 1096
    congenital, 1096
    infection causing, 1096
    inflammatory causes of, 1096–1097
    intestinal, of small intestine, 1097
    radiation-induced, 1097
    traumatic, 1096
    tumors causing, 1097

Fistulas *(Continued)*
staging/classification of, 1097
tracheoesophageal, 15
following esophageal resection with
visceral esophageal substitution,
613
radiographic appearance of, 76, 78f
Fistulography, 1105f, 1105–1106
with anorectal fistulas, 2049
with biliary fistulas, 1542
contrast, 1893
Fistulotomy
for anorectal abscesses, primary versus
delayed, 2054–2055
for anorectal fistulas, 2055
radiofrequency, 2055
for rectovaginal fistulas, 1952
FK506
for inflammatory bowel disease, 2092
for islet transplantation, 1424
mechanism of action of, 2377t
Floating gallbladder, 1450, 1453f
Fluconazole, hepatotoxicity of, 1722
Fluid and electrolyte abnormalities
in biliary tract disease, 1620
in cirrhosis, 1625
with gastrointestinal fistulas, 1098
in liver disease, 1620
Fluid and electrolyte therapy, for
pancreatitis
acute, mild, 1302
severe, necrotizing, 1303
Fluid and electrolyte transport, colonic, 1872
Fluid management, in fulminant hepatic
failure, 1704
Fluoroscopic wire basket stone retrieval,
1484
5-Fluorouracil
for anal intraepithelial neoplasia, 2290
for metastatic colorectal cancer, 2201,
2202
Focal nodular hyperplasia, 1728–1729
diagnosis of, 1728, 1728f
drug-induced, 1723
etiology of, 1728
treatment of, 1728–1729
Focused abdominal sonography for trauma
in abdominal trauma, in pediatric
patients, 1807
in colorectal trauma, 1974–1975
in gastric blunt trauma, 762
in pancreatic trauma, 1401
in small bowel injury, 772
in splenic trauma, 1799
Folate/folic acid
deficiency of, in Crohn's disease, 1054
small intestinal absorption of, 1006,
1007t
Follicular lymphoma, pathology of, 1204
Fontolizumab, mechanism of action of,
2377t
Foods. *See also* Diet; Nutrition.
phytobezoars and, 943, 944, 944t
Foramen of Bochdalek, 36
Foramen of Morgagni, 36–37
Foramen of Winslow, 964, 966f
hernias of, 975, 976, 977f, 1123–1124,
1124f

Foregut. *See also* Esophagus.
cranial segment of
malformations of, 32–33
prenatal development of, 31–33, 33f,
34f
intermediate segment of, prenatal
development of, 33–34
prenatal development of, 29t, 29–31
basic tissue and organ development
and, 30, 30f, 31f
of cardia, 34f–36f, 34–35
congenital anomalies and. *See*
Congenital disorders; *specific
anomalies.*
congenital malformations and
anomalies and, 30
crown-rump length and, 29
of duodenum, 34f–36f, 34–35
of esophagus, 33–34
of hypopharynx, 31–33, 33f, 34f
intraembryonic body cavity
development and, 31
of larynx, 31–33, 33f, 34f
of mediastinum, 35–37, 37f
mesenchymal clefts and, 31
of nervous system, 43–46
of pharynx, 31–33, 33f, 34f
of phrenoesophageal membrane, 36,
36f
of primitive digestive system, 31,
32f
of research system, 31–33, 33f, 34f
of stomach, 34f–36f, 34–35
tissue organization and, 37–46
lamina mucosa, submucosa, and
esophageal lumen formation
and, 37, 39t, 39–42
muscular, 37, 38f
of trachea, 34f, 35, 39f
vascular, 42–43, 43f, 44f
Foreign body ingestion, 940–945
bezoars and, 943–945, 944t
diagnosis of, 944f, 944–945, 945f
signs and symptoms of, 944
treatment of, 945
diagnosis of, 940–941
duodenal injury due to, 1095
management of, 941–943
for button batteries, 942–943
for illicit drugs, 943, 943f
for sharp/pointed or long foreign
bodies, 941–942, 942f
FortaGen, for ventral herniorrhaphy, 676
Fowler-Stevens procedure, 711
Fowler-Weir-Mitchel incision, for
appendectomy, 2145, 2146f
Fox's sign, 1299
Frantz tumors, in pediatric patients, 1411
Free perforation, in Crohn's disease, 1066
"French hernia," 688
Frey procedure
Hamburg modification of, for
pancreatitis, chronic, 1315
in pediatric patients, 1410
"Frozen" abdomen, 1148
FTY720, for islet transplantation, 1428
Fulminant hepatic failure, 1702. *See also*
Liver failure, acute.

Fundic gland polyps (fundic glandular cysts;
fundic hyperplasia), 884, 2162
Fundic gland-type polyps, endoscopic
appearance of, 740, 741f
Fundoplication
Belsey, for esophageal strictures,
241–242
Dor, 276, 277f
for achalasia, 416
for esophageal perforation, 417
laparoscopic
for epiphrenic diverticulum,
435–437, 437f
surgical technique for, 282
results with, 283
laparoscopic
for esophageal strictures, 245, 247,
247f
gastric perforation due to, 1094
Nissen. *See* Nissen fundoplication.
Toupet. *See* Toupet fundoplication.
Watson, 276, 277f, 278
Fungal infections, splenic abscess due to,
1820
Furosemide, for ascites, 1764–1765
Fuykwan procedure, for rectal prolapse,
1961, 1961f, 1964t

G

Galen, 632, 1771, 1813
Gallbladder
agenesis of, 1450
anatomy and embryology of, 1443f,
1443–1444, 1444f
anomalies of, 1448–1451, 1449b
bilobed, 1449, 1451f
diverticulum of, 1449–1450, 1451f
duplication of, 1450, 1452f
floating, 1450, 1453f
function of, 1455–1458
hourglass, 1449, 1451f
injury of, 1663, 1667
intrahepatic, 1450–1451, 1453f
left-sided, 1451
motility of, 1458
retrodisplaced, 1451
rudimentary, 1450
transverse, 1451
Gallbladder cancer, 1519–1526
adjuvant therapy for, 1524
anatomy of, 1520
diagnosis of, 1520–1521, 1521f
epidemiology of, 1519–1520
palliation for, 1524
pathology of, 1520
practical management of, 1524–1525
for cancer diagnosed incidentally
after laparoscopic
cholecystectomy, 1525
for cancer presenting as gallbladder
mass, 1525
for cancer presenting with
obstructive jaundice, 1525
for preoperatively diagnosed
radiographically suspicious
gallbladder polyps, 1524–1525

Gallbladder cancer (Continued)
staging of, 1521, 1522t
surgical treatment of, 1521, 1522f, 1523–1524
technique for, 1525–1526
Gallbladder neoplasms
benign, 1519
malignant. See Gallbladder cancer.
Gallbladder polyps
with primary sclerosing cholangitis, 1565
treatment of, 1567
radiographically suspicious, preoperatively diagnosed, 1524–1525
Gallstone(s). See Cholelithiasis.
Gallstone pancreatitis, 1298
acute, treatment of, 1497–1499
Ganciclovir, for cytomegalovirus infection, in immunocompromised patients, 2382
Ganglia, of gallbladder, 1444
Ganglioneuromas
gastric, 887–888
small intestinal, 900
Gant-Miwa procedure, for solitary rectal ulcer syndrome, 2076
Gardner's syndrome, 2160
small intestinal, 894t, 895
Garengeot, Rene Jacques Croissant de, 688
Gas embolism, with inguinal herniorrhaphy, laparoscopic, 666
Gastrectomy. See also Gastric resection and reconstruction.
for caustic injury, gastric, 763
distal, technique for, 845, 849f–856f
for duodenal ulcers, 795–796, 796f–798f
external biliary fistulas following, etiology and prevention of, 1540
near-total, for gastroparesis, 924, 925
partial
fistulas following, 1093
with Roux-en-Y biliary diversion, for esophageal stricture, 249
postgastrectomy syndromes and. See Postgastrectomy syndromes.
proximal, for foregut reconstruction for benign disease, 302–304, 303f
with Roux gastrojejunostomy, for gastroparesis, 925
subtotal, for gastric adenocarcinoma, 909
reconstruction following, 911
total
for gastric adenocarcinoma, 909
technique for, 847f–860f, 857
vertical, for emetogenic injuries, 763–764
Gastric access, for enteric feeding, 754–755
Gastric acid
functions of, 727
hypersecretion of
in short-bowel syndrome, 1168
in Zollinger-Ellison syndrome. See Zollinger-Ellison syndrome.
secretion of, 724–727
basal or interprandial, 724
cellular basis of, 725–727
nocturnal, 255
pharmacologic regulation of, 727
stimulated, 724

Gastric adenocarcinoma, 904–915
clinical features of, 906
diagnosis of, 907–908
epidemiology of, 904–905
of gastric remnant, reoperative surgery for, 1140
pathology of, 905, 905b
risk factors for, 905–906, 906b
staging of, 908, 908b
treatment of
adjuvant, 912–913
chemoradiotherapy as, 912
chemotherapy as, 912
intraperitoneal, 912–913
for advanced disease, 914
palliative chemotherapy as, 914
palliative endoscopy as, 914
palliative radiotherapy as, 914
palliative surgery as, 914
neoadjuvant, 913–914
chemoradiotherapy as, 913–914
chemotherapy as, 913
radiotherapy as, 913
surgical, 908–912
for distal tumors, 909
endoscopic mucosal resection as, 909
lymphadenectomy extent and, 909–911, 910f, 910t
for midbody tumors, 909
prognostic factors and patterns of failure and, 911–912
for proximal tumors, 908–909
reconstruction after gastrectomy and, 911
Gastric antral vascular ectasia, 886
endoscopic appearance of, 739–740
symptoms and diagnosis of, 886
treatment of, 740, 886
Gastric arteries, 20, 20f, 718, 719f
anatomy of, 1237
aneurysms of, 1282
Gastric banding
adjustable, 934
failed, revision surgery for, 1145
for obesity, 934–935, 935f
Gastric barrier function, 729
Gastric bypass
for foregut reconstruction for benign disease, 302–304, 303f
internal hernias due to, 1124–1126, 1125f
clinical features of, 1125
diagnosis of, 1125–1126
treatment of, 1126
resection of excluded distal gastric remnant after, 304
Roux-en-Y
failed, revision surgery for, 1145–1146
for obesity, 931–934, 932f, 933t
Gastric cancer. See also Gastric adenocarcinoma; Gastric lymphomas.
endoscopic appearance of, 740, 740f
following gastrectomy, 809
treatment of
endoscopic, 744–745
laparoscopic, 745

Gastric carcinoid tumors, 1181
treatment of, 1185
Gastric cysts, esophageal, 525, 525f
Gastric derotation, for gastric volvulus, in pediatric patients, 950
Gastric distention, lower esophageal sphincter and, 227f, 227–229, 228f
Gastric duplication, in pediatric patients, 948
clinical features of, 948
diagnosis of, 948, 950f
incidence and etiology of, 948
management of, 948, 950f
Gastric dysmotility, 730–731
gastroparesis as. See Gastroparesis.
reoperative surgery for, 1139–1140
Roux stasis syndrome as, 809, 880, 925
reoperative surgery for, 1140
Gastric electrical stimulation, for gastroparesis, 921–924
Enterra, 921–923, 922f
postsurgical, 923–924
Gastric emptying, delayed, 185–190
assessment of
antroduodenal manometry and, 186–188, 188f, 188t, 189f, 190, 190t
barium burger studies and, 190
^{13}C breathing test for, 185–186
gastric emptying scintigraphy and, 185, 186f, 187f
in gastroparesis. See Gastroparesis.
Helicobacter pylori and, 730
reoperative surgery for, 1139–1140
Gastric emptying scintigraphy, 185, 186f, 187f
Gastric fistulas, etiology of, 1093–1096
Gastric foreign bodies. See Foreign body ingestion.
Gastric heterotopia, small intestinal, 892
Gastric inhibitory peptide
duodenal function and, 981t, 981–982
small intestinal neuroendocrine function and, 1018
Gastric injuries, 760–764
anatomy and physiology and, 760–761, 761f
blunt, 761–762
diagnosis of, 762–763
treatment of, 763
caustic, 762
diagnosis of, 763
treatment of, 763
complications of, 764
diagnosis of, 762–763
emetogenic, 762
treatment of, 763–764
historical background of, 760
iatrogenic, 762
penetrating, 761
diagnosis of, 762–763
treatment of, 763
treatment of, 763–764
Gastric interposition, for esophageal reconstruction, 249

Gastric juice, 727–728, 728t
  increased esophageal exposure to
    causes of, 141f, 141–142
    tests to detect, 161, 164–168, 165t
      clinical use of, 169–173
      performance of, 165–168
      24-hour esophageal pH
        monitoring as, 164–168
Gastric lymphomas
  diagnosis of, 1207f, 1207–1208, 1208f
  epidemiology of, 1199, 1200t
  treatment of, 1209, 1209t, 1210f
Gastric motility, 729–731
  fasting, 729–730
  normal, 920
  postprandial, 730
Gastric neoplasms. See also specific neoplasms.
  benign
    mesenchymal lesions as, 886–889
    mucosal hypertrophy and
      hyperplasia as, 882–886
      diffuse, 885–886
      focal, 882–885, 883t
  malignant. See Gastric adenocarcinoma;
    Gastric cancer; Gastric lymphomas.
  in pediatric patients, 958–959
    clinical features and diagnosis of,
      958–959
    incidence of, 958
    management of, 959
Gastric outlet obstruction
  following esophageal resection with
    visceral esophageal substitution,
    613–614, 614f
  at gastrojejunostomy site, reoperative
    surgery for, 1137–1138
  in pancreatitis, chronic, 1348–1349,
    1349f
  in pediatric patients, 950–951
    clinical features of, 950–951
    diagnosis of, 951, 951f
    management of, 951–952
    types of, 951, 951f
  in peptic ulcer disease
    emergency surgery for, 806–808
    reoperation for, 1136–1137
    vagotomy and drainage for,
      825–826
Gastric perforation
  in laparoscopic fundoplication, 1094
  in neonates, 957–958
    clinical features and diagnosis of,
      957–958
    etiology of, 957
    incidence of, 957
    management of, 958
  with Nissen fundoplication, 273
  operative, 1094
  treatment of, 1108–1110
Gastric polyps
  adenomatous or neoplastic, 884–885
  benign, 882–885
    adenomatous or neoplastic, 884–885
      flat adenomas as, 885
      papillary adenomas as, 885
    non-neoplastic, 882–884
      adenomyomas as, 884
      Brunner's gland, 884

Gastric polyps (Continued)
      fundic gland, 884
      hamartomatous, 884
      hyperplastic or regenerative,
        883–884
      inflammatory, 884
      pancreatic, heterotopic, 884
    non-neoplastic, 882–884
    retention, 884
Gastric pull-up
  for caustic ingestions, 545
  for foregut reconstruction for benign
    disease, 296, 299
  for gastric adenocarcinoma, 909
Gastric resection. See Gastrectomy.
Gastric resection and reconstruction, 831–857
  postoperative management for, 857
  preoperative preparation for, 831
  procedures for, 831–857
    gastrectomy
      distal, 845, 849f–856f
      total, 857, 857f–860f
    gastrojejunostomy, 845, 846f–848f
    gastrostomy, Stamm, 857, 860f, 861f
    pyloroplasty, 831, 841f–845f
    vagotomy
      gastric, proximal, 831, 835f–838f
      highly selective, 831, 838f–840f
      truncal, 831, 832f–835f
Gastric restrictive operations, for obesity,
  930–931, 931f
Gastric rotation, development of, 35
Gastric stasis, following vagotomy, 874–875
Gastric ulcers, 820f, 820–822
  classification of, 820f, 820–821
  endoscopic appearance of, 737, 737f,
    738f
  intractable, elective surgery for, 798–800,
    799f, 799t
    for type I ulcers, 799–800
    for type II ulcers, 800
    for type III ulcers, 800
    for type IV ulcers, 800, 801f
    for type V ulcers, 800, 801f
  pathogenesis of, 812
  perforated, emergency surgery for, 806,
    808f
Gastric varices, in pancreatitis, chronic,
  1352–1353
Gastric volvulus, 1037–1039
  diagnosis of, 1037–1038, 1038f, 1039f
  etiology of, 1037, 1037f
  in pediatric patients, 950
  treatment of, 1038–1039
Gastrin, 721–722
  hypergastrinemia and, 722
  receptors for, gastric acid secretion and,
    725
  synthesis and action of, 721–722
Gastrinoma(s), 1375
  lymph node primary, 863
  secretin infusion for localization of,
    865
  in Zollinger-Ellison syndrome, 863–864.
    See also Zollinger-Ellison syndrome.
Gastrinoma triangle, 863
Gastrin-releasing peptide, 723
  duodenal function and, 981t, 984

Gastritis, bile reflux
  following gastrectomy, 875–877, 876f–878f
  reoperative surgery for, 1146f,
    1146–1147, 1147f
Gastrocolic fistulas, in Crohn's disease, 1094
Gastrocolic ligament, 717, 718f
Gastrocolic reflex, 1875
Gastrocolic trunk, 968, 972f
Gastroduodenal anastomosis, longitudinal,
  for gastric outlet obstruction, 951
Gastroduodenal artery, 964, 968, 971f
  anatomy of, 1237
  aneurysms of, 1280f, 1280–1282
Gastroduodenal fistulas, treatment of, 1110
Gastroduodenal reflux disease, esophageal
  mucosal injury and, 230–232
  animal studies of, 230
  human studies of, 230–231
  mechanism of, 231–232
Gastroduodenostomy
  Billroth I
    for caustic injury, gastric, 763
    for duodenal ulcers, 795, 796, 796f,
      797f
    following gastrectomy, 911
  Jaboulay, for duodenal ulcers, 795
Gastroepiploic arteries, 718, 719f
  aneurysms of, 1282
  right, 1237
Gastroesophageal barrier, 223–229
  anatomic alterations and, 228
  definition of, 223
  gastroesophageal reflux disease
    pathophysiology and, integrated
    hypothesis of, 228–229
  lower esophageal sphincter and,
    223–226, 224f, 226t
    transient loss of competence of,
      226f–228f, 226–228
Gastroesophageal junction, 334
  cancer at. See also Esophageal cancer.
    staging systems for, 450–451, 452f
  cardiac mucosa at, 344
  endoscopic evaluation of, 100–102, 101f,
    102f
  impedance in, measurement of, in
    esophageal disease, 195
Gastroesophageal reflux
  amount of, determination of, 206
  detection of, barium examination for, 68
  esophageal strictures resulting from. See
    Esophageal strictures.
  following esophageal surgery, 599
  following Heller myotomy, 417
  multichannel intraluminal impedance
    for monitoring, 175–183
    combined with manometry, 175–176,
      178f, 179, 179f
    combined with pH monitoring,
      180f–183f, 180–181
    principles of, 175, 176f–178f
Gastroesophageal reflux disease, 206–221
  adenocarcinoma and, 445, 467
  antireflux surgery for. See Antireflux
    procedures; Nissen fundoplication.
  barium examination in
    to detect esophageal injury, 68–69,
      69f, 70f

Gastroesophageal reflux disease (*Continued*)
to detect gastroesophageal reflux, 68
to evaluate esophageal clearance, 68
to exclude motility disorder, 68
for postoperative complication evaluation, 70
for preoperative planning, 70, 71f
Barrett's esophagus and. *See* Barrett's esophagus.
cardiac mucosa in, at gastroesophageal junction, 344
diagnosis of
of atypical disease, 171–172, 172f
bilirubin monitoring for, 168–169
clinical use of, 169–173
endoscopic, 105–106, 106t, 107f
pH monitoring for, 164–168, 165t
clinical use of, 169–173
test performance for, 165–168
24-hour esophageal pH monitoring and, 164–168
of typical disease, 170–171
duodenogastroesophageal reflux associated with, 194
end-stage, esophageal perforation associated with, 538
epidemiology of, 197–202
based on endoscopic assessment, 199–200, 200t
increasing prevalence and, 201–202
population risk factors and, 200–201, 201f
regional variation in prevalence and, 201
of symptoms, 198t, 198–199, 199f
erosive, natural history of, 202–203
esophageal motility disorders in, 140–142, 141f
gastroesophageal barrier and, 223–229
anatomic alterations and, 228
definition of, 223
integrated hypothesis of gastroesophageal reflux disease pathophysiology and, 228–229
lower esophageal sphincter and, 223–226, 224f, 226t
transient loss of competence of, 226f–228f, 226–228
histologic classification of, 219–221, 220b
histologic grading of, 214–215
imaging in
esophageal, 67–70
barium examination for, 68–70, 69f–71f
gastric, 66
medical therapy for, 252–261
antacids in, 253
for complications, 255–258
Barrett's esophagus as, 257–258
esophagitis as, 255–256, 256f
strictures as, 256–257
evaluation of response to, 173
for extraesophageal manifestations, 258–260
asthma as, 258, 259f, 260f
cough as, 258–259
laryngitis as, 259–260, 261f

Gastroesophageal reflux disease (*Continued*)
histamine₂ receptor antagonists in, 254
lifestyle modifications in, 252–253
nocturnal acid secretion and, 255
promotility agents in, 253–254
proton pump inhibitors in, 254–255, 255f
natural history of, 202–203
of erosive gastroesophageal reflux disease, 202–203
of nonerosive gastroesophageal reflux disease, 202
nonerosive, 211
epidemiology of, 197
natural history of, 202
normal endoscopy and histology and, 207–210, 208b, 208f–210f, 210b
pathology of, 210–218
acid-induced damage and, 210–211, 211f
esophageal squamous epithelium primed by, 211–212
carcinogenesis in intestinal metaplasia and, 217–218
cardiac mucosa and, 213f, 213–215, 215f
columnar transformation and, 212, 212f
intestinal metaplasia and, 215–216
oxyntocardiac mucosa and, 216–217
reversibility of genetic switches and, 217
pathophysiology of, integrated hypothesis of, 228–229
patient approach for, 58–60
refluxate in, 60, 206–207
surgical treatment of. *See also* Antireflux procedures; Nissen fundoplication.
evaluation of response to, 173
symptoms of, typical vs. atypical, 58–59
without Barrett's esophagus, refluxate in, 60
Gastroesophageal scintiscanning, 165t
Gastrointestinal disorders. *See also specific disorders.*
in cirrhosis, 1625
Gastrointestinal perforation
diagnosis of, 1097
steroid-induced, in immuno-compromised patients, 2382
Gastrointestinal stromal tumors, 1189–1197. *See also* Leiomyomas.
adjuvant therapy for, 1196–1197
clinical evaluation of, 1191f, 1191–1192
colorectal, 2314–2317
epidemiology of, 2314
investigation of, 2315, 2315f
management of
medical, 2315
surgical, 2315–2316
pathophysiology and pathology of, 2314f, 2314–2315, 2315f
presentation of, 2315
prognosis of, 2316
esophageal, 520
gastric, endoscopic appearance of, 740–741, 741f

Gastrointestinal stromal tumors (*Continued*)
historical background of, 1189
imaging of, 1195f, 1195–1196
malignant potential of, assessing, 1191
management of
medical, 2315
surgical, 1196, 2315–2316
targeted therapy for, 1193–1195, 1194f
molecular biology of, 1192f, 1192–1193
natural history of, 1189–1190, 1190t
pancreatic, 1359
pathology of, 1190f, 1190–1191, 1191f
Gastrojejunocolic fistulas, internal, 1094
Gastrojejunostomy
Billroth II
bile reflux gastritis following. *See* Bile reflux gastritis.
for caustic injury, gastric, 763
for duodenal ulcers, 795, 796, 796f, 797f
following gastrectomy, 911
gastroparesis following, 923
revision of, for bile reflux gastritis, 877, 878f
for duodenal ulcers, 795
for gastric drainage, 815–816, 817f
gastric outlet obstruction at site of, reoperative surgery for, 1137–1138
technique for, 1138
jejunogastric intussusception following, 879–880
for obesity, 932
pyloric exclusion with, 768–769
for pyloric outflow obstruction, 1137, 1137f
Roux-en-Y
for bile reflux gastritis, 876, 876f
for dumping syndrome, 872f, 872–873
following gastrectomy, 911
technique for, 845, 846f–848f
Gastroparesis, 920–925
postsurgical, 924–925
electrical stimulation for, 923–924
Roux stasis syndrome as, 809, 880, 925
reoperative surgery for, 1140
treatment of
botulinum toxin for, 921
electrical stimulation for, 921–924, 922f
for postsurgical gastroparesis, 923–924
pharmacologic, 921
reoperative surgery for, 1139–1140
surgical, 924
Gastropathy, hypertrophic, 886
Gastropexy
anterior, for gastric volvulus, in pediatric patients, 950
Collis, 599
for gastric volvulus, 1038
Hill
complications of, 598–599
imaging following, 85
for paraesophageal hernia, 559

Gastroplasty
  Collis. *See* Collis gastroplasty.
  endoluminal, 309–314
    advantages of, 313
    complications of, 312–313
    disadvantages of, 313
    efficacy of, 310, 311t, 312, 312f
    endoscopic, physiologic/anatomic
        mechanisms of, 328–329, 330f
    failure of, 313
    histologic changes and, 310, 310f
    historical background of, 309
    plication configuration and number
        and, 312
    procedure for, 309, 309f
    results with, 325, 326t, 327t
    selection criteria for, 312
  for obesity, 930–931, 931f
  vertical banded
    failed, revision surgery for, 1144–1145
    for obesity, 931, 931f
Gastroschisis, intestinal atresia with, 1220
Gastrosplenic ligament, 717–718
Gastrostomy, 755–756
  for gastroduodenal perforations,
      1109
  image-guided, percutaneous, 960
  Janeway
    with hostile abdomen, 1147
    in pediatric patients, 960
  laparoscopic, 755
  laparoscopy-assisted, in pediatric
      patients, 960
  longitudinal, for gastric outlet
      obstruction, 951
  for paraesophageal hernia, 559
  in pediatric patients, 960–961
    complications of, 960–961
    indications for, 960
    types of, 960
  percutaneous, 755–756, 757f
    contraindications to, 750t
    endoscopic
      fistulas due to, 1095
      in pediatric patients, 960
    indications for, 750t
  Stamm, 755, 756f
    contraindications to, 750t
    for esophagocoloplasty, 591
    with hostile abdomen, 1147
    indications for, 750t
    in pediatric patients, 960
    technique for, 857, 860f, 861f
  Witzel, in pediatric patients, 960
Gatekeeper, for endoscopic antireflux
    procedures, 323–325, 325, 326t, 327t
  advantages of, 325
  complications of, 325
  disadvantages of, 325
  efficacy of, 323, 324t, 325
  patient selection for, 323
  physiologic/anatomic mechanisms of,
      330–331
  procedure with, 323, 324f
  results with, 325, 326t, 327t
Gaucher's disease, splenectomy for, 1835
Gefitinib, for colorectal cancer metastases,
    2271

Gemcitabine, for pancreatic and
    periampullary carcinoma, palliative,
    1372–1373
Genetic factors
  in Barrett's esophagus, 343, 348, 349t
  in Crohn's disease, 1042–1043
  gastroesophageal reflux disease and, 200
  groin hernias and, 635
Genetic switches, in gastroesophageal reflux
    disease, 215–218
  intestinal metaplasia as, 215–216
  irreversible, 217–218
  oxyntocardiac mucosa as, 216–217
  reversibility of, 217
Genitofemoral nerve, 657, 658f
Genitourinary anomalies, associated with
    imperforate anus, 2390, 2405–2406
Gentamicin, for cholangitis prophylaxis,
    1550t
GERD. *See* Gastroesophageal reflux disease.
Gerlach's valve, 1862
Ghrelin
  duodenal function and, 981t, 984
  gastric, 723
Ghrelinoma, 1383
GIA staplers, 1086, 1087f
Giant migrating contractions, small
    intestinal, 1017, 1017f
Gibson, Thomas, 563
Gimbernat's ligament, 636
GISTs. *See* Gastrointestinal stromal tumors.
Glands, esophageal, prenatal development
    of, 41, 42f
Glandular cysts, fundic, 884, 2162
Glasgow criteria, modified, for pancreatitis,
    acute, 1300, 1301t
Glisson, Francis, 1751
Glomus tumors, gastric, 887–888
Glucagon-like peptide, small intestinal
    neuroendocrine function and, 1018
Glucagonoma, 1381–1382
  diagnosis of, 1381, 1382f
  therapy of, 1382, 1382f
Glucocorticoids, hepatotoxicity of, 1722
Glucose, small intestinal absorption of, 1003t
Glucose-dependent insulinotropic peptide,
    duodenal function and, 981t, 981–982
Glucose-6-phosphate dehydrogenase
    deficiency, splenectomy for, 1826
Glycoprotein, secretion of, by gallbladder,
    1458
Goblet cells
  in Barrett's esophagus, 341–342, 347
    development of, 347
    intestinalization of cardiac mucosa
        and, 345, 347
  prenatal development of, 40–41, 41f
Goodsall's rule, 2049
Gracilis muscle sling operation, 2405
Graft-versus-host disease, following
    intestinal transplantation, 1177
Granular cell tumors, esophageal, 520–521,
    521f
  endoscopic ultrasonography in, 123
Granulomatous colitis. *See* Crohn's disease.
Gray-scale ultrasonography, 112
Great prosthesis for reinforcement of the
    visceral sac, 652–653

Grey Turner's sign, 1299
GRFoma, 1382
  diagnosis of, 1382
  therapy, 1382
Gridiron incision, for appendectomy, 2145
Griffith's point, 1239, 1868
Groin hernias, 1471–1493. *See also* Femoral
    hernias; Inguinal hernias.
  anatomy and, 635–642
    of anterior abdominal wall, 636–639
      muscles, ligaments, and
          aponeurosis of, 636–639,
          637f–639f
      skin, fascia, vessels, and nerves of,
          636
    of inguinal region, laparoscopic,
        639–642
      of abdominal wall innervation
          and blood supply, 641–642,
          642f
      of deep aspects, 639–640, 640f
      of Hesselbach's triangle and
          spermatic cord, 641
      or transversalis fascia and its
          derivatives, 640–641, 641f
  classification of, 643–644, 644t, 645f
  embryology and, 633–634
  in females, 643
  femoral, 643
  historical background of, 632–633, 633f
  incarceration of, 643
  incidence of, 634
    etiology, biochemical basis, and
        mechanical stress and, 634–635
  indirect, 643
  irreducible, 643
  natural history of, 634
  recurrent, 653–654
  sliding, 643
  strangulation of, as indication for
      surgery, 644
  surgical treatment of, 644–654
    anesthesia for, 646
    combined anterior and
        preperitoneal approaches for,
        647t, 653
    complications of, 653–654
    conventional anterior nonprosthetic
        approach for, 647t, 647–649
    conventional anterior prosthetic
        approach for, 647t, 649, 650f
    conventional preperitoneal
        prosthetic approach for, 647t,
        649, 651–653
    indications and alternatives for,
        644–645, 646f
    preoperative preparation for,
        645–646
    prosthetic material for, 646b,
        646–647
  symptoms and diagnosis of, 642–643
Groin pain
  following hernia surgery, 653
  with inguinal herniorrhaphy,
      laparoscopic, 668
"Ground glass" appearance, in meconium
    ileus, 1224, 1224f
Grynfeltt-Lesshaft hernias, 687

Guanylin, small intestinal neuroendocrine
function and, 1019
Gut-associated lymphoid tissue, small
intestinal immune function and, 1010,
1012f
Gynecologic disorders
following ileal pouch–anal anastomosis,
2117–2118
pruritus ani and, 2068

H

Haemophilus influenzae infection
immunization against
with asplenia, in pediatric patients,
1811
with splenic cysts, 1815
overwhelming postsplenectomy infection
and, 1782
Haight, Cameron, 563
Hair, trichobezoars and, 943, 944, 944t
Hairy cell leukemia, splenectomy for, 1831
HALO system, for Barrett's ablation,
367–370, 368f, 369f
Halothane, fulminant liver failure due to,
1703
Halsted suture, 1085
Hamartomas
in Cowden's disease, 894t, 897, 2159t,
2175–2176
in Peutz-Jeghers syndrome, 2174
Hamartomatous polyps
colorectal, 2157f, 2157–2158, 2158f
gastric, 884
Hand-assisted laparoscopic surgery
for colonic diverticular disease, 2023f,
2023–2024
colorectal, 2353
splenectomy as, 1786
for splenic tumors, 1816
Hanley, Patrick H., 2053
Hannington-Kiff sign, 693
Hardy, Thomas G., Jr., 1089
Harmonic scalpel
for hemorrhoidectomy, 2033
hepatic surgery using, external biliary
fistulas following, etiology and
prevention of, 1540
for splenectomy, partial, 1815
Hartmann procedure, 2330
for colonic diverticular disease, 2025,
2025f
reversal of, 2415, 2416f
Harvey, William, 1751
Hayward, John, 341
Heart. *See also* Cardiovascular disorders.
esophagectomy affecting complications,
480
iron overload and, 1693
Heartburn, in esophageal disease, 56,
57b
achalasia as, 407
motility disorders as, 71
Heineke-Mikulicz cardioplasty, 5
Heineke-Mikulicz pyloroplasty, 816, 818f
for duodenal ulcers, 794–795, 795f
technique for, 841f, 842f

Heineke-Mikulicz stricturoplasty, for
Crohn's disease, 1059, 1059f
Heister, valves of, 1444
Helicobacter pylori infection
adenocarcinoma and, 445–446
Barrett's esophagus and, 334–335
gastric, endoscopic appearance of, 737
gastric adenocarcinoma and, 905, 906
gastric dysmotility associated with,
730–731
gastric lymphoma and, treatment and,
1209
gastric polyps associated with,
hyperplastic, 883
gastroesophageal reflux disease and,
200–201, 201f
MALT lymphoma associated with, 1203
treatment and, 1208
peptic ulcer disease and, in pediatric
patients, 961
reflux carditis and, 213–214
somatostatin and, 722–723
ulcerogenesis and, 811–812
Heliodorus, 632
Heller, Ernst, 5
Heller myotomy, 5
for achalasia, 409
with Dor repair, results with, 283
esophagography following, 85, 86f
laparoscopic
for achalasia, 413–415
antireflux procedure with, 416
complications of, 416–417, 417f
fundoplication technique and,
416
length of myotomy and, 415
operative steps for, 413–414, 414f,
415f
patient positioning and
preparation for, 413
port placement for, 413, 413f
postoperative management for,
414–415
with sigmoid-shaped esophagus
or megaesophagus, 416
for epiphrenic diverticulum,
435–437, 437f
Hemangioendotheliomas, epithelioid,
hepatic, 1748–1749
Hemangiomas
colonic, 1995–1997, 1996f
in blue rubber bleb syndrome, 1997
cavernous, rectal, 1996
in diffuse intestinal
hemangiomatosis, 1997
cutaneous, cavernous, 1997
esophageal, 521–522
endoscopic ultrasonography in, 123
gastric, 887
hepatic, 1726–1728
diagnosis of, 1726–1727, 1727f
etiology of, 1726
giant, 1726
treatment of, 1727–1728
intestinal
cavernous, 1997
small intestinal, 899
rectal, cavernous, 1996

Hemangiomas *(Continued)*
small intestinal, 899
splenic, 1815
Hemangiomatosis, gastrointestinal, diffuse,
small intestinal, 899
Hemangiosarcomas, splenic, primary, 1815
Hematologic disorders, splenectomy for. *See*
Splenectomy, for hematologic disorders.
Hematomas
duodenal, 1095
intramural, 766
Hemiazygos vein, 22
Hemicolectomy, right
for colonic ectasias, 1995
steps for, 2349b, 2349f, 2350f
Hemochromatosis
cardiac iron deposition and, 1693
hepatic laboratory tests in, 1613
Hemodialysis, for liver failure, acute,
1705–1706
Hemofiltration, for liver failure, acute,
1706
Hemoglobinopathies, splenectomy for, 1826
Hemoperfusion, charcoal and resin, for
liver failure, acute, 1706
Hemorrhage. *See also* Bleeding.
with aortoenteric fistulas, 1270–1271
colonic
acute, control of, in colonic ectasia,
1995
diverticular, 2016, 2016f, 2017f
diverticular
colonic, 2016, 2016f, 2017f
duodenal, 780
duodenal, diverticular, 780
as emergency surgical indication, 2102
following antireflux procedures,
609–610
following ileal pouch–anal anastomosis,
2111
with gastrointestinal fistulas, 1098
with ileostomy, 1081
with jejunoileal diverticula, 784–785
with Meckel's diverticulum, 787
with pancreatic pseudocysts, 1343–1344
rectal bleeding and, 1883
upper gastrointestinal, with splenic vein
thrombosis, 1353
Hemorrhagic proctitis, management of,
2321
Hemorrhoid(s), 2029–2035
anatomy and etiology of, 2029
clinical evaluation of, 2029–2030
external, thrombosed, 1887
treatment of
bipolar diathermy for, 2031, 2031f
excisional hemorrhoidectomy for,
2031–2033, 2032f
hemorrhoidal ligation with rubber
bands for, 2031, 2032f
nonexcisional options for, 2030
postoperative management and,
2034
for prolapsing hemorrhoids,
2033–2034, 2035f
rubber band ligation for, 2031,
2032f
sclerotherapy for, 2030f, 2030–2031

Index

Hemorrhoidectomy
    excisional, 2031–2033, 2032f
        instrumentation for, 2033
    nonexcisional, for prolapsing
        hemorrhoids, 2033–2034, 2035f
    postoperative management and, 2034
Hemostasis, with hepatobiliary trauma,
    1664f, 1664–1665, 1667
Henle's trunk, 968, 972f
Hepatectomy
    general maneuvers for, 1676f,
        1676–1677, 1677f
    major, 1677–1680
        left
            extended, 1680, 1682f
            with hilar dissection, 1678–1679,
                1681f
            left lateral sectionectomy and,
                1679–1680
        right
            extended, 1680, 1681f, 1682f
            with hilar dissection, 1678, 1679f,
                1680f
    native, total, 1695
    salvage, for metastatic colorectal cancer,
        2285
Hepatic adenomas, 1729
    diagnosis of, 1729, 1730f
    drug-induced, 1723
    etiology of, 1729
    treatment of, 1729, 1730f
Hepatic angiosarcomas, end-stage liver
    disease due to, 1687
Hepatic arterioportal shunts, 1713f,
    1713–1714
Hepatic arteriovenous shunts, 1713f,
    1713–1714
Hepatic artery(ies), 1445, 1445f, 1446, 1600,
    1602
    anatomy of, 1237, 1237f
    anomalies of, 1753, 1754f
    common, 1292, 1293f, 1600
        absent, 1600
        accessory, 1602
        left, 1602
        replaced, 1600, 1602
        right, 1602
    hepatocellular carcinoma and,
        1732–1733
Hepatic artery aneurysms, 1277–1278,
    1711–1712, 1712f
    clinical findings in, 1278
    diagnosis of, 1278
    false, 1277
    incidence of, 1277
    pathogenesis of, 1277
    treatment of, 1278
Hepatic artery arterioportal and
    arteriovenous shunts, 1713f, 1713–1714
Hepatic artery disorders, 1711–1714. See also
    specific disorders.
Hepatic artery failure, liver transplantation
    and, 1697
Hepatic artery infusion, for metastatic
    colorectal cancer, 2282–2283
Hepatic artery injury, 1712
Hepatic artery ligation, liver necrosis
    following, 1278

Hepatic artery thrombosis, 1712–1713, 1713f
    liver transplantation and, 1698
Hepatic blood flow, 1607
Hepatic cryotherapy, external biliary fistulas
    following, etiology and prevention of,
    1540
Hepatic cyst(s), 1630–1638
    cystic neoplasms and, 1636, 1636f, 1637f
    echinococcal, 1636–1638, 1638f
    in polycystic liver disease, 1634–1635,
        1635f
    solitary, 1630–1633, 1631f–1634f
Hepatic cystadenocarcinomas, 1746–1747
Hepatic ducts, 1602
    anomalies of, 1447–1448, 1448f, 1449f
    confluence of, 1602
Hepatic encephalopathy
    in cirrhosis, 1625
    in end-stage liver disease, 1694, 1694b
    portal hypertension and, 1756
Hepatic fibrosis, congenital, portal
    hypertension and, 1757
Hepatic flexure, 1847, 1863, 1865f
Hepatic functional reserve, 1621
Hepatic laboratory tests, abnormal,
    1610–1616
    albumin and, 1615–1616
    in alcoholic liver disease, 1612
    alkaline phosphatase elevation as,
        1614–1615
    aminotransferase elevations as, 1611b,
        1611–1612
    in autoimmune hepatitis, 1613
    in hemochromatosis, 1613
    in nonalcoholic fatty liver disease,
        1612–1613
    percutaneous liver biopsy and, 1616
    prothrombin time and, 1615
    serum bilirubin elevation as, 1613–1614,
        1614f
    in viral hepatitis, 1612
    in Wilson's disease, 1613
Hepatic lobectomy, for hepatic cysts,
    solitary, 1633
Hepatic metabolism, 1607–1608
Hepatic metastases, of colorectal cancer,
    2274–2287
    cryoablation for, 2283
    hepatic artery infusion for, 2282–2283
    hepatic resection for
        anatomic unisegmental and
            polysegmental, 2278
        anatomy and, 2275–2276, 2276f
        complications of, 2281–2282
        general principles of, 2275
        lobar, 2278–2281, 2279f–2281f
        patient selection for, 2274–2275
        postoperative care for, 2281
        preoperative care for, 2276
        surgical technique for, 2276f–2278f,
            2276–2278
        wedge, 2278
    hyperthermia for, 2284
    prognostic determinants for, 2284, 2285t
    recurrent and repeat hepatic resection
        for, 2285–2287
        prognostic factors affecting
            resectability and, 2285–2286

Hepatic metastases, of colorectal cancer
    (Continued)
        salvage hepatectomy and, 2285
        strategies for improving resectability
            and, 2286–2287
Hepatic neoplasms. See also specific neoplasms.
    benign, 1726–1730
        adenoma as, 1729
            diagnosis of, 1729, 1730f
            etiology of, 1729
            treatment of, 1729, 1730f
        angiomyolipoma as, 1730
        bile duct adenoma as, 1729
        biliary hamartoma as, 1729–1730,
            1730f
        focal nodular hyperplasia as,
            1728–1729
            diagnosis of, 1728, 1728f
            etiology of, 1728
            treatment of, 1728–1729
        hemangioma as, 1726–1728
            diagnosis of, 1726–1727, 1727f
            etiology of, 1726
            treatment of, 1727–1728
        peliosis hepatis as, 1730
    malignant, 1743–1749, 1744b, 1744t
        epithelial, 1743–1747
            hepatic cystadenocarcinoma as,
                1746–1747
            intrahepatic cholangiocarcinoma
                as, 1743–1745, 1745f
            mixed cholangiohepatocellular
                carcinoma as, 1745–1746,
                1746f
            squamous cell carcinoma as,
                1747
        mesenchymal, 1747
            fibrosarcoma as, 1747, 1747f
            leiomyosarcoma as, 1747
            liposarcoma as, 1747
            rhabdomyosarcoma as, 1747
            schwannoma as, 1747
        vascular, 1747–1749
            angiosarcoma as, 1747–1748,
                1748f
            epithelioid
                hemangioendothelioma as,
                1748–1749
Hepatic osteodystrophy, in end-stage liver
    disease, 1693
Hepatic resection
    for hepatocellular carcinoma,
        1738–1739
        liver transplantation vs., 1740
        operative techniques for, 1739
    intraoperative assessment in, 1675f,
        1675–1676, 1676f
    laparoscopic, for hepatic cysts, solitary,
        1633
    for metastatic colorectal cancer. See
        Hepatic metastases, of colorectal
        cancer, hepatic resection for.
    oncologic considerations in, 1674–1675
    postoperative complications with, 1683
    postoperative management of,
        1627–1628, 1683
    segmental, 1680
    wedge, 1683, 1683f

Hepatic reserve, preoperative evaluation of, 1674, 1674t
Hepatic trauma. *See* Hepatobiliary trauma.
Hepatic veins, 1603
  disorders of, Budd-Chiari syndrome as, 1714f, 1714–1715
Hepatic venous pressure gradient, in portal hypertension, 1757–1758
Hepaticojejunostomy
  for biliary atresia, 1548
  for choledochal cysts, 1554–1555
Hepatitis
  autoimmune
    hepatic laboratory tests in, 1613
    in primary sclerosing cholangitis, 1564
  drug-induced
    acute, 1721
    chronic, 1722
  viral, hepatic laboratory tests in, 1612
Hepatitis B
  end-stage liver disease due to, 1686
  fulminant liver failure due to, 1703
  hepatocellular carcinoma and, 1732
Hepatitis C
  end-stage liver disease due to, 1686
  hepatic laboratory tests in, 1612
  hepatocellular carcinoma and, 1732
Hepatitis D, fulminant liver failure due to, 1703
Hepatobiliary cancer
  with choledochal cysts, 1554
  hepatic abscesses associated with, pyogenic, 1642–1643
Hepatobiliary disease. *See also specific disorders.*
  with primary sclerosing cholangitis, treatment of, 1568
Hepatobiliary surgery, with low anterior resection, 2222
Hepatobiliary trauma, 1468, 1659–1668
  biliary system and, 1659, 1661f
  blunt, hepatic, 1662–1663, 1663f
  classification of, 1660, 1662t
  diagnosis of, 1668
  of gallbladder, 1663
  hemostasis and, 1667–1668
  mechanism of injury and, hepatic, 1659–1660
  mobilization of liver and, 1659, 1660f, 1661f
  operative management of, 1664f–1666f, 1664–1667
    for biliary trauma, 1666–1667, 1667f, 1668f
    débridement and, 1666
    for gallbladder injury, 1667
    Gore-Tex grafts for, 1668
    hepatic resection for, total, 1667
  penetrating, diagnostic approach for, 1660, 1662
  shock and, 1668
Hepatoblastoma, in children, alfa-fetoprotein and, 1734
Hepatocellular carcinoma, 1732–1740
  cholangiocarcinoma and, 1534
  clinical presentation of, 1733–1735
    biopsy and, 1734

Hepatocellular carcinoma *(Continued)*
    imaging and, 1734–1735
    laboratory investigation and, 1733–1734
  drug-induced, 1723–1724
  end-stage liver disease due to, 1687
  epidemiology of, 1732, 1733f
  etiology of, 1732
  liver transplantation for, 1692, 1692t
  management of, 1736–1740
    ablative therapies for, 1736–1738
    chemotherapy for, 1736
    resection for, 1738–1739
      transplantation vs. 1740
    transplantation for, 1739–1740
      resection vs., 1740
  pathology of, 1732–1733, 1733f
  risk factors for, 1732, 1733b
  staging of, 1735–1736
    Barcelona Chronic Liver Cancer staging system for, 1735
    Cancer of the Liver Italian Program for, 1736
    Okuda classification for, 1735
    TNM system for, 1735
Hepatocellular necrosis
  zone 1, drug-induced, 1719t, 1720
  zone 3, drug-induced, 1719t, 1719–1720
Hepatoduodenal ligament, 717, 718f
Hepatogastric ligament, 717, 718f
Hepatolithiasis, postoperative, with choledochal cysts, 1555
Hepatologists, on portal hypertension multidisciplinary team, 1767
Hepatoportoenterostomy, for biliary atresia, 1550
Hepatopulmonary syndrome, 1766f, 1766–1767
  clinical presentation of, 1766
  liver transplantation and, 1693
  pathophysiology of, 1766
Hepatorenal syndrome
  in cirrhosis, 1625
  in end-stage liver disease, 1693–1694
Hepatosplenopathy, 1751
Herald bleeding, with aortoenteric fistulas, 1114
Hereditary flat adenoma syndrome, small intestinal, 894t, 896
Hereditary hemorrhagic telangiectasia, colonic, 1999
Hereditary mixed polyposis syndrome, 2159t, 2176–2177
  small intestinal, 894t, 898
Hereditary nonpolyposis colorectal cancer, 2159t, 2169–2173
  clinical considerations in, 2169
  as colorectal cancer risk factor, 2188, 2188b
  diagnosis of, 2171, 2171b, 2172b
  extracolonic cancers and, 2169
  genetic testing and counseling and, 2171–2172
  genetics of, 2169–2171, 2170f
  surgical treatment of, 2172–2173
Hereditary spherocytosis, splenectomy for, 1825–1826, 1826t

Hernias
  diaphragmatic, congenital. *See* Diaphragmatic hernias.
  femoral. *See* Femoral hernias.
  Grynfeltt-Lesshaft, 687
  with ileostomy, 1080–1081
  inguinal, in children, 705–709
    clinical features of, 706
    contralateral inguinal exploration and, 709
    embryology of, 705
    incidence of, 705–706
    indirect, operative management of, 706–708, 707f, 708f
    with undescended testes, 709, 710f
  internal. *See* Internal hernias.
  levator ani, 687
  lumbar, 687–691
    anatomic considerations and, 688, 688f
    classification of, 689–690
    clinical features and diagnosis of, 688–689, 689f
    historical background of, 687–688
    incarceration plus strangulation of, 689
    treatment of, 690f, 690–691
  mesocolic (paraduodenal), 1858, 1861f
  obturator, 691–694
    anatomy and, 691, 692f
    clinical features and diagnosis of, 691, 693, 693f, 694f
    treatment of, 693–694, 694f
  paraesophageal. *See* Paraesophageal hernias.
  parastomal, 2372, 2372f
  perineal (levator), 694–700
    anatomy and, 696, 697f
    classification of, 694–696, 695f, 696f
    clinical features and diagnosis of, 696, 698f, 698–699, 699f
    treatment of, 699–700, 700f–703f
  pudendal, 695, 696f
  sciatic, 700–704
    anatomy and, 701, 703f
    clinical features and diagnosis of, 701–702, 703f
    treatment of, 702–704, 703f
  spigelian, repair of, 682
Herniation, internal, small bowel obstruction due to, 1027
Herniogenetics, 635
Herniorrhaphy
  for groin hernias, 643
  hiatal
    esophageal perforation due to, 606b, 606–607, 607f, 608f, 609–610, 610f
    laparoscopic, complications of, 610–611
  inguinal. *See* Inguinal herniorrhaphy.
  laparoscopic, for umbilical hernias, 681–682
  Lichtenstein, 649, 650f
Herophilus, 632
Herpes simplex virus infection
  achalasia due to, 406
  pruritus ani associated with, 2070

Hesselbach, Franz, 632
Hesselbach's triangle, 641
Heterotropic pancreatic polyps, 884
Hiatal hernias
    Allison repair for, 228
    Barrett's esophagus and, 60
    classification of, 549–550, 550f
    early development of surgery for, 6–7
    evaluation of, barium examination for,
        70
    following esophageal resection with
        visceral esophageal substitution, 614,
        615f
    gastric, endoscopic appearance of,
        737–738, 738f
    gastroesophageal reflux disease and, 200
    imaging of, 87, 88f, 89f
    lower esophageal sphincter competence
        and, 228
    paraesophageal. See Paraesophageal
        hernias.
    prevalence of, 550
    short esophagus, imaging of, 87, 89f
    sliding (type I), imaging of, 87, 88f
    type II, imaging of, 87, 89f
Hiatal herniorrhaphy
    esophageal perforation due to, 606b,
        606–607, 607f, 608f, 609–610, 610f
    laparoscopic, complications of, 610–611
Hiatal obstruction, following esophageal
    resection with visceral esophageal
    substitution, 614, 615f
Hiatus of Schwalbe, 696
Hidradenitis suppurativa, 2076–2078
    clinical presentation of, 2077, 2077f
    pathophysiology of, 2076–2077
    pruritus ani associated with, 2070
    treatment of, 2077–2078
Highly active antiretroviral therapy, 2380
    hepatotoxicity of, 1720
Hilar dissection, hepatectomy with
    left, 1678–1679, 1681f
    right, 1678, 1679f, 1680f
Hilar plate, 1599, 1603
Hill, Lucious, 6
Hill gastropexy
    complications of, 598–599
    imaging following, 85
Hippocrates, 632, 1771
Hirschsprung's disease, 1879, 2392
Histamine, gastric, 723
Histamine₂ receptor antagonists
    for esophageal strictures, 256
    for esophagitis, reflux, 255
    gastric acid secretion and, 727
    for gastroesophageal reflux disease, 254
Histamine receptors, gastric acid secretion
    and, 725
Histiocytoma, malignant fibrous, colorectal,
    2317
Hoarseness, gastroesophageal reflux disease
    associated with, diagnosis of, 171
Hodgkin's disease
    Ann Arbor staging system with Cotswold
        modification for, 1827, 1828t
    splenectomy for, 1827–1829, 1828f,
        1828t
    splenic, 1816

hOKT3-γ1-ala-ala antibody, for islet
    transplantation, 1428
Horizontal mattress suture, 1085
Hormonal disorders, obesity and, bariatric
    surgery and, 938
Hormonal therapy, for carcinoid tumors,
    1186
Hospital costs, for laparoscopic colorectal
    surgery, 2344
Hospital stay, length of, for laparoscopic
    colorectal surgery, 2343
Hostile abdomen, 1147–1148, 1148b
Hourglass gallbladder, 1449, 1451f
Howell-Jolly bodies, 1775
Howship-Romberg sign, 693
Human immunodeficiency virus infection.
    See also Acquired immunodeficiency
    syndrome.
    anal intraepithelial neoplasia and, 2289
    anorectal fistulas in, 2058
    anorectal sepsis in, 2058
    cholangiopathy and, 1615
    splenectomy for, 1825
Human papillomavirus infection, anal
    anal intraepithelial neoplasia and, 2289
    in immunocompromised patients, 2383t,
        2384
Hunter, John, 632, 811
Hunt-Lawrence pouch, for microgastria,
    950
Hurst dilators, 5
Hydatid disease of liver, external biliary
    fistulas associated with, etiology and
    prevention of, 1540, 1540f
Hydrocarbons, fulminant liver failure due
    to, 1703
Hydrocele, with inguinal herniorrhaphy,
    laparoscopic, 668
Hydrocortisone phosphate, pruritus ani
    associated with, 2069
Hydrodissection, 2412
Hydrogen ions, secretion of, by gallbladder,
    1458
Hydropneumothorax, in esophageal
    perforation, 93, 95f
5-Hydroxyindoleacetic acid, carcinoid
    tumors and, 1182–1183
5-Hydroxytryptophan. See Serotonin.
Hydroxyzine, for pruritus, in primary
    sclerosing cholangitis, 1567
Hyperamylasemia, pancreatitis associated
    with, 1299
Hyperbilirubinemia, direct (conjugated)
    alkaline phosphatase level in, 1614–1615
    in infancy, 1545
Hypercalcemia, pancreatitis associated with,
    1299
Hyperemia, intestinal, postprandial,
    1242–1243
Hyperfractionation, 1156
Hypergastrinemia, 722
Hyperglycemia, in short-bowel syndrome,
    1166
Hyperinsulinism, in pediatric patients,
    1408–1409
Hyperlipidemia
    obesity and, bariatric surgery and, 938
    pancreatitis associated with, 1299

Hyperplastic colorectal polyps, 2158, 2158f
Hyper-rotation, duodenal, 1214, 1216f
Hypersplenism, 1777
    partial splenic embolization for,
        1793–1795, 1794f, 1795f
Hypertension
    portal, in pancreatitis, chronic,
        1312–1313
    portopulmonary, 1767, 1767f
Hyperthermia, for metastatic colorectal
    cancer, 2284
Hypogastric nerves, total mesorectal
    excision with autonomic nerve
    preservation and, 2237–2238, 2238f
Hypoglycemia
    factitious, with insulinoma, 1376
    hyperinsulinemic, of infancy, persistent,
        1408–1409
    with insulinoma, management of, 1378
    in short-bowel syndrome, 1166
Hypopharynx, prenatal development of,
    31–33, 33f, 34f
Hyposplenism, 1777

I

Icones Herniarum (Camper), 632
Idiopathic thrombocytopenic purpura,
    splenectomy for, 1822–1824, 1824f
Ileal adenocarcinoma, 916
Ileal artery aneurysms, 1282f, 1283
Ileal atresia, 1219
Ileal carcinoids, treatment of, 1185
Ileal motility, 2105–2106
Ileal pouch–anal anastomosis
    for Crohn's disease, 2130, 2132
        failure of, 2121–2122
    for familial adenomatous polyposis,
        2165, 2165f, 2166t, 2167
    redo, 2417
    revision pouch surgery for, 2118–2120,
        2120f, 2121f
        alternative techniques for pouch
            salvage and, 2119–2120, 2120f,
            2121f
        surgical technique for, 2118–2119,
            2119t
    total proctocolectomy with, for
        ulcerative colitis, 2093–2094
    for ulcerative colitis, 2102–2122
        alternatives to, 2122
        critical level of, 2109–2110
        ileal pouch design for, 2103f,
            2103–2105
            comparative studies of, 2105
            quadruplicated pelvic ileal
                reservoir (W pouch) as, 2105
            three-limbed pelvic ileal reservoir
                (S pouch) as, 2104
            two-limbed pelvic ileal reservoir
                (J pouch) as, 2104–2105
        ileal pouch function and, 2105–2107
            ecology of pouch and, 2107
            efficiency of evacuation and,
                2106
            functional outcome and, 2107
            ileal motility and, 2105–2106

Ileal pouch–anal anastomosis (Continued)
    postprandial pouch tone and,
      2106–2107
    pouch compliance and capacity
      and, 2105
    ileoanal anastomosis and, 2107–2110
      single- or double-stapled
        technique for, 2108–2109,
        2109f
      transanal mucosectomy and,
        2108, 2108f
    laparoscopic, 2102
    operative technique for, 2102f,
      2102–2103
    pouch-specific complications of,
      2111–2122
      age-related, 2118
      anastomotic cuff abscess as, 2111
      Crohn's disease as, 2121–2122
      dysplasia in residual rectal
        mucosa as, 2112
      enterocutaneous fistulas as, 2112
      gynecologic, 2117–2118
      intra-abdominal abscess as, 2111
      neoplastic, 2116–2117
      postoperative hemorrhage as,
        2111
      pouchitis as, 2113, 2115t,
        2115–2116
      pouch-vaginal fistulas as,
        2112–2113, 2114f
      proctitis in residual rectal mucosa
        as, 2112
      quantification of risk of pouch
        failure and, 2120–2121
      revision pouch surgery for,
        2118–2120, 2119f–2121f
      sexual dysfunction as, male, 2117
      small bowel obstruction as, 2111
      stricture at anastomosis as, 2112
    two vs. one stage, 2110
Ileocecal valve
    anatomy of, 1846, 1861, 1862
    on colonoscopy, 1867
    lipohyperplasia (lipomatous
      hypertrophy) of, 900–901
Ileocolic artery, 1849, 1851f, 1852f
Ileocolostomy
    for colorectal cancer, 2331
    end-loop, 2367–2368, 2369f
Ileorectal anastomosis, colectomy with
    for familial adenomatous polyposis,
      2165, 2165t, 2166t, 2166–2167, 2168
    for ulcerative colitis, 2122
Ileorectostomy, colectomy with, for
    intractable constipation, 1880
Ileosigmoid anastomosis, for colonic inertia,
    1934
Ileosigmoid fistulas, in Crohn's disease,
    1064
Ileosigmoid knotting, 1984
Ileostomy, 1070–1081
    complications of, 1078–1081
      bowel obstruction as, 1078–1080
      diarrhea as, 1081
      hemorrhage and peri-ileostomy
        varices as, 1081
      mucocutaneous separation as, 1080

Ileostomy (Continued)
      parastomal hernia as, 1080
      peri-ileostomy fistula as, 1080–1081
      skin problems as, 1081
      stoma necrosis as, 1078
      stoma prolapse as, 1080
      stoma retraction as, 1080
      stoma stenosis as, 1080
    continent, Kock
      for familial adenomatous polyposis,
        2165t, 2165–2166, 2166t
      for ulcerative colitis, 2122
    diverting, for ileal pouch–anal
      anastomosis, 2110
    divided-loop, 1075, 1077f
    end, 1071, 1072f–1074f, 1074–1075,
      2363–2364, 2363f–2366f
      total proctocolectomy with, for
        familial adenomatous polyposis,
        2165, 2165t, 2166t
    end-loop, 1075–1076, 1078f, 2367, 2368f
    historical background of, 1070
    indications for, 1070–1071
    loop, 1075, 1076f, 2366, 2367f
      closure of, 1076–1078, 1079f
      temporary, 1071
    panproctocolectomy with, for ulcerative
      colitis, 2122
    physiology and, 1071
    preoperative preparation for, 1071
    techniques for, 1071
Ileostomy bags, for abscess drainage, 1102,
    1103f
Ileus
    with inguinal herniorrhaphy,
      laparoscopic, 667
    meconium, 1224f, 1224–1225, 1225f
    postoperative, bowel obstruction vs.,
      1028
Iliac artery, deep circumflex, 673
Iliococcygeus muscle, 696
Iliohypogastric nerve, 656
Ilioinguinal nerve, 656
Iliopectineal arch, 656–657
Iliopubic tract, 657
Iliopubic tract hernia repair, 652
Illicit drugs, ingested packages of, 943, 943f
ILS staplers, 1087
Image-guided interventional therapy, for
    spleen. See Spleen, image-guided
    interventional therapy for.
Imaging. See also specific imaging modalities.
    of carcinoid tumors, 1183f, 1183–1184,
      1184f
    for caustic ingestions, 543
    esophageal, 63–95
      in caustic injury, 91
      of diverticula, 94–95, 96f
      of esophageal perforation, 91, 93–94,
        95f
      of esophageal rings and webs, 88f,
        88–89, 90f, 91f
      examination techniques for, 64,
        64f–66f
      in gastroesophageal reflux disease,
        67–70
        barium examination for, 68–70,
          69f–71f

Imaging (Continued)
    of hiatal hernia, 87, 88f, 89f
    in motility disorders, 71–74
      primary, 71–74, 72f, 73f
      secondary, 74
    in neoplastic disease, 74–83
      benign, 81–83, 83f
      malignant, 74–81, 75f–81f
    normal anatomy and function and,
      63
    normal radiographic appearance
      and, 64f–66f, 64–66
    normal variants and, 66–67, 67f
    postoperative, 83–86
      following antireflux procedures,
        85, 86f
      following cardiomyotomy, 85, 86f
      following cricopharyngeal
        myotomy, 84–85, 85f
      following esophageal resection,
        86, 87f, 88f
      goals and techniques of, 83–84,
        84t
    of strictures, 89–91, 92f–94f
    for structural abnormality detection,
      143
    of varices, 95, 97f
    in esophageal spasm, 419, 420f
    in hypertensive lower esophageal
      sphincter, 424
    in nutcracker esophagus, 422
    preoperative, for reoperative pelvic
      surgery, 2410
Imatinib mesylate, for gastrointestinal
    stromal tumors, 1197
[131]I-metaiodobenzylguanidine scans, of
    carcinoid tumors, 1184
Imiquimod, for anal intraepithelial
    neoplasia, 2290
Immune function, in pediatric patients,
    consequences of splenectomy and, 1806
Immune system, small intestinal, 1009–1012
    gut-associated lymphoid tissue and,
      1010, 1012f
    M cells and, 1010, 1012f
    regulation of, 1010
    regulation of gut function by, 1011–1012
    secretory immunoglobulin A and, 1010,
      1011f
Immunoallergy, drug-induced, 1721
Immunocompromised patients, 2375–2384.
    See also Acquired immunodeficiency
    syndrome; Human immunodeficiency
    virus infection.
    colonic diverticular disease in, 2020
    mechanisms of immunodeficiency and,
      2375–2377, 2376b, 2376t
      AIDS as, 2376–2377
      cancer and cancer therapy as, 2376
      malnutrition and injury as, 2376
      pharmacologic, 2375–2376, 2377t
    surgical problems in
      acute appendicitis as, 2381
      anorectal complications as, 2383,
        2383t
      colonic complications as, 2381
      diverticular disease as, 2381
      infectious colitis as, 2381–2382

Immunocompromised patients (Continued)
  malignancies as, 2383–2384
  neutropenic enteritis as, 2382–2383
  steroid-induced gastrointestinal
    perforation as, 2382
  surgical risk assessment in, 2380–2381
  therapeutic approach to, 2377–2381
    altered hormonal response to stress
      and, 2378
    immunosuppression and
      cancer and, 2380
      for inflammatory bowel disease,
        2379–2380
      for transplantation, 2379
    immunosuppression in, 2377–2378
    impaired wound healing and, 2378
    steroids in, 2377
    stress-dose steroids and, 2378–2379,
      2379b, 2379t
Immunodeficiency. See also Acquired
  immunodeficiency syndrome; Human
  immunodeficiency virus infection.
  mechanisms of, 2375–2377, 2376b, 2376t
    AIDS as, 2376–2377
    cancer and cancer therapy as, 2376
    malnutrition and injury as, 2376
    pharmacologic, 2375–2376, 2377t
  pruritus ani associated with, 2070
Immunoglobulin A, secretory, small
  intestinal immune function and, 1010,
  1011f
Immunomodulators, for Crohn's disease,
  1053
Immunosuppression
  for inflammatory bowel disease,
    2091–2092
  for islet transplantation, 1424,
    1428–1429
  for pancreas transplantation, 1418–1419
  steroid-induced, 2377–2378
Immunotherapy. See also
  Immunosuppression.
  for pancreatic and periampullary
    carcinoma, 1373
Impedance testing
  ambulatory, pH monitoring and, for
    esophageal bolus clearance testing,
    158–159, 159f, 160f
  of esophageal bolus clearance, 155–156,
    157f, 158, 158f
Imperforate anus. See also Anorectal
  anomalies.
  anomalies associated with
    genitourinary, 2390
    sacral and spinal, 2390
  high, surgical management of, 2396,
    2398–2402, 2399f
    with cloacal malformation, 2402,
      2403f
    colostomy construction and, 2396,
      2398f
    minimally invasive repair as,
      2400–2402, 2401f, 2402f
    neonatal pull-through procedures
      for, 2400
  low, surgical management of, 2395–2396
    anterior perineal anorectoplasty as,
      2396, 2397f

Imperforate anus (Continued)
    cutback anoplasty as, 2395f, 2395–2396
    transplant anoplasty as, 2396, 2397f
In vitro synthesized protein assay, for APC
  gene mutation screening, 2164
Incision(s)
  abdominal, for Crohn's disease,
    1056–1057, 1057f
  for appendectomy, 2145, 2146f
  closure of, 2329
  for colorectal surgery, 2329
  for esophageal reconstruction, 579–580,
    580f
  for liver surgery, 1671–1673
    midline, 1671
    right thoracoabdominal, 1671, 1673
    subcostal, 1671, 1672f
Incisional hernias, repair of, 682–683, 683f
Inclusion cysts, esophageal, 525
Incontinence. See Fecal incontinence.
Infants
  anorectal fistulas in, 2058
  appendicitis, acute, 2143–2144
  juvenile polyposis syndrome in, 2173
  newborn. See Neonates.
  persistent hyperinsulinemic
    hypoglycemia of infancy and,
    1408–1409
Infections. See also specific infections.
  in cirrhosis, 1626
  following intestinal transplantation, 1176
  with gastrointestinal fistulas, 1098
  hepatic artery aneurysms due to, 1277
  with immunosuppressive therapy,
    following liver transplantation, 1699,
    1699t
  intra-abdominal, hematogenous spread
    of, hepatic abscesses due to,
    pyogenic, 1642
  with pancreatic pseudocysts, 1342–1343,
    1343f
  pruritus ani associated with, 2070
  superior mesenteric artery aneurysms
    due to, 1278
  suture material and, 1084
  systemic, hepatic abscesses due to,
    pyogenic, 1642
  wound, with herniorrhaphy, 654
    inguinal, laparoscopic, 668
Infectious colitis, in immunocompromised
  patients, 2381–2382
Inferior mesenteric artery
  anatomy of, 1238, 1849, 1850, 1851f,
    1867, 1868
    variations in, 1869
  aneurysms of, 1280
  embryology of, 1234, 1236f
  hypogastric communications of, 1239,
    1240f
  in mesenteric ischemia, 1247, 1248f. See
    also Mesenteric ischemia.
  superior mesenteric artery
    communications with, 1239
Inferior mesenteric vein, anatomy of, 1869
Infertility
  with inguinal herniorrhaphy,
    laparoscopic, 667
  obesity and, bariatric surgery and, 938

Inflammation
  cancer and, 348
  local, in pancreatitis, acute, 1297–1298
  in pancreatitis, chronic, 1345
  perineural, in pancreatitis, chronic,
    1345
  systemic, in pancreatitis, acute, 1298
Inflammatory bowel disease, 2080–2096.
  See also Crohn's disease; Ulcerative
  colitis.
  cancer and, 2380
  as colorectal cancer risk factor, 2187
  immunosuppression for, 2379–2380
  in primary sclerosing cholangitis,
    1563–1564
  with primary sclerosing cholangitis, 1693
Inflammatory lesions, gastric, benign, 885
Inflammatory polyps, gastric, 884
Inflammatory processes, small bowel
  obstruction due to, 1027
Inflammatory pseudotumor
  esophageal, 522
  in pancreatitis, chronic, 1312
Infliximab
  for anorectal abscesses, 2057–2058
  for Crohn's disease, 1053, 2128
  for gastrointestinal fistulas, 1105
  for inflammatory bowel disease,
    2092–2093
  mechanism of action of, 2377t
Infrared coagulation, for hemorrhoids,
  2031, 2031f, 2033
Ingelfinger, Franz, 5
Inguinal canal, embryology of, 705
Inguinal hernias, 643–644
  in children, 705–709
    clinical features of, 706
    contralateral inguinal exploration
      and, 709
    embryology of, 705
    incidence of, 705–706
    indirect, operative management of,
      706–708, 707f, 708f
    with undescended testes, 709, 710f
  recurrence of, postoperative, 667
Inguinal herniorrhaphy, 656–668
  anatomy and, 656–657
  laparoscopic, 658–668
    complications of, 665–668, 666t
      associated with hernia repair,
        667–668
      associated with laparoscopic
        approach, 665–667
      associated with patient, 667
    convention herniorrhaphy compared
      with
      operative strategies and, 659,
        661–664
      patient selection and, 659
    conventional herniorrhaphy
      compared with, 658–659, 660t,
        661t, 661–665
Inguinal ligament, 636
Inguinal region, anatomy of, laparoscopic,
  639–642
  of abdominal wall innervation and
    blood supply, 641–642, 642f
  of deep aspects, 639–640, 640f

Inguinal region, anatomy of, laparoscopic (*Continued*)
  of Hesselbach's triangle and spermatic cord, 641
  of transversalis fascia and its derivatives, 640–641, 641f
Inhibitory relaxation wave, swallowing and, 53
Insulinomas, 1375, 1376–1379
  invasive localization studies for, 1377–1378, 1378f
  preoperative localization of, 1377, 1377f
  symptoms and diagnosis of, 1376–1377
  therapy of, 1378–1379, 1379f
Intensity-modulated radiation therapy, 1155
Intercostal trunk, superior, 22
Interdigestive migrating motor complex, 188, 189f
  phasic activity of, disturbance of, detection by antroduodenal manometry, 188
Interferon, for carcinoid tumors, 1186
Internal hernias, 1120–1126
  acquired, 1124–1126, 1125f
    clinical features of, 1125
    diagnosis of, 1125–1126
    treatment of, 1126
  congenital, 1120–1124
    foramen of Winslow, 1123–1124, 1124f
    paraduodenal, 1120–1121, 1121f
      clinical features of, 1121
      diagnosis of, 1121–1122
      treatment of, 1122
    transmesenteric, 1122f, 1122–1123
      clinical features of, 1123
      diagnosis of, 1123
      treatment of, 1123
    transomental, 1123, 1124f
  small bowel obstruction due to, 1120
Internal oblique muscle, 636, 637f, 638
Intersigmoid fossa, 1866
Interstitial cells of Cajal, intestinal motility and, 925
Interventional radiology. *See also specific techniques.*
  biliary
    for benign biliary disease, 1468
    complications of, 1468–1469
    image-guided therapy of malignant biliary disease and, 1466–1468
    percutaneous transhepatic cholangiography and percutaneous biliary drainage and, 1464–1466
    radiologist's role in, 1462–1464, 1463f–1465f
    for stone management, 1466
Intestinal anastomoses, 1083, 2331–2335
  biofragmentable anastomosis ring for, 1089–1090, 1090f
  with colonic J-pouch, 2334
  inverted vs. everted, 1085–1086, 1086f
  with restorative proctocolectomy for familial adenomatous polyposis or ulcerative colitis with dysplasia or cancer, 2335

Intestinal anastomoses (*Continued*)
  stapled, 1086f, 1086–1089, 2333, 2334f–2337f
    hand-sewn vs., 1088–1089
    staplers for, 1086–1087, 1087f
    techniques and pitfalls in, 1087–1088
      functional end-to-end anastomosis and, 1087, 1088f
      stapled end-to-end anastomosis and, 1087–1088, 1088f
  stoma vs., 2335, 2338
  sutured, 1083–1086, 2331, 2331f–2333f, 2333
    hand-sewn vs. stapled anastomoses and, 1088–1089
    methods of, 1084–1086
    suture material and, 1083–1084
      infection and, 1084
      tumor cell adherence and, 1084
  sutureless, 2333–2334
  tissue adhesives for, 1089
Intestinal atresia, in pediatric patients, 1219–1221, 1220f, 1221f
Intestinal bypass, for Crohn's disease, 1063
Intestinal decompression, 750
Intestinal dysmotility, 926–927
  diagnosis of, 926
  treatment of
    pharmacologic, 926
    surgical, 926–927
Intestinal failure. *See* Short-bowel syndrome.
Intestinal fistulas. *See also* Enteric fistulas; *specific sites, e.g.* Anal fistulas.
  in Crohn's disease, surgical treatment of, 2095
Intestinal fluid, small intestinal secretion of, 1008–1009, 1010f
Intestinal ganglioneuromatosis syndrome, small intestinal, 894t, 898
Intestinal hemangiomatosis, diffuse, colonic hemangiomas in, 1997
Intestinal lymphomas
  diagnosis of, 1208, 1208f
  epidemiology of, 1199, 1200t
  treatment of, 1209, 1211f
Intestinal metaplasia
  Barrett's esophagus and, 334–335
  in gastroesophageal reflux disease, 215–216, 217–218
Intestinal motility, 925–926. *See also specific regions of intestine, e.g.* Colonic motility.
  in short-bowel syndrome, 1163–1164
    improving, 1169
Intestinal obstruction. *See also specific regions of intestine, e.g.* Duodenal obstruction.
  with groin hernias, as indication for surgery, 644
  with ileostomy, 1078–1080
  with inguinal herniorrhaphy, laparoscopic, 666
  neonatal, 947–948, 1219
    clinical features and diagnosis of, 948
  with stomas, 2371
Intestinal perforation
  colonic
    as emergency surgical indication, 2102

Intestinal perforation (*Continued*)
  in immunocompromised patients, 2381
  duodenal
    with duodenal diverticula, 779
    treatment of, 1108–1110
  prenatal, meconium peritonitis and, 1225
Intestinal polyposis syndromes. *See also* Familial adenomatous polyposis.
  small intestinal
    attenuated familial adenomatous polyposis as, 894t, 896
    Bannayan-Zonana (Bannayan-Ruvalcaba-Riley) syndrome as, 894t, 897
    Cowden's disease as, 894t, 897
    Cronkhite-Canada syndrome as, 894t, 898
    familial adenomatous polyposis as, 893f, 893–895, 894t
    Gardner's syndrome as, 894t, 895
    hereditary flat adenoma syndrome as, 894t, 896
    hereditary mixed polyposis syndrome as, 894t, 898
    intestinal ganglioneuromatosis syndrome as, 894t, 898
    juvenile polyposis syndrome as, 894t, 896–897
    lymphoid polyposis syndrome as, 894t, 898
    Muir-Torre syndrome as, 894t, 896
    Peutz-Jeghers syndrome as, 894t, 897–898
    Turcot's syndrome as, 894t, 895–896
Intestinal tapering and lengthening procedure, for short-bowel syndrome, 1171–1173, 1172f
Intestinal transit
  colonic
    in constipation, 1931–1932, 1932f
    in rectal prolapse, 1959
    prolonging, in short-bowel syndrome, 1169–1171, 1170f, 1170t
      colon interposition for, 1171
      intestinal pacing for, 1171
      intestinal segment reversal for, 1169–1171
      intestinal valves for, 1171
      recirculating loops for, 1171
  small bowel transit studies and, in constipation, 1932
Intestinal transplantation
  for intestinal dysmotility, 927
  for short-bowel syndrome, 1168, 1173–1177
    indications for, 1173–1174
    operative procedure for, 1174f, 1174–1175
    outcome with, 1175f, 1175–1177, 1176f
Intestinal tubes, for nutrition
  complications of, 758
  management of, 758
Intra-abdominal abscesses
  with appendicitis, 2150
  following ileal pouch–anal anastomosis, 2111

Intra-abdominal fistulas, in colonic diverticular disease, 2021
Intracranial pressure, elevated, in fulminant hepatic failure, management of, 1704
Intraductal papillary mucinous neoplasms, 1359
  pancreatic
    clinical presentation of, 1387–1388
    diagnosis of, 1393–1394, 1395f
    incidence and epidemiology of, 1387
    pathology and biologic behavior of, 1391b, 1391–1392, 1392f
    treatment of, 1397–1398
Intraepithelial carcinoma, colorectal, 2192
Intrahepatic cholangiocarcinoma, 1743–1745, 1745f
Intraoperative radiation therapy, 1156
  for recurrent cancer, 2417–2418
Intraoperative ultrasound, in Zollinger-Ellison syndrome, 865, 865f
Intraperitoneal-only mesh repair, for inguinal hernias, 656, 661, 664, 665t
Intraperitoneal therapy, for gastric adenocarcinoma, adjuvant, 912–913
Intratracheal tubes, development of, 4
Intravenous immunoglobulin, for idiopathic thrombocytopenic purpura, 1824
Intravenous pyelography, with nephroenteric fistulas, 1106
Intrinsic factor, gastric secretion of, 728
Intussusception
  colonic, 1980, 1981f
  jejunogastric, following gastrectomy, 879–880
  in pediatric patients, 1229–1230, 1230f–1232f, 1232
  rectal, surgical treatment of, 1936, 1938f
Invasive radiologic procedures, external biliary fistulas following, etiology and prevention of, 1540–1541
Iodoquinol, for liver abscesses, amebic, 1655
Irinotecan, for metastatic colorectal cancer, 2201
Iron absorption
  duodenal, 979–980, 980f
  small intestinal, 1007t, 1008, 1009f
Iron deficiency anemia
  in Crohn's disease, 1054
  following gastrectomy, 873
Iron overload, cardiac iron deposition and, 1693
Irritable bowel syndrome, diarrhea-predominant, 1879–1880
Ischemia
  colonic. See Colonic ischemia.
  mesenteric, acute, colonic ischemia as manifestation of, management of, 2010
  with stomas, 2372
Ischemic orchitis, following hernia surgery, 654
Island flaps
  for anal stenosis, 2063f, 2063–2064, 2064f
  diamond-shaped, for anal stenosis, 2064, 2064f
  U-shaped, for anal stenosis, 2064
  V-Y, for anal stenosis, 2063f, 2063–2064

Islet cell(s), 1289
  proliferation of, 1290
Islet cell dysmaturation syndrome, 1408–1409
Islet cell tumors, in Zollinger-Ellison syndrome. See Zollinger-Ellison syndrome.
Islet transplantation, 1422–1429
  challenges and emerging opportunities in, 1427–1429, 1428f
    alloimmune and autoimmune drugs as, 1428–1429
    islet protection and regeneration as, 1429
    living donor transplantation as, 1427–1428
    supply and demand as, 1427
  early clinical trials of, 1423–1424
  evaluation and risk assessment for, 1424–1425
  historical background of, 1422–1423, 1423f
  immunosuppression for, 1424
  indications for, 1424
  islet preparation for, 1424, 1425f
  procedure for, 1425
  recent advances in, 1425–1427, 1426f
    outcomes and, 1426–1427, 1427f
  site of, 1423
Isoniazid, hepatotoxicity of, 1722
Isoperistaltic stricturoplasty, side-to-side, for Crohn's disease, 1059, 1062f
Isoproterenol, mesenteric blood flow and, 1243t
Itraconazole, hepatotoxicity of, 1722
Ivor-Lewis esophagogastrectomy, for gastric adenocarcinoma, 909

J

J pouch, 2104–2105, 2334
Jaboulay gastroduodenostomy, for duodenal ulcers, 795
Jaboulay pyloroplasty, 818, 819f
  technique for, 844f
Jaboulay stricturoplasty, for Crohn's disease, 1059, 1062f
Jackson's membrane, 1863
Jamaican bush teas, hepatotoxicity of, 1723
Janeway gastrostomy
  with hostile abdomen, 1147
  in pediatric patients, 960
Japanese Society for Esophageal Diseases staging system, for esophageal cancer, 448, 449, 452f, 453f, 453t, 454t
Jaundice
  with cholangiocarcinoma, palliation for, 1531
  cholestatic, pruritus ani in, 2067
  in newborns, 1545
  obstructive
    gallbladder cancer presenting with, 1525
    in pancreatic and periampullary carcinoma

Jaundice (Continued)
    nonoperative palliation of, 1365
    operative palliation of, 1366, 1366f
  pathophysiology of, 1618–1619
  patient approach for, 1460
Jejunal adenocarcinoma, 916
Jejunal artery aneurysms, 1283
Jejunal atresia, 1219
Jejunal carcinoids, treatment of, 1185
Jejunal interposition
  for bile reflux gastritis, 876–877, 877f
  for dumping syndrome, 872, 872f
Jejunal reservoir, for microgastria, 950
Jejunogastric intussusception, following gastrectomy, 879–880
Jejunoileal atresia, in cystic fibrosis, 1219
Jejunoileal bypass, for obesity, 930, 930f
Jejunoileal diverticula, 783–786
  complications of, 784–785
    hemorrhage as, 784–785
    malabsorption as, 785
    obstruction as, 785
    perforation as, 785
  diagnosis of, 784, 785f
  diseases associated with, 783
  incidence of, 783
  management of, 785–786
    nonoperative, 785
    operative, 785–786
  pathogenesis of, 783–784, 784f
  symptoms of, 784
Jejunojejunostomy, for obesity, 933
Jejunostomy, 757–758, 758f
  contraindications to, 750t
  for esophagogastrostomy, 588
  feeding, for microgastria, 950
  for gastroduodenal perforations, 1109
  indications for, 750t
  Witzel, 757, 758f
Jejunum. See also Small intestine.
  as esophageal substitute, 579
    esophagojejunoplasty and, 592–596
      free transfer and, 595f, 595–596
      interposition and, 593f, 593–594, 594f
      results of, 596t, 596–597
      Roux-en-Y limb and, 594f, 594–595
  for foregut reconstruction for benign disease, 298, 299, 300f
JSED staging system, for esophageal cancer, 448, 449, 452f, 453f, 453t, 454t
Judd stricturoplasty, for Crohn's disease, 1059, 1060f
Juvenile polyposis syndrome, 2159t, 2173–2174
  of colon, 2173
  generalized, 2173
  for hereditary nonpolyposis colorectal cancer, 2188
  of infancy, 2173
  small intestinal, 894t, 896–897
    symptoms and diagnosis of, 897
    treatment of, 897

K

Kaposi's sarcoma, in immunocompromised patients, 2384
Kasabach-Merritt syndrome, 1726
Kegel exercises
for constipation, 1938
for fecal incontinence, 1921–1922
Kelling, G., 4
Ketoconazole, hepatotoxicity of, 1722
Kidney transplantation, with simultaneous pancreas transplantation, 1417f, 1417–1418, 1418f
Killian-Jamison diverticula, 95
Killian's dehiscence, 94
Killian's triangle, 391
KIT molecule, gastrointestinal stromal tumors and, 1192f, 1192–1193
targeted therapy and, 1193–1195, 1194f
Klebsiella pneumoniae, hepatic abscesses and, 1644, 1645
Klippel-Trénaunay-Weber syndrome, colonic involvement in, 1999
Knee-shoulder position, 1886
Kocher maneuver, 579, 964, 966f
with duodenal diverticula, 782, 782f
in duodenal injury, 766, 767f
Kock continent ileostomy
for familial adenomatous polyposis, 2165t, 2165–2166, 2166t
for ulcerative colitis, 2122
Krukenberg tumors, 906
Kugel/Ugahary hernia repair, 651f, 652–653
Kulchitsky cells, 1179, 1182

L

Lacey, Paul E., 1423f
Lacteals, small intestinal, 998
Lactobezoars, 943, 944
in pediatric patients, 960
Lacunar ligament, 636
Ladd, William, 1213
Ladd procedure, 1217, 1218f, 1219f
Ladd's bands, 1214, 1215f, 1857
Laimer's ligament. *See* Phrenoesophageal membrane.
Laird technique, for rectovaginal fistulas, 1948
Lamina mucosa, prenatal development of, 37, 39t, 39–42
ciliated columnar epithelium and, 40–41, 41f
epithelial vacuolization and, 39–40, 40f
goblet cells and, 40–41, 41f
lumen occlusion secondary to vacuoles and, 40, 42f
precursor mucosa proliferation and, 37, 39f
stratified squamous epithelium and, 41
Lamina propria, of gallbladder, 1444
Lamivudine, hepatotoxicity of, 1720
Lanreotide, for carcinoid tumors, 1186

Lansoprazole. *See also* Proton pump inhibitors.
gastric acid secretion and, 727
for laryngitis, 260
Laparoscopic abdominoperineal resection, of rectum, 2239–2241
technique for, 2239–2241, 2240f
Laparoscopic adhesiolysis, for small bowel obstruction, 1032–1033
Laparoscopic appendectomy, 2147, 2149f
Laparoscopic cholecystectomy
for bile duct strictures, 1574, 1575f, 1576
endoscopic retrograde cholangiopancreatography, 1497, 1498f
external biliary fistulas following, etiology and prevention of, 1538, 1539f
gallbladder cancer diagnosed incidentally after, 1525
Laparoscopic colectomy, 2345
Laparoscopic colon resection, 2338
Laparoscopic colorectal surgery, 2340–2358
for cancer
historical data on
prospective, 2346–2347
retrospective, 2346
operative techniques for
for colon, 2347–2348
for rectum, 2348
outcomes with, 2346
preoperative staging and, 2347
randomized trials of, 2345–2346
training and credentialing and, 2353
tumor localization for, 2347
wound implant prevention and, 2348, 2348f–2353f, 2349b, 2351b, 2353
challenges with, 2344–2346
anatomic, 2345
conversions and, 2345–2346
learning curve and, 2345
for Crohn's disease
outcomes of, 2354, 2356, 2356t
technical points for, 2356
for diverticular disease
outcomes of, 2353–2354, 2355t
technical points for, 2354
historical background of, 2340, 2341t–2342f
less common indications for, 2358
outcomes of minimal access techniques and, 2340, 2342–2344
complications and, 2343–2344
hospital costs and, 2343–2344
length of stay and, 2343
operative rime and, 2342
postoperative pain and recovery of pulmonary function and, 2343
quality of life and, 2343–2344
return of bowel activity and resumption of diet and, 2343
for polyps
outcomes of, 2353
technical points for, 2353
for rectal prolapse
outcomes of, 2357, 2357t
technical points for, 2357

Laparoscopic colorectal surgery (*Continued*)
for ulcerative colitis
outcomes of, 2356–2357
technical points for, 2357
Laparoscopic drainage, for splenic abscesses, 1820
Laparoscopic enteroclysis, bowel injury during, 1136
Laparoscopic examination
in gastric adenocarcinoma, 907
in gastric trauma, 763
of liver, 1670–1671
in pancreatic and periampullary carcinoma, for preoperative staging, 1365
small bowel obstruction after, 1027–1028
during splenectomy, 1785
for staging of esophageal cancer, 460
Laparoscopic fundoplication
for esophageal strictures, 245, 247, 247f
gastric perforation due to, 1094
Laparoscopic hepatic resection, for hepatic cysts, solitary, 1633
Laparoscopic hernia repair
for lumbar hernias, 691
for ventral hernias, 678–680, 679f, 680f
Laparoscopic myotomy, 5
Heller. *See* Heller myotomy, laparoscopic.
Laparoscopic splenectomy, 1777, 1780–1788
complications of, 1787–1788
contraindications to, 1781
hand-assisted, 1786
for splenic tumors, 1816
for idiopathic thrombocytopenic purpura, 1823
indications for
elective situations as, 1781, 1781b
emergency situations as, 1780–1781
operative technique for, 1782–1786
anatomic considerations for, 1783
diagnostic laparoscopy and, 1785
division of remaining attachments and placement of spleen in specimen bag and, 1785–1786
division of splenic vessels and, 1785
extraction of spleen from peritoneal cavity and, 1786
inspection of operative field and, 1786
mobilization of spleen with dissection of splenic ligaments and, 1785
positioning and safe access for pneumoperitoneum and, 1783–1785
preliminary steps in, 1783–1786
removal of trocars, desufflation, and closure of port site and, 1786
patient selection for, 1781–1782
portal and splenic vein thrombosis following, 1838
postoperative care for, 1787
preoperative considerations for, 1782
general considerations as, 1782
imaging as, 1782

Laparoscopic splenectomy (*Continued*)
  immunizations against overwhelming
    postsplenectomy infection as,
    1782
  robotic-assisted, 1787
  for splenic trauma, 1802
  for splenic tumors, 1816
Laparoscopic surgery. *See also specific
  procedures.*
  for colon cancer, 2252
  for colonic inertia, 1936
  for Crohn's disease, 1063
  for duodenal ulcers, 798, 799f
  hand-assisted
    for colonic diverticular disease,
      2023f, 2023–2024
    colorectal, 2353
    splenectomy as, 1786
      for splenic tumors, 1816
  for peptic ulcer disease, perforation in,
    823–824
  reoperative, 1135
  technique for, 1135–1136
Laparoscopic therapy
  for choledocholithiasis. *See
    Choledocholithiasis, laparoscopic
    management of.*
  for gastric cancer, 745
  for gastric volvulus, 1038–1039
  for paraesophageal hernia, 554–557
    open repair vs., 558
    technique for, 555, 555f–557f, 557
  for rectal prolapse, 1961
  for undescended testes, 711
Laparoscopic ultrasound, in gastric
  adenocarcinoma, 907–908
Laparoscopically assisted anorectal pull-
  through, for high imperforate anus,
  2400–2402, 2401f 2402f
Laparoscopic-assisted surgery
  for Crohn's disease, 2132
  gastrostomy as, in pediatric patients, 960
Laparotomy
  for caustic injury, gastric, 763
  exploratory, in duodenal injury, 766
  for gastric volvulus, 1038
  with gastrointestinal fistulas, 1106
  small bowel, perforation due to, 770
  ventral hernia following, 674
Lap-Band, 934
Large intestine, 1845. *See also* Colon.
Laryngeal nerves
  inferior
    nonrecurrent, prenatal development
      of, 45
    recurrent, anatomy of, 25–26, 26f,
      27f
  superior, anatomy of, 25–26
Laryngitis
  in gastroesophageal reflux disease,
    medical therapy for, 258–259
  reflux, endoscopic appearance of, 259,
    261f
Larynx, prenatal development of, 31–33,
  33f, 34f
Laser therapy
  ablative, for Barrett's esophagus,
    370–371

Laser therapy (*Continued*)
  for colonic ectasias, 1995
  for hemorrhoids, 2033
  lithotripsy as, for bile duct stones, 1495
  Nd:YAG, for esophageal cancer, 489t,
    492–493
  thermotherapy as, for hepatocellular
    carcinoma, 1738
Lateral decubitus position, 1886, 1886f
Lateral fossa, 639
Leakage
  following cardiomyotomy, 85
  following cricopharyngeal myotomy,
    84–85
  following esophagectomy, 86
  following esophagogastrostomy, 86
LEA29Y, for islet transplantation, 1428
Lecithin, in bile, 1452
Leiomyomas
  colorectal, 2316–2317
  esophageal, 515–520, 516f–519f, 516t,
    518t
    benign, malignant transformation of,
      123
    endoscopic ultrasonography in, 123,
      124f
    imaging of, 81, 82, 83f
  gastric, 888
    endoscopic appearance of, 740–741,
      741f
  small intestinal, 899–900
Leiomyosarcomas
  colorectal, 2316f, 2316–2317
  esophageal, imaging in, 81
  hepatic, 1747
Lembert suture, 1084, 1085f
Leptin, gastric, 723–724
Lesser omentum, 717
Leucovorin, for metastatic colorectal
  cancer, 2201
Leukemia
  anorectal sepsis in, 2058
  splenectomy for, 1830t, 1830–1831
Leukocytosis, following splenectomy, 1777,
  1838
Levator ani muscle complex, 696
Levator hernias, 687, 694–700
  anatomy and, 696, 697f
  classification of, 694–696, 695f, 696f
  clinical features and diagnosis of, 696,
    698f, 698–699, 699f
  treatment of, 699–700, 700f–703f
Levator spasm, 2071
Levator syndrome, 2071
Lewis, double incisions of, 579
Lexipafant, for pancreatitis, severe,
  necrotizing, 1303–1304
Lhermitte-Duclos syndrome, 2175
Lice, pruritus ani associated with, 2070
Lichen planus, esophageal strictures in,
  89–90, 92f
Lichen sclerosus et atrophicus, pruritus ani
  associated with, 2069–2070
Lichtenstein herniorrhaphy, 649, 650f
Liebermann-Meffert, Dorothea, 7
Lifestyle modifications, for
  gastroesophageal reflux disease,
  252–253

Ligament(s)
  anchoring stomach, 717–718, 718f
  associated with external oblique muscle,
    636, 637f
Ligament of Treitz, 968, 970f, 1864
Ligamentum venosum, 1598
Ligature, for Crohn's disease, 1063
Linea alba, 672, 672f
Linear cutters, 1086, 1087f
Linear staplers, 1086, 1087f
Linitis plastica, 905, 906
Lipase, serum
  in pancreatic trauma, 1401
  in pancreatitis, 1299, 1300b
Lipids
  duodenal absorption of, 980
  small intestinal absorption of, 1003t,
    1004–1006, 1005f, 1006f
Lipohyperplasia, of ileocecal valve, 900–901
Lipomas
  esophageal, 522
    endoscopic ultrasonography in, 123
  gastric, 887–888, 888
  small intestinal, 900
Lipomatous hypertrophy, of ileocecal valve,
  900–901
Liposarcomas
  colorectal, 2317
  hepatic, 1747
Lithotripsy, for bile duct stones, 1494–1495
Littre, Alexis, 632
Liver. *See also* Hepatic *entries;* Hepatobiliary
  entries.
  anatomic segments of (Couinaud),
    1604–1607, 1673f, 1673–1674
    left hemiliver (segments II, III, IV,
      and I) and, 1604
    left lobe (segments II and III) and,
      1604–1605
    posterior liver (dorsal liver, sector I)
      and, 1604
    right hemiliver (segments V, VI, VII,
      and VIII) and, 1605f, 1605–1606
    right lateral sector (segments VI and
      VII) and, 1606
    right paramedian sector (segments V
      and VIII) and, 1606
    segment IV and, 1605
    segment VII and, 1606
    segment VIII and, 1607
    segments V and VI and, 1606
  anatomy of, 2275–2276, 2276f
    of cystic veins, 1603
    of cystohepatic ducts, 1603
    of fissures, 1599f, 1602–1603
    functional, 1673f, 1673–1674
    of hepatic arteries, 1600, 1602
    of hepatic ducts, 1602
    of hilar plate, 1599f, 1603
    of hilum, 1602
    lymphatic, 1607
    microscopic, 1607
    neural, 1607
    of parabiliary venous system, 1603
    of portal vein, 1602
    segmental, 1753, 1754f
    of small ducts, 1603
    of sulcus of Rouviere, 1603

Liver (*Continued*)
  of vasculobiliary sheaths, 1599–1600
  venous, 1603–1604
  bile formation and, 1608
  colorectal cancer metastases to. *See*
    Hepatic metastases, of colorectal
    cancer.
  divisions of, 1598–1599
  embryology of, 1598
  metastases to, carcinoid, 1185–1186
  mobilization of, 1659, 1660f, 1661f
  morphology of, 1673f, 1673–1674
  packing of, to control bleeding, 1664f,
    1664–1665
  regeneration of, 1608, 1608f
  trauma to. *See* Hepatobiliary trauma.
  wrapping with absorbable mesh, to
    control bleeding, 1665, 1665f
Liver abscesses, 1640–1657
  amebic, 1650–1657
    complications of, 1654–1655
      pleuropulmonary, 1655
      rupture into pericardium as,
        1655
    demographics of, 1651
    diagnosis of, 1653–1654
      computed tomography in, 1654
      liver scanning in, 1654
      magnetic resonance imaging in,
        1654
      radiography in, 1654
      ultrasonography in, 1654
    etiology and pathogenesis of, 1651
    incidence of, 1650–1651
    location and number of, 1651–1652
    outcome and prognostic factors for,
      1656–1657
    patient presentation and, 1652t,
      1652–1653, 1653t
    treatment of, 1655–1656
      medical, 1655–1656
      percutaneous drainage for,
        1656
      surgical drainage for, 1656
  pyogenic, 1640–1650
    anatomic considerations with, 1654,
      1655t
    demographics of, 1640–1641, 1641t
    diagnosis of, 1646–1647
      cholangiography in, 1646, 1646f
      computed tomography in,
        1646–1647, 1647f
      magnetic resonance imaging in,
        1647, 1648f
      radiography in, 1646
      ultrasonography in, 1646
    etiology and pathogenesis of,
      1641–1642, 1642t
    laboratory analysis for, 1643, 1644t
    management of, 1647–1650
      antibiotics in, 1648–1649
      drainage procedures for, 1649
    microbiology of, 1644–1645
    outcome with, 1650
    presenting signs and symptoms of,
      1643, 1643t, 1652t, 1653t
    prognostic factors for, 1650
    risk factors for, 1642–1643

Liver biopsy, 1670–1671
  in hepatocellular carcinoma, 1734
  laparoscopic, 1670–1671
  open, 1671
  percutaneous, 1616, 1670
  in primary sclerosing cholangitis, 1561
  transjugular, 1670
Liver bud, 1598
Liver disorders. *See also specific disorders.*
  anesthesia in, 1626
  operative considerations in, 1626–1627
  with parenteral nutrition, in short-bowel
    syndrome, 1165, 1167
  perioperative management for,
    1618–1622
    general assessment and preoperative
      preparation and, 1619t,
      1619–1620, 1620t
    hepatic functional reserve and, 1621
    nutritional intervention and,
      1621–1622
    nutritional status and, perioperative
      management for, 1621
  postoperative management in,
    1627–1628
  vascular, 1711–1715
    of hepatic artery, 1711–1714
      aneurysms as, 1711–1712, 1712f
      arterioportal and arteriovenous
        shunts as, 1713f, 1713–1714
      thrombosis as, 1712–1713, 1713f
      traumatic, 1712
    of hepatic vein, Budd-Chiari
      syndrome as, 1714f, 1714–1715
Liver failure
  acute, 1702–1704
    etiology of, 1702–1703
    fulminant, 1702
    treatment of, 1703–1704
      liver transplantation for, 1704
      medical, 1703–1704
  in portal hypertension, 1756
Liver function
  assessment of, in portal hypertension,
    1758
  tests of. *See* Hepatic laboratory tests.
Liver injury, external biliary fistulas
  following, etiology and prevention of,
  1539, 1539f
Liver resection, external biliary fistulas
  following, etiology and prevention of,
  1539–1540
Liver scans, with liver abscesses, amebic,
  1654
Liver support systems, 1704–1708
  biologic, 1706–1707, 1707f
  future of, 1707–1708, 1708f
  need for, 1705
  nonbiologic, 1705–1706
Liver surgery
  incisions for, 1671–1673
    midline, 1671
    right thoracoabdominal, 1671,
      1673
    subcostal, 1671, 1672f
  modern anatomic approach to, 1597,
    1599f–1601f
  transfusion with, 1619–1620

Liver transplantation, 1685–1700, 1686f
  for ascites, 1765
  for biliary atresia, 1550–1551
  candidacy for, 1688–1694
    allocation and, 1691t, 1691–1692,
      1692t
    associated conditions and special
      considerations and, 1692–1694
    contraindications and, 1688–1691,
      1689t, 1690t
    indications for transplantation and,
      1688
  for cholangiocarcinoma, 1530–1531
  complications of
    early, 1698
      biliary, 1698
      hepatic artery thrombosis as,
        1698
      portal vein thrombosis as, 1698
    late, 1699–1700
      of immunosuppressive
        medications, 1699–1700
      rejection as, 1699
  epidemiology of, 1685–1687, 1686t
    causes of end-stage liver disease and,
      1686–1687
  evaluation for, 1687–1688
  external biliary fistulas following,
    etiology and prevention of, 1540
  for fulminant liver failure, 1704
  future directions for, 1700
  for hepatocellular carcinoma,
    1739–1740
    resection vs., 1740
  intraoperative problems and
    graft function and primary
      nonfunction as, 1697–1698
    hepatic artery failure as, 1697
    portal vein thrombosis as, 1697
    split grafts as, 1697
  living donor, 1740
    adult-to-adult, 1694–1695, 1695f
  for metastatic carcinoid, 1186
  Milan criteria for, 1739–1740
  organ shortage and, 1700, 1700b
  for polycystic liver disease, 1635
  for primary sclerosing cholangitis,
    1569–1570, 1588–1589
  procedure for, 1695–1697
    for back table preparation of donor
      organ, 1696
    for biliary reconstruction, 1696–1697
    for implantation, 1696
    reperfusion syndrome and, 1696
    for total native hepatectomy, 1695
    for venovenous bypass, 1695–1696
  split grafts for, 1697
  University of California San Francisco
    criteria for, 1740
Liver–small bowel transplantation, for short-
  bowel syndrome, 1174f, 1174–1175
Longmire-Traverso procedure, for
  pancreatitis, chronic, 1314, 1315
Long-tube decompression, for small bowel
  obstruction, 1032
Loop ileostomy, 2366, 2367f
Loperamide, for fecal incontinence, 1921
Lortat-Jacob, Jean-Louis, 337

Los Angeles classification, for reflux esophagitis, 106, 106t, 107f
Lower esophageal high-pressure zone. *See* Lower esophageal sphincter.
Lower esophageal sphincter, 100
  achalasia and, 405–406, 406f. *See also* Achalasia.
  anatomy of, 17–18, 19f, 63
  failure of, increased esophageal exposure to gastric juice due to, 141, 141f
  gastroesophageal barrier and, 223–228, 224f, 226t
  hypertensive, 423–426
    in achalasia, 407
    examination in, 424
    manometric features of, 420t
    treatment of, 424, 426
  incompetent, Nissen fundoplication for. *See* Nissen fundoplication.
  length of, 224, 225f
  medications relaxing, adenocarcinoma and, 445
  nonrelaxing, 138, 140f
  permanently defective, 225–226, 226t
  position of, 224–225
  pressure and, 224, 225f
  swallowing and, 53–55, 54t, 132–134, 133f
  transient loss of competence of, gastroesophageal barrier and, 226–228, 226f–228f
Lower esophageal sphincter manometry, 165t
Ludlow, Abraham, 5
Lumbar hernias, 687–691
  anatomic considerations and, 688, 688f
  classification of, 689–690
  clinical features and diagnosis of, 688–689, 689f
  historical background of, 687–688
  incarceration plus strangulation of, 689
  treatment of, 690f, 690–691
Lumbar plexus, 657
Lung disease, end-stage, gastroesophageal reflux disease associated with, diagnosis of, 171–172
Lung transplantation, gastroesophageal reflux disease associated with, diagnosis of, 171–172
Luschka, ducts of, 1444
Lyall, Alexander "Sandy," 337
Lye, gastric injury due to, 762
Lymphadenectomy, for gastric adenocarcinoma, extent of, 909–911, 910f, 910t
Lymphangiomas
  gastric, 887
  small intestinal, 899
  splenic, 1815
Lymphocytic leukemia, chronic, splenectomy for, 1830t, 1830–1831, 1831t
Lymphogranuloma venereum, anal, in immunocompromised patients, 2383t
Lymphoid polyposis syndrome, small intestinal, 894t, 898
Lymphoid tumors, splenic, 1815

Lymphomas
  colorectal, 2314
  Hodgkin's, splenic, 1816
  non-Hodgkin's, 1199–1210
    clinical features of, 1199–1200, 1201t
    diagnosis of, 1206–1208
      of gastric lymphoma, 1207f, 1207–1208, 1208f
      of intestinal lymphoma, 1208, 1208f
    epidemiology of, 1199, 1200t
    esophageal, imaging in, 81
    gastric, epidemiology of, 1199, 1200t
    grading of, 1205–1206
    incidence of, 1199
    pancreatic, 1434–1436, 1436f
      in pediatric patients, 1411
    pathology of, 1200, 1201t, 1202t, 1203–1205
      of Burkitt's lymphoma, 1204, 1204f
      of diffuse large B-cell lymphoma, 1200, 1202f, 1203
      of enteropathy-type T-cell lymphoma, 1205, 1205f, 1206t
      of follicular lymphoma, 1204
      of MALT lymphoma, 1203f, 1203–1204, 1204f
      of mantle cell lymphoma, 1204, 1205f
    prognosis of, 1210
    small intestinal, epidemiology of, 1199, 1200t
    splenectomy for, 1829, 1829t, 1830b
    splenic, 1816
    staging of, 1206, 1206b, 1207b
    treatment of, 1208–1209
      of gastric lymphoma, 1209, 1209t, 1210f
      of intestinal lymphoma, 1209, 1211f
Lymphoplasmacytic sclerosing pancreatitis, 1436–1437, 1437f
Lymphoproliferative disorders, splenectomy for, 1827–1831
  for Hodgkin's disease, 1827–1829, 1828f, 1828t
  for leukemias, 1830t, 1830–1831
  for non-Hodgkin's lymphoma, 1829, 1829t, 1830b
Lynch syndrome I, 2169, 2188
Lynch syndrome II, 2169, 2188

M

M cells, small intestinal immune function and, 1010, 1012f
Macrocystic adenomas. *See* Mucinous cystic neoplasms, pancreatic.
Macronutrients, duodenal absorption of, 980
Magnetic resonance cholangiopancreatography
  with alkaline phosphatase elevation, 1615
  with bile duct strictures, 1579
  with biliary fistulas, 1542

Magnetic resonance cholangiopancreatography *(Continued)*
  with choledochal cysts, 1553
  in malignant bile duct obstruction, 1506
  in pancreatic carcinoma, 1354
  with pancreatic cystic neoplasms, 1396
  in pancreatitis
    acute, 1300
    chronic, 1347
Magnetic resonance defecography, in constipation, 1933
Magnetic resonance imaging
  with anorectal abscesses, 2051
  with anorectal fistulas, 2051
  of carcinoid tumors, 1183–1184, 1184f
  with colon, rectal, and anal disorders, 1893, 1895, 1895f
  in Crohn's disease, 1047–1048, 1048f, 1049f
  in gastric adenocarcinoma, 907
  with groin hernias, 643
  with hepatic abscesses, pyogenic, 1647, 1648f
  of hepatic cysts, solitary, 1631, 1632f–1634f
  in hepatocellular carcinoma, 1735, 1735f
  for insulinoma localization, 1377
  in jaundice, obstructive, 1462, 1462f
  with liver abscesses, amebic, 1654
  in mesenteric ischemia, 1253
  in obstructed defecation, 1879
  with pancreatic cystic neoplasms, 1393
  of pancreatic pseudocysts, 1331
  in pancreatitis, chronic, 1347
  in periampullary carcinoma, 1362, 1363f
  of perineal hernias, 699
  in perineal pain syndromes, 2074
  in portal hypertension, 1757
  in primary sclerosing cholangitis, 1562
  with retrorectal tumors, 2301
Magnification endoscopy, in Barrett's esophagus, 104, 105f
Major histocompatibility complex antigens, achalasia due to, 406
Malabsorption, with jejunoileal diverticula, 785
Malago maneuver, 1605
Malaise, in Crohn's disease, 1045
Males
  anorectal anomalies in, 2394, 2394f
  low anterior resection in, 2228–2229, 2229f
  sexual dysfunction in, as ileal pouch–anal anastomosis complication, 2117
Malignancies. *See also* Metastases; *specific malignancies.*
  achalasia due to, 408–409
  in immunocompromised patients, 2383–2384
  immunosuppression due to, 2376
  with immunosuppressive therapy, 2380
    following liver transplantation, 1699–1700
  inflammation and, 348
  reoperative pelvic surgery for, 2417–2418
  in ulcerative colitis, as surgical indication, 2101

Malignant carcinoid syndrome, 1182
Malignant fibrous histiocytoma, colorectal, 2317
Mallory-Weiss tears, 762
Malnutrition
    with gastrointestinal fistulas, 1098
    immunosuppression due to, 2376
Malone antegrade colonic enema procedure, 2405
Maloney dilators, 5
Malrotation, in pediatric patients, 1213–1214, 1214f–1219f, 1216–1217, 1219
MALT lymphoma, pathology of, 1203f, 1203–1204, 1204f
Mannitol, for bowel preparation, 2328
Manometry
    anal, in fecal incontinence, 1919
    anorectal
        in constipation, 1932–1933
        in obstructed defecation, 1879b
    antroduodenal, delayed gastric emptying and, 186–188, 188f, 188t, 189f, 190, 190t
    esophageal
        in achalasia, 407, 408f, 408t, 411
        combined with multichannel intraluminal impedance, 175–176, 178f, 179, 179f
        in esophageal spasm, 419–420, 420t, 421f
        in hypertensive lower esophageal sphincter, 420t, 424, 424f, 425f
        in nutcracker esophagus, 420t, 422f, 422–423, 423f
        with paraesophageal hernia, 552
        24-hour
            ambulatory, 152–154
            stationary, 144–146, 145f–155f, 145t, 150, 152
    lower esophageal sphincter, 165t
    small bowel, in intestinal dysmotility, 926
    sphincter of Oddi, 1492–1493
    for swallowing evaluation, 378
Mantle cell lymphoma
    pathology of, 1204, 1205f
    splenectomy for, 1829
Marginal artery, 1851, 1853f
Marginal zone B-cell lymphoma, splenectomy for, 1829
Markex, 675
MARS, 1705–1706
Marshall, Samuel, 4
Marsupialization
    for pilonidal disease, 1968
    for splenic cysts, 1815
Martin anoplasty, for anal stenosis, 2063
Matrix metalloproteinases, groin hernias and, 635
Matthias, Nicolaus, 1813
Mattress suture, horizontal, 1085
Mayo, William, 681
Mayo repair, 676–677, 677f, 681
McBurney's point, 1846
    tenderness of, in appendicitis, 2142

McVay Cooper's hernia repair, 648
Meandering mesenteric artery, 1239
Meckel's diverticula, 786–789, 1225, 1227, 1227f
    complications of, 787
        diverticulitis as, 787, 789f
        hemorrhage as, 787
        obstruction as, 787, 788f
        umbilical, 787
    diagnosis of, 786f, 786–787
    incidence of, 786
    management of, operative, 787–789
    pathogenesis of, 786
    symptoms of, 786
Meconium, in urine, 2394, 2394f
Meconium cysts, in utero perforation and, 1225, 1225f
Meconium ileus, 1224f, 1224–1225, 1225f
Meconium peritonitis, 1225
Meconium plug syndrome, 1224, 1224f
Meconium syndromes, 1224f, 1224–1225, 1225f
Medial fossa, 639
Mediastinum, prenatal development of, 34f, 35, 39f
Medications. See Drug entries; specific drugs and drug types.
Megacolon
    chronic, 1879
    toxic
        as emergency surgical indication, 2101
        in ulcerative colitis, 2084
Megaesophagus. See Achalasia.
Meglumine diatrizoate studies, in duodenal injury, 765–766
Meissner's plexus, 720
Melanomas
    anal, 2295
    anorectal, pruritus ani and, 2068
    colorectal, 2317–2318, 2318f
    esophageal, imaging in, 81
Melatonin, duodenal function and, 981t, 985
MELD, 1691t, 1691–1692, 1692t
    in portal hypertension, 1758, 1758b
MELS, 1706–1707
MEN. See Multiple endocrine neoplasia; Zollinger-Ellison syndrome.
Ménétrier's disease, 886
Menstrual cycle
    following ileal pouch–anal anastomosis, 2117
    obesity and, bariatric surgery and, 938
Meperidine, for endoscopic retrograde cholangiopancreatography, 1491
6-Mercaptopurine
    for Crohn's disease, 1053, 2128
    for gastrointestinal fistulas, 1105
    for inflammatory bowel disease, 2091–2092
"Mercedes-Benz" sign, 1867
Mesalamine
    for Crohn's disease, 2127
    for inflammatory bowel disease, 2090
Mesenchymal clefts, development of, 31

Mesenteric arteries See also Inferior mesenteric artery; Superior mesenteric artery.
    inferior, 1128
    superior
        anatomy of, 1128, 1129f
        injuries to, 1128–1132
            operative exposure and management decisions regarding, 1128–1130, 1129f–1131f
            treatment results with, 1130t, 1130–1132
Mesenteric arteriography, preoperative, for esophageal replacement, 287–288, 288f
Mesenteric artery endarterectomy, 1258, 1259f
Mesenteric circulation, 1234–1245, 1235f. See also Inferior mesenteric artery; Superior mesenteric artery.
    autoregulatory escape and, 1243
    catecholamines and, 1243t, 1243–1244, 1244f, 1244t
    collaterals of, clinical correlations of, 1234–1245, 1235f
    control mechanisms of, 1241–1242
        extrinsic control of splanchnic blood flow and, 1241
        intrinsic control of splanchnic blood flow and, 1241–1242, 1242b
    digestion and, 1242–1243
    dopamine and, 1243
    embryology of, 1234, 1235f, 1236f
    physiology of, 1240–1241
    resting state and, 1242
Mesenteric cysts, 1860
Mesenteric ischemia, 1247–1261, 1248f
    acute
        arterial, 1248–1255, 1250f–1251f
        colonic ischemia as manifestation of, management of, 2010
        venous, 1255–1257, 1256f
    arterial, acute, 1248–1255, 1250f–1251f
        diagnosis of, 1251–1254
            arteriography for, 1253f, 1253–1254, 1254, 1254f
            computed tomography for, 1252t, 1252–1253
            magnetic resonance imaging for, 1253
            plain films for, 1252
            ultrasonography for, 1252
        embolic occlusion and, 1249b, 1249–1250
        nonocclusive, 1251
        patient management for, 1254f, 1254–1255
        thrombotic occlusion and, 1250
    chronic, 1257–1261
        clinical features and diagnosis of, 1257–1258
        mesenteric revascularization for, 1258–1261
            endovascular, 1260–1261, 1263t, 1264t, 1265f
            surgical, 1258–1260
    venous, acute, 1255–1257, 1256f

Mesenteric revascularization, 1258–1261
  endovascular, 1260–1261, 1263t, 1264t, 1265f
  surgical, 1258–1260
    aortomesenteric bypass for, 1258–1260, 1260f
    mesenteric artery endarterectomy for, 1258, 1259f
    retrograde bypass for, 1260, 1261f, 1262f
Mesenteric vein
  inferior, anatomy of, 1869
  superior, 968, 972f, 1772
    anatomy of, 1869
Mesenteric venous thrombosis
  acute, ischemia due to, 1255–1257, 1256f
  following splenectomy, 1838
Mesh contraction, with inguinal herniorrhaphy, laparoscopic, 668
Mesocolic hernias, 975–976, 976f, 1120–1121, 1121f, 1858, 1861f
  clinical features of, 1121
  diagnosis of, 1121–1122
  treatment of, 1122
Mesomesenteric artery, 1239
Mesorectal excision, total, 2246
  with autonomic nerve preservation, 2236f, 2236–2243
    distal rectal mobilization and, 2239
    hypogastric nerves and pelvic autonomic nerve plexuses and, 2237–2238, 2238f
    initial entry into retrorectal space and, 2236–2237, 2237f
    "lateral ligaments" and, 2238–2239, 2239f
    separation of anterior and posterior compartments and, 2238, 2238f
Metabolic acidosis, in short-bowel syndrome, 1166
Metabolic alkalosis, in short-bowel syndrome, 1166
Metabolic disorders
  following gastrectomy, 873
  following gastric bypass, 934
Metal biliary endoprostheses, for malignant biliary disease, 1466–1468
Metastases
  of anal squamous cell carcinoma, 2294, 2295f
  assessment for, in esophageal carcinoma, 471–472
  carcinoid, surgical therapy for, 1185–1186
  colorectal cancer and. See Colorectal cancer, metastases of; Hepatic metastases, of colorectal cancer.
  to esophagus, imaging in, 81, 82f
  pancreatic, 1437–1439, 1438f, 1439f
  splenic, 1816
    splenectomy for, 1832
  in Zollinger-Ellison syndrome, 868
Methotrexate
  for Crohn's disease, 1053, 2128
  hepatotoxicity of, 1721, 1723
  for inflammatory bowel disease, 2092
Methyldopa, hepatotoxicity of, 1721, 1722

Methylprednisolone
  for cholangitis prophylaxis, 1550t
  for idiopathic thrombocytopenic purpura, 1824
Metoclopramide. See also Prokinetic agents.
  for esophageal strictures, 237
  for gastroesophageal reflux disease, 253
  for gastroparesis, 921
Metronidazole
  for anorectal abscesses, 2057
  for Clostridium difficile colitis, in immunocompromised patients, 2382
  for Crohn's disease, 1052, 2128
  for inflammatory bowel disease, 2091
  for liver abscesses, amebic, 1655–1656
  for lymphoma, 1209t
  preoperative, 2328
Meyers, Willy, 7
MHC antigens, achalasia due to, 406
Microcystic adenomas. See Serous cystic neoplasms, pancreatic.
Microgastria, in pediatric patients, 950
Microsatellite instability, 1360, 2169, 2170–2171
Microsurgery, endoscopic, transanal, for rectal cancer, 2211–2212, 2212f
  outcomes with, 2215, 2216t
Microwave thermotherapy, for hepatocellular carcinoma, 1738
Midesophageal diverticulum, 437–438, 438f, 439f
Midline incision, for appendectomy, 2145
Midpelvic anatomy, transverse, low anterior resection and, 2223, 2224f
Migrating myoelectric complex
  fasting gastric motility and, 730
  gallbladder function and, 1458, 1459
  intestinal motility and, 925
  in short-bowel syndrome, 1163–1164
  small intestinal motility and, 1015f, 1015–1016, 1016f
Milan criteria, for liver transplantation, 1739–1740
Milk, lactobezoars and, 943, 944
Milligan-Morgan hemorrhoidectomy, 2032–2033
Mineral(s), small intestinal absorption of, 1008, 1009f
Mineral oil, pruritus ani associated with, 2069
Minicholecystectomy, 1477
Minnesota Multiphasic Personality Inventory, in constipation, 1934
Minocycline, hepatotoxicity of, 1721, 1722
Mirizzi's syndrome, 1471, 1474, 1526
Mismatch repair gene, 2169–2171, 2170f
Mitochondrial cytopathies, drug-induced, 1719t, 1720
Mixed cholangiohepatocellular carcinoma, 1745–1746, 1746f
Mixed connective tissue disease, esophageal motility disorders in, 140
MMPI, in constipation, 1934
MMR gene, 2169–2171, 2170f
Model for End-Stage Liver Disease, 1691t, 1691–1692, 1692t
  in portal hypertension, 1758, 1758b

Modular Extracorporeal Liver System, 1706–1707
Molecular Adsorbent Recycling System, 1705–1706
Mollard procedure, 2405
Moloney darn, 648
Morbid obesity, surgery for. See Bariatric surgery.
Morgagni, foramen of, 36–37
Morgagni hernias, 561
Moskel-Walske-Neumayer stricturoplasty, for Crohn's disease, 1059, 1060f
Motilin
  duodenal function and, 981t, 982
  small intestinal neuroendocrine function and, 1019
Moynihan, Berkeley, 1296
MRCP. See Magnetic resonance cholangiopancreatography.
MRI. See Magnetic resonance imaging.
Mucinous cystadenocarcinomas, 1391
Mucinous cystadenomas, 1390
Mucinous cystic neoplasms, pancreatic
  clinical presentation of, 1387
  diagnosis of, 1393, 1394f
  incidence and epidemiology of, 1387
  pathology and biologic behavior of, 1389f, 1389–1391, 1390f
  treatment of, 1397
Mucocutaneous pigmentation, in Peutz-Jeghers syndrome, 2174
Mucocutaneous separation, with ileostomy, 1080
Mucosa
  cardiac. See Cardiac mucosa.
  esophageal
    anatomy of, ultrasound, 114–115, 115f
    injury of, duodenal reflux and, 230–232
  small intestinal, 998
Mucosal resection, endoscopic
  for Barrett's esophagus, 370
  for gastric adenocarcinoma, 909
Mucosectomy
  of rectal stump, for coloanal anastomosis, 2247, 2247f, 2248f
  transanal, for ileal pouch–anal anastomosis, 2108, 2108f
Mucus, gastric, 728
Muir-Torre syndrome, 2188
  small intestinal, 894t, 896
"Mules," 943, 943f
Multichannel impedance–esophageal manometry, 136–138, 137t, 138f, 139f
Multichannel intraluminal impedance, 175–183
  combined with manometry, 175–176, 178f, 179, 179f
  combined with pH monitoring, 180–181, 180f–183f
  preoperative, for Nissen fundoplication, 266
  principles of, 175, 176f–178f
Multilumen tubes, 756
Multiorgan Dysfunction Score, for pancreatitis, acute, 1302

Multiple endocrine neoplasia
surgical management for, 866–867, 867f
type 1, 1379–1380
diagnosis of, 1379–1380
prognosis of, 1380
therapy of, 1380
Zollinger-Ellison syndrome and. *See*
Zollinger-Ellison syndrome.
Multiple hamartoma syndrome, 894t, 897,
2159t, 2175–2176
Multiple sclerosis, esophageal motility
disorders in, 140
Multipolar electrocoagulation, for Barrett's
esophagus, 371
Multislice (multidetector) computed
tomography, with pancreatic tumors,
unusual, 1431
Multivisceral transplantation, for intestinal
dysmotility, 927
Muscarinic receptors, gastric acid secretion
and, 725
Muscle(s). *See also specific muscles.*
esophageal
arrangement of, 16, 17f–19f
types of, 17, 19f
foregut, prenatal development of, 37, 38f
Muscle guarding, in appendicitis, 2142
Muscle layer, of gallbladder, 1444
Muscle-splitting incision, for appendectomy,
2145
Muscularis propria
anatomy of, ultrasound, 115f, 115–116
benign tumors of, endoscopic
ultrasonography in, 123, 124f
small intestinal, 998
MUSE classification, for reflux esophagitis,
106t
Mushroom poisoning
fulminant liver failure due to, 1703
liver disease due to, 1720
Mutation cluster region, 2163
Mycobacterium infection
M. avium subspecies *paratuberculosis,* in
Crohn's disease, 2091
splenic abscess due to, 1819, 1820
Mycophenolate mofetil, mechanism of
action of, 2377t
Mycotic infections. *See also specific infections.*
pruritus ani associated with, 2070
Myelofibrosis with myeloid metaplasia,
splenectomy for, 1831
Myelogenous leukemia, chronic,
splenectomy for, 1831
Myeloproliferative disorders, splenectomy
for, 1831–1832
Myenteric plexus, prenatal development of,
46
Myenteric reflex, 1014
MYH polyposis, 2168–2169
Myoblastomas, granular cell, esophageal,
520–521, 521f
Myopectineal orifice, 636
Myoplasty, dynamic, for fecal incontinence,
1923–1924
Myotomy
cricopharyngeal, 378–384
esophageal imaging following, 84–85,
85f

Myotomy (*Continued*)
indications for, 378–379
for myogenic dysphagia, 384, 386,
386f, 387f, 388
for neurologic dysphagia, 382, 384,
385f–386f
operative technique for, 379–380
access to pharyngoesophageal
junction and, 379, 380f, 381f
position and incision and, 379, 379f
for oropharyngeal dysphagia, 382f
complications of, 381–382, 384f
drainage and closure for, 381
idiopathic upper esophageal
sphincter dysfunction and, 388,
388, 389f
mucosal integrity and,
documentation of, 381, 384f
myogenic, 384, 386, 386f, 387f,
388
after neck surgery, 379, 388
postoperative care for, 381
results with, 382, 384, 384b,
385f–386f
Zenker's diverticulum and,
378–379, 381, 383f
for Zenker's diverticulum, 429
methods and results of, 429–431,
430f, 431f
for diffuse esophageal spasm, 421
for esophagogastrostomy, 585
extramucosal, for Zenker's diverticulum,
396–397, 397f, 398f
Heller. *See* Heller myotomy.
for hypertensive lower esophageal
sphincter, 424, 426
laparoscopic, 5
for nutcracker esophagus, 423

N

Naltrexone, for pruritus, in primary
sclerosing cholangitis, 1567
NANC pathway, 720
Nasobiliary tubes, for bile duct stones, 1496,
1496f
Nasoenteric intubation, 749–753
complications of, 753
contraindications to, 750t, 752
indications for, 750t, 750–752
methods of, 752f, 752–753
tubes for, 749–750, 751f
Nasogastric intubation, 749–753
complications of, 753
contraindications to, 750t, 752
esophageal strictures due to, 90
indications for, 750t, 750–752
methods of, 752f, 752–753
tubes for, 749–750, 751f
Natalizumab
for inflammatory bowel disease, 2093
mechanism of action of, 2377t
Nausea, in appendicitis, 2142
NDO plicator, for endoscopic antireflux
procedures, 308b, 314–316
complications of, 316
efficacy of, 315–316, 316t

NDO plicator, for endoscopic antireflux
procedures (*Continued*)
physiologic/anatomic mechanisms of,
329–330, 330f
procedure for, 314f, 314–315, 315f
results with, 325, 326t, 327t
Nd:YAG laser therapy, for esophageal
cancer, 489t, 492–493
Neck
anatomy of, 14–15, 15f
esophageal anchorage in, 12, 13f
Neck surgery, oropharyngeal dysfunction
following, cricopharyngeal myotomy for,
388, 390
Necrolytic migratory erythema, with
glucagonoma, 1381
Necrosectomy
gastroduodenal fistulas after, treatment
of, 1110
for pancreatitis, severe, necrotizing,
1304–1306, 1305f–1307f, 1305t
Necrotizing enterocolitis, in premature
infants, 1227–1229, 1228f, 1229f
Neisseria gonorrhoeae infection, anal, in
immunocompromised patients, 2383t
Neisseria meningitidis infection,
overwhelming postsplenectomy infection
and, 1782
Neomycin
for bowel preparation, 831
preoperative, 2328
Neonates
gastric perforation in, 957–958
clinical features and diagnosis of,
957–958
etiology of, 957
incidence of, 957
management of, 958
hyperbilirubinemia in, 1545
intestinal obstruction in, 947–948, 1219
clinical features and diagnosis of,
948
jaundice in, 1545
Neoplastic disorders. *See also* Malignancies;
Metastases; *specific neoplasms and regions,*
e.g. Esophageal neoplasms.
in ileal pouches, 2116–2117
perineal pain syndromes due to,
2073–2074
Neovesical dysfunction, associated with
imperforate anus, 2406
Nephroenteric fistulas, treatment of, 1113
Nephrolithiasis, in short-bowel syndrome,
1167–1168
Nephrologists, on portal hypertension
multidisciplinary team, 1767
Nerve conduction studies, in perineal pain
syndromes, 2074
Nervous system, foregut, prenatal
development of, 43–46
of cranial nerves, 44
of myenteric plexus, 46
nonrecurrent inferior laryngeal nerve
and, 45
of periesophageal nerves, 46
of phrenic nerve, 45–46
of vagus nerve, 44–45, 45f
Nesidioblastosis, 1408–1409

Neuralgia, obturator, 693
Neurilemomas
  gastric, 887–888
  small intestinal, 900
Neuroblastomas, pancreatic, in pediatric
  patients, 1411, 1411f
Neuroendocrine carcinomas, colorectal,
  2313
Neuroenteric cysts, esophageal, 525
Neurofibromas
  esophageal, endoscopic ultrasonography
    in, 123
  gastric, 887–888
Neurogenic tumors
  gastric
    benign, 888
    retrorectal, 2304
Neurologic disease, intestinal motility and,
  926
Neuropeptide Y, duodenal function and,
  981t
Neurotensin, duodenal function and, 981t,
  983
Neurotensinoma, 1383
Neutropenia, autoimmune, splenectomy
  for, 1827
Neutropenic enteritis, in
  immunocompromised patients,
  2382–2383
Newborns. See Neonates.
Nigro, Norman, 2288
Nissen, Rudolf, 7
Nissen fundoplication, 265–274
  for Barrett's esophagus, 356
    symptomatic outcome with, 356–357,
      357f
  Collis gastroplasty with, for esophageal
    strictures, 244f, 244–245, 246f–248f,
    247–248
  complications of, 598–599, 599f
  dysphagia following, 611
  early development of, 6, 7
  endoscopic examination following, 106,
    108, 108f
  for esophageal strictures, 241–242
  failed, reoperative surgery for, 1141
  gastroparesis following, 923
  hernias following, 560
  historical background of, 265
  for hypertensive lower esophageal
    sphincter, 424
  imaging following, 85, 86f
  indications for, 266b, 266–267
  laparoscopic, 267–271
    for Barrett's esophagus, symptomatic
      outcome with, 367, 367f
    crural closure for, 270, 270f
    dissection for, 268–270
      of crus, 268, 269f
      of fundus and greater curve, 269,
        269f
      of lesser curve, 268
      of mediastinal and posterior
        esophagus, 270, 270f
    for esophageal strictures, 245, 247,
      247f
    exposure for, 268
    fundoplication and, 270–271, 271f

Nissen fundoplication (Continued)
  gastric perforation due to, 1094
  open fundoplication vs., 267
  partial, 280–281, 281f
    surgical technique for, 282, 282f
    position and port placement for,
      267–268, 268f
  "missin'," 106
  open, 271
    exploration and exposure for, 271
    laparoscopic fundoplication vs., 267
    repair and fundoplication and, 271,
      272f
  for paraesophageal hernia, 558
  partial, 276–283
    contraindications to, 279–280
    indications for, 278–279, 279t
    mechanism of, 278, 278f, 279f
    postoperative care for, 283
    preoperative evaluation for, 280, 280t
    results with, 283, 283t, 284t
    surgical technique for, 280–283, 281f,
      281t
      for laparoscopic Dor procedure,
        282
      for laparoscopic Toupet
        procedure, 282, 282f
      for transthoracic Belsey Mark IV
        repair, 282f, 282–283
    types of, 276–278, 277f
  patient selection for, 265
  postoperative care for, 273
  postoperative complications of, 273–274
  preoperative evaluation for, 266
  results with, 274
  with short esophagus, acquired, 272f,
    272–273, 273f
  slipped, 106, 108f, 242, 242f, 598, 599f
  too-generous, 108
Nitric oxide
  duodenal function and, 981t, 983
  gastric innervation and, 720
Nitrofurantoin, hepatotoxicity of, 1721,
  1722
Nitroglycerin
  mesenteric blood flow and, 1243t
  topical, for anal fissures, 2040
Nitroprusside, mesenteric blood flow and,
  1243t
Nixon, H. H., 2400
Nizatidine, 255. See also Histamine₂ receptor
  antagonists.
Nociceptive pain, 668
Nodular regenerative hyperplasia, drug-
  induced, 1723
Nonadrenergic noncholinergic pathway, 720
Nonalcoholic fatty liver disease, hepatic
  laboratory tests in, 1612–1613
Non-Hodgkin lymphomas. See Lymphomas,
  non-Hodgkin's.
Non-meckelian diverticula. See Jejunoileal
  diverticula.
Nonrotation, 1213–1214, 1215f
Nonsteroidal anti-inflammatory drugs
  for Barrett's esophagus, 258
  for desmoids, in familial adenomatous
    polyposis, 2161, 2162
  esophageal cancer and, 445

Norepinephrine, mesenteric blood flow
  and, 1243t
Nuclear medicine. See Scintigraphy.
Nutcracker esophagus, 74, 421–423
  examinations in, 422f, 422–423, 423f
  manometric features of, 420t
  treatment of, 423
Nutrient deficiencies, prevention of, in
  short-bowel syndrome, 1166–1167
Nutrition. See also Diet.
  in Crohn's disease, 1053–1055
    malnutrition and, 1053–1054
    as primary therapy, 1054–1055
  esophageal cancer and, 443, 445
  with gastrointestinal fistulas, 1100–1101
  maintenance of, for caustic ingestions,
    543–544
  for pancreatitis
    acute, mild, 1302
    severe, necrotizing, 1303
  reoperative surgery and, 1136
  in short-bowel syndrome, 1165
Nutritional status
  biliary surgery and, 1621
  liver surgery and, 1621
Nutritional therapy
  for biliary surgery, 1621–1622
  for liver surgery, 1621–1622
Nyhus/Condon hernia repair, 652

O

Obesity
  Barrett's esophagus and, 343
  costs associated with, 929
  esophageal cancer and, 443, 443t, 444f
  esophageal motility disorders associated
    with, 142, 142t
  gastroesophageal reflux disease and,
    200, 253
  health risk and mortality due to,
    928–929, 929f, 929t
  prevention of, 928
  pruritus ani in, 2067
  ventral herniorrhaphy and, 684
Obesity-hypoventilation syndrome, bariatric
  surgery and, 938
Oblique incision, for colorectal surgery,
  2329
Oblique muscle
  external, 672–673, 673f
  internal, 673, 673f
Obstipation, in small bowel obstruction,
  1028
Obturator hernias, 691–694
  anatomy and, 691, 692f
  clinical features and diagnosis of, 691,
    693, 693f, 694f
  treatment of, 693–694, 694f
Obturator neuralgia, 693
Occludin, 999
Octreoscan, for insulinoma localization,
  1377
Octreotide
  for carcinoid tumors, 1186
  for dumping syndrome, 871
  for gastrointestinal fistulas, 1103–1104

Octreotide (*Continued*)
  for intestinal dysmotility, 926
  for pancreatic pseudocysts, 1342
  for variceal bleeding, 1759
Octyl-2-cyanoacrylate, for bowel
    anastomoses, 1089
Oddi, sphincter of, 1444–1445, 1445f
  function of, 1458f, 1458–1459
Ogilvie's syndrome, 1879
Ohsawa, Tatsuo, 4
OISC, 1799
OKT3, mechanism of action of, 2377t
Okuda classification, 1735
Olsalazine, for inflammatory bowel disease,
    2089
Omental cysts, 1223
Omentum, lesser, 717
Omeprazole. *See also* Proton pump
    inhibitors.
  for Barrett's esophagus, 257–258
  for esophageal strictures, 237
  for esophagitis, reflux, 255–256, 256f
  gastric acid secretion and, 727
  for lymphoma, 1209t
  for Zollinger-Ellison syndrome, 866, 866f
Omphalomesenteric duct remnants, 1225,
    1226f, 1227
  Meckel's diverticulum as, 1227, 1227f
  omphalomesenteric band as, 1227
  omphalomesenteric cyst as, 1227
  patent omphalomesenteric duct as,
    1225, 1227
  at umbilicus, 1227
  vitelline blood vessel remnants as, 1227
Onlay patch anastomosis, for rectovaginal
    fistulas, 1954
Opioids, duodenal function and, 981t
Orchitis, ischemic
  following hernia surgery, 654
  with inguinal herniorrhaphy,
    laparoscopic, 668
Organ Injury Scaling Committee, 1799
Orthotopic bypass, esophageal, length of,
    10
Orthotopic liver transplantation. *See* Liver
    transplantation.
Osler-Weber-Rendu syndrome, gastric,
    887
Osseous lesions, retrorectal, 2306
Osteodystrophy, hepatic
  in end-stage liver disease, 1693
  with primary sclerosing cholangitis,
    treatment of, 1568
Ostomies, 2362–2373
  complications of, 2369–2373
    bowel obstruction as, 2371
    high-output state as, 2371
    incidence of, 2370
    ischemia as, 2372
    parastomal hernia as, 2372, 2372f
    peristomal varices as, 2373, 2373f
    prolapse as, 2372–2373, 2373f
    skin irritation and leakage as, 2370f,
      2370–2371
    stenosis as, 2372
  enterostomal therapy for, 2368–2369,
    2369b
  indications for, 2362, 2363b

Ostomies (*Continued*)
  preoperative considerations for,
    2362–2363, 2363f
  types of, 2363–2368
    diverting stomas as, 2365
    end colostomy as, 2364–2365
    end ileostomy as, 2363f–2366f,
      2363–2364
    end-loop, 2366–2368
      end-loop colostomy as, 2367
      end-loop ileocolostomy as,
        2367–2368, 2369f
      end-loop ileostomy as, 2367,
        2368f
    loop colostomy as, 2366
    loop ileostomy as, 2366, 2367f
Ostomy triangle, 2363, 2363f
Outlet bleeding, 1883
Ovarian metastases, of colorectal cancer,
    2270
Overwhelming postsplenectomy infection,
    1778, 1838
  counseling regarding, 1787
  immunizations against, 1782, 1787
  prevention of, 1814
Oxaliplatin, for metastatic colorectal cancer,
    2201, 2202
Oxyntocardiac mucosa, 216–217

P

PACAP, small intestinal neuroendocrine
    function and, 1018
Pacemaker region, duodenal, 1013
Paget's disease
  anal, 2294–2295
  anorectal, 1887
  pruritus ani and, 2068
Pain. *See also specific site.*
  with groin hernias, 642
  nociceptive, 668
  in pancreatic and periampullary
    carcinoma
    nonoperative palliation of, 1366
    operative palliation of, 1367, 1367f
  pancreatic generation of, 1294
Palisade vessels, endoscopic appearance of,
    102, 102f
Pancreas
  acinar cells of, 1291, 1291f
  annular, duodenal obstruction due to,
    953
  blood supply of, 1292–1293, 1293f
  cellular membrane function in, 1292
  ductal epithelial cells of, 1290f,
    1290–1291, 1291f
  dysfunctional cellular changes in,
    1291–1292, 1292f
  embryology of, 1287–1290
    cellular changes and, 1289–1290
    early anatomic formations and,
      1287–1289, 1288f, 1289f
  endocrine, embryology of, 1289
  exocrine, embryology of, 1289
  innervation of, 1293f, 1293–1294, 1294f
  lymphatic system of, 1293
  regulation of, 1294–1295

Pancreas divisum, 1299, 1409–1410
  management of, 1513
Pancreas transplantation, 1415–1420. *See
    also* Islet transplantation.
  immunosuppression for, 1418–1419
  postoperative course with, 1418
  rejection and, 1419
  results of, 1419–1420, 1420f
  with simultaneous kidney
    transplantation, 1417f, 1417–1418,
    1418f
  of vascularized pancreas allograft,
    1415–1418
    cadaveric organ procurement and
      preservation for, 1416–1417
    candidates for, 1415–1416
    living-donor transplant and, 1417
    surgical techniques for, 1417f,
      1417–1418, 1418f
Pancreatectomy
  cadaveric, 1416–1417
  distal
    for living-donor pancreas
      transplantation, 1417
    for pancreatic cancer in body or tail
      complications following,
        1370–1371, 1371t
      technique for, 1370, 1370f
    for pancreatic ductal disruption, 1351
  near-total, for hyperinsulinism, 1409
Pancreatic abscesses, 1329
  definition of, 1296
  with pancreatic pseudocysts, 1342–1343,
    1343f
  with trauma, 1405
Pancreatic adenocarcinoma, 1431
  etiology of diet, 1359t, 1359–1360
    environmental factors in, 1359–1360
    host factors and, 1360
    genetic alterations and, 1360
Pancreatic arteries, 1292, 1293f
  aneurysms of, 1280–1282
Pancreatic ascites, 1349–1352, 1350f–1352f
  in pancreatitis, chronic, 1312
Pancreatic biopsy, in pancreatic and
    periampullary carcinoma, 1363–1364
Pancreatic carcinoma, 1353t, 1353–1354,
    1358–1373. *See also* Pancreatic
    adenocarcinoma.
  adjuvant therapy for, 1372
  clinical findings in, 1360–1361
  etiology of, 1359t, 1359–1360
    genetic alterations and, 1360
    host factors and, 1360
  gastrointestinal stromal tumors as, 1359
  immunotherapy for, 1373
  incidence of, 1358
  intraductal papillary mucinous
    neoplasms as, 1359
  laboratory findings in, 1361
  neoadjuvant therapy for, 1372
  palliation for
    nonoperative, 1365–1366
      chemotherapeutic, 1372–1373
      of duodenal obstruction,
        1365–1366
      of obstructive jaundice, 1365
      of pain, 1366

Pancreatic carcinoma (Continued)
   operative, 1366–1367
      of duodenal obstruction,
         1366–1367
      of obstructive jaundice, 1366,
         1366f
      for pain, 1367, 1367t
   pathology of, 1358–1359
   resection of, 1367–1370
      pancreatectomy for
         for cancer in pancreatic body or
            tail, 1370, 1370f
         complications following,
            1370–1371, 1371t
      pancreaticoduodenectomy for
         complications following,
            1370–1371, 1371t
         operative technique of,
            1367–1370, 1368f, 1369f
   staging of
      clinicopathologic, 1365
      preoperative, 1364–1365
   tissue diagnosis of, 1363–1364
Pancreatic cystic neoplasms, 1387–1398
   clinical presentation of, 1387–1388
   diagnosis of, 1392–1396
      cross-sectional imaging in,
         1393–1394, 1393f–1395f
      endoscopic retrograde
         cholangiopancreatography in,
         1394, 1395f
      endoscopic ultrasonography in,
         1396
      fine-needle aspiration in, 1396
      of intraductal papillary mucinous
         neoplasms, 1393–1394, 1395f
      magnetic resonance cholangiography
         in, 1396
      of mucinous cystic neoplasms, 1393,
         1394f
      of serous cystic neoplasms, 1393,
         1393f
   incidence and epidemiology of, 1387
   pathology and biologic behavior of,
      1388b, 1388–1392
      of intraductal papillary mucinous
         neoplasms, 1391b, 1391–1392,
         1392f
      of mucinous cystic neoplasms, 1389f,
         1389–1391, 1390f
      of serous cystic neoplasms,
         1388–1389, 1389f
   prognosis and follow-up of, 1398
   treatment of, 1396–1398
      of intraductal papillary mucinous
         neoplasms, 1397–1398
      of mucinous cystic neoplasms, 1397
      of serous cystic neoplasms,
         1396–1397
Pancreatic drainage procedures, 1509–1513
   for chronic pancreatitis, 1509
   for pancreatic ductal stones, 1510–1511
   for pancreatic pseudocysts and fistulas,
      1511f, 1511–1513, 1512t
   for pancreatic strictures, 1509–1510
Pancreatic duct
   disruption of, in pancreatitis, chronic,
      1349–1352

Pancreatic duct (Continued)
   pancreatic ascites and pleural
      effusions and, 1349–1352,
      1350f–1352f
   elevated pressure in, in pancreatitis,
      chronic, 1345
   injuries of, in pediatric patients, 1412
Pancreatic duct of Santorini, 964
Pancreatic duct of Wirsung, 964
Pancreatic ductal stones, pancreatic
   drainage procedures for, 1510–1511
Pancreatic fistulas
   external, 1352
   internal, in pancreatitis, chronic, 1311
   management of, 1307–1308
   pancreatic drainage procedures for,
      1511f, 1511–1513, 1512f
   with trauma, 1404
Pancreatic fluid collections, acute, 1296,
   1329
   management of, 1307
Pancreatic insufficiency, endocrine and
   exocrine, management of, 1307
Pancreatic lymphomas, in pediatric
   patients, 1411
Pancreatic necrosis
   definition of, 1296
   infected, 1329
   management of, 1307
   treatment of, 1343, 1343f
Pancreatic neoplasms. See also specific
   neoplasms.
   in pediatric patients, 1410–1411
   unusual, 1431–1439
      acinar cell carcinoma as, 1432, 1433f,
         1434
      diagnostic imaging of, 1431–1432
      lymphoma as, 1434–1436, 1436f
      lymphoplasmacytic sclerosing
         pancreatitis as, 1436–1437, 1437f
      metastatic, 1437–1439, 1438f, 1439f
      solid pseudopapillary tumor as, 1434,
         1435f
Pancreatic neuroblastomas, in pediatric
   patients, 1411, 1411f
Pancreatic neuroendocrine tumors,
   1375–1384, 1376f
   classification of, 1376
   corticotropin-producing tumor as,
      1382–1383
      diagnosis of, 1383
      therapy for, 1383
   diagnosis of, 1381
   ghrelinoma as, 1383
   glucagonoma as, 1381–1382
      diagnosis of, 1381, 1382f
      therapy of, 1382, 1382f
   GRFoma as, 1382
      diagnosis of, 1382
      therapy, 1382
   insulinoma as, 1376–1379
      invasive localization studies for,
         1377–1378, 1378f
      preoperative localization of, 1377,
         1377f
      symptoms and diagnosis of,
         1376–1377
      therapy of, 1378–1379, 1379f

Pancreatic neuroendocrine tumors
   (Continued)
   multiple endocrine neoplasia 1 as,
      1379–1380
      diagnosis of, 1379–1380
      prognosis of, 1380
      therapy of, 1380
   neurotensinoma as, 1383
   nonfunctioning, 1383–1384
      diagnosis of, 1383
      presentation of, 1383, 1384f
      prognosis of, 1383–1384
      therapy of, 1383
   PPoma as, 1383–1384
      diagnosis of, 1383
      presentation of, 1383, 1384f
      prognosis of, 1383–1384
      therapy of, 1383
   presentation of, 1381
   somatostatinoma as, 1380–1381
      diagnosis of, 1380
      presentation of, 1380
      therapy of, 1381
   treatment of, 1381
   tumor-releasing parathyroid hormone–
      related protein and, 1383
   VIPoma as, 1381
Pancreatic polypeptide, duodenal function
   and, 981t, 984
Pancreatic polyps, heterotropic, 884
Pancreatic pseudocysts, 1329–1344, 1330b,
   1330f
   acute, definition of, 1296
   clinical features of, 1330–1331
   complications of, 1342–1344
      hemorrhage as, 1343–1344
      infection as, 1342–1343, 1343f
      obstruction as, 1344
      rupture as, 1344
   diagnosis of, 1331t, 1331–1332
   etiology of, 1330
   management of, 1307, 1307f, 1333b,
      1333–1335, 1335f–1342f, 1339,
      1341–1342
   natural history of, 1332–1333, 1333t
   pancreatic drainage procedures for,
      1511f, 1511–1513, 1512t
   in pediatric patients, drainage of, 1412,
      1412f
   rupture of
      silent, 1344
      spontaneous, 1344
   terminology for, 1329, 1331f
   treatment algorithm for, 1332,
      1332f
Pancreatic pseudopseudocysts, 1329
Pancreatic resection
   duodenum-preserving, operative
      modifications of, 1315–1316
   for pancreatic pseudocysts, 1339,
      1341
   reoperative, 1317
Pancreatic rests, endoscopic appearance of,
   738, 739f
Pancreatic stones
   endotherapy for, results after, 1324
   obstructing calculi and, 1322
   removal of, 1323

Pancreatic strictures
  benign, dilation of, 1323
  chronic, pancreatic drainage procedures
    for, 1509–1510
  inflammatory stenoses and, 1322
  without stones, endotherapy for, results
    after, 1323
Pancreatic tissue, ectopic, small intestinal,
  892
Pancreatic trauma, 1400–1405
  diagnosis of, 1400–1401, 1401f
  intraoperative evaluation of, 1401, 1402f
  operative treatment of, 1402–1404,
    1403f–1405f, 1403t
  postoperative considerations with,
    1404–1405
Pancreaticobiliary union, anomalous,
  treatment of, 1508–1509
Pancreaticoduodenal artery, 1445, 1446
  aneurysms of, 1280–1282, 1281f
  inferior, 968, 971f
  superior, 968, 971f, 1237
Pancreaticoduodenal injuries, 769
Pancreaticoduodenal veins
  anterior inferior, 968, 972f
  posterosuperior, 968, 972f
Pancreaticoduodenectomy, 1341
  for duodenal adenocarcinoma, 915
  for pancreatic and periampullary
    carcinoma
    complications following, 1370–1371,
      1371t
    operative technique of, 1367–1370,
      1368f, 1369f
  for pancreaticoduodenal injury, 769–770
  pylorus-preserving, 1321
    results after, 1325–1327
    results after head resection with,
      1325–1327
    techniques for, 1324, 1325f, 1326f
Pancreaticojejunostomy
  longitudinal, side-to-side, with common
    bile duct strictures, 1348
  Roux-en-Y, for pancreatic ductal
    disruption, 1351, 1351f
Pancreatitis
  acute, 1296–1308
    Atlanta Classification for, 1296, 1297f
    clinical presentation of, 1299
    definition of, 1296
    diagnosis of, 1299–1300
    etiology of, 1298b, 1298–1299
    future directions for, 1308
    gallstone, 1298
    laboratory studies in, 1299, 1300b
    mild
      definition of, 1296
      management of, 1301–1302
    pathogenesis and pathophysiology
      of, 1296–1298
      acinar cell injury in, 1296–1297
      local inflammation in, 1297–1298
      systemic inflammation and
        distant organ injury in, 1298
    postoperative, 1298
    postprocedural, 1298
    prognostic indicators for, 1300,
      1301b, 1301t, 1302

Pancreatitis (Continued)
    radiologic studies in, 1299–1300,
      1300f, 1302f
    sequelae of, management of,
      1307–1308
    severe, definition of, 1296
    severe necrotizing, management of,
      1303t, 1303–1306, 1305f–1307f,
      1305t
  with choledochal cysts, 1554, 1554f
  chronic, 1310–1317, 1344–1354
    clinical features of, 1344–1345,
      1345b
    complications of, 1311–1314,
      1345–1354
      common bile duct obstruction as,
        1345–1348, 1346f
      common bile duct stenosis as,
        1311
      duodenal and gastric outlet
        obstruction as, 1348–1349,
        1349f
      duodenal obstruction as, 1311
      external pancreatic fistula as,
        1352
      internal pancreatic fistulas as,
        1311
      pancreatic cancer as, 1353t,
        1353–1354
      pancreatic ductal disruption as,
        1349–1352
      splenic vein thrombosis as,
        1352–1353
      vascular, 1312–1314
    distal common bile duct strictures
      secondary to, biliary drainage
      procedures for, 1501, 1502f,
      1502t, 1503
    endoscopic treatment of, 1321–1327,
      1322f, 1322t
      results after endotherapy for
        stones, 1324, 1324f
      results after endotherapy for
        stricture without stones, 1323
      results after head resection with
        pylorus-preserving
        pancreaticoduodenectomy,
        1325–1327
      surgical resection techniques and,
        1324, 1325f, 1326f
      techniques for, 1323
    hypertension in, ductal and
      parenchymatous, 1310–1311
    natural course of, 1310
    pain in, pathogenesis of, 1310
    pancreatic drainage procedures for,
      1509
    in pediatric patients,
      pancreaticoenteric procedures
      for, 1410
    small duct disease, 1317
    surgical treatment of, 1314–1317
      indications for drainage
        procedures and, 1316–1317,
        1318f
      modifications of duodenum-
        preserving resectional
        procedures and, 1315–1316

Pancreatitis (Continued)
      rationale for drainage procedures
        and, 1314
      rationale for resectional
        procedures or "extended"
        drainage procedures and,
        1314–1315, 1315f–1317f
      salvage procedures and, 1317
    following esophageal resection with
      visceral esophageal substitution, 615
    gallstone, 1298, 1303
      acute, treatment of, 1497–1499
    sclerosing, lymphoplasmacytic,
      1436–1437, 1437f
Pancreatitis chronic, recurrence following
  surgical treatment of, salvage
  procedures for, 1317
Pancreatoblastoma, in pediatric patients,
  1411
Pancreatography, 1493, 1493f
  in pancreatic trauma, 1403
  with pancreaticoduodenal injury, 769
Pancreozymin, 981
Panitumumab, for colorectal cancer
  metastases, 2271
Panproctocolectomy, with ileostomy, for
  ulcerative colitis, 2122
Pantoprazole. See also Proton pump
  inhibitors.
  for Zollinger-Ellison syndrome, 866, 866f
Pantothenic acid, small intestinal
  absorption of, 1006, 1007t
Papaverine
  mesenteric blood flow and, 1243t
  for mesenteric ischemia, 1254–1255
  for mesenteric venous thrombosis, 1257
Papilla of Vater, 964, 965f
Papillary adenomas, gastric, 885
Papillary cystic tumors, 1434, 1435f
  in pediatric patients, 1411
Papillomas, squamous, esophageal,
  523–524, 524f
Pappenheimer bodies, 1775
Paraduodenal hernias, 975–976, 976f,
  1120–1121, 1121f, 1858, 1861f
  clinical features of, 1121
  diagnosis of, 1121–1122
  treatment of, 1122
Paraesophageal diseases, endoscopic
  ultrasonography in, 125
Paraesophageal hernias, 549–560
  classification and pathophysiology of,
    549–550, 550f, 551f
  diagnosis of, 552
  preoperative evaluation of, 552
  prevalence of, 550
  symptoms of, 550–552, 552t
    bleeding as, 552
    esophageal or gastric compression
      as, 551–552
    incarceration and strangulation as,
      550–551
    pulmonary, 552
  treatment of, 552, 554–557
    esophageal lengthening for, 558–559
    fundoplication for, 558
    gastropexy and gastrostomy for, 559
    indications for, 554

Paraesophageal hernias (Continued)
    laparoscopic approach for, 554–555
    laparoscopic technique for, 555,
        555f–557f, 557
    outcomes of, 557–558
    prosthetic mesh for, 559–560
    surgical approach for, 554
Paraesophageal tissue, anatomy of,
    ultrasound, 116
Parahiatal hernias, 560
Paramedian incision, for colorectal surgery,
    2329
Paraprosthetic-enteric fistulas, 1114
Parasitic infections, pruritus ani associated
    with, 2070
Parastomal hernias, 2372, 2372f
    with ileostomy, 1080
Pare, Ambrose, 632
Parent education, for asplenia, in pediatric
    patients, 1811–1812
Parenteral nutrition, in short-bowel
    syndrome, 1165
Parietal cell(s), gastric acid secretion by,
    725–727, 726f
Parietal cell receptors, gastric acid secretion
    and, 725
Parks postanal repair, 1923
Paromomycin, for liver abscesses, amebic,
    1655
Partial splenic embolization, for
    hypersplenism, 1793–1795, 1794f,
    1795f
Pathologists, on portal hypertension
    multidisciplinary team, 1767
Patient advocate, as clinical nurse specialist
    role, in palliative treatment, for
    esophageal cancer, 497
Patient controlled analgesia, following
    bariatric surgery, 937
Patient education, for asplenia, in pediatric
    patients, 1811–1812
Pediatric End-Stage Liver Disease, 1691,
    1691t
Pediatric patients. See also Infants; Neonates.
    annular pancreas in, 1407–1408, 1408f
    appendicitis in, acute, 2143–2144
    bezoars in, 959–960
        clinical features and diagnosis of,
            959
        management of, 959f, 959–960
        types of, 959
    caustic ingestions in, 540
    chronic pancreatitis in,
        pancreaticoenteric procedures for,
        1410
    colonic intussusception in, 1980
    congenital disorders in
        anorectal. See Anorectal anomalies.
        duodenal obstruction as, 952–954
            clinical features and diagnosis of,
                953, 953f, 954f
            embryology and etiology of, 952
            incidence and epidemiology of,
                952
            management of, 953–954, 955f
        gastric duplication as, 948
            clinical features of, 948
            diagnosis of, 948, 950f

Pediatric patients (Continued)
        incidence and etiology of, 948
            management of, 948, 950f
        gastric outlet obstruction as, 950–951
            clinical features of, 950–951
            diagnosis of, 951, 951f
            management of, 951–952
            types of, 951, 951f
        gastric volvulus as, 950
        intestinal atresia as, 1219–1221,
            1220f, 1221f
        malrotation as, 1213–1214,
            1214f–1219f, 1216–1217, 1219
        meconium syndromes as, 1224f,
            1224–1225, 1225f
        microgastria as, 950
        omphalomesenteric duct remnants
            as, 1225, 1226f, 1227
            Meckel's diverticulum as, 1225,
                1227, 1227f
            omphalomesenteric band as,
                1227
            omphalomesenteric cyst as, 1227
            patent omphalomesenteric duct
                as, 1225, 1227
            at umbilicus, 1227
            vitelline blood vessel remnants as,
                1227
        small intestinal duplications and cysts
            as, 1221–1223, 1222f, 1223f
    diabetes mellitus in, type 1, 1415
        pancreas transplantation for. See
            Pancreas transplantation.
    endoscopic retrograde
        cholangiopancreatography in,
        1412–1413
    femoral hernia in, 712
    foreign bodies in, 959, 959f. See also
        Foreign body ingestion.
    foreign body ingestion in, 940
    gastric perforation in, in neonates,
        957–958
        clinical features and diagnosis of,
            957–958
        etiology of, 957
        incidence of, 957
        management of, 958
    gastric tumors in, 958–959
        clinical features and diagnosis of,
            958–959
        incidence of, 958
        management of, 959
    gastrostomy in, 960–961
        complications of, 960–961
        indications for, 960
        types of, 960
    hepatoblastoma in, alfa-fetoprotein and,
        1734
    hyperinsulinism in, 1408–1409
    inguinal hernia in, 705–709
        clinical features of, 706
        contralateral inguinal exploration
            and, 709
        embryology of, 705
        incidence of, 705–706
        indirect, operative management of,
            706–708, 707f, 708f
        with undescended testes, 709, 710f

Pediatric patients (Continued)
    intestinal obstruction in, in newborn,
        947–948
        clinical features and diagnosis of,
            948
    intussusception as, 1229–1230,
        1230f–1232f, 1232
    Ménétrier's disease in, 886
    necrotizing enterocolitis in, 1227–1229,
        1228f, 1229f
    pancreas divisum in, 1409–1410
    pancreatic duct injuries in, 1412
    pancreatic pseudocysts in, drainage of,
        1412, 1412f
    pancreatic tumors in, 1410–1411
    peptic ulcer disease in, 961–962
        clinical features of, 961
        definition and types of, 961
        diagnosis of, 961
        etiology of, 961
        management of, 961–962
    polyposis in. See Juvenile polyposis
        syndrome.
    pyloric stenosis in, hypertrophic, 954,
        956
        clinical features of, 954, 956
        diagnosis of, 956
        etiology and pathogenesis of, 954
        incidence and epidemiology of, 954
        management, 956, 957f, 958f
    splenic trauma in, 1805–1812
        asplenia prophylaxis for, 1811–1812
        evaluation of, 1806–1808, 1807f,
            1808t, 1809f, 1810f, 1811t
        historical background of, 1805–1806
        immune function and consequences
            of splenectomy and, 1806
        operative management of, 1808,
            1811
    testicular torsion in, 711–712
        operative management of, 711–712
    undescended testes in, operative
        management of, 709–711
Pediculosis pubis, pruritus ani associated
    with, 2070
PELD, 1691, 1691t
Peliosis hepatis, 1730
    drug-induced, 1723
Pelvic abscesses, with appendicitis, 2150
Pelvic anatomy, low anterior resection and,
    2222
Pelvic floor, perineal pain and, 2072
Pelvic floor exercises, for fecal
    incontinence, 1921–1922
Pelvic floor function, tests of, 1897
Pelvic floor retraining, for constipation,
    1938
Pelvic girdle disorders, pain associated with,
    2072
Pelvic muscles, anatomy of, continence and,
    2391–2394
Pelvic organ prolapse, perineal hernias
    associated with, 695–696
Pelvic outlet obstruction, surgical treatment
    of, 1936, 1937f, 1938f
Pelvic pain. See Perineal pain syndromes.
Pelvic pouch procedure, redo, 2415,
    2417

Pelvic splanchnic nerves, 1870
Pelvic surgery
    operative measures to improve ease and
        safety of, 2418
    perineal pain and, 2072
    reoperative. *See* Reoperative surgery,
        pelvic.
Peña procedure, 2387, 2398, 2399f, 2400
    fecal incontinence following, 2405
    postoperative complications of,
        2402–2403
Penicillin V, for asplenia, in pediatric
    patients, 1811
Pepsinogen, gastric secretion of, 728
Peptic ulcer disease
    bleeding ulcers and
        emergency surgery for, 802t,
            802–804, 803f, 804f
            for gastric ulcers, 804
        in pediatric patients, 962
        vagotomy and drainage for, 824–825,
            825f
    duodenal. *See* Duodenal ulcers.
    gastric. *See* Gastric ulcers.
    gastric barrier function and, 729
    intractable, vagotomy and drainage for,
        822–823
    pathogenesis of, 811–812
    in pediatric patients, 961–962
        clinical features of, 961
        definition and types of, 961
        diagnosis of, 961
        etiology of, 961
        management of, 961–962
    perforation of, vagotomy and drainage
        for, 823–824
    recurrent, after vagotomy and drainage,
        826–827
    surgery for, 791–809
        complications of, 808–809
        elective, 792–800
            for intractable duodenal ulcer
                disease, 792–798
            for intractable gastric ulcer
                disease, 798–800, 799f, 799t
        emergency, 800–808
            bleeding lesions and, 802t,
                802–804
            gastric outlet obstruction and,
                806–808
            perforation and, 804–806
        gastric outlet obstruction following,
            reoperation for, 1136–1137
        indications for, 791
        vagotomy and drainage as.
            See Vagotomy, with drainage.
        in Zollinger-Ellison syndrome.
            See Zollinger-Ellison syndrome.
Peptide YY, duodenal function and, 981t,
    984–985
Percutaneous aspiration, of pancreatic
    pseudocysts, 1333
Percutaneous drainage
    biliary
        alkaline phosphatase elevation in,
            1615
        complications of, 1468–1469
        technique of, 1464–1466

Percutaneous drainage *(Continued)*
    of pancreatic pseudocysts, 1333–1334
    for splenic abscesses, 1820
Percutaneous endoscopic gastrostomy
    contraindications to, 750t
    fistulas due to, 1095
    indications for, 750t
    in pediatric patients, 960
Percutaneous transhepatic cholangiography
    with bile duct strictures, 1578–1579
    with biliary fistulas, 1542
    complications of, 1468–1469
    indications for, 1463–1464
    in periampullary carcinoma, 1363,
        1364f
    technique of, 1464–1466
Perhexiline, hepatotoxicity of, 1721
Periampullary carcinoma, 1358–1373
    adjuvant therapy for, 1372
    clinical findings in, 1360–1361
    etiology of, 1360
    imaging studies in, 1361–1363
        on computed tomography,
            1361–1362, 1362f
        on endoscopic retrograde
            cholangiopancreatography,
            1362–1363, 1363f
        on magnetic resonance imaging,
            1362, 1363f
        on percutaneous transhepatic
            cholangiography, 1363, 1364f
        on positron-emission tomography,
            1363
        on right upper quadrant ultrasound,
            1361
        on upper endoscopy and endoscopic
            ultrasonography, 1364, 1364f
    immunotherapy for, 1373
    incidence of, 1358
    laboratory findings in, 1361
    neoadjuvant therapy for, 1372
    palliation for
        chemotherapeutic, 1372–1373
        nonoperative, 1365–1366
            of duodenal obstruction,
                1365–1366
            of obstructive jaundice, 1365
            of pain, 1366
        operative, 1366–1367
            of duodenal obstruction,
                1366–1367
            of obstructive jaundice, 1366,
                1366f
            for pain, 1367, 1367t
    pathology of, 1358–1359
    resection of, 1367–1370
        long-term survival after, 1371f,
            1371–1372
        pancreatectomy for
            for cancer in pancreatic body or
                tail, 1370, 1370f
            complications following,
                1370–1371, 1371t
        pancreaticoduodenectomy for
            complications following,
                1370–1371, 1371t
            operative technique of,
                1367–1370, 1368f, 1369f

Periampullary carcinoma *(Continued)*
    staging of
        clinicopathologic, 1365
        preoperative, 1364–1365
    tissue diagnosis of, 1363–1364
Periampullary diverticula, 780
Perianal abscesses, in Crohn's disease,
    surgical treatment of, 2135, 2136f
Perianal disease, in Crohn's disease, 1045
Perianal lumps, examination of, 1887
Perianal neoplasms, pruritus ani and, 2068
Perianal sepsis, endoanal ultrasound in,
    1911
Periappendiceal abscesses, 2148–2149
Peribiliary venous system of Couinaud, 1603
Pericolic abscesses, 2016–2017
Pericysts, echinococcal, 1637, 1638
Periesophageal nerves, prenatal
    development of, 46
Periesophageal tissue, anatomy of, 11
Peri-ileostomy fistulas, 1080–1081
Perineal abscesses, in Crohn's disease, 2088
Perineal body, 696
Perineal hernias, 694–700
    anatomy and, 696, 697f
    classification of, 694–696, 695f, 696f
    clinical features and diagnosis of, 696,
        698f, 698–699, 699f
    treatment of, 699–700, 700f–703f
Perineal pain syndromes, 2071–2075
    anatomy and, 2072
    causes of, 2072–2074, 2073t
        functional, 2074
        inflammatory diseases as, 2072
        mechanical, 2072–2073
        muscular, 2072
        neoplastic, 2073–2074
        neurologic, 2072, 2074
        orthopedic, 2074
        pelvic, 2072
        spinal, 2072
    evaluation of, 2074
    treatment of, 2074–2075, 2075t
Perineoproctectomy, with layered closure,
    for rectovaginal fistulas, 1952
Perinuclear antineutrophil cytoplasmic
    antibodies, in Crohn's disease, 1046
Peristalsis
    colonic, 1874f, 1874–1875
    esophageal, 51–53, 52f–54f, 130–132,
        132f
        deglutitive inhibition and, 52–53, 54f
        duration response and, 51
        inhibitory relaxation wave and, 53
        primary, 130, 132f
        propulsive force and, 53
        pharyngeal peristaltic contraction and,
            49
Peristaltic reflex, 1014
Peritoneal lavage, diagnostic
    in abdominal trauma, in pediatric
        patients, 1807–1808
    in colorectal trauma, 1974
    in gastric trauma, 762–763
Peritonitis
    in colonic diverticulitis, 2018, 2019f
    diffuse, perforated appendicitis with,
        2149

Permacol, for ventral herniorrhaphy, 676
Persistent hyperinsulinemic hypoglycemia of infancy, 1408–1409
PET scans. *See* Positron-emission tomography.
Petit, Jean Louis, 632
Peutz-Jeghers syndrome, 2159t, 2174–2175
    as risk factor for colorectal cancer, 2188–2189
    small intestinal, 894t, 897–898
        small intestinal
            symptoms and diagnosis of, 897
            treatment of, 898
Pfannensteil incision, for Crohn's disease, 1057, 1057f
pH, of ingested material, in caustic ingestions, 541
pH monitoring
    esophageal, 164–169
        ambulatory esophageal impedance testing and, for esophageal bolus clearance, 158–159, 159f, 160f
        Bravo probe for, 167–168, 168f
        combined with multichannel intraluminal impedance, 180–181, 180f–183f
        instrumentation for
            catheters and probes and, 165, 165f
            data-recording devices and, 165
            software analysis and, 165–166
        integrated ambulatory monitoring and, 173
        with paraesophageal hernia, 552
        preoperative, for esophageal replacement, 287
        protocols for, 166–167
            catheter systems and, 166
            data analysis and, 166–167, 167f, 167t
            diary and, 166
            patient preparation and, 166, 166b
        24-hour, 161
    in esophageal spasm, 420–421
    gastric, 24-hour, for duodenogastro-esophageal reflux, 191f–193f, 191–193, 192t
    in gastroesophageal reflux disease, 231
    in hypertensive lower esophageal sphincter, 424
    24-hour
        in gastroesophageal reflux disease, 59
        preoperative, for Nissen fundoplication, 266
Pharmacobezoars, 943, 944, 944t
Pharyngeal cylinder, valves in, 128–129
Pharyngoesophageal diverticulectomy, for Zenker's diverticulum, methods and results of, 430–431
Pharyngoesophageal diverticulum. *See* Zenker's diverticulum.
Pharyngoesophageal junction, access to, 379, 380f, 381f
Pharyngoesophageal junction disorders, 374–390. *See also* Dysphagia, oropharyngeal.

Pharyngoesophageal transit studies, radionuclide, for swallowing evaluation, 378
Pharynx
    peristaltic contraction of, 49
    prenatal development of, 31–33, 33f, 34f
Phenobarbital, for pruritus, in primary sclerosing cholangitis, 1567
Phenothiazine derivatives, for gastroparesis, 921
Phenylephrine, mesenteric blood flow and, 1243t
Phenytoin, hepatotoxicity of, 1721
Phospholipids, in bile, 1452
Photodynamic therapy
    for anal intraepithelial neoplasia, 2290
    for Barrett's esophagus, 370
    for esophageal cancer, 489t, 493
    for low-grade dysplasia, following antireflux procedures, 360
Phrenic veins, 1604
Phrenoesophageal membrane
    anatomy of, 12–14, 14f
    prenatal development of, 36, 36f
Phrygian cap, 1449, 1450f
Phytobezoars, 943–944, 944t
    in pediatric patients, 960
Pigmentation, mucocutaneous, in Peutz-Jeghers syndrome, 2174
Pilonidal disease, 1966–1970
    clinical presentation of, 1966–1967
    etiology of, 1966, 1967f
    malignant degeneration of, 1969–1970
    pathology of, 1966
    treatment of, 1967–1969
        for acute pilonidal abscess, 1967
            drainage technique for, 1967
        for chronic disease, 1968–1969
            conservative, nonresectional approach for, 1968
            excision with or without closure for, 1968–1969
            incision and curettage with marsupialization or saucerization for, 1968
            midline follicle excision and lateral drainage for, 1968, 1968f
        for recurrent or unhealed disease, 1969
            cleft lip technique for, 1969, 1970f
Pinworms, pruritus ani associated with, 2070
Piperacillin, for cholangitis prophylaxis, 1550t
Piriformis muscle, sciatic hernias and, 701
Pituitary adenylate cyclase activating polypeptide, small intestinal neuroendocrine function and, 1018
Plain radiographs
    abdominal. *See* Abdominal plain films.
    chest. *See* Chest radiography.
    sacral, with retrorectal tumors, 2301
Plasma exchange, for liver failure, acute, 1705
Pleural effusions, pancreatic, 1349–1352, 1350f–1352f

Plexiglas, for endoscopic antireflux procedures, 325
Pliny the Elder, 1813
Plug and patch hernia repair, 649, 650f, 651f
Pneumatic dilatation, for achalasia, 412
Pneumocystis carinii infection, splenic abscess due to, 1820
Pneumonia, following esophageal surgery, 599
Pneumothorax
    following Heller myotomy, 417
    with Nissen fundoplication, 273
Polycystic liver disease, 1634–1635, 1635f
Polydioxanone suture material, for bowel anastomoses, 1083, 1084
Polyester, for ventral herniorrhaphy, 676
Polyethylene glycol, for bowel preparation, 831, 2328
Polyfilament, for groin hernia repair, 646
Polyglycolic mesh, for rectovaginal fistulas, 1952
Polyglyconate suture material, for bowel anastomoses, 1083, 1084
Polymyositis, esophageal motility disorders in, 140
Polyp(s)
    adenomatous. *See also* Familial adenomatous polyposis.
        colorectal. *See* Colorectal polyps, adenomatous.
        endoscopic appearance of, 740, 741f
        gastric, endoscopic appearance of, 740, 741f
    Brunner's gland, 884
    colorectal. *See* Colorectal polyps; Polyposis syndromes; *specific polyposis syndromes*.
    ectopic tissue, small intestinal, 892–893
    esophageal
        endoscopic ultrasonography in, 122–123
        imaging of, 82, 83f
    fibroid, inflammatory, gastric, 884
    fibrovascular, esophageal, 522–523, 523t
    fundic gland, 2162
    fundic gland-type, endoscopic appearance of, 740, 741f
    gallbladder, 1519
        with primary sclerosing cholangitis, 1565
        treatment of, 1567
        radiographically suspicious, preoperatively diagnosed, 1524–1525
    gastric. *See* Gastric polyps.
    hamartomatous
        colorectal, 2157f, 2157–2158, 2158f
        gastric, 884
    inflammatory, gastric, 884
    pancreatic, heterotopic, 884
    retention, 2157
        gastric, 884
    small intestinal. *See also* Intestinal polyposis syndromes.
        neoplastic, 891–893
            Brunner's gland, 892–893
            ectopic tissue, 892–893

Polyp(s) (Continued)
  endometriosis as, 893
    tubular adenomas as, 891–892
    villous adenomas as, 892–893
  non-neoplastic, benign, 891
Polypectomy, colonoscopic, 2157
  complications of, 2157
  for malignant polyps, 2156f, 2156–2157
  for pedunculated polyps, 2155–2156
  for sessile polyps, 2156
Polypoid lesions, gastric, endoscopic
    appearance of, 740, 740f, 741f
Polyposis syndromes, 2158–2177, 2159t
  Cowden's disease as, 2159t, 2175–2176
  Cronkhite-Canada syndrome as, 2159t,
    2176
  familial. See Familial adenomatous
    polyposis.
  hereditary mixed polyposis syndrome as,
    2159t, 2176–2177
  hereditary nonpolyposis colorectal
    cancer as. See Hereditary
    nonpolyposis colorectal cancer.
  juvenile, 2159t, 2173–2174
  Peutz-Jeghers syndrome as, 2159t,
    2174–2175
  Ruvalcaba-Myhre-Smith syndrome as,
    2159t, 2176
Polypropylene
  for groin hernia repair, 646
  mesh for ventral herniorrhaphy and,
    675, 675f
  patches for paraesophageal hernia and,
    559–560
Polysplenia, 1777
Polytetrafluoroethylene
  expanded
    for groin hernia repair, 647
    paraesophageal hernia and, 560
    for ventral herniorrhaphy, 676, 676f
  mesh for paraesophageal hernia and,
    559, 560
Porfimer sodium, for Barrett's esophagus,
    370
Porphyria cutanea tarda, in primary
    sclerosing cholangitis, 1562
Porta hepatis, 1602
Portal fissure, main, 1599f, 1602–1603
Portal hypertension, 1751–1767
  anatomy and, 1752–1753, 1753f, 1754f
  ascites in, 1755–1756, 1763–1765
    diagnosis of, 1764
    management of, 1764–1765, 1765f
    pathophysiology of, 1763–1764,
      1764f
  in cirrhosis, 1624, 1693
  clinical presentation of, 1755–1756
  encephalopathy in, 1756
  etiology of, 1756b, 1756–1757
  evaluation of, 1757b, 1757–1758, 1758b,
    1758t
  hepatocellular carcinoma in, 1756
  historical background of, 1751–1752
  intrahepatic, 1756–1757
  liver failure in, 1756
  multidisciplinary team for, 1767
  noncirrhotic, drug-induced, 1723
  in pancreatitis, chronic, 1312–1313

Portal hypertension (Continued)
  pathophysiology of, 1754–1755, 1755f
  portopulmonary syndromes in, 1756
  posthepatic, 1757
  prehepatic, 1756
  with primary sclerosing cholangitis,
    1566
    treatment of, 1568
  pulmonary syndromes in, 1766t,
    1766–1767
    clinical presentation of, 1766
    hepatopulmonary syndrome as,
      1766f, 1766–1767
    pathophysiology of, 1766
    portopulmonary hypertension as,
      1767, 1767f
  splenectomy for, 1834
  variceal bleeding in. See Esophageal
    varices, bleeding.
Portal pedicle, 1599
Portal vein, 1602, 1772
  anatomy of, 1752–1753, 1753f
  anomalies of, 1602
  hepatocellular carcinoma and, 1733
  preduodenal, 974, 974f
Portal vein thrombosis
  with cavernous transformation, in chronic
    pancreatitis, 1313f, 1313–1314
  following splenectomy, 1838
  liver transplantation and, 1697, 1698
Portal venous sampling, for insulinoma
    localization, 1378
Portocaval shunt, intrahepatic, transjugular
  for ascites, 1765
  for bleeding due to portal hypertension,
    1693
  for bleeding varices, 1693, 1761–1762
    procedure for, 1761f, 1761–1762
  for Budd-Chiari syndrome, 1714, 1715
Portopulmonary hypertension, 1767,
    1767f
  in cirrhosis, 1693, 1693b
  clinical presentation of, 1766
  pathophysiology of, 1766
Portopulmonary syndromes, in portal
    hypertension, 1756
Positron-emission tomography
  of carcinoid tumors, 1184
  with colon, rectal, and anal disorders,
    1895, 1896f
  to detect colorectal cancer tumor
    relapse, 2259
  in esophageal carcinoma
    assessment for metastases using,
      471–472
    for recurrent cancer assessment, 79,
      81
    for staging, 77–78, 81f
      therapy monitoring and, 461
    for treatment selection, 79
  FDG, for staging of esophageal cancer,
    459f, 459–460
  in gastric adenocarcinoma, 907
  of gastrointestinal stromal tumors,
    1195f, 1195–1196
  in pancreatic carcinoma, 1354
  in periampullary carcinoma, 1363
Postanal repair, 1923

Posterior sagittal anorectoplasty, 2387, 2398,
    2399f, 2400
  fecal incontinence following, 2405
  postoperative complications of,
    2402–2403
Postgastrectomy syndromes, 808–809,
    870–880
  afferent loop obstruction as, 809,
    877–879, 879f
  bile reflux gastritis as, 875–877,
    876f–878f
  diarrhea as, 809, 873–874, 874f
    reoperative surgery for, 1138–1139
  dumping syndrome as, 809, 870–873,
    872f
    reoperative surgery for, 1138–1139
  duodenogastroesophageal reflux
    associated with, 190
  early satiety as, 808–809
  efferent loop obstruction as, 809, 877,
    878
  gallstones as, 875
  gastric cancer as, 809
  gastric stasis as, 874–875
  jejunogastric intussusception as, 879–880
  metabolic aberrations as, 873
  reflux gastritis as, alkaline, 809
  Roux stasis syndrome as, 809, 880
    reoperative surgery for, 1140
Postoperative pain, following laparoscopic
    colorectal surgery, 2343
Postpolycythemic myeloid metaplasia,
    splenectomy for, 1831
Post-thrombocytopenic myeloid metaplasia,
    splenectomy for, 1831
Post-transplant hyperproliferative disease,
    following intestinal transplantation,
    1176–1177
Potassium
  absorption of, colonic, 1872
  secretion of, colonic, 1872
Pott, Percivall, 632, 633f
Pouchitis, following ileal pouch-anal
    anastomosis, 2113, 2115t, 2115–2116
    anti-tumor necrosis factor and, 2115
    morphologic changes in ileal pouch
      mucosa and, 2116
      acute, treatment of, 2116
    pathogenesis of, 2115
    severe, 2115–2116
Pouch–vaginal fistulas, following ileal pouch–
    anal anastomosis, 2112–2113, 2114f
PPH staplers, 1087
PPomas, 1383–1384
  diagnosis of, 1383
  presentation of, 1383, 1384f
  prognosis of, 1383–1384
  therapy of, 1383
Prednisone
  for cholangitis prophylaxis, 1550t
  for inflammatory bowel disease, 2090
Pregnancy
  acute fatty liver of, 1703
  appendicitis during, 2144
  gastroesophageal reflux disease and, 200
Prenatal development of, of phrenic nerve,
    45–46
Presacral nerve, 1856

Prevertebral ganglia, 1869
Primary biliary cirrhosis, end-stage liver disease due to, 1686–1687
Primary sclerosing cholangitis, 1560–1570, 1586t, 1586–1589
  biliary drainage procedures for, 1503f, 1503–1504
  biliary tumors vs., 1526
  biochemical and serologic abnormalities in, 1561
  clinical presentation of, 1560, 1587
  complications of, 1564–1565
    non-primary sclerosing cholangitis–associated, 1566
    primary sclerosing cholangitis–associated, 1565–1566
      biliary strictures as, 1565
      cholangiocarcinoma as, 1565–1566
      choledocholithiasis as, 1565
      cholelithiasis as, 1565
      gallbladder polyps as, 1565
  diagnosis of, 1560–1561, 1561b, 1586–1587, 1587f
  diseases associated with, 1563–1564, 1564b
    autoimmune hepatitis as, 1564
    inflammatory bowel disease as, 1563–1564
  end-stage liver disease due to, 1686–1687
  epidemiology of, 1560
  etiopathogenesis of, 1562–1563
  imaging studies in, 1561–1562, 1562f
  inflammatory bowel disease with, 1693
  natural history of, 1564, 1587
  pathogenesis of, 1586
  pathology of, 1562, 1563t, 1586
  treatment of, 1587–1588
    medical, 1567–1568
      for hepatobiliary disease, 1568
      nonoperative dilation therapy for, 1588
      for non-primary sclerosing cholangitis-associated complications, 1567t, 1567–1568, 1568t
      for primary sclerosing cholangitis-associated complications, 1567
    surgical, 1568–1570, 1588f, 1588–1589
      with cholangiocarcinoma, 1570
      liver transplantation as, 1569–1570
      proctocolectomy as, 1570
      reconstructive biliary surgery as, 1568–1569
Primitive neuroectodermal tumors, in pediatric patients, 1411
Pringle maneuver, 1605
  for hepatectomy, 1676, 1677
  in hepatobiliary trauma, 1664
Procedure for prolapsing hemorrhoids, 2034–2035, 2035f
Processus vaginalis, 633–634
Procidentia. See Rectal prolapse.
Proctalgia fugax, 2071

Proctitis
  hemorrhagic, management of, 2321
  radiation, medical management for, 2321–2322
    argon plasma coagulation as, 2322
    formalin instillation as, 2321–2322
    hyperbaric oxygen as, 2322
  in residual rectal mucosa, following ileal pouch–anal anastomosis, 2112
Proctocolectomy
  for primary sclerosing cholangitis, 1570
  total
    with continent ileostomy, for familial adenomatous polyposis, 2165, 2165t, 2166t
    with end ileostomy
      for familial adenomatous polyposis, 2165, 2165t, 2166t
      for ulcerative colitis, 2093
    for familial adenomatous polyposis, 1070
    with ileal pouch–anal anastomosis, for ulcerative colitis, 2093–2094
    for ulcerative colitis, 1070
Proctosigmoidectomy, perineal, for rectal prolapse, 1962, 1964t
Proctosigmoidoscopy
  with colonic vascular ectasias, 1991
  flexible, 1890, 1890f
  rigid, 1889f, 1889–1890
Prokinetic agents
  for cough, in gastroesophageal reflux disease, 259
  for gastroesophageal reflux disease, 253–254
  for gastroparesis, 921
Proliferative mucinous cystic neoplasms, noninvasive, 1390
Prolonged propagated contractions, small intestinal, 1017, 1017f
Promoter of quality care, as clinical nurse specialist role, in palliative treatment, for esophageal cancer, 497–498
Prone jackknife position, 1886, 1886f
Prosthetic materials. See also specific materials.
  for groin hernia surgery, 646b, 646–647
  for hernia repair, complications of, 654
Prosthetic mesh
  for paraesophageal hernia, 559–560
  for ventral herniorrhaphy, 675f, 675–676, 676f
Proteins
  duodenal absorption of, 980
  small intestinal absorption of, 1002–1004, 1003t, 1004f
Prothrombin time, increased, patient approach for, 1615
Proton pump inhibitors. See also specific drugs.
  for asthma, in gastroesophageal reflux disease, 258, 259f, 260f
  for Barrett's esophagus, 257–258
  for cough, in gastroesophageal reflux disease, 259
  for esophageal strictures, 237, 256–257
  for esophagitis, reflux, 255–256, 256f
  evaluation of patients receiving, pH monitoring for, 173
  gastric acid secretion and, 727

Proton pump inhibitors (Continued)
  for gastroesophageal reflux disease, 254–255, 255f
    empirical trials of, 181
  for gastrointestinal fistulas, 1104
  for laryngitis, reflux, 259–260
  maintenance of, 543
Pruritus
  in cholestatic liver disease, 1694
  with primary sclerosing cholangitis, 1566
  treatment of, 1567, 1567t, 1588
Pruritus ani, 1884, 2065–2071
  causes of, 2066–2070, 2068t
    anatomic compromise as, 2067
    dermatologic conditions as, 2069–2070
    diarrhea as, 2068
    dietary, 2068
    drugs as, 2069
    gynecologic, 2068
    infectious, 2070
    neoplastic, 2068
    personal hygiene as, 2066–2067
    psychological, 2069
    radiation as, 2069
    systemic diseases as, 2067–2068
  history in, 2065
  pathophysiology of, 2066
  physical examination in, 2066, 2066f
  treatment of, 2070–2071
Pseudoachalasia, 408–409
  imaging in, 72–73
Pseudoaneurysms
  of hepatic artery, 1711
  of splenic artery, image-guided interventional therapy for, 1791, 1793, 1793f
Pseudocysts
  pancreatic. See Pancreatic pseudocysts.
  splenic, image-guided interventional therapy for, 1795, 1795f
Pseudoepitheliomatous hyperplasia, 1887
Pseudomembranous colitis
  antibiotics and, 2329
  in immunocompromised patients, 2382
Pseudomonas infection, hepatic abscesses and, 1645
Pseudopapillary tumors, solid, in pediatric patients, 1411
Pseudopolyps, 2158, 2159f
  inflammatory, gastric, 884
Pseudopseudocysts, pancreatic, 1329
Pseudotumors, inflammatory
  esophageal, 522
  in pancreatitis, chronic, 1312
Psoas sign, in appendicitis, 2142
Psoriasis, perianal, pruritus ani associated with, 2069
Psychological factors, pruritus ani and, 2069
Psychosocial factors, gastroesophageal reflux disease and, 201
PTEN hamartoma syndrome, 2159t, 2176
Pteroylglutamic acid
  deficiency of, in Crohn's disease, 1054
  small intestinal absorption of, 1006, 1007t

PTFE
expanded
for groin hernia repair, 647
paraesophageal hernia and, 560
for ventral herniorrhaphy, 676,
676f
mesh for paraesophageal hernia and,
559, 560
Pubococcygeus muscle, 696
Puborectalis muscle, 696
paradoxical contraction of, surgical
treatment of, 1936–1938, 1939f,
1940f, 1941t
Puborectalis syndrome, surgical treatment
of, 1936–1938, 1939f, 1940f, 1941t
Pudendal hernias, 695, 696f
Pudendal nerve terminal motor latency
in constipation, 1933–1934
in fecal incontinence, 1919–1920
Puestow procedure, modified, in pediatric
patients, 1410
Pulmonary disorders
in cirrhosis, 1693, 1693b
with paraesophageal hernia, 552
postoperative, following esophageal
surgery, 599
esophagectomy as, 480
resection with visceral esophageal
substitution as, 613
Pulmonary embolism, following bariatric
surgery, 937
Pulmonary function, recovery of, following
laparoscopic colorectal surgery, 2343
Pulmonary metastases, of colorectal cancer,
management of, 2269–2270
patient selection for, 2269
pulmonary resection results and,
2269–2270
Pulmonologists, on portal hypertension
multidisciplinary team, 1767
Pulse-echo technique, 112
Purse-string suture, 1085
Push endoscopy, in Crohn's disease, 1050f,
1050–1051
Pyelography
intravenous, with nephroenteric fistulas,
1106
retrograde, with nephroenteric fistulas,
1106
Pyloric atresia, gastric outlet obstruction
and, 950f, 951
Pyloric exclusion
for gastroduodenal perforations, 1110
with gastrojejunostomy, 768–769
Pyloric reconstruction
for dumping syndrome, 871–872
longitudinal, for gastric outlet
obstruction, 951
Pyloric stenosis
endoscopic appearance of, 738, 739f
hypertrophic, in pediatric patients, 954,
956
clinical features of, 954, 956
diagnosis of, 956
etiology and pathogenesis of, 954
incidence and epidemiology of,
954
management, 956, 957f, 958f

Pyloric ulcers, surgery for, gastric outlet
obstruction following, reoperation for,
1136–1137
Pyloric webs, gastric outlet obstruction and,
951
Pyloromyotomy, for esophagogastrostomy,
585, 585f
Pyloroplasty, 816–818
for duodenal ulcers, 794–795
Finney, 816, 818, 819f
for duodenal ulcers, 795
technique for, 842f
gastroparesis following, 923
Heineke-Mikulicz, 816, 818f
for duodenal ulcers, 794–795,
795f
technique for, 841f, 842f
Jaboulay, 818, 819f
technique for, 844f
longitudinal, for gastric outlet
obstruction, 951
technique for, 831, 841f–845f
Pylorus-preserving pancreaticoduodenectomy, 1321
results after, 1325–1327
results after head resection with,
1325–1327
techniques for, 1324, 1325f, 1326f
Pyoderma gangrenosum, in colonic
diverticular disease, 2021

Q

Quincke, Heinrich Irenaeus, 3, 6, 337–338,
338f
Quinidine, pruritus ani associated with,
2069

R

Rabeprazole. *See also* Proton pump
inhibitors.
gastric acid secretion and, 727
Race, gastroesophageal reflux disease and,
200
Radiation enteritis, 1150–1158
clinical features of, 1153
diagnosis of, 1153–1154
etiology of, 1151
histologic findings in, 1151–1152
early, 1151
late, 1151–1152
historical background of, 1150
incidence of, 1150–1151
management of, 1155–1158
conservative/symptomatic,
1156–1157
novel techniques in radiotherapy
and combined radiotherapy/
chemotherapy for, 1155–1156
prevention and, 1155
surgical, 1157–1158
microcirculation and
molecular biology of, 1152
radiation and, 1152
molecular biology of, 1152

Radiation enteritis *(Continued)*
natural history of, 1152–1153
predisposing risk factors for, 1151
prognosis of, 1154–1155
Radiofrequency ablation
circumferential balloon-based, for
Barrett's esophagus, 367–370, 368f,
369f
for hepatocellular carcinoma,
1737–1738, 1738
transarterial, hepatic abscesses following,
pyogenic, 1642
Radiographic embolization, of injured
spleens, in pediatric patients, 1808,
1810f
Radioisotope-labeled meal, in constipation,
1932
Radiologists, on portal hypertension
multidisciplinary team, 1767
Radiopaque marker method, for colonic
transit measurement, 1873, 1873f
Radioprotectant chemicals, 1155
Radiotherapy. *See also* Chemoradiotherapy.
adjuvant, radiation enteritis and, 1156
for anal squamous cell carcinoma,
2292–2293, 2293t
electron beam, intraoperative delivery
of, for locally recurrent colorectal
cancer, 2265–2267, 2268f
esophageal, esophageal carcinoma and,
466
external beam, for carcinoid tumors,
1187
for gallbladder cancer, 1524
for gastric adenocarcinoma
neoadjuvant, 913
palliative, 914
hormone receptor–mediated, for
carcinoid tumors, 1187
hyperfractionated, 1156
immunosuppression due to, 2376
intraoperative, 1156
for recurrent cancer, 2417–2418
for lymphoma, 1209
in multimodality therapy, for esophageal
cancer, 499–502
postoperative, 501t, 501–502
preoperative, 499–501, 500t
neoadjuvant, radiation enteritis and,
1156
palliative, for esophageal cancer,
493–495
brachytherapy as, 494
combined radiation therapy as,
494–495
external beam radiotherapy as,
494
patient selection for, 493
preoperative
for locally recurrent colorectal
cancer, 2262–2263
with low anterior resection, 2220
pruritus ani due to, 2069
rectal injuries due to. *See* Rectum,
radiation injuries of.
total-body, hepatotoxicity of, 1723
Raloxifene, for desmoids, in familial
adenomatous polyposis, 2162

Ranitidine, 255. *See also* Histamine₂ receptor antagonists.
for esophageal strictures, 237
for gastroesophageal reflux disease, 254
Ranson's criteria, 1300, 1301t
Rapid ACTH stimulation test, for evaluation of response to surgical stress, 2378
Read, Raymond, 674
Read/Rives hernia repair, 651–652
Real-time ultrasonography, 112
Recombinant tissue plasminogen activator, for mesenteric venous thrombosis, 1257
Rectal adenocarcinoma, abdominoperineal resection for, 2235
Rectal bleeding
differential diagnosis of, 1883–1884
examination for, 1887
Rectal cancer. *See also* Colorectal adenocarcinoma; Colorectal cancer; Colorectal carcinoma.
adenocarcinoma as, abdominoperineal resection for, 2235
carcinoids as, treatment of, 1185
local excision of, 2197–2198, 2208–2216
algorithm for, 2215–2216, 2216t
endorectal ultrasound and endorectal magnetic resonance imaging and, 2209
outcomes with, 2212–2215
adjuvant therapy and, 2214t, 2214–2215
prospective studies of, 2215, 2215t
retrospective studies of, 2213t, 2213–2214
with transanal endoscopic microsurgery, 2215, 2216t
preoperative evaluation for, 2208, 2209b
technique for, 2209–2212
transanal, 2209, 2210f
transanal endoscopic microsurgery and, 2211–2212, 2212f
transcoccygeal, 2209–2211, 2210f, 2211f
transsphincteric, 2211
recurrent, reoperative pelvic surgery for, 2417
staging of, endorectal ultrasound for, accuracy of, 1900–1903, 1903t
Rectal carcinoids, treatment of, 1185
Rectal disorders. *See also specific disorders.*
diagnosis of, 1883–1897
examination for, 1885–1888
with anorectal pain or swelling, 1887
for bleeding, 1887
for constipation, 1888
general principles of, 1885–1886
inspection and palpation in, 1886–1887
positioning for, 1886, 1886f
for urgency and incontinence, 1888
history in, 1883
investigation for, 1888–1897
blood and stool testing in, 1888–1889

Rectal disorders (*Continued*)
endoscopy in, 1889f, 1889–1891, 1890f
radiologic tests in, 1891f, 1891–1897, 1892f, 1894f–1897f
symptoms in, 1883–1885
abdominal pain and distention as, 1884
anorectal pain, itching and swelling as, 1884
bleeding as, 1883–1884
constipation as, 1884–1885
diarrhea as, 1885
urgency and incontinence as, 1885
Rectal dyschezia, surgical treatment of, 1936–1938, 1939f, 1940f, 1941t
Rectal examination
in appendicitis, 2142
for small bowel obstruction, 1029
Rectal intussusception, surgical treatment of, 1936, 1938f
Rectal neoplasms. *See also* Colorectal adenocarcinoma; Colorectal cancer; Colorectal carcinoma; Rectal cancer; Retrorectal tumors; *specific neoplasms.*
transanal excision of, 2338
Rectal obstruction, management of, 2220–2221
Rectal pain. *See also* Perineal pain syndromes.
examination for, 1887
idiopathic, chronic, 2071
Rectal prolapse, 1958–1965, 1959f
diagnosis and testing in, 1958–1959
historical background of, 1958
laparoscopic surgery for
outcomes of, 2357, 2357t
technical issues for, 2357
pathophysiology of, 1958
physical examination in, 1918, 1958
treatment of, 1959–1965
acute management for, 1959–1960
results and patient selection for, 1964t, 1965
surgical, 1960–1965
abdominal approaches for, 1960–1961
perineal approaches for, 1961–1965, 1962f
Rectal reconstruction, for radiation injury, 2322–2323
Rectal sensation, determination of, 1919
Rectal stump, identification of, 2413f, 2413–2414
Rectal ulcers
endoanal ultrasound with, 1913–1914, 1914f
solitary, 2075–2076
diagnosis of, 2075–2076, 2076f
treatment of, 2076
Rectoanal inhibitory reflex, 1919
Rectoanal reflex, 2392
Rectocele
repair of, 699, 700f–702f
surgical treatment of, 1936, 1938f

Rectopexy
for rectal prolapse, 1960–1961, 1964t
resection with, for rectal prolapse, 1961, 1961f, 1964t
Rectorectal neoplasms, endoanal ultrasound in, 1913, 1914f
Rectorectal space, initial entry into, for total mesorectal excision with autonomic nerve preservation, 2236–2237, 2237f
Rectourethral fistulas, 1954–1955
meconium in urine and, 2394, 2394f
Rectovaginal fistulas, 1945–1954
clinical presentation of, 1945–1946
in Crohn's disease, 2088
surgical treatment of, 2136, 2138
diagnosis of, 1946
endoanal ultrasound in, 1912
etiology of, 1945
examination of, 1946
local repairs of, 2324–2325
treatment of, 1946–1954, 1947b
abdominal procedures for, 1952, 1954
coloanal anastomosis as, 1952, 1954
diversion and, 1954
onlay patch anastomosis as, 1954
local procedures for
advancement sleeve flap as, 1951, 1951f
autologous fibrin glue for, 1952
fistulotomy as, 1952
perineoproctectomy with layered closure as, 1952
polyglycolic mesh for, 1952
sliding flap repair as, 1947–1950, 1948f–1950f, 1949t
sphincteroplasty as, 1950f, 1950–1951, 1951t
timing of surgery and, 1947
tissue transfer techniques for, 1952
Rectrorectus extraperitoneal repair, for ventral hernias, 677–678, 678f, 679f
Rectum. *See also* Anorectal *entries;* Colorectal *entries;* Rectal *entries.*
abdominoperineal resection of, 2234–2243
for adenocarcinoma of rectum, 2235
adjacent organ involvement and, 2243
closure of pelvic floor and biologic spacers and, 2243
colostomy and, 2242–2243
indications for, 2234
laparoscopic, 2239–2241
technique for, 2239–2241, 2240f
patient preparation for, 2234–2235
bowel preparation and, 2235
consultation with patient and family and, 2234–2235
patient positioning and, 2235
staging and, 2234
perineal dissection and, 2241f, 2241–2243, 2242f
total mesorectal excision with autonomic nerve preservation and, 2236f, 2236–2243
distal rectal mobilization and, 2239

Rectum (Continued)
  hypogastric nerves and pelvic
      autonomic nerve plexuses
      and, 2237–2238, 2238f
  initial entry into retrorectal space
      and, 2236–2237, 2237f
  "lateral ligaments" and,
      2238–2239, 2239f
  separation of anterior and
      posterior compartments and,
      2238, 2238f
  cavernous hemangiomas of, 1996
  radiation injuries of, 2320–2325
      incidence of, 2320–2321
      medical treatment of, 2321
      proctitis due to, medical
          management for, 2321–2322
      reconstructive surgery for, 2322–2323
      rectovaginal fistulas and, local
          repairs of, 2324–2325
      transabdominal approaches for,
          2323–2324
          Bricker-Johnston, 2323
          coloanal anastomosis as,
              2323–2324
          coloplasty as, 2324
          colopouch anal anastomosis as,
              2324
          low anterior resection as, 2323
  vascular supply to, 2223, 2224f
Rectus abdominis muscle, 1290f, 1291–1292
Rectus sheath, 638–639, 639f, 672, 672f
Recurrent laryngeal nerve, injury of, during
    esophageal surgery, 598
Redo pelvic pouch procedure, 2415, 2417
Reflection, in ultrasonography, 111–112
Reflux carditis, 213f, 213–215. See also
    Cardiac mucosa.
    evolution of, 215, 215f
Reflux esophagitis. See also
    Gastroesophageal reflux disease.
    classification of, 105–106, 106, 106t, 107f
    stricture formation due to, 90
    treatment of, 255–256, 256, 256f
Reflux gastritis, alkaline, following
    gastrectomy, 809
Refraction, in ultrasonography, 112
Regeneration, hepatic, 1608, 1608f
Regurgitation
    in achalasia, 407
    with epiphrenic diverticulum, 433
    in esophageal disease, 56–57
    in esophageal motility disorders, 71
    following esophagomyotomy, for
        achalasia, 620
Rejection, of pancreas transplants, 1419
Renal cell carcinoma, metastatic to
    pancreas, 1437–1439, 1438f, 1439f
Renal dysfunction
    in cirrhosis, 1625
    in end-stage liver disease, 1693–1694
Renal failure, chronic, pruritus ani in, 2067
Rendu-Osler-Weber disease, 1713
Renogastric fistulas, 1095
Reoperative surgery, 1133–1136, 1134b
    for adenocarcinoma, of gastric remnant,
        1140
    for afferent limb syndrome, 1147

Reoperative surgery (Continued)
    for anorectal anomalies, 2403
    assessment and counseling for, 1134
    bariatric, 1143–1146
        for failed laparoscopic adjustable
            gastric banding, 1145
        for failed malabsorptive procedures,
            1146
        for failed Roux-en-Y gastric bypass,
            1145–1146
        for failed vertical banded
            gastroplasty, 1144–1145
        patient selection for, 1144
    for bile reflux gastritis, 1146f,
        1146–1147, 1147f
    for desmoid tumors, recurrent, 1141
    for gastric outlet obstruction
        at gastrojejunostomy site, 1137–1138
            operative technique for, 1138
        after pyloric or duodenal ulcer
            surgery, 1136–1137
            operative technique for, 1137,
                1137f
    for gastroesophageal reflux disease,
        1141–1143
        technical aspects of, 1143, 1143b
    for gastroparesis, 1139–1140
    hostile abdomen and, 1147–1148, 1148b
    information preparation for, 1133–1134
    laparoscopic, 1135–1136
        technique for, 1135–1136
            bowel injury during, 1136
    nutritional issues and access for, 1136
    open, 1134–1135
    pelvic, 2409–2418
        anatomy and, 2409, 2410b
        anticipation of problems with,
            2410–2411
        conduction of, 2412, 2412f
        control of bleeding and, 2414–2415
        drainage and, 2415
        identification of pelvic structures
            and, 2412–2414
            of bladder, 2413
            of rectal stump, 2413f, 2413–2414
            of ureters, 2412
            of vagina, 2414
        for malignancies, 2417–2418
        operative measures to make pelvic
            surgery easier and safer and,
            2418
        optimizing visibility and exposure
            for, 2411f, 2411–2412
        patient preparation for, 2410, 2411
        preoperative imaging studies for,
            2410
        preparation for bleeding and, 2410
        to redo pelvic pouch procedure,
            2415, 2417
        for reversal of Hartmann's
            procedure, 2415, 2416f
        timing of, 2409–2410
    for postgastrectomy dumping and
        diarrhea, 1138–1139
    for Roux limb syndrome, 1140
    for stromal cell tumor, recurrent, 1141
Reperfusion syndrome, liver transplantation
    and, 1696

Researcher, as clinical nurse specialist role,
    in palliative treatment, for esophageal
    cancer, 498
Resin hemoperfusion, for liver failure,
    acute, 1706
Resolution, in ultrasonography, 112
Respiratory insufficiency, following
    esophageal resection with visceral
    esophageal substitution, 613
Respiratory system, prenatal development
    of, 31–33, 33f, 34f
Resuscitation
    for caustic ingestions, 543
    for gastrointestinal fistulas, 1099–1100
Retention polyps, 2157
    gastric, 884
Retroduodenal artery, 1445, 1446
    anatomy of, 1237
Retrograde bypass, for mesenteric
    revascularization, 1260, 1261f, 1262f
Retrograde giant contractions, small
    intestinal, 1016–1017
Retrograde pyelography, with
    nephroenteric fistulas, 1106
Retrorectal tumors, 2299–2309
    anatomy and, 2299
    classification of, 2300, 2300b
    clinical findings and diagnosis of,
        2300–2302
        biopsy in, 2301–2302
        of developmental cysts, 2302–2304
            enterogenous, 2302, 2302t
            epidermoid and dermoid, 2302,
                2302t
            tailgut, 2302t, 2302–2304, 2303f
        history and physical examination in,
            2300–2301
        investigations in, 2301
        of neurogenic tumors, 2304
        of osseous lesions, 2306
        of sacrococcygeal chordomas, 2304,
            2304f–2306f
        of teratoma and teratocarcinoma,
            2302t, 2304–2305
    incidence of, 2299–2300
    surgical therapy for, 2306–2309
        multidisciplinary team and, 2306
        rationale for, 2306
        results with, 2309
            for benign tumors, 2309, 2310f
            for malignant tumors, 2309
        surgical approach for, 2307–2309
            combined abdominoperineal
                approach as, 2307–2308, 2308f
            preoperative planning and, 2307
            for tumors located below S3,
                2307, 2307f
Retrosacral fascia, division of, for low
    anterior resection, 2227–2228, 2228f
Reverse rotation, 1214, 1215f, 1216f
Rex's ramus arcuatus, 1606
Rhabdomyomas, esophageal, 522
Rhabdomyosarcomas
    colorectal, 2317
    hepatic, 1747
Riboflavin, small intestinal absorption of,
    1006, 1007t
Ricordi, Camillo, 1424

Riedel's lobe, 1598

Rifampin, for pruritus, in primary sclerosing cholangitis, 1567

Riolan, arch of, 1239

Ripstein procedure
for rectal prolapse, 1960f, 1960–1961
Well's modification of, for rectal prolapse, 1960, 1960f

Rituxumab, for islet transplantation, 1428

Robotic-assisted laparoscopic splenectomy, 1787

Rockey-Davis incision, for appendectomy, 2145, 2146f

Rokitansky-Aschoff sinuses, 1444

Ronsil, Roland Arnaud de, 688

Rosary-bead esophagus, 419, 420f

Rosetti, Franciscus, 1813

Rotational flaps, for anal stenosis, 2064–2065, 2065f

Rouviere, sulcus of, 1603

Roux, Cesar, 4

Roux gastrojejunostomy, gastrectomy with, for gastroparesis, 925

Roux stasis syndrome
following gastrectomy, 809, 880, 925
reoperative surgery for, 1140

Roux-en-Y biliary diversion, partial gastrectomy with, for esophageal stricture, 249

Roux-en-Y choledochojejunostomy, for duodenal diverticula, 782–783, 784f

Roux-en-Y duodenojejunostomy
for duodenal diverticula, 782, 783f
for gastroduodenal fistulas, 1110

Roux-en-Y gastric bypass
for foregut reconstruction for benign disease, 303, 303f
for obesity, 931–934, 932f, 933t

Roux-en-Y gastrojejunostomy
for bile reflux gastritis, 876, 876f
for dumping syndrome, 872f, 872–873
following gastrectomy, 911

Roux-en-Y reconstruction, for duodenal ulcers, 796, 798f

Rubber bands, hemorrhoidal ligation with, 2031, 2032f

Rutkow hernia repair, 649, 650f, 651f

Ruvalcaba-Myhre-Smith (Ruvalcaba-Riley-Smith) syndrome, 894t, 897, 2159t, 2176

S

S pouch, 2104

Sacral anomalies, associated with imperforate anus, 2390

Sacral nerve stimulation, for fecal incontinence, 1925, 1925f

Sacral plain radiographs, with retrorectal tumors, 2301

Sacrococcygeal chordomas, 2304, 2304f–2306f

Sagittal anatomy, low anterior resection and, 2223, 2223f

"Salem sump" tube, 750, 751f

Salmonella, splenic abscess due to, 1819

Salvage surgery, for anal squamous cell carcinoma, 2293–2294, 2294f

Santorini, pancreatic duct of, 964

Sarcoidosis, splenectomy for, 1835

Sarcoptes scabiei infection, pruritus ani associated with, 2070

Satiety, early, following gastrectomy, 808–809

Saucerization, for pilonidal disease, 1968

Savary Miller classification, for reflux esophagitis, 106t

Scabies, pruritus ani associated with, 2070

Scarpa, Antonio, 632

Scarpa's fascia, 636

Schatzki rings
imaging of, 88, 90f
origin of, 229

Schistosomiasis, portal hypertension and, 1756–1757

Schwannomas
esophageal, 520
hepatic, 1747
small intestinal, 900

Sciatic hernias, 700–704
anatomy and, 701, 703f
clinical features and diagnosis of, 701–702, 703f
treatment of, 702–704, 703f

Scintigraphy
in aortoenteric fistulas, 1271f, 1271–1272
with bile duct strictures, 1578
with colon, rectal, and anal disorders, 1895–1896, 1896f
for colonic transit measurement, 1873f, 1873–1874
with colonic vascular ectasias, 1991, 1993
esophageal transit, 154–155
gastric emptying, 185, 186f, 187f
HIDA, with biliary fistulas, 1542
in jaundice, obstructive, 1462, 1463f
somatostatin receptor-based
of carcinoid tumors, 1184, 1184f
for insulinoma localization, 1377
in Zollinger-Ellison syndrome, 864, 865f

Scleroderma, esophageal motility disorder in, imaging in, 74

Sclerotherapy
alcohol, for esophageal cancer, 488, 489t
for gastric bleeding, 742–743
for hemorrhoids, 2030f, 2030–2031
for hepatic cysts, in polycystic liver disease, 1634–1635
for hepatocellular carcinoma, 1737

Scopolamine, for gastroparesis, 921

Seat belt sign, small bowel perforation and, 770, 771, 771f

Seborrheic dermatitis, pruritus ani associated with, 2069

Second messengers, gastric acid secretion and, 725, 725f

Secretin
duodenal function and, 980, 981t
infusion of, for gastrinoma localization, 865
pancreatic cell function and, 1292
small intestinal neuroendocrine function and, 1018

Sectionectomy, left lateral, 1679–1680

Segmental arteries, 1772

Selenium, deficiency of, in Crohn's disease, 1054

Self-expanding metal stents
for colorectal cancer metastases, 2271
for esophageal cancer, 489–492
placement of, 490, 491f, 492, 492f
special considerations with, 492
for esophageal perforation, 532
for gastric bleeding, 743–744, 744f

Sentinel bleeding, with aortoenteric fistulas, 1114

Sepsis
catheter-related, in short-bowel syndrome, 1167
control of, with gastrointestinal fistulas, 1101–1103, 1103f, 1104f
with gastrointestinal fistulas, 1098
with parenteral nutrition, 1165
perianal, endoanal ultrasound in, 1911

Seromas
with inguinal herniorrhaphy, laparoscopic, 668
with ventral herniorrhaphy, laparoscopic, 681

Seromyotomy, lesser curve, anterior, 815, 822

Serosa, small intestinal, 998

Serosal patching, for short-bowel syndrome, 1168–1169, 1169f

Serotonin
carcinoid tumors and, 1183
duodenal function and, 981t, 982–983

Serotonin receptors, intestinal motility and, 926

Serous cystic neoplasms, pancreatic
clinical presentation of, 1387
diagnosis of, 1393, 1393f
incidence and epidemiology of, 1387
pathology and biologic behavior of, 1388–1389, 1389f
treatment of, 1396–1397

SES-CD, 1051

Setons
for anorectal fistulas, 2055f, 2055–2056
for fistula treatment, in Crohn's disease, 2135–2136, 2137f–2138f

Sex
Barrett's esophagus and, 342
drug-induced liver disease and, 1717
esophageal cancer and, 444
gastroesophageal reflux disease and, 200

Sex hormone–binding globulin, obesity and, bariatric surgery and, 938

Sex hormones, hepatotoxicity of, 1721, 1722, 1723, 1724

Sexual dysfunction, following ileal pouch–anal anastomosis, 2117

Sham feeding, to stimulate postoperative gastrointestinal motility, 1028

Shock, with hepatobiliary trauma, 1668

Short chain fatty acids, metabolism of, colonic, 1873

Short esophagus
acquired, Nissen fundoplication for, 272f, 272–273, 273f
definition of, 234

Short esophagus (Continued)
evaluation of, barium examination for, 70, 71f
preoperative assessment of, 237
strictures and. See Esophageal strictures.
Short-bowel syndrome, 1162–1177, 1163b
intestinal adaptation and, 1163–1164, 1164b, 1164f
intestinal remnant length and, 1162
medical management of, 1164–1168
maintenance of nutritional status and, 1165
maximization of enteral nutrient absorption and, 1165–1166, 1166b
prevention of complications and, 1166–1168, 1167f
outcome, factors influencing, 1162–1163, 1163t
prevalence of, 1162
site of resection and, 1162
surgical management of, 1168b, 1168t, 1168–1177
to improve intestinal function, 1169–1171
motility and, 1169
prolonging intestinal transit and, 1169–1171, 1170f, 1170t
to increase absorptive area, 1171–1173, 1172f
intestinal transplantation as, 1173–1177
indications for, 1173–1174
operative procedure for, 1174f, 1174–1175
outcome with, 1175f, 1175–1177, 1176f
to preserve and maximize intestinal remnant, 1168–1169, 1169f
Short-segment colon interposition, 596–597
results of, 596t, 596–597
Shoulder pain, with inguinal herniorrhaphy, laparoscopic, 666–667
Shouldice hernia repair, 633, 648–649
Shrock shunt, 1665
Shunts
arterioportal, hepatic, 1713f, 1713–1714
arteriovenous, hepatic, 1713f, 1713–1714
portocaval, intrahepatic, transjugular
for ascites, 1765
for bleeding due to portal hypertension, 1693
for bleeding varices, 1693, 1761–1762
procedure for, 1761f, 1761–1762
for Budd-Chiari syndrome, 1714, 1715
Shrock, 1665
splenorenal, distal, for bleeding varices, 1762–1763
follow-up for, 1762–1763
management of, 1762
procedure for, 1762, 1762f
Sickle-cell disease, splenectomy for, 1826
Siderotic particles, 1775
Side-to-side isoperistaltic stricturoplasty, for Crohn's disease, 1059, 1062f
Sigmoid arteries, 1850–1851, 1851f

Sigmoidocele, surgical treatment of, 1936, 1937f
Sigmoidoscopy
with anorectal fistulas, 2049
flexible, screening with, for colorectal carcinoma, 2191–2192
rigid, with colonic vascular ectasias, 1991
Sildenafil
for achalasia, 412
for nutcracker esophagus, 423
Silk sutures, for bowel anastomoses, 1083–1084
Simonds, Charter, 743
Simplified Endoscopic Activity Score for Crohn's Disease, 1051
Sims' position, 1886, 1886f
Sirolimus
for islet transplantation, 1424
mechanism of action of, 2377t
Sister Mary Joseph's nodule, 906, 1361
Skin problems
in Crohn's disease, 2087
with stomas, 1081, 2370f, 2370–2371
Skip lesions, in Crohn's disease, 1043
Sleep apnea, obesity and, bariatric surgery and, 938
Sliding flap repair
for rectourethral fistulas, 1955
for rectovaginal fistulas, 1947–1950, 1948f–1949f, 1949t
Sliding hernias, 643
Small bowel
Crohn's disease in, surgical treatment of, 2132
diverticula of. See Duodenal diverticula; Jejunoileal diverticula; Meckel's diverticula.
endoscopic examination of, 745f–747f, 745–747
Small bowel enteroclysis, in Crohn's disease, 1046–1047, 1047f
Small bowel follow-through, in Crohn's disease, 1046–1047, 1047f
Small bowel injury, 770–773
anatomy and physiology and, 770
diagnosis of, 771f, 771–772, 772f
historical background of, 770
mechanism of, 770–771
operative management of, 772
perforation of, 770
postoperative management of, 772–773
Small bowel motility, obstruction and, 1025
Small bowel obstruction, 1025–1033
classification of, 1025, 1026t
clinical findings in, 1028, 1028t
closed-loop, pathophysiology of, 1026–1027, 1027f
complete, 1025
etiology of, 1027
following ileal pouch–anal anastomosis, 2111
functional, 1025
high grade, 1025
internal hernias as cause of, 1120
with jejunoileal diverticula, 785
laboratory tests in, 1029
low grade, 1025
mechanical, 1025

Small bowel obstruction (Continued)
with Meckel's diverticulum, 787, 788f
motility and, 1025
partial, 1025
pathophysiology of, 1025–1027
of closed-loop obstruction, 1026–1027, 1027f
physical examination in, 1028–1029
radiologic investigations in, 1029–1032
computed tomography and, 1030–1032, 1031f
contrast radiographs and, 1030, 1030f
plain radiographs and, 1029, 1029f
risk of, following laparoscopy, 1027–1028
treatment of
medical, 1032
surgical, 1032–1033
adhesion prevention and, 1033
laparoscopic vs. open adhesiolysis for, 1032–1033
operative, 1033
Small bowel resection
for Crohn's disease, 2132, 2133f
for intestinal dysmotility, 927
Small bowel strictures, in Crohn's disease, management of, 1063
Small bowel transit studies, in constipation, 1932
Small bowel transplantation, for intestinal dysmotility, 927
Small bowel volvulus, 1035–1037
diagnosis of, 1036, 1036f
etiology of, 1035–1036, 1036t
treatment of, 1036–1037
Small intestinal adenocarcinoma, 915–916
duodenal, 915–916
ileal, 916
jejunal, 916
pathogenesis of, 915
risk factors for, 915
Small intestinal adenomas
Brunner's gland, 892–893
ectopic tissue, 892–893
Small intestinal cysts, in pediatric patients, 1221–1223, 1222f, 1223f
Small intestinal duplications, in pediatric patients, 1221–1223, 1222f, 1223f
Small intestinal epithelium, 998–1009
architecture of, 998, 999f, 1000f
barrier function of, 998–999, 1000f, 1001
digestion and absorption and, 1001–1008
of bile salts, 1007t, 1008
of carbohydrates, 1002, 1002f, 1003f, 1003t
of lipids and cholesterol, 1003t, 1004–1006, 1005f, 1006f
of minerals, 1008, 1009f
of protein, 1002–1004, 1003t, 1004f
of sodium, 1001–1002, 1002f
of vitamins, 1006–1008, 1007t
of water, 1001, 1001t
intestinal fluid secretion and, 1008–1009, 1010f
Small intestinal fistulas. See Enteric fistulas.

Small intestinal immune system, 1009–1012
  gut-associated lymphoid tissue and, 1010, 1012f
  M cells and, 1010, 1012f
  regulation of, 1010
  regulation of gut function by, 1011–1012
  secretory immunoglobulin A and, 1010, 1011f
Small intestinal lymphomas, epidemiology of, 1199, 1200t
Small intestinal polyps, 891–893
  benign, non-neoplastic, 891
  fibroid, inflammatory, 891
  neoplastic, 891–893
    Brunner's gland, 892–893
    ectopic tissue, 892–893
    endometriosis as, 893
    tubular adenomas as, 891–892
    villous adenomas as, 892–893
Small intestine. See also specific parts, e.g. Duodenum.
  anatomy of, 988, 989f, 990, 990f, 1234, 1236f
  benign neoplasms of, 889–901, 890t
    mesenchymal, 898–901
      congenital, 901
      leiomyomas as, 899–900
      lipomas as, 900–901
      vascular, 898–899
    mucosal, 891–893
    polyposis syndromes and. See Intestinal polyposis syndromes.
    symptoms and diagnosis of, 889–890, 890t
  developmental anomalies of, 994–997
    atresia as, 997, 997f
    duplications as, 994
    internal hernias as, 997
    omphalocele as, 994–995, 995f
    rotational, 995, 996f, 997
    stenosis as, 997
    ventral hernias as, 994–995
    vitelline duct, 994, 995f
  embryology of, 992–993
    gastrulation and, 992–993, 993f, 994f
  foreign bodies in. See Foreign body ingestion.
  histology of, 990, 991f
  innervation of, 990, 992
  lymphoid functions and architecture of, 992
  microvasculature, 992
  motility of, 1012–1017
    intestinal smooth muscle cells and, 1013, 1013f
    organization of contractile activity and, 1015b, 1015–1017
      individual phasic contractions and, 1015
      organized groups of contractions and, 1015f, 1015–1016, 1016f
      special propulsive contractions and, 1016–1017
    patterns of contractions and, 1013–1015
      chemical control and, 1014–1015
      myogenic control and, 1013–1014
      neural control and, 1014

Small intestine (Continued)
  neuroendocrine function of, 1017–1019, 1018b
    cholecystokinin and, 1018
    guanylin and, 1019
    motilin and, 1019
    secretin and related peptides and, 1018
    somatostatin and, 1018–1019
    uroguanylin and, 1019
  physiology of, 997–998
Small-bowel follow-through, in small bowel obstruction, 1030
Smith-Lortat-Jacob, M., 337
Smoking
  cessation of, for gastroesophageal reflux disease, 253
  esophageal cancer and, 444, 466
  pancreatic adenocarcinoma and, 1359
Smooth muscle cells, intestinal, small intestinal motility and, 1013, 1013f
Smooth muscle disease, intestinal motility and, 925–926
Sodium
  absorption of, colonic, 1872
  small intestinal absorption of, 1001–1002, 1002f
Sodium butyrate, for rectal radiation injuries, 2321
Solid pseudopapillary tumors, 1434, 1435f
  in pediatric patients, 1411
Solitary rectal ulcer syndrome, 2075–2076
  diagnosis of, 2075–2076, 2076f
  endoanal ultrasound in, 1913–1914, 1914f
  treatment of, 2075–2076
Somatostatin
  duodenal function and, 981t, 982
  gastric, 722–723
    Helicobacter pylori effects on, 722–723
    synthesis and action of, 722
  small intestinal neuroendocrine function and, 1018–1019
  for variceal bleeding, 1759
Somatostatin receptor(s), gastric acid secretion and, 725
Somatostatin receptor-based scintigraphy
  of carcinoid tumors, 1184, 1184f
  for insulinoma localization, 1377
  in Zollinger-Ellison syndrome, 864, 865f
Somatostatinoma, 1380–1381
  diagnosis of, 1380
  presentation of, 1380
  therapy of, 1381
Spastic pelvic floor syndrome, surgical treatment of, 1936–1938, 1939f, 1940f, 1941t
Speech, preservation of, with oropharyngeal strictures, 546–547
Spencer, Thomas, 1813
Spermatic cord, 641
Sphincter of Oddi, 1444–1445, 1445f
  function of, 1458f, 1458–1459
Sphincter of Oddi manometry, 1492–1493
Sphincteroplasty
  for common bile duct stones, 1594
  for rectovaginal fistulas, 1950f, 1950–1951, 1951t

Sphincteroplasty (Continued)
  transduodenal, for duodenal diverticula, 781, 781f, 782f
Sphincterotomy
  antegrade, 1485
  for common bile duct stones, 1594
  endoscopic, 1493
    complications of, 1494
Sphincter-sparing techniques, for colorectal cancer, 2195, 2197f
Spiegel, Adriaan van der, 682
Spigelian fascia, 672, 673f
Spigelian hernias, repair of, 682
Spinal anomalies, associated with imperforate anus, 2390
Spinal disorders, pain associated with, 2072
Spinal dysraphism, associated with imperforate anus, 2406
Spinal surgery, gastroparesis following, 923
Spindle cells, gastrointestinal stromal tumors and, 1190, 1190f
Spironolactone
  for ascites, 1764
  following distal splenorenal shunt procedure, 1762–1763
Splanchnic autoregulatory, 1243
Splanchnic blood flow
  extrinsic control of, 1241
  intrinsic control of, 1241–1242, 1242b
Splanchnic nerve, 1294
Splanchnicectomy, for pain palliation, in pancreatic and periampullary carcinoma, 1367, 1367f
Spleen
  accessory
    in idiopathic thrombocytopenic purpura, 1823, 1824f
    search for, 1785
  anatomy of, 1771–1772
    of blood supply, 1772, 1773f
    of lymphatic drainage, 1772, 1773f
    neural, 1772, 1773f
  embryology of, 1772, 1772f
  function of, evaluation of, 1775
  functions of, 1772–1773
  histology and immunophenotype of, 1773–1775, 1774f, 1775t, 1776f
  image-guided interventional therapy for, 1788–1795
    for hypersplenism, partial splenic embolization as, 1793–1795, 1794f, 1795f
    for pseudoaneurysm of splenic artery, 1791, 1793, 1793f
    for splenic abscess and pseudocyst, 1795, 1795f
    transarterial splenic embolization as, 1788–1790
      anatomy and, 1788, 1789f, 1790f
      splenic bleeding and, 1790–1791, 1792f
      technique for, 1788–1790, 1790f
  imaging of, 1775–1776
  pathologic findings in, 1776–1777
  red pulp of, 1772
  white pulp of, 1772

Splenectomy, 1777–1778, 1822–1838
for abscesses, 1833
for amyloidosis, 1835
for bleeding varices, 1353
complications of, 1777–1778
consequences of, in pediatric patients, 1806
for cysts, 1832–1833
nonparasitic, 1833
parasitic, 1832
for Gaucher's disease, 1835
for hematologic disorders, 1822–1827
autoimmune neutropenia as, 1827
causing anemia, 1825–1827
hemolytic, acquired, 1826–1827
hereditary, 1825–1826
causing thrombocytopenia, 1822–1825
human immunodeficiency virus as, 1825
idiopathic thrombocytopenic purpura as, 1822–1824, 1824f
systemic lupus erythematosus as, 1824–1825
thrombotic thrombocytopenic purpura as, 1824
Wiskott-Aldrich syndrome as, 1825
Evans's syndrome as, 1827
Felty's syndrome as, 1827
for iatrogenic injury, 1834–1835
indications for, 1777
for lymphoproliferative disorders, 1827–1831
Hodgkin's disease as, 1827–1829, 1828f, 1828t
leukemias as, 1830t, 1830–1831
non-Hodgkin's lymphoma as, 1829, 1829t, 1830b
for myeloproliferative disorders, 1831–1832
nonsurgical, 1353
operative considerations with, 1835–1837, 1836f, 1837f
partial, 1836
operative considerations for, 1836
for splenic cysts, 1815
for splenic tumors, 1816
postoperative course and complications of, 1837–1838
preoperative preparation for, 1835
for sarcoidosis, 1835
for splenic abscesses, 1820
for splenic cysts, 1815
for splenic trauma, 1801
for tumors, 1832
for vascular disorders, 1833–1834
portal hypertension as, 1834
splenic artery aneurysm as, 1833–1834
splenic vein thrombosis as, 1834
"wandering spleen" and splenic torsion as, 1834
Splenic abscesses, 1818–1820
characteristics of, 1819
diagnosis of, 1818, 1819f
image-guided interventional therapy for, 1795, 1795f

Splenic abscesses (Continued)
management of, 1820
presenting signs and symptoms of, 1818
splenectomy for, 1833
Splenic artery, 20, 20f, 21f, 1237, 1292, 1293f
aneurysms of, 1274–1277
clinical findings in, 1275
diagnosis of, 1275, 1276f
incidence of, 1274
pathogenesis of, 1274–1275
splenectomy for, 1833–1834
treatment of, 1275, 1277
pseudoaneurysm of, image-guided interventional therapy for, 1791, 1793, 1793f
Splenic autotransplantation, for splenic trauma
in adults, 1802
in pediatric patients, 1811
Splenic bleeding, transarterial splenic embolization and, 1790–1791, 1792f
Splenic circulation, 1775, 1777f
Splenic cysts, 1813–1815
nonparasitic
congenital, 1814
secondary (false), 1813, 1814
splenectomy for, 1833
parasitic, 1813–1814
splenectomy for, 1832
splenectomy for, 1832–1833
true, 1813
Splenic decapsulization, partial, for splenic cysts, 1815
Splenic embolization
partial, for hypersplenism, 1793–1795, 1794f, 1795f
transarterial, 1788–1790
anatomy and, 1788, 1789f, 1790f
splenic bleeding and, 1790–1791, 1792f
technique for, 1788–1790, 1790f
Splenic flexure, 1847
Splenic flexure volvulus
etiology and pathophysiology of, 1985
treatment of, 1985
outcomes following, 1985
Splenic hypertrophy, 1777
Splenic injury
in adults, 1798–1803
diagnostic modalities for, 1798–1800, 1800t
grading systems for, 1799–1800, 1800t
nonoperative treatment of, 1802–1803
operative treatment of, 1800–1802
autotransplantation as, 1802
general principles of, 1800–1801
laparoscopic splenectomy as, 1802
splenectomy as, 1801
splenorrhaphy as, 1801–1802
rupture following, delayed, 1803
following esophageal resection with visceral esophageal substitution, 615
with Nissen fundoplication, 273

Splenic injury (Continued)
in pediatric patients, 1805–1812
asplenia prophylaxis for, 1811–1812
evaluation of, 1806–1808, 1807f, 1808t, 1809f, 1810f, 1811t
historical background of, 1805–1806
immune function and consequences of splenectomy and, 1806
operative management of, 1808, 1811
Splenic neoplasms
benign, splenectomy for, 1832
solid, 1815–1816
splenectomy for, 1832
Splenic nervous plexus, 1772
Splenic pseudocysts, image-guided interventional therapy for, 1795, 1795f
Splenic torsion, splenectomy for, 1834
Splenic vein, 1772
Splenic vein thrombosis
asymptomatic, 1353
following splenectomy, 1838
in pancreatitis, chronic, 1352–1353
splenectomy for, 1834
Splenomegaly, 1777
massive, 1778
with splenic vein thrombosis, 1353
Splenorenal shunt, distal, for bleeding varices, 1762–1763
follow-up for, 1762–1763
management of, 1762
procedure for, 1762, 1762f
Splenorrhaphy, for splenic trauma, 1801–1802
Sporadic MIS tumors, 2189
Squamocolumnar junction, 19
Barrett's esophagus classification and, 103–104
endoscopic appearance of, 101, 101f
in Barrett's esophagus, 103, 103f, 104f
Squamous cell carcinoma
anal, 2291–2294
clinical features of, 2291
physical examination of, 2291
staging of, 2291, 2292f
therapy of, 2291–2294
combined chemotherapy and radiation therapy for, 2292–2293, 2293t
salvage surgery as, 2293–2294, 2294f
surgical, primary, 2291–2292
colorectal, 2313
esophageal, epidemiology of
age, sex, and race distribution and, 443
risk factors and, 443–445
alcohol as, 443
diet and nutrition as, 443, 445
nonsteroidal anti-inflammatory drugs as, 445
obesity as, 443, 443t, 444f
tobacco as, 443
hepatic, 1747
perianal, pruritus ani and, 2068
Squamous papilloma, esophageal, 523–524, 524f
Stacked coin sign, 765–766

Stamm gastrostomy
  contraindications to, 750t
  for esophagocoloplasty, 591
  with hostile abdomen, 1147
  indications for, 750t
  in pediatric patients, 960
  technique for, 857, 860f, 861f
Staphylococcus aureus infection
  hepatic abscesses and, 1644–1645
  overwhelming postsplenectomy infection
    and, 1782
  splenic abscess due to, 1819
Stapled gastric partitioning, for obesity, 930
Stapled intestinal anastomoses, 2333,
  2334f–2337f
Staplers
  circular (EEA; ILS; PPH), 1087
  GIA, 1086, 1087f
  linear, 1086, 1087f
Stapling, for bowel anastomoses, 1086f,
  1086–1089
  hand-sewn vs. stapled anastomoses and,
    1088–1089
  staplers for, 1086–1087, 1087f
  techniques and pitfalls in, 1087–1088
    functional end-to-end anastomosis
      and, 1087, 1088f
    stapled end-to-end anastomosis and,
      1087–1088, 1088f
Steatohepatitis, drug-induced, 1719t,
  1720–1721
Steatorrhea
  following ileal resection, 1880
  in pancreatitis, chronic, 1345
  with primary sclerosing cholangitis, 1566
    treatment of, 1567, 1588
Stents
  for bile duct stones, 1496
  for caustic ingestions, 543
  for celiac artery aneurysms, 1278–1279
  for colorectal cancer, colonoscopic
    positioning of, 2331
  for gastric bleeding, 743f, 743–744, 744f
  for hepatic artery aneurysms, 1278
  for pancreatitis, chronic, with bile duct
    stricture, 1348
  self-expanding
    for esophageal cancer, 489–492
      placement of, 490, 491f, 492, 492f
      special considerations with, 492
    for esophageal perforation, 532
    metal
      for colorectal cancer metastases,
        2271
      for gastric bleeding, 743–744, 744f
  surgical, for bleeding varices, 1762
STEP procedure, for short-bowel syndrome,
  1171, 1172f, 1173
Steroids. *See also* Corticosteroids.
  anabolic, hepatotoxicity of, 1723
  androgenic, hepatotoxicity of, 1724
  for caustic ingestions, 543
Stoma(s). *See also* Ostomies; *specific
  procedures.*
  anastomosis vs., 2335, 2338
  formation of, for Crohn's disease, 1060,
    1062–1063
  necrosis of, with ileostomy, 1078

Stoma(s) *(Continued)*
  prolapse of, 2372–2373, 2373f
    with ileostomy, 1080
  retraction of, with ileostomy, 1080
  stenosis of, 2372
    with ileostomy, 1080
Stomach. *See also* Gastric *entries;*
  Gastro- *entries.*
  anatomy of, 717–721
    anatomic relationships and, 717–718,
      718f
    of divisions, 717, 718f
    of glandular organization, 721, 721t,
      722f
    of innervation, 719–720, 720f
    lymphatic, 719
    morphology and, 720–721, 721f
    vascular, 718, 719f
  antrum of, 717, 718f
  cardia of, 717, 718f
  compression of, with paraesophageal
    hernia, 551–552
  congenital malformation of, 35
  decompression of, 750
  embryology of, 947
  endoscopy of, diagnostic, 733–741
    in gastric adenocarcinoma, 907
    indications for, 733
    instrumentation for, 733–734
    pathology on, 736–741, 737f–741f
    patient preparation for, 734
    technique for, 734f–736f, 734–736
  as esophageal substitute, 579
    esophagocoloplasty and,
      postoperative care for, 591
    esophagogastrostomy and, 582–588
      anastomosis for, 586–587, 587f,
        588
      drainage of stomach for, 584–585,
        585f
      functional results with, 588
      lengthening of stomach for, 584,
        584f
      mobilization of stomach for,
        582–584, 583f
      transposition of stomach for, 585,
        586f
  foreign bodies in. *See* Foreign body
    ingestion.
  gastric barrier function and, 729
  gastric peptides and, 721–724
  imaging of
    in dysphagia, 66
    in gastroesophageal reflux disease, 66
  ligaments anchoring, 717–718, 718f
  mucosa of, 720–721, 721f
  peptic ulcer disease and. *See* Peptic ulcer
    disease.
  physiologic and pathophysiologic aspects
    of, in esophageal disease, 184–185
  prenatal development of, 34–35, 35f, 36f
  pylorus of, 717, 718f
  secretions of. *See* Gastric acid; Gastric
    juice.
  watermelon, 886
    endoscopic appearance of, 739–740
    symptoms and diagnosis of, 886
    treatment of, 740, 886

Stoppa extraperitoneal repair, for ventral
  hernias, 677–678, 678f, 679f
Streptococcus infection
  group b, overwhelming postsplenectomy
    infection and, 1782
  hepatic abscesses and, 1645
  S. milleri, hepatic abscesses and, 1645
  S. pneumoniae
    immunization against, with splenic
      cysts, 1815
    overwhelming postsplenectomy
      infection and, 1782
    vaccination against, with asplenia, in
      pediatric patients, 1811
  splenic abscess due to, 1819
Stress, surgical, altered hormonal response
  to, 2378
Stretta procedure, 317–320, 325, 326t, 327t
  complications of, 319
  efficacy of, 318f, 318–319, 319t
  failure of, alternatives after, 319–320
  histologic changes and, 318
  patient selection for, 317
  physiologic/anatomic mechanisms of,
    330–331
  precautions recommended for, 319
  procedure for, 317f, 317–318
  results with, 325, 326t, 327t
Strictures. *See also specific sites and conditions,
  e.g.* Biliary strictures.
  following ileal pouch–anal anastomosis,
    2112
Stricturoplasty
  for Crohn's disease, 2132, 2134f–2135f
    bowel resection vs., 1058–1059
    techniques for, 1059, 1059f–1062f
  Finney, for Crohn's disease, 1059, 1061f
  Heineke-Mikulicz, for Crohn's disease,
    1059, 1059f
  isoperistaltic, side-to-side, for Crohn's
    disease, 1059, 1062f
  Jaboulay, for Crohn's disease, 1059,
    1062f
  Judd, for Crohn's disease, 1059, 1060f
  Moskel-Walske-Neumayer, for Crohn's
    disease, 1059, 1060f
  for short-bowel syndrome, 1168, 1169,
    1169f
"String of lakes" appearance, in mesenteric
  ischemia, 1254
Stromal cell tumor, recurrent, reoperative
  surgery for, 1141
Stromayr, Casper, 632
Subcutaneous tissue infections, with
  appendicitis, 2150
Submucosa
  esophageal, anatomy of, ultrasound,
    115, 115f
  small intestinal, 998
Subphrenic abscesses, with appendicitis,
  2150
Subserosa, of gallbladder, 1444
Substance P, duodenal function and, 981t,
  983–984
Sucralfate, for esophageal strictures, 237
Sudek's point, 1868
Suicide attempts, caustic ingestions and,
  540

Sulcus of Rouviere, 1603
Sulfapyridine, plasma, in constipation, 1932
Sulfasalazine
for Crohn's disease, 1052, 2127
for inflammatory bowel disease, 2089
Sulfonamides, hepatotoxicity of, 1721
Sulindac, for desmoids, in familial adenomatous polyposis, 2162
Sump syndrome, biliary drainage procedures for, 1508
Superior mesenteric artery, 968, 971f, 1292, 1293f
anatomy of, 1237–1238, 1238f, 1849, 1851f, 1852f, 1857, 1867
variations in, 1867
aneurysms of, 1278–1279
clinical findings in, 1278
diagnosis of, 1278–1279
incidence of, 1278
pathogenesis of, 1278
treatment of, 1279
balloon dilation of, 1261, 1264t
communications with celiac axis, 1238–1239, 1239f
communications with inferior mesenteric artery, 1239
embolic occlusion of, 1249b, 1249–1250
embryology of, 1234, 1235f
in mesenteric ischemia, 1247, 1248f. See also Mesenteric ischemia.
thrombotic occlusion of, 1250
Superior mesenteric artery syndrome, 974–975, 975f, 976f
Superior mesenteric vein, 968, 972f, 1772
anatomy of, 1869
Superoxide dismutase, for radiation enteritis prevention, 1155
Support, form clinical nurse specialist, in palliative treatment, for esophageal cancer, 497
Suprapubic hernias, repair of, 683–684, 684f
Suprarenal veins, 1603–1604
Supravesical fossa, 639
Surgeons
esophageal, 7–8
on portal hypertension multidisciplinary team, 1767
Surgical stents, for bleeding varices, 1762
Surgical stress, altered hormonal response to, 2378
Surgisis Gold, for ventral herniorrhaphy, 676
Suspicious bleeding, 1883
Suture(s)
Connell, 1085
for esophagogastrostomy, 586, 587f, 588
Halsted, 1085
Lembert, 1084, 1085f
mattress, horizontal, 1085
purse-string, 1085
Suture materials, for bowel anastomosis, 1083–1084
Sutured intestinal anastomoses, 2331, 2331f–2333f, 2333
Sutureless intestinal anastomoses, 2333–2334

Swallowing, 48–55
of air, partial fundoplication for, 279
deglutitive inhibition and, 52–53, 54f
disorders of. See Dysphagia.
duration response and, 51
esophageal phase of, 50–55, 51f, 129–132, 132f
esophageal peristalsis and, 51–53, 52f–54f
lower esophageal sphincter and, 53–55, 54t
esophageal propulsive force and, 53
inhibitory relaxation wave and, 53
lower esophageal high-pressure zone and, 132–134, 133f
normal, 374–377, 376f, 377f
oral phase of, 48, 129, 129f–131f
oropharyngeal phase of, imaging of, 66, 66f
pharyngeal peristaltic contraction and, 49
pharyngeal phase of, 48–50, 49f, 50f, 375
pharyngoesophageal phase of, disorders of, 134–135, 135f, 136f
preservation of, with oropharyngeal strictures, 546–547
studies of, 375, 376f
upper esophageal sphincter and, 49–50, 50f, 375–377, 376f, 377f
Swedish adjustable gastric band, 934
Sweet anastomosis, 586, 587f, 588
Sweet's double-rib resection, 579
Sympathetic nerves, low anterior resection and, 2223, 2225
Sympathetic nervous system, prenatal development of, 45–46
Syphilis, anal, in immunocompromised patients, 2383t
Syphilitic lesions, pruritus ani associated with, 2070
Systemic lupus erythematosus, splenectomy for, 1824–1825

T

Tacrolimus
for inflammatory bowel disease, 2092
for islet transplantation, 1424
mechanism of action of, 2377t
Tamoxifen
for desmoids, in familial adenomatous polyposis, 2162
hepatotoxicity of, 1721, 1723
TA-stapler, for splenectomy, partial, 1815
Tazobactam, for cholangitis prophylaxis, 1550t
Teacher, as clinical nurse specialist role, in palliative treatment, for esophageal cancer, 497
Tegaserod
for gastroesophageal reflux disease, 253
for intestinal dysmotility, 926
Telangiectasia
colonic, 1997, 1999
gastric
acquired, 887
congenital, 887

Telangiectasia (Continued)
hereditary, 1713
small intestinal, 898–899
Tenderness, in appendicitis, 2142
Tensilon test. See Edrophonium test.
Tensor fasciae latae, 687
Teratocarcinoma, retrorectal, 2304–2305
Teratomas
gastric, in pediatric patients, 959
retrorectal, 2302t, 2304–2305
Terbinafine, hepatotoxicity of, 1722
Terminal patients, with esophageal cancer, management of, 497
Testes
blood supply to, injury of, with contralateral inguinal exploration, 709
injury of, with inguinal herniorrhaphy, laparoscopic, 667
undescended, operative management of, 709–711
Testicular descent, with inguinal herniorrhaphy, laparoscopic, 668
Testicular torsion, in children, 711–712
operative management of, 711–712
Tetracyclines
hepatotoxicity of, 1720
for lymphoma, 1209t
pruritus ani associated with, 2069
Thalassemia major, splenectomy for, 1826
Thermotherapy
laser, for hepatocellular carcinoma, 1738
microwave, for hepatocellular carcinoma, 1738
Thiamine, small intestinal absorption of, 1006, 1007t
Thiersch encirclement, for rectal prolapse, 1964f, 1964t, 1964–1965
Third spacing, 1025
Thoracoscopy, for staging of esophageal cancer, 460
Thorium, hepatotoxicity of, 1724
Three-dimensional radiation treatment planning, 1155
Thrombocytopenia
splenectomy for hematologic disorders causing, 1822–1825
human immunodeficiency virus as, 1825
idiopathic thrombocytopenic purpura as, 1822–1824, 1824f
systemic lupus erythematosus as, 1824–1825
thrombotic thrombocytopenic purpura as, 1824
Wiskott-Aldrich syndrome as, 1825
Thromboembolectomy, operative, for mesenteric ischemia, 1255
Thrombosis
deep vein, with inguinal herniorrhaphy, laparoscopic, 667
hepatic artery, 1712–1713, 1713f
liver transplantation and, 1698
mesenteric vein
acute, ischemia due to, 1255–1257, 1256f
following splenectomy, 1838

Thrombosis (*Continued*)
portal vein
with cavernous transformation, in chronic pancreatitis, 1313f, 1313–1314
following splenectomy, 1838
liver transplantation and, 1697, 1698
splenic vein
asymptomatic, 1353
following splenectomy, 1838
in pancreatitis, chronic, 1352–1353
splenectomy for, 1834
Thrombotic thrombocytopenic purpura, splenectomy for, 1824
Thyroid arteries, 20
Tileston, Walter, 338
TIPS. *See* Transjugular intrahepatic portocaval shunt.
Tissue adhesives, for bowel anastomoses, 1089
TNM staging system
for esophageal cancer, 448, 449–450, 450t, 451f, 472t, 472–473, 473t
for residual tumors, 455
for gastric adenocarcinoma, 908, 908b
for hepatocellular carcinoma, 1735
Tobacco use
esophageal cancer and, 444, 466
pancreatic adenocarcinoma and, 1359
smoking cessation for gastroesophageal reflux disease and, 253
Toldt, white line of, 1857, 1860f
Torek, Feranz, 4
Total parenteral nutrition
for biliary surgery, 1622
for liver surgery, 1622
for radiation enteritis, 1157
Total-body irradiation, hepatotoxicity of, 1723
Totally extraperitoneal hernia repair
for femoral hernias, 626, 628–629, 629f
for inguinal hernias, 656, 659, 663–664, 664f, 665t
Toupet fundoplication, 276, 277f
for achalasia, 416
endoscopic examination following, 106
laparoscopic, surgical technique for, 282, 282f
for paraesophageal hernia, 557, 557f
results with, 283, 284t
Toxic megacolon
as emergency surgical indication, 2101
in ulcerative colitis, 2084
Toxins, fulminant liver failure due to, 1703
Trabecular arteries, 1772
Trachea, prenatal development of, 34f, 35, 39f
Tracheal cartilage, 14–15, 15f
Tracheobronchial arteries, 20
Tracheobronchial remnant, 572
Tracheoesophageal atresia, 563–571
abnormalities associated with, 564, 565f
classification of, 564, 565f
clinical findings and diagnostic evaluation of, 565, 566f
development and, 563–564
historical background of, 563
management of, 565–566

Tracheoesophageal atresia (*Continued*)
complications of, 569–571, 571f
operative, 566–569, 567f–570f
recurrent, 570
Tracheoesophageal fistulas, 15
following esophageal resection with visceral esophageal substitution, 613
radiographic appearance of, 76, 78f
Tracheomalacia, with esophageal and tracheoesophageal atresia, 564, 570, 571f
Transabdominal preperitoneal hernia repair
for femoral hernias, 625–626, 628–629
for inguinal hernias, 656, 659, 661–663, 661f–663f, 665t
Transanal endoscopic microsurgery, 2338
for rectal cancer, 2211–2212, 2212f
outcomes with, 2215, 2216t
Transanal excision of rectal tumors, 2338
Transarterial splenic embolization, 1788–1790
anatomy and, 1788, 1789f, 1790f
splenic bleeding and, 1790–1791, 1792f
technique for, 1788–1790, 1790f
Transcatheter arterial embolization/chemoembolization, for hepatocellular carcinoma, 1738
Transducers, for ultrasonography, 111
Transfusion therapy
with biliary surgery, 1619–1620
with liver surgery, 1619–1620
Transhepatic wires, percutaneous, duodenal perforation due to, 1095
Transient lower esophageal sphincter relaxation, 54–55
Transjugular intrahepatic portocaval shunt
for ascites, 1765
for bleeding varices, 1693, 1761–1762
procedure for, 1761f, 1761–1762
for Budd-Chiari syndrome, 1714, 1715
Transmesenteric hernias, 1122f, 1122–1123
clinical features of, 1123
diagnosis of, 1123
treatment of, 1123
Transomental hernias, 1123, 1124f
Transplantation. *See also specific types of transplantation.*
immunosuppression for, 2379
Transversalis fascia, 640–641, 641f, 656–657
Transverse incision
for appendectomy, 2145, 2146f
for colorectal surgery, 2329
Transversus abdominis muscle, 636, 637f, 638, 673, 673f
Trapezoidal flap, for rectovaginal fistulas, 1948–1950, 1949t
Trauma. *See also specific locations, e.g. Gastric injuries.*
esophageal perforation due to, 529
Traumatic hernias, 560
Treatise on Ruptures (Pott), 632
Treitz, ligament of, 968, 970f, 1864
Treves
arch of, 1239
bloodless fold of, 1862
Triangle of doom, 639

Triangle of pain, 639–640
Trichobezoars, 943, 944, 944t, 945
in pediatric patients, 959–960, 960f
Trichophyton infection, pruritus ani associated with, 2070
Trimethoprim/sulfamethoxazole, for cholangitis prophylaxis, 1550t
Triple-tube ostomy, for duodenal injuries, 768
Troglitazone, hepatotoxicity of, 1722
Trusses, for groin hernias, 645, 646f
Tube decompression, for duodenal injuries, 768
Tube feeding, for gastroparesis, 924
Tubular adenomas, small intestinal, 891–892
Tuffier, Theodore, 4
Tumor(s). *See* Malignancies; Metastases; Neoplastic disorders; *specific neoplasms.*
Tumor cell adherence, suture material and, 1084
Tumor markers, for colorectal cancer, 2200–2201
Tumor necrosis factor, for esophageal cancer, 510
Tumor-releasing parathyroid hormone-related protein, pancreatic neuroendocrine tumors and, 1383
Tunica adventitia, esophageal, 16, 16f
Tunica muscularis, esophageal, anatomy of, 16f, 16–17
Turcot's syndrome, 2159t, 2160
small intestinal, 894t, 895–896
Turner, Grey, 4
Turner's syndrome, 887
24-hour esophageal motor activity monitoring, ambulatory, 136
Tylosis, esophageal carcinoma and, 466
Typhlitis, in immunocompromised patients, 2382–2383

U

Ulcer(s)
aphthous, in Crohn's disease, 1043
peptic. *See* Peptic ulcer disease.
Ulcerative colitis, 2080–2085. *See also* Inflammatory bowel disease.
acute, severe, 2084–2085, 2085f
clinical course of, 2081–2082
colorectal cancer and dysplasia and, 2082–2084
Crohn's disease differentiated from, 1050, 1050f
diagnosis of, 2082, 2082f
diarrhea in, 1880
with dysplasia or cancer, surgical management of, restorative proctocolectomy for, 2335
epidemiology and etiopathogenesis of, 2080
fulminant, as emergency surgical indication, 2101
laparoscopic surgery for
outcomes of, 2356–2357
technical points for, 2357
massive hemorrhage in, 2085

Ulcerative colitis (*Continued*)
  medical treatment of, 2089–2093
    5-aminosalicylic acid compounds in, 2089–2090
    antibiotics in, 2090–2091
    biological therapies in, 2092–2093
    corticosteroids in, 2090
    immunosuppressive agents in, 2091–2092
    sulfasalazine in, 2089
  pathologic features of, 2081, 2081t, 2082f
  surgical treatment of, 2101–2122
    colectomy with ileorectal anastomosis for, 2122
    ileal pouch–anal anastomosis for. *See* Ileal pouch–anal anastomosis, for ulcerative colitis.
    indications for, 2101–2102
      for elective surgery, 2101
      for emergency surgery, 2101–2102
    Kick continent ileostomy for, 2122
    panproctocolectomy with ileostomy for, 2122
Ultrasonography
  anorectal
    with anorectal abscesses, 2049–2051, 2050f–2052f
    with anorectal fistulas, 2049–2051, 2050f–2052f
  in aortoenteric fistulas, 1272
  in appendicitis, 2142–2143
  B-mode, 112
  with choledochal cysts, 1553
  in colorectal trauma, 1974
  in Crohn's disease, 1048–1049
  of echinococcal cysts, 1637
  endorectal. *See* Endorectal ultrasound.
  endoscopic. *See* Endoscopic ultrasonography.
  fundamentals of, 111–112
  gray-scale, 112
  with groin hernias, 643
  with hepatic abscesses, pyogenic, 1646
  of hepatic cysts, solitary, 1630, 1631f
  in hepatocellular carcinoma, 1734
  in ileocolic aneurysms, 1282f, 1283
  intraoperative
    in biliary disease, 1627
    in liver disease, 1627
  in jaundice, obstructive, 1460–1461, 1461f
  with liver abscesses, amebic, 1654
  in mesenteric ischemia, 1252
  in mesenteric venous thrombosis, 1256
  in pancreatitis, acute, 1299
  percutaneous, for staging of esophageal cancer, 457
  real-time, 112
  right upper quadrant, in periampullary carcinoma, 1361
  with splenic abscesses, 1818
  with splenic cysts, 1815
  in splenic trauma, 1799
Umbilical anomalies, with Meckel's diverticulum, 787
Umbilical arteries, fetal, 656

Umbilical fissure, 1603
Umbilical folds, 656, 657f
Umbilical hernias
  physiologic, 1857
  repair of, 681–682
Umbilical plate, 1599, 1603
Umbilical vein, extrahepatic, 1598
Umbilicus, 672
United Network of Organ Sharing, 1691
University of California San Francisco criteria, 1740
"Uphill" varices, 95, 97f
Upper esophageal sphincter
  anatomy of, 17
  high-pressure zone of, 376–377, 377f
  idiopathic dysfunction of, cricopharyngeal myotomy for, 388, 389f
  swallowing and, 49–50, 50f, 129, 129f–131f, 375–377, 376f, 377f
  Zenker's diverticulum and, 391–392, 392f, 395
Upper gastrointestinal clinical nurse specialist, role of, in palliative treatment, for esophageal cancer, 497–498
Urachus, 656
Ureter(s), identification of, 2412
Ureteral obstruction, in Crohn's disease, 1065–1066
Urge incontinence, 1885
Urinalysis, in appendicitis, 2143
Urinary retention
  after anorectal surgery, 2057
  with inguinal herniorrhaphy, laparoscopic, 667
Uroguanylin, small intestinal neuroendocrine function and, 1019
Ursodeoxycholic acid
  for cholangitis prophylaxis, 1550t
  for hepatobiliary disease, with primary sclerosing cholangitis, 1568
  hepatotoxicity of, 1722
  for pruritus, in primary sclerosing cholangitis, 1567
U-shaped island flaps, for anal stenosis, 2064

V

VACTERL association, 2391
  with esophageal and tracheoesophageal atresia, 564
Vacuoles, epithelial
  lumen occlusion secondary to, 40, 42f
  in prenatal development, 39–40, 40f
Vagal nerve, injury of, during esophageal surgery, 598
Vagina, identification of, 2414
Vaginal delivery, following ileal pouch–anal anastomosis, 2117–2118
Vaginography, with colon, rectal, and anal disorders, 1893
Vagotomy
  with antrectomy, for duodenal ulcers, 796, 797, 798t
  completion, for gastric outlet obstruction, at gastrojejunostomy site, 1138

Vagotomy (*Continued*)
  definition of, 814
  with drainage, 811–827
    drainage procedures and, 815–818, 817f
    for duodenal ulcers, 796, 798t
    indications for, 822–826
      bleeding ulcers as, 824–825, 825f
      obstruction as, 825–826
      ulcer intractability as, 822–823
      ulcer perforation as, 823–824
    for peptic ulcer disease, 818, 820–822
      gastric, 820f, 820–822
    ulcer recurrence after, 826–827
    vagal anatomy and, 812–813, 813f
    vagal physiology and, 813–814
    vagotomy and, 814f, 814–815
  for duodenal ulcers, 792–794
  gastric, proximal, 814f, 815, 821–822
    technique for, 831, 835f–838f
  gastric dysmotility following, 730, 923
  highly selective
    for duodenal ulcers, 793–794, 794f, 796, 797, 798t
    technique for, 831, 838f–840f
  with long-limb Roux-en-Y gastric bypass, for Barrett's esophagus, 303–304
  minimally invasive versions of, 815
  selective, 814f, 814–815
    for duodenal ulcers, 792–793, 793f
  supradiaphragmatic, for duodenal ulcers, 794
  truncal
    for duodenal ulcers, 792, 793f
    technique for, 831, 832f–835f
    thoracoscopic, for gastroparesis, 924
    transabdominal, 814, 814f
Vagus nerve, 1294
  anatomy of, 25, 719–720, 720f, 812–813, 813f
  intraoperative injury of, during hiatal herniorrhaphy, 609
  physiology of, 813–814
  prenatal development of, 44–45, 45f
Valproic acid, hepatotoxicity of, 1720
Valves of Heister, 1444
Valvular disease, in carcinoid syndrome, 1182
Vancomycin, for *Clostridium difficile* colitis, in immunocompromised patients, 2382
Varices
  bleeding, esophageal. *See* Esophageal varices, bleeding.
  colonic, 1997
  esophageal. *See* Esophageal varices.
  gastric
    endoscopic appearance of, 739, 739f
    in pancreatitis, chronic, 1352–1353
  peri-ileostomy, 1081
  peristomal, 2373, 2373f
Vas deferens, injury of
  with contralateral inguinal exploration, 709
  with inguinal herniorrhaphy, laparoscopic, 667
Vascular compression, esophageal, 573–574, 574f

Vascular disorders. *See also specific disorders.*
  aneurysms as. *See* Aneurysms.
  pseudoaneurysms as. *See*
    Pseudoaneurysms.
  splenectomy for, 1833–1834
    for portal hypertension, 1834
    for splenic artery aneurysm,
      1833–1834
    for splenic vein thrombosis, 1834
    for "wandering spleen" and splenic
      torsion, 1834
  thrombosis as. *See* Thrombosis.
Vascular ectasia
  colonic. *See* Colon, vascular ectasias of.
  gastric antral, 886
    endoscopic appearance of, 739–740
    symptoms and diagnosis of, 886
    treatment of, 740, 886
Vascular injury, with inguinal
  herniorrhaphy, laparoscopic, 665
Vascular lesions, gastric, 886–888
  angiodysplasia as, 739, 887
  Dieulafoy's lesions as, 740, 740f,
    886–887
    symptoms and diagnosis of, 887
    treatment of, 887
  duplication cysts as, 889
  glomus tumors as, 887–888
  hemangiomas as, 887
  lymphangiomas as, 887
  telangiectasia as, 887
    acquired, 887
    congenital, 887
  watermelon stomach as, 886
    endoscopic appearance of, 739–740
    symptoms and diagnosis of, 886
    treatment of, 740, 886
Vascular system, foregut, prenatal
  development of, 42–43, 43f, 44f
Vasculobiliary sheaths, 1599–1600
Vasoactive intestinal peptide
  duodenal function and, 981t, 983
  small intestinal neuroendocrine
    function and, 1018
Vasoconstriction
  mesenteric, control of, 1242b
  splanchnic, mesenteric ischemia due to,
    1251
Vasodilation, mesenteric, control of, 1242b
Vatalanib, for colorectal cancer metastases,
  2271
Vater, papilla of, 964, 965f
Veins. *See specific veins.*
Vena cava
  clamping of, with liver trauma,
    1665–1666, 1666f
  inferior, 1673, 1673f
Veno-occlusive disease, hepatic, drug-
  induced, 1723
Venous plexuses, esophageal, 21, 22f
Venous thromboembolism, postoperative,
  prophylaxis of, 2327, 2328t
Venous thrombosis. *See* Thrombosis.
Venovenous bypass, for liver
  transplantation, 1695–1696
Ventral hernias, 671–684
  anatomy and, 672f, 672–673, 673f
  definition of, 671–672

Ventral hernias *(Continued)*
  etiology of, 673–674
  repair of, obesity and, 684
  surgical treatment of
    indications for, 674
    preparation for, 674–675
    principles of, 676–684, 677f–679f
      components separation and,
        682–683, 683f
      laparoscopic operative method
        and, 678–680, 679f, 680f
      minimally invasive vs. open mesh
        repair and, 680, 680t
      obesity and, 684
      perioperative considerations and,
        680–681
      for spigelian hernias, 682
      for suprapubic hernias, 683–684,
        684f
      for umbilical hernia, 681–682
    prosthetics for, 675f, 675–676, 676f
  symptoms of, 674
  types of, 671
Venules, mesenteric, 1241
Veress needle, 1135
  perforation due to, 1094
Vermiform appendix, anatomy of, 1846,
  1863, 1864f
Verner-Morrison syndrome, 1381
Vertical midline incision, for colorectal
  surgery, 2329
Videocineroentgenography
  for esophageal bolus clearance
    evaluation, 154, 155f, 156f
  for swallowing disorder assessment, 134,
    135f
Videoesophagography, in gastroesophageal
  reflux disease, 59
Videofluoroscopy, for swallowing evaluation,
  377–378
Villi, small intestinal, 998
Villous adenomas, small intestinal, 892–893
Vinyl chloride, hepatotoxicity of, 1723,
  1724
VIPomas, 1381
Virchow's node, 906, 1361
Visilizumab, mechanism of action of,
  2377t
Vitamin(s)
  fat-soluble
    deficiency of, with primary sclerosing
      cholangitis, treatment of, 1568,
      1568t
    for steatorrhea, with primary
      sclerosing cholangitis, 1588
    small intestinal absorption of,
      1006–1008, 1007t
Vitamin A
  deficiency of, in Crohn's disease, 1054
  hepatotoxicity of, 1723
  small intestinal absorption of,
    1006–1007, 1007t
Vitamin B$_{12}$
  deficiency of
    in Crohn's disease, 1054
    following gastrectomy, 873
  small intestinal absorption of, 1006,
    1007t

Vitamin C, small intestinal absorption of,
  1006, 1007t
Vitamin D
  deficiency of, in Crohn's disease, 1054
  small intestinal absorption of, 1006,
    1007, 1007t
Vitamin E
  deficiency of, in Crohn's disease,
    1054
  small intestinal absorption of, 1006,
    1007, 1007t
Vitamin K
  deficiency of, in Crohn's disease, 1054
  small intestinal absorption of, 1006,
    1007t, 1007–1008
Vitelline blood vessel remnants, 1227
Volvulus
  colonic. *See* Colonic volvulus.
  gastric, 1037–1039
    diagnosis of, 1037–1038, 1038f,
      1039f
    etiology of, 1037, 1037f
    in pediatric patients, 950
    treatment of, 1038–1039
  small bowel, 1035–1037
    diagnosis of, 1036, 1036f
    etiology of, 1035–1036, 1036t
    treatment of, 1036–1037
  types of, 550, 551f
Vomiting
  in afferent loop syndrome, 877–878
  in appendicitis, 2142
  in malrotation, 1216
  in small bowel obstruction, 1028
  in small intestinal atresia, 1219
V-Y island flaps, for anal stenosis, 2063f,
  2063–2064

W

W pouch, 2105
Walaean pedicles, 1599
Walaean sheaths, 1599
"Wandering spleen," splenectomy for,
  1834
Wantz, George, 678
Water, small intestinal absorption of, 1001,
  1001t
Watermelon stomach, 886
  endoscopic appearance of, 739–740
  symptoms and diagnosis of, 886
  treatment of, 740, 886
Water-soluble contrast enema, with colon,
  rectal, and anal disorders, 1893
Watson fundoplication, 276, 277f, 278
Wedge resection, hepatic, 1683, 1683f
Weight loss
  in achalasia, 407
  in Crohn's disease, 1045
  in esophageal cancer, 61
  esophageal carcinoma and, 468
  following gastrectomy, 873
  surgery for. *See* Bariatric surgery.
Whipple procedure
  for duodenal adenocarcinoma, 915
  for pancreatitis, chronic, 1314, 1315
  for Zollinger-Ellison syndrome, 868

Whipple's triad, with insulinoma, 1376
Whirl sign
    in colonic volvulus, 1981
    with transmesenteric hernias, 1123
White blood cell count, in appendicitis, 2142–2143
White line of Toldt, 1857, 1860f
Whitehead deformity, 2062
Whitehead hemorrhoidectomy, 2033
Wilke's syndrome, 974–975, 975f, 976f
Willis, Thomas, 405
Wilson's disease
    fulminant liver failure due to, 1703
    hepatic laboratory tests in, 1613
Winslow, foramen of, 964, 966f
Wirsung, pancreatic duct of, 964
Wiskott-Aldrich syndrome, splenectomy for, 1825
Witch hazel, pruritus ani associated with, 2069
Witzel gastrostomy, in pediatric patients, 960
Witzel jejunostomy, 757, 758f
Wound complications
    after anorectal surgery, 2057
    with gastrointestinal fistulas, 1098
    infection as
        with hernia repair, 654
        with inguinal herniorrhaphy, laparoscopic, 668
Wound healing, steroid-induced impairment of, 2378
Wound implants, prevention of, with laparoscopic colorectal surgery, 2348, 2348f–2353f, 2349b, 2351b, 2353
Wound vacuum drainage systems, 1102, 1104f

Y

Yellow phosphorus, hepatotoxicity of, 1720
York-Mason approach, for rectourethral fistulas, 1955
Yo-yo syndrome, 929
Y-V advancement flaps, for anal stenosis, 2063, 2063f

Z

Zacarelli, Adrian, 1813
Zafirlukast, hepatotoxicity of, 1721
ZAP classification, for Barrett's esophagus, 103–104
Zenker, Albert, 6
Zenker's diverticulum, 94–95, 96f, 391–400, 427–433
    pathophysiology of, 427–428
    physiology and pathophysiology of, 391–395, 392f
        contractility studies and, 392, 393f–395f, 393t, 394–395, 395t
    recurrent, reoperation for, 431
    swallowing disorder in, 134–135, 135f, 136f
    symptoms and diagnosis of, 396, 396t, 428, 428f
    treatment of, 396–398, 429–433
        choice of, 400
        cricopharyngeal myotomy for, 378–379, 381
            for established diverticula, 381, 383f

Zenker's diverticulum (Continued)
        for large diverticula, 381, 383f
        for minute diverticula, 381
    diverticulectomy as, 396
    diverticulopexy as, 396
    early development of surgery for, 5–6
    endoscopic, 397–398, 398f
        methods and results of, 431–433, 432f
    evolution of, 429
    myotomy in, 396–397, 397f, 398f
    results of, 398–400, 399t, 400f, 401t–403t
    surgical, methods and results of, 429–431, 430f, 431f
Zidovudine, hepatotoxicity of, 1720
Zinc, deficiency of, in Crohn's disease, 1054
Zinman, Leonard, 1955
Z-line, 19
    Barrett's esophagus classification and, 103–104
    endoscopic appearance of, 101, 101f
        in Barrett's esophagus, 103, 103f, 104f
Zollinger-Ellison syndrome, 862–868
    carcinoids in, 1181
    diagnosis of, 862–863, 863b, 864f
    GRFomas in, 1382
    localization procedures for, 864–865, 865f
    management of
        medical, 866, 866f
        surgical, 866–868, 867f
    metastatic, 868
    in pediatric patients, 961
    signs and symptoms of, 862
    tumor characteristics in, 863–864